BIRTH DEFECTS COMPENDIUM
Second Edition

BIRTH DEFECTS COMPENDIUM
Second Edition

Editor

Daniel Bergsma, MD, MPH
Clinical Professor of Pediatrics
Tufts University, School of Medicine
Boston, Massachusetts

* * *

Published for The National Foundation–March of Dimes
by Alan R. Liss, Inc., New York

To enhance medical communication in the birth defects field, The National Foundation has published the *Birth Defects Compendium, Second Edition, Syndrome Identification, Original Article Series* and developed a series of films and related brochures.

Further information can be obtained from:

The National Foundation — March of Dimes
1275 Mamaroneck Avenue
White Plains, New York 10605

Published by:

Alan R. Liss, Inc.
150 Fifth Avenue
New York, New York 10011

Originally published 1973 as Birth Defects Atlas and Compendium

Reprinted 1973, 1974

Second edition, 1979

Second Printing, November 1979

Figure 113, Birth Defect 8; Figure 114, Birth Defect 9; Figure 115, Birth Defect 10; and Figure 368, Birth Defect 677 have been replaced for the second printing.

Printed in the United States of America.

Library of Congress Cataloging in Publication Data

Main entry under title:

Birth defects compendium.

   First ed., entered under D. Bergsma, published in 1972 under title: Birth defects.
   Includes index.
   1. Abnormalities, Human. 2. Abnormalities, Human—Atlases. I. Bergsma, Daniel. II. Bergsma, Daniel. Birth defects. III. National Foundation.
[DNLM: 1. Abnormalities. 2. Abnormalities — Atlases. QS675 B617]
QM691.B53 1979   616'.043   78-20651
ISBN 0-8451-0203-6

DEDICATED

To each dear little child
    who is in need of special help and care;
to each eager parent
    who is desperately, hopefully seeking help;
to each professional
    who brings understanding, knowledge and skillful care;
to each generous friend
    who assists The National Foundation to help.

D. B.

Preface

Birth defects by whatever definition exhibit noteworthy variety or complexity, and often overlap. Indeed the overlap also frequently involves the areas of concern of two or more medical specialties. Collectively, the diagnosis, treatment and genetic counseling associated with birth defects involve the areas of interest and concern of all health professionals. Accordingly, recorded information about birth defects is widely scattered in multiple journals and books under literally thousands of different names. Even with good library resources available, a select bit of information about a given birth defect is often very difficult and time-consuming to obtain. If the desired bit of data is unknown, and hence unrecorded, the total search effort becomes wasted time.

Accordingly, this Compendium was designed to assemble the more commonly sought after information about birth defects in a standardized format for the convenience of students and practitioners of the health professions. Desired data can usually be found under specific subheadings which have a constant sequence for easier reference. When only fragments of data were available these are provided without further comment; expert opinion is distinguished from confirmed data and, when no information was currently available, a simple "?" is inserted for clarity, brevity and certainty, and also as a kind of index of the clinical research that perhaps should be performed.

For the purpose of this Compendium the term "Birth Defects" includes any anatomic or functional variant from the normal range in homo sapiens which is inherited by any mendelian mode of transmission, or caused by fresh mutation, any chromosomal abnormality, or by any infectious, chemical or physical insult to the embryo or fetus prior to birth.

Certain markers, themselves not birth defects, are included because their genetic transmission is known; they may be distinguished as occurring independently; may be associated with certain birth defects; or may affect a patient's reaction to medication.

For the convenience of physicians who normally use French, German or Spanish as their primary language, the most commonly used other language name for most birth defects and markers described in this Compendium is presented under the subtitle "Includes" in the text and is also placed alphabetically in the index. The second language term was omitted for economic reasons when it was so similar that it was essentially identical. Usually one or more additional English language terms or names were also selected and provided to assist the individual seeking information to find the data desired by use of a presently familiar index term. All other alphabetized indexed information is provided as an aid to differential diagnosis. Accordingly, additional index subject headings relate to anatomic parts, signs or symptoms.

The combination "and/or" is rarely used in the text. The word "or" is used to include *either* or *both*. When mutual exclusion is intended, alternate wording is usually employed such as "either a or b."

For increased clarity of meaning, the same wording is usually used to relay information about risk of recurrence to a patient's sib or child when the defect is being transmitted by a specific mode of mendelian inheritance. This is summarized in Table I, Section III. Furthermore, for economy of space and of printing cost, a reference is made to Table I when two or more modes of mendelian transmission are known, or are thought to occur, for the related defects included in the syndrome. As supplemental etiologic data certain references to McKusick's *Mendelian Inheritance in Man* were included, eg McK *----------.

Certain few birth defects have been presented with the data based upon a single case or kindred identified to date. Experience has shown that not infrequently additional patients with the same or very similar syndrome defects are identified by other clinicians once the syndrome has been given initial description.

Our knowledge of birth defects is such that some present syndrome complexes will one day certainly be recognized as two or more biochemically specific types, some overlapping phenotypes may later be shown to be a single entity as more patients are studied in depth, and surely some as yet unidentified birth defects will be defined.

Certain birth defects or syndrome types, by present knowledge, are so phenotypically similar that they are presented as single entries in this Compendium. This not only reduced cost but also emphasized the known differences by their juxtaposition within the write-up.

Each birth defect textual presentation in Section II has its own Birth Defect Compendium Number which is placed at the top left above the selected English primary name for that birth defect. It will be observed that these numbers were assigned as in the 1st Edition in numerical sequence after the selected primary birth defect names were alphabetized. This permits one to find data about a birth defect directly in Section II by either its prime name or its Compendium Birth Defect Number. For convenience, in the index, each English primary name is in capital letters and followed only by its Compendium Birth Defect Number.

Clinicians dealing with a wide spectrum of birth defects, in the absence of both suitable classification and satisfactory nomenclature, have expressed a strong desire for a "Permanent" Birth Defect Number with which to code each birth defect in their files. Such a "more permanent" number is provided in the Compendium. We utilized a number span of one million and assigned numbers so as to permit alphabetic inclusion not only of all current birth defects but also provided interval spaces for subsequent alphabetized entries. Each such "more permanent" number was designated between 000–001 and 999–999. These new numbers may be useful in computer programming as well as for individual files. In Section II the "more permanent" number for each birth defect has been placed at the top right above the selected primary name for that birth defect.

Tables and diagrams or drawings were provided in Section III to supplement or interrelate certain data contained in the text or index, eg Table II identifies 90 "Metabolic Disorders Where Specific Enzyme Defects Have Been Described," and Table XXIV provides Compendium Birth Defect Number references not only for the Eye as a unit but also for Vision, Nystagmus, Retinal Involvement, etc.

Perpetual clinical curiosity and astute observations are necessary to detect many birth defects. With time this may well be increasingly so in order to delineate between a larger number of similar or overlapping phenotypes. Accordingly, sex, age, biologic parents and ethnic groups are necessary considerations when clinically determining each anatomic feature to be associated with a birth defect in a given patient. The presence of only one or two minor defects especially in adults, is not of great importance but the presence of two or three minor defects in a newborn justifies careful

work-up in search of possible significant internal defects. Similarly a single major defect in a neonate, such as the presence of only one umbilical artery, requires careful study for possible systemic involvement.

In certain instances promised textual material did not arrive by publication date. It is planned that these and new birth defect research data will continually be added to the computer bank and be available day or night by a telephone coupled terminal.

The pictorial display in Section I, which includes 108 pictures in color will hopefully help students in the health professions to identify certain defects more readily and accurately. The textual part of this Compendium (Section II) is provided to indicate the abnormalities which are part of, derived from, or associated with each birth defect. A total of 392 black and white pictures or drawings are also presented to aid in differential diagnosis.

425 authors from 24 countries, 21 Assistant and 22 Associate Editors helped to assemble the data compiled in this opus. They alone deserve all the credit for the useful data contained herein. The Compendium editor initially dreamed of the concept involved and then coordinated the overall effort to achieve this product. Each constructive suggestion by any expert will be carefully and seriously considered and, as may be feasible, such desired improvements will be incorporated promptly into the computer information retrieval system.

The text of this Compendium was set by computer. To save time and expense, when the meaning is clear, incorrect syllabication was not corrected.

About 3,000 references to the literature are provided in the text. These references in turn provide thousands more if desired. However, the student of birth defects would surely find supplemental information of value in the *Birth Defects: Original Article Series* or *Syndrome Identification.*

Acknowledgments

It is a great pleasure to acknowledge the significant suggestions and splendid cooperation of the members of the Editorial Board, the invaluable achievements of each Associate Editor who helped with the difficult problems of nomenclature, who selected and assigned authors for birth defects within designated clusters and who helped to achieve scientific accuracy; and also to the Assistant Editors who served in various capacities to help transmute a dream into the reality of the First Edition and continued their dedicated service to make possible this Second Edition.

Acknowledgment is also given to the authors, the medical periodicals and book publishers that granted permission to reproduce certain previously published original photographs and tables, and to all those who provided unpublished original illustrations or tables. Special thanks is also extended to my friend, Victor McKusick who graciously permitted us to use * number references as recorded in his very helpful book entitled *Mendelian Inheritance in Man* which contains useful etiologic data and numerous additional references to the literature.

Special acknowledgment is made to my friends and colleagues, too numerous to name here, who gave generously of their time and talents at all stages of our efforts, during the preparation of both the First and Second Edition of this Compendium, to sort out from among thousands of names for birth defects those which might best be forgotten, those which perhaps should be used as primary names or, in turn, used as inclusion and index terms for the convenience of persons searching for data in the Compendium.

Thanks are also extended to the devoted efforts of Connie Fisher, Florence Dickman, Sue Greene, Louis Gutentag, Ann Klek, Cynthia Krusen, Marcia MacDonald, Marilyn Orlando, David Pachura, Adam Schneider, Eric Whitney, and especially Jeanne R. Mudge and Seymour Small who were completely untiring and very helpful in various aspects of this task.

Last, but definitely not least, sincere appreciation is felt and grateful thanks is due my wife, Nellie Dorothy, who provided patience and encouragement, and to the spouse of each Associate and Assistant Editor who made various sacrifices while time and energy were devoted to this opus.

D. B.

Assistant Editors

Hugh D. Allen, MD
Associate Professor of Pediatrics (Cardiology)
Department of Pediatrics
Health Sciences Center
University of Arizona
Tucson, AZ 85724

Dr. Salvador Armendares
Sección de Genética
Instituto Mexicano del Seguro Social
Departamento de Investigación Científica
Apartado Postal 73–032
Mexico, 73, D.F., Mexico

Cor W. R. J. Cremers, MD
Department of Otorhinolaryngology
St. Radboud Hospital
University of Nijmegen
Nijmegen, The Netherlands

Larry P. Elliott, MD
Chief and Professor
Division of Cardiovascular Radiology
University of Alabama Medical Center
Birmingham, AL 35233

Peter Farnsworth, MD
Director of Pediatrics
Westchester County Medical Center
Valhalla, NY 10595

Newton Freire-Maia, MD
Departamento de Genética
Instituto de Biología
Caixa Postal AA
80.000 Curitiba, Paraná
Brazil

Jaime L. Frias, MD
Professor of Pediatrics
Chief, Division of Genetics
Department of Pediatrics
University of Florida College of Medicine
Gainesville, FL 32610

Professor Dr. S. J. Geerts
Head, Department of Human Genetics
University of Nijmegen
Faculty of Medicine
Nijmegen, The Netherlands

Ira H. Gessner, MD
Chief, Division of Cardiology
Department of Pediatrics
University of Florida College of Medicine
Gainesville, FL 32610

Stanley J. Goldberg, MD
Professor of Pediatrics (Cardiology)
Department of Pediatrics
Health Sciences Center
University of Arizona
Tucson, AZ 85724

Professor Dr. P. Gruetzner
Univ. – Augenklinik
D-78 Freiburg
Germany

Ronald J. Jorgenson, DDS
Assistant Professor
Department of Pediatric Dentistry
Medical University of South Carolina
Charleston, SC 29401

Oonagh C. Kater
Editorial Assistant
Department of Pediatrics
University of Florida College of Medicine
Gainesville, FL 32610

Professor Jacques LaFourcade
Clinique de Pédiatrie et Génétique Medicale
Hôpital de la Salpetriere
83, bd de l'Hôpital
75013 Paris
France

Pierre Maroteaux, MD
Directeur de Recherche, C.N.R.S.
ER 202 C.N.R.S. and U.12 I.N.S.E.R.M.
Hôpital des Enfants Malades
149 rue de Sèvres
75730 Paris CEDEX 15
France

James J. Nora, MD
Professor of Pediatrics
Director of Pediatric Cardiology
University of Colorado Medical Center
Denver, CO 80220

Professor Jean Rey
Hôpital des Enfants Malades
Clinique de Génétique Medicale
149, Rue de Sèvres
75730 Paris CEDEX 15
France

David J. Sahn, MD
Associate Professor of Pediatrics
Department of Pediatrics
Health Sciences Center
University of Arizona
Tucson, AZ 85724

Morton E. Smith, MD
Professor of Ophthalmology and Pathology
Department of Ophthalmology
Washington University School of Medicine
St. Louis, MO 63110

Docteur Catherine Turleau
Chargée de Recherche C.N.R.S.
ER 149 C.N.R.S. and U. 173 I.N.S.E.R.M.
Hôpital des Enfants Malades
149, rue de Sèvres
75730 Paris CEDEX 15
France

Dr. med. Peter Ude
Oberarzt
der Universitatshautklinik
Kiel, Germany

Dr. med. dent. Werner Utz
Universitatsklinik
fur Zahn, Mund -u. Kieferkrankheiten
Weimarer Strasse 8
23 Kiel, Germany

L. H. S. Van Mierop, MD
Professor of Pediatrics and Pathology
University of Florida College of Medicine
Gainesville, FL 32610

Contributors

Dagfinn Aarskog
Department of Pediatrics
University of Bergen
Bergen, Norway

Donald C. Abele
Department of Dermatology
Medical College of Georgia
Augusta, GA 30904

Donald C. Aberfeld
807 United Nations Plaza
New York, NY 10017

Albert M. Abrams
130 South Saltair Ave.
Los Angeles, CA 90049

M. J. Acquarelli
Department of Otolaryngology
Wadsworth Veterans Administration Hospital
Los Angeles, CA 90073

Hugo Aebi
Medizinisch-Chemisches Institut der
   Universität Bern
3000 Bern, Switzerland

Kyrieckos Aleck
Department of Medical Genetics
Harbor General Hospital
Torrance, CA 90509

Charles A. Alford, Jr.
Department of Pediatrics
University of Alabama School of Medicine
Birmingham, AL 35233

Penelope Witte Allderdice
Faculty of Medicine
Memorial University of New Foundland
St. John's, Newfoundland, Canada A1C 5S7

C. H. Alström
Psykiatriska kliniken
S:t Görans Sjukhus
Stockholm, Sweden

Arthur J. Ammann
Department of Pediatric Immunology
University of California, San Francisco
School of Medicine
San Francisco, CA 94143

Constantine S. Anast
Department of Child Health
University of Missouri School of Medicine
Columbia, MO 65201

René A. Arcilla
Department of Pediatrics
University of Chicago, The Pritzker School of
   Medicine
Chicago, IL 60637

Irwin M. Arias
Department of Medicine
Albert Einstein College of Medicine
Bronx, NY 10461

H. Brock Armstrong
Department of Pediatrics
University of Alberta Medical School
Edmonton 7, Alberta, Canada

Keith W. Ashcraft
4400 Broadway
Kansas City, MO 64111

James H. Austin
Department of Neurology
University of Colorado School of Medicine
Denver, CO 80220

Kalim U. Aziz
Division of Cardiology
The Children's Memorial Hospital
Chicago, IL 60614

Henry W. Baird
St. Christopher's Hospital for Children
Philadelphia, PA 19133

Lewis A. Barness
Department of Pediatrics
University of South Florida
College of Medicine
Tampa, FL 33620

Roger A. Barnhart
Bellingham Medical Center
Bellingham, WA 98225

James L. Barrett
414 E. Main Street
Lancaster, OH 43130

Bruce J. Bart
Department of Dermatology
University of Minnesota
Medical School, Minneapolis
Minneapolis, MN 55455

Robert S. Bart
New York University Medical Center
Skin and Cancer Unit
New York, NY 10016

Louis E. Bartoshesky
New England Medical Center Hospital
Boston, MA 02111

Peter Beighton
Department of Human Genetics
University of Cape Town Medical School
Cape Town, South Africa

H. Bennhold
Medizinsche Universitäts-Klinik
74 Tübingen, West Germany

William R. Bergren
1446 Morada Place
Altadena, CA 91001

Donald R. Bergsma
Department of Ophthalmology
University of Kentucky College of Medicine
Lexington, KY 40506

LaVonne Bergstrom
Division Head & Neck Surgery
UCLA Center for Health Sciences
Los Angeles, CA 90024

Michael A. Berman
Department of Pediatrics
University of Maryland School of Medicine
Baltimore, MD 21201

Joel M. Bernstein
191 West North Street
Buffalo, NY 14201

Frederick R. Bieber
Department of Human Genetics
Medical College of Virginia
Richmond, VA 23298

Nesrin Bingol
New York Medical College
New York, NY 10029

Harry C. Bishop
Department of Pediatric Surgery
University of Pennsylvania School of
   Medicine
Philadelphia, PA 19104

John A. Black
The Children's Hospital
Sheffield S 10 2TH England

Harry M. Blackfield
45 Castro
San Francisco, CA 94114

R. W. Blaine*

John H. Bland
Medical Center Hospital of Vermont
University of Vermont College of Medicine
Burlington, VT 05401

John P. Blass
Neuropsychiatric Institute
UCLA-Center for Health Sciences
Los Angeles, CA 90024

Robert M. Blizzard
Department of Pediatrics
University of Virginia School of Medicine
Charlottesville, VA 22901

William E. Bloomer
3440 Atlantic Avenue
Long Beach, CA 90807

*Present address unknown.

Jessie Bodenhoff
Mycological Department
Statens Seruminstitut
2300 Copenhagen, Denmark

Jan A. Böök
The Institute for Medical Genetics
University of Uppsala
Uppsala, Sweden

Wayne H. Borges
Department of Hematology
The Children's Memorial Hospital
Chicago, IL 60614

Barbara J. Bourland
Department of Pediatrics
Baylor College of Medicine
Houston, TX 77025

Peter Bowen
Department of Pediatrics
University of Alberta Medical School
Edmonton 7, Alberta, Canada

W. Roy Breg
Yale University School of Medicine
New Haven, CT 06510

Richard L. Bucciarelli
Department of Pediatrics (Cardiology)
University of Florida College of Medicine
Gainesville, FL 32610

Marylou Buyse
New England Medical Center Hospital
Boston, MA 02111

Thomas C. Calcaterra
Department of Surgery
University of California, Los Angeles School of
   Medicine
Los Angeles, CA 90024

Richard M. Caplan
Department of Dermatology
University of Iowa College of Medicine
Iowa City, IA 52242

Cedric O. Carter
MRC Clinical Genetics Unit
Institute of Child Health
London, England WC1N 1EH

Vernon H. Carter
455 South Federal Highway
Boca Raton, FL 33432

Suzanne B. Cassidy
4324 NE 44th Street
Seattle, WA 98105

Stephen D. Cederbaum
Neuropsychiatric Institute
UCLA-Center for Health Sciences
Los Angeles, CA 90024

Jaroslav Červenka
Divisions of Oral Pathology & Human
   and Oral Genetics
University of Minnesota School of Dentistry
Minneapolis, MN 55455

Joe C. Christian
Department of Medical Genetics
Indiana University Medical Center
Indianapolis, IN 46202

H. William Clatworthy, Jr.
904 East Broad Street
Columbus, OH 43205

C. C. Clawson
Department of Pediatrics
University of Minnesota Medical School, Minneapolis
Minneapolis, MN 55455

William E. Clendenning
Hitchcock Clinic
Hanover, NH 03755

Hartwig Cleve
Department of Anthropology & Human
   Genetics
University of Munich
8 Munich 2, Germany

Jay T. Cline
Department of Pediatric Dentistry
University of Minnesota School of Dentistry
Minneapolis, MN 55455

David Cogan
Clinical Branch
National Eye Institute
Bethesda, MD 20014

M. Michael Cohen, Jr.
Department of Orthodontics
University of Washington School of
   Dentistry
Seattle, WA 98105

M. Michael Cohen, Sr.
1101 Beacon Street
Brookline, MA 02146

David E. Comings
Department of Medical Genetics
City of Hope Medical Center
Duarte, CA 91010

Louis Z. Cooper
Department of Pediatrics
Roosevelt Hospital
New York, NY 10019

Jean A. Cortner
Children's Hospital
Philadelphia, PA 19104

John C. Crawhall
University of McGill Clinic
Montreal 11, P.Q. Canada

Cor W. R. J. Cremers
Department of Otorhinolaryngology
St. Radboud Hospital
University of Nijmegen
Nijmegen, The Netherlands

Allen C. Crocker
Children's Hospital Medical Center
Boston, MA 02115

Harold E. Cross
Ophthalmology Division
Arizona University Medical Center
Tucson, AZ 85724

Charlotte Cunningham-Rundles
Memorial Sloan-Kettering Cancer Center
New York, NY 10021

Helen Ollendorff Curth
35 East 84th Street
New York, NY 10029

Albert A. Dahlberg
Department of Anthropology
Zoller Memorial Clinic
University of Chicago
Chicago, IL 60637

Joseph Dancis
Department of Pediatrics
New York University School of Medicine
New York, NY 10016

Murray Davidson
Department of Pediatrics
Bronx Lebanon Hospital Center
Bronx, NY 10457

R. G. Davidson
Department of Pediatrics
McMaster University
Hamilton, Ontario, Canada L8S 4J9

Franklin DeBusk
Department of Pediatrics
University of Florida College of Medicine
Gainesville, FL 32610

Leslie J. DeGroot
Department of Medicine
University of Chicago, The Pritzker School
of Medicine
Chicago, IL 60637

Nicholas R. Dennis
MRC Clinical Genetics Unit
Institute of Child Health
London, England WC1N IEH

Eugene L. Derlacki
55 East Washington Street
Chicago, IL 60602

Robert J. Desnick
Department of Pediatrics
Mount Sinai School of Medicine
New York, NY 10029

Loren T. DeWind
9819 Paramount Blvd.
Downey, CA 90240

Liebe Sokol Diamond
833 Park Avenue
Baltimore, MD 21201

Louis K. Diamond
Department of Pediatrics
University of California San Francisco
School of Medicine
San Francisco, CA 94143

David A. Dolowitz
Allergy, Ear, Nose and Throat Clinic of Utah
Salt Lake City, UT 84105

George N. Donnell
Children's Hospital
Los Angeles, CA 90027

Marion P. Downs
Division of Otolaryngology
University of Colorado Medical Center
Denver, CO 80220

Patrick J. Doyle
Division of Otorhinolaryngology
University of British Columbia
Vancouver, B.C. Canada

Edward Drescher‡

Paolo Durand
Third Department of Pediatrics
Giannina Gaslini Institute
Genova, Quarto, Italy

Arndt J. Duvall, III
Department of Otolaryngology
University of Minnesota Health Sciences
Center
Minneapolis, MN 55455

Jesse E. Edwards
Department of Pathology and Clinical
Laboratory
United Hospitals
St. Paul, MN 55102

Lorentz Eldjarn
Institute of Clinical Biochemistry
University of Oslo, Rikshospitalet
Oslo, Norway

Larry P. Elliott
Division of Cardiovascular Radiology
University of Alabama Medical Center
Birmingham, AL 35233

Elliot F. Ellis
Department of Pediatrics
Children's Hospital
Buffalo, NY 14222

Robert M. Ellsworth
Edward S. Harkness Eye Institute
New York, NY 10032

Nabil I. Elsahy
315 Boulevard, N.E.
Atlanta, GA 30312

Eric Engel
Dept. of Medicine/Genetics Division
Vanderbilt University Hospital
Nashville, TN 37232

Gerald M. English
1666 S. University Boulevard
Denver, CO 80210

‡Deceased.

John B. Erich
Section of Publications
Mayo Clinic
Rochester, MN 55901

Franz Escher
Spezialarzt fur Ohren, Nasen-und
Halskrankheiten
Lindenhofspital, Bremgartenstr
CH-3012 Bern, Switzerland

Nyles R. Eskritt*

John R. Esterly
Departments of Pathology and Obstetrics
and Gynecology
University of Chicago, The Pritzker School
of Medicine
Chicago, IL 60637

David A. Price Evans
Department of Medicine
University of Liverpool
Liverpool, England L69 3BX

John A. Ewing
Department of Psychiatry
University of North Carolina School
of Medicine
Chapel Hill, NC 27514

Harold F. Falls
Department of Ophthalmology
University of Michigan Hospitals
Ann Arbor, MI 48104

Blaise E. Favara
Children's Hospital
Denver, CO 80218

Murray Feingold
Tufts-New England Medical Center
Boston, MA 02111

Moshe Feinmesser
Department of Otolaryngology
Hadassah University Hospital
Jerusalem, Israel

R. Storey Fenton
Department of Otolaryngology
St. Michael's Hospital
Toronto, Ontario, Canada M5B 1W8

Malcolm A. Ferguson-Smith
Royal Hospital for Sick Children
Yorkhill
Glasgow, Scotland G3 8SJ

Robert M. Fineman
Department of Pediatrics
University of Utah College of Medicine
Salt Lake City, UT 84132

Delbert A. Fisher
Harbor General Hospital
Torrance, CA 90509

*Present address unknown.

Naomi Fitch
Lady Davis Institute for Medical Research
of Jewish General Hospital
Montreal, Quebec, Canada H3T 1E2

Gordon M. Folger, Jr.
Department of Pediatric Cardiology
Henry Ford Hospital
Detroit, MI 48202

Eric W. Fonkalsrud
Department of Pediatric Surgery
UCLA Medical Center
Los Angeles, CA 90024

Sidney A. Fox
Department of Ophthalmology
New York University School of Medicine
New York, NY 10016

Uta Francke
Department of Pediatrics
Yale University School of Medicine
New Haven, CT 06510

Donald Fraser
Departments of Pediatrics and Physiology
The Research Institute
Hospital for Sick Children
Toronto, Ontario, Canada

F. Clarke Fraser
Department of Biology
McGill University
Montreal, Quebec, Canada H3C 3G1

G. R. Fraser
Faculty of Medicine
Memorial University of Newfoundland
St. John's, Newfoundland, Canada A1C 5S7

Joseph F. Fraumeni, Jr.
Epidemiology Branch
National Cancer Institute
Bethesda, MD 20014

Donald S. Fredrickson
Molecular Disease Branch
National Institutes of Health
Bethesda, MD 20014

John Mark Freeman
The Johns Hopkins University School
of Medicine
Baltimore, MD 21205

Bert C. Frichot, III
University of Nebraska
Omaha, NE 68105

William F. Friedman
Department of Pediatrics
University Hospital
San Diego, CA 92110

George W. Frimpter
Veterans Administration Hospital
7400 Merton Minter Blvd.
San Antonio, TX 78284

E. R. Froesch
Renggerstrasse 31
8000 Zurich, Switzerland

George Gaethe
3439 Prytania Street
New Orleans, LA 70115

Stephen L. Gans
2080 Century Park East
Los Angeles, CA 90067

David W. Gardner
Department of Medicine
University of Missouri School of
Medicine
Columbia, MO 65201

Richard A. Gatti
Departments of Pediatrics, Oncology &
Immunology
Cedars-Sinai Medical Center
Los Angeles, CA 90048

Robert N. Gebhart
UCLA Medical Center
Los Angeles, CA 90024

William C. Gentry, Jr.
Dept. of Dermatology
University of Minnesota Medical School,
Minneapolis
Minneapolis, MN 55455

James L. German, III
Laboratory of Human Genetics
The New York Blood Center
New York, NY 10021

Theo Gerritsen
Organization for Health Research TNO
The Hague, The Netherlands

Ira H. Gessner
Department of Pediatrics (Cardiology)
University of Florida College of Medicine
Gainesville, FL 32610

H. Ghadimi
3612 Bertha Dr.
Baldwin, NY 11510

Samuel T. Giammona
Department of Pediatrics
Children's Hospital of San Francisco
San Francisco, CA 94119

Eloise R. Giblett
King County Central Blood Bank, Inc.
Seattle, WA 98104

Ronald E. Gier
Department of Oral Diagnosis
University of Missouri School of
Dentistry
Kansas City, MO 64108

Enid F. Gilbert
Department of Pathology
University of Wisconsin Medical School
Madison, WI 53706

John W. Gittinger
Department of Ophthalmology
Tufts University School of Medicine
Boston, MA 02111

Richard Gitzelmann
Laboratory for Metabolic Research
University Pediatric Department
Kinderspital
8032 Zurich, Switzerland

Morton F. Goldberg
Department of Ophthalmology
Illinois Eye and Ear Infirmary
Chicago, IL 60612

Robert Goltz
Department of Dermatology
University of Minnesota Medical School,
Minneapolis
Minneapolis, MN 55455

Robert A. Good
Memorial Sloan-Kettering Cancer Center
New York, NY 10021

Richard M. Goodman
Department of Human Genetics
Tel Aviv University Medical School
Tel-Hashomer, Israel

Stephen I. Goodman
Department of Pediatrics
University of Colorado Medical Center
Denver, CO 80220

Thomas F. Goodman, Jr.
501 Stratford Dr.
Augusta, GA 30904

W. S. Goodman
Department of Otolaryngology
University of Toronto
Toronto 2, Ontario, Canada

Robert J. Gorlin
Division of Oral Pathology
University of Minnesota School of
Dentistry
Minneapolis, MN 55455

Thomas P. Graham, Jr.
Division of Pediatric Cardiology
Vanderbilt University Medical Center
Nashville, TN 37232

Jay L. Grosfeld
Department of Surgery
Indiana University Medical Center
Indianapolis, IN 46202

Juan R. Guerrero
Squibb Institute for Medical Research
Princeton, NJ 08540

Paul Guggenheim
Mid-Valley Medical Center
Simi Valley, CA 93065

Sudhir Gupta
Memorial Sloan-Kettering Cancer Center
New York, NY 10021

P. John Hagan
The ENT Surgical Group
Kingston, PA 18704

N. A. Halasz
Department of Surgery
University of California, San Diego
    School of Medicine
La Jolla, CA 92037

Judith G. Hall
Department of Medical Genetics
Children's Orthopedic Hospital &
    Medical Center
Seattle, WA 98105

James W. Hanson
Department of Pediatrics
University of Iowa Hospitals & Clinics
Iowa City, IA 52242

B. Hardcastle
2240 N. W. 19th Lane
Gainesville, FL 32605

Robert H. A. Haslam
Division of Pediatrics
University of Calgary
Alberta, Canada T2N 1N4

Newlin Hastings
1136 W. 6th Street
Los Angeles, CA 90017

Frederick T. Hatch
Lawrence Livermore Laboratory
University of California
Livermore, CA 94550

Irvin F. Hawkins, Jr.
Department of Radiology
University of Florida College of Medicine
Gainesville, FL 32610

Daniel M. Hays
Children's Hospital of Los Angeles
Los Angeles, CA 90054

James R. Hayward
Department of Oral Surgery
University of Michigan Medical Center
Ann Arbor, MI 48104

Frederick Hecht
Southwest Biomedical Research
    Institute
Tempe, AZ 85281

William E. Hellenbrand
Department of Pediatrics
Yale University School of Medicine
New Haven, CT 06510

Jürgen Herrmann
Department of Pediatrics
University of Wisconsin Medical School
Madison, WI 53706

Victor H. Hildyard
Colby Clinic
Colby, KS 67701

Richard E. Hillman
Division of Medical Genetics
Washington University School of Medicine
St. Louis, MO 63110

Raymond L. Hintz
Department of Pediatrics
Stanford University School of Medicine
Stanford, CA 94305

Sølve Hognestad
Horselssentralen, St. Franciscus Hospital
4000 Stavanger
Norway

Thomas M. Holder
4400 Broadway
Kansas City, MO 64111

Paul H. Holinger
700 N. Michigan Avenue
Chicago, IL 60611

David W. Hollister
Departments of Pediatrics and Medicine
Harbor General Hospital
Torrance, CA 90509

Lewis B. Holmes
Genetics Unit
The Massachusetts General Hospital
Boston, MA 02114

Richard Hong
Department of Pediatrics
University of Wisconsin Medical School
Madison, WI 53706

George R. Honig
Department of Hematology
The Children's Memorial Hospital
Chicago, IL 60614

William A. Horton
Department of Medicine
Kansas University Medical Center
Kansas City, KS 66103

Jack Van Doren Hough
3400 N.W. 56th Street
Oklahoma City, OK 73112

Carolyn D. Hudson
Department of Oral Medicine & Pathology
Guy's Hospital Dental School
London, England SE1 9RT

Irene Hussels-Maumenee
The Wilmer Institute
The Johns Hopkins Hospital
Baltimore, MD 21205

Agnes M. Ickenroth
Department of Human Genetics
University of Nijmegen
The Netherlands

Donald Imbrie
Department of Otolaryngology
University of Oregon Medical School
Portland, OR 97201

Kent F. Jacobs*

Egil Jellum
Institute of Clinical Biochemistry
University of Oslo, Rikshospitalet
Oslo 1, Norway

Jan E. Jirásek
Institute for the Care of Mother & Child
Prague-Podoli, Czechoslovakia

Clinton C. Johnson
Dental Service
Veterans Administration Hospital
Dallas, TX 75216

Dale G. Johnson
Department of Surgery
Primary Children's Hospital
Salt Lake City, UT 84103

Waine C. Johnson
Department of Dermatology
The Skin and Cancer Hospital
Philadelphia, PA 19140

William J. Johnson
Department of Internal Medicine
Mayo Clinic
Rochester, MN 55901

Paul W. Johnston
50 Bellefontaine St.
Pasadena, CA 91105

Kenneth Lyons Jones
Clinical Research Center, AID
University Hospital
San Diego, CA 92103

Ronald J. Jorgenson
Department of Pediatric Dentistry
Medical University of South Carolina
Charleston, SC 29401

Herbert L. Joseph
1516 Napa Street
Vallejo, CA 94590

Richard C. Juberg
Children's Medical Center
Dayton, OH 45404

Ilkka I. Kaitila
Children's Hospital
University of Helsinki
Helsinki, Finland SF-00290

Hans Kalmus
Galton Laboratory
University College London
London, England WC1

Harry Irving Katz
4001 Stinson Blvd., NE
Minneapolis, MN 55421

Dennis Kay
Division of Otolaryngology
University of Colorado Medical Center
Denver, CO 80220

*Present address unknown.

B. H. Kean
Department of Medicine
Cornell University Medical Center
New York, NY 10021

Harris J. Keene
Oral Oncology
University of Texas
The Health Science Center at Houston
   Medical School
Houston, TX 77025

Gordon G. Keyes
Department of Oral Pathology
West Virginia University
Morgantown, WV 26506

Anne C. Kimball
Department of Medicine
Cornell University Medical College
New York, NY 10021

Stanley E. Kirkpatrick
Department of Pediatrics
University Hospital
San Diego, CA 92110

Yukio Kitano
Department of Dermatology
University of Osaka
Fukushimaku, Osaka, Japan

Marion A. Koerper
Department of Pediatrics
University of California, San Francisco
School of Medicine
San Francisco, CA 94143

Maurice D. Kogut
Children's Hospital
Los Angeles, CA 90027

Alfried Kohlschütter
Universitatskinderklinik
D-34 Gottingen, Germany

Robert I. Kohut
Department of Surgery
University of California, Irvine,
   College of Medicine
Irvine, CA 92664

Bruce W. Konigsmark ‡

K. S. Kozlowski
Staff Radiologist
Royal Alexandra Hospital for Children
Sydney, Australia 2050

Alex E. Krill‡

Saul Krugman
Department of Pediatrics
New York University Medical Center
New York, NY 10016

Ralph S. Lachman
Department of Radiology
Harbor General Hospital
Torrance, CA 90509

Leonard O. Langer, Jr.
Department of Radiology
University of Wisconsin
   Medical Center
Madison, WI 53706

‡Deceased.

Normand Lapointe
Department of Immunology
Hôpital Sainte Justine
Montreal, Quebec, Canada H3T 1C5

Carl-Bertil Laurell
Department of Clinical Chemistry
University of Lund
S-214 01 Malmö, Sweden

Benjamin C. Leadholm
Division of Otolaryngology
University of Colorado Medical Center
Denver, CO 80220

Robert S. Lees
Clinical Research Center
Massachusetts Institute of Technology
Cambridge, MA 02139

L. Stefan Levin
Department of Otolaryngology
The Johns Hopkins University School of
   Medicine
Baltimore, MD 21205

Robert I. Levy
Molecular Disease Branch
National Heart and Lung Institute
Bethesda, MD 20014

Jack R. Lichtenstein
Washington University School of Medicine
St. Louis, MO 63110

Leonard M. Linde
Los Angeles Pediatric Cardiology Medical
   Group, Inc.
10921 Wilshire Blvd.
Los Angeles, CA 90024

Russell V. Lucas, Jr.
Department of Cardiology
University of Minnesota Medical
   School, Minneapolis
Minneapolis, MN 55455

Thomas J. McCarter
1514 White Bear Avenue
St. Paul, MN 55106

Wallace W. McCrory
Department of Pediatrics
Cornell University Medical College
New York, NY 10021

Barbara J. McGee
AA-5218 Medical Center
Vanderbilt University Hospital
Nashville, TN 37232

Guy M. McKhann
Department of Neurology
The Johns Hopkins University
   School of Medicine
Baltimore, MD 21205

David H. McKibben, Jr.
Cleft Palate Research Center
University of Pittsburgh School of Medi-
   cine
Pittsburgh, PA 15261

Victor A. McKusick
Department of Medicine
The Johns Hopkins University
   School of Medicine
Baltimore, MD 21205

Dan G. McNamara
Section of Cardiology
Texas Children's Hospital
Houston, TX 77030

Ellen Magenis
Department of Medical Genetics
University of Oregon Medical School
Portland, OR 97201

Philip M. Marden
340 E. Summit Avenue
Oconomowoc, WI 53066

Pierre Maroteaux
Assistant Medical Biologist
Hôpital des Enfants Malades
75730 Paris, Cedex 15 France

Henry J. L. Marriott
Department of Clinical Research
St. Anthony's Hospital
St. Petersburg, FL 33705

Yoshinobu Masuda
323–47 Mizonuma
Asaka-shi, Saitama-ken
Japan

Roland S. Medansky
1600 Dempster
Park Ridge, IL 60068

Amir H. Mehregan
415 S. Monroe Street
Monroe, MI 48161

Marvin C. Mengel
115 W. Columbia Street
Orlando, FL 32806

William C. Mentzer, Jr.
Department of Pediatrics
San Francisco General Hospital
San Francisco, CA 94110

Lawrence Meskin
Department of Health Ecology
University of Minnesota School of Dentistry
Minneapolis, MN 55455

Louise Brearley Messer
Department of Pediatric Dentistry
University of Minnesota School of Dentistry
Minneapolis, MN 55455

Irving Meyer
40 Maple Street
Springfield, MA 01103

George R. Mikhail
Department of Dermatology
Henry Ford Hospital
Detroit, MI 48202

B. Lynn Miller
Department of Pediatrics (Cardiology)
University of Florida College of Medicine
Gainesville, FL 32610

Daniel R. Miller
Ear, Nose & Throat-Facial Plastic Surgery
3316 Fourth Street
Lewiston, ID 83501

Michael E. Miller
Department of Pediatric Immunology
University of California School of Medicine
Torrance, CA 90509

Orlando J. Miller
Department of Obstetrics & Gynecology &
　Human Genetics & Development
Columbia University College of Physicians
　& Surgeons
New York, NY 10032

Robert H. Miller
Division of Pediatric Cardiology
University Hospital of Jacksonville
Jacksonville, FL 32209

Robert W. Miller
402 Federal Building
National Cancer Institute
Bethesda, MD 20014

Stephen H. Miller
Department of Surgery
Hershey Medical Center
Hershey, PA 17033

David T. Mininberg
New York Medical College
New York, NY 10029

Narla Mohandas
Cancer Research Institute
University of California Medical Center
San Francisco, CA 94143

James H. Moller
Division of Pediatric Cardiology
University of Minnesota, Medical
　School, Minneapolis
Minneapolis, MN 55455

Merle E. Morris
Division of Pedodontics
University of California School of Dentistry
San Francisco, CA 94143

Grant Morrow, III
Department of Pediatrics
University of Arizona School of Medicine
Tucson, AZ 85724

Edmund J. Moynahan
Department of Dermatology
Guy's Hospital
London, SE 1, England

Thomas J. Muckle
Director of Laboratories
McMaster University Medical School
Hamilton, Ontario, Canada L8N 3L6

Sigfrid A. Muller
Department of Dermatology
Mayo Clinic
Rochester, MN 55901

Charles E. Mullins
Section of Pediatric Cardiology
Texas Children's Hospital
Houston, TX 77030

Roger E. Murken
1067 Bowdain Ave.
St. Paul, MN 55116

Walter E. Nance
Department of Human Genetics
Medical College of Virginia
Richmond, VA 23298

Lewis N. Neblett
1211 S. Glenstone St.
Springfield, MO 65804

Gerhard Neuhäuser
Kinderklinik Universitat
Loschgestrasse 15
D-8520 Erlangen
West Germany

Robert C. Newell
Bellingham Medical Center
Bellingham, WA 98225

Buford L. Nichols
Baylor University
College of Medicine
Houston, TX 77030

Audrey H. Nora
Department of Pediatrics
University of Colorado Medical Center
Denver, CO 80220

James J. Nora
Department of Pediatric Cardiology
University of Colorado Medical Center
Denver, CO 80220

Robert A. Norum
Division of Medical Genetics
Cornell University Medical College
New York, NY 10021

William L. Nyhan
Department of Pediatrics
University of California, San　Diego,
　School of Medicine
La Jolla, CA 92037

Samuel Scott Obenshain
Department of Pediatrics
University of New Mexico School of
　Medicine
Albuquerque, NM 87106

John S. O'Brien
Department of Neurosciences
University of California, San Diego,
　School of Medicine
La Jolla, California 92037

John M. Opitz
Department of Genetics
University of Wisconsin Medical School
Madison, WI 53706

Richard J. O'Reilly
Memorial Sloan-Kettering Cancer Center
New York, NY 10021

Eduardo Orti
Department of Pediatrics
State University of New York
Downstate Medical Center
Brooklyn, NY 11203

John Q. Owsley, Jr.
Franklin Medical Center
San Francisco, CA 94114

Savita Pahwa
Department of Immunology
Memorial-Sloan-Kettering Cancer Center
New York, NY 10021

A. D. Patrick
Institute of Child Health
University of London
London, England WC1N 1EH

Milton H. Paul
Division of Cardiology
The Children's Memorial Hospital
Chicago, IL 60614

Carl M. Pearson
Division of Rheumatology
UCLA School of Medicine
Los Angeles, CA 90024

Thomas L. Perry
Department of Pharmacology
University of British Columbia
Vancouver, Canada

Udo Pfändler
Faculty of Medicine
University of Berne
Berne, Switzerland

Rudolf A. Pfeiffer
Institut fur Humangenetik
Ratzeburger Allee 160
24 Lubeck
Federal Republic of Germany

Michel Philippart
Neuropsychiatric Institute
University of California, Los Angeles,
　School of Medicine
Los Angeles, CA 90024

Lawrence K. Pickett
Department of Surgery
Yale University School of Medicine
New Haven, CT 06510

V. K. Pillay
Orthopaedic Surgery, Singapore Polyclinic
Republic of Singapore

Steven M. Podos
Department of Ophthalmology
Washington University School of Medicine
St. Louis, MO 63110

George Polgar
Department of Physiology
University of Pennsylvania School of
    Medicine
Philadelphia, PA 19104

Philip Posner
Department of Physiology
University of Florida College of Medicine
Gainesville, FL 32610

Marilyn Preus
Department of Medical Genetics
The Montreal Children's Hospital
Montreal, Quebec, Canada H3H 1P3

Bozidar Puretíc‡

Štefanija Puretíc
Petrova 90
41000 Zagreb
Yugoslavia

Qutub H. Qazi
Department of Pediatrics
State University of New York
Downstate Medical Center
Brooklyn, NY 11203

Elsa K. Rahn
Department of Ophthalmology
Nassau County Medical Center
East Meadow, NY 11554

Satish R. Rao
Department of Pediatric Dentistry
Medical University of South Carolina
Charleston, SC 29401

Gerald M. Reaven
Stanford University School of Medicine
Stanford, CA 94305

Robert S. Redman
V. A. Hospital
Denver, CO 80220

William B. Reed‡

Samuel Refetoff
Department of Medicine
University of Chicago, The Pritzker School
    of Medicine
Chicago, IL 60637

William Reichel
Franklin Square Hospital
9000 Franklin Square Drive
Baltimore, MD 21237

J. Sidney Rice
1205 North Center Street
Hickory, NC 28601

Thomas A. Riemenschneider
Department of Pediatrics
University of California at Davis
Sacramento Medical Center
Sacramento, CA 95817

David L. Rimoin
Department of Pediatrics
Harbor General Hospital
Torrance, CA 90509

Donald A. Riopel
Division of Pediatric Cardiology
Medical University of South Carolina
Charleston, SC 29401

Meinhard Robinow
Department of Pediatrics
University of Virginia Medical Center
Charlottesville, VA 22901

Leon E. Rosenberg
Departments of Human Genetics,
    Pediatrics and Medicine
Yale University School of Medicine
New Haven, CT 06510

Nathaniel H. Rowe
Department of Oral Pathology
University of Michigan School of
    Dentistry
Ann Arbor, MI 48104

Jack H. Rubinstein
Children's Neuromuscular Diagnostic
    Center
Cincinnati, OH 45229

Raymond Saddi
Maitre de Recherche CNRS
University Cochin
Paris, XIV France

Inge Sagel
New York Medical College
New York, NY 10029

Isamu Sando
Department of Otopathology
University of Pittsburgh School of
    Medicine
Pittsburgh, PA 15213

John J. Sauk, Jr.
Department of Human and Oral
    Genetics
University of Minnesota Medical School,
    Minneapolis
Minneapolis, MN 55455

Georges Schapira
Universite de Paris
Institut de Pathologie Moleculaire
Paris, XIV France

I. Herbert Scheinberg
Albert Einstein College of Medicine
Bronx, NY 10461

Gerold L. Schiebler
Department of Pediatrics
University of Florida College of Medicine
Gainesville, FL 32610

R. Neil Schimke
Dept. of Medicine and Pediatrics
University of Kansas Medical Center
Kansas City, KS 66103

Jerry A. Schneider
Department of Pediatrics
University of California, San Diego
    School of Medicine
La Jolla, CA 92037

Joseph D. Schulman
National Institute of Child Health &
    Human Development
National Institutes of Health
Bethesda, MD 20014

Robert Schwartz
Department of Pediatric Metabolism
Rhode Island Hospital
Providence, RI 02902

Stanley A. Schwartz
Memorial Sloan-Kettering Cancer Center
New York, NY 10021

Charles I. Scott, Jr.
Department of Pediatrics
University of Texas Medical School
Houston, TX 77025

Charles R. Scriver
Departments of Pediatrics & Biology
The McGill University
Montreal, Quebec H3H 1P3, Canada

Heddie O. Sedano
Department of Oral Pathology
University of Minnesota School of
    Dentistry
Minneapolis, MN 55455

Victor J. Selmanowitz
Orentreich Foundation for the
    Advancement of Science
New York, NY 10021

Larry J. Shapiro
Department of Medical Genetics
Harbor General Hospital
Torrance, CA 90509

Carol S. Shear
University of Miami Mailman Center for
    Child Development
Miami, FL 33152

Madoka Shibuya
New York Hospital Cornell University
    Medical Center
New York, NY 10021

Henry R. Shinefield
Kaiser Foundation Hospital
San Francisco, CA 94119

Stephen B. Shohet
Cancer Research Institute
University of California
San Francisco, CA 94143

Kenneth Shulman
Department of Neurological Surgery
Albert Einstein College of Medicine
Bronx, NY 10461

James B. Sidbury, Jr.
National Institute of Child Health
    and Human Development
NIH
Bethesda, MD 20014

William K. Sieber
3500 Fifth Avenue
Pittsburgh, PA 15213

David C. Siggers
Department of Child Health
Southampton General Hospital
Southampton, SO9 4XY, England

Henry K. Silver
Department of Pediatrics
University of Colorado Medical Center
Denver, CO 80220

Frederic N. Silverman
Department of Radiology
Stanford University Medical Center
Stanford, CA 94305

Olli G. Simell
Children's Hospital
University of Helsinki
Helsinki SF-00290, Finland

Joe Leigh Simpson
Department of Obstetrics and Gynecology
Northwestern University School of
    Medicine
Chicago, IL 60611

John Simpson
Birth Defects Information Office
1720 7th Ave. South
Birmingham, AL 35233

William Singer
Department of Pediatric Neurology
New England Medical Center Hospital
Boston, MA 02111

G. T. Singleton
Shands Teaching Hospital
University of Florida College of Medicine
Gainesville, FL 32610

Howard R. Sloan*

David W. Smith
Department of Pediatrics
The University of Washington School of
    Medicine
Seattle, WA 98105

Morton E. Smith
Department of Ophthalmology
Washington University School of
    Medicine
St. Louis, MO 63110

Raymond O. Smith, Jr.
Department of Otolaryngology
Oklahoma Medical Center
Oklahoma City, OK 73104

Elizabeth M. Smithwick
Memorial Sloan-Kettering Cancer Center
New York, NY 10021

Selma Snyderman
Department of Pediatrics
New York University School of Medicine
New York, NY 10016

*Present address unknown.

Madison S. Spach
Division of Pediatric Cardiology
Duke University Medical Center
Durham, NC 27710

Mark A. Sperling
Endocrinology Division
Children's Hospital Medical Center
Cincinnati, OH 45229

Jürgen W. Spranger
Department of Pediatrics
University Kinderklinik
65 Mainz, Germany

Arthur G. Steinberg
Department of Biology
Case Western Reserve University School
    of Medicine
Cleveland, OH 44106

Daniel Steinberg
Department of Metabolic Disease
University of California, San Diego
School of Medicine
La Jolla, CA 92037

Sandra Stenmark
Children's Hospital
Denver, CO 80218

Roger E. Stevenson
Greenwood Genetics Center
Greenwood, SC 29646

Janet M. Stewart
Department of Pediatrics
University of Colorado Medical Center
Denver, CO 80220

Oddvar Stokke
University of Oslo
Institute of Clinical Biochemistry
Oslo, Norway

Orville J. Stone
Division of Dermatology
University of California, Irvine
California College of Medicine
Irvine, CA 92664

Lotte Strauss
Mount Sinai School of Medicine
New York, NY 10029

Joel Sugar
Department of Ophthalmology
University of Illinois Hospital
Chicago, IL 60612

Mai Park Suhr
240 Sleepy Hollow Terrace
Glendale, CA 91206

Robert L. Summitt
Departments of Pediatrics, Anatomy
    and Child Development
University of Tennessee Center for
    The Health Sciences
Memphis, TN 38163

H. Eldon Sutton
Department of Zoology
University of Texas
Austin, TX 78712

T. Sveger
Department of Clinical Chemistry
University of Lund
S-214 01 Malmö, Sweden

Lawrence Sweetman
Department of Pediatrics
University of California, San Diego
School of Medicine
La Jolla, CA 92037

Chester A. Swinyard
Visiting Professor Emeritus of Surgery
The Children's Hospital at Stanford
Palo Alto, CA 94304

Norman S. Talner
Department of Pediatrics
Yale University School of Medicine
New Haven, CT 06510

Samia A. Temtamy
Department of Human Genetics
National Research Centre
Dokki, Cairo, Egypt

Thomas M. Teree
Department of Pediatrics
Baystate Medical Center
Springfield, MA 01107

Darrell L. Teter
6850 East Hampden Ave.
Denver, CO 80222

E. George Thorne
West 8th Ave. & Cherokee Street
Denver, CO 80204

Paul M. Tocci
University of Miami School of Medicine
Miami, FL 33152

Kathleen Toomey
Department of Pediatrics
University of South Florida College
    of Medicine
Tampa, FL 33612

Robert J. Touloukian
Department of Surgery
Yale University School of Medieine
New Haven, CT 06510

Oscar Touster
Department of Molecular Biology
Vanderbilt University
Nashville, TN 37203

John N. Trodahl
Oral Disease Research Laboratory
V. A. Hospital
Houston, TX 77211

Donald P. Tschudy
National Institutes of Health
Clinical Center
Bethesda, MD 20014

Jouni Uitto
Division of Medical Genetics
Washington University School of Medicine
St. Louis, MO 64110

Robert A. Ulstrom
University of Minnesota Medical School,
Minneapolis
Minneapolis, MN 55455

Paul R. Vandersteen
Department of Dermatology
Fargo Clinic
Fargo, ND 58102

L. H. S. Van Mierop
Department of Pediatrics (Cardiology)
University of Florida College of Medicine
Gainesville, FL 32610

Thomas A. Vargo
Division of Pediatric Cardiology
Baylor College of Medicine
Houston, TX 77025

William F. Via, Jr.
Department of Oral Diagnosis
University of North Carolina School
of Dentistry
Chapel Hill, NC 27514

Robert A. Vickers
Department of Oral Pathology
University of Minnesota School of
Dentistry
Minneapolis, MN 55455

Benjamin E. Victorica
Department of Pediatrics (Cardiology)
University of Florida College of Medicine
Gainesville, FL 32610

William B. Wadlington
2614 Old Lebanon Road
Nashville, TN 37214

Thomas A. Waldmann
Department of Metabolism
National Cancer Institute
Bethesda, MD 20014

Charles A. Waldron
Department of Oral Pathology
Emory University School of Dentistry
Atlanta, GA 30322

Paul O. Walker
Department of Pedodontics
University of Minnesota School of
Dentistry
Minneapolis, MN 55455

I. S. Wallman
111 Barker Road
Subiaco, Australia 6008

Diane W. Wara
Department of Pediatrics
University of California, San Francisco
School of Medicine
San Francisco, CA 94143

Dorothy Warburton
Department of Human Genetics and
Development
Columbia University College of
Physicians and Surgeons
New York, NY 10032

Paul H. Ward
Department of Surgery
UCLA School of Medicine
Los Angeles, CA 90024

Josef Warkany
Department of Research Pediatrics
The Children's Hospital Research
Foundation
Cincinnati, OH 45229

Edward Wasserman
Department of Pediatrics
New York Medical College
New York, NY 10029

David G. Watson
University of Mississippi Medical Center
Jackson, MS 39216

William Watson
Department of Dermatology
Stanford University Medical Center
Stanford, CA 94305

Gary L. Way
Department of Pediatric Cardiology
University of Colorado Medical Center
Aurora, CO 80011

William B. Weil, Jr.
Department of Human Development
Michigan State University
East Lansing, MI 48823

Bernd Weinberg
Audiology and Speech Sciences
Purdue University
West Lafayette, IN 47906

Benjamin T. Wells
411 West 21st Street
Houston, TX 77008

Walter Weyler, Jr.
Department of Pediatrics
University of California, San Diego
School of Medicine
La Jolla, CA 92093

James G. White
Department of Pediatrics
University of Minnesota Medical School,
Minneapolis
Minneapolis, MN 55455

Peter F. Whitington
Department of Pediatrics
University of Wisconsin Medical School
Madison, WI 53706

L. S. Wildervanck
Department of Human Genetics
State University Groningen
Antonius Deusinglaan 4
Groningen, Holland

Robert L. Williams
Section of Pediatrics
Texas Children's Hospital
Houston, TX 77030

R. S. Wilroy, Jr.
Department of Pediatrics
University of Tennessee Center for
The Health Sciences
Memphis, TN 38163

Charles J. Wilson
200 University Boulevard
Galveston, TX 77550

A. M. Winchester
Department of Biological Sciences
College of Arts & Sciences
University of Northern Colorado
Greeley, CO 80631

Carl J. Witkop, Jr.
Division of Human and Oral Genetics
University of Minnesota School of
Dentistry
Minneapolis, MN 55455

Mitchel L. Wolf
Department of Ophthalmology
Washington University School of
Medicine
St. Louis, MO 63110

Raymond P. Wood, II
Department of Otolaryngology
University of Colorado Medical Center
Denver, CO 80220

Morton M. Woolley
Children's Hospital of Los Angeles
Los Angeles, CA 90027

H. M. Worth
Department of Medicine and Radiology
University of British Columbia
Vancouver 8, B.C. Canada

Herman E. Wyandt
Department of Pediatrics
University of Virginia Medical Center
Charlottesville, VA 22901

Sonja R. Wyss
Medizinisch-Chemisches Institut
der Universitat Bern
3000 Bern, Switzerland

Patricia S. Zelkowitz
Borgess Hospital
1521 Gull Road
Kalamazoo, MI 49001

Hans Zellweger
Department of Pediatrics
University of Iowa College of Medicine
Iowa City, IA 52240

William H. Zinkham
The Johns Hopkins University
School of Medicine
Baltimore, MD 21205

Jonathan Zonana
Division of Medical Genetics
Harbor General Hospital
Torrance, CA 90509

Contents

Section I
Atlas

Figure   *Page*

1. Normal disk and vessels. 1
2. Normal disk, vessels and macula 1
3. Drusen of optic nerve head 1
4. Drusen of macula 1
5. Small retinal coloboma 2
6. Coloboma of disk 2
7. Large coloboma of macula 2
8. Severe coloboma of disk and macula 2
9. Choroideremia 3
10. Choroidal nevus 3
11. Ectopic macula 3
12. Retinal fold 3
13. Epipapillary membrane 4
14. Congenital pit of optic nerve 4
15. Myelinated nerve fibers 4
16. Astrocytoma of retina 4
17. Aberrant congenital venous loop 4
18. Retinal vessel tortuosity in sickle cell hemoglobinopathy 4
19. Normal macula of patient with retinitis pigmentosa . . 5
20. Optic disk and vessels of patient with retinitis pigmentosa 5
21. Retinitis pigmentosa in midperiphery 5
22. Retinitis pigmentosa, dense 5
23. Pseudoxanthoma elasticum and angioid streak 5
24. Tay-Sachs disease as seen in retina 5
25. Acute chorioretinitis, toxoplasmic 6
26. Healed chorioretinitis, toxoplasmic 6
27. Microphakia 6
28. Rubella nuclear cataract 6
29. Sickle cell anemia as seen in retina 7
30. Polycythemia vera as seen in retina 7
31. Albinism as seen in retina 7
32. Congenital retinal telangiectasia 7
33. Vitelliruptive macular degeneration 8
34. Tuberous sclerosis as seen in retina 8
35. von Hippel-Lindau syndrome as seen in retina 8
36. Melanocytoma 8
37. Retinal fold, developmental 9
38. Heterochromia, partial 9
39. Cloudy cornea in congenital glaucoma 9
40. Acute angle closure glaucoma 9
41. Asteroid hyalitis 10
42. Cytoid bodies 10
43. Cataract zonularis 10
44. Corneal dystrophy, granular 10
45. Anterior polar cataract, small 10

Figure   *Page*

46. Anterior polar cataract, moderate 10
47. Iris coloboma 11
48. Albinism of iris and skin 11
49. Keratoconus 11
50. Keratoglobus 11
51. Conjunctival melanosis in Negro 11
52. Argyrosis of conjunctiva and eyelids 11
53. Heterochromia 12
54. Microphthalmia with pupillary abnormality and heterochromia 12
55. Cystinosis as seen in corneal stroma 12
56. Neurofibromatosis of upper eyelid 12
57. Kayser-Fleischer ring 12
58. Sunflower cataract 12
59. Aniridia 13
60. Retinoblastoma 13
61. Lens subluxated downward
62. Lens subluxated upward 13
63. Inverse epicanthal fold 14
64. Horner syndrome with heterochromia 14
65. Heterochromia and iris coloboma 14
66. Dermoid cyst of orbit 14
67. Epibulbar dermoid 14
68. Unilateral congenital glaucoma 14
69. Chromosome 21 trisomy syndrome 14
70. Bloom syndrome 14
71. Ochronosis 15
72. Hairy pinna 15
73. Microtia, type I with preauricular appendage 15
74. Microtia, type II 15
75. Microtia, type III with auricular appendage 15
76. Microtia, type III and polyotia 15
77. Aural exostosis 15
78. Primary cholesteatoma of middle ear 15
79. Gustatory sweating 15
80. Enamel hypoplasia and yellow staining from tetracycline 16
81. Incisors, shovel-shaped 16
82. Dentinogenesis imperfecta 16
83. Pegged teeth 16
84. Intraepithelial dyskeratosis 16
85. Odontodysplasia 16
86. Fused lateral and central incisor 17
87. Geminated primary lateral incisors 17
88. Erythropoietic porphyria 17
89. Gingival fibromatosis 17
90. Cleft uvula 17

91. Submucous cleft of soft and hard palate 17
92. Fabry disease as seen on conjunctiva. 18
93. Nasopharyngeal stenois. 18
94. Lingual thyroid. 18
95. Vitiligo on upper eyelid and poliosis. 18
96. Thyroglossal duct cyst. 18
97. Microphthalmia, esotropia and hypoplasia
     of nose with single nostril. 18
98. Keratoacanthoma. 18
99. Macroglossia. 18
100. Hemangioma 18
101. Tyrosinase-positive Caucasian albino. 19

102. Yellow-mutant Caucasian albino. 19
103. Tyrosinase-negative Caucasian albino 19
104. Hermansky-Pudlak syndrome 19
105. Microphthalmic-depigmented child with
     Cross syndrome 19
106. α-Thalassemia (hemoglobin H disease) 19
107. β-Thalassemia trait 19
108. Sickle cell anemia 19
109. Normal eye. 20
110. Normal pinna and nomenclature, microtia by
     type, and anotia 21

Section II
Compendium

Birth Defects Number and Name

1 Aarskog syndrome
2 Abetalipoproteinemia
3 Ablepharon
4 Abnormal fibrinogens
5 Acanthosis nigricans
6 Acatalasemia
7 Acetylator polymorphism (Marker)
8 Achondrogenesis, Langer-Saldino type
9 Achondrogenesis, Parenti-Fraccaro type
10 Achondroplasia
11 Acid maltase deficiency
12 Acoustic neuromata
13 Acrocephalopolysyndactyly
14 Acrocephalosyndactyly
15 Acrodermatitis enteropathica
16 Acrodysostosis
17 Acrofacial dysostosis
18 Acromegaloid phenotype, cutis verticis and gyratacorneal leukoma
19 Acromesomelic dysplasia, Campailla-Martinelli type
20 Acromesomelic dysplasia, Maroteaux type
21 Acro-osteolysis, dominant type
22 Acropectorovertebral dysplasia
23 Adrenal hypoaldosteronism of infancy, transient isolated
24 Adrenal hypoplasia, congenital
25 Adrenocortical unresponsiveness to ACTH, hereditary
26 Adrenocorticotropic hormone deficiency, isolated
27 Agammaglobulinemia, X-linked infantile
28 Agnathia, microstomia and synotia
29 Agonadia
30 Albinism-cutaneous and deafness
31 Albinism-cutaneous without deafness
32 Albinism-ocular
33 Albinism-oculocutaneous, Hermansky-Pudlak type
34 Albinism-oculocutaneous, tyrosinase negative
35 Albinism-oculocutaneous, tyrosinase positive
36 Albinism-oculocutaneous, yellow mutant
37 Alkaptonuria
38 Alopecia areata
39 Alpha$_1$-antitrypsin deficiency
40 Alpha-methyl-acetoacetic aciduria
41 Alström syndrome
42 Amastia
43 Amaurosis congenita of Leber
44 Amelo-cerebro-hypohidrotic syndrome
45 Amelo-onycho-hypohidrotic syndrome
46 Amelogenesis imperfecta
47 Analbuminemia
48 Analphalipoproteinemia
49 Androgen insensitivity syndrome, complete
50 Androgen insensitivity syndrome, incomplete
51 Anemia, hypoplastic congenital
52 Anencephaly
53 Aneurysm of aortic sinus of Valsalva
54 Angioedema, hereditary
55 Angio-osteohypertrophy syndrome
56 Anhidrosis
57 Aniridia
58 Anisocoria
59 Anisometropia
60 Ankyloblepharon
61 Ankyloglossia
62 Annular pancreas
63 Anomalous origin of contralateral subclavian artery
64 Anomalous origin of coronary arteries from pulmonary artery
65 Anonychia and ectrodactyly
66 Anonychia, hereditary
67 Anophthalmia
68 Anorchia
69 Anorectal malformations
70 Anosmia, congenital
71 Antibodies to human allotypes (Markers)
72 Anus-hand-ear syndrome
73 Aorta, coarctation
74 Aortic arch, cervical
75 Aortic arch, double
76 Aortic arch interruption
77 Aortic arch, right
78 Aortic stenosis, supravalvar
79 Aortic valve atresia
80 Aortic valve stenosis
81 Aortic valve, tetracuspid
82 Aortico-left ventricular tunnel
83 Aortico-pulmonary septal defect
84 Aphakia
85 Arachnodactyly, contractural
86 Argininemia
87 Argininosuccinic aciduria
88 Arthrogryposis

89   Arthrogrypotic hand anomaly and
      sensorineural deafness
90   Arthro-ophthalmopathy
91   Asphyxiating thoracic dysplasia
92   Asplenia syndrome
93   Ataxia-hypogonadism syndrome
94   Ataxia-telangiectasia
95   Atransferrinemia
96   Atrial septal defects
97   Auditory canal atresia
98   Auriculo-osteodysplasia
99   Baldness, common
100 Bartter syndrome
101 Basal cell nevus syndrome
102 Basan syndrome
103 Basilar impression, primary
104 Beckwith-Wiedemann syndrome
105 Berlin syndrome
106 Beta-mercaptolactate-cysteine disulfiduria (Marker)
107 Beta-methyl-crotonyl-glycinuria
108 Bicuspid aortic valve
109 Bicuspid pulmonary valve
110 Biliary atresia
111 Blepharochalasis, double lip and nontoxic
      thyroid enlargement
112 Bloom syndrome
113 Blue rubber bleb nevus syndrome
114 Brachydactyly
115 Brain, spongy degeneration
116 Brancher deficiency
117 Branchial cleft cysts or sinuses
118 Branchio-skeleto-genital syndrome
119 Broad thumb-hallux syndrome
120 Bronchial atresia
121 C syndrome
122 Campomelic dysplasia
123 Cardioauditory syndrome
124 Carnitine deficiency of muscle, primary
125 Carnitine palmytl transferase deficiency
126 Carnosinemia
127 Carotid body tumor
128 Carpal-tarsal osteolysis and chronic
      progressive glomerulopathy
129 Carpal-tarsal osteolysis, recessive
130 Caruncle aberrations
131 Cataract and ichthyosis
132 Cataracts, cortical and nuclear
133 Cataracts, polar and capsular
134 Central core disease
135 Centralopathic epilepsy
136 Cerebellar ataxia and chorioretinal degeneration
137 Cerebral gigantism
138 Cerebro-costo-mandibular syndrome
139 Cerebro-hepato-renal syndrome
140 Cerebro-oculo-facio-skeletal syndrome
141 Cerumen variation (Marker)
142 Cervico-oculo-acoustic syndrome
143 Chédiak-Higashi syndrome
144 Cheilitis glandularis
145 Chemodectoma of middle ear
146 Chin fissure
147 Chin, trembling
148 Chloride diarrhea, congenital
149 Choledochal cyst
150 Cholesteatoma of temporal bone

151 Cholesteryl ester storage disease
152 Cholinesterase, atypical
153 Chondrodysplasia punctata, Conradi-Hünermann type
154 Chondrodysplasia punctata, rhizomelic type
155 Chondrodystrophic myotonia
156 Chondroectodermal dysplasia
157 Chromosome eight trisomy syndrome
158 Chromosome eighteen p- syndrome
159 Chromosome eighteen q- syndrome
160 Chromosome eighteen trisomy syndrome
161 Chromosome eleven q- partial trisomy syndrome
162 Chromosome eleven q- syndrome
163 Chromosome five p- syndrome
164 Chromosome four p- syndrome
165 Chromosome fourteen q distal partial trisomy
      syndrome
166 Chromosome fourteen q proximal partial
      trisomy syndrome
167 Chromosome thirteen q- syndrome
168 Chromosome thirteen trisomy syndrome
169 Chromosome triploidy syndrome
170 Chromosome twenty-one monosomy
171 Chromosome twenty-one trisomy syndrome
172 Chromosome twenty-two monosomy
173 Chromosome 45,X/46,XY mosaicism
174 Citrullinemia
175 Clasped thumbs
176 Cleft lip or palate and filiform fusion of eyelids
177 Cleft lip or palate and lip pits or mounds
178 Cleft lip with or without cleft palate
179 Cleft lip-palate, ectodermal dysplasia and syndactyly
180 Cleft palate
181 Cleft palate and persistence of buccopharyngeal
      membrane
182 Cleft palate, micrognathia and glossoptosis
183 Cleft palate, stapes fixation and oligodontia
184 Cleft uvula (Marker)
185 Cleidocranial dysplasia
186 CNS arteriovenous malformation
187 CNS depression, hemorrhage, skeletal syndrome
188 CNS neoplasms
189 Cockayne syndrome
190 Coffin-Lowry syndrome
191 Cogan congenital ocular motor apraxia
192 Colon aganglionosis
193 Colon atresia or stenosis
194 Colon duplication
195 Color blindness, blue monocone-monochromatic
196 Color blindness, red-green deutan series
197 Color blindness, red-green protan series
198 Color blindness, total
199 Color blindness, yellow-blue
200 Common origin of brachiocephalic and
      contralateral carotid artery
201 Cone-rod degeneration
202 Conjoined twins
203 Coproporphyria
204 Cor triatriatum
205 Cornea plana
206 Corneal dystrophy and sensorineural deafness
207 Corneal dystrophy, congenital hereditary
208 Corneal dystrophy, endothelial
209 Corneal dystrophy, granular
210 Corneal dystrophy, juvenile epithelial
211 Corneal dystrophy, lattice

212 Corneal dystrophy, macular
213 Corneal dystrophy, polymorphous posterior
214 Corneal dystrophy, recurrent erosive
215 Corneal dystrophy, Reis-Bücklers
216 Corneal dystrophy, Schnyder crystalline
217 Coronary arterial calcinosis
218 Coronary arteriovenous fistula
219 Coronary artery, single
220 Corpus callosum agenesis
221 Cortical hyperostosis, infantile
222 Corticosteroid-binding globulin abnormalities
223 Cranio-carpo-tarsal dysplasia
224 Craniodiaphyseal dysplasia
225 Craniofacial dysostosis
226 Craniofacial dysostosis with diaphyseal hyperplasia
227 Craniofacial dyssynostosis
228 Craniometaphyseal dysplasia
229 Cranio-oculo-dental syndrome
230 Craniosynostosis
231 Craniosynostosis-radial aplasia syndrome
232 Cryptotia
233 Cutis laxa
234 Cyclopia
235 Cylindromas of scalp
236 Cystathioninuria
237 Cystic fibrosis
238 Cystinosis
239 Cystinuria
240 Cysts of spleen
241 Darwin tubercle (Marker)
242 De Lange syndrome
243 Deaf-mutism, semilethal
244 Deafness and absent incudo-stapedial junction
245 Deafness and atopic dermatitis
246 Deafness and diabetes
247 Deafness and ear pits
248 Deafness and episodic vertigo
249 Deafness and goiter
250 Deafness and metaphyseal dysostosis
251 Deafness and myopia
252 Deafness and onychodystrophy
253 Deafness and progressive optic nerve atrophy
254 Deafness-conductive and malformed low-set ears
255 Deafness, diabetes, photomyoclonus and nephropathy
256 Deafness, dominant low-frequency
257 Deafness, goiter and peripheral resistance to thyroid hormone
258 Deafness, hyperprolinuria and ichthyosis
259 Deafness, keratopachydermia and digital constrictions
260 Deafness, low-tone
261 Deafness, myopia, cataract and saddle nose
262 Deafness, onychodystrophy and digital anomalies
263 Deafness, peripheral pulmonary stenoses and brachy-telephalangy
264 Deafness, renal and digital anomalies
265 Deafness-sensorineural, diverticulitis and neuropathy
266 Deafness-sensorineural, dystonia and retardation
267 Deafness-sensorineural, midfrequency
268 Deafness-sensorineural, polyneuropathy and optic atrophy
269 Deafness-sensorineural, progressive high-tone
270 Deafness-sensorineural, recessive early-onset
271 Deafness-sensorineural, recessive profound
272 Deafness, streptomycin-sensitivity
273 Deafness, tune (Marker)
274 Deafness, unilateral inner ear
275 Deafness, vitiligo and muscle wasting
276 Dens in dente
277 Dentin dysplasia, coronal
278 Dentin dysplasia, radicular
279 Dentinogenesis imperfecta
280 Dentino-osseous dysplasia
281 Dermal hypoplasia, focal
282 Dermo-chondro-corneal dystrophy of François
283 Dermoid cyst or teratoma of head and neck
284 Dermolipoma
285 Dextrocardia, bronchiectasis and sinusitis syndrome
286 Dextroposition of ventricular septum and double inlet left ventricle
287 Diabetes insipidus, vasopressin-resistant
288 Diaphragm, eventration
289 Diaphragmatic hernia
290 Diaphyseal dysplasia
291 Diastema, median incisal (Marker)
292 Diastematomyelia
293 Diastrophic dysplasia
294 Dicarboxylic aminoaciduria
295 Diplegia, spastic
296 Distichiasis
297 Double outlet right ventricle with anterior ventricular septal defect
298 Double outlet right ventricle with posterior ventricular septal defect
299 Dubowitz syndrome
300 Duodenal atresia or stenosis
301 Dupuytren contracture
302 Dwarfism, Laron
303 Dwarfism, panhypopituitary
304 Dwarfism, pituitary with abnormal sella turcica
305 Dwarfism, snub-nose
306 Dyggve-Melchior-Clausen syndrome
307 Dysautonomia
308 Dyschondrosteosis
309 Dyscoria
310 Dysosteosclerosis
311 Dysplasia epiphysealis hemimelica
312 Ear, absent tragus
313 Ear, arteriovenous fistula
314 Ear, cupped
315 Ear dysplasias, inner
316 Ear, ectopic pinna
317 Ear, exchondrosis (Marker)
318 Ear exostoses
319 Ear, hairy
320 Ear lobe, absent
321 Ear lobe, cleft
322 Ear lobe pit (Marker)
323 Ear lobes, attached (Marker)
324 Ear lobes, hypertrophic thickened
325 Ear, long, narrow, posteriorly rotated
326 Ear, lop
327 Ear, low-set
328 Ear, Mozart (Marker)
329 Ear pits (Marker)
330 Ear, prominent anthelix
331 Ear, small with folded-down helix
332 Ebstein anomaly
333 Ectodermal dysplasia, anhidrotic
334 Ectodermal dysplasia, hidrotic
335 Ectopia cordis

336 Ectrodactyly
337 Ectrodactyly-ectodermal dysplasia-clefting syndrome
338 Ehlers-Danlos syndrome
339 Elastosis perforans serpiginosa
340 Enamel and dentin defects from erythroblastosis fetalis
341 Enamel and dentin defects from tetracycline
342 Enamel, hypoplasia
343 Encephalocele
344 Encephalopathy necrotizing
345 Enchondromatosis
346 Enchondromatosis and hemangiomas
347 Endocardial cushion defects
348 Endocardial fibroelastosis of left ventricle
349 Endocardial fibroelastosis of right ventricle
350 Endocrine neoplasia I, multiple
351 Endocrine neoplasia II, multiple
352 Endocrine neoplasia III, multiple
353 Endomyocardial fibrosis of left ventricle
354 Endomyocardial fibrosis of right ventricle
355 Epiblepharon
356 Epicanthus
357 Epimerase deficiency (Marker)
358 Epiphyseal dysplasia, multiple
359 Epithelioma, multiple self-healing squamous
360 Epulis, congenital
361 Erythrokeratoderma, variable
362 Erythropoietic protoporphyria
363 Esophageal achalasia
364 Esophageal atresia
365 Esophageal atresia and tracheoesophageal fistula
366 Esophageal chalasia
367 Esophageal diverticulum
368 Esophageal duplication
369 Esophageal stenosis
370 Eustachian tube defects
371 Eyelid ectropion, congenital
372 Eyelid entropion
373 Fabry disease
374 Facial cleft, lateral
375 Facial cleft, oblique
376 Facial diplegia, congenital
377 Facial palsy, congenital
378 Facial palsy, late-onset
379 Fetal alcohol syndrome
380 Fetal aminopterin syndrome
381 Fetal cytomegalovirus syndrome
382 Fetal hydantoin syndrome
383 Fetal radiation syndrome
384 Fetal rubella syndrome
385 Fetal syphilis syndrome
386 Fetal thalidomide syndrome
387 Fetal toxoplasmosis syndrome
388 Fetal trimethadione syndrome
389 Fetal warfarin syndrome
390 Fibrous dysplasia, monostotic
391 Fibrous dysplasia, polyostotic
392 Fibula dysplasia and brachydactyly
393 Fingerprints absent
394 Frontometaphyseal dysplasia
395 Fructose-1-phosphate aldolase deficiency
396 Fructose-1,6-diphosphatase deficiency
397 Fructosuria (Marker)
398 Fucosidosis
399 Fundus albipunctatus
400 Fundus flavimaculatus
401 G syndrome
402 Galactokinase deficiency
403 Galactosemia
404 Gallbladder anomalies
405 Gastroschisis
406 Gaucher disease
407 Gingival fibromatosis
408 Gingival fibromatosis and corneal dystrophy
409 Gingival fibromatosis and digital anomalies
410 Gingival fibromatosis and hypertrichosis
411 Gingival fibromatosis and multiple hyaline fibromas
412 Gingival fibromatosis, Cowden type
413 Gingival fibromatosis, depigmentation and microphthalmia
414 Glaucoma, congenital
415 Globoid cell leukodystrophy
416 Glomus tumors, multiple
417 Glossitis, median rhomboid
418 Glucoglycinuria (Marker)
419 Glucose-galactose malabsorption
420 Glucose-6-phosphate dehydrogenase deficiency
421 Glutaric aciduria
422 Glutathionuria
423 Gluten-induced enteropathy
424 Glycogen synthetase deficiency
425 Glycogenosis, type I
426 Glycogenosis, type III
427 Glycogenosis, type VI
428 Glycogenosis, type VII
429 Glycogenosis, type VIII
430 Glycogenosis, type IX
431 G_{M1}-gangliosidosis, type 1
432 G_{M1}-gangliosidosis, type 2
433 G_{M2}-gangliosidosis with hexosaminidase A and B deficiency
434 G_{M2}-gangliosidosis with hexosaminidase A deficiency
435 Goiter, goitrogen-induced
436 Gonadal dysgenesis, XX type
437 Gonadal dysgenesis, XY type
438 Gonadotropin deficiency, isolated
439 Goniodysgenesis
440 Gorlin-Chaudhry-Moss syndrome
441 Gout
442 Granulomatous disease of females, chronic
443 Granulomatous disease of males, chronic
444 Granulosis rubra nasi
445 Grebe syndrome
446 Group-specific component (Marker)
447 Growth hormone deficiency, isolated
448 Gustatory sweating
449 Gyrate atrophy
450 Hand muscle wasting and sensorineural deafness
451 Hanhart syndrome
452 Haptoglobin (Marker)
453 Hartnup disorder
454 Heart block, congenital complete
455 Heart-hand syndrome
456 Hemangioma and thrombocytopenia syndrome
457 Hemifacial microsomia
458 Hemihypertrophy
459 Hemimelia and scalp-skull defects
460 Hemochromatosis, idiopathic

461 Hemophilia A
462 Hemophilia B
463 Hepatic agenesis
464 Hepatic arterial anomalies
465 Hepatic cyst, solitary
466 Hepatic hemangiomatosis
467 Hepatic lobes, accessory
468 Hepatic venous anomalies
469 Hepatolenticular degeneration
470 Herrmann-Opitz arthrogryposis syndrome
471 Hiatus hernia
472 Histidinemia
473 Holoprosencephaly
474 Homocystinuria
475 Horner syndrome
476 Human allotypes (Markers)
477 Humeroradial synostosis
478 Huntington chorea
479 Hyaloideoretinal degeneration of Wagner
480 Hydranencephaly
481 Hydrocephaly
482 Hydroxyprolinemia (Marker)
483 Hymen, imperforate
484 Hyperaldosteronism, familial glucocorticoid suppressible
485 Hyperammonemia
486 Hyperbeta-alaninemia
487 Hyperbilirubinemia I (Marker)
488 Hypercholesteremia
489 Hyperchylomicronemia
490 Hypercystinuria (Marker)
491 Hyperdibasic-aminoaciduria
492 Hyperglycinemia, nonketotic
493 Hyperhidrosis, premature hair greying and premolar aplasia
494 Hyperkeratosis palmoplantaris and periodontoclasia
495 Hyperlipoproteinemia III
496 Hyperlipoproteinemia, combined
497 Hyperostosis corticalis generalisata
498 Hyperostosis frontalis interna
499 Hyperparathyroidism, neonatal familial
500 Hyperprebeta-lipoproteinemia
501 Hyperprebeta-lipoproteinemia and hyperchylomicronemia
502 Hyperprolinemia (Marker)
503 Hypersarcosinemia
504 Hypertelorism
505 Hypertelorism-hypospadias syndrome
506 Hypertelorism, microtia, facial clefting and conductive deafness
507 Hypertrichosis lanuginosa
508 Hyperuricemia, deafness and ataxia
509 Hypervalinemia
510 Hypochondroplasia
511 Hypodontia and nail dysgenesis
512 Hypoglycemia, familial neonatal
513 Hypoglycemia, leucine-induced
514 Hypomagnesemia, primary
515 Hypoparathyroidism, X-linked infantile
516 Hypophosphatasia
517 Hypophosphatemia
518 Hypospadias
519 Imidazole aminoaciduria (Marker)
520 Iminoglycinuria (Marker)
521 Immunodeficiency, common variable
522 Immunodeficiency, severe combined
523 Immunodeficiency with Wiskott-Aldrich syndrome
524 Immunodeficiency, X-linked severe combined
525 Immunoglobulin A deficiency
526 Incontinentia pigmenti
527 Independent origin of ipsilateral vertebral artery
528 Inferior vena cava, absent hepatic segment
529 Inguinal hernia
530 Internal carotid artery aneurysm of middle ear
531 Intestinal atresia or stenosis
532 Intestinal duplication
533 Intestinal enterokinase deficiency
534 Intestinal lymphangiectasia
535 Intestinal polyposis I & II
536 Intestinal polyposis III
537 Intestinal rotation, incomplete
538 Intraepithelial dyskeratosis
539 Intraosseous fibrous swelling of jaws
540 Inversion of ventricles with transposition of great arteries
541 Inversion of ventricles without transposition of great arteries
542 Iodide transport defect
543 Iodotyrosine deiodinase deficiency
544 Iris coloboma and anal atresia syndrome
545 Isolated meconium ileus
546 Isolation of subclavian artery from aorta
547 Isovalericacidemia
548 Jaw-winking syndrome
549 Juvenile diabetes mellitus
550 Juvenile diabetes mellitus, optic atrophy and deafness
551 Keloid
552 Keratoconus
553 Keratopathy, band-shaped
554 KGB syndrome
555 Kleeblattschädel anomaly
556 Klinefelter syndrome
557 Kniest dysplasia
558 Knuckle pads, leukonychia and deafness
559 Koilonychia
560 Kuskokwim syndrome
561 Kyrle disease
562 Labyrinth aplasia
563 Lacrimal canaliculus atresia
564 Lacrimal gland, ectopic
565 Lacrimal sac fistula
566 Lactase deficiency, congenital
567 Lactase deficiency, primary
568 Lactate dehydrogenase isozymes
569 Lactose intolerance
570 Larsen syndrome
571 Laryngeal atresia
572 Laryngeal cysts
573 Laryngeal ventricle, prolapse
574 Laryngeal web
575 Laryngocele
576 Laryngomalacia
577 Laryngo-tracheo-esophageal cleft
578 Laurence-Moon-Biedl syndrome
579 Leber optic atrophy
580 Lecithin:cholesterol acyl transferase deficiency
581 Left ventricle, double outlet

582 Left ventricle, single papillary muscle
583 Lens and pupil, ectopic
584 Lens, ectopic
585 Lenticonus
586 Lentigines syndrome, multiple
587 Leprechaunism
588 Lesch-Nyhan syndrome
589 Leukonychia
590 Liddle syndrome
591 Limbal dermoid
592 Limb-oto-cardiac syndrome
593 Linear nevus sebaceous syndrome
594 Lip, double
595 Lip, median cleft of upper
596 Lip pits or mounds (Marker)
597 Lipase deficiency, congenital isolated
598 Lipogranulomatosis
599 Lipoid proteinosis
600 Lipomas, familial symmetric
601 Lipomatosis of face and neck
602 Lipomeningocele
603 Lissencephaly syndrome
604 Liver, hamartoma
605 Liver, polycystic disease
606 Liver transposition
607 Lobodontia
608 Localized absence of skin
609 Localized absence of skin, blistering and nail
     abnormalities
610 Long Qt syndrome without deafness
611 Lung, aberrant lobe
612 Lung lobe sequestration
613 Lymphangioma of alveolar ridges
614 Lymphedema I
615 Lymphedema II
616 Lysinemia
617 Macrodontia
618 Macroglossia
619 Macrotia
620 Macula, heterotopic
621 Macular coloboma and brachydactyly
622 Macular degeneration, vitelliruptive
623 Madarosis
624 Malate dehydrogenase, mitochondrial (Marker)
625 Malate dehydrogenase, soluble (Marker)
626 Mandibular prognathism
627 Mandibulofacial dysostosis
628 Maple syrup urine disease
629 Marden-Walker syndrome
630 Marfan syndrome
631 Maxilla, median alveolar cleft
632 McDonough syndrome
633 Meckel diverticulum
634 Meckel syndrome
635 Median cleft face syndrome
636 Median clefts of lower lip, mandible and tongue
637 Megalocornea
638 Megalocornea-mental retardation syndrome
639 Melanocytoma
640 Melanosis oculi, congenital
641 Melorheostosis
642 Meningocele
643 Menkes syndrome
644 Mesenchymal dysplasia of Puretić
645 Mesenteric cysts

646 Mesomelic dysplasia, Langer type
647 Mesomelic dysplasia, Nievergelt type
648 Mesomelic dysplasia, Reinhardt-Pfeiffer type
649 Mesomelic dysplasia, Werner type
650 Metachondromatosis
651 Metachromatic leukodystrophies
652 Metaphyseal chondrodysplasia, type Jansen
653 Metaphyseal chondrodysplasia, type McKusick
654 Metaphyseal chondrodysplasia, type Schmid
655 Metaphyseal chondrodysplasia with thymolym-
     phopenia
656 Metatropic dysplasia
657 Methionine malabsorption syndrome
658 Methylmalonic acidemia
659 Microcephaly
660 Microdontia (Marker)
661 Microphthalmia
662 Microphthalmia and digital anomalies
663 Microspherophakia
664 Microtia-atresia
665 Mitral valve atresia
666 Mitral valve insufficiency
667 Mitral valve insufficiency, deafness and skeletal
     malformations
668 Mitral valve prolapse
669 Mitral valve stenosis
670 Moynahan syndrome
671 Mucolipidosis I
672 Mucolipidosis II
673 Mucolipidosis III
674 Mucopolysaccharidosis I-H
675 Mucopolysaccharidosis I-S
676 Mucopolysaccharidosis II
677 Mucopolysaccharidosis III
678 Mucopolysaccharidosis IV
679 Mucopolysaccharidosis VI
680 Mucopolysaccharidosis VII
681 Mucosa, white folded dysplasia
682 Müllerian aplasia
683 Müllerian derivatives in males, persistent
684 Müllerian fusion, incomplete
685 Multiple cartilaginous exostoses
686 Muscle hypoplasia, congenital universal
687 Muscular dystrophy, adult pseudohypertrophic
688 Muscular dystrophy, autosomal recessive pseudohyper-
     trophic
689 Muscular dystrophy, childhood pseudohypertrophic
690 Muscular dystrophy, distal
691 Muscular dystrophy, limb-girdle
692 Muscular dystrophy, oculopharyngeal
693 Myelomeningocele
694 Myopathy, mitochondrial
695 Myopathy, myotubular
696 Myopathy, nemaline
697 Myopathy with lactic acidemia
698 Myophosphorylase deficiency
699 Myopia
700 Myositis ossificans
701 Myotonia congenita
702 Myotonic dystrophy
703 Naegeli syndrome
704 Nail-patella syndrome
705 Nasolacrimal duct impatency
706 Nasopharyngeal cysts
707 Nasopharyngeal stenosis

708 Nephritis and nerve deafness, hereditary
709 Nephrosis, congenital
710 Nephrosis, familial
711 Neuroectodermal pigmented tumor
712 Neurofibromatosis
713 Neuronal ceroid-lipofuscinoses
714 Neutropenia, cyclic
715 Nevus flammeus
716 Nevus of Ota
717 Niemann-Pick disease
718 Nightblindness
719 Nightblindness, stationary
720 Noonan syndrome
721 Norrie disease
722 Nose and nasal septum defects
723 Nose, anterior atresia
724 Nose, bifid
725 Nose, duplication
726 Nose, glioma
727 Nose, posterior atresia
728 Nose, transverse groove (Marker)
729 Nucleoside-phosphorylase deficiency
730 Obesity, hyperthermia, oligomenorrhea and parotid swelling
731 Obstruction within right ventricle or its outflow tract
732 Ocular and facial anomalies with proteinuria and deafness
733 Ocular colobomas
734 Ocular drusen
735 Oculo-auriculo-vertebral dysplasia
736 Oculo-cerebro-renal syndrome
737 Oculo-dento-osseous dysplasia
738 Oculo-mandibulo-facial syndrome
739 Odontodysplasia
740 Oguchi disease
741 Oligophrenia, epilepsy and ichthyosis syndrome
742 Olivopontocerebellar atrophy, dominant Menzel type
743 Olivopontocerebellar atrophy, dominant Schut-Haymaker type
744 Olivopontocerebellar atrophy, dominant with ophthalmoplegia
745 Olivopontocerebellar atrophy, dominant with retinal degeneration
746 Olivopontocerebellar atrophy, late-onset
747 Olivopontocerebellar atrophy, recessive Fickler-Winkler type
748 Omphalocele
749 Ophthalmo-mandibulo-melic dysplasia
750 Ophthalmoplegia externa and myopia
751 Ophthalmoplegia, familial static
752 Ophthalmoplegia, progressive external
753 Ophthalmoplegia totalis with ptosis and miosis
754 Opitz-Kaveggia FG syndrome
755 Optic atrophy, infantile heredofamilial
756 Optic disk pits
757 Optic disk, situs inversus
758 Optic nerve hypoplasia
759 Optico-cochleo-dentate degeneration
760 Oral dermoids
761 Orbital and periorbital dermoid cysts
762 Orbital cephaloceles
763 Orbital glioma
764 Orbital hemangioma
765 Orbital lymphangioma
766 Origin of left pulmonary artery from right pulmonary artery
767 Origin of pulmonary artery from ascending aorta
768 Origin of pulmonary artery from ductus arteriosus
769 Oro-cranio-digital syndrome
770 Oro-facio-digital syndrome I
771 Oro-facio-digital syndrome II
772 Oroticaciduria
773 Ossicle and middle ear malformations
774 Osteochondritis dissecans
775 Osteodysplasty
776 Osteoectasia
777 Osteogenesis imperfecta
778 Osteopathia striata
779 Osteopetrosis, dominant
780 Osteopetrosis, recessive
781 Osteopoikilosis
782 Osteoporosis, juvenile idiopathic
783 Osteoporosis-pseudoglioma syndrome
784 Otodental dysplasia
785 Oto-oculo-musculo-skeletal syndrome
786 Oto-palato-digital syndrome
787 Otosclerosis
788 Pachydermoperiostosis
789 Pachyonychia congenita
790 Palate fistula (Marker)
791 Pallister-W syndrome
792 Palmo-plantar erythema
793 Pancreatitis, hereditary
794 Paralysis, hyperkalemic periodic
795 Paralysis, hypokalemic periodic
796 Paramyotonia congenita
797 Paranasal sinuses, absent
798 Parastremmatic dysplasia
799 Parotitis, punctate
800 Patent ductus arteriosus
801 Pectus carinatum
802 Pectus excavatum
803 Pelizaeus-Merzbacher syndrome
804 Pentosuria (Marker)
805 Pericardium agenesis
806 Periodontosis, juvenile
807 Persistent left superior vena cava connected to coronary sinus
808 Phenylketonuria
809 Phenylthiocarbamide tasting (Marker)
810 Phytanic acid storage disease
811 Pityriasis rubra pilaris
812 Plasma-associated defect of phagocytosis
813 Poland syndrome
814 Polydactyly
815 Polymastia
816 Polysplenia syndrome
817 Polysyndactyly
818 Popliteal pterygium syndrome
819 Porokeratosis
820 Porphyria, acute intermittent
821 Porphyria, erythropoietic
822 Porphyria, variegate
823 Prader-Willi syndrome
824 Proboscis lateralis
825 Progeria
826 Propionic acidemia
827 Pruritus, hereditary localized
828 Pseudoachondroplastic dysplasia

829 Pseudohypoaldosteronism
830 Pseudohypoparathyroidism
831 Pseudovaginal perineoscrotal hypospadias
832 Pseudoxanthoma elasticum
833 Psoriasis vulgaris
834 Ptosis, congenital
835 Pulmonary artery coarctation
836 Pulmonary valve absent
837 Pulmonary valve atresia
838 Pulmonary valve incompetence
839 Pulmonary valve stenosis
840 Pulmonary valve, tetracuspid
841 Pulmonary venous connection, partial anomalous
842 Pulmonary venous connection, total anomalous
843 Pulpal dysplasia
844 Puncta and canaliculi, supernumerary
845 Pupillary membrane persistence
846. Pyknodysostosis
847 Pyle disease
848 Pyloric stenosis
849 Pyroglutamic acidemia
850 Pyruvate carboxylase deficiency with lactic acidemia
851 Pyruvate dehydrogenase deficiency
852 Pyruvate kinase deficiency
853 Radial defects
854 Radioulnar synostosis
855 Reifenstein syndrome
856 Renal agenesis, bilateral
857 Renal agenesis, unilateral
858 Renal bicarbonate reabsorptive defect
859 Renal disease, polycystic adult type
860 Renal, genital and middle ear anomalies
861 Renal glycosuria (Marker)
862 Renal tubular acidosis
863 Renal tubular acidosis and sensorineural deafness
864 Renal tubular syndrome, Fanconi
865 Retinal aplasia
866 Retinal dysplasia
867 Retinal fold
868 Retinal telangiectasia and hypogammaglobulinemia
869 Retinitis pigmentosa
870 Retinoblastoma
871 Retinoschisis
872 Retrolental fibroplasia
873 Rickets, vitamin D-dependent
874 Ring constrictions
875 Roberts syndrome
876 Robinow syndrome
877 Sacrococcygeal teratoma
878 Salivary gland, mixed tumor
879 Scimitar syndrome
880 Sclerosteosis
881 Seckel syndrome
882 Short finger-flexor-tendons and inability to open
        mouth fully
883 Short rib-polydactyly syndrome, Majewski type
884 Short rib-polydactyly syndrome, Saldino-Noonan type
885 Shwachman syndrome
886 Sickle cell anemia
887 Silver syndrome
888 Situs inversus viscerum
889 Sixth nerve paralysis
890 Skin leiomyomas, multiple
891 Smith-Lemli-Opitz syndrome
892 Spherocytosis

893 Spherophakia-brachymorphia syndrome
894 Spinal cord, neurenteric cyst
895 Spinal muscular atrophy
896 Spondylocostal dysplasia
897 Spondyloepiphyseal dysplasia congenita
898 Spondyloepiphyseal dysplasia tarda
899 Spondylometaphyseal chondrodysplasia, type Kozlowski
900 Spondylothoracic dysplasia
901 Sprengel deformity
902 Steroid 11 β-hydroxylase deficiency
903 Steroid 17 α-hydroxylase deficiency
904 Steroid 17, 20-desmolase deficiency
905 Steroid 18-hydroxylase deficiency
906 Steroid 18-hydroxysteroid dehydrogenase deficiency
907 Steroid 20-22 desmolase deficiency
908 Steroid 21-hydroxylase deficiency
909 Steroid 3β-hydroxysteroid dehydrogenase deficiency
910 Stomach atresia
911 Stomach diverticulum
912 Stomach duplication
913 Stomach hypoplasia
914 Stomach teratoma
915 Sturge-Weber syndrome
916 Subaortic stenosis, fibrous
917 Subaortic stenosis, muscular
918 Subglottic hemangioma
919 Subglottic stenosis
920 Sucrase-isomaltase deficiency
921 Sulfite oxidase deficiency
922 Supraventricular tachycardias, congenital
923 Syndactyly
924 Syringomyelia
925 Tapetochoroidal dystrophy
926 Taurodontism (Marker)
927 Teeth, ankylosed
928 Teeth, concrescence of roots
929 Teeth, dilacerated
930 Teeth, fused
931 Teeth, geminated
932 Teeth, impacted
933 Teeth, natal or neonatal
934 Teeth, pegged or absent maxillary lateral incisor
935 Teeth, snow-capped
936 Teeth, supernumerary (Marker)
937 Teeth, thistle-shaped pulp chambers
938 Tetralogy of Fallot
939 Thalassemia
940 Thanatophoric dysplasia
941 Thrombocytopenia with absent radius
942 Thrombocytopenic purpura and lipid histiocytosis
943 Thymic agenesis
944 Thymoma and agammaglobulinemia syndrome
945 Thyroglossal duct remnant
946 Thyroid dysgenesis
947 Thyroid peroxidase defect
948 Thyrotropin (TSH) unresponsiveness
949 Thyrotropin deficiency, isolated
950 Thyroxine-binding globulin defects (Marker)
951 Tongue folding or rolling (Markers)
952 Tongue, cleft
953 Tongue, fissured (Marker)
954 Tongue, geographic
955 Tongue, pigmented papillae (Marker)
956 Tongue, plicated (Marker)
957 Torsion dystonia

958   Torus mandibularis
959   Torus palatinus
960   Tracheoesophageal fistula
961   Transglucuronylase, severe deficiency
962   Transposition of great vessels
963   Tremor, duodenal ulceration syndrome
964   Tremor, heredofamilial
965   Tricho-dento-osseous syndrome
966   Tricho-rhino-phalangeal syndrome, type I
967   Tricho-rhino-phalangeal syndrome, type II
968   Tricuspid valve atresia
969   Tricuspid valve insufficiency
970   Tricuspid valve stenosis
971   True hermaphroditism
972   Truncus arteriosus
973   Trypsinogen deficiency
974   Tryptophan malabsorption
975   Tuberous sclerosis
976   Tubular stenosis
977   Turner syndrome
978   Tyrosinemia
979   Uhl anomaly
980   Ulnar drift with digital webs and contractures
981   Ulnar-mammary syndrome, type Pallister

982   Urticaria, deafness and amyloidosis
983   Usher syndrome
984   Vaginal atresia
985   Vaginal septum, transverse
986   Van den Bosch syndrome
987   Vater association
988   Ventricular diverticulum
989   Ventricular septal defect
990   Viscera, fatty metamorphosis
991   Vitamin B_6 dependency
992   Vitamin B_{12} malabsorption
993   Vitiligo
994   Vitreous, persistent hyperplastic primary
995   Von Hippel-Lindau syndrome
996   Von Willebrand disease
997   Waardenburg syndrome
998   Werner syndrome
999   Williams syndrome
1000   Winchester syndrome
1001   WL symphalangism-brachydactyly syndrome
1002   Wolff-Parkinson-White syndrome
1003   Wolman disease
1004   Xeroderma and mental retardation
1005   Xeroderma pigmentosum

Section III
Tables and Diagrams

Table   *Page*

I—Modes of mendelian inheritance 1093

II—Metabolic disorders where specific enzyme defects have been described 1094

III—Metabolic disorders where variants have been described 1095

IV—Metabolic disorders transmitted as autosomal recessives where heterozygotes can be detected by direct measurements 1095

V—Metabolic disorders transmitted as autosomal recessives where heterozygotes can be detected by loading tests 1096

VI—Metabolic disorders transmitted as X-linked recessives where heterozygotes can be detected by direct measurement 1096

VII—Metabolic disorders which can be screened for during newborn period 1096

VIII—Metabolic disorders which can be detected in leukocytes or fibroblasts 1097

IX—Metabolic disorders which theoretically can and which have been detected prenatally 1098

X—Metabolic diseases where specific forms of therapy are available 1099

XI—Clinical and hematologic features of the major forms of thalassemia 1100

XII—Cleft lip with or without cleft palate, derived complications and frequencies . . 1101

XIII—Cleft lip with or without cleft palate, associated complications and frequencies 1101

XIV—Cleft palate, associated complications and frequencies 1102

Table   *Page*

XV—Frequency of cleft lip and/or palate under various conditions 1104

XVI—Adult skeletal elements of the face derived from the frontonasal prominence and the branchial arches 1104

XVII—Natural appositions or junctions of the face along which clefts occur 1104

XVIII—Syndromes with a prominent or forward bulging forehead, as distinguished from high, flat or broad foreheads which do not bulge forward as in acrocephalopolysyndactyly 1104

XIX—Syndromes with large sutures and fontanels or delayed closure 1105

XX—Conditions which may cause the illusion of hypertelorism even though the actual interorbital distance as measured on PA radiographs may be small or normal 1105

XXI—Genetic forms of pituitary dwarfism 1105

XXII—Biologic mother 1106

XXIII—Retardation 1106

XXIV—Birth defects which may involve the Eye . . 1107

XXV—Birth defects which may involve the Ear . . . 1108

XXVI—Birth defects which may involve the Face, Facial Bones, Nose, or Nasopharynx 1108

XXVII—Birth defects which may involve the Oral Cavity, Teeth, Speech, or Neck 1109

XXVIII—Birth defects which may involve Skin, Hair, or Nails 1109

XXIX—Birth defects which may involve the Skeletal System 1110

Table   *Page*

XXX—Birth defects which may involve the
    Muscular System.................... 1111
XXXI—Birth defects which may involve the
    Respiratory System................. 1111
XXXII—Birth defects which may involve the Heart
    or Vessels 1112
XXXIII—Birth defects which may involve the Liver
    or Spleen 1112
XXXIV—Birth defects which may involve the GI
    System 1113
XXXV—Birth defects which may involve the GU
    System 1113
XXXVI—Birth defects which may involve the
    Nervous System 1114

Diagram   *Page*

I—Simplified scheme of steroidogenesis in the
    adrenal gland 1116
II—Role of testosterone and dihydrotestosterone
    in sexual differentiation in utero........ 1116
III—Hypospadias associated with maternal treat-
    ment with progestins.................. 1117
IV—Gonadal dysgenesis and its variants 1117
V—External genital differentiation in the human
    fetus 1118
VI—Sexual differentiation in the human fetus 1119
VII—Allotransplantation in genetic diseases....... 1120
VIII—Hair patterning........................ 1120
IX—Hair patterning........................ 1121
X—Hair patterning........................ 1122

Section I
ATLAS

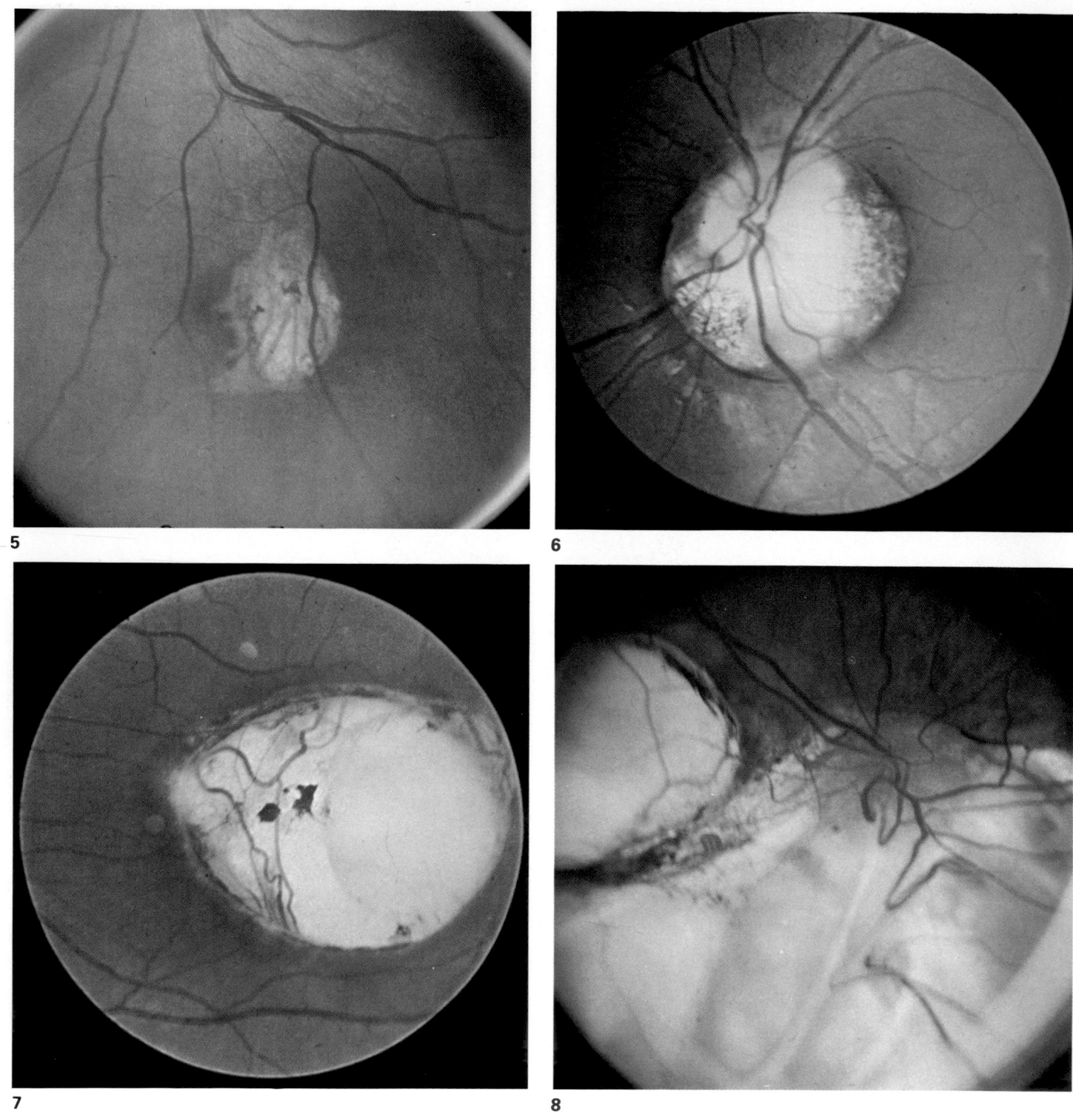

5 Small retinal coloboma (cleft) in inferior midperiphery

6 Coloboma of disk

7 Large coloboma of macula

8 Severe coloboma of disk and macula extending to iris (fellow eye to Fig. 5)

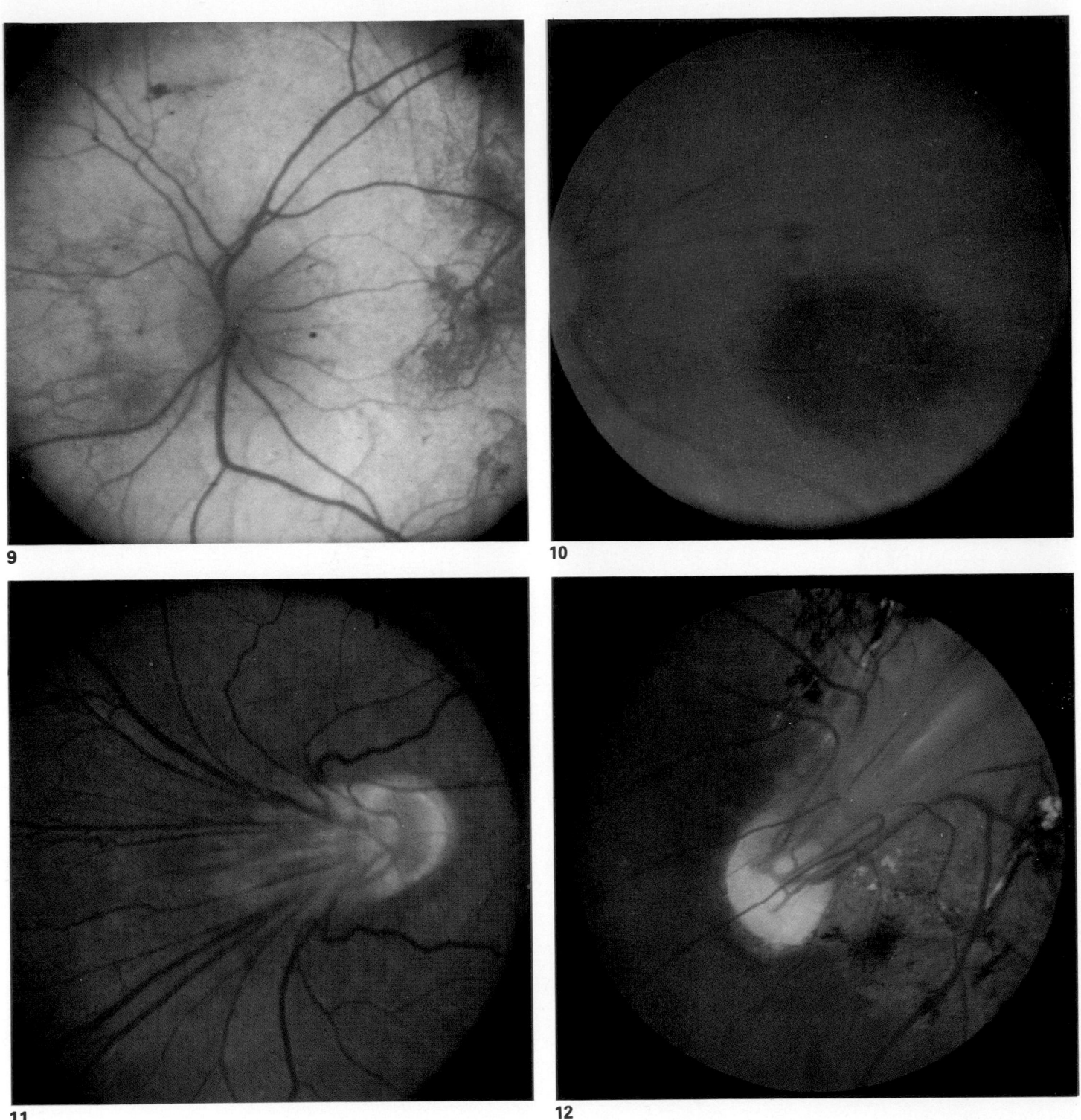

9   Choroideremia

10   Choroidal nevus, benign

11   Ectopic macula. Note vessels dragged from disk toward macula

12   Retinal fold from congenital chorioretinitis

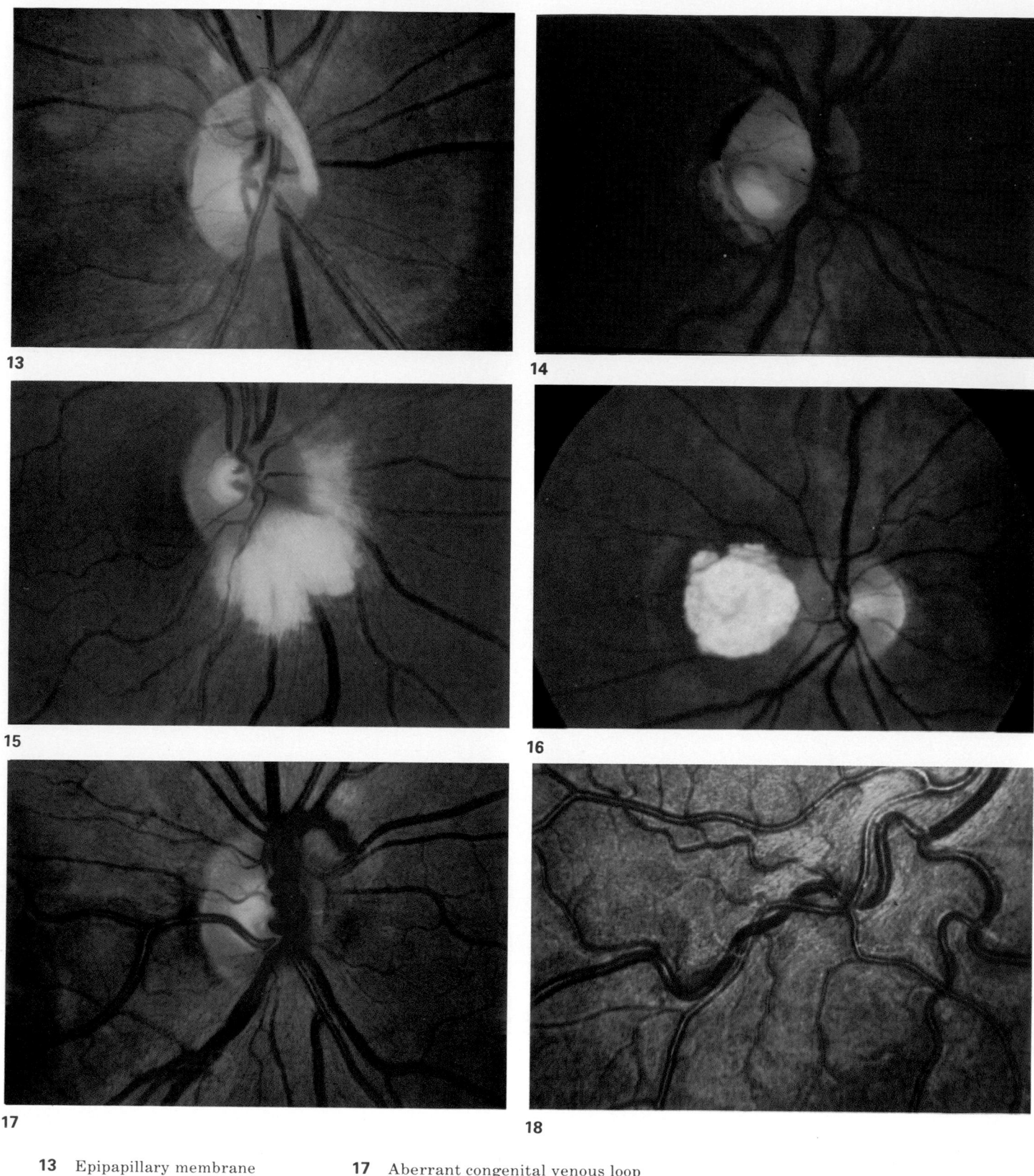

13 Epipapillary membrane

14 Congenital pit of optic nerve

15 Myelinated nerve fibers

16 Astrocytoma of retina

17 Aberrant congenital venous loop

18 Retinal vessel tortuosity in sickle cell hemoglobinopathy

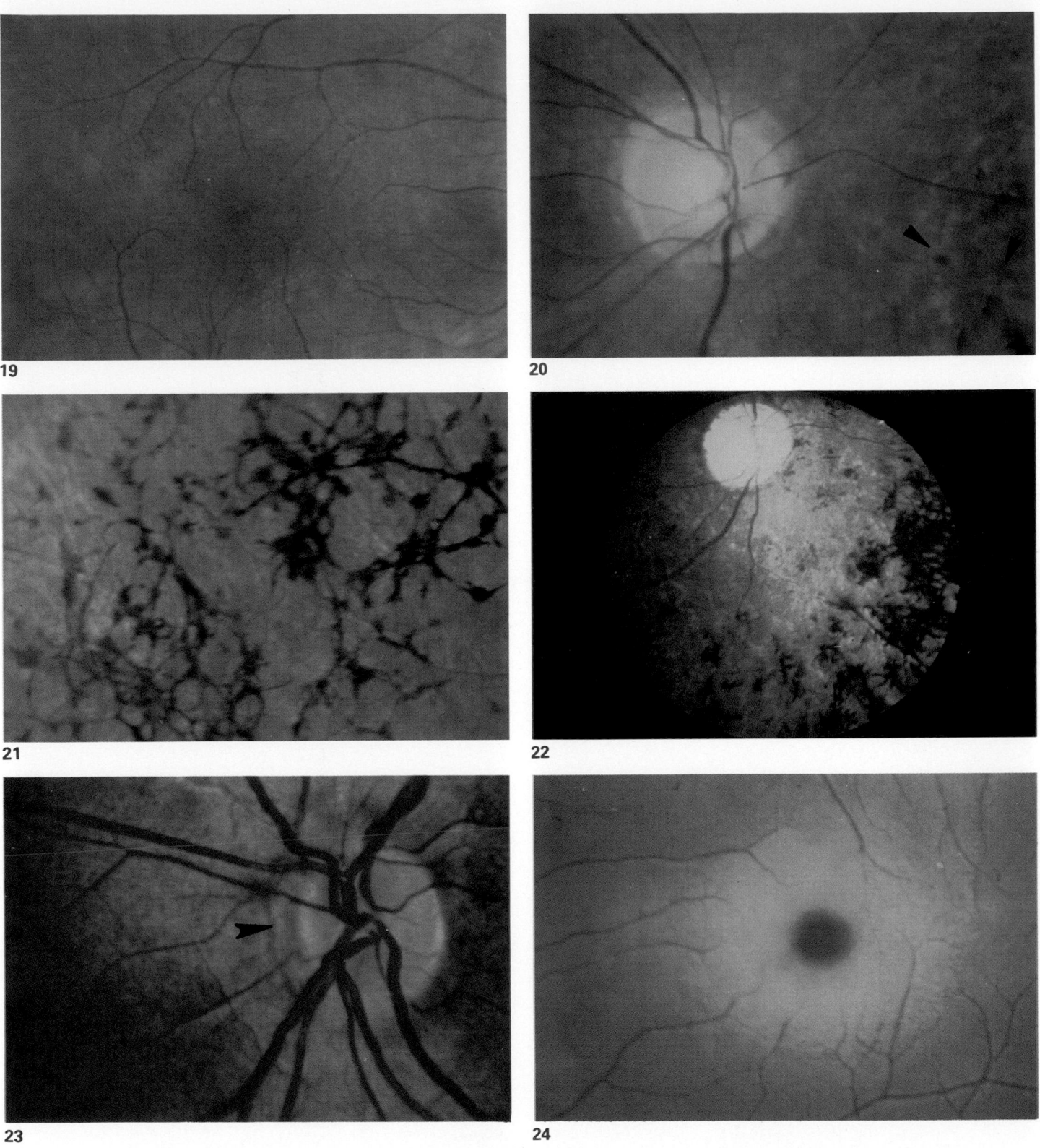

19 Normal macula OD of patient with retinitis pigmentosa. (Figs. 19, 20, and 21 are from same patient)

20 Optic disk and vessels OD of patient with retinitis pigmentosa. Note mild waxy pallor of disk, moderate arterial constriction and pigment clumps in midperiphery as typical

21 Retinitis pigmentosa in midperiphery. Note bone spicule pigmentation

22 Retinitis pigmentosa, dense. Note very dense clumping of pigment

23 Pseudoxanthoma elasticum and angioid streak OD. Note latter parallels outer margin of disk

24 Tay-Sachs disease as seen in the retina. Note cherry red spot in macula

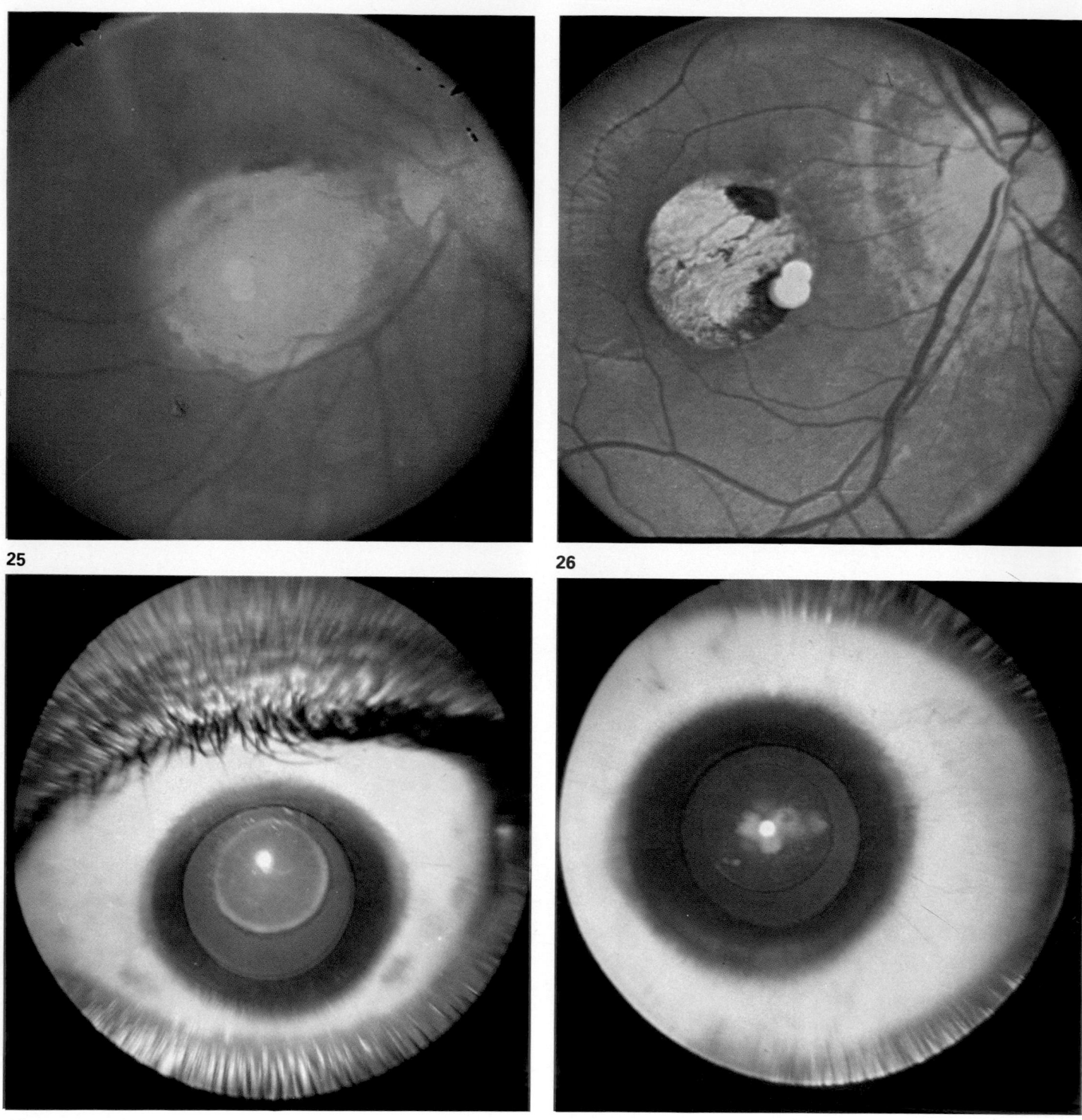

25   Acute chorioretinitis, toxoplasmic. Note generalized mild haze is due to inflammation in vitreous

26   Healed chorioretinitis, toxoplasmic

27   Microphakia. Note microphakic lens which is smaller than pupil area. Small white spot is a light reflection

28   Rubella nuclear cataract. Note, in contrast to Fig. 27, lens is of normal size with red reflex showing through clear periphery of lens. Cataract involves central portion of lens representing size of embryonic lens at time of maternal infection

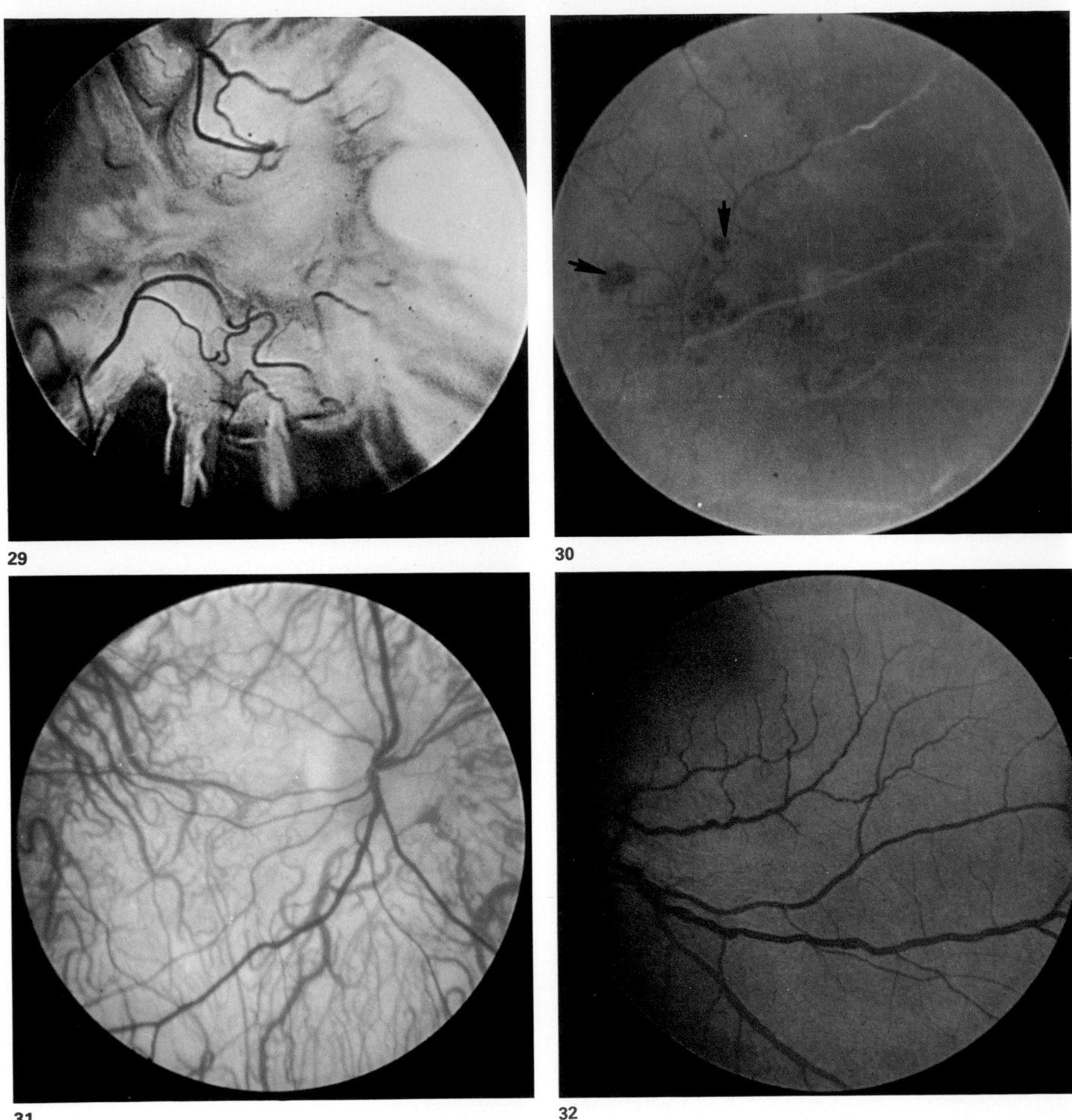

29 Sickle cell anemia as seen in retina. Note retinal changes include vascular and fibrous proliferation and secondary retinal detachment

30 Polycythemia vera as seen in retina. Note hemorrhages, vascular occlusion, retinal edema and neovascularization

31 Albinism as seen in retina. Note absence of retinal epithelial and choroidal pigmentation allowing visualization of choroidal vessels and sclera

32 Congenital retinal telangiectasia

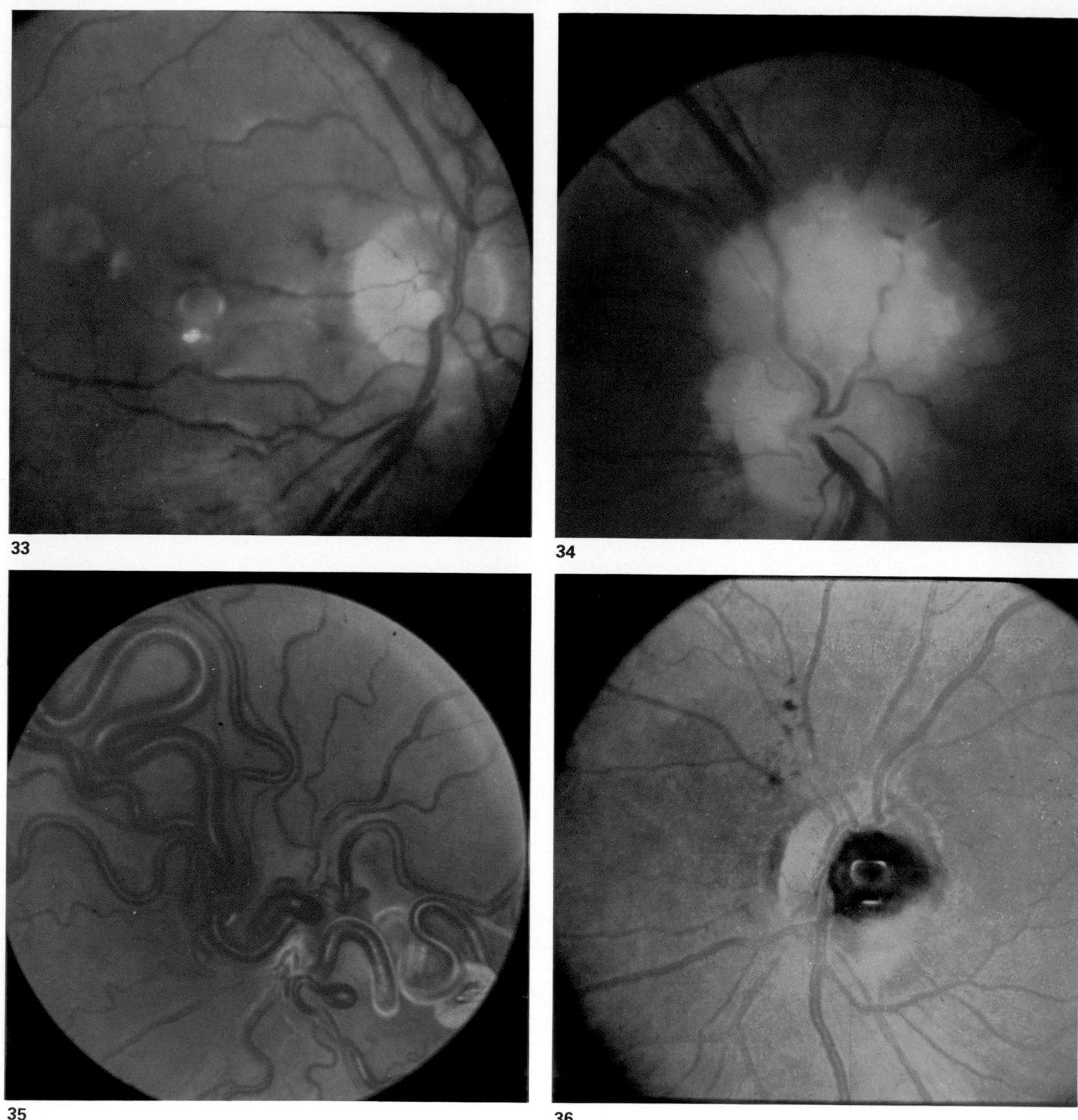

33 Vitelliruptive macular degeneration

34 Tuberous sclerosis as seen in the retina. Note "white refractile mulberry"

35 von Hippel-Lindau syndrome as seen in retina. Note vessels are enlarged and tortuous and usually extend to network in one quadrant

36 Melanocytoma

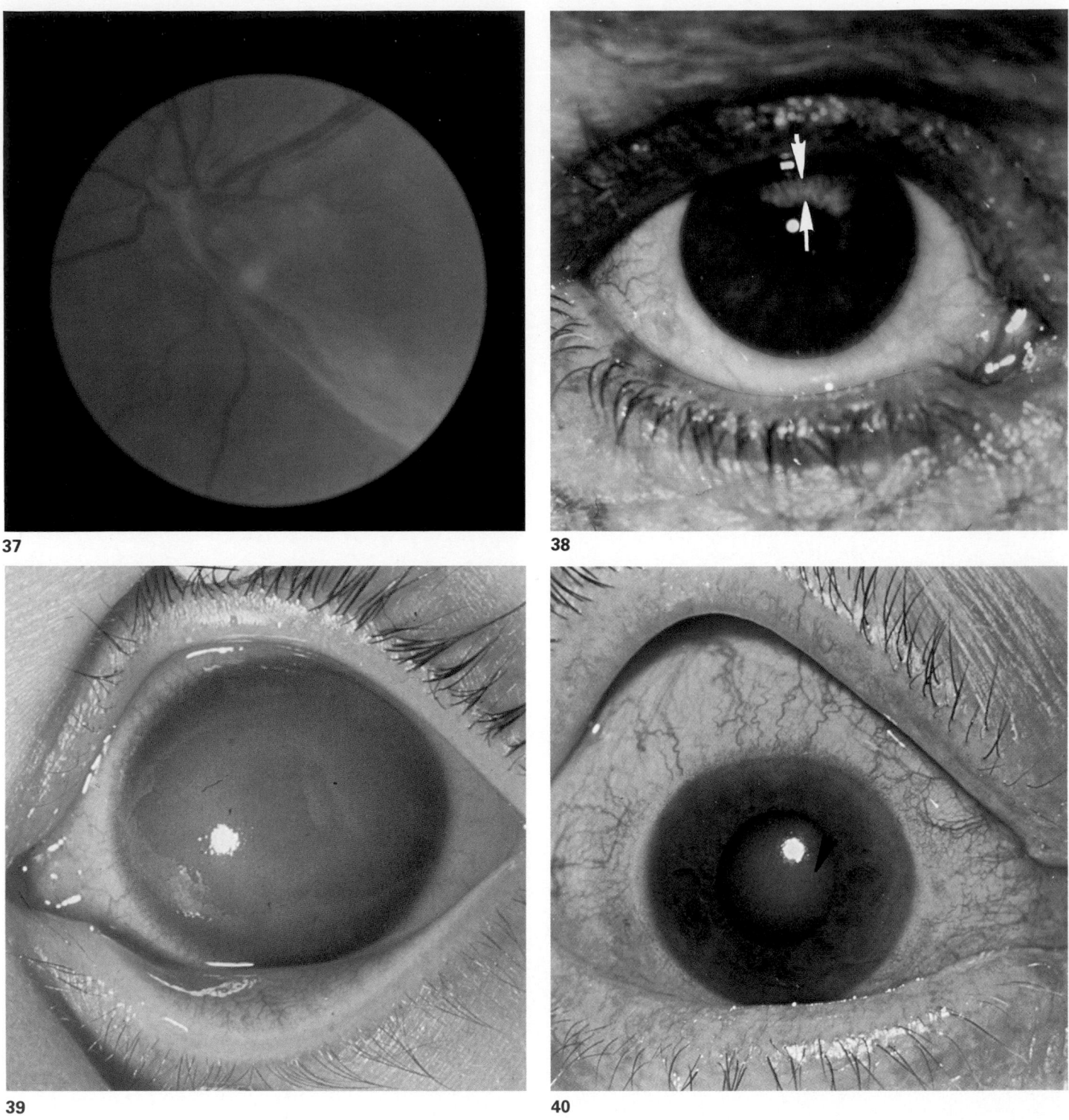

37 Retinal fold, developmental

38 Heterochromia, partial. Note blue sector of iris above pupil

39 Cloudy cornea in congenital glaucoma

40 Acute angle closure glaucoma. Note corneal clouding and congestion of conjunctival and episcleral vessels

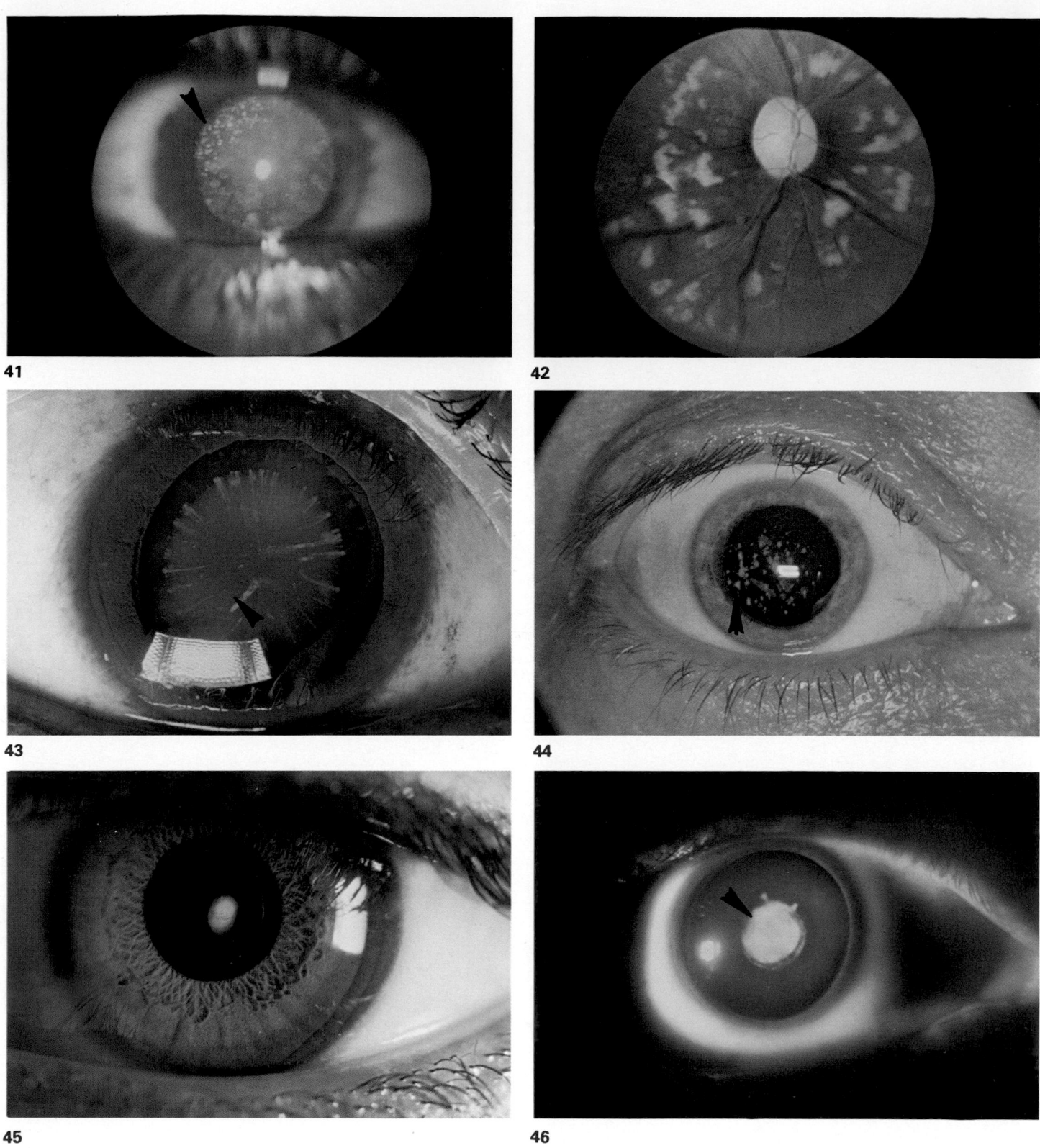

41   Asteroid hyalitis. Note refractile bodies in vitreous as seen through pupillary opening

42   Cytoid bodies. These white areas are infarctions of retina

43   Cataract zonularis. Spoked zonulas are opaque lens fibers

44   Corneal dystrophy, granular

45   Anterior polar cataract, small

46   Anterior polar cataract, moderate

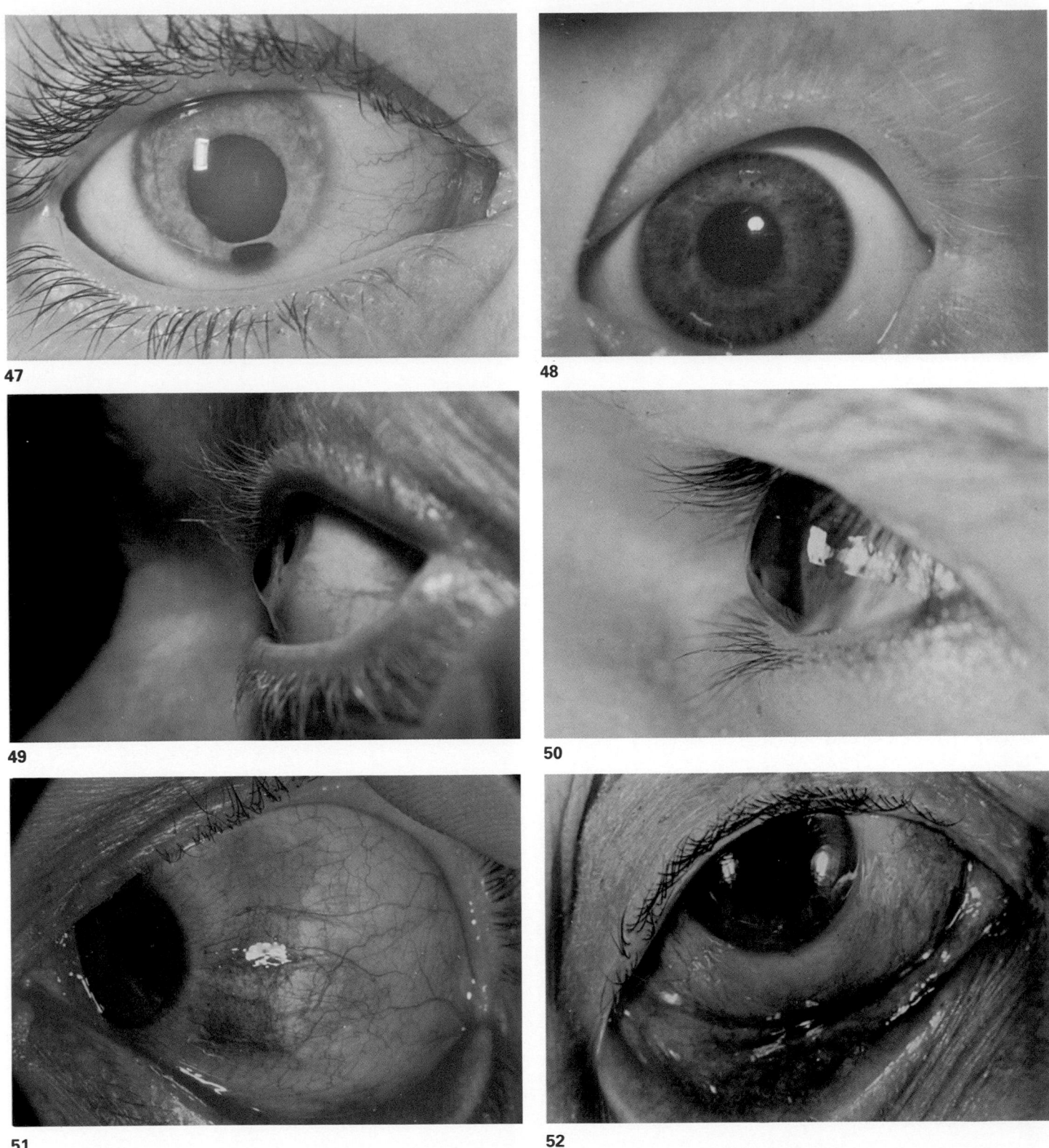

47   Iris coloboma. Note tissue bridge in this patient

48   Albinism of iris and skin. Note prominent red reflex through undilated pupil and depigmentation of iris and skin

49   Keratoconus. Note conical protrusion of cornea and "apparent double pupil" caused by light reflections

50   Keratoglobus. Note general spherical enlargement and protrusion of entire cornea

51   Conjunctival melanosis in Negro. Note, called Nevus of Ota if eyelids are involved

52   Argyrosis of conjunctiva and eyelids (for comparison with melanosis)

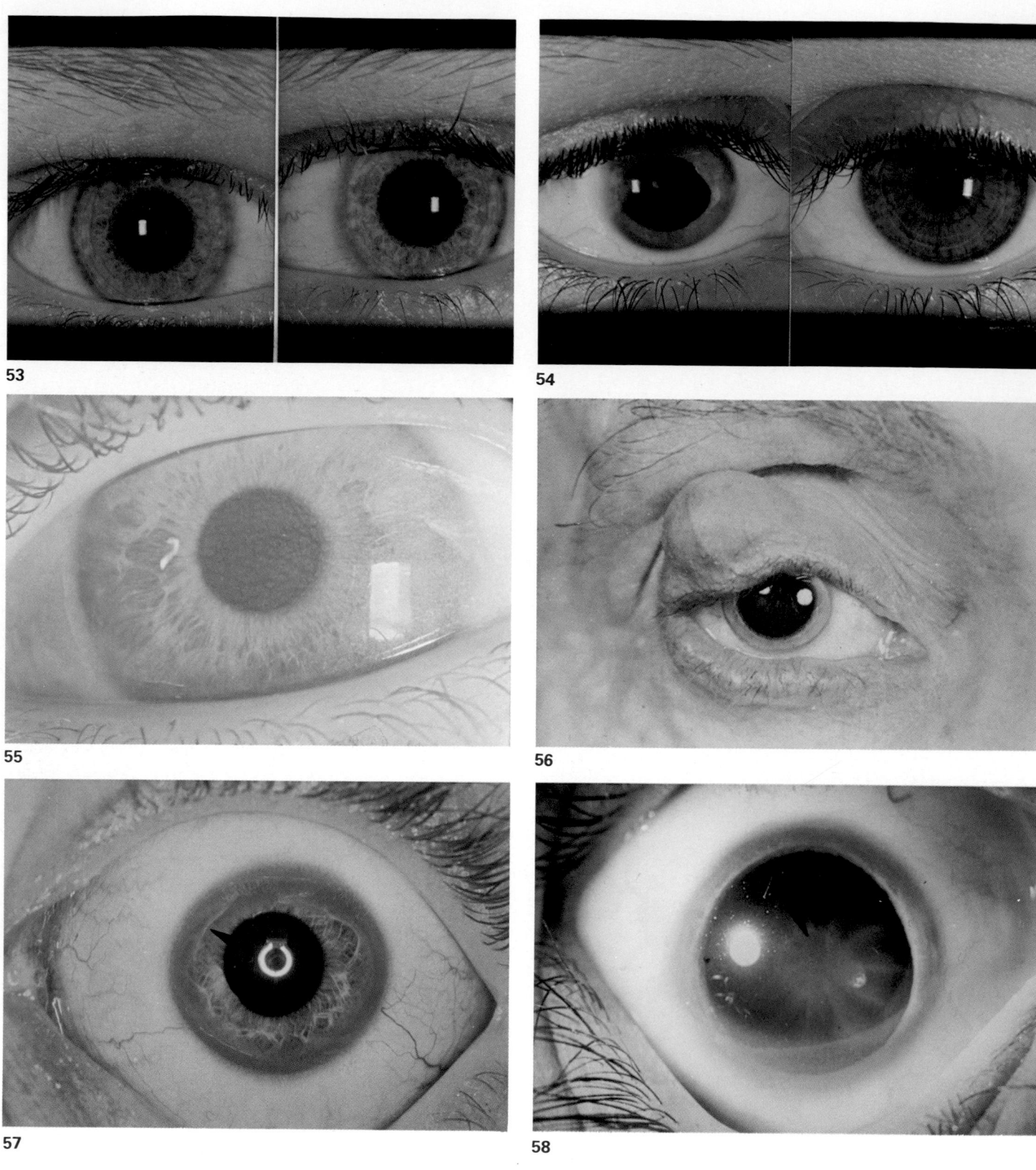

53   Heterochromia

54   Microphthalmia OD, with pupillary abnormality and heterochromia

55   Cystinosis. Note many small granules in corneal stroma, best seen over dark pupil area

56   Neurofibromatosis of upper eyelid

57   Kayser-Fleischer ring. Note golden-brown color in peripheral cornea

58   Sunflower cataract in Wilson disease. Note vague central opacity with spokes

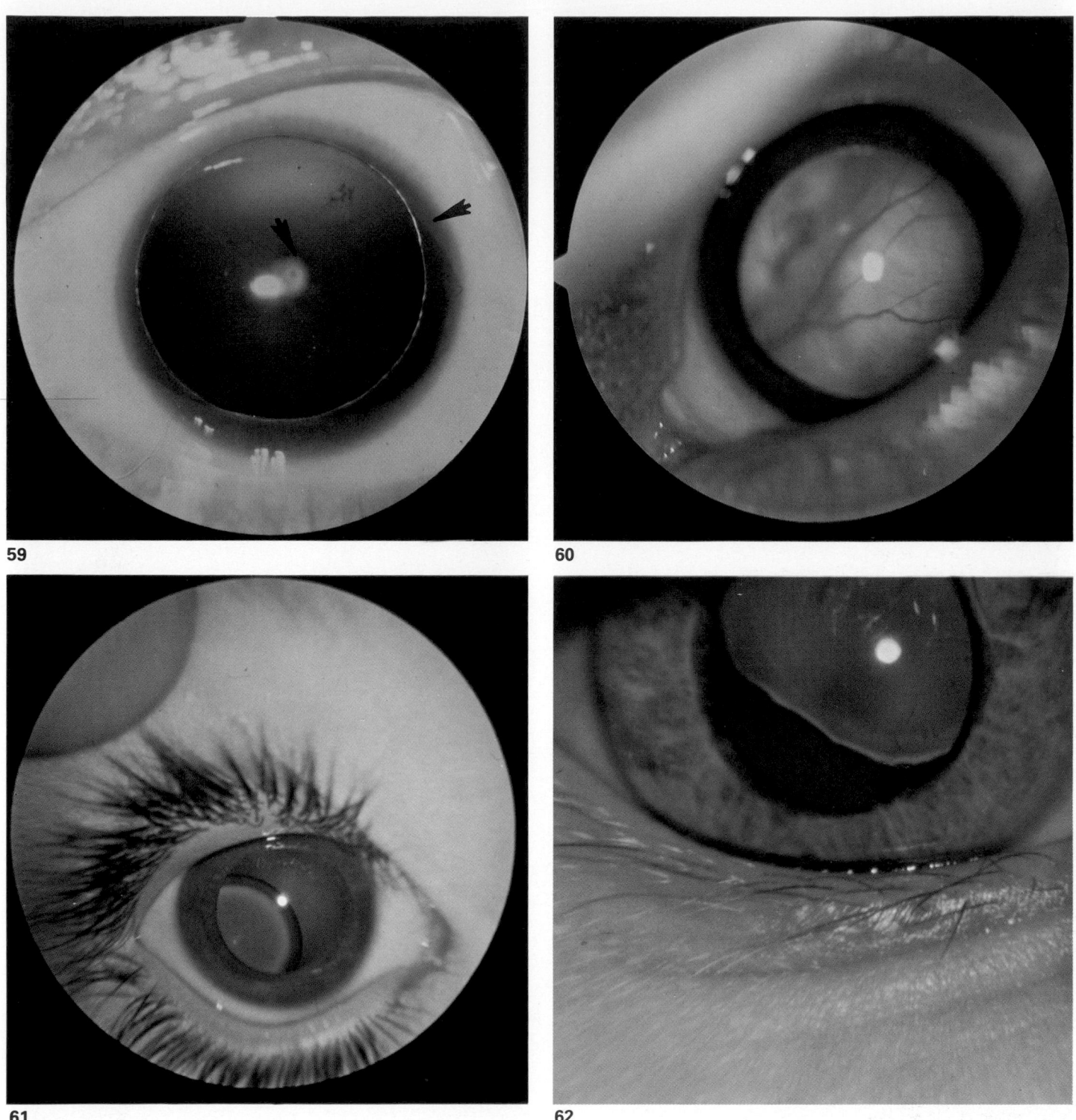

59 Aniridia. Note edge of lens just inside pupil area and also cataract adjacent to light reflection spot

60 Retinoblastoma filling vitreous cavity

61 Lens subluxated downward

62 Lens subluxated upward

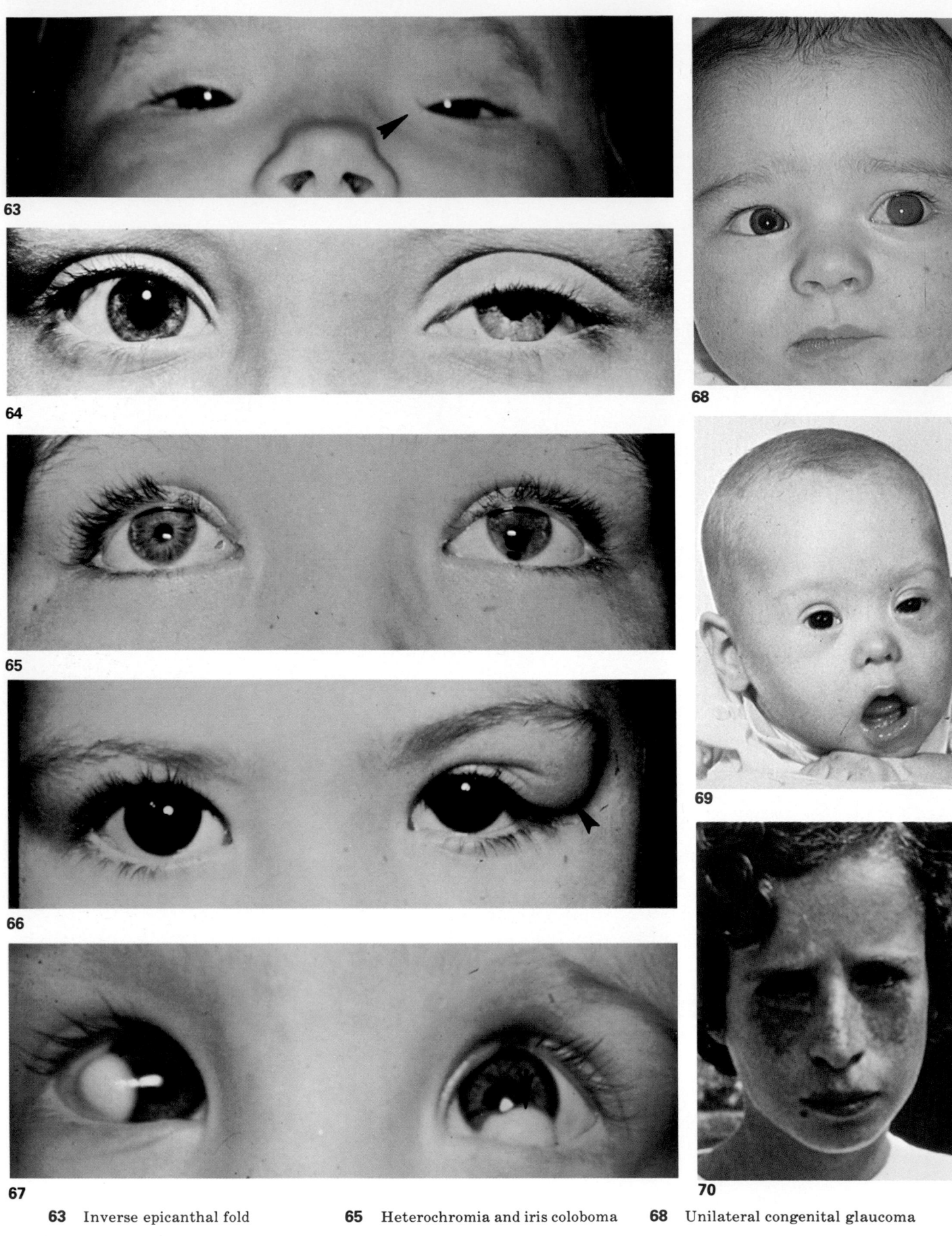

63 Inverse epicanthal fold

64 Horner syndrome with heterochromia

65 Heterochromia and iris coloboma

66 Dermoid cyst of orbit OS

67 Epibulbar dermoid in each lower
lateral quadrant

68 Unilateral congenital glaucoma

69 Chromosome 21 trisomy syndrome

70 Bloom syndrome

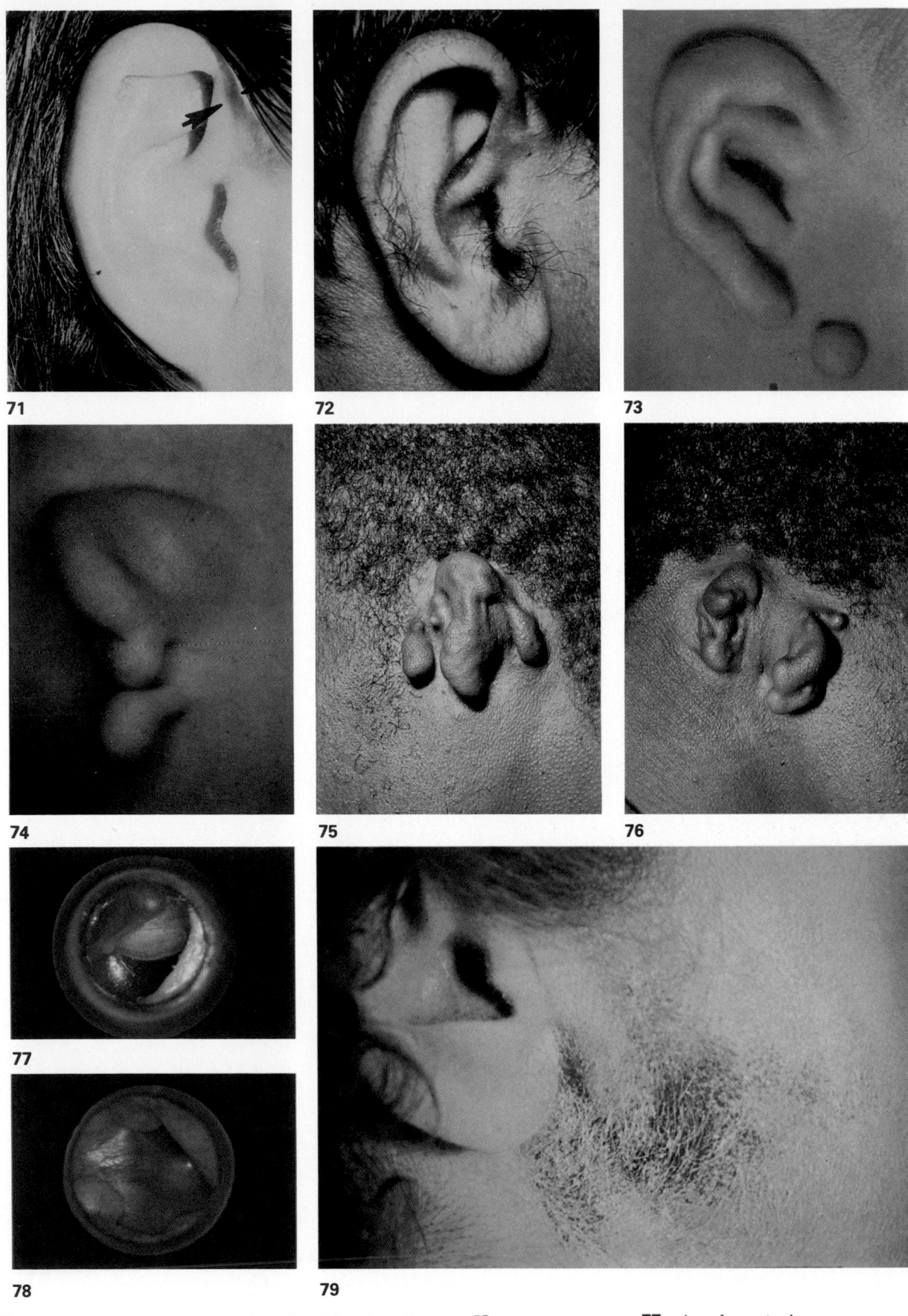

71 Ochronosis. Note pigmentation of auricular cartilage of anterior edge of helix nearest head

72 Hairy pinna (marker)

73 Microtia, type I with preauricular appendage

74 Microtia, type II

75 Microtia, type III with auricular appendages

76 Microtia, type III and polyotia in patient who also had rubella nuclear cataract

77 Aural exostosis

78 Primary cholesteatoma of middle ear

79 Gustatory sweating, anterior to ear, demonstrated by starch–iodine test

15

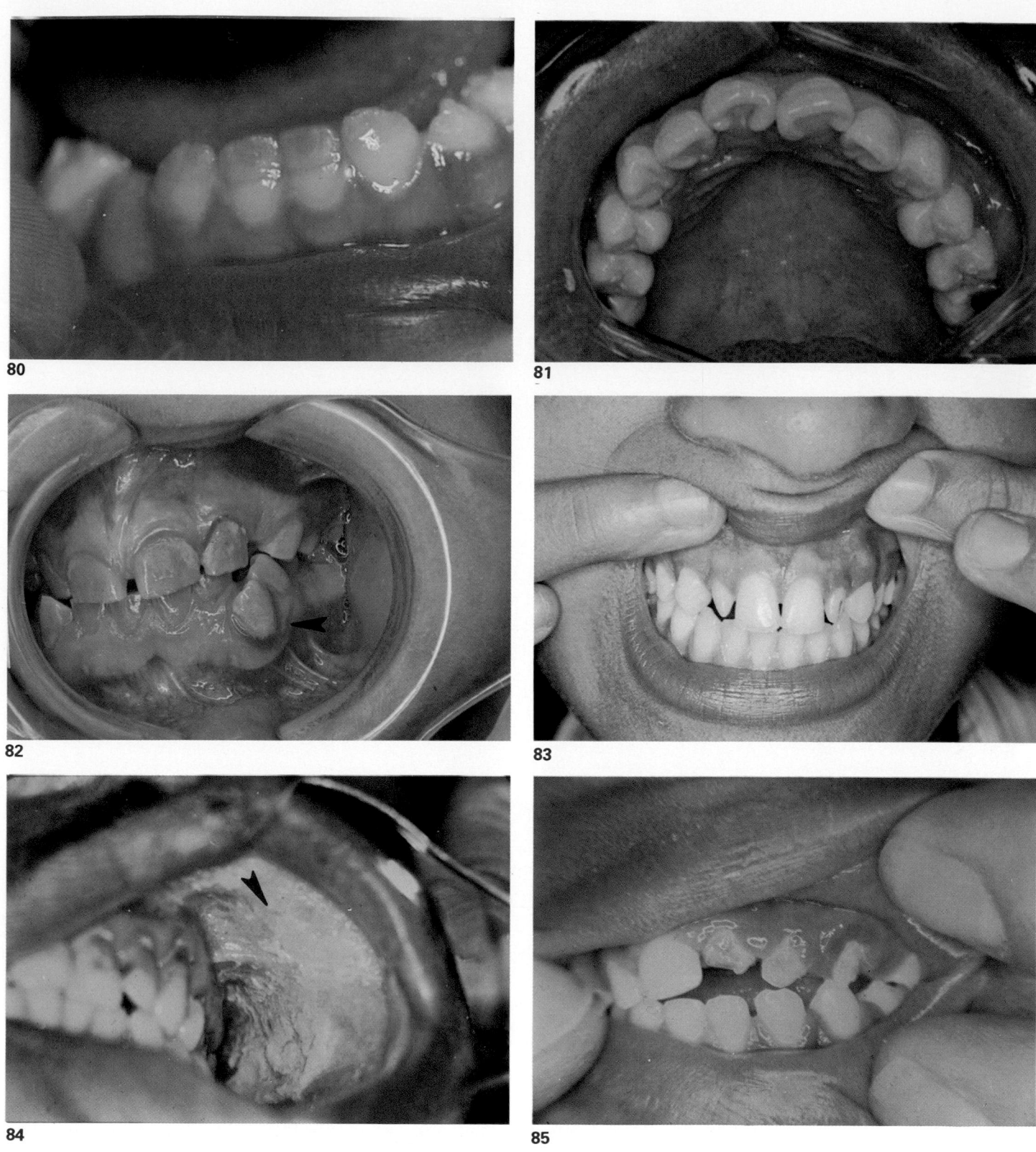

80 Hypoplasia of enamel and yellow staining from tetracycline, primary dentition

81 Incisors, shovel-shaped (marker)

82 Dentinogenesis imperfecta opalescent dentin. Note ectopic eruption of mandibular canine

83 Bilateral permanent maxillary incisors (pegged teeth)

84 Intraepithelial dyskeratosis. Note soft white lesions on oral mucosa. Tooth staining from smoking

85 Odontodysplasia

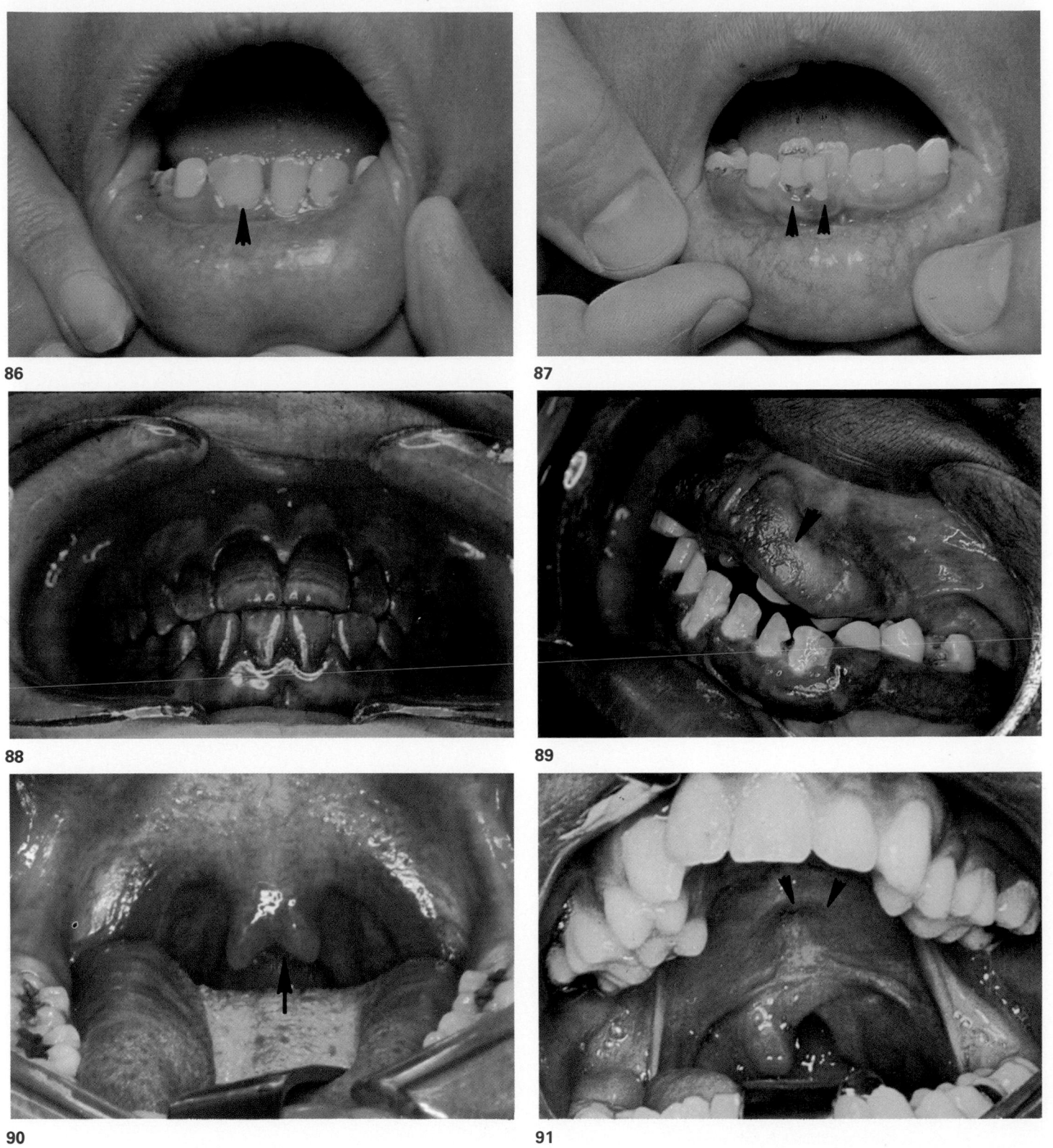

86	Fused lateral and central incisor	**89**	Gingival fibromatosis (Laband syndrome)
87	Geminated primary lateral incisors	**90**	Cleft uvula (marker)
88	Erythropoietic porphyria	**91**	Submucous cleft of soft and hard palate

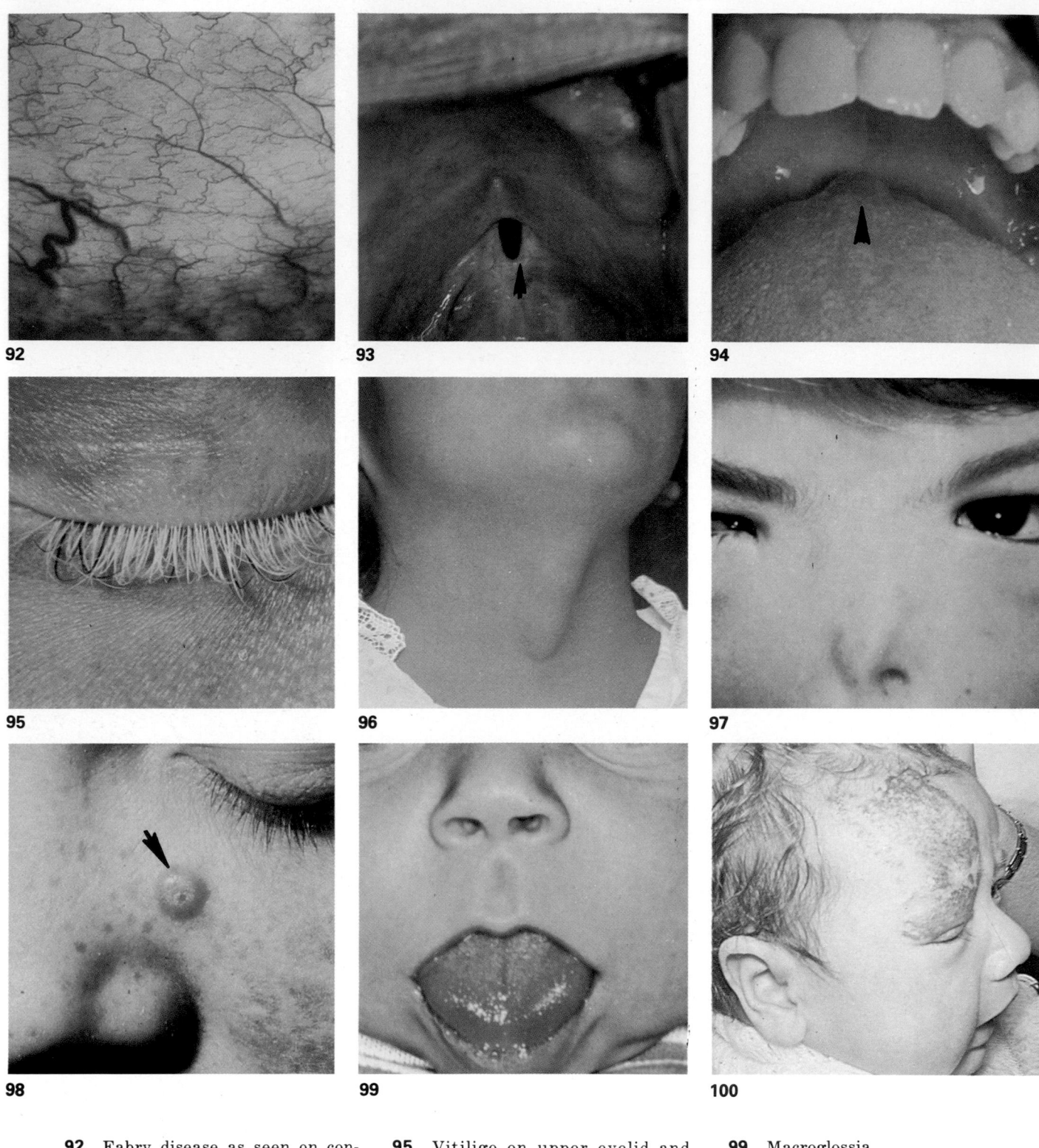

92 Fabry disease as seen on conjunctiva. Note dilated, tortuous, varicose vessels

93 Nasopharyngeal stenosis showing only small communication between oropharynx and nasopharynx

94 Lingual thyroid shown as small elevated area at foramen cecum of tongue

95 Vitiligo on upper eyelid and poliosis

96 Thyroglossal duct cyst

97 Microphthalmia OD, esotropia, hypoplasia of nose with single nostril

98 Keratoacanthoma

99 Macroglossia

100 Hemangioma

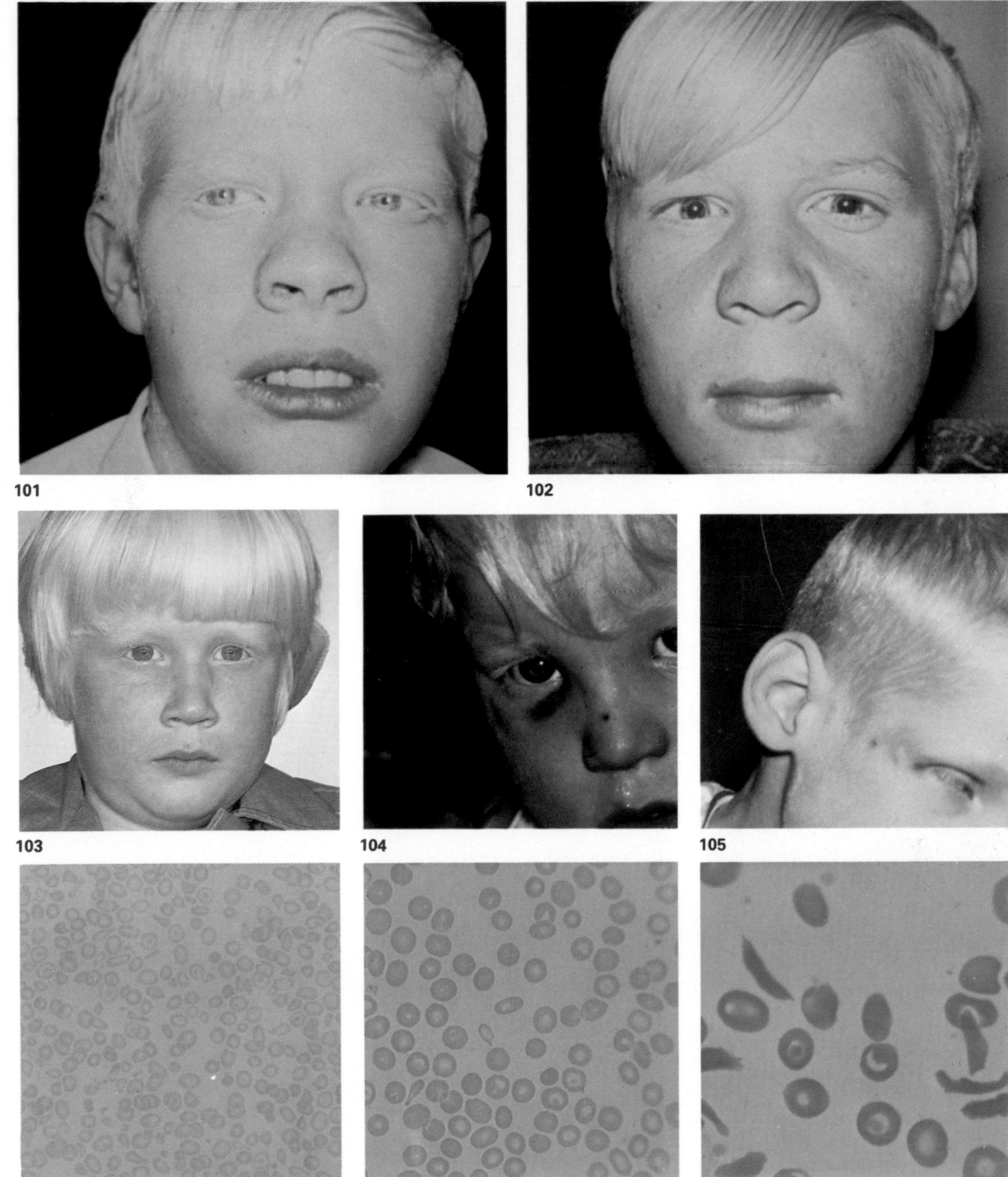

101   Tyrosinase-positive Caucasian albino. Note reddish hue of skin, hair has yellow tinge

102   Yellow-mutant Caucasian albino. Note cream color of skin, hair is deep intense yellow

103   Tyrosinase-negative Caucasian albino. No melanin pigment is discernible in hair, skin or eyes

104   Hermansky-Pudlak syndrome, albino with hemorrhagic diathesis. Note ecchymosis under eye which resulted from relatively minor trauma

105   Microphthalmic depigmented child with Cross syndrome. Note white hair with grey-yellow tinge

106 α-thalassemia (hemoglobin H disease)

107 β-thalassemia trait

108   Sickle cell anemia

19

LACRIMAL CARUNCLE   SEMILUNAR FOLD

LACRIMAL PAPILLAE   LACRIMAL LAKE

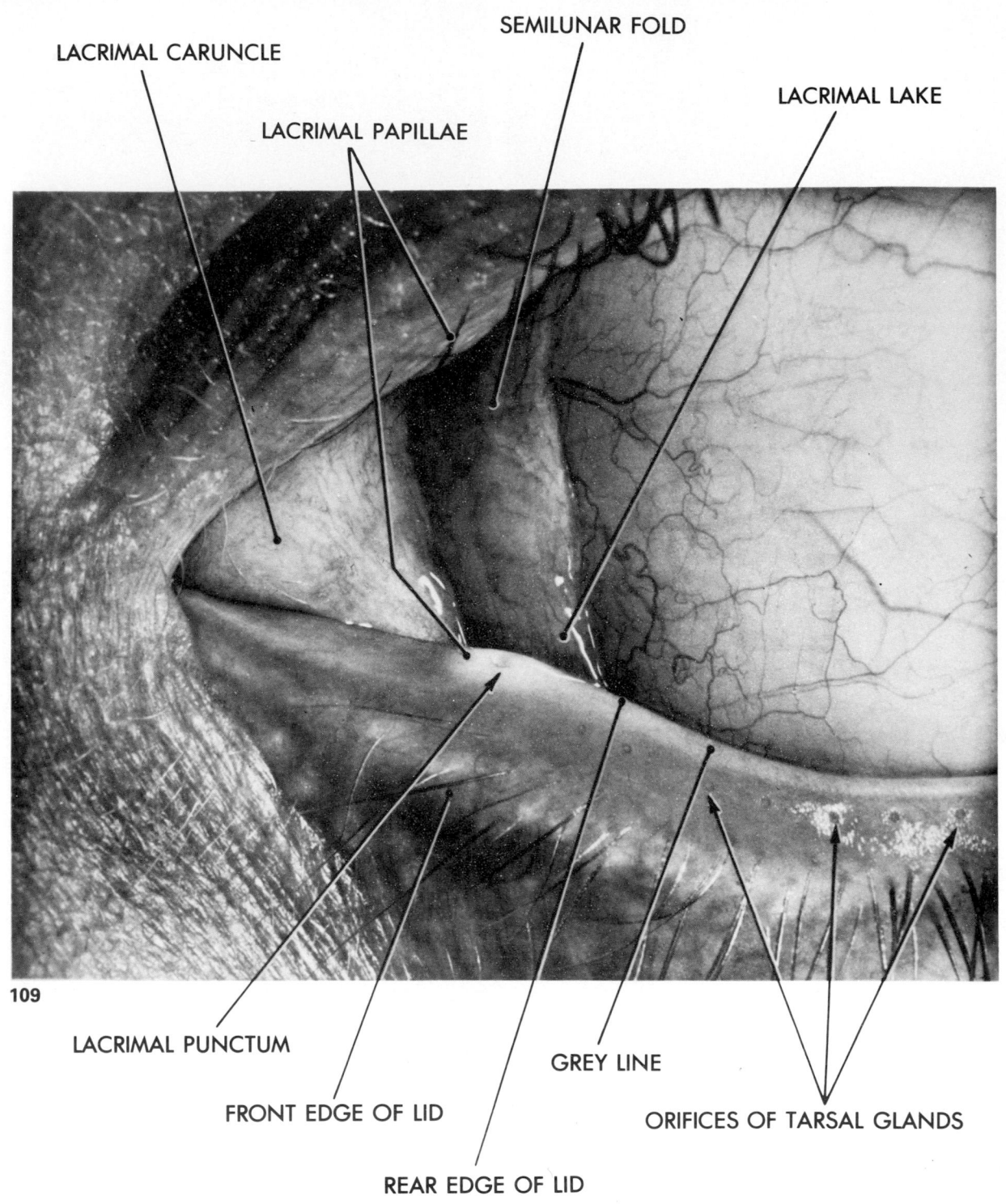

109

LACRIMAL PUNCTUM   GREY LINE   ORIFICES OF TARSAL GLANDS

FRONT EDGE OF LID

REAR EDGE OF LID

109   Normal eye

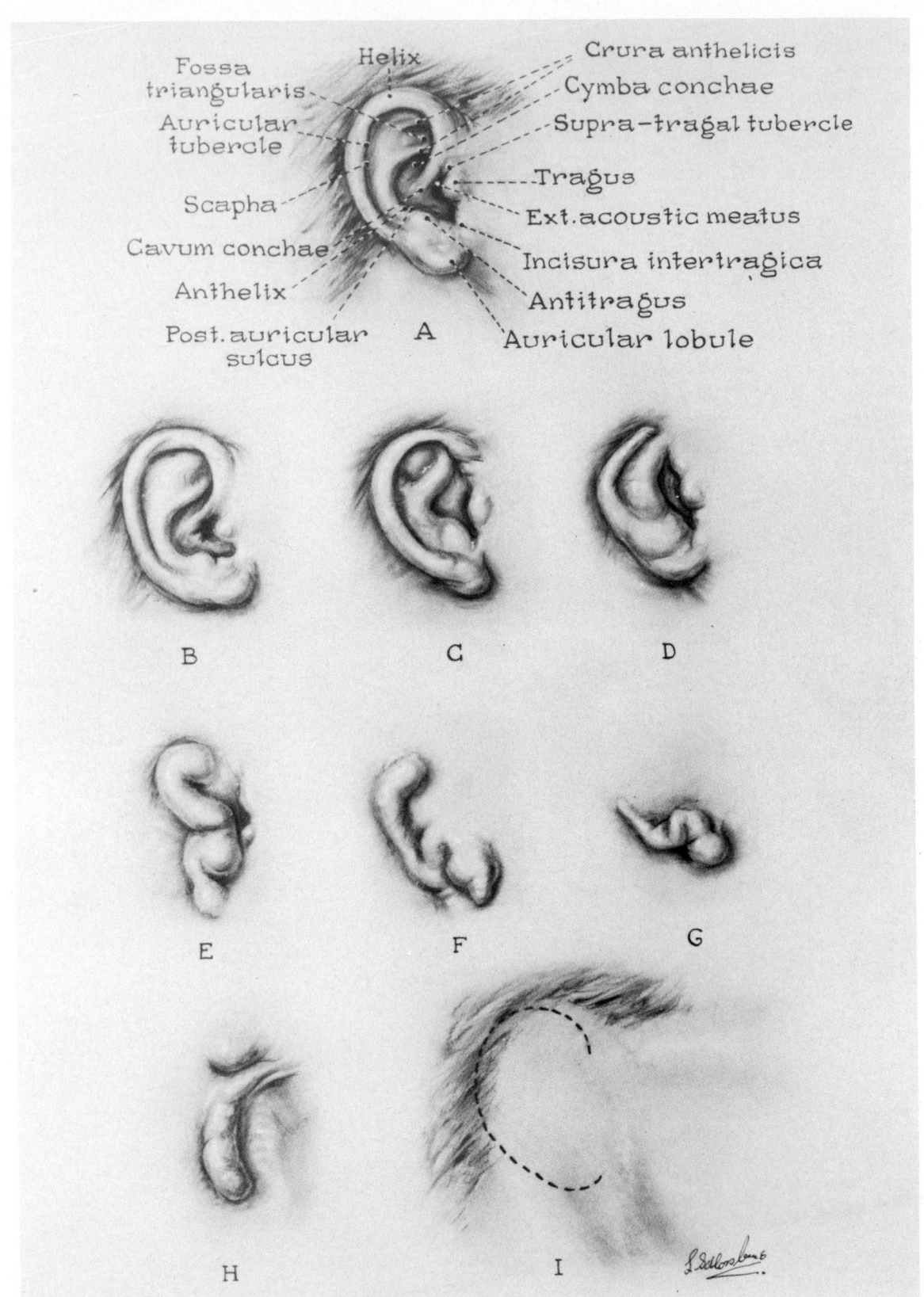

Fossa triangularis — Helix — Crura anthelicis

Auricular tubercle — Cymba conchae — Supra-tragal tubercle

Scapha — Tragus — Ext. acoustic meatus

Cavum conchae — Incisura intertragica

Anthelix — Antitragus

Post. auricular sulcus — A — Auricular lobule

B   C   D

E   F   G

H   I

110 A. Normal, adult pinna and nomenclature. B. Example of a minor malformation. Pinna reveals regular overall dimensions and position, but incomplete differentiation. C. and D. Examples of microtia type I. Auricle is smaller, rudimentary and often located in abnormal position. Different parts of pinna are still discernible. E. and F. Examples of microtia type II. Auricle, besides being smaller and often in abnormal position, is represented by verticle curving ridge, resembling primitive helix. G. and H. Examples of microtia type III. Rudiment of auricle has no resemblance to any portion of pinna. I. Example of anotia (Compendium Birth Defect No. 664)

21

Section II
COMPENDIUM

1
AARSKOG SYNDROME

Includes: Syndrome de Aarskog
Síndrome de Aarskog
Faciodigitogenital syndrome

Excludes: Noonan syndrome (720)

Minimal Diagnostic Criteria: So far, no consistent biochemical abnormality has been discovered and the diagnosis of the syndrome must be made principally on the basis of the clinical phenotype. No one feature of the syndrome is either pathognomonic or obligatory. Thus, only arbitrary minimal diagnostic criteria can be set forth. The diagnosis should be suspected in a male child of short stature who presents with the major facial features and a "shawl" scrotum. Observation of the characteristic positions of the interphalangeal joints when the fingers are extended might be helpful in establishing the diagnosis.

Clinical Findings: Based upon 39 reported cases the principal features of the syndrome are shortness of stature (90%) and facial, digital and genital malformations.

The birthweight is usually normal for gestational age. In cases where the growth pattern could be evaluated, the growth deficiency was evident during the 1st year of life. From 2-4 years of age, growth usually parallels the normal growth curve, but remains at or below the 3rd percentile until puberty. Bone age is retarded and corresponds roughly to height age.†

The major facial features include: widow's peak (60%), hypertelorism (95%), broad nasal bridge (85%), short nose with anteverted nostrils (94%), and long philtrum (97%). Eyelid ptosis has occurred in about half of the cases and usually is pronounced because of the associated antimongoloid obliquity of the palpebral fissures. Ophthalmoplegia, strabismus, hyperopic astigmatism and large corneas may be additional ophthalmic features. Anomalies of the auricles have been noted in 76% of reported cases.

The limb manifestations consist of short and broad hands (88%), short 5th finger with/without single flexion crease (72%), mild cutaneous syndactyly (60%) and simian line (53%). When the fingers are extended at the metacarpophalangeal joints there is marked hyperextensibility of the proximal interphalangeal joints, with concomitant flexion of the distal joints. This sign seems to be fairly characteristic of this syndrome. Broad feet with bulbous toes have been encountered in 75% of cases.

The most characteristic genital manifestation consists of a scrotal fold extending dorsally surrounding the base of the penis (81%). Cryptorchidism has been noted in 75% of cases and inguinal hernia in 66%.

Skeletal features include pectus excavatum (61%), metatarsus adductus and joint laxity.

Although most of the children have normal intelligence (86%), mild mental retardation or learning difficulties apparently occur more often in this group of children than in the general population.

Complications
I   Derived: —
II Associated: —

Etiology: Most probably X-linked recessive; McK *30540

Pathogenesis: ?

Related Facts
I   Sex Ratio: M1:F0
II Risk of Occurrence: ?
III Risk of Recurrence for
    Patient's Sib: If mother is a carrier 1 in 2 (50%) for each

brother to be affected and 1 in 2 for each sister to be a carrier.
    Patient's Child: 1 in 1 (100%) for carrier daughters; not increased for sons unless wife is a carrier.
IV **Age of Detectability:**   At birth
V   **Prevalence:**   ?

Treatment
I   **Primary Prevention:**   Genetic counseling
II **Secondary Prevention:**   —
III **Other Therapy:**   Surgical treatment of possible cryptorchidism and inguinal hernia.

Prognosis: Bone age is delayed. Growth might continue into the late teenage years. Puberty is delayed, but is otherwise normal and accompanied by a growth spurt. With the exception of affected males in 1 French-Canadian family the reported final adult heights have been above 158 cm. The life span appears normal.

Detection of Carrier: Varying degrees of short stature and minor facial and digital anomalies have occurred in 6 mothers and 2 sisters of affected boys.

†**Special Considerations:** Endocrine studies including measurement of serum growth hormone levels have been normal. One patient showed no response to a therapeutic trial with human growth hormone.

References:
Aarskog, D.: A familial syndrome of short stature associated with facial dysplasia and genital anomalies. J. Pediatr. 77:856, 1970.
Berman, M.B. et al: The inheritance of the Aarskog facial-digital-genital syndrome. J. Pediatr. 86:885, 1975.
Furukawa, C.T. et al: The Aarskog syndrome. J. Pediatr. 81:1117, 1972.

Contributor: **Dagfinn Aarskog**

Editor's Computerized Descriptors: Vision, Eye, Ear, Face, Nose, Dermatoglyphic, Hair, Skel., Hernia not CNS, GU.

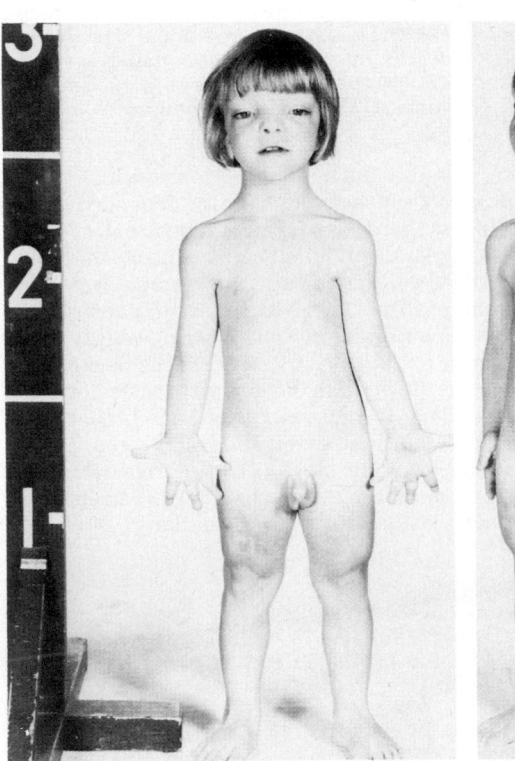

111. Aarskog syndrome

ABETALIPOPROTEINEMIA

Includes: Absence congénitale de bêta-lipoprotéines
Abetalipoproteinämie
Betalipoprotein deficiency
Acanthocytosis
Bassen-Kornzweig syndrome

Excludes: Analphalipoproteinemia (48)

Minimal Diagnostic Criteria: A patient with malabsorption, diffuse CNS signs, and acanthocytes should be studied for this syndrome. A serum immunoelectrophoresis showing absent or greatly reduced betalipoprotein secures the diagnosis.

Clinical Findings: Acanthocytes found in the blood smear. The primary clinical findings are diarrhea, steatorrhea, ataxia, tremor, muscle weakness and an atypical retinal pigmentation. The intestinal symptoms are the earliest and most consistent (>90%). The neurologic signs and symptoms tend to occur later and are less frequent, though progressive. Of these, areflexia, proprioceptive changes and cerebellar symptoms are the most notable, with muscle weakness and sensory changes less prominent. Retinitis pigmentosa eventually occurs in about 50% of the patients. Associated laboratory abnormalities include reduced serum cholesterol and triglycerides. RBC phosphatidyl choline and linoleic acid are reduced, while RBC sphingomyelin is often increased. The red cell peroxide hemolysis test for vitamin E deficiency is positive.†

Complications
I **Derived:** A progressive neurologic handicap develops, reflecting damage to the cerebellum, basal ganglia and posterior columns. Blindness can also develop if the retinopathy involves the macula.
II **Associated:** ^{51}Cr RBC survival may be somewhat shortened, but clinical hemolytic anemia does not occur.

Etiology: Autosomal recessive transmission of reduced betalipoprotein synthesis (referable to the deficiency of the principal apoprotein in the low-density lipoproteins). Recent studies suggest that a variant of abetalipoproteinemia is due to autosomal dominant mode of transmission "familial hypobetalipoproteinemia." McK *20010

Pathogenesis: Possibly the malabsorption results from defective chylomicron synthesis (normally dependent upon betalipoprotein), or there may be an intrinsic defect in the small intestine mucosal cell membrane. A basic abnormality in the red blood cell membrane is presumably responsible for the shortened cell survival; defective phospholipid and cholesterol renewal and increased vulnerability to oxidative stress have both been suggested as the background for the membrane defect. Reduced erythrocyte levels of vitamin E, secondary to malabsorption, are probably responsible for the abnormal sensitivity of the red cells to exposure to peroxide. The mechanism of the neurologic changes remains puzzling; a defect in myelin membrane function has been suggested by some workers.

Related Facts
I **Sex Ratio:** M1:F1
II **Risk of Occurrence:** ? Very low
III **Risk of Recurrence for**
  Patient's Sib: 1 in 4 (25%) for each offspring to be affected
  Patient's Child: Not increased unless mate is carrier or homozygote
IV **Age of Detectability:** Probably at birth or early infancy (blood smear, immunoelectrophoresis)
V **Prevalence:** Rare, less than 40 published cases

Treatment
I **Primary Prevention:** Genetic counseling
II **Secondary Prevention:** Infusions of betalipoprotein preparations have not been of value. A diet substituting medium chain length fatty acids (in triglycerides) has had some success in Isselbacher's hands. It is assumed that lipid of this sort can be absorbed without the need for chylomicron formation. Although weight gain and reduction in steatorrhea has occurred, the red blood cell and neurologic changes have not been reversed. Parenteral vitamin E or massive oral vitamin E may inhibit erythrocyte peroxide sensitivity in vitro. Though clinical usefulness has not been definitively established, long-term vitamin E therapy seems reasonable.
III **Other Therapy:** As required for progressive ataxia and other neurologic manifestations.

Prognosis: Up to this time deaths have been rare, and patients are known who have survived to the 4th decade.

Detection of Carrier: In the variant with autosomal dominant mode of transmission "familial hypobetalipoproteinemia," the parents of patients with homozygous abetalipoproteinemia are heterozygous carriers with reduced levels of lipoproteins.

†Special Considerations: This rare disorder has special interest because of the multiple systems involved. The common denominator for all of the manifestations appears to be cell membrane deficiencies. Nerve cells, retinal pigment cells, red blood cells, and intestinal mucosa cells are all affected. The possibility that the membranes of these cells are handicapped because of a lack of lipid-carrying protein is intriguing. It does not seem unreasonable that membrane renewal and maintenance could be partially dependent upon such a protein.

References:
Bassen, F.A. and Kornzweig, A.L.: Malformation of erythrocytes in a case of atypical retinitis pigmentosa. Blood 5:381, 1950.
Biemer, J.J. and McCammon, R.E.: The genetic relationship of abetalipoproteinemia and hypobetalipoproteinemia: A report of the occurrence of both diseases within the same family. J. Lab. Clin. Med. 85:556, 1976.
Cottrill, C. et al: Familial homozygous hypobetalipoproteinemia. Metabolism 23:779, 1974.
Gotto, A.M. et al: On the protein defect in abetalipoproteinemia. N. Engl. J. Med. 284:813, 1971.
Isselbacher, K.J. et al: Congenital betalipoprotein deficiency; an hereditary disorder involving a defect in the absorption and transport of lipids. Medicine 43:347, 1964.
Kayden, H.J.: Abetalipopoproteinemia. Annu. Rev. Med. 23:285, 1972.
Lees, R. and Ahrens, E.H., Jr.: Fat transport in abetalipoproteinemia; the effects of repeated infusions of β-lipoprotein-rich plasma. N. Engl. J. Med. 280:1261, 1969.

Contributors: **Stephen B. Shohet**
Narla Mohandas

Editor's Computerized Descriptors: Vision, Eye, Muscle, GI, Nerve

ABLEPHARON

Includes: Ablépharie
Ablefarón
Cryptophthalmus
Eyelid, absent

Excludes: Ankyloblepharon (60)

Minimal Diagnostic Criteria: Absence of eyelid

Clinical Findings: In the most severe form it is bilateral without recognizable differentiation of the lids and its associated structures of lashes and brows. The skin of the forehead and face are fused with an occasionally visible horizontal line within the area of the absent eyelids. In its less severe form ablepharon may be unilateral, or incomplete, in which case only the upper or lower lid is lacking.

Complications
I   **Derived:** —
II **Associated:** Lid colobomas in unilateral involvement, absent lacrimal glands, ocular deformities such as anophthalmos, microphthalmos and anterior segment abnormalities, dermoids, cleft lip and palate, umbilical hernia, ear and nose aberrations, laryngeal atresia, syndactylism, malformations of urogenitalia, ventral hernias, meningoencephalocele, basal encephalocele, tricuspid atresia, ventricular and atrial septal defects, transposition of great vessels, right aortic arch and aberrant right subclavian artery.

Etiology: Suggestion of autosomal recessive inheritance although most cases occur sporadically.

Pathogenesis: Controversial. May be due to agenesis from a primary failure in induction, or secondary to abnormal intrauterine factors such as increased amniotic pressure causing localized obstruction, or response to infectious or other teratogenic substances.

Related Facts
I   **Sex Ratio:** M1:F1
II **Risk of Occurrence:** Rare, about 50 reported cases
III **Risk of Recurrence for**
    Patient's Sib: When autosomal recessive, 1 in 4 (25%) for each offspring to be affected.
    Patient's Child: Not increased unless mate is carrier or homozygote
IV **Age of Detectability:** At birth
V   **Prevalence:** Rare

Treatment
I   **Primary Prevention:** Genetic counseling. Avoidance during pregnancy of infectious exposure and ingestion of possible teratogenic substances.
II **Secondary Prevention:** If laryngeal atresia is present, immediate tracheotomy for relief of airway obstruction. Surgical restoration of existing anatomy of eyelids in partial cases, protection against exposure and further destruction of remaining eye structures, cosmetic and functional repair of other malformations.
III **Other Therapy:** —

Prognosis: Poor for vision on affected side. Life expectancy related to severity of associated anomalies.

Detection of Carrier: —

Special Considerations: —

References:
Duke-Elder, S.: System of Ophthalmology, vol. 3, part 2. Congenital Deformities. London:Henry Kimpton, 1964, p. 829.
Goldhammer, Y. and Smith, J. L.: Cryptophthalmos syndrome with basal encephalocele. Am. J. Ophthalmol. 80:146, 1975.
Gorlin, R. J. and Červenka, J.: Syndromes of facial clefting. Scand. J. Plast. Reconstr. Surg. 8:13, 1974.
Rahn, E. K. and Scheie, H. G.: The eye. In Rubin, A. (ed.): Handbook of Congenital Malformations. Philadelphia: W. B. Saunders, 1967, p. 179.
Waring, G.O. and Shields, J.A.: Partial unilateral cryptophthalmos with syndactyly, brachycephaly, and renal anomalies. Am. J. Ophthalmol. 79:437, 1975.

Contributor: **Elsa K. Rahn**

Editor's Computerized Descriptors: Eye, Hair

ABNORMAL FIBRINOGENS

003-500

Diath. Haemorrh. 39 (Suppl.) 307, 1970.

Contributors: **Marion A. Koerper**
Louis K. Diamond

Editor's Computerized Descriptor: —

Includes: Anomalies du fibrinogéne
Dysfibrinogenämie
Fibrinogenos anormales
Congenital dysfibrinogenemia†
Fibrinogens, abnormal

Excludes: Hemorrhagic diseases of the newborn

Minimal Diagnostic Criteria: A discrepancy between the fibrinogen determination based on activity and that based upon the quantity of fibrinogen present, ie a low level of fibrinogen, suggested by the slow rate of fibrin formation after addition of thrombin but a normal concentration of fibrinogen determined by immunologic techniques.

Clinical Findings: Clinical manifestations of bleeding or bruising are extremely variable and may be entirely absent. A bleeding tendency may be observed in the newborn after circumcision; however, some patients tolerate surgical procedures without unusual bleeding. Recurrent thromboembolism and abnormal wound healing have been observed in some individuals. The diagnosis may be suspected with an unexplained prolongation of the one-stage prothrombin time or the partial thromboplastin time (PTT).

Complications
I **Derived:** See Clinical Findings.
II **Associated:** —

Etiology: Autosomal dominant; McK *13480

Pathogenesis: Molecular abnormalities probably account for the aberrant function of these fibrinogens. In one case, an amino acid substitution (arginine to serine) has been documented. To date, at least 25 abnormal fibrinogens have been described.

Related Facts
I **Sex Ratio:** M1:F1
II **Risk of Occurrence:** ?
III **Risk of Recurrence for**
   Patient's Sib: If parent is affected, 1 in 2 (50%) for each offspring to be affected; otherwise not increased
   Patient's Child: 1 in 2
IV **Age of Detectability:** Probably at birth
V **Prevalence:** Clinically evident cases are rare compared to other congenital clotting disorders such as hemophilia A.

Treatment
I **Primary Prevention:** Genetic counseling but manifestations in most cases are mild and variable.
II **Secondary Prevention:** Administration of a concentrate of human fibrinogen will always correct clotting abnormalities and should be considered before elective surgical procedures especially in patients who have a history of previous bleeding episodes.
III **Other Therapy:** Treatment with concentrates of human fibrinogen may rarely be required, but the bleeding tendency is mild in cases described to date. A single adequate dose of 100-200 mg/kg should be effective since the half-life of fibrinogen is about 5 days.

Prognosis: Most patients are not substantially handicapped by the defect.

Detection of Carrier: The simplest screening procedures include a prothrombin time and a thrombin clotting time.

†Special Considerations: Some cases now designated as afibrinogenemia may subsequently prove to be abnormal fibrinogens.

References:
Brinkhous, K.M. (Ed.): Hemophilia and New Hemorrhagic States, 2nd Ed. Chapel Hill: Univ. of North Carolina Press, 1975.
Ménache, D.: Congenitally abnormal fibrinogens. Thromb.

ACANTHOSIS NIGRICANS

Includes: Acantosis nigricans
Benign acanthosis nigricans
Juvenile acanthosis nigricans

Excludes: Pseudo acanthosis nigricans
Malignant acanthosis nigricans

Minimal Diagnostic Criteria: Cutaneous changes in the armpits

Clinical Findings: The dermatosis is characterized by dark, hyperpigmented, confluent and raised areas involving principally the axillae and other body folds. Although the nipples and umbilicus are affected, it is rare to find the entire body involved.

Acanthosis nigricans per se may be present at birth, but usually presents in childhood or at puberty. After puberty it usually regresses or becomes stationary. Sex hormones seem to stimulate the epidermal hyperplasia. The age of onset and the duration of the dermatosis varies, dependent upon an associated syndrome.

Complications
I **Derived:** Heat prostration, patients with widespread dermatosis may not sweat.
II **Associated:** Craniofacial dysostosis, diabetes mellitus, mental retardation, lipodystrophy

Etiology: Autosomal dominant with variable expression; McK *10060

Pathogenesis: ?

Related Facts
I **Sex Ratio:** M1:F1
II **Risk of Occurrence:** Very uncommon
III **Risk of Recurrence for**
   Patient's Sib: If parent is affected < 1 in 2 (< 50%) for each offspring to be affected; otherwise not increased.
   Patient's Child: < 1 in 2
IV **Age of Detectability:** Occasionally at birth, usually in childhood or at puberty.
V **Prevalence:** Rare; has been observed in both Caucasians and Negroes.

Treatment
I **Primary Prevention:** Genetic counseling
II **Secondary Prevention:** —
III **Other Therapy:** Dermabrasion, surgical shaving, topical cortisone preparations

Prognosis: Normal life span, if disease is not part of other syndrome.

Detection of Carrier: —

Special Considerations: —

References:
Brubaker, M.M. et al: Acanthosis nigricans and congenital total lipodystrophy; associated anomalies observed in two siblings. Arch. Dermatol. 91:320, 1965.
Curth, H.O.: Acanthosis nigricans. In Jadassohn, J. (ed.): Hanbuch de haut-und geschlechtskrankheiten. New York: Springer-Verlag, 1966, vol. 7, p. 799.
Curth, H.O.: The necessity of distinguishing four types of acanthosis nigricans. 13th Congr. Intern. Dermatol., Munich, 1967. New York: Springer-Verlag, 1968, p. 557.
Reed, W.B. et al: Congenital lipodystrophic diabetes with acanthosis nigricans; the Seip-Lawrence syndrome. Arch. Dermatol. 91:326, 1965.

Contributor: **Helen Ollendorff Curth**

Editor's Computerized Descriptors: Skin, Sweating

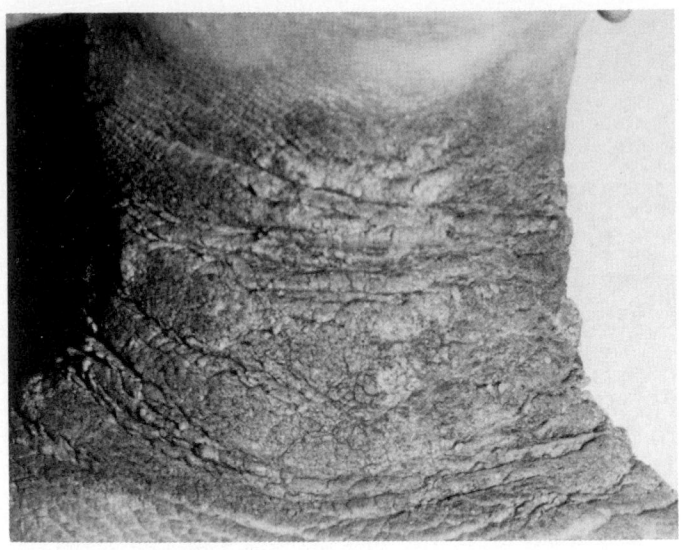

112. Note raised, hyperpigmented lesion

ACATALASEMIA

Includes: Acatalasemie
Akatalasaemie
Acatalasia
Takahara syndrome
Acatalasemia Type I (Japanese variant of low specific activity)
Acatalasemia Type II (Swiss variant of low stability)

Excludes: Allocatalasia†
Other catalase variants with approximately normal activity

Minimal Diagnostic Criteria: Proof that catalase in blood is virtually absent.

Clinical Findings: Clinical evidence of acatalasemia (Takahara syndrome) occurs in the mouth only when the hydrogen peroxide concentration in the mucosa is persistently and sufficiently high to injure exposed cells. Progressive gangrenous lesions may involve the gingiva and alveolar bone with loss of teeth.

Catalase activity is almost completely absent in the blood of homozygotes. The level of catalase in tissues is also reduced, but apparently to a variable degree. The red cells have a high sensitivity towards reagent-H_2O_2, agents generating peroxides, and to x irradiation. Detection of homozygous and heterozygous individuals can be accomplished only by screening.

Absence of catalase in blood can be proved by adding a drop of blood to 2 ml of 2% H_2O_2. If the sample contains a normal amount of catalase, there is immediate foaming, but no change in color. If the sample contains less than about 5% of the normal catalase concentration, no foaming occurs, however, the color rapidly changes to brown and then to white due to hemoglobin oxidation. Leukocytes and cultured skin fibroblasts are also deficient in catalase.

Complications
I **Derived:** A special form of gangrene similar to noma. Frequency in Japanese homozygotes about 50%; children are especially affected.
II **Associated:** —

Etiology: Autosomal recessive enzyme defect; McK *20020. Also occurs in mice and guinea pigs.

Pathogenesis: Deficiency of catalase in blood and tissue. Instead of the normal enzyme, a variant of very low specific activity (Type I) or an unstable variant (Type II) are synthesized. Oral organisms produce H_2O_2 which accumulates and injures exposed tissues by oxidation.

Related Facts
I **Sex Ratio:** M1:F1
II **Risk of Occurrence:** The gene(s) responsible for acatalasemia are rare but highly variable in occurrence, eg in a screening covering 73,661 individuals in Switzerland 3 homozygotes were detected. From this figure an average gene frequency of 0.0064 was calculated. No homozygote has been reported from the U.S.A.
III **Risk of Recurrence for**
   Patient's Sib: 1 in 4 (25%) for each offspring to be affected
   Patient's Child: Not increased, unless mate is carrier or homozygote.
IV **Age of Detectability:** ?
V **Prevalence:** Large-scale screening in East Asia revealed considerable variation as to frequency of heterozygotes for acatalasemia Type I, namely 1 in 77 in North Korea, 1 in 115 in North China, 1 in 323 in Taiwan and 1 in 400 in Japan. Based on these data a total average gene frequency of 0.00083 was calculated.

Treatment

I **Primary Prevention:** Genetic counseling. Careful oral and dental hygiene, good nutrition.
II **Secondary Prevention:** Excision of oral gangrenous lesions, extraction of involved teeth and systemic antibiotic treatment. (Healing capability of tissue is normal.)
III **Other Therapy:** —

Prognosis: Normal life span unless sepsis is untreated.

Detection of Carrier: The heterozygote carrier state for acatalasemia can be detected by measuring catalase activity in blood (Type I) or by means of a heat stability test and electrophoretic mobility (Type II). Depending on the type of acatalasemia the level of activity in blood of heterozygotes varies between 35-60% (Type I) or 60-100% (Type II).

†Special Considerations: There are now 96 individuals known to be homozygous for acatalasemia (84 in Japan, 11 in Switzerland, 1 in Israel). Heterogeneity must be assumed because several types of acatalasemia can be distinguished: Variations are found in the level of residual catalase activity in blood of homozygotes and heterozygotes, in cellular distribution of residual activity among the red cell population, in the frequency of Takahara syndrome and, finally, in the combination with another enzyme deficiency (eg G-6-PD).

In allocatalasia a normal level of catalase activity in blood is associated with an unusually fast electrophoretic mobility of the enzyme. Here, apparently a variant catalase exerting normal activity and stability is synthesized. Detection and investigation of more individuals homozygous for acatalasemia are desirable for practical reasons: Most likely catalase-deficient cells (notably erythrocytes) have an increased sensitivity towards x irradiation or towards certain drugs producing oxidizing radicals, eg hydrazine derivatives. On the other hand their ability to oxidize methanol is probably reduced.

References:
Aebi, H. and Wyss, S.R.: Acatalasemia. In Stanbury, J.B. et al (eds.): The Metabolic Basis of Inherited Disease, 4th Ed. New York: McGraw-Hill, 1976.
Aebi, H. and Suter, H.: Acatalasemia. In Harris, H. and Hirschhorn, K. (eds.): Advances in Human Genetics. New York: Plenum Press, 1971, vol. 2.
Aebi, H. et al: Acatalas(em)ia in Switzerland. In Beutler, E. (ed.): Hereditary Disorders of Erythrocyte Metabolism. New York:-Grune and Stratton, 1968, p. 41.
Aebi, H. et al: Heterogeneity of erythrocyte catalase II. Eur. J. Biochem. 48:137, 1974.
Feinstein, R.N. et al: Acatalasemic and hypocatalasemic mouse mutants. Genetics 53:923, 1966.
Feinstein, R.N. et al: Acatalasemic mice. Proc. Natl. Acad. Sci. USA 52:661, 1964.
Radev, T.: Inheritance of hypocatalasemia in guinea pigs. J. Genet. 57:169, 1960.
Takahara, S.: Acatalasemia in Japan. In Beutler, E. (ed.): Hereditary Disorders of Erythrocyte Metabolism. New York: Grune and Stratton, 1968, p. 21.
Takahara, S.: Acatalasemia and hypocatalasemia in the Orient. Semin. Hematol. 8:397, 1971.
Wyss, S.R. and Aebi, H.: Properties of leukocyte catalase in Swiss type acatalasemia: A comparative study of normals, heterozygotes and homozygotes. Enzyme 20:257, 1975.

Contributors: **Hugo Aebi**
Sonja R. Wyss

Editor's Computerized Descriptors: Oral, Teeth

ACETYLATOR POLYMORPHISM (MARKER)

Includes: Inactivation de l'isoniazide
Isoniazid-Inaktivierung
Inactivación de la isoniacida (Marcador)
Rapid izoniazid (INH) inactivation
Hyperacetylation
Hypoacetylation
Isoniazid inactivation

Excludes: —

Minimal Diagnostic Criteria: Plasma isoniazid half-life after IV dose of isoniazid.

Plasma concentration isoniazid, eg 6 hours after 10 mg oral isoniazid per kg body weight, > about 2.5 μg/ml = slow acetylation, whereas < 2.5 μg/ml = rapid acetylation.

Ratio urinary acetylisoniazid to acid-labile isoniazid in urine, eg 3 hours after 5 mg IV/kg.

Percentage sulfamethazine in the acetylated form in a) one-hour urine collection 5 to 6 hours after drug ingestion, and b) serum collected 6 hours after ingestion of 40 mg sulfamethazine per kg metabolically active mass (= weight to the power of 0.7). Doses vary between 500 and 1000 mg. Analyses can be automated.

Sulfapyridine can be used instead of sulfamethazine (above).

All these procedures give a bimodal frequency distribution (or a 2 cloud scatterogram) separating persons into rapid and slow acetylators.

It is also possible to perform phenotyping using dapsone (Gelber et al, 1971; Ellard et al, 1974) and hydralazine (Reidenberg et al, 1973).

Clinical Findings: This genetic polymorphism like the ABO blood groups and other polymorphisms occurs in normal healthy persons. The medical importance of this polymorphism lies in its influence on the outcome of medical treatments.

The existence of polymorphic acetylation has been demonstrated for isoniazid, phenelzine, hydralazine, salicylazosulfapyridine, dapsone, sulfamethazine, procaine amide and the amino metabolite of nitrazepam.

Slow acetylators are more prone than rapid acetylators to: peripheral neuropathy on conventional doses of isoniazid; phenotoin toxicity when also on isoniazid; various adverse reactions when under treatment with hydralazine, dapsone, salicylazosulfapyridine and phenelzine.

Rapid acetylators have a) less favorable results when open tuberculosis is treated with a once-weekly isoniazid dosage regime; b) higher incidence of isoniazid-hepatitis; c) significantly less improvement of depression on standard dosages of phenelzine; d) require higher doses of hydralazine to control hypertension, and of dapsone to control dermatitis herpetiformis.

Complications
I   **Derived:** Drug toxicity or ineffectiveness
II   **Associated:** —

Etiology: Populations are polymorphic for acetylation. Individuals are either slow or rapid acetylators. Slow acetylators are recessive homozygotes. The dominant rapid acetylator phenotype includes both heterozygous and homozygous rapid acetylator genotypes. McK *24340

Pathogenesis: —

Related Facts
I   **Sex Ratio:** M1:F1

II   **Risk of Occurrence:** Not applicable
III   **Risk of Recurrence for**
    Patient's Sib: Not applicable
    Patient's Child: Not applicable
IV   **Age of Detectability:** Difficult below 4 or 5 years with most of the above phenotyping procedures.
V   **Prevalence:** About 35-50% of Caucasian and African populations and about 90% of the Japanese are rapid acetylators.

Treatment
I   **Primary Prevention:** Not applicable
II   **Secondary Prevention:** Not applicable
III   **Other Therapy:** Not applicable

Prognosis: It has been suggested that slow acetylators are more prone than rapid acetylators to develop spontaneous systemic lupus erythematosus. (Reidenberg and Martin, 1974).

Detection of Carrier: There is as yet no reliable and universally applicable method of identifying heterozygotes.

Special Considerations: —

References:
Eze, L.C. and Evans, D.A.P.: The use of the autoanalyser to determine the acetylator phenotype. J. Med. Genet. 9:57-59, 1972.
Gelber, R. et al: The polymorphic acetylation of dapsone in man. Clin. Pharmacol. Ther. 12:225-238, 1971.
Jeanes, C.W.L. et al: Inactivation of isoniazid by Canadian Eskimos and Indians. Can. Med. Assoc. J. 19:335, 1973.
Karim, A.K.M.B. and Evans, D.A.P.: Polymorphic acetylation of nitrazepam. J. Med. Genet. 13:17-19, 1976.
Karlsson, E. and Molin, L.: Polymorphic acetylation of procaine amide in healthy subjects. Acta Med. Scand. 197:299-302, 1975.
Reidenberg, M.M. et al: Hydralazine elimination in man. Clin. Pharmacol. Ther. 14:970-977, 1973.
Schroder, H. and Evans, D.A.P.: The polymorphic acetylation of sulfapyridine in man. J. Med. Genet. 9:168-171, 1972.

Contributor: **David A. Price Evans**

Editor's Computerized Descriptors: Liver, Nerve

ACHONDROGENESIS, LANGER-SALDINO TYPE

Includes: Achondrogénèse type II
Acondrogénesis tipo II
Achondrogenesis Type II

Excludes: Achondrogenesis, Parenti-Fraccaro type (9)
Grebe syndrome (445)

Minimal Diagnostic Criteria: Lethal neonatal dwarfism with characteristic clinical, radiologic and pathologic features.

Clinical Findings: This form of neonatal dwarfism is often associated with prematurity and hydrops. It is characterized by a very large head and severe shortening of the limbs, neck, and trunk which is often square in shape. Radiologically, there is poor to absent calcification of the lumbar vertebrae and complete lack of ossification of the sacrum and pubis. Although enlarged, the skull is normally ossified. The ribs are severely shortened as are the long tubular bones which are not bowed but have an irregular metaphyseal border. Shortening of ribs and long bones is not as severe in this disorder as in the Parenti-Fraccaro form of achondrogenesis.

Complications
I **Derived:** Intrauterine or neonatal death
II **Associated:** —

Etiology: Autosomal recessive; McK *20061

Pathogenesis: The characteristic histopathologic abnormalities at the growth plate, ie hypertrophic chondrocytes with little intervening matrix, suggest a defect in synthesis or secretion of cartilage matrix.

Related Facts
I   **Sex Ratio:** M1:F1
II **Risk of Occurrence:** ? Very low
III **Risk of Recurrence for**
    Patient's Sib: 1 in 4 (25%) for each offspring to be affected
    Patient's Child: Patients die neonatally.
IV **Age of Detectability:** At birth†
V   **Prevalence:** ?

Treatment
I   **Primary Prevention:** Genetic counseling†
II **Secondary Prevention:** —
III **Other Therapy:** —

Prognosis: Fatal in neonatal period

Detection of Carrier: —

†**Special Considerations:** Prenatal diagnosis through midtrimester xrays potentially available.

References:
Rimoin, D.L.: The chondrodystrophies. Adv. Hum. Genet. 5:1, 1975.
Spranger, J.W. et al: Bone Dysplasias: An Atlas of Constitutional Disorders of Skeletal Development. Philadelphia: W.B. Saunders, 1974, p. 26.
Yang, S.S. et al: Lethal short-limbed chondrodysplasia in early infancy. Perspect. Pediatr. Pathol. 3:1, 1976.

Contributor: William A. Horton

Editor's Computerized Descriptor: Skel.

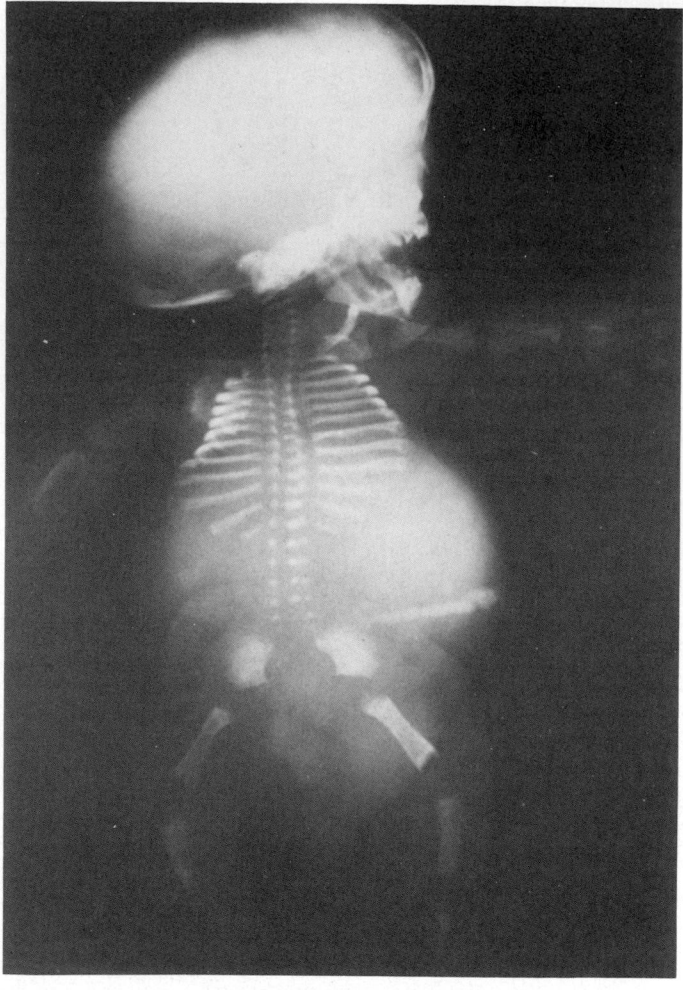

113. In radiograph of stillborn note deficient ossification in the lumbar vertebrae, absent ossification in the sacral, pubic and ischial bones, and flared proximal and distal metaphyses of the humeri

ACHONDROGENESIS, PARENTI-FRACCARO TYPE

Includes: Achondrogénèse type I
Acondrogénesis tipo I
Achondrogenesis Type I

Excludes: Achondrogenesis, Langer-Saldino type (8)
Grebe syndrome (445)

Minimal Diagnostic Criteria: Lethal neonatal dwarfism with characteristic clinical radiologic and histopathologic features.

Clinical Findings: This disorder is a form of neonatal dwarfism associated with prematurity, fetal hydrops and death either in utero or shortly thereafter. The neck is shortened, trunk barrel-shaped, and there is extreme shortening of the limbs. Although the head may be very soft, it is normal in size. Radiologically, there is a complete lack of ossification of the vertebral bodies, although the pedicles in the lumbar area do ossify. Similarly, the pelvis ossifies poorly, while the skull ossification is variable. The ribs are very short with expanded costochondral junctions and may be fractured. The long tubular bones are extremely short and bowed, and longitudinally projecting spurs occur at the borders of the expanded metaphyses. The rib and long bone shortening is much more severe in this disorder than in the Langer-Saldino form of achondrogenesis.

Complications
I **Derived:** Intrauterine or neonatal death
II **Associated:** —

Etiology: Autosomal recessive; McK *20060

Pathogenesis: Pathologic examination of cartilage has demonstrated abnormal resting chondrocytes containing unusual inclusion bodies.

Related Facts
I **Sex Ratio:** M1:F1
II **Risk of Occurrence:** ? Very low
III **Risk of Recurrence for**
    Patient's Sib: 1 in 4 (25%) for each offspring to be affected
    Patient's Child: Patients die neonatally.
IV **Age of Detectability:** At birth†
V **Prevalence:** ? Very rare

Treatment
I **Primary Prevention:** Genetic counseling†
II **Secondary Prevention:** —
III **Other Therapy:** —

Prognosis: Fatal in neonatal period

Detection of Carrier: —

†**Special Considerations:** Prenatal diagnosis through midtrimester xray is potentially available.

References:
Rimoin, D.L.: The chondrodystrophies. Adv. Hum. Genet. 5:1, 1975.
Spranger, J.W. et al: Bone Dysplasias. An Atlas of Constitutional Disorders of Skeletal Development. Philadelphia: W.B. Saunders, 1974, p. 24.
Yang, S.S. et al: Lethal short-limbed chondrodysplasia in early infancy. Perspect. Pediatr. Pathol. 3:1, 1976.

Contributor: **William A. Horton**

Editor's Computerized Descriptors: Face, Nose, Neck, Skin, Skel.

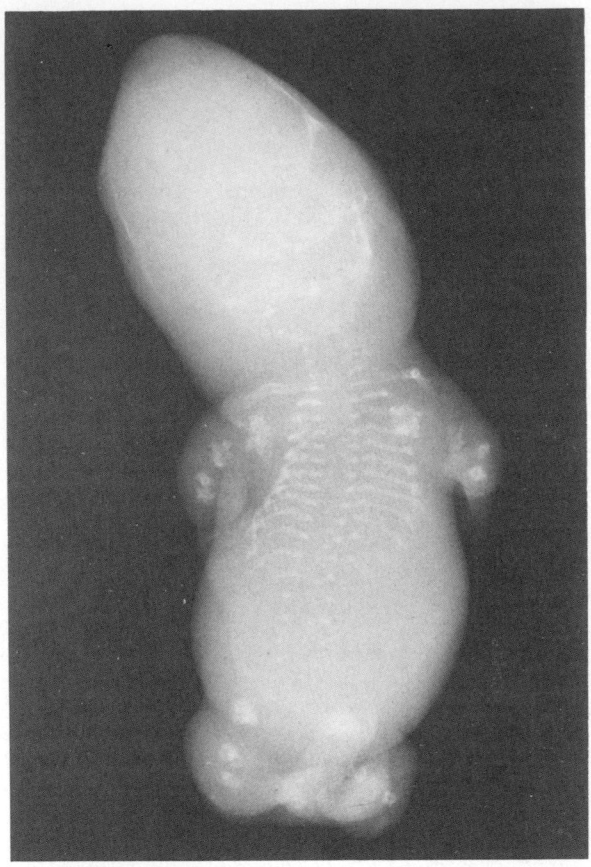

114. Achondrogenesis (Parenti type). Roentgenogram of fetus at 18 weeks' gestation

ACHONDROPLASIA

Includes: Achondroplasie
Acondroplasia
Chondrodystrophia foetalis
Chondrodystrophy

Excludes: Hypochondroplasia (510)
Thanatophoric dysplasia (940)
Other forms of short-limb dwarfism

Minimal Diagnostic Criteria: Radiographic criteria for pelvis, spine and limbs for infancy, pelvis and spine for childhood and adulthood as outlined below.

Only constant clinical finding is disproportionate short-limb dwarfism.†

Clinical Findings: At all ages, newborn through adulthood, radiographic findings are diagnostic of achondroplasia. In most instances, the diagnosis is strongly suggested on clinical inspection, but some affected individuals do not have large heads with prominent foreheads, depressed nasal bridges, or trident hands. In these individuals, achondroplasia cannot be differentiated clinically from other short-limb dwarf conditions.

Length at birth is usually 46-48 cm. Limbs are disproportionately short in relation to trunk. Head usually disproportionately large with prominent forehead, depressed nasal bridge, "button nose." Shallow thoracic cage. Motor milestones in infancy are retarded. Mentality is normal in most instances, (no data on IQ testing available in statistically significant groups at any age).

Childhood: Small stature with disproportionately short limbs with rhizomelia especially of upper limbs. Buttocks prominent and abdomen protuberant because of pelvic tilt. Shallow thoracic cage, head unusually large and brachycephalic, nasal bridge depressed, inability to approximate sides of distal ends of all fingers in extension (trident hand). Limitation of motion at elbows, fibulae disproportionately long, commonly associated with bowlegs. Adults show same findings as children but pelvic tilt increases and prognathism is common. Mean adult height, 132 cm in males, 123 cm in females. Normal head size and normal bridge of nose in 2-3%, absence of trident hands in 5%.

Radiographic diagnostic criteria vary with age. Infants show roughly square ilia, small sacrosciatic notches, short pubic and ischial bones (frontal projection), lack of normal increase in interpediculate distance from L1-L5 (frontal projection), decreased anteroposterior diameter of ossified proximal femora (abnormal lucency in frontal projection), broad, relatively short proximal and middle phalanges in hands (frontal projection), and small foramen magnum. Children have roughly square ilia, small sacrosciatic notches, narrow sacrum which articulates low in relation to iliac crests (frontal projection), narrowing of interpediculate distance from L1-L5 (frontal projection), short pedicles in lumbar spine (lateral projection), limbs are short, so visual impression is that of widened diaphyses and flared metaphyses. Shortening is most marked in humerus. In early childhood, there is V-shaped indentation of distal femoral and proximal tibial metaphyses with small centrally located epiphyses (ball and socket) appearance. Fibulae are disproportionately long. Base of the skull is short, the foramen magnum small. The cranial vault is usually brachycephalic with prominence of frontal, parietal and occipital regions. The adult reveals less than normal flare of iliac crests, small sacrosciatic notches, narrow sacrum which articulates low in relation to iliac crests (frontal projection), abnormally horizontal orientation of sacrum (lateral projection), narrowing of interpediculate distance from L1-L5 (frontal projection), short pedicles and concave configuration of backs of lumbar vertebrae (lateral projection), short limbs, so diaphyses appear wide and metaphyses flared. Shortening is most marked in humerus. Sites of muscle attachment are prominent. Fibulae are disproportionately long. The skull is the same as in childhood.

Conductive or sensorineural deafness may be present. There are no abnormal laboratory findings.

Complications
I **Derived:** In infancy spinal cord compression at foramen magnum (very rare, < 1%), poor respiratory reserve with superimposed pulmonary abnormality (rarely fatal in antibiotic era). In childhood and adulthood cauda equina claudication, frequency increases with age. Relatively common in older age group. (50% of small group examined). Rootlet irritation due to pressure from osteophyte formation and disk herniation, frequency increases with age (approximately 10% of small group examined). Cord compression if thoracolumbar gibbus present, relatively rare (3-5%). Cord compression at foramen magnum, very rare (< 1%).
II **Associated:** Recurrent otitis media due to narrow nasopharynx.

Etiology: Autosomal dominant (over 80% of cases are due to fresh mutation, both parents being normal.)
The incidence of sporadic achondroplastic births increases with paternal age. McK *10080

Pathogenesis: Decreased rate of endochondral ossification with normal membranous ossification leading to the short, squat long bones and disproportion between the base of the skull and the calvarium. Histopathology and ultrastructure of chondroosseous tissue is relatively normal.

Related Facts
I **Sex Ratio:** M1:F1
II **Risk of Occurrence:** Figures of approximately 1 in 10,000 live births in literature are inaccurate because of lack of differentiation between achondroplasia and other forms of short-limb dwarfism in these series.
III **Risk of Recurrence for**
Patient's Sib: If parent is affected, 1 in 2 (50%) for each offspring to be affected; otherwise not increased. If both parents are achondroplastic 1 in 2 (50%) for heterozygous and 1 in 4 (25%) for homozygous achondroplasia; no homozygous achondroplasts are known to have survived infancy.
Patient's Child: 1 in 2 (50%) if mate not affected
IV **Age of Detectability:** Newborn by radiographic examination
V **Prevalence:** No accurate information, same objection to published figures as cited above.

Treatment
I **Primary Prevention:** Genetic counseling
II **Secondary Prevention:** Osteotomies for bowleg deformity when functionally or cosmetically indicated. Decompression procedures, eg laminectomies, suboccipital craniotomies when indicated by neurologic symptoms and signs. Early treatment of otitis media, and surgical treatment as indicated for conductive hearing loss.
III **Other Therapy:** Cesarean section is necessary for delivery in pregnant achondroplasts.

Prognosis: Life span is normal in absence of serious complications listed above.

Detection of Carrier: —

†Special Considerations: Exaggerated increase in head size in the first 3 years of life is normal in achondroplasia. In the absence of symptoms and signs of increased intracranial pressure, shunting procedures do not appear to be indicated. Signs of increased intracranial pressure are usually associated with findings of cord compression at the foramen magnum. The ventricular system is frequently borderline dilated by normal standards in achondroplasia without loss of brain substance. The large head and delayed motor milestones in infancy may give a false impression of neurologic disease.

References:

Langer, L.O., Jr. et al: Achondroplasia. Am. J. Roentgenol. Radium Ther. Nucl. Med. 100:12, 1967.

Langer, L.O., Jr.: Achondroplasia: Clinical radiologic features with comment on genetic implications. Clin. Pediatr. (Phila.) 7:474, 1968.

Rimoin, D.L. et al: Endochondral ossification in achondroplastic dwarfism. N. Engl. J. Med. 283:728, 1970.

Scott, C.I.: Achondroplastic and hypochondroplastic dwarfism. Clin. Orthop. 114:18, 1976.

Silverman, F.N.: Achondroplasia. In Cooke, R.E. (ed): The Biologic Basis of Pediatric Practice. New York: McGraw-Hill, 1968, p. 154.

Contributors: **Leonard O. Langer, Jr.**
                    David L. Rimoin

Editor's Computerized Descriptors: Hearing, Face, Nose, Skel., Nerve

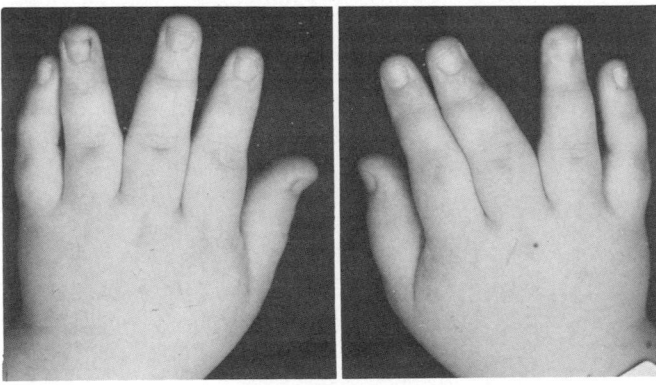

115. Hands in classic achondroplasia showing trident hands and short metacarpals

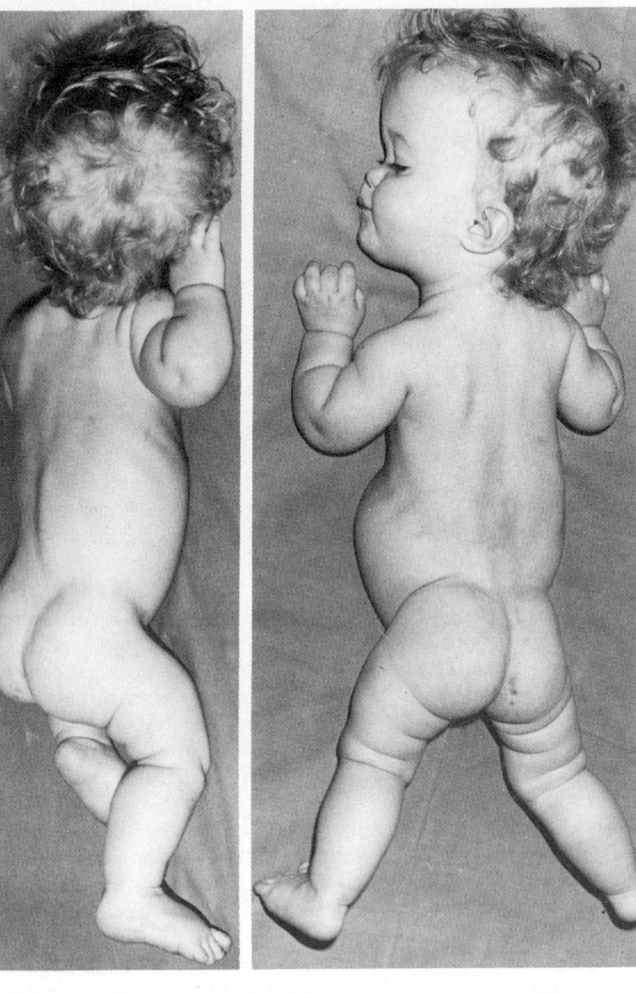

116. Note large head, depressed nasal bridge, short limbs and lumbar kyphosis

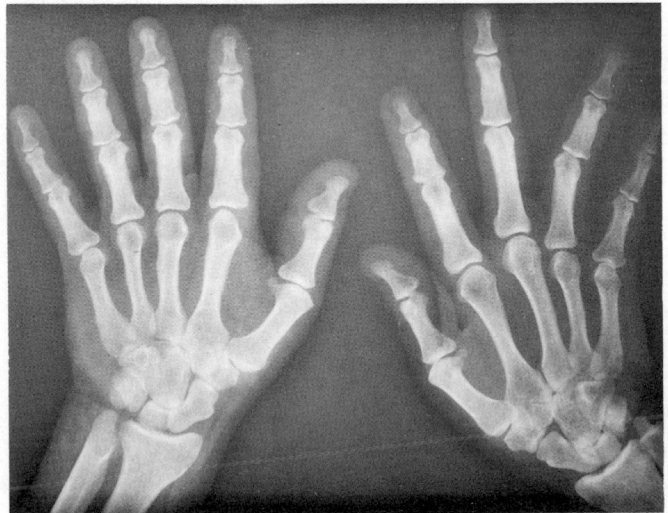

117. Note achondroplastic changes in right hand; normal appearance of metacarpals and phalanges of 2nd—5th fingers of left hand

ACID MALTASE DEFICIENCY

Includes: Déficit en maltase acide
Pompesche Krankheit
Deficiencia en maltasa ácida
Glycogen storage disease, type II
Glycogenosis II
Pompe disease
Alpha 1, 4-glucosidase deficiency
Heart disease, glycogen

Excludes: All other forms of glycogen storage disease

Minimal Diagnostic Criteria: Progressive dyspnea, cardiomegaly, congestive failure or pulmonary infection and frequently muscular weakness during infancy. Demonstration of absence of the lysosomal enzyme acid maltase in a variety of tissues and the accumulation of normally structured glycogen.

Clinical Findings: This disorder is caused by a generalized accumulation of glycogen in all body tissues, but both clinically and at autopsy the picture is usually dominated by massive accumulations of glycogen in the heart muscle. The condition commonly manifests itself in infants of 2 to 5 months of age, by dyspnea and cyanosis. Death from cardiac failure or pulmonary infection usually occurs between 12 and 18 months. Occasionally cardiomegaly is not a prominent feature and central nervous and neuromuscular involvement may lead to a picture like that of infantile spinal muscular atrophy (Werdnig-Hoffmann disease). In this situation there may be profound muscular weakness and hypotonia.

The laboratory features that assist in the diagnosis of this condition consist of demonstration of an absence of acid maltase in the affected tissues including muscle, and more recently a similar deficiency in blood leukocytes. The glycogen content of muscle is often very markedly raised and may reach 12% (normal less than 1%). The glycogen is normal in structure, it is contained within large vacuoles in muscle and other tissues and its presence progressively compromises the structure of all tissues so affected.

Complications
I **Derived:** Congestive heart failure, pulmonary infection, macroglossia, muscular weakness, aspiration pneumonitis
II **Associated:** —

Etiology: Autosomal recessive. Absence of the lysosomal enzyme acid maltase (alpha 1, 4-glucosidase). McK *23230

Pathogenesis: Pathologic accumulation of massive amounts of normally structured glycogen in many body tissues leading to cardiac failure, muscular weakness, nervous system defects and other organ-system deficiencies. Most glycogen is accumulated within lysosomes, but, in the later stages of the disease, there is a large quantity of extra-lysosomal glycogen also accumulated.

Related Facts
I **Sex Ratio:** M1:F1
II **Risk of Occurrence:** ?
III **Risk of Recurrence for**
  Patient's Sib: 1 in 4 (25%) for each offspring to be affected
  Patient's Child: Not increased unless mate is carrier or homozygote
IV **Age of Detectability:** Usually before the 6th month of life and potentially at birth
V **Prevalence:** Essentially zero among population over 2 years of age

Treatment
I **Primary Prevention:** Genetic counseling
II **Secondary Prevention:** —
III **Other Therapy:** Supportive as indicated

Prognosis: The outlook is extremely grim, death usually occurs from cardiac failure or pulmonary infection before 12 to 18 months and survival to 2 years of age is extremely rare. One family has been described in which 2 male sibs, both of whom lacked acid maltase in their muscles, survived at least to ages 15 years and 4 years. Neither showed accumulation of glycogen in other tissues.

Detection of Carrier: ?

Special Considerations: —

References:
Cori, G. T.: Biochemical aspects of glycogen deposition diseases. Mod. Probl. Pädiatr. 3:344, 1957.
Hers, H. G.: Alpha-glucosidase deficiency in generalized glycogen-storage disease (Pompe's disease). Biochem. J. 86:11, 1963.
Zellweger, H. et al: A mild form of muscular glycogenosis in two brothers with alpha-1, 4-glucosidase deficiency. Ann. Paediatr. (Basel) 205:413, 1965.

Contributor: **Carl M. Pearson**

Editor's Computerized Descriptors: Muscle, CV. Resp., Nerve

12

ACOUSTIC NEUROMATA

Includes: Neuromes auditifs bilatéraux
Beidseitiges Acusticus-Neurinom
Neuroma acústico bilateral
Bilateral acoustic neurofibromata
Central neurofibromatosis

Excludes: Unilateral neuroma, peripheral fibroblastoma
Peripheral and mixed neurofibromatosis

Minimal Diagnostic Criteria: Abnormalities in audiometric or vestibular testing, showing progressive auditory and vestibular dysfunction, in a family with a previously diagnosed case.

Clinical Findings: Early symptoms are referable to abnormalities of auditory or vestibular function: marked hearing loss, tinnitus, imbalance and, less commonly, vertigo. Relatively early mild cerebellar ataxia and corneal reflex depression are seen. Other complaints may be facial weakness, pain or numbness, headache, nausea and vomiting, severe visual loss progressing to blindness, emotional or mental changes, diplopia, dysphagia and dysarthria. Cafe-au-lait spots and skin tumors are rare findings. Central nervous tumors (eg meningioma, cystic astrocytoma) will be present in many cases. Increased symptomatology or actual precipitation of symptoms is noted during late pregnancy. At onset, symptoms may occur unilaterally, and involvement of the opposite side will appear within 2 years. Electrocochleography can be of diagnostic value, as polytomography and meatography of internal acoustic meatus. Computerized axial tomography can diagnose lesions smaller than those usually seen on brain scan. Tomographs of the auditory canal may be necessary in some cases.

Complications
I **Derived:** Tumor growth may cause impaired blood supply to the inner ear, being responsible for secondary degenerative changes in the sensory apparatus. Facial paralysis may be present.
II **Associated:** Fatal accidents, drowning, and suicide are reported.

Etiology: Autosomal dominant with high penetrance.† McK
*10100

Pathogenesis: Neurofibromas with palisade cells and tumor penetrating nerve fibers are found, mostly arising from the vestibular part of the 8th nerve.

Related Facts
I **Sex Ratio:** M1:F1
II **Risk of Occurrence:** 8% of CNS tumors are acoustic neuromas, 5% of them being bilateral.
III **Risk of Recurrence for**
  Patient's Sib: If parent is affected 1 in 2 (50%) for each offsrping to be affected; otherwise not increased.
  Patient's Child: 1 in 2
IV **Age of Detectability:** Generally, about 20 years.
V **Prevalence:** Rare

Treatment
I **Primary Prevention:** Early and periodic screening studies of relatives.
II **Secondary Prevention:** Operative approaches: possibly the translabyrinthine or middle fossa approach, otherwise suboccipital decompression followed by translabyrinthine approach.
III **Other Therapy:** —

Prognosis: Rate of progression is variable. Survival after onset of symptoms ranges from 2-40 years with an average of about 20 years.

Detection of Carrier: —

†**Special Considerations:** This condition may appear familially or sporadically. The latter will occur later; in the sporadic cases a new mutation is suggested. Bilateral tumors appear to be distinct from unilateral neuromas, which are generally sporadic, occur later and have a more rapid course.

Recently virus particles have been described in 6 acoustic neuroma specimens and the relationship of this finding to the etiology of unilateral and bilateral cases should be explored.

References:
Allen, J.C. et al: Early-onset acoustic neuroma: Genetic, clinical and nosologic aspects. In Bergsma, D. (ed.): Medical Genetics Today. Birth Defects: Orig. Art. Ser., vol. X, no. 10. Baltimore: The Johns Hopkins University Press for The National Foundation-March of Dimes, 1974, p. 171.
Gardner, W.J. and Frazier, C.M.: Bilateral acoustic neurofibromas. Arch. Neurol. Psychiatr. 23:266, 1930.
Gardner, W.J. and Turner, O.: Bilateral acoustic neurofibromas. Arch. Neurol Psychiatr. 44:76, 1940.
Moyes, P.D.: Familial bilateral acoustic neuromas affecting 14 members from four generations. J. Neurosurg. 29:78, 1968.
Perez De Moura, L.F. et al: Bilateral acoustic neurinoma and neurofibromatosis. Arch. Otolaryngol. 90:28, 1969.
Young, D.F. et al: Hereditary bilateral acoustic neuroma. In Bergsma, D. (ed.): Part IX. Ear. Birth Defects: Orig. Art. Ser., vol. VII, no. 4. Baltimore: Williams & Wilkins for The National Foundation-March of Dimes, 1971, p. 73.

Contributors: **Agnes M. Ickenroth**
Cor W.R.J. Cremers

Editor's Computerized Descriptors: Vision, Eye, Hearing, Ear, Speech, Skin, Muscle, GI., Nerve

ACROCEPHALOPOLYSYNDACTYLY

Includes: Acrocéphalopolysyndactylie
Akrozephalopolysyndaktylie
Acrocéfalopolisindactilia
Acrocephalopolysyndactyly (ACPS) types I, II, and III
ACPS type I
ACPS type II
ACPS type III
Noack syndrome
Carpenter syndrome
Sakati syndrome

Excludes: Acrocephalosyndactyly (14)
Polysyndactyly associated with peculiar skull shape
Laurence-Moon-Biedl syndrome (578)

Minimal Diagnostic Criteria: Typical x-ray findings

Clinical Findings: The main features are acrocephaly and polysyndactyly of the feet (preaxial polydactyly associated with syndactyly).

Three clinical and genetic types are recognized:

ACPS type I, (Noack syndrome) is characterized by the association of acrocephaly of a moderate degree with enlarged thumbs and duplicated great toes, without mental retardation, obesity, or hypogenitalism, and is of autosomal dominant transmission. This may not be distinct from acrocephalosyndactyly V (Pfeiffer type).

In ACPS type II (Carpenter syndrome) the skull malformation is acrocephaly of a severe degree due to premature synostosis of all the cranial sutures associated with a characteristic facies due to lateral displacement of both medial canthi and epicanthic folds, "down-thrust" eyes, rather flat nasal bridge, broad cheeks, relatively low-set ears and hypoplastic mandible. The limb malformation is symmetric. The hand malformation is soft tissue syndactyly affecting mainly the 3rd and 4th digits, and brachymesophalangy. A characteristic finding is that the proximal phalanx of the thumb has 2 ossification centers in childhood, represented as duplication of the thumb in adult affected cases.

In the feet the digital malformation is polysyndactyly (the association of syndactyly with preaxial polydactyly). Other features are coxa valga, pes varus, mild obesity, mental retardation, large abdominal hernias, and hypogenitalism as shown in older affected males.

In ACPS type III (Sakati syndrome) in addition to acrocephaly and polysyndactyly, the legs are very short, the femora bowed laterally, the tibiae hypoplastic, and the fibulae deformed and dyplastic. Associated anomalies are dyplastic ears, alopecia, and skin atrophy, linear scar lesions in submental area, cryptorchidism, small phallus, inguinal hernia, and congenital heart disease.

Complications
I **Derived:** —
II **Associated:** —

Etiology: ACPS type I (Noack syndrome) autosomal dominant
ACPS type II (Carpenter syndrome) autosomal recessive: McK *20100
ACPS type III etiology not known (? dominant mutation)

Pathogenesis: ?

Related Facts
I **Sex Ratio:** M1:F1
II **Risk of Occurrence:** ?
III **Risk of Recurrence for**
Patient's Sib: ACPS type I, see Table I AD; ACPS type II, see Table I AR.

Patient's Child: ACPS type I, see Table I AD; ACPS type II, see Table I AR. However, the reproductive fitness in cases with ACPS type II (Carpenter syndrome) must be low because of the severe malformation in females and the hypogenitalism in males.
IV **Age of Detectability:** At birth
V **Prevalence:** ?

Treatment
I **Primary Prevention:** Genetic counseling
II **Secondary Prevention:** Surgical correction of malformation, particularly early management of the cranial synostosis in Carpenter syndrome, and of large umbilical defects, and of the congenital heart disease.
III **Other Therapy:** ?

Prognosis: The skull and digital malformations do not affect life span. However, cases with ACPS type II who have congenital heart disease or large umbilical defects (omphalocele major) have a shorter life expectancy. The oldest reported case among the 25 cases known to date in the world literature was 25 years of age.

Detection of Carrier: —

Special Considerations: —

References:
Sakati, N. et al: A new syndrome with acrocephalopolysyndactyly, cardiac disease, and distinctive defect of the ear, skin, and lower limbs. J. Pediatr. 79:104, 1971.
Schönenberg, H. and Scheidhauer, E.: Über zwei ungewöhnliche Dyscranio-Dysphalangien bei Geschwistern (Atypische Akrocephalosyndactylie und fragliche Dysencephalia splanchocystica). Monatsschr. Kinderheilkd. 114:322, 1966.
Temtamy, S.A.: Carpenter's syndrome: Acrocephalopolsyndactyly; an autosomal recessive syndrome. J. Pediatr. 69:111, 1966.
Temtamy, S.A.: Genetic factors in hand malformations. Unpublished doctoral dissertation, Johns Hopkins University, 1966.
Temtamy, S.A. and McKusick, V.A: The Genetics of Hand Malformations. Birth Defects: Orig. Art. Ser., Bergsma, D. (ed.). New York: Alan Liss, Inc. for The National Foundation-March of Dimes. 1978, vol. XIV, no. 3.

Contributor: **Samia A. Temtamy**

Editor's Computerized Descriptors: Eye, Ear, Face, Nose, Skin, Hair, Skel., Hernia not CNS, GU., Nerve

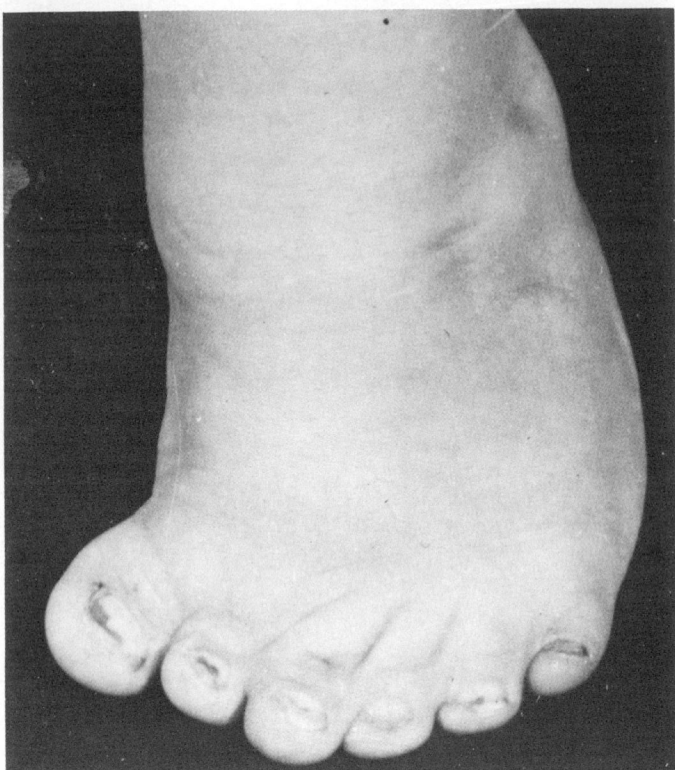

118. Polysyndactyly of foot

14   **013-500**

ACROCEPHALOSYNDACTYLY

Includes: Acrocéphalosyndactylie
 Akrozephalosyndaktylie
 Acrocéfalosindactilia
 Apert syndrome
 Apert-Crouzon disease or Vogt cephalodactyly
 Saethre-Chotzen syndrome
 Pfeiffer syndrome
 Acrocephalosyndactyly, Waardenburg type
 Acrocephalosyndactyly, Summitt type
 Acrocephalosyndactyly, Herrmann-Opitz type

Excludes: Cranio-oculo-dental syndrome (229)
 Acrocephalopolysyndactyly (13)

Minimal Diagnostic Criteria: Acrocephaly and variable degrees
 of syndactyly

Clinical Findings: *Apert syndrome:* The skull malformation is cranial synostosis of variable degrees affecting mainly the coronal sutures and associated with sphenoethmoidomaxillary hypoplasia of the basis cranii. The malformation leads to a facies characterized by flat forehead, hypertelorism, depressed nasal bridge and relative prognathism. The digital malformation is characterized by complete syndactyly involving the 2nd to 5th digits of the hands and feet, sometimes with synonychia and synostosis. *Apert-Crouzon* type or *Vogt cephalodactyly* is probably the same entity with more severe craniofacial involvement.

 Saethre-Chotzen syndrome The skull malformation is craniosynostosis of variable degrees that is usually asymmetric leading to plagiocephaly. Other craniofacial anomalies include frontal and parietal bossing, ptosis of eyelids, hypertelorism, esotropia and exotropia. The digital malformation is usually mild and incomplete soft tissue syndactyly most often involving the 2nd and 3rd digits of the hands and feet, and brachydactyly.

 Waardenburg type: Acrocephaly is associated with beaked pointed nose, hypertelorism, cleft palate, bilateral hydrophthalmos, congenital heart disease and pseudohermaphroditism. Limb anomalies include contractures of elbows and knees, soft tissue syndactyly of digits, absent 1st metatarsal and great toe, and bifid distal phalanx of index. Only 1 sporadic case was reported by Waardenburg (1934).

 Pfeiffer syndrome: Acrocephaly is associated with broad thumbs, great toes, and mild syndactyly. In a few cases, duplication of the 1st metatarsal and proximal phalanx of the great toe were noted.

 Summitt type: The features are acrocephaly, peculiar facies, syndactyly of hands and feet, obesity, genu valgum, hypogenitalism and normal intelligence. The only report of the syndrome was by Summitt (1969) in brothers, the offspring of normal 1st cousins.

 Herrmann-Opitz type: Main features are acrocephaly, brachysyndactyly of the hands, monodactyly of the feet, reduced stature, mental retardation and cryptorchidism. Only 1 sporadic case was reported by Herrmann and Opitz (1969).

Complications
 I **Derived:** Mental retardation of variable degrees has been attributed to associated dilatation of the lateral ventricles.
 II **Associated:** In almost all ACS types, visceral and other skeletal anomalies, and deafness have been noted.

Etiology: Apert syndrome (McK *10120) is dominant, either autosomal or X-linked. Saethre-Chotzen and Pfeiffer syndromes (McK *10140, *10160) are autosomal dominant, Summitt type is autosomal recessive, Waardenburg type and Herrmann-Opitz type are sporadic with unknown etiology.

Pathogenesis: —

Related Facts

I Sex Ratio: M1:F1

II Risk of Occurrence: 1 in 160,000 births for Apert syndrome in the English population

III Risk of Recurrence for

Patient's Sib: In Apert, Saethre-Chotzen and Pfeiffer syndromes: if parent is affected 1 in 2 (50%) for each offspring to be affected; otherwise not increased. In Summitt type: 1 in 4 (25%).

Patient's Child: In Saethre-Chotzen, Pfeiffer and Apert syndromes: 1 in 2 (50%). (However, reproductive fitness is very low in cases with Apert syndrome). Summitt type: 0 unless mate were to be a carrier. In Waardenburg and Herrmann-Opitz types the risk is unknown.

IV Age of Detectability: At birth

V Prevalence: ?

Treatment

I Primary Prevention: Genetic counseling

II Secondary Prevention: Surgical correction of skull and digital anomalies.

III Other Therapy: Hearing aid for hearing loss. Early detection and management of internal hydrocephalus.

Prognosis: Malformations do not affect life span except when associated with serious visceral involvement.

Detection of Carrier: —

Special Considerations: —

References:

Cohen, M.M., Jr.: An etiologic and nosologic overview of craniosynostosis syndromes. In Bergsma, D. (ed.): Malformation Syndromes. Birth Defects: Orig. Art. Ser., vol. XI, no. 2. Amsterdam: Excerpta Medica for The National Foundation-March of Dimes, 1975, p. 137.

Herrmann, J. and Opitz, J.M.: An unusual form of acrocephalosyndactyly. In Bergsma, D. (ed.): Part III. Limb Malformations. Birth Defects: Orig. Art. Ser., vol. V, no. 3. White Plains: The National Foundation-March of Dimes, 1969, p. 39.

Summitt, R.L.: Recessive acrocephalosyndactyly with normal intelligence. Ibid, p. 35.

Temtamy, S.A.: Genetic Factors in Hand Malformations. Unpublished doctoral dissertation, Johns Hopkins University, 1966.

Temtamy, S.A. and McKusick, V.A.: The Genetics of Hand Malformations. Birth Defects: Orig. Art. Ser., Bergsma, D. (ed.). New York: Alan R. Liss for The National Foundation-March of Dimes, 1978, vol XIV, no. 3.

Waardenburg, P.J.: Eine merkwürdige Kombination von angeborenen Missbildungen: doppelseitiger Hydrophthalmus verbunden mit Akrocephalosyndaktylie, Herzfehler, Pseudohermaphroditismus und anderen Abweichungen. Klin. Monatsbl. Augenheilkd. 92:29, 1934.

Contributor: **Samia A. Temtamy**

Editor's Computerized Descriptors: Eye, Hearing, Face, Nose, Skel., CV., GI.

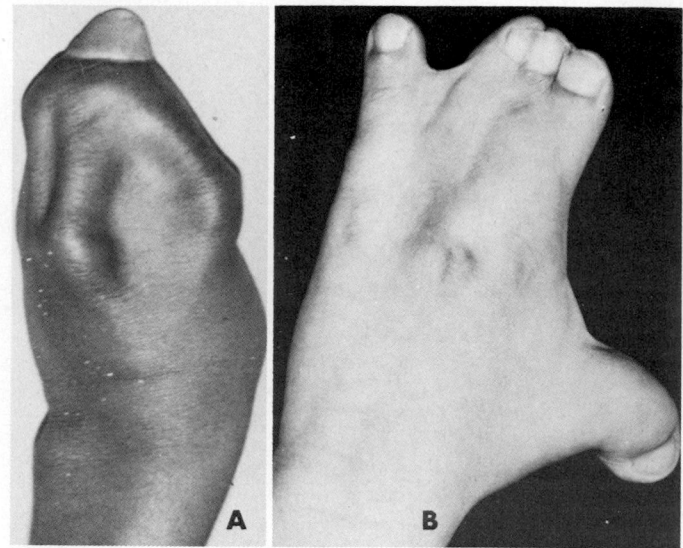

119. A) Stocking syndactyly with single nail; B) syndactyly with radial deviation of thumb

ACRODERMATITIS ENTEROPATHICA

Includes: Acrodermatite entéropathique
Acrodermatitis enteropática

Excludes: Gluten-induced enteropathy (423)
Chronic monilial granuloma

Minimal Diagnostic Criteria: Diagnosis thus far is clinical and should include skin eruption, alopecia or diarrhea with at least some of the associated abnormalities to substantiate the clinical impression. The dramatic response to therapy which has been reported in most cases helps to clarify the diagnosis.

Clinical Findings: A peculiar skin eruption that consists of lesions varying from bullae to verrucous plaques and has a predilection for the distal portions of the limbs, the perioral region and the perineum, 100%; diarrhea, 91%; alopecia, 98%.

In addition, these patients also may have glossitis and stomatitis, photophobia, conjunctivitis, paronychia, dystrophy of the nails, perlèche, irritability and emotional disturbances, as well as frequent secondary infection of the skin and mucous membrane with Candida albicans, or bacteria, or both.

Infants who are destined to have the disease rarely give evidence of an abnormality at birth. The disorder begins insidiously between the ages of 3 weeks and 10 years with an average age of onset of 9 months, frequently at the time of weaning. The first indication of the disease is usually the appearance of a skin eruption, localized to the body orifices and limbs, which is accompanied by or followed shortly afterward by alopecia and GI symptoms. The sequence of appearance of symptoms is not consistent. The alopecia is usually total but in 13% of cases it has been diffuse. The diarrhea may be severe or mild and in 10% of cases it has not been a prominent feature of the disease. The primary skin lesions are usually vesicobullous in type. They appear in groups and are located symmetrically about the body orifices, eyes, occiput, elbows, knees, hands and feet. The lesions are especially prone to occur around the nails and between the fingers and toes. The trunk is usually not involved. After a time the lesions begin to dry and crust and with the occurrence of lamellar scaling they develop a psoriasiform appearance. Lesions in various stages of development may be present simultaneously and the appearance may be further altered by the occurrence of bacterial infection or monilial infection or both, common features of this condition. Any stage of development may predominate and in many instances the vesicular phase is not observed at all. The heavily scaled psoriasiform lesions seem to dominate the picture in many instances. Resolution of the skin lesions leaves no scarring or atrophy. In general the baldness, skin eruption and dejected attitude of afflicted children produce a striking uniformity of appearance. If unrecognized or untreated, the disease follows an intermittent but relentlessly progressive course that may eventuate in death from general debility or intercurrent infection or both. Short lived spontaneous remissions are followed by relapses which are increasingly more severe and in many instances are related to intercurrent infection.

Complications
I **Derived:** Intercurrent infection, particularly of the respiratory tract and general debility.
II **Associated:** —

Etiology: Presumably autosomal recessive; 65% of the reported cases had affected sibs. McK *20110

Pathogenesis: The primary abnormality appears to be in the GI phase of the disease although there has been no consistently demonstrable bowel change in afflicted patients. Reportedly a deficiency of succinic dehydrogenase in intestinal mucosal cells was noted. The most recently proposed theory is that the disease is due to an alteration of tryptophan metabolism which leads to production of a metabolite with toxic effects on the cutaneous and intestinal epithelium.

Related Facts
I **Sex Ratio:** M1:F1
II **Risk of Occurrence:** ?
III **Risk of Recurrence for**
  Patient's Sib: 1 in 4 (25%) for each offspring to be affected
  Patient's Child: Not increased unless mate is carrier or homozygote
IV **Age of Detectability:** —
V **Prevalence:** —

Treatment
I **Primary Prevention:** Genetic counseling
II **Secondary Prevention:** Dramatic response to therapy with diiodohydroxyquin. Enterovioform and Chloroquin also have been used successfully. Recent success with human milk feedings has been reported.
  Successful treatment seems to include both the quinoline compounds and human milk and it is possible that either alone may not be satisfactory. The key to successful treatment of the disease is early diagnosis no matter what modality is used, for the prompt institution of therapy may be lifesaving.
III **Other Therapy:** Control of infection as may be indicated.

Prognosis: Untreated, outlook is death at an early age. Treated, patients may develop into normal individuals with a normal life span. There seems to be some evidence that there is a tendency for spontaneous involution at puberty, if the patient can be carried to that point by adequate therapy. Cases of the disease in adults have been reported but they may represent a forme fruste or atypical variation of acrodermatitis enteropathica.

Detection of Carrier: ?

Special Considerations: —

References:
Danbolt, N. and Closs, K.: Akrodermatitis enteropathica. Acta Derm. Venereol. (Stockh.) 23:127, 1942.
Dillaha, C.J. et al: Acrodermatitis enteropathica; review of literature and report of case successfully treated with diodoquin. JAMA 152:509, 1953.
Wells, B.T. and Winkelmann, R.K.: Acrodermatitis enteropathica, report of six cases. Arch. Dermatol. 84:40, 1961.

Contributor: **Benjamin T. Wells**

***

Editor's Computerized Descriptors: Eye, Oral, Skin, Hair, Nails, GI., Nerve

16
ACRODYSOSTOSIS

Includes: Acrodysostose
Acrodisostosis
Peripheral dysostosis, nasal hypoplasia and mental retardation syndrome (PNM)
PNM

Excludes: Pseudohypoparathyroidism (830)
Brachydactyly (114)
Other forms of acrodysplasia

Minimal Diagnostic Criteria: The diagnosis of this syndrome depends on clinical and radiographic criteria. Peripheral dysostosis, nasal hypoplasia, and mental retardation are found in almost all cases; and at least 2 of these features should be present to make a diagnosis. This syndrome must be distinguished from other disorders included in the heterogeneous group of "peripheral dysostosis." Lack of alterations in calcium and phosphorus metabolism and the presence of generalized brachymetacarpaly with severely shortened phalanges distinguishes this syndrome from Albright osteodystrophy.†

Clinical Findings: The major features of this syndrome are peripheral dysostosis, nasal hypoplasia, mental retardation, and short stature. The hands and feet are short with stubby fingers and toes and broad short nails. These patients are short at birth and growth retardation is progressive. This shortening is acromesomelic with short forearms and limitation of motion at the elbows. The facies is characteristic with marked nasal hypoplasia; the nasal bridge is low, the nose is flat and short, and the nasal tip is broad and somewhat dimpled with anteverted nostrils and a long philtrum. Maxillary hypoplasia, hypertelorism, epicanthal folds, and malocclusion are often present. Almost all of the reported patients have had some degree of mental retardation.

Radiographs reveal severe shortening of the metacarpals and phalanges. The epiphyses are deformed in the metacarpals and cone-shaped in the phalanges. The carpal bones may be small and the distal radius and ulna are often malformed. There is premature fusion of the epiphyses of the hands, feet, and elbows. Changes in the feet are comparable to those of the hands. Radiographic changes suggestive of juvenile spondylitis have been described in several cases. The skull is usually brachycephalic and may show thickening of the calvaria.

Complications
I   **Derived:** Difficulty with manual skills due to shortened fingers, limitation of motion in the elbows and spine; arthritic symptoms in the hands and feet may occur with age.
II **Associated:** —

Etiology: ? All reported cases to date have been sporadic. No parental consanguinity has been reported.

Pathogenesis: ? Premature epiphyseal fusion may partially account for the severe shortening of the hands and feet, but there is also generalized growth retardation involving many bones whose epiphyses are radiographically normal.

Related Facts
I   **Sex Ratio:** M1:F2
II **Risk of Occurrence:** ?
III **Risk of Recurrence for**
   Patient's Sib: ? All reported cases were sporadic.
   Patient's Child: ? (None of the reported cases have reproduced to date.)
IV **Age of Detectability:** Usually detectable at birth or early infancy by the clinical features
V   **Prevalence:** ?

Treatment

I   **Primary Prevention:** —
II **Secondary Prevention:** Plastic surgery may be required in severe cases to improve the facial appearance.
III **Other Therapy:** —

Prognosis: Apparently normal for life span, poor for intelligence and reduced function of hands, feet and elbows

Detection of Carrier: —

†Special Considerations: This syndrome must be differentiated from other disorders which are associated with "peripheral dysostosis," a descriptive term which simply refers to shortening and deformity of the bones of the hands and feet. This can be seen in pseudohypoparathyroidism, the trichorhinophalangeal syndrome, as part of the various brachydactyly syndromes, and as an isolated phenomenon. Bachman and Norman have described peripheral dysostosis in a woman and her 2 children, but these patients did not have the peculiar facial appearance and were mentally normal, ruling out acrodysostosis. A number of experts in the field now feel that acrodysostosis may be simply a form of pseudohypoparathyroidism.

References:
Bachman, R.K. and Norman, A.P.: Hereditary peripheral dysostosis (3 cases). Proc. R. Soc. Med. 60:21, 1967.
Maroteaux, P. and Malamut, G.: L'Acrodysostose. Presse Med. 76:2189, 1968.
Robinow, M. et al: Acrodysostosis. A syndrome of peripheral dysostosis, nasal hypoplasia, and mental retardation. Am. J. Dis. Child. 121:195, 1971.

Contributors: **David L. Rimoin**
David W. Hollister

Editor's Computerized Descriptors: Eye, Face, Teeth, Nose, Nails, Skel., Nerve

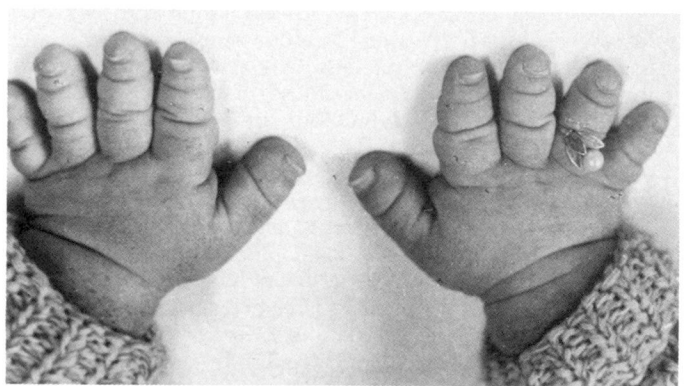

120. Note very short broad digits with short nails

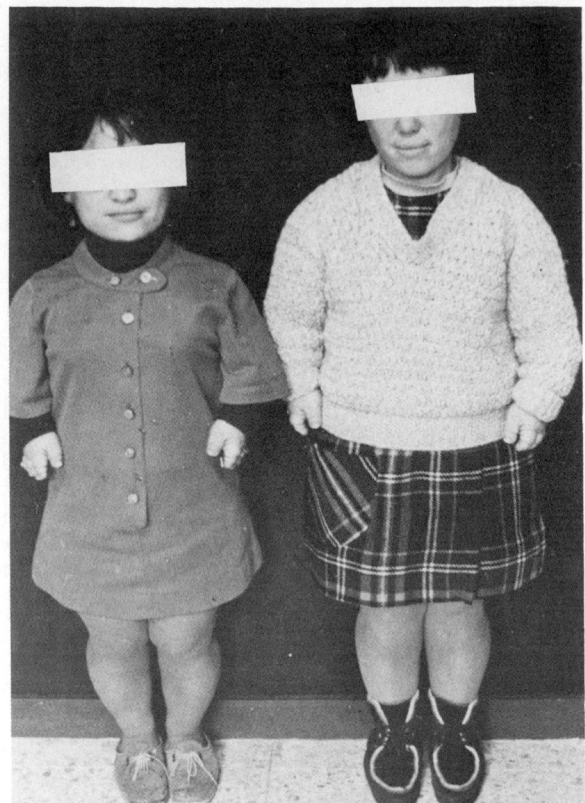

121. Note very short stature, semiflexed position of the arms, and extremely short fingers

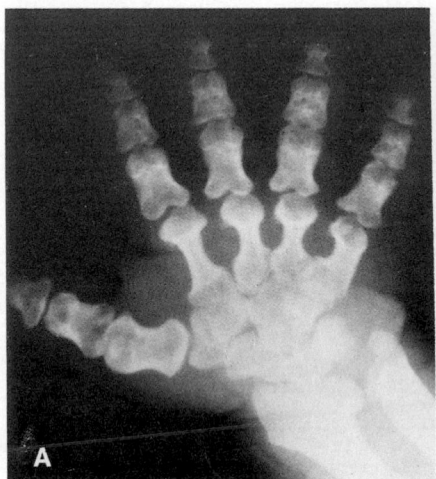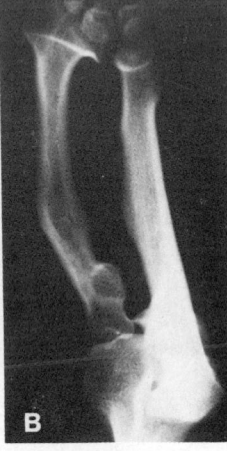

122. A) Note extremely short metacarpals, cone-shaped phalangeal epiphyses and flaring of distal metaphyseal portion of radius; B) bowing of radius

17

17
ACROFACIAL DYSOSTOSIS

Includes: Dysostose acro-faciale
Dysostosis acrofacialis
Disostosis acrofacial
Dysostosis, acrofacial

Excludes: Acrofacial dysostosis of Nager (17)
Isolated postaxial hexadactyly
Median clefts of lower lip mandible and tongue (636)
Ectodermal dysplasia (Robinson type)
Chondroectodermal dysplasia (156)
Oro-facio-digital syndrome II (771)
Other syndromes with polydactyly
Isolated cleft chin

Minimal Diagnostic Criteria: Postaxial hexadactyly and bony cleft of mandibular symphysis or anomalies of lower central incisors.

Clinical Findings: Postaxial hexadactyly of both hands and feet with synostosis of metacarpals (metatarsals) V and VI have been observed in all reported cases. Bony cleft of mandibular symphysis, anomalies of lower central incisors ranging from peg-shaped teeth to complete aplasia especially in the permanent dentition, and peg-shaped or missing lateral incisors have also been noted frequently.

The oral vestibule is absent in the anterior mandibular region. Occasionally this feature is present also in the anterior maxillary region often associated with persistent folds at the borders of the premaxilla.†

Complications
I **Derived:** Early loss of malformed teeth leading to malocclusion
II **Associated:** See Clinical Findings

Etiology: Autosomal dominant with variable expressivity and incomplete penetrance

Pathogenesis: Limb abnormalities and mandibular clefting arise during the 5th and 6th week of embryogenesis.

Related Facts
I **Sex Ratio:** Both sexes are affected. Too few cases reported to know sex ratio.
II **Risk of Occurrence:** ?
III **Risk of Recurrence for**
Patient's Sib: If parent is affected < 1 in 2 (< 50%) for each offspring to be affected; otherwise not increased.
Patient's Child: < 1 in 2. Probably lower for full syndrome.
IV **Age of Detectability:** At birth by clinical evaluation (including radiologic examination of mandible)
V **Prevalence:** ? Very rare disorder

Treatment
I **Primary Prevention:** Genetic counseling
II **Secondary Prevention:** Excision of extra digits, surgical repair of mandibular symphysial cleft, prosthodontic treatment for missing or malformed teeth.
III **Other Therapy:** —

Prognosis: Good. Not known if longevity is reduced.

Detection of Carrier: —

†Special Considerations: The full spectrum is not yet certain because too few cases have been reported. Patients and first-degree relatives should be carefully examined for other possible features and minor malformations of the syndrome.

References:
Weyers, H.: Hexadactylie, Unterkieferspalt und Oligodontie, ein neuer Symptomenkomplex. Dysostosis acro-facialis. Ann. Paediatr. (Basel) 181:45, 1953.
Weyers, H.: Zur Kenntnis der Chondroektodermaldysplasie (Ellis-van Creveld); Bericht über 2 Beobachtungen. Z. Kinderheilkd.

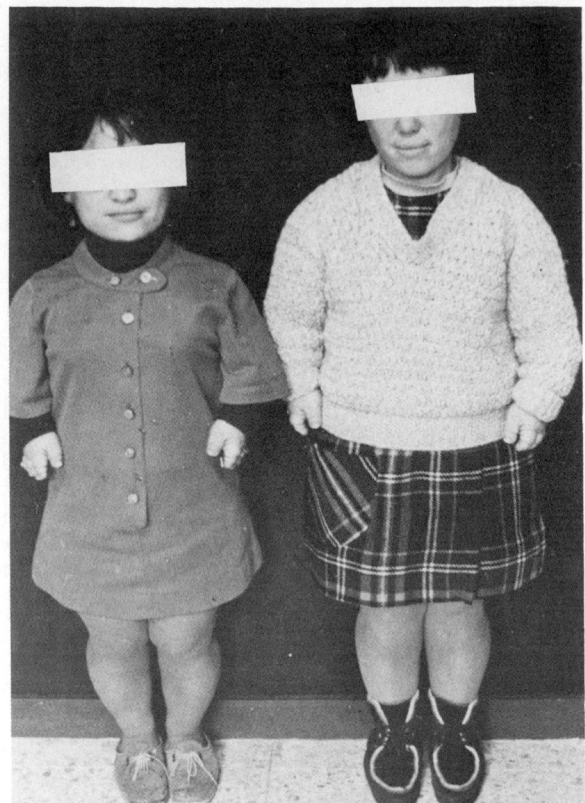

121. Note very short stature, semiflexed position of the arms, and extremely short fingers

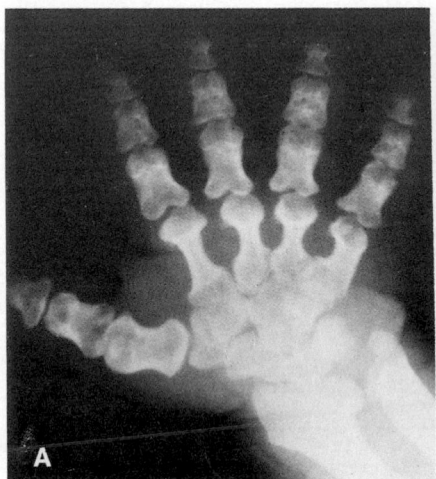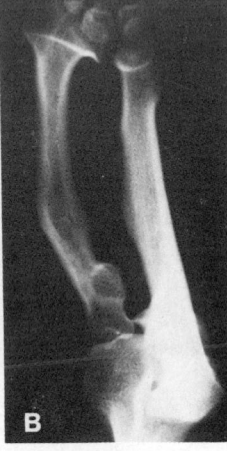

122. A) Note extremely short metacarpals, cone-shaped phalangeal epiphyses and flaring of distal metaphyseal portion of radius; B) bowing of radius

78:111, 1956.

Contributors: **Gordon G. Keyes**
Heddie O. Sedano

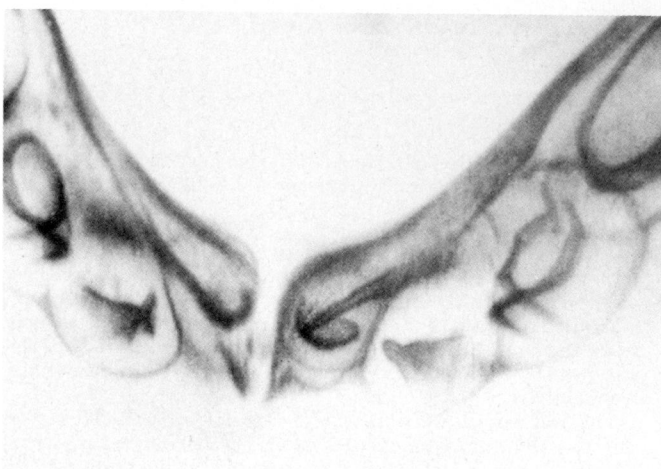

123. Cleft of mandibular symphysis

ACROMEGALOID PHENOTYPE, CUTIS VERTICIS AND GYRATACORNEAL LEUKOMA

Includes: Acromégalie avec cutis verticis gyrata et leucome de la cornée
Acromegaloider Habitus-Cutis verticis gyrata und Hornhaut-Leukom
Fenotipo acromegaloide, cutis verticis gyrata y leucoma corneano
Gyratacorneal leukoma, acromegaloid phenotype and cutis verticis

Excludes: Acromegaly
Acromegaly associated with cutis verticis gyrata

Minimal Diagnostic Criteria: Progressive leukoma formation and gyrate convolutions of the scalp in association with a somatotype suggesting acromegaly.

Clinical Findings: Acromegaloid features include large bones, eg the jaw, but the sella turcica is normal in size. The lateral half of the supraorbital arch of the frontal bone is particularly enlarged. The scalp is also enlarged, causing gyrus-like formations of skin over the surface of the skull. There is longitudinal splitting of dermal ridges in the palms. During the first decade of life, unilateral or bilateral progressive opacification of the cornea occurs. It characteristically begins in the inferonasal quadrant of the corneal epithelium as a flat, then raised, leukoma, which subsequently becomes slightly elevated (about 1/2 mm) and considerably more widespread, leading to blindness. The peripheral 1 mm of the cornea is usually spared.

Complications
I **Derived:** Blindness due to corneal opacification
II **Associated:** —

Etiology: Autosomal dominant; McK *10210

Pathogenesis: ?

Related Facts
I **Sex Ratio:** M1:F1
II **Risk of Occurrence:** —
III **Risk of Recurrence for**
  Patient's Sib: 1 in 2, (50%) for each offspring to be affected
  Patient's Child: 1 in 2
IV **Age of Detectability:** —
V **Prevalence:** —

Treatment
I **Primary Prevention:** Genetic counseling
II **Secondary Prevention:** —
III **Other Therapy:** Optical iridectomy

Prognosis: Normal for life, probably poor for vision. ? normal for intelligence

Detection of Carrier: —

Special Considerations: —

References:
Rosenthal, J.W. and Kloepfer, H.W.: An acromegaloid cutis verticis gyrata, corneal leukoma syndrome: A new medical entity. Arch. Ophthalmol. 68:722, 1962.

Contributor: **Morton F. Goldberg**

ACROMESOMELIC DYSPLASIA, CAMPAILLA-MARTINELLI TYPE

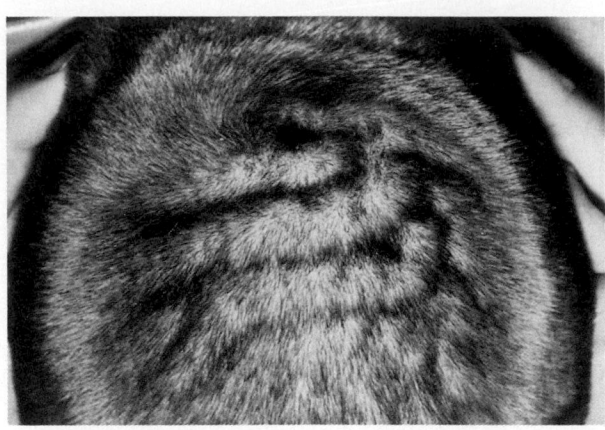

124. Gyrate scalp folds

Includes: Dysplasie acromésomélique type Campailla-Martinelli
Akromesomele Dysplasie, Typ Campailla-Martinelli
Displasia acromesomiélica tipo, Campailla-Martinelli

Excludes: Acromesomelic dysplasia, Maroteaux type (20)
Chondroectodermal dysplasia (156)
Acrodysostosis (16)
All forms of mesomelic dysplasia
Dyschondrosteosis (308)

Minimal Diagnostic Criteria: Moderate-to-marked short stature with a profound shortening of the middle and especially distal segments of the limbs and the characteristic radiographic changes in the limbs.

Clinical Findings: Disproportionate dwarfism with short distal limbs. The digits are short and stubby with normal nails. The range of movement of all joints, the skull, and intelligence are normal. The adult height is about 127-137 cm. Radiographically the tubular bones of the forearms and the lower legs are short and thick. The radius is laterally curved with a mild Madelung deformity at the wrists. The proximal fibula and the distal ulna are hypoplastic. The middle and terminal phalanges in the hands and feet are short and squared as are the 4th and 5th metatarsals. At the wrists there is fusion of the capitate and hamate bones. Scoliosis, pes planus and hallux valgus deformities may be present.

Complications
I **Derived:** Scoliosis
II **Associated:** —

Etiology: Autosomal recessive; McK *20125

Pathogenesis: Retarded growth of the tubular bones at the growth plates of the distal limbs.

Related Facts
I   **Sex Ratio:** M1:F1
II **Risk of Occurrence:** ?
III **Risk of Recurrence for**
      Patient's Sib: 1 in 4 (25%) for each offspring to be affected
      Patient's Child: Not increased unless mate is carrier or homozygote
IV **Age of Detectability:** At birth
V   **Prevalence:** ?

Treatment
I   **Primary Prevention:** Genetic counseling
II **Secondary Prevention:** Physiotherapy; orthopedic surgery may be needed for correction of the scoliosis.
III **Other Therapy:** —

Prognosis: Probably normal life span

Detection of Carrier: —

Special Considerations: —

References:
Beighton, P.: Autosomal recessive inheritance in the mesomelic dwarfism of Campailla and Martinelli. Clin. Genet. 5:363, 1974.
Campailla, E. and Martinelli, B: Deficit staturale con micromesomelia. Minerva Ortop. 22:180, 1971.
Kaitila, I.I. et al: Mesomelic skeletal dysplasias. Clin. Orthop. 114:94, 1976.

Contributor: **Ilkka I. Kaitila**

Editor's Computerized Descriptor: Skel.

ACROMESOMELIC DYSPLASIA, MAROTEAUX TYPE

Includes: Dysplasie acromésomélique, type Maroteaux
Akromesomele Dysplasie, Typ Maroteaux
Displasia acromesomiélica, tipo Maroteaux

Excludes: Acromesomelic dysplasia, Campailla-Martinelli type (19)
Dyschondrosteosis (308)
Acrodysostosis (16)
Chondroectodermal dysplasia (156)
All forms of mesomelic dysplasia

Minimal Diagnostic Criteria: Disproportionate short stature at birth with marked distal shortening of the limbs and the characteristic radiographic appearance of the radius, ulna, short tubular bones and phalanges.

Clinical Findings: The patients present with marked disproportionate dwarfism resulting from short distal limbs. The face is normal but the skull appears slightly scaphocephalic. All long bones are disproportionately short compared to the trunk. The hands are broad and short with short and stubby fingers. There are limitations of pronation-supination and extension at the elbows. The lower legs are short and straight; the feet are short, flat, and square with stubby toes. Lumbar lordosis is mild. Adult height ranges from 110-120 cm. Intelligence is normal.

Radiologically, all long bones are short with exaggerated outlines, particularly at the sites of muscular attachments. The distal ulna is hypoplastic and the shortness is further augmented by the marked curve in midshaft. The radius is slightly shortened, often bent and the proximal head is dislocated. The metacarpals, metatarsals, and especially the phalanges, are short and square in form. Early epiphyseal fusion occurs in the tubular bones of the hands and feet. The fibula is short in relation to the tibia and its proximal end remains at the level of the growth plate of the tibia. The skull is slightly scaphocephalic due to mild bossing of the frontal bones. The basal angle of the skull is larger than normal (135-140°). The heights of the vertebrae are slightly reduced and there may be some narrowing of the interpedicular distance towards the last lumbar vertebrae.

Complications
I   **Derived:** —
II **Associated:** —

Etiology: Autosomal recessive; McK *20125

Pathogenesis: The shortness of the distal limbs may partly result from early fusion of the growth plates.

Related Facts
I   **Sex Ratio:** M1:F1
II   **Risk of Occurrence:** ?
III **Risk of Recurrence for**
    Patient's Sib: 1 in 4 (25%) for each offspring to be affected
    Patient's Child: Not increased unless mate is carrier or homozygote
IV **Age of Detectability:** At birth
V   **Prevalence:** ?

Treatment
I   **Primary Prevention:** Genetic counseling
II   **Secondary Prevention:** —
III **Other Therapy:** —

Prognosis: Probably normal life span

Detection of Carrier: —

Special Considerations: —

References:
Kaitila, I.I. et al: Mesomelic skeletal dysplasias. Clin. Orthop. 114:94, 1976.
Maroteaux, P. et al: Le nanisme acromésomélique. Presse Méd. 79:1839, 1971.

Contributor: **Ilkka I. Kaitila**

Editor's Computerized Descriptor: Skel.

ACRO-OSTEOLYSIS, DOMINANT TYPE

Includes: Acro-ostéolyse
Akroosteolyse
Acro-osteolisis
Acroosteolysis without neuropathy

Excludes: Pyknodysostosis (846)
Oculo-auriculo-vertebral dysplasia (735)
Mesenchymal dysplasia of Puretić (644)
Cheney syndrome
Various sensory neuropathy-acroosteolysis syndromes (dominant and recessive)
"Vinyl chloride" acroosteolysis
Dactylolysis spontanea (ainhum)
Hyperparathyroidism
Leprosy
Sclerodactyly
Various carpal-tarsal osteolysis syndromes
Raynaud disease

Minimal Diagnostic Criteria: Osteolysis of phalanges, especially in the distal phalanges, with a compatible clinical course and absence of sensory deficits, cutaneous changes, vertebral, skull, or mandibular skeletal defects, osteoporosis or osteosclerosis, abnormal facies, or exposure to the vinyl chloride polymerization process.†

Clinical Findings: The term "acroosteolysis" has been used to designate a variety of syndromes which have as a prominent feature osteolysis of the distal bones of a limb. "Acroosteolysis" in the present usage refers to osteolysis predominantly involving, but not necessarily limited to, the phalanges without neuropathic changes.

The following clinical description is based on 2 cases reported by Lamy and Maroteaux:

Beginning in early childhood, essentially asymptomatic osteolysis of the distal phalanges of the fingers and toes develops. Insidious shortening of the digits occurs without functional disability, loss of sensation, or cutaneous ulceration or atrophy. The nails are present although somewhat shortened and elliptical in shape. There are no associated skeletal deformities and the facies is normal.

Radiographs disclose osteolysis of the phalangeal tufts with subsequent extension to the diaphyses of the terminal phalanges. The distal phalanx of the thumb is also involved. In the 4th and 5th digits of the hands and feet, however, the osteolytic process may commence in the proximal or middle phalanges, leaving the terminal phalanx intact.

The osteolysis is a chronic, very slowly progressive affliction; in the most advanced case (age 34) there was significant shortening of the digits, some of which were reduced to wrinkled nubbins of tissue, especially those digits with more proximal osteolysis.

Radiographically, the distal phalanges were either absent or reduced to small fragments. Occasionally, the lytic process extended past the proximal interphalangeal joint to involve the adjacent middle phalanx. Those digits involved in the more proximal osteolysis exhibited variable loss of all phalanges with marked tapering and shortening of adjacent metacarpals and metatarsals ("sucked candy" appearance). Lateral erosion of the bases of metacarpals and metatarsals was evident with moderate irregularity and loss of outline of carpal and tarsal bones.

No pathologic examination of affected tissues was reported.

The laboratory examination was completely normal including normal calcium, phosphorus, and alkaline phosphatase. Calcium balance studies were normal.

Complications
I **Derived:** Mild-to-moderate manual disability secondary to loss of finger length.
II **Associated:** —

Etiology: Autosomal dominant or X-linked dominant

Pathogenesis: ?

Related Facts
I **Sex Ratio:** Approximately M1:F1
II **Risk of Occurrence:** ?
III **Risk of Recurrence for**
    Patient's Sib: When autosomal dominant or X-linked dominant, see Table I AD or X-linked D, respectively.
    Patient's Child: When autosomal dominant or X-linked dominant, see Table I AD or X-linked D, respectively.
IV **Age of Detectability:** Early-to-late childhood by clinical and radiographic examination
V **Prevalence:** ? Rare

Treatment
I **Primary Prevention:** Genetic counseling
II **Secondary Prevention:** —
III **Other Therapy:** —

Prognosis: Apparently good for life span, apparently normal for intelligence, with mild-to-moderate manual disability.

Detection of Carrier: —

†Special Considerations: Differentiation of dominant acroosteolysis from the many syndromes in which acroosteolysis is a prominent feature requires thorough clinical and laboratory evaluation. Absence of sensory deficits and cutaneous ulcerations or atrophy tends to rule out leprosy, sclerodactyly, Raynaud disease, and the sensory neuropathy-acroosteolysis syndromes. A radiographic survey disclosing normal carpal-tarsal bones, long tubular bones, vertebrae, skull, and mandible without osteoporosis or osteosclerosis, rules out the Puretić syndrome, Cheney syndrome, pyknodysostosis, and various carpal-tarsal osteolysis syndromes. Normal facies without eye or ear malformations or vertebral defects rules out oculoauriculovertebral dysplasia. The pattern of bone resorption, absence of other skeletal changes, and lack of alterations in calcium and phosphorus metabolism separates this syndrome from advanced hyperparathyroidism. Dactylolysis spontanea (ainhum) affects a limited number of digits of the feet only. "Vinyl chloride" acroosteolysis has been confined to individuals employed in cleaning polymerization vats; there is a notable lack of this problem in individuals participating in the further manufacture of polyvinyl chloride products.

References:
Lamy, M. and Maroteaux, P.: Acro-osteolyse dominante. Arch. Fr. Pediatr. 18:693, 1961.

Contributors: **David W. Hollister**
David L. Rimoin

Editor's Computerized Descriptors: Nails, Skel.

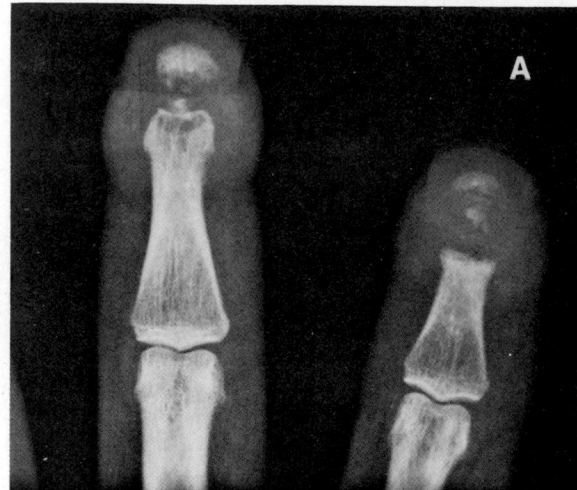

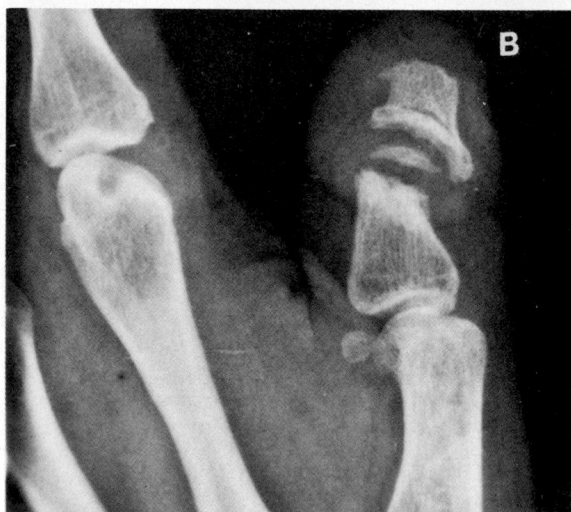

125. A) Left fingers 2 and 3; B) left thumb

ACROPECTOROVERTEBRAL DYSPLASIA

Includes: Dysplasie acropectoro-vertébrale
Displasia acro-péctoro-vertebral
F syndrome

Excludes: —

Minimal Diagnostic Criteria: Hypoplasia of 1st digits, partial webbing of 1st and 2nd digits, carpal and tarsal synostoses.

Clinical Findings: The syndrome most prominently affects the hands and feet. Major anomalies include extensive carpal and tarsal synostoses, prominence of the sternum with a more or less extensive pectus excavatum component, and spina bifida occulta of L5 or S1. Characteristically the broad, short and malformed thumbs show incipient distal phalangeal duplication and are, to a variable degree, webbed with the index finger which is radially deviated, particularly when the webbing is extensive. An extra bone may be present in the web; it seems to be derived from thumb phalanges and is associated with the formation of a bony bridge between the tip of the thumb and a radial projection from the distal end of the 1st phalanx of the index finger. When the web between the first 2 fingers is complete, the 2 distal phalanges of the index are hypoplastic and form part of a bony "chain" connecting the tips of the thumb and index finger. The capitate and hamate are fused; other carpals may also be incorporated into the fusion. Clinodactyly of the 5th finger occurs commonly.

The first 2 toes generally consist of 2 phalanges; they are more or less webbed and are associated with a single broad and short metatarsal. One accessory bone which extends laterally from the tip of the "common metatarsal" to the proximal end of the adjacent 1st phalanx is frequently present and may perhaps represent the head of an incompletely formed 2nd metatarsal. Camptodactyly, partial or complete postaxial polydactly, polysyndactyly or syndactyly occur infrequently in other toes. The 2 lateral metatarsals are always fused at their base, and the 3 lateral metatarsals are proximally fused when the "3rd" metatarsal is involved in the synostotic process, or when 1 of the 2 lateral metatarsals is partially duplicated distally. Extensive tarsal fusion never involves the 1st cuneiform bone.

Minor craniofacial anomalies (highly arched palate with or without broad alveolar ridges, highly bridged nose, long and broad uvula) and apparent predisposition to middle ear infection may be manifestations or coincidental findings in the 1 known family. Affected individuals generally obtained lower mean scores on tests of psychometric intelligence, academic achievement and psychomotor and motor proficiency than their unaffected relatives.

Complications
I **Derived:** Inability to use hands properly; difficulties in fitting shoes; at times pain in walking.
II **Associated:** Slightly reduced intelligence?

Etiology: Autosomal dominant mutation with complete penetrance and variable expressivity. McK *10251

Pathogenesis: ?

Related Facts
I **Sex Ratio:** M1:F1
II **Risk of Occurrence:** ?
III **Risk of Recurrence for**
  Patient's Sib: If one parent affected, 50%; if parents and all other relatives are unaffected, presumably negligible.
  Patient's Child: 50%
IV **Age of Detectability:** At birth

V Prevalence: ?

Treatment
I   **Primary Prevention:** Genetic counseling
II   **Secondary Prevention:** —
III **Other Therapy:** —

Prognosis: Functional impairment of hand

Detection of Carrier: —

Special Considerations: —

References:
Grosse, F.R. et al: The *F*-form of acro-pectoro-vertebral dysplasia: The *F*-syndrome. In Bergsma, D. (ed.): Part III. Limb Malformations. Birth Defects: Orig. Art. Ser., vol. V, no.3. White Plains: The National Foundation-March of Dimes, 1969, pp. 48-63.
Trites, R.L. and Matthews, C.G.: Psychological test findings in the *F*-form of acro-pectoro-vertebral dysplasia: The *F*-syndrome. Ibid pp. 64-67.

Contributor: **John M. Opitz**

———————————

Editor's Computerized Descriptors: Oral, Nose, Skel.

ADRENAL HYPOALDOSTERONISM OF INFANCY, TRANSIENT ISOLATED

Includes: Hypoaldostéronisme isolé et transitoire du nourrison Passagerer, isolierter Hypoaldosteronismus des Säuglingsalters Hipoaldosteronismo aislado transitorio de la infancia Transient adrenocortical insufficiency of infancy Delayed biochemical maturation of 18-oxidation

Excludes: Steroid 18-hydroxylase deficiency (905) Steroid 18-hydroxysteroid dehydrogenase deficiency (906) Salt-losing congenital adrenal hyperplasia Adrenal hypoplasia, congenital (24)

Minimal Diagnostic Criteria: Clinical features of aldosterone deficiency confirmed by appropriate studies in plasma or urine. Adrenal secretion of other steroids and response to ACTH must be normal. A deficiency of 18-hydroxylase or 18-OH dehydrogenase cannot be excluded initially but should not persist beyond the early childhood years, to fulfill the criterion of transience.

Clinical Findings: This syndrome is characterized by renal salt-wasting, hyponatremia, hyperkalemia, vomiting, dehydration and failure to thrive in infancy. Urinary excretion of aldosterone is negligible, and does not increase following salt deprivation or the administration of ACTH. However, urinary excretion of 17-ketosteroids and 17-hydroxycorticosteroids is normal and rises significantly following ACTH. The external genitalia are normal in males and females, thereby excluding defects early in steroidogenesis. There is an excellent response to salt-retaining steroids such as deoxycorticosterone (DOC) and supplemental salt. As affected infants grow, the symptoms spontaneously ameliorate, so that therapy may gradually be diminished and may frequently be discontinued in the 2nd year of life. Reinvestigation of an affected infant at age 5 years revealed normal secretion rates of cortisol and aldosterone and an appropriate response to administration of ACTH and salt deprivation. Definitive steroid studies have not been performed; consequently a maturational defect or an enzyme block in the final 2 steps of aldosterone biosynthesis have not been excluded. One report concerned sibs, raising the possibility of an inherited enzyme defect.

Complications
I   **Derived:** These are related to the degree of electrolyte disturbance and dehydration, as described in Clinical Findings; all are avoidable by recognition of the disorder and therapy with supplemental salt and mineralocorticoids.
II   **Associated:** —

Etiology: It is not entirely resolved whether this is a separate entity representing maturational delay in aldosterone biosynthesis, or poorly documented enzyme deficiencies. Since affected sibs have been described, the possibility of an autosomal recessively inherited enzyme defect affecting aldosterone biosynthesis cannot be excluded (see Steroid 18-Hydroxylase Deficiency and Steroid 18-Hydroxysteroid Dehydrogenase Deficiency).

Pathogenesis: In all forms of aldosterone deficiency, there is a tendency for the severity of symptoms and urinary salt-wasting to improve with increasing age. Thus, the transient nature of this disorder of hypoaldosteronism in infancy may represent the amelioration of an inadequately documented enzyme deficiency in aldosterone biosynthesis. Alternatively, the syndrome may represent a true maturational delay in the zona glomerulosa of the adrenal, or a delay in the biochemical maturation of the final 2 enzyme steps of aldosterone biosynthesis, namely 18-hydroxylase and 18-OH-dehydrogenase. Apart from these 2 enzyme deficiencies, affecting aldosterone synthesis only, all other adrenal enzyme deficiencies, and diseases involving the entire adrenal cortex, also affect some steps in glucocorticoid or sex steriod synthesis, a useful point in differential diagnosis.

Related Facts
I **Sex Ratio:** M1:F1
II **Risk of Occurrence:** ?
III **Risk of Recurrence for**
  Patient's Sib: If autosomal recessive 1 in 4 for each offspring to be affected. Otherwise?
  Patient's Child: If autosomal recessive not increased unless mate is carrier or homozygote. Otherwise?
IV **Age of Detectability:** Neonatal period-symptoms and signs ameliorate after the 2nd year and may normalize by the 5th year.
V **Prevalence:** ?

Treatment
I **Primary Prevention:** ?
II **Secondary Prevention:** Recognition of aldosterone deficiency with salt and mineralocorticoid supplementation is essential. Other enzyme deficiencies must be excluded.
III **Other Therapy:** —

Prognosis: Normal for life and intelligence if recognized and treated in the neonatal period. In addition, the transience of the disorder assures an excellent prognosis in later life.

Detection of Carrier: —

Special Considerations: —

References:
Royer, P. et al: Hypoaldosteronisme familiale chronique à début néonatal. Ann. Pediatr. 39:596, 1963.
Russell, A. et al: A reversible salt-wasting syndrome of the newborn and infant. Possible infantile hypoaldosteronism. Arch. Dis. Child. 38:313, 1963.
Visser, H.K.A.: Hypoadrenocorticism. In Gardner, L.I. (ed.): Endocrine and Genetic Diseases of Childhood. Philadelphia: W.B. Saunders, 1969, p. 447.

Contributor: **Mark A. Sperling**

Editor's Computerized Descriptor: GI.

ADRENAL HYPOPLASIA, CONGENITAL

Includes: Hypoplasie congénitale des surrénales
Angeborene Nebennieren-Hypoplasie
Hipoplasia suprarrenal congénita
Congenital adrenal hypoplasia associated with congenital hypoplasia of the pituitary gland
Adrenal hypoplasia, congenital-autosomal recessive form
Adrenal hypoplasia, congenital-X-linked form

Excludes: Addison disease
Adrenocortical unresponsiveness to ACTH
Enzyme defects in adrenal steroid biosynthesis

Minimal Diagnostic Criteria: Clinical and biochemical features of adrenal insufficiency, with low plasma or urinary concentrations of all adrenal steroids and no response to administered ACTH. A family history is helpful in suspecting the diagnosis, particularly when affecting males. Adrenal hemorrhage, calcification or cysts can be excluded by radiologic techniques; definitive diagnosis may require arteriography. Gonadal function and external genitalia are normal.†

Clinical Findings: This is a disorder in which there is hypoplasia or aplasia of the adrenal glands. The clinical features result from the deficiency of glucocorticoids and mineralocorticoids and may include cyanosis, apneic spells, hypoglycemia, vascular collapse, and seizures shortly after birth. Death may occur within 72 hours; electrolyte disturbances consisting of hyponatremia and hyperkalemia may be profound, reflecting the deficiency of mineralocorticoids. However, affected individuals have been known to survive and to present later in infancy or childhood with feeding difficulties, vomiting, growth retardation, hypoglycemia, and melanodermia.†

Laboratory findings reveal low or undetectable plasma concentrations or urinary excretion of cortisol, 17-hydroxycorticosteroids, 17 ketosteroids and aldosterone. In those without pituitary hypoplasia there is no response to stimulation by ACTH, dietary manipulation of sodium, and changes in posture. Pituitary ACTH and growth hormone secretion in response to insulin-induced hypoglycemia were reported to be normal in affected identical twins; the plasma concentration of luteinizing hormone was appropriate for the degree of pubertal development, and plasma thyroid stimulating hormone was normal in these patients. The birth of an affected male had been anticipated; at delivery, cortisol, corticosterone sulfate and aldosterone were low or undetectable in cord blood. Estrone and estradiol concentrations were also low in maternal and cord serum, consistent with the absence of fetal adrenal provision of DHEA sulfate as precursor for these steroids.

Complications
I **Derived:** —
II **Associated:** —

Etiology: Most cases are sporadic but solid evidence exists for autosomal recessive and X-linked recessive forms of inheritance. The basic defect in embryogenesis is unknown. Adrenal hypoplasia associated with pituitary hypoplasia suggests that ACTH may be important in determining fetal adrenal growth. Pituitary hypoplasia has also been described in familial aggregates. McK *30020

Pathogenesis: ? In those cases with pituitary hypoplasia and in the autosomal recessive form the adrenal histology is of the immature adult type with a well-differentiated permanent cortex, and diminished or absent fetal cortex. In contrast, in the X-linked form, the adrenal cortex is disorganized and composed of large cells resembling the cells of the fetal cortex. Occasionally, adrenal tissue has been identified in conjunction with the ovary or testis, or diffusely scattered throughout the retroperitoneum; rarely, no adrenal tissue is found.

Related Facts
I   **Sex Ratio:** M3:F1
II **Risk of Occurrence:** ?
III **Risk of Recurrence for**
    Patient's Sib: 1 in 4 (25%) in autosomal recessive form; 1 in 2 (50%) for males and zero for females in X-linked recessive form. In sporadic cases, these figures should be provided to parents as possible risk figures.
    Patient's Child: ?
IV **Age of Detectability:** May be detected from birth to adult life with the most frequent age of detection birth to 2 years.
V   **Prevalence:** ?

Treatment
I   **Primary Prevention:** Genetic counseling
II **Secondary Prevention:** Prompt recognition of adrenal insufficiency and appropriate replacement with gluco- and mineralocorticoids prevent death and can result in normal growth and development. Lifelong treatment is essential to ensure normal growth and development; surgical or other stress may require additional supplemental steroids to prevent collapse from adrenal insufficiency.
III **Other Therapy:** If associated with pituitary hypoplasia, and pituitary hormone insufficiency is confirmed, replacement with thyroid, growth hormone and sex steroids or chorionic gonadotropin may be indicated.

Prognosis: Excellent if condition is recognized and treated.

Detection of Carrier: —

†**Special Considerations:** A 20-22 desmolase deficiency will mimic all the biochemical features. In that deficiency however, the adrenals are large and lipid laden, and the defect also involves the gonads causing genital ambiguity in males.

References:
Moncriete, M.W. et al: Congenital absence of pituitary gland and adrenal hypoplasia. Arch. Dis. Child. 47:136, 1972.
Pakravan, P. et al: Familial congenital absence of adrenal glands; evaluation of glucocorticoid, mineralocorticoid, and estrogen metabolism in the perinatal period. J. Pediatr. 84:74, 1974.
Rimoin, D.L. and Schimke, R.N.: Genetic Disorders of the Endocrine Gland. St. Louis: C.V. Mosby Co., 1971, p. 219.
Sperling, M.A. et al: Congenital adrenal hypoplasia: An isolated defect of organogenesis. J. Pediatr. 82:444, 1973.
Weiss, L. and Mellinger, R.C.: Congenital adrenal hypoplasia- an X-linked disease. J. Med. Genet. 7:27, 1970.

Contributor: **Mark A. Sperling**

Editor's Computerized Descriptors: Skin, Resp., CV., GI., Nerve

ADRENOCORTICAL UNRESPONSIVENESS TO ACTH, HEREDITARY

Includes: Insensibilité surrénalienne congénitale à l'ACTH
Hereditäre ACTH-Unempfindlichkeit der Nebennierenrinde
Falta de respuesta suprarrenal al ACTH hereditaria
Migeon syndrome
Familial Addison disease
Familial isolated glucocorticoid deficiency

Excludes: Addison disease associated with multiple endocrine deficiency and autoantibodies
Adrenal hypoplasia, congenital (24)
Adrenal hyperplasia, congenital, with enzymatic defect in steroidogenesis

Minimal Diagnostic Criteria: Documented glucocorticoid deficiency unresponsive to ACTH administration with normal serum electrolytes, normal aldosterone secretion as reflected by plasma concentration and urinary excretion, and renal conservation of salt during a low sodium diet. Hypoglycemia and hyperpigmentation are characteristic. Genitalia are appropriate for chromosomal sex.

Clinical Findings: This inherited defect affects 1 of the sites of ACTH action on glucocorticoid biosynthesis. However, mineralocorticoids, produced in the zona glomerulosa, are not affected, suggesting a normal adrenocortical response to angiotensin. Lack of feedback inhibition by cortisol leads to high levels of ACTH. Symptoms and signs are related to severe cortisol deficiency and the MSH-like activity inherent in ACTH, without disturbances in serum electrolytes. Affected individuals commonly present in late infancy or early childhood with lethargy, feeding problems, hyperpigmentation of the skin or gums, and recurrent episodes of hypoglycemia. Seizures of the grand mal or minor motor type may occur during the hypoglycemia episodes and may result in permanent impairment of brain function. Thus, developmental milestones may be delayed, and seizures may continue in the absence of hypoglycemia. Occasionally blood glucose concentration is normal while cerebrospinal fluid glucose concentration is clearly in the hypoglycemic range. Despite glucocorticoid deficiency, growth and weight gain are frequently normal or supranormal and bone age is appropriate for chronologic age. Pulse, blood pressure, and degree of hydration remain normal. If unrecognized and untreated, sudden death can occur during periods of stress such as infection or surgery; a history of sudden death in 1 or more sibs has been recorded. Laboratory investigation reveals normal serum concentrations of electrolytes. Plasma cortisol concentration and production rate are low or undetectable, while aldosterone, deoxycorticosterone and corticosterone levels and production rates are normal or high. Similarly, urinary excretion of 17-hydroxycorticosteroids, 17 ketosteroids and pregnanetriol is low or undetectable, while aldosterone excretion is normal or high. Endogenous plasma ACTH concentration is strikingly elevated and there is no response in plasma or urinary cortisol, 17-OHCS, and 17-KS to acute or prolonged administration of ACTH in pharmacologic doses. In contrast, aldosterone levels and secretions rise promptly, and renal conservation of sodium is demonstrable following the institution of a salt restricted diet. Antibodies to adrenal tissue are not present in affected patients.

Complications
I   **Derived:** Hypoglycemic seizures may lead to permanent impairment of brain function, resulting in persistence of seizure activity or psychomotor retardation.

II Associated: —

Etiology: The syndrome is inherited in an autosomal recessive or X-linked recessive manner.† McK *20220

Pathogenesis: The adrenal glands are usually small, and histologically show marked atrophy of the adrenal cortex but relative sparing of the zona glomerulosa. The high endogenous ACTH concentration and lack of response to administered ACTH, with normal mineralocorticoid production by the zona glomerulosa clearly implicate unresponsiveness of the zona fasciculata and reticularis to the action of ACTH. The mechanism of action of ACTH has been reviewed recently; it involves attachment of ACTH to a specific cell membrane receptor, activation of cyclic 3'5'-adenosine monophosphate (cAMP) and a subsequent series of intracellular events. Theoretically, a defect in any of these sites is possible; however in vitro incubation of adrenal slices from an affected individual in the presence of added cAMP produced no change in cortisol production but did increase corticosterone synthesis. Thus, in this instance the defect in cortisol synthesis resided in steps beyond the membrane activation of cAMP. Investigation of parents and sibs suggests potential for recognizing the heterozygote by virtue of low normal plasma cortisol and subnormal cortisol response following ACTH.

Glucocorticoid deficiency is responsible for the hypoglycemia by virtue of cortisol's effect on gluconeogenesis.

Related Facts
I **Sex Ratio:** Males predominate because of the X-linked form
II **Risk of Occurrence:** ?
III **Risk of Recurrence for**
  Patient's Sib: When autosomal recessive or X-linked recessive, see Table I AR or X-linked R, respectively.
  Patient's Child: When autosomal recessive or X-linked recessive, see Table I AR or X-linked R, respectively.
IV **Age of Detectability:** Birth to adult life with most frequent presentation from 6 months to 5 years of age.
V **Prevalence:** ?

Treatment
I **Primary Prevention:** Once an index case is identified parents can be informed of risk factors. Intrauterine diagnosis is not currently feasible.
II **Secondary Prevention:** Replacement with cortisol 15 mg/M^2/day results in disappearance of hypoglycemia and reduction of pigmentation. Salt and mineralocorticoid replacement are not required.
III **Other Therapy:** —

Prognosis: The prognosis is excellent if treated with glucocorticoids before permanent CNS sequelae arise from hypoglycemia.

Detection of Carrier: Potentially feasible by ascertaining plasma cortisol and response to ACTH as reported.

†Special Considerations: In the deceased sib of 1 well-documented case of adrenocortical unresponsiveness to ACTH, where enzyme deficiency early in adrenal steroid biosynthesis was excluded, the adrenals were large, hyperplastic and lipid-laden. Thus, there is heterogeneity in this syndrome with regard to the effects of ACTH on steroidogenesis and adrenal growth-promoting activity. Further evidence for heterogeneity comes from genetic analyses of affected pedigrees, suggesting that the inheritance of the disorder may be either autosomal recessive or X-linked recessive.

References:
Franks, R.C. and Nance, W.E.: Hereditary adrenocortical unresponsiveness to ACTH. Pediatrics 45:43, 1970.
Gill, G.M.: Mechanism of ACTH action. Metabolism 21:571, 1972.
Kelch, R.P. et al: Hereditary adrenocortical unresponsiveness to adrenocorticotropic hormone. J. Pediatr. 81:726, 1972.
Migeon, C.J. et al: The syndrome of congenital adrenocortical unresponsiveness to ACTH: Report of six cases. Pediatr. Res. 2:501, 1968.

Contributor: **Mark A. Sperling**

Editor's Computerized Descriptors: Oral, Skin, Skel., GI., GU., Nerve

ADRENOCORTICOTROPIC HORMONE DEFICIENCY, ISOLATED

Includes: Déficit isolé en hormone adrénocorticotrope
Isolierter ACTH-Mangel
Deficiencia aislada de hormona adrenocorticotrópica

Excludes: Panhypopituitary dwarfism, familial
Adrenal hypoplasia, congenital (24)
Adrenal hyperplasia, congenital
Adrenocortical unresponsiveness to ACTH

Minimal Diagnostic Criteria: Evidence of ACTH deficiency, ie low serum cortisol and urinary 17-hydroxy steroids confirmed by abnormal metapyrone test with otherwise normal pituitary function. Undetectable plasma ACTH.

Clinical Findings: Clinical features of isolated adrenocorticotropic hormone (ACTH) deficiency are those of adrenal insufficiency with weight loss, anorexia, weakness, nausea and vomiting and hypotension. Hypoglycemia, hyponatremia and hyperkalemia often occur. Although males have a normal hair pattern, females have very little pubic or axillary hair. Skin pigmentation is usually decreased but may be normal or increased. Except for 2 children, all reported cases have been diagnosed in adulthood. Specific endocrine abnormalities include a low circulating cortisol concentration, low urinary 17-hydroxy- and 17-ketosteroids, lack of normal response to metapyrone and undetectable circulating levels of ACTH.

Complications
I   **Derived:** See Clinical Findings
II **Associated:** —

Etiology: All cases appear to be sporadic.

Pathogenesis: Defects in the hypothalamic-pituitary axis have been postulated.

Related Facts
I   **Sex Ratio:** M1:F1
II   **Risk of Occurrence:** Very low
III **Risk of Recurrence for**
     Patient's Sib: Negligible
     Patient's Child: Negligible
IV   **Age of Detectability:** Usually not suspected until adulthood but may be diagnosed biochemically in infancy.
V   **Prevalence:** —

Treatment
I   **Primary Prevention:** —
II   **Secondary Prevention:** Replacement with either cortisone or synthetic ACTH. Although the former is more convenient, it is less physiologic than the latter.
III **Other Therapy:** —

Prognosis: Probably normal life with therapy.

Detection of Carrier: —

Special Considerations: —

References:
Hung, W. and Migeon, C.J.: Hypoglycemia in a two year old boy with adrenalcortiocotropic hormone (ACTH) deficiency (probably isolated) and adrenal medullary unresponsiveness to insulin-induced hypoglycemia. J. Clin. Endocrinol. Metab. 28:146, 1968.
Odell, W.D.: Isolated deficiencies of anterior pituitary hormones. JAMA 197:1006, 1966.
Rimoin, D.L. and Schimke, R.N.: Genetic Disorders of the Endocrine Gland. St. Louis:C.V. Mosby, 1971, p. 11.

Contributors: **William A. Horton**
                   David L. Rimoin

AGAMMAGLOBULINEMIA, X-LINKED INFANTILE

Includes: Agammaglobulinémie liée au sexe
Geschlechtsgebundene Agammaglobulinämie
Agamaglobulinemia ligada al sexo
Bruton agammaglobulinemia
Congenital agammaglobulinemia

Excludes: Immunodeficiency, common variable (521)
Immunodeficiency, X-linked severe combined (524)
Thymoma and agammaglobulinemia syndrome (944)
Deficiencies not involving all classes of immunoglobulins
Immunoglobulin A deficiency (525)
Secondary immunoglobulin deficiency

Minimal Diagnostic Criteria: Boys with absent or severely diminished peripheral and intestinal lymphoid tissue, as demonstrable for instance by absence of tonsils and adenoids. Histologically, plasma cells and germinal centers of lymphoid tissue are absent with or without antigenic stimulation. B lymphocytes are absent. Absent or very diminished Ig and antibody response to administered antigens. Frequency and severity of bacterial infections starting toward the end of the 1st half year of life, involving respiratory tract and sinuses, GI tract and skin.†

Clinical Findings: Age of onset of manifestations usually between 3-6 months, boys with repeated bouts of purulent conjunctivitis, otitis media, recurrent upper respiratory infections and bronchitis as well as skin infections. Early sinusitis is frequent, pneumonias begin during the 1st year of life and often lead to bronchiectasis. Recurrent episodes of septicemia are added, and meningitis attacks may be seen repeatedly. There is a propensity to contract infectious hepatitis which not infrequently becomes a fatal disease in these patients. Varicella is the other virus disease known to be more severe in these children both by recurrence and occasional accompanying pneumonia. Tonsillar and adenoid tissues are absent. Xrays reveal clouding of the sinuses with evident infection, obliteration and destruction of the mastoid air cells, minimal hilar shadows, pulmonary infiltrates, segmental atelectasis and areas of bronchiectasis, wasting of the tissues and gaseous distention of the abdomen. Laboratory findings reveal diminished immunoglobulins (Ig), less than 100 mg%, IgM and IgA absent, IgG normal at birth, drops to less than 100 mg% in first 6 months. The peripheral blood picture is normal, but sometimes there is periodic neutropenia, transient eosinophilia or monocytosis. B lymphocytes are absent from the blood and lymphoid tissues. The bone marrow reveals absence or severe paucity of plasma cells. Bacteriologic investigation of infections demonstrates recurrently: diplococcus pneumonias, hemophilus infl., meningococcus, streptococcus, and after antibiotic therapy, usually pseudomonas, ASOT remains negative in spite of documented streptococcal infections. Isoagglutinins are absent, and there is failure to respond to injected antigens such as DPT immunization with production of antibodies.

Complications
I   **Derived:** Stunting of growth, wasting, clubbing of the fingers and toes, erythema nodosum, potbelly, septicemias, bronchiectasis, pulmonary fibrosis and cor pulmonale, cholesteatoma, conductive hearing loss, anemia, diarrhea, hypocalcemia, protein-losing enteropathy, ulcerative colitis and regional enteritis.
II **Associated:** Arthritis of rheumatoid type in 20-40%, later a dermatomyositis-like illness, agranulocytosis, thrombocytopenia, autoimmune diseases, malabsorption, amyloidosis.

Etiology: Genetically determined defect in immunoglobulin synthesis or of B-lymphocyte differentiation inherited in an X-linked recessive manner. McK *30030

Pathogenesis: The inability to muster a humoral antibody response to pyogenic organisms which surround the infant leads to severe infections as soon as the maternal complement of immunoglobulins to newborn is exhausted. Pneumococcus, H. influenzae, meningococcus, and streptococcus are the most successful invaders under these conditions, spreading from the natural portals of entry inward without effective host resistance. Thus recurrent and later chronic sinopulmonary disease is the outstanding clinical event, together with pyoderma, purulent conjunctivitis and purulent otitis media. Further uncontrolled spread and dissemination are manifested by septicemias, meningitis, deep abscesses, osteomyelitis and other parenchymatous pyogenic involvement. Progressive pulmonary impairment with bronchiectasis, fibrosis and eventual right heart overload from increasing pulmonary vascular resistance are later sequelae. Intestinal involvement with diarrhea bouts, protein-losing enteropathy and development of regional enteritis and ulcerative colitis are probably consequences of the absence of plasma cells and lymphoid tissue aggregates normally responsible for host resistance in this area. The susceptibility to severe infectious hepatitis and recurrent varicella indicates that B-cell function or antibodies are involved in defense against these organisms. Long-range effects of the chronic infectious processes are physical underdevelopment, amyloidosis and possible CNS damage. Survival beyond early childhood with his underlying deficiency makes this patient susceptible to rheumatoid arthritis, dermatomyositis-like illness and autoimmune disease. The pathogenesis of these complications is not understood but their occurrence in this pure antibody deficiency state indicates that cell-mediated immunity attributed to T lymphocytes can be responsible for some of the manifestations of autoimmune disease.

Related Facts
I   **Sex Ratio:**   M1:F0
II   **Risk of Occurrence:**   ?
III **Risk of Recurrence for**
   Patient's Sib: If mother is a carrier, 1 in 2 (50%) for each brother to be affected and 1 in 2 for each sister to be a carrier.
   Patient's Child: 1 in 1 (100%) for carrier daughters; not increased for sons unless wife is a carrier; (few patients have reached adulthood).
IV   **Age of Detectability:**   Neonatal period with study of blood lymphocytes, bone marrow or lymph node cells.
V   **Prevalence:**   Rare

Treatment
I   **Primary Prevention:**   Genetic counseling
II   **Secondary Prevention:**   IM immunoglobulin injection, 0.6 cc/kg/month, or 0.3 cc/kg/2 weeks, or plasma from hepatitis-free donors, or papain digest or disaggregated products of immunoglobulin, avoidance of exposure to infections, regular follow-up.
III **Other Therapy:**   Vigorous antibiotic therapy at earliest signs of infection.

Prognosis: Progressive sinopulmonary disease is still a major problem. Untreated cases rarely survive infancy or early childhood. With good medical attention and preventive immunoglobulin therapy, outlook is fair. Long-range survivors are now reaching adulthood.

Detection of Carrier: Not yet possible by laboratory testing.

†Special Considerations: This defect has many clinical and laboratory features in common with common variable immunodeficiency. However, the clear-cut defect in the humoral antibody producing capacity without any thymic-mediated involvement makes it possible to distinguish clinically with the help of laboratory evidence. Lymphoreticular malignancy may be increased although carcinoma and sarcoma are not known to be increased, an important prognostic consideration.

References:
Good, R.A. et al: Consideration of some questions asked by patients with an attempt at classification. In Bergsma, D. and Good, R.A. (eds.): Immunologic Deficiency Diseases in Man. Birth Defects: Orig. Art. Ser., vol. IV, no. 1. White Plains: The National Foundation - March of Dimes, 1968, p. 17.
Rosen, F. S. and Janeway, C. A.: Diagnosis and treatment of antibody deficiency syndromes. Postgrad. Med. 43:188, 1968.
Seligmann, M. et al: A proposed classification of primary immunologic deficiencies. (Editorial) Am. J. Med. 45:817, 1968.

Contributor: **Robert A. Good**

Editor's Computerized Descriptors: Eye, Hearing, Nasoph., Skin, Nails, Skel., Resp., GI, Liver, Nerve

AGNATHIA, MICROSTOMIA AND SYNOTIA

Includes: Agnathie, microstomie et synotie
Agnathie, Mikrostomie und Synotie
Agnatia, microstomia y sinotía
Otocephaly
Synotia, agnathia and microstomia
Microstomia, agnathia and synotia

Excludes: Hypognathic cyclopism
Micrognathia and limb anomalies
Hanhart syndrome (451)
Cleft palate (180)
Glossoptosis
Micrognathia (Marker)

Minimal Diagnostic Criteria: Agnathia, extremely low-set or fused ears, and microstomia

Clinical Findings: Agnathia (although anatomic dissection usually reveals a small fragment of mandibular bone in the midline); extremely low-set ears which are sometimes fused in the midline; there may be fusions of the auditory canals, tympanic cavities, and mallei; microstomia or astomia; oral cavity is usually a cul-de-sac with no pharyngeal connection; small, posteriorly positioned tongue; tongue and hyoid bone may be absent in some cases; deformities of the auditory ossicles, temporal bone, palate, maxilla, and sphenoid may occur; associated anomalies may include transposition of the viscera, congenital heart defects, and anomalies of the limbs.

Complications
I   Derived: —
II   Associated: †

Etiology: ?

Pathogenesis: Branchial arch embryopathy with developmental field effects†

Related Facts
I   **Sex Ratio:**   ?
II   **Risk of Occurrence:**   ?
III   **Risk of Recurrence for**
     Patient's Sib: ?
     Patient's Child: ?
IV   **Age of Detectability:**   At birth by clinical evaluation
V   **Prevalence:**   Very rare

Treatment
I   **Primary Prevention:**   —
II   **Secondary Prevention:**   —
III   **Other Therapy:**   Condition incompatible with life

Prognosis: Very poor

Detection of Carrier: —

†**Special Considerations:** Since extracephalic anomalies such as transposition of the viscera may occur, this disorder is probably more dysmorphogenetically complex than a simple isolated branchial arch embryopathy. In all cases, careful genetic and prenatal history, autopsy, and complete anatomic dissection should be carried out.

References:
Ballantyne, J.W.: Manual of Antenatal Pathology and Hygiene. Edinburgh: William Green and Sons, 1904, p. 428.
Johnson, W.W. and Cook, J.B., 3rd: Agnathia associated with pharyngeal isthmus atresia and hydramnios. Arch. Pediatr. 78:211, 1961.

Contributor: **M. Michael Cohen, Jr.**

AGONADIA

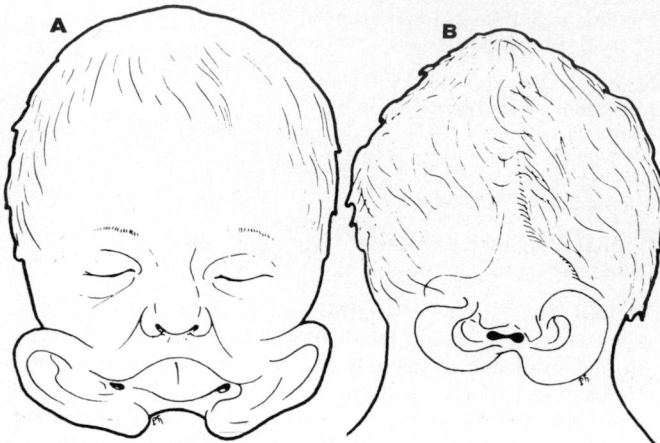

126. Otocephaly: A) Moderate; B) marked

Includes: Agonadie
Gonadenaplasie
Gonadal agenesis
True agonadism

Excludes: Gonodal dysgenesis, XY type (437)
Anorchia (68)†
Chromosome 45,X/46,XY mosaicism (173)
All other forms of male pseudohermaphroditism

Minimal Diagnostic Criteria: Surgically verified absence of gonads in a 46,XY individual with abnormal external genitalia and absence of all but rudimentary müllerian or wolffian derivatives.

Clinical Findings: Individuals with agonadia have abnormal external genitalia, rudimentary müllerian and wolffian derivatives, and no detectable gonads. Mental retardation may coexist with craniofacial, vertebral, and dermatoglyphic anomalies. External genitalia usually consist of a small phallus about the size of a clitoris, underdeveloped labia majora, and sometimes nearly complete fusion of the labioscrotal folds. The sex of rearing is usually female. By definition, no gonadal tissue is present. Sex steroid secretion is thus decreased, and gonadotropin secretion is increased. Although neither normal müllerian nor normal wolffian derivatives are present, structures resembling a rudimentary fallopian tube, an epioophoron, or an epididymis may be present along the lateral pelvic wall. Affected individuals are usually ascertained at birth because of genital ambiguity, but some were ascertained only after secondary sexual development failed to occur at puberty.

Complications
I **Derived:** Lack of secondary sexual development; infertility.
II **Associated:** Vertebral anomalies, craniofacial anomalies, and possibly mental retardation.

Etiology: ? In 1 and possibly 2 kindreds multiple sibs were affected, suggesting autosomal recessive inheritance.

Pathogenesis: Any explanation for agonadia must account not only for the absence of gonads, but also for abnormal genital development and lack of normal internal ductal derivatives. The fetal testes might have functioned long enough to inhibit müllerian development, yet not sufficiently long to produce genital virilization. Teratogenic factors or defective connective tissue could also play roles.

Related Facts
I **Sex Ratio:** M1:F0†
II **Risk of Occurrence:** ?
III **Risk of Recurrence for**
Patient's Sib: ? possibly as high as 1 in 4 for 46,XY sibs and 1 in 8 for all sibs.†
Patient's Child: All patients are infertile.
IV **Age of Detectability:** Usually at birth because of genital ambiguity, but sometimes not until puberty.
V **Prevalence:** ? But rare; about 15 cases have been reported.

Treatment
I **Primary Prevention:** Genetic counseling
II **Secondary Prevention:** Hormone replacement. Surgical creation of vagina. Detection and treatment of craniofacial and vertebral abnormalities.
III **Other Therapy:** —

Prognosis: Normal life span provided associated somatic abnormalities are not serious.

Detection of Carrier: —

†Special Considerations: This condition should be distinguished from anorchia, a condition in which gonads are also absent but well-differentiated male external genitalia are present. In addition, at least two 46,XX individuals have shown features of agonadism.

References:
Duck, S.C. et al: Pseudohermaphroditism with testes and a 46,XX karyotype. J. Pediatr. 87:58, 1975.
Parks, G.A. et al: "True agonadism": A misnomer? J. Pediatr. 84:375, 1975.
Sarto, G.E. and Opitz, J.M.: The XY gonadal agenesis syndrome. J. Med. Genet. 10:288, 1973.
Simpson, J.L.: Disorders of Sexual Differentiation: Etiology and Clinical Delineation. New York: Academic Press, 1976.

Contributor: **Joe Leigh Simpson**

Editor's Computerized Descriptors: Face, Dermatoglyphic, Skel., GU., Nerve

ALBINISM-CUTANEOUS AND DEAFNESS

Includes: Albinisme avec surdi-mutité
Albinismus mit Schwerhörigkeit
Albinismo cutáneo y sordomudez
Albinism, cutaneous and deaf-mutism
Deaf-mutism and cutaneous albinism

Excludes: Waardenburg syndrome (997)
Total albinism with deafness
Piebaldness with deafness

Minimal Diagnostic Criteria: ?

Clinical Findings: Sensorineural deafness, areas of hypomelanosis and hypermelanosis of skin in a symmetric distribution. Pigmentation of genital and scrotal regions. Scalp hair - white sometimes with patches of pigmentation. Few show heterochromia of iris.

Complications
I   Derived: —
II Associated: —

Etiology: X-linked inheritance. A 6-generation Sephardic Jewish family was reported. McK *30070

Pathogenesis: An unknown disturbance of melanocyte migration to skin and ear

Related Facts
I   Sex Ratio: M1:F0
II Risk of Occurrence: Very rare
III Risk of Recurrence for
  Patient's Sib: If mother is a carrier, 1 in 2 (50%) for each brother to be affected and 1 in 2 for each sister to be a carrier
  Patient's Child: 1 in 1 (100%) for carrier daughters; not increased for sons unless wife is a carrier
IV Age of Detectability: Neonatal period
V   Prevalence: Rare. But many may be misdiagnosed as Waardenburg syndrome or unusual piebaldness with deafness.

Treatment
I   Primary Prevention: Genetic counseling
II Secondary Prevention: Hearing aid and special training
III Other Therapy: —

Prognosis: —

Detection of Carrier: —

Special Considerations: —

References:
Margolis, E.: A new hereditary syndrome—sex linked deaf-mutism associated with total albinism. Acta Genet. (Basel) 12:12, 1962.
Reed, W.B. et al: Pigmentary disorders in association with congenital deafness. Arch. Dermatol. 95:176, 1967.
Ziprkowski, L. et al: Partial albinism and deaf-mutism due to a recessive sex-linked gene. Arch. Dermatol. 86:530, 1962.

Contributor: **William B. Reed‡**

Editor's Computerized Descriptors: Eye, Hearing, Skin, Hair, GU.

ALBINISM-CUTANEOUS WITHOUT DEAFNESS

Includes: Albinisme cutané sans surdité
Albinismus ohne Schwerhörigkeit
Albinismo cutáneo sin sordera
Piebaldness
Piebaldism with white forelock
White forelock without deafness
Piebalds
Cutaneous albinism without deafness

Excludes: Waardenburg syndrome (997)
Isolated heterochromia
Vitiligo (993)

Minimal Diagnostic Criteria: Albinism restricted to the ventral portions of the body, normal pigmentation of the middorsal surfaces of the back and neck, present since birth.†

Clinical Findings: Absence of skin pigmentation primarily on the ventral surfaces of the body. This includes such characteristics as a frontal blaze of white hair (white forelock), absence of pigmentation of the central portion of the forehead, the medial portion of the eyebrows and portions of the nose and chin, and to a variable degree the ventral portion of the chest, abdomen and ventral surfaces of arms and legs. The wrists, hands, ankles and feet are often fully pigmented. The occiput, back of the neck, and middorsal surface of the trunk are fully pigmented. Islands of pigmentation may occur within the nonpigmented areas. The borders between normally pigmented and unpigmented skin are usually hyperpigmented. Heterochromia is occasionally present.

Complications
I **Derived:** —
II **Associated:** —

Etiology: Autosomal dominant with full penetrance; McK *17280

Pathogenesis: Electron microscopy of the affected skin shows an absence of melanoblasts but presence of Langerhans cells. The defect could be explained by incomplete migration of melanoblasts to the ventral midline or by a defect in differentiation of ventral melanoblasts. The relationship between Langerhans cells and melanoblasts, the similarity in the electron microscopic picture with that of acquired vitiligo, and transplantation studies of piebald spotting in mice all suggest that an inherited defect in melanoblast differentiation is the most likely cause.

Related Facts
I   **Sex Ratio:** M1:F1
II **Risk of Occurrence:** Rare
III **Risk of Recurrence for**
    Patient's Sib: If parent is affected, 1 in 2 (50%) for each offspring to be affected; otherwise not increased.
    Patient's Child: 1 in 2
IV **Age of Detectability:** At birth
V   **Prevalence:** ?

Treatment
I   **Primary Prevention:** Genetic counseling
II **Secondary Prevention:** For cosmetic problem, hair dye and skin cosmetics may be used.
III **Other Therapy:** —

Prognosis: Normal life span. There is no associated mortality or morbidity.

Detection of Carrier: —

†**Special Considerations:** It is most likely to be confused with Waardenburg syndrome in which a white forelock with occasional depigmentation of the medial portions of the eyebrows and heterochromia iridum are also common.

References:
Comings, D.E. and Odland, G.F.: Partial albinism. JAMA 195:519, 1966.
Cooke, J.V.: Familial white skin spotting (piebaldness) ("partial albinism") with white forelock. J. Pediatr. 41:1, 1952.

Contributor: **David E. Comings**

Editor's Computerized Descriptors: Eye, Skin, Hair

ALBINISM-OCULAR

Includes: Albinisme oculaire
Okulärer Albinismus
Albinismo ocular
Ocular albinism

Excludes: Generalized albinism
Oculocutaneous albinism
Chédiak-Higashi syndrome (143)
Waardenburg syndrome (997)

Minimal Diagnostic Criteria: Deficiency of uveal pigmentation with photophobia, nystagmus, and decreased vision in males and variable coarse mottling and stippled appearance of ocular fundus in female carriers.

Clinical Findings: Photophobia, nystagmus, and decreased vision are usually present in males. The degree of pigmentation present is variable. In infants the iris is light grey and in adults blue-grey and translucent. A red pupil glow may be present. The fundus is bright red-orange with prominent vessels and the macula is pink and often devoid of yellow pigment. Retinal pigment is usually completely absent and uveal pigment variable. In Negroes more pigmentation may be present. Central scotomas and poor visual acuity relate to the degree of pigment left and maldevelopment of the fovea centralis. Laboratory tests are normal.

Complications
I **Derived:** Foveal aplasia, decreased visual acuity, nystagmus, head nod, strabismus, poor pupillary responses
II **Associated:** Partial aniridia, ocular colobomas, astigmatism

Etiology: X-linked recessive; McK *30050

Pathogenesis: For the ocular form less information is available than for generalized albinism. In the latter case melanocytes are present and the defect is metabolic not structural. Serum tyrosine is normal but melanocytes produce less than normal amounts of melanin either due to a deficiency of the enzyme tyrosinase or insufficient amounts of tyrosine locally. A rabbit model of ocular albinism occurs which is autosomal recessive.

Related Facts
I **Sex Ratio:** M1:F0. Rare homozygous females have been reported.
II **Risk of Occurrence:** ?
III **Risk of Recurrence for**
Patient's Sib: If mother is a carrier, 1 in 2 (50%) for each brother to be affected and 1 in 2 for each sister to be a carrier.
Patient's Child: 1 in 1 (100%) for carrier daughters; not increased for sons unless wife is a carrier.
IV **Age of Detectability:** At birth
V **Prevalence:** ?

Treatment
I **Primary Prevention:** Genetic counseling
II **Secondary Prevention:** Colored glasses, artificial pupil, scleral contact lenses and corneal tattooing have been employed.
III **Other Therapy:** —

Prognosis: Normal life span but poor visual prognosis

Detection of Carrier: Although variably affected and usually functionally normal, the female heterozygote has a translucent iris, coarse pigment stippling of the macula and islands of brown pigment clusters alternating with deep depigmentation in the near periphery. In known pedigrees, some carriers can be identified by determination of their Xg status, since this locus is closely linked to that of the ocular albinism locus.

Special Considerations: —

References:
Falls, H. F.: Sex-linked ocular albinism displaying typical fundus

changes in female heterozygote. Am. J. Ophthalmol. 34 (part 2):41, 1951.
Fitzpatrick, T. B. and Quevedo, W. C.: Albinism. In Stanbury, J. B. et al (eds.): The Metabolic Basis of Inherited Disease. New York:McGraw-Hill, 1966. P. 324.
Nance, W.E. et al: Genetic and biochemical evidence for two forms of oculocutaneous albinism in man. In Bergsma, D. (ed.): Part VIII. Eye. Birth Defects: Orig Art. Ser., vol. VII, no. 3. Baltimore: Williams and Wilkins for The National Foundation-March of Dimes, 1971, p. 125.
Waardenburg, P.J. et al: Genetics and Ophthalmology Netherlands:C. C Thomas, 1961, p. 715

Contributor: **Harold E. Cross**

Editor's Computerized Descriptors: Vision, Eye

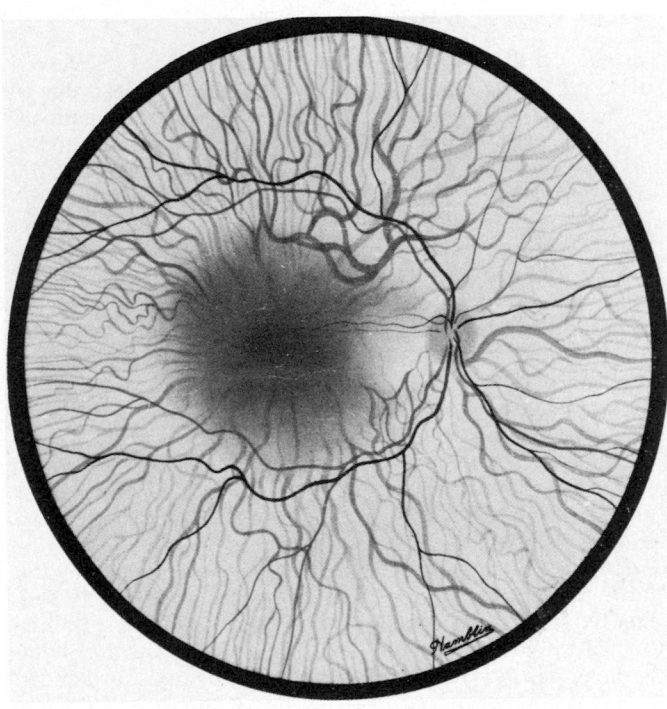

127. Retina in ocular albinism

ALBINISM-OCULOCUTANEOUS, HERMANSKY-PUDLAK TYPE

Includes: Albinisme oculo-cutané, Hermansky-Pudlak type
Albinismus Okulokutaner, Hermansky-Pudlak typ
Albinismo oculocutáneo, Hermansky-Pudlak tipo
Hermansky-Pudlak syndrome
Albinism, hemorrhagic diathesis and pigmented reticuloendo-
thelial cells

Excludes: Chédiak-Higashi syndrome (143)
Albinism-oculocutaneous, tyrosinase-negative (34)
Albinism-oculocutaneous, tyrosinase-positive (35)
Albinism-oculocutaneous, yellow mutant (36)
Other storage pool deficient platelet disorders

Minimal Diagnostic Criteria: A tyrosinase-positive form of
oculocutaneous albinism, abnormal platelet aggregation in an as-
pirin-free patient and presence of yellow UV fluorescing material
in urine sediment or bone marrow.

Clinical Findings: Originally described by Hermansky
and Pudlak as albinism with hemorrhagic diathesis due to
a vascular hemophilia and storage of ceroid in reticuloendothelial cells of lung, liver, bone marrow, lymph nodes,
and bladder. The condition is now known to consist of the
triad of a tyrosinase-positive form of oculocutaneous albinism; storage pool deficient platelets with a marked decrease in dense bodies, adenosine diphosphate and serotonin; and accumulation of a yellow granular substance in
reticuloendothelial cells, circulating macrophages, urine
sediment and oral mucosal cells. Phenotypically, patients
may resemble tyrosinase-negative or tyrosinase-positive
oculocutaneous albinos depending upon the racial and pigmentary background of the parents. Patients have moderate-to-severe photophobia, nystagmus, decreased visual
acuity and about 30% have strabismus. With age, some
pigment accumulates at the limbus and pupillary border
giving a cartwheel effect on transillumination of the
irides.†

Hair color may vary from white to reddish-brown, the
latter in patients from darkly pigmented populations. Pigmented nevi may be frequent. Patients usually give a history of mild-to-moderate bleeding episodes (but fatal hemorrhage has occurred), of bruisability, epistaxis, prolonged
bleeding following tooth extraction or delivery. With few
exceptions, menses have not been unusual. Bleeding time
may be prolonged or fall within the upper limits of normal.
Aspirin markedly prolongs bleeding time, usually over 30
minutes. Chest radiographs of older patients frequently
show diffuse streaking and dense nodular radiopaque areas
due to storage material. Palatal lesions in older patients
are small papules with white centers resembling gouti tophi. The storage material is not ceroid. It is found in bone
marrow, lung, liver, spleen, kidney, bladder, urine sediment, and oral epithelium as a yellow granular pigment
which fluoresces bright yellow under UV light.

Complications
I **Derived:** Death from hemorrhage especially in patients taking aspirin or aspirin-like drugs blocking prostaglandin synthesis following minor surgery such as tooth extraction or
delivery. Several patients have developed a severe fatal colitis, especially after taking proprietary antacid containing
aspirin. Gastric bleeding is frequent following aspirin ingestion; severe sunburn following solar exposure. Degenerative
skin changes, solar keratoses, basal cell and squamous cell
carcinomas occur in patients over 30 years of age following
prolonged solar exposure.
II **Associated:** —

Etiology: Autosomal recessive; McK *20330

Pathogenesis: ? The pleiotropic effect of a gene involving
a metabolic step affecting pigmentation, the platelet storage pool and accumulation of an unidentified storage
material. Ultra microscopic specimens of hairbulbs show
pheomelanosomes with uneven pigmentation but tyrosinase activity in the Golgi. Hairbulbs incubated in 1-tyro-
sine or 1-dopa show increased pigmentation and tyrosinase
assay falls within normal. Platelet rich plasma exposed to
aggregating agents such as collagen and epinephrine show
lack of secondary aggregation on nephalometry, have less
than 1 dense body per 70 platelets (normal 1.4 dense bodies
per platelet), have less than 10% normal levels of ADP and
serotonin, but have a normal prostaglandin endoperoxide
generating system. Serotonin uptake by platelets is initally
normal but is rapidly lost. The storage material is not ceroid, does not increase in urine following ingestion of high
polyunsaturated fat diet and does not have an elemental
analysis compatible with a lipid. Vitamins C and E levels
in serum are normal. Circulating macrophages contain 2
types of inclusions, the yellow granular UV fluorescing
material and a membrane-bound particle with a dense core
and radiating fibular material similar to a "new" pigment
described in a species of tree frogs.

Related Facts
I **Sex Ratio:** Ml:Fl
II **Risk of Occurrence:** ?
III **Risk of Recurrence for**
Patient's Sib: 1 in 4 (25%) for each offspring to be affected
Patient's Child: Not increased unless mate is carrier or
homozygote.
IV **Age of Detectability:** Childhood
V **Prevalence:** Rare. The condition has been reported or ob-
served in over 100 patients. All Puerto Rican albinos but 2
tested to date have this disorder. In Arecebo-Aguadilla area
of Puerto Rico, about 1:2000. Occurs with high frequency in
residents and families who trace ancestry to Appledorn, Holland or Madras, India.

Treatment
I **Primary Prevention:** Genetic counseling
II **Secondary Prevention:** These patients must avoid drugs
that inhibit prostaglandin synthesis: such as aspirin and en-
domethacin. *Fatal bleeding has occurred after use of aspirin.*
Platelet transfusion for surgery. Avoidance of sun exposure,
use of sunscreens and visual aids.
III **Other Therapy:** —

Prognosis: With avoidance of solar exposure and aspirin-like
drugs and treatment of premalignant skin lesions, prognosis is
fair for a normal life span.

Detection of Carrier: Obligate heterozygotes have statistically
significant lower levels of serotonin in platelets. The test is not
reliable, however, for about 40% overlap the lower range of normal.

†Special Considerations: The majority of retinofugal optic neurons that in normals arise in the temporal retina and course to the
same side of the brain as the eye of origin do not do so in these
patients but cross to the opposite side. They tend to have a completely crossed optic neuronal system. They lack the mechanism
for binocular vision and do not benefit from early strabismus
surgery which in pigmented persons preserves a degree of
binocularity of vision.

References:
Hermansky, F. and Pudlak, P.: Albinism associated with hemorrhagic diathesis and unusual pigmented reticular cells in the
bone marrow: Report of two cases with histochemical studies.
Blood 14:162, 1959.
White, J.G. and Witkop, C.J., Jr.: Effects of normal and aspirin
platelets on defective aggregation in the Hermansky-Pudlak syndrome: A test for storage pool deficient platelets. Am. J. Pathol.

68:57, 1972

White, J.G. et al: The Hermansky-Pudlak syndrome: Inclusions in circulating leucocytes. Br. J. Haematol. 24;761, 1973.
Witkop, C.J., Jr. et al: Oculocutaneous albinism. In Nyhan, W.L. (ed.): Heritable Disorders of Amino Acid Metabolism: Patterns of Clinical Expression and Genetic Variation. New York: John Wiley and Sons, 1974, p. 177.
Witkop, C.J., Jr. et al: Albinism. In Stanbury, J.B. et al (eds.): The Metabolic Basis of Inherited Disease. New York: McGraw-Hill, 1978, p. 283.

Contributors: **Carl J. Witkop, Jr.**
James G. White

Editor's Computerized Descriptors: Vision, Eye, Skin, Hair
Also see Section I, Fig. 104

ALBINISM-OCULOCUTANEOUS, TYROSINASE NEGATIVE

Includes: Albinisme oculocutané avec absence de tyrosinase
Tyrosinase-negativer okulo-kutaner Albinismus
Albinismo óculocutaneo tirosinasa negativa
Albinism, tyrosinase negative oculocutaneous
Tyrosinase negative oculocutaneous albinism

Excludes: Albinism-oculocutaneous, tyrosinase positive (35)
Albinism-oculocutaneous, yellow mutant (36)
Gingival fibromatosis, depigmentation and microphthalmia (413)
Albinism-ocular (32)
Albinism-cutaneous without deafness (31)
Chédiak-Higashi syndrome (143)
Albinism-oculocutaneous, Hermansky-Pudlak type (33)

Minimal Diagnostic Criteria: Depigmentation of all of the skin, hair, and eyes with nystagmus, photophobia and a red reflex in a patient whose hairbulbs do not form pigment when incubated in 1-tyrosine solution.

Clinical Findings: Marked depigmentation is found in all of the skin, hair, and eyes with nystagmus, photophobia and a prominent red reflex. There is no visible pigment in these structures, the fundus is unpigmented and the iris diaphanous without a cartwheel effect on transillumination. Iris color is blue to grey-blue in oblique light but may have a pinkish color when viewed in light reflected from the fundus. Hair, skin, and eye color is the same in all racial backgrounds and does not change with age. Hair is dead white but may have a light yellow cast after exposure to sunlight. Skin is pink-red and shows no tanning. A prominent red reflex is present and does not vary with age or race of the subject. Pigmented nevi and freckles are absent. Nystagmus and photophobia are severe. Visual acuity is impaired for both near and far vision usually 20/200 or worse and does not improve with age. Other eye abnormalities occur but their exact frequency in the ty-neg albino must be reevaluated. (See Albinism-Oculocutaneous Tyrosinase Positive.) The macular reflex is usually absent. This phenotype cannot always be distinguished from some Caucasian ty-pos albinos by clinical criteria. Patients lack binocular vision.†

Complications
I **Derived:** Susceptibility to skin cancer, basal cell, squamous cell or basosquamous carcinoma
II **Associated:** Albinos have been reported with a number of anomalies such as cleft palate, pretragal ear pits, deafness, sickle cell trait, and oligophrenia, or have developed malignant melanomas but these traits either segregate separately in kindreds or do not appear in albinos in a frequency greater than chance expectation.

Etiology: Autosomal recessive

Pathogenesis: Absence of the enzyme tyrosinase in melanocytes causing a block in the pathway for melanogenesis at the steps 1-tyrosine→1-dopa→dopaquinone which results in the production of unpigmented premelanosomes (premelanosomes Stage II) but none beyond this stage. Stage II unpigmented premalanosomes are passed to keratinocytes but are not effective in increasing protective pigmentation.

Related Facts
I **Sex Ratio:** M1:F1
II **Risk of Occurrence:** Caucasians 1 in 39,000, American Negroes 1 in 28,000. Not observed to date in American Indians.
III **Risk of Recurrence for**
  Patient's Sib: 1 in 4 (25%) for each offspring to be affected
  Patient's Child: Not increased unless mate is carrier or

homozygote. (Chances 1 in 99 Caucasian, 1 in 84 American Negro)

IV **Age of Detectability:** At birth by physical examination and hairbulb incubation test

V **Prevalence:** 1 in 39,000 Caucasian, 1 in 28,000 American Negro

Treatment

I **Primary Prevention:** Genetic counseling

II **Secondary Prevention:** —

III **Other Therapy:** Avoidance of exposure to sunlight, protective clothing and sun screen lotions. Tinted glasses or contact lenses

Prognosis: Is compatible with long life but longevity is probably reduced somewhat in general due to susceptibility to skin cancer and higher risk for accidents due to poor vision. Many are legally blind with visual acuity 20/200 or worse.

Detection of Carrier: Tyrosinase activity in hairbulbs half or less than half of normal in heterozygote.

†**Special Considerations:** Oculocutaneous albinos of all types have absent or decreased ipsilateral retinogeniculate nerve tracts resulting in absent or decreased binocular vision.

References:

Creel, D. et al: Asymmetric visually evoked potentials in various types of human oculocutaneous albinos: Evidence for anatomic abnormalities of the optic tract. Invest. Ophthalmol. 13:430, 1974.

Guillery, R.W. et al: Abnormal visual pathways in the brain of a human albino. Brain Res. 96:373, 1975.

King, R.A. and Witkop, C.J., Jr.: Detection of heterozygotes for tyrosinase-negative oculocutaneous albinism by hairbulb tyrosinase assay. Am. J. Hum. Genet. 29:164, 1977.

Witkop, C.J., Jr.: Albinism. In Harris, H. and Hirschhorn, K. (eds.): Advances in Human Genetics. New York:Plenum Press, 1971, p. 61.

Witkop, C.J., Jr. et al: Autosomal recessive oculocutaneous albinism in man: Evidence for genetic heterogeneity. Am. J. Hum. Genet. 22:55, 1970.

Witkop, C.J., Jr. et al: Oculocutaneous albinism. In Nyhan, W.L. (ed.): Heritable Disorders of Amino Acid Metabolism: Patterns of Clinical Expression and Genetic Variation. New York:John Wiley & Sons, 1974, p. 177.

Contributor: **Carl J. Witkop, Jr.**

Editor's Computerized Descriptors: Vision, Eye, Skin, Hair
Also see Section I, Fig. 103

ALBINISM-OCULOCUTANEOUS, TYROSINASE POSITIVE

Includes: Albinisme oculocutané avec tyrosinase
Tyrosinase-positiver okulo-kutaner Albinismus
Albinismo óculocutaneo tirosinasa positiva
Albinism, tyrosinase positive oculocutaneous
Tyrosinase positive oculocutaneous albinism

Excludes: Albinism-oculocutaneous, tyrosinase negative (34)
Albinism-oculocutaneous, yellow mutant (36)
Gingival fibromatosis, depigmentation, and microphthalmia (413)
Albinism-ocular (32)
Chédiak-Higashi syndrome (143)
Albinism-cutaneous without deafness (31)
Albinism-oculocutaneous, Hermansky-Pudlak type (33)

Minimal Diagnostic Criteria: Decreased pigment in all of the skin, hair, and eyes with nystagmus and photophobia in a patient whose hairbulbs form pigment when incubated in tyrosine solution.

Clinical Findings: Decreased pigment is found in all of the skin, hair, and eyes in a patient with horizontal nystagmus and photophobia. The amount of visible pigment in this type of albino varies with age and race. The clinical pigment characteristics overlap those of the tyrosinase-negative (ty-neg) albino on the one hand and the yellow mutant and normal lightly pigmented individuals on the other. There is a gradual accumulation of pigment with age so that the patient may give a history of a change in eye color from blue to yellow-hazel or brown, and in hair color from white to cream, tan, yellow-red or light brown. Nystagmus and photophobia are marked but less severe than in the ty-neg type. In all infants a red reflex is easily elicited which is lost in older children from deeply pigmented populations but may be retained in adult Caucasians. Funduscopically the retina of infants, children and adult Caucasians appears to have no pigment, but in older children and adults from deeply pigmented populations appears typically blond. Diaphanous irides are present in all patients and on transillumination, a cartwheel effect may be noted due to pigment at the pupil border and limbus. Visual acuity is decreased usually 20/200 or worse in children but may improve with age so adults may have 20/100 or better. Increased frequency of eye defects are found in this type:

Absent or markedly diminished macular reflex	90%
Mesodermal remnants on anterior suface of iris and posterior suface of corneal	25%
Strabismus, usually esotropia	20%
High-grade myopia	20%
Pigmented nevi and freckles	60%
Absent binocular vision†	100%

Complications

I **Derived:** Susceptibility to skin neoplasia, basal cell, squamous cell and basosquamous carcinomas

II **Associated:** Albinos have been reported with a number of other anomalies such as cleft palate, pretragal ear pits, deafness, sickle cell trait, and oligophrenia, or have developed malignant melanomas. These traits either segregate in kindreds or do not appear in albinos in a frequency greater than chance expectation.

Etiology: Autosomal recessive

Pathogenesis: ? Melanocytes can utilize tyrosine to form normal appearing pigment in vitro. Serum tyrosine levels are normal. Proposed site of block has been in substrate utilization possibly due to a defect in premelanosome membranes or due to an inhibitor.

Related Facts

I **Sex Ratio:** M1:F1

II **Risk of Occurrence:** Caucasian 1 in 40,000, American Negro 1 in 15,000, American Indian varies by tribe from 1 in 85 to 1 in 6500 at birth in southern and southwestern tribes. Nigerians (Ibo) 1 in 1000.

III **Risk of Recurrence for**

   Patient's Sib: 1 in 4 (25%) for each offspring to be affected.

   Patient's Child: Not increased unless mate is carrier or homozygote

IV **Age of Detectability:** At birth to neonatal period by clinical examination and hairbulb incubation test

V **Prevalence:** Same as Risk of Occurrence

Treatment

I **Primary Prevention:** Genetic counseling

II **Secondary Prevention:** —

III **Other Therapy:** Avoidance of exposure to sunlight. Protective skin creams and clothing. Tinted glasses or contact lenses with tinted iris.

Prognosis: Good. Most are legally blind exceeding 20/200 in childhood but may improve with age. Longevity probably somewhat reduced by susceptibility to skin cancer and accidents secondary to poor vision.

Detection of Carrier: ? Obligate carriers as a group do not have a higher frequency of diaphanous irides on transillumination than controls.

†**Special Considerations:** Oculocutaneous albinos of all types have absent or decreased ipsilateral retinogeniculate nerve tracts resulting in absent or decreased binocular vision.

References:

Creel, D. et al: Asymmetric visually evoked potentials in various types of human oculocutaneous albinos: Evidence for anatomic abnormalities of the optic tract. Invest. Ophthalmol. 13:430, 1974.

Guillery, R.W. et al: Abnormal visual pathways in the brain of a human albino. Brain Res. 96:373, 1975.

Witkop, C.J., Jr.: Albinism. In Harris, H. and Hirschhorn, K. (eds.): Advances in Human Genetics. New York:Plenum Press, 1971, p. 61.

Witkop, C.J., Jr. et al: Autosomal recessive oculocutaneous albinism in man: Evidence for genetic heterogeneity. Am. J. Hum. Genet. 22:55, 1970.

Witkop, C.J., Jr. et al: Oculocutaneous albinism. In Nyhan, W.L. (ed.): Heritable Disorders of Amino Acid Metabolism: Patterns of Clinical Expression and Genetic Variation. New York:John Wiley & Sons, 1974, p. 177.

Contributor: **Carl J. Witkop, Jr.**

Editor's Computerized Descriptors: Vision, Eye, Skin, Hair
Also see Section I, Fig. 101

ALBINISM-OCULOCUTANEOUS, YELLOW MUTANT

Includes: Albinisme oculocutanée, mutant jaune
Okulokutaner Albinismus - gelbe mutante
Albinismo óculocutáneo mutante amarillo
Albinism, yellow mutant oculocutaneous
Amish albinism
Yellow mutant oculocutaneous albinism

Excludes: Albinism-oculocutaneous, tyrosinase negative (34)
Albinism-oculocutaneous, tyrosinase positive (35)
Gingival fibromatosis, depigmentation, and microphthalmia (413)
Albinism-ocular (32)
Chédiak-Higashi syndrome (143)
Albinism-cutaneous without deafness (31)
Albinism-oculocutaneous-Hermansky-Pudlak type (33)

Minimal Diagnostic Criteria: Depigmentation of all of the skin, hair and eyes in a patient with nystagmus and photophobia whose hairbulbs contain some pigment but do not increase in pigment upon incubation in 1-tyrosine solution.

Clinical Findings: Depigmentation of all of the skin, hair, and eyes with nystagmus and photophobia. At birth, children have snow-white hair, pink skin, grey-blue translucent irides, a prominent red reflex and a pigment-free fundus. At this time, they have a marked photophobia and nystagmus. During the first few months of life there is a gradual increase in pigment so that by 2 years of age the hair is flaxen yellow to bright yellow-brown often with a red tint. Older children have a mild-to-moderate horizontal or rotary nystagmus, profound retinal depigmentation, and a prominent red reflex. The eye color darkens with age so adults may have dark blue irides. Skin tanning occurs after 2 years of age but is less than that of most normal red-haired individuals. Skin sensitivity to actinic radiation is not a marked feature of this type. Negro children have very light cream-brown hair at birth which rapidly becomes light brown to light reddish brown by 1 year of age. Older children and adults have brown eyes with diaphanous irides, moderate nystagmus and photophobia, and light brown skin. Eye color darkens with age from a yellow or yellow-brown to brown. Visual acuity is markedly defective usually from 20/200 to 20/400. Older children and adults are frequently mistaken for ocular albinos. Absent or markedly decreased binocular vision is found in subjects tested.†

Complications

I **Derived:** ? Probably susceptibility to skin cancer, but not enough subjects have been observed to substantiate this.

II **Associated:** Probably none; 1 of 14 subjects had a ventricular septal defect.

Etiology: Autosomal recessive

Pathogenesis: Essentially unknown. Patients have peripheral melanocytes which appear to be normal in number and distribution. Melanocytes contain numerous round-to-ovoid and also elongated Stage III premelanosomes showing irregular pigmentation of matrix resembling that seen in normal yellow and red hair. Hairbulbs do not form black eumelanin when incubated with various combinations of tyrosine, dopa or copper. When cysteine and tyrosine are added, there is an intensification of yellow color. The block has been suggested to be at or beyond the step dopaquinone →leukodopachrome but evidence is inconclusive.

Related Facts

I **Sex Ratio:** M1:F1

II **Risk of Occurrence:** Unknown, rare, by indirect estimates 1 in 125,000

III **Risk of Recurrence for**

Patient's Sib: 1 in 4 (25%) for each offspring to be affected
Patient's Child: Not increased unless mate is carrier or homozygote
IV **Age of Detectability:**   At birth by physical examination and hairbulb incubation test
V **Prevalence:**   ? By indirect estimates about 1 in 125,000. High frequency among Amish.

Treatment
I **Primary Prevention:**   Genetic counseling
II **Secondary Prevention:**   None
III **Other Therapy:**   Tinted glasses or contact lenses

Prognosis: Essentially unknown; probably slight reduction in longevity. Most patients legally blind, 20/200 or worse.

Detection of Carrier: ? Abnormal iris translucency not found in majority of heterozygotes. Kindreds suggest ym is allelic with ty-neg.

†**Special Considerations:**   Oculocutaneous albinos of all types have absent or decreased ipsilateral retinogeniculate nerve tracts resulting in absent or decreased binocular vision.

References:
Creel, D. et al: Asymmetric visually evoked potentials in various types of human oculocutaneous albinos: Evidence for anatomic abnormalities of the optic tract. Invest. Ophthalmol. 13:430, 1974.
Nance, W.E. et al: Amish albinism: A distinctive autosomal recessive phenotype. Am. J. Hum. Genet. 22:597, 1970.
Witkop, C.J., Jr.: Albinism. In Harris, H. and Hirschhorn, K. (eds.): Advances in Human Genetics. New York:Plenum Press, 1971, p. 61.
Witkop, C.J., Jr. et al: Oculocutaneous albinism. In Nyhan, W.L. (ed.): Heritable Disorders of Amino Acid Metabolism: Patterns of Clinical Expression and Genetic Variation. New York:John Wiley & Sons, 1974, p. 177.

Contributor: **Carl J. Witkop, Jr.**

———————————

Editor's Computerized Descriptors: Vision, Eye, Skin, Hair
Also see Section I, Fig. 102

ALKAPTONURIA

Includes: Alcaptonurie
Alkaptonurie
Alcaptonuria
Ochronosis
Ochronotic arthritis
Homogentisic aciduria

Excludes: Osteoarthritis
Rheumatoid arthritis
Acquired ochronosis from exogenous chemicals or drugs

Minimal Diagnostic Criteria: Homogentisic acid can be documented by paper chromatography; alkalinization of the urine results in the appearance of black pigment.

Clinical Findings: Children and young adults usually have no symptoms. The urine is usually clear when passed but on standing or alkalinization it turns brown or black. Patients may never have recognized this. The urine is also positive for reducing substance and reacts with ferric chloride. With age patients develop pigmentation of the sclerae, cartilages, or other fibrous tissue. The sweat may be dark and the cerumen is often brown or black. There may be widespread dusky pigmentation of the skin, particularly over the cheeks, forehead, axillae and genital regions. The buccal mucosa and nails may be brown. Marked darkening of tissues is seen on exposure to air at surgery. Later the patients develop an arthritis which resembles osteoarthritis roentgenographically but has some inflammatory features resembling rheumatoid arthritis. Some degree of limitation of motion is usually the ultimate result and complete ankylosis is common.

Complications
I **Derived:**   Ruptured intervertebral disk.
II **Associated:**   Cardiovascular disease, prostatitis, renal stones

Etiology: Autosomal recessive enzyme defect; McK*20350

Pathogenesis: Deficiency of hepatic homogentisic acid oxidase

Related Facts
I **Sex Ratio:**   M1:F1
II **Risk of Occurrence:**   ?
III **Risk of Recurrence for**
   Patient's Sib: 1 in 4 (25%) for each offspring to be affected
   Patient's Child: Not increased unless mate is carrier or homozygote
IV **Age of Detectability:**   At birth
V **Prevalence:**   ?

Treatment
I **Primary Prevention:**   Genetic counseling
II **Secondary Prevention:**   —
III **Other Therapy:**   Dependent on arthritic condition

Prognosis: Normal for life span and intelligence but function may be reduced because of arthritis.

Detection of Carrier: ?

Special Considerations: —

References:
Garrod, A.E.: Inborn Errors of Metabolism. London:Oxford University Press, 1923.
Garrod, A.E.: The incidence of alkaptonuria: A study in chemical individuality. Lancet 2:1616, 1902.
LaDu, B.N. et al: The nature of the defect in tyrosine metabolism in alkaptonuria. J. Biol. Chem. 230:251, 1958.

Contributor: **William L. Nyhan**

Editor's Computerized Descriptors: Eye, Oral, Skin, Sweating, Nails, Skel., CV., GU.
Also see Section I, Fig. 71

ALOPECIA AREATA

Includes: Alopécie en aires
Alopecia totalis
Alopecia universalis
Ophiasis

Excludes: Congenital alopecia
Congenital absence of scalp

Minimal Diagnostic Criteria: Presence of circumscribed or extensive areas of complete nonscarring alopecia affecting the scalp, beard, or other hairy skin including eyebrows or eyelashes.

Clinical Findings: Single or multiple, discrete or confluent plaques of asymptomatic, nonscarring alopecia are most commonly seen on the scalp, but hairy skin anywhere may be affected. Occasionally the condition may progress to generalized hairlessness. The majority of cases are mild, however, and normal regrowth usually occurs after a few months, although initial attempts at formation of hair produce fine nonpigmented hairs. Exclamation point hairs are usually seen in variable numbers at the margins of the bald areas. They are distinctive, short, and pigmented, tapering down to atrophic roots. Dystrophic changes in fingernails, usually pitting or longitudinal ridging of the nail plates, are commonly seen. Shedding of the nails rarely occurs.

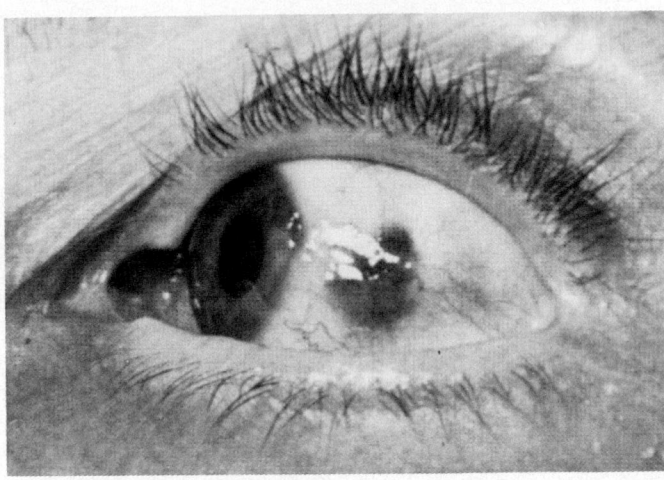

128. Note dark pigmentation of sclera

Complications
I **Derived:** Cataracts rarely have been reported but may be a coincidental finding.
II **Associated:** Vitiligo and thyroid disorders and probably atopic dermatitis.

Etiology: ?

Pathogenesis: Growth of hair is restrained in the growth period (anagen) of the hair cycle, which is characteristic. This can be seen in the shed hairs as tapering, depigmented hair roots. The number of telogen (resting) hairs is also increased, probably as a secondary phenomenon. Characteristic microscopic features are lymphocytic inflammatory infiltration of the connective tissue sheath enveloping affected hair bulbs and atrophic anagen hairs. Lymphocytic involvement, favorable response to corticosteroid therapy, and increased frequency of association with certain conditions suggest that allergic, possibly autoimmune, mechanisms may be at fault.

Related Facts
I **Sex Ratio:** M1:F1
II **Risk of Occurrence:** ?
III **Risk of Recurrence for**
    Patient's Sib: ?† Studies show a familial incidence of approximately 10% for this disorder and of 20% for alopecia totalis.
    Patient's Child: ?†
IV **Age of Detectability:** Anytime after birth but most commonly in the 3rd, 4th, or 5th decades. The average age at onset is 30 years, but 20% of patients are children. Detected by clinical evaluation, which may include gross and microscopic examination of the scalp and hairs.
V **Prevalence:** Estimates in a Swedish population are 1 in 3300 to 1 in 1000.

Treatment
I **Primary Prevention:** —
II **Secondary Prevention:** —
III **Other Therapy:** Systemic corticosteroid therapy frequently will cause regrowth of hair, but the effects are usually temporary. Intralesional injections of triamcinolone acetonide into affected scalp areas may result in regrowth of hair in

stable, limited disease. A wig may aid psychosocial adjustment to the loss of hair.

Prognosis: Normal life span and general health. In mild disease, regrowth of hair usually occurs spontaneously within a few months although recurrences are not uncommon. Progression to alopecia totalis is more common among children or when loss of hair is severe or widespread. Estimates of progression to alopecia totalis vary from 5-30% depending on the selection of cases and length of follow-up. Permanent regrowth of hair after the development of alopecia totalis is infrequent.

Detection of Carrier: —

†Special Considerations: Estimates indicate that the probability of an affected patient having an affected relative is approximately 100 times greater than in the general population. In a few families, however, twins, sibs or consecutive members of 3 generations have been affected. A number of disorders have been related to the onset of alopecia areata, but they are either incidental or nonspecific precipitating factors. These include errors of refraction, foci of infection, psychic trauma and anxiety, physical trauma, or allergic reactions.

References:
Gip, L. et al: Alopecia areata: A follow-up investigation of outpatient material. Acta Derm. Venerol. (Stochk.) 49:180, 1969.
Muller, S. A. and Winkelmann, R. K.: Alopecia areata: An evaluation of 736 patients. Arch. Dermatol. 88:290, 1963.
Van Scott, E. J.: Morphologic changes in pilosebaceous units and anagen hairs in alopecia areata. J. Invest. Dermatol. 31:35, 1958.

Contributor: **Sigfrid A. Muller**

Editor's Computerized Descriptors: Hair, Nails

39
038-500
ALPHA₁-ANTITRYPSIN DEFICIENCY

Includes: Emphysème familial
Familiärer Emphysem
Enfisema familial
Familial emphysema
Familial chronic obstructive lung disease
Prolonged obstructive jaundice
Neonatal hepatitis
Juvenile cirrhosis
Adult liver fibrosis and cirrhosis
Pi phenotype ZZ, SZ, -Z and —

Excludes: Nonfamilial idiopathic chronic pulmonary obstructive disease
Neonatal hepatitis and juvenile cirrhosis of other origin
Other Pi phenotypes with slightly decreased serum content of α_1-antitrypsin (α_1-AT)

Minimal Diagnostic Criteria: Clinical evidence of obstructive lung disease and low α_1-AT concentration of serum. Prolonged obstructive jaundice or cirrhosis and α_1-AT deficiency. Pi-typing necessary to ascertain Pi phenotype.

Clinical Findings: In adult PI ZZ individuals, a severe and characteristic form of obstructive lung disease may develop by the 3rd or 4th decade of life. The presenting symptom is shortness of breath at rest or on minimal exertion. The productive cough of chronic bronchitis is uncommon. Cyanosis is rarely present initially but may become a prominent feature as the disease progresses. This form of chronic obstructive lung disease develops earlier in life than idiopathic emphysema and, in further contrast, has a M1:F1 sex ratio.

Physical examination reveals an asthenic, malnourished-appearing individual, who is dyspneic at rest. There is clinical evidence of generalized overinflation of the lungs and decreased or absent breath sounds at the bases. Respiratory failure or cor pulmonale is a late manifestation of the disease. The chest roentgenogram typically shows generalized overinflation of the lungs with diffuse loss of vascular markings over the lower lung fields. Lung scanning confirms a bilateral decrease in lower zone perfusion.

In symptomatic individuals, pulmonary function studies are generally compatible with obstructive lung disease. In younger homozygotes, pulmonary function may be normal or near normal. Blood gas studies are normal for a long time in the course of the disease. There is rarely CO_2-retention. In individuals heterozygous for the Pi^Z gene slightly decreased lung recoil may be found.

Clinical manifestations of pulmonary disease in children have been observed in phenotype Pi — and is exceptionally rare.

Liver Disease: In children as well as in adults the major abnormality is the presence of deposits, PAS-positive globules, in the hepatocytes. The inclusion bodies contain aggregated α_1-AT and both homozygous and heterozygous individuals for the Pi^Z allele have these inclusion bodies in some of their periportal hepatocytes. The number increases with age. Pi — individuals have no inclusion bodies.

During the 1st year of life, slight liver cell lesion is the most common disorder associated with α_1-AT deficiency, but giant cell neonatal hepatitis may also be present. Prolonged obstructive jaundice with hepatomegaly appears during the 1st year of life in about 10% of the Pi ZZ children. Cholestasis may be marked and biliary atresia suspected. Usually the cholestatic symptoms gradually subside within weeks or a few months. The development of cirrhosis and the appearance of clinical symptoms in these earlier cholestatic children may be noted after a variable time interval. The natural history of the disease in children is not clearly delineated. Children with cholestasis or cirrhosis have the Pi ZZ type. Pi SZ individuals apparently have no clinical liver disease (except in 2 reported cases). In adults, liver studies in patients with emphysema have not shown any sign of clinical liver disease in most cases. Morphologically, however, the pulmonary lesion is regularly associated with portal fibrosis or cirrhosis. Cirrhosis may also be the only manifestation of α_1-AT deficiency. It has been observed in homozygous Pi ZZ individuals.

α_1-AT, a glycoprotein with a molecular weight of about 54,000, is the dominating protease inhibitor of plasma. It is the major component of the α_1-globulin band on serum electrophoresis. The different α_1-AT variants are included in the Pi protease inhibitor system.

The normal mean plasma level for Pi ZZ is 15%, Pi SZ 38%, Pi MZ 58% and the normal Pi MM phenotype 100%. A rare allele with no detectable α_1-AT *Pi* has also been described. The mean normal plasma level is 2.0—2.2 gm/1 and the SD $\pm$ 0.4 gm/1.

Complications
I **Derived:** Respiratory failure, cor pulmonale and heart failure. Cirrhosis, liver failure, bleeding from varices.
II **Associated:** —

Etiology: Autosomal recessive. α_1-AT deficiency is genetically determined by 23 autosomal codominant alleles. The most important Pi alleles have the following production rate of α_1-AT compared to Pi^M 1.0: $Pi^{.}$ 0, Pi^Z 0.15 and Pi^S 0.60.

Pathogenesis: A major biologic function attributed to α_1-AT is the inactivation of proteases released mainly intercellularly during the activity of granulocytes. The lung capillaries serve as a storage place for circulating leukocytes, and some migrate out into the alveoli. With deficient α_1-AT level the endopeptidases have a greater chance to injure the elastin fibers supporting the alveoli. The result is decreased lung recoil. There is no explanation for the development of liver disease.

Related Facts
I **Sex Ratio:** M1:F1
II **Risk of Occurrence:** 1 in 1400 births in Swedish neonates.
III **Risk of Recurrence for**
  Patient's Sib: 1 in 4 (25%) for each offspring to be affected.
  Patient's Child: Not increased unless mate is carrier or homozygote.
IV **Age of Detectability:** A simple screening method for the detection of Pi ZZ individuals at birth is available. Estimation of α_1-AT level and Pi-typing can be accomplished throughout life. Symptoms of liver disease may develop during the 1st months of life while patients generally do not develop symptoms of lung disease before the 3rd or 4th decade.
V **Prevalence:** α_1-AT deficiency Pi ZZ with a level 20% or less of normal occurs in about 0.1-0.05% of the population. Such individuals have about a 10% risk of developing signs of cholestasis and juvenile cirrhosis and about 60-70% risk of chronic obstructive lung disease.

Treatment
I **Primary Prevention:** Genetic counseling
II **Secondary Prevention:** It is recommended that patients with α_1-AT deficiency not smoke, not work in a polluted environment and that pulmonary infection be treated early. These precautions hopefully will modify the progression and severity of the obstructive lung disease. No prevention for the occurrence of liver disease is so far available. Surgery in those with prolonged obstructive jaundice should be avoided.
III **Other Therapy:** Obstructive pulmonary disease and cirrhosis are treated symptomatically.

Prognosis: In the homozygote who develops obstructive lung dis-

ease, the life span is shortened from 10-30 years. Our current hypothesis suggests that early detection of individuals with severe deficiencies (Pi -Z, Pi ZZ and Pi SZ) would benefit from environmental counseling.

Detection of Carrier: —

Special Considerations: —

References:
Berg, N.O. and Eriksson, S.: Liver disease in adults with α_1-antitrypsin deficiency. N. Engl. J. Med. 287:1264, 1972.
Eriksson, S.: Studies in α_1-antitrypsin deficiency. Acta Med. Scand. (Suppl.) 177:1, 1965.
Fagerhol, M.K. and Laurell, C.-B.: The Pi-system of inherited variants of serum α_1-antitrypsin. Prog. Med. Genet. 7:96, 1970.
Laurell, C.-B. and Jeppsson, J.O.: α_1-antitrypsin, α_2-macroglobulin and other α_1-globulins with antiprotease activity. In Putnam, F.W. (ed.): Plasma Proteins, 2nd Ed. New York: Academic Press, 1975.
Laurell, C.-B. and Sveger, T.: Mass-screening of newborn Swedish infants for α_1-antitrypsin deficiency. Am. J. Hum. Gent. 27:213, 1975.
Lieberman, J.: α_1-antitrypsin deficiency. Med. Clin. North Am. 57:691, 1973.
Sharp, H.L. et al: Cirrhosis associated with α_1-antitrypsin deficiency: A previously unrecognized inherited disorder. J. Lab. Clin. Med. 73:934, 1969.
Talamo, R.C. et al: α_1-antitrypsin deficiency: A variant with no detectable α_1-antitrypsin. Science 181:70, 1973.

Contributors: **C.-B. Laurell**
T. Sveger

Editor's Computerized Descriptors: Skel., Resp., CV., Liver

039-500

ALPHA-METHYL-ACETOACETIC ACIDURIA

Includes: Acidurie α-méthyl-acétoacétique
α-Methyl-Acetoacetacidurie
Aciduria α-metil acetoacética
β-Ketothiolase deficiency
α-Methyl-β-hydroxybutyric aciduria

Excludes: Propionic acidemia (826)
Methylmalonic acidemia (658)
Hyperglycinemia, nonketotic (492)

Minimal Diagnostic Criteria: Recurrent episodes of ketoacidosis and vomiting. Increased excretion of α-methylacetoacetic acid and α-methyl-β-hydroxybutyric acid. Normal oxidation of propionate by white cells or fibroblasts but decreased oxidation of isoleucine.

Clinical Findings: The patient described by Hillman and Keating was indistinguishable clinically from patients described with propionic acidemia. This patient presented in early life with episodes of vomiting, ketoacidosis, neutropenia, thrombocytopenia, hyperammonemia, and coma. Serum and urine glycine concentrations were elevated. The patients described by Daum et al presented at 1-4 years of age with episodes of vomiting, ketoacidosis, and coma. Glycine concentrations were not elevated. Some of their patients had histories of feeding difficulties and vomiting early in life. A consanguineous marriage had occurred in 1 of their families. The patient reported by Gompertz et al had had repeated episodes of vomiting and abdominal pain throughout childhood but did not present in coma until age 7 years. Glycine concentrations were elevated in serum and urine. All of the patients described have excreted excess amounts of α-methyl-β-hydroxybutyric acid, α-methylacetoacetic acid, and butanone in their urine. All but one excreted tiglyl glycine. Propionic acid levels in serum when measured were low or normal. Mental retardation occurred in some of the patients, presumably secondary to the episodes of ketoacidosis and coma.

Complications
I **Derived:** Mental retardation and early death.
II **Associated:** Hyperglycinemia and hyperglycinuria.

Etiology: Probably autosomal recessive; McK *20375

Pathogenesis: Probably a defect in the β-ketothiolase reaction which cleaves α-methyl-acetoacetyl CoA to propionyl CoA and acetyl CoA.†

Related Facts
I **Sex Ratio:** M1:F1
II **Risk of Occurrence:** ?
III **Risk of Recurrence for**
    Patient's Sib: Probably 1 in 4 (25%) for each offspring to be affected.
    Patient's Child: Probably not increased unless mate is carrier or homozygote
IV **Age of Detectability:** Birth to several days. Method: quantitative assay of urinary metabolites.
V **Prevalence:** ?

Treatment
I **Primary Prevention:** Genetic counseling
II **Secondary Prevention:** The more mildly affected patients may only require therapy during periods of infection or unexplained ketoacidosis. The more severely affected patients must be treated with a low-protein (0.5-1 gm/kg) diet. These patients are abnormally sensitive to isoleucine, but not to leucine, valine, threonine, or methionine.
III **Other Therapy:** Deletion of protein-containing foods and the use of electrolyte-containing solutions in the presence of ketosis.

Prognosis: One patient died at 1 year of age and 2 have had cardiorespiratory arrests. At least 2 patients suffer from mental retardation. The other reported cases were apparently well except during periods of ketoacidosis or coma. Long-term longitudinal data are not available on any of the patients.

Detection of Carrier: No simple methods are available. Daum reported increased excretion of α-methyl-β-hydroxybutyrate in some presumed heterozygotes.

†Special Considerations: Although the evidence for a defect in the β-ketothiolase reaction is quite strong, a direct definition of the enzymatic defect has not been made. Optimal therapy will vary depending on the severity of the defect.

References:
Daum, R.S. et al: A "new" disorder of isoleucine catabolism. Lancet 2:1289, 1971.
Daum, R.S. et al: An inherited disorder of isoleucine catabolism causing accumulation of α-methylacetoacetate and α-methyl-β-hydroxybutyrate, and intermittent metabolic acidosis. Pediatr. Res. 7:149, 1973.
Gompertz, D. et al: A defect in L-isoleucine metabolism associated with α-methyl-β-hydroxybutyric and α-methylacetoacetic aciduria: Quantitation in vivo and in vitro studies. Clin. Chim. Acta 57:269, 1974.
Hillman, R.E. and Keating, J.P.: Beta-ketothiolase deficiency as a cause of the "ketotic hyperglycinemia" syndrome. Pediatrics 53:221, 1974.

Contributor: **Richard E. Hillman**

Editor's Computerized Descriptors: GI., Nerve

ALSTRÖM SYNDROME

Includes: Syndrome d'Alström
Síndrome de Alström
Alström-Hallgren syndrome

Excludes: Laurence-Moon-Biedl syndrome (578)
Weiss syndrome
Klein syndrome

Minimal Diagnostic Criteria: All 3 cases show marked similarity in the clinical picture. Since the 1st year of life retinal degeneration has been progressive, making school education at the State Institute for the Blind necessary at age 7 years. All 3 have general obesity since infancy without demonstrable underdevelopment of external genitalia during puberty and with normal secondary sex characteristics. Progressive neurosensory hearing loss begins at about 10 years of age and results in clinical deafness during adolescence. Diabetes mellitus first occurs during puberty. Mental development is normal with good intelligence.†

Clinical Findings: The findings included here are based upon 3 reported cases belonging to 2 families - a brother and sister and their second cousin, a male - born within a limited geographic area of isolate character. Clinical findings and symptom development, identical in all 3 cases, include the following: obesity since infancy (3), nystagmus and sensitivity to light since the 1st year of life (3), progressive central and peripheral impairment of vision with insignificant vision remaining at 7 years of age (3), pale papillae and attenuation of retinal vessels, but no pigment changes, increasing atypical small retinal pigmentations observable after puberty (3), no bone corpuscles (3), posterior cataracts of moderate degree (3) and ERG extinguished (3). Hearing was normal at the age of entrance into school; the first signs of neurosensory hearing loss appeared in the next few years (3). After puberty manifest diabetes mellitus was discovered (2) and in the 3rd case the IV glucose tolerance test initially showed only a diabetic curve but the patient later also developed manifest diabetes mellitus.

Mental and intellectual development were normal, as was the neurologic examination. Sexual development was normal (3) but testicular biopsy in one male at 25 years of age showed "germinal cell aplasia with varying degree of tubular sclerosis and slight immaturity" and increased urinary gonadotropins.

Complications
I **Derived:** The female died at age 16, with symptoms of serious kidney defect. At autopsy the kidneys were macroscopically normal, but microscopically heavily fibrous with clear lobular spreading. Within these areas glomerulosclerosis was found along with heavily hyalinized arterioles. Ovaries and endocrine organs were macroscopically and microscopically normal. The brain was macroscopically and microscopically normal. Her brother died at age 32 at home with symptoms of renal disease and diabetes mellitus. No autopsy was performed.

II **Associated:** —

Etiology: This disease probably is the homozygous manifestation of a single recessive autosomal gene mutation which apparently occurred not later than in the 17th century within the isolate area where the 3 probands belonging to 2 families of the same pedigree were born. Four hundred and thirteen ancestors were traced and of the ancestors, 74% were born within the isolate. The mothers of the 2 families are first cousins; the fathers of the 2 families are also related; the parents of the one male are third cousins. McK *20380

Pathogenesis: —

Related Facts

I **Sex Ratio:** M2:F1
II **Risk of Occurrence:** Extremely rare; cases reported are of Swedish derivation
III **Risk of Recurrence for**
Patient's Sib: 1 in 4 (25%) for each sib
Patient's Child: Negligible theoretically in nonconsanguineous marriage, high if marriage is consanguineous and mates are from the Swedish isolate area. No probands have reproduced.
IV **Age of Detectability:** Complete syndrome is developed after puberty. Obesity and impaired vision appear in the 1st year of life.
V **Prevalence:** Rare; for comparison less than 1-2% of the prevalence for heredoretinopathia congenitalis, a recessive autosomal disease (investigated by Alström and Olson at the same period of time), which for the Swedish population had a prevalence of $2.5\text{-}3 \times 10^{-5}$.

Treatment
I **Primary Prevention:** Genetic counseling. (In one family the children born 2nd and 3rd of a sibship of 8 were affected. Their younger second cousin was a single child, his parents desisted from further children after his birth.)
II **Secondary Prevention:** Treatment of diabetes mellitus
III **Other Therapy:** A hearing aid, sign language, finger spelling. (The visual defect would preclude teaching lip-reading or other visual forms of communication.)

Prognosis: For life: In general, life expectancy is shortened, death being due to diabetes mellitus or renal disease. For intelligence: No effect upon intelligence. For function: Blindness and deafness are progressive. Diabetes mellitus may also impair function.

Detection of Carrier: Parents of both proband families are healthy. They had normal hearing, but the mothers of the 2 families showed slight neurosensory hearing impairment with the Bekesy audiogram, one father had a normal audiogram; the other refused investigation. Both parents in one family showed impaired glucose tolerance; the parents belonging to the other family had normal glucose tolerance tests.

†Special Considerations: The diagnosis of the Alström syndrome is necessarily clinical. It is easy to distinguish from the Laurence-Moon-Biedl syndrome because of the absence in the latter of neurosensory deafness and diabetes mellitus; and from the Weiss syndrome because of the absence in the latter of ocular signs. Furthermore the Alström syndrome should not be confused with the Klein syndrome. Klein (1968) reported 2 Swiss brothers, who showed: 1) obesity since infancy, 2) impaired vision and retinal degeneration since the 1st year of life, 3) neurosensory deafness since school age, 4) decreased glucose tolerance, 5) genital hypoplasia with underdevelopment of both external genitalia and secondary sex-characteristics, and increased urinary gonadotropin excretion. These 2 brothers also had glaucoma, acanthosis nigricans, muscular spasticity, pronounced lordosis, kyphosis and scoliosis; intelligence was normal. The clinical picture was identical in the 2 brothers.

References:
Alström, C.H. and Olson, O.: Heredo-retinopathia congenitalis: Monohybrida recessiva autosomalis. A genetical-statistical study. Hereditas 43:1, 1957.
Alström, C.H. et al: Retinal degeneration combined with obesity, diabetes mellitus and neurogenous deafness: A specific syndrome (not hitherto described): Distinct from the Laurence-Moon-Bardet-Biedl syndrome. A clinical, endocrinological and genetic examination based on a large pedigree. Acta Psychiatr. Scand. (Suppl. 34) 129:1, 1959.
Cohen, S. S. and Weiss, E: Dystrophia adiposogenitalis, with atypical retinitis pigmentosa and mental deficiency, possibly of cerebral origin. (Abstract) Trans. Assoc. Am. Physicians 39:356, 1924.
Johnson, J.: Diabetes, neurogenous deafness, and retinal degenera-

tion. Br. Med. J. 2:646, 1961.

Klein,D.: Sur quelques variétés cliniques et génétiques du syndrome de Bardet-Biedl. Rev. Otoneuroophtalmol. 40(3):125, 1968.

Lista, G.A. et al: El sindrome de Alström. Pren. Med. Argent. 59:253, 1972.

Weiss, E.: Cerebral adiposity with nerve deafness, mental deficiency and genital dystrophy: Variant of the Laurence-Biedl syndrome. Am. J. Med. Sci. 183:268, 1932.

Contributor: **C. H. Alström**

Editor's Computerized Descriptors: Vision, Eye, Hearing

AMASTIA

Includes: Amastie

Congenital hereditary absence of breast tissue and nipple either unilateral or bilateral, with no associated endocrine or chromosomal disorder

Excludes: Absence of the breast or breasts associated with X-linked ectodermal dysplasia

Minimal Diagnostic Criteria: Absence of at least 1 mamma with or without musculoskeletal abnormalities.

Clinical Findings: Absence of nipples, unilateral or bilateral, from birth; lack of breast development at puberty or during pregnancy; no abnormality of other secondary sexual characteristics; normal fertility.

Complications
I **Derived:** Lack of lactation
II **Associated:** Unilateral amastia is frequently associated with absence of corresponding pectoral muscles. Nearly 40% of cases of bilateral absence of breasts have multiple congenital anomalies: skeletal anomalies, cleft or high-arched palate, hypertelorism, etc.

Etiology: It has been reported as an autosomal dominant and also as an autosomal recessive trait. When one member of a given pedigree shows bilateral amastia, absence is bilateral in all other members.

Pathogenesis: Absence of breast results from failure of the pectoral portions of the mammary ridges to develop. There is lack of breast enlargement in the affected female at puberty and during pregnancy. No relationship has been described with the use of teratogenic agents.

Related Facts
I   **Sex Ratio:** Nearly M1:F5 has been reported in both unilateral and bilateral cases. However, the very small number of published cases do not allow such a conclusion.
II **Risk of Occurrence:** Extremely rare
III **Risk of Recurrence for**
    Patient's Sib: When autosomal recessive or autosomal dominant, see Table I AR or AD, respectively.
    Patient's Child: When autosomal recessive or autosomal dominant, see Table I AR or AD, respectively.
IV **Age of Detectability:** At birth
V   **Prevalence:** Extremely rare

Treatment
I   **Primary Prevention:** Genetic counseling
II **Secondary Prevention:** —
III **Other Therapy:** Tattooing of the nipples or grafting of the skin from labia minora or scrotum to simulate the nipple. Injection of plastic materials (silastic gel or equivalent) to produce protuberance of the breast in pubertal female.

Prognosis: Normal life span and reproductive fitness.

Detection of Carrier: —

Special Considerations: —

References:
Kowlessar, M. and Orti, E.: Complete breast absence in siblings. Am. J. Dis. Child. 115:91, 1968.

Tawil, H. M. and Najjar, S. S.: Congenital absence of the breasts. J. Pediatr. 73:751, 1968.

Trier, W. C.: Complete breast absence: Case report and review of the literature. Plast. Reconstr. Surg. 36:431, 1965.

Contributors: **Eduardo Orti**
Qutub H. Qazi

Editor's Computerized Descriptor: GU.

AMAUROSIS CONGENITA OF LEBER

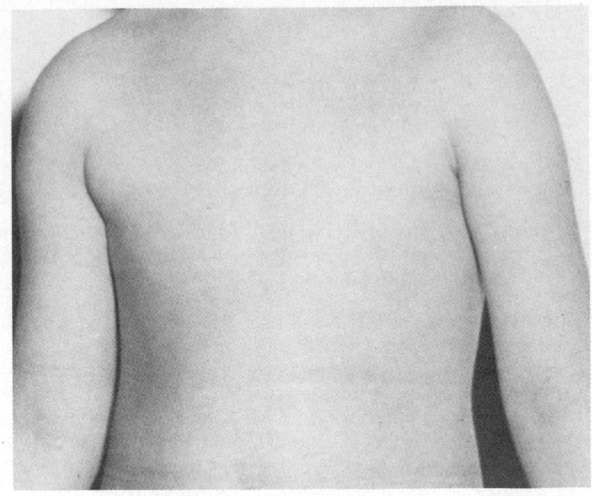

129. Note absence of nipples

Includes: Maladie de Leber
 Lebersche congenitale Atrophie
 Amaurosis congénita de Leber
 Amaurosis congenita of Leber, types I and II
 Congenital amaurosis of retinal origin
 Pigmentary retinitis with congenital amaurosis
 Heredoretinopathy congenitalis monohybrida recessiva autoso-
  malis
 Dysgenesis neuroepithelialis retinae
 Congenital retinal degeneration
 Hereditary retinal aplasia
 Optic atrophy and pigmentary stippling

Excludes: Color blindness, total (198)
 Nightblindness, stationary (719)
 Albinism-ocular (32)
 Retinal degeneration of childhood or adult onset (retinitis pigmen-
  tosa)

Minimal Diagnostic Criteria: A moderately to severely blind
 infant with no or minimal eyeground changes characterized by an
 ERG with either minimal or completely absent responses.

Clinical Findings: The advent of clinical ERG proved that
 diffuse retinal disease can exist without ophthalmoscopic
 evidence as in amaurosis congenita of Leber. Frequently
 signs of poor vision are noted in the 1st few months after
 birth. Occasionally onset occurs after the 1st year of life.
 The initial ocular findings may include minimal or absent
 pupillary reflexes, pendular nystagmus, cataracts, strabismus, and early signs of keratoglobus or keratoconus (although this is usually more evident later in life). The eyegrounds may be normal but frequently minimal and occasionally moderately severe changes are noted. The reported changes include: a loss of foveal light reflexes, pigmentary stippling or salt and pepper-like deposits, particularly in the periphery but sometimes over the entire eyegrounds, typical bone corpuscle-like pigmentation, narrow
 retinal vessels, pale optic nerves, pseudopapillitis and
 choroidal sclerosis. The 2 most common changes are pigmentary stippling and optic atrophy.
  The disease usually progresses but occasionally remains
 stationary. With progression the eyegrounds eventually
 show typical changes of retinitis pigmentosa between 8 and
 14 years of age. The stationary form may remain with only
 minimal or no eyeground changes.†
  Often the infants will be found rubbing their eyes (the
 "oculodigital" sign) perhaps in an attempt to produce
 visual phosphenes. This "gouging" may be marked enough
 to cause enophthalmos.

Complications
I **Derived:** —
II **Associated:** Neurologic findings such as mental retardation,
   epilepsy, hydrocephaly, muscular hypotonia and deaf-mutism.

Etiology: Autosomal recessive transmission with the possibility of
 several different genetic types; McK *20400, *20410

Pathogenesis: Abnormalities of the receptor layer have been
 found, but these have been variable in degree. The descriptions
 include a complete absence of rods and cones, a single layer of cells
 or the presence of normal receptors in the posterior pole with a
 shortening of the structures away from this area. It has been
 difficult to make clinical and pathologic correlations, but it has
 been suggested that the eye evaluated with only minimal receptor
 layer changes represents the stationary form of the disease and
 the other eyes probably represent the more common progressive
 form in various stages.

Related Facts
I   **Sex Ratio:** M1:F1
II **Risk of Occurrence:** 1 in 33,000
III **Risk of Recurrence for**
       Patient's Sib: 1 in 4 (25%) for each offspring to be affected
       Patient's Child: Not increased unless mate is carrier or homozygote.
IV **Age of Detectability:** Usually 1st year of life
V   **Prevalence:** 3 in 100,000. It has been observed in all races.

Treatment
I   **Primary Prevention:** Genetic counseling
II **Secondary Prevention:** Hearing aid, lip and speech reading, manual language for the deafness
III **Other Therapy:** —

Prognosis: Normal life span unless severe associated neurologic abnormality results in early death. Most patients ultimately have severe blindness, but a few patients with the stationary form of the disease retain fairly good acuity, fields and night vision.

Detection of Carrier: —

†Special Considerations: Because of the 2 different courses of patients with amaurosis congenita of Leber, it has been speculated that this category actually includes 2 different diseases. All patients with the diagnosis have a markedly abnormal ERG but Henkes has noted 2 distinct electrooculogram patterns in these children. He suggests that the EOG is normal in those with the stationary condition and abnormal in those with the more common progressive disease. Visual fields are usually markedly abnormal when testing can be done. Dark-adaptation with markedly elevated thresholds have usually been described.

References:

Alström, C.H. and Olson, O.: Heredo-retinopathia congenitalis-monohybrida recessiva autosomalis. Hereditas 43:1, 1957.

Dekeban, A. and Carr, R.: Congenital amaurosis of retinal origin: Frequent association with neurological disorders. Arch. Neurol. 14:294, 1966.

Deutman, A.F.: Rod-cone dystrophy: Primary, hereditary pigmentary retinopathy, retinitis pigmentosa. In Krill, A.E. and Archer, D.B. (eds.): Krill's Hereditary Retinal and Choroidal Diseases. Hagerstown: Harper and Row, 1977, vol. II

Krill, A.E.: Congenital retinal degenerations. In Franceschetti, A. (ed.): Symposium on Surgical and Medical Management of Congenital Anomalies of the Eye. St. Louis: C.V. Mosby Co. , 1968.

Schappert-Kimmijser, J. et al: Amaurosis congenital (Leber). Arch. Ophthalmol. 61:211, 1959.

Tipton, R.E.: Leber's congenital amaurosis and mental retardation. (Case report). In Bergsma, D. (ed.): Part VIII. The Eye. Birth Defects: Orig. Art. Ser., vol. VII, no. 3. Baltimore: Williams & Wilkins for The National Foundation March of Dimes, 1971, p. 198.

Contributors: **Alex E. Krill‡**
                    Donald R. Bergsma
                    Mitchel L. Wolf

———————————

Editor's Computerized Descriptors: Vision, Eye

AMELO-CEREBRO-HYPOHIDROTIC SYNDROME

Includes: Syndrome amélocérébrohypohydrotique
Amelocerebrohypohydrotisches Syndrom
Síndrome amielo-cerebro hipohidrótico
Kohlschütter syndrome

Excludes: Amelo-onycho-hypohidrotic syndrome (45)
Ectodermal dysplasia, anhidrotic (333)

Minimal Diagnostic Criteria: Thin hypoplastic enamel on all teeth in a patient with seizures, spasticity, progressive oligophrenia and hypohidrosis.

Clinical Findings: The syndrome is characterized by thin hypoplastic enamel on teeth of both dentitions, severe epileptiform seizures usually appearing between 11 months and 4 years of age, muscle spasticity, progressive mental retardation, and hypohidrosis. Peripheral nerve conduction velocities are normal and EEG is diffusely abnormal. Decreased numbers of sweat and sebaceous glands, and increased sweat potassium have been found. Brain histology shows diminished number of neurons, small glial cells, ballooning of axons and lipid-filled pericytes.

Complications
I   **Derived:** Sensitivity of teeth to thermal changes. Psychosocial changes with oligophrenia.
II **Associated:** —

Etiology: ? All affected patients have been male. Possibly X-linked.†

Pathogenesis: ?

Related Facts
I   **Sex Ratio:** ?
II **Risk of Occurrence:** ?
III **Risk of Recurrence for**
       Patient's Sib: If X-linked and mother is a carrier, 1 in 2 (50%) for each brother to be affected and 1 in 2 (50%) for each sister to be a carrier.
       Patient's Child: ?
IV **Age of Detectability:** For tooth defect: at time of eruption of primary teeth (6 months-1 year). For spasticity: 11 months-4 years.
V   **Prevalence:** Rare. Occurs in isolates in Switzerland and Germany.

Treatment
I   **Primary Prevention:** Genetic counseling
II **Secondary Prevention:** Crowning and reconstruction of teeth; prevention of seizures by anticonvulsant drugs.
III **Other Therapy:** —

Prognosis: Guarded. Most affected males have died in 1st decade.

Detection of Carrier: —

†Special Considerations: Autosomal recessive inheritance has not been excluded, as all cases in 4 kindreds have been from isolate populations in Switzerland and Germany.

References:

Kohlschütter, A. et al: Familial epilepsy and yellow teeth- a disease of the CNS associated with enamel hypoplasia. Helv. Paediatr. Acta 29:283, 1974

Witkop, C.J., Jr. and Sauk, J.J., Jr.: Defects of enamel. In Stewart, R.E. and Prescott, G.H. (eds.): Oralfacial Genetics. St. Louis: C.V. Mosby, 1976.

Contributors: **Carl J. Witkop, Jr.**
                    Alfried Kohlschütter

———————————

Editor's Computerized Descriptors: Teeth, Sweating, Nerve

AMELO-ONYCHO-HYPOHIDROTIC SYNDROME

Includes: Hypocalcification de l'émail avec oncholyse et hypohydrose

Zahnschmelzhypoplasie, Oncholyse und Hypohidrose

Hipocalcificación del esmalte, onicolisis e hipodrosis

Amelogenesis imperfecta with onycholysis, hypohidrosis, rough skin and seborrhea of scalp

Onycholysis, hypohidrosis and enamel hypocalcification

Hypohidrosis, onycholysis and enamel hypocalcification

Ameloonycholyticdyshidrotic syndrome

Ameloonychodyshidrotic syndrome

Enamel hypocalcification, onycholysis and hypohidrosis

Excludes: Amelogenesis imperfecta (46)

Onycholysis

Ectodermal dysplasia, anhidrotic (333)

Anhidrosis (56)

Anhidrosis and neurolabyrinthitis

Tricho-dento-osseous syndrome (965)

Minimal Diagnostic Criteria: In 1 kindred all 12 affected members had all 5 signs. In another kindred, 4 affected patients lacked seborrheic dermatitis of scalp.

Clinical Findings: The condition is characterized by the association of 5 distinctive features:

1) A hypocalcified-hypoplastic enamel which is brown, pitted, thin and soft. Many teeth fail to erupt in the permanent dentition and undergo resorption of enamel of the incisal edges. Enamel at the cervical of the crown is usually better formed, approaching normal thickness and mineralization.

2) Onycholysis of finger and toe nails involve from 1/4 to 1/2 of the distal portion of the nail separating the nail from the nail bed with a thin layer of subungual hyperkeratosis. The surface of the nail is smooth.

3) Hypohidrosis. The number of sweat gland openings on dermal ridges is normal but the response of the glands to heat by secreting sweat is markedly diminished. Rectal temperatures may be slightly elevated.

4) Skin is rough and dry, particularly on the volar surfaces, back and upper arm.

5) Seborrheic dermatitis of scalp.

Complications

I   **Derived:** Premature loss of teeth, impacted teeth with radiolucent lesions of jaws and intraalveolar resorption of teeth

II   **Associated:** —

Etiology: Autosomal dominant

Pathogenesis: ? Possibly a defect in keratin-producing cells

Related Facts

I   **Sex Ratio:** M1:F1

II   **Risk of Occurrence:** ? Very rare, 2 kindreds known

III   **Risk of Recurrence for**

     Patient's Sib: 1 in 2 (50%) for each offspring to be affected; otherwise not increased.

     Patient's Child: 1 in 2

IV   **Age of Detectability:** Six to 12 months of age with eruption of teeth. Nail and skin involvement become apparent later at 2-3 years of age.

V   **Prevalence:** ? Very rare

Treatment

I   **Primary Prevention:** Genetic counseling

II   **Secondary Prevention:** Jacket crowns or prosthetic restoration of teeth.

III   **Other Therapy:** —

Prognosis: Does not appear to reduce longevity or fertility.

Premature loss of teeth.

Detection of Carrier: —

Special Considerations: —

References:

Witkop, C.J., Jr. et al: Hypoplastic enamel, oncholysis and hypohidrosis inherited as an autosomal dominant trait. A review of the ectodermal dysplasia syndromes. Oral Surg. 39:71, 1975.

Contributor: **Carl J. Witkop, Jr.**

Editor's Computerized Descriptors: Teeth, Skin, Nails

AMELOGENESIS IMPERFECTA

Includes: Défaut héréditaire de l'émail
Amelogenesis imperfecta:
    Type—hypoplastic, pitted autosomal dominant
    Type—hypoplastic, rough autosomal dominant
    Type—hypoplastic, rough autosomal recessive
    Type—hypoplastic, smooth autosomal dominant
    Type—hypoplastic, local autosomal dominant
    Type—hypoplastic, smooth X-linked dominant
    Type—hypocalcified, autosomal dominant
    Type—hypocalcified, autosomal recessive
    Type—hypomaturation, pigmented autosomal recessive
    Type—hypomaturation, X-linked recessive

Excludes: Enamel defects associated with syndromes, generalized diseases and extrinsic causes
Isolated taurodontism

Minimal Diagnostic Criteria: All or nearly all teeth show enamel defect in patient without disease or syndrome.

Clinical Findings: Clinical, roentgenologic and histologic features vary according to type of amelogenesis. Both primary and permanent dentitions affected unless otherwise noted.

Type—hypoplastic, pitted autosomal dominant. Enamel is thin with random pits from pinpoint to pinhead size primarily on labial or buccal surfaces in permanent teeth. Some teeth may appear normal in both dentitions. Normal contrast between enamel and dentin on xray.

Type—hypoplastic, rough autosomal dominant. Enamel is thin, brown, very hard, with granular vitreous surface. Lack of contact between adjacent teeth. On xray, teeth outlined by thin layer of enamel. High contrast between enamel and dentin.

Type—hypoplastic, rough autosomal recessive. Tooth surface is rough, granular and light yellow-brown in color. Lack of contact between adjacent teeth. There is no radiographic evidence of enamel and many teeth are unerupted and partially resorbed in the alveolus. Histologically, only evidence of enamel is laminated agate-like vitreous calcification on dentin surface.

Type—hypoplastic, smooth autosomal dominant. Enamel is thin, brown, smooth and glossy except where hypocalcified at contact points. Lack of contact between adjacent teeth. On xray, many teeth unerupted with resorption of crowns. Small calcified bodies may be seen adjacent to unerupted teeth.

Type—hypoplastic, local autosomal dominant. Only primary teeth may be affected. Pits and grooves of hypoplastic enamel in a horizontal fashion across middle third of tooth. All or only some teeth show defect. Most frequently affected teeth are incisors, premolars or primary molars.

Type—hypoplastic, smooth X-linked dominant. Males—enamel thin, brown to yellow-brown, smooth and shiny. Females—show alternating vertical bands of normal and abnormal enamel (Lyon effect). Xrays of females show vertical banding of enamel.

Type—hypocalcified, autosomal dominant. Unerupted and newly erupted teeth are covered by a light yellow-brown enamel of normal thickness. After eruption, enamel becomes brown to black from food stains. Enamel is friable, soft and rapidly lost by attrition so by 10-12 years only dentin cores remain. Cervical enamel may be better calcified. Anterior open bite frequently associated 12:16. Teeth sensitive to temperature changes. On xray, enamel less radiopaque than dentin. Moth-eaten appearance of crown with radiodense line of calcified enamel at cervical.

Type—hypocalcified, autosomal recessive. Essentially the same clinical findings as in the dominant type but with a greater degree of severity.

Type—hypomaturation, pigmented autosomal recessive. Clear to cloudy agar-brown enamel of normal thickness. Enamel fractures from dentin. Enamel softer than normal will admit probe point under pressure. On xray, lack of contrast between enamel and dentin.

Type—hypomaturation, X-linked recessive. Males—enamel of primary teeth ground glass white. Enamel of permanent teeth mottled yellow. Enamel soft will admit point of probe under pressure. Females—enamel of primary teeth shows random alternating vertical bands of abnormal ground glass white enamel with bands of translucent normal enamel. Enamel of permanent teeth shows random alternating vertical bands of either opaque white or opaque yellow enamel with bands of translucent normal enamel. Transillumination aid to diagnosis in females. On xray: males—contrast between enamel and dentin reduced from normal; females—no defects observed.

Complications
I Derived: Among 50 patients: psychic changes secondary to unsightly teeth 40/50; early tooth loss 46/50; prone to periodontal disease 25/50; sensitivity to hot and cold 24/50; pulpal exposure from attrition 8/50; anterior open bite Type—hypocalcified autosomal dominant 12/16; Type—hypoplastic, rough X-linked dominant males 22/22, females 18/30; Type—hypoplastic, rough autosomal dominant 15/29.
II Associated: —

Etiology: Genetic traits which may be transmitted as autosomal dominant, autosomal recessive or X-linked depending upon type. It is not known whether the autosomal traits and the X-linked traits represent genes at different loci or if they represent alleles. McK *10450, *10453, *20470, *30110

Pathogenesis: Structural defects in enamel formation. The primary protein defect is unknown. In the hypoplastic forms there is a failure of ameloblasts to lay down an enamel matrix of full thickness. It is my opinion that in the thin enamel type the defect is primarily in the ameloblast while in the pitted forms the defect may be in a vascular defect of the enamel organ. In the hypocalcified types full thickness of enamel matrix is produced but fails to calcify normally. Scanning electron microscopy shows defect in so-called enamel sheath in hypomaturation types.

Related Facts
I Sex Ratio: Autosomal dominant and recessive types M1:F1; X-linked dominant type M1:F2; X-linked recessive type M1:F0 (if females who have mild defect detectable by special examination are included M1:F2).
II Risk of Occurrence: ?
III Risk of Recurrence for
    Patient's Sib: When autosomal dominant, autosomal recessive, X-linked recessive or X-linked dominant, see Table I AD, AR, X-linked R or X-linked D, respectively.
    Patient's Child: When autosomal dominant, autosomal recessive, X-linked recessive or X-linked dominant, see Table I, AD, AR, X-linked R or X-linked D, respectively.
IV Age of Detectability: At the time of eruption of teeth; 1-2 years by visual examination.
V Prevalence: 1 in 16,000 in North American Caucasians of which Type—hypocalcified, autosomal dominant accounts for about 40%.

Treatment
I Primary Prevention: Genetic counseling
II Secondary Prevention: Excellent results in all types with full crown restorations and orthodontic procedure for open bite.†
III Other Therapy: Desensitizing tooth paste

Prognosis: Early loss of teeth by attrition, pulp exposure and periodontal disease if untreated. With restoration, normal life span of teeth can be maintained.

Detection of Carrier: In recessive type—none. In X-linked recessive type—alternating vertical stripes of normal translucent enamel and opaque yellow-white abnormal enamel. Can best be seen on transillumination.

†Special Considerations: Dental restoration at early age recommended to prevent further psychosocial trauma. Nearly all patients (80 of the 100 patients seen to date) have shown marked psychosocial changes from their unsightly teeth. With treatment there has been a marked improvement in their personality and social relations with others; however, a few individuals who had used their defect to elicit attention from family members had negative reactions after restoration.

References:
Weinmann, J.P. et al: Hereditary disturbances of enamel formation and calcification. J. Am. Dent. Assoc. 32:397, 1945.

Witkop, C.J., Jr. and Rao, S.R.: Inherited defects in tooth structure. In Bergsma, D. (ed.): Part XI. Orofacial Structures. Birth Defects: Orig. Art. Ser., vol. VII, no. 7. Baltimore: Williams and Wilkins Co. for The National Foundation-March of Dimes, 1971, p. 153.

Witkop, C.J., Jr. and Sauk, J.J., Jr.: Defects of enamel. In Stewart, R.E. and Prescott, G.H. (eds.): Oral Facial Genetics. St. Louis: C.V. Mosby Co., 1976.

Contributor: **Carl J. Witkop, Jr.**

Editor's Computerized Descriptor: Teeth

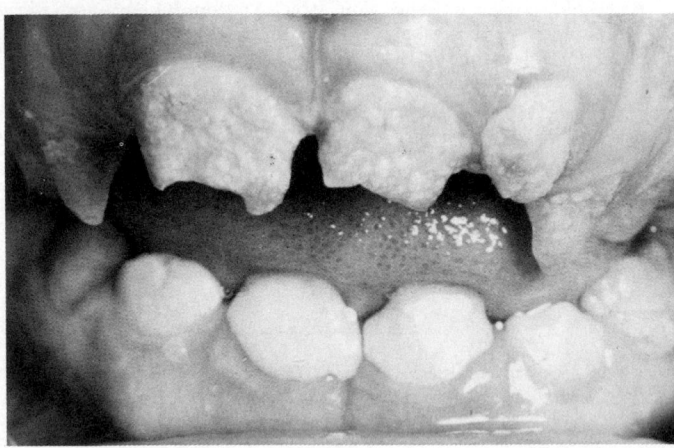

130. Amelogenesis imperfecta, hypocalcified type

ANALBUMINEMIA

Includes: Analbuminémie
Analbuminämie
Anabolic idiopathic hypoalbuminemias

Excludes: Nephrosis
Exudative enteropathy
Protein-losing gastroenteropathy
Hypercatabolic idiopathic hypoalbuminemias
Essential hypoproteinemia with a specific decrease of albumins and gamma globulins

Minimal Diagnostic Criteria: Plasma albumin concentration is less than 100 mg% (values gained by immunochemical means). High cholesterol concentration in the blood; much accelerated sedimentation of the erythrocytes. Slight edema in the region of the ankles or the legs.

Clinical Findings: The decisive finding is a nearly complete lack of albumins in the plasma. The typical concentration lies between 4 and 100 mg%. By precipitation methods, according to Howe, small amounts of globulins remain unprecipitated which lead to too high albumin values.

Most of the patients have no complaints. Some mention slight rheumatic pains. More often a patient complains of getting tired very quickly by physical work. Edema may occur, especially in female patients and then mostly in the premenstruum. In other cases no edema was ever observed nor physical weakness. One such patient did very hard agricultural work, in winter even felling of trees, with only 10 mg% of albumin in his blood.

Further symptoms: A lowered level of the total serum protein. Higher levels up to the double of the alpha- and beta-globulins, as well as of the gamma-M-globulins. The sedimentation of the erythrocytes is always much accelerated. The concentration of calcium and bilirubin may be abnormally low. The cholesterol and transferrin values are always distinctly higher than normal. The blood pressure often is low. In some cases slight endocrine disturbance: for instance, atrophy of the testicles, gynecomastia, osteoporosis. In the eyes: sludge phenomenon in the blood vessels of the retina; pterygia and pinguecula are seen in the conjunctiva. In female patients remarkable lipodystrophy in the pelvic girdle may occur. Liver tissue shows no pathologic findings by light microscopy; the electron microscopic method shows no certain defect of ribosomes, but a very important lack of liposomes as the only anomaly.†

Complications
I **Derived:** ?
II **Associated:** ?

Etiology: Autosomal recessive; McK *20530

Pathogenesis: The anomaly of analbuminemia is mostly diagnosed in adults. The youngest patient was 10 years old when the analbuminemia was ascertained; the oldest patients were a 55-year-old woman in England and possibly a 61-year-old Negro man in the United States. The latter case, however, was atypical: the albumin concentration was 600 mg% but gained by the method of Howe. (Probably the precipitate contained small portions of globulin.) This patient also suffered from severe rheumatic arthritis and rheumatic cardiopathy. In this case it is remarkable that the cholesterol values were normal. In this it differs from all other cases observed.

Related Facts
I **Sex Ratio:** M6:F5 (11 cases)
II **Risk of Occurrence:** ?

III Risk of Recurrence for
Patient's Sib: 1 in 4 (25%) for each offspring to be affected

Patient's Child: Nothing is known of offspring of analbuminemic patients.

IV Age of Detectability:
? Probably after 2 months. It is improbable that in the 1st weeks of life the analbuminemia is already present. A lack of albumins in the 1st weeks of life would almost inevitably lead to bilirubin intoxication and to kernicterus.

V Prevalence:
The 11 cases of analbuminemia come from all parts of the world: from the German Federal Republic, Switzerland, England, the United States, the Caucasus, Yugoslavia, Ireland and Algeria. The Algerian patients are 2 brothers and a sister in a family of 6 children. The 3 other children and the parents had normal albumin values.

Treatment
I Primary Prevention: —

II Secondary Prevention: IV infusions of human albumin are not of vital importance; they can, however, improve the general physical condition. In case of intercurrent illnesses they are advisable, especially if the compatibility with albumin has been previously ascertained. Even with repeated applications of albumin infusions there is no danger of allergic reactions. The IV application of drugs with great affinity to bind albumin needs much caution. An accelerated delivery from the circulating blood and an abundant afflux of high concentrated free and active drugs to the sites of efficacy in the tissue must be expected. Collapse can occur after smallest intravenously injected doses of sulphonamides. Among others for instance suramin, tolbutamides, cumarin derivates, etc seem to be especially dangerous in analbuminemic patients. In cases in which the application of such medicaments is very necessary, a slow IV infusion of albumin should be given beforehand.

III Other Therapy: —

Prognosis: Good as far as this can be said, after only 17 years of experience and only 11 cases. Theoretically, the constantly high hypercholesterinemia might become a risk in old age.

Up to now, 1 of the analbuminemic patients died at age 61 years of rheumatic arthritis and rheumatic cardiopathy.

Detection of Carrier: The heterozygotes have normal concentration of immunochemical identical albumin; they have 1 silent and 1 normal gene.

†Special Considerations: Considering the almost complete lack of the largest fraction of the serum proteins we might expect a number of deficiencies in important functions and of manifest illnesses. In most of the observed analbuminemic patients nothing of the sort occurred. They consult the doctor for some trifling complaints. The constantly high erythrocyte sedimentation rate without any plausible explanation leads to a clinical examination including electrophoresis. The resulting pathologic laboratory findings can either be caused directly by the albumin deficiency or by mobilized compensatory mechanisms of the organism.

Among the first is the very much accelerated erythrocyte sedimentation rate, as well as the very pathologic Congo red test (disappearance rate of 72%h). After albumin infusion, it is normalized to 16%. The lowering of the colloid osmotic pressure must also be mentioned, as well as the low bilirubin level of 0.09-0.2 mg%; perhaps also the lowered calcium level in the blood. The most fatal consequence of the very much reduced vehicle function of the albumins is the lowering of the colloid osmotic pressure to half of the normal.

The following symptoms may be considered to be compensating mechanisms: hypotonia of arteries and capillaries, the augmentation of the alpha- beta and gamma-M globulins up to about twice normal. Transferrin participates to a high degree in the increase of the globulins. After albumin infusions the transferrin level falls to about normal, and rises again with the decreasing albumin level in the plasma. The pathologically increased cholesterol has the same interdependence with the changing albumin level. In analbuminemia the catabolic rate of albumin is distinctly diminished (prolonged half-life time) but increases after each albumin infusion. The hypercatabolic group, the most important form of which is the protein-losing enteropathy, shows contrary reactions.

In analbuminemia the kidneys have the following important peculiarities. The glomerulus filtration (C_{IN}) is not increased- as might be expected in view of the low colloid osmotic pressure, but even somewhat diminished on account of a remarkable clearance of the renal plasma flow (C_{PAH}). Probably a preglomerular throttling of the arterioles of the kidney in analbuminemic patients is the most plausible explanation of this reaction of the plasma flow.

The filtration fraction is increased. The tubular reabsorption of water is lowered from the normal of 99.5 to 95.1%.

In the vehicle function of the albumins regarding hormones, metals, bile acids and fatty acids as well as drugs, globulins under certain conditions can act as supplementary vehicles. These bindings to the globulins often have stronger and more specific binding capacities.

The sum of all these supplementary mechanisms elucidates the fact that analbuminemic patients can be in good health and have the normal life expectation.

References:

Bennhold, H. S. and Scheurlen, P. G.: Analbuninaemie und deren Auswirkung auf die Nierenfunktion. In Pathogenese und Therapie der Ödeme. Proc. 6th Int. Cong. of Internal Medicine, Basel, 1960. Basel: Benno Schwabe & Co. 1961.

Freeman, T. R.: Analbuminaemia: A study of albumin and transferrin metabolism. In Birke, G. et al (eds.): Physiology and Pathophysiology of Plasma Protein Metabolism. New York:Pergamon Press, 1969, p. 75.

Waldmann, T.A. et al: Studies on the metabolism of the serum proteins and lipids in a patient with analbuminemia. Am. J. Med. 37:960, 1964.

Contributor: **H. Bennhold**

Editor's Computerized Descriptors: Eye, Skin, Skel., Muscle, CV., GU.

ANALPHALIPOPROTEINEMIA

Includes: Maladie de Tangier
Mb. Tangier
Analfalipoproteinemia
Tangier disease
Alphalipoprotein deficiency
Familial high density lipoprotein deficiency

Excludes: Cholesteryl ester storage disease (151)
Lecithin:cholesterol acyl transferase deficiency (580)

Minimal Diagnostic Criteria: Demonstration by immunochemical means that plasma HDL are less than 10% of normal in presence of low cholesterol, normal or high glycerides, and usual ratio of free to esterified cholesterol.

Specific immunochemical tests now exist for the apolipoproteins A-I and A-II which constitute the bulk of HDL apolipoproteins. The level of each in plasma is about 1% of normal in Tangier disease.

Further support is obtained by demonstrating that cholesteryl ester storage is occurring in tonsil or rectal biopsy specimens.

Clinical Findings: An abnormally low plasma cholesterol level (below 120 mg%), and near absence of α or high density lipoproteins (HDL) are invariable. Elevated plasma triglyceride levels are usual. A red-orange abnormal coloration of the tonsils is characteristic, splenomegaly commonly found, but enlargement of the liver or lymph nodes infrequent. Foam cells may be found in the bone marrow. When looked for, orange spots are seen on the rectal mucosa, corresponding to foam cell aggregations in the lamina propria. Neurologic signs occur in more than half of the patients, including cutaneous sensory losses with paresthesia, decreased deep tendon reflexes, muscle wasting and weakness (with electromyographic and biopsy changes of "denervation"). In adults one finds corneal infiltrations visible by slit lamp, and skin deposition of cholesteryl esters (seen on biopsy).

Complications

I **Derived:** Recurrent peripheral neuropathy is the most serious. Hypersplenism occasionally seen; possibly associated is accelerated atherosclerosis.

II **Associated:** Of possible chance association are the infrequently found anemia or jaundice.

Etiology: Autosomal recessive mode of transmission. The homozygote is unable to synthesize or retain any normal HDL in plasma. This is believed most likely due to synthesis of a structurally abnormal apolipoprotein A-II. A small HDL particle containing only apolipoprotein A-II exists in plasma. There is also absolute deficiency of C-apolipoproteins, for which HDL normally provides a reserve pool, and of low density lipoproteins. Abnormal chylomicrons and triglyceride-rich particles circulate in plasma after meals. McK *20540

Pathogenesis: The primary defect, absence of normal HDL, is presumably present at birth. This appears to interfere with metabolism of chylomicrons which are ingested by macrophages in the reticuloendothelial system. Progressive storage of cholesteryl esters then occurs in tonsils, spleen, bone marrow, lymph nodes, and liver. Most of the stored lipid is not bound by lysosomal membranes. Foam cells may be demonstrated which stain well with Sudan, Oil-red-O, and Schultz procedures, but not with Baker or PAS techniques. Electron microscopy shows lipid storage within Schwann cells of peripheral nerves. Oil-red-O positive, anisotropic infiltration is found in the skin, as well as changes in muscle suggestive of denervation.

The patients do absorb dietary fat, and make chylomicrons but there is a delay in the clearance of exogenous triglycerides from the plasma.

Related Facts

I **Sex Ratio:** M1:F1 in the >20 known cases

II **Risk of Occurrence:** All patients Caucasian thus far except for single Australian aboriginal.

III **Risk of Recurrence for**
Patient's Sib: 1 in 4 (25%) for each offspring to be affected
Patient's Child: Not increased unless mate is carrier or homozygote

IV **Age of Detectability:** Probably at birth, by immunologic measurement

V **Prevalence:** < 1 in 100,000

Treatment

I **Primary Prevention:** Genetic counseling

II **Secondary Prevention:** —

III **Other Therapy:** Possible splenectomy if hypersplenism is present

Prognosis: Fair to good. Two of >20 patients have died, possibly of unrelated causes.

Detection of Carrier: Heterozygotes have about half the normal α-lipoprotein levels (concentrations in the plasma at the level of the lowest 5% of the population). Eventually, measurement of HDL apolipoproteins (A-I and A-II) should provide certain identification of heterozygotes.

Special Considerations: —

References:
Ferrans, V.J. and Frederickson, D.S.: The pathology of Tangier disease. Am. J. Pathol. 78:101, 1975.
Herbert, P.N. et al: Familial lipoprotein deficiency. In Stanbury, J.B. et al (eds.) The Metabolic Basis of Inherited Disease. 4th Ed., New York: McGraw-Hill, 1978, p. 544.

Contributor: **Donald S. Fredrickson**

Editor's Computerized Descriptors: Eye, Muscle, Lymphatic, Spleen, GI., Liver, Nerve

ANDROGEN INSENSITIVITY SYNDROME, COMPLETE

Includes: Syndrome de féminisation testiculaire
Testikuläre Feminisierung
Síndrome del testículo feminizante
Testicular feminization syndrome, complete
Feminizing testes syndrome

Excludes: Androgen insensitivity syndrome, incomplete (50)
Pseudovaginal perineoscrotal hypospadias (831)
Reifenstein syndrome (855)
All forms of male pseudohermaphroditism producing a female genital phenotype caused by defects in testosterone biosynthesis† including:
Defect in conversion of cholesterol to δ^5 pregnenolone due to defect in enzyme system which includes 20α-hydroxylase, 22R-hydroxylase and 20,22-desmolase.
Steroid 17α-hydroxylase deficiency (903)
Steroid 17,20-desmolase deficiency (904)
Male psuedohermaphroditism with female genital phenotype caused by Leydig cell agenesis.
Müllerian derivatives in males, persistent (683)
Gonadal dysgenesis, XX type (436)
Gonadal dysgenesis, XY type (437)

Minimal Diagnostic Criteria: The diagnosis of the complete androgen insensitivity syndrome requires the following:
Female external genital phenotype
Absence of müllerian and wolffian duct derivatives
Primary amenorrhea
46,XY karyotype (can be 47,XXY or 47,XYY)
Presence of testicles
Feminization at puberty
No demonstrable defect in testosterone biosynthesis or in the conversion of testosterone to dihydrotestosterone
Absence of effects following administration of androgens, as determined by lack of virilization and lack of nitrogen retention
A defect in androgen cytosol-binding protein may be demonstrable in cultured genital skin fibroblasts from affected patients

Clinical Findings: The patient with the complete androgen insensitivity syndrome has an unambiguously female external genital phenotype. Thus, the sex assignment in the affected newborn is correctly female. The diagnosis is not ordinarily suspected in the infant. The clitoris is not enlarged, labia majora and minora appear normal, and separate urethral and vaginal orifices are present. The vagina is a few millimeters to several centimeters in depth. Müllerian duct derivatives are absent, so the affected patient has no cervix, uterus or fallopian tubes. Wolffian duct derivatives are also absent, so no internal ductal structures are present. The gonads are testicles. Prior to puberty they are histologically normal or similar to those in cryptorchid males. After puberty abnormalities include small seminiferous tubules made up mostly of Sertoli cells, deficient spermatogonia and absence of spermatozoa, and Leydig cell hyperplasia with presence of clusters of Leydig cells. The testicles may be located intraabdominally, along the pathway of testicular descent, or in the labia.

The complete androgen insensitivity syndrome produces no symptoms in infancy or childhood with 1 notable exception. About half of affected patients have inguinal herniae. The herniae are found at surgery to contain testicles. The complete androgen insensitivity syndrome should be suspected, and appropriate diagnostic tests undertaken in any female child with an inguinal hernia.

At puberty, feminization occurs with normal female breast development. The affected adult has a normal female external genital phenotype except for a paucity of pubic and other body hair. Primary amenorrhea is the most common presenting complaint in this condition, and by definition occurs in all cases. Body proportions are ordinarily normal for an adult female. Affected patients are sterile.

No other somatic features are encountered in the complete androgen insensitivity syndrome.

Complications
I **Derived:** Primary amenorrhea and sterility are part and parcel of the syndrome. The risk of gonadal neoplasia is increased, with estimates that 5-20% of affected patients will have a gonadal neoplasm. The lower figure is probably nearer the correct incidence. This may or may not be simply a reflection of the location of the testicles, similar to the situation in cryptorchid males. Tumors include benign tubular adenomas and seminomas. Psychologic problems may occur if patient is not handled intelligently. Menopausal symptoms following orchiectomy unless estrogen substitution therapy is initiated.

II **Associated:** —

Etiology: An X-linked recessive mutant allele (or an autosomal dominant, male sex-limited mutant allele). A genetically and endocrinologically similar condition in several other mammals is inherited in an X-linked recessive manner. This is evidence in favor of an X-linked recessive mode of inheritance in the human. Whether the responsible mutant allele is allelic to that responsible for the incomplete androgen insensitivity syndrome remains to be proved. It is tempting to speculate that it is. McK *31370

Pathogenesis: Evidence available for some time has implicated a target tissue unresponsiveness to intrinsically synthesized and externally administered testosterone. A defect in the conversion of testosterone to dihydrotestosterone has been discounted because affected patients are also unresponsive to administered dihydrotestosterone. Testosterone concentration in peripheral and testicular vein plasma is at least that of the normal male of the age at which the determination is made. Testosterone and androstenedione secretion rates are normal. Plasma estrogen concentrations are within the low normal female range in affected patients.

Recent work has indicated that a specific protein is necessary for the specific target cell binding of testosterone (T) and dihydrotestosterone (DHT). This protein actively binds T and DHT at the plasma membrane of target cells and transports the androgen to the nucleus where it binds to the nuclear chromatin and performs its inductive functions. A defect in the specific cytosol-binding protein has been postulated as the pathogenetic mechanism in the androgen insensitivity syndrome. Available data indicate either an absence of or a functional defect in specific androgen cytosol-binding protein in at least some affected patients with this condition. Whether this is the primary pathogenetic mechanism in all affected patients remains to be proved.

In the normal female fetus (in whom testicles are absent), wolffian ducts regress and leave only rudiments in the differentiated female. At the same time, müllerian ducts differentiate to form the fallopian tubes, uterus and cephalad portion of the vagina. Also, in the absence of a testicle, the bipotential primitive external genitalia differentiate into the definitive external genitalia of the female. The presence of a testicle is necessary for male sex differentiation. This testicle-dependent male sex differentiation is mediated apparently through 2 compounds: Androgens synthesized by the Leydig cells induce wolffian duct differentiation to form epididymides, vasa deferentia and seminal vesicles. Androgens also are responsible for masculinization of the bipotential primitive external genitalia to form penis and scrotum. The 2nd testicular-derived substance, apparently a high molecular weight peptide, is called *müllerian suppressive factor*. It may be a product of the Sertoli cells. It functions to cause regression of the müllerian duct system in the male fetus. Thus, normal male sex differentiation depends upon the action of 2 testicular-derived substances: the androgens, testosterone and dihydrotestosterone, and müllerian suppressive factor.

In the complete androgen insensitivity syndrome, target cells cannot respond to normally secreted amounts of biologically active androgens. The results are failure of induction of the wolffian duct system with absence of epididymides, vasa deferentia and seminal vesicles; and failure of masculinization of the bipotential primitive external genitalia. The latter leads to unambiguously female external genitalia in the affected patient. At the same time, the fetal testis produces müllerian suppressive factor to which the target cells can respond. The result is active suppression of all müllerian duct derivatives. Thus, the affected patient has no internal male duct structures, no fallopian tubes, no uterus, and a shallow, blind-ending vaginal vault; ie only that caudad portion of the vagina derived from the urogenital sinus is formed. The pelvis of the affected patient is empty of internal genital ductal structures. In addition, failure of response of target cells to androgens postnatally results in paucity of body hair, absence of beard, failure of nitrogen response to administered androgens, and failure of all other androgen-dependent functions.

The testicle in normal males elaborates estrogens as well as androgens. Apparently, the action of these estrogens, unopposed by androgen counterbalance, is responsible for breast development in patients with the complete androgen insensitivity syndrome.

Related Facts
I **Sex Ratio:** M1:F0
II **Risk of Occurrence:** ? Relatively rare. One estimate puts the incidence at 1 in 62,400 liveborn males.
III **Risk of Recurrence for**
    Patient's Sib: 1 in 2 (50%) for 46,XY sib to be affected, 1 in 4 (25%) for all sibs, assuming mother is heterozygous for X-linked recessive or autosomal dominant (male-sex-limited) mutant allele.
    Patient's Child: All patients are sterile.
IV **Age of Detectability:** The diagnosis is made in infancy only if it is suspected on the basis of a positive family history, or if the infant has an inguinal hernia. The diagnosis is made usually at puberty because of primary amenorrhea.
V **Prevalence:** ? Relatively rare. See Risk of Occurrence above.

Treatment
I **Primary Prevention:** Genetic counseling, possibly intrauterine diagnosis on the basis of 46,XY fetal karyotype plus the demonstration of a defect in androgen cytosol-binding protein in cultured amniotic cells.
II **Secondary Prevention:** The risk of gonadal neoplasia dictates that gonadectomy be done in all affected patients. The age at which this should be done is controversial. Neoplasms do not occur prior to puberty. If gonadectomy is delayed until after puberty, the patient will feminize without treatment. This may constitute a psychologic advantage for the patient. If gonadectomy is done prior to puberty, then estrogen substitution therapy will be necessary beginning in the 2nd decade of life. Estrogen substitution therapy is necessary following gonadectomy if it is delayed until after puberty.

No treatment can alter the primary amenorrhea or sterility. Supportive counseling is indicated regarding these features.

Vaginoplasty may be necessary for the deepening of the vaginal vault to make intercourse possible.

Inguinal hernia repair if indicated.

III **Other Therapy:** —

Prognosis: Presumably normal life span provided gonadal neoplasia does not supervene and shorten life. As mentioned, all patients are sterile. Intelligence is not affected.

Detection of Carrier: It is said that some of the mothers of patients have less than normal amounts of axillary and pubic hair and experience on the average a later onset of menarche. Other investigators have been unable to confirm this.

†**Special Considerations:** The syndrome of Leydig cell agenesis and several defects in testosterone biosynthesis may produce a female external genital phenotype. However, such conditions involve not only a defect in androgen biosynthesis, but also a defect in estrogen biosynthesis. Thus, in affected patients feminization does not occur at puberty. In addition, if the enzymatic defect in androgen biosynthesis is at a step shared by corticoid biosynthesis, signs and symptoms of adrenal failure will occur. Thus, it should be possible in all cases to differentiate these conditions from the complete androgen insensitivity syndrome. Appropriate diagnostic studies should be undertaken in any 46,XY individual with a female external genital phenotype. These studies should investigate the possibility of XY gonadal dysgenesis, of a defect in testosterone and corticoid biosynthesis, of Leydig cell agenesis, of a lack of response to administered androgens, and of defects in androgen cytosol-binding protein in cultured fibroblasts from genital skin biopsy.

The extent of information provided to patients and families regarding genetic sex and the nature of gonads in affected patients must be formulated on an individual basis, and depends, in the judgment of the responsible physician, on the ability of the patient and family to comprehend such information.

References:
Crawford, J.D. et al: Syndromes of testicular feminization. Clin. Pediatr. 9:165, 1970.
Kaufman, M. et al: Specific 5α-dihydrotestosterone binding in labial skin fibroblasts cultured from patients with male pseudohermaphroditism. Clin. Genet. 9:567, 1976.
Keenan, B.S. et al: Syndrome of androgen insensitivity in man: Absence of 5α-dihydrotestosterone binding protein in skin fibroblasts. J. Clin. Endocrinol. Metab. 38:1143, 1974.
Ohno, S. et al: Molecular biology of sex differentiation. Hereditas 69:107, 1971.
Rosenfield, R.L. et al: Androgens and androgen responsiveness in the feminizing testis syndrome. Comparison of complete and "incomplete" forms. J. Clin. Endocrinol. Metab 32:625, 1971.
Simpson, J.L.: Disorders of Sexual Differentiation. New York: Academic Press, 1977, p. 199.
Summitt, R.L.: Disorders of sex differentiation. In Givens, J.R. (ed.): Gynecologic Endocrinology. Chicago:Year Book Publishers, 1977, p. 69.

Contributor: **Robert L. Summitt**

Editor's Computerized Descriptors: Hair, Hernia not CNS, GU.

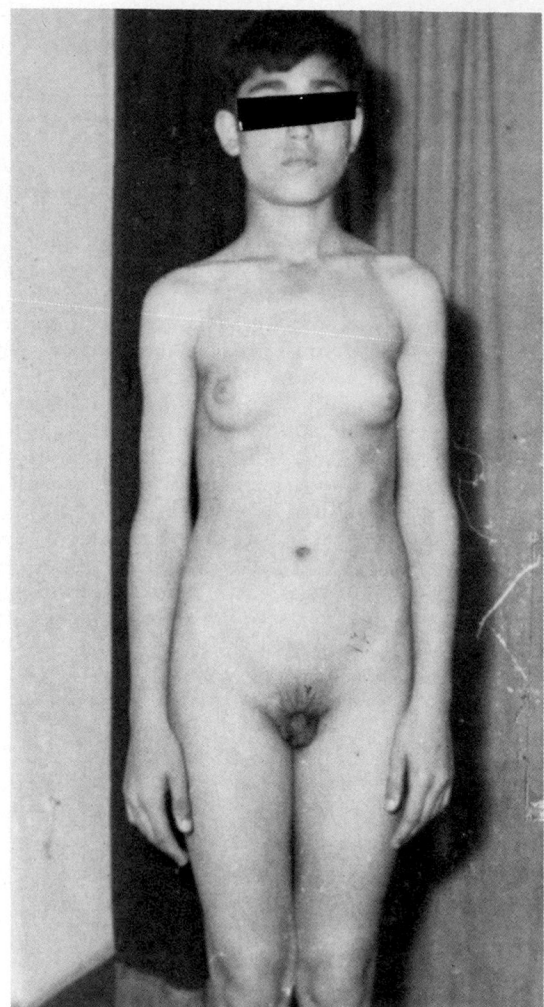

131. Note breast development at age 15

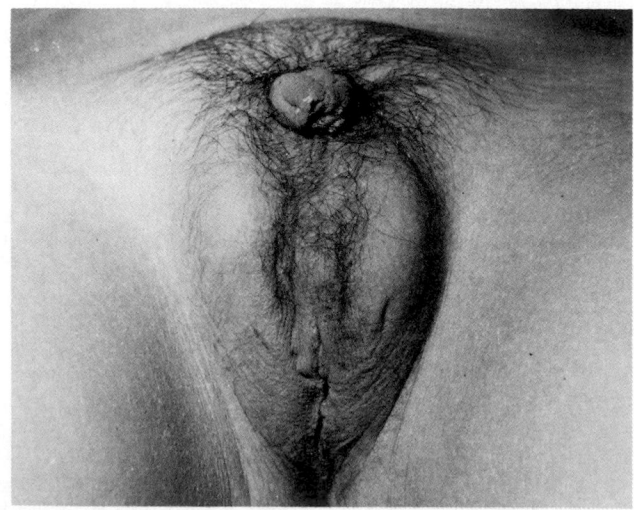

132. Note hypoplastic phallus and feminine distribution of hair

ANDROGEN INSENSITIVITY SYNDROME, INCOMPLETE

Includes: Syndrome de féminisation testículaire incompléte
Inkomplette testikuläre Feminisierung
Síndrome de feminizacion testicular incompleto
Incomplete male pseudohermaphroditism type 1 (Wilson and Goldstein)†
Feminizing male pseudohermpahroditism (Jones)†
Incomplete testicular feminization syndrome†
Incomplete feminizing testes syndrome†
Lubs syndrome†
Gilbert-Dreyfus syndrome†
Note: See Reifenstein syndrome (855)

Excludes: Androgen insensitivity syndrome, complete (49)
Chromosome 45,X/46/XY mosaicism (173)
Adrenal lipoid hyperplasia
3β-ol-dehydrogenase deficiency
Steroid 17α-hydroxylase deficiency (903)
Pseudovaginal perineoscrotal hypospadias (831)
Steroid 17,20-desmolase deficiency (904)
17-ketosteroid reductase deficiency
Müllerian derivatives in males, persistent (683)

Minimal Diagnostic Criteria: Male pseudohermaphroditism in which the phenotype includes intersex external genitalia (clitoromegaly with varying degrees of labioscrotal fusion), normal sized intraabdominal or inguinal testes, a 46,XY karyotype (could be 47,XXY or 47,XYY), absent or hypoplastic wolffian duct derivatives, absent müllerian duct derivatives, and breast development with variably defective virilization at puberty. Plasma testosterone is normal, and no error in androgen biosynthesis is demonstrable. The administration of androgens in doses that ordinarily produce normal adult plasma testosterone levels fails to induce virilization or nitrogen retention. The demonstration of a defect in androgen cytosol receptor protein in cultured genital fibroblasts from an affected patient strongly supports the diagnosis.

Clinical Findings: Certain 46,XY individuals with testes who feminize at puberty have been shown to have partial or incomplete androgen insensitivity (androgen hyposensitivity). Such patients have intersex external genitalia characterized by phallic enlargement (clitoromegaly) and partial labioscrotal fusion. Somatic anomalies are absent. This incomplete androgen insensitivity syndrome shares the following features with the complete androgen insensitivity syndrome: bilateral testes with similar histologic features, absence of müllerian duct derivatives, absence or hypoplasia of wolffian duct derivatives, puberal breast development, defective puberal virilization, normal male plasma testosterone levels, normal response to HCG and ACTH, and failure to show an anabolic response (eg nitrogen retention) following testosterone administration in usual doses. Testes are usually cryptorchid (intraabdominal) or in inguinal canals; pubic hair is present. The incomplete and complete androgen insensitivity syndromes differ only in that in the incomplete androgen insensitivity syndrome, the external genitalia show partial labioscrotal fusion and clitoromegaly. Some individuals with the incomplete androgen insensitivity syndrome have wolffian duct derivatives, namely epididymides and vasa deferentia; however, such derivatives are not consistently present. No evidence of enzymatic deficiency in testosterone biosynthesis or conversion of testosterone to dihydrotestosterone is present in these individuals, although they may show an abnormality of the target-cell cytosol receptor protein for androgens (androgen-binding protein).

Complications
I **Derived:** Neoplastic transformation of cryptorchid or inguinal testes; infertility.
II **Associated:** —

Etiology: This condition is inherited in the fashion of an X-linked recessive or male-limited autosomal dominant disorder. Whether the mutant allele is allelic to that for the complete androgen insensitivity syndrome remains to be proved, but it is tempting to speculate that it is. McK *31370

Pathogenesis: The incomplete androgen insensitivity syndrome is NOT the result of a defect in testosterone biosynthesis or in the conversion of testosterone to dihydrotestosterone. Currently available information implicates target cell hyporesponsiveness to testosterone and dihydrotestosterone. In some cases of the complete androgen insensitivity syndrome (see discussion of that disorder), a defect in the cytosol binding protein that binds testosterone and dihydrotestosterone to target cells and transports these androgens to the nuclei has been demonstrated. Limited data further suggest that a similar but less severe defect is responsible for at least some cases of the incomplete androgen insensitivity syndrome. Whether this mechanism explains all such cases remains to be determined. Appropriate studies are mandatory in all patients in whom a presumptive diagnosis of incomplete androgen insensitivity syndrome is made.

Related Facts
I **Sex Ratio:** M1:F0
II **Risk of Occurrence:** ? Relatively rare
III **Risk of Recurrence for**
  Patient's Sib: 1 in 2 (50%) for each 46,XY sib to be affected; 1 in 4 (25%) for all sibs, assuming the mother is heterozygous for the responsible mutant allele.
  Patient's Child: All patients are infertile
IV **Age of Detectability:** Usually at birth because of genital ambiguity, but occasionally not until puberty because of primary amenorrhea.
V **Prevalence:** ? Rare. Many affected kindreds have been reported, but in most, defects in testosterone biosynthesis or its conversion to dihydrotestosterone were not excluded.

Treatment
I **Primary Prevention:** Genetic counseling. Prenatal diagnosis may be possible on the basis of the demonstration of an androgen cytosol binding protein defect in cultured amniotic cells.
II **Secondary Prevention:** Assignment of a female sex of rearing with orchiectomy and surgical construction of female external genitalia. Construction of an artificial vagina may be necessary, but this is preferably performed in the 2nd decade of life. Estrogen substitution therapy should be initiated in the 2nd decade of life and continued until the usual age of menopause.
III **Other Therapy:** —

Prognosis: Presumably normal lifespan, provided neoplastic transformation of testes does not occur.

Detection of Carrier: Not currently available, but studies of receptor function in cells cloned from potential (female) heterozygotes might be informative.

†Special Considerations: Androgen hyposensitivity should be demonstrated either clinically, by showing deficient nitrogen retention following androgen administration, or biochemically by demonstration of a defect in cytosol androgen receptor protein activity. Individuals who on the basis of the external appearance could be said to have the incomplete androgen insensitivity syndrome may actually represent a heterogeneous sample. For example, genital development similar to that of the incomplete androgen

insensitivity syndrome may occur in 17α-hydroxylase deficiency and sometimes 17-ketosteroid reductase deficiency. Thus, the absence of a defect in testosterone biosynthesis is mandatory in making the diagnosis of the incomplete androgen insensitivity syndrome.

Many individuals said to have the Reifenstein syndrome differ in no important way from patients with the incomplete androgen insensitivity syndrome. As appropriate studies are performed on more patients heretofore said to have the Reifenstein syndrome, hyposensitivity to androgen will probably be demonstrated. The same is probable for the so-called Lubs syndrome and the so-called syndrome of Gilbert-Dreyfus. Prior to puberty individuals with the condition called pseudovaginal perineoscrotal hypospadias (PPSH), also a heterogeneous group of disorders, may be clinically indistinguishable from those with incomplete testicular feminization (see discussion of PPSH). Finally, to prevent nosologic confusion, it should be mentioned that Wilson et al reported a family in which there appeared to be segregating a variably expressed X-linked recessive or male-limited autosomal dominant gene capable of producing phenotypes consistent with either the incomplete androgen insensitivity syndrome or the Reifenstein syndrome; those authors concluded that both conditions resulted from a single mutant gene, and designated the condition, "incomplete male pseudohermaphroditism, type 1." Affected individuals in the kindred reported by Wilson et al have the incomplete androgen insensitivity syndrome, and in 3 members of that family a defect has been demonstrated in the binding of dihydrotestosterone to cultured genital skin fibroblasts. The family reported by Wilson et al demonstrates the clinical variablity possible in a single kindred in which the incomplete androgen insensitivity syndrome is segregating.

References:
Griffin, J.E. et al: Dihydrotestosterone binding to cultured human fibroblasts. Comparison of cells from control subjects and from patients with hereditary male pseudohermaphroditism due to androgen resistance. J. Clin. Invest. 57:1343, 1976.
Inhorn, S.L. and Opitz, J.M.: Abnormalities of sex development. In Bloodworth, J.M.B., Jr., (ed.): Endocrine Pathology. Baltimore: Williams & Wilkins, 1968, p. 529.
Opitz, J.M. et al: Pseudovaginal perineoscrotal hypospadias. Clin. Genet. 3:1, 1972.
Simpson, J.L.: Disorders of Sexual Differentiation: Etiology and Clinical Delineation. New York: Academic Press, 1976.
Summitt, R.L.: Disorders of sex differentiation. In Givens, J.R., (ed.): Gynecologic Endocrinology. Chicago:Year Book Publishers, 1977, p. 69.
Wilson, J.D. et al: Familial incomplete male pseudohermaphroditism, type 1. N. Engl. J. Med. 290:1097, 1974.

Contributors: **Joe Leigh Simpson**
Robert L. Summitt

Editor's Computerized Descriptor: GU.

ANEMIA, HYPOPLASTIC CONGENITAL

Includes: Anémie hypoplastique congénitale
Angeborene hypoplastische Anämie
Anemia hipoplástica congénita
Congenital erythroid hypoplastic anemia
Erythrogenesis imperfecta
Diamond-Blackfan syndrome
Hypoplastic anemia, congenital
Congenital red cell aregenerative anemia

Excludes: Secondary hypoplastic anemia associated with toxin, drug, infection or thymoma
Aplastic phase of hemolytic anemia
Aplastic anemia with leukopenia or thrombocytopenia
Fanconi hypoplastic anemia

Minimal Diagnostic Criteria: Moderate-to-severe anemia with reticulocytopenia beginning in early infancy and without serious leukopenia or thrombocytopenia. Bone marrow cytology showing normal white cell production but virtual absence of recognizable erythroid cells.

Clinical Findings: The patient gradually becomes pale usually before age 3 months, but sometimes shortly after birth, and rarely after 6-12 months. The pulse becomes rapid as anemia increases, and cardiac enlargement and dilatation may develop. Heart failure and secondary pneumonia may ensue as the anemia becomes profound. A preagonal level as low as 1 gm% hemoglobin has been seen. The white cells and platelets are not affected; therefore neither recurrent infections nor petechiae and ecchymoses are ordinarily to be expected. The plasma immunoglobulins are normal. The spleen and liver are usually not enlarged except in association with hemosiderosis after many transfusions. In a number of cases, accessory or triphalangeal thumbs have been found. Webbed neck may be present but abnormal karyotypes have not been found. The red cells generally are fairly normal in appearance but there often is a distinct macrocytosis; reticulocytes are few or absent. The bone marrow shows a paucity or a virtual absence of recognizable erythroid elements only. There may be a few clusters of small lymphoid-looking cells, not "blast-forms," but possibly erythroid precursors. Red cell survival in the circulation is usually normal or only slightly shortened. The percent of fetal hemoglobin may be high.

Complications

I   **Derived:** Generalized hemosiderosis involving the skin and viscera caused by repeated transfusions. Of the latter, the liver, kidneys, spleen, and heart are early sites of excessive pigment deposits from the destruction of infused red cells which have suffered storage lesions of varying severity. Continued transfusions, usually numbering in the hundreds, may lead to allosensitization against rare red cell antigens (blood groups) foreign to the patient. Also, white cell, platelet, and even plasma factors may initiate antibody responses and cause subsequent troublesome transfusion reactions. In such cases, washed red cells may be required for each transfusion. Cirrhosis and liver failure can result from the increasing pigment accumulation. Viral hepatitis may occur in patients receiving multiple blood transfusions and has complicated the course of the disease. Growth retardation occurs in the multitransfused patients, possibly as a result of a combination of chronic anemia, liver insufficiency and unknown metabolic deficiencies.

II **Associated:** —

Etiology: May be both autosomal recessive and autosomal dominant. Two typical sib cases have been recorded in about a quarter of the families. Relatives with the same condition have rarely been found (3-4 possible cases) and related blood dyscrasias have rarely been found in family members in contrast to the situation in Fanconi aplastic anemia. Recently, however, a few families with possible cases in 2 or 3 generations have been reported. These may represent autosomal dominant variants or the disorder may prove to be a dominant trait with variable penetrance, the underlying defect yet to be found. Once this defect is discovered, the carriers may be identifiable.

Pathogenesis: The disorder probably is due to an end-organ failure of erythrogenesis beginning late in fetal life or early in infancy. The extent varies considerably from patient to patient but usually is alike in sibs. That some enzymatic abnormality or defect is present has been suggested by the corrective effect of adrenal corticosteroid therapy in most patients when it is begun early. In most of these children the sensitivity of erythrogenesis to small changes, even 2.5 - 5 mg/week in prednisone dosage, is extraordinary. Spontaneous remissions have occurred, usually after puberty and even after years of transfusion therapy.

Related Facts

I   **Sex Ratio:** M1:F1
II **Risk of Occurrence:** Very rare. Only about 150 verified cases reported or recognized since first described in 1938.
III **Risk of Recurrence for**
    Patient's Sib: When autosomal dominant or autosomal recessive, see Table I AD or AR, respectively.
    Patient's Child: When autosomal dominant or autosomal recessive see Table I AD or AR, respectively.
IV **Age of Detectability:** Usually before age of 3 months.
V   **Prevalence:** No racial or ethnic association. No parental consanguinity noted. A very rare disease.

Treatment

I   **Primary Prevention:** Genetic counseling
II **Secondary Prevention:** As soon as diagnosis is established by blood and bone marrow examinations, as well as by exclusion of other causes, adrenal corticosteroid therapy should be started in order to increase the likelihood of a favorable response; most infants under 4 months have shown rapid restoration of red cell levels whereas only half of those who have been treated by transfusions for a year or more have responded to corticosteroids thereafter. Usually oral prednisone is given 2-3 mg/kg/day for 7-10 days. Responders will show increase in erythroblasts and normoblasts in bone marrow aspirates within 4-5 days and fairly brisk reticulocytosis in the peripheral blood shortly thereafter with a rise in hemoglobin or hematocrit levels following. If there is no response within 3-4 weeks, it is wiser to stop the drug lest its side effects become troublesome and to delay another drug trial for a few months, using red cell transfusion when the hematocrit becomes dangerously low. After several months, corticosteroid may be tried again at a high dosage level for a few weeks.

In the responders, the hemoglobin is permitted to climb to a normal level of 11-12 gm% or more, using intermittent corticosteroid therapy (every other day or 3 consecutive days per week, etc) The dosage is then slowly diminished on a weekly basis until the hemoglobin value levels off at about 11 gm%. Once responsiveness to corticosteroid has begun, it generally continues even if the drug is stopped for a time and then resumed. In only a few cases have the patients become refractory to adrenal corticosteroid and for no known reason. Any infection, overt or occult, may produce exacerbation of erythroid hypoplasia with recurrence of anemia requiring increase in corticosteroid dosage temporarily or even transfusion until the marrow recovers.

III **Other Therapy:** When the disorder is unresponsive to adrenal corticosteroids, transfusions must be given every 6-10 weeks.

Prognosis: If treatment is successful, patient's future health seems to be unimpaired. However, most of the patients successfully treated are still under 25 years of age.

Detection of Carrier: —

Special Considerations: —

References:
Diamond, L.K. and Blackfan, K.D.: Hypoplastic anemia. Am. J. Dis. Child. 56:464, 1938.
Diamond, L.K. et al: Congenital (erythroid) hypoplastic anemia. Am. J. Dis. Child. 102:403, 1961.
Gasser, C.: Aplastische Anämie chronische Erythroblastophthise und Cortison. Schweiz. Med. Wochenschr. 81:1214, 1951.

Contributor: **Louis K. Diamond**

Editor's Computerized Descriptors: Skin, Skel., Resp., CV.

ANENCEPHALY

Includes: Anencéphalie
Anenzephalie
Anencefalia
Acrania
Craniorachischisis
Exencephaly
Hemicrania

Excludes: Hydranencephaly (480)

Minimal Diagnostic Criteria: At birth by inspection. Anencephaly should be suspected when hydramnios develops.

Clinical Findings: Cranial vault deficient with frontal, parietal and occipital bones present only in their basal portions. Basal bones are abnormal with small orbits causing protrusion of eyes. Exposed neural tissue pervaded by angiomatous stroma filling the open cranial defect, usually covered by a thin membrane (? arachnoid) continuous with surrounding hair-bearing skin. Generally stillborn or short-lived.

Complications
I   **Derived:** —
II **Associated:** Absence of ganglia cells of retina, pituitary gland represented by anterior lobe only, adrenal cortex of adult type with high pressor amine content, amyelia, spina bifida.

Etiology: In doubt, but appears to be multifactorial. Genetic factors seem important by the familial incidence while geographic variation suggests an environmental cause. Causative factors act on developing embryo between 16th and 26th day after conception. Concordance and discordance have occurred in monozygous twins.

Pathogenesis: Secondary necrosis of developing cerebral hemispheres.

Related Facts
I   **Sex Ratio:** M1:F3 to 7
II **Risk of Occurrence:** Variable, 1 in 1000 live births to as high as 1 in 105 births in South Wales
III **Risk of Recurrence for**
    Patient's Sib: 1 in 20 (5%)
    Patient's Child: Affected die in utero or at birth.
IV **Age of Detectability:** At birth
V   **Prevalence:** —

Treatment
I   **Primary Prevention:** Genetic counseling
II **Secondary Prevention:** —
III **Other Therapy:** —

Prognosis: Stillborn or die at birth.

Detection of Carrier: ?

Special Considerations: —

References:
Carter, C.O. et al: The genetics of the major central nervous system malformations, based on the South Wales socio-genetic investigation. Dev. Med. Child. Neurol. (Suppl.) 13:30, 1967.
Carter, C.O.: Multifactorial inheritance revisited. In Congenital Malformations. Amsterdam:Excerpta Medica, 1969, p. 227.
deBellefeville, P.: Contrib. a l'étiologie de l'encephalie par l'étude des jumeaux. L'Union Med. Canada 98:437, 1969.
Laurence, K.M.: The recurrence risk in spina bifida cystica and anencephaly. Dev. Med. Child. Neurol. (Suppl.) 20:23, 1969.

Contributor: **Kenneth Shulman**

Editor's Computerized Descriptors: Eye, Skel.

ANEURYSM OF AORTIC SINUS OF VALSALVA

Includes: Anévrisme du sinus de Valsalva
Aneurysma des Sinus Valsalva
Aneurisma del seno aórtico de Valsalva
Congenital aortic sinus aneurysm with or without rupture

Excludes: Acquired aortic sinus aneurysm
Cystic medial necrosis with aneurysmal dilatation of aortic root
Congenital aorticocardiac fistula

Minimal Diagnostic Criteria: The diagnosis may be strongly suspected from the clinical picture of the previously healthy individual with a loud, continuous murmur at the lower precordial area in whom cardiac catheterization reveals left-to-right shunting at the ventricular or atrial level. To confirm the diagnosis, retrograde aortography with injection of the contrast medium at the region of the ascending aorta is necessary. This clearly outlines the aortic sinus aneurysm, the fistulous communication into the right heart chamber, and the normal course of the coronary arteries.

Clinical Findings: The pathologic anatomy consists of aneurysmal dilatation of an aortic sinus due to defective development of the aortic root. The aneurysm generally involves 1 sinus only—the right coronary sinus in about 70%, the noncoronary sinus in 22% and the left coronary sinus in about 4%. Congenital aneurysm of more than 1 aortic sinus is observed only in about 3%. The aneurysm grows insidiously and gradually bulges into the adjoining low-pressure right heart chambers. Eventually, its protruding weakest point ruptures, resulting in an aorticocardiac fistula. The receiving chamber is either the right ventricle or the right atrium in almost all cases. Right coronary sinus aneurysms rupture into the right ventricle in more than 70%, and into the right atrium in about 25%. The ones that open into the latter chamber are generally those that originate from the posterior portion of the right coronary sinus; those that rupture into the right ventricle usually arise from the left or medial third of the same sinus. Noncoronary sinus aneurysms rupture into the right atrium in 85%, and into the right ventricle in 11%. The rare left coronary sinus aneurysms may rupture into the right atrium or left atrium.

An associated ventricular septal defect is observed in more than a third of the cases. It is especially common (80%) in aneurysms of the right coronary sinus. The septal defect tends to be situated immediately beneath the pulmonary valve. Congenital aortic sinus aneurysms may sometimes be accompanied by coarctation of the aorta. The unruptured aneurysm generally does not become large enough to cause significant hemodynamic changes. It is, therefore, a clinically silent lesion. Occasionally, it may cause some right ventricular outflow obstruction as it protrudes into the subpulmonary conus. An ejection systolic murmur at the upper left sternal border and moderate splitting of the second sound, simulating the findings of mild pulmonary stenosis, may then be observed. In the presence of associated ventricular septal defect, a typical harsh pansystolic murmur and thrill at the left lower sternal border, due to the septal defect, is present. Heart size may be normal or enlarged depending upon the size of the ventricular defect.

When rupture of the aortic sinus aneurysm occurs, an aorticocardiac fistula suddenly develops, resulting in continuous runoff of blood from the aorta to the receiving chamber during systole and diastole. Acute symptoms may accompany this episode, such as severe chest or right upper abdominal pain, weakness, nausea or emesis, and shortness of breath. These symptoms may last several minutes to an hour. An intervening period lasting for several weeks or months then follows, during which time exertional dyspnea, palpitation, fatigability and angina are observed. Eventually, congestive heart failure develops, leading to death after several months. Rarely, death may occur immediately following the rupture. The intervening period may also occasionally last for several years before heart failure finally supervenes. In rare cases rupture has occurred before birth.

The striking clinical finding is a loud, continuous, machinery-like murmur along the left or right sternal border. Unlike the continuous murmur of patent ductus arteriosus which has its peak intensity at the time of the second sound, the systolic component of the murmur reveals accentuation in the midsystole. The diastolic component may or may not be louder than the systolic one. In addition, the continuous murmur is usually maximally heard at the lower left or right sternal border where a thrill is often present. The arterial pulses are bounding due to a wide pulse pressure. The cardiac apical impulse is hyperactive and is accompanied by a prominent lower left parasternal heave, compatible with combined ventricular volume overload. The chest roentgenograms in isolated unruptured congenital aortic sinus aneurysms are normal as long as the aortic valve remains competent. The aneurysm is intracardiac and not sufficiently large to cause distortion of the cardiac silhouette. Among cases with unruptured aortic sinus aneurysm and an associated ventricular septal defect, there is shunt vascularity, left atrial enlargement and combined ventricular enlargement. After rupture has occurred in patients without an associated shunt (ventricular septal defect), there is enlargement of the right atrium and right ventricle. If aortico-right atrial or right ventricular communication is of a moderate to large size, the pulmonary vascularity is increased as well.

The ECG in unruptured aneurysms is normal. Following rupture, combined ventricular hypertrophy with, usually, left ventricular preponderance appears. Right ventricular hypertrophy is usually manifested by RSR complexes in the right precordial tracings. Disturbances in conduction, such as varying forms of A-V block and right bundle branch block, may occur in those where the aneurysm projects just above or below the tricuspid valve in the area of the A-V node and bundle of His. This is likely to be observed in aneurysms arising from the posterior portion of the right coronary sinus or from the noncoronary sinus where rupture tends to be into the right atrium. It may be observed also in those where the aortic sinus encroaches into or involves the ventricular septum.

Cardiac catheterization demonstrates a left-to-right shunt to be at the ventricular or, less frequently, at the atrial level. The magnitude of the shunt varies. Pulmonary hypertension is rather uncommon and pulmonary vascular resistance is normal. A pressure gradient across the right ventricular outflow tract may sometimes be present.

Complications
I **Derived:** Aortic insufficiency is common particularly in those where there is associated ventricular septal defect. Bacterial endocarditis is not uncommon. Eventually, congestive heart failure terminating in death develops usually within a period of 1 year following rupture. Hemorrhage into extracardiac tissues resulting in hemopericardium or hemothorax does not occur.
II **Associated:** Marfan syndrome

Etiology: Sporadic and syndrome associated cases (Marfan syndrome).

Pathogenesis: The aneurysm is presumed to be secondary to the presence of a weak point in the aortic root resulting from congenital separation or discontinuity of the aortic media and annulus fibrosus. Inadequate fusion of the bulbar septum has also been incriminated for this tissue defect. As the weak aortic root segment becomes constantly exposed to the left ventricular ejectile force and high aortic pressures, it gradually bulges toward the low pressure right heart chambers, becoming aneurysmal as it increases in size and finally rupturing at its weakest point. If a high ventricular septal defect is present, the aneurysm protrudes across the defect into the right ventricular outflow tract resulting in functional reduction of the size of the septal defect and occurrence of aortic insufficiency and some right ventricular outflow obstruction. Fibrosis with focal or diffuse chronic inflammatory reaction may also be noted in the wall of the aneurysm as well as in the adjoining myocardium. Some right ventricular outflow narrowing occurs as the aneurysm protrudes into the subpulmonary conus. Following rupture, continuous systolic and diastolic runoff of blood from aorta to the receiving right heart chamber occurs, with consequent volume overload of both ventricular chambers.

Related Facts
I   **Sex Ratio:**   M3:F1
II **Risk of Occurrence:**   Less than 1 in 20,000 (less than 0.5% of CHD)
III **Risk of Recurrence for**
      Patient's Sib: Depends on etiology
      Patient's Child: Depends on etiology
IV **Age of Detectability:**   From infancy on, if ruptured, by aortography or selective angiography. In unruptured aneurysms, the diagnosis is incidental during angiocardiography for other suspected congenital heart defects (eg ventricular septal defect, coarctation of the aorta).
V   **Prevalence:**   ?

Treatment
I   **Primary Prevention:**   —
II **Secondary Prevention:**   Irrespective of whether the aneurysm is ruptured or unruptured, surgical occlusion of the fistula or aneurysm and reconstruction of aortic root is indicated. This is accomplished with the aid of cardiopulmonary bypass, alone or with additional hypothermia.
III **Other Therapy:**   In unruptured aneurysms not yet surgically corrected, chemoprophylaxis for bacterial endocarditis is most important. In ruptured aneurysms with heart failure, the usual medical therapy consisting of digitalis, diuretics, oxygen and antibiotics for accompanying pulmonary infection is indicated.

Prognosis: Although hemodynamically benign, the solitary aneurysm is a serious condition due to its inherent tendency to rupture. Following the latter complication, death from congestive heart failure generally occurs within about a year. The time of rupture varies but is uncommon in childhood and rare in utero . Most frequently, it occurs during the 4th decade. The risk of bacterial endocarditis is also considerably higher in this condition than it is in most other congenital heart defects.

Detection of Carrier: —

Special Considerations: —

References:
Morch, J. E. and Greenwood, W. F.: Rupture of the sinus of Valsalva: A study of eight cases with discussion on the differential diagnosis of continuous murmurs. Am. J. Cardiol. 18:827, 1966.
Sakakibara, S. and Konno, S.: Congenital aneurysm of the sinus of Valsalva: Anatomy and classification. Am. Heart J. 63:405, 1962.

Contributor: **René A. Arcilla**

Editor's Computerized Descriptor: CV.

ANGIOEDEMA, HEREDITARY

Includes: Oédème angioneurotique héréditaire
Hereditäres angioneurotisches Ödem
Angioedema hereditario
Hereditary angioneurotic edema
Complement C'1 esterase inhibitor deficiency
Complement C'1 esterase inhibitor dysfunction

Excludes: All forms of nonhereditary angioedema

Minimal Diagnostic Criteria: History of recurrent self-limiting episodes of edema or abdominal pain. Demonstration of either the deficiency of the C'1 esterase inhibitor in serum or the presence of a nonfunctional C_1 inhibitor immunochemically identical with the normal inhibitor.

Clinical Findings: Usually a family history or individual history of recurrent episodes of localized peripheral subcutaneous edema, usually without apparent precipitating event, though sometimes associated with menses, extremes of temperature; physical trauma or emotional distress. Any area of the body may be affected. Attacks are self-limiting lasting 6 to 72 hours; recurrent episodes of self-limited abdominal pain and vomiting, episodes of pharyngeal and laryngeal edema. Peripheral edema involving any part of the body is noninflammatory, nonpitting and usually nonpuritic and nonpainful. During episodes of abdominal pain, the abdomen may be diffusely tender but no localization is apparent. The abdomen may be distended. This clinical picture may be confused with other causes of acute abdomen. Facial edema may progress to involve mucosa of the mouth, the soft palate, epiglottis and laryngeal mucous membrane. This has led to fatality in 10-30% of affected individuals. Attacks are occasionally preceded by or associated with a transient salmon pink serpiginous skin eruption. The only primary abnormality is deficiency (quantitative or functional) of the C'1 esterase inhibitor, an alpha 2 globulin which normally prevents formation of C'1 esterase and the reaction with its natural substrates.

Secondary depletion of serum C'_4 and C'_2. C_4 titers are consistently depressed becoming more so during symptomatic period. However, C_2 titers are sometimes normal in the intervals between attacks of angioedema. Xrays reveal persistent narrowing of lumen of small bowel segment presumably due to mucosal edema, during abdominal pain distended loops of intestine and increased thickness of the intestinal wall.

Complications
I **Derived:** Death from laryngeal edema in approximately 10-30% of affected individuals. Unnecessary abdominal surgery. Pulmonary edema.
II **Associated:** —

Etiology: Autosomal dominant transmission of biochemical deficiency. Though this deficiency of C'1 esterase inhibitor (an alpha 2 globulin, an inhibitor of the esterase activity of the first component of serum complement which also inhibits other factors which affect vascular permeability) is present continuously through life, the symptoms often become more frequent and severe at adolescence, are episodic in nature and self-limiting. The exact relationship of the biochemical deficiency to the symptoms has not been clarified. McK *10610

Pathogenesis: It is believed, though not substantiated, that the edema in these patients results from an uninhibited enzyme activity leading directly or indirectly to the release of permeability factors from complement components, kinin precursors or other similar substances. It is reported that the ultimate mediation of the symptoms in angioedema is probably perpetrated by a vasoactive, kinin-like peptide, probably derived from C_2 and not by bradykinin. The resulting edema may be due to increased vascular permeability at the time of enhanced enzyme activity.

Related Facts
I **Sex Ratio:** M1:F1
II **Risk of Occurrence:** ?
III **Risk of Recurrence for**
Patient's Sib: If parent is affected, 1 in 2 (50%) for each offspring to be affected; otherwise not increased.
Patient's Child: 1 in 2
IV **Age of Detectability:** In infancy by deficiency of C'1 esterase inhibitor. Subsides in the 5th decade.
V **Prevalence:** ? The disorder has been observed in a large number of ethnic groups. Affected kindreds have been found to originate in Northern Europe, the Mediterranean area, and Africa.

Treatment
I **Primary Prevention:** Genetic counseling
II **Secondary Prevention:** a) There is some recent evidence that Epsilon aminocaproic acid may reduce the frequency of attacks of edema. b) An analog, tranexamic acid has proved effective in aborting attacks of angioedema. The drug has not yet been released by the F.D.A. c) Recently Damazol, a derivative of ethinyltestosterone, has been shown to prevent attack of hereditary angioedema and acts to correct the underlying biochemical abnormality. Side effects are minimal. d) If possible, affected members should carry information indicating the nature of their disease in order to avoid unnecessary abdominal surgery and to alert physicians of the possible need for tracheotomy when edema of the face and oral mucosa occurs.
III **Other Therapy:** Careful observation in hospital, if possible, during episodes of facial and oral edema since swelling can extend to the larynx rapidly. Tracheotomy is often necessary; the need should be anticipated.

Analgesia may be helpful if abdominal pain is severe. Hospitalization and IV fluid therapy may be necessary if vomiting is excessive.

There is some suggestion that administration of fresh plasma may stop progress of the edema and perhaps prevent need for tracheotomy or terminate abdominal pain in selective instances. This effect is thought to be dependent upon replacement of C'1 esterase inhibitor by plasma; however its value is questionable.

Prognosis: The degree of disruption of normal daily living depends on the frequency of attacks. Some individuals have one attack of peripheral edema in a lifetime. Others are troubled by frequent episodes of peripheral edema or abdominal pain which may cause frequent work loss and some individuals have had repeated tracheotomies. Deaths from respiratory obstruction secondary to laryngeal edema occur in 10-30% of affected individuals in different reported series.

Detection of Carrier: —

Special Considerations: —

References:
Donaldson, V. H. and Rosen, F. S.: Hereditary angioneurotic edema: A clinical survey. Pediatrics 37:1017, 1966.
Donaldson, V.H. et al: Permeability-increasing activities in hereditary angioneurotic edema plasma. J. Clin. Invest. 48:642, 1969.
Gelfand, J.A. et al: Treatment of hereditary angioedema with damazol. N. Engl. J. Med. 295:1444, 1976.
Landerman, M. S.: Hereditary angioneurotic edema. I. Case reports and review of the literature. J. Allergy 33:316, 1962.
Pickering, R.J. et al: Replacement therapy in hereditary angioedema: Successful treatment of two patients with fresh frozen plasma. Lancet 1:326, 1969.
Rosen, F.S. et al: Hereditary angioneurotic edema: Two genetic variants. Science 148:957, 1965.

Contributor: **Sudhir Gupta**

ANGIO-OSTEOHYPERTROPHY SYNDROME

Includes: Syndrome ostéo-angio-hypertrophique
Klippel-Trénaunay-Syndrom
Síndrome de angio-osteohipertrófico
Hemangiectatic hypertrophy
Nevus varicosus osteohypertrophicus

Excludes: Sturge-Weber syndrome (915)
Isolated cutaneous hemangiomatosis
Hemihypertrophy (458)

Minimal Diagnostic Criteria: Cutaneous hemangiomatous lesions, varicosities, soft tissue, and bony hypertrophy. Venograms are necessary to rule out compression or absence of the deep venous channels of the leg. Arteriovenous fistula is ruled out by arteriogram.

Clinical Findings: The main features include cutaneous hemangiomatous lesions, varicose veins, soft tissue, and bony hypertrophy. Most cases present unilateral involvement, and the long bones are affected in 90% of cases. Occasionally, bilateral involvement occurs. Rarely may be combined with features of the Sturge-Weber syndrome. Other findings may include compression of the deep venous channels of the leg by a fibrous cord or by an aberrant artery, absence of the normal deep venous channels of the leg, arteriovenous fistula, orofacial involvement (without other features of the Sturge-Weber syndrome), and visceral hemangiomatosis.

Complications
I **Derived:** If arteriovenous fistula is present, arterial insufficiency and secondary heart disease may ensue. Persistent hemorrhage and thrombocytopenia are possible if visceral hemangiomatosis is present. A protein-losing enteropathy has been observed in 1 case associated with intestinal lymphangiectasia.
II **Associated:** Intestinal lymphangiectasia, syndactyly, polydactyly

Etiology: Autosomal dominant and autosomal recessive modes of inheritance with modifying genes have been postulated.

Pathogenesis: It has been suggested that hypertrophy may be attributed to abnormal vascular development with associated one-sided increase in the blood supply. However, the sites of angiomatosis and hypertrophy are not always concordant, suggesting that this relationship is not one of cause and effect. Rather, angiomatosis and hypertrophy may be 2 concomitant manifestations of the same morbid cause. A disturbance of neurovegetative regulation also has been advanced as a common pathogenic mechanism.

Related Facts
I **Sex Ratio:** M1:F1
II **Risk of Occurrence:** ?
III **Risk of Recurrence for**
    Patient's Sib: When autosomal dominant or autosomal recessive, see Table I AD or AR, respectively.
    Patient's Child: When autosomal dominant or autosomal recessive, see Table I AD or AR, respectively.
IV **Age of Detectability:** Hemangiomatosis present at birth; varicosities and hypertrophy develop during infancy.
V **Prevalence:** Rare

Treatment
I **Primary Prevention:** Genetic counseling
II **Secondary Prevention:** Some vascular anomalies are amenable to surgical correction. If the deep venous channels of the leg are compressed or absent, stripping of varicosities is not recommended.
III **Other Therapy:** Elastic hose may be worn if there is dependent edema. Plastic surgical procedures can be utilized in

cases of limited hemangiomatous involvement.

Prognosis: Fair. Depends on type and extent of involvement.

Detection of Carrier: —

Special Considerations: —

References:
Caplan, D.B. et al: Angioosteohypertrophy syndrome with protein-losing enteropathy. J. Pediatr. 74:119, 1969.
Haberland, C. and Perou, M.: Bone involvement in Sturge-Weber-Dimitri syndrome: Combined Sturge-Weber-Dimitri and Klippel-Trénaunay-Weber syndrome. Confin. Neurol. 28:413, 1966.
Koch, G.: Zur Klinik Symptomatologie, Pathogenese und Erbpathologie des Klippel-Trénaunay-Weberschen syndroms. Acta Genet. Med. Gemellol. (Roma)5:(Suppl.) 1:326, 1956.
Kuffer, F.R. et al: Klippel-Trénaunay syndrome, visceral angiomatosis and thrombocytopenia. J. Pediatr. Surg. 3:65, 1968.
Lindenauer, S.M.: The Klippel-Trénaunay syndrome: Varicosity, hypertrophy and hemangioma with no arteriovenous fistula. Ann. Surg. 162:303, 1965.

Contributor: **M. Michael Cohen, Jr.**

Editor's Computerized Descriptors: Skin, Skel., CV., Lymphatic, GI.

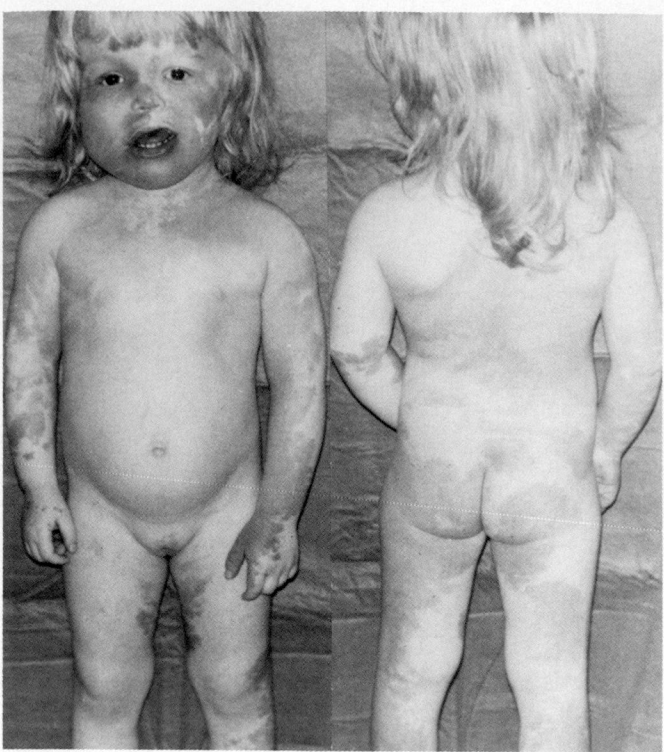

134. Note extensive hemangiomas and facial asymmetry. Patient has Sturge-Weber syndrome as part of angio-osteohypertrophy syndrome

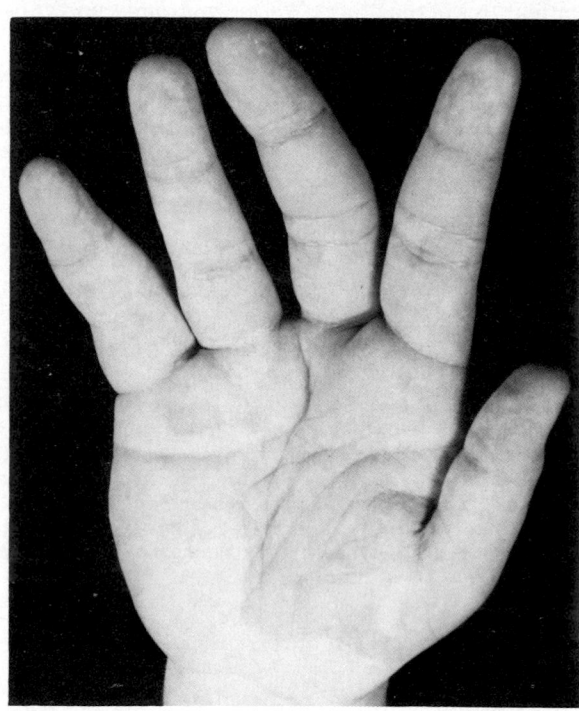

133. Hand in angio-osteohypertrophy. Note macrodactyly associated with hemangioma

ANHIDROSIS

Includes: Anhydrose
Anhydrose
Simple anhidrosis
Congenital anhidrosis
Familial anhidrosis

Excludes: Ectodermal dysplasia, anhidrotic (333)
Congenital familial anhidrosis and neurolabyrinthitis

Minimal Diagnostic Criteria: Inability to tolerate heat, skin biopsy of the anterior axilla showing absence of sweat glands, no other associated abnormalities.

Clinical Findings: There have been 3 clinically very similar cases all recorded in 1 Iranian family. Inability to tolerate exposure to heat (ie become markedly flushed, uncomfortable, restless and frightened; drinking vast quantities of water with only slight relief). Dry skin with thickened palms and soles but no other clinical abnormality. Biopsy of skin (in anterior axilla) reveals complete absence of sweat glands. Urinalysis, whole blood count and chest xray within normal limits. Test for presence of electrolytes in a filter paper attached to the skin during a heating experiment revealed no activity.

Complications
I   **Derived:**   ?
II **Associated:**   ?

Etiology: Probably autosomal recessive; McK *20660

Pathogenesis: ?

Related Facts
I   **Sex Ratio:**   ? M1:F1 probably; (2 males and 1 female to date)
II   **Risk of Occurrence:**   ? Very rare
III **Risk of Recurrence for**
     Patient's Sib: If autosomal recessive, 1 in 4 (25%) for each offspring to be affected.
     Patient's Child: Not increased unless mate is carrier or homozygote.
IV   **Age of Detectability:**   Infancy
V   **Prevalence:**   ? Very rare, identified in only 1 Iranian family.

Treatment
I   **Primary Prevention:**   Genetic counseling
II   **Secondary Prevention:**   Avoidance of exposure to extreme heat
III **Other Therapy:**   —

Prognosis: ?

Detection of Carrier: ?

Special Considerations: —

References:
Mahloudji, M. and Livingston, K.E.: Familial and congenital simple anhidrosis. Am. J. Dis. Child. 113:477, 1967.

Contributor: **Bert C. Frichot, III**

Editor's Computerized Descriptor: Skin

ANIRIDIA

Includes: Aniridie
Simple iris coloboma
Hypoplasia of iris with rudimentary root†

Excludes: Ocular colobomas (733)
Wilms tumor-aniridia syndrome

Minimal Diagnostic Criteria: Congenital absence of all or part of iris

Clinical Findings: In aniridia a rudimentary stump of iris, often visible only on slit-lamp examination, is usually present at birth. The anomaly is generally bilateral (50:1). On examination the pupil is large and the lens edge, zonules and ciliary body may be visible. Photophobia, poor vision and nystagmus are very common, frequencies over 50%. Cataracts are said to be present in about 66% of cases. A secondary glaucoma due to structural angle changes is frequently seen. Structural deformities of the cornea and progressive opacification are frequently present.

Complications
I   **Derived:**   Glaucoma (54/122 in one series)
II **Associated:**   Microphthalmia, ectopia lentis, coloboma of lens and choroid, persistence of pupillary membrane.†

Etiology: Autosomal dominant with about 85% penetrance. Heterogeneity exists. Care must be taken to distinguish this disorder from sporadic cases of aniridia associated with Wilms tumor, hemiatrophy, GU tract anomalies, mental retardation and skeletal malformations. Only one familial case of aniridia with Wilms tumor has been reported. McK *10620

Pathogenesis: Two of the theories suggested are defective neural ectoderm development and aberrant or persistent vascular mesoderm of the lens tunica vasculosa at the anterior optic cup preventing the normal growth of the iris. These have not been documented.

Related Facts
I   **Sex Ratio:**   M1:F1
II   **Risk of Occurrence:**   —
III **Risk of Recurrence for**
     Patient's Sib: If parent is affected <1 in 2 (<50%) for each offspring to be affected; otherwise not increased. (In one series the ratio was 38:62 affected to normal children in segregating sibships).
     Patient's Child: <1 in 2
IV   **Age of Detectability:**   Usually at birth
V   **Prevalence:**   1 in 100,000 to 1 in 200,000

Treatment
I   **Primary Prevention:**   Genetic counseling
II   **Secondary Prevention:**   Cataract extraction and glaucoma therapy as indicated; some evidence for the beneficial use of artificial pupil contact lenses.
III **Other Therapy:**   All sporadic cases should have evaluation for Wilms tumor and other malformations.

Prognosis: Life span and intelligence normal; ocular prognosis poor

Detection of Carrier: —

†Special Considerations: Simple or atypical iris colobomas (not embryonic fissure derived) are very common congenital abnormalities that occur in all sectors of the iris, complete or incomplete, total or partial. These are also autosomal dominant. The theories of formation are the same as those for aniridia.

Six cases of aniridia among 440 patients with Wilms tumor emphasize this recently described association. Two of the children had residual iris tags visible on external examination, 4 had cataract and 1 glaucoma. Ear deformities were present in 3. None had a parent with aniridia. Nonocular associated defects are more common in those patients with aniridia and Wilms tumor.

References:

Duke-Elder, S.: System of Ophthalmology, vol. 3, part 2. Congenital Deformities. London: Henry Kimpton, 1964, p. 566.

Fraumeni, J.F., Jr.: The aniridia - Wilms' tumor syndrome. In Bergsma, D. (ed.): Part II. Malformation Syndromes. Birth Defects: Orig. Art. Ser. vol. V, no. 2. New York: The National Foundation-March of Dimes, 1969, pp. 198-201.

Miller, R.W. et al: Association of Wilms' tumor with aniridia, hemihypertrophy and other congenital malformations. N. Engl. J. Med. 270:922, 1964.

Shaw, M.W. et al: Congenital aniridia. Am. J. Hum. Genet. 12:389, 1960.

Contributor: **Harold E. Cross**

Editor's Computerized Descriptors: Vision, Eye
Also see Section I, Fig. 59

ANISOCORIA

Includes: Anisocorie
Anisokorie

Excludes: Acquired anisocoria

Minimal Diagnostic Criteria: Pupillary inequality greater than 20%

Clinical Findings: Defining the upper limit of normal pupillary inequality at 20%, then 2% of the population have anisocoria ranging from .5 to 2.0 mm.

Complications
I   **Derived:** —
II   **Associated:** —

Etiology: Heterogeneity exists. Possibly sometimes autosomal dominant. Other disorders such as Rieger syndrome, iris atrophy and stromal hypoplasia must be excluded as causes.

Pathogenesis: ?

Related Facts
I   **Sex Ratio:** Ml:Fl
II   **Risk of Occurrence:** 1 in 50 live births
III   **Risk of Recurrence for**
     Patient's Sib: When autosomal dominant if parent is affected 1 in 2 (50%) for each offspring to be affected; otherwise not increased
     Patient's Child: When autosomal dominant 1 in 2
IV   **Age of Detectability:** Childhood
V   **Prevalence:** 1 in 50

Treatment
I   **Primary Prevention:** Genetic counseling when autosomal dominant
II   **Secondary Prevention:** —
III   **Other Therapy:** —

Prognosis: Normal for life span and intelligence. Visual prognosis good.

Detection of Carrier: —

Special Considerations: —

References:

Duke-Elder, S.: System of Ophthalmology, vol. 3, part 2. Congenital Deformities. London: Henry Kimpton, 1964, p. 592.

Contributor: **Harold E. Cross**

Editor's Computerized Descriptor: Eye

59
ANISOMETROPIA

Includes: Anisométropie
Myopia unilateral
Bilateral myopia with marked difference between eyes
Unilateral hyperopia
Bilateral hyperopia with marked difference between eyes

Excludes: Keratoconus (552)
Unilateral microphthalmos
Tumors distorting shape of eyeball
Unilateral refractive error secondary to disease†
Unilateral aphakia

Minimal Diagnostic Criteria: It is difficult to set a functional lower limit on the refractive difference between a pair of eyes which is significant, because patients vary tremendously in their awareness of symptoms. Corneal, lenticular and neoplastic factors mentioned below should be excluded.

Clinical Findings: A difference of greater than 2 or 3 diopters in the spheric refraction of a patient's eyes. Usually the corneal curvature and lenses are identical but the axial length of 1 eye is greater than the other. Patients often complain of visual fatigue and perception of tilting of space. The condition is most frequent in myopic individuals and may be progressive.

Complications
I **Derived:** Aniseikonia. (Unequal retinal images in the 2 eyes.) Asthenopia. (Visual fatigue) Amblyopia and strabismus secondary to suppression to eliminate the symptoms. Pathologic retinal and optic disk changes of severe high myopia.
II **Associated:** —

Etiology: The specific etiology is unknown in most cases. Examples of apparent autosomal dominant and autosomal recessive inheritance of anisometropia in families have been reported. High myopia per se is usually inherited as an autosomal recessive. The evidence is in favor of an inherited multifactorial etiology for severe (pathologic) myopia which progresses with age, particularly during the growing years. Some observers feel, however, that close work influences progression of myopia. Dietary deficiencies or collagen disorders may influence some cases.

Pathogenesis: The specific pathogenesis is unknown. Structural weakness of the sclera may be a significant mechanical cause. The degree of expression of any inherited and environmental influences on axial length of the eye is obviously greater on 1 side than the other when anisometropia occurs. Embryologically, the sclera is formed about the posterior optic vesicle (where abnormal lengthening occurs) very late in development.

Related Facts
I **Sex Ratio:** Ml:Fl
II **Risk of Occurrence:** ? Considered uncommon, not rare.
III **Risk of Recurrence for**
   Patient's Sib: When autosomal recessive or autosomal dominant, see Table I AR or AD, respectively.
   Patient's Child: When autosomal recessive or autosomal dominant, see Table I AR or AD, respectively.
IV **Age of Detectability:** During the 1st month of life by objective refraction if suspected, but most go undetected for years or arise later.
V **Prevalence:** ?

Treatment
I **Primary Prevention:** Genetic counseling
II **Secondary Prevention:** Appropriate spectacle correction decreases symptoms and, if instituted early enough, helps to prevent amblyopia. Amblyopia per se should be treated early.
III **Other Therapy:** Special procedures are occasionally warranted to control retinal damage in severe myopia.

Prognosis: Varies with age of onset, severity of myopia, severity of anisometropia and severity of symptoms.

Detection of Carrier: ? However, it should be noted that high myopia per se is hereditary.

†Special Considerations: The conditions listed as exclusions do, of course, frequently cause anisometropia by definition. They have been excluded because they are etiologically unrelated and usually easily identifiable.

References:
François, J.: Refraction errors. In Heredity in Ophthalmology. St. Louis: C.V. Mosby Co., 1961, p. 186.
Nordlöw, W.: Anisometropia, induced aniseikonia and estimated correction with iseikonic lenses in four-year-olds. Acta Ophthalmol. 48:959, 1970.
Waardenburg, P.J. et al: Genetics in Ophthalmology. Oxford: Blackwell Scientific Publications, Ltd., 1961, vol. 2. p. 1261.

Contributor: **Donald R. Bergsma**

Editor's Computerized Descriptors: Vision, Eye, Nerve

ANKYLOBLEPHARON

Includes: Ankyloblépharie
Anquiloblefarón
Internal ankyloblepharon
External ankyloblepharon
Ankyloblepharon filiforme adnatum
Eyelid fusion

Excludes: —

Minimal Diagnostic Criteria: Partial adhesion of the ciliary edges of the eyelids.

Clinical Findings: Ankyloblepharon is a condition in which the lid margins are variably fused. Internal ankyloblepharon is characterized by failure of separation of the lid borders medially thereby shortening the interpalpebral fissure. In external ankyloblepharon the lid fusion is at the lateral canthus. Ankyloblepharon filiforme adnatum consists of one or more stretchable bands of tissue which connect the upper and lower edges of the lids at the grey line restricting the opening of the interpalpebral fissure. These strands are composed of fibrovascular connective tissue surrounded by epithelium without inflammatory alteration. Sebaceous glands and hair follicles may also be found within them.

Complications
I **Derived:** —
II **Associated:** Cleft palate, harelip, anophthalmia, microphthalmia, ptosis, microcephaly, patent ductus arteriosus, lower lip fistula, interventricular septal defect, syndactyly, ear anomalies and Waardenburg syndrome

Etiology: Autosomal dominant transmission has been noted in some instances of ankyloblepharon. Autosomal recessive transmission is suggested in Khanna's report of ankyloblepharon filiforme adnatum although most cases are seen sporadically.

Pathogenesis: Believed to arise from aberration of mesodermal or ectodermal origin during lid fusion. Theories of intrauterine inflammation or trauma from fingernails have been refuted.

Related Facts
I **Sex Ratio:** Ml:Fl
II **Risk of Occurrence:** Rare
III **Risk of Recurrence for**
  Patient's Sib: When autosomal dominant or autosomal recessive, see Table I AD or AR, respectively.
  Patient's Child: When autosomal dominant or autosomal recessive, see Table I AD or AR, respectively.
IV **Age of Detectability:** At birth
V **Prevalence:** Rare

Treatment
I **Primary Prevention:** Genetic counseling
II **Secondary Prevention:** The shortened interpalpebral fissure can be lengthened by plastic surgery of the fused canthal areas. This is seldom necessary, unless extreme, since the cosmetic appearance tends to improve with age. The adhesions in ankyloblepharon filiforme adnatum may be broken with a muscle hook if thin and narrow. Broader and thicker bands are excised with scissors.
III **Other Therapy:** —

Prognosis: No deterrent to health or function

Detection of Carrier: —

Special Considerations: —

References:
Gorlin, R. J. and Červenka, J.: Syndromes of facial clefting. Scand. J. Plast. Reconstr. Surg. 8:13-25, 1974.

Khanna, V. D.: Ankyloblepharon filiforme adnatum. Am. J. Ophthalmol. 43:774, 1957.
Long, J. C. and Blandford, S. E.: Ankyloblepharon filiforme adnatum with cleft lip and palate. Am. J. Ophthalmol. 53:126, 1962.
Sood, N. N. et al: Ankyloblepharon filiforme adnatum with cleft lip and palate. J. Pediatr. Ophthalmol. 5:30, 1968.

Contributor: **Elsa K. Rahn**

Editor's Computerized Descriptor: Eye

ANKYLOGLOSSIA

Includes: Ankyloglossie
Anquiloglosia
Tongue-tie

Excludes: Hanhart syndrome (451)

Minimal Diagnostic Criteria: Tongue movement is restricted so that with the mouth opened to its fullest extent, effort to raise the tongue tip fails to bring it above the level of a line between the commissures of the mouth. Upon forward protrusive effort the tip of the tongue demonstrates a central groove.

Clinical Findings: A variation of the lingual frenum resulting in an elevated and short band-like structure adherent at a higher than normal position of attachment on the alveolar ridge behind the central incisors causing a restriction of elevation and protrusion of tongue.

Complications
I   **Derived:** Some varieties may produce spacing of mandibular central incisors, periodontal disease, and some limitations in cleansing excursions of the tongue. There is no interference with infant nursing or later masticatory functions. If any disorder in speech is produced by ankyloglossia, it is extremely minor.
II **Associated:** —

Etiology: ? Evidence suggests autosomal dominant mode of inheritance although further data are needed for support.

Pathogenesis: A developmental variation in the lingual frenum of the tongue such that the fibrous band of the midline raphe of the tongue, which anteriorly forms the lingual frenum, attaches anteriorly to tongue tip and high onto the alveolar process.

Related Facts
I   **Sex Ratio:** M1:F1
II **Risk of Occurrence:** 1 in 330
III **Risk of Recurrence for**
    Patient's Sib: ?
    Patient's Child: ?
IV **Age of Detectability:** At birth
V   **Prevalence:** 1 in 330 (approximate)

Treatment
I   **Primary Prevention:** —
II **Secondary Prevention:** Frenulotomy†
III **Other Therapy:** —

Prognosis: Excellent

Detection of Carrier: —

†Special Considerations: Principal motivation for surgical removal should be based upon associated dental disorders or dental prosthetic needs. Speech benefits for articulatory movements should not be overestimated since the role is probably not significant. Under special considerations of musical wind instrument players, there may be further indication for surgical release.

References:
Block, J.R.: The role of the speech clinician in determining indications for frenulotomy in cases of ankyloglossia. NY State Dent. J. 34:479, 1968.
McEnery, E.T. and Gaines, F.P.: Tongue-tie in infants and children. J. Pediatr. 18:252, 1941.
Witkop, C.J., Jr. and Barros, L.: Oral and genetic studies of Chileans, 1960. I. Oral anomalies. Am. J. Phys. Anthropol. 21:15, 1963.

Contributor: **James R. Hayward**

Editor's Computerized Descriptor: Oral

ANNULAR PANCREAS

Includes: Pancreas annulaire
Pankreas annulare
Páncreas anular
Pancreas, annular
Malrotation of pancreas

Excludes: Duodenal atresia or stenosis (300)

Minimal Diagnostic Criteria: Intestinal obstruction, "double bubble" gas pattern by xray, ultimately collar of pancreas surrounding duodenum at laparotomy.

Clinical Findings: All grades of obstruction from complete duodenal obstruction in neonate, associated with maternal hyperhydramnios with bile-stained vomiting, to intermittent vomiting and failure to thrive. Nonobstructing forms may be found at operation or autopsy without symptoms.†

Complications
I   **Derived:** Defective pancreatic drainage with pancreatitis later in life, occasional stasis ulcer of duodenum with perforation into annular pancreas, failure to thrive secondary to occasional vomiting.
II **Associated:** Chromosome 21 trisomy—20-30%; other remote anomalies in 40-50% of cases (Rickham).

Etiology: ?

Pathogenesis: Several versions of basic incomplete rotation of dorsal and ventral anlage of pancreas so that portions of pancreas remain on both sides of the 2nd duodenum. Exact mode of formation of defect not known; perhaps several different variations of rotation may cause some resultant annular rings of pancreas and various diagnoses of obstruction.

Related Facts
I   **Sex Ratio:** M?:F?
II **Risk of Occurrence:** 1 in 10,000 live births
III **Risk of Recurrence for**
    Patient's Sib: ?
    Patient's Child: ?
IV **Age of Detectability:** Any age from birth on where symptomatic
V   **Prevalence:** ?

Treatment
I   **Primary Prevention:** —
II **Secondary Prevention:** Generally duodenojejunostomy or duodenoduodenostomy should be performed. Cutting pancreatic substance is dangerous in causing pancreatic fistula and not relieving permanent stenosis.
III **Other Therapy:** —

Prognosis: Excellent for relief of obstruction. Normal life expectancy except for rare pancreatitis or biliary tract disease in later life.

Detection of Carrier: —

†Special Considerations: Vomiting may not be bile-stained when obstruction is preampullary. Differential diagnosis then must include pyloric stenosis, or with "double bubble" appearance by xray, biliary atresia before jaundice appears.

References:
Rickham, P.P.: Duodenal atresia and stenosis; annular pancreas. In Rickham, P.P. and Johnston, J.H. (eds.): Neonatal Surgery. New York: Appleton-Century-Crofts, 1969. p. 286.

Contributor: **Lawrence K. Pickett**

Editor's Computerized Descriptor: GI.

ANOMALOUS ORIGIN OF CONTRALATERAL SUBCLAVIAN ARTERY

Includes: Origine contra-latérale de l'artère sous-clavière
Atypischer Abgang der aa. subclaviae
Origen contralateral de las arterias subclavias
Anomalous origin of left subclavian artery from right aortic arch
Anomalous origin of right subclavian artery from left aortic arch
Subclavian artery, anomalous origin of contralateral

Excludes: Isolation of subclavian artery from aorta (546)
Common origin of ipsilateral (to arch) common carotid and subclavian artery

Minimal Diagnostic Criteria: An esophagram in the PA, lateral and both oblique views is necessary to suspect the anomalous vessel. However, an aortic root aortogram may be necessary to demonstrate associated anomalies in the symptomatic case.

Clinical Findings: The anomaly, regardless of side, is usually an incidental finding on barium esophagram, on angiocardiography, during cardiac surgery for other anomalies or at autopsy. Occasionally, the anomalous vessel will be related to dysphagia. In the case of the anomalous left subclavian artery with a right aortic arch, this is commonly associated with a left ductus arteriosus or ligamentum arteriosus which completes a true vascular ring. In the case of anomalous right subclavian artery with a left aortic arch, recent evidence has related the symptomatic cases to associated anomalous origin of the carotid vessels. This is either an unusual closeness of their origins from the arch, or even a true common origin. This anomalous origin of the carotids creates an anterior sling which prevents the trachea and esophagus from bending away from the posterior compression of the anomalous right subclavian artery. This combined anomaly occasionally also causes tracheal compression and resultant respiratory symptoms.

For either the anomalous right or left subclavian artery, barium esophagram demonstrates a posterior and sharp oblique (running cephalad to the side contralateral to the arch) indentation in the esophagus. An aortic root angiocardiogram will confirm this anomaly.

Complications
I   Derived: Rarely, dysphagia will occur. Minimal dysphagia or stridor occurs more often, but considering the frequency of the defect, this is still a rare occurrence.
II Associated: Contralateral origin of the right subclavian artery is frequently found with other congenital heart defects, especially tetralogy of Fallot and coarctation of the aorta. It is also found quite often in chromosome 21 trisomy.†

Etiology: ?

Pathogenesis: The contralateral origin of the subclavian artery results from the early obliteration of the contralateral embryonic 4th arch and the corresponding distal dorsal aorta is retained to form the 1st part of the anomalous vessel. This explains why such a subclavian artery passes behind the esophagus.

Related Facts
I   Sex Ratio: M1:F1
II   Risk of Occurrence: ? Anomalous origin of contralateral right subclavian artery occurs in approximately 1 in 200 live births. Anomalous origin of contralateral left subclavian artery occurs in approximately 1 in 5000 to 1 in 6000 live births. Right aortic arch occurs in approximately 1 in 2500 live births.
III Risk of Recurrence for
    Patient's Sib: ?
    Patient's Child: ?
IV   Age of Detectability: If symptomatic, usually found during infancy, otherwise detectable at any age or at necropsy.

V   Prevalence: Anomalous origin of right subclavian artery with left aortic arch < 1 in 2000 persons of all studied populations. Isolated right arch is probably < 1 in 2500 persons. However, most of these without heart defects have contralateral origin of left subclavian artery, ie 40-50%. Anomalous origin of left subclavian with right aortic arch in approximately 1 in 5000 to 1 in 6000.

Treatment
I   Primary Prevention: ?
II Secondary Prevention: ?
III Other Therapy: Usually none required. Occasionally (rarely), a division of the right subclavian or of the left ligamentum with anomalous left subclavian will be necessary to relieve dysphagia. It is important to note the presence of the contralateral origin of the subclavian prior to cardiac catheterization or when associated with other congenital heart lesions, particularly when a subclavian to pulmonary artery shunt is under consideration. Use of such an anomalous left subclavian artery to left pulmonary artery anastomosis with a right aortic arch would produce a vascular ring.

Prognosis: The anomaly is compatible with normal life expectancy in the great majority of cases. Death, when it occurs, is either nonrelated or secondary to associated congenital heart disease.

Detection of Carrier: —

†Special Considerations: Right aortic arch has high correlation with certain congenital heart defects, especially tetralogy of Fallot, truncus arteriosus and, less frequently, tricuspid atresia. On the other hand, many patients with a right aortic arch and anomalous origin of left subclavian artery do not have other congenital heart defects.

References:

Klinkhamer, A.C.: Aberrant right subclavian artery (clinical and roentgenologic aspects). Am. J. Roentgen. Radium Ther. Nucl. Med. 97:438, 1966.
Stewart, J.R. et al: An Atlas of Vascular Rings and Related Malformations of the Aortic Arch System. Springfield: Charles C Thomas, 1964.
Stewart, J.R. et al: Right aortic arch: Plain film diagnosis and significance. Am. J. Roentgen. Radium Ther. Nucl. Med. 97:377, 1966.

Contributors: **Charles E. Mullins**
                      Dan G. McNamara

Editor's Computerized Descriptors: GI., CV.

ANOMALOUS ORIGIN OF CORONARY ARTERIES FROM PULMONARY ARTERY

Includes: Origine anormale des coronaires naissant de l'artère pulmonaire
Atypischer Ursprung der Koronararterien aus der Pulmonararterie
Origen anormal de las coronarias en la arteria pulmonar
Anomalous origin of left coronary artery from pulmonary artery
Anomalous origin of right coronary artery from pulmonary artery
Anomalous origin of both coronary arteries from pulmonary artery
Coronary arteries, anomalous origin from pulmonary artery

Excludes: Coronary arteriovenous fistula (218)
Coronary artery, single (219)

Minimal Diagnostic Criteria: Aortic root angiography is diagnostic and is the procedure of choice to confirm the diagnosis and to differentiate anomalous left coronary artery from endocardial fibroelastosis, myocarditis, glycogen storage disease, congenital mitral insufficiency, and cardiomyopathy of unknown cause.

Clinical Findings: *Anomalous origin of the left coronary artery from the pulmonary artery:* This lesion is characterized by a normal right coronary artery arising from the aorta, while the left coronary artery arises wholly from the pulmonary trunk. There is no intrauterine disturbance of myocardial blood supply since pulmonary artery and aortic pressures, as well as oxygen contents, are similar. With the normal drop in pulmonary vascular resistance after birth, however, perfusion pressure in the left coronary artery will become insufficient for antegrade flow. As a consequence of this decrease in pulmonary artery pressure, perfusion of the myocardium supplied by the left coronary artery will be dependent on adequate anastomoses between the right and left coronary arteries. Thus the left coronary artery can be filled retrogradely and the direction of the blood flow will then be out into the pulmonary artery. The presence or absence of symptoms or signs of this defect then will be related to the adequacy of myocardial perfusion which in turn will be related to intercoronary anastomoses, intracoronary vascular resistance, aortic pressure, pulmonary pressure and cardiac metabolic demands.

The majority of patients will present with symptoms during the first 6 months of life. The typical history is one of gradually increasing irritability, sweating, tachypnea, dyspnea and excessive crying as if in pain. The onset of these symptoms has been reported as early as the 1st month of life. A small number of children will present after infancy with only mild symptoms of exercise intolerance. Asymptomatic adults have been reported and may comprise 10-15% of patients with this lesion.

Physical examination in the sick infant will reveal signs of congestive heart failure. Cardiac examination generally reveals cardiomegaly and a prominent third sound. Mitral insufficiency is a common finding in infants as well as older children. Older children and adults may have diastolic or continuous murmurs.

Cardiac roentgenograms usually show severe left ventricular enlargement with a small aorta. The left atrium may be normal in size unless there is mitral insufficiency. Signs of pulmonary venous congestion of the lungs are almost invariably present. The ECG is the key to the diagnosis and classically shows signs of anterolateral myocardial infarction with broad deep Q waves in I, aVL and left precordial leads. In addition there may be decreased anterior-lateral QRS forces with poor progression of R wave with ST elevation or T wave inversion over the left precordium. The pattern of anteroseptal infarction with Q in V$_5$ greater than Q in V$_6$ has also been reported as well as a reversed Q loop. In addition, criteria for left ventricular hypertrophy generally are present.

Cardiac catheterization usually fails to reveal oximetry evidence of a left-to-right shunt in infants but may do so in adults. Left ventricular end diastolic pressure is elevated and left ventricular angiocardiography reveals a poorly contracting ventricle. Mitral insufficiency will be evident in many patients. Pulmonary artery angiography may reveal transient filling of the proximal part of the anomalous vessel. Aortic root angiography is diagnostic and reveals a single right coronary artery arising from the aorta and usually sequential retrograde filling of the left coronary and pulmonary artery. Rarely, patients with sparse collaterals fail to show this retrograde filling, and these infants generally have the most severe symptoms.

Anomalous origin of the right coronary artery from the pulmonary artery: This lesion has been discovered as an incidental finding at surgery or autopsy, and there have been no cases reported with symptoms related to its presence. The vessel frequently is thin walled and suggestive evidence of retrograde flow has been shown in 1 case at surgery. Physical examination, roentgenogram and ECG are generally normal.

Anomalous origin of both coronary arteries from the pulmonary artery: This lesion is felt to be incompatible with life after pulmonary artery pressure declines postnatally. Eight patients have been reported with age at death ranging from 8 hours-10 days.

The coronary origin cannot be imaged by M-mode echocardiography. Echocardiographic findings are of infarction. These include dilatation of the left ventricle with areas of akinesis or dyskinesis. Since the problem is frequently a segmental one, two-dimensional high resolution examination is required in most instances to image these abnormalities.

Symptoms include early onset of congestive failure of increasing severity with marked cardiomegaly. Murmurs have not been reported and an ECG has not been recorded in an infant with this lesion.

Complications
I Derived: Anomalous left coronary artery—myocardial ischemia and infarction, papillary muscle dysfunction, mitral insufficiency and congestive heart failure. Anomalous right coronary artery—none known. Anomalous origin of both coronaries—progressive myocardial ischemia, congestive heart failure and death.
II Associated: Anomalous left coronary artery—none known. Anomalous right coronary artery—insufficient number of cases to establish. Anomalous origin of both coronaries—insufficient number of cases to establish.

Etiology: ?

Pathogenesis: Unknown, but 2 theories have been proposed. The first states that either the truncus arteriosus is abnormally divided so that one or both coronary anlagen are included in the pulmonary artery or that a coronary bud arises in an anomalous position from a part of the truncus which will become the pulmonary artery. An alternate theory proposes that there are 6 coronary anlagen from the truncus, each of which is related to a portion which will become an aortic or pulmonary sinus of Valsalva. Normally all but 2 anlagen involute but variations in involution and persistence of such anlagen could explain the known anomalous origins of coronary arteries.

Related Facts

I **Sex Ratio:** Anomalous left coronary artery—M1:F1; anomalous right coronary artery—not established; anomalous origin of both coronaries—not established (M1:F1 in 8 cases).

II **Risk of Occurrence:** Anomalous left coronary artery <3 in 1000 cases of congenital heart disease; anomalous right coronary artery—not established; anomalous origin both coronaries—exceedingly rare.

III **Risk of Recurrence for**
Patient's Sib: None reported
Patient's Child: None reported

IV **Age of Detectability:** Anomalous left coronary is detectable from birth by aortic root angiography: As soon as pulmonary vascular resistance falls, retrograde filling of the left coronary may be evident (normally by 1-3 months); anomalous right coronary artery—detectable from birth by proximal aortography; anomalous origin of both coronaries—from birth by selective pulmonary arteriogram.

V **Prevalence:** ?

Treatment
I **Primary Prevention:** —
II **Secondary Prevention:** Anomalous left coronary artery—some groups advocate surgical ligation of left coronary artery in infancy when catheterization data indicate coronary flow into the pulmonary artery. Others feel that surgery should be avoided in infancy; but if deemed necessary by the infant's clinical course, an attempt at reconstruction of a 2-coronary artery system is preferable to ligation. Anomalous right coronary artery—surgery probably not indicated in asymptomatic patients. Ligation has been performed in a patient with retrograde flow. Alternate therapy as above; anomalous origin of both coronaries—surgery has not been attempted. Theoretic considerations include prosthetic or venous graft for anastomosis of one or both vessels to the aorta in early infancy.

III **Other Therapy:** —

Prognosis: Prognosis in general is very poor in patients with anomalous left coronary artery, a few infants survive with or without medical management to an age when reconstruction of a 2-coronary artery system can be accomplished.

The long-term prognosis of associated mitral insufficiency is unknown. In older children and adults with minimal symptoms, prognosis is good. Anomalous right coronary artery—excellent untreated; anomalous origin of both coronaries—uniformly fatal in infancy.

Detection of Carrier: —

Special Considerations: —

References:
Corya, B.C. et al: Echocardiographic examination of the anterior left ventricular wall in patients with coronary artery disease. Am. J. Cardiol. 33:132, 1974.
Nora, J.J. and McNamara, D.C.: Anomalies of the coronary arteries and coronary artery fistula. In Watson, H. (ed.): Paediatric Cardiology. St. Louis: C.V. Mosby, 1968, p. 295.
Roberts, W.C.: Anomalous origin of both coronary arteries from the pulmonary artery. Am. J. Cardiol. 10:595, 1962.
Sabiston, D.C.,Jr. et al: The direction of blood flow in anomalous left coronary artery arising from the pulmonary artery. Circulation 22:591, 1960.
Wesselhoeft, H. et al: Anomalous origin of the left coronary artery from the pulmonary trunk. Circulation 38:403, 1968.

Contributor: **Thomas P. Graham, Jr.**

Editor's Computerized Descriptors: CV., Resp.

ANONYCHIA AND ECTRODACTYLY

Includes: Anonychie avec ectrodactylie
Anonychie mit Ektrodaktylie
Anoniquia y ectrodactilia
Ectrodactyly and anonychia

Excludes: Anonychia, hereditary (66)
Nail-patella syndrome (704)
Anonychia with congenital localized absence of skin and blistering of skin and mucous membranes

Minimal Diagnostic Criteria: Characteristic anonychia and digital abnormalities. See below.

Clinical Findings: Characterized by nail anomalies-usually complete absence of nail and nail bed with index and middle fingers commonly affected. Thumb nail often present only on the proximal, lateral corners of the nail fold; radial half of the ring fingernail usually absent; little fingernail usually normal; toe anonychia parallels the anonychia in corresponding fingers.

The nail anomaly is usually present from birth, non-progressive and symmetric digitally.

Digital anomalies occur in about one-third of the affected individuals. They are nearly always asymmetric and often restricted to 1 hand or 1 foot. The digital anomalies are bizarre including absence of 1 or more digits, absence of corresponding metacarpal bones, syndactyly or polydactyly.

Complications
I **Derived:** —
II **Associated:** —

Etiology: Autosomal dominant (nonallelism of this syndrome and nail-patella genes)† McK *10690

Pathogenesis: ?

Related Facts
I **Sex Ratio:** M1:F1
II **Risk of Occurrence:** Very rare
III **Risk of Recurrence for**
Patient's Sib: If parent is affected 1 in 2 (50%) for each offspring to be affected; otherwise not increased
Patient's Child: 1 in 2
IV **Age of Detectability:** At birth
V **Prevalence:** Very rare

Treatment
I **Primary Prevention:** Genetic counseling
II **Secondary Prevention:** —
III **Other Therapy:** Occupational and physical therapy (appliances, etc) as needed

Prognosis: Does not appear to affect normal life span

Detection of Carrier: —

†**Special Considerations:** Gene for this trait may be linked with that for the Lutheran Blood Group.

References:
Lees, D.H. et al: Anonychia with ectrodactyly. Ann. Hum. Genet. 22:69, 1957.

Contributor: **Nyles R. Eskritt**

Editor's Computerized Descriptors: Nails, Skel.

ANONYCHIA, HEREDITARY

Includes: Anonychie héréditaire
Hereditäre Anonychie
Anoniquia hereditaria
Anonychia
Congenital absence of nails
Anonychia totalis congenital
Hereditary onychial dysplasia
Nail absent

Excludes: Nail-patella syndrome (704)
Anonychia and ectrodactyly (65)
Localized absence of skin, blistering and nail abnormalities (609)

Minimal Diagnostic Criteria: Partial or total absence of nails

Clinical Findings: Characterized by various abnormalities of finger or toenails and phalanges including complete absence of nail, rudimentary nail matrix at proximal or lateral edge of nail bed, large pointed lunulae, longitudinal furrowing, thinning or thickening of nail plate. Usually symmetric. May be present at birth or develop at a later age. Nail beds are present. X-ray studies occasionally show tapering and spatulation of distal phalanges and shortening of phalanges and metacarpal bones.

Complications
I   **Derived:** —
II   **Associated:** —

Etiology: Both autosomal dominant and autosomal recessive inheritance have been reported. McK *20680

Pathogenesis: ?

Related Facts
I   **Sex Ratio:** ?
II   **Risk of Occurrence:** Very rare
III   **Risk of Recurrence for**
   Patient's Sib: When autosomal dominant or autosomal recessive, see Table I AD or AR, respectively
   Patient's Child: When autosomal dominant or autosomal recessive, see Table I AD or AR, respectively
IV   **Age of Detectability:** At birth or later
V   **Prevalence:** ?

Treatment
I   **Primary Prevention:** Genetic counseling
II   **Secondary Prevention:** —
III   **Other Therapy:** —

Prognosis: No effect on average life span or intelligence

Detection of Carrier: ?

Special Considerations: —

References:
Hobbs, M.D.: Hereditary onychial dysplasia. Am. J. Med. Sci. 190:200, 1935.
Littman, A. and Levin, S.: Anonychia as a recessive autosomal trait in man. J. Invest. Dermatol. 42:177, 1964.
Strandskov, H.H.: Inheritance of absence of thumb nails. J. Hered. 30:53, 1939.

Contributor: **Nyles R. Eskritt**

Editor's Computerized Descriptors: Nails, Skel.

ANOPHTHALMIA

Includes: Anophtalmie
Anophthalmie
Anoftalmia
True or primary anophthalmos
Clinical anophthalmia
Eye absent

Excludes: Severe microphthalmia
Secondary anophthalmia
Degenerative or consecutive anophthalmia
Surgical anophthalmia

Minimal Diagnostic Criteria: Anophthalmia is clinically suspected and is diagnostically confirmed microscopically.

Clinical Findings: Anophthalmia, strictly speaking, means the total absence of eye tissue. This is rare. It occurs if there is complete failure of formation of the primary optic vesicle in which case it is called a true or primary anophthalmia. It is usually bilateral. Only upon histologic examination of the entire orbital contents can the absence of all ocular tissue be ascertained.

The ocular adnexa are usually present, structurally intact, but smaller than normal. Tears are produced upon crying from functionally normal lacrimal glands. The orbit is shallow and lined with conjunctiva. The ophthalmic artery is the only structure ordinarily observed to course through the underdeveloped optic foramen.

Complications
I   **Derived:** —
II   **Associated:** Chromosomal aberrations (eg chromosome 13 trisomy syndrome), developmental disturbances including absence of the lower optic pathways and lacrimal puncta, ankyloblepharon, microphthalmia of opposite eye, malformations of the brain, face and limbs, posterior orbital encephalocele, and congenital cyst of the orbit; also seen in the Villaret, Weyers-Thier oculovertebral and Klinefelter syndromes.

Etiology: Autosomal recessive. In conjunction with other defects it can be transmitted as an autosomal dominant, X-linked recessive, or found sporadically with a chromosomal aberration. McK *20690

Pathogenesis: Ectodermal elements of the eye are missing; minute traces of mesodermal elements may be present. Lack of differentiation of the optic plate following the development of the rudimentary forebrain which results in failure of formation of the optic vesicle. One theory postulates pressure upon the head of the embryo by thickened amnion with suppression of growth of the optic vesicles.

Related Facts
I   **Sex Ratio:** M1:F1
II   **Risk of Occurrence:** Rare
III   **Risk of Recurrence for**
   Patient's Sib: If isolated defect, 1 in 4 (25%) for each offspring to be affected.
   Patient's Child: Not increased unless mate is a heterozygote.
IV   **Age of Detectability:** At birth
V   **Prevalence:** Rare

Treatment
I   **Primary Prevention:** Genetic counseling
II   **Secondary Prevention:** —
III   **Other Therapy:** Cosmetic improvement through progressive dilatation of the orbit by successive implants of increasingly larger size during the period of rapid growth for proper development and for maintenance of a prosthesis. Surgical reconstruction of the sockets is done only if neces-

Prognosis: Good when defect is isolated; dependent upon the severity of the coexistent findings when part of other syndromes.

Detection of Carrier: —

Special Considerations: —

References:

Fargueta, J.S. et al: Posterior orbital encephalocele with anophthalmos and other brain malformations. J. Neurosurg. 38:215, 1973.

Ingle, V.N. et al: Bilateral congenital anophthalmos. Indian J. Pediatr. 33:149, 1966.

Roy, F.H.: Cosmetic treatment of bilateral anophthalmos. Am. J. Ophthalmol. 67:580, 1969.

Welter, D.A. et al: Klinefelter's syndrome with anophthalmos. Am. J. Ophthalmol. 77:895, 1974.

Contributor: **Elsa K. Rahn**

——————————

Editor's Computerized Descriptors: Eye, Hair

ANORCHIA

Includes: Anorchie
Anorquia
Congenital absence of testes

Excludes: Agonadia† (29)
Hypogonadotropic hypogonadism
All other forms of male pseudohermaphroditism

Minimal Diagnostic Criteria: Surgically verified absence of testes in a 46,XY individual with well-differentiated male external genitalia.

Clinical Findings: Males with anorchia have well-differentiated male external genitalia, normal wolffian derivatives, but absent müllerian derivatives and absent testes. No somatic anomalies are present. To verify the diagnosis a surgeon should explore the scrotum, inguinal canal, and entire path along which the testes descend during embryogenesis. Vasa differentia terminate blindly, often at the same location as spermatic vessels. Individuals with anorchia appear normal at birth except for absence of scrotal testes, and during the 1st decade development is completely normal. Anorchia may be unilateral or bilateral; the latter is much more rare. The diagnosis of congenital anorchia may not be made until virilization fails to occur at puberty, despite androgen-sensitivity; unilateral anorchia may not be recognized until even later.

Complications

I **Derived:** Lack of secondary sexual development, if bilateral; infertility.

II **Associated:** —

Etiology: The etiology is uncertain, although familial tendencies exist. Monozygotic twins concordant for anorchia have been reported, and in several kindreds multiple family members were affected. In other families 1 sib had bilateral anorchia and another sib had unilateral anorchia. On the other hand, monozygotic twins have been discordant for anorchia, indicating that genetic factors are not operative in all cases.

Pathogenesis: In anorchic individuals the fetal testes presumably secreted hormones necessary for external genital virilization, wolffian differentiation, and müllerian inhibition. Testicular tissue thus probably persisted until at least 14-20 weeks of embryonic development, after which time the fetal testes could have undergone atrophy to produce the anorchic phenotype.

Related Facts

I **Sex Ratio:** M1:F0

II **Risk of Occurrence:** ?

III **Risk of Recurrence for**
Patient's Sib: Presumably zero for 46,XX sibs; increased to a small but unknown magnitude in 46,XY sibs.
Patient's Child: All patients are infertile.

IV **Age of Detectability:** During infancy because of absence of testes or at puberty because of lack of secondary sexual development (bilateral cases).

V **Prevalence:** ? At least 100 cases of bilateral anorchia have been reported; unilateral anorchia is more commmon.

Treatment

I **Primary Prevention:** Genetic counseling

II **Secondary Prevention:** Treatment of hypogonadism

III **Other Therapy:** —

Prognosis: Presumably normal life span; infertility in bilateral but not in unilateral anorchia.

Detection of Carrier: —

†Special Considerations: Anorchia should be distinguished from agonadia, a condition in which not only are gonads absent but genital and ductal differentiation is abnormal.

References:

Hall, J.G. et al: Familial congenital anorchia. In Bergsma, D.(ed.): Genetic Forms of Hypogonadism. Birth Defects: Orig. Art. Ser., vol XI, no. 4. Miami: Symposia Specialists for The National Foundation-March of Dimes, 1975, p. 115.

Simpson, J.L. et al: Bilateral anorchia: Discordance in monozygotic twins. In Bergsma, D. (ed.): Part X. The Endocrine System. Birth Defects: Orig. Art. Ser., vol. VII, no. 6. Baltimore: Williams & Wilkins for The National Foundation-March of Dimes, 1971, p. 196.

Simpson, J.L.: Disorders of Sexual Differentiation: Etiology and Clinical Delineation. New York: Academic Press, 1976.

Contributor: **Joe Leigh Simpson**

Editor's Computerized Descriptor: GU.

ANORECTAL MALFORMATIONS

Includes: Malformations ano-rectales
Fehlbildungen von Anus und Rektum
Malformaciónes anorectales
Imperforate anus
Anal atresia or stenosis
Anal membrane
Ectopic anus
Perineal anus
Anoperineal fistula
Rectoperineal fistula
"High" and "low" imperforate anus

Excludes: Colon atresia or stenosis (193)

Minimal Diagnostic Criteria: An International Classification which integrates the clinical and anatomic features of all anorectal anomalies previously described has been proposed. In 41.3% of males, the bowel traversed the puborectalis sling of the levator ani muscle and an external opening was present at the normal anal site (10.3%) or in the perineum (31%). In 51.2% of male patients the termination of the bowel was above the puborectalis sling ending with a urinary fistula to the posterior urethra or bladder in 40.3% of cases. The bowel terminated in an intermediate position between the supralevator and infralevator groups in the remaining 7.5% of male patients. The bowel terminated below the puborectalis sling in 59.4% of female patients and an external opening was identified at the normal anal site (4.7%), in the perineum (26.6%), or vulva (28.1%). Supralevator anomalies were less common in females (17.8%) than in males (51.2%). In 19.0% of the remaining 22.8% of female patients the bowel terminated in an intermediate position with an external opening in the vestibule or the lower portion of the vagina.

Clinical Findings: Imperforate anus is the traditional descriptive term for a large number of anorectal malformations resulting from a defect in the embryologic development of the terminal portion of the hindgut. The external opening of the terminal bowel is 1) normal in location but smaller than normal in size, or 2) occupies an ectopic site in the perineum, scrotum, vulva, vestibule or vagina, or 3) is not visible on examination. The majority of infants with anorectal malformations will show signs of low intestinal obstruction within 24 hours of birth because of the incomplete evacuation of meconium. In the male, pneumaturia or the passage of meconium in the urine indicates a rectourinary fistula. Constipation is the 1st symptom developing several days or weeks after birth if the external opening is of nearly normal size. The diagnosis in these patients is evident by digital examination of the anus.

Complications
I   **Derived:** The untreated patient having an external opening of inadequate size gradually develops signs of low intestinal obstruction or constipation. Rectal bleeding from fissuring of the anal canal, buttock and perineal excoriation from paradoxical diarrhea with fecal impaction, and acquired megacolon are findings secondary to constipation in patients having an external orifice.
II   **Associated:** Anomalies occur in 48% of all patients with anorectal malformation. These are subclassified as: a) skeletal (30%) usually lumbosacral (agenesis; dysplasia; hemivertebrae; malsegmentation), b) GU (38%) renal agenesis and ectopia, vesicoureteral reflux and obstruction, c) esophageal atresia with tracheoesophageal fistula (9.6%), d) CNS (9.0%), e) cardiovascular (5.6%), f) other GI (4.7%), g) miscellaneous (13%).

Etiology: Anorectal malformations are chance occurrences in the great majority of cases. An autosomal recessive inheritance is strongly suggested in studies of 7 of 10 families having more than 1 sib with an anorectal malformation.

Pathogenesis: Anorectal malformations result from a defect or arrest in the embryologic development of the terminal hindgut, 1) during the initial cloacal stage, or 2) when the cloaca is separated into a urogenital sinus and rectum by the urorectal septum, 3) during the posterior migration of the rectum, or 4) at the final stage of anal perforation. Infants with anorectal agenesis and urinary, cloacal, or high vaginal fistulae have anomalies related to the 1st and 2nd stage of hindgut development. Infants having an abnormal external opening in the perineum, scrotum, vulva, vestibule or lower vagina manifest an arrest in posterior migration of the rectum and belong to the intermediate or infralevator group of anorectal malformations. Completely covered anus and anal stenosis are examples of abnormalities in anal perforation.

Related Facts
I **Sex Ratio:** M6:F4
II **Risk of Occurrence:** 1 in 5000 live births (U.S.A.)
III **Risk of Recurrence for**
    Patient's Sib: When autosomal recessive, 1 in 4 (25%) for each offspring to be affected.
    Patient's Child: Not increased, unless mate is carrier or homozygote.
IV **Age of Detectability:** Detection of all anorectal malformations may be made by careful examination of the newborn.
V **Prevalence:** ? No racial or ethnic predilection is known.

Treatment
I **Primary Prevention:** Genetic counseling when autosomal recessive
II **Secondary Prevention:** Operative treatment of the newborn is directed to adequate decompression of the colon either by a) dilatation of the external orifice, b) enlargement of the external orifice by anoplasty procedure, c) temporary defunctionalizing double-barrelled colostomy in infants without a visible external orifice or when an external opening is present but anoplasty procedure is not suitable. Definitive operative treatment by perineal anoplasty or by combined abdominoperineal pull-through or sacroabdominal pull-through is deferred until 1 year of age.†
III **Other Therapy:** —

Prognosis: The overall mortality rate varies from 9.1 to 30% in reported cases. Over 90% of the deaths were attributed to major associated anomalies; these occurred more commonly in the group with supralevator anorectal malformations. The functional results are related to the inherent sensory neural and motor components left undisturbed by the embryologic defects, as well as the expertise of the anorectal reconstruction. Impairment of normal defecation occurs in approximately 50% of the supralevator group following anorectal reconstruction.

Detection of Carrier: —

†**Special Considerations:** Dilatation of anal stenosis constitutes complete treatment. Dilatation of ectopic anal openings to allow decompression may precede definitive anoplasty procedures in selected patients. The risk of constipation in this group is high. Anoplasty procedures, usually by the "cut-back" techniques, are performed when the ectopic external opening is in the perineum, scrotum, vulva or vestibule. If the external opening is in the vagina, colostomy is recommended. An adequate perineal body must be constructed at definitive perineal anoplasty procedure. Transverse or sigmoid colostomy should be performed promptly in all newborn infants without a visible external opening instead of attempting anoplasty by perineal exploration since the risk of recurrent fistulae, undetected

fistulae, nerve injury, anal stenosis and fecal incontinence is increased by this treatment. Definitive anorectal reconstruction for infants not having a visible external opening and those infants with a vaginal orifice should be deferred until approximately 1 year of age. Male patients in this group require combined abdominoperineal pull-through operation with special attention directed to division of the existing urinary communications, preservation of the pelvic parasympathetic nerve plexus, precise placement of the rectum through the puborectalis sling, and creation of a skin-lined anal orifice surrounded by external sphincter muscle.

References:
Bill, A.H., Jr. and Johnson, R.J: Failure of migration of the rectal opening as a cause for most cases of imperforate anus. Surg. Gynecol. Obstet. 106:643, 1958.
Santulli, T.V. et al: Ano-rectal anomalies: A suggested international classification. J. Pediatr. Surg. 5:281, 1970.
Touloukian, R. J. and Pickett, L. K.: Management of the newborn with imperforate anus. Clin. Pediatr. (Phila.) 8:38, 1969.

Contributor: **Robert J. Touloukian**

Editor's Computerized Descriptors: Skel., CV., GI., GU., Nerve

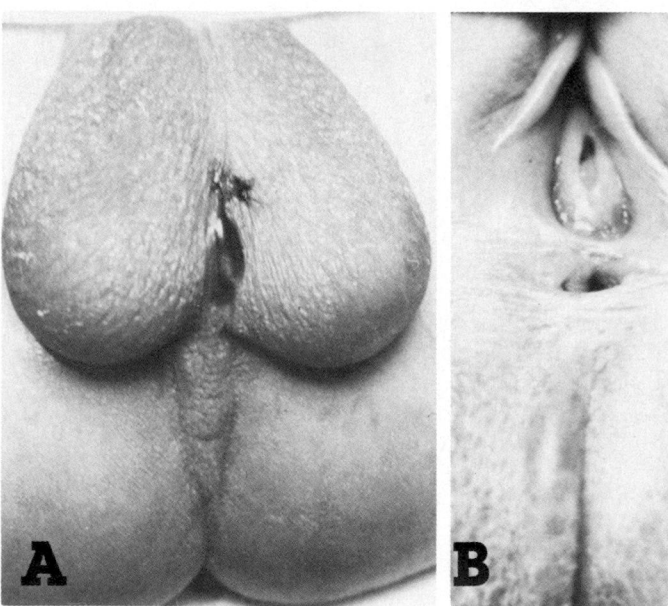

135. A) Covered anus in newborn male with meconium in scrotal raphe; B) anterior perineal anus in newborn female

ANOSMIA, CONGENITAL

Includes: Anosmie congénitale
Angeborene anosmie
Anosmia congénita
Anosmia, isolated
Hyposmia
Selective anosmia
Smelling loss, congenital
Olfaction loss, congenital

Excludes: Acquired anosmia
Hyposmia or anosmia associated with various syndromes

Minimal Diagnostic Criteria: None are as yet established for hyposmia or anosmia; (the mercaptans and potassium cyanide have been most commonly used in the past as olfactory stimulants. Delineation of hyposmic entities have been discussed by Henkin.)

Clinical Findings: Congenital anosmia and congenital hyposmia include a group of individuals with an inability to smell certain or all odors.

Except for the group with congenital craniofacial defects and those with endocrinologic disabilities—pseudohypoparathyroidism and hypogonadotropic hypogonadism—most persons with isolated anosmia are detected by clinical surveys.

It has been noted that certain individuals are anosmic to certain odors of which most persons are aware. However, these same patients are acutely sensitive to other odors; suggesting a selective anosmia or hyposmia. These patients were not found to fall into the above cephalometric or endocrine categories. Perhaps, because the above information is relatively new, they were not studied for these abnormalities.

Complications
I   Derived: —
II   **Associated:** Hypogonadotropic hypogonadism, pseudohypoparathyroidism, craniofacial defect, and Usher syndrome of congenital deafness, retinitis pigmentosa and progressive blindness.

Etiology: ? It is the hypothesis of many that anosmia and hyposmia are developmental abnormalities when trauma, neoplasia, inflammation, hypovitaminosis A can be ruled out. There are numerous examples in the literature of familial isolated anosmia.

Pathogenesis: Agenesis of the olfactory system, especially in the region of the olfactory bulb.†

Related Facts
I   **Sex Ratio:** ? Documentation is very limited
II   **Risk of Occurrence:** ?
III **Risk of Recurrence for**
      Patient's Sib: ?
      Patient's Child: ?
IV   **Age of Detectability:** Childhood. Dependent upon subject communication.
V   **Prevalence:** ?

Treatment
I   **Primary Prevention:** Not indicated
II   **Secondary Prevention:** (It appears that specific therapy for endocrine abnormalities as noted above does not alter the olfactory function.)
III **Other Therapy:** —

Prognosis: Normal for life span and intelligence

Detection of Carrier: —

†**Special Considerations:** In the early 1900s, when investigation was first recorded on this subject, flowers, such as verbena, were utilized to differentiate between normal function, anosmia, or hyposmia. Subsequent to this time, multiple substances such as hydrogen cyanide, alcohol, ether, chloroform, isobutyric acid, thymol, heliotrope, methyl salicilate, many of the mercaptans, especially butyl mercaptan (skunk), pyridine, and thiophene have been used as olfactory stimuli for purposes of differentiation.

Much recent interest in and development of theories of chemoreception have made feasible experimentation into hyposmia and anosmia. Amoore has described 7 basic molecular configurations which stimulate a particular subjective olfactory response. He has further demonstrated combinations of these as producing another specific response. The responses are dependent upon morphologic character of the molecule and, hence, increase the potential objectivity of studies into this field.

References:
Amoore, J.E.: Specific anosmia: A clue to the olfactory code. Nature 214:1095, 1967.
DeMorsier, G.: Études sure les dysraphies crânioencéphaliques. Schweiz. Arch. Neurol. Psychiatr. 74:309, 1954.
Henkin, R.I.: Impairment of olfaction and of the tastes of sour and bitter in pseudohypoparathyroidism. J. Clin. Endocrinol. 28:624, 1968.

Contributors: Roger A. Barnhart
                    LaVonne Bergstrom

_____

Editor's Computerized Descriptors: Vision, Eye, Hearing, Nasoph., Neck, GU.

ANTIBODIES TO HUMAN ALLOTYPES (MARKERS)

Includes: Anticorps contre les allotypes
Antikörper gegen menschliche Allotypen
Anticuerpos contra los alotipos humanos (Marcadores)
Rheumatoid agglutinators (Raggs)
Serum normal agglutinants (SNaggs)
Allotypes, antibodies to human

Excludes: —

Minimal Diagnostic Criteria: Ability of the serum to cause sensitized red blood cells to agglutinate and for the agglutinating activity to be inhibitable by some serum samples and not others.

Clinical Findings: Ragg antibodies against gamma globulin (Gm) antigens are frequently found in the serum of patients with rheumatoid arthritis. These antibodies are carried by IgM, ie the same molecules that carry the rheumatoid factor. Ragg antibodies almost invariably act against 2 or more of the Gm antigens. While they generally have a high titer they are difficult to use, because they are inhibited by all serum samples if the samples are not diluted more than one-fourth, hence the difference between a positive serum and a negative serum is one of titer. Furthermore, it is a common finding that the specificity of the antibody varies during the course of the patient's disease. Thus far no Ragg antibody against the Inv antigens has been found. SNagg (from the French, *Serum Normal agg*lutinant) antibodies against Gm and Inv antigens are found in the serum of healthy individuals. Although these antibodies are almost invariably IgM they are, with rare exceptions, unispecific. While they are generally of low titer they have the great virtue of not reacting with negative serum samples even in the undiluted state. In the majority of cases SNagg antibodies seem to result from an immune reaction by the fetus against the mother's IgG when the latter carries an antigen not present in the genotype of the fetus. The frequency with which these antibodies are detected in healthy individuals depends upon the IgG employed to coat the red blood cells used in the test and upon the age of the donors being tested. In one study, 11% of children between 6 months and 5 years of age were found to have antibodies, while older children and adults had antibodies in approximately 5% of the cases. SNagg antibodies may be induced by repeated transfusions. Antibodies against Gm antigens but not against the Inv antigens have been raised in many kinds of animals, including rabbits and rhesus monkeys.

Antibodies against alpha globulin allotypes (Am) have been found in patients who have experienced transfusion reactions. These antibodies, unlike those against the Gm and Inv allotypes, are IgG.

Complications

I   **Derived:** Gm and Inv antibodies: No complications are ordinarily associated with the presence of antibodies against the Gm or Inv allotypes, however, 1 volunteer in whom an antibody had been induced by repeated transfusions showed a reaction to a massive infusion of incompatible plasma, and a patient, with a presumably normally induced antibody, has been reported to have suffered a transfusion reaction.

Am antibodies: As indicated above, antibodies against the Am allotypes are IgG and may cause transfusion reactions.

II **Associated:** —

Etiology: Antigen-antibody interaction

Pathogenesis: ?

Related Facts

I   **Sex Ratio:** ?
II   **Risk of Occurrence:** ?
III **Risk of Recurrence for**
     Patient's Sib: ?
     Patient's Child: ?
IV **Age of Detectability:** ?
V   **Prevalence:** ?

Treatment

I   **Primary Prevention:** —
II   **Secondary Prevention:** —
III **Other Therapy:** —

Prognosis: Normal for life span, intelligence and function

Detection of Carrier: —

Special Considerations: —

References:
Giblett, E.R.: Genetic Markers in Human Blood. Philadelphia:F.A. Davis Co., 1969.
Steinberg, A.G.: Globulin polymorphism in man. Annu. Rev. Genet. 3:25, 1969.
Vyas, G.N. and Fudenberg, H.H.: Immunobiology of human anti-IgA: A serologic and immunogenetic study of immunization to IgA in transfusion and pregnancy. Clin. Genet. 1:45, 1970.

Contributor: **Arthur G. Steinberg**

Editor's Computerized Descriptor: —

ANUS-HAND-EAR SYNDROME

Includes: Imperforation de l'anus, triphalangie du pouce, décollement du pavillon de l'oreille et surdité de perception
Analatresie, dreigliedrige Daumen, abstehende Ohren, Innenohr-Schwerhörigkeit
Ano imperforado, pulgares trifalángicos, orejas en asa y pérdida de la audición neurosensorial
Townes syndrome

Excludes: Isolated anorectal malformations
Recessive onychodystrophy, triphalangeal thumbs and halluces, mental retardation, seizures and congenital sensorineural deafness
Triphalangeal or bifid thumb as an isolated trait in association with Holt-Oram syndrome

Minimal Diagnostic Criteria: Imperforate anus, triphalangeal thumbs, lop ears and sensorineural hearing loss.

Clinical Findings: One kindred is reported in which 5 of 7 sibs and their father showed signs of this syndrome. All affected persons had imperforate anus. Pes planus was present in 5/6, triphalangeal thumbs in 3/6, a bifid triphalangeal thumb in 2/6, supernumerary thumbs in 1/6, bilateral clinodactyly of the 5th toe in 4/6, "satyr" ears in 6/6 and a mild-to-moderate sensorineural hearing loss in 4/6.

Complications
I   **Derived:** Rectovaginal or rectoperitoneal fistula
II **Associated:** —

Etiology: Autosomal dominant

Pathogenesis: ?

Related Facts
I   **Sex Ratio:** M4:F2
II **Risk of Occurrence:** ?
III **Risk of Recurrence for**
    Patient's Sib: If parent is affected 1 in 2 (50%) for each offspring to be affected.
    Patient's Child: 1 in 2 (50%)
IV **Age of Detectability:** Early childhood
V **Prevalence:** ? Single reported family with 6 affected members in 2 generations.

Treatment
I   **Primary Prevention:** Genetic counseling
II **Secondary Prevention:** Surgical treatment of anorectal anomalies; hearing aid in case of moderate sensorineural hearing loss; surgical correction of triphalangeal thumbs and lop ears.
III **Other Therapy:** —

Prognosis: Probably good for normal life span

Detection of Carrier: The affected patient is heterozygous for the dominant mutant gene.

Special Considerations: —

References:
Townes, P.L. and Brocks, E.R.: Hereditary syndrome of imperforate anus with hand, foot and ear anomalies. J. Pediatr. 81:321, 1972.

Contributor: **Cor W.R.J. Cremers**

Editor's Computerized Descriptors: Hearing, Ear, Skel., GI, GU.

AORTA, COARCTATION

Includes: Coarctation de l'aorte
Aortenisthmusstenose
Coartación de la aorta
Preductal coarctation
Postductal coarctation
Coarctation of lower thoracic aorta
Coarctation of abdominal aorta
Aortic coarctation

Excludes: Aortic hypoplasia
Hypoplasia of aortic arch
Aortic arch interruption (76)
Absence of aortic arch
Pseudocoarctation cervical arch

Minimal Diagnostic Criteria: A blood pressure difference between the upper and lower limbs is diagnostic. Typical roentgenographic findings and aortography are confirmatory.

Clinical Findings: The typical thoracic coarctation consists of a localized area of narrowing just distal to the left subclavian artery and situated just proximal to, opposite or distal to the insertion of the ductus arteriosus. Collateral circulation arises primarily from the subclavian artery and its branches and includes upper intercostal, internal mammary, scapular, lateral thoracic, transverse cervical and anterior spinal arteries. Associated cardiovascular malformations may include: patent ductus arteriosus (40% of preductal coarctations), bicuspid aortic valve (up to 85% of the cases), ventricular septal defect, anomalous origin of the right subclavian artery above or below the coarctation, stenosis or atresia of the left subclavian artery.

Approximately 2% of aortic coarctations are situated in atypical locations in the thoracic or abdominal aorta and may be localized or involve a larger segment of the aorta. Coarctation of the abdominal aorta is more frequently located above or at the level of the renal arteries and may involve these vessels as well as the celiac and superior mesenteric vessels. Significant collateral circulation may be present through anastomoses of the middle colic branch of the inferior mesenteric artery. Associated cardiovascular lesions occur infrequently.

The infant with coarctation of the aorta often develops congestive heart failure between 2 and 6 weeks of age. An additional cardiovascular lesion such as patent ductus arteriosus or ventricular septal defect, may frequently be present. The older child with coarctation usually presents with findings of a heart murmur, absent or diminished and delayed femoral pulses together with a significant pressure gradient between the upper and lower limbs and frequently, a systolic suprasternal notch thrill. A mid-to-late systolic murmur is best heard along the left sternal border. Posteriorly, between the scapulae, this systolic murmur may extend past the second sound. In older children, systolic or continuous bruits are related to the presence of collateral circulation. A high-pitched decrescendo diastolic murmur at the 3rd left intracostal space suggests the association of aortic insufficiency due to a bicuspid valve. An aortic systolic click may be encountered, especially in the presence of a bicuspid aortic valve. A murmur in the epigastric and lumbar areas suggests a lower thoracic or abdominal coarctation.

The ECG frequently demonstrates right ventricular hypertrophy in the infant, especially in the presence of an associated lesion. In the absence of associated lesions, most children over 6 months of age demonstrate left ventricular hypertrophy. The thoracic roentgenogram is usually diagnostic once the patient is beyond the infant age range. The two primary signs are: 1) notching of the inferior margin of the ribs (usually the 3rd rib through the 8th). The finding, however, is not commonly seen in children less than 4 years of age, is not always present, and is usually confined to the posterior aspect of the ribs. 2) Some distortion or disfigurement of the aortic knob is present in the vast majority of cases. This distortion may result in densities in this region which resemble a "figure of three." The remainder of findings involving the heart and great vessels may be identical to any condition which places the left ventricle under an obstructive stress. When this occurs, the heart assumes a left ventricular configuration. If the left ventricle maintains compensation, the vasculature is normal and the heart is normal sized. With left ventricular failure, there are signs of pulmonary venous obstruction and left atrial enlargement. The ascending aorta is prominent in nearly all cases. In an atypical coarctation, thoracic roentgenograms fail to demonstrate indentation of the aortic isthmus. Rib-notching is absent or confined to the lower ribs. Cardiac catheterization generally demonstrates hypertension above the site of the coarctation, while below the lesion, aortic pressure is decreased and the pressure curve reveals a narrow pulse pressure, slow rise and delay of peak pressure. Aortography demonstrates the site, severity and extent of the coarctation, together with the degree of collateral circulation. Injection of contrast material in the ascending aorta demonstrates the presence or absence of a bicuspid aortic valve. When aortography indicates that an abdominal coarctation involves one or both renal arteries, individual renal function studies are indicated.

Echocardiographically detectable abnormalities associated with coarctation of the aorta such as bicuspid aortic valve, parachute deformity of the mitral valve or the presence of left ventricular hypertrophy can aid in the serial follow-up of these patients. Infants with clinical findings of coarctation should be screened for hypoplastic left heart syndrome. The area of coarctation has not been imaged noninvasively.

Complications
I **Derived:** Congestive heart failure is common in infancy (2-4 weeks), especially when a patent ductus arteriosus, ventricular septal defect or other cardiovascular lesion is present.
II **Associated:** The most common cardiovascular anomaly in patients with gonadal dysgenesis is coarctation of the aorta. Aneurysms of the cerebral vasculature may be present and may rupture at some time in life.

Etiology: Presumably multifactorial inheritance

Pathogenesis: Has been related to the presence of ductal tissue in the wall of the aorta at the site of the coarctation. May be caused by exaggeration of the normal infolding of the wall of the aorta distal to the left subclavian artery producing a "subclavian shelf." Coarctation may be present at birth or occasionally may develop postnatally. Abdominal coarctation may be congenital or acquired, and has been reported in patients with neurofibromatosis, pulseless disease, and certain infectious diseases.

Related Facts
I **Sex Ratio:** M2:F1
II **Risk of Occurrence:** 1 in 1600 live births
III **Risk of Recurrence for**
   Patient's Sib: Predicted risk 2.4%; empiric risk 1.8%
   Patient's Child: Predicted risk 2.4%; empiric risk 2.7%
IV **Age of Detectability:** From birth by selective angiography
V **Prevalence:** Less than 1 in 2000 in the pediatric population

Treatment
I **Primary Prevention:** Genetic counseling

II **Secondary Prevention:** Thoracic coarctation—resection and end-to-end anastomosis or graft (preferable after 3 years of age). Abdominal coarctation—resection or bypass graft. Correction of associated renal vascular abnormality by bypass graft or resection.†
III **Other Therapy:** Symptomatic therapy for hypertension and congestive heart failure. The infant with congestive heart failure and isolated coarctation usually responds to medical management and does not require immediate operation. When heart failure is unresponsive to medical management in complicated coarctation, operation is indicated.

Prognosis: The average age of death in untreated coarctation is 35 years, due to cerebral hemorrhage, aortic rupture, progressive aortic insufficiency with congestive heart failure or subacute bacterial endocarditis. Prognosis is much improved in surgically treated coarctation with decrease in hypertension often to normal levels. Surgical correction in infancy may provide initial improvement, but can result in later development of obstruction as the anastomotic site fails to keep up with growth of the aorta.

Detection of Carrier: —

†Special Considerations: Postoperative complications: hemorrhage from anastomotic site, pulmonary infection, paradoxical hypertension, necrotizing arteritis of the GI tract blood vessels. Paradoxical hypertension occurring in the first 24 to 36 hours postoperatively usually does not require treatment. Delayed hypertension may occur 48 hours after surgery and last for 7 to 14 days. Necrotizing arteritis of the GI tract blood vessels may occur in up to 19% of patients undergoing repair of coarctation. On about the 4th postoperative day there is onset of abdominal pain and distention, fever, vomiting, and melena associated with leukocytosis. Conservative management is usually recommended with sympatholytics, intestinal antibiotics and decompression. The hypertension occurring with coarctation of the aorta has been attributed to mechanical obstruction and to the development of humoral factors. More recent reports have implicated the renin-angiotensin-aldosterone mechanism as the basis of a humoral involvement, or to increased sympathetic nerve activity. Prognosis in coarctation of the aorta is also affected by the presence of the associated defects, particularly by a bicuspid aortic valve. This, in later life, may become insufficient or stenotic.

References:
Duffie, E.R. and Wilson, J.F.: Coarctation of the aorta. In Moss, A.J. and Adams, F.H. (eds.): Heart Disease in Infants, Children, and Adolescents. Baltimore: Williams and Wilkins, 1968, p. 384.
McNamara, D.G. and Rosenberg, H.S.: Coarctation of the aorta. In Watson, H. (ed.): Paediatric Cardiology. St. Louis: C.V. Mosby, 1968, p. 175.
Riemenschneider, T.A. et al: Coarctation of the abdominal aorta in children: Report of three cases and review of the literature. Pediatrics 44:716, 1969.
Williams, D.E. et al: Cross-sectional echocardiographic localization of the sites of left ventricular outflow tract obstruction. Am. J. Cardiol. 37(2):250, 1976.

Contributors: **Thomas A. Riemenschneider**
Leonard M. Linde

Editor's Computerized Descriptors: Skel., CV.

AORTIC ARCH, CERVICAL

Includes: Arche aortique cervicale
Zervikaler Aortenbogen
Arco aórtico cervical
Persistence of third aortic arch
Cervical aortic arch

Excludes: Congenitally unwound aorta
Pseudocoarctation
Aneurysms or pathologic elongation of individual brachiocephalic vessels

Minimal Diagnostic Criteria: Pulsating mass in supraclavicular area, compression of which will diminish the femoral pulses. The mass may be on either side.

Clinical Findings: What appears to be the aortic arch is located much higher than the normal aortic arch in the lower neck. The striking clinical feature of this anomaly is the presence of a large pulsating mass in either the right or left supraclavicular region. This mass may extend as high as the hyoid bone (the 5th or 6th cervical vertebra). The mass may be associated with symptoms of a vascular ring, ie dysphagia or airway obstruction, or it may be completely asymptomatic. Several cases reported have discrepancies in the pulses and blood pressures in the upper limbs. The diminution of the femoral pulses by compression of the pulsating mass against the adjacent vertebra provides a pathognomonic clinical maneuver. On plain PA chest roentgenogram, there is an asymmetric widening of the superior mediastinal shadow and the aortic arch is inconspicuous. On barium swallow there is a large posterior indentation of the esophagus at the level of the usual position of the aortic arch. This is a result of the retroesophageal passage of the descending limb of the cervical aorta.

Complications
I **Derived:** May cause symptoms of vascular ring (in 3/8). Long-term effects of vascular aging process on the tortuous aorta are unknown.
II **Associated:** —

Etiology: ?

Pathogenesis: Most likely represents a persistence of the 3rd aortic arch (instead of the usual 4th) and the ductus caroticus (segment of the dorsal aorta between the 3rd and 4th arches). A similar anomaly may involve the contralateral subclavian artery which then arises from the innominate artery at a much higher level than normal.

Related Facts
I **Sex Ratio:** M1:F1
II **Risk of Occurrence:** Only 8 cases recorded in the literature
III **Risk of Recurrence for**
　Patient's Sib: ?
　Patient's Child: ?
IV **Age of Detectability:** From birth
V **Prevalence:** Extremely rare

Treatment
I **Primary Prevention:** —
II **Secondary Prevention:** Surgical relief of encircling structures such as contralateral ductus or ligamentum arteriosus when symptoms of vascular ring are present.
III **Other Therapy:** —

Prognosis: ? Probably benign

Detection of Carrier: —

Special Considerations: —

References:
deJong, I. H. and Klinkhamer, A. C.: Left-sided cervical aortic arch. Am. J. Cardiol. 23:285, 1969.
Harley, H. R.: The development and anomalies of the aortic arch and its branches with the report of a case of right cervical aortic arch and intrathoracic vascular ring. Br. J. Surg. 46:561, 1959.
Lipchik, E. O. and Young, L. W.: Unusual symptomatic aortic arch anomalies. Radiology 89:85, 1967.
Sissman, N. J.: Anomalies of the aortic arch complex. In Moss, A.J. and Adams, F.H. (eds.): Heart Disease in Infants, Children, and Adolescents. Baltimore:Williams and Wilkins, 1968, p. 400.

Contributors:　　**Charles E. Mullins**
　　　　　　　　　　Dan G. McNamara

Editor's Computerized Descriptors: Resp., CV., GI.

AORTIC ARCH, DOUBLE

Includes: Arche aortique double
Doppelter Aortenbogen
Arco aórtico doble
Bilateral aortic arch with left or right descending aorta
Double aortic arch

Excludes: Other forms of aortic arch anomalies causing the vascular ring syndrome

Minimal Diagnostic Criteria: Characteristic indentations of the barium-filled esophagus and air-filled trachea in infants with symptoms and signs of upper airway obstruction. Aortography is confirmatory.

Clinical Findings: An aortic arch is present on each side of the trachea and esophagus. Both arise anteriorly from the ascending aorta, encircle the trachea and esophagus and join posteriorly to continue as descending aorta. The descending aorta is usually located on the left side but is on the right side in some cases. The right posterior aortic arch is generally (80%) the larger, but in 20% of the cases, it may be the smaller of the 2, or the 2 arches are of approximately equal size. Each of the 2 arches gives rise to the ipsilateral common carotid and subclavian arteries.

In the great majority of patients the encirclement of the trachea and esophagus by the 2 arches causes significant symptoms, usually appearing in infancy. Occasionally, symptoms do not occur until later in childhood, or, rarely, in adults. The severity of the symptoms is directly related to the degree of obstruction to the trachea and esophagus. In infants, the most obvious and sometimes alarming symptom is severe inspiratory stridor associated with wheezing and a hacking cough. Respiratory tract infections are common, not only due to airway obstruction, but also to obstruction of the esophagus leading to aspiration. Hyperextension of the head alleviates the respiratory symptoms more or less successfully and this position is usually assumed by the child as being the most comfortable. In older children or adults, the only symptom may be dysphagia.

Cardiac murmurs are not present unless there are associated cardiovascular anomalies. The findings on physical examination are dominated by those caused by upper airway obstruction. Unless other cardiovascular anomalies are present, the ECG is normal. Plain xrays of the chest may show a widened upper mediastinum and direct or indirect evidence of airway obstruction such as hyperaeration, atelectasis and pneumonic infiltrates. In the most common type of double aortic arch in which the right posterior arch is the larger of the 2, this arch will cause a large indentation in the right lateral wall of the barium-filled esophagus. A similar but smaller indentation may be visible on the left side of the barium-filled esophagus. The air-filled trachea almost invariably shows an anterior indentation from the anterior arch. Aortography will confirm the diagnosis and reveal the precise anatomy and relative size of the 2 arches.

Complications
I **Derived:** Hyperaeration of the lungs, atelectasis, pneumonia and dysphagia
II **Associated:** —

Etiology: ?

Pathogenesis: In cases of double aortic arch, both dorsal aortae persist rather than only the usual left.

Related Facts
I **Sex Ratio:** M1:F1

II **Risk of Occurrence:** Approximately 1 in 20,000 live births
III **Risk of Recurrence for**
  Patient's Sib: Predicted risk 1:100; empiric risk: ?
  Patient's Child: Predicted risk 1:100; empiric risk: ?
IV **Age of Detectability:** Neonatal period
V **Prevalence:** Approximately 5 in 100,000

Treatment
I **Primary Prevention:** —
II **Secondary Prevention:** In patients in whom the presence of a double aortic arch causes symptoms, the treatment is surgical and consists of division of the minor of the 2 arches.
III **Other Therapy:** —

Prognosis: In symptomatic patients, particularly infants, the prognosis without surgical treatment is poor.

Detection of Carrier: —

Special Considerations: —

References:
Hewitt, R.L. et al: Aortic arch anomalies. J. Thorac. Cardiovasc. Surg. 160:746, 1970.
Netter, F.H. (ed.): Ciba Collection of Medical Illustrations. The Heart. Summit, N.J.: Ciba Publishing Co., 1969, vol. 5.
Nora, J.J. and McNamara, D.G.: Vascular rings and related anomalies. In Watson, H. (ed.): Paediatric Cardiology. St. Louis: C.V. Mosby Co., 1968, p. 233.
Stewart, J.R. et al: An Atlas of Vascular Rings and Related Malformations of the Aortic Arch System. Springfield: Charles C Thomas, 1964.

Contributors: **James J. Nora**
Gary L. Way

Editor's Computerized Descriptors: Resp., GI.

AORTIC ARCH INTERRUPTION

Includes: Interruption de la crosse aortique
Unterbrechung des Aortenbogens
Interrupción del arco aórtico
Absence of left or both aortic fourth arches

Excludes: Coarctation of aorta with or without complete occlusion

Minimal Diagnostic Criteria: Selective aortography may be diagnostic, but in some cases even this may fail to differentiate interruption of the aortic arch from the most extreme form of coarctation of the aorta in the living patient.

Clinical Findings: Most commonly the ascending aorta, which is somewhat smaller than normal, divides into the right and left common carotid arteries and does not continue to form the normal aortic arch. Both subclavian arteries arise from the proximal descending aorta just beyond the entrance of a very large ductus arteriosus which connects the pulmonary trunk with the descending aorta and forms its only blood supply. In a smaller number of cases, the ascending aorta terminates into an innominate and left common carotid artery.

Only 4% of patients have no additional cardiac anomaly other than the obligatory patent ductus arteriosus. In 60% of the cases a ventricular septal defect is the only associated lesion, but other cardiovascular anomalies, such as transposition of the great arteries, aortic valve stenosis and truncus arteriosus, are not uncommon. In the few cases where the interrupted arch is the only malformation, the symptoms and signs are similar to those seen in severe preductal coarctation of the aorta, and differential cyanosis, as evidenced by cyanosis of only the lower body and lower limbs, may be present. In cases with associated ventricular septal defect, the signs and symptoms are those seen in any patient with a large left-to-right shunt at the ventricular or great arterial level. In such cases differential cyanosis is not usually apparent because of the relatively high oxygen content of the right ventricular blood.

In most patients the pressures in ascending and descending aorta are approximately equal. In others the patent ductus arteriosus may become small enough so that diminished pulses and lower arterial pressure in the lower limbs may lead to the erroneous diagnosis of coarctation of the aorta.

Thoracic roentgenograms usually show hypervascular lungs, cardiomegaly and left atrial enlargement. The linear density formed by the upper descending thoracic aorta is almost invariably absent. The ECG may be normal but usually shows right, left or combined ventricular hypertrophy. The diagnosis of interrupted aortic arch and clarification of any associated cardiovascular malformations necessitate cardiac catheterization and angiocardiography.

Complications
I **Derived:** Dyspnea and congestive heart failure as seen in other types of congenital heart disease with large left-to-right shunt associated with left ventricular outflow obstruction.
II **Associated:** These are almost always present and usually consist of a large ventricular septal defect. Frequently associated with thymic aplasia and immunodeficiency (DiGeorge syndrome).

Etiology: Teratogenic exposure documented in some cases, suggestion of multifactorial inheritance in others.

Pathogenesis: In cases where the right subclavian artery originates normally from the innominate artery, interruption of the aortic arch is due to early disappearance of the left 4th branchial arch. If both 4th arches disappear, the result is interruption of the aortic arch in which the right subclavian artery originates from the descending aorta.

Related Facts
I **Sex Ratio:** M1:F1
II **Risk of Occurrence:** ?
III **Risk of Recurrence for**
   Patient's Sib: ?
   Patient's Child: ?
IV **Age of Detectability:** From birth
V **Prevalence:** ?

Treatment
I **Primary Prevention:** —
II **Secondary Prevention:** Medical treatment is unsatisfactory and surgery is indicated in virtually all cases. An attempt is made to reestablish continuity between the ascending aorta and the descending aorta with division of the patent ductus arteriosus. Since most cases are associated with ventricular septal defect, it is probably advisable initially to also carry out pulmonary arterial banding. In patients in whom the associated cardiovascular malformations are hopelessly complex, surgery should probably not be attempted.
III **Other Therapy:** —

Prognosis: The prognosis without surgical treatment is extremely poor. Approximately 90% of patients die within the first year of life, and of these the great majority die within the first 20 days.

Detection of Carrier: —

Special Considerations: —

References:
McNamara, D.G. and Rosenberg, H.S.: Interruption of the aortic arch. In Watson, H. (ed.): Paediatric Cardiology. St. Louis:C.V. Mosby Co., 1968, p. 224.
Roberts, W.C. et al: Complete interruption of the aortic arch. Circulation 26:39, 1962.
Stewart, J.R. et al: An Atlas of Vascular Rings and Related Malformations of the Aortic Arch System. Springfield:Charles C. Thomas, 1964.

Contributors: **Robert L. Williams**
                    Dan G. McNamara

Editor's Computerized Descriptors: Resp., CV.

AORTIC ARCH, RIGHT

Includes: Syndrome de l'arche aortique droite
Rechtsaortenbogen
Arco aórtico derecho
Right aortic arch types I, II and III
Right aortic arch with or without retroesophageal anomalous subclavian artery

Excludes: Aortic arch, double (75)

Minimal Diagnostic Criteria: Right aortic arch is easily distinguishable on plain films. A barium esophagram is necessary to distinguish Types I and II arches. Type III arch (isolation of the left subclavian) is recognizable by the combination of xray signs of right arch plus decreased amplitude of the arterial pulses of the left arm. Thoracic aortography is definitive.

Clinical Findings: Right aortic arch is defined as the transverse aortic arch coursing to the right of the trachea. This anomaly is usually asymptomatic and therefore diagnosed incidentally on chest xray. The most reliable xray sign is a concave deformity on the right side of the trachea. Additional signs are an aortic knob on the right side of the dorsal spine, a clear space on the left side of the dorsal spine, the superior vena cava deviated to the right, the descending thoracic aorta coursing inferiorly along the right side of the spine and signs on the esophagram of an aberrant left subclavian artery if present. When the right arch is present it has 1 of 2 relationships to the esophagus. In 1 form the arch occupies a retroesophageal position. In the other form it does not pass behind the esophagus but remains to the right of it. By far, the most common form is the right aortic arch without a retroesophageal aortic segment.

For practical purposes, there are three main types of right aortic arch without a retroesophageal segment:

Type I: Mirror Image Branching: In this type the aortic arch passes over the right main stem bronchus and connects with a right-sided proximal aorta. This form demonstrates mirror image branching of the major arteries from that observed in the normal left aortic arch. The first branch of the arch is the left innominate artery and is followed by the right carotid and the right subclavian arteries, in that order. It is the most common right-sided arch and has a very high incidence of congenital heart disease with tetralogy of Fallot being the most common.

Type II: Aberrant Left Subclavian Artery: The aortic arch in this type has a similar course to type I with the same reversal of branches. In this type, however, the left subclavian, instead of coming off the left innominate, comes off distal to the right subclavian. It courses toward the left arm by crossing the midline behind the esophagus, and subsequently causes an indentation in the posterior esophagus. In contrast to what formerly was suspected, this type may have a high incidence of cardiac anomalies. When there is a left-sided ductus arteriosus (or ligamentum arteriosum) present there may be significant compression of the trachea and the esophagus. In elderly adults, the bulbous origin of the left subclavian may project to the left of the spine and be misinterpreted as a nonvascular mass.

Both types I and II right aortic arches are easily recognizable and distinguishable on chest xrays with barium in the esophagus. In the type II aortic arch, if the ductus arteriosus is on the left, the retroesophageal component produces a wide, concave compression on the esophagus. Uncommonly, when the ductus arteriosus is on the right, the retroesophageal compression is smaller, shallower and angles upward from right to left at approximately 70° from the horizontal. These findings are caused by the anomalous left subclavian arising directly from the aortic arch below the right subclavian.

Type III: Isolation of the Left Subclavian Artery†: In this type of right aortic arch the configuration of the arch and descending aorta is similar to types I and II. As before, the 3 branches from the arch are reversed with the left common carotid coming off first, then the right carotid and then the right subclavian. The left subclavian artery is not attached to the aorta but is connected to the left pulmonary artery through a ductus arteriosus or ligamentum arteriosum. In the latter, the left subclavian and brachial artery are perfused by the left vertebral artery; so-called "subclavian steal." The pulses in the left arm are diminished when compared with the right. This type of right aortic arch is extremely rare.

Right arch with retroesophageal aortic segment is an uncommon form of right aortic arch. In this type, the aortic arch occupies a retroesophageal position. The solitary arch passes over the right main bronchus to the right of the trachea and esophagus. It then turns abruptly toward the left behind the esophagus and upon reaching the left side of the esophagus it joins the proximal end of a left-sided descending aorta. A left-sided ductus arteriosus commonly attaches to a diverticula at the junction of the arch and the descending aorta and thus creates a vascular ring. The ring is comprised of the right arch to the right, its retroesophageal segment posteriorly, the PA to the left and the pulmonary arterial bifurcation anteriorly.

In a case of congenital heart disease having a right aortic arch, a number of conditions should be considered as they frequently occur together. The approximate incidence of right aortic arch occurring in each condition is:

Tetralogy of Fallot - 25%: The more severe the degree of obstruction to pulmonary flow, the higher the incidence of right arch. End-stage tetralogy has an incidence for right arch of nearly 50%.

Persistent truncus arteriosus - 35%

Complete transposition with ventricular septal defect and pulmonary stenosis - 25%

Tricuspid atresia - 8%

Isolated ventricular septal defect, usually Eisenmenger anatomy in type - 2%

Complications
I **Derived:** A vascular ring may be created with either a left posterior ligamentum arteriosum or an aberrant left subclavian artery.
II **Associated:** Cardiovascular defects as cited in Clinical Findings.

Etiology: Presumably multifactorial inheritance.

Pathogenesis: A right aortic arch in situs solitus is due to retention of the right dorsal aorta rather than the left.

Related Facts
I **Sex Ratio:** M1:F1
II **Risk of Occurrence:** 1 in 2500
III **Risk of Recurrence for**
  Patient's Sib: ?
  Patient's Child: ?
IV **Age of Detectability:** From birth
V **Prevalence:** 1 in 2500

Treatment
I **Primary Prevention:** —
II **Secondary Prevention:** When a retroesophageal component creates a vascular ring, surgical intervention may be necessary to alleviate the obstruction. The left ligamentum or ductus may be divided. Occasionally, division of the left subclavian is necessary.

III Other Therapy: —

Prognosis: Without associated cardiac defects or retroesophageal component, the prognosis is normal. With an associated cardiac defect, the prognosis would be dependent only on the cardiac defect. When there is a retroesophageal component, a vascular ring may occur which may be relieved by surgical intervention.

Detection of Carrier: —

†Special Considerations: See Isolation of Subclavian Artery from Aorta. (546)

References:

Knight, L. and Edwards, J.E.: Right aortic arch: Types and associated cardiac anomalies. Circulation 50:1047, 1974.

Matthew, R. et al: The significance of right aortic arch in D-transposition of the great arteries. Am. J. Cardiol. 87(3):314, 1974.

Nora, J.J. and McNamara, D.G.: Vascular rings and related anomalies. In Watson, H. (ed.): Paediatric Cardiology. St. Louis: C.V. Mosby, 1968, p. 233.

Sissman, N.J.: Anomalies of the aortic arch complex. In Moss, A.J. and Adams, F.H. (eds.): Heart Disease in Infants, Children, and Adolescents. Baltimore:Williams and Wilkins, 1968, p. 400.

Contributors: **Gary L. Way**
James J. Nora

Editor's Computerized Descriptors: Resp., CV.

AORTIC STENOSIS, SUPRAVALVAR

Includes: Sténose aortique supra-valvulaire
Supravalvuläre Aortenstenose
Estenosis aórtica supravalvular
Supraaortic stenosis
Supravalvar aortic stenosis

Excludes: Aorta, coarctation (73)
Aortic hypoplasia
Aortic valve stenosis (80)

Minimal Diagnostic Criteria: The diagnosis is usually suspected on the basis of the typical clinical features described below. However, definitive localization of the site of left ventricular outflow obstruction requires the demonstration of a pressure gradient a short distance beyond the aortic valve via left heart catheterization.

Clinical Findings: Supravalvar aortic stenosis is a congenital narrowing of the ascending aorta, either localized or diffuse, originating at the superior margin of the sinuses of Valsalva just above the level of the coronary arteries. It may be separated anatomically into 3 categories, although any specific patient may demonstrate pathologic findings characteristic of more than 1 type. Most common is the hour-glass type, in which a constricting annular ridge at the superior margin of the sinuses of Valsalva is produced by extreme thickening and disorganization of the aortic media. Although the lumen of the aorta is reduced, the constriction may not be evident on gross inspection of the external surface of the vessel. It has been suggested that this lesion results from a developmental exaggeration of the normal transverse supravalvar aortic plica. The membranous type is produced by a fibrous or fibromuscular diaphragm with a small central opening stretched across the lumen of the aorta. The hypoplastic type is characterized by uniform hypoplasia of the ascending aorta. In the older cardiovascular literature, a 4th anomaly, consisting of a nonobstructing band or cord stretched across the lumen of the aorta at the level of the aortic leaflets, was designated supravalvar aortic stenosis, although it most likely has no functional significance.

In contrast to other forms of aortic stenosis, in the supravalvar variety the coronary arteries arise proximal to the site of outflow obstruction and are subjected to the elevated pressure that exists within the left ventricle. These vessels are often dilated and tortuous and coronary arteriosclerosis has been observed, even in children. In addition, if the free edges of some or all of the aortic cusps are adherent to the site of supravalvar stenosis, there may be interference with coronary arterial flow. The clinical picture of supravalvar aortic stenosis differs from that observed in other forms of left ventricular outflow obstruction. Chief among these differences is the association of supravalvar aortic stenosis with early hypercalcemia syndrome (Williams syndrome). The designation supravalvar aortic stenosis syndrome has been applied to the distinctive clinical picture produced by coexistence of the cardiac and metabolic disorder. Patients with this syndrome have mental retardation, characteristic facial features, and anomalies in dentition. Most commonly, supravalvar aortic stenosis is a feature of the distinctive syndrome described above. However, the aortic anomaly and peripheral pulmonary arterial stenosis are also seen in familial and sporadic forms unassociated with the other features of the syndrome. Occasionally, there is moderate thickening of the aortic cusps, and valvar pulmonary stenosis may occur in association with the narrowing of peripheral pulmonary arteries. Rare patients may have mitral valve abnormalities with prolapse and mitral regurgitation.

A positive family history in a patient with a normal appearance and clinical signs suggesting left ventricular outflow obstruction should alert the physician to a diagnosis of either supravalvar aortic stenosis or muscular subaortic stenosis.

With a few exceptions, the major physical findings resemble those observed in patients with stenosis of aortic valve. Among these exceptions are the frequent accentuations of the sound of aortic valve closure due to the elevated pressure in the aorta proximal to the stenosis, the infrequency of an ejection sound, and the more prominent transmission of the thrill and murmur into the jugular notch and along the carotid vessels. Occasionally, there is an early diastolic decrescendo blowing murmur of aortic regurgitation, due to the fusion of 1 or more cusps to the area of stenosis. The narrowing of the peripheral pulmonary arteries that frequently coexists in these patients may produce a continuous murmur that may help distinguish this anomaly from stenosis of the aortic valve. The latter distinction is reinforced by the frequent finding of a significant disparity between the arterial pressures in the upper limbs in supravalvar aortic stenosis; the systolic pressure in the right arm tends to be the higher of the 2 and may even exceed that in the femoral arteries. When obstruction is severe, the ECG reveals left ventricular hypertrophy. However, biventricular, or even right ventricular hypertrophy may be observed if significant narrowing of the peripheral pulmonary arteries coexists. Roentgenographically, in contrast to valvar and discrete subvalvar aortic stenosis, poststenotic dilatation of the ascending aorta is rarely seen. Most often the sinuses of Valsalva are dilated and the ascending aorta and the aortic arch are of normal size or appear small. Retrograde arterial catheterization is the most valuable technique for localizing the site of obstruction to the supravalvar area and to assess the degree of hemodynamic abnormality. The diagnosis is confirmed by the demonstration of a pressure gradient just above the aortic valve and a constriction at this level by aortography. The angiogram may also permit visualization of narrowed segments of the aorta or great vessels distal to the obstruction. At right heart catheterization the presence of stenosis of peripheral pulmonary arteries may be detected by continually recording pressure as a catheter is withdrawn from a peripheral artery to the main pulmonary artery and by right ventricular or pulmonary artery angiocardiography.

The demonstration of supravalvular aortic narrowing in the aorta above the sinus of Valsalva has been reported echocardiographically in at least 2 series. Nevertheless, the difficulty of ascertaining precise aortic alignment above the aortic valve makes this a difficult procedure. If, on continued sweep, one cannot identify a normally dimensioned aortic root above the valve, supravalvular aortic stenosis may be diagnosed. The M-mode echo picture seems to underestimate the severity of angiographic stenosis. Two-dimensional techniques may increase the reliability of echo diagnosis.

Complications
I **Derived:** Syncope, aortic regurgitation, congestive heart failure, bacterial endocarditis, premature coronary arteriosclerosis, sudden unexpected death.
II **Associated:** A high incidence of narrowing of peripheral pulmonary arteries is seen (80%). Commonly, there is narrowing of the peripheral systemic arteries, including renal and carotid arteries. Mild degrees of pulmonary and aortic valvular stenosis, as well as coarctation of the aorta, and mitral valve prolapse may also be observed.

Etiology: Genetic studies suggest that when the anomaly is familial it is transmitted as an autosomal dominant trait with variable expression. Some family members may have supravalvar pulmonic stenosis either as an isolated lesion or in combination with supravalvar aortic stenosis. McK *18550

The multiple system involvement observed when supravalvar aortic stenosis is associated with early hypercalcemia syndrome may be related to a derangement of vitamin D (metabolism in the mother or fetus during pregnancy). The creation of hypervitaminosis D in the pregnant rabbit has resulted in cardiovascular and craniofacial malformations in the offspring resembling those observed in the supravalvar aortic stenosis syndrome.

Pathogenesis: ?

Related Facts
I **Sex Ratio:** Ml:Fl
II **Risk of Occurrence:** ?
III **Risk of Recurrence for**
  Patient's Sib: Unknown except that the risk approaches 1 in 2 in the genetic type.
  Patient's Child: Unknown except that the risk approaches 1 in 2 in the genetic type.
IV **Age of Detectability:** From birth by typical clinical features, left heart catheterization and selective left ventricular or aortic angiocardiography.
V **Prevalence:** ?

Treatment
I **Primary Prevention:** Genetic counseling
II **Secondary Prevention:** Early recognition of the distinctive supravalvar aortic stenosis syndrome may prove to be a prerequisite to successful medical management, insofar as prompt diagnosis and treatment of the idiopathic hypercalcemia in infancy may possibly retard the progression of the cardiovascular lesions. Supravalvar aortic stenosis is often amenable to operative treatment. The lumen of the aorta at the supravalvar level may be widened effectively by the insertion of an oval or diamond-shaped fabric prosthesis only in those patients with a normal ascending aorta. If the aorta is hypoplastic, this procedure merely displaces the pressure gradient distally, without abolishing the obstruction. Under these circumstances, totally effective surgical treatment may necessitate replacement or widening of the entire hypoplastic aorta with an appropriate prosthesis.
III **Other Therapy:** —

Prognosis: The prognosis depends upon the severity of obstruction, the extent of the aortic wall and other great vessels involved by the pathologic process, the degree of coronary arteriosclerosis and the severity of the associated peripheral pulmonary or peripheral arterial stenoses.

Detection of Carrier: —

Special Considerations: —

References:
Bolen, J. et al: Echocardiographic features of supravalvular aortic stenosis. Circulation 52:817, 1975.
Friedman, W.F.: Vitamin D and the supravalvular aortic stenosis syndrome. In Woollam, D.H.M. (ed.): Advances in Teratology. New York:Academic Press, 1968, vol. 3, p. 85.
Friedman, W.F. and Mills, L.F.: The relationship between vitamin D and the craniofacial and dental anomalies of the supravalvular aortic stenosis syndrome. Pediatrics 43:12, 1969.
Kahler, R.L. et al: Familial congenital heart disease; familial occurrence of atrial septal defect with a-v conduction abnormalities; supravalvular aortic and pulmonic stenosis, and ventricular septal defect. Am. J. Med. 40:384, 1966.
Usher, B.W. et al: Echocardiographic detection of supravalvular

aortic stenosis. Circulation 49:1257, 1974.
Williams, D.E. et al: Cross-sectional echocardiographic localization of the sites of left ventricular outflow tract obstructions. Am. J. Cardiol. 37(2):250, 1976.

Contributors: **William F. Friedman**
Stanley E. Kirkpatrick

Editor's Computerized Descriptors: Face, Teeth, CV.

AORTIC VALVE ATRESIA

Includes: Atrésie des valvules aortiques
Aortenklappen-Atresie
Atresia de la válvula aórtica
Aortic atresia
Atresia of aortic valve

Excludes: Aortic valve stenosis (80)
Coarctation of the aorta and other forms of the hypoplastic left heart syndrome in which the aortic valve is patent

Minimal Diagnostic Criteria: Cardiomegaly and congestive heart failure during the 1st week of life in a mildly to moderately cyanotic infant with weak or absent pulses and marked right ventricular hypertrophy on the ECG strongly suggest the diagnosis. Angiocardiography with demonstration of retrograde filling of the proximal aorta is confirmatory.

Clinical Findings: Aortic valve maldevelopment varies from complete absence of identifiable valve tissue, through the appearance of definite raphae, to the formation of an imperforate dome. The coronary arteries arise from the base of the aorta, which is hypoplastic in the ascending portion and the arch. The left atrium and ventricle are hypoplastic and may exhibit endocardial fibroelastosis; the mitral valve is hypoplastic or atretic. An interatrial opening is usually present. The right atrium, right ventricle, and pulmonary arteries are enlarged and there is always a large patent ductus. A ventricular septal defect is uncommon and complete transposition of the great arteries is rare.

The pulmonary venous blood does not enter the left ventricle from the left atrium, but passes to the right atrium, right ventricle, pulmonary artery and then not only to the lungs, but also via the patent ductus to both the ascending and descending aorta. The pressure in the pulmonary arteries is at systemic level.

Aortic atresia is the most common cause of heart failure in the 1st week of life. Failure tends to occur early and to progress rapidly. Cyanosis occurs in nearly all cases, with an average age of onset at 2 days, but may be delayed in appearance. The peripheral pulses may be weak or absent and blood pressures, when obtained, are lower than normal. More than half the patients have grade 1-4/6 systolic murmurs along the sternal border, probably due to increased pulmonary valve flow or to tricuspid insufficiency. Systolic ejection clicks and middiastolic murmurs may occur, but thrills are rare.

Thoracic roentgenograms show prominent pulmonary vasculature in nearly all cases. In most cases vasculature is of the shunt type, whereas the remainder show severe pulmonary venous obstruction. A prominent main pulmonary artery helps distinguish this defect from transposition of the great arteries. The heart is usually moderately enlarged. The "ductus infundibulum" is evident in the aortic knob region in at least half the cases. The ECG usually shows right axis deviation, but left axis deviation has been reported. Two-thirds show right atrial hypertrophy, and most show right ventricular hypertrophy, often with a qR pattern or upright T waves in the right precordial leads. In the left precordial leads, ST-T abnormalities are frequent, and the q wave is often absent.

The echocardiogram in aortic valve atresia shows little or no motion in the area of the aortic valve. The aorta is hypoplastic as viewed in both the anterior-posterior and superior-inferior axes. The mitral valve echo is usually absent and the left ventricular cavity is slit-like. The left atrium may be dilated. The right ventricle is dilated, as is the pulmonary artery (suprasternal), and tricuspid motion is excessive.

Cardiac catheterization shows reduced oxygen saturation in the venae cavae, with a rise in the right atrium. The oxygen saturation and systolic pressure in the right ventricle is similar to those in the aorta and systemic arteries. A right-sided angiocardiogram can show the right-to-left flow through the patent ductus with retrograde filling of the hypoplastic descending aorta. These structures may also be shown by thoracic aortography.

Complications
I **Derived:** Death from congestive heart failure or hypoxia. Myocardial infarction has been reported.
II **Associated:** Extracardiac anomalies (mostly minor GU malformations) occur in approximately 25% of the cases.

Etiology: ?

Pathogenesis:
This is poorly understood. The basic defect may be faulty early development of the outflow portion of the left ventricle, probably between the 5th and 8th weeks of fetal life.

Related Facts
I **Sex Ratio:** Estimated to be M2:F1
II **Risk of Occurrence:** ? Probably < 1 in 100 cases of congenital heart disease
III **Risk of Recurrence for**
    Patient's Sib: ?
    Patient's Child: Patients have never reached the reproductive age
IV **Age of Detectability:** From birth by selective angiocardiography
V **Prevalence:** Beyond 7 months, zero

Treatment
I **Primary Prevention:** —
II **Secondary Prevention:** Although no palliative procedures are generally accepted, balloon atrial septostomy, surgical creation of an atrial septal defect, and aortic-right pulmonary artery anastomosis with bilateral distal pulmonary artery banding have been tried. Reconstructive surgery may be possible for those few with an adequate left ventricle.
III **Other Therapy:** Symptomatic therapy if indicated

Prognosis:
Uniformly fatal, usually within the 1st week. Two cases have been known to survive for 7 months.

Detection of Carrier: —

Special Considerations: —

References:
Deely, W.J. et al: Hypoplastic left heart syndrome. Am. J. Dis Child. 121:168, 1971.
Meyer, R.A. and Kaplan, S.: Echocardiography in the diagnosis of hypoplasia of the left or right ventricle in the neonate. Circulation 46:55, 1972.
Moodie, D.S. et al: Congenital aortic atresia: Report of long survival and some speculations about surgical approaches. J. Thorac. Cardiovasc. Surg. 63:726, 1972.
Watson, D.G. and Rowe, R.D.: Aortic-valve atresia: Report of 43 cases. JAMA 179:14, 1962.

Contributor: **David G. Watson**

Editor's Computerized Descriptors: Resp., CV.

AORTIC VALVE STENOSIS

Includes: Sténose des valves aortiques
Valvuläre Aortenstenose
Estenosis de la válvula aórtica
Valvar aortic stenosis
Stenotic bicuspid aortic valve
Unicommissural aortic valve stenosis
Incomplete tricuspid aortic valve
Stenosis of aortic valve

Excludes: Hypoplastic left heart syndrome
Aortic valve atresia (79)
Aortic hypoplasia
Subaortic stenosis, fibrous (916)
Aortic stenosis, supravalvar (78)

Minimal Diagnostic Criteria: Left heart catheterization establishes the site and severity of obstruction. The essential hemodynamic abnormality produced by the obstruction to left ventricular outflow is the pressure gradient between the left ventricle and aorta during the systolic ejection period localized to the level of the aortic valve.

Clinical Findings: In approximately 65% of patients the aortic valve is bicuspid with a single, fused commissure and an eccentrically placed orifice; a 3rd incomplete or rudimentary commissure may sometimes be apparent. About 15% of patients have an aortic valve in which each of the commissures is partially fused. In 10-20% of patients, especially symptomatic infants, the stenotic aortic valve is unicommissural, possesses only a single leaflet, and is dome-shaped. The aortic valve ring may be relatively underdeveloped in infants and young children with severe stenosis of the aortic valve, a lesion which represents a segment of the spectrum extending to the hypoplastic left heart syndrome and the aortic hypoplasia and atresia complexes. The dynamics of blood flow associated with a congenitally deformed aortic valve commonly lead to thickening of the cusps and ultimately to calcification in later life. Secondary calcification of the valve is extremely rare in childhood. When the obstruction is hemodynamically significant, concentric hypertrophy of the left ventricular wall and dilatation of the ascending aorta occur.

Congenital aortic stenosis may be responsible for severe obstruction to left ventricular outflow without the clinical symptoms of diminished cardiac reserve that are so frequent in other forms of congenital heart disease. Conversely, in an occasional patient with mild obstruction, the clinical findings may be striking. Most children with congenital aortic stenosis are asymptomatic and grow and develop normally. Initial attention is usually called to these children only when a murmur is detected on a routine examination. When symptoms do occur, those most commonly noted are fatigability, exertional dyspnea, angina pectoris and syncope. Rarely described are abdominal pain, profuse sweating and epistaxis. The obstruction is at least moderately severe if there is a definite history of fatigability and exertional dyspnea. Exertional syncope occurs usually only in patients with gradients exceeding 50 mm Hg and is related to inability of the left ventricle to increase its output and to maintain cerebral flow during exercise. The disparity between the oxygen supply to the left ventricle and myocardial oxygen requirements is responsible for anginal pain. The diminished perfusion pressure and the increased duration of left ventricular systole limit coronary blood flow, while the elevated tension developed by myocardial fibers and the increased left ventricular mass increase the oxygen requirements of the heart.

When the degree of aortic stenosis is significant, a left

ventricular lift is usually palpable. If the systolic pressure gradient across the aortic valve exceeds approximately 25 mm Hg, a precordial systolic thrill is often palpated over the base of the heart with transmission to the jugular notch and along the carotid arteries. Ordinarily, the obstruction is mild if neither a left ventricular lift nor a thrill are present. The increased force of left atrial contraction in the presence of left ventricular hypertrophy results in a palpable presystolic expansion. The latter sign is almost always associated with a severe degree of obstruction and an elevated left ventricular end diastolic pressure.

A systolic aortic ejection sound (click) may be heard at the cardiac apex when the valve is mobile; and it is more often heard in patients with mild or moderate stenosis than in those with severe stenosis. In most instances the opening of the aortic valves is responsible for the ejection sound. Prolongation of left ventricular emptying and delayed closure of the aortic valve may lead to a single or a closely split second heart sound. With increasingly more severe degrees of obstruction the aortic closure sound may follow the pulmonic sound during expiration; ie paradoxical splitting is present. The systolic murmur which is characteristic of valvar aortic stenosis starts after the completion of left ventricular isometric contraction or with the ejection sound, and is diamond-shaped, loud, harsh, and best heard at the base of the heart. The murmur, like the thrill, radiates to the jugular notch and carotid vessels as well as to the apex. In approximately one-fourth of the patients with stenosis of the aortic valve an early diastolic blowing murmur of aortic regurgitation is present. Since the degree of regurgitation is usually not hemodynamically significant, the diastolic murmur is faint and the arterial pulse pressure is normal or decreased.

Although it is true that the ECG findings in congenital aortic stenosis often vary with the severity of obstruction, a normal or near normal ECG does not exclude severe stenosis. The findings that tend to accompany severe obstruction are T wave vectors in the frontal plane to the left of -40°, widening of the angle between the mean QRS and T forces in the frontal plane in excess of 100°, an S wave in V_1 greater than 20 mm and an R wave in V_6 exceeding 30 mm. Perhaps the most reliable index of the severity of obstruction in patients not receiving digitalis is the left ventricular "strain pattern" which consists of the findings of left ventricular hypertrophy combined with ST segment depressions and T wave flattening or inversion in the left precordial leads. This pattern generally, but not always, indicates that severe aortic stenosis is present. The vectorcardiogram best demonstrates the major influences of the left ventricular wall in the later phases of the QRS loop, and left ventricular hypertrophy is reflected in the abnormal displacement of the mean spatial QRS vector in a posterior, superior and leftward direction, maximal QRS spatial vector exceeding 1.4 mv and a QRS-T angle exceeding 60°.

A good relationship appears to exist between exercise induced ECG changes and the severity of obstruction. Thus, the development during exercise of ischemic ST-segment changes has been observed in patients with normal resting cardiac indices and transvalvar pressure differences in excess of 50 mm Hg.

On chest roentgenograms the overall heart size is usually normal or the degree of enlargement is minimal. However, concentric left ventricular hypertrophy accompanies moderate or severe obstruction and is manifested by rounding of the cardiac apex in the frontal projection. More striking left ventricular enlargement may exist in the presence of severe obstruction. Left atrial enlargement and evidence of

pulmonary venous obstruction strongly suggest that a severe degree of stenosis exists. Poststenotic dilatation of the ascending aorta is a common finding in patients with valvar aortic stenosis. Roentgenographic evidence of calcification of the valve does not usually occur in the pediatric age group but is a relatively common finding in adults with congenital aortic stenosis.

The single crystal ultrasound findings that may suggest a diagnosis of aortic valve stenosis include multiple diastolic closure lines, or a single eccentrically placed diastolic closure line in the lumen of the aorta, with or without thickening of the left ventricular posterior wall. Real-time cross-sectional echocardiography reveals impaired mobility of cusp tissue, an alteration in the phasic movement of the aortic valve with reduced lateral and increased superior excursions of valve echoes, and an increase in the internal aortic root dimension beyond the level of the valve annulus. Although the latter findings may accurately localize the site of left ventricular outflow tract obstruction, they have not yet been shown to correlate with the severity of stenosis. (See Bicuspid Aortic Valve)

The malformation may create unique problems in infants and the clinical picture in this group therefore deserves special comment. Although isolated stenosis of the aortic valve seldom causes symptoms in infancy, occasionally the lesion is responsible for profound and intractable congestive heart failure. In spite of apparently normal coronary arteries, infarction of the left ventricular papillary muscles may occur in some of these infants, resulting in an acquired form of mitral valvar regurgitation, which intensifies the heart failure state. Moreover, endocardial fibroelastosis often results from reduced subendocardial oxygen delivery and myocardial degeneration may be prominent. The symptomatic infant with isolated valvar aortic stenosis is irritable, pale and hypotensive. Presenting manifestations include tachycardia, cardiomegaly and pulmonary venous congestion, manifested by dyspnea, tachypnea, subcostal retractions and diffuse rales. Cyanosis secondary to pulmonary venous unsaturation may be observed. The systolic murmur is often atypical, particularly when the infant is suffering from heart failure. The murmur is frequently best heard at the apex or along the lower left sternal border and may be confused with that caused by a ventricular septal defect. In some infants with heart failure, the murmur may be absent or extremely soft, but it becomes louder when myocardial contractility is improved with digitalis therapy and other medical measures. Often, however, the response to medical management of the infant with congestive heart failure is poor.

The ECG findings in infants may not be characteristic; left ventricular hypertrophy with strain as well as right atrial enlargement and right ventricular hypertrophy may be detected shortly after birth. The ECG signs of right heart involvement result from pulmonary hypertension secondary to elevated left ventricular diastolic and left atrial pressures and volume loading of the right ventricle due to left-to-right shunting across the foramen ovale.

Complications
I   **Derived:** Left ventricular failure, aortic regurgitation (25%), sudden death. (The world's literature yields values ranging from 1-18%. Clearly, a large number of factors regarding selection are operative in providing this range of numbers.) Bacterial endocarditis (4%).
II **Associated:** As many as 20% of patients may have associated cardiovascular anomalies. Patent ductus arteriosus and coarctation of the aorta occur most frequently and all 3 lesions may coexist in the same patient. Less often, a ventricular septal defect and pulmonic stenosis are associated mal-

formations.

Etiology: Multifactorial inheritance

Pathogenesis: In a true bicuspid valve, 1 of the valve anlagen presumably has never formed. In other cases, 2 of the cusps have fused, forming a functional, single cusp containing a raphe (incomplete tricuspid valve). If 2 commissures have fused completely, a so-called unicuspid valve is formed. Rarely, there is partial fusion of all 3 commissures, resulting in a stenotic tricuspid valve.

Related Facts
I   **Sex Ratio:**   M4:F1
II   **Risk of Occurrence:**   1 in 2000 (5% of patients with congenital heart disease).
III   **Risk of Recurrence for**
  Patient's Sib: Predicted - 2.2 in 100; empiric - 2.2 in 100
  Patient's Child: Predicted - 2.2 in 100; empiric - 3.9 in 100
IV   **Age of Detectability:**   From birth by left heart catheterization and angiography.
V   **Prevalence:**   1 in 2000

Treatment
I   **Primary Prevention:**   Genetic counseling
II   **Secondary Prevention:**   Since the malformed aortic valve is a potential site of bacterial infection, careful prophylaxis against this complication should be followed in all patients, regardless of the severity of obstruction. Strict avoidance of strenuous physical activity is advised even when the patient is asymptomatic if severe aortic stenosis is present. Participation in competitive sports should probably also be restricted in patients with milder degrees of obstruction. Digitalis should be administered to patients with symptoms of diminished cardiac reserve.

  The most critical decision concerns the advisability of surgical treatment. Among the factors influencing the indications, techniques and results of operation are the patient's age, the nature of the valvar deformity and the experience of the surgical team. The decision to advise operation depends primarily on the presence of severe obstruction rather than on the symptoms described by the patient. At the present time, operation is recommended for any child with critical stenosis, ie peak systolic pressure gradient exceeding 75 mm Hg, measured in the basal state when the cardiac output is normal, or calculated effective orifice less than 0.5 cm^2 per M^2 of body surface area. At operation, the fused commissures are opened. When this is done precisely and judiciously, the commissural incision enlarges the valvar orifice appreciably and does not result in significant aortic regurgitation. Complete or almost complete relief of obstruction occurs in the majority of patients unless the valve ring is hypoplastic.

  Following commissurotomy, the valve leaflets remain somewhat deformed, and it is possible that further degenerative changes, including calcification, will lead to significant stenosis in later years. Because the valves are not rendered normal anatomically, antibiotic prophylaxis is indicated in the postoperative patient, even if the systolic pressure gradient has been completely abolished.

  Special mention of the treatment of aortic stenosis in infancy is important. The seriously ill newborn with congenital aortic stenosis must be considered to be a medical emergency. Because imminent death may be anticipated unless surgical treatment is undertaken promptly, definitive establishment of the diagnosis and valvotomy are usually justified, despite the high risk.
III   **Other Therapy:**   —

Prognosis: The prognosis varies with the degree of obstruction. Mild aortic stenosis is compatible with a nearly normal life span. However, even when the obstruction is mild, the potential hazard of bacterial endocarditis remains and there is a tendency for sclerosis and calcification of the aortic valve to develop in later life so that a note of caution regarding prognosis is necessary. Not only may sclerosis

lead to further diminution of the valve orifice with age, but the increase in the cardiac output and participation in strenuous athletic activities accompanying adolescence may also lead to a markedly elevated left ventricular systolic pressure. Moreover, although sudden death usually occurs in patients with the clinical signs of severe obstruction, this type of demise rarely occurs unexpectedly even in patients who are relatively asymptomatic.

  The worst prognosis is encountered in infants in congestive heart failure whose clinical course can usually be improved only if operative relief of the obstruction is accomplished. With the exception of infants, death is rarely due to congestive heart failure in the pediatric age group. Rather, ventricular arrhythmias are probably the most common cause of fatal outcome.

Detection of Carrier: —

Special Considerations: —

References:
Braunwald, E. et al: Congenital aortic stenosis. I. Clinical and hemodynamic findings in 100 patients. Circulation 27:426, 1963.
Friedman, W.F.: Congenital aortic valve disease. Natural history indications and results of surgery. In Goldberg, H. and Morse, D. (eds.): Important Topics in Congenital, Valvular and Coronary Artery Disease. Mt. Kisco, New York: Futura Publishing, 1975, p. 43.
Friedman, W.F. and Braunwald, E.: Congenital aortic stenosis. In Moss, A.J. and Adams, F.H. (eds.): Heart Disease in Infants, Children and Adolescents. Baltimore: Williams & Wilkins Co., 1968, p. 358.
Friedman, W.F. and Pappelbaum, S.J.: Indications for hemodynamic evaluation and surgery in congenital aortic stenosis. Pediatr. Clin. North Am. 18:1207, 1971.
Nanda, N.C. et al: Echocardiographic recognition of congenital bicuspid aortic valve. Circulation 49:870, 1974.
Weymann, A.E. et al: Cross-sectional echocardiography in assessing the severity of valvular aortic stenosis. Circulation 52:828, 1975.
Williams, D.E. et al: Cross-sectional echocardiographic localization of the site of left ventricular outflow tract obstruction. Am. J. Cardiol. 37(2):250, 1976.

Contributors: **William F. Friedman**
Stanley E. Kirkpatrick

Editor's Computerized Descriptors: Muscle, Resp., CV., Nerve

AORTIC VALVE, TETRACUSPID

Includes: Valve aortique tétracuspide
Vierklappiges Aortenostium
Válvula aórtica tetracuspídea
Quadricuspid aortic valve
Four-cusped aortic valve

Excludes: Four-cusped truncal valve associated with persistent truncus arteriosus
Aortic valve incompetence

Minimal Diagnostic Criteria: Four distinct aortic valve cusps may be noted at cardiac operation. Angiographic visualization, although possible, is difficult.

Clinical Findings: Usually, the tetracuspid aortic valve is a random finding at autopsy. Rarely, symptoms and signs of aortic incompetence may occur.

Complications
I **Derived:** Aortic insufficiency (20%).
II **Associated:** Displacement of the coronary orifice above the aortic ring.

Etiology: ?

Pathogenesis: This anomaly probably results from the formation of an additional intercalated valve swelling.

Related Facts
I **Sex Ratio:** Ml:Fl probable
II **Risk of Occurrence:** Rare (10 cases reported in the world literature)
III **Risk of Recurrence for**
    Patient's Sib: ?
    Patient's Child: ?
IV **Age of Detectability:** From birth by aortography in cases with insufficiency
V **Prevalence:** ? Extremely rare

Treatment
I **Primary Prevention:** —
II **Secondary Prevention:** Antibiotic prophylaxis for dental procedure if clinical diagnosis is established.
III **Other Therapy:** —

Prognosis: Excellent, unless complicated by development of aortic incompetence.

Detection of Carrier: —

Special Considerations: —

References:
McRonald, R. E. and Dean, D. C.: Congenital quadricuspid aortic valve. Am. J. Cardiol. 18:761, 1966.
Peretz, D.I. et al: Four-cusped aortic valve with significant hemodynamic abnormality. Am. J. Cardiol. 23:291, 1969.
Robicsek, F. et al: Congenital quadricuspid aortic valve with displacement of the left coronary orifice. Am. J. Cardiol. 23:288, 1969.

Contributors: **William F. Friedman**
Stanley E. Kirkpatrick

Editor's Computerized Descriptor: CV.

AORTICO-LEFT VENTRICULAR TUNNEL

Includes: Tunnel aortico-ventriculaire gauche
Aorto-linksventrikuläre Tunnelung
Túnel aórtico-ventricular izquierdo

Excludes: Acquired aneurysms
Coronary artery anomalies
Other forms of aortic valvular incompetence
Aneurysm of aortic sinus of Valsalva (53)

Minimal Diagnostic Criteria: In individuals with a general state of aortic regurgitation, aortography reveals the tunnel itself arising from the anterior aspect of the ascending aorta, beginning above the level of the origin of the right coronary artery and associated with early opacification of the left ventricle.

Clinical Findings: Clinical findings are those of aortic insufficiency with left ventricular strain. This condition also may be seen in the newborn period. Left ventricular enlargement is present and prominent pericardial bulge is commmon, as is a systolic thrill over "aortic area" and a diastolic thrill maximal along the left sternal border. Loud, harsh systolic and blowing diastolic murmurs are present in areas corresponding to those of thrills. Murmurs are separate, and do not resemble the continuous murmur of patent ductus arteriosus. Wide pulse pressure is a feature. There are ECG signs of left ventricular hypertrophy and strain. Radiologically, if the left ventricle fails, the pulmonary vascularity shows pulmonary congestion. The left ventricle is almost invariably enlarged with a prominent ascending aorta. Aortography shows enlargement of aorta with early opacification of left ventricle. In frontal projections, a tubular-like density, which represents the tunnel, projects from the anterior aspect of the ascending aorta in the region of the pulmonary trunk without opacification of the latter. In lateral views the tunnel projects anteriorly above the level of the right coronary arterial origin, and terminates in the left ventricle. The latter becomes densely opacified. The coronary arteries are normal. The aortic valve may appear stenotic.

Complications
I **Derived:** Left ventricular failure. Bacterial endocarditis in the tract is a theoretic possibility.
II **Associated:** —

Etiology: ?

Pathogenesis: ? The tract beginning in the aorta may be an accessory coronary artery which, in the ventricular septum, has direct communication with myocardial sinusoids.

Related Facts
I **Sex Ratio:** Favors male
II **Risk of Occurrence:** Rare
III **Risk of Recurrence for**
    Patient's Sib: ?
    Patient's Child: ?
IV **Age of Detectability:** From birth
V **Prevalence:** 1 per 1000 cases of congenital heart disease

Treatment
I **Primary Prevention:** Surgical obliteration of fistula. Early operation advisable.
II **Secondary Prevention:** —
III **Other Therapy:** —

Prognosis: In general, good to excellent. Aortic valvular insufficiency may be observed postoperatively in some cases.

Detection of Carrier: —

Special Considerations: —

References:
Levy, M.J. et al: Aortico-left ventricular tunnel. Circulation 27:841, 1963.
Nichols, G.M. et al.: Aortico-left ventricular tunnel. Recognition and repair in infancy. Chest 70:74, 1976.
Okoroma, E.O. et al.: Aortico-left ventricular tunnel. Clinical profile, diagnostic features, and surgical considerations. J. Thorac. Cardiovasc. Surg. 71:238, 1976.
Somerville, J. et al: Aortico-left ventricular tunnel. Clinical features and surgical management. Br. Heart J. 36:321, 1974.

Contributor: **Jesse E. Edwards**

Editor's Computerized Descriptor: CV.

AORTICO-PULMONARY SEPTAL DEFECT

Includes: Anomalie du septum aortico-pulmonaire
Aortopulmonaler Septumdefekt
Defecto del tabique aórtico pulmonar
Aorticopulmonary fistula
Aorticopulmonary fenestration
Aorticopulmonary window
Aortic septal defect
Aortopulmonary defect

Excludes: Truncus arteriosus (972)
Isolated right pulmonary artery arising from aorta
Large short patent ductus arteriosus simulating aorticopulmonary window

Minimal Diagnostic Criteria: Root of aorta aortography best delineates the abnormal communication between the ascending aorta and the main pulmonary artery, and is the diagnostic procedure of choice. Right ventriculography will reveal a normally formed infundibulum, a finding not present in truncus arteriosus.

Clinical Findings: The pathologic anatomy of aorticopulmonary septal defect consists of a window-like communication between the ascending aorta and main pulmonary artery. The defect is usually large and oval shaped with its lower margin lying at, or a few millimeters above, the normal pulmonary and aortic valve rings. The defect is rarely small. Approximately 25% of patients will have additional cardiovascular anomalies, the most common of which are patent ductus arteriosus, coarctation of the aorta, right aortic arch and ventricular septal defect.

The hemodynamic abnormalities in patients with aorticopulmonary window result from a large left-to-right shunt at the level of the great vessels. Because of the large size of the defect, the magnitude of the shunt and the clinical presentation depend almost entirely upon the relationship between pulmonary and systemic vascular resistances. The usual auscultatory findings consist of a loud systolic ejection murmur along the upper left sternal border that ends before the second sound. In less than 20% of patients there is a continuous murmur similar to a patent ductus arteriosus. When a continuous murmur is present, one can be sure that the defect is relatively small. Approximately 45% of patients will also have a low-pitched mid and late diastolic mitral flow murmur over the midprecordium and apex. As pulmonary vascular resistance increases, the systolic murmur may eventually disappear. Under such circumstances a loud, narrowly split second sound becomes the most prominent auscultatory finding with an increased intensity of the pulmonic component followed by a high-pitched diastolic murmur of pulmonic valve insufficiency. At this stage with pulmonary vascular hyperresistance, mild cyanosis is common secondary to some right-to-left shunting at the site of the defect (Eisenmenger physiology). Differential cyanosis of upper and lower limbs is not seen with right-to-left shunting in this lesion, as might be seen with a reversing ductus arteriosus and pulmonary hyperresistance, since with an A-P window desaturated blood flows directly into the ascending aorta, and is distributed to the entire body.

Thoracic roentgenologic findings are nonspecific and are consistent with any number of lesions that produce left-to-right shunting at the level of the ventricles or great vessels. Prominence of the main pulmonary arteries, increased pulmonary arterial vascularity, biventricular enlargement and left atrial enlargement are usually present. ECG findings vary and are directly related to the presence and severity of pulmonary hypertension and pulmonary vascular resistance. The majority of patients will present with a combination of right ventricular hypertrophy of the pressure overload variety and left ventricular hypertrophy of the volume overload type. Right ventricular hypertrophy alone is detected when the "Eisenmenger physiology" is present. Cardiac catheterization reveals a large shunt at the level of the great vessels just above the aortic valve. At times the catheter can be passed through the defect between the great vessels.

Complications
I **Derived:** Frequent development of marked pulmonary vascular obstructive disease (Eisenmenger physiology). Death from congestive heart failure or bacterial endocarditis.
II **Associated:** —

Etiology: Presumably multifactorial inheritance

Pathogenesis: Aorticopulmonary septal defect appears to result from a failure of fusion of the embryonic aorticopulmonary septum and truncus septum. This would account for the persistent communication between the ascending aorta and pulmonary trunk in the presence of normally developed arterial roots. In cases where the defect is large, the aorticopulmonary septum is probably hypoplastic as well.

Related Facts
I **Sex Ratio:** M1.5:F1
II **Risk of Occurrence:** ? Less than 125 cases have been reported in the English and European literature
III **Risk of Recurrence for**
    Patient's Sib: ?
    Patient's Child: ?
IV **Age of Detectability:** From birth by selective angiocardiography
V **Prevalence:** ?

Treatment
I **Primary Prevention:** —
II **Secondary Prevention:** Repair of the defect utilizing total cardiopulmonary bypass
III **Other Therapy:** Treatment for congestive heart failure or bacterial endocarditis

Prognosis: In the presence of a large defect, the prognosis is poor unless repair of the defect is accomplished early in childhood. Many patients will die in the neonatal period and virtually all by the 4th or 5th decade. With early repair, patients should have restoration of normal hemodynamics with minimal risk of residual pulmonary hypertension.

Detection of Carrier: —

Special Considerations: —

References:
Morrow, A.G. et al: Congenital aortopulmonary septal defect: Clinical and hemodynamic findings, surgical technique, and results of operative correction. Circulation 25:463, 1962.
Neufeld, H.N. et al: Aorticopulmonary septal defect. Am. J. Cardiol. 9:12, 1962.
Perloff, J.K.: The Clinical Recognition of Congenital Heart Disease. Philadelphia: W.B. Saunders Co., 1970, pp. 442-445.
Wright, J.G. et al: Aortopulmonary fenestration. A technique of surgical management. J. Thorac. Cardiovasc. Surg. 55:280, 1968.

Contributors: **Richard L. Bucciarelli**
Gerold L. Schiebler

Editor's Computerized Descriptor: CV.

APHAKIA

Includes: Aphakie
Afaquia
Primary aphakia
Secondary or apparent aphakia

Excludes: Surgical aphakia

Minimal Diagnostic Criteria: Presence of lens remnants or complete absence of the lens

Clinical Findings: Aphakia or absence of the lens, may be divided into primary and secondary types. Primary aphakia is very rare and more serious than the secondary form because it is usually accompanied by gross malformations of the eye such as aplasia of the anterior segment, severe microphthalmia or anophthalmia.
Secondary aphakia implies degeneration or rupture and absorption of the lens. This may occur without other eye disorders. Lens capsule remnants, often vascularized with fibrous tissue formation, are visualized along with ill-formed zonules within the pupil which generally dilates poorly.

Complications
I **Derived:** —
II **Associated:** Anterior segment anomalies, microphthalmia, anophthalmia, cataract in the opposite eye, facial malformations, retinal colobomas, nystagmus, congenital retinal folds, harelip, cleft palate, strabismus and mental retardation; also seen in the Hallermann-Streiff syndrome and chromosomal aberrations.

Etiology: ? Possible intrauterine inflammation, teratogenic agents or chromosomal abnormality. Occurs in rats and pigs.

Pathogenesis: In primary aphakia an arrest or failure of development of the lens plate has been postulated. Secondary aphakia results from reabsorption of the lens. This may follow spontaneous rupture of an abnormally thin lens capsule or abnormality in either the surface ectoderm or lens fibers.

Related Facts
I **Sex Ratio:** ?
II **Risk of Occurrence:** Primary: Rare. Secondary: Also rare but more common than primary.
III **Risk of Recurrence for**
    Patient's Sib: ?
    Patient's Child: ?
IV **Age of Detectability:** Primary: At birth. Secondary: At birth or postnatal.
V **Prevalence:** Very rare

Treatment
I **Primary Prevention:** —
II **Secondary Prevention:** Correct refractive error whenever possible. Enucleation may be necessary if eye is grossly abnormal and cosmetically disfiguring. An oculoprothesis is inserted after enucleation.
III **Other Therapy:** —

Prognosis: Vision adequate-to-good in the presence of an otherwise normal eye. Vision guarded-to-poor dependent upon associated eye anomalies.

Detection of Carrier: —

Special Considerations: —

References:
Mann, I.: Developmental Abnormalities of the Eye. Philadelphia:J.B. Lippincott Co., 1957, p.301.
Manschot, W.A.: Primary congenital aphakia. Arch. Ophthalmol. 69:571, 1963.
Pratt, J.C. and Richards, R.D.: Bilateral secondary congenital aphakia. Arch. Ophthalmol. 80:420, 1968.

Contributor: **Elsa K. Rahn**

ARACHNODACTYLY, CONTRACTURAL

Includes: Arachnodactylie avec contractions
Kontrakturelle Arachnodaktylie
Aracnodactilia con contracturas
Congenital contractural arachnodactyly
Hereditary dysplasia of bone with kyphoscoliosis, contractures and
   abnormally shaped ears
Beals-Hecht syndrome
Contractures, multiple with arachnodactyly

Excludes: Marfan syndrome† (630)
Achard syndrome
Homocystinuria (474)
Arachnodactyly, cataracts and mental retardation
Arthrogryposis (88)

Minimal Diagnostic Criteria: Arachnodactyly with multiple congenital contractures of limbs.

Clinical Findings: Multiple congenital joint contractures of fingers, knees, hips, elbows and ankles. There may be limitation of elbow extension. Fingers are usually long and narrow at birth with flexion contractures of the proximal interphalangeal joints. Thumb tends to be adducted onto palm. Ankles, usually valgus, have excessive dorsiflexion. Toes are long and often slightly incurving. Contractures improve spontaneously. Arachnodactyly is present with particularly long, thin feet and elongation of proximal phalanges of digits. Most affected individuals are taller than average. Pectus excavatum and carinatum are seen. "Crumpled" ears are almost always present with flattened top of helix, "crumpled" anthelix and partial obliteration of the concha. Kyphoscoliosis is an inconstant feature. It may be present in infancy and progresses with age, becoming quite severe in older affected individuals. Eyes, heart, and intelligence are normal.

Complications
I   **Derived:** Knee contractures may persist but are responsive to physical therapy. Scoliosis may become worse with age.
II **Associated:** Affected individuals are frequently breech deliveries. They may have delayed motor development because of contractures and hypotonia. There may be limited jaw movement and mild retrognathia. Congenital heart disease has been reported in a few cases.

Etiology: Autosomal dominant inheritance with variable expression. McK *12105

Pathogenesis: This condition would appear to be a generalized connective tissue disorder affecting connective tissue in utero, and improving with age in most cases.

Related Facts
I   **Sex Ratio:** M1:F1
II **Risk of Occurrence:** ?
III **Risk of Recurrence for**
    Patient's Sib: If parent affected 1 in 2 (50%) for each offspring to be affected; otherwise not increased.
    Patient's Child: 1 in 2 (50%)
IV **Age of Detectability:** At birth
V   **Prevalence:** ?

Treatment
I   **Primary Prevention:** Genetic counseling
II **Secondary Prevention:** Physical therapy; surgery rarely needed.
III **Other Therapy:** —

Prognosis: Normal life span with improvement of contractures by adulthood.

Detection of Carrier: Adults may appear almost normal with regard to contractures, but abnormal ear shape may help identify affected adults.

†**Special Considerations:** Marfan's original patient may have had this condition rather than what we now recognize as the Marfan syndrome.

References:
Beals, R.K. et al: Congenital contractural arachnodactyly. J. Bone Joint Surg. 53A:987, 1971.
Lipson, E.H. et al: The clinical spectrum of congenital contractural arachnodactyly. Z. Kinderheilkd. 118:1, 1974.
McLeod, P.M. et al: Congenital contractural arachnodactyly. Am. J. Dis. Child. 126:810, 1973.

Contributor: **Judith G. Hall**

_____

Editor's Computerized Descriptors: Ear, Skel.

ARGININEMIA

Includes: Argininémie
Argininämie
Arginase deficiency
Some forms of atypical cystinuria

Excludes: Argininosuccinic aciduria (87)
Dibasicaminoaciduria
Hyperammonemia (485)

Minimal Diagnostic Criteria: Elevated levels of arginine in the blood; absent or reduced levels of arginase in red blood cell lysates.†

Clinical Findings: The onset seemed delayed in some patients who appeared normal for the first 2-3 years of life, while others were considered to be retarded and to have had neurologic impairment in the first 6 months. Increasing clumsiness, spastic quadriplegia (lower limbs more than upper limbs) and loss of language and intellectual ability have been noted. Three patients from 6-12 years of age have lost the ability to walk and virtually all ability to speak. Seizures and EEG abnormalities have occurred in most of the patients. Periodic lethargy and irritability have been present in 5 of 6 patients.

 Blood arginine has been elevated in all cases, usually to levels > 10 mg/dl. Other blood amino acids usually have been normal. Urea has been at the lower end of the normal range. Urinary amino acid excretion may be normal on a low or moderate protein intake, but an atypical cystinuric pattern with arginine predominating has been seen in all patients at some time. Arginine also has been elevated in the CSF. Intermittent elevation of blood ammonia with lethargy, irritability, and in some cases, vomiting has been seen in 5 of 6 patients.

Complications
I **Derived:** Progressively more severe mental retardation and neurologic impairment.
II **Associated:** —

Etiology: Autosomal recessive; McK *20780

Pathogenesis: The diminution of arginase in red blood cells and presumably liver is the probable cause of arginine accumulation in the blood, CSF, and usually the urine. Impairment of urea synthesis is suggested by the persistently low blood levels and the intermittent hyperammonemia which may result from increased protein intake, intercurrent infection, or other stress.†

Related Facts
I **Sex Ratio:** M1:F1
II **Risk of Occurrence:** ?
III **Risk of Recurrence for**
  Patient's Sib: 1 in 4 (25%) for each offspring to be affected.
  Patient's Child: None of the patients described has reached reproductive age; the severity of their impairment will likely preclude reproduction.
IV **Age of Detectability:** At birth with assay of red cell arginase levels in cord blood.
V **Prevalence:** ?

Treatment
I **Primary Prevention:** Genetic counseling
II **Secondary Prevention:** Decreased protein intake will diminish the ammonia load to the impaired urea cycle and has been shown to lower blood ammonia and blood arginine. The use of keto acid analogs of essential amino acids may also be helpful. Therapy has not yet been shown to influence the course of the disease.
III **Other Therapy:** Physical therapy to mitigate the impact of increasing spasticity; nonprotein, high carbohydrate fluids

to treat the signs and symptoms of hyperammonemia.

Prognosis: The oldest known patient is 12 years of age. Clinical deterioration in this child and 4 other patients has been continuous. The effect of therapy, if any, is unknown.

Detection of Carrier: Red blood cell arginase levels in 5 carriers were at least 2.5 SD below the mean.

†Special Considerations: A normal urinary amino acid excretion pattern is seen at some time in all patients. The abnormal urinary amino acid pattern might be considered to be coincidental cystinuria.

References:
Cederbaum, S.D. et al: Argininemia with red blood cell arginase deficiency. Am. J. Hum. Genet. 25:200, 1973.
Cederbaum, S.D. et al: Argininemia with red blood cell arginase deficiency in two siblings. Pediatr. Res. 10:363, 1976.
Terhaggen, H.G. et al: Hyperargininämie mit Arginasedefekt: Ein neue familiäre Stoffwechselstörung. I. Klinische Befunde; II. Biochemische Untersuchungen. Z. Kinderheilkd. 107:293-312, 313-323, 1970.
Terhaggen, H.G. et al: Familial hyperargininemia. Arch. Dis. Child. 50:57, 1975.
Walser, M.: Nutritional effects of nitrogen-free analogues of essential amino acids. Life Sci. 17:1011, 1975.

Contributor: **Stephen D. Cederbaum**

Editor's Computerized Descriptors: GI., Nerve

ARGININOSUCCINIC ACIDURIA

Includes: Argininosuccinurie
Arginosuccinurie
Arginosuccinuria
Argininosuccinuria

Excludes: Hyperammonemia (485)
Citrullinemia (174)

Minimal Diagnostic Criteria: Presence of argininosuccinic acid in the urine, blood or cerebrospinal fluid

Clinical Findings: More than 2 dozen cases of argininosuccinuria have been reported. One form of the disease presents in the neonatal period with a rapidly fatal course. Most children are diagnosed at a later age and usually have severe mental retardation. Associated findings are seizures, ataxia, abnormal EEGs and trichorrhexis nodosa. Except for an enlarged liver, no other abnormal characteristic physical findings are noted.

Urinary excretion of argininosuccinic acid (ASA) ranges from 2.2 to > 20 gm/day. Concentrations of ASA in the CSF exceed that in the blood.† Normally there are only trace amounts of ASA in urine, blood or spinal fluid. Urinary excretion of ASA varies directly with protein intake. Urinary citrulline, as well as postprandial blood ammonia levels, are increased.

Complications
I **Derived:** Mental retardation is very common; ammonia toxicity with coma.
II **Associated:** —

Etiology: Autosomal recessive biochemical defect; McK *20790

Pathogenesis: Deficiency of liver argininosuccinase.†

Related Facts
I **Sex Ratio:** M1:F1
II **Risk of Occurrence:** Rare
III **Risk of Recurrence for**
   Patient's Sib: 1 in 4 (25%) for each offspring to be affected
   Patient's Child: Not increased, unless mate is carrier or homozygote
IV **Age of Detectability:** Presumably in the nursery by measuring urinary argininosuccinic acid after the beginning of milk feedings. Earliest patient diagnosed at 4 days of age. Measurement of argininosuccinic acid in amniotic fluid or argininosuccinase in cultured amniotic cells can diagnose an affected fetus.
V **Prevalence:** Rare

Treatment
I **Primary Prevention:** Genetic counseling
II **Secondary Prevention:** Dietary protein restriction to prevent ammonia intoxication.
III **Other Therapy:** Keto analogs of essential amino acids in the diet may reduce ammonia toxicity.

Prognosis: Severe mental retardation is very likely. Effect on life span unknown.

Detection of Carrier: Red blood cell argininosuccinase activity in the heterozygote is below normal values. Urine ASA may be slightly above normal in the carrier state.

†Special Considerations: Argininosuccinic acid (ASA) is rapidly cleared by the kidney so that the absolute plasma levels are not as elevated as in other aminoacidopathies. Since CSF concentrations are higher than blood values, ASA is presumably produced in the CNS where its abnormal accumulation may relate to the clinical findings.

Fasting blood ammonia values may be in the normal range whereas 1 1/2 -2 hour postprandial specimens are usually abnor-

range whereas 1 1/2 -2 hour postprandial specimens are usually abnormal.

Liver enzyme studies from 2 patients revealed essentially no argininosuccinase activity.

References:
Batshaw, M. et al: Treatment of carbamyl phosphate synthetase deficiency with keto anologues of essential amino acids. N. Engl. J. Med. 292:21, 1975.
Goodman, S.I. et al: Antenatal diagnosis of argininosuccinic aciduria. Clin. Genet. 4:236, 1973.
Hambraeus, L. et al: Arginosuccinic aciduria: Report of three cases and the effect of high and reduced protein intake on the clinical state. Acta Paediatr. Scand. 63:525, 1974.
Moser, H.W. et al: Argininosuccinic aciduria: Report of two new cases and demonstration of intermittent elevation of blood ammonia. Am. J. Med. 42:9, 1967.
Palmer, T. et al: Urinary excretion of arginonosuccinic acid. Clin. Chim. Acta 47:443, 1973.

Contributor: **Grant Morrow, III**

Editor's Computerized Descriptors: Liver, Nerve

ARTHROGRYPOSIS

Includes: Arthrogrypose multiple congénitale
Arthrogryposis multiplex congenita
Artrogriposis múltiple congénita
Multiple congenital articular rigidities
Guérin-Stern syndrome
Amyoplasia congenita

Excludes: Chromosome eighteen trisomy syndrome (160)
Pseudotrismus camptodactyly
Arachnodactyly, contractural (85)
Pterygium syndrome
Diastrophic dysplasia (293)

Minimal Diagnostic Criteria: Congenital nonprogressive limitation of joint movement in multiple sites.

Clinical Findings: Heterogeneous group of conditions all with congenital nonprogressive limitation of movement in 2 or more joints in 2 or more body areas. Multiple congenital contractures are also seen in a number of etiologically distinguishable conditions (Trisomy 18, Potter syndrome, congenital myotonic dystrophy, meningomyelocele, diastrophic dwarfism, etc). All combinations of flexion and extension deformities of joints can be found. Absence of normal skin creases and the presence of dimpling and webs over joints are commonly seen.

Three categories of arthrogryposis not secondary to recognizable syndromes can be distinguished: 1) primarily limb involvement, 2) limb joint limitation plus scoliosis, ptosis, cleft palate, generalized weakness or other malformations and, 3) limitation of joint movement associated with severe CNS disturbance. Individuals in category #1 are clinically similar with limbs usually in extension or mild flexion, internal rotation of shoulders, equinovarus feet, wrist and hand flexion, amyoplasia of limb and limb girdle muscles. Intelligence is normal, deformities are usually symmetric and involving all 4 limbs, but only arms or only legs can be involved. Category #2 is heterogeneous and undoubtedly represents several etiologic entities. Limbs are usually in flexion with feet in either calcaneous valgus or equinovarus. Muscles may be doughy or woody. Mild mental retardation may be seen. Elevated CPK, aldolase and abnormal EMGs are sometimes seen. In category #3 severe mental retardation often with microcephaly is seen. Limbs are always flexed and may be spastic.

Complications
I   Derived: Skeletal changes secondary to the original deformities, ie scoliosis and changes in shapes of carpal and tarsal bones. Delayed developmental landmarks because of limitation of movement. Breech presentation at birth. External genitalia may be abnormal depending on hip position (ie cryptorchid, or absent labia major).
II Associated: Anomalies are seen almost entirely in categories #2 and #3.

Etiology: Category #1 appears to be sporadic with a very small (< 1%) risk for recurrence. Category #2 is heterogeneous; all reported familial cases fall into this category. 1/3 of all cases have a family history. Autosomal dominant and autosomal recessive families have been well documented. 3/4 of reported familial cases are autosomal recessive.† McK *20810

Pathogenesis: Apparently anything causing decreased or absent movement in utero (neurogenic, myogenic, connective tissue, infection, space limitation, drugs) can lead to congenital contractures.

Related Facts
I   Sex Ratio: M1:F1

II Risk of Occurrence: Rare

III Risk of Recurrence for
  Patient's Sib: Category #1 - extremely low, category #2 - depends on family history, category #3 - ?
  Patient's Child: Category #1 - extremely low, category #2 - depends on family history, category #3 - ?

IV Age of Detectability: At birth

V Prevalence: 1-3 per 10,000

Treatment

I Primary Prevention: Category #1 & #3 - ?, category #2 - genetic counseling

II Secondary Prevention: Aggressive physical therapy and multiple orthopedic procedures often necessary. In category #1 contractures are very resistant to physical therapy, often requiring radical surgery. In category #2, contractures often respond well to physical therapy. In category #3, surgery to place limbs in position for care required. Poorly responsive to any therapy.

III Other Therapy: —

Prognosis: Life span may be normal, but probably related to degree of severity of involvement and number of other malformations. Scoliosis may compromise respiratory function. Functional prognosis depends on persistence and emotional support by family and physician. Patients can do surprisingly well and live independently.

Detection of Carrier: —

†**Special Considerations:** Arthrogryposis is a term which has been used loosely in the past to refer to any congenital contracture. Etiologic heterogeneity is definitely present. It is most important to make an attempt to recognize and distinguish known syndromes for prognosis and genetic counseling.

References:

Daentl, D.L. et al: A new familial arthrogryposis without weakness. Neurology (Minneap.) 24(1):55, 1974.

Fisher, R.L. et al: AMC: A clinical investigation. J. Pediatr. 76:255, 1970.

Hall, J.G. et al: Clinical delineation of arthrogryposis. Clin. Res. In press.

Lloyd-Roberts, G.C. and Lettin, A.W.F.: Arthrogryposis multiplex congenita. J. Bone Joint Surg. 52B:494, 1970.

Contributor: **Judith G. Hall**

Editor's Computerized Descriptors: Eye·, Oral, Skin, Skel., Muscle, CV., GU.

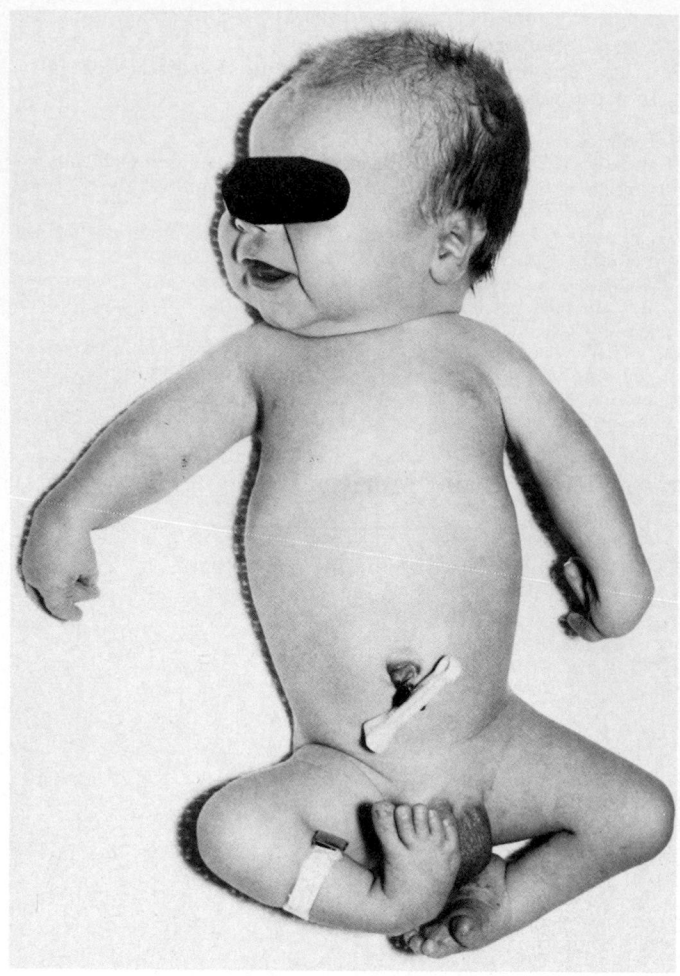

136. Note multiple joint deformities

ARTHROGRYPOTIC HAND ANOMALY AND SENSORINEURAL DEAFNESS

088-500

Includes: Arthrogrypose de la main et surdité de perception
Arthrogrypose der Hand mit Innenohr-Schwerhörigkeit
Malformacíon artrogripótica de la mano y sordera neurosensorial

Excludes: Arthrogryposis, isolated or in association with several syndromes
Cranio-carpo-tarsal dysplasia (223)

Minimal Diagnostic Criteria: Sensorineural hearing loss and arthrogrypotic hand anomaly

Clinical Findings: A family has been reported with an arthrogrypotic-like hand anomaly. Seven of the 12 affected persons in 5 generations have an associated sensorineural hearing loss. There is considerable variation in the severity of both the hand anomaly and the hearing loss. The degree of hearing loss varied from moderate to profound deafness with unilateral hearing loss in some family members. Height and weight of the affected persons were usually < 10th percentile. There was limitation of both active and passive flexion and extension of the fingers, and the flexion creases over both proximal and distal interphalangeal joints were absent. The thenar, hypothenar and interosseous muscle masses were decreased. Ulnar deviation of the wrist and of the fingers at the proximal interphalangeal joint was noted. Dorsiflexion of the wrist was limited. Contractures of the lateral and collateral ligaments of the interphalangeal joints were present. Muscle weakness was most marked in the distribution of the ulnar nerve. Limitation of elbow extension and flexion of the toes were noted in some individuals. Other patients showed limitation of pronation and supination of the hands. Roentgenograms indicated no underlying bone or joint pathology. Nerve conduction studies of the ulnar nerve were normal. Electromyography did not eliminate either a neurogenic or myogenic basis for this defect. Palmar dermatoglyphics demonstrated striking vertical orientation of the dermal ridges, absent digital triradii, and absent axial triradii.

Complications
I Derived: —
II Associated: —

Etiology: Autosomal dominant

Pathogenesis: ?

Related Facts
I Sex Ratio: M4:F8
II Risk of Occurrence: ?
III Risk of Recurrence for
   Patient's Sib: If parent is affected 1 in 2 (50%) for each offspring to be affected; otherwise not increased.
   Patient's Child: 1 in 2
IV Age of Detectability: Early childhood
V Prevalence: ?

Treatment
I Primary Prevention: Genetic counseling
II Secondary Prevention: Hearing aid in case of severe hearing loss in addition to supportive educational measures.
III Other Therapy: —

Prognosis: Probably good for normal life span

Detection of Carrier: —

Special Considerations: —

References:

Drachman, D.B. and Banker, B.Q.: Arthrogryposis multiplex congenita. Arch. Neurol. 5:77, 1961.
Stewart, J.M. and Bergstrom, L.: Familial hand abnormality and sensorineural deafness: A new syndrome. J. Pediatr. 78:102, 1971.

Contributor: **Cor W.R.J. Cremers**

Editor's Computerized Descriptors: Hearing, Skin, Dermatoglyphic, Skel., Muscle, Nerve

ARTHRO-OPHTHALMOPATHY

Includes: Arthro-ophtalmopathie
Arthro-ophthalmopathie
Artro-oftalmopatía
Progressive arthroophthalmopathy
Ophthalmoarthropathy
Stickler syndrome
Epiphyseal changes and high myopia

Excludes: Ehlers-Danlos syndrome (338)
Wagner syndrome
Marfan syndrome (630)
Epiphyseal dysplasias, multiple (358)
Spondyloepiphyseal dysplasias
Kniest dysplasia (557)

Minimal Diagnostic Criteria: Congenital high myopia and epiphyseal changes on xrays, in a nondwarfed individual who may have Pierre-Robin anomaly.

Clinical Findings: The primary feature is the high degree of myopia (ranging from 8-18 diopters) and moderately high myopic astigmatism. There are chorioretinal pigmentary changes and myopic crescents at the disks, premature vitreous liquefaction and peripheral condensation. Spontaneous total retinal detachments can occur in the 1st decade of life.

The associated joint manifestations are recognizable at birth by bony enlargement of certain joints, especially ankles, knees, and wrists. During childhood, stiffness and soreness occur after overuse; swelling, redness and heat occur occasionally, leading to crepitation and temporary locking of joints. The most severely involved joints are hips and knees. Slight joint hypermobility is observed in the majority of patients. On xrays there is unusual irregularity of the articular surfaces of many joints including the vertebral column and the knees which are commonly involved. Subluxation of the hips is a frequent finding. Abnormal development of the epiphyseal plate and loose intraarticular osteocartilaginous bodies are frequently encountered. The skin is normal histologically and laboratory findings are within normal limits. Cleft palate and micrognathia (Pierre-Robin anomaly) are common.† Many individuals have a Marfanoid habitus.

Complications
I **Derived:** Total blindness after the 1st decade and progressive moderate arthropathy
II **Associated:** Sensorineural hearing deficit in some patients; also cleft palate.

Etiology: Autosomal dominant with some variable expressivity; McK *10830

Pathogenesis: This is possibly a connective tissue disease.

Related Facts
I **Sex Ratio:** M1:F1
II **Risk of Occurrence:** ? Rare
III **Risk of Recurrence for**
Patient's Sib: If one parent is affected, 1 in 2 (50%) for each offspring to be affected; otherwise not increased.
Patient's Child: 1 in 2
IV **Age of Detectability:** Shortly after birth in case of positive family history, or Pierre-Robin anomaly.
V **Prevalence:** ?

Treatment
I **Primary Prevention:** Genetic counseling
II **Secondary Prevention:** Avoidance of excessive exertion including contact sports.
III **Other Therapy:** Enucleation of glaucomatous eyes

Prognosis: Normal for life span and intelligence. Disability exists in the majority of cases after age 10 years; ambulation mobility is preserved life long.

Detection of Carrier: —

†Special Considerations: Opitz has postulated that Stickler syndrome is one of the most common causes of severe myopia and Pierre-Robin anomaly.

References:
Knobloch, W.H. and Layer, J.M.: Clefting syndromes associated with retinal detachment. Am. J. Ophthalmol. 73:517, 1972.
Opitz, J.M.: Ocular anomalies in malformation syndromes. Trans. Am. Acad. Ophthalmol. Otolaryngol. 76:1193, 1972.
Opitz, J.M. et al: The Stickler syndrome. N. Engl. J. Med. 286:546, 1972.
Stickler, G.B. et al: Hereditary progressive arthroophthalmopathy. Mayo Clin. Proc. 40:433, 1965.
Stickler, G.B. and Pugh, D.G.: Hereditary progressive arthro-ophthalmopathy II. Additional observations on vertebral abnormalities, a hearing defect, and a report of a similar case. Mayo Clin. Proc. 42:495, 1967.

Contributor: **Irene Hussels-Maumenee**

Editor's Computerized Descriptors: Vision, Eye, Face, Oral, Skel.

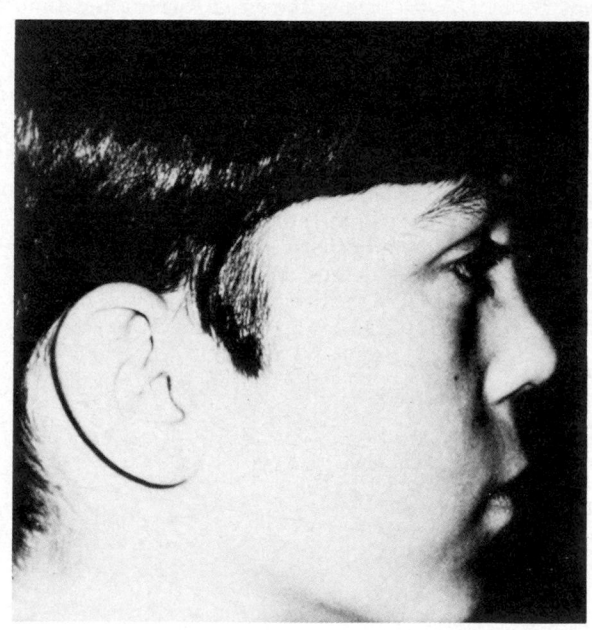

137. Note flat midface.

ASPHYXIATING THORACIC DYSPLASIA

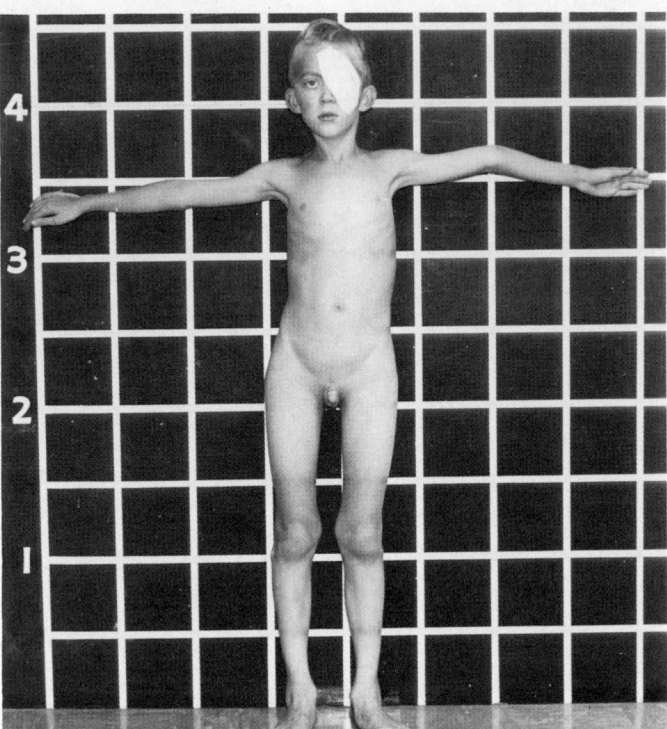

138. Note slender body build, joint hyperextensibility and genu valgum. Left eye retinal detachment bandaged postoperatively

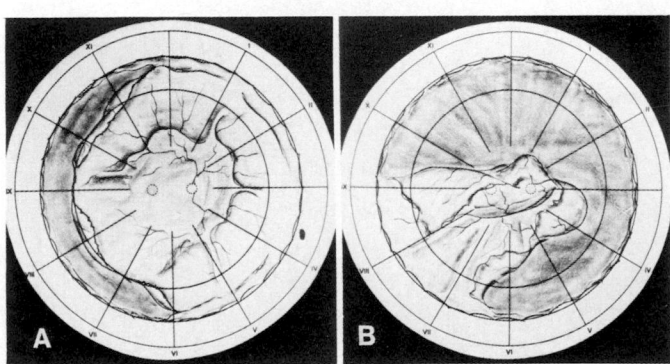

139. Retinal sketches: A) Rolled over temporal edges with 180° of disinsertion on right; B) rolled over retina with 270° disinsertion on left

Includes: Dysplasie thoracique asphyxiante
Asphyxierende Thoraxidystrophie
Displasia toráxica asfixiante
Thoracic dysplasia, asphyxiating

Excludes: Chondroectodermal dysplasia (156)
Thanatophoric dysplasia (940)
Metatropic dysplasia (656)

Minimal Diagnostic Criteria: The diagnosis can be made only by careful roentgenologic study of the thorax, pelvis and long bones. Although involvement of the pelvis may not be a consistent finding, its absence must cast some doubt upon the diagnosis.†

Clinical Findings: Asphyxiating thoracic dysplasia can be diagnosed at birth by a careful physical examination and a high index of suspicion. Findings include a narrow thorax which is in contrast to the shortness of the limbs. However, diagnosis of the condition is more often not made until the onset of respiratory distress, which usually occurs in the early months of life in association with an upper respiratory infection. The narrowness and immobility of the thorax lead to tachypnea and cyanosis. Expandability of the thorax is so severely limited that respiration is diaphragmatic. The limbs appear short in comparison to the trunk, but the morphology of the limbs is not otherwise altered. The craniofacial morphology is also normal. In an occasional case, polydactyly may be observed.

Asphyxiating thoracic dysplasia is often rapidly fatal in spite of intensive therapeutic measures. However, some less severe cases do survive. Sometimes, functional respiratory problems do not occur. In such cases, the diagnosis is possible only upon roentgenologic study. The roentgenogram reveals shortening of the ribs which is particularly evident on the lateral view of the thorax. The ribs are horizontal, short and stubby, and the anterior portions of the ribs are widened.

The characteristic appearance of the pelvis aids in confirmation of the diagnosis of asphyxiating thoracic dysplasia. The iliac wings are square, the roof of the acetabulum is horizontal, and its medial portion is deformed by a rounded protuberance limited on each side by a spur-shaped projection.

The long bones are in some cases somewhat short and stubby and the metaphyseal ends may be irregular. Often a small spine may be visible roentgenographically on the distal metaphysis of the humerus or on the proximal end of the tibia. The bones of the hands and feet are minimally involved, however, cone-shaped epiphyses may be observed. In patients who survive, the metaphyseal lesions of the long bones usually become more apparent, especially at the proximal end of the femur. On the other hand, asymmetry of the tibial plateau and fusion of the carpal bones is not observed as it is in chondroectodermal dysplasia.

Complications
I   **Derived:** In addition to the severe respiratory problems which are characteristic of the condition, Herdman and Langer have noted the occurrence of complicating renal insufficiency with albuminuria and hypertension in surviving patients.
II **Associated:** —

Etiology: Autosomal recessive; McK *20850

Pathogenesis: ? The functional respiratory problems are the result of a structural defect involving narrowness and immobility of the thoracic cage. Histologic study of the costochondral junctions reveals an oblique growth line with alteration of the cartilaginous portion. These alterations allow the condition to be classed as a form of chondrodysplasia. The lesion of the kidney first involves the tubules and interstitial tissues; glomerular lesions occur later.

Related Facts
I **Sex Ratio:** M1:F1
II **Risk of Occurrence:** ?
III **Risk of Recurrence for**
  Patient's Sib: 1 in 4 (25%) for each sib to be affected.
  Patient's Child: Not increased, unless mate is carrier or homozygote
IV **Age of Detectability:** The condition may be recognized in the newborn period by careful clinical and roentgenographic examination.
V **Prevalence:** Limited for the most part to the Caucasian race

Treatment
I **Primary Prevention:** Genetic counseling
II **Secondary Prevention:** No means known
III **Other Therapy:** Respiratory infections should be treated promptly and vigorously. Antibiotics and oxygen therapy should be used along with endotracheal aspiration and postural drainage when indicated. Maintenance of adequate nutrition may require feeding by nasogastric tube or even by gastrostomy. Affected infants should be immunized early against such diseases as influenza, measles and pertussis.

Prognosis: For life: Most affected infants do not survive early infancy. If the patient does survive the first months of life, death may result later from renal involvement. For intelligence: No effect upon intelligence in patients who survive. For function: In surviving patients, the growth of long bones is not markedly altered. Respiratory problems become less severe, but the thoracic malformation persists. Impaired renal function may occur.

Detection of Carrier: ?

†**Special Considerations:** The relationship of asphyxiating thoracic dysplasia to chondroectodermal dysplasia has been a point of discussion for several years. Indeed, the roentgenologic features of the 2 conditions are very similar, particularly those of the pelvis. Narrowness of the thorax, at times very pronounced, is not rare in chondroectodermal dysplasia. Moreover, the presence of polydactyly and dental anomalies have been observed in asphyxiating thoracic dysplasia, further illustrating its resemblance to chondroectodermal dysplasia. Despite these similarities, the 2 conditions are probably due to 2 different gene mutations, the modes of action and end results of which are similar.

Asphyxiating thoracic dysplasia of the newborn is not to be confused with another chondrodystrophy, thanatophoric dwarfism, which is incompatible with life, leading to death in the 1st few hours or days of life. The reduction in the height of the vertebral bodies seen in thanatophoric dwarfism allows its differentiation from asphyxiating thoracic dysplasia.

While asphyxiating thoracic dysplasia may be confused in the newborn with other conditions, including metrophic dwarfism and mucolipidosis II, differences in the alterations in the vertebrae, pelvis, and long bones allow distinction. In metatropic dwarfism, the ends of the long bones exhibit a dumbbell contour and the height of the vertebral bodies is reduced. In mucolipidosis II, the metaphyses of the long bones are irregular, simulating osteomalacia.

References:
Burkle, F. M., Jr. and Bravo, A. J.: Asphyxiating thoracic dystrophy: Malformation of the newborn. Clin. Pediatr. (Phila.) 8:165, 1969.
Herdman, R. C. and Langer, L. O.: The thoracic asphyxiant dystrophy and renal disease. Am. J. Dis. Child. 116:192, 1968.
Maroteaux, P. and Savart, P.: La dystrophie thoracique asphyxiante. Étude radiologique et rapports avec le syndrome d'Ellis et van Creveld. Ann. Radiol. (Paris) 7:332, 1964.

Contributor: **Pierre Maroteaux**

Editor's Computerized Descriptors: Skel., Resp., CV., GU.

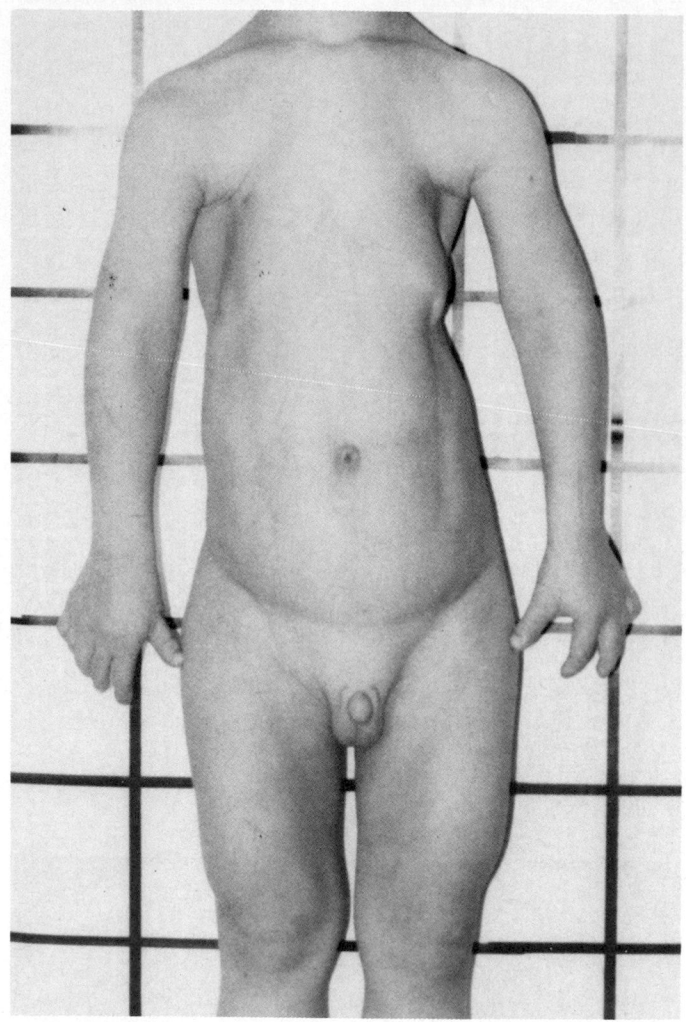

140. Note narrow thorax and short limbs

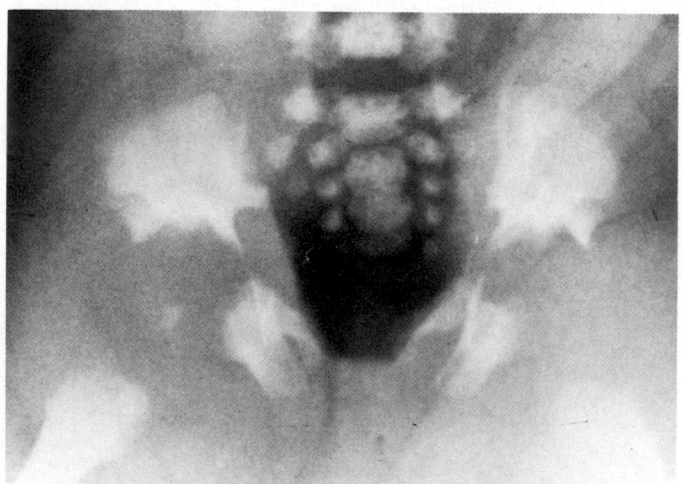

141. Note trident, short ilia; symmetric defect at lateral side of iliac bones above lateral articular margin in newborn at 32 weeks' gestational age

ASPLENIA SYNDROME

Includes: Agènèsie de la rate
Asplenie-Syndrom
Síndrome asplénico
Syndrome of bilateral right-sidedness
Teratologic syndrome of visceral heterotaxy
Splenic agenesis

Excludes: Isolated congenital splenic agenesis
Polysplenia syndrome† (816)

Minimal Diagnostic Criteria: Evidence for partial visceral heterotaxy and presence of Howell-Jolly bodies in the blood smear in an infant with (cyanotic) congenital heart disease. Radiographically, dextrocardia in combination with signs of severe pulmonary venous hypertension is virtually pathognomonic.

Clinical Findings: Asplenia rarely occurs as an isolated defect. Asplenia syndrome indicates a characteristic constellation of visceral anomalies of which the outstanding feature, in addition to the splenic agenesis, is a strong tendency for normally asymmetric organs or pairs of organs to develop more or less symmetrically. The left-sided organs or members of pairs of organs assume the morphologic characteristics of their right-sided counterparts, but in mirror image (isomerism). In at least 90% of cases an eparterial bronchus is present bilaterally, and the lobation of both lungs resembles that of a normal trilobed right lung. Accessory pulmonary fissures are common. The right and left lobes of the liver are about equal in size in 40% of cases and the lower edge of the liver is essentially horizontal. The stomach is located on the right side in about half the cases. Occasionally the stomach has retained a midline position with a proximthel portion located in the posterior mediastinum. Usually the intestinal tract has failed to rotate in which case the colon lies behind and below the small bowel and the mesentery is free and its root located in the midline. In rare cases a hypoplastic spleen may be present.

The echocardiographic findings are directly related to the specific associated lesions. Bilateral superior vena cava will not be appreciated by echocardiography. The total anomalous pulmonary venous connection may be found if the collecting chamber is posterior to the left atrium. See Total Anomalous Pulmonary Venous Connection.

Absence of the coronary sinus has not been appreciated by M-mode echocardiography. If an endocardial cushion defect is present, it will be associated with the usual findings. See Endocardial Cushion Defect, complete.

Right ventricular outflow tract obstruction will demonstrate its usual echocardiographic characteristics.

Children with this anomaly have very complex cardiac defects, and a 2-dimensional echocardiographic examination is warranted in most instances.

Complex cardiovascular anomalies are almost always present. Bilateral superior venae cavae are common, as is a common hepatic vein, contralateral to the inferior vena cava, draining the corresponding liver lobe. Some form of total anomalous pulmonary venous connection is found in almost all cases, at least 10% of these are of the infradiaphragmatic type. There is isomerism of the atria, ie both atria morphologically resemble right atria. The atrial septum in most cases is absent except for a peculiar triangularly shaped band of muscle which crosses the atrial cavity. The coronary sinus is absent. Some form of endocardial cushion defect, usually of the complete type, is present in the great majority of cases and generally there is only one functioning ventricle. Partial or complete obstruction to pulmonary arterial blood flow is found in at least 70% of

the cases and the great arteries, as a rule, are transposed. The cardiac apex may be directed to either side.

Clinically children with asplenia syndrome generally present themselves within days or weeks after birth with marked cyanosis, respiratory distress, feeding difficulties and congestive heart failure. Early death is common and infants who survive for any length of time often fail to thrive and tend to suffer from cutaneous, respiratory, and other infections. Peripheral blood usually shows the presence of polycythemia, Howell-Jolly bodies, Heinz bodies, siderocytes, target cells and normoblasts. The P vector may be abnormal, or change from time to time. Left axis deviation is common as might be expected, considering the high incidence of endocardial cushion defects; otherwise, the ECG varies so much from case to case as to be of little help. Radiographs commonly demonstrate partial visceral heterotaxy and the liver shadow may be evenly distributed bilaterally. There is a high incidence of dextrocardia. Because severe pulmonary stenosis or atresia is almost invariably present, the pulmonary vascularity is usually diminished. Occasionally, the airfilled tracheobronchial tree may be seen to be symmetric. Cardiac catheterization is of limited value, but angiocardiography will show the complexity of the cardiovascular lesions. Probably the most important angiographic finding is the disclosure that the abdominal aorta and inferior vena cava are found together on the same side of the spine.

Complications
I   **Derived:** Persistent or recurrent, difficult to treat infections. Volvulus has been reported.
II **Associated:** —

Etiology: ?

Pathogenesis: The spleen first appears in human embryos of 10 mm C-R length, ie about 36-37 days of gestation. Splenic agenesis must therefore be determined by the 34th-36th day. The conotruncal structures of the heart, abnormalities of which are so constantly associated with splenic agenesis, develop a day or two later and, therefore, some common factors acting at this period in gestation may be responsible for both anomalies. It has also been proposed that splenic agenesis and symmetric liver may be produced by vascular changes associated with partial situs inversus. The cause of the latter is unknown.

Related Facts
I   **Sex Ratio:** M2:F1 In some series, male predominance is much more pronounced.
II **Risk of Occurrence:** Exact figures are not available, but the syndrome is being recognized with increasing frequency and is not as rare as originally thought.
III **Risk of Recurrence for**
    Patient's Sib: Probably negligible
    Patient's Child: Patients have never reached the reproductive age.
IV **Age of Detectability:** Shortly after birth, by examination of peripheral blood smear
V   **Prevalence:** Very low due to extremely high, early mortality.

Treatment
I   **Primary Prevention:** —
II **Secondary Prevention:** Because of the extreme complexity of the malformations and the poor prognosis, therapy including palliative surgery is of little value.
III **Other Therapy:** —

Prognosis: Extremely poor, more than 90% of infants die during the 1st year of life because of associated defects or infection.

Detection of Carrier: —

†Special Considerations: While asplenia syndrome is very probably in some way related etiologically and pathogenetically to polysplenia syndrome, the 2 syndromes should be considered distinct entities.

References:
Goldberg, S.J. et al: Pediatric and Adolescent Echocardiography: A Handbook. Chicago: Year Book Medical Publishers, 1975.
Ivemark, B.I.: Implications of agenesis of spleen on pathogenesis of cono-truncus anomalies in childhood; analysis of heart malformations in splenic agenesis syndrome with 14 new cases. Acta Paediatr. (Uppsala) 44:Suppl. 104:1, 1955.
Putschar, W.G. and Manion, W.C.: Congenital absence of the spleen and associated anomalies. Am. J. Clin. Pathol. 26:429, 1956.
Ruttenberg, H.D. et al: Syndrome of congenital cardiac disease with asplenia: Distinction from other forms of congenital cyanotic cardiac disease. Am. J. Cardiol. 13:387, 1964.
Van Mierop, L.H.S. and Wiglesworth, F.W.: Isomerism of the cardiac atria in the asplenia syndrome. Lab. Invest. 11:1303, 1962.
Van Mierop, L.H.S. et al: Asplenia and polysplenia syndrome. In Bergsma, D. (ed.): Congenital Cardiac Defects - Recent Advances. Birth Defects: Orig. Art. Ser., vol. VIII, no. 1. Baltimore: Williams & Wilkins Co., for The National Foundation-March of Dimes, 1972, p. 74.

Contributors: **L. H. S. Van Mierop**
Elliot F. Ellis

Editor's Computerized Descriptors: Resp., CV., GI.

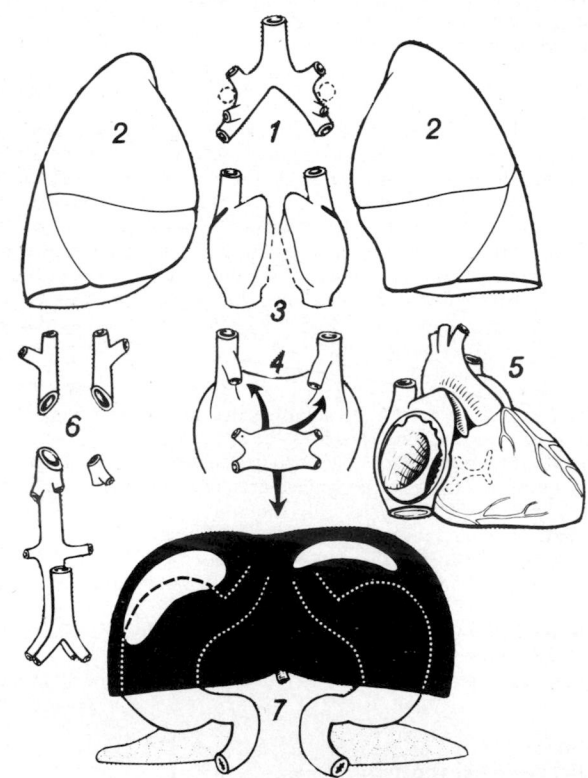

142. Note partial or complete failure of bowel rotation: 1) Bilateral eparterial bronchi; 2) bilateral trilobed lungs; 3) bilateral morphologic right atria; 4) pulmonary venous anomalies; 5) cardiac malformations; 6) systemic venous anomalies; 7) symmetric liver and right- or left-sided stomach

ATAXIA-HYPOGONADISM SYNDROME

Includes: Syndrome d'ataxie et hypogonadisme
Syndrom von Ataxie und Hypogonadismus
Sindrome de hipogonadismo y ataxia
Syndrome of cerebellar ataxia and hypogonadotropic hypogonadism

Excludes: Hypogonadism in other hereditary ataxias
Ataxia and hypergonadotropic hypogonadism

Minimal Diagnostic Criteria: Cerebellar ataxia and hypogonadotropic hypogonadism

Clinical Findings: Cerebellar ataxia, predominantly of truncal type, occurs in adolescence or early adulthood, usually accompanied by nystagmus, muscular hypotonia, rebound phenomenon, dysdiadochokinesia, tremor. Incoordination and dysarthric speech become more pronounced with advancing age. Signs of peripheral neuropathy may be present. External and internal genitalia are hypoplastic. There is no breast development or menses in female patients. Eunuchoid body habitus, gynecomastia and infertility are features in affected males. Emotional disturbance and personality disorders may be seen. Endocrine studies reveal the hypogonadism to be of hypogonadotropic origin.

Complications
I   **Derived:** Physical handicap because of difficulties in walking and manipulation; speech disorder; infertility.
II **Associated:** Macular degeneration and mental deterioration observed in some patients.

Etiology: Autosomal dominant male sex-limited (X-linked recessive?); in some families autosomal recessive (occurrence in both sexes, parental consanguinity).†

Pathogenesis: ?

Related Facts
I   **Sex Ratio:** ?
II   **Risk of Occurrence:**   ?
III **Risk of Recurrence for**
     Patient's Sib: 25% (50% for males in autosomal dominant, male sex-limited sibships)
     Patient's Child: 0 (Infertility)
IV   **Age of Detectability:** Puberty (hypogonadism); adolescence or early adulthood (20-30 years) for ataxia.
V   **Prevalence:** ? Rare

Treatment
I   **Primary Prevention:** Genetic counseling
II   **Secondary Prevention:** —
III **Other Therapy:** Physiotherapy, hormone therapy may be helpful.

Prognosis: Ataxia is slowly progressive in most patients; life expectancy may be reduced.

Detection of Carrier: ?

†Special Considerations: Sporadic and familial cases of hypogonadotropic hypogonadism and cerebellar ataxia were described predominantly in male patients; in a small number of sibships both sexes were affected suggesting autosomal recessive inheritance. The ataxia syndrome is not fully comparable with other forms of hereditary ataxia, but this suggestion deserves further studies. Endocrine dysfunctions are not uncommon in patients with hereditary ataxias or ataxia syndromes; however, hypergonadotropic hypogonadism usually is found. Extensive endocrinologic studies in such patients are necessary for clarification. Hypogonadism may be caused by the CNS defect, but more likely it is an expression of pleiotropic gene effects.

References:

Neuhäuser, G. and Opitz, J.M.: Autosomal recessive syndrome of cerebellar ataxia and hypogonadotropic hypogonadism. Clin. Genet. 7:426, 1975.

Rimoin, D.L. and Schimke, R.N.: Genetic Disorders of the Endocrine Glands, St. Louis: C.V. Mosby Co., 1971.

Skre, H. et al: Cerebellar ataxia and hypergonadotropic hypogonadism in two kindreds. Chance concurrence, pleiotropism or linkage? Clin. Genet. 9:234, 1976.

Contributor: **Gerhard Neuhäuser**

Editor's Computerized Descriptors: Eye, Speech, Muscle, GU., Nerve

ATAXIA-TELANGIECTASIA

Includes: Ataxie télangiectasie
Ataxie-Teleangiektasie
Boder-Sedgwick Syndrome
Louis-Bar syndrome
Telangiectasia and ataxia

Excludes: Ataxia without immunologic deficiency
Telangiectasis without immunologic deficiency
Immunoglobulin A deficiency (525)

Minimal Diagnostic Criteria: Cerebellar ataxia, oculocutaneous telangiectasis, sinopulmonary infections, decreased-to-absent serum or secretory IgA, immunodeficiency.†

Clinical Findings: Cerebellar ataxia becomes evident in infancy when the child first begins to walk between 7 and 14 months of age. Commencing as a truncal ataxia manifested by swaying of the head and trunk, slow progression subsequently involves the gait with later development of intention tremor and choreoathetosis. Characteristic oculomotor signs are: apraxia of eye movements, fixation nystagmus and strabismus. Telangiectasis of the bulbar conjunctiva may not become apparent until 2 to 6 years of age and frequently extends from the conjunctivae to the malar area and the pinnae. Faint telangiectasia may also appear on other exposed skin areas. Sinopulmonary infections of viral or bacterial etiology are the 3rd major component of the syndrome and are indicative of an underlying immunodeficiency. These may be radiographically evidenced as clouding of the sinuses, and acute and chronic changes in the lung fields. Defects of humoral immunity, notably decreased or absent serum IgA have been noted in 70-80% of patients studied. Reports of increased levels of IgM may be complicated by the finding of low molecular weight IgM in the serum of A-T patients which may erroneously appear as higher concentrations of the normal macroglobulin in several assay systems. Other immunoglobulin deficiencies include serum or secretory IgA deficiency and depressed-to-absent serum IgE levels. Cell-mediated immunodeficiencies have been evidenced by diminished cutaneous delayed hypersensitivity responses to common antigens and challenge with DNCB. Skin allograft rejection is also markedly prolonged. In vitro lymphocyte responses to several mitogens were found to be inhibited in many patients, but this could be reversed in some individuals by culturing their cells in normal human plasma, suggesting the presence of a circulating inhibitor substance. Histopathology of the lymphoid tissues reveals lymphocyte depletion in peripheral nodes contrasted with reticulum cell hyperplasia. Hypocellularity of the spleen and other sites of lymphoid tissue, notably along the gut, has also been reported. Autopsy studies have demonstrated that the thymus is often aplastic or rudimentary coinciding with frequent failure to visualize same on antemorten chest xrays. On microscopic examination, lymphocytes are sparse, the Hassall corpuscles are rare or absent, and reticular-epithelial stromal cells predominate. The major neuropathologic lesion is a diffuse atrophy of the Purkinje and granular cells of the cerebellar cortex and an associated degeneration of the olivary and dentate nuclei. Findings in the CNS have included diffuse demyelination and axonal degeneration of the posterior columns, partial demyelination of the spinocerebellar tracts, degeneration of anterior horn cells and axonal swellings in the tegmentum of the medulla. Ovarian agenesis or hypoplasia has also been found at autopsy. Other endocrinopathies include decreased 17-ketosteroid excretion consistent with gonadal dysgenesis, abnormal glucose metabolism associated with elevated plasma insulin levels and growth retardation as a possible consequence of pituitary dysfunction. A striking finding has been extensive nucleomegalic aneuploidy involving most of the organ systems and tissues of the body. A distinctive cytogenetic finding has been the emergence of clones of abnormal lymphocytes often involving a group D chromosome, identified as No. 14 in several cases. Other chromosomal aberrations including breaks, gaps and rearrangements have been reported to involve groups B,D,F, and G. Progeric integumentary changes in A-T patients, consisting of greying of the hair, and atrophy and increased pigmentation of the skin are suggestive of a sensitivity to actinic damage. Recent studies have shown that cells from A-T patients are highly radiosensitive, developing numerous chromosomal aberrations which are poorly repaired after irradiation. A high incidence of lymphoreticular and other neoplasms is associated with A-T and in fact, is the 2nd most frequent cause of death in these patients.

Complications
I **Derived:** Ataxia 100%, choreoathetosis 90-100%, nystagmus 90-100%, ocular apraxia 80-90%, dysarthria, recurrent sinopulmonary infections 60-80%, lymphoreticular malignancies 10-30%, other neoplasms.
II **Associated:** Ovarian dysgenesis, testicular atrophy, growth retardation, abnormal carbohydrate metabolism, hepatic dysfunction.

Etiology: Autosomal recessive; McK *20890

Pathogenesis: Onset of the syndrome is heralded by early ataxia. It has been suggested that the demyelinating process may have an autoimmune basis with sensitization occurring via low grade infection of the CNS as a consequence of an associated immunodeficiency. Neurologic dysfunction is followed by extension of telangiectases from the bulbar conjunctivae to the eyelids, malar area, exposed surfaces of the skin and outer ears. Progressive sinopulmonary infections and their severity appear directly related to the extent of the immunologic defect. Potential for neoplastic disease increases steadily with age and may be associated with an alteration in the proposed normal immune surveillance mechanism. It is also possible that this disease syndrome may predispose to a high rate of development of primary malignancies.

Related Facts
I **Sex Ratio:** M1:F1
II **Risk of Occurrence:** 2 to 3 in 100,000 live births
III **Risk of Recurrence for**
   Patient's Sib: 1 in 4 (25%) for each offspring to be affected
   Patient's Child: Patients have not had children.
IV **Age of Detectability:** 2-6 years if major clinical manifestations are present; diagnosis may be hastened and assisted if humoral or cellular immunodeficiency demonstrated.
V **Prevalence:** Equals incidence up to adolescence and declines as patients die. Longest survival to date is 46 years.

Treatment
I **Primary Prevention:** Genetic counseling
II **Secondary Prevention:** Avoidance of contact with respiratory pathogens; cultures and appropriate antibiotic therapy of respiratory illnesses; aggressive pulmonary toilet; immunization with killed vaccines only; physical therapy appropriate to neurologic dysfunction.
III **Other Therapy:** Treatment with intramuscular immune serum globulin is ineffective for IgA deficiency, but should be considered if IgG and specific antibody levels are significantly depressed. Frozen plasma has not been effective for the infectious complications of IgA deficiency. Oral treatment with fresh bovine colostrum is presently being studied as a source of IgA replacement. Use of radiotherapy or radiomimetic drugs in the treatment of associated malignancies should proceed with caution in view of the reports of significant radiosensitivity in several A-T patients.

Prognosis: Complete neurologic incapacitation usually occurs by 10-11 years followed by death due to sinopulmonary infection or lymphoreticular malignancy by midadolescence. Patients without pulmonary or neoplastic disease may expect survival to the 5th decade.

Detection of Carrier: In one study approximately half of the parents and normal sibs of A-T patients were found to be anergic or have depressed delayed hypersensitivity responses; another investigation demonstrated that 60% of the healthy family members of affected individuals had IgE deficiencies. Such findings may be suggestive of a carrier state.

†**Special Considerations:** Immunologic evaluations should be performed periodically as progressive immunologic deterioration including IgA deficiency, may not occur until late in the course of the syndrome.

References:
Biggar, W.D. and Good, R.A.: Immunodeficiency in ataxia telangiectasia. In Bergsma, D. et al (eds.): Immunodeficiency in Man and Animals. Birth Defects: Orig. Art. Ser., vol. XI, no. 1. Sunderland, MA:Sinauer Associates, Inc., for The National Foundation-March of Dimes, 1975, p. 271.
Boder, E.: Ataxia-telangiectasia: Some historic, clinical and pathologic observations. Ibid, p. 255.
McFarlin, D.E. et al: Ataxia-telangiectasia. Medicine 51:281, 1972.

Contributors: **Stanley A. Schwartz**
Robert A. Good

Editor's Computerized Descriptors: Eye, Speech, Skin, Skel., Nerve, Resp.

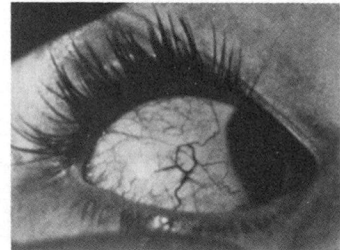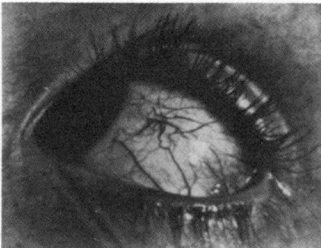

143. Note telangiectasia of the bulbar conjunctiva

ATRANSFERRINEMIA

Includes: Absence de transférrine
Atransferrinämie
Transferrin variant markers
Siderophilin
Iron-binding β-globulin deficiency

Excludes: Ferritin
Ferridoxin

Minimal Diagnostic Criteria: Diagnosis of atransferrinemia depends on demonstration of markedly decreased levels of transferrin or serum iron-binding capacity. The patient reported had low serum iron of 9-14 μg/100 ml and unsaturated iron-binding capacity of 19 μg/100 ml.

Recognition of transferrin variants depends on altered electrophoretic mobility. Acrylamide gel and starch-gel electrophoresis at pH 8-9 are the most widely used techniques, although some variants can only be discriminated at lower pH values, eg 6.5.

Clinical Findings: One case of apparently hereditary atransferrinemia has been reported in a 7-year-old girl who had severe hypochromic, microcytic anemia. At autopsy, there was hemosiderosis of the heart and liver, death having resulted from cardiac muscle damage. Low normal transferrin levels were found in both parents.

Transferrin from most persons consists of a single electrophoretic type, designated Tf C. Some 20 inherited electrophoretic variants are known, the group designation Tf B being used for variants more negatively charged than Tf C, and Tf D being used for variants more positively charged. Each variant corresponds to a separate Tf allele, all apparently at the same locus. Most variant transferrins are found in heterozygous combination with the common Tf C, both forms being produced. No clinical abnormality has been associated with electrophoretic variants of transferrin. They are widespread among animals.

Complications
I **Derived:** For atransferrinemia, the complications are those of hemosiderosis. For electrophoretic variants, there are none.
II **Associated:** —

Etiology: Autosomal recessive transmission for atransferrinemia. Autosomal dominant transmission for transferrin electromobility variants.† McK *20930

Pathogenesis: The chemical events leading to atransferrinemia are unknown.

Variant gene structures result in differences in the primary amino acid structure and hence in variations in transferrin electromobility.

Related Facts
I **Sex Ratio:** M1:F1
II **Risk of Occurrence:** ?
III **Risk of Recurrence for**
Patient's Sib: For atransferrinemia, 1 in 4 (25%) for each offspring to be affected.
For transferrin variants, 1 in 2 (50%) for each offspring
Patient's Child: For atransferrinemia, not increased unless mate is carrier or homozygote.
For transferrin variants, 1 in 2
IV **Age of Detectability:** At birth by electrophoresis
V **Prevalence:** Among American Negroes, certain African groups and Australian aborigines, the frequency of Tf D$_1$ heterozygotes may reach 10%. Tf D Chi occurs in approximately 5% of Orientals. Tf B$_2$ has been reported in approximately 1% of Western Europeans. Other variants are less frequent, many being very rare.

Treatment

I **Primary Prevention:** Genetic counseling
II **Secondary Prevention:** For atransferrinemia, transfusion. Pure transferrin is now commercially available but has not been tested. For electrophoretic variants, none required.
III **Other Therapy:** —

Prognosis: For atransferrinemia, shortened life span from effects of hemosiderosis. For electrophoretic variants, normal life span.

Detection of Carrier: Presumed carriers of atransferrinemia have low normal transferrin values and cannot be identified specifically. Electrophoretic variants are dominant and can be recognized by serum electrophoresis.

†Special Considerations: The structural locus for transferrin has been shown to be closely linked to the structural locus for serum cholinesterase.

References:

Giblett, E. R.: Genetic Markers in Human Blood. Oxford:Blackwell Scientific Publications, 1969, pp.126-159.
Heilmeyer, L. et al: Kongenitale Atransferrinämie bei einem sieben Jahre alten Kind. Dtsch. Med. Wochenschr. 86:1745, 1961.
Sutton, H. E. and Jamieson, G. A.: Plasma glycoproteins: Transferrins, haptoglobin, and ceruloplasmin. In Gottschalk, A. (ed.): The Glycoproteins, 2nd Ed. Amsterdam:Elsevier, 1972, pp. 653-689.

Contributor: **H. Eldon Sutton**

Editor's Computerized Descriptor: CV.

ATRIAL SEPTAL DEFECTS

Includes: Communication interauriculaire
Vorhofseptum-Defekte
Anomalías del tabique interauricular
High sinus venosus type defect with or without partial pulmonary
venous connection
Low sinus venosus type defect
Ostium secundum
Atrial septal defect at fossa ovalis
Absent atrial septum
Common atrium

Excludes: Endocardial cushion defects (347)
Pulmonary venous connection, total anomalous (842)
Lesions in which atrial septal defect is anatomically or physiologi-
cally a relatively insignificant part of the total clinical picture

Minimal Diagnostic Criteria: The clinical findings of pulmonary
ejection systolic murmur, tricuspid inflow diastolic murmur,
widely split and relatively fixed second sound with an accentuated
pulmonic component when combined with confirmatory ECG,
vectorcardiogram, and roentgenogram allow surgical intervention without further testing by catheterization and angiocardiography.

Clinical Findings: Atrial septal defect (ASD) as an independent lesion comprises 10% of all congenital heart
anomalies. Although the size of the defect affects the
amount of shunting, the defect is usually large and the
shunt therefore depends on the relative compliance of the
left and right ventricles. The most common anatomic type
is the large, central fossa ovalis variety, but ASD may also
occur at the entrance of the superior vena cava and more
rarely at the inferior vena cava entrance. In the former,
partial anomalous right pulmonary venous connection
may be an associated abnormality. In the early weeks of
life, the persistence of increased pulmonary vascular resistance and the thick-walled, relatively noncompliant right
ventricle limit left-to-right shunting. With increasing age,
pulmonary vascular resistance and the right ventricular
thickness decrease and the left-to-right shunt increases. It
is at this time that the murmurs and the clinical and
laboratory consequences of increased right heart flow become evident and the diagnosis is made.

Although the left atrial pressure is only slightly higher
than the right atrial pressure, a left-to-right shunt is
present and the pulmonary blood flow may exceed the systemic blood flow by 3-4 times. This flow produces the characteristic systolic ejection murmur of relative pulmonary
stenosis. The usual absence of a thrill is a helpful clinical
finding. Right ventricular systolic pressure is seldom more
than 50 mm Hg in an uncomplicated case of ASD and a
systolic gradient as high as 20 mm Hg may be present
across the pulmonary valve related to excessive flow across
a normal outflow tract. With large flow (eg exceeding 2:1
ratio of pulmonary:systemic blood flow) a diastolic inflow
murmur is heard from relative tricuspid stenosis. Wide and
relatively fixed splitting of the second sound with a late
loud pulmonary component is the most valuable and consistent diagnostic finding. A precordial bulge and right ventricular hyperactivity may be observed and palpated. The
presence of partial anomalous pulmonary venous connection as an associated defect does not significantly alter the
clinical picture.

Roentgenographic findings include increased pulmonary
blood flow, enlargement of the right atrium, right ventricle
and main pulmonary artery. In contrast to lesions with left-
to-right shunting at the ventricular and the great vessel
level, left atrial enlargement is absent. The ECG commonly

shows moderate right ventricular enlargement in the form
of the rSR[1] pattern. Some cardiographic evidence of right
atrial enlargement is seen in about 25%. The PR interval
is at the upper limits of normal except in sinus venosus
defects which are often accompanied by first degree heart
block. Axis is normal or rightward, and rarely may be leftward. In these latter cases, it is necessary to differentiate
an ostium secundum atrial defect from the ostium primum
variety in which left axis deviation and first degree heart
block are characteristic. The vectorcardiogram shows right
ventricular hypertrophy consistently with increased terminal rightward and anterior QRS forces.

The atrial septal defect itself usually cannot be imaged
by conventional M-mode echocardiographic technique, but
changes in blood flow which result from the defect can be
observed. The right ventricular cavity is enlarged with respect to normal and the septum may exhibit paradoxical
motion. Valvular motions are usually normal.

Right ventricular anterior wall thickness is usually normal. These individual findings are not exclusive for ASD
but, when all are combined, a right ventricular volume
overload is suggested.

Cardiac catheterization data show an increase in oxygen
saturation at the atrial level. Right ventricular systolic
pressure is usually mildly elevated. Tiny defects requiring
detection by more sensitive methods (eg hydrogen electrode) are rare. Angiocardiographic demonstration can be
accomplished by injection into the main pulmonary artery
with the shunt seen in the anterior-posterior view right
after pulmonary venous return into the left atrium. The
ASD can be more precisely delineated with left atrial injection with the patient in the LAO position. The diagnosis of
partial anomalous pulmonary venous connection as an alternate or accompanying cause of increased oxygen saturation of the right atrium can be made by selective pulmonary artery angiocardiography or indicator dilution techniques.

Complications
I **Derived:** Congestive heart failure, when present, develops
only with large shunts, usually in infancy or in adult life.
Pneumonia may occur. Bacterial endocarditis is very rare in
unoperated ostium secundum defects. Pulmonary hypertension with later development of the Eisenmenger physiology
usually does not occur until after the 2nd decade.

II **Associated:** —

Etiology: Multifactorial inheritance in the majority of cases. Also
associated with certain single mutant gene syndromes such as
Holt-Oram and Ellis-van Creveld. McK *10880

Pathogenesis: Defects at the fossa ovalis may be due to overab-
sorption of septum primum or hypoplasia of the septum secundum, or both. The pathogenesis of the sinus venosus defect is
unknown.

Related Facts
I **Sex Ratio:** M1:F2
II **Risk of Occurrence:** Approximately 1 in 1000
III **Risk of Recurrence for**
   Patient's Sib: Predicted Risk - 3.2 in 100; empiric risk - 3.2
   in 100
   Patient's Child: Predicted Risk - 3.2 in 100; empiric risk -
   2.5 in 100
IV **Age of Detectability:** The ASD may be diagnosed in early
infancy but more typically becomes apparent between 6
months and 3 years.
V **Prevalence:** 1 in 1000 in the pediatric population

Treatment
I **Primary Prevention:** —
II **Secondary Prevention:** Open heart surgery, formerly done

under hypothermia and inflow occlusion, is now usually performed with the heart-lung machine and cardiopulmonary bypass. The operation can be performed whenever the child is of sufficient size (usually 30 pounds is quite safe), and is done if the pulmonary blood flow is twice that of the systemic flow. Usually direct suture closure is feasible, but occasionally a prosthetic patch may be needed. Septal repositioning may be necessary with partial anomalous pulmonary venous connection and with sinus venosus type defects.†

III Other Therapy: Medical management until age 3 years. Usually this consists of observation alone, but rarely, treatment for congestive heart failure is necessary.

Closure of small atrial septal defects has recently been accomplished by threading an umbrella-like device into the heart by catheter technique. This method has been used successfully and safely in a few patients and may eliminate the need for thoracotomy in ASD repair in selected individuals.

Prognosis: Small secundum type atrial septal defects are compatible with a long life. Spontaneous closure of secundum atrial septal defects may rarely occur, particularly early in life.

Death in early infancy is rare but it has been reported, usually from congestive failure. Pneumonia is also a rare cause of mortality, but death from all causes is rare before the 4th decade. In later life, patients with an ASD have a higher incidence of arrhythmias and unoperated cases may die from progressive pulmonary vascular disease.

Detection of Carrier: —

†Special Considerations: Larger defects with cardiomegaly and clinical symptoms require operative closure. Closure should be accomplished before pulmonary hypertension occurs. This usually does not occur until early adult life and the occurrence then of cyanosis with right-to-left shunting implies inoperability. Patients with small defects without clinical symptoms, without cardiomegaly and without pulmonary vascular disease can probably live a full lifetime without operation. On the other hand, operation in the pediatric age group carries a mortality which is less than 0.5%, so that some cardiologists advise operation more freely in milder cases.

References:

Diamond, M.A. et al: Echocardiographic features of atrial septal defect. Circulation 43:129, 1971.

Goldberg, S.J. et al: Pediatric and Adolescent Echocardiography. Chicago:Year Book Medical Publishers, 1975.

Keith, J.D. et al: Atrial septal defect. In Heart Disease in Infancy and Childhood, 2nd Ed. New York:Macmillan Co., 1967, p. 392.

Krovetz, L.J. et al: Atrial septal defect: Ostium secundum. In Handbook of Pediatric Cardiology. New York:Harper and Row, 1969.

Weidman, W.H. and DuShane, J.W.: Defects of the atrial septum and endocardial cushion. In Moss, A.J. and Adams, F.H. (eds.): Heart Disease in Infants, Children, and Adolescents. Baltimore:Williams & Wilkins, 1968, p. 297.

Contributor: **Leonard M. Linde**

_____

Editor's Computerized Descriptors: Resp., CV.

AUDITORY CANAL ATRESIA

Includes: Atrésie du conduit auditif externe
Gehörgangsatresie
Atresia del conducto auditivo externo
Atresia of auditory canal

Excludes: Microtia-atresia (664)
Postsurgical or posttraumatic stenosis of external auditory canal

Minimal Diagnostic Criteria: Atresia of external auditory canal

Clinical Findings: The appearance of the pinna is not diagnostic. The patient may have a normal pinna or one that is somewhat low set, large, small or with a minor variation such as a prominent anthelix or folded-over helix. The canal may be completely atretic without a visible meatus or may appear patent only to funnel down to complete atresia at about the osseous-cartilaginous junction of the ear canal. Membranous occlusion has also been reported. Limited information is available regarding polytomography or other roentgenographic findings in the ears. In general, xrays have been normal except for 1 report in which the middle ear in the unilateral case was smaller than that on the normal side. Vestibular testing by rotation has been done in a few cases and reported to be normal. At surgical exploration 1 or more of the following middle ear anomalies have been noted: fixation of the malleus to the tympanic plate, stapes footplate fixation, fusion of the malleus and incus, abnormal course of the facial nerve, hypoplasia of the middle ear space, retrodisplacement of the ossicles in reference to the bony posterior canal wall, and absence of the anulus tympanicus.

Most patients with external auditory canal atresia are otherwise normal.

Complications
I Derived: Maximum conductive hearing loss with significant speech and language handicap if bilateral.
II Associated: Somatic malformations, mild hypertelorism, epicanthal folds, flattened midface, submucous cleft palate, micrognathia, mild syndactyly of some of the toes and fingers, clubfoot, congenital dislocation of the hip, cardiac anomalies, hydronephrosis, hypospadias, mental retardation, microcephaly, frontal bossing, ptosis, chromosome 18q-, absent IgA.

Etiology: ?

Pathogenesis: ? There may be failure of recanalization of the primitive auditory canal, or recanalization may be partial.

Related Facts
I Sex Ratio: M1:F1
II Risk of Occurrence: ?
III Risk of Recurrence for
    Patient's Sib: ?
    Patient's Child: ?
IV Age of Detectability: Potentially at birth, but if a careful newborn physical examination is not performed, it may be missed since the meatus and cartilaginous canal may appear normal. In these instances the defect may not be known until the hearing loss is discovered.
V Prevalence: ?

Treatment
I Primary Prevention: —
II Secondary Prevention: If the atresia is bilateral the infant should be fitted with a hearing aid. At about age 4 or 5 years corrective surgery to create a canal and correct middle ear malformations should be done on 1 side unless petrous pyramid polytomography shows that there is a coincidental inner ear malformation or that the middle ear malformation is so

severe that it precludes successful surgery. If the atresia is unilateral, surgery should be deferred until adult life when the individual can decide whether or not he wishes to undergo surgery, fully understanding the risks involved.

III Other Therapy: —

Prognosis: Generally good for life unless the patient has serious concomitant defects.

Fair for obtaining serviceable hearing after surgery. Possible complications of surgery include failure to have improvement in hearing, otitis media and perforation of the tympanic membrane graft, injury to the inner ear with loss of hearing, injury to the facial nerve resulting in facial palsy or paralysis, persistent perilymph leak from the oval window if a fixed stapes and abnormally patent cochlear aqueduct coexist, and recurrent meningitis if a perilymph fistula persists.

Detection of Carrier: —

Special Considerations: —

References:
Colver, B.N.: Bilateral atresia of external auditory canal without malformation of concha; report of case with surgical relief. Arch Otolaryngol. 17:476, 1933.

Crabtree, J.A.: Tympanoplastic techniques in congenital atresia. Arch. Otolaryngol. 88:63, 1968.

Hall, C: Unilateral atresia of auditory canal without external deformity; case. Ann. Otol. Rhinol. Laryngol. 43:306, 1934.

Hooft, C. et al: Chromosome 18 en anneau. (Ring chromosome). Acta Paediatr. Belg. 22:Fasc. 2, 69, 1968.

Stewart, J.M. et al: Absent IgA and deletions of chromosome 18. J. Med. Genet. 7:11, 1970.

Contributor: LaVonne Bergstrom

Editor's Computerized Descriptors: Eye, Hearing, Ear, Face, Oral, Speech, Skel., CV., GU., Nerve

AURICULO-OSTEODYSPLASIA

Includes: Auriculo-osteodysplasie
Osteodisplasia auricular
Short stature, elongated ear lobe, elbow-hip dislocation

Excludes: Nail-patella syndrome (704)

Minimal Diagnostic Criteria: Abnormal shape of the ear lobes, short stature and dysplasia or dislocation of the elbows and hips.

Clinical Findings: Short stature with all affected individuals below the 50th% for height. The external ear is distinguishing as it shows elongated lobes, attached and accompanied by a small, slight posterior lobule. They may also be small and flattened superiorly. A number of skeletal abnormalities are found. The elbows vary from mild radial head dysplasia to dislocation, always bilaterally and there is associated limited range of movement. Similar though less frequent changes are seen in the hips. Other skeletal features include minor anomalies of the scapula, clavicles and wrists. The nails, teeth and hair are normal. Intelligence is also normal.

Complications
I Derived: Degenerative joint disease may occur in dysplastic or dislocated hips.
II Associated: —

Etiology: Autosomal dominant with full penetrance but variability in expression; McK *10900

Pathogenesis: ?

Related Facts
I Sex Ratio: M1:F1
II Risk of Occurrence: ? Rare
III Risk of Recurrence for
    Patient's Sib: If parent is affected, 1 in 2 (50%) for each offspring to be affected; otherwise not increased.
    Patient's Child: 1 in 2
IV Age of Detectability: At birth by physical and radiographic examination
V Prevalence: ? Rare, only 2 kindreds reported in the literature

Treatment
I Primary Prevention: Genetic counseling
II Secondary Prevention: By early recognition and care of the hips for dysplasia or dislocation
III Other Therapy: —

Prognosis: Normal for life span and intelligence. Limb function variable.

Detection of Carrier: —

Special Considerations: —

References:
Beals, R.K.: Auriculo-osteodysplasia. A syndrome of multiple osseous dysplasia, ear anomaly, and short stature. J. Bone Joint Surg. 49-A:1541, 1967.

Contributor: Charles I. Scott, Jr.

Editor's Computerized Descriptors: Ear, Skel.

Includes: Calvitie commune
Kahlköpfigkeit
Calvicie común
Alopecia, male or female pattern
Premature alopecia
Androgenetic alopecia
Androgen-genetic regional alopecia
Seborrheic alopecia
Chronic diffuse alopecia

Excludes: Other congenital alopecias
Alopecia areata (38)

Minimal Diagnostic Criteria: Chronic or progressive postpubertal loss of hair on scalp

Clinical Findings: An M-shaped frontal recession of the hair margin is usually followed by the development of a bald spot on the posterior crown in men. Enlargement and confluence of these bald areas may progress to a final stage where only a peripheral fringe of scalp hair remains on the temporal and occipital portions of the scalp. Women with masculinizing syndromes or idiopathic hirsutism may have a similar loss of hair. However, common baldness in women is usually quite different clinically, in that alopecia is more diffuse and severe in the frontocentral scalp and only rarely, if ever, progresses to a smooth pate. Seborrhea and tenderness or discomfort of the scalp may be experienced.

Complications
I **Derived:** Actinic keratosis and epitheliomas of scalp caused by sunlight
II **Associated:** —

Etiology: Mode of transmission is not certain. Has been thought to be autosomal dominant in males and autosomal recessive in females who are bald only if homozygous. Some reports suggest autosomal dominant inheritance with incomplete penetrance and variable expressivity. Men are more commonly and severely affected than women. Androgens are necessary for phenotypic expression, as is aging. McK *10920

Pathogenesis: Most likely there is a single pathogenic entity in men and women. Usually the onset is gradual with increased loss of hair and thinning of the frontal and vertical scalp regions. The shed hairs are all telogen (resting) hairs and tend to be short and thinned because the anagen (growth) phase progressively shortens. An ascending obliterative fibrosis of the follicular connective tissue sheaths is seen histologically.

Related Facts
I   **Sex Ratio:** ? M1.5-2:F1
II **Risk of Occurrence:** ?
III **Risk of Recurrence for**
    Patient's Sib: If autosomal dominant or autosomal recessive, see Table I AD or AR, respectively.
    Patient's Child: If autosomal dominant or autosomal recessive, see Table I AD or AR, respectively.
IV **Age of Detectability:** Average age at onset in Caucasian men is in early 20s and in women a decade later. Detection by clinical evaluation including gross and microscopic examination of the scalp and hairs.†
V   **Prevalence:** Precise data are not available. Current estimates are at least 50% of men and 25% of women of Caucasian ancestry will be affected. Negroes are less commonly affected, and American Indians and Orientals least of all.

Treatment
I **Primary Prevention:** ? Genetic counseling
II **Secondary Prevention:** Punch or strip autografts of the peripheral unaffected fringe of occipital and temporal scalp may be used to repopulate the bald areas with permanently growing hairs.
III **Other Therapy:** —

Prognosis: Normal life span, intelligence, and fertility. The end stages of the condition where only a peripheral fringe of normal scalp hair outlines a bald pate will develop in at least 15% of Caucasian men. Degrees of baldness in women are rarely as severe as those that develop in men.

Detection of Carrier: —

†**Special Considerations:** Delayed onset and variable expression make ascertainment difficult to determine. The distinction between normal growth of scalp hair and mild common baldness may be difficult to determine. Also, expression of the disorder will be more apparent in later decades but will merge with loss of hair thought to be unrelated and normal for aged persons.

References:
Barman, J.M. et al: Biological basis of the inception and evolution of baldness. J. Gerontol. 24:163, 1969.
Hamilton, J. B.: Patterned loss of hair in man: Types and incidence. Ann. N. Y. Acad. Sci. 53:708, 1951.
Salamon, T.: Genetic factors in male pattern alopecia. In Baccaredda-Boy, A. et al (eds.): Biopathology of Pattern Alopecia. New York:S.Karger, 1968, p. 39.

Contributor: **Sigfrid A. Muller**

————————————

Editor's Computerized Descriptor: Hair

BARTTER SYNDROME

Includes: Syndrome de Bartter
Sindrome de Bartter
Pseudohypoadrenocorticism

Excludes: Secondary hyperaldosteronism due to
a) medullary cystic disease of kidney
b) juvenile nephrophthisis
c) chronic laxative abuse
d) chronic diuretic abuse

Minimal Diagnostic Criteria: The term Bartter syndrome should be restricted to those patients having hypokalemic alkalosis, normotension, hyperaldosteronism, and juxtaglomerular hyperplasia without a primary renal, GI, or drug-induced cause.

Clinical Findings: This syndrome most commonly presents in late infancy or early childhood, and is characterized by hypokalemia, hypochloremia, alkalosis, normal blood pressure, hyperaldosteronism and hyperplasia of the juxtaglomerular apparatus. Other features include growth retardation, muscle weakness, mental retardation, and polyuria with inability to concentrate urine. Edema is not present. Plasma renin and angiotensin levels are elevated. The pressor response to infused angiotensin is diminished, as is the rise in aldosterone following infusion of renin.

Adolescents and young adults with this syndrome also have been reported. In these cases intellect and stature have been normal, periods of severe weakness have even been diagnosed as periodic paralysis, and weight loss with vomiting has been ascribed to psychologic disturbances including anorexia nervosa.

Chronic abuse of diuretics and purgatives may mimic this condition: indeed chronic sodium depletion of various etiologies may mimic the findings by its effect of stimulating the renin-angiotensin-aldosterone system and the juxtaglomerular renal apparatus. Consequently renal diseases such as medullary cystic disease and juvenile nephronophthisis may simulate the Bartter syndrome.

Complications
I **Derived:** The complications are predominantly due to the effects of hypokalemia; and have been described above.
II **Associated:** Erythropoietin overproduction and erythrocytosis have been described. Also, capillary basement membrane thickening has been described in the renal glomeruli.

Etiology: The precise etiology of this defect remains unknown. In the full blown syndrome, male and female sibs have been reported and consanguinity has been recorded suggesting autosomal recessive inheritance. McK *24120

Pathogenesis: The precise pathogenesis of Bartter syndrome is not known. There may be a defect in renal tubular reabsorption of sodium or a defect in the conversion of angiotensin I to angiotensin II, as a result of deficiency in renin substrate. Expansion of the plasma volume by sodium loading does not lower aldosterone excretion in Bartter syndrome, whereas expansion of plasma volume will lower aldosterone secretion when the syndrome is simulated by renal, GI or drug-induced causes.

Related Facts
I **Sex Ratio:** M1:F1
II **Risk of Occurrence:** ?
III **Risk of Recurrence for**
Patient's Sib: If autosomal recessive 1 in 4 (25%) for each offspring to be affected.
Patient's Child: Not increased unless mate is carrier or homozygote.
IV **Age of Detectability:** May be detected in infancy to adult life, most commonly in early childhood.
V **Prevalence:** ?

Treatment
I **Primary Prevention:** The likelihood of autosomal recessive inheritance permits genetic counseling and evaluation of sibs.
II **Secondary Prevention:** Aldosterone antagonists such as spironolactone or triamterene in association with supplementation by large doses of potassium have tended to correct the hyperkalemia in some patients. The beta-adrenergic blocking agent propranolol which can inhibit the production of renin, when given in conjunction with spironolactone, has also proven efficacious.
III **Other Therapy:** Secondary causes such as diuretic abuse should be eliminated.

Prognosis: Guarded for normal life span.

Detection of Carrier: —

Special Considerations: —

References:
Bartter, F.C. et al: Hyperplasia of the juxtaglomerular complex with hyperaldosteronism and hypokalemic alkalosis: A new syndrome. Am. J. Med. 33:811, 1962.
Gardner, J.D. et al: Altered membrane sodium transport in Bartter's syndrome. J. Clin Invest. 51:1565, 1972.
Glaz, E. and Vecsei, P. (eds): Aldosterone. Budapest:Akademiai Kiado, 1971, p. 216.
Goodman, A.D. et al: Pathogenesis of Bartter's syndrome. N. Engl. J. Med. 281:1435, 1969.
Modlinger, R.S. et al: Some observations on the pathogenesis of Bartter's syndrome. N. Engl. J. Med. 289:1022, 1973.
Rimoin, D.L. and Schimke, R.N.: Genetic Disorders of the Endocrine Glands. St. Louis:C.V. Mosby, 1971, p. 238.
Tarm, F. et al: Bartter's syndrome: An unusual presentation. Mayo Clin. Proc. 48:280, 1973.

Contributor: **Mark A. Sperling**

Editor's Computerized Descriptors: Skel., Muscle, GI.

BASAL CELL NEVUS SYNDROME

Includes: Naevi à cellules basales
Basalzell naevus-Syndrom
Síndrome de nevus a células basales
Nevoid basal cell carcinoma syndrome
Gorlin syndrome
Fifth phacomatosis
Hereditary cutaneomandibular polyoncosis

Excludes: Melanocytic nevi
Cylindromas of scalp (235)
Syringoma

Minimal Diagnostic Criteria: Major features are basal cell carcinomas, jaw cysts, skeletal anomalies, ectopic calcification and pits of hands and feet. (The pits on the hands and feet may be pathognomonic.) In the absence of a positive family history, any 2 major features may be sufficient for diagnosis. With a positive family history any of the major or a combination of minor anomalies indicates some expression of the syndrome.†

Clinical Findings:

Cutaneous:

Basal cell carcinomas	75%
Keratin defects on hands and feet	65%
Epithelial cysts, milia, lipomas, fibromas	20-40%

Osseous:

Jaw cysts (mandibular and maxillary)	80%
Sellar bridging	75%
Vertebral anomalies (spina bifida occulta, scoliosis)	65%
Rib anomalies (bifidness, splaying, synostoses)	60%
Subcortical cystic changes (long bones and phalanges)	45%
Brachymetacarpalism	30%
Sprengel deformity	5%
Defective dentition	?
Frontal and biparietal bossing	?
Mandibular prognathism	?

Neurologic:

Calcification of the falx cerebri, tentorium cerebelli, and petroclinoid ligaments	80%
Mental aberration, retardation	1-10%
EEG changes (nonspecific), various neurologic defects	1-10%
Medulloblastoma	1-5%

Ophthalmologic:

Hypertelorism, dystopia canthorum	25-50%
Strabismus	25%
Congenital blindness (colobomas, cataracts, glaucoma)	5-10%

Reproductive:

Ovarian fibromas	?
Hypogonadism	?

Miscellaneous:

Fibrosarcomas and squamous cell carcinomas of jaws	1-2%
Adenocarcinomas of ovary	1-2%
Lymphatic mesenteric cysts	?

Complications

I Derived: Hemorrhage from basal cell carcinomas, destruction of soft and osseous tissues from local invasion of tumors, infection in jaw cysts, pain and swelling from expanding jaw cysts, early loss of teeth, strangulation of mesenteric cysts, and death from medulloblastoma, fibrosarcoma, squamous cell carcinoma or ovarian adenocarcinoma.

II Associated: Pseudohypoparathyroidism, Marfan syndrome, neurofibromatosis, Turner syndrome, intestinal polyposis III, spherophakia-brachymorphia syndrome

Etiology: Autosomal dominant with high penetrance of gene (97%) and variable expressivity. Syndrome gene locus shows possible linkage with Rh blood group locus. McK *10940

Pathogenesis: ?

Related Facts

I Sex Ratio: M1:F1

II Risk of Occurrence: ?

III Risk of Recurrence for
    Patient's Sib: If parent is affected 1 in 2 (50%) for each offspring to be affected; otherwise not increased.
    Patient's Child: 1 in 2

IV Age of Detectability: At birth, by skeletal anomalies; in childhood, by jaw cysts, defective dentition, skeletal anomalies or medulloblastoma. In early adult life, by basal cell carcinomas or jaw cysts.

V Prevalence: ? Over 300 cases reported in past decade.

Treatment

I Primary Prevention: Genetic counseling

II Secondary Prevention: Early removal of basal cell carcinomas by various surgical methods, including excision, curettage and electrocautery. Radiation, dermabrasion and chemotherapy (ie 5-fluorouracil) not recommended.

III Other Therapy: —

Prognosis: Generally good for an average life span, but variable dependent on location and invasiveness of the basal cell carcinomas and the less common tumors.

Detection of Carrier: —

†Special Considerations: Syndrome may have little or delayed expressivity. Xrays of skull, mandible, maxilla, ribs, vertebrae and hands may be helpful in identifying the syndrome, particularly in children, before the basal cell carcinomas become manifest. Anthropometrics of skull identifies carriers in 85-90% of cases.

References:

Anderson, D. E. et al: The nevoid basal cell carcinoma syndrome. Am. J. Hum. Genet. 19:12, 1967.

Basal cell nevus syndrome. Combined clinical staff conference at the National Institute of Health. Ann. Intern. Med. 64:403, 1966.

Gorlin, R. J. et al: Multiple basal-cell nevi syndrome: An analysis of a syndrome consisting of multiple nevoid basal-cell carcinoma, jaw cysts, skeletal anomalies, medulloblastoma and hyporesponsiveness to parathormone. Cancer 18:89, 1965.

Jackson, R. and Gardere, S.: Nevoid basal cell carcinoma syndrome. Can. Med. Assoc. J. 125:850, 1971.

Contributor: **William E. Clendenning**

Editor's Computerized Descriptors: Vision, Eye, Face, Skin, Skel., GU., Nerve

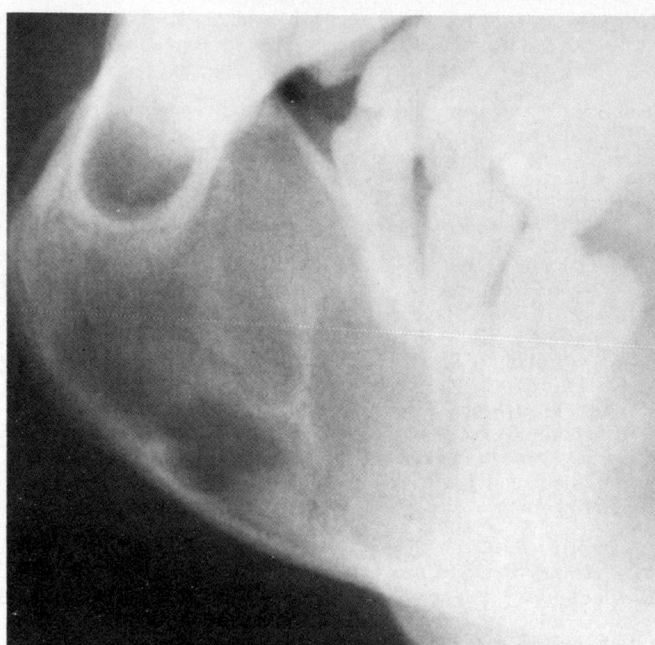

144. Cysts of mandible

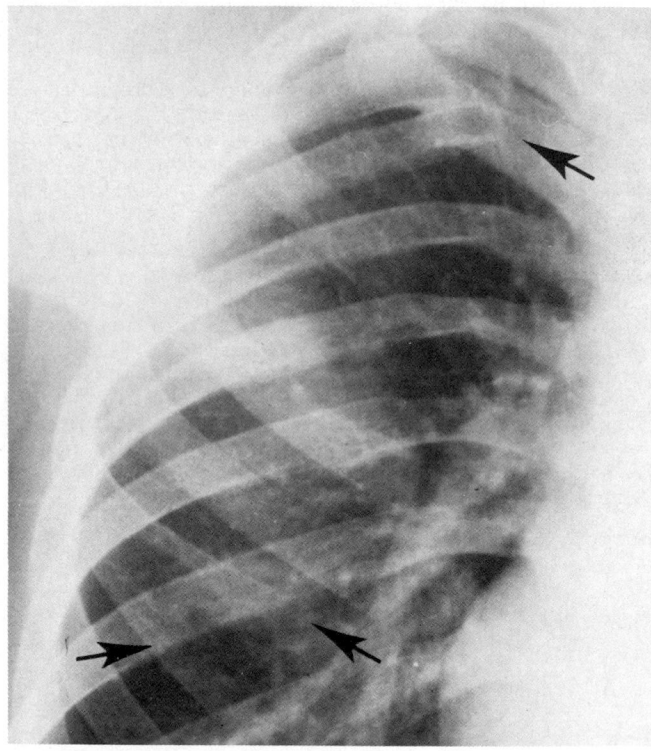

145. Note posterior fusion of ribs 3 and 4 and anterior bifurcation of rib 5

BASAN SYNDROME

Includes: Syndrome de Basan
Ektodermale Dysplasie mit fehlendes Papillarmuster, Nagelveranderungen und Vierfingerfurche
Síndrome de Basan
Ectodermal dysplasia with hypotrichosis, hypohidrosis, defective teeth and unusual dermatoglyphics

Excludes: Clouston syndrome
Ectodermal dysplasia, anhidrotic (333)
Dyskeratosis congenita

Minimal Diagnostic Criteria: Hypohidrosis, hypotrichosis, very fine dermal ridges over the hands and feet, single palmar flexion creases and dysplastic nails.

Clinical Findings: The major characteristics of this syndrome are dry skin over the entire body, very fine dermal ridges over the hands and feet, single palmar flexion creases, short fingernails and toenails with thick longitudinal ridges, hypotrichosis, hypohidrosis and dry mucosa. Body hair, eyebrows and eyelashes are sparse from birth on. Scalp hair in members of 1 family was normally thick at birth, but was coarse and grew slowly; it was shed rapidly toward the end of the 2nd decade of life. Affected individuals sweat evenly over their entire bodies, although the amount of sweat is less than normal. The conjunctivae are dry and conjunctivitis is frequent.

Facial features of affected members of 1 family were strikingly similar, characterized by thin alae nasi, long philtrums and thin upper lips. Teeth of these individuals were lost early in life because of uncontrollable decay. The enamel appeared to be normal in thickness and density, but reportedly developed brown spots that eventually coalesced and decayed over the labial and buccal surfaces.

Complications
I   **Derived:** Nausea and flushing due to hypohidrosis; inability to tolerate heat; decreased libido.
II   **Associated:** —

Etiology: Autosomal dominant; McK *12920

Pathogenesis: Defective formation of several derivatives of the embryonic ectoderm suggest that this disorder may be properly classified as an ectodermal dysplasia. The onset of the dysplasia is probably later than that of several others of this set of disorders since it is the late forming structures only that are affected. The late age of hair loss is unexplained, but the associated dental decay may be secondary to sparse oral secretions.

Related Facts
I   **Sex Ratio:** M1:F1
II   **Risk of Occurrence:** ?
III **Risk of Recurrence for**
     Patient's Sib: If parent is affected 1 in 2 (50%) for each offspring to be affected; otherwise not increased.
     Patient's Child: 1 in 2
IV   **Age of Detectability:** At birth
V   **Prevalence:** Rare, only 2 families reported

Treatment
I   **Primary Prevention:** Genetic counseling
II   **Secondary Prevention:** Avoidance of heat; lacrimal duct expansion may aid tearing; salves and creams keep mucosa moist.
III **Other Therapy:** Wigs are necessary in early adult life; early aggressive dental care to reduce spread of caries.

Prognosis: Good. The sweating dysfunction is not severe enough to cause excessive problems. Vision is the most severely compromised function.

Detection of Carrier: —

Special Considerations: —

References:
Basan, M.: Ektodermale Dysplasie: Fehlendes Papillarmuster, Nagelveranderungen und Vierfingerfurche. Arch. Clin. Exp. Derm. 222:546, 1965.
Jorgenson, R.J.: Ectodermal dysplasia with hypotrichosis, hypohidrosis, defective teeth and unusual dermatoglyphics (Basan syndrome?). In Bergsma, D. (ed.): Part XVI. Urinary System and Others. Birth Defects: Orig. Art. Ser., vol X, no. 4. Baltimore: Williams & Wilkins for The National Foundation-March of Dimes, 1974, p. 323.

Contributor: **Ronald J. Jorgenson**

Editor's Computerized Descriptors: Eye, Face, Teeth, Nose, Skin, Sweating, Dermatoglyphic, Hair, Nails

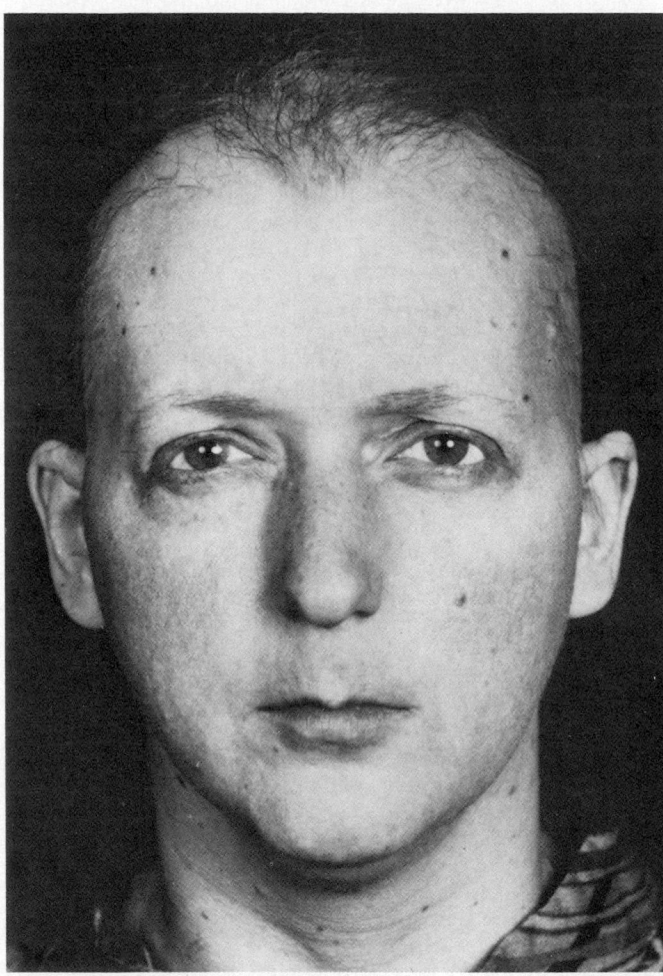

146. Note characteristic facies including narrow nose, long philtrum, thin vermilion border of upper lip, and sparse lashes, brows and scalp hair

BASILAR IMPRESSION, PRIMARY

Includes: Impression basilaire primitive
Platybasie
Impresión basilar primaria
Primary basilar impression

Excludes: Secondary basilar impression

Minimal Diagnostic Criteria: Demonstrated congenital bony abnormality in the occipitocervical region associated with progressive neurologic signs.

Clinical Findings: Symptoms usually begin insidiously in the 3rd or 4th decade. The patient may complain of occipital headaches, neck stiffness, dysphagia, aphonia, diplopia, trigeminal pain, mental deterioration, unsteady gait and various sensory disturbances. Examination may reveal a short neck with restricted movements. Dorsal kyphosis with increased cervical lordosis is common. The neurologic findings may include increased intracranial pressure, signs of compression of the medulla and pons, cerebellar signs as well as evidence of spinal cord compression producing long tract and sensory disturbances. Examination of the CSF reveals, in most cases, a modest elevation of protein. Occasionally a block is demonstrated by the Queckenstedt test or by myelography. The radiologic criteria for diagnosis are debatable but commonly include abnormalities in position of the atlas and odontoid process in relation to the Chamberlain line.

Complications
I **Derived:** Directly related to the bony deformities at the base of the skull in which there is upward displacement of the floor of the posterior fossa, producing combinations of the following: a) may be pressure on cranial nerves, brainstem, cerebellum or cervical cord; b) altered blood supply to these structures because of direct pressure or adhesions; c) interference with CSF flow producing hydrocephalus.
II **Associated:** Abnormally small foramen magnum defects of the atlas, Klippel-Feil syndrome, Arnold-Chiari malformation, as well as vascular anomalies particularly of the vertebral artery, which may in part explain some of the symptoms and signs.

Etiology: Possibly autosomal dominant

Pathogenesis: There is evidence to suggest that primary basilar impression is the result of a defect in embryogenesis.

Related Facts
I **Sex Ratio:** M1:F1
II **Risk of Occurrence:** ?
III **Risk of Recurrence for**
Patient's Sib: When autosomal dominant and if parent is affected, 1 in 2 (50%) for each offspring to be affected; otherwise not increased.
Patient's Child: When dominant, 1 in 2
IV **Age of Detectability:** 1st decade by means of radiographs, 3rd or 4th decade by onset of neurologic signs.
V **Prevalence:** 1 in 3300. Russell reported a high incidence of basilar impression in Eskimos; others in poorly documented studies, have noticed an increase in the Netherlands and Northern Brazil.

Treatment
I **Primary Prevention:** Genetic counseling
II **Secondary Prevention:** Most patients asymptomatic. Immobilization or limited use. Surgical decompression should be approached with considerable caution. Shunting procedures may be contemplated for those with progressive hydrocephaly.
III **Other Therapy:** —

Prognosis: Extremely variable, death may occur in 4th or 5th decade or patient may be totally asymptomatic.

Detection of Carrier: Secondary basilar impression may be the result of bone diseases such as Paget disease, rickets, osteomalacia, osteoporosis, cleidocranial dysostosis, Morquio disease, syphilis, tuberculosis; or possibly from carrying heavy loads upon the head.

Special Considerations: —

References:
Bull, J.W.D. et al: Radiological criteria and familial occurrence of primary basilar impression. Brain 78:229, 1955.
List, C.F.: Neurologic syndromes accompanying developmental anomalies of occipital bone, atlas and axis. Arch. Neurol. Psychiatr. 45:577, 1941.
Russell, F.: Studies in cranial variation. Am. Natural 34:737, 1900.

Contributor: **Robert H. A. Haslam**

Editor's Computerized Descriptors: Vision, Speech, Neck, Skel., Nerve

BECKWITH-WIEDEMANN SYNDROME

Includes: Viscéromégalie, omphalocèle et macroglossie
Exomphalos-Makroglossie-Gigantismus-Syndrom
Síndrome de visceromegalia, onfalocele y macroglosia
Macroglossia, omphalocele and visceromegaly syndrome
EMG syndrome
Visceromegaly, umbilical hernia and macroglossia
Wiedemann-Beckwith syndrome
Omphalocele, visceromegaly and macroglossia syndrome

Excludes: Macroglossia (618)
Omphalocele (748)
Hypoglycemia, familial neonatal (512)

Minimal Diagnostic Criteria: The syndrome has no obligatory anomalies and clinical findings may be quite variable. The syndrome has been observed in patients without macroglossia or omphalocele in whom the visceral histologic lesions have been florid. Any infant with macroglossia and omphalocele (or umbilical hernia) should be evaluated for neonatal hypoglycemia. Ear lobe grooves or circular depressions on the posterior helices, when present, are especially significant for diagnosis.

Clinical Findings: Macroglossia and omphalocele (umbilical hernia or diastasis recti in some cases) seem to be the most frequent anomalies. Other defects include anomalies of intestinal rotation or fixation, visceromegaly (hepatomegaly, nephromegaly, pancreatomegaly and in some cases, cardiomegaly), neonatal hypoglycemia, polycythemia, somatic gigantism (not evident at birth in some cases), advanced bone age, ear lobe grooves, circular depressions on the posterior helix, facial nevus flammeus, microcephaly, and maxillary hypoplasia with relative mandibular prognathism. Hemihypertrophy has been observed in some cases. Malignant tumors have occurred in approximately 5% of the patients. Mental retardation may occur. Other findings can include diaphragmatic eventration (occasionally diaphragmatic hernia), hyperplastic uterus, thymus and bladder, clitoromegaly, bicornuate uterus, undescended testes, hydrocephaly and other anomalies. Hyperlipemia, hypercholesterolemia, and hypocalcemia have been noted in a few instances. Severe combined immunodeficiency has been associated as has a zoster-like rash at birth.

Chemical or clinical hypoglycemia occurs in 50% or more of the infants within 2 days after birth. This hypoglycemia is due to relative hyperinsulinemia (leucine sensitive) associated with pancreatic islet hyperplasia (nesidioblastosis) and is most common in those infants with high birthweight (> 4000 gm) who have other findings of the syndrome. Persistence of the tendency to become hypoglycemic may remain for up to 33 months, although most recover earlier. The hypoglycemia tends to be severe and resists simple treatment (frequent feedings, IV glucose). A nonketogenic diet high in calories and low in protein (leucine) should be used. Diazoxide(R), long acting epinephrine, corticosteroids or ACTH also may be necessary. Partial pancreatectomy may be necessary.

Complications
I Derived: Mental retardation when present, may possibly result from undetected neonatal hypoglycemia.
II Associated: Wilms tumor and adrenal cortical carcinoma occur in 5% of reported cases. Hepatoblastoma, glioma, embryonal rhabdomyosarcoma, carcinoid tumor, myxoma, and fibroma have been noted rarely. The presence of hemihypertrophy in the syndrome does not increase the risk for malignancy. Gonadal interstitial cell hyperplasia occurs in males. This may be due to elevated serum gonadotropin levels.

Etiology: ? Most cases are sporadic. Affected sibs occur occasionally and consanguinity has been established in 1 case. Several cases have occurred in more than 1 sibship in the same kindred. Based on familial cases, autosomal recessive, autosomal dominant, polygenic, and autosomal dominant sex-dependent inheritance have been proposed. Etiologic heterogeneity also is possible. McK *22560

Pathogenesis: Altered placental endocrine physiology may play a role in producing many of the features found during the neonatal period. Omphalocele, anomalies of intestinal rotation and fixation, and diaphragmatic eventration may be secondary to early visceromegaly.

Related Facts
I **Sex Ratio:** M1:F1 in sporadic cases; males predominantly affected in most familial instances.
II **Risk of Occurrence:** ? (1 in 13,700 live births in the West Indies)
III **Risk of Recurrence for**
Patient's Sib: ? Recurrence risk negligible in sporadic instances
Patient's Child: ?
IV **Age of Detectability:** At birth by clinical evaluation
V **Prevalence:** ? (rare)

Treatment
I **Primary Prevention:** —
II **Secondary Prevention:** Omphalocele repair, treat neonatal hypoglycemia. Partial glossectomy may be indicated if macroglossia persists.
III **Other Therapy:** Orthognathic surgery, orthodontic and speech therapy

Prognosis: Fair. A number of patients have died during infancy from complications of the syndrome.

Detection of Carrier: —

Special Considerations: —

References:
Beckwith, J.B.: Macroglossia, omphalocele, adrenal cytomegaly, gigantism and hyperplastic visceromegaly. In Bergsma, D. (ed.): Part II. Malformation Syndromes, Birth Defects: Orig. Art. Ser., vol. V, no. 2. White Plains: The National Foundation-March of Dimes, 1969, p. 188.
Cohen, M.M., Jr. et al: The Beckwith-Wiedemann syndrome: Seven new cases. Am. J. Dis. Child. 122:515, 1971.
Gorlin, R.J. et al: Syndromes of the Head and Neck, 2nd Ed. New York: McGraw-Hill Co., 1976.

Contributors: **M. Michael Cohen, Jr.**
Robert A. Ulstrom

Editor's Computerized Descriptors: Ear, Face, Oral, Skin, Skel., Hernia not CNS, CV., Thymus, GI., Liver, GU., Nerve

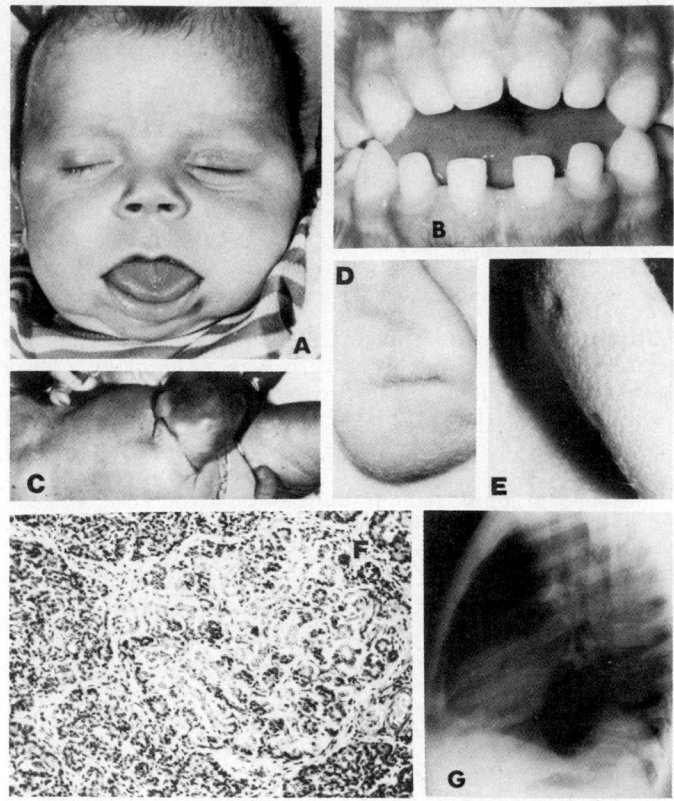

147. A) Macroglossia; B) anterior open bite; C) omphalocele; D) ear lobe groove; E) circular depression on posterior rim of helix; F) hyperplasia of ducts and acini in pancreas; G) diaphragmatic eventration

BERLIN SYNDROME

Includes: Syndrome de Berlin
Síndrome de Berlín
Ectodermal dysplasia, Berlin type

Excludes: Ectodermal dysplasia without pigmentary changes
Incontinentia pigmenti (526)
Werner syndrome (998)
Rothmund syndrome

Minimal Diagnostic Criteria: Still uncertain

Clinical Findings: This rare form of ectodermal dysplasia is characterized by short stature, slender build with "bird-like" legs, moderate hyperflexibility of fingers, sparse eyebrows with absence of the lateral parts, flat saddle-shaped nose, deep furrows about the eyes and mouth, generalized melanoleukoderma (leopard skin), anetopoikilodermatous lesion over joints, palmar and plantar hyperkeratoses, underdevelopment of the pilosebaceous apparatus with complete absence of lanugo hair, moustache in both sexes, delayed 1st and 2nd dentition, hypodontia, sexual underdevelopment in males (hypospadias, small penis, scrotum and testes, absence of secondary characteristics), mental retardation.

Complications
I   **Derived:** Kidney stones
II   **Associated:** —

Etiology: Apparently autosomal recessive. This is perhaps an incomplete and mixed type of an ectodermal hypoplasia. It may represent pituitary dwarfism.†

Pathogenesis: ? Apparently normal at birth. In early childhood onset of pigmentary, dental, mental and other changes.

Related Facts
I   **Sex Ratio:** M1:F1
II   **Risk of Occurrence:** Very rare
III **Risk of Recurrence for**
     Patient's Sib: Presumably 1 in 4 (25%) for each offspring to be affected
     Patient's Child: Male patients are sexually underdeveloped and have no offspring. Female patients who may be heterozygotes show normal sexual development and have offspring.
IV   **Age of Detectability:** Early childhood
V   **Prevalence:** Only 1 family known (Iranians living in Israel).

Treatment
I   **Primary Prevention:** Genetic counseling
II   **Secondary Prevention:** —
III **Other Therapy:** As may be indicated

Prognosis: Normal life span. Patients are mentally retarded but even-tempered and industrious. Males are sexually underdeveloped.

Detection of Carrier: ?

†Special Considerations: In the only known family, the affected children are the product of a cousin marriage.

References:
Berlin, C.: Congenital generalized melanoleucoderma associated with hypodontia, hypotrichosis, stunted growth and mental retardation occurring in two brothers and two sisters. Dermatologica 123:227, 1961.

Contributor: **Helen Ollendorff Curth**

Editor's Computerized Descriptors: Eye, Face, Teeth, Nose,

105-500

BETA-MERCAPTOLACTATE-CYSTEINE DISULFIDURIA (MARKER)

Acta 158:493, 1968.

Contributor: **John C. Crawhall**

Editor's Computerized Descriptors: Eye, Skel., Nerve

Includes: Excrétion urinaire du disulfide β mercaptolactate-cystéine

Beta-Mercaptolaktat-Cystein-Disulfidurie

Beta mercaptolactato-cisteín disulfiduria (Marcador)

Excludes: —

Minimal Diagnostic Criteria: Urine positive to the nitroprusside test. Chromatography of the urinary amino acids shows the presence of a characteristic spot which can be revealed by the following reagents: ninhydrin, iodoplatinic acid and cyanide-nitroprusside.

Clinical Findings: Four patients have been identified. The first was a 46-year-old American male with severe lifelong mental retardation. The parents were sibs. The 2nd and 3rd were 2 Swiss female sibs identified by a screening program. They were mentally and physically normal. The parents were unrelated. The 4th was a 16-year-old Scottish male with severe mental retardation. The parents were 1st cousins.

Complications
I   Derived: —
II Associated: Mental retardation 2 cases.† Chronic otitis media with subsequent deafness 1 case. Obesity, hypogonadism, valgus deformity of both knees, severe pes planus, bilateral congenital cataract with nystagmus - 1 case

Etiology: Probably autosomal recessive; McK *25205

Pathogenesis: A deficiency of the enzyme β-mercaptopyruvate sulfur transferase has been identified in the erythrocytes from the 1st patient described.

Related Facts
I   Sex Ratio: M1:F1 (of 4 cases reported)
II   Risk of Occurrence: Very rare
III Risk of Recurrence for
    Patient's Sib: ?
    Patient's Child: ?
IV Age of Detectability: Has been detected in childhood and adult life. Probably present from infancy.
V   Prevalence: Very rare

Treatment
I   Primary Prevention: —
II   Secondary Prevention: —
III Other Therapy: —

Prognosis: Life span may be normal but mental retardation appears to be unchanged through life.

Detection of Carrier: No carriers identified. This amino acid has been described in small quantities in the urine of normal people.

†Special Considerations: On the basis of the 4 cases currently known, it is not possible to be certain that the metabolic abnormality and the mental retardation are causally related.

References:
Ampola, M.G. et al: Mental deficiency and a new aminoaciduria. Am. J. Dis. Child. 117:66, 1969.
Crawhall, J. C. et al: β-mercaptolactate cysteine disulfide in the urine of a mentally retarded patient. Am. J. Dis. Child. 117:71, 1969.
Niederwieser, A. et al: β-mercaptolactate cysteine disulfiduria in two normal sisters. Isolation and characterization of β-mercaptolactate cysteine disulfide. Clin. Chim. Acta 43:405, 1973.
Shih, V.E. et al: β-mercaptopyruvate sulfur transferase deficiency. The enzyme defect in β-mercaptolactate-cysteine disulfiduria. Pediatr. Res. 11:464, 1977.
Ubuka, T. et al: S-(2-hydroxy-2-carboxyethylthio) cysteine and S-(carboxymethylthio) cysteine in human urine. Biochim. Biophys.

BETA-METHYL-CROTONYL-GLYCINURIA

Includes: β-Methylcrotonylglicinurie
β-Metilcrotonilglicinuria
β-hydroxyisovaleric aciduria
Biotin-responsive β-methylcrotonylglycinuria

Excludes: Isovalericacidemia (547)

Minimal Diagnostic Criteria: Detection of β-hydroxyisovaleric acid and β-methylcrotonylglycine in the urine. The odor of the urine may be helpful.

Clinical Findings: Clinical manifestations varied in the 3 known patients. One had a picture similar to infantile spinal muscular atrophy with severe hypotonia, atrophy of muscle, and absence of deep tendon reflexes without ketosis or acidosis. The urine had an odor resembling that of cat's urine. The 2nd patient had intermittent vomiting from birth and erythematous skin lesions. He developed attacks of persistent vomiting, deep rapid respirations, ketosis and metabolic acidosis. Odor of the urine also resembled cat's urine. The 3rd patient developed high fever at 9 months of age. Delay in motor development was noted. Ketosis was not present.

All 3 patients had abnormal amounts of β-hydroxyisovaleric acid and β-methylcrotonylglycine in the urine, up to 490 and 270 mg per day, respectively. These 2 metabolites were not detected in blood.

Complications
I **Derived:** Retarded motor development, possible early death.
II **Associated:** —

Etiology: Probably autosomal recessive; McK *21020

Pathogenesis: Defect in the metabolism of leucine involving the carboxylation of 3-methylcrotonyl CoA to 3-methylglutaconyl CoA, which may be secondary to deranged metabolism or transport of biotin.†

Related Facts
I **Sex Ratio:** M1:F1
II **Risk of Occurrence:** ?
III **Risk of Recurrence for**
  Patient's Sib: Probably 1 in 4 (25%) for each offspring to be affected.
  Patient's Child: Probably not increased unless mate is carrier or homozygote
IV **Age of Detectability:** Probably from birth. Possibly at 6-8 weeks in the biotin-responsive patient. Prenatal diagnosis is possible
V **Prevalence:** ?

Treatment
I **Primary Prevention:** Genetic counseling
II **Secondary Prevention:** Leucine is toxic to these patients, therefore, diets restricted in this amino acid are helpful. Two patients responded well to treatment with 10 mg of biotin per day. The 1st patient did not respond to biotin treatment.
III **Other Therapy:** The use of electroyte-containing solutions in the presence of ketosis.

Prognosis: If biotin-responsive, normal development may be expected. The biotin-nonresponsive patient died at 9 months.

Detection of Carrier: Method not available

†Special Considerations: The 3 patients described are heterogeneous. This probably reflects molecular heterogeneity in the enzymatic block.

References:
Gompertz, D. et al: Biotin-responsive β-methylcrotonylglycinuria. Lancet 2:22, 1971.

Gompertz, D. et al: Child with a defect in leucine metabolism associated with β-hydroxyisovaleric aciduria and β-methylcrotonylglycinuria. Arch. Dis. Child. 48:975, 1973.
Stokke, O. et al: Organic acidurias. In Stern, J. and Toothill, C. (eds.): Proc. 9th Symp. Soc. for Study of Inborn Errors of Metabolism. Edinburgh and London: Livingstone, 1972.
Tanaka, K.: Disorders of organic acid metabolism. In Gaull, G.E. (ed.): Biology of Brain Dysfunction. New York: Plenum Publishing Corp, 1975, vol. 3.

Contributors: **Walter Weyler, Jr.**
                      Lawrence Sweetman

Editor's Computerized Descriptors: Skin, Muscle, Resp., GI.

BICUSPID AORTIC VALVE

Includes: Valvule aortique bucuspidé
Bikuspidale Aortenklappe
Válvula aórtica bicúspide
Congenital bicuspid aortic valve
Aortic valve, bicuspid

Excludes: Aortic valve stenosis (80)
Aortic valve incompetence
Bicuspid aortic valve, acquired

Minimal Diagnostic Criteria: No reliable clinical criteria exist to establish a diagnosis of a bicuspid aortic valve in the absence of left ventricular outflow obstruction or aortic valve incompetence. If selective left ventriculography or thoracic aortography is performed during cardiac catheterization for other cardiovascular anomalies, the bicuspid aortic valve may be an incidental finding.

Clinical Findings: The uncomplicated bicuspid aortic valve may be undetected in early life and produce no hemodynamic abnormality until it becomes stenotic and of clinical significance in adult life. When stenosis occurs in childhood, there is usually an aortic systolic ejection murmur, often preceded by an ejection click. A congenital bicuspid aortic valve should be suspected when bacterial endocarditis occurs in a child previously thought to be normal. An increased incidence of bacterial endocarditis occurs in patients with a bicuspid aortic valve, even in the absence of stenosis. Among cases of isolated, calcified aortic stenosis in adults, the congenital bicuspid aortic valve is often the underlying lesion. Rarely, at any age, prolapse of 1 cusp may result in valvar incompetence. The chest film may show a prominent ascending aorta 2° to poststenotic dilatation. The aortic valva is calcified in a large majority of adults over the age of 30.

Echocardiographically, abnormal aortic valves when they are bicuspid can sometimes be identified by the asymmetric placement of the diastolic closure line within the aortic root. Aortic root enlargement is often seen in such patients. Great variability often exists in the position of diastolic aortic closure, even in normals. Nevertheless, if multiple redundant echoes are consistently asymmetrically placed within the aortic root, the diagnosis of bicuspid aortic valve stenosis can be made. The severity of aortic stenosis is most easily judged by the detection and serial follow-up of left ventricular hypertrophy on the echocardiogram. Suprasternal notch echo demonstration of a dilated aortic arch can often be achieved. Cross-sectional echo studies delineating abnormal leaflet motion (doming) or the presence of poststenotic dilation are of assistance in making this diagnosis. The presence of fluttering of the mitral valve in patients suspected of having a bicuspid aortic valve is usually confirmatory of aortic insufficiency.

Complications

I **Derived:** Aortic incompetence secondary to cusp prolapse; sclerosis and calcification resulting in aortic stenosis; bacterial endocarditis.

II **Associated:** Coarctation of the aorta (20%)

Etiology: Presumably multifactorial inheritance

Pathogenesis: The pathologic anatomy is the presence of 2, rather than 3, aortic valve cusps. The cusps may be equal in size but, more commonly, are unequal. Usually, 1 of the 2 cusps is divided by a vertical raphe into 2 segments. Progressive trauma to the valve may lead to the typical appearance of calcific aortic stenosis in adulthood.

Related Facts

I **Sex Ratio:** M4:F1

II **Risk of Occurrence:** Still controversial. Some authorities believe it may be as high as 1 in 250.

III **Risk of Recurrence for**
   Patient's Sib: ?
   Patient's Child: ?

IV **Age of Detectability:** Beyond the 3rd decade by clinical findings of aortic stenosis or aortic incompetence. Definitive diagnosis may be made by ascending aorta angiography at any age.

V **Prevalence:** ? †

Treatment

I **Primary Prevention:** —

II **Secondary Prevention:** Institution of appropriate prophylaxis for bacterial endocarditis.

III **Other Therapy:** As required for various degrees of complicating aortic stenosis and aortic incompetence.

Prognosis: The prognosis is directly related to the nature and severity of the complications. These include aortic stenosis, aortic incompetence and bacterial endocarditis. By the 5th decade, sclerotic and calcific changes almost always occur in the bicuspid valve.

Detection of Carrier: —

†**Special Considerations:** This defect may represent the most common congenital cardiovascular malformation. In the past, even in the absence of a history of rheumatic fever, when isolated aortic stenosis was first detected after age 15 years, the lesion was considered to be of rheumatic etiology. It is now apparent that as many as 70% of these patients have congenital bicuspid aortic valve.

References:

Edwards, J.E.: The congenital bicuspid aortic valve. Circulation 23:485, 1961.
Gould, S.E.: Pathology of the Heart and Blood Vessels, 3rd Ed. Springfield:Charles C Thomas, 1968.
Nanda, N.C. et al: Echocardiographic recognition of the congenital bicuspid aortic valve. Circulation 48:870, 1974.
Roberts, W.E.: The congenitally bicuspid aortic valve. A study of 85 autopsy cases. Am. J. Cardiol. 26:72, 1970.
Williams, D.E. et al: Cross-sectional echocardiographic localization of the sites of left ventricular outflow tract obstructions. Am. J. Cardiol. 37(2):250, 1976.

Contributors: **William F. Friedman**
Stanley E. Kirkpatrick

Editor's Computerized Descriptor: CV.

BICUSPID PULMONARY VALVE

Includes: Valvule pulmonaire bicuspidé
Bikuspidale Pulmonalklappe
Válvula pulmonar bicúspide
Bicuspid pulmonary valve with or without a raphe
Pulmonary valve, bicuspid

Excludes: Pulmonary valve stenosis (839)
Pulmonary valve atresia (837)

Minimal Diagnostic Criteria: Physical findings suggesting a pulmonary valve lesion not associated with electrocardiographic or vectorcardiographic abnormalities of any kind may suggest the lesion.

Clinical Findings: Two functional pulmonary valve cusps are present rather than 3. The 2 cusps may be approximately equal in size in which case there usually is no raphe in either sinus of Valsalva. Both sinuses of Valsalva, while larger than normal, are well-formed. More commonly, however, one of the cusps is somewhat larger than the other and contains a raphe which partially divides the sinus of Valsalva into more or less shallow components. Since by definition neither stenosis nor incompetence is present, the lesion is asymptomatic. Even in nonstenotic bicuspid valves, however, turbulence is usually produced which is responsible for the soft or moderately loud systolic ejection type murmur usually present in these patients. A suprasternal systolic thrill may be present.

The ECG and vectorcardiogram are normal in uncomplicated simple bicuspid pulmonary valve. Xrays of the chest may show some "poststenotic" dilatation of the pulmonary trunk. At cardiac catheterization, no pressure difference is found across the valve and the physiologic findings are normal. A pulmonary arterial angiogram or ventriculogram may demonstrate the true nature of the anomaly.

Complications
I   **Derived:** Calcification of the bicuspid pulmonary valve is unusual, as is bacterial endocarditis.
II **Associated:** A bicuspid pulmonary valve is commonly associated with tetralogy of Fallot, in which case it does not have to be stenotic but may be hypoplastic. Any other cardiovascular lesion may be present.

Etiology: Presumably multifactorial inheritance

Pathogenesis: True bicuspid pulmonary valve without a raphe is probably due to absence of one of the pulmonary valve cusp anlagen. This may be the intercalated valve swelling of either of the anlagen derived from the truncus septum. Bicuspid pulmonary valve with a raphe: all 3 anlagen are present, 2 of these have fused to form a functionally single cusp and 2 poorly developed sinuses of Valsalva separated by a raphe.

Related Facts
I   **Sex Ratio:** M1:F1
II **Risk of Occurrence:** ?
III **Risk of Recurrence for**
     Patient's Sib: ?
     Patient's Child: ?
IV **Age of Detectability:** Probably in early childhood, if all soft pulmonic murmurs are investigated.
V   **Prevalence:** ?

Treatment
I   **Primary Prevention:** —
II **Secondary Prevention:** —
III **Other Therapy:** —

Prognosis: The prognosis of bicuspid pulmonary valve is excellent, if it occurs as an isolated lesion. If other congenital cardiac defects are present, the prognosis is determined by the associated lesion.

Detection of Carrier: —

Special Considerations: —

References:
Ford, A.B. et al: Isolated congenital bicuspid pulmonary valve: Clinical and pathologic study. Am. J. Med. 20:474, 1956.
Koletsky, S.: Congenital bicuspid pulmonary valve. Arch. Pathol. 31:338 1941.

Contributor: **James H. Moller**

Editor's Computerized Descriptor: CV.

BILIARY ATRESIA

Includes: Atrésie des voies biliaires
Gallengangsatresie
Atresia biliar
Extrahepatic biliary atresia with discontinuity of bile duct (correctable)
"Noncorrectable" extrahepatic biliary atresia
Intrahepatic biliary atresia

Excludes: Choledochal cyst (149)
Inspissated bile syndrome
Hepatic agenesis (463)

Minimal Diagnostic Criteria: An infant with clay-colored stools and evidence of obstruction on Rose Bengal scan should be considered to have a variant of biliary atresia until ruled otherwise.

Clinical Findings: Infants with biliary atresia are not jaundiced at birth because of maternal clearance of bilirubin via the placenta. Jaundice usually occurs sometime after the 2nd or 3rd day of life. The infant's stools become bulky, malodorous, clay-colored, and contain no bile. The urine is dark, contains bile but no urobilinogen. The serum bilirubin is elevated (predominantly direct) with levels usually above 6.0 mg%. Enzyme levels (SGOT/PT, IDH, alkaline phosphatase) may be elevated. Hepatomegaly is usually present, and the spleen may also be palpable. Hepatic scintiscan with Rose Bengal I^{131} or I^{123} shows biliary obstruction, with only trace amounts noted in the stools (less than 5%). Except for absence of bile in the stools and an obstructed scan, the majority of biochemical tests are of little diagnostic value in differentiating various causes of obstruction in the early neonatal period. Even the test for bile in the stool may be falsely positive in certain cases of complete obstruction where the bilirubin levels are high and traces of bile pigments are found due to desquamation of intestinal mucosal cells.

Complications
I **Derived:** Persistent biliary obstruction progresses to biliary cirrhosis which may begin at 1 month of age, progress, and be irreversible by 3 months. Portal hypertension, splenomegaly, ascites formation, and hemorrhage from esophageal varices are frequent complications. Respiratory distress from an elevated right diaphragm or ascites is common. Irritability and pruritis due to bile pigment deposition in the skin occurs later in the disease. Hypoprothrombinemia, anemia, and malnutrition eventually occur. Although growth and development are normal early in the disease, growth retardation is apparent as the disease progresses.
II **Associated:** —

Etiology: This anomaly has long been thought to represent a failure of recanalization of the obliterative solid stage of bile-duct formation. The current popular theory concerning the etiology of biliary atresia involves an ongoing, dynamic, inflammatory process (a form of cholangitis) resulting in sequential obliterative changes of the extra- and intrahepatic ducts as well as surrounding tissues. Varying involvement may result in a wide spectrum of clinical findings including what previously were classically described as neonatal hepatitis (nonobstructive and obstructive forms), biliary hypoplasia, extrahepatic biliary atresia amenable to surgical correction (extrahepatic duct discontinuity), "noncorrectable" extrahepatic biliary atresia, and intrahepatic biliary atresia. It is suggested that all of these variants are due to a single acquired disease process, perhaps of viral etiology, in which biliary atresia in the classic "noncorrectable" form represents 1 phase of a broad spectrum of defects.

Pathogenesis: Grossly, the liver is hard, enlarged, and green in color. The gallbladder may be present or absent. The outstanding microscopic feature of biliary atresia is extensive fibrosis within the portal triads in which proliferating ducts are embedded with bile stasis. At times, the histologic evaluation is quite difficult to distinguish forms of biliary atresia from what was previously considered neonatal hepatitis. Giant cells and various degrees of fibrosis have been observed in both instances of biliary atresia and neonatal hepatitis, which also supports the single acquired disease process theory. Histologic appearance of the liver changes with age with decrease in the number of giant cells and giant cell nuclei associated with increasing fibrosis and diminution of numbers of bile ducts within the liver with time. Bile duct hyperplasia is prominent up to 3 months of age, at which time this decreases significantly with excessive deposition of fibrous tissue. Serial sections of the atretic ducts often demonstrate an inflammatory process with granulation tissue, fibrosis, and inflammatory cells with minute biliary ducts often documented only by microscopic evaluation. Current reappraisal of the etiology and pathophysiology indicates that a new nomenclature for these disorders will probably be forthcoming.

Related Facts
I **Sex Ratio:** M1:F1
II **Risk of Occurrence:** 1 in 16,000 live births (Note: NOT seen in embryos, stillborns, or in premature infants.) Increased incidence in Japanese and Hawaiians of Chinese ancestry. More common in instances of situs inversus and in patients with anterior portal vein.
III **Risk of Recurrence for**
Patient's Sib: ? Although rare, occasional instances of familial occurrence have been observed.
Patient's Child: ?
IV **Age of Detectability:** Jaundice that persists for longer than 2 weeks in the newborn is pathologic, usually obstructive in nature, and demands a thorough evaluation.
V **Prevalence:** ?

Treatment
I **Primary Prevention:** —
II **Secondary Prevention:** The importance of arriving at the proper diagnosis in instances of obstructive jaundice is of the utmost importance. Despite the myriad of studies, frequently one cannot differentiate between obstructive forms of what was previously called neonatal hepatitis or biliary atresia. An open liver biopsy and cholangiogram are performed between the 4th and 6th week of life. If cholangiography demonstrates an intact biliary tree with minute ducts, the diagnosis is either hypoplasia of the bile ducts or neonatal hepatitis. If contrast material passes easily into the liver as well as the duodenum, no further surgical intervention is indicated at this time. If, however, over a 4-week period, no improvement of the obstruction occurs, hepatoportoenterostomy may be indicated. Rarely at operation a choledochal cyst may be observed even in this infant age group and appropriate operative therapy should be undertaken either by end-to-side Roux-Y choledocyst jejunostomy, cholecyst duodenostomy, or primary resection and hepatoportoenterostomy. If no gallbladder is found, or if on cholangiography, the gallbladder does not empty into an intact biliary tree, serial sections of the atretic ducts should be taken at the porta hepatis and evaluated by frozen section analysis for the presence of minute biliary ducts. If patent ducts > 70-100 µ are observed, a Japanese type of modified hepatoportoenterostomy as championed by Kasai and other Japanese investigators is indicated. In the absence of microscopic ducts, this operation should not be performed and the abdomen closed. In instances of extrahepatic biliary atresia with discontinuity (a correctable situation) a bulbus common bile

duct distal to the entrance of the cystic duct from the gallbladder is observed and a Roux-Y hepatoportoenterostomy is also indicated.

III Other Therapy: Vitamin-K, diuretics, albumin for ascites, and whole blood for hemorrhage from varices may be necessary. Portosystemic shunting procedures for bleeding varices are limited to children over 5 years old.

Cholestyramine has been useful in certain children with high cholesterol levels.

Antibiotics are employed when episodes of cholangitis or sepsis occur.

Recent therapy with hepatic transplantation have not been particularly encouraging.

Prognosis: In the past, the majority of infants with biliary atresia succumbed to their underlying disorder within the first 2 years of life because of sequelae of advanced cirrhosis. Even in cases that were correctable, operation was not synonomous with salvage when operation was performed after 3 months of age because of the irreversible biliary damage.

A correctable form (biliary discontinuity) is present in approximately 10-12% of cases and these should do well following appropriate drainage if done early. Even in the noncorrectable forms, which represent the majority of cases, 15% of the children will have a successful outcome if the operation is performed prior to irreversible damage. Improved survival data will be dependent on early diagnosis and corrective surgery prior to the development of these irreversible changes.†

Detection of Carrier: —

†Special Considerations: The traditional concepts concerning the etiology, pathology, and the role of surgical therapy for biliary atresia are currently undergoing considerable reappraisal. Although controversy still exists (particularly in regard to why only 25% of uncorrectable cases respond to the Japanese type operations and how a nonmucosal anastomosis can function well) this still allows one-fourth of the children previously considered hopeless to have an opportunity for survival. Improved survival in these infants has been confirmed by workers in this country as well. Successful outcome depends upon a liver with intact intrahepatic ducts, presence of microscopic bile ducts at the porta hepatis, a successful anastomosis to a Roux-Y segment of jejunum, a cutaneous enterostomy to prevent postoperative cholangitis, flow of bile, relief of jaundice, and eventual enlargement of the ducts. Success is age related and has never been achieved in patients over 4 months of age and is unusual after 3 months. These recent data suggest that clinical work-up for jaundice be initiated at 1 month of age and operation performed prior to age 3 months in each instance. Although controversy still exists as to the long-term efficacy of these operations, the potential for quality survival in 15% of cases previously considered hopeless indicates the operation should be offered to any infant under the age of 3 months with "noncorrectable" biliary atresia and *may be useful* in those cases of hypoplasia of the bile ducts or neonatal hepatitis with obstructive symptoms that do not respond to observation and remain jaundiced. These recent observations seriously question withholding operation in infants with obstructive jaundice until after 4 months of age as has been popularly practiced by many segments of the pediatric physician population in the past. The progression of disease appears to be age related and operative success has not been achieved in patients over the previously recommended age of 4 months. This indicates changing to an early operative intervention program is advisable. There is very little to offer infants with noncorrectable forms of atresia, that have no microscopic bile ducts visible on frozen section analysis at the porta hepatis. There is no evidence to support the efficacy of intrahepatic manipulations and intubations with synthetic cannulas nor attempts at lymphatic diversion of bile by anastomosis of thoracic duct to esophagus or portohepatolymphaticojejunostomy. Liver allotransplantation has been employed in instances of noncorrectable biliary atresia and in some cases has been successful.

References:

Hays, D.M.: Biliary atresia: The current state of confusion. Surg. Clin. North Am. 53:1257, 1973.

Kasai, M.: Treatment of biliary atresia with special reference to hepatic portoenterostomy and its modifications. Prog. Pediatr. Surg. 6:5, 1974.

Koop, C.E.: Biliary obstruction in the newborn. Surg. Clin. North Am. 66:373, 1976.

Landing, B.: Changing approaches to neonatal hepatitis and biliary atresia. Pediatrics 53:647, 1974.

Lilly, J.R.: The Japanese operation for biliary atresia: Remedy or mischief? Pediatrics 55:12, 1975.

Contributors: **Jay L. Grosfeld**
H. William Clatworthy, Jr.

Editor's Computerized Descriptors: Spleen, GI., Liver

BLEPHAROCHALASIS, DOUBLE LIP AND NONTOXIC THYROID ENLARGEMENT

Includes: Blépharochalasis, dédoublement de la lèvre et goitre non toxique
Blepharochalasis, Doppellippe und Struma
Bléfarocalasia, labio doble y tiroidea notóxica tumefacción
Ascher syndrome
Double lip, blepharochalasis and nontoxic thyroid enlargement

Excludes: Lip, double (594)

Minimal Diagnostic Criteria: Blepharochalasis and double lip

Clinical Findings: Upper lip defect (rarely lower lip), in which the pars villosa sags below the pars glabrosa, appears in infancy or early childhood. Sagging of the upper eyelids (rarely lower lids) usually appears at puberty, but may occur earlier in some cases. Nontoxic goiter is a variable feature which appears following eyelid involvement.

Complications
I   **Derived:** —
II   **Associated:** —

Etiology: Probably autosomal dominant; McK *10990

Pathogenesis: Lip develops excessive areolar tissue and hyperplastic mucous glands. Eyelid develops prolapsed orbital fat and hyperplastic lacrimal tissue.

Related Facts
I   **Sex Ratio:** M1:F1 (approximately)
II   **Risk of Occurrence:** —
III   **Risk of Recurrence for**
    Patient's Sib: If one parent affected, 1 in 2 (50%) for each offspring; otherwise not increased.
    Patient's Child: 1 in 2
IV   **Age of Detectability:** In infancy or early childhood, by clinical evaluation
V   **Prevalence:** More than 1 in 4000 in Utah children

Treatment
I   **Primary Prevention:** Genetic counseling
II   **Secondary Prevention:** Cosmetic surgery for redundant labial and eyelid tissue
III   **Other Therapy:** —

Prognosis: Excellent

Detection of Carrier: Affected individuals show syndrome features.

Special Considerations: —

References:
Findlay, G. H.: Idiopathic enlargements of lips: Cheilitis granulomatosa, Ascher's syndrome and double lip. Br. J. Dermatol. 66:129, 1954.
Franceschetti, A.: Cas observé: Manifestation de blépharochalasis chez le père associe à des doubles lèvres apparaissant également chez sa fillette âgée d'un mois. J. Génét. Hum. 4:181, 1955.
Panneton, P.: Le blepharo-chalasis: À propos de 51 cas dans une même famille. Arch. Ophtalmol. (Paris) 53:729, 1936.

Contributor: **M. Michael Cohen, Jr.**

Editor's Computerized Descriptors: Eye, Face, Oral, Neck

BLOOM SYNDROME

Includes: Syndrome de Bloom
Síndrome de Bloom
Congenital telangiectatic erythema and stunted growth

Excludes: Rothmund syndrome
Thomson syndrome

Minimal Diagnostic Criteria: Proportionate short stature, the characteristic facial lesion, or both, plus the characteristic increase in sister-chromatid exchange.

Clinical Findings: The major features are small size at birth subsequent dwarfing with normal body proportions; dolichocephaly and characteristic facies (narrow, with nasal prominence associated with hypoplastic malar areas); and, a sun-sensitive telangiectatic erythema affecting almost exclusively the face, particularly the butterfly area, the lower eyelids, and the lower lip. A predisposition to infections usually exists (ear, upper and lower respiratory tract), and bouts of infantile diarrhea are common. Both improve with age.

A marked increase in the number of exchanges between both sister and nonsister-but-homologous chromatids in cultured cells is consistent and apparently unique, being therefore of great diagnostic value.

Complications
I   **Derived:** —
II   **Associated:** Minor developmental defects appear to be increased in frequency, and mild mental retardation has occasionally existed. Malignancies of various types tend to occur at earlier than normal ages.

Etiology: Autosomal recessive; McK *21090

Pathogenesis: Increased infection is associated with defective immune function. The predisposition to malignancy may be related to chromosome "instability," but possibly also to the immune defect.

Related Facts
I   **Sex Ratio:** M1:F4
II   **Risk of Occurrence:** Rare in Ashkenazic Jews, very rare in other groups.
III   **Risk of Recurrence for**
    Patient's Sib: 1 in 4 (25%) for each offspring to be affected
    Patient's Child: Not increased unless mate is carrier or homozygote
IV   **Age of Detectability:** Theoretically at birth. Practically, diagnosis is usually made only after skin lesion appears, at least in the first affected in a sibship.
V   **Prevalence:** > in 100,000 Ashkenazic Jews

Treatment
I   **Primary Prevention:** Genetic counseling and prenatal diagnosis for parents of an affected individual.
II   **Secondary Prevention:** Intrauterine diagnosis using cytogenetic and sonographic techniques is possible theoretically.
III   **Other Therapy:** Antibiotics for infections

Prognosis: Adult height is rarely 5 feet or more. Males have small testes, and those tested have been infertile. Postpubertal females menstruate, but their fertility status is unknown. The risk of malignancy at a relatively early age is increased.

Detection of Carrier: Not possible at present, except by having an affected child.

Special Considerations: —

References:
German, J.: Bloom's syndrome. I. Genetical and clinical observations in the first twenty-seven patients. Am.J. Hum. Genet.

21:196, 1969.
German, J.: Bloom's syndrome. II. The prototype of human genetic disorders predisposing to chromosome instability and cancer. In German, J. (ed.): Chromosomes and Cancer. New York: John Wiley and Sons, 1974, p. 601.

Contributor: James L. German, III

Editor's Computerized Descriptors: Face, Nose, Skin, Skel., GI.
Also see Section I, Fig. 70

BLUE RUBBER BLEB NEVUS SYNDROME

Includes: Angiomatose cutanée et digestive
Haemangiomatosis cutis et visceralis cavernosa
Síndrome de nevus vesiculosos azulados
Hemangiomatosis generalized cavernous
Hamartoma, venous
Blue rubber bleb nevus of skin and gastrointestinal tract
Multiple hemangiomas of skin and internal organs

Excludes: Fabry disease (373)
Familial hemorrhagic telangiectasia
Solitary cavernous hemangioma
Enchondromatosis and hemangiomas (346)

Minimal Diagnostic Criteria: Multiple cavernous hemangiomas of the skin, 0.2-4 cm in diameter, bluish to purplish-red to black, sometimes lobulated, spongy and compressible, rumpled in appearance when partially emptied by squeezing and slowly refilling when pressure is released, associated with cavernous hemangiomas of one or more internal organs, very frequently associated with GI bleeding.

Clinical Findings: Multiple cavernous hemangiomas of the skin (100%), GI tract (90%), subcutaneous tissue, mucous membranes, lungs, liver, skeletal muscle, thyroid, brain, spinal cord, meninges, cranial bones, spleen, heart, kidney.

Complications
I **Derived:**   Serious spontaneous GI bleeding (frequent), anemia (frequent). Spontaneous bleeding of the skin lesions is rare, but they may bleed from injury. The cosmetic defect of the skin lesions may be severe. Lesions of the soles may interfere with walking. Oozing, irritation, and offensive odor from genital area and perianal area may occur.
II **Associated:** Meningioma, medulloblastoma, osteoma, syringomyelia and cysts of many organs have been reported.

Etiology: ? In some reported instances, the disease did not appear to be hereditary. However, Berlyne reported a case in which he traced the family history in 5 generations, and he stated it was transmitted as an autosomal dominant trait. McK *11220

Pathogenesis: Microscopically the lesions are thin-walled and filled with blood, with the walls resembling those of veins.

Related Facts
I **Sex Ratio:**   ? Probably M1:F1
II **Risk of Occurrence:**   ? Very low. Reported in various races.
III **Risk of Recurrence for**
   Patient's Sib: ? When autosomal dominant and if parent is affected 1 in 2 (50%) for each offspring to be affected; otherwise not increased.
   Patient's Child: When autosomal dominant, 1 in 2
IV **Age of Detectability:**   At birth, lesions will usually be visible
V **Prevalence:**   ? Extremely low

Treatment
I **Primary Prevention:**   Genetic counseling when autosomal dominant
II **Secondary Prevention:**   Some of the most troublesome skin lesions may be excised.
III **Other Therapy:**   Treatment of anemia due to bleeding from GI lesions.

Prognosis: May live a normal life span or may die earlier in adult life from associated conditions or from internal hemorrhage.

Detection of Carrier: —

Special Considerations: —

References:
Berlyne, G. M. and Berlyne, N.: Anaemia due to "blue rubber-bleb" naevus disease. Lancet 2:1275, 1960.
Jaffe, R. H.: Multiple hemangiomas of skin and of internal organs. Arch. Pathol. 7:44, 1929.

Rice, J. S. and Fischer, D. S.: Blue rubber-bleb nevus syndrome: Generalized cavernous hemangiomatosis or venous hamartoma with medulloblastoma of the cerebellum; case report and review of the literature Arch. Dermatol. 86:503, 1962.

Contributor: **J. Sidney Rice**

Editor's Computerized Descriptors: Oral, Skin, Muscle, GI., Nerve

BRACHYDACTYLY

Includes: Brachydactylie
Brachydaktylie
Braquidactilia
Brachydactyly types A_1, A_2, A_3, B, C, D, and E
Brachydactyly type A_1 (Farabee type)
Brachydactyly type A_2 (brachymesophalangy II, Mohr-Wriedt type)
Brachydactyly type A_3 (brachymesophalangy V, clinodactyly)
Brachydactyly type B
Brachydactyly type C
Brachydactyly type D ("stub thumb")
Brachydactyly type E (brachymesophalangy and brachymetapody)

Excludes: Turner syndrome (977)
Chromosome 21 trisomy syndrome (171)
Macular coloboma and brachydactyly (621)
Broad thumb-hallux syndrome (119)
Tabatznik syndrome
Poland syndrome (813)
Pseudohypoparathyroidism (830)
Numerous other syndromes with brachydactyly

Minimal Diagnostic Criteria: See below by type

Clinical Findings: Brachydactyly is shortening of the fingers due to shortening of any of its components, the metacarpals or phalanges. Brachydactyly has been classified into 7 genetic types according to the inheritance of selective and specific shortening of certain parts of the digits consistently within families. In types A_1, A_2, and A_3 brachydactyly, shortening is confined to the middle phalanges.

In type A_1 (Farabee type) it affects all the middle phalanges, which are rudimentary and sometimes fused with the terminal phalanges. The proximal phalanges of the thumbs and big toes are short. The subjects are short of stature.

In type A_2 shortening of the middle phalanges is confined to the index finger and the 2nd toe with the other digits being more or less normal. Because of a rhomboid or triangular shape of the affected middle phalanx, the end of the 2nd finger usually deviates radially.

In type A_3 shortening affects the middle phalanx of the 5th digit.

In type B brachydactyly, the middle phalanges are also short but in addition, the terminal phalanges are rudimentary or absent. Thumbs and big toes are usually deformed. Symphalangism is also a feature. The absence of distal phalanges has led some authors to define this malformation as ectrodactyly and as apical dystrophy. The association with syndactyly has led some authors to describe it as symbrachydactyly.

In type C brachydactyly, the middle phalanges as well as some metacarpals are shortened. The characteristic change is a deformity of the middle and proximal phalanges of the 2nd and 3rd digits (index and middle fingers), sometimes with hypersegmentation of the proximal phalanx. The ring finger may be essentially normal and, therefore, is the longest digit.

Type D brachydactyly is characterized by short and broad terminal phalanges of the thumbs and big toes.

Type E brachydactyly is due mainly to shortening of the metacarpals and metatarsals. Wide variability in the number of digits affected occurs from person to person even in the same family. The patients are moderately short of stature and have a round face but do not have ectopic calcification or mental retardation or cataract as occurs in pseudohypoparathyroidism.

Complications
I   **Derived:** —
II **Associated:** —

Etiology: Each of the different types of brachydactyly as isolated malformations has autosomal dominant transmission. McK *11250, *11260, *11270, *11300, *11310, *11320, *11330

Pathogenesis: ?

Related Facts
I   **Sex Ratio:** M1:F1
II **Risk of Occurrence:** ?
III **Risk of Recurrence for**
    Patient's Sib: If parent is affected, 1 in 2 (50%) for each offspring to be affected; otherwise not increased.
    Patient's Child: 1 in 2. (Extreme variability in lesion from very mild to very severe should be considered.)
IV **Age of Detectability:** From birth to late in childhood
V   **Prevalence:** While types A_1, A_2, B, C, and E are rather rare, types A_3 (5th finger clinodactyly) and D ("stub thumb") are common and can be considered as normal variations.

Treatment
I   **Primary Prevention:** Genetic counseling
II **Secondary Prevention:** Surgical intervention is recommended in type A_2, when syndactyly is an associated malformation, and in some cases with type C brachydactyly when talipes is an associated malformation.
III **Other Therapy:** —

Prognosis: Brachydactyly as an isolated malformation does not affect life span.

Detection of Carrier: —

Special Considerations: —

References:
Haws, D.V. and McKusick, V. A.: Farabee's brachydactylous kindred revisited. Bull. Johns Hopk. Hosp. 113:20, 1963.
McKusick, V.A. and Milch, R.A.: The clinical behavior of genetic diseases: Selected aspects. Clin. Orthop. 33:22, 1964.
Temtamy, S.A.: Genetic factors in hand malformations. Unpublished doctoral dissertation, Johns Hopkins University, 1966.
Temtamy, S.A. and McKusick, V.A.: The Genetics of Hand Malformations. Birth Defects: Orig. Art. Ser., Bergsma, D. (ed.). New York: Alan Liss, Inc. for The National Foundation-March of Dimes. l978, vol XIV, no. 3.

Contributor: **Samia A. Temtamy**

Editor's Computerized Descriptors: Face, Skel.

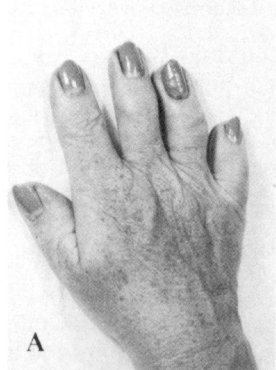
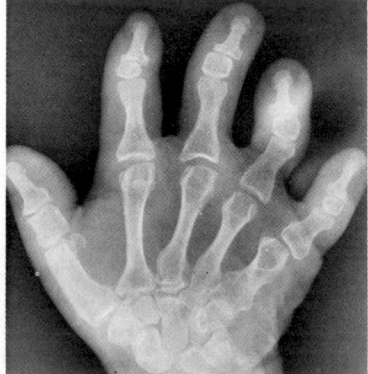

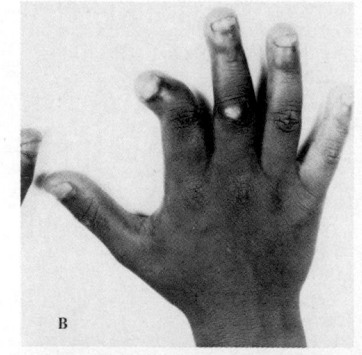
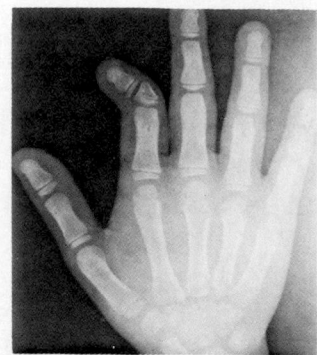
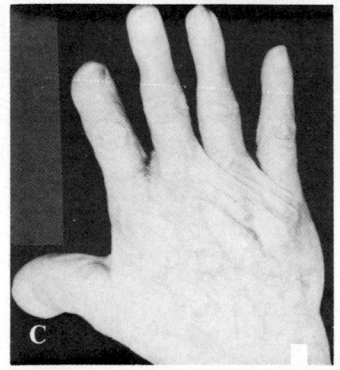
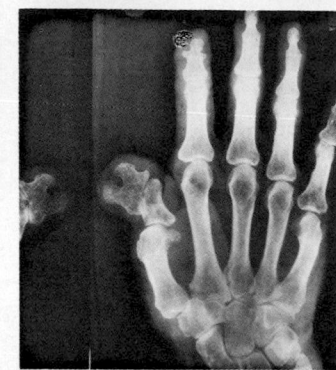
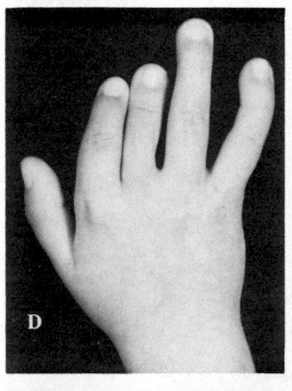
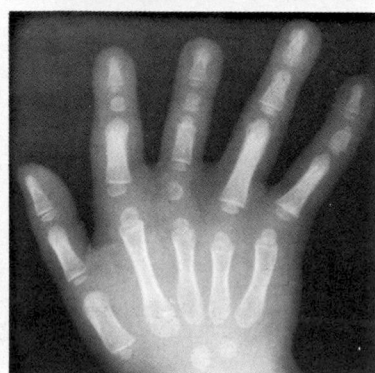
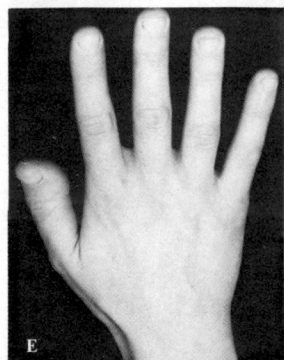
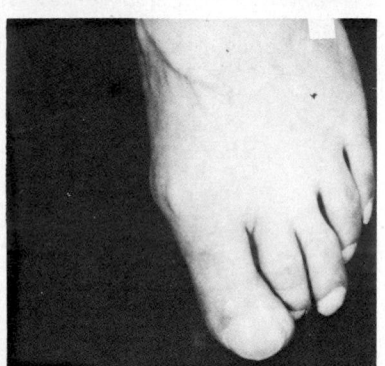
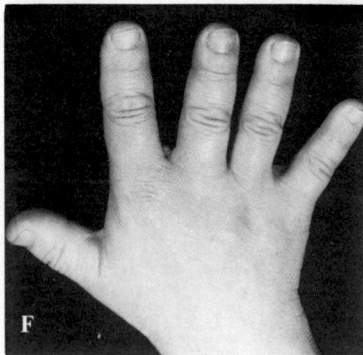
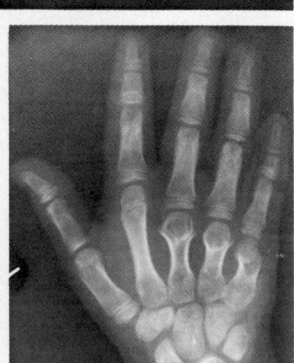

148, 149. Brachydactyly: A) Type A_1; B) Type A_2; C) Type B; D) Type C; E) Type D; F) Type E

BRAIN, SPONGY DEGENERATION

Includes: Dégénérescence spongieuse de la substance blanche
Spongiöse Dystrophie der weissen Hirnsubstanz
Degeneración esponjosa de la substancia blanca cerebral
Cerebral white matter, spongy degeneration
Canavan disease
Spongy degeneration of brain

Excludes: Schilder disease
Other leukodystrophies
Hydrocephaly (481)
Diffuse degeneration of cerebral gray matter

Minimal Diagnostic Criteria: The early onset with optic atrophy, hypotonia turning to intermittent hypertonia and megacephaly can strongly suggest a diagnosis. There are no laboratory tests which can confirm the diagnosis. The diagnosis may be confirmed by brain biopsy.

Clinical Findings: This disease develops from the first 2 months of life and is marked by failure to develop motor or psychosocial milestones. Initially the children are quite hypotonic but later become hypertonic. This hypertonicity may be quite intermittent. Optic atrophy and blindness occur later in the disease. Megacephaly may be striking. The life expectancy is 2-3 years. In the terminal stages the children may be almost indistinguishable from children with globoid cell leukodystrophy, the leukodystrophy with hyaline deposits, or G_{M2}-gangliosidosis with hexosaminidase A deficiency.

Complications
I **Derived:** Feeding disorders, seizures, and aspiration pneumonia
II **Associated:** —

Etiology: Appears to be autosomal recessive. McK *27190

Pathogenesis: The disease appears to be an error of metabolism of myelin but no characteristic biochemical findings have been detected. The CSF, blood and urinalyses are all normal. The histopathology is distinctive in the appearance of a spongiform degeneration of both gray and white matter in the presence of a large brain. This spongy appearance is most prominent in deeper layers of cortex and subcortical white matter but there are also large astrocytes of the types seen in chronic liver disease (Alzheimer type 2 cells). There is a lack of sudanophilic or other products of myelin breakdown.

Related Facts
I **Sex Ratio:** M1:F1
II **Risk of Occurrence:** ? This disease occurs primarily in Jewish Ashkenazi families. There have, however, been a few cases in non-Jewish families.
III **Risk of Recurrence for**
    Patient's Sib: Presumably 1 in 4 (25%) for each offspring to be affected
    Patient's Child: (Condition is lethal for patient.)
IV **Age of Detectability:** 4-6 months on the basis of clinical criteria
V **Prevalence:** ?

Treatment
I **Primary Prevention:** Genetic counseling
II **Secondary Prevention:** —
III **Other Therapy:** Supportive measures to prevent complications of pneumonia

Prognosis: The usual age of death is 2-3 years.

Detection of Carrier: —

Special Considerations: —

References:
Hogan, G.R. and Richardson, E.P., Jr.: Spongy degeneration of the nervous system (Canavan's disease). Pediatrics 35:284, 1965.

Van Bogaert, L.: Spongy degeneration of the brain. In Vinken, P.J. et al (eds.): Handbook of Clinical Neurology. Amsterdam: North Holland Publishing Co., 1970 vol. 10, p. 203.

Contributor: **Guy M. McKhann**

Editor's Computerized Descriptors: Eye, Skel., Muscle

BRANCHER DEFICIENCY

Includes: Déficit en enzyme branchante (glycogénose type IV)
Glykogenose, Typ IV
Deficiencia de brancher
Glycogen storage disease, type IV
Amylopectinosis
Andersen disease
Glycogenosis IV

Excludes: All other forms of glycogen storage disease

Minimal Diagnostic Criteria: Progressive liver failure with jaundice in infancy, hepatomegaly, ascites, moderate muscular weakness and demonstration of abnormal glycogen accumulations and abnormal glycogen structure in liver and other tissues.

Clinical Findings: Patients usually present as infants with cirrhosis of the liver and storage of abnormal glycogen. Occasionally muscular weakness is present and, in addition, muscular contractures. Hence, although cirrhosis with associated hepatic failure is the most characteristic feature, in conjunction with progressive accumulating ascites, muscular weakness may occur in an occasional infant.

Laboratory features are those of progressive hepatic failure with cirrhosis, deepening icterus and associated severe chronic illness. Liver biopsy will demonstrate accumulation of glycogen in the range of 2 to 4 gm%, with lesser amounts of glycogen in muscle and other tissues. The glycogen is abnormal in its structure with a reduced number of 1,6 branch points. The glycogen resembles amylopectins of plant starch.

Complications
I **Derived:** Hepatic failure, occasionally congestive heart failure or renal failure due to accumulation of glycogen or to an unusual foreign body reaction to an abnormal polysaccharide component.
II **Associated:** —

Etiology: Probably autosomal recessive. Absence of brancher enzyme in liver and other tissues due to a genetic deletion. Brancher enzyme is also identified as amylo-(1,4 to 1,6) transglucosidase. McK *23250

Pathogenesis: Accumulation of abnormal structured polysaccharide quite similar to an amylopectin in liver, muscle, kidney and other tissues. Probably there is a foreign body reaction to the accumulation of this unusual polysaccharide component which leads to significant hepatic fibrosis and advanced cirrhosis in the patients so affected.

Related Facts
I   **Sex Ratio:** ? Probably M1:F1
II **Risk of Occurrence:** Very rare
III **Risk of Recurrence for**
    Patient's Sib: 1 in 4 (25%) for each offspring to be affected.
    Patient's Child: Not increased unless mate is carrier or homozygote.
IV **Age of Detectability:** Usually before 1 year of age associated with lethargy and progressive hepatic failure.
V   **Prevalence:** Extremely rare

Treatment
I   **Primary Prevention:** Genetic counseling
II **Secondary Prevention:** —
III **Other Therapy:** —

Prognosis: Extremely poor with death usually occurring from hepatic failure before the 3rd year of life.

Detection of Carrier: ?

Special Considerations: —

References:
Andersen, D. H.: Studies on glycogen disease with report of a case in which the glycogen was abnormal. In Najjar, V.A. (ed.), Carbohydrate Metabolism: A Symposium on the Clinical and Biochemical Aspects of Carbohydrate Utilization in Health and Disease. Baltimore: Johns Hopkins Press, 1953, p. 28.
Holleman, L.W.J. et al: Type IV glycogenosis. Lab. Invest. 15:357, 1966.
Sidbury, J.B., Jr. et al: Type IV glycogenosis: Report of a case proven by characterization of glycogen and studied at necropsy. Bull. Johns Hopk. Hosp. 111:157, 1962.

Contributor: **Carl M. Pearson**

Editor's Computerized Descriptors: Muscle, CV., Liver, GU.

BRANCHIAL CLEFT CYSTS OR SINUSES

Includes: Kyste bronchogénique
Branchiogene Zyste, branchiogene Sinus
Quistes o senos de las hendiduras branquiales
Pharyngeal cyst or fistula
Cervical cyst or sinus
Branchial cleft fistula

Excludes: Laryngocele (575)
Pharyngocele
Cervical adenopathy
Solitary lymph cysts
Cavernous hemangioma of neck
Dermoid cyst or teratoma of head and neck (283)
Thyroid cyst
Thyroglossal duct remnant (945)
Thymic cyst

Minimal Diagnostic Criteria: Histopathologic examination

Clinical Findings: Either a cyst or a sinus or both can result from abnormal development of the pharyngeal pouches or cervical sinus. These lesions appear along the anterior border of the sternocleidomastoid muscle or medial to this muscle.

The branchial cyst is a slowly enlarging, painless mass in the neck that may be present at birth. Pressure and a sense of fullness in the neck with mild dysphagia and hoarseness are frequent symptoms. Children with large cysts may have stridorous breathing and cyanosis. Uncomplicated cysts are characteristically soft, mobile and transparent when transilluminated. The cyst may vary in size, increasing with infection and decreasing as infection subsides. Neck injuries may cause the cyst to become enlarged, tense and painful.

Small cysts may be difficult to palpate, particularly those lying medial to the sternocleidomastoid muscle. These may be detected by having the patient push his chin firmly against the examiner's palm. Needle aspiration yields a mucoid material.

A typical sinus has an external opening at the junction of the lower third and upper two-thirds of the sterno-cleidomastoid muscle. This small pinpoint opening may not be noticed until mucoid material or food particles pass from it. Symptoms of vagal irritation such as cough, hoarseness, pallor, bradycardia, sweating and faintness have been elicited by probing the sinus. Persistent cough, drainage into the pharynx and pain from repeated infections of the external openings are unusual symptoms of a cervical sinus. X-ray examination after injecting the sinus with radiopaque oil will reveal a typical smooth-walled tract. A cyst may develop at any point along the sinus tract.†

Complications
I   **Derived:** Upper airway obstruction, aspiration, infection of cyst or sinus, malignant tumor formation.
II **Associated:** —

Etiology: Unknown, but anomalous development of the branchial clefts and pharyngeal pouches is the most popular theory. McK *11360

Pathogenesis: Pharyngeal pouches and branchial grooves are present for only a short time during embryonic life. Epithelial rests, incomplete closure of the branchial grooves, rupture of the closing membranes between the pharyngeal pouches and branchial grooves, and persistence of the cervical sinus are thought to be responsible for these abnormalities. The constant relationship between the cyst or sinus and anatomic structures normally formed by the branchial apparatus substantiates this concept.†

Related Facts

I   **Sex Ratio:** M3:F1
II **Risk of Occurrence:** ?
III **Risk of Recurrence for**
    Patient's Sib: ?
    Patient's Child: About 5%
IV **Age of Detectability:** From birth through adulthood, depending upon the occurrence of symptoms and clinical findings.
V   **Prevalence:** ?

Treatment
I   **Primary Prevention:** —
II **Secondary Prevention:** Total excision of the cyst and sinus tract will give the patient a complete cure. Stepladder incisions may be indicated removing the entire sinus tract. When the sinus originates from the tonsillar fossa, a tonsillectomy must be performed to ensure complete excision of the tract.
III **Other Therapy:** —

Prognosis: Normal life span unless rare malignancy occurs.

Detection of Carrier: —

†**Special Considerations:** The knowledge of embryologic development and related anatomy is essential for understanding branchial cysts and sinuses.

A 1st cleft fistula will be entirely above the hyoid bone with its upper end opening into the external auditory canal. The tract is superficial to the mandible and passes through the parotid gland. It may lie deep or superficial to the facial nerve.

The 2nd arch sinus begins in the tonsillar fossa. It extends between the internal and external carotid arteries above and superficial to the hypoglossal nerve, glossopharyngeal nerve, and stylopharyngeus muscle. The sinus opens onto the skin along the anterior border of the sternocleidomastoid muscle. The junction of the lower and middle thirds of the muscle is the most common site for this opening. This 2nd arch sinus is the most commonly seen of these abnormalities.

A sinus formed from *the 3rd branchial cleft* opens in the same area as the 2nd branchial sinus. This tract passes deep to the platysma muscle along the sheath of the common carotid artery, but extends behind the internal carotid artery. The tract is superficial to the vagus nerve and crosses the hypoglossal nerve, but does not ascend above the glossopharyngeal nerve or stylopharyngeus muscle. The internal opening is in the pyriform sinus.

Cysts or sinuses of *the 4th branchial cleft* are theoretically possible, but very few have been reported. The tract would have to course below the aorta on the left and the subclavian artery on the right, ascend into the neck to empty into the upper esophagus after crossing the hypoglossal nerve. Downey and Ward have described a mediastinal cyst they believe originated from a 4th branchial cleft. This cyst was lined with squamous and transitional epithelium with islands of lymphoid tissue in its wall.

References:
Davies, J.: Embryology of the Head and Neck in Relation to the Practice of Otolaryngology. Department of Anatomy, Washington University, St. Louis, Missouri.
Downey, W. L. and Ward, P. H.: Branchial cleft cysts in the mediastinum. Arch. Otolaryngol. 89:762, 1969.
Proctor, B. and Proctor, C.: Congenital lesions of the head and neck. Otolaryngol. Clin. North Am. 3:221, 1970.
Simpson, R. A.: Lateral cervical cysts and fistulas. Laryngoscope. 79:30, 1969.

Contributors: **Gerald M. English**
                    Dennis Kay

BRANCHIO-SKELETO-GENITAL SYNDROME

Includes: Syndrome branchio-squeletto-génital
Branchyskeletogenitales Syndrom
Síndrome génito-branquio-esquelético
Genito-oculo-oligophrenic-dento-skeleto syndrome (GOODS)
Elsahy-Waters syndrome†

Excludes: Spherophakia-branchymorphia syndrome (893)
Oculo-mandibulo-facial syndrome (738)

Minimal Diagnostic Criteria: Hypoplasia of the maxilla and relative prognathism, cleft palate or uvula, hypertelorism, brachycephaly, pectus excavatum and hypospadias.

Clinical Findings:

Branchial arch (1st and 2nd) anomalies:

Maxilla:	hypoplasia, multiple dentigerous cysts and unerupted teeth
Mandible:	relative prognathism, multiple dentigerous cysts and unerupted teeth, dentin dysplasia, radicular type teeth with demilune or obliterated chambers with abnormal and short roots
Palate:	bifid uvula, high-arched, cleft palate
Mastoid bone:	undeveloped
Nose:	broad and flat with wide nasal tip and flared alar cartilages
Eyes:	hypertelorism, strabismus, ptosis, nystagmus.

Skeletal anomalies:

Skull:	brachycephalic, (mental retardation)
Vertebral column:	fusion of 2nd and 3rd cervical spinous processes, Schmorl nodes in lumbar vertebrae
Sternum:	pectus excavatum

Genital anomalies:	penoscrotal hypospadias

Complications
I **Derived:** Mental retardation, convulsions, nasal speech, destruction of mandible and maxilla from cyst expansion.
II **Associated:** Difficult sexual activity because of hypospadias.

Etiology: Probably autosomal recessive trait. Unaffected parents were 1st cousins.

Pathogenesis: Defect appears to be a midline clefting syndrome, ie hypertelorism, cleft palate, pectus excavatum, hypospadias, probably indicating an embryonic somite fusion defect involving the embryologic origin of the head and neck (namely the 1st and 2nd branchial arch derivatives, the forebrain, skull, and cervical vertebrae) and the rest of the body. Histologic changes in teeth are identical to those of radicular dentin dysplasia.

Related Facts
I **Sex Ratio:** Probably M1:F1, actually M3:F0
II **Risk of Occurrence:** ?
III **Risk of Recurrence for**

Patient's Sib: If autosomal recessive, 1 in 4 (25%) for each offspring to be affected.

Patient's Child: If autosomal recessive, not increased unless mate is a carrier or homozygote.

IV Age of Detectability: At birth by clinical and radiologic examination.

V Prevalence: Very rare. One sibship reported.

Treatment

I Primary Prevention: Genetic counseling

II Secondary Prevention: Surgical repair of anatomic defects of palate, teeth, and genitalia

III Other Therapy: —

Prognosis: Poor. Patients have survived to adulthood but are psychosocially retarded.

Detection of Carrier: ?

†Special Considerations: This syndrome was originally described by Elsahy and Waters in 1971 as the branchio-skeleto-genital syndrome. This same family was subsequently inadvertently designated Unger-Trott syndrome by Witkop. The histologic pictures of the tooth defect in the paper by Elsahy and Waters had been erroneously replaced by a picture of Witkop's patient with fibrous dysplasia of dentin.

References:

Elsahy, N.I. and Waters, W.R.: The branchio-skeleto-genital syndrome: A new hereditary syndrome. Plast. Reconstr. Surg. 58:542, 1971.

Elsahy, N.I. and Vistnes, L.M.: Anomalies of the head and neck-An attempt at classification. Acta Chir. Plast. (Praha) 14:1, 1972.

Witkop, C.J., Jr. and Rao, S.: Inherited defects in tooth structure. In Bergsma, D. (ed.): Part XI. Orofacial Structures. Birth Defects: Orig. Art. Ser., vol. VII, no. 7. Baltimore Williams & Wilkins for The National Foundation-March of Dimes, 1971, p. 153.

Witkop, C.J., Jr.: Genetics. Schweiz. Monatsschr. Zahnheilkd. 82:917, 1972.

Witkop, C.J., Jr.: Hereditary defects of dentin. Dent. Clin. North Am. 19:25, 1975.

Contributors: **Nabil I. Elsahy**
Carl J. Witkop, Jr.

Editor's Computerized Descriptors: Eye, Face, Oral, Teeth, Speech, Skel., Muscle, GU., Nerve

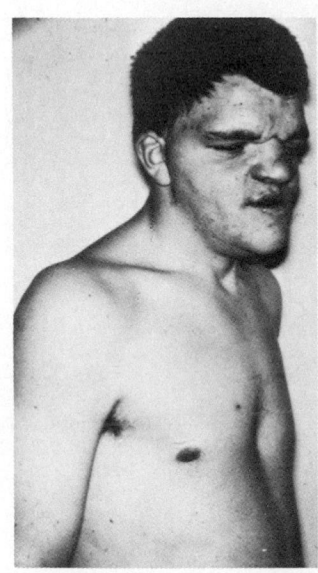
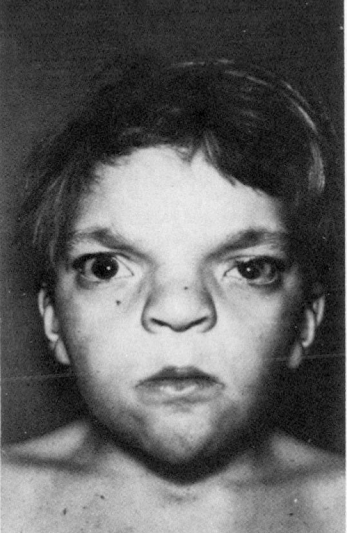

150. Note hypertelorism; broad, flat nose with wide nasal tip; prognathism

BROAD THUMB-HALLUX SYNDROME

Includes: Syndrome de Rubinstein-Taybi
Syndrom der breiten Daumen und Grosszehen
Síndrome de pulgar y dedo gordo del pie ancho
Rubinstein-Taybi syndrome
Broad thumbs syndrome
Brachydactyly, peculiar facies and mental retardation syndrome
Digitofacial-mental retardation syndrome

Excludes: Brachydactyly, type D without associated facial characteristics or mental retardation
Acrocephalosyndactyly, type VI

Minimal Diagnostic Criteria: No pathognomonic criterion yet exists. However, a syndrome of developmental retardation, broad terminal phalanges of thumbs and halluces, characteristic facial "gestalt", with stature, head circumference and bone age below 50th percentile and incomplete or delayed descent of testes in males are very significant.†

Clinical Findings: Broad terminal phalanges of thumb and hallux 114/114, broad terminal phalanges of other fingers 63/87, overlapping toes 35/65, clinodactyly of 5th finger 29/54, angulation deformity of thumb with abnormal shape of proximal phalanx 35/91, angulation deformity of hallux with abnormal shape of proximal phalanx or 1st metatarsal 15/75, duplicated distal phalanx of hallux 8/59, duplicated proximal phalanx of hallux 6/58.

Head circumference below 50th percentile 93/96, (28 in 10th to 3rd percentile, 54 in the 3rd percentile or below) large foramen magnum 15/23, large anterior fontanel or delay in its closing 28/44, prominent forehead 41/81, parietal foramina 16/42. Antimongoloid slant of palpebral fissures 104/111, "apparent hypertelorism", probably secondary to broad nasal bridge and epicanthi, but not necessarily confirmable by measurement of interpupillary or interorbital distance 78/90, strabismus 74/97, refractive error 29/46, eyebrows heavy or highly arched 57/102, epicanthi 54/100, long eyelashes 15/34, nasolacrimal duct obstruction 13/36, ptosis 18/93. Minimal abnormalities in ear position, rotation, size or shape 66/99. Beaked or straight nasal appearance 97/111, nasal septum extending below alae 62/84, broad nasal bridge 70/102. Highly-arched palate 99/103, grimacing or unusual smile 22/31, mild retrognathia 54/79, somewhat small appearing mouth 37/84.

Mental, motor, language or social retardation 108/108, below 50 IQ 74/89, EEG abnormalities 27/38, absence of corpus callosum by pneumoencephalography or autopsy 5/12. Stature below 50th percentile 102/105 (81 at the 3rd percentile or below), bone age below the 50th percentile 47/54, abnormal stiff gait 40/56, abnormalities of the pelvis 13/19 (eg reduction in the acetabular and iliac angles, etc), vertebral anomalies 31/50 (eg scoliosis, kyphosis, etc), sternal or rib anomalies 35/63 (eg pectus excavatum, etc).

Heart murmur 28/91, heart disease 16/60 (eg patent ductus arteriosus, etc). Azygous lobe or other anomalous lung lobation 8/15. Supernumerary nipples 8/61. Incomplete or delayed descent of testes in males 44/51, anomalies or disease of urinary tract 18/37 (eg duplicated kidney and ureter, etc).

Nevus flammeus of forehead, nape of neck, or back 36/79, hirsutism of trunk and limbs at all ages and of the face in infants 46/72. High incidence of dermatoglyphic loops or whorls often with a large pattern on thenar or 1st interdigital area of 1 or both palms, slightly increased incidence of distal loops in 3rd interdigital area, patterns in hypothenar area, distal axial triradius tendency to an increased maximal *atd* angle, rare whorls with mainly arches and loops on fingertips, double pattern on the thumb, extra triradius on the enlarged thumb tip near the nail, small total ridge count. Simian line 29/66. Large hallucal loop with laterally displaced f triradius with or without an associated e' triradius or a distal loop opening to the 1st interdigital space associated with a more proximal fibular loop. Deep plantar crease in 1st interdigital area 10/19.

Complications
I **Derived:** Presumably mental retardation, feeding difficulties in infancy, respiratory distress and recurrent infections
II **Associated:** Uncertain, possibly 6th toe on fibular side of foot, lack of mandibular prominence, irregular and crowded teeth, abnormalities in cytoarchitecture of cerebral cortex, genu valgum, valgus foot, angulated penis and others of lesser frequency

Etiology: ? No consistent metabolic, genetic or cytogenetic findings have been found. There is no apparent relation to maternal or paternal age.

Pathogenesis: ?

Related Facts
I **Sex Ratio:** M1:F1
II **Risk of Occurrence:** ?
III **Risk of Recurrence for**
Patient's Sib: ?
Patient's Child: ? No individual with the syndrome has reportedly had children.
IV **Age of Detectability:** Syndrome can be detected in the newborn period by characteristic thumb, hallux and facial abnormalities, confirmed by roentgenographic findings of hands, feet and pelvis.
V **Prevalence:** Unknown for general population. Varies in diagnostic clinic and mental retardation groups from 1 in 720 to 1 in 300. Reported among Caucasians, Orientals (Japanese) and Negroes.

Treatment
I **Primary Prevention:** ?
II **Secondary Prevention:** Appropriate management of retardation. Medical or surgical management of improvable defects.
III **Other Therapy:** Antibiotics for infections and anticonvulsants for seizures

Prognosis: Of the 114 known cases, the oldest was 49 years old. Ten of the patients are known to have expired. The cause of death and age at the time of death were: respiratory distress syndrome at 8 days, meningitis at 2 weeks, bronchopneumonia at 2 weeks, bronchopneumonia and congestive failure at 5 1/2 months, pneumonitis and "sudden death syndrome" at 18 months, pneumonia at 22 months, fulminant enteritis at 6 years, trauma and respiratory infection at 9 years, brain tumor (ectopic pinealoma) at 14 years and acute leukemia at 17 years.

Detection of Carrier: —

†**Special Considerations:** At the present time, broad thumbs and halluces along with the facial gestalt have been taken as essential findings in the syndrome. If some basic pathognomonic finding, clinical or laboratory, is uncovered, it might well prove that these are really not essential features. Until such time, however, questionable cases that do not truly meet these minimal requirements would probably best not be diagnosed as examples of the syndrome. Mental retardation has not been an essential requirement; however, the nature of the populations that have been studied have biased the findings. No one finding that has been found is pathognomonic of the broad thumb syndrome and each may be found in other clinical entities. It is possible that with further delineation of the syndrome

or with the discovery of an etiologic factor or factors, several distinct entities may emerge out of what presently is being considered a single entity.

References:
Rubinstein, J. H.: The broad thumbs syndrome- progress report 1968. In Bergsma, D. (ed.): Part II. Malformation Syndromes. Birth Defects: Orig. Art. Ser., vol. V, no. 2. New York: The National Foundation- March of Dimes, 1969, p. 25.
Rubinstein, J. H. and Taybi, H.: Broad thumbs and toes and facial abnormalities: A possible mental retardation syndrome. Am. J. Dis. Child. 105:588, 1963.
Rubinstein, J.H. et al: The Rubinstein-Taybi syndrome. In Richards, B.W. (ed.): 1st Congr. Int. Ass. Scientific Study of Mental Deficiency, France, 1967. Surrey, England: Michael Jackson Publishing Co., Ltd., 1968, p. 588.

Contributor: **Jack H. Rubinstein**

Editor's Computerized Descriptors: Eye, Oral, Nasoph., Nose, Skin, Dermatoglyphic, Hair, Skel., GU. CV., Nerve

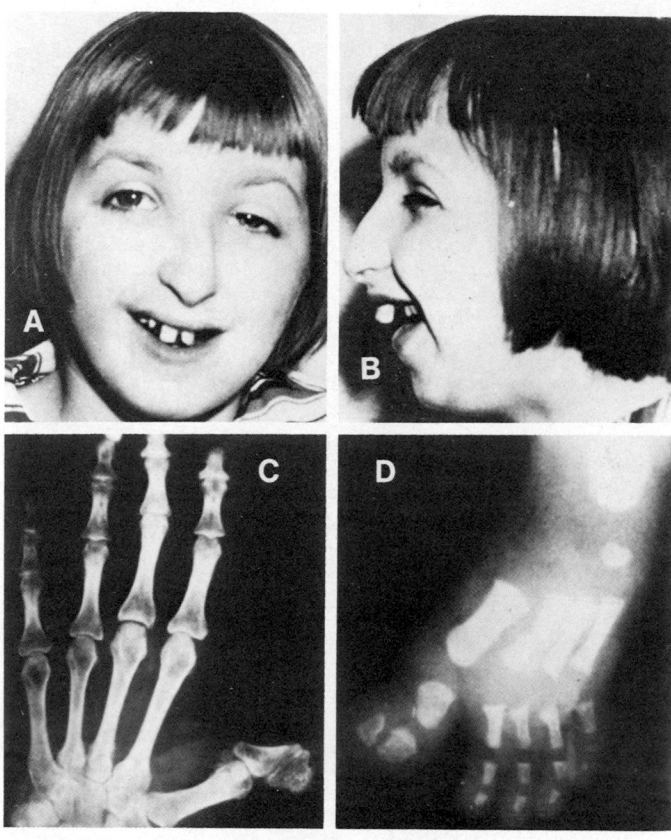

151. A) Frontal view; B) lateral view; C) triangular and spatulate deformities of proximal and terminal phalanges of thumb; D) broad great toe with duplication of terminal phalanx

BRONCHIAL ATRESIA

Includes: Atrésie bronchique
Bronchialatresie
Atresia bronquial
Bronchial atresia of posterior apical segment left upper lobe
Atresia, bronchial

Excludes: Tracheoesophageal fistula (960)

Minimal Diagnostic Criteria: Emphysema of left upper lobe on chest xray. Bronchogram demonstrates the atresia.†

Clinical Findings: Usually asymptomatic. Most cases have been diagnosed on routine chest xray during childhood or early adulthood. Local emphysema or hyperlucency in a portion of the left upper lobe has been a common finding in the reported cases. Bronchogram demonstrates atresia of the bronchus to the apical posterior segment of the left upper lobe. Occasionally a homogeneous well-circumscribed mass within the hyperlucent area has been seen on the xray. Cystic areas with air-fluid levels may also appear within the hyperlucent lung. On physical examination the only finding is diminished breath sounds in the area of the left upper lobe.

Complications
I   **Derived:**   Infrequent infection
II **Associated:**   Anatomic variations of left upper lobe bronchi

Etiology: ?

Pathogenesis: There is occlusion of the bronchus to the posterior apical segment of the left upper lobe. Immediately beyond the atresia, the bronchus is cystic with roughly peripheral bronchi distributed into aerated alveoli which are greatly enlarged. There are normal mucous secreting glands within the bronchial epithelium distal to the atresia. Local emphysema is characteristic and is thought to be due to air entering the lung segment via small anomalous communications existing between alveoli in the abnormal segment and distal bronchi in adjacent normal lung. The egress of air is impaired.†

Related Facts
I   **Sex Ratio:**   ?
II   **Risk of Occurrence:**   ?
III **Risk of Recurrence for**
      Patient's Sib: ?
      Patient's Child: ?
IV   **Age of Detectability:**   Variable—probably in infancy if a chest xray is taken.
V   **Prevalence:**   ? Approximately 10 reported cases

Treatment
I   **Primary Prevention:**   —
II   **Secondary Prevention:**   —
III **Other Therapy:**   Treatment of intermittent pulmonary infection

Prognosis: Normal for life span, intelligence and function

Detection of Carrier: —

†**Special Considerations:**   One theory of the cause of the atresia has been that an occlusion of a bronchial artery to the affected area occurs after branching of bronchi has occurred - after the 15th week of gestation. This syndrome must be differentiated from other causes of unilateral hyperlucent lung.

References:
Curry, T. S., 3d. and Curry, G. C.: Atresia of the bronchus to the apical-posterior segment of the left upper lobe. Am. J. Roentgenol. Radium Ther. Nucl. Med. 98:350, 1966.

Contributor: **Patricia S. Zelkowitz**

Includes: Syndrome C
Síndrome C
Opitz trigonocephaly syndrome

Excludes: —

Minimal Diagnostic Criteria: Impossible to define on the basis of 5 known patients; see Clinical Findings.

Clinical Findings: Based on data from 5 published cases, the C syndrome is a sublethal condition. The sibs initially reported by Opitz et al became jaundiced about the 5th or 6th day (highest total bilirubin levels 21-25 mg%). The girl died suddenly at 8 days of life, cause of death unknown. The boy sucked poorly, was lethargic, showed no sign of psychomotor maturation and failed to thrive. He died of pneumonia at 13 weeks. Patient 1 of Preus et al died at 15 months, 8 days after right hemicolectomy for cecal volvulus; the patient of Oberklaid and Danks died at 2 weeks of unknown cause.

General findings included strikingly abnormal appearance, with abnormal body proportions (some total body shortness, a nearly normal sized to small head, slightly short trunk and very short limbs) with short fingers and toes, unusual hyperextensibility of the joints of the limbs. Skull is trigonocephalic with prominent metopic suture, premature closure of anterior fontanel; flat supraorbital ridges and bridge of nose, upward slanting of palpebral fissures, Brushfield spots, extremely thick and prominent, complete inner epicanthic folds; diffuse and spotty capillary hemangiomata of nose and glabellar region, anterior "cowlick," small, incompletely differentiated, possibly low-set, posteriorly angulated auricles apparently devoid of cartilage; small nares, relatively long philtrum, large mouth, and micrognathia with somewhat puckered lips. Alveolar ridges are wide, the palate highly arched with multiple frenula between alveolar ridges and buccal mucosa. In the case of Oberklaid and Danks the palate appeared flat, continuous with alveolar ridges and upper lip, and had a deep midline fissure (not cleft). Skin of the entire body markedly redundant; nipples widely spaced; diastasis recti; pilonidal dimple and sinus in the girl; cryptorchidism of right testis in her brother. Clinodactyly of index fingers, bridged palmar creases, postaxial hexadactyly with extensive cutaneous webbing of the toes. Nails normal. Patient 1 of Preus et al and the patient of Oberklaid and Danks did not have polydactyly, but the latter had flexion deformities at elbows, wrists and fingers.

Skeletal findings included complex arthro-osteodysplasia with dyschondroplastic body proportions, crepitation of right elbow in 1 sib, hyperextensible joints of limbs with anterior displacement or dislocation of the legs (1 sib was born with legs hyperextended at the knees and folded onto the thighs and abdomen). Dissection of 1 knee joint showed weak posterior and cruciate ligaments. Other findings at autopsy included trigonocephaly with shallow anterior fossa, and deep, funnel-shaped posterior fossa, platybasia; bone defects over the cribriform plate, ethmoid sinuses and absence of bone between the superior portions of the orbits; short sternum with reduced number of ossification centers but long xiphisternum, deformity of ribs; severe shortness of all metacarpals. Patient of Oberklaid and Danks had bilateral dislocation of head of radius. In the patients of Preus et al knees and elbows could be rotated excessively.

Visceral and cardiovascular anomalies included hepato-

megaly, free floating cecum and ascending colon combined within the mesentery of the ileum (leading to cecal volvulus in patient 1 of Preus et al); prominent fetal lobulations of the kidneys, histologic immaturity of lung and kidneys, extensive fibrosis of pancreas. Patent ductus arteriosus, separate origin of left internal and external carotids from the aorta, thin-walled pulmonary arteries, congenital heart disease of unspecified type in both patients of Preus et al.

Central nervous system findings included incomplete development of tentorium, many foci of cerebral, cerebellar and meningeal hemorrhage, poor myelinization of the brain. The patient of Oberklaid and Danks had a macroscopically normal brain, persistent pupillary membranes, central hyaloid arteries and a coloboma of the optic disks. Patient 1 of Preus et al had glaucoma requiring goniotomy.

Complications
I **Derived:** See Clinical Findings
II **Associated:** See Clinical Findings

Etiology: Probably homozygous state of autosomal recessive mutant gene

Pathogenesis: ?

Related Facts
I **Sex Ratio:** Presumably M1:F1
II **Risk of Occurrence:** ?
III **Risk of Recurrence for**
Patient's Sib: 1 in 4 (25%) for each sib
Patient's Child: ?
IV **Age of Detectability:** At birth, by physical examination
V **Prevalence:** ?

Treatment
I **Primary Prevention:** —
II **Secondary Prevention:** —
III **Other Therapy:** As may be indicated

Prognosis: Lethal in infancy in 4/5 cases

Detection of Carrier: —

Special Considerations: —

References:
Oberklaid, F. and Danks, D.M.: The Opitz trigonocephaly syndrome; a case report. Am. J. Dis. Child. 129:1348-1349, 1975.
Opitz, J.M. et al: The C syndrome of multiple congenital anomalies. In Bergsma, D. (ed.): Part II. Malformation Syndromes. Birth Defects: Orig. Art. Ser., vol. V, no. 2. White Plains: The National Foundation -March of Dimes, 1969, p. 161.
Preus, M. et al: The C syndrome. In Bergsma, D. (ed.): Malformation Syndromes. Birth Defects: Orig. Art. Ser., vol. XI, no. 2. Amsterdam: Excerpta Medica for The National Foundation-March of Dimes, 1975, p. 58.

Contributor: **John M. Opitz**

Editor's Computerized Descriptors: Eye, Ear, Face, Oral, Nose, Skin, Hair, Skel., Muscle, Resp., CV., GI., Liver, GU., Nerve

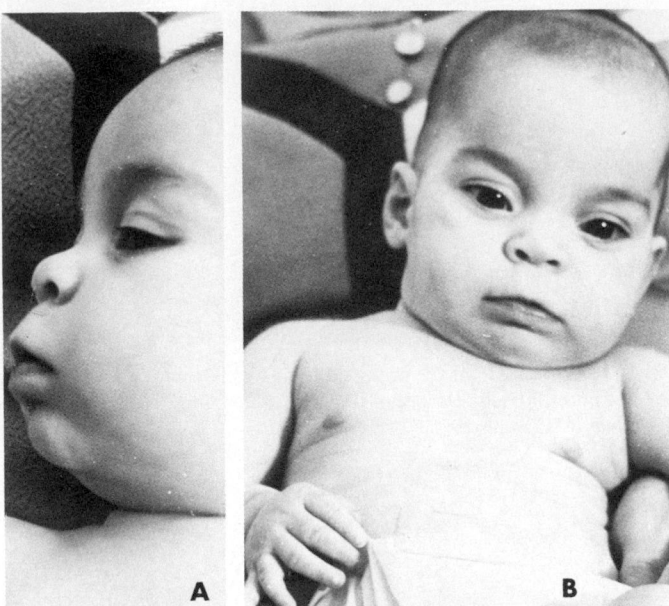

152. A) Note short nose, prominent maxilla and slightly receding chin; B) upward slant of palpebral fissures, broad nose, wide mouth, short neck, widely spaced nipples and postaxial hand polydactyly

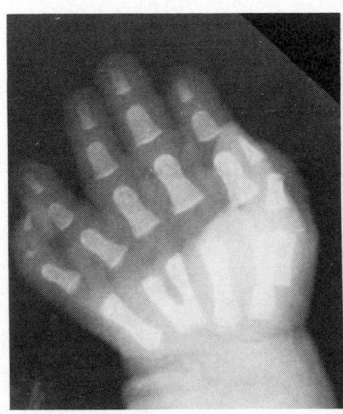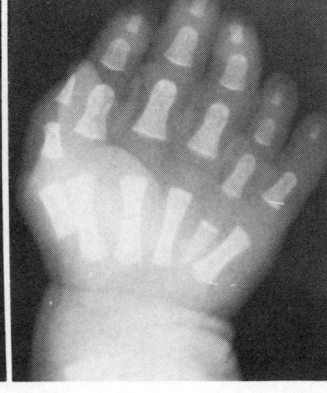

153. Note polydactyly, metacarpal fusion and hypoplasia of terminal phalanges

CAMPOMELIC DYSPLASIA

Includes: Syndrome campomélique
Kampomeles Syndrom
Síndrome campomiélico
Campomelic dwarfism
Camptomelic syndrome
Congenital bowing of the limbs

Excludes: Short limb varieties of campomelia
Other forms of congenital bowing of the limbs

Minimal Diagnostic Criteria: Congenital bowing of the long bones in a short-limbed dwarf, in whom the bent femur is relatively long and slender.†

Clinical Findings: The typical campomelic syndrome is associated with short-limbed dwarfism affecting selectively the lower limbs with anterior bending of the femur and tibia over which there are pretibial skin dimples. The calvarium is large with disproportionately small facies. The ears are low-set and there is micrognathia and hypertelorism. The facies appear flat with a depressed nasal root and a posterior cleft palate is usually present. Hypotonia and absence of olfactory nerves have been found, and death usually results in the neonatal period secondary to respiratory distress. Radiographically in the classic form of campomelic syndrome the bent long bones are fairly long and slender. There is femoral and tibial bowing and hypoplastic fibulae. Eleven pairs of ribs have been described in these patients with hypoplasia of the scapulae. The ribs are narrow and wavy and the clavicles slender. There is scoliosis or kyphoscoliosis. The pelvis is high and narrow with hypoplasia of the ischiopubic rami, and the ischia appear vertical in their orientation.

Complications
I **Derived:** Respiratory distress secondary to decreased rib cage size and tracheal cartilage abnormalities.
II **Associated:** —

Etiology: ? Autosomal recessive. One pair of affected sibs with the typical form of the disease has been described. McK *21135

Pathogenesis: Histologic examination of the site of bowing of the long bones shows parallel masses of periosteal new bone extending into the medullary cavity at right angles to the axis of the bone. This is probably secondary to the stress that produced the bending of the bone.

Related Facts
I **Sex Ratio:** Approximately M1:F2
II **Risk of Occurrence:** Rare
III **Risk of Recurrence for**
    Patient's Sib: Uncertain. If it is autosomal recessive this could be 1 in 4 (25%)
    Patient's Child: These individuals usually do not live past the neonatal period.
IV **Age of Detectability:** Newborn
V **Prevalence:** ?

Treatment
I **Primary Prevention:** Genetic counseling, if autosomal recessive hypothesis proves correct.
II **Secondary Prevention:** Support of respiratory function in the newborn.
III **Other Therapy:** —

Prognosis: Almost all result in neonatal or infant death.

Detection of Carrier: —

†**Special Considerations:** Campomelia, or bending of the long bones can be produced by a heterogeneous group of

disorders. This classic or long bone variety of campomelic dwarfism must be distinguished from various generalized bone dysplasias that can produce bending of the long bones, such as osteogenesis imperfecta and hypophosphatasia, as well as several recently described rare conditions. Thus, the campomelic syndrome appears to be a well-defined distinct disorder that can be delineated by a variety of radiographic findings, including the long slender bent bones. Two apparently distinct syndromes which have been termed "short bone varieties" of campomelic dwarfism, have recently been described. These include: a) the *short bone craniostenotic type,* in which one has campomelic limbs with short bent bones with normal metaphyses; gross skull deformity with craniostenosis and hydrocephalus (Kleeblattschädel) and facial hypoplasia with micrognathia; slender ribs and hypoplastic scapula; radioulnar synostosis and precocious ossification of the carpal bones. The vertebral bodies appear square with stellate fissured centers and there is an abnormal pelvis. The etiology of this syndrome is unknown. b) *Short bone normocephalic type,* in which the campomelic limbs are also short and broad but there is metaphyseal flaring and irregularity. The upper limbs are frequently bowed as well and there are 11 pairs of ribs. One pair of sibs has been reported with this syndrome suggesting autosomal recessive inheritance. Both of these short bone varieties also result in neonatal death.

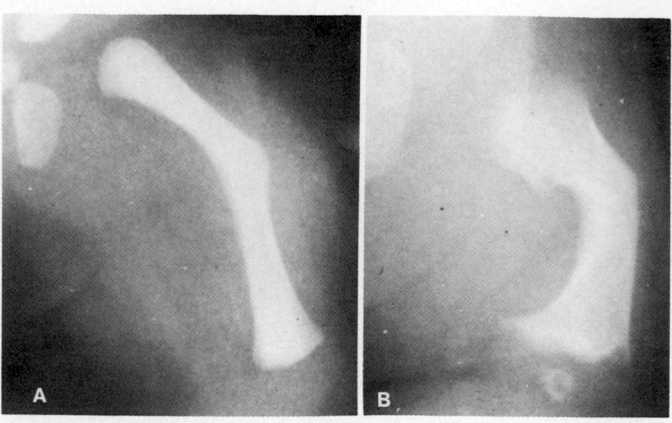

154. Note angulation of the proximal femoral shaft with apex directed anteriorly and laterally; B) marked shortening of shaft and flaring of distal epiphysis

References:

Becker, M.H. et al: Campomelic dwarfism. In Bergsma. D. (ed.): Disorders of Connective Tissue. Birth Defects: Orig. Art. Ser., vol. XI, no. 6. Miami: Symposia Specialists for The National Foundation-March of Dimes, 1975, p. 113.

Bound, J. et al: Congenital anterior angulation of the tibia. Arch. Dis. Child. 27:179, 1952.

Kahajavi, A. et al: Heterogeneity in the campomelic syndromes: Long and short bone varieties. In Bergsma, D. (ed.): Growth Problems and Clinical Advances. Birth Defects: Orig. Art. Ser., vol. XII, no. 6. New York: Alan R. Liss for The National Foundation-March of Dimes, 1976, p. 93.

Lee, F.A. et al: The "Campomelic" syndrome. Am. J. Dis. Child. 24:485, 1972.

Thurmon, T.F. et al: Familial camptomelic dwarfism. J. Pediatr. 83:841, 1973.

Contributors: **Ralph S. Lachman**
David L. Rimoin

Editor's Computerized Descriptors: Eye, Ear, Face, Oral, Nose, Skin, Skel., Muscle, Resp.

CARDIOAUDITORY SYNDROME

Includes: Syndrome de Jervell-Nielsen
Kardioauriculäres Syndrom
Síndrome cardioauditivo
Surdocardiac syndrome
Deafness and functional heart disease
Jervell and Lange-Nielsen syndrome

Excludes: Cardiac conduction defects without deafness

Minimal Diagnostic Criteria: Sensorineural deafness, characteristic ECG findings

Clinical Findings: Characterized by deafness, cardiac conduction abnormalities and syncopal attacks.

The deafness is congenital or at least of very early onset and probably not progressive. It is perceptive and of profound degree; the hearing loss is symmetric. There is variable preservation of hearing in the low tones but this is insufficient for the normal learning of speech, and special education is necessary. No results of tests of vestibular function are available.

The fainting attacks may begin in infancy or childhood and are usually precipitated by nervousness or physical exertion; sometimes they are first noticed when the child begins to walk. These attacks may be mild, or so severe as to produce loss of consciousness for 5-10 minutes, with temporary residual disorientation. They may be frequent so that several occur in a day, or infrequent so that months or years elapse between them. If the true cause is unsuspected they may be mistaken for epilepsy or even hysterical episodes.

The ECG is abnormal with large T-waves which may be upright, biphasic or inverted, and a prolonged QT interval indicating abnormal ventricular repolarization. In some instances, however, the T-waves may be normal and the QT prolongation less marked. In general, the degree of the QT prolongation varies greatly between different affected individuals and in the same individual at different times.

Death may occur in one of the syncopal attacks and is probably due to ventricular fibrillation. There is some evidence that if affected persons survive adolescence, adaptation of the abnormal situation takes place, the attacks become less frequent and the prognosis improves.

A mild hypochromic anemia may be an additional feature of the syndrome.

Complications
I Derived: Deafness in infancy or childhood is common; sudden death.
II Associated: —

Etiology: Autosomal recessive; McK *22040

Pathogenesis: ? Microscopic changes have been found at autopsy both in the ear (organ of Corti) and in the heart (Purkinje fibers and arteries supplying the sinuatrial node).

Related Facts
I Sex Ratio: M1:F1
II Risk of Occurrence: May be of the order of 1 in 100,000 to 1 in 200,000 births.
III Risk of Recurrence for
Patient's Sib: 1 in 4 (25%) for each offspring to be affected
Patient's Child: Not increased unless mate is carrier or homozygote.
(The reproductive fitness of affected individuals is much reduced because of the high risk of early death. If survival to the reproductive age occurs, then probably fitness is similar to that of other deaf persons-ie up to 75% of normal-but no example of a documented case having offspring has

in fact been recorded.)
IV Age of Detectability: Deafness: early infancy (though often not detected until later). The condition could probably be detected at birth or even in utero by ECG examination.
V Prevalence: Low and falls rapidly with age. The condition has been described in many populations of European origin and seems to be especially common in Norway. No data are available concerning populations of non-European origin.

Treatment
I Primary Prevention: Genetic counseling
II Secondary Prevention: It has been suggested that digitalization makes the ECG less abnormal and improves the prognosis. Beta-adrenergic blockade with propanolol has been used with encouraging results, and it has also been suggested that phenobarbitone and phenytoin sodium, either in combination or separately, are effective in reducing the frequency of fainting attacks. Perhaps a pacemaker could be considred as a temporary measure when attacks are frequent and life-threatening, but meager practical experience with the use of such a technique has not been encouraging from the point of view of long-term application.
III Other Therapy: Hearing aids and rehabilitative measures for the sensorineural hearing loss.

Prognosis: Poor. It is difficult to make accurate estimates but possibly 50% or more of cases die before adolescence.

Detection of Carrier: ? Moderate prolongation of the QT interval may be present in the ECG of a proportion of carriers.

Special Considerations: —

References:
Fraser, G.R. et al: Congenital deafness associated with electrocardiographic abnormalities, fainting attacks and sudden deaths; a recessive syndrome. Q.J. Med. 33:361, 1964.
Friedmann, I. et al: Pathology of the ear in the cardio-auditory syndrome of Jervell and Lange-Nielsen: Report of a third case with an appendix on possible linkage with the Rh blood group locus. J. Laryngol. 82:882, 1968.
Jervell, A. et al: The surdo-cardiac syndrome: Three new cases of congenital deafness with syncopal attacks and Q-T prolongation in the electrocardiogram. Am. Heart J. 72:582, 1966.

Contributor: **G.R. Fraser**

Editor's Computerized Descriptors: Hearing, Speech, CV., Nerve

CARNITINE DEFICIENCY OF MUSCLE, PRIMARY

Includes: Déficit musculaire en carnitine
Primärer Carnitinmangel der Muskulatur
Deficiencia primaria muscular de carnitina

Excludes: Some slowly progressive muscular dystrophies
Lipoidosis of muscle from a variety of causes
A number of early-onset forms of progressive weakness

Minimal Diagnostic Criteria: Lowered plasma carnitine; generalized muscle weakness; liver tenderness

Clinical Findings: The first examples of this condition were described by A.G. Engel and others. The 1st patient they saw was 19 years of age; no family history was available. She had been well until age 16 but could never sit up without using her hands, and she slept with her eyes open.

In subsequent years there was progression of her muscle weakness so that she became bedfast and the liver became tender. Myographic studies revealed myopathic features and some elevation of serum enzymes, including CPK. Liver function tests were moderately abnormal. Muscle biopsies showed vacuolization of many muscle fibers with lipid accumulation.

Complications
I **Derived:**   Uncertain, but probably progressive muscle and liver damage.
II **Associated:**   ?

Etiology: ?

Pathogenesis: Deficiency of carnitine, which is a regulator of the cellular rate of long-chain fatty acid oxidation. Deficiency of carnitine in muscle can result in impaired fatty acid oxidation by mitochondria, increased triglyceride synthesis, lipid storage myopathy, and muscle weakness. Muscle carnitine deficiency may be the result of impaired carnitine uptake by the muscle fiber (due to a defect in active transport or lack of a hypothetic receptor substance), or it may result from impaired hepatic carnitine synthesis. It is not clear which of these mechanisms is involved.

Related Facts
I **Sex Ratio:**   ?
II **Risk of Occurrence:**   ?
III **Risk of Recurrence for**
   Patient's Sib: ?
   Patient's Child: ?
IV **Age of Detectability:**   By the 2nd decade or earlier
V **Prevalence:**   ?

Treatment
I **Primary Prevention:**   ?
II **Secondary Prevention:**   Therapy with corticosteroids
III **Other Therapy:**   —

Prognosis: Apparently progressive muscular weakness occurs in individuals with this condition, but ultimate outcome has not yet been determined.

Detection of Carrier: —

Special Considerations: —

References:
Engel, A.G. and Angelini, C.: Carnitine deficiency of human skeletal muscle with associated lipid storage myopathy: A new syndrome. Science 179;899, 1973.
Engel, A.G. et al: Identification of carnitine deficiency as a cause of human lipid storage myopathy. In Milhorat, A.T. (ed.): Exploratory Concepts in Muscular Dystrophy II. Amsterdam: Excerpta Medica, 1974, p. 601.

Contributor: **Carl M. Pearson**

CARNITINE PALMITYL TRANSFERASE DEFICIENCY

Includes: Déficit en carnitine palmityl transférase
Carnitinpalmityl-Transferase-Mangel
Deficiencia de carnitina palmitil transferase
Inability to utilize long-chain fatty acids as a source of energy in muscle
Idiopathic recurrent myoglobinuria

Excludes: Other congenital myopathies, other forms of muscle weakness, and other causes of myoglobinuria which follow exertion.

Minimal Diagnostic Criteria: Muscle cramps following exercise, starvation, or a high fat diet. Possible family history of similar disease. Myoglobinuria of unexplained cause.

Clinical Findings: Muscle carnitine palmityl transferase (CPT) deficiency is a rare disorder that was first described by Engel and his colleagues in 1970 in two 18-year-old girls, identical twins, who suffered from "intermittent muscle cramps" and recurrent myoglobinuria associated with either exercise, ingestion of a high-fat diet, or fasting and the induction of ketosis. The symptoms of cramping, etc are almost invariably associated with or follow exercise, whether prolonged or strenuous. The symptoms appear in the exercised muscles only, and if strenuous exercise is undertaken, cramping, muscle necrosis, and myoglobinuria, as well as elevation of serum enzymes, invariably appear. The precise deficiency of the enzyme CPT was first defined by DiMauro and DiMauro.

Little more is known about this condition except for the fact that CPT is an enzyme that handles long-chain fatty acids and allows them to pass across the mitochondrial membranes where the fatty acids are received by another enzyme, palmityl-CoA synthetase. The DiMauros describe this syndrome in a 29-year-old man with a similar history of muscle stress after exercise or starvation. Recently, Reza et al found 3 additional unrelated cases in muscle frozen in storage during the past 15 years. All 12 samples were obtained from persons with exertional myoglobinuria of unknown cause.

Aside from muscle necrosis after exercise, there is nothing histologically characteristic of uninvolved muscles, and at rest there are no abnormal electrical findings in muscle.

Complications
I   **Derived:** Potential acute renal tubular necrosis associated with massive myoglobinuria. Fibrosis of muscle following repeated attacks.
II   **Associated:** —

Etiology: ? McK *25510

Pathogenesis: Profound deficiency or absence of the enzyme carnitine palmityl transferase resulting in deficient utilization of long-chain fatty acids as a source for energy in exercise in muscle.

Related Facts
I   **Sex Ratio:** ?
II   **Risk of Occurrence:** Minimal
III   **Risk of Recurrence for**
    Patient's Sib: ?
    Patient's Child: ?
IV   **Age of Detectability:** 15 to 30 years of age (possibly lower). Depends upon suspicion of disease and myoglobinuria, as well as availability of specific biochemical test procedures. Theoretically, could be detected soon after birth.
V   **Prevalence:** Very rare

Treatment

I   **Primary Prevention:** Avoidance of excessive or strenuous exertion. Avoidance of diet primarily limited to fats. Avoidance of starvation or fasting.
II   **Secondary Prevention:** —
III   **Other Therapy:** —

Prognosis: Probably normal life span if above procedures are followed. Adequate numbers of cases have not been detailed in the literature to make a definitive statement on this point.

Detection of Carrier: ?

Special Considerations: —

References:
DiMauro, S. and DiMauro, P.M.: Muscle carnitine palmityltransferase deficiency and myoglobinuria. Science 182:929, 1973.
Engel, W.K. et al: A skeletal-muscle disorder associated with intermittent symptoms and a possible defect of lipid metabolism. N. Engl. J. Med. 282:697, 1970.
Reza, M.J. et al: Three additional cases of carnitine palmityltransferase deficiency in association with exertional myoglobinuria. Ann. Intern. Med. In press.

Contributor: **Carl M. Pearson**

Editor's Computerized Descriptors: Muscle, GU.

CARNOSINEMIA

Includes: Carnosinémie
Karnosinämie
Bound-β-alanine metabolism, disorders of
Serum carnosinase deficiency

Excludes: Dietary carnosinuria
Imidazole aminoaciduria (519)

Minimal Diagnostic Criteria: Persistent carnosinuria while on a diet which excludes carnosine. Absence of 1-methylhistidine from the urine, coupled with presence of anserine in the urine, following the oral ingestion of anserine (as in chicken breast). Serum carnosinase activity markedly lower than age-matched control subjects.

Clinical Findings: Seven patients belonging to 4 unrelated pedigrees have been described. Five of these patients developed progressive neurologic deterioration commencing in early infancy. They had myoclonic and later generalized seizures, spasticity, and became severely mentally retarded. All 5 had abnormal EEG patterns. One patient died at 10 months, and a second died at 7 1/2 years. One patient with carnosinemia was clinically normal at the age of 6 years, and one infant was normal when last described at the age of 2 months.†

Biochemical studies have shown persistent excretion of carnosine in the urine, generally 0.5 to 1.0 mmole/g creatinine. Carnosinuria persists even when all sources of this dipeptide (meat and poultry) are excluded from the diet. Carnosine has been irregularly detectable in the fasting plasma of patients, reaching as high as 4 μmole/l while on a carnosine-free diet.

Serum carnosinase activity is markedly reduced.

Complications
I **Derived:** Relationship of biochemical abnormalities to clinical findings has not been established.†
II **Associated:** —

Etiology: Probably autosomal recessive enzyme defect.† Mck *21220

Pathogenesis: Deficiency of serum carnosinase activity.†

Related Facts
I **Sex Ratio:** M1:F1 probable
II **Risk of Occurrence:** Very rare
III **Risk of Recurrence for**
  Patient's Sib: ? Possibly 1 in 4 (25%) for each offspring to be affected
  Patient's Child: Probably not increased unless mate is carrier or homozygote
IV **Age of Detectability:** Early infancy
V **Prevalence:** Very rare

Treatment
I **Primary Prevention:** —
II **Secondary Prevention:** —
III **Other Therapy:** —

Prognosis: At least 5 of the 7 described patients have been severely damaged neurologically; one died at age 10 months, and one died at age 7 1/2 years. However, one patient was physically and intellectually normal at age 6 years.†

Detection of Carrier: Not established; but serum carnosinase activity was low in both parents in one pedigree, and in one of the parents in 2 additional pedigrees.

†Special Considerations: It is not clear whether the degenerative neurologic disease observed in 5 of the 7 described patients with carnosinemia is related in any way to their deficiency in serum carnosinase activity. The good health of one patient at the age of 6 years suggests the possibility that serum carnosinase deficiency and the presence of elevated carnosine concentrations in plasma are entirely harmless, and that the neurologic disease(s) described and the biochemical abnormality are merely a chance association.

Carnosine content was normal in skeletal muscle obtained at autopsy from one of the patients, and tissue carnosinase activity was present in muscle of both patients who died. Since carnosine is not normally detectable in human brain, and since the related dipeptide homocarnosine was present in normal amounts in the brain of one patient who died, it is difficult to see why a deficiency of serum carnosinase activity should produce any neurologic abnormalities.

References:
Perry, T.L.: Carnosinemia. In Nyhan, W.L. (ed.): Heritable Disorders of Amino Acid Metabolism. New York:John Wiley & Sons, 1974, p. 293.
Perry, T. L. et al: Carnosinemia: A new metabolic disorder associated with neurologic disease and mental defect. N. Engl. J. Med. 277:1219, 1967.
Van Munster, P.J.J. et al: A new sensitive method for the determination of serum carnosinase activity using L-carnosine-(1-^{14}C)-β-alanyl as substrate. Clin. Chim. Acta 29:243, 1970.

Contributor: **Thomas L. Perry**

Editor's Computerized Descriptor: Nerve

CAROTID BODY TUMOR

Includes: Tumeur du cortuscule carotidien
Glomus caroticum Tumor
Tumor del cuerdo carotídeo
Chemodectoma of neck
Ganglion nodosum tumor
Juxtavagal tumor

Excludes: Chemodectoma of middle ear (145)
Aortic body tumor
Chemodectoma located elsewhere in the body

Minimal Diagnostic Criteria: Presence of a mass in the region of the carotid bifurcation and a positive tumor flush by arteriography. Biopsy should be avoided if possible but if tissue is obtained the findings are characteristic.

Clinical Findings: A painless neck mass is found which may or may not be associated with a bruit. The mass can be moved laterally but not vertically. Dysphagia, hoarseness or cough, syncope with carotid sinus syndrome, headache, occasionally pain or tenderness may be seen. Tumors may present in the lateral pharyngeal wall. Also paralysis of one or more of the IXth, Xth, XIth and XIIth cranial nerves may occur. If these tumors are of a secreting nature, laboratory findings would be those of a pheochromocytoma, namely elevated catecholamines in the blood and urine. However, the incidence of secreting chemodectomas of the neck is only about 1 or 2%. Arteriography provides significant information. A typical tumor flush is seen and venous studies may show obstruction of the internal jugular vein or the jugular bulb. It is possible to have multiple tumors which could be bilateral and involve other areas.

Complications
I **Derived:** Local mass or pressure effects, including obstruction of the carotid vessel or internal jugular vein. Present 15% of the time are cranial nerve paralysis, Xth nerve first, then XIth and XIIth nerves followed by the IXth nerve. Rare tumors secrete norepinephrine and are associated with hypertension.
II **Associated:** Chemodectomas may be multiple: occurring in the neck, ear, thorax or abdomen.

Etiology: Unknown except for familial pattern

Pathogenesis: Tumor growth by one or more elements of chemoreceptor tissue. Primarily these are locally invasive tumors. Incidence of malignancy is undetermined. Probably 3-4% develop metastasis. Multicentric location is at least 5%, going up to 26% in familial cases.

Related Facts
I **Sex Ratio:** M1:F1
II **Risk of Occurrence:** ?
III **Risk of Recurrence for**
   Patient's Sib: ? Incidence of multiple chemodectomas is highest in carotid body tumors and approaches 5%. Where there is a positive family history, the incidence of multiple tumors as distinct from a single carotid body tumor increases to 26%.
   Patient's Child: ? See for Patient's Sib.
IV **Age of Detectability:** Most commonly noted in the 3rd and 4th decades, however, 1 case has been reported at birth. Somewhat younger average age of detection in families with positive history.
V **Prevalence:** Unknown; there are well over 500 cases of carotid body tumors reported.

Treatment
I **Primary Prevention:** —
II **Secondary Prevention:** Early diagnosis and surgical excision whenever possible, which leaves a low incidence of local recurrence. Careful arteriography will lead to the discovery of multiple tumors.
III **Other Therapy:** For large, unresectable lesions or poor surgical risks, radiation therapy in the range of 4000 to 6000 rads.

Prognosis: Fortunately the majority of patients have a slow growing tumor. The incidence of metastases is low. Small tumors have a very good prognosis with surgical excision. Large tumors carry fair to poor prognosis over a long duration. Because of the slow growth of these tumors, survival is usually of long duration.

Detection of Carrier: —

Special Considerations: —

References:
Akkary, S.: Malignant carotid body tumor in the neck of a newborn infant. Arch. Dis. Child. 39:194, 1964.
Berman, S.O.: Chemoreceptor system and its tumor - the chemodectoma. Int. Abstr. Surg. 102:330, 1956.
Grimley, P.M. and Glenner, G.G.: Ultrastructure of the human carotid body: A perspective on the mode of chemoreception. Circulation 37:648, 1968.
Resler, D. R. et al: Multiplicity and familial incidence of carotid body and glomus jugulare tumors. Ann. Otol. Rhinol. Laryngol. 75:114, 1966.
Rush, B.F., Jr.: Familial bilateral carotid body tumors. Ann. Surg. 157:633, 1963.

Contributor: **Robert C. Newell**

Editor's Computerized Descriptors: Speech, Neck, CV., Nerve

CARPAL-TARSAL OSTEOLYSIS AND CHRONIC PROGRESSIVE GLOMERULOPATHY

Includes: Ostéolyse carpo-tarsienne
Karpo-tarsale Osteolyse
Osteolisis carpo-tarsal
Essential osteolysis and nephropathy
Essential hereditary osteolysis
Osteolysis and proteinuria
Proteinuria and osteolysis

Excludes: Carpal-tarsal osteolysis, recessive (129)
Carpal-tarsal osteolysis, dominant
Various aseptic necrosis syndromes
Acroosteolysis syndromes
Osteoarthropathy of Schinz and Furtwaengler
Rheumatoid arthritis

Minimal Diagnostic Criteria: Osteolysis of carpal and tarsal bones associated with moderate-to-marked involvement of adjacent tubular bones, proteinuria and microscopic hematuria.†

Clinical Findings: Osteolysis of carpal and tarsal bones begins in the 1st decade, usually before age 5. It may occur in the absence of notable symptomatology or may be accompanied by tenderness, swelling, and painful limitation of motion of ankle or wrist. As a rule, osteolysis is bilaterally symmetric and progresses slowly to complete dissolution of carpal and tarsal bones. Adjacent tubular bones are shortened with marked tapering resembling a "sucked candy" appearance radiographically. Progressive shortening of the forearms is noted, and lytic involvement of the elbow leads to loss of mobility and function. Cortical thinning of the nonaxial tubular bones also becomes evident. Other nonprogressive skeletal defects have been associated with this syndrome.

Progressive proteinuria with onset at about the end of the 1st decade, associated with microscopic hematuria, is found. Azotemia is usually manifested by the late 2nd or early 3rd decade; nonoliguric renal insufficiency (with the nephrotic syndrome) rapidly progresses to frank renal failure and death.

Pathologic examination of affected wrists has revealed replacement of bone and cartilage by fibrofatty tissue, and a notable lack of inflammatory response or vascular or hemangiomatous changes. Arrest of endochondral bone formation and areas of fibrocartilaginous metaplasia have been observed. Both percutaneous biopsy and autopsy specimens of kidney have demonstrated a proliferative glomerulopathy with epithelial crescent formation and numerous hyalinized glomeruli. Unusual neovascularization of glomeruli by capillary ingrowths from the Bowman capsule have been observed. No immunopathologic studies have been reported.

Laboratory evaluations early in the course of this syndrome are normal; ESR, latex fixation, and LE preparations are normal. Somewhat later, proteinuria and hematuria are found; and finally, the chemical disarray of uremia and massive proteinuria becomes manifest.

Complications
I **Derived:** Painful limitation of motion of affected areas with progressive dysfunction due to loss of bone and resultant deformity (volar subluxation of hands, flexion contractures of elbows and pes cavum). Marked muscle atrophy without neurologic deficit is presumably due to loss of bony insertions. Progressive chronic renal insufficiency results in early death.
II **Associated:** —

Etiology: Autosomal dominant; McK *16630

Pathogenesis: ?

Related Facts
I **Sex Ratio:** Approximately M1:F1
II **Risk of Occurrence:** ?
III **Risk of Recurrence for**
  Patient's Sib: If parent is affected 1 in 2 (50%) for each offspring to be affected; otherwise not increased.
  Patient's Child: 1 in 2
IV **Age of Detectability:** 1st decade
V **Prevalence:** ? Rare

Treatment
I **Primary Prevention:** Genetic counseling
II **Secondary Prevention:** —
III **Other Therapy:** Symptomatic treatment with mild analgesics for wrist and ankle pain. Supportive therapy for chronic renal failure. There is no reported experience with immunosuppressive agents.

Prognosis: Death in uremia in late 2nd and early 3rd decade. One of 4 patients had microcephaly and mental retardation. Function is variable depending on degree and extent of osteolysis.

Detection of Carrier: —

†Special Considerations: Whether carpal-tarsal osteolysis without glomerulopathy and with extensive lytic involvement of adjacent tubular bones and elbow joints is a separate entity is not clear. This syndrome is easily distinguished from recessive carpal-tarsal osteolysis by the above criteria and the notable osteoporosis, cortical thinning and especially increased caliber of phalanges and metacarpals found in the recessive syndrome. The syndrome is easily distinguished from the various acroosteolysis syndromes and aseptic necrosis syndromes by distribution of the lesions. The lack of acute phase reactants, systemic illness and inflammatory reaction in biopsy material serve to distinguish this syndrome from rheumatoid arthritis. The lack of generalized joint stiffness and other skeletal disorders separates this syndrome from osteoarthropathy of Schinz and Furtwaengler.

References:
Lagier, R. and Rutishauser, E.: Osteoarticular changes in a case of essential osteolysis. J. Bone Joint Surg. 47B:339, 1965.
Marie, J. et al: Acro-osteolyse essentielle compliquée d'insuffisance renal d'evolution fatale. Presse Med. 71:249, 1963.
Shurtleff, D.B. et al: Hereditary osteolysis with hypertension and nephropathy. JAMA 188:363, 1964.
Torg, J.S. and Steel, H.H.: Essential osteolysis with nephropathy. J. Bone Joint Surg. 50A:1629, 1968.

Contributors: **David W. Hollister**
David L. Rimoin

Editor's Computerized Descriptors: Skel., GU.

CARPAL-TARSAL OSTEOLYSIS, RECESSIVE

Includes: Ostéolyse carpo-tarsienne (récessive)
Rezessiv erbliche Carpo-tarsale Osteolyse
Osteolisis carpo-tarsal recesiva
Hereditary multicentric osteolysis with recessive transmission
Recessive carpal-tarsal osteolysis

Excludes: Carpal-tarsal osteolysis, dominant
Carpal-tarsal osteolysis and chronic progressive glomerulopathy (128)
Various aseptic necrosis syndromes
Acroosteolysis syndromes
Osteoarthropathy of Schinz and Furtwaengler
Rheumatoid arthritis

Minimal Diagnostic Criteria: Osteolysis of carpal and tarsal bones accompanied by a compatible clinical course with osteoporosis, cortical thinning and increased caliber of nonaxial tubular bones.†

Clinical Findings: A single pedigree with 3 young affected members has been described. Beginning in early childhood, onset of a progressive osteolysis of the carpal and tarsal bones occurs, usually accompanied by swelling, tenderness and painful limitation of motion of the affected area. Fusiform swelling of the fingers may be observed with deformity of the proximal interphalangeal joints. In at least 1 case, nontender subcutaneous nodules on knees, feet, elbows and fingers were observed and "hyperpigmented and erythematous" skin lesions noted.

Radiographs prior to the onset of osteolysis demonstrate decreased mineralization of the bones of the hand and increased caliber of phalanges, metacarpals, and long tubular bones of the upper limb with thinning of cortical bone. Osteolysis of carpal and tarsal bones is usually bilaterally symmetric, but may be unilateral. In the most advanced case (age 10 years), complete loss of all carpal bones and extensive lysis of tarsal bones was found with increased caliber, osteoporosis and cortical thinning of nonaxial tubular bones. The phalanges demonstrated focal areas of resorption. There was a notable lack of metacarpal erosion or resorption of long tubular bone excepting the distal epiphyses of radius and ulna.

Length discrepancies of a limb may develop, apparently secondary to involvement of epiphyses of long tubular bones. In addition to the deformities due to bony loss at the wrist and ankle, flexion contractures of elbows and knees, and deformities of metacarpophalangeal and interphalangeal joints gradually develop.

Biopsy of a metacarpal bone demonstrated only hypomineralization; the subcutaneous nodules showed only normal fibrofatty tissue, and the hyperpigmented skin lesions demonstrated normal histology.

Laboratory studies in a 7-year-old boy revealed increased ESR and +1 latex fixation; all other blood and urine studies were normal.

Complications
I   **Derived:** Limb length discrepancies and contractures at multiple small and large joints may occur. Painful limitation of motion may compromise function as does deformity secondary to bony loss (volar subluxation of the hand and pes cavum).
II **Associated:** —

Etiology: The pattern of inheritance is consistent with either autosomal recessive or X-linked recessive. McK *25960

Pathogenesis: ?

Related Facts

I   **Sex Ratio:** M3:F0 (Only 1 family reported)
II   **Risk of Occurrence:** ?
III **Risk of Recurrence for**
     Patient's Sib: When autosomal recessive or X-linked recessive, see Table I AR or X-linked R, respectively.
     Patient's Child: When autosomal recessive or X-linked recessive, see Table I AR or X-linked R, respectively.
IV   **Age of Detectability:** 2 to 6 years by clinical and radiographic examination
V   **Prevalence:** ? Rare

Treatment
I   **Primary Prevention:** Genetic counseling
II   **Secondary Prevention:** —
III **Other Therapy:** Analgesics

Prognosis: Unknown for life span (oldest reported case-10 years), apparently normal for intelligence, variable for function but probably poor for hand and foot function depending on degree and extent of osteolysis.

Detection of Carrier: —

†**Special Considerations:** Differentiation of this syndrome from dominant carpal-tarsal osteolysis depends on family history and demonstration of osteoporosis, cortical thinning and especially increased caliber of nonaxial tubular bones. This syndrome is distinguished from carpal-tarsal osteolysis and chronic progressive glomerulopathy by the above criteria and by the extensive lytic involvement of adjacent tubular bones, proteinuria and hematuria of more advanced cases of the latter syndrome. The various aseptic necrosis syndromes and acroosteolysis syndromes are distinguished by the distribution and extent of the lesions. Subcutaneous nodules, elevated ESR, swelling and tenderness, and a positive latex fixation may suggest rheumatoid arthritis, but biopsy materials fail to reveal the characteristic pathologic changes. The lack of generalized joint stiffness and other skeletal disorders separates this syndrome from the osteoarthropathy of Schinz and Furtwaengler.

References:
Torg, J.S. et al: Hereditary multicentric osteolysis with recessive transmission: A new syndrome. J. Pediatr. 75:243, 1969.

Contributors: **David W. Hollister**
David L. Rimoin

Editor's Computerized Descriptors: Skin, Skel.

CARUNCLE ABERRATIONS

Includes: Anomalies de la caroncule
Fehlbildungen der Carunculi lacrimales
Anomalías de la carúncula
Absence of caruncle
Anomalies of caruncle
Hyperplasia of caruncle
Hypoplasia of caruncle
Notch or cleavage of caruncle
Supernumerary caruncle

Excludes: Melanosis of caruncle
Orbital and periorbital dermoid cysts (761)

Minimal Diagnostic Criteria: Anatomic variation from normal caruncle is the sole criterion.

Clinical Findings: The caruncle is the fold of opaque pink tissue located at the inner canthus. Developmental anomalies of the caruncle are usually associated with anomalies of the plica semilunaris (the fold of translucent tissue) on the same side. As indicated above, the anatomic findings are highly variable. They are present from birth, although minor anomalies may remain undetected for years. Unless associated with other anomalies, they are inconsequential.†

Complications
I   **Derived:** Occasionally hairs on abnormal caruncular tissue irritate the eye.
II **Associated:** Absence or hypoplasia usually occurs in association with other congenital anomalies such as epicanthus, dystopia canthorum, ankyloblepharon, coloboma of the lid or abnormal extraocular muscles. Cleavage of the caruncle has occurred in association with mandibulofacial dysostosis.

Etiology: ?

Pathogenesis: The caruncle develops as an outgrowth from the posterior surface of the lower lid. Specific factors causing maldevelopment are unknown.

Related Facts
I   **Sex Ratio:** ?
II   **Risk of Occurrence:** Not known precisely, but rare
III **Risk of Recurrence for**
     Patient's Sib: ?
     Patient's Child: ?
IV   **Age of Detectability:** At birth, although frequently unnoticed initially.
V   **Prevalence:** ?

Treatment
I   **Primary Prevention:** —
II   **Secondary Prevention:** Plastic surgery
III **Other Therapy:** —

Prognosis: Nonprogressive

Detection of Carrier: —

†**Special Considerations:** The caruncle and plica semilunaris correspond to the nictitating membrane found in many animals.

References:
Duke-Elder, S.: System of Ophthalmology. Vol. 3, Part 2. Congenital Deformities. St. Louis: C.V. Mosby Co., 1963, p. 860.

Contributor: **Donald R. Bergsma**

Editor's Computerized Descriptor: Eye

CATARACT AND ICHTHYOSIS

Includes: Syndrome cataracte-ichtyose
Katarakt-Ichthyosis-Syndrom
Síndrome de cataratas e ictiosis
Ichthyosis and cataract

Excludes: Ichthyosis simplex
Bullous ichthyosiform erythroderma
Sjögren-Larsson syndrome
Phytanic acid storage disease (810)
X-linked ichthyosis

Minimal Diagnostic Criteria: The clinical picture enhanced by dermal biopsy is the basis of the diagnosis.

Clinical Findings: The skin changes are present at birth or shortly thereafter. Hyperkeratosis of the horny layer produces dry, fissured, thick, leathery, scaly skin with cornified masses. Sweat glands are aplastic. Diffuse erythema is common. The palms, soles and skin creases are predominantly affected along with nail hypertrophy. Although the lens opacities may vary, at least one family has been reported to have cortical cataracts.

Complications
I   **Derived:** Ectropion of the lids, conjunctivitis, deep stromal corneal opacities
II **Associated:** —

Etiology: Autosomal recessive; McK *21240

Pathogenesis: ?

Related Facts
I   **Sex Ratio:** ?
II   **Risk of Occurrence:** Very rare
III **Risk of Recurrence for**
     Patient's Sib: Probably 1 in 4 (25%) for each offspring to be affected
     Patient's Child: Probably not increased unless mate is carrier or homozygote
IV   **Age of Detectability:** Neonatal in early onset cases
V   **Prevalence:** Very rare

Treatment
I   **Primary Prevention:** Genetic counseling
II   **Secondary Prevention:** —
III **Other Therapy:** Local amelioration

Prognosis: Fatal in most severe early cases but normal life span in the mild and late onset cases.

Detection of Carrier: —

Special Considerations: —

References:
François, J.: Congenital Cataracts. Netherlands: C. C Thomas, 1963, p. 309.
Jay, B. et al: Ocular manifestations of ichthyosis. Br. J. Ophthalmol. 52:217, 1968.
Pinkerton, O.D.: Cataract associated with congenital ichthyosis. Arch. Ophthalmol. 60:393, 1958.
Wells, R.S. and Kerr, C.B.: Genetic classification of ichthyosis. Arch. Dermatol. 92:1, 1965.

Contributor: **Harold E. Cross**

Editor's Computerized Descriptors: Eye, Skin, Nails

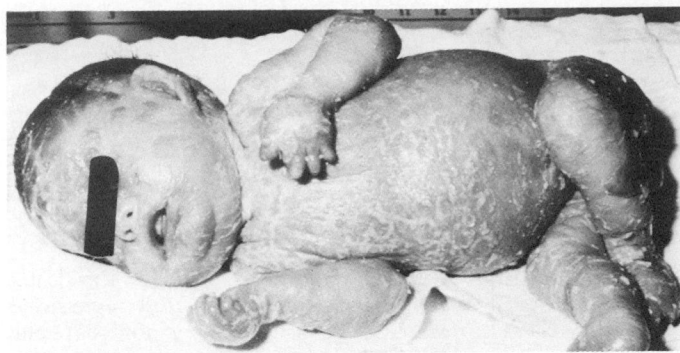

155. Congenital ichthyosis

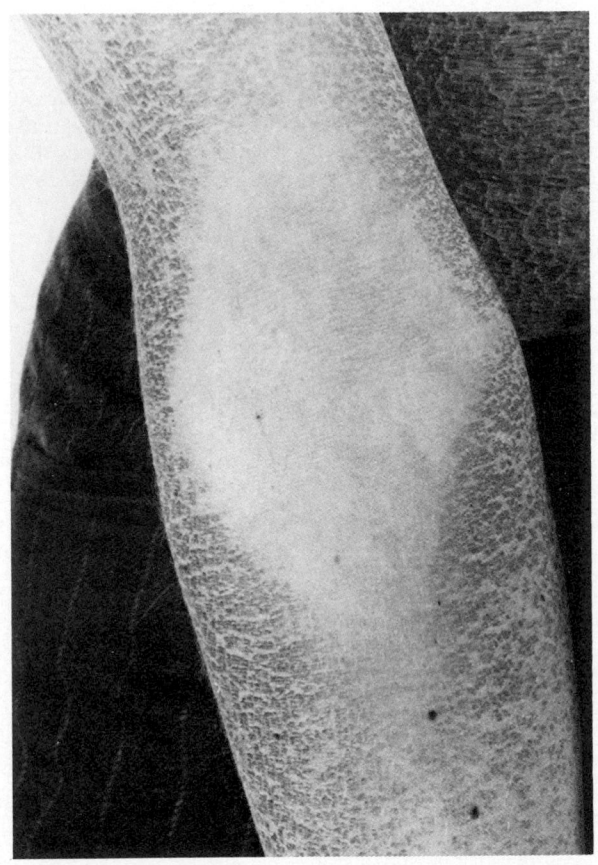

156. Ichthyosis

CATARACTS, CORTICAL AND NUCLEAR

Includes: Cataractes corticales et nucléaires
Rand-und Kern-Katarakte
Cataratas corticales y nucleares
Lenticular cataract
Zonular cataract
Lamellar cataract
Sutural cataract
Total cataract
Congenital cataracts
Nuclear cataract
Cortical and nuclear cataracts

Excludes: Cataracts, polar and capsular (133)

Minimal Diagnostic Criteria: Opacities by slit-lamp examination with pupil dilated.

Clinical Findings: The clinical picture varies from functionally insignificant, minute opacities to a variety of rarer and sometimes vision-affecting opacifications to the totally opacified lens. Duke-Elder divides these into those cataracts affecting a particular zone, those not so limited, and those affecting most of the lens. Combinations of types occur. In central pulverulent cataract the embryonic nucleus has many small white dots. Vision is rarely disturbed and the condition is usually bilateral and nonprogressive. Total nuclear cataract accounts for about 25% of all congenital cataracts and appears as a large white opacity of the embryonic and infantile nuclei. It occurs bilaterally and affects vision, sometimes seriously. Zones of opacity between the embryonic nucleus and cortex are called lamellar cataracts. The more central the affected concentric zone, the earlier the insult in embryogenesis. The condition is usually bilateral and the visual disability is variable, depending upon the degree of opacification. This form of congenital cataract is said to account for 40% of all types. It may be slowly progressive and quite disabling. Cataracts may affect just the Y sutures. Others form discrete opacities particularly in the axial region of the lens affecting several layers. They are usually bilateral, nonprogressive and do not affect vision. Morphologic types include anterior axial embryonic cataract, floriform cataract (resemble flower petals), dilacerated cataract (mossy) or punctate or blue dot cataract (affects fetal nucleus). Crystalline forms include coralliform cataract (resemble coral) and spear-shaped cataract (resemble grains of wheat). Much or all of the lens is affected in total cataract. In disk-shaped cataract the nucleus is missing, and in membranous cataract the lens is mostly resorbed. Vision is severely impaired in these forms.

Complications
I   **Derived:** Nystagmus and strabismus each in about 30% of cases if visual impairment is present.
II **Associated:** Combinations of the above occur especially with lamellar cataract. In axial fusiform cataract, opacities of the nucleus may combine with polar cataracts. In membranous cataract, other sequelae of intrauterine inflammation may be present. Almost all other ocular anomalies can be found in conjunction with congenital cataract, particularly the more severe lens afflictions. Microphthalmia is said to occur in about 25% of unilateral and 11% of bilateral cases of congenital cataract. Colobomata, aniridia, ectopia lentis, persistent hyperplastic primary vitreous and vasculosa lentis are not uncommon. Possibly one-half the cases of congenital cataract have other ocular defects. Many syndromes include congenital cataract ie rubella embryopathy, galactosemia.

Etiology: About 25% of cases represent an hereditary influence, such as a genetically determined defect in embryogenesis. Most of these appear to be autosomal dominant. Recessive pedigrees are uncommon. Cases related to systemic syndromes follow their modes of inheritance. Well-documented hereditary dominant pedigrees are noted for central pulverulent cataract, total nuclear cataract, lamellar cataract and coralliform cataract. Total cataract may be transmitted hereditarily in a number of fashions. A few dominant pedigrees have been documented for the axial type cataracts. Sporadic cases, possibly due to environmental causes, have been seen in all forms but are prevalent in total cataract, disk-shaped cataract and membranous cataract. In sporadic cases of lamellar cataract, biochemical disturbances have been implicated. Thus exogenous factors, both constitutional and local, either hereditary or not, play a role in the majority of congenital cataracts. McK *30220

Pathogenesis: Little is known about the pathogenesis of congenital cataracts. Discrete opacities may be poorly formed lens fibers which have degenerated as in the punctate cataract. Some crystalline opacities have been found to be cysteine, tyrosine and calcium salt. Disk-shaped cataracts may result from interferences with development about the 5th fetal month. Total cataract could relate to persistence of the hyaloid artery, faulty lens vesicle separation or intrauterine inflammation. Genetic influence on embryogenesis may play a role. Environmental factors such as toxins and their direct effect or their effect on induction are exemplified by viral infections such as rubella. Metabolic factors include a potential defect in calcium metabolism, as suggested in lamellar cataracts where hypocalcemia and tetany are known to be deleterious, and carbohydrate metabolism such as in galactosemia and galactokinase deficiency. These may have a hereditary basis. Finally local changes induced by intrauterine inflammation could produce sporadic abnormalities.

Related Facts
I   **Sex Ratio:** M1:F1 (Males are more frequently affected than females in lamellar cataract.)
II **Risk of Occurrence:** ?
III **Risk of Recurrence:**
   Patient's Sib: When autosomal dominant or autosomal recessive, see Table I AD or AR, respectively.
   Patient's Child: When autosomal dominant or autosomal recessive, see Table I AD or AR, respectively.
IV **Age of Detectability:** —
V   **Prevalence:** Minute opacities in the lens present in over 90% of children. Anterior axial embryonic cataract occurs in 20-30% of children as does blue-dot cataract.

Treatment
I   **Primary Prevention:** Genetic counseling
II **Secondary Prevention:** —
III **Other Therapy:** Cataract extraction where indicated

Prognosis: Normal life span, ocular prognosis generally good unless associated defects are present.

Detection of Carrier: —

Special Considerations: —

References:
Duke-Elder, S.: System of Ophthalmology, vol. 3, part 2. Congenital Deformities. London:Henry Kimpton, 1964, p. 726.
François, J.: Congenital Cataracts. Netherlands:C.C Thomas, 1963.

Contributor: **Harold E. Cross**

Editor's Computerized Descriptors: Vision, Eye

CATARACTS, POLAR AND CAPSULAR

Includes: Cataractes polaires et capsulaires
  Pol-und Kapsel-Katarakte
  Cataratas polar y capsular
  Capsulolenticular cataract
  Capsular and polar cataracts
  Polar and capsular cataracts

Excludes: Cataracts, cortical and nuclear (132)
  Pupillary membrane persistence (845)

Minimal Diagnostic Criteria: As per slit-lamp examination

Clinical Findings: Capsular cataracts, anterior and posterior, are small discrete flecks of opacity and pigmented satellite formations in the lens epithelium and capsule, usually less than 1 mm which do not interfere with vision.

Polar cataracts involve the lens capsule, epithelium and underlying lens fibers. The anterior variety assumes a multitude of shapes and sizes. Anterior protrusion leads to the pyramidal form. After formation, normal lens fibers may develop between the cortical and capsular opacities (reduplication). The changes are usually bilateral, stationary and functionally insignificant.

Posterior polar cataracts occur as the above described entities in a stationary form present at birth with a variety of opaque bodies in the posterior pole of the lens, and also in a progressive variety where radiating opacities form in the posterior lens cortex resulting in progressive decrease of vision.

Complications
I   **Derived:** —
II **Associated:** Persistence of pupillary membrane and hyaloid vascular system, corneal opacities, anterior lenticonus, axial fusiform cataract (whereby a central nuclear cataract connects to one or both poles).

Etiology: A defect in embryogenesis with a strong hereditary tendency of autosomal dominant transmission has been described. Intrauterine inflammation is a possibility in other cases, especially those with corneal opacities.

Pathogenesis: Intrauterine inflammation produced by a corneal perforation or adhesion to the lens could lead to anterior polar lens changes. Adhesions of the tunica vasculosa lentis or pupillary membrane to the lens in the anterior polar cataracts, and adhesion or invasion of the posterior lens by the fetal vascular system in the posterior polar cataracts are the usually given explanations.

Related Facts
I   **Sex Ratio:** M1:F1
II **Risk of Occurrence:** ?
III **Risk of Recurrence for**
   Patient's Sib: When autosomal dominant and if parent is affected, 1 in 2 (50%) for each offspring to be affected; otherwise not increased.
   Patient's Child: 1 in 2 if autosomal dominant
IV **Age of Detectability:** At birth
V   **Prevalence:** ?

Treatment
I   **Primary Prevention:** Genetic counseling
II **Secondary Prevention:** —
III **Other Therapy:** Cataract extraction when indicated

Prognosis: Normal life span with ocular prognosis variable according to degree of defect

Detection of Carrier: Affected parent and patient when autosomal dominant

Special Considerations: —

References:
Duke-Elder, S.: System of Ophthalmology, vol. 3, part 2. Congenital Deformities. London:Henry Kimpton, 1964, p. 716.
François, J.: Congenital Cataracts. Netherlands:C. C Thomas, 1963.

Contributor: **Harold E. Cross**

Editor's Computerized Descriptors: Vision, Eye
Also see Section I, Figs. 45, 46

CENTRAL CORE DISEASE

Includes: Zentralfibrillen-Myopathie
Enfermedad del grupo central de miofibrillas de la fibra muscular esquelética
Shy-Magee disease
Muscular central core disease
Hypotonia and weakness

Excludes: Muscular dystrophy, childhood pseudohypertrophic (689)
Myopathy, nemaline (696)
All other forms of nonprogressive congenital myopathy

Minimal Diagnostic Criteria: This disorder can be diagnosed only by muscle biopsy and muscle histochemistry.†

Clinical Findings: Hypotonia and weakness occur in infants with this condition. In one reported case there were also diminished fetal movements. Weakness is noted usually early in infancy. It is diffuse and it involves all striated muscular tissue in almost equal proportion. The distribution of muscular weakness in its early stages resembles that found in childhood pseudohypertrophic muscular dystrophy (Duchenne) but progressive deterioration does not occur. Tendon reflexes are preserved and the serum level of muscle enzymes such as creatine phosphokinase (CPK) are not elevated. Muscular wasting is not marked and the condition is not progressive.

Complications
I   **Derived:** Generalized moderate muscular weakness
II **Associated:** —

Etiology: ? McK *11700

Pathogenesis: ? There are multiple metabolic deficiencies within the central cores of muscle fibers due to an absence of mitochondria and oxidative metabolism in these cores or zones.

Related Facts
I   **Sex Ratio:** ?
II   **Risk of Occurrence:** ?
III **Risk of Recurrence for**
      Patient's Sib: ?
      Patient's Child: ?
IV   **Age of Detectability:** Usually within the 1st year of life due to congenital hypotonia and failure of normal maturation of muscle function.
V   **Prevalence:** Extremely rare

Treatment
I   **Primary Prevention:** —
II   **Secondary Prevention:** —
III **Other Therapy:** —

Prognosis: Generally good for life with nonprogressive condition leading to a static diffuse weakness

Detection of Carrier: —

†**Special Considerations:** Examination of striated muscle fibers demonstrates that the fibers are large and that a central "core" of fibrils have different staining properties from the fibrils around the margins. The central core is devoid of oxidative enzymes and phosphorylase activity and it suggests that these cores are nonfunctioning. Utilizing the trichrome stain, the central cores stain blue, whereas the periphery stains red. The periodic acid Schiff reaction (PAS) is more strongly positive in the core than in the rest of the muscle fiber. However, this reaction was not influenced by prior treatment with diastase, and therefore is probably not due to the presence of glycogen.
In central core disease the cores are much more readily

discernible with the enzyme techniques than with the routine histologic stains. This is particularly so with the phosphorylase reaction, which is thus a useful and quick screening test for central core disease in the biopsy from a patient with infantile hypotonia or of a nonprogressive myopathy. Ultrastructural analysis demonstrates that within the central cores there is a gross disruption of the normal fibrillar architecture which contains no normal cytoplasmic organelles, such as sarcoplasmic reticulum or mitochondria. Deficiency of the latter is reflected by the failure of histochemical stains to show any evidence of oxidative enzyme activity in the central core regions.

References:
Dubowitz, V. and Platts, M.: Central core disease of muscle with focal wasting. J. Neurol. Neurosurg. Psychiatry 28:432, 1965.

Seitelberger, F. et al: The muscle fiber in central core disease: Histochemical and electron microscopic observations. Acta Neuropathol. (Berl.) 1:223, 1961.

Shy, G. M. and Magee, K. R.: A new congenital nonprogressive myopathy. Brain 79:610, 1956.

Contributor: **Carl M. Pearson**

Editor's Computerized Descriptor: Muscle

CENTRALOPATHIC EPILEPSY

Includes: Épilepsie d'origine centrale
Zentrenzephale Epilepsie
Epilepsia centropática
Epilepsy, centrencephalic
Genetic epilepsy
Petit mal lapse ("absence")
Petit mal automatism
Automatisms and psychopathic behavior
Myoclonic petit mal
Alkinetic or atonic "drop" seizures
Petit mal-grand mal epilepsy
Grand mal epilepsy
Epilepsy centralopathic

Excludes: Myoclonic epilepsy I, II and III
Epilepsy due to focal cortical lesion

Minimal Diagnostic Criteria: The typical, abnormal, bilaterally synchronous EEG is used to identify centralopathic epilepsy. The patient may have the EEG abnormality but remain asymptomatic.

Clinical Findings: Penfield classified a group of seizure disorders that have in common the origination of the epileptogenic discharges within the central integrating system of the brainstem. This system has connections with both cerebral hemispheres. The EEG therefore reveals bilateral synchronous abnormalities.

Petit Mal Lapse ("Absence"): This seizure may be so mild as to escape routine notice. There may be a slight pause, blinking of the eyes, a brief stare and then resumption of activity. There may be urinary incontinence. Gross motor movements do not occur and the patient does not fall or cry. The diagnosis is made by the history and the typical EEG finding of regular spike-and-wave rhythm at 3 per second.

Petit Mal Automatism: Infrequently, some patients have a seizure pattern characterized by lip smacking, fumbling hand movements suggestive of a temporal lobe origin. The EEG, however, may show the typical bilaterally synchronous 3 per second spike-and-wave, without evidence of temporal lobe involvement.

Automatisms and Psychopathic Behavior: Seizures which may be preceded by an aura, followed by crying, screaming, negativism, running, hallucinations, flushing or pallor, difficulty in learning or concentrating, asocial behavior and frank major motor seizures. The EEG is characterized by bilaterally synchronous theta (4-7 per second) rhythm appearing in the temporal regions.

Myoclonic Petit Mal: A seizure disorder characterized by "absence" attacks and in addition myoclonic jerks usually involving the muscles of the face and arms in a symmetric fashion. The EEG is characterized by bilaterally synchronous multiple spike-and-wave discharges, a short burst of spikes followed by a series of slow waves.

Akinetic or Atonic "Drop" Seizures: Seizures characterized by sudden loss of muscle tone causing the patient to fall. They may or may not be associated with loss of consciousness. Major motor seizures may occur as well. Penfield did not recognize a specific EEG pattern in these patients.

Petit Mal-Grand Mal Epilepsy: Some patients with "absence" attacks may develop major motor seizures. It is suggested that on occasion the cortex is activated to produce seizures by discharges originating in subcortical regions.

Grand Mal Epilepsy: Rarely, there are patients with major motor seizures in which the EEG displays diffuse paroxysmal rapid waves of 25-30 per second.

Complications

I **Derived:** Only those complications of seizures, namely prolonged anoxia, rarely cardiac standstill and airway obstruction.

II **Associated:** —

Etiology: Autosomal dominant† McK *11710

Pathogenesis: ?

Related Facts
I **Sex Ratio:** M1:F1
II **Risk of Occurrence:** ?
III **Risk of Recurrence for**
  Patient's Sib: If parent is affected, 1 in 2 (50%) for each offspring to be affected; otherwise not increased.†
  Patient's Child: 1 in 2†
IV **Age of Detectability:** Most readily detected between ages 4 and 16
V **Prevalence:** 1 in 200

Treatment
I **Primary Prevention:** Genetic counseling
II **Secondary Prevention:** The use of specific drugs such as the barbiturates, hydantoins and the ethosuximides.
III **Other Therapy:** —

Prognosis: Generally good. Depends largely on the type of epilepsy. Some more responsive to drug management.

Detection of Carrier: By EEG

†**Special Considerations:** Centralopathic epilepsy is probably the result of an autosomal dominant gene which has low penetrance at birth, but gains almost complete penetrance between the ages of 4 and 16 and then rather rapidly declines.

Twin studies have shown that when 1 monozygotic twin develops seizures, the chance of the other twin being affected is 60-70%. Dizygotic twins show only a 10% concordance. Monozygotic twins also show a high degree of concordance as to the age of onset of seizures, type of seizure, as well as EEG pattern.

References:
Lennox, W.G.: Heredity of epilepsy as told by relatives and twins. JAMA 146:529, 1951.
Metrakos, K. and Metrakos, J.D.: Genetics of convulsive disorders: II. Genetic and electroencephalographic studies in centrencephalic epilepsy. Neurology 11:474, 1961.
Penfield, W. and Jasper, H.: Epilepsy and the Functional Anatomy of the Human Brain. Boston: Little, Brown and Co., 1954.

Contributor: **Robert H. A. Haslam**

Editor's Computerized Descriptor: Nerve

CEREBELLAR ATAXIA AND CHORIORETINAL DEGENERATION

Includes: Ataxie cérébelleuse avec dégénérescence chorio-rétinienne
Zerebellëre Ataxie und Chorioretinale Degeneration
Ataxia cerebelosa y degeneración corioretineana
Ataxia and tapetoretinal degeneration
Chorioretinal degeneration and ataxia
Tapetoretinal degeneration and ataxia

Excludes: Friedreich ataxia
Marie ataxia
Retinal aplasia (865)

Minimal Diagnostic Criteria: Evidence of both ataxia and tapetoretinal degeneration

Clinical Findings: Heredoataxias are characterized chiefly by progressive disturbance of equilibrium and motion and pathologically by lesions of nuclei and tracts subserving these functions. Characteristic of this group of diseases is that the dividing line between the more closely related entities seems to be blurred by the high incidence of borderline or transitional cases.

The ocular manifestations in ataxias include: ocular palsies especially of upward gaze, pupillary disturbances, nystagmus especially in extremes of gaze and retrobulbar neuritis or optic atrophy.

Chorioretinal degeneration (tapetoretinal) may occur both in Friedreich ataxia and Marie ataxia but in higher incidence in the latter. In most individuals affected with cerebellar ataxia and chorioretinal degeneration, the retinal and neurologic changes have nearly similar age onsets and seem to develop simultaneously. These ocular changes have a certain intrafamilial similarity but variation in expressivity is to be expected and includes: macular degeneration, advancing choroidal sclerosis, punctata albescens, and retinitis pigmentosa.†

Complications
I **Derived:** Dementia, severe disabling limb contractures, urinary incontinence and intercurrent respiratory disease
II **Associated:** —

Etiology: Heterogeneity exists among the heredoataxias. Monozygotic twins with the same disease, age of onset and course have been reported. The majority of these diseases are transmitted as autosomal recessive, however, regular or irregular dominant transmission is fairly commonly encountered (Marie ataxia). Even a few X-linked recessive pedigrees have been reported.†

Pathogenesis: ? Usually appears as simple neuronal atrophy.

Related Facts
I **Sex Ratio:** M1:F1 usually
II **Risk of Occurrence:** Rare
III **Risk of Recurrence for**
  Patient's Sib: When autosomal recessive, autosomal dominant or X-linked recessive see Table I AR, AD or X-linked R, respectively.
  Patient's Child: When autosomal recessive, autosomal dominant or X-linked recessive see Table I AR, AD or X-linked R, respectively.
IV **Age of Detectability:** Varies greatly from family to family and by defect or cluster of defects but, in general, has a certain intrafamilial constancy.
V **Prevalence:** ? Rare

Treatment
I **Primary Prevention:** Genetic counseling
II **Secondary Prevention:** ?
III **Other Therapy:** ?

Prognosis: Usually progressive leading to extreme disability or death.

Detection of Carrier: Within families it is not infrequent to encounter individuals exhibiting isolated retinal or neural signs, or symptoms which may or may not constitute carrier states in heterozygotes.†

†Special Considerations: Klein and Franceschetti reported intrafamilial alternation between the heredoataxias and chorioretinal degeneration which they found, in the now famous Glaser family. These authors reported 21 members with Friedreich ataxia, 4 cases of macular degeneration, 4 cases of retinitis pigmentosa and 2 cases of punctata albescens all being transmitted recessively and found in different branches of the family.

It is important to stress that one may encounter within the same family combined neuroretinal expression, isolated neurologic changes or isolated retinal degeneration.

References:
Blackwood, W. et al (eds.): Greenfield's Neuropathology. Baltimore: Williams & Wilkins, 1963, p. 586.

Ford, F.R.: Diseases of the Nervous System in Infancy, Childhood and Adolescence, 3rd Ed. Springfield: Charles C Thomas, 1952, p. 396.

Franceschetti, A. and Klein, D.: Ueber das Vorkommen von hereditärer juveniler Maculadegeneration (Typ Stargardt) bei zwei Geschwisterpaaren der Friedreich-Sippe "Glaser" (mit kasuistische Beiträgen von Retinitis pigmentosa und dominanter labyrinthärer Schwerhörigkeit). Arch. Klaus-Stift. Vereb-Forch. 16:469, 1941.

Franceschetti, A. et al: Tapeto-retinal degeneration. Acta 16 Conc. Ophthalmol. Br. 1:158, 1950.

François, J.: Heredity in Ophthalmology. St. Louis: C.V. Mosby, 1961, p. 552.

Klein, D.: Genetic approach to the nosology of retinal disorders. In Bergsma, D. (ed.): Part VIII. Eye. Birth Defects: Orig. Art. Ser., vol. VII, no. 3. Baltimore: Williams & Wilkins for the National Foundation-March of Dimes, 1971, p. 52.

Contributor: **Harold F. Falls**

Editor's Computerized Descriptors: Eye, Nerve, Skel., Resp., GU.

CEREBRAL GIGANTISM

Includes: Gigantisme cérébral
Zerebraler Gigantismus
Gigantismo cerebral
Sotos syndrome
Gigantism, cerebral

Excludes: Acrocephaly

Minimal Diagnostic Criteria: Characteristic facial appearance, large size, large hands and feet and mental retardation are all nonprogressive.

Clinical Findings: Excessive growth usually over 90th percentile of height or weight at birth and continuing to be excessively large. Mental retardation is usually mild, but may be profound. Acromegalic features including large head, frontal bossing, prognathism, large hands and feet. Moderately dilated ventricles on pneumoencephalogram without increased intracranial pressure. Bone age is 2 - 4 years advanced. Patient has unusual dermatoglyphics and exhibits clumsiness. Extensive endocrinologic evaluation including growth hormone urinary steroid excretion, adrenopituitary interrelationships, glucose and fatty acid metabolism have shown no consistent abnormalities.

Complications
I   **Derived:** —
II **Associated:** —

Etiology: ?†

Pathogenesis: ? Abnormalities of hypothalamic anterior pituitary axis have been postulated.

Related Facts
I   **Sex Ratio:** M1:F1
II   **Risk of Occurrence:** ? Appears to be uncommon but not rare
III **Risk of Recurrence for**
     Patient's Sib: Not increased
     Patient's Child: Not increased
IV   **Age of Detectability:** Large size at birth may raise suspicion; usually can be diagnosed by 2 or 3 years of age.
V   **Prevalence:** ?

Treatment
I   **Primary Prevention:** —
II **Secondary Prevention:** —
III **Other Therapy:** —

Prognosis: Appears good within limits of the mental retardation

Detection of Carrier: —

†Special Considerations: The etiology of the syndrome is unknown, but it is tempting to tie the excessive growth to the ventricular dilatation and mental retardation. Cortical effects on growth are seen in the decreased size of a hemiparetic limb and hemihypertrophy could be the converse of this. Whether cerebral gigantism represents bilateral hemihypertrophy of cortical origin, or is truly hypothalamic in origin remains to be determined.

References:
Bejar, R.L. et al: Cerebral gigantism: Concentration of amino acids in plasma and muscle. J. Pediatr. 76:105, 1970.

Gardner-Medwin, D.: Cerebral gigantism. Dev. Med. Child. Neurol. 11:796, 1969.

Hook, E. B. and Reynolds, J. W.: Cerebral gigantism; endocrinological and clinical observations of six patients including a congenital giant, concordant monozygotic twins, and a child who achieved adult gigantic size. J. Pediatr. 70:900, 1967.

Contributor: **John Mark Freeman**

Editor's Computerized Descriptors: Face, Dermatoglyphic, Skel., Nerve

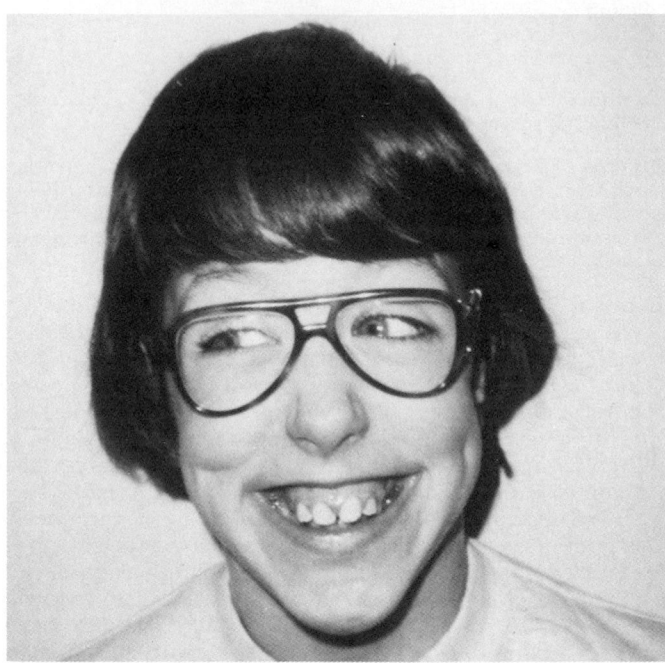

157. Cerebral gigantism

CEREBRO-COSTO-MANDIBULAR SYNDROME

Includes: Syndrome cérébro-costo-mandibulaire
Cerebro-costo-mandibuläres Syndrom
Síndrome cerebro-costo-mandibular
Rib gap defects with micrognathia

Excludes: Other conditions with severe micrognathia
Other syndromes with the Pierre Robin anomaly

Minimal Diagnostic Criteria: Combination of microcephaly, micrognathia and posterior rib gap defects.

Clinical Findings: Severe micrognathia, glossoptosis, cleft palate, posterior rib gap defects, microcephaly and mental retardation. The rib defects consist of replacement of bone by fibroconnective tissue in the posterior paravertebral portions of the ribs. The lesions are bilateral, but not necessarily symmetric and they may involve all or only some ribs, particularly the 4th and 5th pairs. Cartilage or bone may be abnormal in other areas (trachea, hip, elbow). The combination of micrognathia, glossoptosis and "flat chest" causes severe respiratory distress. Mortality in early infancy is high.

Complications
I **Derived:** Respiratory distress, respiratory infection, feeding difficulties, failure to thrive, mental retardation, speech delay, high infant mortality.
II **Associated:** Ventricular septal defect, polycystic kidneys.

Etiology: Probably autosomal recessive; McK *21400

Pathogenesis: ?

Related Facts
I **Sex Ratio:** M1:F1
II **Risk of Occurrence:** Small
III **Risk of Recurrence for**
Patient's Sib: 1 in 4 (25%) for each offspring to be affected
Patient's Child: None has reproduced; theoretically zero unless mate is heterozygote.
IV **Age of Detectability:** At birth; prenatal diagnosis may be possible.
V **Prevalence:** Condition is rare but was observed in different (Caucasian) populations.

Treatment
I **Primary Prevention:** Genetic counseling
II **Secondary Prevention:** Intensive care for respiratory distress, feeding difficulty and infection. Cleft palate repair.
III **Other Therapy:** Special education

Prognosis: Of the 8 reported patients, 4 died neonatally, 3 died before age 1 and one was still alive at age 4 years.

Detection of Carrier: —

Special Considerations: —

References:
Langer, L.O., Jr. and Herrmann, J.: The cerebrocostomandibular syndrome. In Bergsma, D. (ed.): Malformation Syndromes, Birth Defects: Orig. Art. Ser., vol. X, no. 7. Miami: Symposia Specialists for The National Foundation-March of Dimes, 1974, p. 167.
McNicholl, B. et al: Cerebro-costo-mandibular syndrome. Arch. Dis. Child. 45:521, 1970.
Smith, D.W. et al: Rib-gap defect with micrognathia, malformed tracheal cartilages, and redundant skin: A new pattern of defective development. J. Pediatr. 69:799, 1966.

Contributor: **Jürgen Herrmann**

Editor's Computerized Descriptors: Face, Oral, Speech, Skel., Resp., CV., GI., Nerve

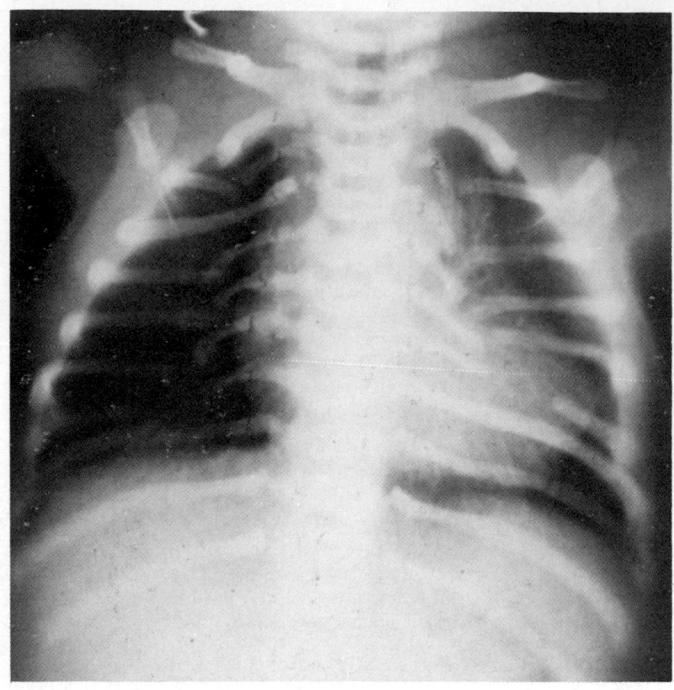

158. Multiple posterior rib defects bilaterally

CEREBRO-HEPATO-RENAL SYNDROME

Includes: Syndrome cérébro-hépato-rénal
Cerebro-hepato-renales Syndrom
Síndrome cerebro-hepato-renal
Bowen syndrome
Zellweger syndrome
Hypotonia and craniofacial dysmorphia

Excludes: Other forms of the floppy infant syndrome
Chondrodysplasia punctata

Minimal Diagnostic Criteria: Profound muscular hypotonia with decreased or absent reflexes, hepatomegaly, typical craniofacial dysmorphy and such inconsistent symptoms as elevated serum iron and copper, stippling of patella, glaucoma and cataracts.

Clinical Findings: Prenatal history is unrevealing, yet prenatal growth failure is often encountered. About 50% of cases have a birthweight below 3,000 gm and about 25% have a birthweight below 2,500 gm in spite of a normal duration of gestation. The syndrome can be recognized at birth or soon thereafter. Profound muscular hypotonia or even atonia is present in all cases. Most patients are motionless, with weak or absent Moro response, tendon, suck and swallowing reflexes. Gavage feeding over many weeks is often necessary. These patients display a typical craniofacial dysmorphy with a high and bulging forehead, brachyturricephaly, widely patent sutures including the metopic suture, widened fontanels, puffy eyelids, poorly developed supraorbital ridges, ocular hypertelorism, mongoloid slant of the orbital fissures, epicanthic folds, Brushfield spots, glaucoma, corneal cloudiness, cataracts, low-set ears, high-arched palate, rounded face and micrognathia. Congenital heart lesions are rare, but septal defects and delayed closure of ductus arteriosus and foramen ovale may occur. Hepatomegaly is a nearly constant finding. Jaundice and bleeding due to hypoprothrombinemia can occur after the 1st week of life. Boys are frequently cryptorchid and clitoral hypertrophy may be observed in girls. Limb anomalies such as cubitus valgus, four-finger line, camptodactyly, metatarsus adductus and talipes equinovarus occur. Dermatoglyphic changes are nonspecific, ridge counts often are low, ulnar loops prevail in some cases and some patients show an unusual number of whorls. Failure to thrive is conspicuous. Psychomotor development is very limited and convulsions with abnormal EEG and paroxysmal discharges are frequent. Life expectancy is severely curtailed, 70% of the infants die within the first 3 months of life and to date none of the hitherto reported cases has reached an age of 1 year.

Complications
I **Derived:** Aspiration due to feeding difficulties, repeated respiratory infections.
II **Associated:** A certain immunodeficiency connected with the occasionally noticed thymus hypoplasia may have an effect on the outcome of the infections.

Etiology: Autosomal recessive inheritance. Parental consanguinity present in 4 of 33 families with 1 or more affected sibs. Chromosomal studies yield a normal karyotype and allow the exclusion of a cytogenetic disorder. McK *21410

Pathogenesis: The profound muscular hypotonia, lack of psychomotor development and the occurrence of convulsions are explained by a primary dysgenesis of the CNS. Neuropathologic studies indicate that the early differentiation of the neuraxis, closure of the neural groove, formation of the major brain vesicles and prosencephalic cleavage are essentially undisturbed. The developmental abnormalities involve the finer differentiation of CNS structures which take place during the 4th-6th month of gestation. They result in pachygyria, micropolygyria, hypoplasia of midline structures such as corpus callosum, olivary dysplasia, dystopias, formation of paraventricular cysts, defective neuronal myelination and gliosis. Lissencephaly is rare.

The liver is regularly increased in size and shows considerable architectural disorganization with abnormal liver lobules, dysgenesis of the biliary system and intralobular and periportal fibrosis. The kidneys show dysgenesis of the parenchyma and multiple small subcortical cysts. Hypoplasia of the thymus is found in some cases, and hypoplasia of the lung is a frequent finding. Hemosiderosis and increased iron deposits are found in various organs, notably bone marrow and liver. These changes are not due to hemolysis but rather suggest a disturbance of iron transfer in utero. Serum iron is often, though not regularly and not persistently, increased; iron-binding capacity is high normal in most instances. An increase of serum copper is likewise found. Pancreatic islets may be hyperplastic perhaps explaining the occasional hypoglycemia. Nonspecific aminoaciduria is found in some cases. A disturbance of pipecolic acid metabolism with increased serum level, and increased urinary excretion of pipecolic acid has been observed. Another study revealed a mitochondrial dysfunction in various organs and absence of the peroxisomes in hepatocytes and renal tubular epithelia. Oxygen consumption studies of the mitochondrial function suggest a defect in the electron transport system prior to the cytochromes.

While it is difficult to correlate understandably the various chemical, pathologic and neuropathologic findings, a genetically determined teratogenic factor acting during the postorganogenic period of gestational life might be postulated.

Related Facts
I   Sex Ratio: M1:F2 (actual M16:F30)
II   Risk of Occurrence: Incidence 1 in 100,000 live births in Victoria, Australia, but may be higher if correctly diagnosed.
III Risk of Recurrence for
   Patient's Sib: 1 in 4 (25%) for each offspring to be affected
   Patient's Child: No patient has lived long enough to reproduce
IV   Age of Detectability: In newborn period or early infancy
V   Prevalence: Over 50 cases are known and probably a considerable number go undetected. In several families, the condition was recognized only after the birth of a 2nd or 3rd affected child.

Treatment
I   Primary Prevention: Genetic counseling
II   Secondary Prevention: —
III Other Therapy: No specific therapy. Vitamin K for hypoprothrombinemia. EDTA therapy has been attempted in cases with hypersideremia without influencing the clinical course of the condition.

Prognosis: Fatal within 1st year

Detection of Carrier: —

Special Considerations: —

References:
Danks, D.M. et al: Cerebro-hepato-renal syndrome of Zellweger. J. Pediatr. 86:382, 1975.
Gilchrist, K.W. et al: Studies of malformation syndromes of man XIB: The cerebro-hepato-renal syndrome of Zellweger: Comparative Pathology. Eur. J. Pediatr. 121:99, 1976.
Goldfischer, S. et al: Peroxisomal and mitochondrial defects in the cerebro-hepato-renal syndrome. Science 182:62, 1973.
Patton, R.G. et al: Cerebro-hepato-renal syndrome of Zellweger. Am. J. Dis. Child. 124:840, 1972.
Torii, S. and Furuta, M.: An autopsy case of cerebro-hepato-renal syndrome. Teratology 6:122, 1972.
Volpe, J.J. and Adams, R.D.: Cerebro-hepato-renal syndrome of Zellweger: An inherited disorder of neuronal migration. Acta Neuropathol. (Berl.) 20:175, 1972.

Contributor: Hans Zellweger

Editor's Computerized Descriptors: Eye, Ear, Face, Oral, Dermatoglyphic, Skel., Muscle, Resp., CV., Thymus, GI., Liver, GU., Nerve

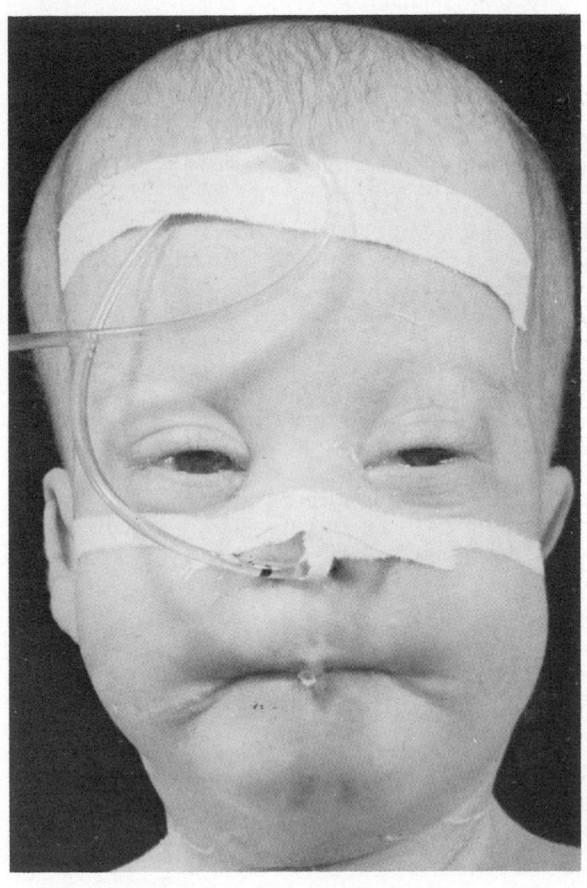

159. Note high forehead, epicanthal folds, ptosis and rounded face

CEREBRO-OCULO-FACIO-SKELETAL SYNDROME

Includes: Syndrome cérébro-oculo-facio-squelettique
Cerebro-oculo-facio-ossäres Syndrom
Síndrome cerebro-óculo-facio-esquelético
Lethal syndrome of microcephaly with multiple congenital anomalies
COFS syndrome

Excludes: Arthrogryposis (88)
Oculo-mandibulo-facial syndrome (738)
Oculo-auriculo-vertebral dysplasia (735)
Cerebro-hepato-renal syndrome (139)
Cerebro-costo-mandibular syndrome (138)
Oculo-cerebro-renal syndrome (736)
Chromosome abnormalities
Viral infections
Fetal rubella syndrome (384)

Minimal Diagnostic Criteria: This syndrome has not been sufficiently delineated to establish minimal diagnostic criteria. However, the diagnosis should be suspected in patients with some combination of the clinical findings listed below.†

Clinical Findings: The cerebral feature is microcephaly, sometimes with a sloping forehead; the ocular features are cataract, microphthalmia, and narrow palpebral fissures; the facial features are high nasal bridge with a prominent saddle-like bony ridge, large ears, upper lip overhanging the lower, and micro- or retrognathia; and the skeletal features are kyphosis, scoliosis, hip dislocation or acetabular dysplasia, narrow pelvis, coxa valga, flexion contractures of the limbs and digits, rocker bottom feet and osteoporosis. In addition, affected infants are usually small for dates and they may have renal anomalies, short neck, widely spaced nipples, simian creases, a longitudinal foot groove and hypotonia.†

Complications
I **Derived:** Feeding difficulty, respiratory distress, repeated lower respiratory infections.
II **Associated:** —

Etiology: Autosomal recessive inheritance strongly suggested by pedigree analysis and by consanguinity in parents. McK *21415

Pathogenesis: ?

Related Facts
I **Sex Ratio:** M1:F1
II **Risk of Occurrence:** ? Probably rare
III **Risk of Recurrence for**
   Patient's Sib: Probably 1 in 4 (25%) for each offspring to be affected
   Patient's Child: Probably not applicable because of reproductive unfitness
IV **Age of Detectability:** At birth
V **Prevalence:** ? Probably rare

Treatment
I **Primary Prevention:** Genetic counseling
II **Secondary Prevention:** —
III **Other Therapy:** —

Prognosis: Most patients die within the first 3 years of life. The cause of death has been respiratory failure, in some instances due to repeated lower respiratory infections.

Detection of Carrier: —

†Special Considerations: Detailed gross and microscopic examination of the eyes in 1 patient revealed microphthalmia, incomplete cleavage of the chamber angle, persistent pupillary membrane, partial detachment and absence of the corneal endothelium and corneal edema, and cataract. Ganglion cell and nerve fiber layers of the retina were absent and there were intraretinal hemorrhages with decreased presence of retinal blood vessels, exudates in the anterior and posterior chambers, vitreous cavity and subretinal space, and optic atrophy. Whether all patients referenced here represent a homogeneous disorder is, of course, debatable at this stage of delineation of the syndrome.

References:
Lowry, R.B. et al: Cataracts, microcephaly, kyphosis, and limited joint movement in two siblings: A new syndrome. J. Pediatr. 79:282, 1971.
Neu, R.L. et al: A lethal syndrome of microcephaly with multiple congenital anomalies in three siblings. Pediatrics 47:610, 1971.
Pena, S.D. J. and Shokeir, M.H.K.: Autosomal recessive cerebro-oculo-facio-skeletal (COFS) syndrome. Clin. Genet. 5:285, 1974.
Preus, M. and Fraser, F.C.: The cerebro-oculo-facio-skeletal syndrome. Clin. Genet. 5:294, 1974.
Preus, M. et al: Renal anomalies and oligohydramnios in the cerebro-oculo-facio-skeletal syndrome. Am. J. Dis. Child. 131:62, 1977.

Contributor: **Marilyn Preus**

Editor's Computerized Descriptors: Eye, Ear, Face, Nose, Neck, Skin, Dermatoglyphic, Skel., Muscle, Resp., GI., GU.

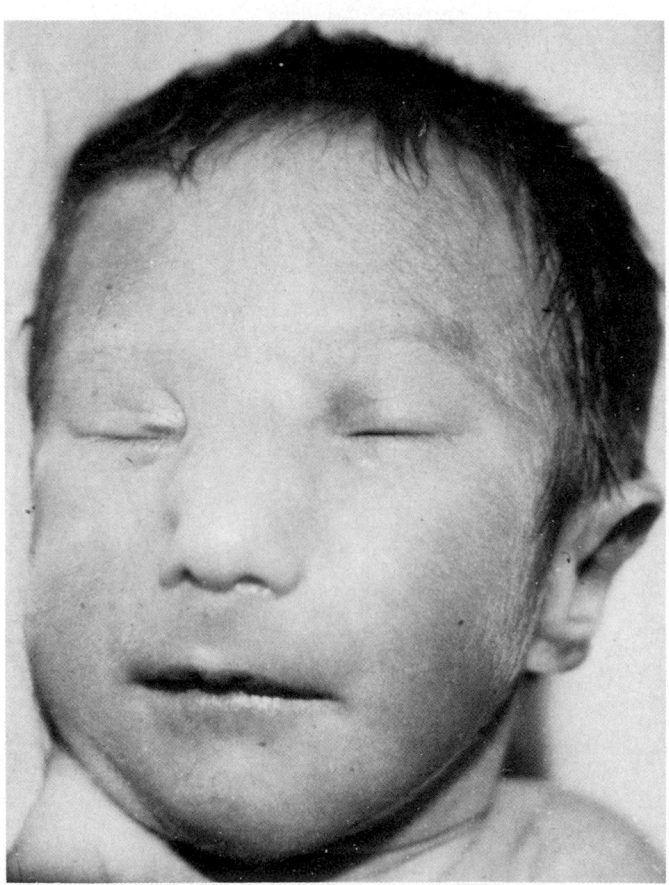

160. Note sloping forehead, microphthalmia and high nasal bridge

CERUMEN VARIATION (MARKER)

Includes: Variations dans le cérumen
Ceruminalformen
Variación del cerumen (Marcador)
Ear wax grey or brown

Excludes: —

Minimal Diagnostic Criteria: Identification of cerumen in the cartilaginous portion of the human ear canal as the grey, brittle and dry type or the brown, sticky and wet type.

Clinical Findings: There are 2 distinct types of normal human cerumen: one is grey, brittle and dry; the other type is brown, sticky and wet. These types of cerumen are manifest soon after birth. Cerumen is mainly a mixture of the secretions of ceruminous and sebaceous glands that are found in the cartilaginous portion of the human ear canal. Desquamated epithelial cells, dust, shed hair and other small foreign bodies that enter the external auditory canal are mixed into the cerumen. Biochemical studies show that no qualitative and quantitative differences in chemical composition have been identified except that the dry type is composed of more free amino acid than the wet type. Histologically there are abundant lipid droplets and pigment granules in the cytoplasm of the secretory cells in persons with wet cerumen. In persons with dry cerumen these cytoplasmic components are very scarce. The striated cuticular borders of the secretory cells are found in nearly every cell in persons with wet cerumen, but are rare in persons with dry cerumen.

Complications
I **Derived:** Loss of hearing acuity if either type accumulates and occludes the external auditory canal. Coughing may be associated with movement of dry, hard cerumen within ear canal. About 83.4% of wet type is observed to be associated with axillary odor.

II **Associated:** —

Etiology: † McK *11780

Pathogenesis: —

Related Facts
I **Sex Ratio:** M1:F1
II **Risk of Occurrence:** Frequencies in 1000 live births in different ethnic groups:

	WET TYPE	DRY TYPE
Koreans	76	934
Japanese	163	847
American Indians	431	659
American Whites	975	25
American Negroes	995	5

III **Risk of Recurrence for**
Patient's Sib: —
Patient's Child: May be calculated by types of matings. Frequencies of alleles for ear wax types in different ethnic groups:

	WET TYPE	DRY TYPE
Koreans	0.0378	0.9622
Japanese	0.0850	0.9150
American Indians	0.2485	0.7515
American Whites	0.8420	0.1580
American Negroes	0.9306	0.0694

IV **Age of Detectability:** Neonatal period

V **Prevalence:** Add two zeroes to figures for Risk of Occurrence for prevalence in 100,000 population.

Treatment
I **Primary Prevention:** —
II **Secondary Prevention:** Removal of excess cerumen is best done with instruments under direct observation (using operating microscope). The most useful instruments are wire loops, dull curettes, and Hartmann forceps. Irrigation and suctioning are also used.
III **Other Therapy:** —

Prognosis: Normal for life span, intelligence and function

Detection of Carrier: Person, who is phenotypically an Oriental and perhaps also a person who is phenotypically an American Indian, who has wet ear wax by definition is heterozygous and therefore a carrier of the recessive trait (dry wax).

†**Special Considerations:** The incidence of ear wax types is highly variable among different ethnic groups. This may be considered to be due to several factors, selection, racial intermixture and random genetic drift which is of particular significance when a population of small size is isolated or immigrated. However, the distinct differences for Caucasians, Negroes and Asian races in the frequencies of ear wax types cannot be accounted for by random genetic drift or racial intermixture alone but may be explained by considering the effect of natural selection.

References:
Kataura, A. and Kataura, K.: The comparison of free and bound amino acids between dry and wet types of cerumen. Tohoku J. Exp. Med. 91:215, 1967.
Kataura, A. and Kataura, K.: The comparison of lipids between dry and wet types of cerumen. Tohoku J. Exp. Med. 91:227, 1967.
Matsunaga, E.: The dimorphism in human normal cerumen. Ann. Hum. Genet. 25 :273, 1962.
Nagashima, T.: Über Ceruminaldrüse und Cerumen, besonders die Beziegung derselben zu Osmidrosis axillaris bei Japaneren. (Abstract) Jpn. J. Dermatol. Urol. 36 :118, 1934.
Petrakis, N. L. et al: Cerumen in American Indians: Genetic implications of sticky and dry types. Science 158:1192, 1967.

Contributors: **Isamu Sando**
Yoshinobu Masuda

Editor's Computerized Descriptor: Hearing

CERVICO-OCULO-ACOUSTIC SYNDROME

Editor's Computerized Descriptors: Eye, Hearing, Ear, Dermatoglyphic, Skel.

Includes: Dystrophie cervico-oculo-faciale
Zervico-Oculo-Acusticus Syndrom
Síndrome cérvico-óculo-acústico
Wildervanck syndrome
Cervicooculofacial dystrophy

Excludes: Hemifacial microsomia (457)
Oculo-auriculo-vertebral dysplasia (735)

Minimal Diagnostic Criteria: Clear evidence of involvement in all 3 areas (ear, eye and neck)

Clinical Findings: Patients present with severe congenital inner ear deafness. Roentgenologic findings include constricted internal auditory meatus, underdevelopment of cochlea and vestibular structures, often absence of semicircular canals. Absence of caloric response, retraction of eyeball, abducens palsy, often with limited adduction, plus the clinical features of cervical vertebral fusion.

Complications
I   **Derived:** —
II   **Associated:** In some cases epibulbar dermoid, facial asymmetry, pterygium colli, deformed auricle, atresia auris and mental retardation with normal dermatoglyphics.

Etiology: ? Possibly X-linked dominant with lethality in the hemizygous male, as nearly only females are clinically affected. Another possibility is a polygenic heritability by a pleiotropic gene with sex-limitation to the female.

Pathogenesis: ?

Related Facts
I   **Sex Ratio:** M6:F82
II   **Risk of Occurrence:** ?
III   **Risk of Recurrence for**
     Patient's Sib: Not increased
     Patient's Child: Not increased
IV   **Age of Detectability:** Clinically about one-half to 1 year
V   **Prevalence:** 0.8 to 1% of all deaf children (the Netherlands, England)

Treatment
I   **Primary Prevention:** —
II   **Secondary Prevention:** If the deafness is detected early and is not complete, early habilitation with amplification, speech and auditory training may be of benefit.
III   **Other Therapy:** Special education for the deaf. As the deafness is nearly complete, hearing aids are of no use.

Prognosis: Normal for life span

Detection of Carrier: —

Special Considerations: —

References:
Fraser, W.I. and MacGillivray, R.C.: Cervico-oculo-dysplasia ("the syndrome of Wildervanck"). J. Ment. Defic. Res. 12:322, 1968.
Linsay, J.R.: Inner ear histopatholgy in genetically determined congenital deafness. In Bergsma, D. (ed.): Part IX. Ear, Birth Defects: Orig. Art. Ser., vol. VII, no. 4. Baltimore: Williams & Wilkins Co., for The National Foundation-March of Dimes, 1971, p. 22.
McLay, K. and Maran, A.G.: Deafness and the Klippel-Feil syndrome. J. Laryngol. 83:175, 1969.
Wildervanck, L.S. et al: Radiological examination of the inner ear of deaf-mutes presenting the cervico-oculo-acusticus syndrome. Acta Otolaryngol. (Stockh.) 61:445, 1966.
Wildervanck, L.S.: A cervico-oculo-acusticus syndrome belonging to the status dysraphicus. Proc. 2nd Int. Congr. Hum. Genet., Rome, 1961. Rome: Instituto G. Mendel, 1963, p. 1409.

Contributor: **L. S. Wildervanck**

CHÉDIAK-HIGASHI SYNDROME

Includes: Syndrome de Chédiak-Higashi
Síndrome de Chédiak-Higashi
Anomalous panleukocytic granulation
Béguez César-Steinbrinck-Chédiak-Higashi syndrome
Chédiak anomaly, syndrome or disease
Chédiak-Steinbrinck anomaly, disease or syndrome
Congenital gigantism of peroxidase granules
Constitutional granular gigantism
Granulation anomaly of leukocytes
Hereditary constitutional giant granulations of leukocytes
Hereditary gigantism of cytoplasmic organelles
Incomplete oculocutaneous albinism

Excludes: May-Hegglin anomaly
Dohle bodies
Alder-Reilly anomaly
Riley bodies

Minimal Diagnostic Criteria: The pathognomonic feature of the Chédiak-Higashi syndrome is the presence of giant granules in the leukocytes of the peripheral blood in patients with recurrent infections and the characteristic depigmentation of skin, hair, and eyes.†

Clinical Findings: The skin is light cream to slate grey; may approach albinism in offspring of pale individuals. After exposure to sunlight, skin may show papillary or hyperpigmented lesions. The hair is very light blond to brunette with prominent frosted-grey sheen; the eyes have decreased-to-absent uveal pigment and also may show variable photophobia, nystagmus and squint. Neuropathy includes progressive cranial and peripheral neuropathy, muscle weakness, foot drop and decreased muscle stretch reflexes. The patient may have convulsions or mental retardation and may have decreased motor nerve conduction velocity. Hepatosplenomegaly and jaundice are variable and seen especially terminally. Lymphadenopathy is common especially terminally. Hematologic findings include granulocytes with giant granules (some up to 10 times normal size). Not all cells contain these granules and there may be normal appearing granules in the same cell with one or more giant granules. Lymphocytes and monocytes may also contain one or more azurophilic giant granules. Anemia occurs in over 80% of cases; thrombocytopenia in about 50% of cases; leukopenia in about 40% of cases and lymphocytosis is relative. Giant granules have also been observed in granulocyte and erythroid precursors of the bone marrow, plasma cells, histiocytes, reticular cells, hepatocytes, adrenal cortex, anterior pituitary, vascular endothelium and pericytes, neurons and Schwann cells, renal tubules, gut epithelium, fibroblasts in tissue culture and melanocytes.

The immunologic status is normal for humoral antibodies and immunoglobulin levels, capacity for delayed hypersensitivity, inflammatory cycle and in vitro bacterial phagocytosis approximates the normal. Phagocytic killing especially by mononuclear cells may be defective. In spite of the apparently normal parameters of specific immunity these patients have frequent recurrent infections, especially of the GI tract, skin, and respiratory tract, fevers of unknown origin and ulcerations of the oral mucosa. These are usually not to the severe degree seen in agammaglobulinemic children.

Roentgenologic findings are normal.

Complications
I   **Derived:** Reported cases have had frequent recurrent severe infections, especially of the GI tract, skin, and respiratory

tract, fevers of unknown origin and ulceration of the oral mucosa. Lymphoreticular malignancy and neuropathy may also occur in very high frequency.
II **Associated:** A form of familial hyperlipoproteinemia has been reported in a few cases of Chédiak-Higashi syndrome. This probably represents a chance association as it is not present in the great majority of cases.

Etiology: Autosomal recessive transmission of single defective gene. The primary lesion of this syndrome appears to reside in the granular cytoplasmic inclusions of a variety of cell types including especially the granulocytes of the blood. The biochemical basis of this lesion is unknown. McK *21450.

Pathogenesis: Giant cytoplasmic granulations appear in infancy in a variety of cell types. In general these granulations resemble the normal granules of the specific cell type in both fine structure and cytochemical staining reactions. The mechanism by which the presence of these giant granules leads to the decreased resistance to infection, the lymphoreticular malignancy, or the neuropathy is unknown. It has been postulated that many forms of the giant granules are lysosomes and that their large size reflects a functional abnormality leading to the improper handling for distribution of the normal lysosomal enzymes. Recent studies show that microtubules are poorly developed in the cells of patients with this defect.

Related Facts
I   **Sex Ratio:** M1:F1
II **Risk of Occurrence:** Very rare; most have been of European ancestry especially Spanish, but cases have been reported from other regions including Japan.
III **Risk of Recurrence for**
    Patient's Sib: 1 in 4 (25%) for each offspring to be affected
    Patient's Child: Not increased unless mate is carrier, (50% will be heterozygous asymptomatic carriers of the trait). Most of the patients have not lived to reproductive age.
IV **Age of Detectability:** Birth to a few months of life by examination of peripheral blood smear for presence of giant granules.
V   **Prevalence:** Very rare

Treatment
I   **Primary Prevention:** Genetic counseling
II **Secondary Prevention:** —
III **Other Therapy:** Diligent treatment of infections, and such preventive or prophylactic measures as seem warranted for the avoidance of infections. Splenectomy has been reported to provide some temporary relief in the progression of the disease. This is not well substantiated. Corticosteroids as a known stabilizer of lysosomal membranes may have some rationale as a form of supportive therapy. Steroids have been used in conjunction with alkylating agents in the production of remission in at least one case of the malignant transformation in Chédiak-Higashi disease. Recent evidence indicates that ascorbic acid treatment in vitro or in vivo has corrected phagocytic and chemotactic abnormality of the leukocytes.

Prognosis: The prognosis is uniformly grave. Most cases have died in childhood. There has been only a single report of 2 individuals who lived beyond 20 years of age. In younger children, death is usually the result of infection while those who survive beyond the early years often die of a fulminant illness malignant in character.

Detection of Carrier: Heterozygotic carriers may often, but not uniformly, be identified by the presence of occasional giant granules in the peripheral blood cells on a standard microscopic smear preparation.

†**Special Considerations:** The same or very similar anomaly of cellular granules has been described in Aleutian mink, Hereford cattle, Biege mice, and even a killer whale.

References:

Dent, P. B. et al: Chédiak-Higashi syndrome: Observations on the nature of the associated malignancy. Lab. Invest. 15:1634, 1966.

Lockman, L. A. et al: The Chédiak-Higashi syndrome: Electrophysiologic and electron microscopic observations on the peripheral neuropathy. J. Pediatr. 70:942, 1967.

Windhorst, D.B. et al: The Chédiak-Higashi anomaly and the aleutian trait in mink: Homologous defects of lysosomal structure. Ann. N.Y. Acad. Sci. 155:818, 1968.

Contributors: C. C. Clawson
Robert A. Good

Editor's Computerized Descriptors: Vision, Eye, Oral, Skin, Hair, Muscle, Lymphatic, Liver, Nerve

CHEILITIS GLANDULARIS

Includes: Cheilite glandulaire
Queilitis glandular
Cheilitis glandularis apostematosa
Baelz syndrome
Lip, enlargement of lower

Excludes: Cheilitis granulomatosis
Blepharochalasis, double lip and nontoxic thyroid enlargement (111)
Cheilitis exfolitiva

Minimal Diagnostic Criteria: Enlargement of lower lip, increased secretion of mucous, vesicle-like lesions or palpable enlargement of mucous glands.

Clinical Findings: There is enlargement of the lower lip, and increased secretion of mucous on the lower lip resulting in a wet, sticky lip; collection of mucous in dilated mucous ducts beneath the mucosa gives vesicle-like cystic lesions; protrusion and eversion of the lower lip; and nodular enlargement of mucous glands of the lip can be detected by palpation. All of these features are present in the well-developed stage but earlier changes consist of enlargement of the lower lip and excess mucous secretion with or without vesicle-like lesions.

Complications

I **Derived:** Mucous cyst (mucocele) formation is due to traumatic rupture of mucous ducts and this complication is common. In Caucasians, 18 to 35% of patients reported with cheilitis glandularis have developed squamous cell carcinoma. This complication is due presumably to protrusion of the lip making it susceptible to solar radiation and other irritations such as smoking. Secondary bacterial infection may occur with fistula formation.

II **Associated:** —

Etiology: Autosomal dominant†

Pathogenesis: The gross structural defect in the fully developed condition includes enlargement of lower lip 2-4 times normal size, enlargement of mucous glands up to 12 mm in size and dilatation of the mucous ducts in the mucosa or submucosa, a marked hypertrophy of the mucous glands, chronic inflammation involving the stroma of the mucous glands consisting mainly of plasma cells and fibrosis and edema of the stroma. It is probable that the glandular hypertrophy with increased mucous secretion occurs as the initial change with secondary changes of partial obstruction resulting in dilatation of ducts and inflammation.

Related Facts

I **Sex Ratio:** M1:F1 (Probably, but males predominate in reported cases.)
II **Risk of Occurrence:** ? Rare
III **Risk of Recurrence for**
Patient's Sib: If parent is affected, 1 in 2 (50%) for each offspring to be affected; otherwise not increased
Patient's Child: 1 in 2
IV **Age of Detectability:** Usually between 5 and 10 years by enlargement of lower lip, increased mucous secretion of lip and vesicle-like lesions.
V **Prevalence:** ? Uncommon, 100 cases reported by 1970.

Treatment

I **Primary Prevention:** Genetic counseling
II **Secondary Prevention:** Partial excision of the lower lip with removal of enlarged mucous glands. This will prevent complications and give a cosmetically and functionally satisfactory result.
III **Other Therapy:** —

Prognosis: If treated, there is minimal morbidity and normal life span. If untreated, complications may cause moderate morbidity and if squamous cell carcinoma develops and is not treated, death may occur.

Detection of Carrier: —

†**Special Considerations:** The majority of patients with cheilitis glandularis recognized in the past have not been reported as having a hereditary form of the disease.

References:
Doku, H. C. et al: Cheilitis glandularis. Oral Surg. 20:563, 1965.
Sutton, R. L.: Cheilitis glandularis apostematosa. J. Cutan. Dis. 27:150, 1909.
Weir, T. W. and Johnson, W. C.: Cheilitis glandularis. Arch. Dermatol. 103:433, 1971.

Contributor: **Waine C. Johnson**

Editor's Computerized Descriptor: Face

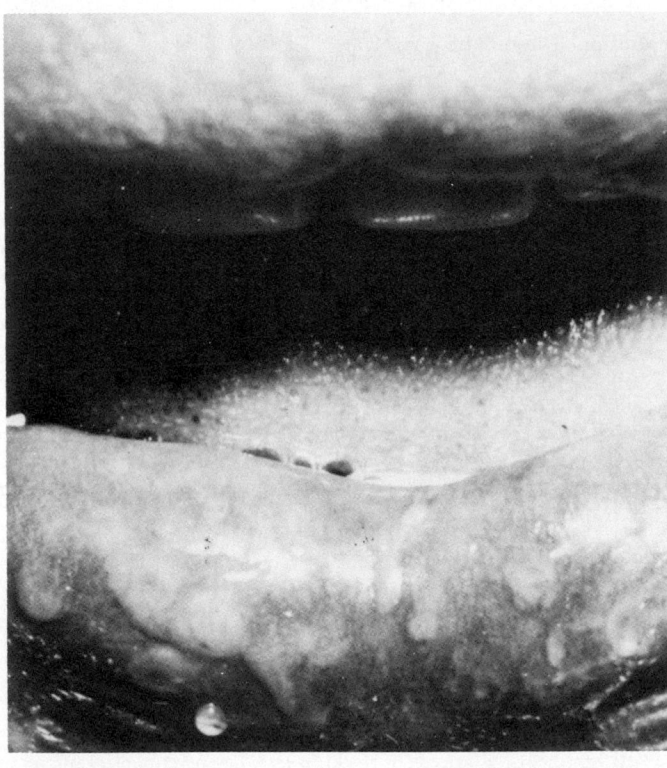

161. Cheilitis glandularis

CHEMODECTOMA OF MIDDLE EAR

Includes: Chémodectomie de l'oreille moyenne
Glomus jugulare Tumor
Quemodectoma del oído medio
Middle ear chemodectoma
Glomus tympanicum tumor
Glomus jugulare of middle ear
Nonchromaffin paragangliomata of middle ear

Excludes: Carotid body tumor (127)

Minimal Diagnostic Criteria: Positive biopsy of middle ear tumor. Eosinophilic epithelioid cells in large groups, with granular cytoplasm and hyperchromatic nuclei. Cells are seen adjacent to thin-walled capillaries. Mitoses are rare.

Clinical Findings: Fleshy red or bluish, pulsatile mass in the middle ear with or without intact tympanic membrane. Most common presenting complaint is hearing loss (91%). Pulsatile tinnitus also occurs, as may aural discharge, hemorrhage, and vertigo. Lesions may be diagnosed from early adulthood on, although these tumors have usually been seen in middle-aged women. A red or bluish mass in the middle ear which blanches with pneumatic compression and pulsates upon gradual release of pressure (Brown's sign) is suggestive. Xrays may reveal areas of bony erosion. Carotid arteriograms with subtraction studies help in diagnosis and determining the extent of lesion. Blood biochemical tests are equivocal.

Complications
I **Derived:** Otitis media, hemorrhage, functional deficits of cranial nerves VII, VIII, IX, X, XI, & XII. Erosion of petrous bone and base of skull, brain invasion, meningitis, etc.
II **Associated:** Possibly carotid body tumors

Etiology: ?

Pathogenesis: ?

Related Facts
I **Sex Ratio:** M1:F3 (4 known cases)
II **Risk of Occurrence:** ?
III **Risk of Recurrence for**
    Patient's Sib: ?
    Patient's Child: ?
IV **Age of Detectability:** Early adulthood
V **Prevalence:** Very rare; 4 cases reported.

Treatment
I **Primary Prevention:** —
II **Secondary Prevention:** Surgical excision, if small
III **Other Therapy:** If lesion is very large or recurs, cobalt teletherapy-5000 rads or greater tumor dose. (Tumors fairly radio-resistant)

Prognosis: For small, readily excised tumors, excellent. For large tumors with neurologic findings, poor.

Detection of Carrier: —

Special Considerations: —

References:
Alford, B.R. and Guilford, F.R.: A comprehensive study of tumors of the glomus jugulare. Laryngoscope 72:765, 1962.
Geokoop, Von C.: Fibro-haemangiom des Felsenbeines und des Mittelohres bei drei Schwestern. Acta Otolaryngol. (Stockh.) 18:153, 1933.
Resler, D. R. et al: Multiplicity and familial incidence of carotid body and glomus jugulare tumors. Ann. Otol. Rhinol. Laryngol. 75:114, 1966.

Contributor: **Raymond P. Wood, II**

CHIN FISSURE

Includes: Fissure mentonnière
  Kinngrübchen
  Fisura del mentón
  Sulcus mentalis
  Incisura mentalis Types I, II, III, & IV
  Chin groove or furrow
  Chin dimple
  Y-shaped fissure of chin
  Chin cleft
  Fovea mentalis

Excludes: Mental fold
  Syndromes related to cleft tongue
  Median clefts of lower lip mandible and tongue (636)
  Acrofacial dysostosis (17)
  Chin furrows in Hallermann-Streiff syndrome
  Cranio-carpo-tarsal dysplasia (223)

Minimal Diagnostic Criteria: Constant depression of the soft tissue part of the chin

Clinical Findings: Chin fissures are single visible depressions of the soft tissue part of the chin. Four different types of chin fissures can be distinguished clinically and genetically. The most common type is a perpendicular furrow in the midline of the chin (incisura mentalis) ranging from a superficial depression in the area of the gnathion to a more pronounced furrow. Less commonly a steep fissure (sulcus mentalis) or a round dimple with a center of various depth (fovea mentalis) is observed. Very rarely a Y-shaped fissure in the middle of the chin is found. Bony defects of the underlying mental tubercle may or may not be associated with fissures in the soft tissues and may even be present without a furrow of the overlying skin. Fissures of the chin may not be present at birth but arise later during childhood or early adulthood. They may disappear later in life or after trauma.†

Complications
I   **Derived:** —
II **Associated:** In one family reported by Günther, 4 of 6 individuals had preauricular fistulas in addition to a Y-shaped fissure of the chin.†

Etiology: Autosomal dominant with high degree of penetrance and variable expressivity for all types. McK *11900

Pathogenesis: Fissures of the chin may occur by partial fusion of the mental muscles with the overlying skin. Local absence of subcutaneous fat and muscular tissue in the area of the gnathion may cause an adhesion of the dermis to the periosteum by means of collagen bundles or even a ligament. These developmental variations leading to chin furrows may be determined around the end of the first trimester.

Related Facts
I   **Sex Ratio:** About M2:F1. Strong male predominance. Figures might be biased by sex influence on expressivity.
II   **Risk of Occurrence:** No figures available
III **Risk of Recurrence for**
   Patient's Sib: If parent is affected, 1 in 2 (50%) for each offspring to be affected; otherwise not increased.
   Patient's Child: 1 in 2
IV   **Age of Detectability:** Fissures are sometimes present at birth, more commonly become visible in childhood or early adulthood.
V   **Prevalence:** About 14 to 21% in males and 9 to 15% in females in German populations. The first type (incisura mentalis) was 8.4% in males and 4.2% in females. The second type (sulcus mentalis) was present in 0.73% and 0.04%, fovea mentalis was found in 0.27% and 0.16% and the Y-shaped fissure in 0.15% and 0.08%, respectively.†

Treatment

I Primary Prevention: Genetic counseling

II Secondary Prevention: Plastic surgery only to reduce cosmetic concern.

III Other Therapy: —

Prognosis: Furrows may disappear with aging or after trauma. No effect on longevity or function.

Detection of Carrier: —

†Special Considerations: Chin fissures, especially the first type (sulcus mentalis), are a common finding in the general population and should be considered as normal variations of chin form. The steep furrow (sulcus mentalis) resembling a cleft of the soft tissue part of the chin may only represent a more pronounced expression of the common furrow. Günther reported 4 out of 6 individuals of one family having in addition to a Y-shaped fissure preauricular fistulas suggesting a specific syndrome. However, this association was probably caused by 2 different traits (preauricular fistulas are also known to be transmitted in an autosomal dominant pattern).

References:

Günther, H.: Anomalien und Anomalienkomplexe in der Gegend des ersten Schlundbogens. Z. Menchl. Vererb. -Konstit. -Lehre 23:43, 1939.

Lebow, M.R. and Swain, P.B.: Inheritance of human facial features; pedigree study involving length of face, prominent ears and chin cleft. J. Hered. 32:127, 1941.

Pfannenstiel, D.: Zur Morphologie und Genetik der Mund- und Kinnregion. Arch. Julius Klaus-Stift. Vererb. -Forsch. 27:1, 1952.

Contributor: **Gordon G. Keyes**

Editor's Computerized Descriptor: Face

CHIN, TREMBLING

Includes: Trémulation du menton
Wackelkinn
Mentón trémulo
Hereditary quivering of chin
Chin, quivering

Excludes: Facial tics
Facial myokymia

Minimal Diagnostic Criteria: The presence of a trembling chin in a patient who has a positive family history.

Clinical Findings: Trembling of the patient's chin may last for a few seconds or for several minutes. The tremor may be either fine or coarse movements and not particularly related to the precipitating cause. The trembling of the chin is perpendicular and at a rate of 2 or 3 times per second. In most cases an emotional stimulus is the trigger mechanism, but it may occur during sleep. EEG studies are not helpful.

Complications

I Derived: —

II Associated: Horizontal nystagmus

Etiology: Autosomal dominant with almost complete penetrance; McK *19010

Pathogenesis: Electromyographic studies suggest that the chin movement is due to a rapid rhythmic simultaneous discharge of a number of motor units, producing virtually a tetanic twitch.

Related Facts

I Sex Ratio: M1:F1

II Risk of Occurrence: ? Rare

III Risk of Recurrence for
Patient's Sib: If parent is affected, 1 in 2 (50%) for each offspring to be affected; otherwise not increased
Patient's Child: 1 in 2

IV Age of Detectability: Noted frequently in the first few weeks of life

V Prevalence: ? Rare

Treatment

I Primary Prevention: Genetic counseling

II Secondary Prevention: Avoidance of known precipitating factors (anger, rapid eye movement, etc)

III Other Therapy: The occasional intermittent use of tranquilizing drugs may be justified in patients where anxiety and tension are the sole precipitating factors. Long-term drug therapy is not indicated for this benign condition.

Prognosis: Excellent. There is usually a lessening severity of the trembling with increasing age. One case followed by the author stopped quivering spontaneously. Another reported case was "cured" by a blow on the chin.

Detection of Carrier: —

Special Considerations: —

References:

Frey, E.: Ein streng dominant erbliches Kinnmuskelzittern (Beitrag zur Erforschung der menschlichen Affektäusserungen. Dtsch. Z. Nervenheilk. 115:9, 1930.

Laurance, B.M. et al: Hereditary quivering of the chin. Arch. Dis. Child. 43:249, 1968.

Wadlington, W.B.: Familial trembling of the chin. J. Pediatr. 53:316, 1958.

Contributor: **William B. Wadlington**

Editor's Computerized Descriptors: Eye, Face, Nerve

CHLORIDE DIARRHEA, CONGENITAL

Includes: Diarrhée chlorée
Chlorid-Diarrhoe
Clorurorrea
Alkalosis with diarrhea
Diarrhea, congenital chloride

Excludes: Infectious gastroenteridides
Mucous colitis

Minimal Diagnostic Criteria: Fecal chloride concentration above 60 meq/l in the newborn and above 100 meq/l later. Stools are solid and Cl⁻ concentrations < 60 meq/l only in chronic dehydration. Serum and urinary Cl⁻ concentrations are very low.

Clinical Findings: The pregnancy is uniformly complicated by hydramnios, and the child is often premature. Watery diarrhea begins from the first day of life. Abdomen is often distended. Meconium usually cannot be found.

Complications
I **Derived:** Excessive neonatal loss of weight with dehydration and jaundice. Hyponatremia and hypochloridemia develop rapidly and, later, hypokalemia and metabolic alkalosis.
II **Associated:** —

Etiology: Autosomal recessive defect probably causing a defect in the Cl⁻/HCO₃⁻ exchange mechanism in the distal ileum and the colon.† McK *21470

Pathogenesis: Impairment or net Cl⁻ reabsorption in ileum and colon apparently responsible for osmotic diarrhea with high Cl⁻ concentration, low net fecal HCO₃⁻ excretion is associated with metabolic alkalosis.

Related Facts
I   **Sex Ratio:** Probably M1:F1; 2 or more affected sibs in at least 1 family
II   **Risk of Occurrence:** 1 in 30,000 live births in Finland: rarer elsewhere
III **Risk of Recurrence for**
     Patient's Sib: Probably 1 in 4 (25%) for each offspring to be affected.
     Patient's Child: Not increased, unless mate is carrier or homozygote.
IV   **Age of Detectability:** At birth or as neonate
V   **Prevalence:** Twenty probands outside Finland; 21 others in Finland.

Treatment
I   **Primary Prevention:** Genetic counseling
II   **Secondary Prevention:** In the newborn, give extra free water (150ml/day per infant) together with 10 meq of Cl⁻/kg (approximately 2 meq as KCl, the rest as NaCl). Later adjust the daily intake of additional salt solution (both NaCl and KCl; Na:K = 5:1 - 1:1) so that serum potassium and acid-base balance are normal and Cl⁻ is excreted into the urine. Early treatment is life saving.
III **Other Therapy:** —

Prognosis: Patients have died from superimposed infection during the first few years of life; growth failure and retarded mental development have been noted as well. Aggressive treatment from birth compatible with normal development.

Detection of Carrier: Parents of affected patients have no diarrhea or excessive fecal chloride concentration.

†Special Considerations: Must be thought of in any patient with neonatal diarrhea; demonstrates that chloride transport in intestine is genetically controlled and chemically mediated. No associated defect in renal handling of chloride indicating that renal tubular reabsorptive mechanism for chloride is distinct from that in intestine.

References:
Darrow, D. C.: Congenital alkalosis with diarrhea. J. Pediatr. 26:519, 1945.
Gamble, J.L. et al: Congenital alkalosis with diarrhea. J. Pediatr. 26:509, 1945.
Holmberg, C. et al: Colonic electrolyte transport in health and in congenital chloride diarrhea. J. Clin. Invest. 56:302, 1975.
Norio, R. et al: Congenital chloride diarrhea, an autosomal recessive disease: Genetics of 14 Finnish and 12 other families. Clin. Genet. 2:182, 1971.
Perheentupa, J. et al: Familial chloride diarrhoea ("congenital alkalosis with diarrhoea"). Acta Paediatr. (Uppsala) Suppl. 159:119, 1965.

Contributors: **Leon E. Rosenberg**
                      Olli G. Simell

Editor's Computerized Descriptor: GI.

CHOLEDOCHAL CYST

Includes: Kyste du chólédoque
Choledochus-zyste
Quiste del colédoco
Congenital cystic dilation of common duct
Diverticulum of common bile duct
Choledochocele
Intrahepatic cystic dilatation of bile ducts
Bile duct cyst

Excludes: Hepatic cyst, solitary (465)
Liver, polycystic disease (605)
Pancreatic pseudocyst
Gallbladder anomalies (404)
Mesenteric cysts (645)
Liver hamartoma (604)
Parasitic hepatic cyst

Minimal Diagnostic Criteria: Suspect choledochal cyst when a right upper quadrant mass presents in a female child or young adult with a history of recurrent intermittent pain and jaundice.†

Clinical Findings: Right upper quadrant mass (80%), jaundice (75%), and pain (60%) are common findings with the entire triad present in 60% of cases. Intermittent episodes of pain and jaundice associated with chills and fever may occur repeatedly. Leukocytosis, elevated bilirubin, and alkaline phosphatase, acholic stools, and dark urine may be observed during such episodes. In the absence of jaundice, IV cholangiography may be diagnostic. Barium swallow may be helpful in delineating a mass or displacement of the duodenum (anteriorly or to the left), the colon, or stomach. Percutaneous transhepatic cholangiography, ultrasound, and I^{131} or I^{123} Rose Bengal excretion tests may also be useful in achieving a diagnosis, whereas oral cholecystograms rarely show the dilatation due to failure of concentration of the dye.

Complications
I **Derived:** Cholangitis, biliary cirrhosis, portal hypertension and varices. Obstruction of adjacent structures (eg duodenum) by enlarging cysts, pancreatitis, and malignant degeneration to carcinoma.

II **Associated:** —

Etiology: The exact cause is obscure. However, the cyst appears to be of congenital origin, most likely representing an embryologic weakness in the bile duct wall. Some investigators believe cystic dilatation of the common duct is related to a variant of biliary atresia and hypoplasia (see Biliary Atresia).

Pathogenesis: The wall of the cyst is composed of fibrous tissue with occasional smooth muscle or elastic fibers noted. The inner lining is often devoid of epithelium. Common duct proximal to the cyst may be dilated whereas distally the common bile duct is narrow. Stasis and intermittent obstruction result in cholangitis and biliary cirrhosis.

Related Facts
I **Sex Ratio:** M1:F4
II **Risk of Occurrence:** Unknown, but appears more common in Japanese patients.
III **Risk of Recurrence for**
 Patient's Sib: Not increased
 Patient's Child: Not increased
IV **Age of Detectability:** 22% in 1st year, 33% between 1-10 years, with 80% of all cases presenting in the first 30 years of life.
V **Prevalence:** Only 500+ cases reported; 1 in 13,500 hospital admissions

Treatment
I **Primary Prevention:** —

II **Secondary Prevention:** Surgical: biliary-intestinal drainage procedure (cyst-duodenostomy, cyst Roux-Y jejunostomy, or cyst resection and anastomosis). Close follow-up after initial operation for anastomotic stricture, cholangitis, and calculous formation.†

III **Other Therapy:** Antibiotics for cholangitis

Prognosis: If untreated, this defect is lethal with death eventually due to cholangitis and biliary cirrhosis (29 of 30 dead by age 32).
 Life expectancy of many of these children (25-35%) is adversely affected by this anomaly. Drainage procedures carried out in childhood may be followed by a protracted life-limiting chronic hepatobiliary disease process. Improved results may be expected in those instances which are diagnosed early, operated upon with cyst resection, and subsequent hepatojejunostomy or cystojejunostomy (Roux-Y type) as the initial procedure.

Detection of Carrier: —

†Special Considerations: The diagnosis of choledochal cyst should be entertained whenever the triad of pain, jaundice, and right upper quadrant mass present in a girl, characterized by repeated episodes of chills and fever. In many instances only one of the major triad components exists. The treatment of choice is surgical. At the time of operation, cholangiography is a very helpful diagnostic adjunct. The procedure of choice in most centers is biliary-intestinal drainage. In past years cyst duodenostomy was the most popular operation employed. Recent reports, however, stress the occurrence of postoperative complications after this procedure requiring revision to a cyst Roux-Y jejunostomy. A few centers in Japan and Switzerland, as well as in this country, regard complete cyst excision (when possible) and hepatoenterostomy to be the therapy of choice. The cyst has little or no epithelial lining, is fibrotic, with disruption of elastic fibers in the wall, has poor motility, and therefore has the potential for stasis. Stasis and inappropriate cyst-duodenostomy are probably why, in the past, chronic hepatobiliary disease in children with choledochal cysts was observed even after drainage operations. Many of these former cases developed biliary calculi and evidence of permanent hepatic damage from instances of recurrent cholangitis and biliary cirrhosis which adversely affected the life expectancy of these children. It is obvious that early intervention and long-term follow-up in these cases is most essential.

References:
Fonkalsrud, E. W. and Boles, E. T., Jr.: Choledochal cysts in infancy and childhood. Surg. Gynecol. Obstet. 121:733, 1965.
Hays, D.M. et al: Congenital cystic dilatation of the common bile duct. Arch. Surg. 98:457, 1969.
Mahour, G. H. and Lynn, H. B.: Choledochal cyst in children. Surgery 65:967, 1969.
Saito, S. and Ishida, M.: Congenital choledochal cyst (cystic dilatation of common bile duct). Prog. Pediatr. Surg. 6:63, 1974.

Contributors: **Jay L. Grosfeld**
H. William Clatworthy, Jr.

Editor's Computerized Descriptors: GI., Liver

CHOLESTEATOMA OF TEMPORAL BONE

Includes: Cholestéatome de l'os temporal
Cholesteatom
Colesteatoma del hueso temporal
Temporal bone cholesteatoma
Petrous pyramid cholesteatoma
Congenital cholesteatoma
Primary cholesteatoma
True cholesteatoma

Excludes: Acquired cholesteatoma

Minimal Diagnostic Criteria: Otoscopic examination revealing a whitish mass, either circumscribed or filling the middle ear space, behind an intact tympanic membrane or a gradually progressive facial nerve palsy in the absence of chronic ear infection.†

Clinical Findings: Vary according to site of lesion.

Middle ear or mastoid cholesteatoma is usually seen in children. Most show a conductive hearing loss but occasionally hearing is normal. In 80% of cases the otoscopic examination has revealed a whitish mass, either circumscribed or totally filling the middle ear space, behind an intact tympanic membrane. The age of the patient at discovery is usually between 3-14 years.

Primary cholesteatoma originating in the petrous pyramid is detected in about 90% of cases because of a facial palsy of gradual onset and progression. There is usually a homolateral profound sensorineural deafness, and a loss of caloric response. The patient's age at discovery of the cholesteatoma is usually between 35-55.

Polytome radiography of the temporal bone has proved decidedly superior to conventional x-ray examination in defining the exact location of the lesion and the extent of bone erosion.

Complications
I **Derived:** Conductive hearing loss in about three-fourths of primary cholesteatoma of the middle ear and mastoid; a slowly progressive facial palsy and a profound sensorineural hearing loss in about 90% of petrous pyramid cholesteatomata.
II **Associated:** —

Etiology: ?

Pathogenesis: The consensus of opinion assumes the presence of an embryonic epidermal rest within the middle ear, attic, mastoid or petrous pyramid. Once this stratified squamous epithelium starts to grow it sloughs off in layers as a normal growth process. This results in a gradually enlarging enclosed mass of desquamated keratinized epithelium. Whether necrosis of contiguous bony structures results from the pressure of an expansile mass or from a chemical and enzymatic lysis is an unsettled question.

Related Facts
I **Sex Ratio:** M1:F1
II **Risk of Occurrence:** ?
III **Risk of Recurrence for**
   Patient's Sib: ?
   Patient's Child: ?
IV **Age of Detectability:** Middle ear and mastoid 3-14 years; petrous pyramid 35-55 years.
V **Prevalence:** ?

Treatment
I **Primary Prevention:** —
II **Secondary Prevention:** Complete surgical excision
III **Other Therapy:** Periodic postoperative recheck for early detection of any residual or recurrent cholesteatoma which will require secondary excision.

Prognosis: Normal life span for treated cases. Unknown for untreated cases.

Detection of Carrier: —

†Special Considerations: Polytomography provides accurate information regarding ossicular destruction and is helpful in differentiating primary from acquired cholesteatoma.

References:
Cawthorne, T. and Griffith, A.: Primary cholesteatomata of the temporal bone. Arch. Otolaryngol. 73:252, 1961.
Derlacki, E. L. and Clemis, J. D.: Congenital cholesteatoma of the middle ear and mastoid. Ann. Otol. Rhinol. Laryngol. 74:706, 1965.
Derlacki, E. L. et al: Congenital cholesteatoma of the middle ear and mastoid: A second report presenting seven additional cases. Laryngoscope 78:1050, 1968.

Contributor: **Eugene L. Derlacki**

Editor's Computerized Descriptors: Hearing, Ear, Skel., Nerve

CHOLESTERYL ESTER STORAGE DISEASE

Includes: Lipidose à ester du cholestérol
Cholesterinester-Speicherkrankheit
Tesaurismosis hepática de ésteres del colesterol
Hepatic cholesteryl ester storage disease
CESD
Polycorie cholestérolique
Liver, cholesteryl ester storage

Excludes: Analphalipoproteinemia (48)
Wolman disease (1003)

Minimal Diagnostic Criteria: Demonstration of elevated concentrations of cholesteryl esters in the liver and markedly reduced (almost absent) levels of acid (lysosomal) cholesteryl ester hydrolase activity in the liver and spleen. Acid (lysosomal) triglyceride hydrolase activity is also greatly reduced in these tissues.

Clinical Findings: A remarkably high concentration (up to 18% of the wet weight of the liver) of cholesteryl ester has been found in the 3 patients whose livers have been examined chemically; liver glycerides are also moderately increased. Hepatomegaly is a constant feature; splenomegaly has also been observed (2 of 5). Hyperlipemia was found in 4 of the 5 patients and plasma lipids were at the upper limits of normal in the fifth. Foam cells may be found in the bone marrow. Lipids also may accumulate in the lamina propria of the intestine. There are no neurologic symptoms.

Complications
I **Derived:** Possibly accelerated atherosclerosis. One patient died at the age of 24 days of "respiratory distress"; the twin sister of this patient died at 21 years of age of severe aortic stenosis. She also had advanced coronary atherosclerosis.
II **Associated:** —

Etiology: Autosomal recessive mode of transmission. The homozygote apparently cannot make the enzyme (or the normal enzyme) acid (lysosomal) cholesteryl ester hydrolase. There is also apparently a deficient activity of acid (lysosomal) triglyceride hydrolase.

Pathogenesis: The decreased activity of acid cholesteryl ester hydrolase results in the accumulation of cholesteryl ester in the liver, spleen and intestine. In spite of the depressed activity of the acid triglyceride lipase, the accumulation of glycerides is only modest. There is no adequate explanation for the hyperlipemia.

Related Facts
I **Sex Ratio:** M2:F3 in the 5 known cases
II **Risk of Occurrence:** ? All patients Caucasian thus far
III **Risk of Recurrence for**
    Patient's Sib: 1 in 4 (25%) for each offspring to be affected
    Patient's Child: Not increased unless mate is carrier or homozygote. (Probands may survive to childbearing age.)
IV **Age of Detectability:** Presumably at birth, by determination of the level of acid cholesteryl ester hydrolase and acid triglyceride hydrolase in liver.
V **Prevalence:** < 1 in 100,000

Treatment
I **Primary Prevention:** Genetic counseling
II **Secondary Prevention:** —
III **Other Therapy:** —

Prognosis: Guarded: One of the 5 patients died in infancy; the cause of death was not fully established. Her twin sister died at age 21 of severe aortic valvular stenosis; the 3 other living patients with cholesteryl ester storage disease do not have aortic stenosis. The patient who died at 21 years of age also had severe coronary atherosclerosis; premature coronary vascular disease may be a feature of cholesteryl ester storage disease.

Detection of Carrier: ?

Special Considerations: —

References:
Infante, R. et al: Polycorie cholestérolique de l'adulte, II. Étude biochimique. Presse Méd. 75:2829, 1967.
Schiff, L. et al: Hepatic cholesterol ester storage disease, a familial disorder. I. Clinical aspects. Am. J. Med. 44:538, 1968.
Sloan, H.R. and Fredrickson, D.S.: Rare familial diseases with neutral lipid storage. In Stanbury, J.B. et al (eds.): The Metabolic Basis of Inherited Disease, 3rd Ed. New York:McGraw-Hill, 1972, p.808.

Contributor: **Howard R. Sloan**

Editor's Computerized Descriptors: Spleen, Liver

CHOLINESTERASE, ATYPICAL

Includes: Cholinestérase atypique
Atypische Plasma-Cholinesterase
Colinesterasa plasmática atípica
Acylcholine acyl-hydrolase EC 3.1.1.8
Anectine apnea
Succinylcholine apnea
Pseudocholinesterase defect
Suxamethonium sensitivity
Plasma cholinesterase, atypical

Excludes: Apnea after use of succinylcholine in patients for whom laboratory evaluation of plasma cholinesterase gives normal values

Minimal Diagnostic Criteria: No physical findings prior to apnea. Occurrence of prolonged apnea after succinylcholine administration. Detecting the occurrence of prolonged apnea is dependent upon the amount and anticipated duration of the drug in relation to the total anesthesia procedure. Apnea lasting longer than 10 minutes is considered abnormal. A peripheral nerve stimulator may aid confirmation of diagnosis by demonstrating flaccidity of hand muscles. Confirmation of clinical diagnosis by laboratory tests.†

Clinical Findings: Prolonged apnea after succinylcholine administration. Apnea lasting longer than 10 minutes in absence of significant amounts of depressant premedication, anesthetic agent or neurologic defect. Prolonged recovery of adequate spontaneous ventilation, with obvious persistent weakness of intercostal and cervical musculature, eg inability to raise head while supine.

Complications
I **Derived:** Complications may include hypoxia (may lead to cardiac arrest), hypercarbia (acidosis—both respiratory and metabolic), dehydration and postoperative psychologic disturbances (failure to keep patient asleep during apnea).
II **Associated:** —

Etiology: Autosomal recessive

Pathogenesis: Succinylcholine is a skeletal muscle relaxant which acts at the neuromuscular junction to provide alteration in sensitivity to acetylcholine, the transmitter substance. The circulating drug molecules have a short route from the blood to their site of action, and onset of paralysis after IV injection of the drug is rapid. The high concentration of drug in plasma immediately after IV injection falls very quickly in the normal individual because of the rapid action of plasma cholinesterase. The prolonged effect of succinylcholine in persons with atypical plasma cholinesterase is considered to be due to an excessive amount of the drug reaching the endplate. Not all cases of prolonged apnea during anesthesia are associated with atypical cholinesterase, but it should be recognized that the atypical homozygote is always at risk of a prolonged effect of succinylcholine.†

Related Facts
I **Sex Ratio:** M1:F1
II **Risk of Occurrence:** The occurrence of atypical homozygotes for the dibucaine-resistant form has been estimated to be from 1 in 2000 to 1 in 4000 in various populations. The fluoride-resistant atypical form and the silent gene variant are much rarer.
III **Risk of Recurrence for**
Patient's Sib: 1 in 4 (25%) for each offspring to be affected
Patient's Child: Not increased unless mate is carrier or homozygote.
IV **Age of Detectability:** On theoretic grounds it is possible to detect atypical homozygous individuals by inhibition studies at any age. The relatively low plasma cholinesterase activity

in the neonate may prejudice screening tests dependent only on enzyme activity measurement.
V **Prevalence:** The gene for dibucaine-resistant atypical cholinesterase appears to be widely distributed. An unusually high rate has been reported among Jews from Iran and Iraq, but a low incidence in Jews from North Africa. Low carrier rates have been found in Orientals and Negroes. An unusually high rate of occurrence of silent gene has been described in southern Eskimos.

Treatment
I **Primary Prevention:** Genetic counseling
II **Secondary Prevention:** It is essential in taking the history to elicit information concerning a previous occurrence of apnea in the patient or in the family and, pending biochemical evaluation, to avoid the use of succinylcholine with an individual possibly at risk.
III **Other Therapy:** The essential therapy is assisted respiration and associated care during the period of apnea. Because of the risk of psychic trauma associated with consciousness of the patient during a part of the period of paralysis, it is advisable to administer an agent such as nitrous oxide as soon as the fact of the existence of apnea is recognized. The infusion of normal plasma as a source of normal cholinesterase has been advocated as a means of shortening the period of paralysis, but this treatment has not come into general use. Injection of normal purified plasma cholinesterase before and after injection of succinylcholine has been advocated for control of apnea.

Prognosis: Good, providing the apnea is recognized early and appropriate therapy is given.

Detection of Carrier: Identification of the heterozygous state on clinical grounds is uncertain. Some individuals experiencing apnea of short duration have been shown to be heterozygotes by biochemical studies. Detection of the heterozygote state by biochemical means depends upon studying inhibition of plasma cholinesterase activity.

†**Special Considerations:** Women of childbearing age using oral contraceptives have reduced plasma cholinesterase levels.

Atypical forms of plasma cholinesterase are not as efficient as the normal enzyme in destroying succinylcholine used intravenously as a muscle relaxant. In affected individuals the action of the drug is prolonged markedly. The effect is immediate and dose-related.

Biochemical abnormalities are indicated by the presence of atypical enzymes which have different properties with respect to substrates than the normal form of plasma cholinesterase. Atypical plasma cholinesterase can be detected by inhibition studies with compounds such as dibucaine and sodium fluoride.

Electrophoresis: Migration in starch gels of plasma cholinesterase in 4 or more separate activity bands can be demonstrated. No differences have been reported to date between the normal form and atypical cholinesterase. Separation of normal and atypical forms of plasma cholinesterase has been demonstrated on chromatographic columns.

References:
Goedde, H.W. et al: Pseudocholinesterasen: Pharmakogenetik Biochemie Klinik. Berlin:Springer-Verlag, 1967.
Harris, H. and Whittaker, M.: The genetics of drug sensitivity with special reference to suxamethonium. In Mongar, J.L. and de Reuck, A.V.S. (eds.): Ciba Foundation Symposium on Enzymes and Drug Action. Boston:Little Brown and Co., 1962.
Kalow, W.: Pharmacogenetics; Heredity and the Response to Drugs. Philadelphia:W.B. Saunders, 1962.

Contributors: **William R. Bergren**
George N. Donnell
Mai Park Suhr

CHONDRODYSPLASIA PUNCTATA, CONRADI-HÜNERMANN TYPE

Includes: Chondrodysplasie ponctuée, type Conradi-Hünermann
Condrodisplasia punctata, tipo Conradi-Hünermann
Chondrodystrophia calcificans
Dysplasia epiphysealis punctata (congenita)
Punctate epiphyseal dysplasia
Conradi-Hünermann syndrome

Excludes: Chondrodysplasia punctata, rhizomelic type (154)
Epiphyseal dysplasia, multiple (358)
Fetal warfarin syndrome (389)

Minimal Diagnostic Criteria: Flat facial features, limb shortening and multiple punctate calcifications in an infant without coronal clefts of the vertebral bodies. Prenatal history should exclude in utero exposure to warfarin.†

Clinical Findings: This skeletal dysplasia is characterized by frequent asymmetry of limbs, flat facies with depressed nasal bridge and punctate skeletal calcifications. Scoliosis may develop in the 1st year of life as may contractures of the large joints (approximately 30%), cataracts (20%), ichthyosiform skin changes or alopecia (20%).

Radiographs show punctate calcifications affecting primarily the ends of the long bones, carpal and tarsal regions, processes of the vertebrae, and ischiopubic bones; irregular deformities of the vertebral bodies and usually unilateral shortening of the tubular bones. In childhood and adulthood there is usually asymmetric shortening of the long tubular and metacarpal bones with epiphyseal deformities in areas in which punctate calcifications were present in infancy. Scoliosis and irregular deformities of the vertebral bodies are frequently present.

Complications
I   Derived: Severely affected patients may be stillborn or die during the 1st week of life. Hydramnios and hydrops are frequent in severe cases. Orthopedic problems may arise from asymmetric shortening of the limbs or from scoliosis. The epiphyseal deformities predispose to precocious arthritic changes in the affected joints.
II Associated: Congenital heart disease, hydronephrosis, optic atrophy, herniae.

Etiology: Autosomal dominant with considerable variability in phenotypic expression. Genetic heterogeneity is not excluded. McK *11865

Pathogenesis: ? Pathohistologic studies of epiphyseal cartilage show areas of "mucoid degeneration," cyst formation and calcification with invasion of highly vascularized fibrous tissue. Focal disruption of the growth plate by fibrous tissue has been observed in the rib.

Related Facts
I   Sex Ratio: ?
II Risk of Occurrence: ?
III Risk of Recurrence for
    Patient's Sib: If parent is affected 1 in 2 (50%) for each offspring to be affected: otherwise not increased.
    Patient's Child: 1 in 2
IV Age of Detectability: At birth
V   Prevalence: ?

Treatment
I   Primary Prevention: —
II Secondary Prevention: —
III Other Therapy: Appropriate for orthopedic problems, cataracts, and skin changes.

Prognosis: After the first weeks, life expectancy and mental development are normal. The adult height is usually above 130 cm.

The calcific stippling disappears during infancy.

Detection of Carrier: —

†**Special Considerations:** Calcific stippling in the newborn is a nonspecific finding. It has been observed in the Zellweger syndrome, G$_{M1}$ gangliosidosis, De Barsy syndrome, anencephaly, trisomy 21, trisomy 17, Smith-Lemli-Opitz syndrome and particularly after maternal coumadin ingestion during pregnancy. Intrauterine infection may cause neonatal calcific stippling. There may be additional genetic and environmental disorders mimicking the Conradi-Hünermann type of chondrodysplasia punctata.

References:
Spranger, J. et al: Heterogeneity of chondrodysplasia punctata. Humangenetik 11:190, 1971.

Contributor: **Jürgen W. Spranger**

Editor's Computerized Descriptors: Eye, Face, Nose, Skin, Hair, Skel.

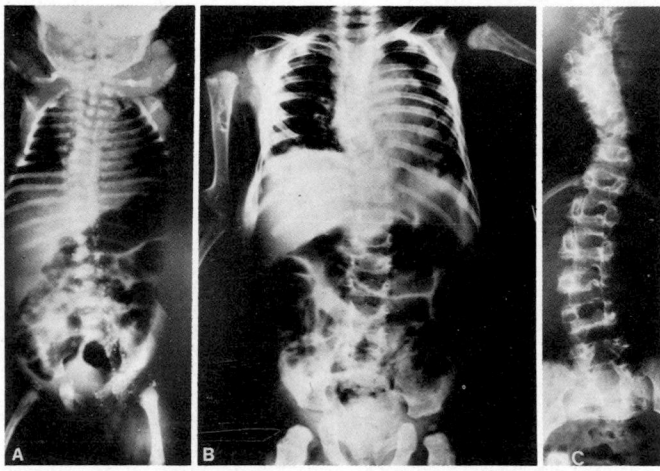

162. A) Newborn: Note widespread stippling; B) 9 months: Stippling no longer seen; short and deformed right humerus; C) 11 years: Marked scoliosis; irregular end plates of lumbar vertebrae

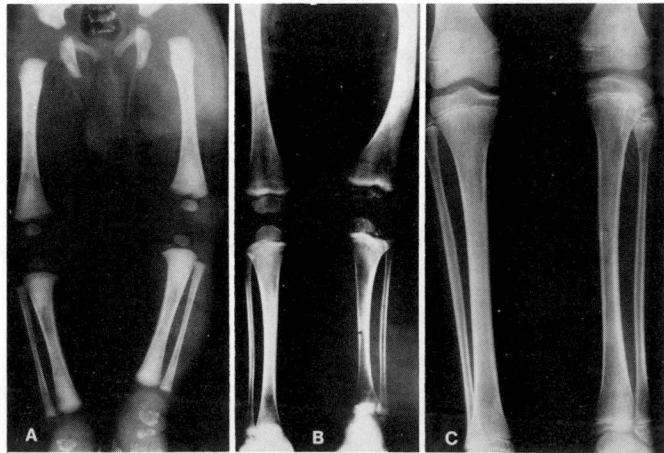

163. A) Newborn: Note discrete stippling in sacral spine, greater trochanters and tarsal bones; B) 2 years: Left leg shorter than right; external bowing of small, deformed left femur; C) 11 years: Short left tibia and fibula

CHONDRODYSPLASIA PUNCTATA, RHIZOMELIC TYPE

Includes: Chondrodysplasie ponctuée, type rhizomélique
Chondrodysplasia punctata, rhizomele Form
Condrodisplasia punctata, tipo rizomiélica

Excludes: Chondrodysplasia punctata, Conradi-Hünermann type (153)
Fetal warfarin syndrome (389)
Other, nonspecific forms of calcific stippling in the newborn
Cerebro-hepato-renal syndrome (139)

Minimal Diagnostic Criteria: Coronal clefts in lateral radiographic views of the vertebral bodies and shortening of the humeri or femora. The coronal clefts affect all or most of the vertebral bodies.

Clinical Findings: Disproportionate shortness of stature affecting primarily the proximal parts of the limbs; microcephaly in most cases; flat face with upward slanting of the palpebral fissures, lymphedema of the cheeks ("chipmunk" appearance) in the newborn; bilateral cataracts (approximately 80% of cases); ichthyosiform skin changes, alopecia (27%), contractures of multiple joints (60%).

Radiographs show dorsal and ventral ossification centers of the vertebral bodies in lateral views of the spine; symmetric shortening and metaphyseal irregularities of the humeri or femora; extracartilaginous and epiphyseal stippling in most cases; a trapezoid shape of the iliac bones in AP projections of the pelvis. Stippling is not a condition sine qua non. It disappears during the 1st year of life. The ossification centers of the vertebral bodies fuse during later infancy.

Complications
I **Derived:** Cerebral hypoplasia; severe mental deficiency; spastic quadriplegia in survivors with the syndrome
II **Associated:** Congenital heart disease; optic atrophy

Etiology: Autosomal recessive

Pathogenesis: ? Pathohistologic examination of the long bones shows disruption of the growth plates, foci of calcification, ossification, cyst formation and zones of inflammation. The changes possibly reflect some damage during development with subsequent healing of the cartilage by fibrosis, calcification and ossification. The clefts of the vertebral bodies are due to an embryonic arrest of development. The microcephaly is related to a decrease in the number of nerve cells found in neurohistologic examinations. Its cause is unknown.

Related Facts
I **Sex Ratio:** M1:F1
II **Risk of Occurrence:** Rare
III **Risk of Recurrence for**
　　Patient's Sib: Theoretically, 1 in 4 for each offspring to be affected; empirically 3 in 27
　　Patient's Child: Not increased unless mate is carrier or homozygote
IV **Age of Detectability:** At birth
V **Prevalence:** Very rare

Treatment
I **Primary Prevention:** Genetic counseling
II **Secondary Prevention:** —
III **Other Therapy:** Supportive

Prognosis: Lethal condition. Affected infants fail to thrive and usually die in the 1st weeks of life from recurrent infections. Patients who survive their 1st year of life are severely retarded in psychomotor development. They usually die before the age of 10 years.

Detection of Carrier: —

References:
Spranger, J. et al: Heterogeneity of chondrodysplasia punctata. Humangenetik 11:190, 1970.
Visekul,C. et al: Pathology of chondrodysplasia punctata, rhizomelic type. In Bergsma, D. (ed.): Skeletal Dysplasias. Birth Defects: Orig. Art. Ser., vol. 10, no. 12. Amsterdam: Excerpta Medica, for The National Foundation-March of Dimes. 1974, p. 327.

Contributor: **Jürgen W. Spranger**

Editor's Computerized Descriptors: Eye, Face, Skin, Hair, Skel., CV., Nerve

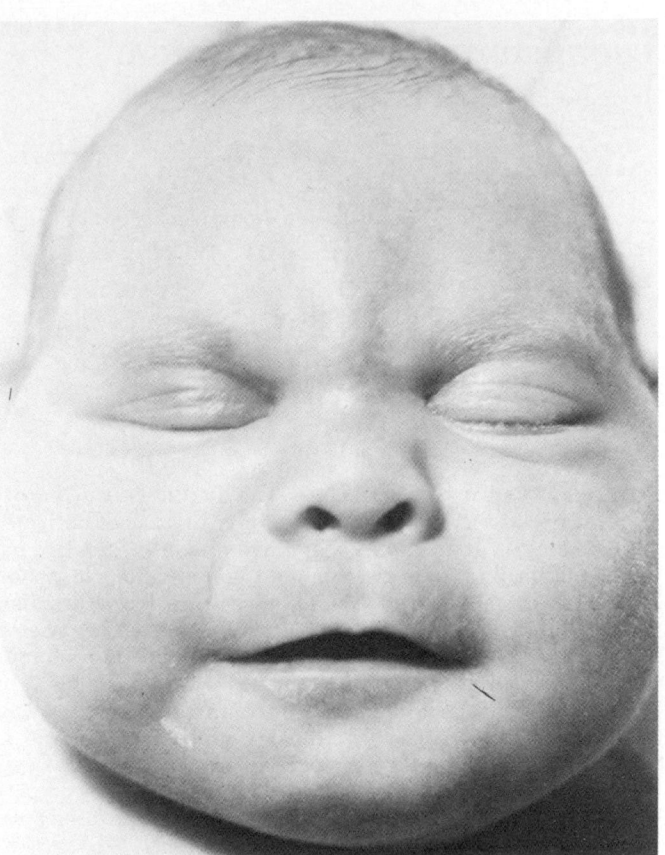

165. Facial features demonstrate a remarkable lymphedema of cheeks imparting chipmunk-like appearance

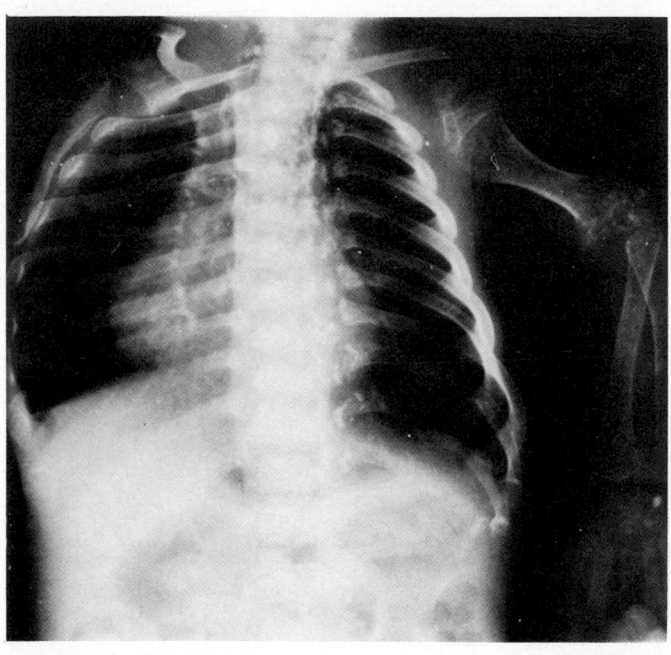

164. Note stippled calcifications at base of ribs, sternum and elbow; short humerus with widened metaphysis

CHONDRODYSTROPHIC MYOTONIA

Includes: Syndrome d'Aberfeld
Síndrome de Aberfeld
Dysostosis enchondralis meta epiphysaria (Catel-Hempel type)
Aberfeld syndrome
Schwartz-Jampel syndrome
Myotonic myopathy, dwarfism, chondrodystrophy, ocular and facial abnormalities

Excludes: Mucopolysaccharidoses
Arthrogryposis (88)
Cranio-carpo-tarsal dysplasia (223)
Seckel syndrome (881)
Mandibular arch syndrome with dwarfism
Myotonia congenita (701)
Myotonic dystrophy (702)
Heredofamilial myosclerosis (Löwenthal)

Minimal Diagnostic Criteria: The diagnosis is primarily clinical and the presence of myotonia has to be confirmed electromyographically. Biochemical abnormalities are not detectable and radiographic and histopathologic abnormalities are not characteristic. The association of dwarfism with skeletal deformities and myotonia of early onset is characteristic of the syndrome. Facial and ocular anomalies are always present but their severity is variable. The association of myotonia with short stature, > 2 SD below the mean for the age in children, and under 150 cm in adults has apparently not been reported outside this syndrome. In familial cases, a pattern of inheritance compatible with autosomal recessive transmission helps to substantiate the diagnosis.†

Clinical Findings: The birthweight is normal (2/4) or low (2/4). The first symptoms and signs appear at the end of the 1st year or during the 2nd year of life. Motor development is abnormally slow, growth falls below the normal range, skeletal deformities become apparent, the facial features change and myotonia is diagnosed after age 2 years. The disease is stationary after the 2nd year, motor function improves and, in 1 patient followed for over 5 years, myotonia diminished. Mental development was normal.

Eight patients with this syndrome, 4 of whom were studied personally and reported, had dwarfism, multiple skeletal deformities and myotonia. Based upon the 4 reported cases and 1 unreported case, the clinical findings also include the following: Skeletal deformities: short neck (5), pigeon breast deformity (5), kyphoscoliosis (5), hip dysplasia (4), joint contractures (5). Anomalies of the face: flattened face, relatively small in relation to the normal size of the skull (5), small mouth (5), small chin (5), fixed facial expression (5). Anomalies of the eyes: short and narrow palpebral apertures (5), shortening of the distance between the outer angles of the eyes in relation to the distance between the inner angles (5), increased distance between the inner angles of the eyes (1), intermittent, unilateral ptosis (2), microcornea, probable microphthalmus and bilateral pseudoptosis (3), severe myopia (2), juvenile cataract (1), eyelashes inserted in 2 or several rows instead of 1 row, as normal (3). Abnormalities of the skeletal muscles: increased consistency of the muscles (5), small muscles (2), generalized muscular hypertrophy (1), suspected muscular hypertrophy (1).

Other associated abnormalities include: transient lactosuria (1), umbilical and inguinal hernia (1), abnormally small testicles (1), patency of the anal sphincter (1), indistinct speech and drooling persisting after age 2 years.

Complications

I **Derived:** Inability to ambulate independently because of hip dysplasia. Limitation of movement because of joint contractures and myotonia. Impaired vision because of narrowing of the palpebral apertures, myopia or juvenile cataract. Psychologic abnormalities related to crippling by the disease and repeated or prolonged hospitalization.
II **Associated:** The number of patients studied is too small and the component features of the syndrome cannot be separated from the "associated defect."

Etiology: Autosomal recessive; Mck *25580

Pathogenesis: The primary effect of the mutant autosomal gene is not known and is apparently confined to tissues derived from the mesoderm. Bone biopsy was performed in 1 instance and revealed changes suggestive of abnormal ossification of the proximal epiphyseal cartilage plate of the femur. A generalized defect of enchondral ossification is perhaps responsible for the retarded growth rate and the anomalies of the facial and body skeleton. Of the 4 cases studied personally, the muscle biopsy was examined only with light microscopy in 2, and revealed diffuse muscle fiber atrophy with preservation of cross striation, increase of sarcolemmal nuclei and proliferation of fat and connective tissue, but no inflammatory changes. In the 2 remaining cases, studies of the muscle biopsy with light microscopy were normal, but electron microscopy revealed extensive vacuolation of the muscle fibers.

Related Facts
I **Sex Ratio:** M1:F1
II **Risk of Occurrence:** Rare, with no reliable occurrence figures. Two reported pairs were affected sibs.
III **Risk of Recurrence for**
  Patient's Sib: 1 in 4 (25%) for each sib
  Patient's Child: Not increased unless mate is carrier or homozygote. (None of the patients has yet reached reproductive age.)
IV **Age of Detectability:** Ordinarily in the 2nd year of life the condition can be suspected clinically.
V **Prevalence:** Rare, specific figures are not available. One affected pair of sibs was of Italian descent, the other of Irish descent.

Treatment
I **Primary Prevention:** Genetic counseling
II **Secondary Prevention:** Surgical widening of the palpebral apertures; orthopedic treatment for joint contractures and hip dysplasia; correction of refractive errors with glasses.
III **Other Therapy:** —

Prognosis: For life: There is no evidence that life expectancy is shortened. All but 1 patient, who died accidentally, are still alive. For intelligence: All patients have had normal intelligence. For function: Satisfactory, provided that adequate corrective measures are taken for the ocular and orthopedic abnormalities.

Detection of Carrier: —

†**Special Considerations:** The diagnosis of this syndrome is necessarily clinical since it is not known to be associated with specific biochemical, cytogenetic or histopathologic changes. The presence of muscle disease with myotonia is one of the essential features of the syndrome, but can easily be overlooked because skeletal and oculofacial abnormalities dominate the clinical picture. The patients in whom this syndrome was first identified were believed to have congenital blepharophimosis and a unique generalized myopathy due to discrepancy between the skeletal growth and growth of the muscles. They were not known to have diffuse bone disease or myotonia and the growth retardation was not considered a significant feature. There is at least one much earlier report describing similarly affected

patients in whom the presence of myotonia was not investigated, although the patients were known to have muscle disease. The correct diagnosis cannot be made without the use of electromyography because abnormally slow muscle relaxation, as in myotonia, is a nonspecific clinical abnormality.

References:
Aberfeld, D.C. et al: Myotonia, dwarfism, diffuse bone disease and unusual ocular and facial abnormalities (a new syndrome). Brain 88:313, 1965.
Aberfeld, D.C. et al: Chondrodystrophic myotonia: Report of two new cases; myotonia, dwarfism, diffuse bone disease and unusual ocular and facial abnormalities. Arch. Neurol. 22:455, 1970.
Catel, W.: Differentialdiagnostische Symptomatologie von Krankheiten des Kindesalters. 2nd Ed. Stuttgart:Georg Thieme Verlag, 1951, p. 58.
Fowler, W.M., Jr. et al: The Schwartz-Jampel syndrome. Its clinical, physiological and histological expressions. J. Neurol. Sci. 22:127, 1974.
Huttenlocher, P.R. et al: Osteo-chondro-muscular dystrophy: A disorder manifested by multiple skeletal deformities, myotonia and dystrophic changes in muscle. Pediatrics 44:945, 1969.
Pavone, L. et al: Schwartz-Jampel syndrome in two daughters of first cousins. J. Neurol. Neurosurg. Psychiatry, 41:161, 1978.

Contributor: **Donald C. Aberfeld**

Editor's Computerized Descriptors: Vision, Eye, Face, Speech, Neck, Hair, Skel., Muscle, Hernia not CNS, GU.

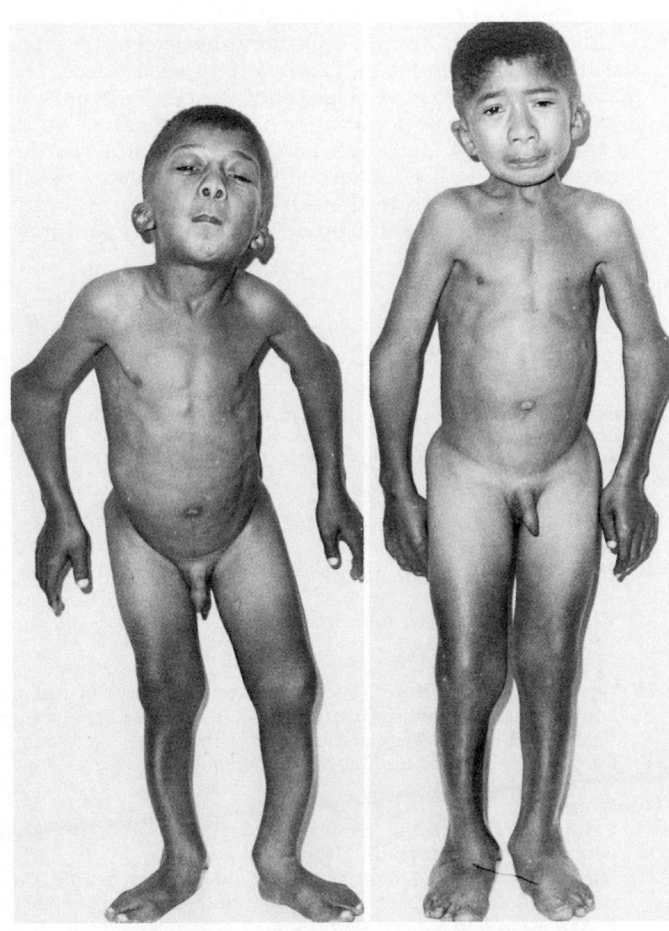

166. Note short neck, joint contractures, fixed facial expression, small mouth and ptosis

CHONDROECTODERMAL DYSPLASIA

Includes: Dysplasie chondro-ectodermique
Chondroektodermale Dysplasie
Displasia condroectodérmica
Ellis-van Creveld syndrome
Mesoectodermal dysplasia
Six-fingered dwarfism
Polydactyly and chondrodystrophy
Dwarfism, polydactly and dysplastic nails

Excludes: Asphyxiating thoracic dysplasia (91)
Other short-limb dwarfism detectable at birth

Minimal Diagnostic Criteria: Postaxial polydactyly of the hands with short-limbed dwarfism and dysplastic fingernails

Clinical Findings: Short-limb dwarfism and postaxial polydactyly permit recognition at birth. All cases have postaxial polydactyly of the hands. Polydactyly of the feet occurs in a minority of cases, perhaps 10%. The extra fingers are rather well developed. All cases have dysplasia of the fingernails which are underdeveloped. So-called partial harelip is usual and consists of a midline puckering of the upper lip with prominent frenulum. This condition is associated with natal teeth that erupt and exfoliate very early.

The shortening of the limbs is more striking in the distal portion, eg forearms and legs, rather than the proximal parts; in the fingers the proximal phalanges are longer than the middle and distal phalanges so that the patient cannot make a tight fist.

Genu valgum is always present and by age 5 or 6 typical x-ray changes consist of erosion of the lateral aspect of the proximal tibial metaphysis. X-ray views of the pelvis show a trident configuration over the acetabulum rather like that of asphyxiating thoracic dysplasia. A characteristic x-ray finding in the wrist is fusion of the hamate and capitate bones.

Over half the patients have congenital malformation of the heart, usually large atrial septal defect either ostium primum or ostium secundum type, more often the former. Occasionally the patient is cyanotic.

Complications
I **Derived:** Heart failure, respiratory failure from thoracic and tracheobronchial abnormalities, severe leg deformity especially knock-knees.
II **Associated:** Natal teeth, precocious exfoliation of teeth, epispadias

Etiology: Autosomal recessive†; McK *22550

Pathogenesis: ?

Related Facts
I **Sex Ratio:** M1:F1
II **Risk of Occurrence:** Ordinarily very rare, no racial predilection. Very frequent in one Amish group.
III **Risk of Recurrence for**
  Patient's Sib: 1 in 4 (25%) for each offspring to be affected
  Patient's Child: Not increased unless spouse is carrier in which case risk is 1 in 2.
IV **Age of Detectability:** At birth
V **Prevalence:** Very low†

Treatment
I **Primary Prevention:** Genetic counseling
II **Secondary Prevention:** Orthopedic correction of genu valgum, amputation of extra digits and surgical repair of cardiac malformation.
III **Other Therapy:** —

Prognosis: In about one-third of cases death occurs under 6

months of age. Survival to adulthood occurs, especially in those patients who are free of cardiac malformation.

Detection of Carrier: ?

†Special Considerations: Among the Old Order Amish of Lancaster County, Pennsylvania, over 80 cases in 40 sibships have been observed. Founder effect, endogamy and consanguinity and perhaps random genetic drift are factors responsible for the high frequency of the condition in this group. It has been reported rarely in many other ethnic groups.

References:

McKusick, F.A. et al: Dwarfism in the Amish. I. The Ellis-ven Crevald syndrome. Bull. Johns Hopk. Hosp. 115:306, 1964.

Murdoch, J.L. and Walker, B.A.: Ellis-van Creveld syndrome. In Bergsma, D. (ed.): Part IV. Skeletal Dysplasias. Birth Defects: Orig. Art. Ser., vol. V. no. 4. New York: The National Foundation-March of Dimes, 1969, p. 279.

Contributor: **Victor A. McKusick**

Editor's Computerized Descriptors: Face, Oral, Teeth, Nails, Skel., Resp., CV., GU.

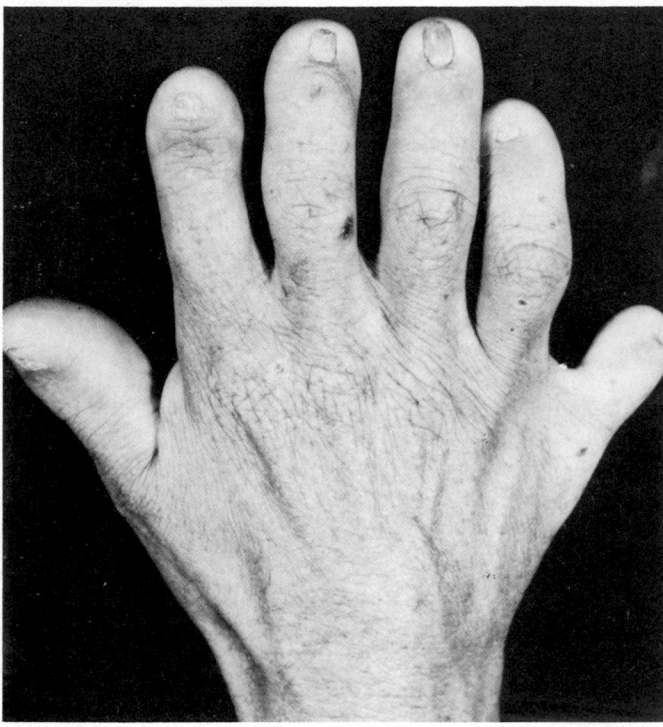

167. Note polydactyly, brachydactyly and nail hypoplasia

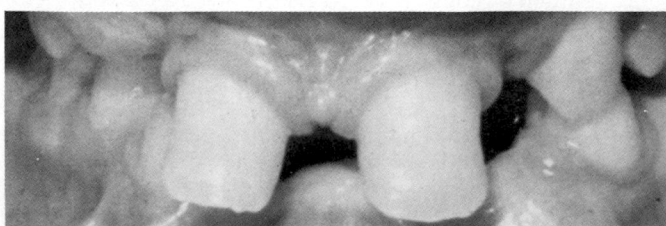

168. Hypertrophied frenula; note barrel-shaped incisors

CHROMOSOME EIGHT TRISOMY SYNDROME

Includes: Trisomie 8
Síndrome de la trisomía 8
Trisomy-8/normal diploid mosaicism

Excludes: Other C trisomies not involving 8

Minimal Diagnostic Criteria: Normal stature, long, narrow trunk with multiple joint retractions, rib and vertebral anomalies, deep palmar and plantar furrows, and a trisomy of chromosome 8, as shown by banding techniques.†

Clinical Findings: Birthweight and stature are normal.

There is moderate psychomotor retardation, particularly speech which is often delayed and poorly articulated; a slender build with narrow shoulder and pelvic girdle; joint contractures and deviations, particularly of the fingers and toes (clinodactyly and camptodactyly); and other skeletal anomalies, especially of ribs and vertebrae. Kyphoscoliosis is common in older patients. The face is often asymmetric with a sharp or broad-based pug nose, an everted lower lip, and a high-arched or cleft palate. The ears may be large and malformed, often with a prominent anthelix which is fused to the descending portion of the helix, and a large, rotated lobule. Other striking features include a short neck, absence or hypoplasia of the patellae, and deep palmar or plantar furrows.

Visceral anomalies consist of congenital heart malformations, particularly septal defects and large vessel anomalies; renal defects, often hydronephrosis and ureteral reflux; and agenesis of the corpus callosum.

Laboratory findings are unremarkable except for a partial deficit of coagulation factor VII in some cases. Dermatoglyphics reveal low ridge counts, excessive number of arches or the unusual association of both arches and whorls on the fingertips, and high palmar and plantar pattern intensity. Focal EEG abnormalities are common. Roentgenograms demonstrate the skeletal contractures or anomalies, in particular spina bifida occulta and supernumerary vertebrae and ribs.

Complications
I   **Derived:**   Based largely on the problems arising from musculoskeletal and visceral malformations.
II **Associated:** —

Etiology: Chromosome nondisjunction, due to unknown factors.

Pathogenesis: Most probably genetic overdosage interfering with ontogenic process.

Related Facts
I   **Sex Ratio:**   M12:F5
II   **Risk of Occurrence:**   Undetermined. A number of cases may be unrecognized.
III **Risk of Recurrence for**
     Patient's Sib: ?
     Patient's Child: ?
IV   **Age of Detectability:**   Usually in the first days of life, or incidentally by amniotic fluid cell culture and karyotyping. May fail to be recognized until later in life.
V   **Prevalence:**   Reliable figures unavailable.†

Treatment
I   **Primary Prevention:**   Antenatal diagnosis
II   **Secondary Prevention:**   None
III **Other Therapy:**   Symptomatic and aimed at correcting anatomic defects or alleviating their manifestations. Special education and speech therapy may prove beneficial.

Prognosis: Life span unknown. Adult patients have been identified.

Detection of Carrier: —

†**Special Considerations:** Clinical familiarity with this syndrome will possibly reveal it to be more common than heretofore recognized.

References:
Atkins, L. et al: Trisomy 8. J. Pediatr. 84:302 1974.
Cassidy, S.B. et al: Trisomy 8 syndrome. Pediatrics 56:826, 1975.
Crandall, B.F. et al: The trisomy 8 syndrome: Two additional mosaic cases. J. Med. Genet. 11:393, 1974.
Jacobsen, P. et al: The trisomy 8 syndrome: Report of two further cases. Ann. Genet. 17:87, 1974.
Van Eys, J. et al: C autosomal trisomy with mosaicism: A new syndrome? Pediatrics 45:665, 1970.

Contributors: **Suzanne B. Cassidy**
Barbara J. McGee
Eric Engel

Editor's Computerized Descriptors: Ear, Face, Oral, Nose, Speech, Neck, Skin, Dermatoglyphic, Skel., CV., GU., Nerve

---

CHROMOSOME EIGHTEEN p- SYNDROME

Includes: Amputation (délétion) du bras court du chromosome 18
Síndrome de la delección 18p

Excludes: Chromosome eighteen q- syndrome (159)
Turner syndrome (977)

Minimal Diagnostic Criteria: Typically, one finds an individual with mental retardation, short stature, facial dysmorphy, skeletal abnormalities and severe dental caries. A deletion involving the short arm of chromosome 18 should be demonstrated in at least a proportion of dividing cells.

Clinical Findings: This summary is based on 67 cases. In addition to low birthweight, there may be webbing of the neck, lymphedema, shield chest and widely spaced nipples. Short stature is very common, as well as mental retardation of extremely variable degree. Hypertelorism, epicanthic folds, strabismus and ptosis are common, and the nasal bridge is generally flattened or broad. Nasal bones were absent in 1 case. The ears tend to be large, floppy, poorly formed and may be low set. A small mandible and severe dental caries are common. Stubby hands with short fingers, high-set thumbs, and partial syndactyly of the toes are seen. Less common malformations include microcephaly, cataract, cebocephaly, arhinencephaly, cleft lip and palate, cyclops deformity, and congenital alopecia. Mental retardation, ranging from borderline to profound, is present in virtually all patients. Among the mentally retarded patients, one also finds aphasia or dysphasia.

Negative findings of note are the absence of cardiac, renal or GI malformations, or characteristic dermatoglyphic changes.

Complications
I   **Derived:** —
II **Associated:** —

Etiology: Deletion of part or all of the short arm of 1 chromosome 18†

Pathogenesis: ?

Related Facts
I   **Sex Ratio:** M8:F15
II   **Risk of Occurrence:** ?
III **Risk of Recurrence for**
    Patient's Sib: Very low except when a parent has a balanced translocation (5 of 67 cases), when the recurrence risk may be as high as 1 in 4, or mosaicism (3 of 67 cases), with a similar though probably somewhat lower risk.
    Patient's Child: —
IV   **Age of Detectability:** At birth or prenatally by karyotype study of fetal cells
V   **Prevalence:** ?

Treatment
I   **Primary Prevention:** Genetic counseling
II   **Secondary Prevention:** —
III **Other Therapy:** —

Prognosis: Dependent on severity of associated defects; otherwise life span not decreased.

Detection of Carrier: Balanced translocation carrier or mosaic, recognizable only by karyotype analysis; at present, this would be looked for only after the birth of an affected child.

†**Special Considerations:** Maternal and paternal ages tend to be advanced in contrast to the findings in other types of structural chromosomal abnormalities.

References:

de Grouchy, J.: The 18p-, 18q- and 18r syndromes. In Bergsma, D.
(ed.): Part V. Phenotypic Aspects of Chromosomal Aberrations.
Birth Defects: Orig. Art. Ser.,vol. V., no. 5, New York: The National Foundation-March of Dimes, 1969, p. 74.

Lurie, I. and Lazjuk, G.: Partial monosomies 18. Humangenetik
15:203, 1972.

Contributor: **Orlando J. Miller**

Editor's Computerized Descriptors: Eye, Ear, Face, Oral, Teeth,
Nose, Neck, Skin, Skel., Muscle, Hernia not CNS, Nerve

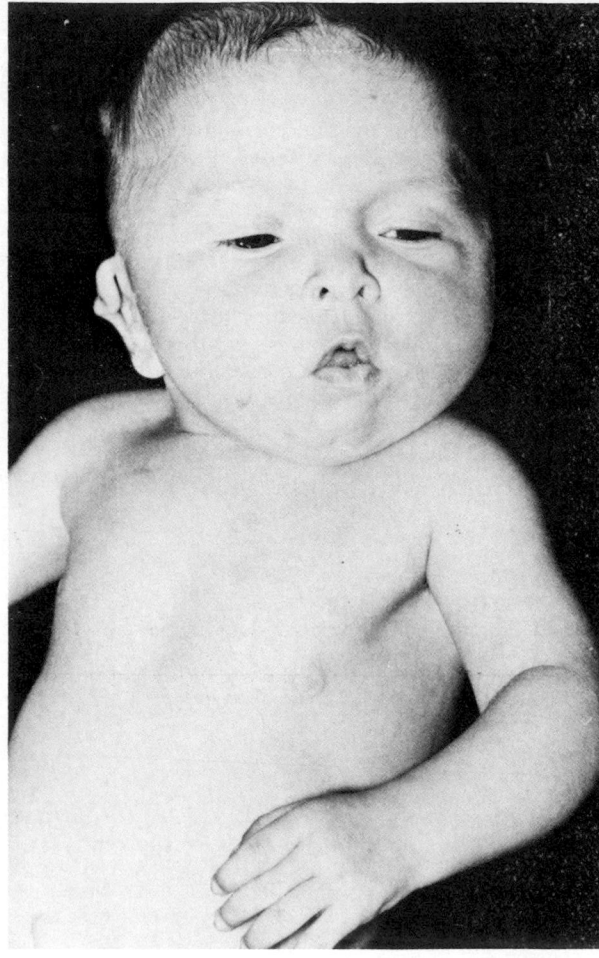

169. Note large floppy ear and facial features of chromosome
18p– syndrome

CHROMOSOME EIGHTEEN q- SYNDROME

Includes: Amputation (délétion) du bras long du chromosome 18
Síndrome de la delección 18q
Chromosome 18r syndrome (most cases)

Excludes: Chromosome eighteen p- syndrome (158)

Minimal Diagnostic Criteria: The characteristic facial dysmorphism, skeletal and ophthalmologic abnormalities should be seen.
Demonstration of a deletion (18q- or 18r) is confirmatory.

Clinical Findings: Study of 95 cases indicates there is a
characteristic syndrome, characterized by low birthweight,
short stature, microcephaly, midface dysplasia, carp-
shaped mouth, prominent anthelix and antitragus, atretic
ear canals, widely spaced nipples, very conspicuous suba-
cromial dimples and dimples on the epitrochlea, the sides
of the patellae and on the back of the hands. Long tapering
fingertips are common, as is clubfoot. Hypotonia is common, and mental retardation is usually profound. Eye defects include nystagmus, strabismus, glaucoma, tapetoretinal degeneration and bilateral optic atrophy. Congenital
heart disease and renal malformations are sometimes seen.
Whorl dermal patterns on the digits of the hands are often
found.

Complications
I **Derived:** Seizures occur in a minority of cases.
II **Associated:** Congenital heart disease and renal malforma-
tions

Etiology: Deletion of part of the long arm of chromosome 18

Pathogenesis: ?

Related Facts
I **Sex Ratio:** M10:F14
II **Risk of Occurrence:** ?
III **Risk of Recurrence for**
Patient's Sib: Low, except when either parent is a balanced
translocation carrier (5 of 57 families), where the risk may
approach 1 in 4, or a mosaic (6 of 57 families) where the risk
may be somewhat less.
Patient's Child: ? Oldest known patient is 11 years old.
IV **Age of Detectability:** At birth, or by karyotype analysis of
fetal cells
V **Prevalence:** ?

Treatment
I **Primary Prevention:** Genetic counseling
II **Secondary Prevention:** Prenatal karyotype analysis of fetal
cells when either parent is a translocation carrier or mosaic.
III **Other Therapy:** —

Prognosis: Severe mental retardation expected. Oldest patient is
11 years old.

Detection of Carrier: Balanced translocation carrier or mosaic,
recognizable by karyotype analysis; at present, screening is not
carried out and carriers are only identified after the birth of an
affected child.

Special Considerations: —

References:

de Grouchy, J.: The 18p-, 18q- and 18r syndromes. In Bergsma, D.
(ed.): Part V. Phenotypic Aspects of Chromosomal Aberrations.
Birth Defects: Orig. Art. Ser., vol. 5, no. 5., New York:The National Foundation-March of Dimes, 1969, p. 74.

Lurie, I. and Lazjuk, G.: Partial monosomies 18. Humangenetik
15:203, 1972.

Contributor: **Orlando J. Miller**

Editor's Computerized Descriptors: Eye, Hearing, Ear, Face, Oral, Nose, Skin, Dermatoglyphic, Skel., Muscle, CV., GU.

CHROMOSOME EIGHTEEN TRISOMY SYNDROME

Includes: Syndrome d'Edwards
Trisomie 18
Síndrome de la trisomía 18
Edwards syndrome
Chromosome trisomy 17-18 syndrome
Chromosome E1-trisomy syndrome
Chromosome trisomy 17 syndrome
Chromosome partial 17 trisomy

Excludes: Chromosome thirteen trisomy syndrome (168)

Minimal Diagnostic Criteria: Eighteen trisomy syndrome should be suspected when patient has 5 or more clinical findings listed below with frequency of 50% or more. Chromosomal study is urged in every instance because of very serious implications.

Certain features help to delineate this syndrome from the 13 trisomy syndrome, particularly those features, for example, which occur 50% more commonly in 18 trisomy than in 13 trisomy: hypertonia, cat-like cry, prominent occiput, superficially normal brain, meningomyelocele, webbed neck, short sternum, eventration (thinning) of the diaphragm, pyloric stenosis, horseshoe kidney, hydronephrosis and hydroureter, Meckel diverticulum, limited hip abduction, distally implanted thumb, retroflexible thumb, partial syndactyly, hypoplasia of nails, simple arches of fingertips, short dorsiflexed big toe, talipes equinovalgus, and prominent calcaneus.

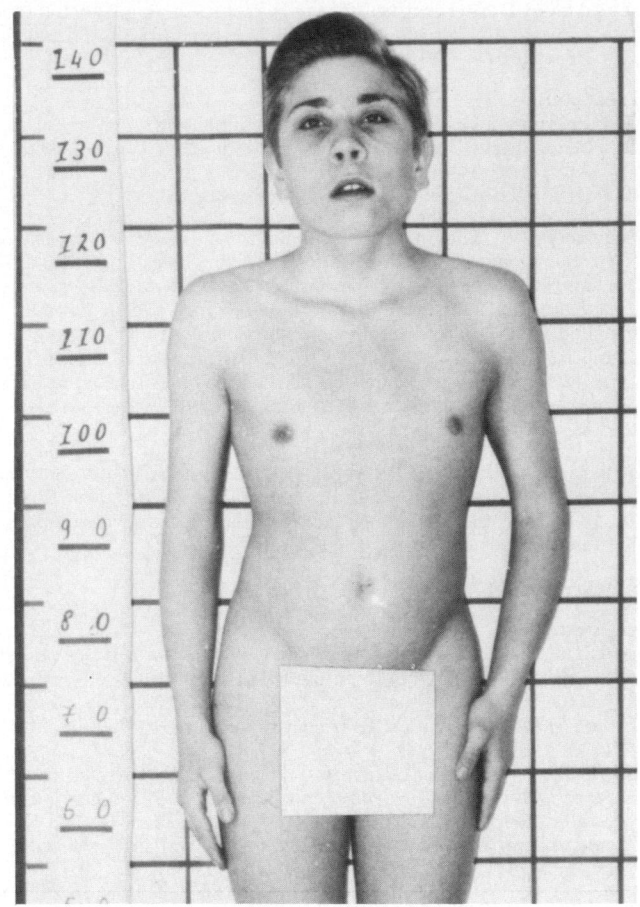

170. Chromosome 18r syndrome in young adult male. Note carp-shaped mouth

Clinical Findings:

Developmental and mental retardation	100%
Failure to thrive	100%
Cryptorchidism	100%
Difficulty feeding with poor suck	> 95%
Congenital heart disease (especially ventricular septal defect and patent ductus)	> 95%
Low-set, malformed ears	> 80%
Prominent occiput with elongated skull	> 80%
Narrow palatal arch	> 80%
Micrognathia	> 80%
Short sternum	> 80%
Single umbilical artery	> 80%
Flexion deformity of fingers	> 80%
Overlapping fingers	> 80%
Simple arches on 6 or more digits	> 80%
Small pelvis	> 80%
Limited hip abduction	> 80%
Hypotonia followed by hypertonia	50-80%
Short neck	50-80%
Heart murmur	50-80%
Inguinal or umbilical hernia	50-80%
Distal t triradius	50-80%
Short, dorsiflexed big toe	50-80%
Prominent calcaneus	50-80%
Renal malformations, especially horseshoe kidney and hydronephrosis and hydroureter	50-80%
Retroflexible thumb	40-60%
Distally implanted thumb	40-60%
Extra skin nape of neck	40-60%

Calcaneovalgus feet	40-60%
Meckel diverticulum	40-60%
Eventration of diaphragm	10-50%
Ptosis of eyelids	10-50%
Epicanthal folds	10-50%
Corneal opacities	10-50%
Microphthalmos	10-50%
Short upper lip	10-50%
Brain or spinal cord malformation	10-50%
Webbed neck	10-50%
Widely spaced nipples	10-50%
Pyloric stenosis	10-50%
Partial syndactyly	10-50%
Ulnar or radial deviation of hands	10-50%
Single palmar creases	10-50%
Single crease of 5th finger	10-50%
Hypoplastic finger and toe nails	10-50%
Cat-like cry	10-50%
Malrotation of the bowel	10-20%
Neonatal jaundice	10-20%
Meningomyelocele	10-20%
Cleft lip or palate	10-20%
Choanal atresia	< 10%
Tracheoesophageal fistula	< 10%
Pyloric stenosis	< 10%
Fibular S hallucal pattern	< 10%
Prominent clitoris	?
Bifid uterus	?
Ovarian hypoplasia	?
Imperforate anus	?
Malformed funnel-shaped anus	?
Dislocation of hips	?
Lobster-claw deformity	?
Phocomelia	?
External auditory canal stenosis and hearing loss	?

Complications

I **Derived:** See Clinical Findings

II **Associated:** Severe feeding and respiratory (aspiration) problems

Etiology: The cause of 18 trisomy with 47 chromosomes is thought to be nondisjunction during meiosis. Cases of 18 trisomy/normal mosaicism involve, at least in addition, postzygotic nondisjunction or anaphase lag. The causes of meiotic and mitotic nondisjunction involving chromosome 18 are unknown. The factors by which advancing maternal age increase the risk of meiotic nondisjunction are also unknown. Eighteen trisomy syndrome results from triplication of part or all of chromosome 18 in some or all of the patient's cells. This may be due to trisomy/normal mosaicism, or a translocation resulting in partial trisomy. Except in the case of inherited translocations, the parent donating the extra chromosome material has not been identified, although the association between 18 trisomy and increasing maternal age makes it likely that the mother is the more common contributor of the extra chromosome.

Pathogenesis: ?

Related Facts

I **Sex Ratio:** At birth M1:F1.8, after 3 months M1:F2.9

II **Risk of Occurrence:** 1 in 6600 live births in North America and Great Britian

III **Risk of Recurrence for**
  Patient's Sib: Probably no greater than 2-3%
  Patient's Child: ? No patient has reproduced.

IV **Age of Detectability:** Early in gestation, in suspected cases, by amniocentesis, cell culture and chromosomal analysis

V **Prevalence:** Very low

Treatment

I **Primary Prevention:** Genetic counseling

II **Secondary Prevention:** Amniocentesis, culture and karyotypic study of fetal cells, if parent is a carrier

III **Other Therapy:** As may be indicated

Prognosis: The diagnosis should be carefully confirmed chromosomally since the prognosis is grim: 30% of patients die by 1 month of age, 50% by 2 months, 70% by 3 months, 90% by 1 year, and 99% before age 10. The survivors are profoundly retarded in motor and intellectual development. None have been able to walk, talk or procreate. The usual causes of death are aspiration, apnea or congenital heart disease. The prognosis may, however, be significantly better in patients with mosaicism or translocations.

Detection of Carrier: Parents or sibs of an affected child may have a balanced translocation or mosaicism. High-risk families may also be identifiable by careful pedigree and chromosomal studies.

Special Considerations: —

References:

Hecht, F. et al: The No. 17-18 trisomy syndrome. Studies on cytogenetics, dermatoglyphics, parental age and linkage. J. Pediatr. 63:605, 1963.

Smith, D.W. et al: The no. 18 trisomy syndrome. J. Pediatr. 60:513, 1962.

Taylor, A.I.: Autosomal trisomy syndromes: A detailed study of 27 cases of Edwards' syndrome and 27 cases of Patau's syndrome. J. Med. Genet. 5:227, 1968.

Yunis, J.J. et al: Deoxyribose-nucleic-acid replication pattern of trisomy 18. Lancet 2:286, 1964.

Contributor: **Frederick Hecht**

Editor's Computerized Descriptors: Eye, Ear, Face, Oral, Skin, Nails, Skel., Muscle, Hernia not CNS, CV., GI., Liver, GU., Nerve

CHROMOSOME ELEVEN q PARTIAL TRISOMY SYNDROME

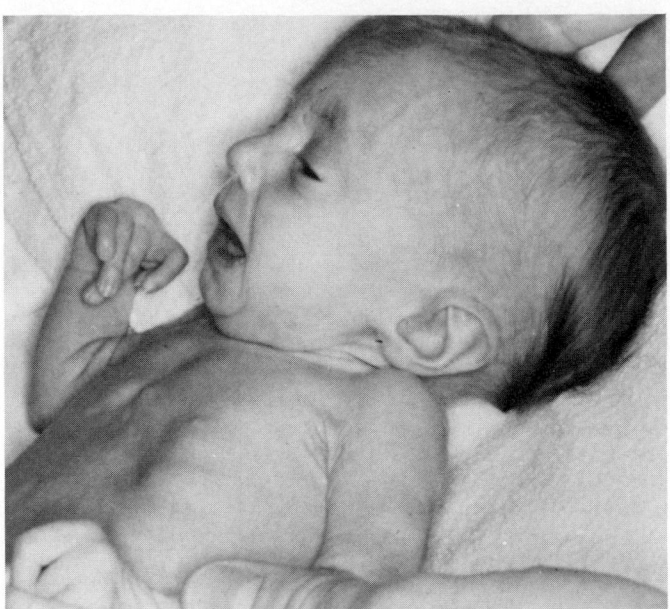

171. Characteristic facies and hand position in trisomy 18

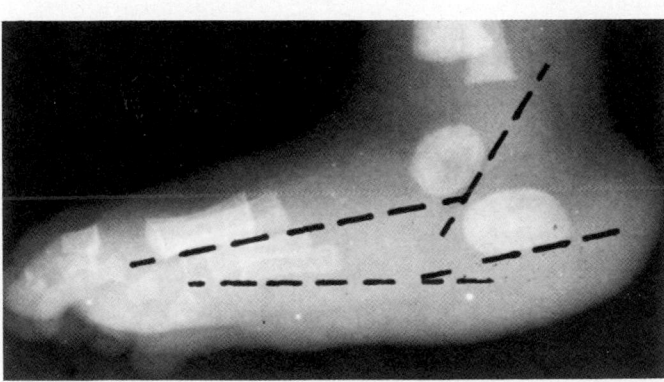

172. Rockerbottom foot deformity. Note reversal of angle between talus and 5th metatarsal, and angle between calcaneous and 1st metatarsal

Includes: Partielle Trisomie 11q
Síndrome de trisomía parcial del cromosoma 11q
Duplication of distal 11q

Excludes: —

Minimal Diagnostic Criteria: Pre- and postnatal growth deficiency, psychomotor retardation, short nose and long philtrum, microretrognathia, clavicular defect, micropenis, congenital heart defect and demonstration of the cytogenetic abnormality.

Clinical Findings: (Based on 13 chromosomally proven cases.) Moderate prenatal and postnatal growth deficiency (12/13); moderate-to-profound psychomotor retardation (5/5); microcephaly (8/10); short nose and long philtrum (11/11); microretrognathia (13/13); retracted lower lip (10/12); low-set ears (9/12); poorly developed helix and prominent anthelix (7/8); cleft palate (6/13). In the newborn, hypotonia of the trunk is combined with hypertonic limbs, feeding difficulties, and cutis laxa. Skeletal defects include dysplastic acetabulum: dislocated hip (4/5); talipes equinovarus (4/6); and clavicular defects (3/3). Congenital cardiac defects are most often septal defect or patent ductus arteriosus (11/11). Males have micropenis without hypospadias (6/7). Occasional visceral defects include inguinal and umbilical herniae and urinary tract malformations. CNS malformations include neural tube closure defects (2/2), and agenesis of corpus callosum (2/2).

Dermatoglyphics show high ridge counts on fingertips, frequent interdigital patterns and radial displacement of the palmar triradius a (3/13).†

Complications
I   **Derived:** Cardiac or renal failure
II **Associated:** —

Etiology: Duplication of the distal 1/3 to 2/3 of the long arm of chromosome 11 (region 11q21, q22, or q23→11qter) usually derived from a balanced reciprocal translocation in either parent. In the 13 reported cases, the unbalanced chromosome was maternally derived in 10 and paternally in 3.

Pathogenesis: ?

Related Facts
I   **Sex Ratio:** M7:F6
II   **Risk of Occurrence:** Rare
III **Risk of Recurrence for**
    Patient's Sib: Estimated to be between 15 and 33% depending upon sex of translocation carrier parent and on nature of translocation.
    Patient's Child: ?
IV **Age of Detectability:** At birth; prenatally by amniotic fluid cell culture and karyotyping.
V   **Prevalence:** ?

Treatment
I   **Primary Prevention:** Genetic counseling for translocation carriers
II   **Secondary Prevention:** Prenatal diagnosis by chromosome analysis of cultured amniotic fluid cells, if a parent has a balanced translocation.
III **Other Therapy:** Symptomatic for congenital defects; special education.

Prognosis: 6/13 died in 1st year of life; oldest survivor is 11 years old.†

Detection of Carrier: Chromosome analysis

†Special Considerations: Severity of manifestations and prognosis are related to the extent of the duplicated segment of 11q.

References:
Aurias, A. and Laurent, C.: Trisomie 11q. Individualisation d'un nouveau syndrome. Ann. Génét. 18:189, 1975.
Francke, U. et al: Duplication 11(q21 to 23→qter) syndrome. In Bergsma, D. (ed.): New Syndromes. Birth Defects: Orig. Art. Ser., vol. XIII, no. 3B New York: Alan R. Liss, Inc. for The National Foundation-March of Dimes, 1977, p. 167.
Giraud, F. et al: Trisomie partielle 11q et translocation familiale 11-22. Hum. Genet. 28:343, 1975.

Contributor: **Uta Francke**

Editor's Computerized Descriptors: Ear, Face, Nose, Skin, Dermatoglyphic, Skel., Muscle, Hernia not CNS, CV., GI., GU., Nerve

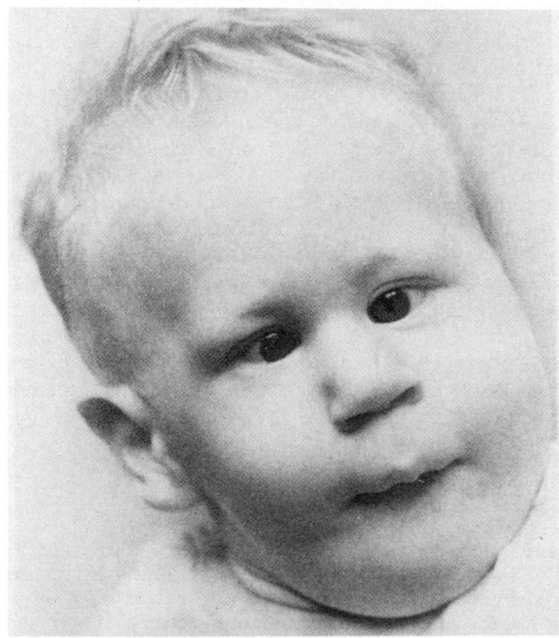
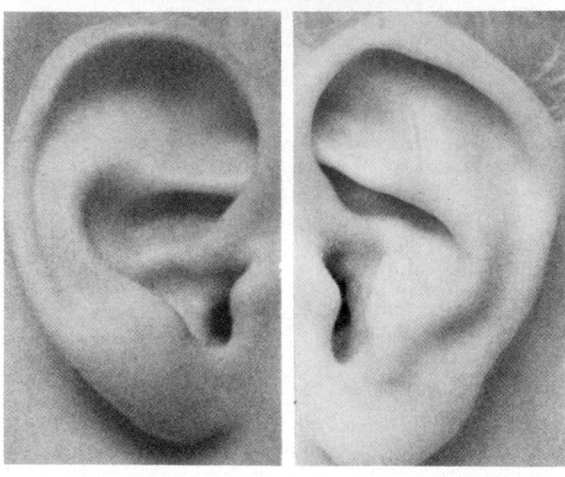

173. Chromosome 11q partial trisomy syndrome. Note differing shapes of auricles

CHROMOSOME ELEVEN q- SYNDROME

Includes: Monosomie partielle 11q
Síndrome del cromosoma 11q-
Partial monosomy of distal 11q

Excludes: Partial monosomy for proximal 11q
Proximal 11q- syndrome

Minimal Diagnostic Criteria: Growth and developmental delay, scaphocephaly, characteristic facies, shortening of fingers and toes, and demonstration of cytogenetic defect.

Clinical Findings: (Based on 10 cases). Intrauterine growth retardation present in 3/10; postnatal growth retardation present in 10/10; psychomotor retardation ranges from mild to profound; speech defect is severe. Scaphocephaly or trigonocephaly is present with premature fusion of metopic suture. Most have hypertelorism and epicanthus, a short broad nose with anteverted nares, a poorly formed or absent philtrum, a thin upper lip and microretrognathia. Palpebral fissures are horizontal in 5/10, upslanting in 3/10 and downslanting in 2/10. Ocular findings include ptosis 3/10, iris coloboma 2/10, notch in upper eyelid 1/10. The external ears are often low-set and unusually shaped with prominent anthelix, and small or absent lobes. Digital abnormalities include irregular and asymmetric shortening of fingers and toes, and clinodactyly.

Congenital heart defects (predominantly ventricular septal defect) and hypospadias have been reported infrequently, as have renal duplication, hydronephrosis, pyloric stenosis, deafness, inguinal hernia and spina bifida occulta.

Complications
I   Derived: —
II Associated: —

Etiology: Deletion of distal 1/3-1/2 of the long arm of chromosome 11 (region 11q22 or q23→11qter), either due to a de novo breakage event during gametogenesis or a balanced translocation in either parent.

Pathogenesis: ?

Related Facts
I   Sex Ratio: Ml:Fl
II   Risk of Occurrence: Rare
III Risk of Recurrence for
      Patient's Sib: High if a parent is balanced translocation carrier; otherwise probably negligible.
      Patient's Child: Theoretically 50% risk.
IV   Age of Detectability: At birth or prenatally during 2nd trimester by amniotic fluid cell culture and karyotyping.
V   Prevalence: —

Treatment
I   Primary Prevention: Genetic counseling
II   Secondary Prevention: Prenatal diagnosis by chromosome analysis of cultured amniotic fluid cells, if a parent has a balanced translocation.
III Other Therapy: Symptomatic for congenital defects, special education.

Prognosis: ?

Detection of Carrier: By chromosome analysis

Special Considerations: —

References:
Engel, E. et al: Chromosome 11 long arm partial deletion: A new syndrome. Am. J. Ment. Defic. 80;473, 1976.
Francke, U.: Abnormalities of chromosomes 11 and 20. In Yunis J. (ed.): New Chromosomal Syndromes. New York: Academic Press, 1977.

Larson, S.A. et al: Deletion of 11q: Report of two cases and a review. In Bergsma, D. (ed.): Cytogenetics, Environment and Malformation Syndromes. Birth Defects: Orig. Art. Ser., vol XII, no. 5. New York: Alan R. Liss for The National Foundation-March of Dimes, 1976, p. 125.

Turleau, C. et al: Monosomie partielle 11q et trigonocephalie - un noveau syndrome. Ann Génét. (Paris) 18:257, 1975.

Contributor: **Uta Francke**

Editor's Computerized Descriptors: Eye, Hearing, Ear, Face, Nose, Speech, Skel., Hernia not CNS, CV., GU.

CHROMOSOME FIVE p- SYNDROME

Includes: Syndrome de délétion 5p
Katzenschreisyndrom
Síndrome de la deleción 5p
Cri du chat syndrome
Cat cry syndrome

Excludes: Chromosome four p- syndrome (164)

Minimal Diagnostic Criteria: The diagnosis is suspected on the basis of the more common features noted below. Although none is diagnostic, the characteristic cry in the younger patients is the most important feature. Confirmation is made by demonstrating a deletion involving the short arm of chromosome 5.

Clinical Findings: The most common, and therefore characteristic features are the cat-like, weak or high-pitched cry in infancy; growth failure; microcephaly; facial abnormalities including hypertelorism, downward slanting palpebral fissures, and micrognathia; and severe mental retardation. The more common features and their approximate frequencies are:

General:

Mental retardation (usually profound; IQ rarely above 35)	100%
Low birthweight (< 2,600 gm)	50%
Slow growth, height < 3rd percentile	85%
Feeding difficulties in infancy	>50%
Abnormal cry, usually cat-like, occasionally weak or high-pitched, in infancy (normalizes with age)	98%
Abnormal larynx	55-65%
Hypotonia (infancy) or poor muscular development (older)	60-80%

Craniofacial:

Microcephaly	98%
Face: round in infants, thin in adults	70%
Facial asymmetry (older patients)	25%
Broad base of nose (infancy) (less frequent in adults)	85%
Ears low-set or poorly formed	85%
Preauricular tags	40%
Micrognathia (infancy) (less common in adults)	75-85%
Prognathism in adults	Occasional
Malocclusion (older patients)	70-80%
Palate abnormal (either high and narrow or broad and flat)	50-75%
Frontal sinuses large (adults)	85-90%

Eye:

Hypertelorism (young patients) (less frequent in adults)	90-95%
Hypotelorism	Occasional
Epicanthal folds (young patients) (less frequent in adults)	85-90%
Oblique palpebral fissures (usually slant downward, occasionally upward)	75-85%
Strabismus, usually divergent, after infancy	60-70%
Deficient tears (Schirmer test) (adults)	6/6
Increased sensitivity of pupil to	

methacholine (adults)	5/5
Tortuous retinal vessels (adults)	6/6
Optic atrophy (adults)	2/6

Heart:

Congenital defects, types variable, patent ductus arteriosus most common	15-30%

Abdomen:

Inguinal hernia	25-30%
Diastasis recti	30-35%
Renal anomalies	Occasional

Limbs:

Short metacarpals or metatarsals (adult)	65-75%
Simian crease	80-90%
Distal axial triradius (t' or t'')	80-90%
Partial syndactyly	25-30%
Pes planus (older)	65-75%
Clinodactyly	Occasional

Skeletal:

Small wings of the ilia or increased iliac angle	70-80%
Scoliosis (adults)	55-65%

Other:

Short neck	45-65%
Premature greying of hair (adults)	30-35%
Cryptorchidism	Occasional

Complications

I **Derived:** Severe respiratory and feeding problems soon after birth

II **Associated:** —

Etiology: In most cases there is simple deletion of the short arm of chromosome 5 which presumably occurs during gametogenesis. The particular segment, loss of which results in the characteristic features, appears to be the distal portion of band p14 or proximal part of band p15. A 5p chromosome is usually present in every cell although there have been infrequent reports of cases with mosaicism in which normal cells are also found. Very occasionally the deletion results from ring formation or a de novo translocation (unbalanced).

The etiology of the chromosomal abnormality is usually not known; average parental age is not increased. However, between 10-15% of cases have inherited the 5p- chromosome from a parent who is heterozygous for a reciprocal translocation involving the short arm of 5. Very infrequently the deleted chromosome may be attributed to a pericentric inversion of chromosome 5 or mosaicism with normal and 5p- cells in a parent.

Pathogenesis: ?

Related Facts

I **Sex Ratio:** There has been a preponderance of females among infants and young children. The sex ratio is more nearly equal in the patients identified in later life. These differences may reflect a bias in ascertainment.

II **Risk of Occurrence:** Of 59,452 unselected newborns studied cytogenetically 3 (or 1 per 20,000) had deletion of the short arm of chromosome 5. One of these cases was a mosaic with normal and 5p- cells.

III **Risk of Recurrence for**

Patient's Sib: Appears to be low (exact figure not available) unless a parent is a carrier of a reciprocal translocation of an inversion involving chromosome 5 or is a mosaic with normal or 5p- cells. In cases with a parental translocation the risk appears to be between 15-25%. Because of the rarity of cases with parental inversion or mosaicism the risk is unknown, but is presumed to be increased.

Patient's Child: ? No known reproduction by a patient. If reproduction were to occur, risk could be up to 50%.

IV **Age of Detectability:** At birth or prenatally by karyotype analysis

V **Prevalence:** General population unknown. Up to 1% of profoundly retarded (IQ < 20) individuals have this syndrome.

Treatment

I **Primary Prevention:** Genetic counseling

II **Secondary Prevention:** Prenatal diagnosis when a parent is a translocation or inversion carrier or is a mosaic. Although recurrence risk appears to be "low" when parental karyotypes are normal, prenatal diagnosis may still be warranted since an exact risk figure has not been established.

III **Other Therapy:** Symptomatic only

Prognosis: Diminished life span, but many of these patients survive into adulthood. Survival to 56 years of age recorded.

Detection of Carrier: Karyotype studies of the parents

Special Considerations: —

References:

Breg, W.R.: Abnormalities of chromosomes 4 and 5. In Gardner, L.I. (ed.): Endocrine and Genetic Diseases of Childhood and Adolescence, 2nd Ed. Philadelphia: W.B. Saunders, 1975.

Breg, W.R. et al: The cri du chat syndrome in adolescents and adults: Clinical findings in 13 older patients with partial deletion of the short arm of chromosome No. 5(5p-). J. Pediatr. 77:782, 1970.

De Capoa, A. et al: Translocation heterozygosis: A cause of five cases of the cri du chat syndrome and two cases with a duplication of chromosome number five in three families. Am. J. Hum. Genet. 19:586, 1967.

Howard, R.O.: Ocular abnormalities in the cri du chat syndrome. Am. J. Ophthalmol. 73:949, 1972.

Labrune, M. et al: Étude des signes radiologiques de la maladie du cri du chat. Ann. Radiol. 10:303, 1967.

Niebuhr, E.: Localization of the deleted segment in the cri-du-chat syndrome. Humangenetik 16:357, 1972.

Ward, P.H. et al: The larynx in the cri du chat (cat cry) syndrome. Laryngoscope 78:1716, 1968.

Contributor: **W. Roy Breg**

Editor's Computerized Descriptors: Eye, Ear, Face, Oral, Teeth, Nose, Larynx, Speech, Neck, Dermatoglyphic, Hair, Skel., Muscle, Hernia not CNS, CV., GI., GU. Nerve

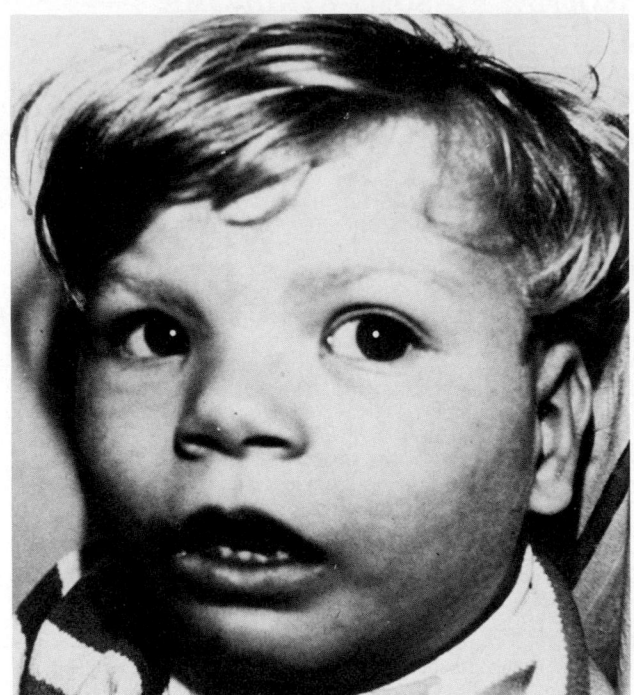

174. Chromosome 5p− syndrome. Note rounded facies

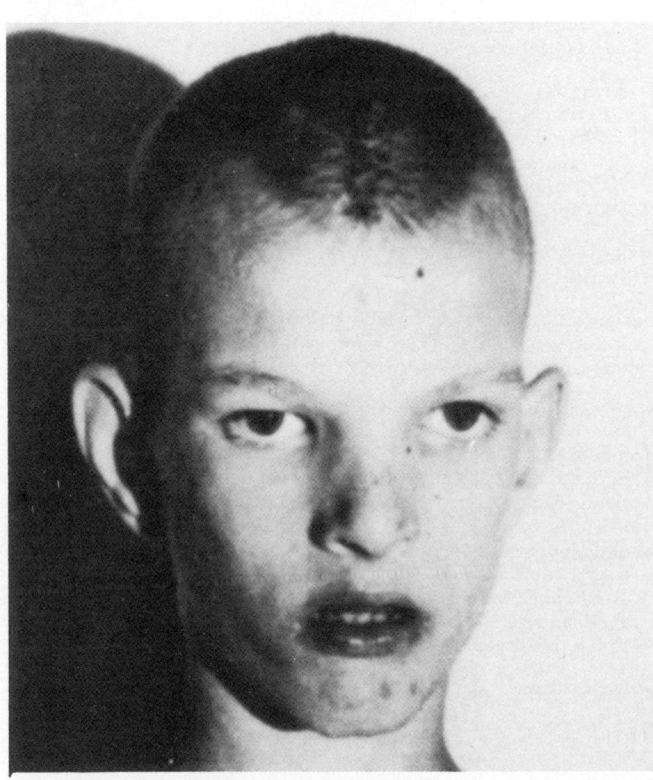

175. Chromosome 5p− syndrome in adolescent

CHROMOSOME FOUR p- SYNDROME

Includes: Délétion du bras court du chromosome 4
Síndrome del cromosoma 4p-
Wolf syndrome
Partial chromosome 4 deletion syndrome

Excludes: Chromosome five p- syndrome (163)
Chromosome thirteen trisomy syndrome (168)

Minimal Diagnostic Criteria: The presence in a profoundly retarded individual of low birthweight, microcephaly, hypertelorism and downward slanting palpebral fissures is suggestive of a short arm deletion of a B-group chromosome. Absence of a cat-like cry in early infancy, and the presence of cleft palate, beaked nose, carp-like mouth, preauricular dimples, underdeveloped dermal ridges, hypospadias in males and delay in ossification of the carpals and pelvis are indications that the deletion involves chromosome 4. Chromosomal studies and identification of the deleted chromosome as a number 4 are necessary to confirm the diagnosis. When midline scalp defect, cleft lip and palate and coloboma are present, the 4 p- syndrome may be confused with the 13 trisomy syndrome clinically, although polydactyly has been reported in only 1 case of 4 p- syndrome with an atypical karyotype.

Clinical Findings: In over 50% of cases there is low birthweight with normal gestation (mean birthweight of 25 cases was 2015 gm), severe psychomotor retardation, growth retardation, microcephaly, hypertelorism, broad beaked nose, low-set simple ears, micrognathia, hypoplastic dermal ridges, seizures and hypospadias in males. 10-50% of cases have epicanthus, antimongoloid slant to the eyes, colobomata, strabismus, cleft lip, palate or uvula, preauricular sinus, midline scalp defect, hemangioma of the forehead, low ridge count on the fingers (< 100), delayed bone age, heart defect and orthopedic deformities.

Complications
I **Derived:** —
II **Associated:** —

Etiology: The syndrome is the result of the deletion of some of the genetic material of the short arm of chromosome number 4. Chromosome breakage during gametogenesis leads to a reciprocal translocation and subsequent segregation of the chromosomes at meiosis gives rise to a gamete with a deletion. A balanced translocation carrier may also be produced in this way; he or she can then have offspring who are balanced carriers, or have a deletion (thus the 4p-syndrome), or have a duplication of chromosome material. Chromosome deletion may also occur without translocation, with loss of the deleted segment, either from the end of the chromosome or interstitially. Of about 40 reported cases, 3 have had a visible translocation associated with the deletion. Two of these were inherited from a parent. Several cases have also been reported with ring chromosome 4.

Pathogenesis: Although many factors such as chemicals and radiation are known to be capable of breaking chromosomes, factors which influence breakage in the human in vivo are unknown. Maternal and paternal ages do not seem to be a factor.

Related Facts
I **Sex Ratio:** Appears to be M1:F1
II **Risk of Occurrence:** Very rare, less common than 5p-
III **Risk of Recurrence for**
    Patient's Sib: If parent is a translocation carrier, risk is high
    Patient's Child: No known reproduction by a patient
IV **Age of Detectability:** Prenatally

V   **Prevalence:** —

Treatment
I   **Primary Prevention:**   Genetic counseling
II **Secondary Prevention:**   If a parent is a translocation carrier at risk for having a child with the 4p- syndrome, the presence of the deletion may be diagnosed after amniocentesis.
III **Other Therapy:** —

Prognosis: The average life span is not known. The oldest known living patient is 25 years old. Ten of the 40 described patients are known to have died, most within the 1st year. One stillbirth has been reported, but no spontaneously aborted fetuses have been found so far with this karyotype.

Detection of Carrier: Balanced translocation carriers may be recognized by chromosomal studies.

Special Considerations: —

References:
Centerwall, W.R. et al: Translocation 4p- syndrome. Am. J. Dis. Child. 129:366-370, 1975
Fryns, J.P. et al: The 4p- syndrome, with a report of 2 new cases. Humangenetik 19:99-109, 1973.
Miller, O.J. et al: Partial deletion of the short arm of chromosome No. 4 (4p-): Clinical studies in five unrelated patients. J. Pediatr. 77:792, 1970.

Contributor: **Dorothy Warburton**

Editor's Computerized Descriptors: Eye, Ear, Face, Oral, Nose, Skin, Dermatoglyphic, Skel., CV., GU., Nerve

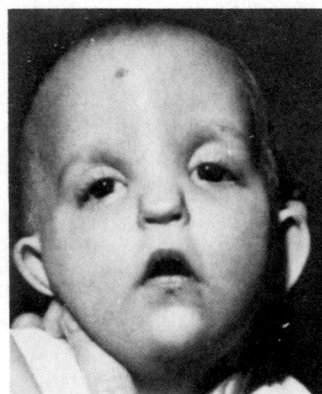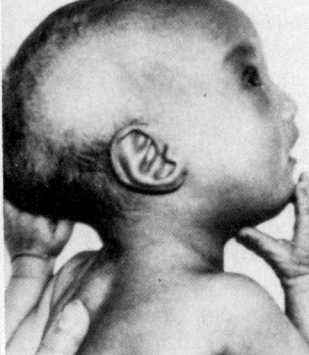

176. Note ocular hypertelorism, carp-like mouth and prominent glabella

CHROMOSOME FOURTEEN q DISTAL PARTIAL TRISOMY SYNDROME

Includes: Trisomie distal 14q
Síndrome de trisomía parcial del cromosoma 14q tipo II
Duplication of distal 14q

Excludes: Chromosome fourteen q proximal partial trisomy syndrome (166)

Minimal Diagnostic Criteria: Dysmorphic features and demonstration of duplication of the distal half of 14q.

Clinical Findings: This is the 2nd syndrome associated with partial trisomy of the long arm (q) of chromosome 14. It involves duplication of the distal portion of 14q and is here termed 14q distal partial trisomy syndrome.
   Study of 3 cases has disclosed the following features: normal birthweight, motor and mental retardation, hyper- or hypotonia, microcephaly, high forehead, epicanthal folds, antimongoloid slant to palpebral fissures, low-set ears, high-arched or cleft palate, protruding upper lip, buccal fat pad, micrognathia, camptodactyly, congenital heart disease (in all 3 patients), anomalous blood vessels, cyanosis, and hypoplasia of the 12th rib.

Complications
I   **Derived:**   None known
II **Associated:**   Congenital heart disease

Etiology: Partial trisomy (duplication) of the distal half of the long arm (q) of chromosome 14.

Pathogenesis: —

Related Facts
I   **Sex Ratio:**   ?
II **Risk of Occurrence:**   ?
III **Risk of Recurrence for**
   Patient's Sib: Low, except when 1 of the parents is carrying a balanced translocation.
   Patient's Child: ?
IV **Age of Detectability:**   At birth or prenatally by amniotic fluid cell culture and karyotyping.
V   **Prevalence:**   ?

Treatment
I   **Primary Prevention:**   Genetic counseling
II **Secondary Prevention:**   Prenatal chromosome studies of amniotic fluid cells when a parent has a balanced translocation or mosaicism with the translocation.
III **Other Therapy:** —

Prognosis: Severe mental retardation. Oldest patient is 15 months.

Detection of Carrier: The balanced translocation carrier or mosaic is recognizable by karyotype analysis. This has only been done to date after the birth of an affected child.

Special Considerations: —

References:
Pfeiffer, R.A. et al: Partial trisomy 14. Following a balanced reciprocal translocation t(14q-; 21q+). Humangenetik 20:187, 1973.
Reiss, J.A. et al: Mosaicism with translocation: Autoradiographic and fluorescent studies of an inherited reciprocal translocation t(2q+; 14q-). J. Med. Genet. 9:280, 1972.
Wyandt, H.E. et al: Abnormal chromosomes 14 and 15 in abortions, syndromes and malignancy. In Yunis, J.J. (ed.): New Chromosomal Syndromes. New York: Academic Press, 1977.

Contributors: **Frederick Hecht**
Herman E. Wyandt

Editor's Computerized Descriptors: Eye, Ear, Face, Oral, Skin,

CHROMOSOME FOURTEEN q PROXIMAL PARTIAL TRISOMY SYNDROME

Includes: Trisomie proximale 14q
Síndrome de trisomía parcial del cromosoma 14q tipo I
Duplication of proximal 14q

Excludes: Chromosome fourteen q distal partial trisomy syndrome (165)

Minimal Diagnostic Criteria: The characteristic facial dysmorphia and generalized retardation of growth, hand and other minor skeletal abnormalities, and demonstration of a duplication of the proximal half of 14q.

Clinical Findings: There are at least 2 distinct syndromes due to partial trisomy of the long arm (q) of chromosome 14. One syndrome is associated with partial trisomy of the proximal portion and is here termed chromosome 14q proximal partial trisomy syndrome.

Study of 9 cases to date has shown the following features: low birthweight (1800-2600 gm), motor and mental retardation, growth retardation, seizures or hypertonia, microcephaly (and sometimes brachycephaly), low anterior hairline, ocular hyper- or hypotelorism, occasional ptosis of the eyelids with antimongoloid slant of the palpebral fissures, small palpebral fissures, microphthalmia or strabismus. The external ears may be low-set or malformed. The nose has a broad base and a prominent tip. The palate is high-arched or cleft. Prominent philtrum and micrognathia may be present. The neck is short. The fingers are long and tapered and clinodactyly or camptodactyly are usually present. Other reported skeletal anomalies include kyphosis, hypoplastic 12th ribs, missing or hypoplastic radius, dislocated or dysplastic hips, and clubfeet. Three of 9 patients have had congenital heart malformations, and 2 have had mild genital malformations.

Complications
I   **Derived:** Seizures
II **Associated:** Congenital heart disease and genital malformations.

Etiology: Partial trisomy (duplication) of the proximal half of the long arm of chromosome 14.

Pathogenesis: —

Related Facts
I   **Sex Ratio:** M1:F1
II   **Risk of Occurrence:** ?
III **Risk of Recurrence for**
     Patient's Sib: Low, except when 1 of the parents has a balanced translocation.
     Patient's Child: ?
IV   **Age of Detectability:** At birth or prenatally by amniotic fluid cell culture and karyotyping
V   **Prevalence:** ?

Treatment
I   **Primary Prevention:** Genetic counseling
II   **Secondary Prevention:** Prenatal chromosomal studies of amniotic fluid cells when a parent has a balanced translocation or mosaicism with the translocation.
III **Other Therapy:** —

Prognosis: Moderate mental retardation. Oldest patient is 7 years old.

Detection of Carrier: The balanced translocation carrier or mosaic is recognizable by karyotype analysis. To the present this has been done only after birth of an affected child.

Special Considerations: —

References:

Allderdice, P.W. et al: Familial translocation involving chromosomes 6, 14, and 20, identified by quinacrine fluorescence. Humangenetik 13:205, 1971.

Fawcett, W.A. et al: Trisomy 14q-. In Bergsma, D. (ed.): New Chromosomal and Malformation Syndromes, Birth Defects: Orig. Art. Ser., vol. XI, no. 5. Miami: Symposia Specialists for The National Foundation-March of Dimes, 1975, p. 223.

Laurent, C. et al: Translocation t(14q-; 21q+) chez le pere. Trisomie 14 et monosomie 21 partielle chez la fille. Ann. Génét. 16:281, 1973.

Reiss, J.A. et al: Mosaicism with translocation: Autoradiographic and fluorescent studies of an inherited reciprocal translocation t(2q+; 14q-). J. Med. Genet. 9:280, 1972.

Contributors: **Frederick Hecht**
Herman E. Wyandt

Editor's Computerized Descriptors: Eye, Ear, Face, Oral, Nose, Neck, Skin, Hair, Skel., Muscle, CV., GU., Nerve

CHROMOSOME THIRTEEN q- SYNDROME

Includes: Délétion du bras long du chromosome 13
Síndrome del cromosoma 13q-
Chromosome 13r syndrome

Excludes: —

Minimal Diagnostic Criteria: Low birthweight for length of gestation, microcephaly, wide prominent nasal bridge, protruding upper maxilla; eye abnormalities such as ptosis, microphthalmia, colobomata, retinoblastoma. Large, malformed ears. Combinations of other clinical findings as listed below. Karyotypic analysis with banded chromosomes is essential if accurate subdivisions of the syndrome are to be made in the future.

Clinical Findings: Among a total of 32 patients for whom the 13r or 13q- chromosome was identified by autoradiography or chromosome banding techniques:

Psychomotor retardation	31 of 32
Microcephaly	27 of 30
Birthweight under 3000 gm	25 of 27
Broad prominent nasal bridge (Greek profile)	23 of 27
Low-set, abnormal ears	24 of 28
Protruding upper maxilla	15 of 19
Genital malformation in males	14 of 22
Trigonocephaly	11 of 24
Microphthalmia	10 of 24
Heart disease	10 of 28
Anal atresia	8 of 30
Retinoblastoma	3 of 27
Colobomata	6 of 32
Absent thumbs	3 of 32

Complications

I Derived: See Clinical Findings

II Associated: Feeding difficulties, failure to thrive. Transient hyperglycemia or symptoms of diabetes insipidus was observed in 2 infants.

Etiology: The 13q- syndrome results from partial monosomy for a segment of the long arm of one chromosome 13. In at least 22 cases the ring or deleted chromosome has been identified as a chromosome 13 by autoradiography. In 10 cases the ring or deleted chromosome 13 has been identified in banded karyotypes.

If the 13q- or 13r chromosome is present in every cell, the marker chromosome was most likely produced after chromosome breakage during gametogenesis. If the individual is a mosaic, breakage and chromosome segment loss probably occurred during embryogenesis. A balanced translocation in a parent could result in either: 1) balanced translocation carrier children, 2) offspring with partial monosomy 13q-, 3) individuals with trisomy for a long arm distal segment of chromosome 13, or 4) through nondisjunction, infants trisomic for segments of the long arm of chromosome 13. Maternal or paternal ages do not seem to be factors.

Pathogenesis: The syndrome develops during the embryogenesis of a zygote with a 46, 13q- or 46, 13r chromosome complement. Evidence from the 10 cases with banded karyotypes suggests that the phenotype resulting from a terminal long arm deletion such as that resulting in the formation of a ring 13, frequently includes hypoplastic or absent thumbs, and other skeletal anomalies, genital malformation, anal atresia, and microphthalmia and colobomata. The cases with monosomy for an interstitial segment of a chromosome 13 long arm share a characteristic facies with microcephaly, a broad prominent nasal bridge, protruding maxilla and large abnormal ears. They are less likely to have hypoplastic or absent thumbs, or anal atresia. Facial asymmetry has been observed in both groups. The phenotypic similarity between patients with the 13q- and the 13r syndrome suggests that disturbance of embryologic development, rather than deletion of specific genes results in the overlapping 13q- and 13r phenotypes.

Related Facts
I **Sex Ratio:** 46,13r: M13:F9; 46,13q-: M5:F4 based on 31 cases.
II **Risk of Occurrence:** ?
III **Risk of Recurrence for**
   Patient's Sib: The risk will vary with the specific balanced translocation carried by a parent
   Patient's Child: There is no report of a child with the 13q-syndrome reproducing
IV **Age of Detectability:** In utero by amniocentesis
V **Prevalence:** Rare

Treatment
I **Primary Prevention:** Genetic counseling
II **Secondary Prevention:** Amniocentesis, culture, and karyotypic analysis of banded chromosomes if one parent is a balanced translocation carrier.
III **Other Therapy:** As may be indicated

Prognosis: The average life span is unknown. In 1971 the oldest reported patient was then 25 years of age (Lehrke et al, 1971).

Detection of Carrier: Carriers may be identified if there is a deletion of a segment from the long arm of a chromosome 13.

Special Considerations: —

References:
Howard, R.O. et al: Retinoblastoma and chromosome abnormality. Arch. Ophthalmol. 92:490, 1974.
Magenis, R.E. et al: Parental origin of a ring 13 chromosome in a female with multiple anomalies. Humangenetik 33:181, 1976.
Niebuhr, E. and Ottosen, J.: Ring chromosome D(13) associated with multiple congenital malformations. Ann. Génét. 16(3):157, 1973.
Noel, B. et al: Partial deletions and trisomies of chromosome 13: Mapping of bands associated with particular malformations. Clin. Genet. 9:593, 1976.

Contributor: **Penelope Witte Allderdice**

Editor's Computerized Descriptors: Eye, Ear, Face, Nose, Skel., CV., GI., GU.

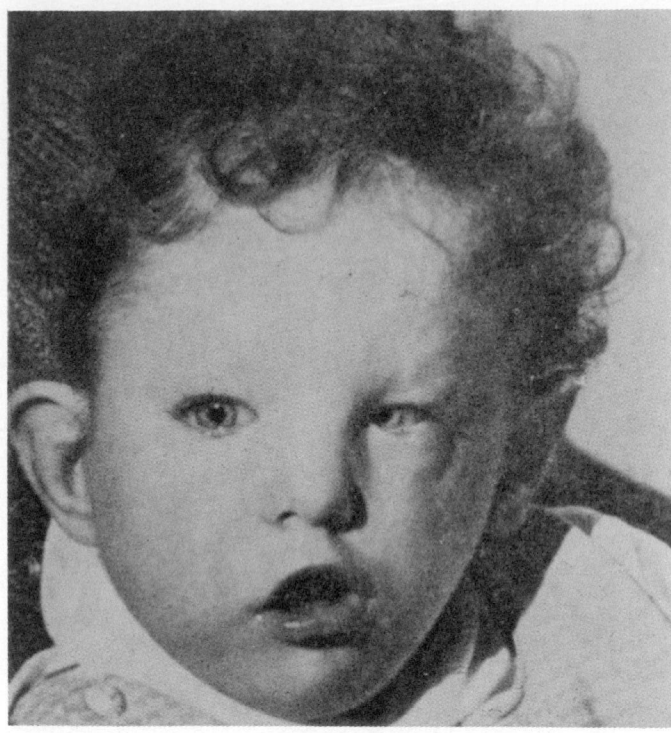

177. Chromosome 13r syndrome in child. Note broad nasal bridge

CHROMOSOME THIRTEEN TRISOMY SYNDROME

Includes: Trisomie 13-15
Trisomie 13
Síndrome de la trisomía 13
Trisomy 13-15 syndrome
D Trisomy syndrome
Partial 13 trisomy
Patau syndrome
Trisomy D1 syndrome

Excludes: Chromosome eighteen trisomy syndrome (160)
Chromosome four p- syndrome (164)

Minimal Diagnostic Criteria: The 13 trisomy patient characteristically shows a triad of microphthalmia, cleft lip and palate, and polydactyly in addition to a number of other abnormalities. One or all of the triad may be absent; however, the syndrome can still be suspected when the patient shows a constellation of other findings mentioned below. Chromosomal study is required.†

Clinical Findings:

Developmental retardation	100%
Undescended testes	100%
Ocular hypertelorism	> 80%
Low-set ears	> 80%
Malformed ears	> 80%
Distal axial triradius	> 80%
Jitteriness and apneic spells	50-80%
Microcephaly	50-80%
Microphthalmia	50-80%
Cleft lip or palate	50-80%
Polydactyly	50-80%
Congenital heart disease	50-80%
Epicanthal folds	50-80%
Presumptive deafness	50-80%
Micrognathia	50-80%
Extra skin nape of neck	50-80%
Short neck	50-80%
Capillary hemangioma	50-80%
Long hyperconvex nails	50-80%
Retroflexible thumbs	50-80%
Flexion deformity of fingers	50-80%
Single palmar crease	50-80%
Tibial loop hallucal pattern	50-80%
Prominent calcaneus	50-80%
Hypotonia	40-50%
Hypertonia	20-30%
Seizures	20-30%
Scalp defects	10-50%
Absent eyebrows	10-50%
Shallow supraorbital ridges	10-50%
Iris colobomata	10-50%
Inguinal or umbilical hernia	10-50%
Single umbilical artery	10-50%
Pilonidal pit	10-50%
Hypoplastic nails	10-50%
Three or more simple arches on digits	10-50%
Fibular S arch hallucal pattern	10-50%
Short dorsiflexed big toe	10-50%
Omphalocele	10-20%
Limited hip abduction	10-20%
Equinovarus deformity of feet	10-20%
Calcaneovalgus deformity of feet	< 10%

Radiologic:

Anomalies of rib number or morphology	?
Low acetabular angles	?

Laboratory:

Elevation of fetal hemoglobin during infancy	100%
Persistence of Gower-2 embryonic hemoglobin to birth	?
Elevation of hemoglobin Portland$_1$, at birth	?
Delayed rise of hemoglobin A_2 to adult levels	?
Increased number of nuclear projections in polymorphonuclear leukocytes	?
Delayed maturation of the I blood group system	?
Delayed maturation of erythrocyte carbonic anhydrase B	?

Autopsy Findings:

Congenital heart defects	> 80%
Ventricular septal defect	50-60%
Patent ductus arteriosus	50-60%
Atrial septal defect	40-50%
Dextroposition	20-50%
Coarctation of the aorta	10-20%
Renal anomalies	> 80%
Multiple small renal cortical cysts	40-50%
Duplication of renal pelvis	10-20%
Hydronephrosis and hydroureter	10-20%
Brain abnormalities	70-80%
Agenesis of olfactory bulbs	60-70%
Agenesis of corpus callosum	?
Failure of hemispheral cleavage	?
Cerebellar hypoplasia	?
Hydrocephaly	?
Reproductive system abnormalities	50-100%
Bicornuate uterus	50-80%
Bifid vagina	?
Hypoplastic ovaries	?
Abnormal fallopian tubes	?
Gastrointestinal system abnormalities	50-80%
Malrotation of the intestine	20-30%
Meckel diverticulum	10-20%
Unattached mesentery	?
Elongated gallbladder	?
Hypoplastic bile ducts	?
Accessory spleens	?
Temporal bone	
Degenerataion of cochlea and saccule	
Organ of Corti absent or replaced by fibrous tissue	
Tectorial membrane, Peissner membrane and stria vascularis degenerated	

Complications

I   Derived: Feeding difficulties > 80%, failure to thrive > 80%, jitteriness and apneic spells 50-80%, hypotonia 40-50%, jaundice 40-50%, hypertonia 20-30% and seizures 20-30%

II Associated: —

Etiology: Meiotic nondisjunction is thought to be the cause of 13 trisomy syndrome with 47 chromosomes. Thirteen trisomy syndrome with 47 chromosomes is also associated with increased maternal age. There are no other known factors. Postzygotic nondisjunction of the 13 trisomy or double fertilization is postulated to cause 13 trisomy/normal mosaicism. 13 trisomy syndrome results from triplication of chromosome 13. The triplication most often is found as a complete extra chromosome 13 in all cells; however 13 trisomy/normal mosaicism may occur. The extra material may also be translocated to another chromosome in varying amounts, giving rise to partial trisomy.

Pathogenesis: ?

Related Facts
I **Sex Ratio:** M1.2:F1
II **Risk of Occurrence:** About 1 in 5000 live births
III **Risk of Recurrence for**
    Patient's Sib: If parent is carrier 1 in 10
    Patient's Child: No known patient has reproduced.
IV **Age of Detectability:** Newborn by clinical examination and chromosomal analysis
V **Prevalence:** —

Treatment
I **Primary Prevention:** Genetic counseling
II **Secondary Prevention:** Amniocentesis, culture and karyotypic study of fetal cells, if parent is a carrier.
III **Other Therapy:** As may be indicated

Prognosis: The prognosis is extremely poor. One-half the patients with 47 chromosomes die by 1 month of age, 65% by 3 months, and about 95% by 3 years. Cases with translocation and with normal/13 trisomy mosaicism have a somewhat better prognosis. All patients have been profoundly retarded. No adult patients are known.

Detection of Carrier: A small proportion of 13 trisomy patients have been shown to have a translocation; in a few of these a parent, most often a mother, has been shown to be a carrier. Further family studies then have revealed members who are also translocation carriers, and who are thus at risk. No cases of parental 13 trisomy/normal mosaicism are yet known.

†**Special Considerations:** Phenocopies have occurred in this syndrome in which a typical 13 trisomy syndrome picture is associated with apparently normal chromosomes. The cause of these is unknown. There is much overlap of clinical findings with the 18 trisomy syndrome, so that patients with "intermediate" features may be confused.

References:
Magenis, R.E. et al: Trisomy 13(D) syndrome: Studies on parental age, sex ratio, and survival. J. Pediatr. 73:222, 1968.
Taylor, A.I.: Autosomal trisomy syndromes: A detailed study of 27 cases of Edwards' syndrome and 27 cases of Patau's syndrome. J. Med. Genet. 5:227, 1968.

Contributors: **Ellen Magenis**
                Frederick Hecht

Editor's Computerized Descriptors: Eye, Hearing, Ear, Face, Oral, Nose, Skin, Dermatoglyphic, Nails, Skel., Hernia not CNS, CV., GI., GU., Nerve

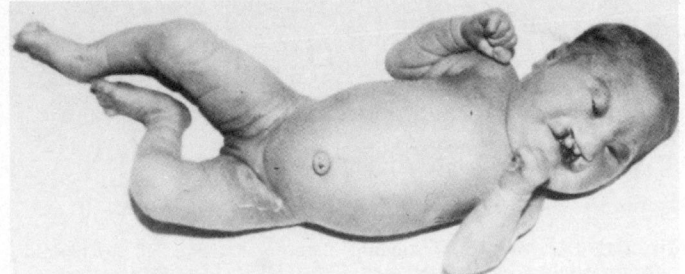

178. Infant with trisomy 13

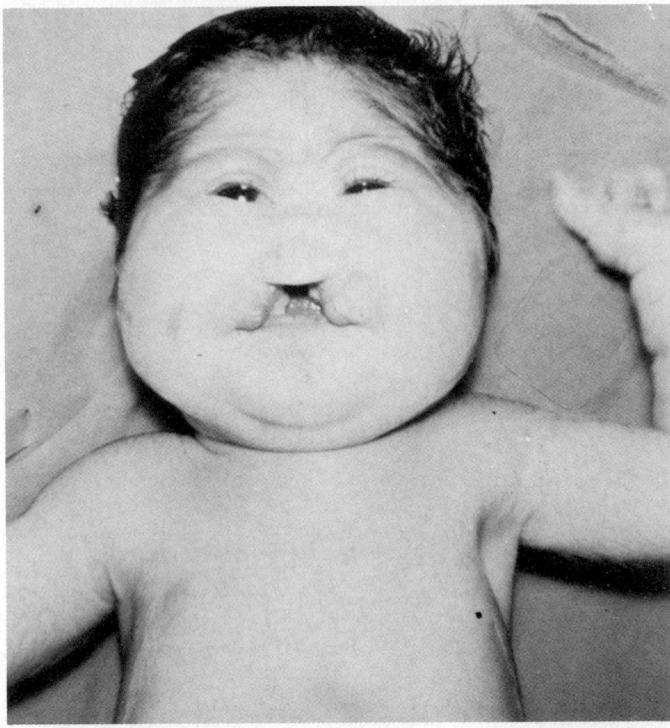

179. Trisomy 13 in infant with premaxillary agenesis

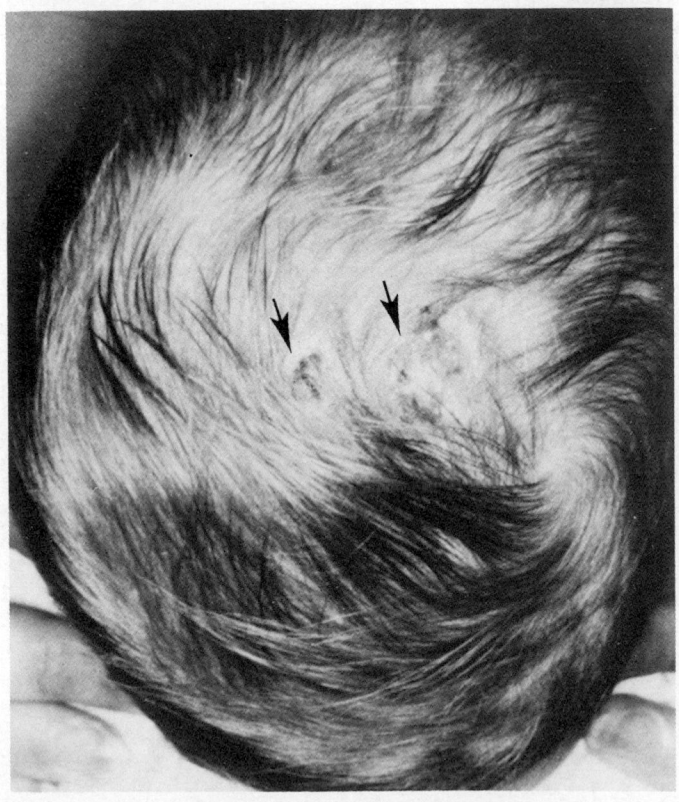

180. Scalp defect in trisomy 13 syndrome

213

CHROMOSOME TRIPLOIDY SYNDROME

Includes: Triploidie
Síndrome de triploidía
Triploid/diploid mosaicism

Excludes: —

Minimal Diagnostic Criteria: Demonstration of a triploid chromosome complement

Clinical Findings: Very low birthweight, premature birth, developmental retardation, extremely low viability, cutaneous syndactyly of 3rd and 4th fingers, coloboma of iris (and sometimes of all structures of the eyeball), hypospadias and testicular germinal cell hypoplasia are very common. Otherwise, the clinical picture is quite variable. Hemiatrophy has been observed in triploid/diploid mosaic individuals.

Complications
I   **Derived:** Early death has occurred in all cases except one.
II **Associated:** —

Etiology: Presence of 3 complete sets of chromosomes instead of the normal 2

Pathogenesis: ? †

Related Facts
I   **Sex Ratio:** Unknown, but both male and female triploids have occurred. The males are either 69,XXY or 69,XYY, while the females have been 69,XXX.
II **Risk of Occurrence:** Although about 1 early embryo in 200 are triploid, most of these are aborted spontaneously. Only 9 triploid and 8 triploid/diploid mosaic infants have been born alive, and several of these quite prematurely.
III **Risk of Recurrence for**
    Patient's Sib: Very small
    Patient's Child: Patients die in infancy.
IV **Age of Detectability:** At birth, or midtrimester by prenatal diagnosis based on chromosomal studies on cultured amniotic fluid cells
V   **Prevalence:** No known cases in the general population

Treatment
I   **Primary Prevention:** —
II **Secondary Prevention:** —
III **Other Therapy:** As may be indicated

Prognosis: Death in the neonatal period, although some triploid/diploid mosaic individuals may survive for several years.

Detection of Carrier: —

†**Special Considerations:** The vast majority of triploid fetuses are aborted early in pregnancy. There is some evidence that the proportion of triploid abortuses is higher in pregnancies which occur soon after oral contraceptives are stopped.

References:
Fryns, J.P. et al: Unusually long survival in a case of full triploidy of maternal origin. Hum. Genet. 38:147, 1977.
Schindler, A.M. and Mikamo, K.: Triploidy in man: Report of a case and a discussion on etiology. Cytogenetics (Basel) 9:ll6, 1970.
Wertelecki, W. et al: The clinical syndrome of triploidy. Obstet. Gynecol. 47:69, 1976.

Contributor: **Orlando J. Miller**

Editor's Computerized Descriptors: Eye, Skel., GU.

CHROMOSOME TWENTY-ONE MONOSOMY

Includes: Monosomie G de type I
Síndrome de la monosomía G tipo I
Partial monosomy G
Antimongolism
Monosomy-G syndrome type I

Excludes: Chromosome twenty-two monosomy (172)

Minimal Diagnostic Criteria: In the absence of pathognomonic signs, the diagnosis rests upon finding a complete or partial monosomy G, plus several of the more common clinical features.

Clinical Findings: Low birthweight, even when full-term, physical and mental retardation, prominent nose and wide nasal bridge, large, low-set ears, microcephaly, micrognathia, epicanthus, downward slant of the palpebral fissures, hypertonia, hypospadias, inguinal hernia and undescended testes, t'axial triradius and simian crease but otherwise normal dermatoglyphics, cataracts, congenital heart disease, renal dysplasia and Potter facies, increased iliac index, pes equinovarus or clubfoot, blepharochalasis, strabismus, and thrombocytopenia.

Complications
I   **Derived:** —
II **Associated:** —

Etiology: Thought to be the result of a deletion of all or part of the long arm of chromosome 21.

Pathogenesis: ?

Related Facts
I   **Sex Ratio:** ? But both sexes are involved
II **Risk of Occurrence:** ?
III **Risk of Recurrence for**
    Patient's Sib: ?
    Patient's Child: ?
IV **Age of Detectability:** At birth
V   **Prevalence:** ? But rare

Treatment
I   **Primary Prevention:** —
II **Secondary Prevention:** —
III **Other Therapy:** —

Prognosis: ? Mental retardation appears to be a constant finding.

Detection of Carrier: —

Special Considerations: —

References:
Mikkelsen, M. and Vestermark, S.: Karyotype 45,XX,-21/46,XX,21q- in an infant with symptoms of G- deletion syndrome I. J. Med. Genet. 11:389, 1974.

Contributor: **Orlando J. Miller**

Editor's Computerized Descriptors: Eye, Ear, Face, Nose, Dermatoglyphic, Skel., Muscle, Hernia not CNS, CV., GU.

CHROMOSOME TWENTY-ONE TRISOMY SYNDROME

Includes: Trisomie 21
Síndrome de la trisomía 21
Trisomy G syndrome
Translocation 21 syndrome
Mosaic 21 syndrome
Down syndrome
Mongolism

Excludes: —

Minimal Diagnostic Criteria: Diagnosis usually definite with 8 or more of the Clinical Findings listed below. In questionable cases demonstration of 1 of the below chromosomal abnormalities may be necessary for diagnosis.

Clinical Findings:

Chromosomal abnormality	99%
Twenty-one trisomy	94%
Translocation trisomy	3-4%
Mosaicism	1-2%
10 ulnar loops or 8-9 with a radial loop, 4th finger	90%
t'axial triradius	?
Flattened facial features	90%
Oblique palpebral fissures	80%
Flat occiput	78%
Brachycephaly	75%
Short limbs	70%
Short, broad hands, short fingers, especially the 5th	70%
High-arched, narrow palate	70%
Short 5th middle phalanx	62%
Hyperextensibility or hyperflexibility	47-77%
Hypotonia	21-77%
Depressed nasal bridge	60%
Speckled iris	50%
Dysplastic ears	50%
Incurved 5th finger	50%
Congenital heart defects	40-60%
Tibial arch in hallucal area	50%
Transverse palmar crease	48%
Increased space between 1st and 2nd toes	45%
Epicanthic folds	40%
Small nose	?
Plantar furrow between 1st and 2nd toes	28%
Single flexion crease, 5th finger	20%
Small or absent nasal bones	?

Additional characteristics useful in newborns or in early childhood:

Absent Moro reflex	82%
Excess skin at nape of neck	81%
Dysplastic pelvis by xray	67%

Additional characteristics useful in older children and adults:

Mental retardation	99%
Mouth usually open	65%
Dental abnormalities	65%
Blepharitis	?
Rhagades	56%
Furrowed tongue	50%
Short broad neck	45%
Strabismus	14-23%

Complications
I **Derived:** See Clinical Findings
II **Associated:** Respiratory infections, epilepsy (10%), duodenal obstruction (8%), leukemia

Etiology: Presence of an additional chromosome number 21 or part of its long arm, including band q22.1 in all or some of the body cells

Pathogenesis: Chromosomal imbalance leads to multiple malformations, mental retardation and growth retardation by unknown mechanisms.

Related Facts
I **Sex Ratio:** Slight male preponderance
II **Risk of Occurrence:** About 1 in 770 live births in Caucasian, American Negro and Japanese populations. Strongly maternal-age-dependent, with 1 in 2500 births in mothers age 20 or less, and 1 in 55 in mothers age 45 or more. Risk of occurrence rises rapidly after maternal age 35.
III **Risk of Recurrence for**
  Patient's Sib: Less than 1% for about 96% of patients; 5-20% for about 4%, ie those with t(21q22q) or most other translocations in 1 parent or, similarly, for 21 trisomy/normal mosaicism in a parent; 100% for much less than 1% of patients, ie those with a t(21q21q) translocation of isochromosome in either parent.
  Patient's Child: 1 in 2 (50%)
IV **Age of Detectability:** At birth, by clinical evaluation, supplemented in doubtful cases by chromosomal analysis. Prenatal diagnosis possible by chromosomal analysis.
V **Prevalence:** 1 in 1000 in 1st year of life; 1 in 1400 by school age; 1 in 2200 in 10-14 year group; 1 in 3300 to 1 in 2000 in the general population.

Treatment
I **Primary Prevention:** Genetic counseling
II **Secondary Prevention:** —
III **Other Therapy:** As may be indicated

Prognosis: Shortened life expectancy-about one-third die during 1st year; one-half by age 3 or 4; remainder's life expectancy about 30 years. Congenital heart disease, a major cause of early death, may be correctable by surgery. Mental retardation at moderate or severe level is almost universal, even in cases with mosaicism. Rarely, higher intelligence levels are seen and, in a rare mosaic, intelligence may reach the normal level.

Detection of Carrier: Balanced translocation: usually t(DqGq) or t(GqGq) type identified by presence of specific translocation. Detectability possible from birth, but only practicable in families where chromosome 21 trisomy syndrome has occurred.

If t(DqGq) in mother, 10-20% risk in each pregnancy for child to have chromosome 21 trisomy syndrome; if t(DqGq) in father, 2-5% risk of same; if t(GqGq) in either parent, possibility of 100% risk if no normal children; otherwise, risk similar to that with t(DqGq) translocation.

Mosaicism includes trisomy and normal cells. Phenotype variable. Such an individual can have the complete 21 trisomy syndrome, can be completely normal, or can have (and usually does have) an intermediate range of clinical findings. Identified by cytogenetic demonstration of significant numbers of both normal and 21 trisomic cells, plus either the birth of an affected child or the presence of several clinical signs of 21 trisomy syndrome. Detectable prenatally. The risk of having a child with chromosome 21 trisomy syndrome appears to be increased, though not to its theoretic maximum of 50%.

Special Considerations: —

References:
Hagemeijer, A. and Smit, E.M.E.: Partial trisomy 21. Further evidence that trisomy of band 22q22 is essential for Down's phenotype. Hum. Genet.38:15, 1977.
Hamerton, J.L.: Robertsonian translocations in man: Evidence for prezygotic selection. Cytogenetics 7:260, 1968.
Penrose, L.S. and Smith, G.F.: Down's Anomaly. London: J. & A. Churchill, 1966.

Contributor: **Orlando J. Miller**

Editor's Computerized Descriptors: Eye, Ear, Face, Oral, Nose, Speech, Neck, Skin, Dermatoglyphic, Hair, Skel., Muscle, CV., GU., Nerve
Also see Section I, Fig. 69

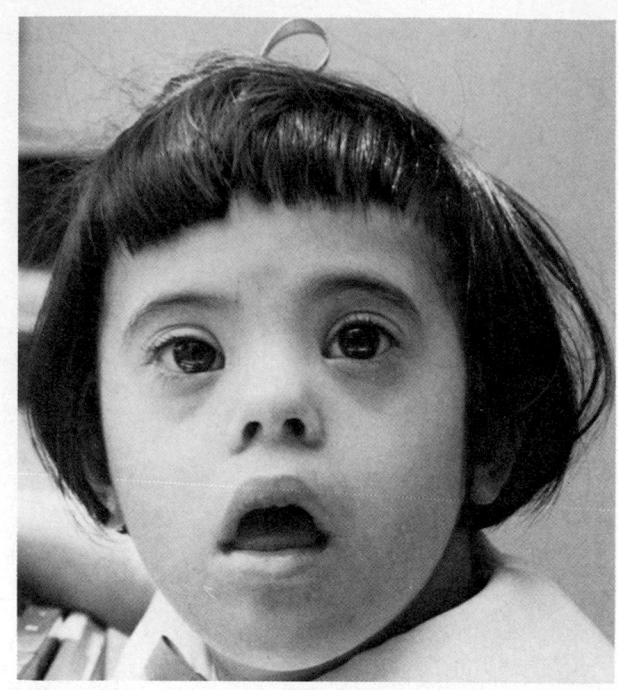

182. Note flat facial features, epicanthal fold and broad depressed nasal bridge

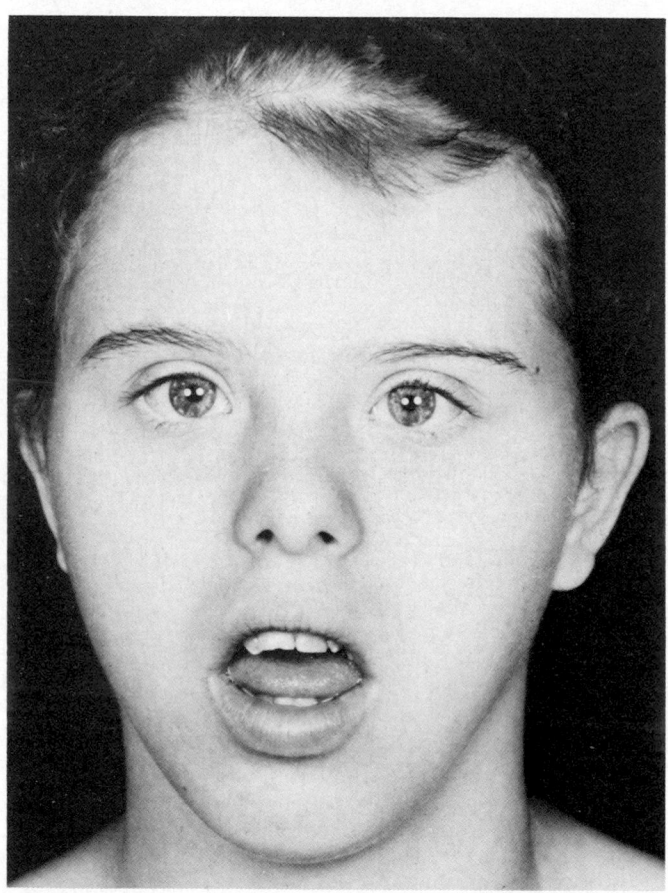

181. Down syndrome in young adult

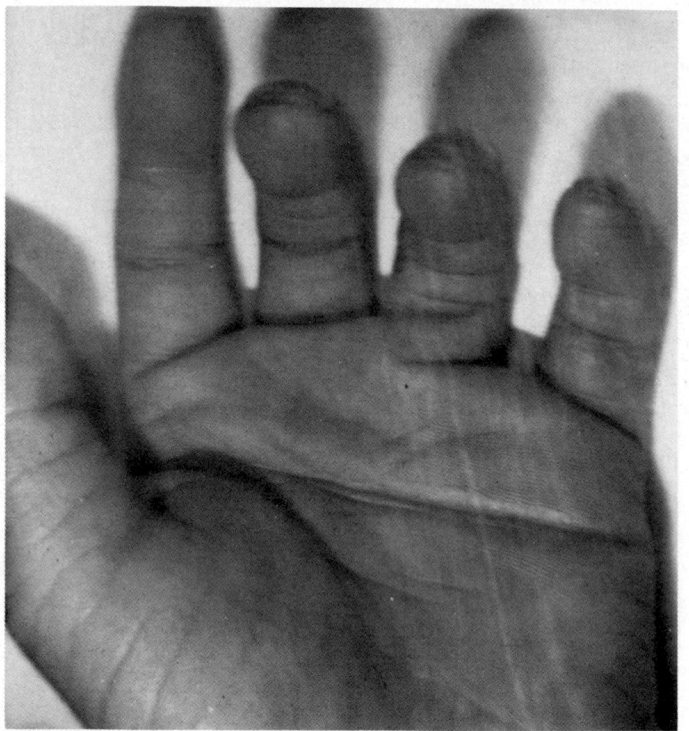

183. Simian crease

CHROMOSOME TWENTY-TWO MONOSOMY

Includes: Monosomie G de type II
Síndrome de la monosomía G tipo II
Monosomy-G syndrome type II

Excludes: Chromosome twenty-one monosomy (170)

Minimal Diagnostic Criteria: Demonstration of complete or partial monosomy 22, plus several of the more common clinical features

Clinical Findings: Low birthweight, growth and developmental retardation, microcephaly, seizures, hypotonia, ptosis, hypertelorism, epicanthus, flat nasal bridge, bifid uvula, large low-set ears, cutaneous syndactyly of toes, increased acetabular or iliac angles, cardiac anomalies

Complications
I   **Derived:**   Mental retardation usual
II **Associated:**   —

Etiology: Presumably due to deletion of all or part of the long arm of chromosome 22.

Pathogenesis: ?

Related Facts
I   **Sex Ratio:**   ? But both sexes affected
II   **Risk of Occurrence:**   —
III **Risk of Recurrence for**
    Patient's Sib: ?
    Patient's Child: ?
IV **Age of Detectability:**   At birth
V   **Prevalence:**   ? Although rare

Treatment
I   **Primary Prevention:**   —
II   **Secondary Prevention:**   —
III **Other Therapy:**   —

Prognosis: ?

Detection of Carrier: —

Special Considerations: —

References:
Warren, R. et al: Identification by fluorescent microscopy of the abnormal chromosomes associated with the G-deletion syndromes. Am. J. Hum. Genet. 25:77, 1973.

Contributor: **Orlando J. Miller**

Editor's Computerized Descriptors: Eye, Ear, Oral, Nose, Skel., Muscle, CV., Nerve

CHROMOSOME 45,X/46,XY MOSAICISM

Includes: Intersexualité par aberration des gonosomes
Gonosomale Intersexualität
Intersexualidad gonosómica
Gonosomal intersexuality
Mixed gonadal dysgenesis
Asymmetric gonadal dysgenesis
Mosaic gonadal dysgenesis
45,X/46,XY mosaicism

Excludes: True hermaphroditism (971)
Gonadal dysgenesis, XY type (437)
Reifenstein syndrome (855)
Androgen insensitivity syndrome, incomplete (50)
Pseudovaginal perineoscrotal hypospadias (831)
All other forms of male pseudohermaphroditism

Minimal Diagnostic Criteria: A mosaic 45,X/46,XY chromosome complement: The diagnosis may be assumed if an individual has a unilateral streak gonad and a contralateral testis, or bilateral dysgenetic testes and müllerian derivatives. If lymphocyte cultures of an individual with ambiguous external genitalia, a unilateral streak gonad, a contralateral testis, and a uterus are 46,XY, it is reasonable to assume the presence of 45,X/46,XY mosaicism because the only form of genetic male pseudohermaphroditism associated with müllerian derivatives is persistence of müllerian derivatives in otherwise normal males. Normal testicular differentiation need not be present, but recognizable seminiferous tubules should be. By contrast, if oocytes are present, a diagnosis of true hermaphroditism is appropriate.

Clinical Findings: In individuals with a 45,X cell line and at least 1 cell line containing a Y chromosome, the phenotype ranges from almost normal males with cryptorchidism or penile hypospadias to females indistinguishable from those with the 45,X Turner syndrome.

45,X/46,XY individuals may be grouped into 1 of 3 clinical categories, namely those with 1)unambiguous female external genitalia, 2) ambiguous external genitalia (sex of rearing in doubt), or 3) almost normal male external genitalia. The spectrum of phenotypes is continuous, however, because no sharp demarcation between categories is possible. Somatic features of the Turner syndrome may be present in any 45,X/46,XY individual. The anomalies present cover the same spectrum as in 45,X individuals, but usually fewer anomalies are detected. It is important to exclude cardiac, vertebral, renal and auditory abnormalities.

1) *Female external genitalia.* About 5% of patients with gonadal dysgenesis and unambiguous external genitalia have 45,X cells and cells containing a Y chromosome. These 45,X/46,XY individuals have well-differentiated female external genitalia, vagina, and müllerian derivatives. At puberty they fail to undergo normal secondary sex development. Gonadoblastomas and dysgerminomas may develop from the dysgenetic gonads.

2) *Ambiguous external genitalia.* Most 45,X/46,XY individuals have ambiguous external genitalia, specifically phallic enlargement, posterior labioscrotal fusion and a urogenital orifice leading superiorly to the urethra and inferiorly to a vagina. An important diagnostic feature is that müllerian derivatives (cervix, uterine corpus and fallopian tubes) are usually present; these are absent in most genetic forms of male pseudohermaphroditism. Occasionally the uterus is rudimentary or a fallopian tube fails to develop on the side on which a testis is present; however,

a fallopian tube is usually present on the side containing the streak gonad. Most 45,X/46,XY individuals with ambiguous external genitalia have gonads consisting of a unilateral streak gonad and a contralateral dysgenetic testis (mixed or asymmetric gonadal dysgenesis). The streak gonads are usually similar in appearance to those of 45,X individuals, although sometimes relatively more mesonephric remnants or hilar cells are present. The testicular tissue is rarely normal in amount or in histologic appearance. However, few seminiferous tubules can usually be identified. The likelihood that a gonad of such a patient will undergo neoplastic transformation is about 15-20%. Breast development in a 45,X/46,XY individual with ambiguous external genitalia suggests the presence of a gonadoblastoma or dysgerminoma, tumors that may produce hormones.

3) *Almost normal male external genitalia.* Some 45,X/46,XY patients may have almost normal male external genitalia, the only abnormalities being hypospadias or unilateral cryptorchidism. Compared with other 45,X/46,XY individuals, testicular development is relatively more normal, wolffian derivatives more normal, and müllerian derivatives less likely to be present. Puberal virilization may occur, and fertility seems possible.

Complications
I **Derived:** Neoplastic transformation of the streak gonad or dysgenetic testis. Secondary sex development is usually not normal; infertility.
II **Associated:** Somatic features of the Turner syndrome.

Etiology: 45,X/46,XY mosaicism is usually believed to arise by mitotic nondisjunction. In addition, structural abnormalities of the Y chromosome are often present. These abnormalities (eg ring or dicentric chromosomes) suggest that the mosaicism may sometimes be initiated through formation of a structurally abnormal Y chromosome, with the 45,X line arising only secondarily. The line containing the structurally abnormal line may or may not persist.†

Pathogenesis: The various associated phenotypes may reflect different tissue distributions of the 45,X and 46,XY cell lines. A streak gonad would thus presumably reflect the presence of 45,X cells, whereas a testis might more likely reflect 46,XY cells. However, this logical assumption has not been proved.

Related Facts
I **Sex Ratio:** Not applicable
II **Risk of Occurrence:** ?
III **Risk of Recurrence for**
 Patient's Sib: Probably negligible.
 Patient's Child: Patients are usually infertile.
IV **Age of Detectability:** At birth if ambiguous external genitalia are present; otherwise at puberty because of lack of normal secondary sex development.
V **Prevalence:** ? Perhaps 200 cases have been reported.

Treatment
I **Primary Prevention:** —
II **Secondary Prevention:** External genital reconstruction may be necessary, particularly if a child has genital ambiguity. Streak gonads and dysgenetic testes should be removed because of the danger of neoplastic transformation. This procedure should be undertaken without delay once the diagnosis is made. In 45,X/46,XY individuals with almost normal male external genitalia, scrotal testes should probably be retained. However, such individuals may or may not have an increased risk for neoplastic transformation and, hence, should be followed carefully. Hormone administration may be necessary. Individuals reared as females require estrogens; individuals reared as males may require androgens.
III **Other Therapy:** —

Prognosis: Presumably normal life span, provided life-threatening anomalies do not coexist or a malignant neoplasm does not supervene. Infertility.

Detection of Carrier: Not applicable

†**Special Considerations:** 45,X/46,XY mosaicism is usually believed to arise by mitotic nondisjunction. Familial recurrences are rare; however, in at least 1 family 45,X/47,XYY mosaicism was detected in 2 and perhaps 3 sibs whose parents were consanguineous.

References:
German, J.: Abnormalities of human sex chromosomes. V. A unifying concept in relation to the gonadal dysgeneses. Clin. Genet. 1:15, 1970.
Hsu, L.Y.F. et al: Familial chromosomal mosaicism, genetic aspects. Ann. Hum. Genet. 33:343, 1970.
Pfeiffer, R.A. et al: Die nosologische Sellung, des XO/XY-Mosaizimus. Arch. Gynaekol. 206:369, 1968.
Simpson, J.L. and Photopulos, G: The relationship of neoplasia to disorders of abnormal sexual differentiation. In Bergsma, D. (ed.): Cancer and Genetics. Birth Defects: Orig. Art. Ser., vol. XII, no. 1. New York: Alan R. Liss for The National Foundation-March of Dimes, 1976, p. 15.
Simpson, J.L.: Disorders of Sexual Differentiation: Etiology and Clinical Delineation. New York: Academic Press, 1976.

Contributor: **Joe Leigh Simpson**

Editor's Computerized Descriptors: Skel., CV., GU.

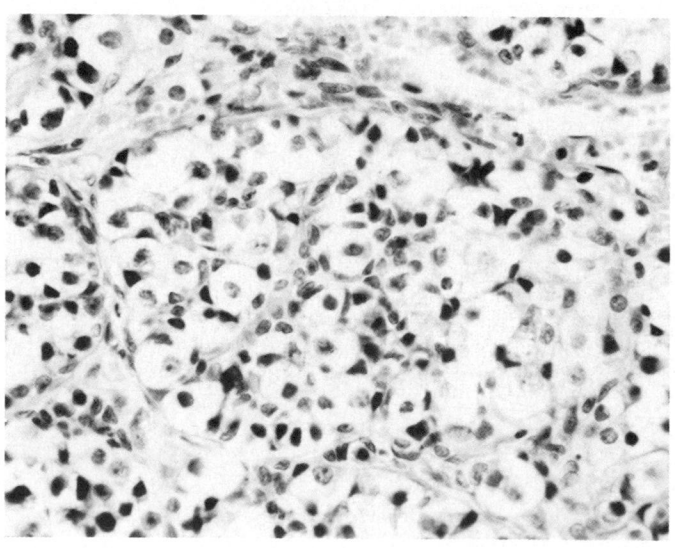

184. Gonadoblastoma. A large tumor with large rounded cells, clear cytoplasm and central nuclei (germ cells); smaller cells with scant cytoplasm and oval nuclei (immature cells of Sertoli or granulosa type) (original magnification, × 490)

CITRULLINEMIA

Includes: Citrullinémie
Citrullinämie
Citrullinuria

Excludes: Argininosuccinic aciduria (87)

Minimal Diagnostic Criteria: Persistent elevation of plasma or urinary citrulline.†

Clinical Findings: Approximately 12 with citrullinemia have been described. Clinically they may develop a rapidly fatal neonatal course or appear normal for several months. After that time severe vomiting with coma and seizures develop. There are no distinguishing physical findings suggestive of the diagnosis although microcephaly and severe mental retardation are present (IQ values of less than 40). Physical growth normal.

Plasma citrulline values range up to 25-35 mg/100 ml (normal less than 1 mg/100 ml) whereas urinary excretion was from 450-2500 mg/day (normal less than 10 mg). Other amino acids are normal. However, one child, a female, had a persistently low BUN. During the initial hospitalization she had evidence of a generalized defect in protein synthesis ie low serum and spinal fluid protein, PTC deficiency and osteoporosis which all reverted to normal on a low-protein diet. Postprandial blood ammonia values are markedly elevated (up to 1,000 µg/100 ml).†

Complications
I **Derived:** Mental retardation common. Ammonia toxicity with coma.
II **Associated:** —

Etiology: Probably autosomal recessive enzyme defect; McK *21570

Pathogenesis: Deficiency of liver argininosuccinic acid synthetase in first patient and in skin fibroblast-like cells cultured from second patient.

Related Facts
I **Sex Ratio:** M1:F1
II **Risk of Occurrence:** Very rare
III **Risk of Recurrence for**
   Patient's Sib: Probably 1 in 4 (25%) for each offspring to be affected
   Patient's Child: Not increased unless mate is carrier or homozygote
IV **Age of Detectability:** Presumably after the beginning of milk feedings in the nursery by measuring plasma citrulline. Prenatal Diagnosis: Enzymatic analysis of amniotic cells for ASA synthesis can detect affected fetus. Autoradiographic methods are also available.
V **Prevalence:** Very rare

Treatment
I **Primary Prevention:** Genetic counseling
II **Secondary Prevention:** Dietary protein restriction to prevent ammonia intoxication
III **Other Therapy:** Keto analogs of essential amino acids in the diet may also reduce ammonia toxicity.

Prognosis: Severe retardation with apparently normal life span.

Detection of Carrier: ? None at present. Fasting amino acids of the parents were normal. Citrulline loading of the parents did not distinguish them from controls.

†**Special Considerations:** Because fasting blood ammonia levels may be normal (< 100 µg/100 ml), it is important to measure postprandial specimens for confirmation of the diagnosis.

Citrullinuria may be found in cystinuric patients because of the intestinal flora's ability to degrade arginine directly to citrulline. This situation must be differentiated from that of true citrullinemia.

References:
Batshaw, M. et al: Treatment of carbamyl phosphate synthetase deficiency with keto analogues of essential amino acids. N. Engl. J. Med. 292:21, 1975.
Danks, D. M. et al: Severe neonatal citrullinaemia. Arch. Dis. Child. 49:579, 1974.
Hill, H.Z. and Goodman, S.I.: Detection of inborn errors of metabolism. III. Defects in urea cycle metabolism. Clin. Genet. 6:79, 1974.
Morrow, G. III et al: Citrullinemia with defective urea production. Pediatrics 40:565, 1967.
Tedesco, T. A. and Mellman, W. J.: Argininosuccinate synthetase activity and citrulline metabolism in cells cultured from a citrullinemic subject. Proc. Natl. Acad. Sci. USA 57:829, 1967.

Contributor: **Grant Morrow, III**

Editor's Computerized Descriptors: Skel., GI, Nerve

CLASPED THUMBS

Includes: Pouce en griffe
Syndrom des eingeschlagenen Daumens
Pulgar en gancho
Adducted thumbs
Thumb extensors, aplasia or hypoplasia
Extensor pollicis brevis or longus, aplasia or hypoplasia
Thumbs clasped

Excludes: Arthrogryposis (88)
"Cortical" thumbs
Radial defects (853)
Adducted thumb syndrome
MASA syndrome
Cranio-carpo-tarsal dysplasia (223)
X-linked hydrocephalus

Minimal Diagnostic Criteria: An isolated inability to extend the thumb, secondary to hypoplasia or aplasia of the extensor muscles and tendons.

Clinical Findings: An isolated aplasia or hypoplasia, usually bilateral, of the extensor muscles and tendons of the thumb, resulting in a persistently flexed or adducted position across the palm. Most common defect involves the extensor pollicis brevis, with an accompanying impairment of extension at the metacarpophalangeal joint. Defects of the extensor pollicis longus have also been described.

Since persistent adduction of the thumb may result from any imbalance in extension and flexion forces, due to structural or neurologic defects, it may be observed in conjunction with generalized joint abnormalities, or as part of other distinct syndromes.†

Complications
I   **Derived:** Without treatment, atrophy of the intrinsic thumb muscles and soft tissue contractures occur, resulting in limited function.
II **Associated:** —

Etiology: Genetic. Familial cases described; mode of inheritance unclear. One pedigree possibly consistent with an X-linked recessive inheritance.

Pathogenesis: ?

Related Facts
I   **Sex Ratio:** M1:F<1 ?
II **Risk of Occurrence:** Rare
III **Risk of Recurrence for**
    Patient's Sib: ?
    Patient's Child: ?
IV **Age of Detectability:** At birth or during infancy.
V   **Prevalence:** ?

Treatment
I   **Primary Prevention:** Genetic counseling when mode of inheritance apparent.
II **Secondary Prevention:** Early splinting of the thumb in extension and abduction may give good results.
III **Other Therapy:** Unresponsive or untreated cases may need surgery for release of soft tissues or tendon transplants or transfers.

Prognosis: Mild-to-moderate impairment in function, improved with early treatment.

Detection of Carrier: ?

†**Special Considerations:** Adducted thumbs may occur with other phalangeal extensor defects and clubfeet, with an apparent dominant inheritance, or in generalized arthrogryposis. Hypoplasia of the radial ray, or neurologic impairment may result in an adducted thumb, as seen in X-linked hydrocephalus. It has also been noted in the adducted thumbs syndrome with cleft palate, microcephaly and dysmyelination; the MASA syndrome with mental retardation, aphasia and shuffling gait; and craniocarpo-tarsal dystrophy.

References:
Fitch, N. and Levy, E.P.: Adducted thumb syndromes. Clin. Genet. 8:190, 1975.
Weckesser, E.C. et al: Congenital clasped thumb (congenital flexion - adduction deformity of the thumb). A syndrome not a specific entity. J. Bone Joint Surg. 50A:1417, 1968.

Contributor: **Jonathan Zonana**

Editor's Computerized Descriptors: Skel., Muscle

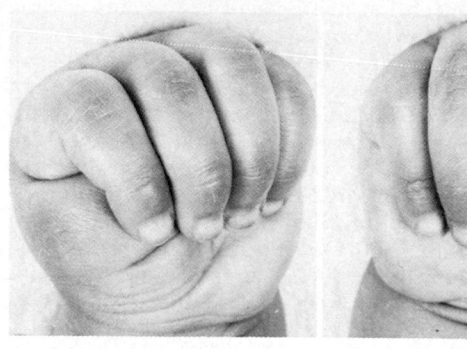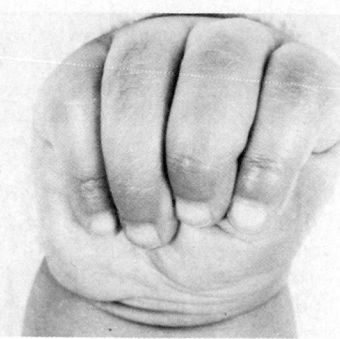

185. Deformity of thumb at age 1 year

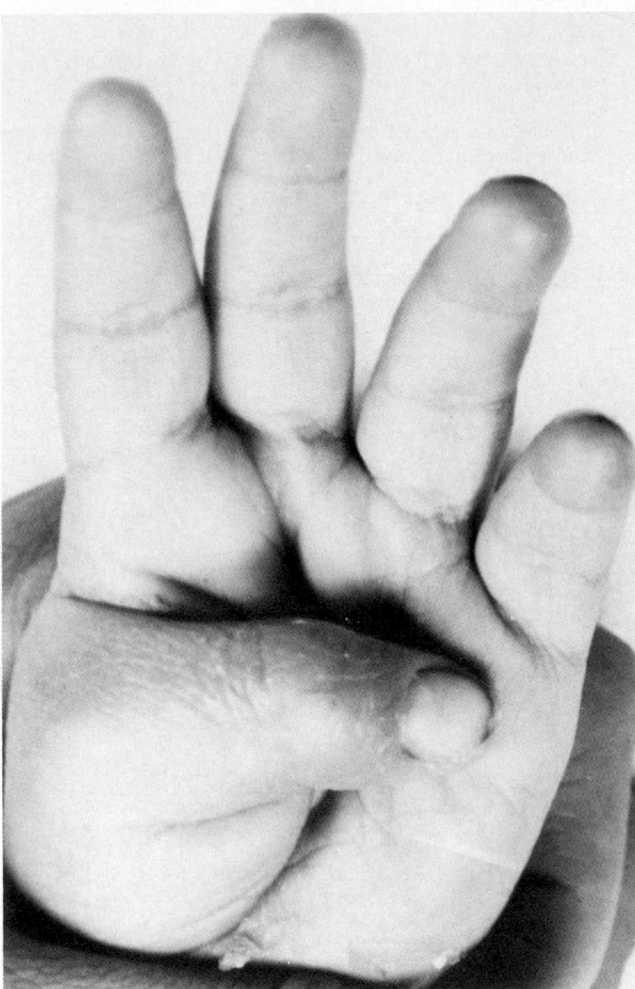

186. Clasped thumb

CLEFT LIP OR PALATE AND FILIFORM FUSION OF EYELIDS

Includes: Fissure labio-palatine avec blépharophimosis
Lippen-oder Gaumenspalte und filiforme Fusion der Augenlider
Fisura labial o palatina con fusión filiforme de los párpados
Eyelid fusion and cleft lip or palate

Excludes: Cleft lip or palate and lip pits or mounds (177)
Popliteal pterygium syndrome (818)

Minimal Diagnostic Criteria: Cleft lip or cleft palate with filiform fusion of the eyelids

Clinical Findings: Multiple connective tissue bands, 0.3-5.0 mm in width, extend from the white line of one lid to that of the other lid, posterior to the cilia and anterior to the meibomian orifices. No associated anomalies are found in the globes. In a few cases, there has been an associated patent ductus arteriosus.

There are various combinations to consider. Filiform fusion of the eyelids may be an isolated phenomenon or it may be seen with cleft lip or cleft palate. In other cases, pits of the lower lip have been found. May also be seen with popliteal pterygium syndrome.

Complications
I   **Derived:** Those usually associated with the clefts since the lid adhesions are corrected by simply severing the attachments.
II **Associated:** A few have had patent ductus arteriosus.

Etiology: Autosomal dominant

Pathogenesis: Unknown, but apparently not related to the simple persistence of normal union of the lids. Failure of fusion of primary and secondary palate.

Related Facts
I   **Sex Ratio:** M1:F1
II   **Risk of Occurrence:** ? Rare
III **Risk of Recurrence for**
     Patient's Sib: If parent is affected, 1 in 2 (50%) for each offspring to be affected; otherwise not increased
       Patient's Child: 1 in 2
IV   **Age of Detectability:** At birth by physical examination
V   **Prevalence:** Less than 30 cases recorded

Treatment
I   **Primary Prevention:** Genetic counseling
II   **Secondary Prevention:** Surgical repair of clefts. Snip filiform adhesions of lids at birth.
III **Other Therapy:** Speech therapy and orthodontic treatment

Prognosis: Excellent. Does not appear to diminish longevity.

Detection of Carrier: —

Special Considerations: —

References:
Lemtis, H. and Neubauer, H.: Ankyloblepharon filiforme et membraniforme adnatum. Klin. Monatsbl. Augenheilkd. 135:510, 1959.
Long, J.C. and Blandford, S.E.: Ankyloblepharon filiforme adnatum with cleft lip and palate. Am. J. Ophthalmol. 53:126, 1962.
Sood, N.N. et al: Ankyloblepharon filiforme adnatum with cleft lip and palate. J. Pediatr. Ophthalmol. 5:30, 1968.

Contributor: Robert J. Gorlin

Editor's Computerized Descriptors: Eye, Face, Oral, CV.

CLEFT LIP OR PALATE AND LIP PITS OR MOUNDS

Includes: Division palatine ou bec-de-lièvre et fossettes des lèvres
Lippen-oder Gaumenspalte und Lippengrübchen
Fisura labial o palatina con fóveas labiales
Lip pits and cleft lip or palate
Van der Woude syndrome

Excludes: Cleft lip or palate without lip pits or mounds
Popliteal pterygium syndrome (818)
Oro-facio-digital syndrome I (770)

Minimal Diagnostic Criteria: Pits of the lower lip associated with cleft lip or palate, or pits in the proband and cleft occurrence in pedigree, or cleft in the proband and occurrence of pits in pedigree.†

Clinical Findings: Most frequently found are two paramedian fistulas or pits on the lower lip, sometimes secreting small amounts of viscous saliva. Some are mere depressions while others are channels 10-15 mm deep. Rarely only one pit is present, which may be either centrally located or lateral to the midline of the lower lip. Pits are frequently associated with cleft of the lip, or cleft palate, or total cleft lip and palate. Frequency of the association is unknown; the estimation is as high as 80%.

Complications
I   Derived: Feeding, respiratory and speech problems associated with oral clefts in untreated cases
II Associated: Rarely syndactyly of hands, popliteal pterygia, ankyloglossia, symblepharon, cleft uvula. Frequently associated with missing or peg lateral upper incisors, if cleft lip present. Missing premolars and bilateral clubfeet described.

Etiology: Pleiotropic autosomal dominant transmission with 80% penetrance. Expressivity is variable: pits (69.6%) and clefts (36%) of affected persons and there is significant association between the types of clefts in parents and their children. Possibly the development of clefts in this syndrome is influenced by modifying genes or by different mutant alleles with a predilection for the different types of cleft. McK *11930

Pathogenesis: Small invaginations appearing on the embryonal mandibular process, "lateral sulci," could be identified in normal embryos 7.5-12.5 mm long. An aberrant mutant prevents the normal obliteration of these "lateral sulci," which results in labial pits. The same mutant gene prevents closure of primary or secondary palate.

Related Facts
I   Sex Ratio: M1:F1 (Caucasians)
II Risk of Occurrence: ?
III Risk of Recurrence for
   Patient's Sib: (Of either pits only, or pits and cleft, or cleft only) 38.5%
   Patient's Child: 50% (Patient with pits only - his child affected in 46.2%, patient with pits and cleft - his child affected in 59.8%, patient with cleft only but having parent or sib with pits - his child affected in 48.5%.)
IV Age of Detectability: At birth
V   Prevalence: 1 in 100,000 to 1 in 80,000 (Caucasians-Czech and U. S. population) (Estimation based on hospital records)

Treatment
I   Primary Prevention: Genetic counseling†
II Secondary Prevention: Plastic surgery on lip pits and clefts
III Other Therapy: Speech therapy and orthodontic treatment

Prognosis: By means of plastic surgery, satisfactory results are achieved to enable affected individuals normal social intercourse and marriage with healthy persons. Average life span seems not to be affected.

Detection of Carrier: —

†Special Considerations: As the risk for clefts is considerably higher in this syndrome, genetic counseling is markedly different from genetic advice given in "common" cleft lip or palate. In each case of facial cleft, inquiry about occurrence of lip pits in family should be made.

References:
Červenka, J. et al: The syndrome of pits of the lower lip and cleft lip and/or palate: Genetic considerations. Am. J. Hum. Genet. 19:416, 1967.
van der Woude, A.: Fistula labii inferioris congenita and its association with cleft lip and palate. Am. J. Hum. Genet. 6:244, 1954.

Contributor: Jaroslav Červenka

Editor's Computerized Descriptors: Eye, Face, Oral, Teeth, Skel.

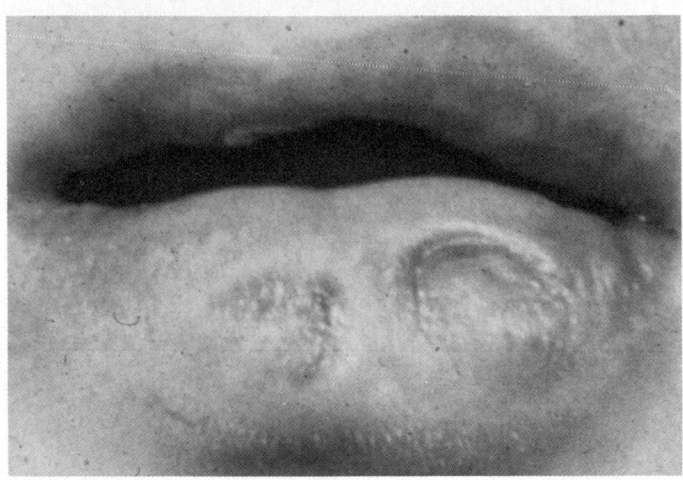

187. Lip pits

CLEFT LIP WITH OR WITHOUT CLEFT PALATE

Includes: Bec-de-lièvre-avec ou sans fente palatine
Lippenspalte mit oder ohne Gaumenspalte
Labio leporino con o sin paladar hendido
Cleft palate and cleft lip
Cheiloschisis
Cheilopalatoschisis
Harelip
Indentations of upper lip
Intrauterine healed clefts

Excludes: Cleft palate (180)
Cleft lip-palate, ectodermal dysplasia and syndactyly (179)
Cleft lip or palate and lip pits or mounds (177)
Cleft lip or palate and filiform fusion of eyelids (176)
Median clefts of lower lip mandible and tongue (636)
Maxillary median alveolar cleft (631)
Lip, median cleft of upper (595)
Median cleft of upper lip with hexadactyly
Ectrodactyly-ectodermal dysplasia-clefting syndrome (337)
Roberts syndrome (875)

Minimal Diagnostic Criteria: Unilateral partial cleft involving the lip

Clinical Findings: Partial or complete clefts of the upper lip which may be unilateral or bilateral and may extend a variable distance posteriorly to include all or part of the maxillary alveolar process, hard and soft palate and superiorly to include the nose. Concave profile, retruded maxilla and lingually tipped incisors most commonly found.

Complications
I   **Derived:** See Table XII.
II   **Associated:** At birth, at least 7 to 13% of patients with isolated cleft lip have associated anomalies and 11 to 14% of patients with cleft lip with cleft palate have associated defects. The frequency of associated defects drops to 2% in those surviving neonatal period. They are more frequent in infants with bilateral clefts than those with unilateral clefts. Clubfoot is the most common defect in isolated cleft lip, polydactyly the most common defect in cleft lip with cleft palate, after anomalies of the cervical vertebra. See Table XIII.

Etiology: Unknown in most cases. It may be one sign associated with a number of causes. Some single gene substitution syndromes occur in which the risk for recurrence is high while in other syndromes the recurrence risk is low. (See Exclusions and Associated Defects). When unassociated with syndromes, probably multifactorial involving both environmental and genetic factors. Present hypothesis is that trait is polygenic with a threshold effect such that the number of genes needed to exceed the developmental threshold and produce cleft is greater in females than in males; such that affected females have a greater risk for having affected children, with boys being at greatest risk, than affected males for having affected offspring. Concordance for cleft lip in monozygotic twins (33%) is greater than for isolated cleft palate (18.2% for monozygotic and 15.3% for dizygotic twins).†

Pathogenesis: Primary palate is formed by the penetration and obliteration of the ectodermal grooves by the 3 mesodermal masses consisting of 1 central mass and 2 lateral ones. Absence or deficiency of these masses, which roughly correspond to the Hisian globular and maxillary processes, or failure of penetration, leads to breakdown of ectoderm and the formation of clefts. The primary palate forms the central portion of upper lip and premaxilla so clefts in this area can extend posteriorly as far as the inci-

sive papillae. When palate is involved a somewhat different process is involved. The palatal shelves develop downward alongside the tongue. Beginning posteriorly they assume a horizontal position, approximate and fuse with each other and the nasal septum beginning at the incisive papillae and progressing posteriorly. One theory suggests that the "shelf force" required to approximate processes is defective, another suggests that the tongue acts as a barrier. Failure of programmed epithelial cell death interfering with fusion has been suggested, as well as a disparity of head width and palatal process size. Soft palate and uvula are probably formed by posterior extension of mesoderm from fused palatine processes.

Related Facts
I   **Sex Ratio:** Depends on ethnic background and severity of defect. Note: the more severe the clefting the greater the male preponderance

Caucasians:	CL only M62:F38
	CL with CP M66:F34
Japanese:	CL only M45:F55
	CL with CP M66:F34
American Negro:	CL only M39:F61
	CL with CP M48:F52

Note: Tentative data indicates that proportion of affected males decreases with increasing number of affected sibs such that when 3 are affected in sibship, the ratio is M48:F52.

II   **Risk of Occurrence:** Note: These are underestimates. See Age of Detectability:

Caucasian:	1 in 1063 live births
Japanese:	1 in 584 live births
American Negro:	1 in 2273 live births
Amerindian:	1 in 1000 to 1 in 234

live births; varies by tribe. Highest reported Haliwa Indians of North Carolina 1 in 234 live births †

III   **Risk of Recurrence for**
     Patient's Sib: —
     Patient's Child: See Exclusions table and Special Considerations for risks when inherited as part of a syndrome

Affected Parents	Affected Sibs	Affected Relatives	Percent Risk For Each Subsequent Child
None	None	None	0.1
None	1	None	4.0
None	1	1	4.0
None	2	None	9.0
1	None	None	4.0
1	1	None	17.0

Risk is increased if affected parent is mother or if first affected child is female, and also with severity of cleft.†

IV   **Age of Detectability:** At birth by inspection. However an error in birth records is noted which is directly related to extent of cleft. Meskin (1966) showed that the proportion of clefts reported on birth certificates to be: Cleft lip 0.65, Cleft lip and palate 0.87

V   **Prevalence:** Unknown, but is probably considerably less than true Risk of Occurrence. Approximately a 10 to 20% mortality in 1st year of life.

Treatment
I   **Primary Prevention:** Genetic counseling
II   **Secondary Prevention:** Surgical repair of lip and palate and associated defects when present.
III **Other Therapy:** Prosthetic replacement of teeth and obturators to close palatal defect, orthodontic therapy, speech therapy, special nursing and feeding devices.

Prognosis: Depends to some extent on type and number of associated defects. Approximately 10 to 20% do not survive 1st year of life. Good to excellent with adequate early therapy in majority of instances.

Detection of Carrier: —

†**Special Considerations:** *Etiology:* Evidence from animal experiments indicates that rates of closure of primary palate (lip and alveolus) and secondary palate (hard and soft palates) are quasicontinuous variables, and that a threshold exists beyond which an individual becomes affected. Evidence for such a system operating in human CL/CP is as follows: 1) Excess of males with more severe defects. 2) Trait frequency in first-degree relatives approximates the square root of the population frequency. 3) Trait frequency drops between first-degree and second-degree relatives. 4) Increasing risk of recurrence with each affected child. 5) Frequency of the trait in first-degree relatives of a cleft patient is higher when the patient is of the sex less often affected (in this case female).

Type of Cleft: Irrespective of race, clefts of lip, lip and palate and of palate only are distributed approximately as follows: CL -25% CL/CP -50% CP -25% Cleft lip may be unilateral or bilateral Unilateral - 80% (of which 70% extend to include palate) Right side - 30% (extent the same for both right and left) Left side - 70% Bilateral - 20% (of which 80% extend to include palate) *Risk:* Risk figures given are for CL/CP when unassociated with a syndrome. While syndromes probably account for less than 10% of all cases of CL/CP, they must be ruled out before applying the risk figures above for counseling purposes, as risk may be as high as 1 in 2. Further, while most studies indicate that in the common forms of CL/CP there is no greater risk for CP and vice versa and, hence, is evidence for the independence of the two traits, in certain syndromes this is not the case.

References:

Gorlin, R. J.: Developmental anomalies of the face and oral structures. In Gorlin, R.J. and Goldman, H.M. (eds.): Thoma's Oral Pathology, 6th Ed. St. Louis:C.V. Mosby Co., 1970, p. 21.

Gorlin, R.J. et al: Facial clefting and its syndromes. In Bergsma, D. (ed.): Part XI. Orofacial Structures. Birth Defects: Orig. Art. Ser., vol. VII, no. 7. Baltimore: Williams & Wilkins for The National Foundation-March of Dimes, 1971, p. 3.

Ross, R. B. and Johnston, M. C.: Cleft Lip and Palate. Baltimore:-Williams & Wilkins, 1972.

Contributor: **Carl J. Witkop, Jr.**

Editor's Computerized Descriptors: Face, Oral, Teeth, Skel.

CLEFT LIP-PALATE, ECTODERMAL DYSPLASIA AND SYNDACTYLY

Includes: Fissure labiale et palatine-dysplasie ectodermique-anomalies des extrémités-oligophrénie
Lippen-Kiefer-Gaumenspalte, ektodermale Dysplasie, Hand-und Fussfehlbildungen, Oligophrenie
Fisura labio-palatina-displasia ectodérmica-anomalías de manos y pies y oligofrenia
Ectodermal dysplasia and cleft lip
Cleft lip-palate, ectodermal dysplasia, hand-foot anomalies and oligophrenia

Excludes: Popliteal pterygium syndrome (818)
Cranio-oculo-dental syndrome (229)
Oro-facio-digital syndrome I (770)
Oro-facio-digital syndrome II (771)
Arthrogryposis (88)
Acrocephalosyndactyly (14)

Minimal Diagnostic Criteria: Cleft lip and evidence of ectodermal dysplasia

Clinical Findings:

Mental retardation	3/3
Alopecia (scarring type)	3/3
Deformed nails	3/3
Cleft palate	3/3
Genital hypoplasia	3/3
Cleft lip	2/3
Photophobia	2/3
Adhesions between eyelids	2/3
Syndactyly -	
toes	2/3
fingers	0/3
Hypoplasia of enamel, missing teeth	3/3
Hidrosis	3/3
Abnormal EEG	2/3

Complications
I **Derived:** Chronic scalp infection, decubitus ulcer, blepharitis
II **Associated:** —

Etiology: The occurrence of the identical syndrome in 3 of 10 sibs whose parents were not affected suggests autosomal recessive inheritance, although proof of this must await further genetic analysis. Parental consanguinity was denied in this family. A recurring, nongenetic factor has not been excluded.†

Pathogenesis: ? The physical defects are present at birth, while developmental retardation is usually obvious within the first few weeks of life. Persistent low-grade inflammation of scalp results in a chronic scarring process and gradual loss of hair from central area of scalp. Growth of nails is slow and irregular. Sweat glands, hair follicles and sebaceous glands are present. In the affected area of scalp the hair follicles and sebaceous glands are absent, rete pegs poorly developed and epidermis thin, with, however, some sweat glands evident.

Related Facts
I **Sex Ratio:** All 3 affected sibs were females.
II **Risk of Occurrence:** ?
III **Risk of Recurrence for**
  Patient's Sib: If autosomal recessive, 1 in 4 (25%) for each offspring to be affected.
  Patient's Child: If autosomal recessive, not increased unless mate is carrier or homozygote.
IV **Age of Detectability:** At birth, on basis of obvious physical characteristics
V **Prevalence:** ?

Treatment
I **Primary Prevention:** Genetic counseling.

II **Secondary Prevention:** Surgical correction of cleft palate and lip is indicated in view of overall prognosis.

III **Other Therapy:** Appropriate hygienic measures to reduce risk of secondary infection of scalp and eyelids. Care in institution may be indicated in view of severe mental retardation compounded by other problems such as chronic scalp infection and blepharitis.

Prognosis: Life expectancy may be normal or only slightly reduced if infancy is survived.

Detection of Carrier: ?

†**Special Considerations:** In spite of many similarities between this syndrome and the popliteal pterygium syndrome, the absence of the pterygia and the presence of mental retardation in all 3 affected sibs in this family strongly suggest genetic heterogeneity, as does the recessive pattern of inheritance.

References:
Bowen, P. and Armstrong, H. B.: Ectodermal dysplasia, mental retardation, cleft lip/palate and other anomalies in three sibs. Clin. Genet. 9:35, 1976.
Gorlin, R. J. et al: Popliteal pterygium syndrome: A syndrome comprising cleft lip-palate, popliteal and intercrural pterygia, digital and genital anomalies. Pediatrics 41:503, 1968.
Rosselli, D. and Gulienetti, R.: Ectodermal dysplasia. Br. J. Plast. Surg. 14:190, 1961.

Contributors: **Peter Bowen**
H. Brock Armstrong

Editor's Computerized Descriptors: Vision, Eye, Face, Oral, Teeth, Sweating, Hair, Nails, Skel. Nerve, GU.

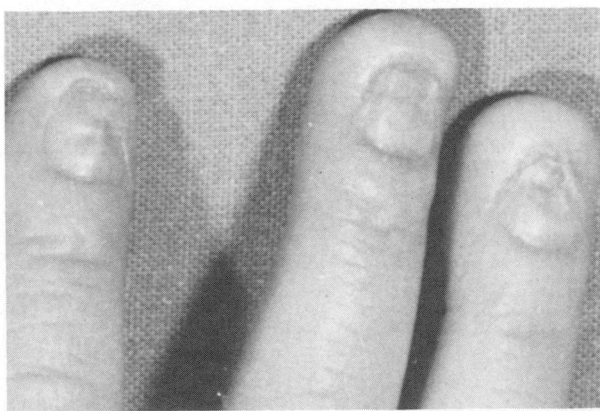

188. Nail dysplasia. Note small, irregular nails

CLEFT PALATE

Includes: Fente palatine
Gaumenspalte
Paladar hendido
Palatoschisis
Cleft of soft palate
Cleft of soft and hard palate
Submucous cleft palate

Excludes: Cleft lip with or without cleft palate (178)
Cleft lip or palate and lip pits or mounds (177)
Cleft uvula (Marker) (184)
Cleft palate and multiple dislocations
Cleft palate and persistence of buccopharyngeal membrane (181)
Cleft palate, micrognathia and glossoptosis (182)
Cleft lip or palate and filiform fusion of eyelids (176)
Popliteal pterygium syndrome (818)
Cervico-oculo-acoustic syndrome (142)
Diastrophic dysplasia (293)
Chondrodysplasia punctata
Arthroophthalmopathy (90)
Cleft palate, retinal detachment and myopia
Cleft palate, retinal detachment and joint hypermobility
Acrocephalosyndactyly (14)
Chromosomal defects: 4p-, 5p-, C trisomy, ring C (Cr), 14q-, 18 trisomy, 18p-, 18q-, 21 trisomy, XXXXY syndrome, various translocations, G trisomy, mosaicism and triploidy
Marfan syndrome (630)
Orofaciodigital syndromes I and II (770 and 771)
Waardenburg syndrome (997)
Smith-Lemli-Opitz syndrome (891)
Spondyloepiphyseal dysplasia, tarda (898)
Mandibulofacial dysostosis (627)
Meckel syndrome (634)
Oculoauriculovertebral dysplasia (735)
Micrognathia, talipes equinovarus, atrial septal defect, and persistence of left superior vena cava
Micrognathia, glossoptosis, pectus carinatum and accessory metacarpal of index finger
Camptodactyly and clubfoot
Stapes fixation and oligodontia
Failure of fusion of anterior fontanel, atypical dentin dysplasia and failure of eruption of teeth, pectus excavatum, diastasis recti, hypospadias and oligophrenia
Hanhart syndrome (451)

Minimal Diagnostic Criteria: A submucous cleft of the palate. Functional short palate and clefts of uvula probably are microforms of cleft palate.

Clinical Findings: A variable-sized congenital cleft extending through the hard palate, soft palate, or both, or a submucous cleft in which there is a thin medium raphe covered by mucosa but with failure of fusion of the underlying mesodermal elements. In this latter instance, there is frequently a notch in the position usually occupied by the posterior palatal spine. Transillumination with a light probe aids in diagnosis of submucous cleft. Clefts may extend through hard or soft palate with closure of palate posteriorly so that an ovoid rather than a V-shaped cleft results. Palatal clefts are frequently associated with abnormalities in the shape of the maxillary dental arch, such as the so-called Byzantine-arch palate in which the palatine processes of the maxilla are incompletely fused with the nasal spine. The vomer may lie unattached or be attached to either of the palatal processes. As a group, head size is usually slightly smaller, cranial base slightly shorter, and nasopharyngeal width greater than in normal individuals. Posterior facial height is reduced with a short mandibular ramus and obtuse gonial angle. Isolated cleft uvula and some types of congenital pharyngeal incompetence are probably an incomplete form of cleft palate.

Complications
I Derived: Difficulty in nursing, swallowing, respiration and phonation. Aspiration leading to lung disease.

II Associated: Approximately 35-50% of patients at birth with cleft palate have associated anomalies of which the most common are umbilical hernia, clubfoot, and deformities of limbs and ears. This falls to 13-25% in surgical series, many with gross abnormalities not surviving neonatal period. Sibs and relatives do not have an increased incidence of these anomalies other than cleft palate.

In many syndromes, cleft palate is one manifestation of the disorder. For those which have a greater than chance association with cleft palate see Table XIV.

Etiology: Unknown in most cases. Cleft palate is a sign that may result from a number of causes. It can occur as a result of either genetic or nongenetic causes and, from animal models, as a result of both environmental and genetic factors together. In some instances, it is one sign found in single gene substitution syndromes where the recurrence risk is high depending upon the mode of inheritance of the syndrome. It is also found as one feature in many nongenetic "developmental" syndromes in which the recurrence risk is very low. (See also Exclusions and Associated Complications.) When unassociated with syndromes, the most widely held hypothesis is that it is a polygenic trait which appears when a normal developmental threshold is not reached. Evidence for the role of genetic factors in cleft palate is less than in cleft lip/palate on the basis of twin studies where the concordance rate for cleft palate is: monozygotic 28.5%; dizygotic 10.5%.†

Pathogenesis: Several hypotheses concerning the development of cleft palate are current. Some evidence can be presented for each in individual experimental or clinical conditions, so that cleft palate may have several modes of development. In normal palatal formation the paired palatal shelves of the maxilla develop downward alongside the tongue. Later, beginning posteriorly they rapidly assume a horizontal position by snapping into the approximating position with each other and the nasal septum. They fuse with each other beginning at the incisive papillae and progressing posteriorly. Soft palate is formed by a posterior extension of mesoderm of fused palatine processes. One theory for CP suggests that the "shelf force" required to approximate the processes is defective. Another proposes that the tongue acts as a barrier. A disparity of head width and palatal size appears to be involved in some types. Failure of programmed epithelial cell death interfering with mesodermal fusion has been suggested.

Related Facts
I Sex Ratio:

Japanese	M34:F66
Caucasians	M43:F57
American Negroes	M52:F48

II Risk of Occurrence: Note: these are underestimates. See Age of Detectability.

American Negroes	1 in 5263
Caucasians	1 in 2702
Japanese	1 in 1587

Amerindian varies with tribe from about 1 in 1600 to 1 in 125. Highest known rate is 1 in 125 Haliwa of North Carolina.

III Risk of Recurrence for
Patient's Sib: —
Patient's Child:

Affected Parents	Affected Sibs	Affected Relatives	Percent Risk for Each Subsequent Child
None	None	None	0.04
None	1	None	2
None	1	1	7
None	2	None	1
1	None	None	6
1	1	None	15†

IV Age of Detectability: At birth by inspection of oral cavity. Note: the under-reporting of cleft palate at birth is considerable and is proportional to the severity of cleft. Meskin (1966) demonstrated the proportion of clefts reported on birth certificates by extent of clefts to be:

Complete cleft of hard palate	0.63
Incomplete cleft of hard palate	0.59
Complete cleft of soft palate	0.50
Incomplete cleft of soft palate	0.14
Submucous and regular clefts of soft palate only	0.05
Other submucous combinations	0.05
Total clefts of palate	0.47

V Prevalence: Unknown but up to 60% greater than reported incidence due to under-reporting on birth certificates.

Treatment
I Primary Prevention: Genetic counseling
II Secondary Prevention: Surgical closure of palate. Prosthetic restoration of palatal defect with obturator. Orthodontic treatment
III Other Therapy: Speech therapy

Prognosis: Depends upon associated anomalies or other features when associated with a syndrome. About 5-10% die in first year. With adequate early therapy, fair to excellent.

Detection of Carrier: —

†Special Considerations: Risk figures given are for CP when unassociated with a syndrome. Risk may approach 1 in 2 when associated with syndromes. See Cleft Lip With or Without Cleft Palate for more data.

References:
Gorlin, R. J.: Developmental anomalies of the face and oral structures. In Gorlin, R.J. and Goldman, H. M. (eds.): Thoma's Oral Pathology, 6th Ed. St. Louis:C.V. Mosby Co., 1970, p. 21.
Gorlin, R. J. et al: Facial clefting and its syndromes. In Bergsma, D. (ed.): Part XI. Orofacial Structures. Birth Defects: Orig. Art. Ser., vol. VII no. 7. Baltimore:Williams & Wilkins for The National Foundation-March of Dimes, 1971, p. 3.
Ross, R.B. and Johnston, M.C.: Cleft Lip and Palate. Baltimore:Williams & Wilkins, 1972.

Contributor: **Carl J. Witkop, Jr.**

Editor's Computerized Descriptors: Face, Oral, Nasoph., Speech, Skel., Hernia not CNS, Resp., Nerve.

CLEFT PALATE AND PERSISTENCE OF BUCCOPHARYNGEAL MEMBRANE

Editor's Computerized Descriptors: Oral, Neck, Skel., Resp., CV., GU., Nerve

Includes: Fente palatine avec persistance de la membrane bucco-pharyngée
Gaumenspalte und persistierende bucco-pharingeale Membran
Fisura palatina y persistencia de la membrana bucofaríngea
Congenital pharyngopalatinal diaphragm
Congenital syngnathism
Congenital atresia of nasopharynx
Intraoral bands with cleft uvula

Excludes: Laryngeal atresia (571)
Dermoid cyst or teratoma of head and neck (283)

Minimal Diagnostic Criteria: Intraoral bands associated with cleft uvula or both uvula and palate

Clinical Findings: Partial or complete closure of the oral cavity (and nasopharynx in some cases) associated with cleft palate of different degree.
  Type I: Intraoral bands or septum are located in the area of tuberculum cecum of the tongue.
  Type II: Intraoral bands connect the sublingual plica with oropharynx leaving tongue behind the bands or medial to the bands.
  Type III: Intraoral septum and absence of the tongue.

Complications
I   **Derived:** Dysphagia, suffocation
II **Associated:** Extra digits, heart anomalies, adrenal neuroblastoma and absence of thyroid

Etiology: ?

Pathogenesis: Persistence of the buccopharyngeal membrane separating the ectodermal and entodermal part and closing the primitive oral cavity in embryos 2-3 mm long. The tongue normally develops and the palatine shelves fuse after the disappearance of the buccopharyngeal membrane.

Related Facts
I   **Sex Ratio:** ?
II   **Risk of Occurrence:** Very rare
III **Risk of Recurrence for**
     Patient's Sib: ?
     Patient's Child: ?
IV   **Age of Detectability:** At birth by physical examination of pharynx
V   **Prevalence:** ?

Treatment
I   **Primary Prevention:** ?
II   **Secondary Prevention:** Surgical
III **Other Therapy:** Speech therapy and orthodontic treatment indicated in some cases.

Prognosis: In severe cases, poor

Detection of Carrier: —

Special Considerations: —

References:
Gorlin, R. J. and Pindborg, J. J.: Syndromes of the Head and Neck. New York:McGraw-Hill, 1964.
Hayward, J. R. and Avery, J. K.: Variation in cleft palate. J. Oral Surg. 15:320, 1957.
Hub, M. and Jirásek, J. E.: Persistence of the central part of the membrane buccopharyngicae. Čas. Lék. Česk. 99:1297, 1960.
Kouyoumdjian, A. O. and McDonald, J. J.: Association of congenital adrenal neuroblastoma with multiple anomalies including an unusual oropharyngeal cavity (imperforate buccopharyngeal membrane?). Cancer 4:784, 1951.

Contributor: **Jan E. Jirásek**

182

181-500

CLEFT PALATE, MICROGNATHIA AND GLOSSOPTOSIS

Includes: Division palatine, micrognathie et glossoptosis
Pierre Robin-Syndrom
Paladar hendido, micrognatia y glosoptosis
Robin anomaly
Micrognathia and glossoptosis syndrome

Excludes: First and second branchial arch syndrome
Mandibulofacial dysostosis (627)
Micrognathia
Cleft palate (180)

Minimal Diagnostic Criteria: Cleft palate, micrognathia, and glossoptosis are facultative and not obligatory. Thus, an occasional case may be missing one of these features.

Clinical Findings: Oral findings include cleft palate, micrognathia, and glossoptosis. The condition is etiologically heterogeneous. Approximately 25% of all cases are associated with other abnormalities constituting known genesis syndromes. The most common is the Stickler syndrome, but other syndromes may have the Robin anomaly. It is a common finding in the campomelic syndrome, cerebrocostomandibular syndrome, and persistent left superior vena cava syndrome. Uncommonly or rarely it may be associated with the Beckwith-Wiedemann syndrome, diastrophic dwarfism, femoral hypoplasia—unusual facies syndrome, myotonic dystrophy, radiohumeral synostosis syndrome, spondyloepiphyseal dysplasia congenita, trisomy 11q, fetal alcohol syndrome, fetal hydantoin syndrome, and fetal trimethadione syndrome.

Approximately 36% of all patients with the Robin anomaly have associated defects but are not recognized as having known genesis syndromes. A great variety of cardiac anomalies have been reported including patent ductus arteriosus, atrial septal defect, ventricular septal defect, patent foramen ovale, dextrocardia, tetralogy of Fallot, cor triloculare, coarctation of the aorta, and pulmonary artery atresia. Various eye anomalies, ear anomalies, and skeletal defects have also been reported. Mental deficiency is another commonly reported association.

Approximately 39% of all patients with the Robin anomaly have no associated defects.

Complications
I **Derived:** Respiratory distress and cyanosis. Feeding difficulties.
II **Associated:** See Clinical Findings.

Etiology: The Robin anomaly is etiologically heterogeneous. For known genetic syndromes, the mode of inheritance is that of the particular syndrome with which the anomaly is associated. The Robin anomaly may also be observed with congenital hypotonia, arthrogryposis, oligohydramnios, and various connective tissue dysplasias. Since the Robin anomaly occurs with a variety of associated defects producing many syndromes of unknown genesis, further delineation of many of these conditions is necessary.

Pathogenesis: Based on arrested development of the mandible which prevents normal descent of the tongue between the palatal shelves, obstructing closure. In this connection, the palate in the Robin anomaly is U-shaped (presumably caused by interference of the tongue) in contrast to the more frequently observed V-shaped cleft palate.

Related Facts
I **Sex Ratio:** Approximately M1:F1
II **Risk of Occurrence:** Approximately 1 in 30,000 live births
III **Risk of Recurrence for**
Patient's Sib: See Etiology and Clinical Findings

Patient's Child: See Etiology and Clinical Fingings
IV **Age of Detectability:** At birth, by clinical examination
V **Prevalence:** ?

Treatment
I **Primary Prevention:** Genetic counseling. See Clinical Findings and Etiology.
II **Secondary Prevention:** Early feeding and airway maintenance are of critical importance during infancy. In some cases, simply keeping the infant in a prone position serves to keep the tongue forward. In other cases, the tongue is temporarily sutured to the lower lip or a Kirshner wire is inserted from the angle of the mandible on one side through the posterior part of the tongue to the angle of the mandible on the other side. In severe cases with pronounced cyanosis, tracheostomy may be necessary.

The cleft palate should be surgically repaired. Mandibular growth catches up with maxillary growth in most cases and by 4-6 years of age, the profile is almost normal. Orthognathic surgery is, therefore, not necessary unless the condyles are ankylosed or in the uncommon case in which mandibular advancement is necessary.
III **Other Therapy:** Orthodontic treatment and speech therapy may be necessary.

Prognosis: Good, if patient survives infancy. Depends on associated abnormalities and overall diagnosis.

Detection of Carrier: See Etiology and Clinical Findings

Special Considerations: —

References:
Cohen, M.M., Jr.: The Robin anomaly - its nonspecificity and associated syndromes. J. Oral Surg. 34:587, 1976.
Hanson, J.W. and Smith, D.W.: U-shaped palatal defect in the Robin anomaly: Developmental and clinical relevance. J. Pediatr. 87:30, 1975.
Smith, J.L. and Stowe, F.R.: The Pierre Robin syndrome (glossoptosis, micrognathia, cleft palate): A review of 39 cases with emphasis on associated ocular lesions. Pediatrics 27:128, 1961.

Contributor: **M. Michael Cohen, Jr.**

Editor's Computerized Descriptors: Vision, Eye, Hearing, Ear, Face, Oral, Skel., CV., Nerve

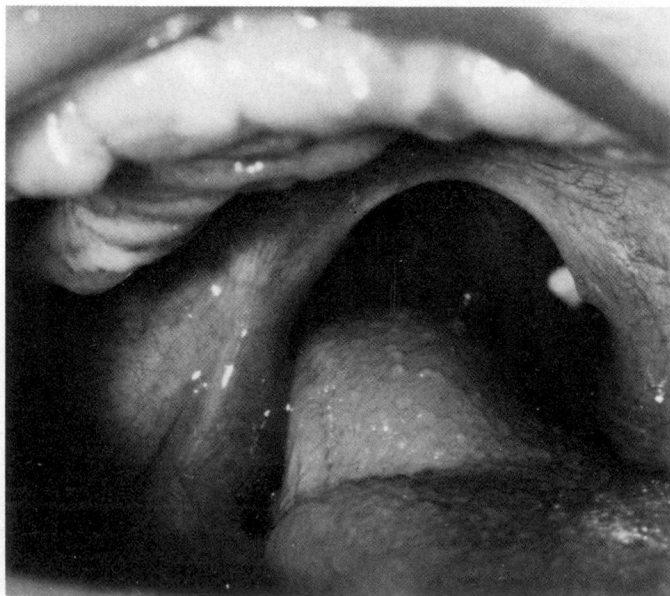

189. U-shaped cleft palate

CLEFT PALATE, STAPES FIXATION AND OLIGODONTIA

Editor's Computerized Descriptors: Eye, Hearing, Ear, Oral, Teeth, Skel., Resp.

Includes: Anomalies du carpe et du tarse, fissure palatine, oligodontie et surdité par ankylose de l'étrier

Carpotarsale Anomalien, Gaumenspalte, Oligodontie und Schwerhörigkeit mit Stapes-Fixation

Anomalías carpo-tarsales, paladar hendido, oligodoncia y sordera por fijación del estribo

Excludes: Dominant symphalangism and stapes fixation

Minimal Diagnostic Criteria: Cleft palate, stapes fixation, oligodontia and carpal and tarsal anomalies.

Clinical Findings: A kindred has been reported in which 2 of 4 sibs have this syndrome. The parents were 2nd cousins. Both female sibs had cleft soft palate, which had been repaired at about 10 years of age and both exhibited mild primary telecanthus. Neither girl had more than 3-4 deciduous teeth and neither had permanent dentition.

Hearing loss was noted prior to puberty and audiometric testing demonstrated a bilateral conductive hearing loss. Exploratory surgery revealed bilateral fixation of the stapes footplate in both girls. The hearing loss in each patient was satisfactorily corrected by stapedectomy. Radiographic examination of the hands and feet showed the following: the 3rd toe was the longest on both feet; there was shortening of the 1st metatarsal which was fused with the navicular bone. The 2nd and 3rd cuneiforms, the talus and navicular, and the talus and calcaneus were fused. The talus was malformed and there was underdevelopment of the joint surface of the tibia. In the hands there was underdevelopment of the navicular bones bilaterally.

Complications
I **Derived:** —
II **Associated:** —

Etiology: ? Autosomal recessive

Pathogenesis: ?

Related Facts
I **Sex Ratio:** M0:F2
II **Risk of Occurrence:** ?
III **Risk of Recurrence for**
  Patient's Sib: 1 in 4 (25%) for each offspring to be affected
  Patient's Child: Not increased unless mate is carrier or homozygote
IV **Age of Detectability:** Childhood
V **Prevalence:** ? Single reported family with 2 affected sibs

Treatment
I **Primary Prevention:** Genetic counseling
II **Secondary Prevention:** Hearing aid or stapes surgery
III **Other Therapy:** Dentures for oligodontia; surgery for cleft palate

Prognosis: Good for normal life span

Detection of Carrier: ?

Special Considerations: —

References:
Gorlin, R.J. et al: Cleft palate, stapes fixation and oligodontia: A new autosomal recessively inherited syndrome. In Bergsma, D. (ed.): Part XI. Orofacial Structures. Birth Defects: Orig. Art. Ser., vol. VII, no. 7. Baltimore: Williams & Wilkins for The National Foundation-March of Dimes, 1971, p. 87.

Contributor: Cor W.R.J. Cremers

CLEFT UVULA (MARKER)

Includes: Luette bifide
Gespaltene Uvula
Uvula hendida (Marcador)
Bifid uvula
Uvula, cleft

Excludes: Palatal insufficiency

Minimal Diagnostic Criteria: Diagnosis based on bilateral separation of uvula on clinical manipulation.

Clinical Findings: Cleft uvula varies from a notching of uvula to complete cleft of uvula extending to posterior border of soft palate.

Complications
I Derived: —
II Associated: Submucous cleft palate

Etiology: Occasionally surgical. Otherwise essentially unknown but thought to be conditioned by minor gene(s) similar to that of cleft palate.†

Pathogenesis: Failure of complete fusion of the uvular portion of the lateral halves of the soft palate during embryogenesis. May be part of the palatal insufficiency syndrome wherein there is incomplete closure of soft palate and pharynx during phonation leading to hypernasality, or minimal closure that results in hypernasality following removal of tonsils and adenoids.

Related Facts
I Sex Ratio: M1.2:F1
II Risk of Occurrence: Greater in families with a child with cleft palate. Otherwise 1 in 77 to 1 in 66 Caucasian live births; less in Negroes; greater in Asiatics, 1 in 10 to 1 in 5.
III Risk of Recurrence for
  Patient's Sib: With an affected parent 30%; without an affected parent 10%
  Patient's Child: 30%
IV Age of Detectability: At birth, by visual examination
V Prevalence: Entity is noted in approximately 1 in 71 of Caucasian populations. The notching accounts for 1 in 83, with more severe clefts approximately 1 in 330. In Asiatic populations, 1 in 10 to 1 in 5.

Treatment
I Primary Prevention: —
II Secondary Prevention: †
III Other Therapy: —

Prognosis: Normal life span

Detection of Carrier: —

†Special Considerations: This anatomic defect can be considered a microform of the cleft palate portion of facial clefts. It can be used as a genetic and anthropologic marker in this context. It may also serve as a marker to indicate a tendency towards a hypernasality speech defect called palatal insufficiency or congenital palatopharyngeal incompetence. In persons with cleft uvula the complete removal of the adenoid pad in the tonsillectomy and adenoidectomy operation may produce hypernasality of speech.

References:
Meskin, L.H. et al: Abnormal morphology of the soft palate: I. The prevalence of cleft uvula. Cleft Palate J. 1:342, 1964.
Meskin, L.H. et al: Abnormal morphology of the soft palate: II. The genetics of cleft uvula. Cleft Palate J. 2:40, 1965.
Meskin, L.H. et al: Cleft uvula- a microform of cleft palate. Acta Chir. Plast. (Praha) 8:91, 1966.

Contributor: **Lawrence Meskin**

Editor's Computerized Descriptors: Oral, Speech
Also see Section I, Fig. 90

CLEIDOCRANIAL DYSPLASIA

Includes: Dysplasie cléidocranienne
Dysplasia cleidocranialis
Displasia cleidocraniana
Cleidocranial dysostosis
Dysplasia, osteodental
Marie-Sainton disease

Excludes: Pyknodysostosis (846)
Craniofacial dysostosis (225)

Minimal Diagnostic Criteria: Brachycephaly and bossing of the cranium with evidence of delayed closure of the fontanels and sutures. Aplasia of all or a part of one or both clavicles and abnormal shoulder movements. Dental anomalies including maleruption or supernumerary dentition.†

Clinical Findings: Proportionate mild-to-moderate short stature with narrow, drooping shoulders. The skull is brachycephalic, there is bossing of the frontal, parietal and occipital areas and there is failure or delayed closure of the fontanels and sutures. Wormian bones may be present. The accessory sinuses and mastoids may be late or hypoplastic in development. Oral features include a high-arched palate with or without cleft; nonunion of the mandibular symphysis; delayed eruption or failure of eruption of the deciduous and permanent teeth, and supernumerary teeth. Mentality is usually normal. Partial or complete aplasia of the clavicles unilaterally or bilaterally with associated muscle defects allows a remarkable range of shoulder movements - many individuals can approximate the shoulders in front of their chest. The hands may show a number of anomalies: asymmetric length of fingers with long 2nd metacarpals, tapering distal phalanges and accessory proximal metacarpal epiphyses. Other skeletal deformities include delayed ossification of the pubic bone, coxa vara or valga, genu valgum, scoliosis, cervical ribs, vertebral malformations and small scapula. A host of other minor anomalies have been reported.

Complications
I Derived: Cyst formation around unerupted, often inverted or displaced teeth may of itself cause problems, as well as lead to gross destruction and pathologic fracture. Pregnancy usually requires cesarean section because of pelvic dysplasia.
II Associated: —

Etiology: Autosomal dominant with wide variability in expression but high penetrance. About one-third of the cases appears to represent new mutations. McK *11960

Pathogenesis: ?

Related Facts
I Sex Ratio: M1:F1
II Risk of Occurrence: ?
III Risk of Recurrence for
  Patient's Sib: If parent is affected, 1 in 2 (50%) for each offspring to be affected; otherwise not increased.
  Patient's Child: 1 in 2
IV Age of Detectability: At birth by physical and radiographic examination
V Prevalence: ? Over 500 cases have appeared in medical literature.

Treatment
I Primary Prevention: Genetic counseling
II Secondary Prevention: Protective head gear while fontanels remain open. Appropriate dental management and surgical closure of cleft palate when indicated
III Other Therapy: —

Prognosis: Normal life span

Detection of Carrier: —

†**Special Considerations:** Because of the wide variability in clinical expression, it may be necessary to obtain selected xrays in order to detect affected cases in which expressivity is low. Pyknodysostosis shows wide skull sutures and delayed closure of the fontanels as in cleidocranial dysplasia but is differentiated by the presence of acroosteolysis, generalized skeletal sclerosis with a tendency to fractures and by an autosomal recessive mode of inheritance. Crouzon disease is distinguished by craniosynostosis, a parrot-beaked nose, normal clavicles and symphysis pubis.

References:

Forland, M.: Cleidocranial dysostosis; a review of the syndrome and report of a sporadic case with hereditary transmission. Am. J. Med. 33:792, 1962.

Gorlin, R.J. and Pindborg, J.J.: Syndromes of the Head and Neck. New York: McGraw-Hill, 1964.

Kalliala, E. and Taskinen, P.J.: Cleidocranial dysostosis: Report of six typical cases and one atypical case. Oral Surg. 15:808, 1962.

Spranger, J.W. et al: Bone Dysplasias. Philadelphia: W.B. Saunders, 1974.

Contributor: **Charles I. Scott, Jr.**

———————————

Editor's Computerized Descriptors: Face, Oral, Teeth, Skel.

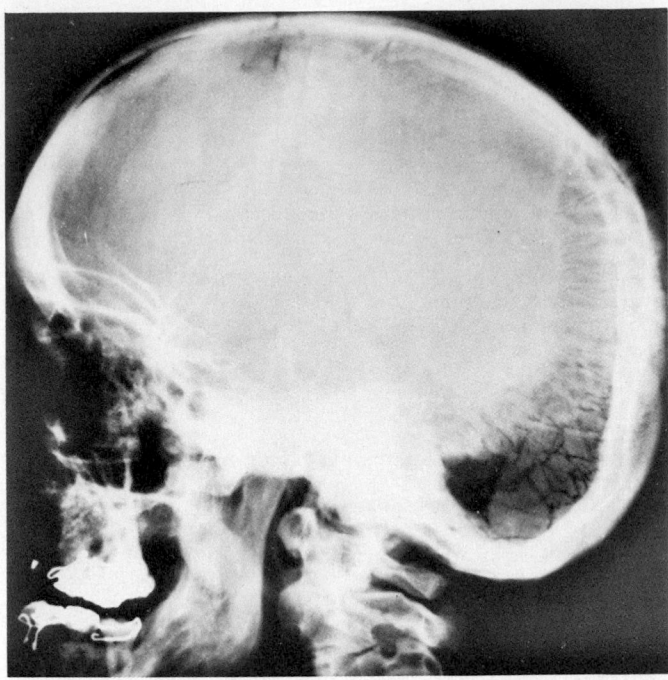

191. Note multiple wormian bones in posterior lateral fontanel, a diamond-shaped defect in metopic suture and settling of occipital bone about cervical spine

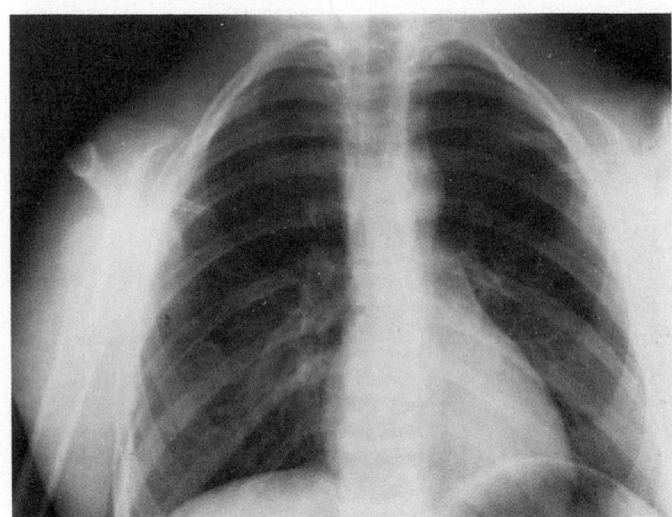

192. Note defect of clavicles

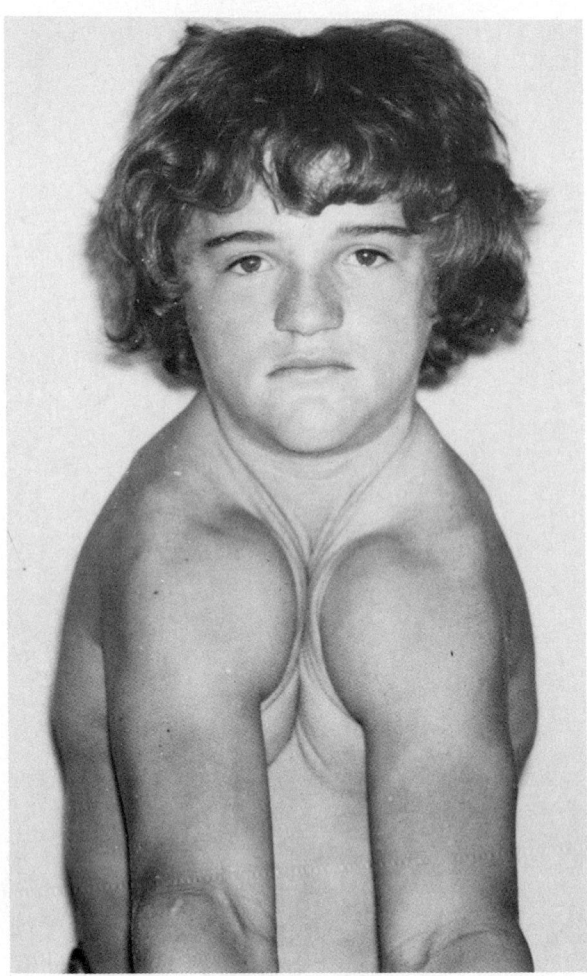

190. Note approximation of shoulders

CNS ARTERIOVENOUS MALFORMATION

Includes: Malformation artério-veineuse
Arteriovenöse Fehlbildungen des Zentralnervensystem
SNC-malformación arteriovenosa
Vein of Galen aneurysm
Cystic arteriovenous malformations
Arteriovenous malformations, spinal, cortical, cerebellar
Central nervous system arteriovenous malformation

Excludes: Intracranial aneurysm of childhood
Sturge-Weber syndrome (915)
von Hippel-Lindau syndrome (995)
Hemangioblastoma

Minimal Diagnostic Criteria: Demonstration of abnormal CNS vasculature by angiogram

Clinical Findings: *Intracranial arteriovenous malformation* (AVM)
Intracranial hemorrhage 40%
Seizures 30%
Hemiparesis or other neurologic defect 33%
Headache 14%
Bruit 22%
Intraspinal (AVM)
Subarachnoid hemorrhage with back pain and sudden onset of paraplegia. Bruit may be heard over spine.
Vein of Galen aneurysm.
Heart failure in newborn; hydrocephaly in infancy

Complications
I **Derived:** Neurologic deficit from bleeding of AVM or from cerebral anoxia of subarachnoid adjacent brain tissue. Repeated bleeding may lead to communicating hydrocephaly.
II **Associated:** —

Etiology: ?

Pathogenesis: There exists a direct artery to vein connection without an intervening capillary bed. Blood shunted through the malformation leading to anoxia of adjacent brain, producing epileptogenic cortex.

Related Facts
I **Sex Ratio:** ?
II **Risk of Occurrence:** ?
III **Risk of Recurrence for**
  Patient's Sib: ?
  Patient's Child: ?
IV **Age of Detectability:** 20% become symptomatic in 1st decade
V **Prevalence:** 5-10% of patients with subarachnoid hemorrhage

Treatment
I **Primary Prevention:** —
II **Secondary Prevention:** Surgical excision. Control of seizures with anticonvulsants.†
III **Other Therapy:** —

Prognosis: Once symptomatic approximately 15% risk of death. Vein of Galen aneurysm usually fatal in newborn period.

Detection of Carrier: —

†Special Considerations: Management of a child with AVM depends upon the accessibility of the lesion and the symptom complex produced.

References:
Bartal, A.D. et al: Excision of the vein of Galen complicated by congestive heart failure. Neurochirurgia 17:16, 1974.
Boynton, R.C. and Morgan, B.C.: Cerebral arteriovenous fistula with possible hereditary telangiectasia. Am. J. Dis. Child. 125:99, 1973.
Matson, D.D.: Neurosurgery of Infancy and Childhood, 2nd Ed. Springfield: Charles C Thomas, 1969.
Perret, G. and Nishioka, H.: Report on the Cooperative Study of Intracranial Aneurysms and Subarachnoid Hemorrhage. Section IV. Arteriovenous Malformation. An analysis of 545 cases of craniocerebral arteriovenous malformations and fistulae reported to the Cooperative Study. J. Neurosurg. 25:467, 1966.

Contributor: **Kenneth Shulman**

Editor's Computerized Descriptors: CV., Nerve

CNS DEPRESSION, HEMORRHAGE, SKELETAL SYNDROME

Includes: Placenta circumvallata
Syndrom der Placenta circumvallata
Síndrome de placenta circumvalada
Circumvallate placenta syndrome

Excludes: —

Minimal Diagnostic Criteria: Polyhydramnios, CNS depression, neonatal hemorrhage and skeletal abnormalities.

Clinical Findings: Neonatal death occurred in 3 sibs due to respiratory insufficiency. All 3 pregnancies were complicated by polyhdramnios and each infant showed cutaneous and intracranial hemorrhage, marked CNS depression and skeletal abnormalities, including thin ribs and overtubulation of long bones. Other findings include brachycephaly, frontal bossing, flat nasal bridge, hyperextensible joints and hyperelastic skin. No specific coagulation defect was found and electron microscopy did not reveal a morphologic defect of capillaries. There was no disease in the mother to explain polyhydramnios. The placenta of only 1 of the 3 cases was examined and it was reported to be circumvallate with characteristic fibrin deposition.

Complications
I **Derived:** Neonatal hemorrhage, aspiration pneumonia, respiratory distress, cardiac arrest and neonatal death.
II **Associated:** —

Etiology: Occurrence in 3 sibs suggests the homozygous state of an autosomal recessive gene. A genetically determined, but as yet unrecognized maternofetal incompatibility leading to fibrin deposition and formation of a circumvallate placenta, remains another possibility, or repeated marginal placental hemorrhages leading to circumvallate placenta.

Pathogenesis: ?

Related Facts
I **Sex Ratio:** M0:F3
II **Risk of Occurrence:** ?
III **Risk of Recurrence for**
    Patient's Sib: If autosomal recessive 1 in 4 (25%) for each offspring to be affected. Possibly 100% if a maternofetal incompatibility.
    Patient's Child: Not increased unless mate is carrier or homozygote
IV **Age of Detectability:** At birth
V **Prevalence:** Single occurrence in 3 sibs thus far reported.

Treatment
I **Primary Prevention:** Genetic counseling
II **Secondary Prevention:** Careful surveillance of such mothers for polyhydramnios and circumvallate placenta and their infants for CNS depression, skeletal anomalies and neonatal hemorrhage. Treatment of anoxia and hemorrhage.
III **Other Therapy:** Supportive measures to prevent further CNS depression and hemorrhage.

Prognosis: —

Detection of Carrier: —

Special Considerations: —

References:
Deacon, J.S.R. et al: Polyhydramnios and neonatal hemorrhage in three sisters. A circumvallate placenta syndrome? In Bergsma, D. (ed.): Malformation Syndromes, Birth Defects: Orig. Art. Ser., vol. X, no. 7. Miami: Symposia Specialists for The National Foundation-March of Dimes, 1974, p. 41.

Morgan, J.: Circumvallate placenta. J. Obstet. Gynaecol. Br. Commwlth. 62:899, 1955.
Naftolin, F. et al: The syndrome of chronic abruptio placentae, hydrorrhea and circumvallate placenta. Am. J. Obstet. Gynecol. 116:347, 1973.

Contributor: **Enid F. Gilbert**

Editor's Computerized Descriptors: Skel., Resp., Nerve Nose, Skin

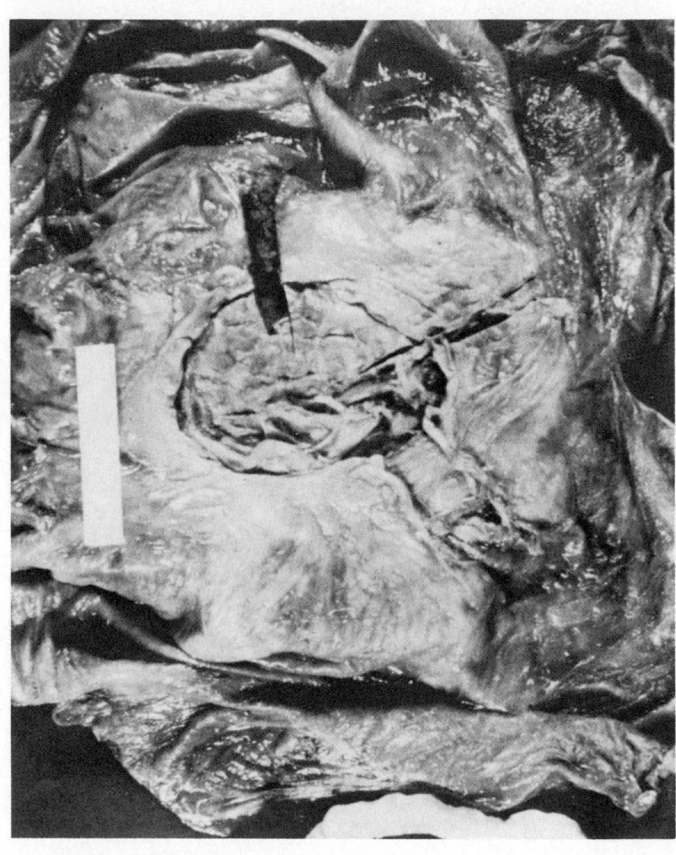

193. Circumvallate placenta

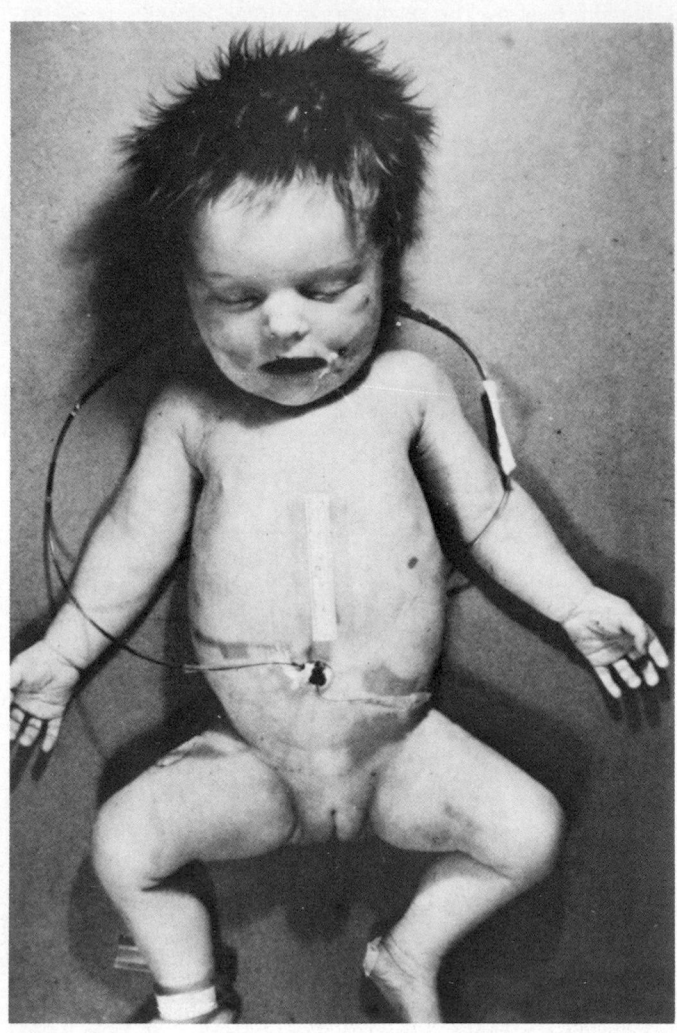

194. Physical appearance immediately after death

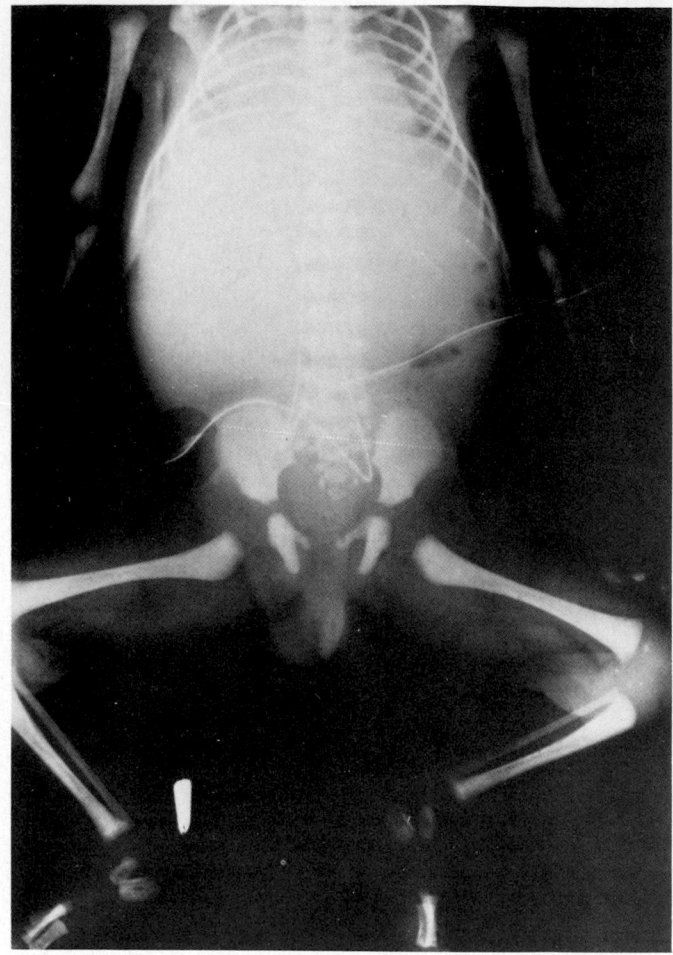

195. Bell-shaped thoracic cage with thin, gracile ribs. Limbs show overtubulation

CNS NEOPLASMS

Includes: Tumeurs du système nerveux central
Hirntumoren
Neoplasmas del SNC
Hamartoma of CNS
Ependymoma
Astrocytoma including optic nerve glioma
Medulloblastoma
Papilloma of choroid plexus
Central nervous system neoplasms
Germinomas
Ectopic pinealomas
Neoplasms of CNS

Excludes: Tumors rising in greatest preponderance after the age of puberty

Minimal Diagnostic Criteria: In all tumors except optic gliomas and in some tumors involving the pineal, tumor biopsy or biopsy during tumor removal for microscopic identification is essential. Diagnosis of optic glioma (associated with von Recklinghausen disease) can be made with an enlarged optic foramen and typical EMI or air study.

Clinical Findings: As the most frequent solid tumor occurring in childhood, brain tumors constitute an important segment of pediatric oncology. Neurologic manifestations may be mild and easily overlooked or misinterpreted, particularly in the very young, because of the remarkable plasticity of the immature nervous system and the expandability of the infant skull. The majority of tumors produce increased intracranial pressure, usually the consequence of obstructive hydrocephalus. Specific neurologic deficits correspond to tumor location. The posterior fossa harbors two-thirds of childhood tumors, and each of the 4 common tumors in this location produces a characteristic syndrome. Supratentorial tumors occupy the cerebral hemisphere, the suprasellar area and the pineal gland. The tumor presentation during the 1st year of life is ordinarily as megalocephaly due to obstructive hydrocephalus. Finding of papilledema and an enlarging head should make one suspect a tumor rather than congenital hydrocephalus. After the age of 1 year, signs of increased intracranial pressure, nausea, vomiting and lethargy predominate, with the gradual development of neurologic signs consistent with the tumor's location. Papilledema provides unequivocal evidence of increased intracranial pressure. Decreased visual acuity as a consequence of long-standing papilledema may be noticed by an observant parent or often as failing vision in school. Abducens palsy, either unilateral or bilateral, may not lead to the complaint of diplopia. An uncorrectable refractive error in a child indicates a tumor of the optic nerve or chiasm or tract. Generalized convulsions are relatively infrequent because of the posterior fossa localization of the tumor.

Focal neurologic abnormalities: Posterior fossa tumors predominate.

1) Cerebellar astrocytomas are the most frequent posterior fossa tumors preferentially involving the cerebellar hemispheres. About 50% of these tumors have an associated cyst within which a neoplastic mass may be confined to a relatively small nodule. A minority involve the vermis. Cerebellar hemisphere dysfunction is represented by ipsilateral hypotonia, incoordination and intention tremor and nystagmus. With unilateral herniation of the ipsilateral cerebellar tonsil, stiff neck and head tilt ensue.

2) Medulloblastoma has a decided predilection for males, occupying the cerebellar vermis and producing a syndrome of truncal ataxia. Because of the rapid growth of the tumor and the early obstruction of the 4th ventricle, increased intracranial pressure occurs early.

3) Brain-stem gliomas present in contradistinction without increased intracranial pressure. Histologically these tumors are low-grade astrocytomas, diffusely involving fiber tracts of the medulla and pons. The hallmark of brain-stem glioma is cranial nerve involvement, at first unilateral, but soon thereafter bilateral. Most frequently the 7th and the 6th nerves are involved, followed by 9th and 10th, with 5th and 8th last. There is associated cerebellar dysmetria and hemiparesis on the basis of cortical spine tract involvement.

4) Ependymomas originate within the 4th ventricle, obstructing it and producing intracranial pressure. These tumors by compressing the floor of the 4th ventricle in the region of the area postrema can produce intractable vomiting.

5) Tumors of the cerebral hemisphere. Several glial tumors arise in the cerebral hemispheres: astrocytomas, ependymomas, subependymal giant cell astrocytomas. Seizures are an early finding, frequently focal motor, with gradual hemiparesis and hemianopsia.

6) Suprasellar tumors. By either compressing or invading structures lying above and within the sella turcica, suprasellar tumors involve the optic chiasm, hypothalamus, 3rd ventricle, and pituitary gland. Frequent tumors are craniopharyngioma, astrocytomas arising from the optic chiasm and optic nerve and germinomas (ectopic pinealomas). Impairment of hypothalamic function may cause a variety of clinical abnormalities. One interesting syndrome is the diencephalic syndrome with growth failure, cachexia and dwarfism. Diabetes insipidus, visual failure and hypopituitarism are characteristic of germinomas. The most frequent tumor, craniopharyngioma, ordinarily presents as visual loss and headaches.

7) Pinealomas represent a clinically distinct syndrome of paresis of upward gaze, the so-called Parinaud syndrome. The pathology in the region of the pineal may include astrocytoma, true pineal tumors or germinomas and mixed teratomas.

8) Papillomas of choroid plexus arise in the plexus of the lateral ventricles (L 7 R) and produce increased intracranial pressure and hydrocephalus due to oversecretion of CSF and recurrent bleeding, which causes obstruction of absorbing mechanisms. Surgical removal and cure is possible.

The diagnosis and management of CNS neoplasms have been revolutionized by the development of computerized axial tomography. This procedure which can be done without risk and discomfort permits imaging of the brain, with tumor density clearly standing apart.

In addition plain skull xrays, radionucleotide scanning, and EEG are useful. As a preoperative assessment, angiography to visualize the blood supply of the tumor and adjacent blood vessels is useful. Pneumoencephalography and ventriculography have been largely put aside with the development of the computerized axial tomography mode of diagnosis.

Complications
I **Derived:** Progressive neurologic deficit; progressive increase in intracranial pressure; visual loss; hypopituitary growth failure.
II **Associated:** Neurofibromatosis is frequently present in children with gliomas of the optic nerve and cerebral gliomas. Tuberous sclerosis is associated with subependymal giant cell astrocytomas.

Etiology: ? Embryonic cell rests lead to hamartomas. Persistence of granular layer may lead to medulloblastoma. This is similarly questionable. Pathogenesis of tumor type is unknown.

Pathogenesis: ?†

Related Facts
I **Sex Ratio:** M1:F1
II **Risk of Occurrence:** ?
III **Risk of Recurrence for**
  Patient's Sib: ?
  Patient's Child: ?
IV **Age of Detectability:** Have been detected in premature newborns.
V **Prevalence:** Second most common neoplasms of children.

Treatment
I **Primary Prevention:** ?
II **Secondary Prevention:** ?
III **Other Therapy:** Surgical removal for craniopharyngioma, supratentorial gliomas, cerebellar astrocytomas and medulloblastomas. Radiotherapy for pineal tumors, germinomas and postop medulloblastoma, supratentorial glioma. Chemotherapy possible.

Prognosis: Best in isolated gliomas, particularly those that are cystic of the cerebellum and optic nerve tumors, an 80-90% cure rate can be effected. Worst in medulloblastoma with tendency to seed throughout the subarachnoid space. With radical surgical removal and total CNS radiation, a 30% - 5 year survival may be obtained.

Detection of Carrier: —

†Special Considerations: Papilloma of the choroid plexus can lead to hydrocephaly on the basis of overproduction of CSF.

References:
Bartlett, J.R.: Craniopharyngiomas - an analysis of some aspects of symptomatology. Radiology and histology. Brain 94:725, 1971.
Bernell, W.R.: Late malignant recurrence of childhood cerebellar astrocytoma - report of two cases. J. Neurosurg. 37:470, 1972.
Bloom, H.J.G. et al: The treatment and prognosis of medulloblastoma in children. Am. J. Roentgenol. Radium Ther. Nucl. Med. 105:43, 1969.
Bouchard, J.L.: Radiation Therapy of Tumors and Diseases of the Nervous System. Philadelphia:Lea & Febiger, 1966.
Bucy, P.C. and Thieman, P.W.: Astrocytomas of the cerebellum - a study of a series of patients operated upon over 28 years ago. Arch. Neurol. 18:14, 1968.
DeGirolami, U. and Schmidek, H.: Clinicopathological study of 53 tumors of the pineal region. J. Neurosurg. 39:455, 1973.
Golden, G.S. et al: Malignant glioma of the brain-stem. J. Neurol. Neurosurg. Psychiatry 35:732, 1972.
Matson, D.D.: Neurosurgery of Infancy and Childhood, 2nd Ed. Springfield: Charles C Thomas, 1969.
Wilson, C.B.: Diagnosis and surgical treatment of childhood brain tumors. Cancer 35:950, 1975.

Contributor: **Kenneth Shulman**

Editor's Computerized Descriptors: Vision, Eye, Neck, Skel., Muscle, GI., Nerve

COCKAYNE SYNDROME

Includes: Syndrome de Cockayne
Síndrome de Cockayne
Neill-Dingwall syndrome

Excludes: Progeria (825)
Seckel syndrome (881)
Bloom syndrome (112)
Dubowitz syndrome (299)
Leprechaunism (587)

Minimal Diagnostic Criteria: Diagnosis must be made primarily upon clinical grounds since no consistent biochemical abnormality has been discovered in the 40 reported patients. One must bear in mind when evaluating possible affected individuals that no 2 patients with any syndrome are identical, although often 2 unrelated affected individuals resemble each other more than either resembles his unaffected sibs. Also, few patients can be expected to manifest all of the "classic" features of a syndrome; no one feature of a syndrome is either syndrome-specific or essential for the diagnosis of that syndrome. With these points in mind, only arbitrary minimal diagnostic criteria can be mentioned.

A combination of most of the following features probably should be present for a clinical diagnosis of the Cockayne syndrome to be strongly suspected: 1) normal 1st year with onset of symptoms in the 2nd year; 2) dwarfism (present in all cases reported); 3) typical facies as previously noted (present in all cases reported); 4) retinal degeneration; 5) microcephaly; 6) cataracts; 7) neurologic impairment including mental deficiency, progressive (present in all cases reported); 8) disproportionately long limbs with large hands and feet; 9) flexion deformities and exaggerated dorsal kyphosis; 10) photosensitive skin rash leading to scarring and pigmentation; and, 11) x-ray findings including thickening of the calvarium, intracranial calcifications, short metacarpals and phalanges, vertebral notching, and minor abnormalities of the pelvis.†

Clinical Findings: Birthweight is not low. Growth and development proceed normally in the 1st year of life. The 1st symptoms and signs usually appear during the 2nd year. Growth falls below the normal range and mental-motor development becomes abnormal. Dwarfism, mental deficiency and other signs of neurologic abnormality (unsteady gait, microcephaly and sensorineural hearing deficit) become more prominent with time.

Based upon 4 personally observed and 36 published cases, clinical findings include the above points with variable combinations of pinched facies, sunken eyes, thin nose and prognathism which become progressively more abnormal with advancing age (all 40); cataracts (13); hypermetropia (9); retinal degeneration (32) as manifested by retinal pigmentation, optic atrophy and attenuation of retinal vessels; extensive dental caries (25); photosensitive skin rash which heals with scarring (30); cryptorchidism (15 of 28 males); disproportionately long limbs with large hands and feet (26); flexion deformities of the joints (29); cold, blue limbs (12); and exaggerated dorsal kyphosis (19). Less frequent findings include hydrocephalus, decreased pupillary response to mydriatic agents, corneal dystrophy, narrowly arched palate, sparse hair, decreased sweating, hepatosplenomegaly, short metacarpals and phalanges, and signs of impaired renal function. Eight of the 40 patients have died, ages at death ranging from 7-31 years.

Roentgenographic features include thickening of the calvarium, intracranial calcifications, anterior notching of vertebral bodies, minor anomalies of the pelvis, slender shafts of long bones with expanded metaphyses and epiphyses, large carpal and tarsal bones, and osteoporosis.

Complications
I   **Derived:** Severe cutaneous reaction to minimal exposure to ultraviolet radiation; deficient perspiration may lead to heat prostration; injuries due to unsteady gait; visual impairment; apparent susceptibility to infections; tendency to rapid dehydration and electrolyte imbalance with gastroenteritis.
II **Associated:** At present the delineation of the Cockayne syndrome is preliminary, so that the separation of component features from "associated defects" is impossible.

Etiology: Autosomal recessive mutant allele; McK *21640

Pathogenesis: The primary effect of the mutant allele is not known. No chromosome abnormality has been identified, and limited results have not revealed an increased tendency to chromosome damage in cultured cells. No common biochemical defect is discernible, although isolated reports of IgA-IgE deficiency are available, as are those of prediabetic glucose tolerance curves, ACTH unresponsiveness by the adrenal gland, and signs of altered renal function such as azotemia, decreased creatinine clearance and hyperchloremic acidosis. In a study of 1 patient Cotton and his associates demonstrated hyperglycemia in the presence of hyperinsulinism. In addition, a dramatic increase in plasma growth hormone followed an insulin challenge, even though the decrease in blood glucose was minimal. On the basis of these observations the authors suggested that excessive growth hormone secretion occurs in the Cockayne syndrome. One might thus speculate that a target cell resistance to growth hormone or that an alteration in the biologic activity of growth hormone is a possible etiologic mechanism in this condition.

Neuropathologic investigations have pointed to neuronal degeneration in the cerebrum, cerebellum and anterior horn cells of the spinal cord, along with patchy but extensive demyelination in the CNS and in peripheral nerves. Extensive mineralization in the walls of small vessels and perivascular spaces has been observed in the CNS.

Other morbid pathologic alterations have included pancreatic islet hyperplasia and secretory inactivity of the adrenal cortex. Ovarian changes have consisted of atrophy, fibrosis and decreased numbers of germ cells. In the kidneys, glomerular hyalinization, tubular atrophy and interstitial fibrosis have been described.

Related Facts
I   **Sex Ratio:** M28:F12
II   **Risk of Occurrence:** Rare, with no reliable occurrence figures
III **Risk of Recurrence for**
     Patient's Sib: 1 in 4 (25%) for each offspring to be affected
     Patient's Child: Negligible theoretically, although no reports exist of a patient having reproduced.
IV   **Age of Detectability:** Ordinarily in the 2nd year of life the condition can be suspected clinically
V   **Prevalence:** Rare; specific figures not available.

Treatment
I   **Primary Prevention:** No measures known other than intelligent preventive genetic counseling for couples who have previously produced an affected offspring.
II   **Secondary Prevention:** No measures known, except that the avoidance of ultraviolet irradiation will minimize skin changes. Surgical removal of cataracts in appropriate cases.
III **Other Therapy:** —

Prognosis: In general, life expectancy is shortened; the oldest reported patient died at 31 years of age. Progressive impairment leading to severe mental defect by 2nd decade of life. Blindness and deafness are usually progressive, with severe flexion contractures, leading to total invalidism.

Detection of Carrier: —

†**Special Considerations:** The diagnosis of the Cockayne syndrome is necessarily clinical. No specific biochemical, cytogenetic or histologic feature is known. Attention has been called to the fact that several other conditions involving mental defect and dyskeratosis are known, including some forms of xeroderma pigmentosum and the Hartnup disease. Also the dwarfism of the Cockayne syndrome, with its somewhat senile facies, has been compared with that of progeria and leprechaunism. However, the photosensitive skin rash, mental deficiency, ocular involvement and deafness of the Cockayne syndrome would serve to differentiate it with certainty from progeria; and its later onset and longer life span differentiate it from leprechaunism. Although suggestions have been made that the Cockayne syndrome and leprechaunism might represent different expressions of the same basic defect, no report has described both conditions in the same sibship. Thus, no real evidence exists to indicate that they are different expressions of the same gene mutation, even though hyperinsulinism has been described in some patients with each condition.

References:
Cotton, R.B. et al: Abnormal blood glucose regulation in Cockayne's syndrome. Pediatrics 46:54, 1970.
Gamstorp, I.: Donohue's syndrome-leprechaunism-Cockayne's syndrome. Eur. Neurol. 7:26, 1972.
MacDonald, W.B. et al: Cockayne's syndrome: An heredofamilial disorder of growth and development. Pediatrics 25:997, 1960.
Moosa, A. and Dubowitz, V.: Peripheral neuropathy in Cockayne's syndrome. Arch. Dis. Child. 45:674, 1970.
Moossy, J.: The neuropathology of Cockayne's syndrome. J. Neuropathol. Exp. Neurol. 26:654, 1967.
Paddison, R.M. et al: Cockayne's syndrome: A report of five new cases with biochemical, chromosomal, dermatologic, genetic and neuropathologic observations. Derm. Trop. 2:195, 1963.
Sugarman, G.I. et al: Cockayne syndrome: Clinical study of two patients and neuropathologic findings in one. Clin. Pediatr. 16:225, 1977.

Contributor: **Robert L. Summitt**

Editor's Computerized Descriptors: Vision, Eye, Hearing, Face, Teeth, Nose, Skin, Sweating, Hair, Skel., Resp., Spleen, Liver, GU.

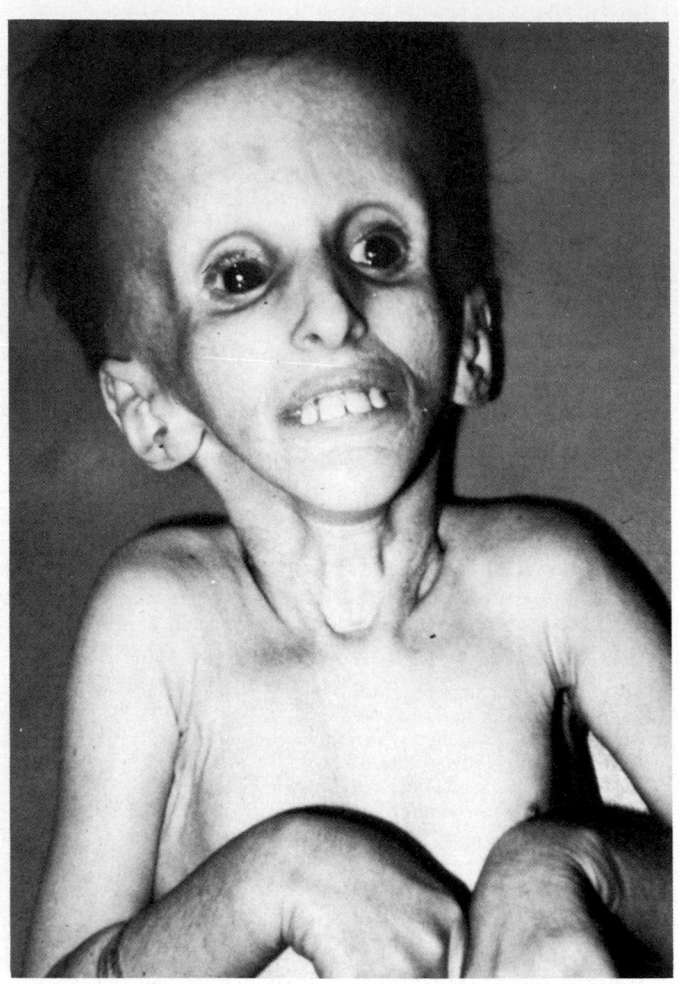

196. Note pinched facies, sunken eyes, thin nose and sparse hair.

COFFIN-LOWRY SYNDROME

Includes: Syndrome de Coffin-Lowry
Síndrome de Coffin-Lowry
Mental retardation with osteocartilaginous anomalies
Coffin syndrome

Excludes: Coffin-Siris syndrome

Minimal Diagnostic Criteria: Unknown, but characteristic craniofacial defects, severe mental retardation, short stature and hand anomalies seem to be minimal criteria in males. Clinical and radiographic manifestations are more variable and less severe in females.

Clinical Findings: The features of this disorder are more severe in males and progress with age. Characteristic facies includes a square forehead with prominent outer lateral aspects, bitemporal narrowing, thickened supraorbital ridges, downslanting palpebral fissures, hypertelorism, thickened upper eyelids, broad nasal bridge with thick nasal septum and anteverted nostrils, thickened prominent lips with pouty lower lip, open mouth facies, thick prominent chin and prominent ears. Limb anomalies include large soft hands with hyperextensible thick fingers that taper distally, a transverse hypothenar crease and a short great toe. The skin in males is loose and easily stretched.

All affected males have been severely mentally deficient with IQ less than 50. The majority of affected females have had mild mental retardation. A clumsy, broad-based gait has been a consistent feature in both males and females. All affected individuals have had shortness of stature.

Roentgenologic features include thickened facial bones, hyperostosis frontalis interna, kyphoscoliosis, narrowed intervertebral spaces, short distal phalanges with prominent tufting, lack of modeling of bases of middle phalanges, shortening of long bones of legs and of the metacarpals and great toe, short wide femoral necks, coxa valga, lower limb length discrepancy and sternal defects including pectus carinatum or excavatum.

Complications
I   Derived: —
II   Associated: —

Etiology: A dominant trait with males more severely affected and no affected male has reproduced. X-linked inheritance is suggested by the fact that males are consistently more severely affected than females. McK *30360

Pathogenesis: ? However, conjunctival and skin biopsy specimens from 1 affected male revealed hypercellularity of the subepithelial connective tissue. Many of these cells were filled with small intracytoplasmic inclusions which by EM, appeared as single-membrane limited inclusions with either fine granular or electron-dense globular contents suggestive of a lysosomal storage disorder.

Related Facts
I   **Sex Ratio:** M1:F1
II   **Risk of Occurrence:** ?
III **Risk of Recurrence for**
       Patient's Sib: If affected parent is female 1 in 2 (50%) for each sib to be affected. If affected parent is male 1 in 1 (100%) for each sister to be affected; not increased for brothers.
       Patient's Child: No affected male has reproduced. However, recurrence risk for offspring of affected females is 50%.
IV   **Age of Detectability:** ?
V   **Prevalence:** ?

Treatment

I   **Primary Prevention:**   Genetic counseling
II   **Secondary Prevention:**   —
III   **Other Therapy:**   —

Prognosis: The majority of males have severe mental retardation with some evidence of progressive deterioration.

Detection of Carrier: —

Special Considerations: —

References:
Coffin, G.S. et al: Mental retardation with osteocartilaginous anomalies. Am. J. Dis. Child. 112:205, 1966.
Lowry, B. et al: A new dominant gene mental retardation syndrome. Am. J. Dis. Child. 121:496, 1971.
Temtamy, S.A. et al: The Coffin-Lowry syndrome: An inherited faciodigital mental retardation syndrome. J. Pediatr. 86:724, 1975.

Contributor: **Kenneth Lyons Jones**

Editor's Computerized Descriptors: Eye, Ear, Face, Nasoph., Nose, Skin, Dermatoglyphic, Skel., Nerve

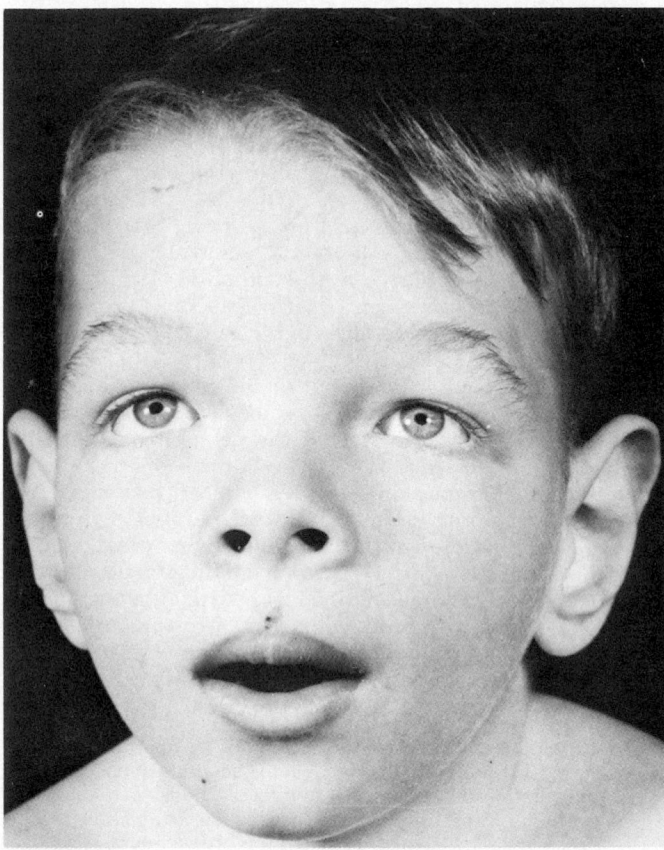

197. Note hypertelorism, prominent supraorbital ridges, broad nasal bridge, anteverted nostrils, open mouth facies with pouty lower lip, protuberant ears.

COGAN CONGENITAL OCULAR MOTOR APRAXIA

Includes: Apraxie oculomotrice congénitale
Angeborene oculäre motorische Apraxie
Apraxia óculomotora congénita
Ocular motor apraxia, congenital

Excludes: Ataxia-telangiectasia (94)

Minimal Diagnostic Criteria: See Clinical Findings below.

Clinical Findings: Congenital ocular motor apraxia is a defect in the horizontal eye movements involved in voluntary gaze and in the fast phase of both vestibular and optokinetic nystagmus.

Compensatory head thrusts on attempting to fixate on object to either side is the most obvious clinical sign. Being unable to initiate the eye movement readily, the subject rotates the head toward the object of regard. But, due to the associated defect in initiating the fast phase of the vestibular response, the eyes show a contraversive deviation during the rotation necessitating a momentary overshoot of the head for fixation. This head thrust is highly characteristic of the abnormality. Also characteristic is the maintained deviation of the eyes when the patient is rotated about a vertical axis.

In contrast to the defect in voluntary eye movement and in tracking a target, the patient makes normal random movements of the eyes when not alerted to make a voluntary fixation. Also, contrasting with the defect of horizontal gaze are the normal vertical movements for all parameters of stimulation.

The head thrusts are usually noted about 3 months of age when the child first begins to hold his head erect. Prior to this, the failure to fixate an object may be misinterpreted as blindness or cerebral palsy. General development is typically normal but the child tends to be clumsy in sports and to be a poor reader in the 1st few years of school. The signs and symptoms progressively improve during the first 2 decades of life and are not known to cause any functional deficit in the adult.

Nothing is known of the responsible lesion. A few familial cases have been documented suggesting an hereditary basis.

Similar head thrusts and defects of the vestibular and optokinetic reflexes are seen with ataxia-telangiectasia and possibly with other defects of the saccadic system but, unlike congenital ocular motor apraxia, these involve the vertical as well as the horizontal eye movements.

Complications
I   **Derived:**   —
II   **Associated:**   Children tend to be clumsy and are poor readers in the 1st few years of school.

Etiology: ? A few familial cases have been documented, suggesting an hereditary basis. McK *21650

Pathogenesis: —

Related Facts
I   **Sex Ratio:**   ?
II   **Risk of Occurrence:**   ?
III   **Risk of Recurrence for**
    Patient's Sib: ?
    Patient's Child: ?
IV   **Age of Detectability:**   Childhood
V   **Prevalence:**   ?

Treatment

I   Primary Prevention: —
II Secondary Prevention: —
III Other Therapy: —

Prognosis: Good. Symptoms progressively improve during the first 2 decades of life and are not known to cause any functional deficit in the adult.

Detection of Carrier: —

Special Considerations: —

References:
Altrocchi, P.H. and Menkes, J.H.: Congenital ocular motor apraxia. Brain 83:579, 1960.
Cogan, D.G.: A type of congenital ocular motor apraxia presenting jerky head movements. Trans. Am. Acad. Ophthalmol. Otolaryngol. 56:853, 1952.
Cogan, D.G.: Heredity of congenital ocular motor apraxia. Trans. Am. Acad. Ophthalmol. Otolaryngol. 76:60, 1972.

Contributor: **David Cogan**

Editor's Computerized Descriptors: Eye, Nerve

COLON AGANGLIONOSIS

Includes: Aganglionose colique
Mb. Hirschsprung
Aganglionosis del colon
Hirschsprung disease
Aganglionic megacolon
Rectal aganglionosis
Anal aganglionosis

Excludes: Functional megacolon
Psychogenic megacolon
Pseudo-Hirschsprung disease

Minimal Diagnostic Criteria: The diagnosis of aganglionic megacolon is based on a combination of physical and roentgenographic findings as cited below and the absence of submucosal and myenteric ganglion cells by full thickness rectal muscle biopsy or seromuscular biopsy of the narrowed distal colon. (Deficiency of ganglion cells is observed in the transitional segment and proliferation or normal distribution of ganglion cells is observed in the colon proximal to the transitional zone.)

Clinical Findings: Constipation occurs in all patients (100%) varying in severity from a) inadequate or delayed passage of meconium to evidence of complete intestinal obstruction in the neonate, b) chronic constipation in the absence of fecal soiling in the infant and child. Days or weeks may lapse before spontaneous defecation occurs. Obstipation accompanies constipation in 28% of patients, abdominal distention (85%). The degree of distention depends upon the adequacy of fecal decompression; vomiting (45%); nonbilious or bilious vomiting depending upon the degree of obstruction.

Physical examination: rectum is "snug" and empty by digital examination. A fecal mass may be palpated on bimanual examination or at the end of the examining finger. Explosive evacuation of fecal fluid and air on withdrawal of the finger is suggestive of rectal or rectosigmoid aganglionosis.

Roentgenography: intestinal distention is evident on 3 positional abdominal films. Absence of the normal rectal gas pattern on lateral films of the pelvis is suggestive of colonic aganglionosis. The classic barium enema appearance of colonic aganglionosis is the demonstration of a narrowed distal aganglionic segment with a proximal dilated (ganglionic) segment. Barium enema is diagnostic in 81.5%, suggestive in 14.6%, and nondiagnostic in 4.9%. Plain abdominal films obtained 24 hours following barium enema demonstrate retained barium. This examination is suggestive of aganglionosis in the neonate who does not have dilatation of the proximal (ganglionic) colon.

Complications
I   **Derived:** a) Enterocolitis (infants 35%; overall 14%). Enterocolitis is characterized by marked dilatation of the colon with retention of air and liquid feces. Diarrhea may or may not be present. Infants are lethargic, febrile and dehydrated. Perforation is rare. b) Physical underdevelopment or signs of malnutrition (18%). Characteristic features are muscular wasting of the limbs and hypoproteinemia. In severe cases infants may have dependent edema or anasarca. c) Obstructive uropathy (11%). Ureterovesical obstruction is a pressure phenomena usually associated with a feces-filled rectosigmoid. d) Melena (5%). This is related to stercoral trauma.
II **Associated:** Imperforate anus (3%). (Aganglionosis associated with imperforate anus is probably secondary to vascular impairment of the colon following the pull-through procedure with a secondary resorption of ganglion cells.)

Etiology: Congenital absence of the intramural myenteric parasympathetic nerve ganglia and sympathetic nerve plexus in a segment of colon that extends proximally from the anus for a varying distance. Aganglionosis is limited to the rectosigmoid in 70% and distal to the splenic flexure in 84% of cases. Total colonic aganglionosis and small intestinal aganglionosis occur in 1-10% of various series.

Pathogenesis: The aganglionic colon is unable to transmit the coordinated peristaltic waves from the proximal colon producing variable degrees of physiologic intestinal obstruction. Hyperperistaltic activity results in increasing hypertrophy and dilatation of the normal colon and possible enterocolitis, if the obstruction is unrelieved.

Related Facts
I   **Sex Ratio:** M2 or 3:F1; Caucasian 90%; Black less than 10%
II   **Risk of Occurrence:** 1 in 8000 live births
III **Risk of Recurrence for**
    Patient's Sib: Familial frequency, 6%
    Patient's Child: Familial frequency, 6%
IV   **Age of Detectability:** Neonatal period 40%; infancy 40%; childhood and adulthood 20%.
V   **Prevalence:** ?

Treatment
I   **Primary Prevention:** —
II   **Secondary Prevention:** Definitive treatment is surgical. Diverting enterostomy in the proximal ganglionic zone is advised for the neonate or infant to allow complete decompression of the obstructed intestine. Patients with enterocolitis must be decompressed by colonic irrigation using saline prior to operation. Definitive surgical reconstruction is performed following restoration of normal colonic function by 1) resection of aganglionic colon and abdominoperineal pull-through (Swenson) procedure; or 2) modification of the Swenson operation to avoid the tedious pelvic dissection, risk of parasympathetic nerve injury, and direct colonic anastomosis (Duhamel and Soave procedures).
III **Other Therapy:** —

Prognosis: Mortality during infancy 20%. Mortality is secondary to combination of findings: a) late diagnosis with nutritional fluid and electrolyte complications, b) enterocolitis during infancy, and c) surgical complications. Following successful surgical reconstruction the life expectancy is normal.

Detection of Carrier: —

Special Considerations: —

References:
Kottmeier, P. K. and Clatworthy, H. W., Jr.: Aganglionic and functional megacolon in children- a diagnostic dilemma. Pediatrics 36:572, 1965.
Shim, W. K. and Swenson, O.: Treatment of congenital megacolon in 50 infants. Pediatrics 38:185, 1966.
Swenson, O. and Davidson, F. Z.: Similarities of mechanical intestinal obstruction and aganglionic megacolon in the newborn infant: A review of 64 cases. N. Engl. J. Med. 262:64, 1960.

Contributor: **Robert J. Touloukian**

Editor's Computerized Descriptors: GI., GU.

COLON ATRESIA OR STENOSIS

Includes: Atrésie ou sténose colique
Kolonatresie oder-stenose
Atresia o estenosis del colon
Colon agenesis
Colon absence
Rectal atresia or stenosis
Exstrophy of the cloaca

Excludes: Intestinal atresia and imperforate anus
Colonic atresia or stenosis associated with aganglionosis and gastroschisis

Minimal Diagnostic Criteria: Intestinal obstruction of colon with x-ray confirmation

Clinical Findings: Signs of low intestinal obstruction with abdominal distention and obstipation. Bile vomiting is a later finding. Stenosis may become clinically apparent later in infancy with constipation the paramount symptom. Plain roentgenographic findings of mechanical intestinal obstruction. Barium enema demonstrates unused colon ("microcolon") distal to the site of atresia. Complete or partial occlusion of the lumen of the colon by a) internal diaphragm (29%); b) separation of the proximal and distal blind ends of the colon by a cord-like remnant of the bowel. The mesentery may or may not be intact (18%); c) complete separation of the proximal and distal ends with defect in the mesentery (53%). Stenosis is relatively uncommon. Proximal and distal colon atresia are of equal frequency. Distal colonic atresia may be associated with severe malformation of the lower abdominal wall, pubis, anus and rectum, with exstrophy of the bladder and cecovesical fistula ("exstrophy of the cloaca"). Duplication of the appendix, a portion of the colon, and terminal ileum occur also with exstrophy of the cloaca.

Complications
I   **Derived:** Perforation a) antenatal with meconium peritonitis but no demonstrable intestinal perforation at the time of birth (10%), b) proximal dilated colon segment at birth either with or without volvulus and infarction (10%), c) of distal colon segment coincident to barium enema examination (10%)
II   **Associated:** Exstrophy of the cloaca; gastroschisis

Etiology: Atresia is secondary to ischemia of the colon during the 2nd or 3rd trimester of pregnancy following mesenteric vascular injury or occlusion.

Pathogenesis: Vascular injury to the inferior mesenteric artery results in segmental atresia with normal rectum and perineum. Exstrophy of the cloaca results from combination of embryologic defect in hindgut development during the 1st trimester and vascular accident with resorption of colon. Rectal atresia has been produced in experimental animals (rabbits) by mesenteric vascular occlusion.

Related Facts
I   **Sex Ratio:** M1:F1
II   **Risk of Occurrence:** 10.5% of atresia involve the colon. Incidence: 1 in 1500 to 1 in 20,000 live births.
III **Risk of Recurrence for**
    Patient's Sib: Not increased
    Patient's Child: Not increased
IV   **Age of Detectability:** Symptoms and signs of intestinal obstruction secondary to atresia are recognized at birth or during the initial week of life. Stenosis may be first detected in childhood or even adulthood.
V   **Prevalence:** ?

Treatment
I   **Primary Prevention:** —

II Secondary Prevention: Surgical correction of intestinal defect with restoration of continuity; temporary enterostomy precedes abdominoperineal pull-through procedure.†

III Other Therapy: —

Prognosis: Normal life span except for late intestinal complications of primary or secondary operations. Chronic urinary tract infection, secondary megacolon and fecal or urinary incontinence frequently occur with exstrophy of the cloaca.

Detection of Carrier: —

†Special Considerations: Surgeon must resect dilated bulbous obstructed proximal colon in attempts to preserve the ileocecal valve and avoid water and electrolyte losses and nutritional complications. This consideration is particularly important for exstrophy of the cloaca where cutaneous enterostomy precedes definitive abdominoperineal pull-through operation.

References:
Benson, C.D. et al: Congenital atresia and stenosis of the colon. J. Pediatr. Surg. 3:253, 1968.
Boles, E.T. et al: Atresia of the colon. J. Pediatr. Surg. 11:69, 1976.
Erskine, J. M.: Colonic stenosis in the newborn: The possible thromboembolic etiology of intestinal stenosis and atresia. J. Pediatr. Surg. 5:321, 1970.

Contributor: **Robert J. Touloukian**

Editor's Computerized Descriptors: Skel., GI., GU.

COLON DUPLICATION

Includes: Duplication colique
Kolon-Duplikation
Duplicacíon del colon
Colonic "cyst"
Rectal duplication

Excludes: Colon diverticulum

Minimal Diagnostic Criteria: Palpable mass or caudal twinning

Clinical Findings: Variable, presenting either in the newborn period or later in infancy and childhood. The common findings are: a) palpable abdominal or rectal mass with or without abdominal distention (40%), b) intestinal obstruction with bile vomiting and abdominal distention (20%), c) rectal bleeding (10%), d) duplication of external genitalia and anal orifice associated with tubular duplication of the colon, terminal ileal duplication, double bladder and urethra (about 30%).

Complications
I Derived: Presacral rectal duplication causes pressure symptoms, rectal prolapse, or bleeding. Tubular duplications of the colon fill with feces, become dilated and compress the normal colon and urinary tract structures.
II Associated: Tubular duplications of the entire colon and rectum represent abortive twinning and are accompanied by duplication of the external genitalia, anus, bladder and urethra (about 90%).

Etiology: The etiology of spherical and tubular duplications of the colon are not well explained by either the "solid core" theory or "diverticulum" theory of an embryologic defect in hindgut development. Complete duplication of the colon and rectum with doubling of the genitalia, bladder and urethra represents a caudal twinning with duplication of the hindgut, genital and lower urinary tracts.†

Pathogenesis: Duplications of the colon arise from the mesenteric surface of the normal colon and have a) colonic mucosal (90%) or heterotopic mucosal lining, usually gastric (about 10%), b) smooth muscle coat shared with a segment of the parent colon, c) a common mesentery, d) an internal communication with the parent colonic lumen (80%), a blind duplication (20%).

Related Facts
I Sex Ratio: M1:F2
II Risk of Occurrence: ?
III Risk of Recurrence for
   Patient's Sib: ?
   Patient's Child: ?
IV Age of Detectability: Caudal twinning of colon duplication is recognized at birth. Other forms of colon duplication present either at birth or in childhood.
V Prevalence: 30% of all duplications in the alimentary tract arise from the colon.

Treatment
I Primary Prevention: —
II Secondary Prevention: Surgical correction, either 1) by total excision of the duplications; 2) partial excision of the duplication and stripping of the mucosa; 3) a reentry procedure to relieve signs of intestinal obstruction and provide adequate internal drainage of the duplication.†
III Other Therapy: —

Prognosis: Normal life span except for late intestinal complications of primary or secondary operations.

Detection of Carrier: —

†Special Considerations: Emphasis is placed on avoiding major resection of normal colon with long tubular duplications, since adequate internal drainage is obtained by partial resection and reentry procedure. Patients with complete tubular duplications of the colon should also be investigated for associated urinary tract duplications or anomalies. "Solid core" theory: growth of the hindgut accelerates during the 6th or 7th week of gestation with proliferation of epithelial cells and occlusion of the lumen. Vacuolation and coalescence of these cells fail to occur normally, leaving a cyst or tube which eventually becomes a duplication. "Diverticulum" theory: a bud of intestinal epithelium penetrates the subepithelial connective tissue in the 4-23 mm embryo, forming a secondary lumen, eventually lined by colonic epithelium and a smooth muscle layer.

References:

Grosfeld, J.L. et al: Enteric duplications in infancy and childhood: An 18-year review. Ann. Surg. 172:83, 1970.

McPherson, A.G. et al: Duplication of the colon. Br. J. Surg. 56:138, 1969.

Ravitch, M.M.: Hindgut duplication—doubling of colon and genital urinary tract. Ann. Surg. 137:588, 1953.

Soper, R. T.: Tubular duplication of the colon and distal ileum: Case report and discussion. Surgery 63:998, 1968.

Contributor: **Robert J. Touloukian**

Editor's Computerized Descriptors: GI., GU.

COLOR BLINDNESS, BLUE MONOCONE-MONOCHROMATIC

Includes: Monochromasie
Monochromatische Blau-Blindheit
Ceguera-monocónica-monocromática al color azul
Blue monocone-monochromatic, color blindness
Cone monochromatism

Excludes: Color blindness, total (198)

Minimal Diagnostic Criteria: Luminosity, foveal dark adaptation and acuity data indicate the presence of blue sensitive cones with a maximum sensitivity at about 440 Mu, and foveal rods.

Clinical Findings: Congenital reduced distance visual acuity 20/200 - 2/80, better near vision (Jaeger 1-4 print), with or without nystagmus and essentially normal ophthalmoscopic findings (rarely minimal pigment clumping in macular area).

These individuals function as rod monochromats in low luminance levels, at high luminance levels as blue-cone monochromats.

Complications
I   **Derived:** Affected individuals, as for rod monochromacy, are seriously handicapped in their environment.
II **Associated:** —

Etiology: X-linked recessive; McK *30370

Pathogenesis: Presumed absence of red and green cones.†

Related Facts
I   **Sex Ratio:** M1:F0 (Affected males are hemizygous; no homozygous females reported.)
II   **Risk of Occurrence:** Extremely rare
III **Risk of Recurrence for**
     Patient's Sib: If mother is a carrier, 1 in 2 (50%) for each brother to be affected and 1 in 2 for each sister to be a carrier.
     Patient's Child: 1 in 1 (100%) for carrier daughters; not increased for sons unless wife is a carrier.
IV   **Age of Detectability:** Age of usual color detection, 2-3 years.
V   **Prevalence:** Extremely rare, perhaps 1 in 300,000 to 1 in 500,000

Treatment
I   **Primary Prevention:** Genetic counseling
II   **Secondary Prevention:** Education in color and brightness interpretation
III **Other Therapy:** —

Prognosis: Nonprogressive

Detection of Carrier: Female heterozygotes, by the Lyon hypothesis, should display varying degrees of color interpretation or brightness anomalies. Aside from relatively minor errors in color interpretation, most carrier females have not demonstrated any suggestive anomaloscope or luminosity curve defects.

†**Special Considerations:** The discovery of blue-cone monochromatism lends credence to and supports the hypothesis that normal color vision, at the receptor level, depends upon 3 different kinds of cone pigment (red-green-blue). It is assumed that blue-cone monochromats have the normal allotment of normal blue cones (and normal rods) and lack the green and red pigment-bearing cones.

References:

Alpern, M. et al: Pi-1 cone monochromatism. Arch. Ophthalmol. 74:334, 1965.

Blackwell, H.R. and Blackwell, O.M.: Rod and cone receptor mechanisms in typical and atypical congenital achromatopsia. Vision Res. 1:62, 1961.

Contributor: **Harold F. Falls**

COLOR BLINDNESS, RED-GREEN DEUTAN SERIES

Includes: Deutéranomalie
Deutanformen der Rot-Grün Blindheit
Deuteranomalía
A red-green deutan allelic series of mutations listed in order of their severity as follows: normal, deuteranomaly, extreme deuteranomaly
Deuteranopia
Red-green deutan series color blindness

Excludes: Color blindness, red-green protan series (197)

Minimal Diagnostic Criteria: The clinical evaluation is usually a screening test employing pseudoisochromatic plates by which to isolate color defectives. Diagnosis and classification are then dependent upon more definitive laboratory color tests.

The pseudoisochromatic plates depend upon the color defective patient confusing a symbol or number to be identified with a particular background. The Ishihara plates are so constructed that the colors of the test symbols and of the background are of such saturation, hue and brightness that they are easily confused by the deutan.

The 1957 revised Hardy-Rand-Ritter (H-R-R) plates present 4 demonstration, 6 screening and 14 diagnostic plates. These plates test for both blue-yellow and red-green defects and also undertake to grade the severity of either defect.

The Farnsworth dichotomous test (D-15 test) utilized 16 colored paper disks-1 cm in diameter-and mounted in black plastic containers. Starting with a fixed blue-violet disk the subject is challenged to arrange the remaining disks in order. This test identifies individuals with a relatively marked color defect. The errors are charted and the axes of such classify the subject as a tritan, protan or possibly a totally color blind.

The anomaloscope, however, is the only instrument by which an exact diagnosis of color vision aberration (red-green) can be made. This test presents a bipartite circular field divided into a yellow half and the other half having a red-green mixture, the relative proportion of which can be varied. The examiner sets various known red-green mixtures which the subjects attempt to match both in brightness and color by varying the intensity of the yellow half of the field.

Clinical Findings: Deuteranomalous individuals have normal visual acuity and frequently are unaware of their color deficiency. In contrast to dichromats such anomalous trichromats have no neutral points under favorable situations of brightness with large stimuli. In comparison, however, to the normal trichromat these individuals can distinguish only 5-25 hues against the 150 or more for the normal. On the anomaloscope the deuteranomal, like the normal has a relatively narrow range of brightness and color match, yet requires at least 4 times more green than the normal in their Rayleigh equations. Deuteranomalous individuals may have a deficiency in quantity of the cone green pigment chlorolabe.

The dichromat-deuteranope also has normal visual acuity but frequently makes errors in his apparel color combinations. This individual can match all the colors he experiences with suitable mixture of 2 colors actually interpreted, however, as various saturations of the hues blue and yellow. The neutral point for the deuteranope is 500 M μ and its complementary. In general, the deuteranope confuses red and green with yellow of varying brightness and saturation.

The extreme deuteranomalous individual is usually somewhat intermediate in his degree of red-green confusion between the deuteranomalous and deuteranopic person.

Complications

I **Derived:** Most deuteranomalous and deuteranopic subjects have but few problems, as far as they are concerned, with gross color interpretation in their ordinary daily life. In fact adjustment is rapid to most color challenges through experience and education. Certain occupations however require *normal* trichromatic vision because of the use of color codes, for example, to differentiate different wires or resistors in a complex electronic circuit.

II **Associated:** —

Etiology: The normal-deuteranomaly-extreme deuteranomaly-and deuteranopia complex of alleles is inherited in an X-linked recessive pattern. The normal gene for trichromatism, however, is dominant to the deuteranomalous allelic gene which, in turn, is dominant to the extreme deuteranomalous allele and so on (the severity of expressivity has the same sequence). Deuteranopes have the normal red and blue cone pigments but lack the normal green cone pigment. Deuteranomals also have the normal red and blue cone pigments and a "green" cone pigment with an action spectrum different from that of the normal, though its precise form is unidentified.†

Pathogenesis: —

Related Facts

I **Sex Ratio:** M > 16:F1. (All red-green color deficient Caucasian males constitute 8% of the population in contrast to 0.4-0.5% of affected females.)

II **Risk of Occurrence:** Deuteranomalous trichromats, 4.9% of the male and 0.38% of the female population. Deuteranopia dichromats, about 1.1% of the females. The incidence is less common among the Japanese (3.9%) and even much lower (1%) among Fiji Islanders and Eskimos.

III **Risk of Recurrence for**
   Patient's Sib: 1 in 2 for brothers; very small for sisters unless father is affected, in which case risk to sisters is 1 in 2.
   Patient's Child: Nil for sons but all of the patient's daughters will be carriers. They, in turn, can transmit the gene to their male (hemizygous) and their female (heterozygous) offspring on a 1 in 2 ratio.

IV **Age of Detectability:** Actually depends upon environmental challenges and the severity of the gene defect.

V **Prevalence:** —

Treatment

I **Primary Prevention:** Genetic counseling
II **Secondary Prevention:** —
III **Other Therapy:** —

Prognosis: Stationary throughout life unless secondary (acquired) retinal or optic nerve disease is encountered.

Detection of Carrier: A female homozygous for the same allelic gene will be color defective similar to an affected male (hemizygous). Color defects have been detected in heterozygous females through red-green flicker photometry. Deutan heterozygotes require significantly more green than the normal subject for minimum flicker.†

†Special Considerations: The marked variablility and infrequent incidence of color defect in females (heterozygous) is explained by some authorities on the basis of the Lyon hypothesis, if applicable, and certainly much more study is necessary. One should anticipate finding heterozygous females who present profound variability from those closely simulating the male picture

or having no effect (detectable by presently available tests).

References:
Alpern, M.: Sensory Processes. Belmont, CA: Brooks-Cole, 1967, p. 36.
Alpern, M. and Torii, S.: The luminosity curve of the deuteranomalous fovea. J. Gen. Physiol. 52:738, 1968.
Kalmus, H.: Diagnosis and Genetics of Defective Colour Vision. Oxford: Pergamon Press, 1965.
Krill, A.E.: Congenital color-vision defects: A symposium on surgical and medical management of congenital anomalies of the eye. Trans. New Orleans Acad. Ophthalmol. St. Louis: C.V. Mosby, 1968, p. 422.

Contributor: **Harold F. Falls**

Editor's Computerized Descriptor: Vision

COLOR BLINDNESS, RED-GREEN PROTAN SERIES

Includes: Daltonisme-protanomalie-protanopie
Protanformen der Rot-Grün Blindheit
Daltonismo-protanomalía-protanopía
A red-green protan allelic series of mutations listed in order of their severity of expressivity as follows: normal, protanomaly, extreme protanomaly
Protanopia
Red-green protan series color blindness

Excludes: Color blindness, red-green deutan series (196)

Minimal Diagnostic Criteria: There is no single clinical instrument or test that is infallible in detecting defective color vision. Most tests, such as the popular charts, are merely screening mechanisms which permit the separation of the defective from the normal. Diagnosis and classification of the defect is dependent upon more sophisticated testing in the laboratory (anomaloscope or densitometer).

Clinical Findings: Protanomalous individuals (trichromats) have normal visual acuity, normal ocular functions but have trouble identifying certain pastel color shades as evidenced in their clothing selections.

When protanomalous individuals are subjected to color testing, they require a larger than normal amount of red in a red-green anomaloscope mixture matched to yellow (Rayleigh equation).

When protanopic individuals await change in car traffic signals, they have a most difficult time in determining whether the "red light is working or not."

Protanopic individuals confuse red and green color to a moderate or severe degree. Protanopes apparently lack the red-absorbing cone pigment (erythrolabe).

Extreme protanomalous individuals are intermediate in their degree of red-green confusion between protanomalous and protanopia men. All protan defectives show a loss of luminosity in the red end of the visible spectrum.

Complications
I **Derived:** None except embarrassing errors in color matching, identification of objects and lights, instrumentation or appliances
II **Associated:** —

Etiology: X-linked recessive. The series of polyalleles, however, are dominant to each other in the following order: normal-protanomaly-extreme protanomalous and protanopia.† (The severity of expressivity has the same sequence.)

Pathogenesis: ? Presumably the gene responsible for the presence of erythrolabe is nonfunctioning (protanopia).†

Related Facts
I **Sex Ratio:** M > 16:F1 for Caucasians
II **Risk of Occurrence:** Protanomalous trichromats 1 in 100 male and 1 in 5000 female Caucasian births. Protanopia dichromats 1 in 100 male and 1 in 500 female Caucasian births.
III **Risk of Recurrence for**
Patient's Sib: If mother is a carrier 1 in 2 (50%) for each brother to be affected and 1 in 2 for each sister to be a carrier.
Patient's Child: 1 in 1 (100%) for carrier daughters; not increased for sons unless wife is a carrier.
IV **Age of Detectability:** Actually depends upon environmental challenges and the severity of the gene's effect.
V **Prevalence:** Protanomalous trichromats 1 in 100 male and 1 in 5000 female Caucasian population. Protanopia dichromats 1 in 100 male and 1 in 500 female Caucasian population.

Treatment
I **Primary Prevention:** Genetic counseling
II **Secondary Prevention:** —
III **Other Therapy:** —

Prognosis: Normal life span and stationary for color blindness

Detection of Carrier: A female homozygous for an allelic pair of genes will be color defective similar to an affected male (hemizygous). Color defects have been detected in heterozygous females and include: moderate to severe decrease in sensitivity to red light (protan series) manifested by an increase in the relative amount of red needed in a red-green flicker photometry or a displacement of the luminosity maximum towards the short waves (Schmidt sign).

†Special Considerations: The variability exhibited by heterozygous carrier females can perhaps be explained by the Lyon hypothesis, namely, that early in embryonic life in each cell in the female 1 of the 2 X chromosomes randomly becomes inactivated (Barr body). Thus in the heterozygous female, the tissues are mosaics comprised of cells bearing either the X chromosome bearing the normal gene or the X chromosome carrying the mutant gene for defective color vision. The size of the resultant clonal growth of either of these cells determines the extent or degree of involvement, or lack of involvement, as expressed in the female.

References:
Adam, A.: Focal red-green ratios of normal color blinds and heterozygotes. Proc. Tel Hashomer. Hosp. 8:2, 1969.
Wald, G.: Defective color vision and its inheritance. Proc. Natl. Acad. Sci. USA 55:1347, 1966.

Contributor: **Harold F. Falls**

Editor's Computerized Descriptor: Vision

Includes: Cécité aux couleurs
Komplette Farbenblindheit
Ceguera al color total
Rod monochromatism
Achromatopsia with amblyopia
Achromatism

Excludes: Color blindness, blue monocone-monochromatic (195)

Minimal Diagnostic Criteria: Colors are interpreted by rod monochromats only as shades of grey. Affected individuals, however, through experience and education learn to interpret certain colors through association with objects or brightness differences.

Clinical Findings: Monochromats have no color vision. To them color TV appears the same as the black and white. In addition, such individuals have photophobia, nystagmus and a serious reduction of visual acuity (20/200). In general, the ophthalmoscopic appearance of the retina is normal or presents minute pigment clumping in or about the macular area, as well as a loss of the fovea reflex. Peripheral visual fields may be normal or slightly constricted especially to colored targets. Central visual fields may present, on occasion, a small central scotoma.

Complications
I **Derived:** Affected individuals, with occasional exceptions, are seriously handicapped in their daily socioeconomic activities. The intelligence is unaffected. Most affected individuals, if sufficiently motivated and intelligent, can usually secure an adequate education and livelihood.
II **Associated:** —

Etiology: Autosomal recessive; McK *21690

Pathogenesis: ? There seems to be an actual deficiency in the number and variety of the cones in the retina of affected individuals. A few histologic specimens have revealed the presence of some cones either normal or abnormal in size and shape.†

Related Facts
I **Sex Ratio:** Nearly M1:F1
II **Risk of Occurrence:** Relatively higher where high incidence of consanguinity exists but in general very rare.
III **Risk of Recurrence for**
  Patient's Sib: 1 in 4 (25%) for each offspring to be affected
  Patient's Child: Not increased unless mate is carrier or homozygote
IV **Age of Detectability:** Usually not until the child is old enough to respond to color tests. The presence of congenital nystagmus and photophobia should certainly arouse suspicion of the diagnosis, particularly if other sibs are affected.
V **Prevalence:** Europe 0.00025 to 0.00055; Japan 0.0041 to 0.0069

Treatment
I **Primary Prevention:** Genetic counseling
II **Secondary Prevention:** —
III **Other Therapy:** —

Prognosis: Continued improvement in environmental adjustments through education and experience. The ocular status is stationary.

Detection of Carrier: ?

†**Special Considerations:** Typical total color blindness is an enigma in that studies suggest that there are 2 types of photoreceptors in such eyes, 1 type functioning at high levels of illumination and having some characteristics of normal cones but no action spectrum of rods, the other type functioning at low levels of illumination (normal rods).

References:
Alpern, M. et al: The enigma of total typical monochromacy. Am. J. Ophthalmol. 50:996, 1960.

François, J.: Heredity in Ophthalmology. St. Louis: C.V. Mosby, 1961, p. 404.

Contributor: **Harold F. Falls**

Editor's Computerized Descriptors: Vision, Eye

COLOR BLINDNESS, YELLOW-BLUE

Includes: Cécité pour le bleu et le jaune
Gelb-blau Blindheit
Ceguera al color amarillo-azul
Tritanopia
Tritanomaly
Yellow-blue color blindness

Excludes: Other color blindness

Minimal Diagnostic Criteria: Neither tritanopia nor tritanomaly can be discovered with the Ishihara charts or by the ordinary anomaloscope. According to Kalmus it is necessary to use special plates especially designed by Kalmus and Farnsworth in order to detect such affected individuals.

Clinical Findings: Affected tritanopia individuals have relatively normal vision but have color confusion with blue-green and orange-pink shades. It is presumed that affected individuals lack the cyanolabe pigment (blue pigment).

Complications
I Derived: —
II Associated: —

Etiology: Tritanopia is hereditary and according to Kalmus is transmitted in an autosomal dominant mode. An interesting variability in expressivity and even decreased penetrance is observed. Tritanomaly is believed, "more or less," to be an X-linked recessive trait.† McK *30400

Pathogenesis: Unknown, there is presumed to be an absence of the blue pigment (cyanolabe) in the cones of the tritanopic patient. This absence, however, has not yet been disclosed with the densitometer.

Related Facts
I Sex Ratio: Tritanopia M1:F1. Tritanomaly M1:F? (for affected homozygous females)
II Risk of Occurrence: 1 in 2000 to 1 in 10,000 Caucasian male births
III Risk of Recurrence for
Patient's Sib: For tritanopia: if parent is affected, 1 in 2 (50%) for each offspring to be affected; otherwise not increased. For tritanomaly: if X-linked recessive and if mother is a carrier, 1 in 2 (50%) for each brother to be affected and 1 in 2 for each sister to be a carrier.
Patient's Child: For tritanopia: 1 in 2. For tritanomaly: if X-linked recessive, 1 in 1 (100%) for carrier daughters; not increased for sons unless wife is a carrier.
IV Age of Detectability: Affected individuals especially tritanomalous subjects are rarely aware of their color vision aberration unless challenged during test or stress situations.
V Prevalence: 1 in 2000 to 1 in 10,000 Caucasian males

Treatment
I Primary Prevention: Genetic counseling
II Secondary Prevention: —
III Other Therapy: —

Prognosis: A congenital and stationary aberration of color interpretation

Detection of Carrier: —

†Special Considerations: The genetics of tritanopia is still in dispute. Much is needed to be learned and physicians should be on the lookout for such individuals.

References:
Kalmus, H.: Diagnosis and Genetics of Defective Colour Vision. Oxford: Pergamon Press, 1965.
Wright, W.D.: Characteristics of tritanopia. J. Opt. Soc. Am. 42:509, 1952.

Contributor: **Harold F. Falls**

COMMON ORIGIN OF BRACHIOCEPHALIC AND CONTRALATERAL CAROTID ARTERY

Includes: Origine commune du tronc brachiocéphalique et de l'artère carotide gauche

Gemeinsamer Ursprung der A. brachiocephalica und der gegenseitigen A. carotis

Origen común del tronco braquiocefálico y de la carótida interna

Left common carotid artery arising from innominate artery

Right common carotid artery originating from left innominate artery in cases with a right-sided aortic arch

Carotid artery, common origin of brachiocephalic and contralateral

Excludes: Abnormality in which all branches arise from a common stem which in turn originates from aortic arch

Minimal Diagnostic Criteria: Arch aortography is definitive

Clinical Findings: The brachiocephalic and contralateral common carotid arteries arise from the aortic arch with a common stem. The abnormally originating carotid artery crosses in front of the trachea as it courses to the opposite side and may compress the trachea. When the contralateral common carotid artery originates as a branch of the brachiocephalic (innominate) artery it crosses the trachea anteriorly.

The clinical manifestations vary with the degree of tracheal compression. Most patients are asymptomatic, but there may be respiratory distress with stridor or crowing during inspiration and a predisposition to respiratory infections. Dysphagia is not present. The esophagram is usually normal. In the rare case associated with tracheal compression, plain films show indentation or grooving in the anterior tracheal surface. This is best seen in the lateral projection.

Complications
I   Derived: ?
II Associated: ?

Etiology: ?

Pathogenesis: ?

Related Facts
I   Sex Ratio: ?
II   Risk of Occurrence: ?
III Risk of Recurrence for
      Patient's Sib: ?
      Patient's Child: ?
IV Age of Detectability: At any age by arch aortography
V   Prevalence: ?

Treatment
I   Primary Prevention: —
II   Secondary Prevention: In symptomatic cases, the anomalous vessel may be sutured to the posterior aspect of the sternum.
III Other Therapy: —

Prognosis: Excellent. In asymptomatic patients it has no effect on life expectancy. In those with tracheal compression, once surgically relieved, they should have a normal life expectancy.

Detection of Carrier; —

Special Considerations: —

References:
Bosniak, M. A.: An analysis of some anatomic-roentgenologic aspects of the brachiocephalic vessels. Am. J. Roentgenol. Radium Ther. Nucl. Med. 91:1222, 1964.

Gross, R. E.: Arterial malformations which cause compression of trachea and esophagus. Circulation 11:124, 1955.

Liechty, J.D. et al: Variations pertaining to the aortic arches and their branches Q. Bull. Northw. Univ. Med. Sch. 31:136, 1957.

Contributors: Juan R. Guerrero
Charles E. Mullins
Dan G. McNamara

Editor's Computerized Descriptor: Resp.

CONE-ROD DEGENERATION

Includes: Dégénérescence des cones et bâtonnets
Degeneration von Zäpfchen und Stäbchen
Degeneración de conos y bastones
Progressive cone-rod degeneration
Atypical retinitis pigmentosa (some forms)
Tapetoretinal degeneration (some forms)

Excludes: Retinitis pigmentosa (869)
Pure cone degeneration
Gyrate atrophy (449)
Malignant myopia
Choroidal sclerosis
Nightblindness, stationary (719)
Tapetochoroidal dystrophy (925)
Retinitis punctata albescens

Minimal Diagnostic Criteria: Evidence of diffuse cone degeneration greater than or prior to rod degeneration as described below. ERG is needed if clinical findings are equivocal. Pigmentary changes in the fundus are not mandatory for the diagnosis. Heavy antimalarial use (as for arthritis therapy) must be excluded.

Clinical Findings: Decreased central vision associated with pigmentary changes in the fundi and evidence of diffuse cone and to a lesser extent, rod involvement are present in the midcourse of this form of progressive retinal degeneration. Evidence of diffuse cone involvment includes photophobia, central visual field loss over a greater area than in macular degeneration, widespread retinal depigmentation, salt and pepper changes or frank spicules, abnormal cone dark adaptation, color vision impairment, and subnormal cone responses on electroretinography (ERG). Evidence of diffuse rod involvement is usually more subtle and includes peripheral visual loss, retinal pigmentary changes, abnormal rod dark adaptation and subnormal rod responses on ERG.

Cone-rod degeneration must be differentiated on one hand from the pure cone degenerations and on the other hand from retinitis pigmentosa (rod-cone degeneration). The onset may occur at any age from childhood to late adulthood. It typically is brought to medical attention in the 2nd or 3rd decades. The rate of progression and ultimate severity are variable even within families. Early and mild cases are often difficult to distinguish from pure cone degenerations, whereas endstage cases mimic typical retinitis pigmentosa even to the extent of having extinguished ERG response to both cone and rod stimuli. History which implicates loss of cone vision before loss of rod vision favors the diagnosis of cone-rod degeneration.

Cone-rod degeneration is inherited in some families as autosomal dominant and in others as autosomal recessive. Sporadic cases, which may be autosomal recessive, occur. There is some evidence that the atypical retinitis pigmentosa occurring in some syndromes such as Lawrence-Moon-Biedl is of the cone-rod type. Care must be taken to exclude heavy use of antimalarials by history, since the clinical characteristics of chloroquine retinopathy are similar to that of cone-rod degeneration. Indeed, in both these conditions the rod dark adaptation curve may be grossly normal in the face of other evidence of rod degeneration.

Complications
I **Derived:** —
II **Associated:** Ocular: Posterior polar cataracts; Extraocular: Cone-rod degeneration sometimes occurs as part of a syndrome eg Lawrence-Moon-Biedl, cerebellar atrophy with retinal degeneration, etc.

Etiology: ? Autosomal recessive and dominant familial patterns occur.

Pathogenesis: ?

Related Facts
I **Sex Ratio:** M1:F1
II **Risk of Occurrence:** ? Less common than retinitis pigmentosa.
III **Risk of Recurrence for**
 Patient's Sib: When autosomal dominant or autosomal recessive, see Table I AD or AR, respectively.
 Patient's Child: When autosomal dominant or autosomal recessive, see Table I AD or AR, respectively.
IV **Age of Detectability:** Any age, most frequently 1st, 2nd or 3rd decades.
V **Prevalence:** ? Uncommon but not rare.

Treatment
I **Primary Prevention:** Genetic counseling
II **Secondary Prevention:** —
III **Other Therapy:** Visual aids including TV image intensifiers in advanced cases. Protecting the retina from light by sunglasses may slow the progression (or, conversely, excessive light exposure may hasten the course).

Prognosis: Normal life span unless part of a systemic syndrome. Visual impairment varies markedly from inconsequential to legal blindness. Most patients are handicapped for driving and require visual aids for reading.

Detection of Carrier: Carriers in the true sense cannot be detected with present methods. However, mildly affected individuals who might otherwise be called carriers can be detected with the clinical methods described above. Pedigree analysis may reveal obligate and potential carriers.

Special Considerations: —

References:
Berson, E.L. et al: Progressive cone-rod degeneration. Arch. Ophthalmol. 80:68, 1968.
Franceschetti, A. et al: Chorioretinal Heredodegenerations. Springfield: Charles C Thomas, 1974.
Krill, A.E.: Cone-degenerations. In Krill, A.E. and Archer, D.B. (eds.): Krill's Hereditary Retinal and Choroidal Diseases. Hagerstown: Harper and Row, 1977, vol. II.

Contributor: **Donald R. Bergsma**

Editor's Computerized Descriptors: Vision, Eye

CONJOINED TWINS

Includes: Frères Siamois
Siamesische Zwillinge
Gemelos siameses
Siamese twins

Excludes: Parasitic monsters

Minimal Diagnostic Criteria: Fusion of some portion of monovular or monozygotic twins.

Clinical Findings: Diagnosis evident by physical examination. The visceral conjunction between the co-twins requires x-ray, isotope and ultrasound techniques to outline anatomic and functional interdependence. Diagnosis can be made in utero by the use of x-ray or ultrasound techniques.

Terata Catadidymus - fusion caudally
    Diprosopus - single trunk and limbs, varying duplication of face and head
    Dicephalus - single trunk and limbs, duplication of head
    Ischiopagus - Fusion at ischia, the axis of the 2 bodies being at 180° - 6%+
    Pygopagus - fusion in sacral region - 19%+
Terata Anadidymus - fusion in cephalic region
    Dipygus - fusion limited to region proximal to pelvis
    Syncephalus - Single head, separation below head
    Craniopagus - fusion at the head - 2%+
Terata Anacatadidymus - fusion in midportion of body
    Thoracopagus - fusion in sternal region - 74%+
    Omphalopagus - fusion in abdominal region
    Rachipagus - fusion back to back in sagittal plane, fusion limited to upper trunk and cervical region

Rudolph et al reviewed 117 cases; the basic problem in thoracopagus is whether separate hearts allow surgery. In ischiopagus, pygopagus and craniopagus decisions need to be made concerning which twin will benefit from single shared organs.

Complications

I Derived: All cases with conjoined hearts have died with or without the aid of surgery. Unexplained postoperative deaths have occurred, therefore, careful postoperative monitoring is required.

II Associated: —

Etiology: Conjoined twins are the product of a single ovum. They are monovular or monozygotic twins. Teratogenesis occurs by incomplete fission during the process of twinning.

Pathogenesis: According to Zimmermann, the morula becomes a blastocyst on day 6 of ovulation age. Within this vesicle, 0.2-0.3 mm in length, the inner cell mass develops at one pole. The inner cell mass is totipotent for morphogenesis and organogenesis. For a short time, this cell mass has the potentialities of forming a single or dual embryologic primordium or germinal disk. The caudal end, appearing between 15 and 18 days of embryonic age, represents the primitive streak which is the primordium of all intraembryogenic mesoderm. Terata are the result either of disordered morphogenesis or organogenesis. By day 20 the process of either normal twinning or conjoined twinning will be initiated. The end of the 3rd week of development age marks the end of the period of incomplete fission. The anomalous twinning can occur at any point of incomplete division of the inner cell mass accounting for the variations in types of conjoined twins.

Related Facts

I **Sex Ratio:** M3:F7
II **Risk of Occurrence:** 0.06:1000 live births in India and Africa; 0.004:1000 live births in Europe and the Americas
III **Risk of Recurrence for**
    Patient's Sib: No case of recurrence ever reported
    Patient's Child: No case of recurrence ever reported.
IV **Age of Detectability:** Birth or prenatally
V **Prevalence:** Rare

Treatment

I **Primary Prevention:** None
II **Secondary Prevention:** Extent of cardiac anomalies not detectable before 8 weeks of fetal development. The presence of twins with a single fetal ECG is the most serious condition.
III **Other Therapy:** Surgical separations have been successfully performed on all conjoined twins with exception of those thoracopagus with conjoined hearts. Although experience is scanty, it is probable that other anomalies of fission can be managed by existing rehabilitation procedures.†

Prognosis: Although conjoined twins have lived as long as 63 years without separation, surgical separation is the management of choice. Psychologic studies of unoperated twins reveal serious limitations to the quality of life. The rehabilitation of any postoperative defects due to incomplete fission of shared organs and tissues is vital to the success of the surgical approach. The general experience has been that optimal surgical management requires a well-rehearsed surgical and pediatric team. In the absence of a single heart, the procedure should not be carried out under emergency conditions. At present, there are no survivors following division of a single heart, however, it is expected that this will become possible with continuing advances in cardiovascular surgery.

Detection of Carrier: None

†Special Considerations: Steps in evaluation of operability: 1) Physical examination to differentiate thoracopagus and omphalopagus twins; operative separation of omphalopagus twins. 2) ECG with standard leads to determine ventricular independence; operative separation of those with separate QRS complexes (25%). 3) Angiography with physiologic study to determine great vessel and atrial communication; operative separation of conjoined atrium (10%) and 4) Ethical considerations whether 1 twin is salvageable with existing shared ventricular structure (68%).

References:
Nichols, B.L. et al: General clinical management of thoracopagus twins. In Bergsma, D.(ed.): Conjoined Twins. Birth Defects: Orig. Art. Ser., vol. III, no. 1. White Plains: The National Foundation-March of Dimes, 1967, p. 28.
Rudolph, A.J. et al: Obstetric management of conjoined twins. Ibid, p. 38.
Zimmermann, A.A.: Embryologic and anatomic considerations of conjoined twins. Ibid, p. 18.

Contributor: **Buford L. Nichols**

Editor's Computerized Descriptor: Skel.

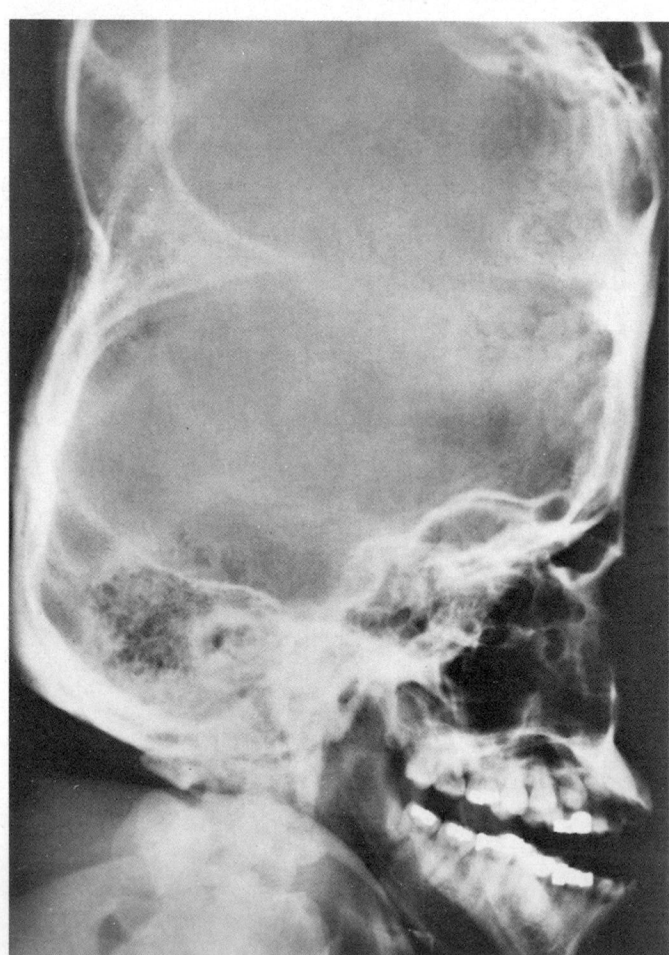

198. Lateral view of thoracopagus twins.

199. Craniopagus twinning with nonseparation of bony calvarium along saggital suture

COPROPORPHYRIA

Includes: Coproporphyrie héréditaire
Hereditäre Koproporphyrie
Coproporfiria hereditaria
Hereditary coproporphyria
Porphyria

Excludes: Other forms of hepatic porphyria

Minimal Diagnostic Criteria: Increased fecal coproporphyrin with slight or no increase of fecal protoporphyrin. Urinary porphobilinogen is increased during acute attacks of neurologic dysfunction. Urinary coproporphyrin may or may not be increased, but this finding by itself is not diagnostic.

Clinical Findings: About half of these patients experience acute attacks of neurologic dysfunction as described for acute intermittent porphyria. Only 1 of 30 experienced photosensitivity and about half of these were asymptomatic. In 4 of the 30 only psychiatric symptoms occurred.†

Complications
I   **Derived:** Chronic pain syndrome (peripheral or abdominal), motor paralysis (including respiratory paralysis), seizures, organic brain syndrome, depression, photosensitivity
II **Associated:** —

Etiology: Autosomal dominant biochemical defect; McK *12130

Pathogenesis: ?

Related Facts
I   **Sex Ratio:** M1:F1
II   **Risk of Occurrence:** ?
III **Risk of Recurrence for**
     Patient's Sib: If parent is affected, 1 in 2 (50%) for each offspring to be affected; otherwise not increased.
     Patient's Child: 1 in 2
IV **Age of Detectability:** —
V   **Prevalence:** ?

Treatment
I   **Primary Prevention:** Genetic counseling
II   **Secondary Prevention:** †
III **Other Therapy:** —

Prognosis: Probably a mortality rate of 24% over a 5-year observation period.

Detection of Carrier: —

†**Special Considerations:** See Porphyria, Acute Intermittent for more detailed Clinical Findings and for Treatment II Secondary Prevention.

References:
Goldberg, A. et al: Hereditary coproporphyria. Lancet 1:532, 1967.
Watson, C.J. et al: Studies of coproporphyrin; idiopathic coproporphyrinuria; a hitherto unrecognized form characterized by lack of symptoms in spite of excretion of large amounts of coproporphyrin. J. Clin. Invest. 28:465, 1949.

Contributor: **Donald P. Tschudy**

Editor's Computerized Descriptors: Skin, Resp., Nerve

COR TRIATRIATUM

Includes: Cor triatum
Estenosis de la vena pulmonar
Stenosis of the common pulmonary vein
Cor triatriatum sinistrum

Excludes: Subtotal cor triatriatum
Cor triatriatum dextrum

Minimal Diagnostic Criteria: Elevation of pulmonary artery wedge pressure and selective pulmonary arteriography

Clinical Findings: Anatomy: Cor triatriatum is a rare cardiac anomaly wherein the left atrium is divided by a fibromuscular septum, having the shape of a windsock, into 2 chambers, distal and proximal. The more distal part of the left atrium receives the pulmonary veins and the more proximal part communicates with the mitral valve, left atrial appendage and the foramen ovale. There may be defects in the atrial septum allowing communication of either the proximal or, more rarely, the distal left atrial chamber with the right atrium. Right ventricular hypertrophy and dilatation are almost invariably found. A large number of variants of cor triatriatum have been described, including the association of cor triatriatum with total anomalous pulmonary venous connection and partial anomalous pulmonary venous connection. Cor triatriatum may be associated with other obstructive lesions on the left side of the heart, including coarctation of the aorta, aortic stenosis, bicuspid aortic valve, parachute mitral valve, supravalvar stenosis of the left atrium and stenosis of the pulmonary veins.

Physiology: In those anatomic defects wherein the blood from the distal atrial chamber enters into the right atrium directly or indirectly, hemodynamics are comparable to those in total anomalous pulmonary venous connection. When there are additional left-sided obstructive lesions the hemodynamic alterations are related to the combination of obstructive lesions. In the classic form of cor triatriatum the obstructive left atrial membrane results in elevated pressure in the accessory left atrial chamber which is transmitted to the pulmonary veins. This pressure is freely transmitted to the pulmonary capillary bed and results in pulmonary edema. Reflex pulmonary arteriolar constriction then reduces blood flow into the pulmonary capillary bed and also results in pulmonary arterial hypertension, right ventricular hypertrophy and ultimately right ventricular failure.

Clinically, most patients with classic cor triatriatum have the onset of symptoms within the 1st years of life. A significant number of patients, however, are asymptomatic until the 2nd or 3rd decades of life. Symptoms include dyspnea, frequent respiratory infections and pneumonia. The signs of pulmonary hypertension, including loud pulmonary component of the second heart sound, right ventricular heave and pulmonary ejection systolic click are invariably present. Right heart failure is often seen and reflected by hepatomegaly, distended neck veins and peripheral edema. Pulmonary rales are often present. A soft blowing systolic murmur is often heard along the left sternal border, less often a diastolic murmur is detected at the mitral area or a continuous murmur is heard. Rarely, a murmur is absent.

The ECG reflects systolic pressure overload of the right ventricle (tall R waves in the right precordial leads) and tall peaked P waves are usual. Occasionally, the P wave is also broad and notched. The chest roentgenogram reflects pulmonary venous obstruction. Fine diffuse reticular pulmonary markings fan out from the pulmonary hilus; Kerley B lines may be present. The main pulmonary artery and major branches are dilated. There are signs of right ventricular and right atrial enlargement.

Echocardiographic features are not pathognomonic because of the multiple anatomic expressions of cor triatriatum. An abnormal left atrial echo may be seen anterior and in proximity to the mitral valve. This echo moves briskly with atrial events. It is similar to the left atrial echo seen in TAPVC to coronary sinus and persistent LSVC connecting to coronary sinus. Cor triatriatum may produce mid left atrial echo with slight motion. The left atrial echo may be thin and intermittent in cor triatriatum or may be absent.

At cardiac catheterization significant pulmonary hypertension is routinely found. A shunt may be detected in the presence of a communication between the proximal and distal left atrial chambers and the right atrium. An elevated pulmonary artery wedge pressure is invariably present.

The precise diagnosis is defined by selective pulmonary arteriography. Films must be programmed to accommodate the prolonged pulmonary transit time. As the pulmonary veins opacify, they drain into the accessory left atrial chamber and a significant delay is noted between the opacification of this chamber and of the true left atrium and left ventricle. The obstructive membrane is best seen in the anterior-posterior view.

Complications
I **Derived:** Death from pulmonary edema and right heart failure, pulmonary congestive symptoms, medial hypertrophy of the pulmonary arterioles occurs but is reversible after surgery.
II **Associated:** —

Etiology: ?

Pathogenesis: ? One view suggests that the anomaly results from a faulty development of the atrial septum. The currently accepted theory is that the common pulmonary vein has failed to become incorporated into the left atrium in a normal fashion. However, the diversity of cor triatriatum variants favors multiple embryologic bases.

Related Facts
I **Sex Ratio:** M1:F1
II **Risk of Occurrence:** ? 0.2% of congenital heart disease
III **Risk of Recurrence for**
    Patient's Sib: ?
    Patient's Child: ?
IV **Age of Detectability:** From birth by selective angiography
V **Prevalence:** ?

Treatment
I **Primary Prevention:** —
II **Secondary Prevention:** Resection of the obstructing left atrial membrane. A closed operation utilizing inflow occlusion has advantages in the infant who tolerates cardiopulmonary bypass poorly. However, the great anatomic variety that may be encountered in patients with cor triatriatum makes utilization of cardiopulmonary bypass and correction by direct vision desirable.
III **Other Therapy:** Symptomatic therapy for heart failure and pneumonia should be instituted. However, once heart failure occurs, the patient follows a relentless course unaffected by medical management and surgical intervention should be performed as soon as possible.

Prognosis: Is related to the size of orifice in the obstructing membrane. (Survival 3 months if orifice < 3 mm^2, 16 years if > 3 mm^2.) Postoperative prognosis approaches normal.

Detection of Carrier: —

Special Considerations: —

References:

Edwards, J.E.: Malformation of the thoracic veins. In Gould, S.E. (ed.): Pathology of the Heart, 2nd Ed. Springfield: Charles C Thomas, 1960, p. 484.

Lucas, R.V., Jr. and Schmidt, R.E.: Anomalous venous connection, pulmonary and systemic. In Moss, A.J. and Adams, F.H. (eds.): Heart Disease in Infants, Children, and Adolescents. Baltimore: Williams and Wilkins, 1968, p. 672.

Niwayama, G.: Cor triatriatum. Am. Heart J. 59:291, 1960.

Contributor: **Russell V. Lucas, Jr.**

Editor's Computerized Descriptors: Liver, Resp., CV.

CORNEA PLANA

Includes: Cornée plane
Sclerocornea

Excludes: Inflammatory keratopathies

Minimal Diagnostic Criteria: Nonprogressive noninflammatory flattened cornea

Clinical Findings: Corneal curvature is less than normal. The stroma usually demonstrates diffuse opacification, frequently more marked posteriorly and centrally, although opacities range from minimal peripheral opacification to total opacification of the cornea resembling the appearance of sclera. There is scleralization of the limbus and absence of a defined corneoscleral interface so that the diameter of the cornea appears subnormal. The flattened cornea results in a shallow anterior chamber. The lid may appear ptotic (Streiff sign). The iris pattern may be absent or abnormal. Other extensive abnormalities of the eye may coexist causing certain authors to classify cornea plana with anterior chamber cleavage syndromes (including Rieger syndrome).

Complications

I **Derived:** Reduced visual acuity due to stromal opacification, abnormal refractive error, angle closure, glaucoma

II **Associated:** Posterior embryotoxon, iris coloboma and stromal abnormalities, abnormally shaped pupils, congenital cataract, retinal coloboma, glaucoma, strabismus, and bony and tooth abnormalities

Etiology: Usually autosomal dominant transmission; less commonly autosomal recessive. Single case reports exist of association with 17p,10q translocation and trisomy 18. McK *12140, *21730

Pathogenesis: Failure of normal "cleavage" of the anterior chamber structures during embryonic life

Related Facts

I **Sex Ratio:** M1:F1
II **Risk of Occurrence:** ?
III **Risk of Recurrence for**
    Patient's Sib: When autosomal dominant or autosomal recessive, see Table I AD or AR, respectively.
    Patient's Child: 1 in 2 for autosomal dominant; not increased for autosomal recessive unless mate is carrier or homozygote.
IV **Age of Detectability:** ?
V **Prevalence:** ?

Treatment

I **Primary Prevention:** Genetic counseling
II **Secondary Prevention:** Surgery for cataract, glaucoma and corneal opacification, as indicated
III **Other Therapy:** —

Prognosis: Poor for vision

Detection of Carrier: —

Special Considerations: —

References:

Bloch, W.: Different types of sclerocornea, their hereditary modes and concomitant congenital malformations. J. Genet. Hum. 14:133, 1965.

Duke-Elder, S.: System of Ophthalmology, vol. 3, pt. 2. Congenital Deformities. London:Henry Kimpton, 1964.

Goldstein, J. E. and Cogan, D. G.: Sclerocornea and associated congenital anomalies. Arch. Ophthalmol. 67:761, 1962.

Henkind, P. et al: Mesodermal dysgenesis of the anterior segment: Rieger's anomaly. Arch. Ophthalmol. 73:810, 1965.

Howard, R.D. and Abrahams, I.W.: Sclerocornea. Am. J. Ophthalmol. 71.:1254, 1971.

Reese, A. B. and Ellsworth, R. M.: The anterior chamber cleavage syndrome. Arch. Ophthalmol. 75:307, 1966.

Contributors: **Morton F. Goldberg**
Joel Sugar

Editor's Computerized Descriptor: Eye

CORNEAL DYSTROPHY AND SENSORINEURAL DEAFNESS

Includes: Dystrophie cornéene et surdité de perception progressive
Hornhautdystrophie mit progressiver Innenohr-Schwerhörigkeit
Distrofia corneana y pérdida de la audición neurosensorial progresiva
Sensorineural deafness and corneal dystrophy

Excludes: Mucopolysaccharidosis I-H (674)
Glaucoma, congenital (414)
Avascular syphilitic intrastitial keratosis
Corneal dystrophy, macular (212)

Minimal Diagnostic Criteria: Corneal dystrophy and sensorineural hearing loss

Clinical Findings: Three patients, 2 sisters and their half-brother have been described. The parents in both marriages, in which the father was the same, were 1st cousins. All 3 patients presented with diffuse bluish-white opacities of the cornea and decreased vision from birth. The corneal epithelium seemed to be rough in 1/3 and bedewed in 2/3; the stroma was diffusely edematous and thickened in 3/3. The cornea was not vascularized in 3/3. Audiometry showed bilateral progressive sensorineural hearing loss, especially for the high tones in 2/3.

Complications
I **Derived:** —
II **Associated:** Intraocular pressure was elevated in 1/3. Recurrent bilateral otitis media was seen in 1/3.

Etiology: Autosomal recessive inheritance is very probable.

Pathogenesis: An increased diameter of collagen fibrils in the stroma, a thinned Descemet membrane and ultrastructural anomalies suggestive of defective endothelium were revealed. Considering the hearing defect, a marked degeneration of the stria vascularis and loss of ganglion cells were noted.

Related Facts
I **Sex Ratio:** M1:F2
II **Risk of Occurrence:** —
III **Risk of Recurrence for**
   Patient's Sib: If autosomal recessive, 1 in 4 (25%) for each offspring to be affected.
   Patient's Child: If autosomal recessive, not increased unless mate is carrier or homozygote.
IV **Age of Detectability:** May be in early adolescence.
V **Prevalence:** One reported family with 3 affected individuals

Treatment
I **Primary Prevention:** Genetic counseling
II **Secondary Prevention:** Treatment of glaucoma and perhaps corneal transplants
III **Other Therapy:** Glycerin instillation to improve vision

Prognosis: Vision will deteriorate

Detection of Carrier: —

Special Considerations: —

References:
Harboyan, G. et al: Congenital corneal dystrophy, progressive sensorineural deafness in a family. Arch. Ophthalmol. 85:27, 1971.

Contributors: **Agnes M. Ickenroth**
Cor W.R.J. Cremers

Editor's Computerized Descriptors: Vision, Eye, Hearing

CORNEAL DYSTROPHY, CONGENITAL HEREDITARY

Includes: Dystrophie cornéenne congénitale héréditaire
Angeborene hereditäre Hornhautdystrophie
Distrofia corneana congénita hereditaria
Congenital hereditary endothelial dystrophy
Congenital hereditary stationary dystrophy
Maumenee syndrome
Congenital hereditary corneal dystrophy

Excludes: Corneal dystrophy, endothelial† (208)
Corneal dystrophy, polymorphous posterior† (213)

Minimal Diagnostic Criteria: Corneal stromal edema in the absence of elevated intraocular pressure or excrescences on Descemet membrane.

Clinical Findings: Diffuse clouding and thickening of the corneal stroma are present at birth and may progress slowly, while in some cases they may be stable from birth. Epithelial irregularity occurs but large bullae and corneal vascularization usually are not seen. Excrescences are not seen in Descemet membrane.

Complications
I   **Derived:** Reduced visual acuity, nystagmus (infrequent).
II   **Associated:** —

Etiology: Autosomal dominant or autosomal recessive; McK *21770

Pathogenesis: Decreased-to-absent endothelial cells.

Related Facts
I   **Sex Ratio:** M1:F1
II   **Risk of Occurrence:** ?
III   **Risk of Recurrence for**
    Patient's Sib: When autosomal dominant or autosomal recessive see Table I AD or AR, respectively.
    Patient's Child: When autosomal dominant or autosomal recessive see Table I AD or AR, respectively.
IV   **Age of Detectability:** At birth
V   **Prevalence:** ?

Treatment
I   **Primary Prevention:** Genetic counseling
II   **Secondary Prevention:** Penetrating keratoplasty
III   **Other Therapy:** —

Prognosis: Normal for life and intelligence. Fair for vision depending on degree of involvement.

Detection of Carrier: —

†Special Considerations: Three different endothelial dystrophies have been described. (See also Corneal Dystrophy, Endothelial, and Corneal Dystrophy, Polymorphous Posterior.)

References:
Maumenee, A.E.: Congenital hereditary corneal dystrophy. Am. J. Ophthalmol. 50:1114, 1960.
Pearce, W.G. et al: Congenital endothelial corneal dystrophy: Clinical, pathological and genetic study. Br. J. Ophthalmol. 53:577, 1969.

Contributors: **Joel Sugar**
                     Morton F. Goldberg

Editor's Computerized Descriptors: Vision, Eye

CORNEAL DYSTROPHY, ENDOTHELIAL

Includes: Dystrophie endothéliale de la cornée
Endotheliale Hornhautdystrophie
Distrofia corneana endotelial
Endothelial corneal dystrophy
Fuchs endothelial dystrophy
Cornea guttata
Congenital endothelial dystrophy of cornea

Excludes: Corneal dystrophy, polymorphous posterior (213)†
Corneal dystrophy, congenital hereditary (207)†

Minimal Diagnostic Criteria: Many tiny excrescences on Descemet membrane

Clinical Findings: This disorder biomicroscopically resembles adult senile Fuchs endothelial dystrophy in that there are numerous tiny (0.04 - 0.08 mm) tightly packed distributed excrescences on Descemet membrane, which give an appearance of endothelial dimples. They may first appear during adolescence. Vision is rarely affected.

Complications
I   **Derived:** Reduced visual acuity (infrequent)
II   **Associated:** Anterior polar cataract

Etiology: Possibly autosomal dominant; McK *12170

Pathogenesis: May be related to abnormal calcium metabolism

Related Facts
I   **Sex Ratio:** M1:F1
II   **Risk of Occurrence:** ?
III   **Risk of Recurrence for**
    Patient's Sib: If autosomal dominant and if parent is affected, 1 in 2 (50%) for each offspring to be affected; otherwise not increased
    Patient's Child: If autosomal dominant, 1 in 2
IV   **Age of Detectability:** Adolescence
V   **Prevalence:** ?

Treatment
I   **Primary Prevention:** Genetic counseling
II   **Secondary Prevention:** —
III   **Other Therapy:** None usually indicated; rarely, penetrating keratoplasty

Prognosis: Normal for life and intelligence. Usually good for vision.

Detection of Carrier: —

†Special Considerations: Three different endothelial dystrophies have been described. (See also Corneal Dystrophy, Polymorphous Posterior and Corneal Dystrophy, Congenital Hereditary.)

References:
Dohlman, C. H.: Familial congenital cornea guttata in association with anterior polar cataract. Acta Ophthalmol. (Kbh.) 29:445, 1951.
Duke-Elder, S.: System of Ophthalmology, vol. 3, part 2. Congenital Deformities. London:Henry Kimpton, 1964.
Duke-Elder, S.: System of Ophthalmology, vol. 8, part 2. Diseases of the Outer Eye. London:Henry Kimpton, 1965.
Hogan, M. J. and Bietti, G.: Hereditary deep dystrophy of the cornea (polymorphous). Trans. Am. Ophthalmol. Soc. 67:234, 1969.
Maumenee, A. E.: An introduction to corneal dystrophies. In Bergsma, D. (ed.): Part VIII. Eye, Birth Defects: Orig. Art. Ser., vol. VII, no. 3. Baltimore:Williams and Wilkins Co. for The National Foundation-March of Dimes, 1971, p. 3.
Theodore, F. H.: Congenital type of endothelial dystrophy. Arch. Ophthalmol. 21:626, 1939.

Contributors: **Morton F. Goldberg**
                     Joel Sugar

CORNEAL DYSTROPHY, GRANULAR

Includes: Dystrophie granulaire de la cornée
Granuläre Hornhautdystrophie
Distrofia granular de la córnea
Groenouw type I corneal dystrophy
Granular corneal dystrophy

Excludes: Corneal dystrophy, lattice (211)
Corneal dystrophy, macular (212)
Corneal dystrophy, Reis-Bücklers (215)

Minimal Diagnostic Criteria: Slit-lamp appearance of discrete, white opacities in anterior, axial, corneal stroma

Clinical Findings: Juvenile onset of multiple, bilateral, progressive, central, anterior, stromal opacities, which are usually grey or white and sharply defined. They may take the form of small disks, doughnuts, clubs, nodules, dots, etc. The peripheral cornea remains uninvolved. Recurrent painful epithelial erosions with secondary opacification and vascularization may occur. Decreased visual acuity often occurs between the 3rd to the 5th decades of life.

Complications
I **Derived:** Decreased corneal transparency
II **Associated:** —

Etiology: Autosomal dominant; McK *12190

Pathogenesis: Hyaline degeneration of the corneal stroma

Related Facts
I   **Sex Ratio:** M1:F1
II **Risk of Occurrence:** ?
III **Risk of Recurrence for**
    Patient's Sib: If parent is affected, 1 in 2 (50%) for each offspring to be affected; otherwise not increased
    Patient's Child: 1 in 2
IV **Age of Detectability:** ?
V   **Prevalence:** ?

Treatment
I   **Primary Prevention:** Genetic counseling
II **Secondary Prevention:** —
III **Other Therapy:** Lamellar, or occasionally penetrating, keratoplasty, depending on depth of stromal opacities.

Prognosis: Good for successful keratoplasty, though recurrences have been reported.

Detection of Carrier: Affected parent and patient

Special Considerations: —

References:
Brownstein, S. et al: Granular dystrophy of the cornea. Am. J. Ophthalmol. 77:701, 1974.
François, J.: Heredofamilial corneal dystrophies. In Symposium on Surgical and Medical Management of Congenital Anomalies of the Eye. St. Louis:C.V. Mosby Co., 1968.
Herman, S.J. and Hughes, W.F.: Recurrence of hereditary corneal dystrophy following keratoplasty. Am. J. Ophthalmol. 75:689, 1973.
Maumenee, A. E.: An introduction to corneal dystrophies. In Bergsma, D. (ed.): Part VIII. Eye. Birth Defects: Orig. Art. Ser., vol. VII, no. 3. Baltimore:Williams and Wilkins Co. for The National Foundation-March of Dimes, 1971, p. 3.
Sornson, E. T.: Granular dystrophy of the cornea: An electron microscopic study. Am. J. Ophthalmol. 59:1001, 1965.
Teng, C. C.: Granular dystrophy of the cornea: A histochemical and electron microscopic study. Am. J. Ophthalmol. 63:772, 1967.

Contributors: **Morton F. Goldberg**
Joel Sugar

CORNEAL DYSTROPHY, JUVENILE EPITHELIAL

Includes: Dystrophie épithéliale de la cornée
Epitheliale Hornhautdystrophie
Distrofia epitelial de la córnea
Juvenile epithelial degeneration of cornea
Hereditary epithelial corneal dystrophy
Juvenile epithelial corneal dystrophy
Meesmann corneal dystrophy

Excludes: Corneal dystrophy, recurrent erosive (214)
Whorl-like corneal dystrophy
Microcystic epithelial dystrophy of Cogan

Minimal Diagnostic Criteria: The appearance of fine vesicles in the corneal epithelium

Clinical Findings: Fine punctate opacities, seen only with magnification, appear in the corneal epithelium bilaterally during the first few years of life. They frequently remain asymptomatic, but may cause an irritative sensation and may stain with topically applied fluorescein solution. Vision may be slightly reduced, due to corneal astigmatism or mild scarring. The opacities are diffusely located in the central area of the corneal epithelium and, in reflected light, resemble tiny vesicles or droplets. In advanced cases, the droplets may assume a vortex or whorl pattern.

Complications
I **Derived:** Corneal scarring with reduced visual acuity
II **Associated:** —

Etiology: Autosomal dominant; McK *12210

Pathogenesis: ?

Related Facts
I **Sex Ratio:** M1:F1
II **Risk of Occurrence:** ?
III **Risk of Recurrence for**
Patient's Sib: If parent is affected, 1 in 2 (50%) for each offspring to be affected; otherwise not increased.
Patient's Child: 1 in 2
IV **Age of Detectability:** First few years
V **Prevalence:** ?

Treatment
I **Primary Prevention:** Genetic counseling
II **Secondary Prevention:** —
III **Other Therapy:** Lamellar or penetrating keratoplasty in advanced cases

Prognosis: Vision is sometimes significantly affected in adult, advanced cases. Prognosis for keratoplasty is guarded.

Detection of Carrier: —

Special Considerations: —

References:
Alkemade, P.P. and van Balen, A.T.: Hereditary epithelial dystrophy of the cornea: Meesmann type. Br. J. Ophthalmol. 50:603, 1966.
Kuwabara, T. and Ciccarelli, E.C.: Meesmann's corneal dystrophy: A pathological study. Arch. Ophthalmol. 71:672, 1964.
Maumenee. A.E.: An introduction to corneal dystrophies. In Bergsma, D. (ed.): Part VIII. Eye. Birth Defects: Orig. Art. Ser., vol. VII, no. 3. Baltimore: Williams and Wilkins Co. for The National Foundation-March of Dimes, 1971, p. 3.
Snyder, W.B.: Hereditary epithelial corneal dystrophy. Am. J. Ophthalmol. 55:56, 1963.

Contributors: **Morton F. Goldberg**
Joel Sugar

Editor's Computerized Descriptors: Vision, Eye

CORNEAL DYSTROPHY, LATTICE

Includes: Dystrophie cornéenne (en réseau)
Gitterförmige Hornhautdystrophie
Distrofia corneana en enrejado
Biber-Haab-Dimmer degeneration
Lattice corneal dystrophy†

Excludes: Interstitial keratitis
Prominent corneal nerves
Corneal dystrophy, granular (209)
Corneal dystrophy, macular (212)

Minimal Diagnostic Criteria: Slit-lamp appearance of opaque and translucent stromal lines

Clinical Findings: Progressive, bilateral opacifications of the corneal stroma, having the form of fine lines or dots, particularly occupying the midperiphery and the anterior portions of the stroma. The process begins at about age 5, causing significant loss of vision by age 40 to 60. Corneal sensitivity is diminished, and recurrent painful erosions are common.

Complications
I **Derived:** Reduced visual acuity due to decreased corneal transparency
II **Associated:** —

Etiology: Autosomal dominant; McK *12220

Pathogenesis: ? Possibly amyloid degeneration in the cornea of the stroma or corneal nerves. Cystine crystals have been reported to precede the amyloid deposition, but this has not been validated.

Related Facts
I **Sex Ratio:** M1:F1
II **Risk of Occurrence:** ?
III **Risk of Recurrence for**
  Patient's Sib: If parent is affected, 1 in 2 (50%) for each offspring to be affected; otherwise not increased.
  Patient's Child: 1 in 2
IV **Age of Detectability:** About 5th year
V **Prevalence:** ?

Treatment
I **Primary Prevention:** Genetic counseling
II **Secondary Prevention:** —
III **Other Therapy:** Keratoplasty, lamellar or penetrating, depending on depth and severity of stromal opacities; soft contact lenses. Recurrences have been noted in corneal grafts.

Prognosis: Good for successful keratoplasty

Detection of Carrier: Affected parent and patient

†Special Considerations: Two types of lattice corneal dystrophy occur. Those with systemic amyloidosis are later in onset, corneal opacities are fewer and more peripheral. Those without systemic amyloidosis are earlier in onset, corneal opacities are more numerous and central. Unilateral corneal involvement in family members of individuals with bilateral involvement as well as unilateral sporadic cases have been reported.

References:
Franceschetti, A. and Forni, S.: Clinical and hereditary aspects of familial degenerations of the cornea. Acta 16 Conc. Ophthalmol. Br. 1:194, 1951.
Herman, S.J. and Hughes, W.F.: Recurrence of hereditary corneal dystrophy following keratoplasty. Am. J. Ophthalmol. 75.689, 1973.
Kaunisto, N.: Lattice dystrophy of the cornea. Acta Ophthalmol. (Kbh.) 51:335, 1973.
Klintworth, G. K.: Lattice corneal dystrophy: An inherited variety of amyloidosis restricted to the cornea. Am. J. Pathol. 50:371, 1967.
Klintworth, G. K.: Current concepts on the ultrastructural pathogenesis of macular and lattice corneal dystrophies. In Bergsma, D. (ed.): Part VIII. Eye, Birth Defects: Orig. Art. Ser., vol. VII, no. 3. Baltimore:Williams and Wilkins Co., for The National Foundation-March of Dimes, 1971, p. 27.
Maumenee, A. E.: An introduction to corneal dystrophies. Ibid p. 3.
Meretoja, J.: Comparative histopathological and clinical findings in eyes with lattice corneal dystrophy of two different types. Ophthalmologica 165:15, 1972.
Rabb, M.F. et al: Unilateral lattice dystrophy of the cornea. Trans. Am. Acad. Ophthalmol. Otolaryngol. 78:440, 1974.
Smith, M. E. and Zimmerman, L. E.: Amyloid in corneal dystrophies: Differentiation of lattice from granular and macular dystrophies. Arch. Ophthalmol. 79:407, 1968.

Contributors: **Morton F. Goldberg**
Joel Sugar

Editor's Computerized Descriptors: Vision, Eye

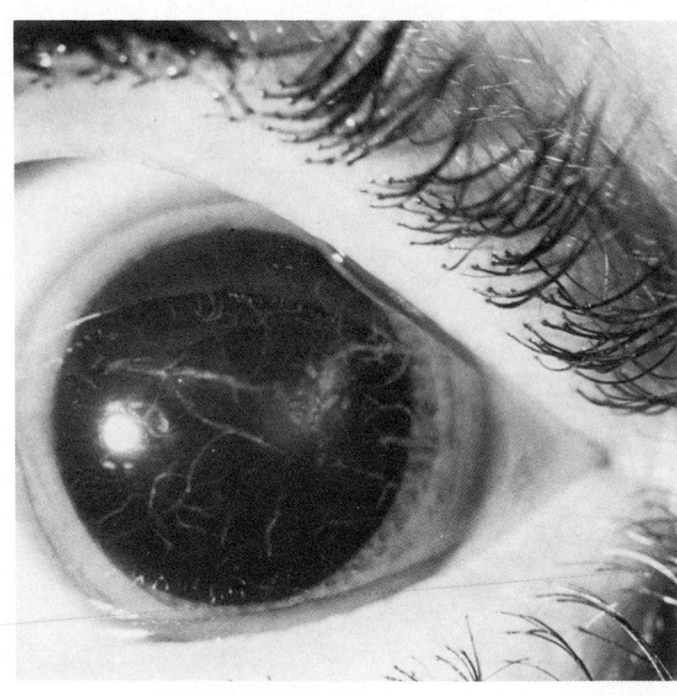

200. Lattice corneal dystrophy

CORNEAL DYSTROPHY, MACULAR

Includes: Dystrophie maculaire de la cornée
Makuläre Hornhautdystrophie
Distrofia macular de la córnea
Groenouw type II corneal dystrophy
Fehr corneal dystrophy
Spotted corneal dystrophy
Macular corneal dystrophy

Excludes: Corneal dystrophy, granular (209)
Corneal dystrophy, lattice (211)
Systemic mucopolysaccharidoses

Minimal Diagnostic Criteria: Slit-lamp evidence that the irregular clouding involves all layers of the corneal stroma with extension from limbus to limbus. The anterior and posterior limiting membranes of the cornea are normal.

Clinical Findings: Variably dense, progressive, bilateral clouding of the corneal stroma begins between the ages of 5 and 9, and extends diffusely from the Bowman to Descemet membrane and from limbus to limbus. There are ill-defined stromal accentuations of the cloudiness called macules. Sensitivity of the cornea may be reduced, and recurrent epithelial erosions can cause photophobia and painful episodes. Visual acuity is significantly reduced by the 4th decade of life.

Complications
I   **Derived:** Decreased visual acuity due to corneal opacities
II   **Associated:** —

Etiology: Autosomal recessive; McK *21780

Pathogenesis: Either a primary storage disease of the corneal fibroblast (keratocyte), involving abnormal mucopolysaccharide metabolism, or a mucoid degeneration of the stromal collagen with secondary accumulation of acid mucopolysaccharide in the keratocytes.

Related Facts
I   **Sex Ratio:** M1:F1
II   **Risk of Occurrence:** ?
III   **Risk of Recurrence for**
    Patient's Sib: 1 in 4 (25%) for each offspring to be affected
    Patient's Child: Not increased unless mate is carrier or homozygote
IV   **Age of Detectability:** 5th to 9th year
V   **Prevalence:** ?

Treatment
I   **Primary Prevention:** Genetic counseling
II   **Secondary Prevention:** ?
III   **Other Therapy:** Lamellar, or (more usually) penetrating keratoplasty

Prognosis: Good for successful keratoplasty

Detection of Carrier: —

Special Considerations: —

References:
Duke-Elder, S.: System of Ophthalmology, vol. 8, part 2. Diseases of the Outer Eye. London:Henry Kimpton, 1965.
Goldberg, M.F. et al: Corneal dystrophies associated with abnormalities of mucopolysaccharide metabolism. Arch. Ophthalmol. 74:516, 1965.
Klintworth, G. K.: Current concepts on the ultrastructural pathogenesis of macular and lattice corneal dystrophies. In Bergsma, D. (ed.): Part VIII. Eye. Birth Defects: Orig. Art. Ser., vol. VII, no. 3. Baltimore:Williams and Wilkins Co. for The National Foundation-March of Dimes, 1971, p. 27.
Klintworth, G.K. and Vogel S.: Macular corneal dystrophy: An inherited acid mucopolysaccharide storage disease of the corneal fibroblast. Am. J. Pathol. 45:565, 1964.
Maumenee, A.E.: An introduction to corneal dystrophies. In Bergsma, D. (ed.): Part VIII. Eye. op. cit. p. 3.
Morgan, G.: Macular dystrophy of the cornea. Br. J. Ophthalmol. 50:57, 1966.
Teng, C.C.: Macular dystrophy of the cornea: A histochemical and electron microscopic study. Am. J. Ophthalmol. 62:436, 1966.

Contributors: **Morton F. Goldberg**
                Joel Sugar

Editor's Computerized Descriptors: Vision, Eye

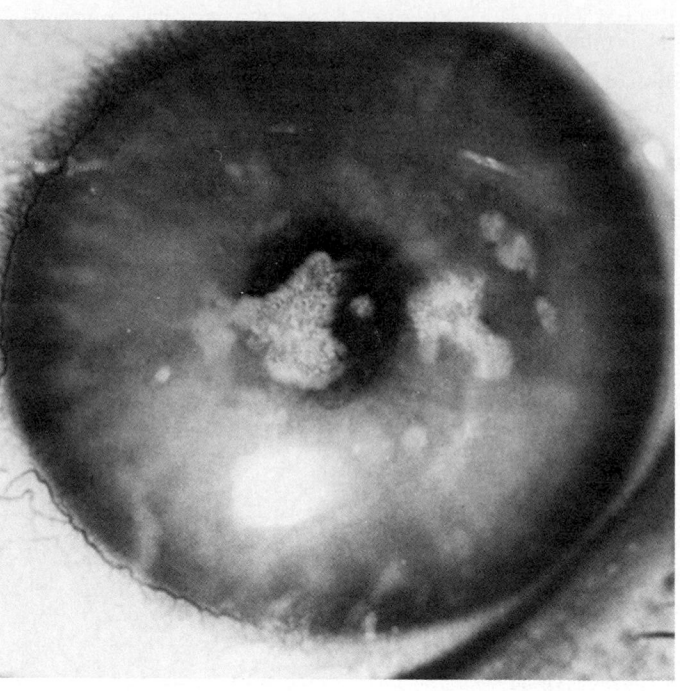

201. Macular corneal dystrophy

CORNEAL DYSTROPHY, POLYMORPHOUS POSTERIOR

Includes: Dystrophie polymorphe postérieure de la cornée
Polymorphe hintere Hornhautdystrophie
Distrofia corneana posterior polimórfica
Hereditary deep corneal dystrophy
Schlichting syndrome
Polymorphous posterior corneal dystrophy

Excludes: Corneal dystrophy, endothelial† (208)
Corneal dystrophy, congenital hereditary (207)†

Minimal Diagnostic Criteria: The slit-lamp appearance of "vesicles" in the posterior limiting membranes of the cornea.

Clinical Findings: Small, bilateral, congenital, nonprogressive "vesicular" lesions in the region of the corneal endothelium and Descemet membrane. These lesions appear clinically to be endothelial depressions or vesicles as in endothelial corneal dystrophy, but these histologically involve the Descemet membrane and the deep stroma, are fewer and larger (about 0.2 mm average with largest diameter about 0.75 mm) and also more irregular in size. There are usually no other symptoms.

Complications
I   **Derived:** Usually none; rarely, diffuse corneal edema
II **Associated:** —

Etiology: Autosomal dominant. Sporadic cases occur. McK *12200

Pathogenesis: ? May be related to abnormal calcium metabolism.

Related Facts
I   **Sex Ratio:** M1:F1
II   **Risk of Occurrence:**   ?
III **Risk of Recurrence for**
     Patient's Sib: When autosomal dominant and if parent is affected, 1 in 2 (50%) for each offspring to be affected; otherwise not increased.
     Patient's Child: 1 in 2 when autosomal dominant
IV   **Age of Detectability:** —
V   **Prevalence:** ?

Treatment
I   **Primary Prevention:** Genetic counseling
II   **Secondary Prevention:**   Usually none required; rarely, penetrating keratoplasty
III **Other Therapy:** —

Prognosis: Normal for life and intelligence. Vision may be variably reduced.

Detection of Carrier: Affected parent and patient

†Special Considerations: Three different endothelial dystrophies have been described. (See also Corneal Dystrophy, Endothelial and Corneal Dystrophy, Congenital Hereditary.)

References:
Hogan, M. J. and Bietti, G.: Hereditary deep dystrophy of the cornea (polymorphous). Trans. Am. Ophthalmol. Soc. 67:234, 1969.
Morgan, G. and Patterson, A.: Pathology of posterior polymorphous degeneration of the cornea. Br. J. Ophthalmol. 51:443, 1967.
Rodriguez, M.M. et al: Endothelial alterations in congenital corneal dystrophies. Am. J. Ophthalmol. 80:678, 1975.
Rubenstein, R. A. and Silverman, J. J.: Hereditary deep dystrophy of the cornea associated with glaucoma and ruptures in Descemet's membrane. Arch. Ophthalmol. 79:123, 1968.
Strachan, I. M. and Maclean, H.: Posterior polymorphous dystrophy of the cornea. Br. J. Ophthalmol. 52:270, 1968.

Contributors: **Morton F. Goldberg**
                     Joel Sugar

CORNEAL DYSTROPHY, RECURRENT EROSIVE

Includes: Dystrophie cornéenne érosive, à rechutes
Rezidivierende erosive Hornhautdystrophie
Distrofia corneana erosiva recurrente
Hereditary recurrent erosive corneal dystrophy
Recurent erosive corneal dystrophy

Excludes: Primary stromal corneal dystrophies with secondary erosions
Epithelial erosions secondary to corneal trauma
Fuchs combined epithelial-endothelial dystrophy

Minimal Diagnostic Criteria: Small (1-2 mm) epithelial erosions without stromal dystrophies or antecedent corneal trauma

Clinical Findings: Between the ages of 4 and 6 years, the onset of recurrent painful desquamation of the corneal epithelium occurs.

Vision and corneal sensation are rarely impaired, but a foreign body sensation, epithelial filaments, small patches of epithelial edema, and fluorescein staining may all occur. Pain may occur just upon awakening, at the time of lid opening. Small epithelial cysts are seen preceding erosive symptoms.

Complications
I   **Derived:** Corneal infection
II **Associated:** —

Etiology: Autosomal dominant; McK *12240

Pathogenesis: ?

Related Facts
I   **Sex Ratio:** M1:F1
II   **Risk of Occurrence:** ?
III **Risk of Recurrence for**
     Patient's Sib: If parent is affected, 1 in 2 (50%) for each offspring to be affected; otherwise not increased.
     Patient's Child: 1 in 2
IV   **Age of Detectability:** Four to six years
V   **Prevalence:** ?

Treatment
I   **Primary Prevention:** Genetic counseling
II   **Secondary Prevention:** An emollient at night to prevent adhesion of the lid to the cornea, nocturnal use of a hypertonic ointment to prevent epithelial edema.
III **Other Therapy:** Topical antibiotics and cycloplegics and firm bandaging when indicated

Prognosis: Good in most cases

Detection of Carrier: Affected parent and patient

Special Considerations: —

References:
Bron, A.J. and Tripathi, R.: Cystic disorders of the corneal epithelium. Br. J. Ophthalmol. 57:361, 1973.
Duke-Elder, S.: System of Ophthalmology, vol. 8, part 2. Diseases of the Outer Eye. London:Henry Kimpton, 1965.
Valle, O.: Hereditary recurring corneal erosions: A familial study with special reference to Fuchs' dystrophy. Acta Ophthalmol. (Kbh.) 45:829, 1967.

**Contributors: Morton F. Goldberg
Joel Sugar**

Editor's Computerized Descriptor: Eye

CORNEAL DYSTROPHY, REIS-BÜCKLERS

Includes: Dystrophie cornéenne type Reis-Bücklers
Reis-Bücklersche Hornhautdystrophie
Distrofia corneana de Reis-Bücklers
Ring-like corneal dystrophy
Annular corneal dystrophy
Reis-Bücklers corneal dystrophy

Excludes: Neuroparalytic keratitis
Corneal dystrophy, granular (209)
Corneal dystrophy, recurrent erosive (214)

Minimal Diagnostic Criteria: The appearance of ring-like or annular opacities in the region of Bowman membrane

Clinical Findings: The juvenile onset of painful, recurring, bilateral desquamations of the cornea is followed by annular opacifications of Bowman membrane. Corneal sensitivity and visual acuity are reduced. There may be a remission in early adult life, followed by a later relapse.

Complications
I   **Derived:** Reduced visual acuity due to corneal opacities
II **Associated:** —

Etiology: Autosomal dominant; McK *12150

Pathogenesis: Basement membrane and hemidesmosomes are absent over areas of destruction of the Bowman layer.

Related Facts
I   **Sex Ratio:** M1:F1
II   **Risk of Occurrence:** —
III **Risk of Recurrence for**
     Patient's Sib: If parent is affected, 1 in 2 (50%) for each offspring to be affected; otherwise not increased
     Patient's Child: 1 in 2
IV   **Age of Detectability:** 5 years
V   **Prevalence:** ?

Treatment
I   **Primary Prevention:** Genetic counseling
II   **Secondary Prevention:** —
III **Other Therapy:** Lamellar keratoplasty

Prognosis: Good, following keratoplasty

Detection of Carrier: Affected parent and patient

Special Considerations: —

References:
Bron, A.J. and Tripathi, R.C.: Corneal disorders. In Goldberg, M.F. (ed.): Genetic and Metabolic Eye Disease. Boston: Little, Brown, and Co., 1974.
Franceschetti, A. and Forni, S.: Clinical and hereditary aspects of familial degenerations of the cornea. Acta 16 Conc. Ophthalmol. Br. 1:194, 1951.
Griffith, D. G. and Fine, B. S.: Light and electron microscopic observations in a superficial corneal dystrophy: Probable early Reis-Bücklers' type. Am. J. Ophthalmol. 63:1659, 1967.
Maumenee, A. E.: An introduction to corneal dystrophies. In Bergsma, D. (ed.): Part VIII. Eye. Birth Defects: Orig. Art. Ser., vol. VII, no. 3. Baltimore: Williams and Wilkins Co. for The National Foundation-March of Dimes, 1971, p. 3.
Paufique, L. and Bonnet, M.: La dystrophie cornéenne hérédo-familiale de Reis-Bücklers. Ann. Oculist. (Paris) 199:14, 1966.

**Contributors: Morton F. Goldberg
Joel Sugar**

Editor's Computerized Descriptors: Vision, Eye

CORNEAL DYSTROPHY, SCHNYDER CRYSTALLINE

215-500

Includes: Dépôts cristallins dans la cornée
Kristalline Form der Hornhautdystrophie (Schnyder)
Distrofia cristalina-corneana de Schnyder
Hereditary crystalline corneal dystrophy
Crystalline corneal dystrophy
Corneal dystrophy, crystalline
Central crystalline corneal dystrophy
Schnyder crystalline corneal dystrophy

Excludes: Cystinosis (238)
Dysproteinemias
Cornea urica
Bietti marginal crystalline dystrophy
(All of foregoing have corneal crystals but of different appearance)

Minimal Diagnostic Criteria: The appearance of needle-shaped crystals in the subepithelial area of the corneal stroma in a circular pattern.

Clinical Findings: Infantile, slowly progressive (or stationary), bilateral, needle-shaped crystals collect in the subepithelial region of the cornea. These crystals are distributed centrally or paracentrally in a circular or disk-shaped pattern and may be white or variegated, dull or scintillating. There is minimal irritation or loss of vision. Xanthelasmata, arcus juvenilis or senilis, and Vogt limbal girdles may coexist. Occasionally, hypercholesterolemia may be found. At least 2 different pedigrees have been reported with associated dystrophies of long bones. Genu valgum is a prominent finding in these cases.

Complications
I **Derived:** Infrequently, decreased visual acuity occurs if the opacities overlie the visual axis
II **Associated:** Abnormalities of the joints

Etiology: Autosomal dominant; McK *12180

Pathogenesis: Unknown, possibly related to abnormal lipid metabolism. Crystals are cholesterol.

Related Facts
I **Sex Ratio:** M1:F1
II **Risk of Occurrence:** ?
III **Risk of Recurrence for**
 Patient's Sib: If parent is affected, 1 in 2 (50%) for each offspring to be affected; otherwise not increased.
 Patient's Child: 1 in 2
IV **Age of Detectability:** Infancy
V **Prevalence:** ?

Treatment
I **Primary Prevention:** Genetic counseling
II **Secondary Prevention:** —
III **Other Therapy:** Corneal grafting and surgery of the knees, when indicated

Prognosis: Usually good for vision; keratoplasty usually successful if required.

Detection of Carrier: Affected parent and patient

Special Considerations: —

References:
Delleman, J. W. and Winkelman, J. E.: Degeneratio cornea cristallinea hereditaria: A clinical, genetic, and histologic study. Ophthalmologica 155:409, 1968.
Fry, W. E. and Pickett, W. E.: Crystalline dystrophy of cornea. Trans. Am. Ophthalmol. Soc. 48:220, 1950.
Goldberg, M. F.: A review of selected inherited corneal dystrophies associated with systemic diseases. In Bergsma, D. (ed.): Part VIII. Eye. Birth Defects: Orig. Art. Ser., vol VII, no. 3. Baltimore:Williams and Wilkins Co. for The National Foundation-March of Dimes, 1971, p. 13.
Luxenberg, M.: Hereditary crystalline dystrophy of the cornea. Am. J. Ophthalmol. 63:507, 1967.
Malbran, J.L. et al: Hereditary crystalline degeneration of cornea. Ophthalmologica 126:369, 1953.

Contributors: **Morton F. Goldberg**
Joel Sugar

Editor's Computerized Descriptors: Eye, Skel.

216-500

CORONARY ARTERIAL CALCINOSIS

Includes: Calcinose des artères coronaires
Kalzinose der Koronararterien
Calcinosis de las coronarias
Coronary artery sclerosis
Juvenile or infantile coronary sclerosis
Coronary calcification of infancy
Congenital medial sclerosis of coronary arteries

Excludes: Coronary atherosclerosis of infancy or childhood

Minimal Diagnostic Criteria: This syndrome cannot at present be diagnosed antemortem. The typical clinical picture, plus roentgenographic proof of arterial calcification, would be highly suggestive.

Clinical Findings: Coronary calcinosis undoubtedly encompasses a number of conditions with varying etiologies. The common finding is one of interruption of normal myocardial blood flow by extensive generalized narrowing of coronary arteries with calcification. Both the intima and media are involved without atheroma. This is a disease of infancy with the vast majority of patients dying before age 6 months.

The classic clinical picture is one of acute onset of pallor, dyspnea, and signs of congestive heart failure which rapidly progress to death in several hours to several days. There may be a recent history of viral infection or even an intercurrent viral illness. There is also a less fulminant form of the disease characterized by more gradual onset of congestive failure with death in a period of weeks or months. There are no heart murmurs.

The ECG in the few patients in whom it has been obtained has shown ischemia or infarction. Progressive heart block also has been reported. Chest roentgenograms show cardiomegaly and pulmonary venous congestion. Some patients will have generalized arterial calcification, and films of the neck may prove useful in delineating thyroid artery or carotid artery calcification.

Complications
I **Derived:** Myocardial infarction, arrhythmias, congestive heart failure and death
II **Associated:** As mentioned above, some patients may have generalized arterial calcification.

Etiology: An autosomal recessive disorder presumably involving a defect of elastic fibers. Probably important environmental component. McK *20800

Pathogenesis: It is undetermined whether or not many of the infants involved with this syndrome are affected pre- or postnatally. Intrauterine insults such as rubella and other viremias may play a role in some patients. Altered calcium metabolism also may play a role in certain patients. Extrauterine infections, as well as anoxia, may be capable of producing coronary arterial medial necrosis with subsequent fibrous proliferation accounting for the pathologic findings.

Related Facts
I **Sex Ratio:** Ml:Fl
II **Risk of Occurrence:** ? < 1 in 1000 cases of congenital heart disease
III **Risk of Recurrence for**
  Patient's Sib: ? Two of 44 reported cases occurred in sibs
  Patient's Child: ?
IV **Age of Detectability:** Antemortem diagnosis is not possible
V **Prevalence:** ?

Treatment
I **Primary Prevention:** —
II **Secondary Prevention:** —

III **Other Therapy:** Supportive only

Prognosis: Uniformly fatal in our limited knowledge of this disease

Detection of Carrier: —

Special Considerations: —

References:
Bird, T.: Idiopathic arterial calcification in infancy. Arch. Dis. Child. 49:82, 1974.
Moran, J.J. and Becker, S.M.: Idiopathic arterial calcification of infancy. Am. J. Clin. Pathol. 31:517, 1959.
Nora, J.J. and McNamara, D.G.: Coronary artery sclerosis. In Watson, H. (ed.) Paediatric Cardiology. St. Louis: C.V. Mosby Co., 1968, p. 311.

Contributor: **Thomas P. Graham, Jr.**

Editor's Computerized Descriptors: Resp., CV.

CORONARY ARTERIOVENOUS FISTULA

Includes: Fistule coronaire artério-veineuse
Arteriovenöse Koronarfistel
Fistula arterio-venosa coronaria
Coronary artery-cameral shunt

Excludes: Anomalous origin of coronary arteries from pulmonary artery (64)

Minimal Diagnostic Criteria: Aortic root angiography is necessary to make the definitive diagnosis of coronary arteriovenous fistula.

Clinical Findings: A coronary arteriovenous fistula is characterized by a single or multiple channel communicating between one or both coronary arteries and a cardiac chamber or pulmonary artery. The most common site of communication is the right heart (90%). This includes the right ventricle (45%), followed in order by the right atrium (including coronary sinus) (30%), and the pulmonary artery (15%). In less than 10% of the cases, the communication is into the left atrium or the left ventricle. The right coronary artery alone is most commonly involved (60%), but the anomaly may occur in both right and left coronary arteries. Rarely, an extra coronary artery may be involved. The hemodynamic findings are related to the magnitude of flow through the fistula. Congestive heart failure has been reported in 21 of 150 patients (14%), usually in infancy or in late adult life.

Physical examination is variable, depending upon the magnitude and point of egress of the shunt. In the common variety (ie into the right heart) there is usually a continuous murmur and thrill maximally along the lower sternal border, either on the right or left side. The murmur may be loud, harsh and machinery-like with a superficial high-pitched quality. The continuous murmur may be differentiated from a patent ductus arteriosus by its location. In addition, it usually peaks near the first heart sound, the diastolic component may be louder than the systolic component. Atrioventricular valve flow murmurs are usually obscured by the continuous murmur. With a large shunt causing considerable aortic run-off, the increased pulse pressure manifests itself as bounding peripheral arterial pulses.

The thoracic roentgenogram generally reveals increased shunt vascularity and cardiomegaly in patients with large shunts to the right heart or pulmonary artery. In patients with small left-to-right shunts, the roentgen findings are normal. The ECG is usually normal. With large left-to-right shunts, left or biventricular hypertrophy is present.

Cardiac catheterization will reveal a left-to-right shunt when a large communication enters the right heart. Right pressures may be elevated. Aortic root angiography is the definitive procedure and will reveal a dilated coronary vessel(s) communicating with a cardiac chamber or vessel.

Complications
I **Derived:** Congestive heart failure, subacute bacterial endocarditis, development of a coronary artery aneurysm, formation of mural thrombi within tortuous coronary artery.
II **Associated:** —

Etiology: ?

Pathogenesis: In normal embryologic development of the coronary arteries, angioblastic buds arise from the truncus arteriosus, acquire lumens, and proliferate through the myocardium connecting through capillary beds with the coronary veins. The veins form also as buds from the caudal end of the primitive cardiac tube at a slightly earlier stage of development. During early development of the coronary arteries, there are communications with muscular intratrabecular spaces which may become lined with endothelium. Persistence of such channels provides a plausible explanation for intracardiac arteriovenous fistula.

Related Facts
I **Sex Ratio:** ? Probably M1:F1
II **Risk of Occurrence:** ? < 4 in 1000 cases of congenital heart disease
III **Risk of Recurrence for**
   Patient's Sib: Recurrence not reported
   Patient's Child: Recurrence not reported
IV **Age of Detectability:** From birth by selective angiography
V **Prevalence:** ?

Treatment
I **Primary Prevention:** —
II **Secondary Prevention:** Surgery on fistula obliterating left-to-right shunt.
III **Other Therapy:** Symptomatic for congestive heart failure, appropriate antibiotic prophylaxis to prevent subacute bacterial endocarditis.

Prognosis: The prognosis is excellent for patients who are detected and have surgical correction. Patients with congestive failure require digitalis followed by surgical therapy. Asymptomatic patients should in most cases have ligation unless the fistula is quite small or other considerations supervene.

Detection of Carrier: —

Special Considerations: —

References:
Gasul, B.M. et al: Systemic arteriovenous fistula. In Gasul, B.M. et al (eds.): Heart Disease in Children: Diagnosis and Treatment. Philadelphia:J.B. Lippincott, 1966, p. 442.
Nora, J. J. and McNamara, D. G.: Anomalies of the coronary arteries and coronary artery fistula. In Watson, H. (ed.), Paediatric Cardiology. London:Lloyd-Luke, 1968, p. 295.
Sabiston, D.C., Jr. et al: Surgical management of congenital lesions of the coronary circulation. Ann. Surg. 157:908, 1963.

Contributor: **Thomas P. Graham, Jr.**

Editor's Computerized Descriptors: Resp., CV.

CORONARY ARTERY, SINGLE

Includes: Artère coronaire unique
Singuläre Koronararterie
Arteria coronaria única
Single left or right coronary artery

Excludes: Anomalous origin of coronary arteries from pulmonary artery (64)

Minimal Diagnostic Criteria: Diagnosis can be made with aortic root angiography or cineangiography at the time of cardiac catheterization.

Clinical Findings: This entity is defined as a single coronary artery arising from the aorta by a single ostium. In 22 of 37 cases with data available, the single artery had the origin of a left coronary artery, while the remaining 15 had the origin of a right coronary artery.

Three anatomic types have been described with approximately one-third of patients falling into each category. Type I includes cases in which the single vessel follows the course of either the normal right or left coronary and supplies the remainder of the heart by extension of those branches. Type II includes cases in which the single artery branches into 2 vessels shortly after its origin, and these 2 vessels then follow the normal right and left artery distributions. Type III includes all cases in which the coronary distribution is atypical of either a normal right or left coronary pattern.

This anomaly occurring as an isolated cardiac defect causes no hemodynamic abnormalities. Because of the few reported cases, it is not known whether the patient is more vulnerable to coronary occlusive disease in later life.

The ECG and roentgenogram are normal in isolated, uncomplicated single coronary artery.

Complications

I Derived: In 4 of 27 adults with single coronary artery examined at necropsy, myocardial infarction was found. These 4 patients were ages 38, 46, 46 and 62. The relationship of the single coronary artery to the myocardial infarcts in these patients is unknown. There is an increase in the incidence of myocardial ischemia and infarction when the main left coronary artery or the anterior descending coronary artery courses between the aorta and the pulmonary trunk even in the absence of atherosclerotic disease. The reason for this complication remains unknown at the present time.

II Associated: There is a high percentage of associated cardiac defects in children with proven single coronary arteries. In 16 of 20 such patients, there were symptoms referable to the associated lesions. These associated defects include common ventricle (4), bicuspid aortic valve (3), fistulous communication with the right ventricle (2) and truncus arteriosus (2).

Etiology: ?

Pathogenesis: The pathogenesis is unknown. Several possibilities seem reasonable. First, there could be an absence of 1 coronary anlage or a development and subsequent involution of 1 anlage. The single artery which develops then would supply the entire myocardium by extension of and addition to its normal branches. Another possibility would be the development of 2 coronary artery anlagen in close proximity with gradual fusing of the 2 into 1 ostium with growth.

Related Facts

I Sex Ratio: Approximately M1:F1

II Risk of Occurrence: ? Probably < 1 in 200 cases of congenital heart disease

III Risk of Recurrence for
Patient's Sib: ?
Patient's Child: ?

IV Age of Detectability: From birth by aortic root angiography

V Prevalence: ?

Treatment

I Primary Prevention: ?

II Secondary Prevention: ?

III Other Therapy: None indicated for isolated condition

Prognosis: The prognosis is excellent for the isolated condition. Prognosis for patients with associated cardiac defects is entirely related to the severity of these defects. Relationship to development of coronary atherosclerosis is undetermined.

Detection of Carrier: —

Special Considerations: —

References:
Chaitman, B.R. et al: Clinical, angiographic and hemodynamic findings in patients with anomalous origin of the coronary arteries. Circulation 53:122, 1976.

Nora, J.J. and McNamara, D.G.: Anomalies of the coronary arteries and coronary artery fistula. In Watson, H. (ed.): Paediatric Cardiology. London:Lloyd-Luke, 1968, p. 295.

Smith, J.C.: Review of a single coronary artery with report of two cases. Circulation 1:1168, 1950.

Contributor: **Thomas P. Graham, Jr.**

Editor's Computerized Descriptor: CV.

CORPUS CALLOSUM AGENESIS

Includes: Agénésie du corps calleux
Agenesie des Corpus callosum
Agenesia del cuerpo calloso
Partial agenesis of corpus callosum
Agenesis of corpus callosum

Excludes: Forebrain defects

Minimal Diagnostic Criteria: Depends upon pneumoencephalographic studies showing a large dorsal displaced 3rd ventricle separating the lateral ventricles so that they assume a "bat-wing" appearance. Computerized axial tomogram shows separation of lateral ventricles.

Clinical Findings: Diagnosed in childhood in the work-up of mental retardation or macrocephaly. Most show severe, but nonprogressive retardation, not incompatible with life. Abnormalities of cerebral spinal fluid circulation are present in a large number with hydrocephaly. Rare association with cleft palate or lip. If corpus callosum is partially developed, this will occur anterior with the defects posterior. The septum pellucidum is absent and the fornix abnormal with a well-developed longitudinal bundle.

Complications
I   **Derived:** Hydrocephaly is usually of the communicating variety.
II   **Associated:** A small brain is a common associated defect in mentally retarded patients. The interhemispheric defect may be filled by a lipoma or cyst derived from the 3rd ventricle or arachnoid membranes. Hypocampal commissure absent, anterior commissure present.

Etiology: Mendelian inheritance or chromosomal defects have not been shown to play a part in man. In the mouse, absence of the corpus callosum and the presence of a longitudinal callosal bundle may be autosomal recessive. McK *21800

Pathogenesis: The corpus callosum does not develop until the 12th week, when the first fibers appear anteriorly near the lamina terminalis. Crossing of fibers is complete by 22 weeks. A vascular cause has been suggested but if this were acting, much more widespread defects of the hemispheres would be anticipated. An interference with this process would account for the pathology.†

Related Facts
I   **Sex Ratio:**   ?
II   **Risk of Occurrence:**   ?
III   **Risk of Recurrence for**
   Patient's Sib: ?
   Patient's Child: ?
IV   **Age of Detectability:**   Variable; 1st year 82%, 2nd year 6.5%(Probst), nearly 90% in first 2 years of life
V   **Prevalence:**   ?

Treatment
I   **Primary Prevention:**   —
II   **Secondary Prevention:**   —
III   **Other Therapy:**   Treatment of hydrocephaly if present and seizures if they occur.

Prognosis: Most patients do not die because of the absence of the corpus callosum. Mental retardation is nonprogressive.

Detection of Carrier: ?

†**Special Considerations:** Secondary loss of the corpus callosum occurs in extreme degrees of hydrocephaly and may also be found in cases of spina bifida with multiple coincidental malformations of brain and viscera.

References:
Davidoff, L.M. and Dyke, C.D.: Agenesis of the corpus callosum. Its diagnosis by encephalography. Am. J. Roentgenol. Radium. Ther. Nucl. Med. 32:1, 1934.
DeLange, D.: On brains with total and partial lack of the corpus callosum and on the nature of the longitudinal callosal bundle. J. Nerv. Ment. Dis. 62:449, 1925.
Hankinson, J. and Amador, L.V.: Agenesis of the corpus callosum diagnosed by pneumoencephalography. Br. J. Radiol. 30:200, 1957.
Kinal, M.E. et al: Lipoma of the corpus callosum. J. Neuropathol. Clin. Neurol. 1:168, 1951.
Lehman, R.A.: Motor co-ordination and hand preference after lesions of the visual pathway and corpus callosum. Brain 91:525, 1968.
Loeser, J.D. and Alvord, E.C., Jr.: Clinicopathological correlations in agenesis of the corpus callosum. Neurology 18:745, 1968.
Marburg, O.: So-called agenesia of the corpus callosum (callosal defect) anterior cerebral dysraphism. Arch. Neurol. Psychiatry 61:297,1949.
Probst, F.P.: Congenital defects of the corpus callosum. Morphology and encephalographic appearances. Acta Radiol. (Diag.) (Suppl.) (Stockh.) 1-152, 1973.
Zingesser, L. et al: Agenesis of the corpus callosum associated with an interhemispheric arachnoid cyst. Br. J. Radiol. 37:905, 1964.

Contributor: **Kenneth Shulman**

Editor's Computerized Descriptors: Face, Oral, Nerve, Skel.

CORTICAL HYPEROSTOSIS, INFANTILE

Includes: Hyperostose corticale infantile
Infantile kortikale Hyperostose
Hiperostosis cortical infantil
Caffey disease

Excludes: Secondary hyperostoses, eg hypervitaminosis A

Minimal Diagnostic Criteria: Onset under 5 months and subperiosteal new bone formation on xray, especially with mandibular involvement, alone or in combination.

Clinical Findings: Onset under 5 months of age; may be prenatal. Hyperirritability, swelling of soft tissues, especially overlying the mandible. Swellings are tender but not warm or discolored. Onset generally sudden in original sites and in recurrences; may resolve in 1 site while appearing in another. Mild-to-moderate temperature elevation. Spontaneous resolution usual in weeks to months. White blood cell response is variable and not diagnostic. Hemoglobin usually slightly low; erythrocyte sedimentation rate elevated and alkaline phosphatase frequently elevated. Radiographically the soft tissue swelling is all that is visible initially; cortical hyperostoses may be present at clinical onset indicating prior disease. Progressive, variable, external cortical thickening of the affected bones. One bone may show severe alteration while an adjacent one is unaffected. In mandible, massive thickening resembles structureless appearance of fibrous dysplasia, but serial subperiosteal layers of new bone may be identified in appropriate projections. In scapulae, may simulate neoplasia. May produce proptosis if orbital bones are affected. All bones affected except phalanges and vertebrae - mandible, clavicle and ulna most common.

Complications
I   **Derived:** Radioulnar synostosis with radial head dislocation. Bony bridging of adjacent affected ribs. Mistaken diagnosis of malignant neoplasm. Proptosis; exophthalmos (rare); ipsilateral diaphragmatic paralysis associated with scapular involvement. Bowing of affected bones after recovery. Pleural reactions when ribs are involved.

II **Associated:** —

Etiology: ? Viral agent suspected because of inflammatory changes on biopsy, apparent early immunity, and failure of response to anti-infectious agents. Milk allergy postulated but unproved. Collagen disease suggested. Familial and prenatal cases suggest genetic factors.†

Pathogenesis: ? Early inflammatory reaction of periosteum with polymorphonuclear infiltration. Periosteal fibrous layers lose definition and merge with adjacent soft tissue while inflammatory reaction extends into it and contiguous muscles. Some focal resorption of cortical bone observed histologically but not radiographically. Subsequent production of subperiosteal new bone. Obliterating intimal proliferation in small arteries of affected bone and fascia has been described.†

Related Facts
I   **Sex Ratio:** M1:F1
II **Risk of Occurrence:** ?
III **Risk of Recurrence for**
    Patient's Sib: ?
    Patient's Child: ?
IV **Age of Detectability:** Onset almost invariably before 5 months of age. Usually detected within the 1st half of 1st year and recovery by the end of the 1st year.
V   **Prevalence:** One report indicates 3/1000 patients under 6 months in hospitals and clinics. A series of cases may be observed over a period of several months, but years may pass before another is identified. Eleven cases reported in 2 generations of 1 family.†

Treatment
I   **Primary Prevention:** ?
II **Secondary Prevention:** Symptomatic treatment for fever, irritability, etc. In progressive or severe cases, steroids produce remission within 3 days; relapses after cessation of treatment for 10 days are not uncommon.
III **Other Therapy:** ?

Prognosis: Good. Rare chronic cases are described. Extremely rare deaths have occurred but the relationship of death to the primary disease is uncertain.

Detection of Carrier: —

†Special Considerations: The disease is frequently familial, occasionally prenatal but generally sporadic. The genetic character is unproved, and an infection is very likely though careful studies have failed to identify bacterial or viral causes.

References:
Caffey, J.: Infantile cortical hyperostosis: A review of the clinical and radiographic features. Proc. R. Soc. Med. 50:347, 1957.
Finsterbusch, A. and Rang, M.: Infantile cortical hyperostosis. Follow-up of 29 cases. Acta Paediatr. Scand. 216:727, 1975.
Holman, G.H.: Infantile cortical hyperostosis: A review. Q. Rev. Pediatr: 17:24, 1962.
Van Buskirk, F.W. et al: Infantile cortical hyperostosis. An inquiry into its familail aspects. Am. J. Roentgenol. Radium Ther. Nucl. Med. 85:613, 1961.

Contributor: **Frederic N. Silverman**

Editor's Computerized Descriptors: Eye, Skin, Skel., Muscle, Nerve

CORTICOSTEROID-BINDING GLOBULIN ABNORMALITIES

Includes: Anomalies de la globuline transporteuse du cortisol (CBG-transcortine)
Anomalien des Kortikoid-bindenden Globulins
Anomalías de la unión corticosteroide globulina
Decreased corticosteroid-binding globulin
Increased corticosteroid-binding globulin
CBG-transcortin

Excludes: Drug-induced changes in CBG
Disease-induced changes in CBG

Minimal Diagnostic Criteria: Low or elevated total plasma cortisol with normal amount of free cortisol in plasma and urine in the absence of symptoms and in absence of diseases or drugs affecting CBG. Measurement of free cortisol in urine, or determination of binding capacity of plasma for radioactively labeled cortisol akin to the T3 resin uptake test may be required.

Clinical Findings: Congenital abnormalities in cortisol-binding globulin (CBG) do not reflect a disease state and are not associated with any abnormality in adrenal function or symptomatology. They are detected as laboratory findings in individuals who have low or high concentrations of cortisol in plasma, but are otherwise normal. However, the laboratory findings may suggest hyper-or hypofunction of the adrenal and spur unnecessary investigations.

Complications
I   **Derived:**   —
II **Associated:**   —

Etiology: CBG deficiency is familial and transmitted as an autosomal dominant or X-linked recessive trait. CBG excess is also familial but the mode of transmission is uncertain.

Pathogenesis: Cortisol-binding globulin (CBG-transcortin) is a plasma glycoprotein with high affinity for cortisol as well as progesterone, desoxycorticosterone, corticosterone and some synthetic glucocorticoids. About 75% of plasma cortisol is reversibly bound by CBG, 15% is bound to albumin, and about 10% remains free and biologically active, being constantly replenished from CBG. Decreased CBG is associated with a low total cortisol, and increased CBG with a high total cortisol; in both circumstances, free cortisol remains normal, urinary excretion of free cortisol is also normal, and cortisol production and the response to ACTH remain normal. In liver disease and nephrotic syndrome, CBG, and consequently total cortisol, are low; in pregnancy and with estrogen therapy CBG and total cortisol are high.†

Related Facts
I   **Sex Ratio:**   M > F in CBG deficiency, M1:F1 CBG excess
II **Risk of Occurrence:**   ?
III **Risk of Recurrence for**
    Patient's Sib: For CBG deficiency, if autosomal dominant or X-linked recessive, see Table 1 AD or X-linked R, respectively. For CBG excess:?
    Patient's Child: For CBG deficiency, if autosomal dominant or X-linked recessive, see Table 1 AD or X-linked R, respectively. For CBG excess:?
IV **Age of Detectability:**   Any age from birth onwards
V   **Prevalence:**   ?

Treatment
I   **Primary Prevention:**   —
II **Secondary Prevention:**   —
III **Other Therapy:**   —

Prognosis: Excellent

Detection of Carrier: —

†Special Considerations: The most common cause of CBG excess is pregnancy and estrogen-containing medication.

References:
Doe, R.P. et al: Familial decrease in corticosteroid-binding globulin. Metabolism 14:940, 1965.
Lohrenz, F.N. et al: Adrenal function and serum protein concentrations in a kindred with decreased corticosteroid-binding globulin (CBG) concentration. J. Clin. Endocrinol. Metab. 27:966, 1967.
Lohrenz, F.N. et al: Idiopathic or genetic elevation of corticosteroid-binding globulin? J. Clin. Endocrinol. Metab. 28:1073, 1968.
Rosner, W.: Interaction of adrenal and gonadal steroids with proteins in human plasma. N. Engl. J. Med. 281:658, 1969.

Contributor: **Mark A. Sperling**

Editor's Computerized Descriptor: —

CRANIO-CARPO-TARSAL DYSPLASIA

Includes: Dysplasie cranio-carpo-tarsienne
Kraniokarpotarsale Dysplasie
Displasia cráneo-carpo-tarsal
Whistling face syndrome
Freeman-Sheldon syndrome
Carpotarsal and cranial dystrophy

Excludes: —

Minimal Diagnostic Criteria: Characteristic face described below with ulnar deviation of hands and finger contractures.

Clinical Findings: Flat, stiff, immobile face with sunken eyes. Hypertelorism, convergent strabismus and a mild degree of blepharophimosis. Antimongoloid obliquity of the eyelids. Small nose with long philtrum. Narrow nostrils. The central parts of the cheek bulge excessively, resembling that seen when whistling, due to what appears to be a muscle deficiency. Microstomia and high-arched palate. A fibrous band or elevation which is demarcated by 2 paramedian grooves, forming an H- or V-shaped scar-like structure extending from the middle of the lower lip to the chin. Retarded growth, flexion contractures of the fingers, especially the metacarpophalangeal joint of the thumbs. Bilateral or unilateral talipes equinovarus.

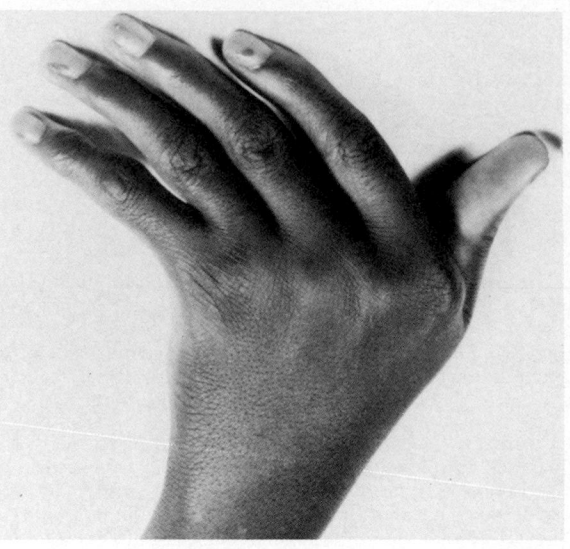

202. Windmill vane hand

Complications
I   **Derived:** Walking difficulties. Growth retardation. Slight speech impairment.
II   **Associated:** —

Etiology: Probably autosomal dominant; McK *19370

Pathogenesis: ?

Related Facts
I   **Sex Ratio:** M1:F1
II   **Risk of Occurrence:** Very rare
III   **Risk of Recurrence for**
     Patient's Sib: If parent is affected 1 in 2 (50%) for each offspring to be affected; otherwise not increased.
     Patient's Child: Probably 1 in 2
IV   **Age of Detectability:** Neonatal
V   **Prevalence:** Very rare

Treatment
I   **Primary Prevention:** Genetic counseling
II   **Secondary Prevention:** Plastic reparative surgery for talipes equinovarus and other defects as may be necessary.
III   **Other Therapy:** —

Prognosis: After surgery, walking improves. General health is not impaired.

Detection of Carrier: —

Special Considerations: —

References:
Cervenka, J. et al: Craniocarpotarsal dysplasia or whistling face syndrome. Arch. Otolaryngol. 91:183, 1970.
Fraser, F.C. et al: Cranio-carpal-tarsal dysplasia: Report of a case in father and son. JAMA 211:1374, 1970.
Sauk, J.J., Jr. et al: Electromyography of oral-facial musculature in craniocarpotarsal dysplasia (Freeman-Sheldon syndrome). Clin. Genet. 6:132, 1974.
Weinstein, S. and Gorlin, R. J.: Cranio-carpo-tarsal dysplasia or the whistling face syndrome. I. Clinical considerations. Am. J. Dis. Child. 117:427, 1969.

Contributor: **Heddie O. Sedano**

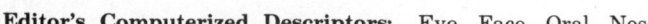

Editor's Computerized Descriptors: Eye, Face, Oral, Nose,

CRANIODIAPHYSEAL DYSPLASIA

Includes: Dysplasie cranio-diaphysaire
Kraniodiaphysäre Dysplasie
Displasia cráneo-diafisial
Dysplasia, craniodiaphyseal
Diaphyseal and cranial dysplasia

Excludes: Pyle disease (847)
Craniometaphyseal dysplasia (228)
Frontometaphyseal dysplasia (394)
Sclerosteosis (880)
Diaphyseal dysplasia (290)

Minimal Diagnostic Criteria: Severe hyperostosis and sclerosis
of the skull bones including the mandible. Diaphyseal widening
and sclerosis of the tubular bones, ribs and clavicles.

Clinical Findings: Severe craniofacial dysmorphism (leontiasis
ossea) caused by thickening of the cranial bones, and small stature. Roentgenologically cranial hyperostosis and sclerosis with
diaphyseal distention of the tubular bones.

Complications
I   **Derived:** Nasal obstruction, symptoms of cranial nerve compression leading to failure of vision, deafness, facial paralysis, mental retardation, seizures.
II **Associated:** —

Etiology: Autosomal recessive; McK *21830

Pathogenesis: On cross-section the bone is dense and the spongiosa is reduced in amount. Increased amounts of dense lamellated
bone are found but the intrinsic structure of the compact bone is
normal.

Related Facts
I   **Sex Ratio:** M1:F1
II   **Risk of Occurrence:** ?
III **Risk of Recurrence for**
Patient's Sib: 1 in 4 (25%) for each offspring to be affected
Patient's Child: Not increased, unless mate is carrier or
homozygote.
IV **Age of Detectability:** Early infancy by roentgenograms of
the skull and long bones
V   **Prevalence:** ?

Treatment
I   **Primary Prevention:** Genetic counseling
II   **Secondary Prevention:** —
III **Other Therapy:** Supportive

Prognosis: The disease is progressive, leading to early death in
the 2nd or 3rd decade of life.

Detection of Carrier: —

Special Considerations: —

References:
Halliday, J.: Rare case of bone dystrophy. Br. J. Surg. 37:52, 1949.
Joseph, R. et al: Dysplasie craniodiaphysaire progressive. Ses rela-
tions avec la dysplasie diaphysaire progressive de Camurati-
Engelmann. Ann. Radiol. (Paris) 1:477, 1958.

Contributor: **Jürgen W. Spranger**

Editor's Computerized Descriptors: Vision, Hearing, Face, Nasoph., Skel., Nerve

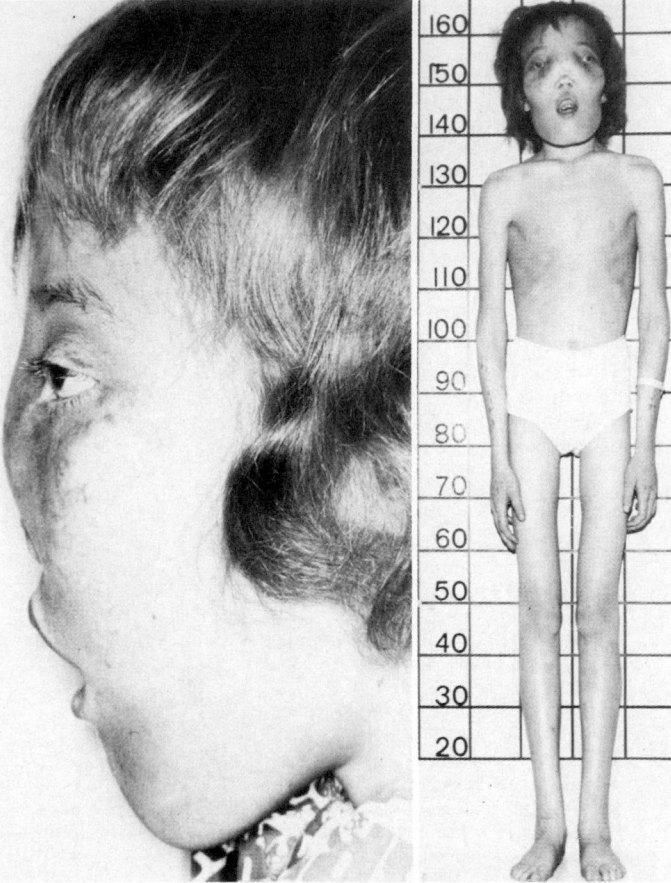

203. Enlarged head and facial features in tall, thin 12-year-old; subcutaneous tissue is reduced and muscles appear hypoplastic

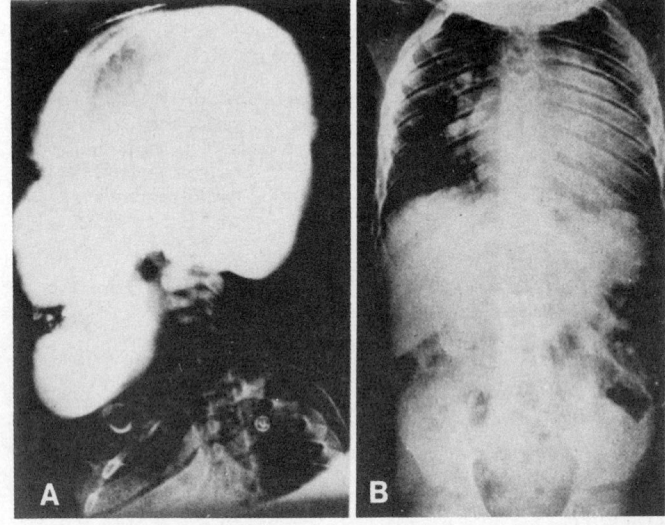

204. A) Marked sclerosis of facial and skull bones; B) enlargement
of ribs and cardiac dilation

CRANIOFACIAL DYSOSTOSIS

Includes: Dysostose cranio-faciale
Dysostosis craniofacialis
Disostosis cráneo-facial
Crouzon syndrome
Facial and cranial dysostosis

Excludes: Acrocephalosyndactyly (14)
Various types of isolated craniostenosis and craniostenosis syndromes†

Minimal Diagnostic Criteria: Brachycephalic cranial deformity resulting from premature craniosynostosis, especially of the coronal and sagittal sutures, exophthalmos with shallow orbits, maxillary hypoplasia with relative mandibular prognathism

Clinical Findings: Common Features: Craniosynostosis especially of the coronal, sagittal, and occasionally lambdoidal sutures with palpable ridging and digital impressions radiographically.†
Widening of the hypophyseal fossa and small paranasal sinuses may be observed in some cases.
Brachycephaly
Ocular hypertelorism
Exophthalmos with shallow orbits
Divergent strabismus, nystagmus, and optic nerve damage
Psitticorhina, deviated septum
Maxillary hypoplasia with relative mandibular prognathism
Short upper lip
Class III malocclusion with V-shaped maxillary dental arch and maxillary anterior crowding
  Occasional Findings:
Mental retardation
Bifid uvula or cleft palate
Bilateral atresia of the auditory meatus
Spontaneous luxation of the eyes
Bilateral anterior subluxation of the head of the radius
A variety of other low frequency anomalies may be observed including Kleeblattschädel anomaly

Complications
I **Derived:** Increased intracranial pressure, mental retardation, optic atrophy, spontaneous luxation of the eyes
II **Associated:** See Clinical Findings.

Etiology: Autosomal dominant transmission with complete penetrance and variable expressivity. Approximately one-fourth of reported cases arise as fresh mutations.† McK *12350

Pathogenesis: Premature synostosis of the coronal, sagittal, and sometimes lambdoidal sutures together with sphenobasilar synchondrosis. Order and rate of progression determine degree of deformity and disability produced. Premature synostosis commences during the 1st year of life and is usually complete by 2-3 years in most instances.

Related Facts
I **Sex Ratio:** M1:F1
II **Risk of Occurrence:** ? Low
III **Risk of Recurrence for**
  Patient's Sib: If parent is affected 1 in 2 (50%) for each offspring to be affected; otherwise not increased
  Patient's Child: 1 in 2
IV **Age of Detectability:** At birth or during the 1st year of life, by physical and roentgenographic examination.
V **Prevalence:** ? Uncommon

Treatment
I **Primary Prevention:** Genetic counseling
II **Secondary Prevention:** Surgical intervention mandatory in cases with rapid progression (increased intracranial pressure, progressive mental retardation, optic nerve involvement)
III **Other Therapy:** Cosmetic surgery in selected cases

Prognosis: Normal for life span

Detection of Carrier: Since expressivity is variable, some individuals may have only minimal involvement. Roentgenograms of the skull should detect premature synostosis in minimally affected family members by age 10.

†Special Considerations: Although the skull is brachycephalic, cranial deformity is variable, depending on the order and rate of progression of sutural involvement. Craniostenosis without the features of craniofacial dysostosis has been observed to follow an autosomal dominant mode of transmission in some instances. Other forms of craniostenosis and craniostenosis syndromes, both genetic and nongenetic, are known to occur. The use of the term pseudo-Crouzon syndrome to describe isolated cases of craniostenosis without the other features of craniofacial dysostosis should be avoided. Cases of so-called Vogt cephalosyndactyly, a condition in which Crouzon syndrome is said to be combined with Apert syndrome, are simply cases of Apert type acrocephalosyndactyly.

References:
Bertelson, T. I.: The premature synostosis of the cranial sutures. Acta Ophthalmol. (Kbh.) Suppl. 51, 1958.
Cohen, M.M., Jr.: An etiologic and nosologic overview of craniosynostosis syndromes. In Bergsma, D. (ed.): Malformation Syndromes. Birth Defects: Orig. Art. Ser., vol. XI, no. 2. Amsterdam: Excerpta Medica for The National Foundation-March of Dimes, 1975, p. 137.
Gorlin, R. J. and Pindborg, J. J.: Syndromes of the Head and Neck. New York: McGraw-Hill, 1964. p. 172.
Vulliamy, D. G. and Normandale, P. A.: Craniofacial dysostosis in a Dorset family. Arch. Dis. Child. 41:375, 1966.

Contributor: **Carolyn D. Hudson**

Editor's Computerized Descriptors: Eye, Ear, Face, Oral, Teeth, Nasoph., Skel.,Nerve

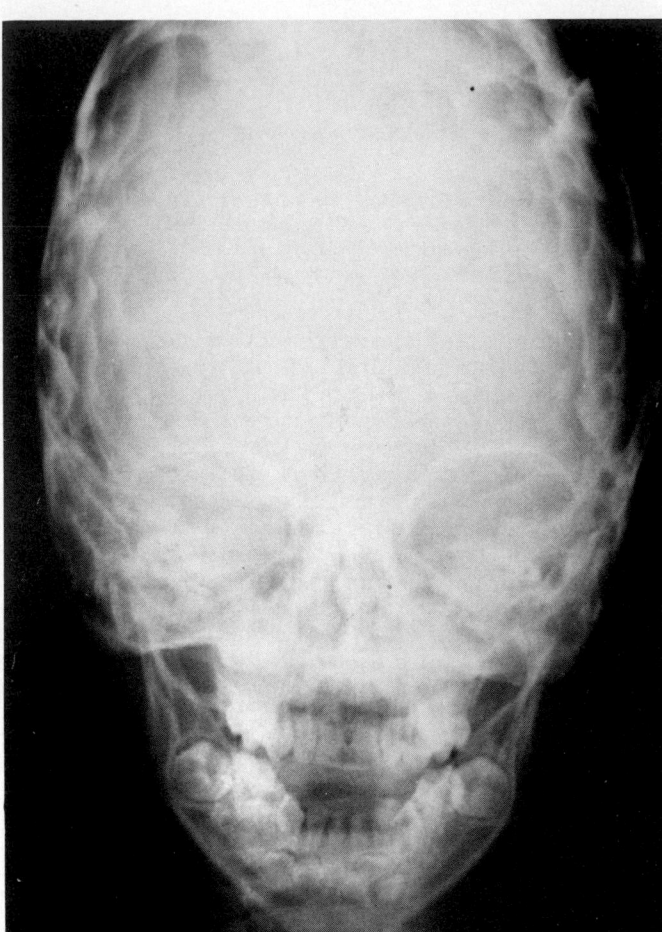

205. Skull in Crouzon syndrome. Note high vertex; increased digital markings; premature suture synostosis; ocular hypertelorism; large, shallow orbits

CRANIOFACIAL DYSOSTOSIS WITH DIAPHYSEAL HYPERPLASIA

Includes: Hyperplasie diaphysaire avec dysostose cranio-faciale
Craniofaciale Dysostosie mit diaphysärer Hyperplasie
Disostosis cráneo-facial con hiperplasia diafisaria
Stanesco dysostosis

Excludes: Craniodiaphyseal dysplasia (224)
Pyknodysostosis (846)
Tubular stenosis (976)

Minimal Diagnostic Criteria: Thick cortices of long bones, small skull with thin cranium, short stature.†

Clinical Findings: Craniofacial dysostosis with small, brachycephalic skull, thin cranial bones with lack of pneumatization, depressions over frontoparietal and occipitoparietal sutures, narrow maxilla with obtuse angle, small mandible, shallow orbits with prominent eyes, rather bulbous nose. Mild-moderate short stature with disproportionately short lower segment and upper arm, and dense long bones with thick cortices. Hands are short without cone epiphyses or osteolysis of phalanges. Teeth are small and crowded with enamel hypoplasia. Some affected individuals had flat roof of palate, sacralization of S-1, exostoses and fractures. Intelligence has been normal.

Complications
I   **Derived:** Short stature, increased thickening of cortices with age
II **Associated:** ?

Etiology: Apparently autosomal dominant inheritance

Pathogenesis: Affected individuals may be short at birth. Stature remains below normal. Cortical thickness increases with age. Histology unknown.

Related Facts
I   **Sex Ratio:** M1:F1
II   **Risk of Occurrence:** Rare
III **Risk of Recurrence for**
     Patient's Sib: If parent affected, 1 in 2 (50%) for each offspring to be affected; otherwise not increased.
     Patient's Child: 1 in 2 (50%)
IV   **Age of Detectability:** Probably at birth; definitely during early childhood.
V   **Prevalence:** Rare

Treatment
I   **Primary Prevention:** Genetic counseling
II   **Secondary Prevention:** —
III **Other Therapy:** —

Prognosis: Apparently normal life span

Detection of Carrier: —

†**Special Considerations:** This condition appears to be distinct because of normal phalanges. An interesting feature is the depressed sutures.

References:
Hall, J.G.: Craniofacial dysostosis-either Stanesco dysostosis or a new entity. In Bergsma, D. (ed.): Skeletal Dysplasias. Birth Defects: Orig. Art. Ser., vol. X, no. 12. Amsterdam: Excerpta Medica for The National Foundation-March of Dimes, 1974, p. 521.
Smith, D.W.: Recognizable Patterns of Human Malformation, 2nd Ed. Philadelphia: W.B. Saunders, 1976, p. 232.
Stanesco, V.: Syndrome hereditarie dominant, reunissant une dysostose craniofaciale de type particulier, une insuffisance de croissance d'aspect chondrodystrophique et un epaississement massif de la corticale des os longs. Rev. Fr. Endocrinol. Clin. 4:219, 1963.

CRANIOFACIAL DYSSYNOSTOSIS

Includes: Dyssynostose cranio-faciale
Kraniofaziale Dyssynostose
Disinostosis cráneo facial
Craniosynostosis-craniofacial dysostosis syndrome with mental retardation and other malformations

Excludes: Other craniosynostosis syndromes and craniofacial dysostoses

Minimal Diagnostic Criteria: Premature synostosis of lambdoid sutures and of posterior part of sagittal suture causing deformity of the skull with prominent forehead and small, flat (or bulging) occiput. Dysostosis of basal structures of the skull causing (secondary) anomalies of the face.

Clinical Findings: Dolichocephalic or brachyturricephalic configuration of the skull is present from birth, with protuberant forehead and small, flat or bulging occiput. The deformity becomes more pronounced during infancy. Osseous ridges are palpable over the lambdoid sutures and posterior part of the sagittal suture suggesting premature closure. The coronal suture may close prematurely, contributing to asymmetry of skull and face. Microcephaly is less often seen than macrocephaly; abnormal hair pattern may be present. Facial appearance is characterized by hypoplastic supraorbital ridges, antimongoloid slanting of palpebral fissures, anteverted nostrils, short maxilla, micrognathia and posteriorly rotated, sometimes dysplastic auricles. The palate usually is high and narrowly arched. Ocular signs include strabismus, nystagmus and optic atrophy. Shortness of stature was seen in all patients except one. Motor development is delayed; mental retardation is seen in most affected children. Seizures may occur; EEG recordings are abnormal. Radiographic findings include brachycephaly, frontal bossing, synostosis of lambdoid sutures and posterior part of sagittal suture, posteriorly located anterior fontanel, short base of skull, steep slope of base of anterior fossa, small posterior fossa. Cerebral malformation (agenesis of the corpus callosum) and hydrocephalus have been reported.

Complications
I   **Derived:** Increased intracranial pressure from craniosynostosis or hydrocephalus soon after birth; mental retardation, seizures, cerebral palsy.
II **Associated:** Congenital heart defect; other anomalies.

Etiology: Autosomal recessive †

Pathogenesis: ?

Related Facts
I   **Sex Ratio:** M1:F1 (in the cases reported)
II   **Risk of Occurrence:** ?
III **Risk of Recurrence for**
     Patient's Sib: 1 in 4 (25%) for each offspring to be affected
     Patient's Child: Not increased unless mate is carrier or homozygote
IV   **Age of Detectability:** Infancy
V   **Prevalence:** Rare; possibly more common in populations of Spanish ancestry

Treatment
I   **Primary Prevention:** Genetic counseling
II   **Secondary Prevention:** Craniosynostectomy at an early age; shunting procedures for progressive hydrocephalus
III **Other Therapy:** Anticonvulsants, physiotherapy, special education

Prognosis: Development may be normal following surgical intervention. Hydrocephalus sometimes arrests spontaneously. Associated anomalies change the outcome.

Detection of Carrier: ?

†**Special Considerations:**   The condition probably reflects an etiologically heterogeneous but pathogenetically similar group of disorders. It is not possible to decide at the present stage of knowledge if the syndrome represents a dysostosis of cranial and facial structures or a dysmorphic syndrome with mental retardation. The mental retardation observed in the patients reported may represent ascertainment bias.

References:
Neuhäuser, G. et al: Studies of malformation syndromes of man XXXIX: A craniosynostosis-craniofacial dysostosis syndrome with mental retardation and other malformations: "Craniofacial dyssynostosis". Eur. J. Pediatr. 123:15, 1976.

Contributor: **Gerhard Neuhäuser**

Editor's Computerized Descriptors: Eye, Ear, Face, Oral, Nose, Hair, Skel., Nerve

CRANIOMETAPHYSEAL DYSPLASIA

Includes: Dysplasie cranio-métaphysaire
Kraniometaphysäre Dysplasie
Displasia cráneo metafisial
Dysplasia, craniometaphyseal

Excludes: Pyle disease (847)
Craniodiaphyseal dysplasia (224)
Frontometaphyseal dysplasia (394)
Sclerosteosis (880)
Diaphyseal dysplasia (290)

Minimal Diagnostic Criteria: Hyperostosis or sclerosis of the cranial bones, especially the frontal and occipital parts of the cranial vault, club-shaped metaphyseal flare of the tubular bones. Metaphyseal undermodeling is minimal in the 1st year of life. Varying degrees of diaphyseal sclerosis are present at this period.†

Clinical Findings: Facial dysmorphism with frontonasal swelling, hypertelorism, mandibular enlargement. Roentgenologically cranial hyperostosis and metaphyseal undermodeling.

Complications
I **Derived:** Nasal obstruction, symptoms of cranial nerve compression such as conductive hearing loss, optic atrophy, facial paralysis. Perceptive hearing loss occurs as well.
II **Associated:** —

Etiology: Genetic heterogeneity is present. Cases with autosomal dominant inheritance are clinically and radiologically less severely affected than cases in which autosomal recessive transmission must be assumed. McK *12300, *21840

Pathogenesis: ? Failure to resorb newly formed bone

Related Facts
I **Sex Ratio:** M1:F1
II **Risk of Occurrence:** ?
III **Risk of Recurrence for**
     Patient's Sib: When autosomal dominant or autosomal recessive, see Table I AD or AR, respectively.
     Patient's Child: When autosomal dominant or autosomal recessive, see Table I AR or AD, respectively.
IV **Age of Detectability:** Early infancy by roentgenogram of skull and long bones
V **Prevalence:** ?

Treatment
I **Primary Prevention:** Genetic counseling
II **Secondary Prevention:** —
III **Other Therapy:** Operative removal of hyperostotic tissue for cosmetic purposes, hearing aids, supportive treatment

Prognosis: Normal life expectancy, but incapacitating progressive hyperostosis of the skull bones and ensuing cranial nerve compression. Normal adult body height. Regression of cranial hyperostosis has also been observed in adolescence and early adulthood.

Detection of Carrier: Unknown for autosomal recessive genotype

†**Special Considerations:**   Craniometaphyseal dysplasia, dominant, must not be confused with Pyle disease in which the skull is only minimally affected.
    Craniometaphyseal dysplasia, recessive, must not be confused with craniodiaphyseal dysplasia in which the skull shows even more sclerosis and in which there is no metaphyseal modeling defect.

References:
Holt, J.F.: The evolution of craniometaphyseal dysplasia. Ann. Radiol. (Paris) 9:209, 1966.
Millard, D.R., Jr. et al: Craniofacial surgery in craniometaphyseal dysplasia. Am. J. Surg. 113:615, 1967.

Spranger, J. et al: Die kraniometaphysäre Dysplasie (Pyle). Z. Kinderheilkd. 93:64, 1965.

Contributor: **Jürgen W. Spranger**

Editor's Computerized Descriptors: Eye, Hearing, Face, Nasoph., Nose, Skel., Nerve

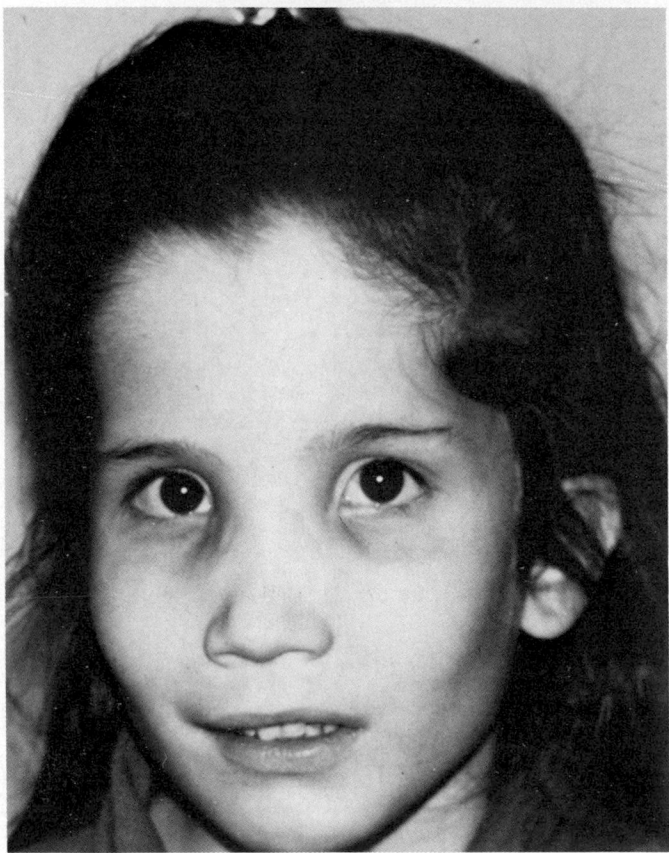

206. Note frontonasal swelling and ocular hypertelorism

CRANIO-OCULO-DENTAL SYNDROME

Includes: Syndrome cranio-oculo-dentaire
Kranio-okulo-dentales Syndrom
Síndrome cráneo-óculo-dental
Oculocraniodental syndrome
Dentocranioocular syndrome

Excludes: Acrocephalosyndactyly (14)
Oro-facio-digital syndrome I (770)
Orocraniodigital dysostosis
Oculo-dento-osseous dysplasia (737)
Craniofacial dysostosis (225)
Oro-facio-digital syndrome II (771)

Minimal Diagnostic Criteria: Frequent findings are partial premature closure of cranial sutures, low hairline, nasal septum deviation, brachydactyly, ptosis of eyelids. These findings are not obligatory but facultative.†

Clinical Findings: The facial appearance is characteristic because of the asymmetry of the face, low hairline, uni- or bilateral ptosis of eyelids, parrot-beaked nose with septum deviation. The nasal bridge tends to be high. Time of onset later and degree of craniostenosis less severe than in acrocephalosyndactyly (Apert syndrome). Coronal or sphenobasilar sutures are involved in an asymmetric fashion in most cases, giving rise to minor bilateral parietal bossing and facial asymmetry. The skull is brachiocephalic with decreased frontooccipital and increased bitemporal diameters, and reduced circumference.

Ptosis of one or both eyelids is frequently observed, sometimes associated with mild hypertelorism and strabismus, myopia or hyperopia, paralysis of superior rectus or inferior oblique muscles. In some patients stenosis or atresia of the tear ducts has been observed. Atrophy of the optic nerve may be observed but with less frequency than in other craniostenotic disorders.

The external ears may be low set with small or folded pinnae. Minor degree of conductive hearing loss is frequent. Brachydactyly is an almost constant finding in the affected individuals, sometimes associated with clinodactyly of the 5th finger. The fingers may show soft tissue syndactyly 2-3 or sometimes 2-3-4.

Hallux valgus has been noted frequently. Partial soft tissue syndactyly may occur between the 2nd and 3rd or the 4th and 5th toes. Simian crease is present in more than half of the affected individuals. The ridge count is low, peculiar thenar and hypothenar loop and whorl patterns have been demonstrated.

High-arched palate is frequent, in some cases cleft palate was noted. The maxilla tends to be somewhat hypoplastic giving rise to a mild relative prognathism. Ankylosis of mandibular condyle has been observed. Peg-shaped or missing upper lateral incisor or duplication have been noted in some cases.

A variety of accompanying anomalies have been encountered like mental retardation, epilepsy and schizophrenia, cryptorchism and renal anomalies.

Complications
I   **Derived:** Early closure of cranial sutures may lead to mental retardation and optic nerve atrophy. Tear duct stenosis leads to tearing and susceptibility to eye infection.
II **Associated:** —

Etiology: Autosomal dominant mode of transmission with wide range in expressivity and high degree of penetrance. Advanced parental age may be contributory in the etiology of newly observed cases.

Pathogenesis: ? The findings in the head and neck area seem to be due to the pleiotropic effect of a single gene rather than being the sequelae of the premature closure of the cranial sutures. The closure of the sutures may start before or after birth and may be minute.

Related Facts
I **Sex Ratio:** M1:F1
II **Risk of Occurrence:** ?
III **Risk of Recurrence for**
  Patient's Sib: If parent is affected 1 in 2 (50%) for each offspring to be affected; otherwise not increased
  Patient's Child: 1 in 2
IV **Age of Detectability:** Usually at birth
V **Prevalence:** ?

Treatment
I **Primary Prevention:** Genetic counseling
II **Secondary Prevention:** Craniotomy and prevention of closure of cranial sutures. Plastic surgery for ptosis and tear duct anomalies. Correction of septum deviation may be necessary to prevent ascending ear infections.
III **Other Therapy:** Glasses for refractive errors and dental restorations

Prognosis: Not known if longevity is reduced.

Detection of Carrier: —

†**Special Considerations:** This syndrome is frequently mistaken as atypical cases of Apert or Crouzon syndrome because of great overlap of manifestations.
  Many other cases in the literature reported under a variety of terms may in fact belong to this syndrome.
  The wide range in expressivity may account for the nosologic splitting.

References:
McKusick, V. A.: Mendelian Inheritance in Man. 3rd Ed. Baltimore:Johns Hopkins Press, 1971.
Waardenburg, P. J.: Orbital and interorbital region. In Waardenburg, P.J. et al (eds.): Genetics and Ophthalmology. Assen, Netherlands: Van Gorcum and Co., 1961, p. 301.

Contributor: **Carl J. Witkop, Jr.**

Editor's Computerized Descriptors: Vision, Eye, Hearing, Ear, Face, Oral, Teeth, Nasoph., Nose, Dermatoglyphic, Hair, Skel., GU., Nerve

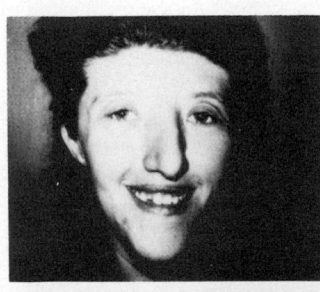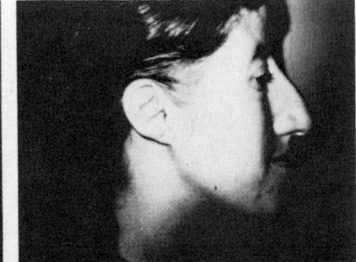
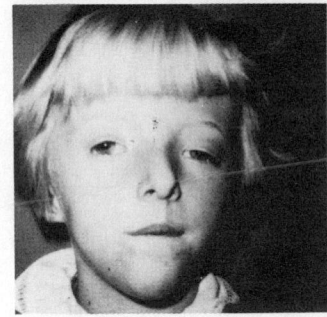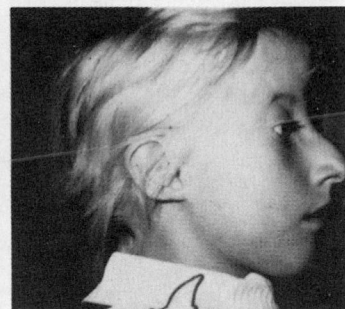

207. Facial features in Saethre-Chotzen

CRANIOSYNOSTOSIS

Includes: Craniosynostose
Kraniosynostose
Cráneosinostosis
Craniostenosis
Scaphocephaly
Brachycephaly
Plagiocephaly
Turricephaly
Premature lambdoid suture closure

Excludes: Craniofacial dysostosis (225)
Acrocephalosyndactyly (14)

Minimal Diagnostic Criteria: Abnormally shaped head with suture closed on x-ray examination.

Clinical Findings: A disorder of shape or form rather than size of cranial vault. The skull cannot enlarge at right angles to the prematurely closed suture. Rather it expands parallel to such a closed suture with compensatory growth at the site of patent sutures, producing a long narrow head with sagittal suture closure (scaphocephaly). Plagiocephaly is unilateral coronal closure. Turricephaly represents a closure of both coronal and sagittal suture with bony growth at the fontanel producing a pointed skull. All premature closures are present at birth, but accentuated by cranial growth during the first months of life. Closed suture tends to be ridged and palpable.

Complications
I **Derived:** Mental subnormality rare in sagittal closure, more frequent in untreated bilateral coronal or multiple suture closure. Papilledema and secondary optic atrophy may also complicate the latter.
II **Associated:** Cleft palate, spina bifida

Etiology: Both autosomal recessive and autosomal dominant transmission reported. McK *12310, *21850

Pathogenesis: Fusion of cranial suture, may possibly be due to increased tension on underlying dura matter produced by a deformity of skull base. Presumably defect involves mesenchyme separating growing bony plates.

Related Facts
I **Sex Ratio:** M > F; sagittal closure more common in males
II **Risk of Occurrence:** ?
III **Risk of Recurrence for**
  Patient's Sib: When autosomal recessive or autosomal dominant, see Table I AR or AD, respectively.
  Patient's Child: When autosomal recessive or autosomal dominant, see Table I AR or AD, respectively. AD.
IV **Age of Detectability:** Newborn to 1st year of life
V **Prevalence:** ?

Treatment
I **Primary Prevention:** Genetic counseling
II **Secondary Prevention:** Surgical repair is indicated in all multiple suture closures to prevent mental retardation and increased pressure. In sagittal synostosis, surgery indicated up to one year of age for cosmetic effect.†
III **Other Therapy:** —

Prognosis: Good with appropriate therapy. 75% of children have satisfactory result.

Detection of Carrier: —

†**Special Considerations:** Recent controversy in literature with regard to surgical indications because of tendency to group all varieties of synostosis. The most prevalent form, sagittal synostosis, does not have high risk of increased pressure or mental retardation. However, surgical repair is indicated in sagittal closure

for cosmetic reasons in those centers where pediatric neurosurgery is performed.

References:
Freeman, J. M. and Borkowf, S. B.: Craniostenosis; review of literature and report of 34 cases. Pediatrics 30:57, 1962.

Matson, D. D.: Neurosurgery of Infancy and Childhood, 2nd Ed. Springfield:Charles C Thomas, 1969.

Moss, M. L.: The pathogenesis of premature cranial synostosis in man. Acta Anat. (Basel) 37:351, 1959.

Shillito, J., Jr. and Matson, D. D.: Craniosynostosis; a review of 519 surgical patients. Pediatrics 42:829, 1969.

Contributor: **Kenneth Shulman**

Editor's Computerized Descriptors: Eye, Oral, Skel.

CRANIOSYNOSTOSIS-RADIAL APLASIA SYNDROME

Includes: Craniosynostose avec aplasie radiale
Craniosynostose-Radiusaplasie-Syndrom
Síndrome de cráneosinostosis y aplasia radial
Baller-Gerold syndrome

Excludes: Fanconi anemia
Thrombocytopenia with absent radius (941)
Acrocephalosyndactyly (14)

Minimal Diagnostic Criteria: Craniosynostosis of one or more sutures and radial aplasia (probably bilateral).

Clinical Findings: Craniosynostosis involving coronal and metopic sutures is always present. Turribrachycephaly with steep forehead, high nasal bridge and prominent mandible have been described. Epicanthal folds, ocular hypotelorism and small dysplastic ears have been present. Radial aplasia is present bilaterally in all cases. The thumb is hypoplastic or absent. Metacarpal and carpal bones are fused, hypoplastic or absent. Ulna is short and curved with radial deviation of the hand. A vertebral anomaly was present in 1 case. Intelligence is normal. One child had sudden unexplained death and at autopsy polymicrogyria of the brain and subaortic valvular hypertrophy were present.

Complications
I   **Derived:** Craniosynostosis can lead to brain compression, but in this condition it is not clear whether the anomaly of the calvaria is primary or secondary to a deficit in brain growth. Delayed fine motor development in hands may occur because of arm and hand anomalies.

II **Associated:** —

Etiology: Presumably an autosomal recessive trait. Consanguinity was present in 1 family and a male and female were affected in another family. McK *21860

Pathogenesis: ?

Related Facts
I   **Sex Ratio:**   ?
II   **Risk of Occurrence:**   Very rare
III **Risk of Recurrence for**
      Patient's Sib: Presumed 1 in 4 (25%) for each offspring to be affected.
      Patient's Child: Not increased unless mate is carrier or homozygote
IV   **Age of Detectability:**   At birth
V   **Prevalence:**   Only 4 cases reported

Treatment
I   **Primary Prevention:**   Genetic counseling
II   **Secondary Prevention:**   Prenatal diagnosis may be possible at 18-20 weeks (looking for radius). Surgical correction of synostosis if signs of increased cranial pressures or for cosmetic indications.
III **Other Therapy:**   Corrective orthopedic surgery, physical and occupational therapy.

Prognosis: Would appear to be good if CNS normal

Detection of Carrier: None known

Special Considerations: —

References:
Baller, F.: Radiusaplasie und Insucht. Z. Menschl. Vererb. Konstit. Lehre 29:782, 1950.

Cohen, M.M.: An etiologic and nosologic overview of craniosynostosis syndromes. In Bergsma, D. (ed.): Malformation Syndromes. Birth Defects: Orig. Art. Ser., vol. XI, no. 2. Amsterdam: Excerpta Medica for The National Foundation-March of Dimes, 1975, p. 137.

Gerold, M.: Frakturheilung bei einem seltenen Fall kongenitaler Anomalie der oberen Gliedmassen. Zentralbl. Chir. 84:831, 1959.

Greitzer, L.J. et al: Craniosynostosis-radial aplasia syndrome. J. Pediatr. 84:723, 1974.

Contributor: **Judith G. Hall**

Editor's Computerized Descriptors: Eye, Ear, Face, Nose, Skel.

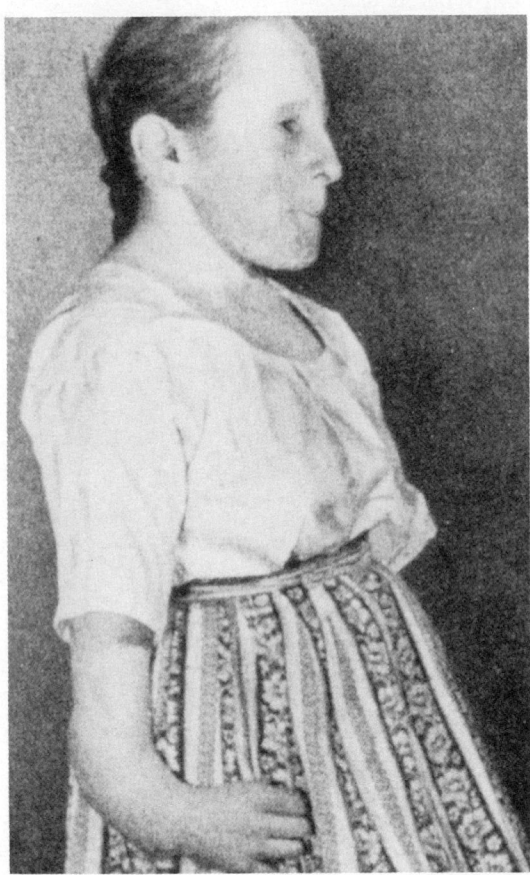

208. Note turribrachycephaly, steep forehead, high nasal bridge, long philtrum, prominent mandible, short curved forearm and absent thumb

CRYPTOTIA

Includes: Agénésie de l'oreille
Kryptotie
Criptotia

Excludes: Microtia-atresia (664)
Atresia alone
Deafness and ear pits (247)
Darwin tubercle (Marker) (241)
Ear lobe pit (Marker) (322)
Ear flare

Minimal Diagnostic Criteria: The upper margin of the pinna is buried under the scalp.†

Clinical Findings: The superior portion of the auricle is covered with scalp. Usually the cartilaginous framework and remainder of the ear are intact and said to be fairly normal. The anomaly is usually unilateral.

Complications
I   Derived: —
II Associated: —

Etiology: ?

Pathogenesis: ?

Related Facts
I   Sex Ratio: ?
II Risk of Occurrence: ?
III Risk of Recurrence for
      Patient's Sib: ?
      Patient's Child: ?
IV Age of Detectability: At birth
V   Prevalence: ?

Treatment
I   Primary Prevention: —
II Secondary Prevention: Plastic surgical repair may be indicated.
III Other Therapy: —

Prognosis: Good for life span, intelligence and function if isolated defect of outer ear, otherwise dependent upon concomitant defects.

Detection of Carrier: —

†**Special Considerations:** Anomalies of the external ear should suggest the possibility of an anomaly of the middle ear as well. Hearing should be assessed as soon as possible and appropriate therapy instituted. The anatomy of the middle and inner ear should be determined by petrous pyramid polytomography.

References:
Converse, J.M. (ed.): Reconstructive Plastic Surgery. Philadelphia:W.B. Saunders Co., 1964, vol. 3.
Rubin, A.: Handbook of Congenital Malformations. Philadelphia:W.B. Saunders Co., 1967.

Contributor: **LaVonne Bergstrom**

Editor's Computerized Descriptor: Ear

CUTIS LAXA

Includes: Congenital generalized cutaneous elastolysis
Chalasoderma
Dermatochalasia
Dermatomegaly†

Excludes: Ehlers-Danlos syndrome (338)
Circumscribed cutaneous elastolysis
Acquired or secondary cutaneous elastolysis

Minimal Diagnostic Criteria: Generalized cutaneous laxity with typical changes in the elastin in skin biopsy specimens.†

Clinical Findings: This systemic disease has a reduction of elastin fibers with laxity of the skin, which hangs in loose folds in all areas. "Hound-dog facies". Deep voice. Dermal changes are usually apparent at birth, or develop during infancy. Late onset has been reported in a few cases. The dermal changes may remain static or may progress. Cardiac and pulmonary involvement is not uncommon. Skin biopsy shows reduced numbers of elastin fibers, which are fragmented and granular.

Complications
I **Derived:** Cardiac failure due to gross pulmonary emphysema or structural cardiac abnormalities, liability to chest infections, diverticulae of the gut and bladder, blepharochalasis, ectropion, external hernia, rectal and vaginal prolapse, lax vocal cords.
II **Associated:** A nasal abnormality consisting of a short columella and a hooked nose is frequently present.

Etiology: It is probable that there are 2 separate genetic forms of the condition—a "benign" autosomal dominant with variable penetrance, and a "malignant" autosomal recessive. These have not yet been completely delineated. McK *12370, *21910

Pathogenesis: The dermal and visceral changes are due to the abnormality of elastin. It is not known whether this is the basic defect or merely a reflection of an underlying biochemical lesion. Diminution in absolute numbers of elastic fibers in the skin and viscera occurs. These fibers are fragmented, granular, have increased thickness and electron density with marked granularity. Gross pulmonary emphysema may lead to cor pulmonale.

Related Facts
I **Sex Ratio:** M1:F1
II **Risk of Occurrence:** ?
III **Risk of Recurrence for**
  Patient's Sib: When autosomal dominant or autosomal recessive, see Table I AD or AR, respectively.
  Patient's Child: When autosomal dominant or autosomal recessive, see Table I AD or AR, respectively.
IV **Age of Detectability:** Usually at birth or in infancy. A few cases of late onset have been reported.
V **Prevalence:** Very rare. There are only about 40 cases reported in the world literature. Except for one American Negro, all of these have been Caucasians.

Treatment
I **Primary Prevention:** Genetic counseling
II **Secondary Prevention:** —
III **Other Therapy:** Plastic surgery may be required to correct the dermal changes. The initial results are usually good, but repeated operations may be required.

Prognosis: Normal intelligence. Probably normal life span if there is no cardiac or pulmonary involvement. Death may occur in childhood if these complications are severe or progressive.

Detection of Carrier: —

†**Special Considerations:** Cutis laxa has been the source of great semantic confusion, as this name has also been applied to the Ehlers-Danlos syndrome and to various localized or secondary forms of lax skin.

When further genetic evidence becomes available, both dominant and recessive forms of the condition may well be delineated. It is likely that the incidence of internal ramifications and complications is quite different in these 2 entities.

There are scattered reports of infants with lax skin, associated with articular and skeletal abnormalities. These probably represent further separate genetic entities, which are excessively rare and poorly understood.

References:
Beighton, P.: The dominant and recessive forms of cutis laxa. J. Med. Genet. 9:216, 1972.
Goltz, R.W. et al: Cutis laxa - a manifestation of generalized elastolysis. Arch. Dermatol. 92:373, 1965.
Marshall, J. et al: Post-inflammatory elastolysis and cutis laxa: A report on a new variety of this phenomenon and a discussion of some syndromes characterized by elastolysis. S. Afr. Med. J. 40:1016, 1966.

Contributor: **Peter Beighton**

Editor's Computerized Descriptors: Speech, Skin, Resp., CV.

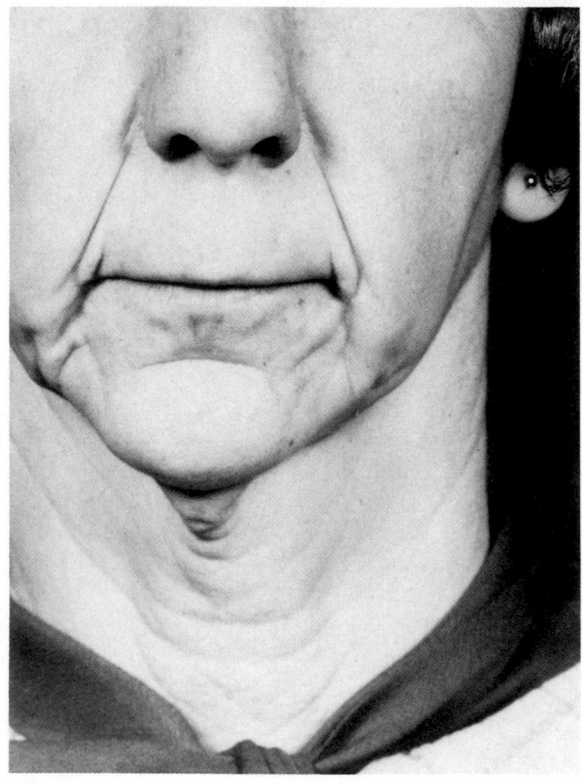

209. Cutis laxa in a 16-year-old

CYCLOPIA

Includes: Cyclopie
Zyklopie
Ciclopía
Synopthalmia
Cebocephaly
Ethmocephaly

Excludes: Aprosopia (complete failure of development of most of the brain and face)
Cephalopagus (twins joined at the head) with fused eyes
Holoprosencephaly (473)

Minimal Diagnostic Criteria: Fusion (to variable degree) of the optic vesicles

Clinical Findings: Cyclopia is part of a complex of anomalies resulting from maldevelopment of the embryonic forebrain. Any degree of fusion of the optic vesicles may occur. The nose is usually either absent or replaced by a proboscis-like structure above the eye. There is a single central bony cavity, the pseudoorbit. There are variable degrees of malformation of the brain, particularly failure of division of the telencephalon. Variable degrees of fusion of the eyelids and lacrimal structures occur. Transitional malformations between synophthalmos and arrhinencephalia are sometimes broadly classified under the term holoprosencephaly.

Complications
I   **Derived:** See Clinical Findings.
II **Associated:** Polydactyly, sirenomelia, umbilical hernia, cleft lip and palate, spina bifida, anencephaly, hydrocephaly

Etiology: ? Although evidence points to diverse causation, eg autosomal recessive gene(s), chromosome 18p-, chromosome 13 trisomy, maternal disease (particularly viral or toxic exposure during the 1st month of pregnancy). Numerous noxious stimuli during early embryonic development have caused cyclopia in experimental animals.†

Pathogenesis: Disturbance in the activity of the prosencephalic organizing center of the embryo resulting in failure of development of the anterior end of the neural tube and of the frontonasal process.

Related Facts
I   **Sex Ratio:** ? But no deviation from M1:F1 has been reported.
II **Risk of Occurrence:** ?
III **Risk of Recurrence for**
    Patient's Sib: ? Rare, but an increased incidence of spontaneous abortions occurs in families producing cyclopia.
    Patient's Child: Precluded by early death of patients.
IV **Age of Detectability:** At birth or, if suspected, by xray in utero after calcification of the skull.
V   **Prevalence:** Essentially zero

Treatment
I   **Primary Prevention:** Genetic counseling when autosomal recessive or associated with chromosome 18p- or chromosome 13 trisomy
II **Secondary Prevention:** —
III **Other Therapy:** —

Prognosis: Most die at birth or within a few hours, although 1 reported case survived 10 years.

Detection of Carrier: —

†**Special Considerations:** Because of tentative evidence for both genetic and environmental etiologies, the reporting of cases of synophthalmos is encouraged.

References:

Cohen, M.M., Jr. and Gorlin, R.J.: Genetic considerations in a sibship of cyclopia and clefts. In Bergsma, D. (ed.): Part II. Malformation Syndromes. Birth Defects: Orig. Art. Ser., vol. V. no. 2. New York: The National Foundation-March of Dimes, 1969, p. 113.
Duke-Elder, S.: System of Ophthalmology. vol. 3, pt. 2. Congenital Deformities. St. Louis: C.V. Mosby, Co., 1963, p. 429.
Johnston, M.C. et al: Abnormal organogenesis of facial structures. In Wilson, J.G. and Fraser, F.C. (eds.): Handbook of Teratology, Vol. 2. Mechanisms and Pathogenesis. New York: Plenum Press, 1977, p. 421.

Contributor: **Donald R. Bergsma**

Editor's Computerized Descriptors: Eye, Nose, Nerve

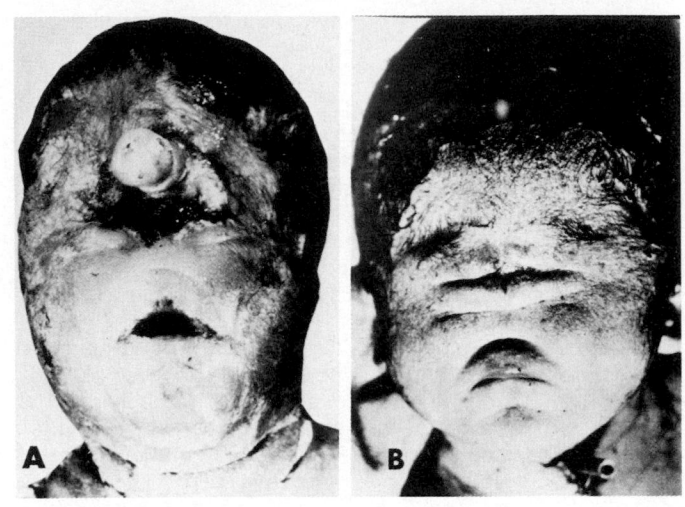

210. Cyclopia: A) With proboscis; B) without proboscis

CYLINDROMAS OF SCALP

Includes: Cylindrome du cuir chevelu
Turbantumoren
Cilindromas del cuero cabelludo
Scalp cylindroma types I and II
Familial cylindroma of scalp
Syphonoma
Tomato tumor
Hydradenoma
Neuroepithelioma adenoids
Epithelioma adenoids cysticum
Nonpapillary hyalinizing hydradenoma
Multiple familial benign nodular intraepidermal basal cell epithelioma
Endothelioma capitis of Kaposi
Cylindromatosis
Turban tumors of scalp

Excludes: Gingival fibromatosis and multiple hyaline fibromas (411)

Minimal Diagnostic Criteria: Clinical picture as below plus biopsy showing 1 of 2 types.

Type I - cylindromatous lesion consisting of close-packed masses of cells of basal type with peripheral palisading. The basal ends of cells rest on a thick hyaline membrane, with scattered masses of hyaline material in midst of tumor masses. Occasional duct-like spaces lined by 1 or 2 layers of flattened cells.

Type II - adenomatous lesion made up of larger less chromatophilic cells than Type I with peripheral palisading, but no limiting hyaline membrane. The border of clumps of cells is wavy with strands of interspersed collagen, there are nodular hyalinized cysts and mucinous cysts. No intracellular mucin nor hyaline is seen.

Clinical Findings: These ectodermal overgrowths are usually multiple, sessile or pedunculated tumors of scalp, face and neck. Sometimes they occur on the trunk, groin and genitalia. Almost always appearing after puberty, these lesions may grow to be very large. They are covered with smooth epithelium but sometimes are accompanied by pain and bleeding.

Complications
I **Derived:** Local infection may occur. Bleeding is usually minimal. There may be a conductive hearing loss due to obstruction of the external auditory canal. Metastases have been reported. Recurrence following excision is common.
II **Associated:** —

Etiology: Thought to be autosomal dominant with variable penetrance.

Pathogenesis: ? local enlargement, frequent recurrence following excision and some reports of metastases. (Follow-ups reported are relatively short.)

Related Facts
I **Sex Ratio:** M1:F1
II **Risk of Occurrence:** ?
III **Risk of Recurrence for**
    Patient's Sib: Probably autosomal dominant. If parent is affected, < 1 in 2 (< 50%) for each offspring to be affected; otherwise not increased.
    Patient's Child: Probably autosomal dominant. < 1 in 2
IV **Age of Detectability:** During puberty
V **Prevalence:** ?

Treatment
I **Primary Prevention:** Genetic counseling
II **Secondary Prevention:** Surgical excision with margin of surrounding skin. Sometimes requires excision of complete scalp with skin graft. Irradiation is ineffective and dangerous.
III **Other Therapy:** —

Prognosis: Appears good for small tumors if widely excised, but limited follow-up on reported cases should cause guarded prognosis because of tendency for late recurrence of tumors of similar histologic types. Also, the few cases of metastases reported should cast doubt on the reportedly benign character of these tumors.

Detection of Carrier: —

Special Considerations: —

References:
Blandy, J. P. et al: Turban tumors in brother and sister. Br. J. Surg. 49:136, 1961.

Contributor: **Raymond P. Wood, II**

Editor's Computerized Descriptor: Skin

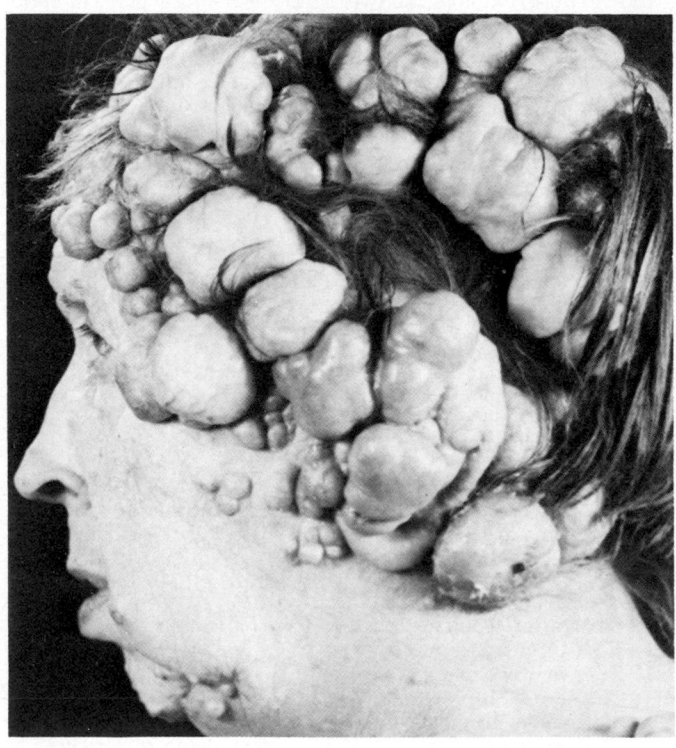

211. Cylindromatosis

CYSTATHIONINURIA

Includes: Cystathioninurie
Zystathioninurie
Cistationinuria
Cystathioninemia

Excludes: Cystathioninuria due to neuroblastoma or hypothyroidism

Minimal Diagnostic Criteria: Persistently elevated blood and urine cystathionine concentrations. Acquired cystathioninuria due to neuroblastoma or, rarely, hypothyroidism should be excluded by clinical studies.†

Clinical Findings: A wide spectrum of findings ranging from multiple congenital defects, thrombocytopenia, endocrinopathy, variable mental retardation to no disease at all. Two patients have been reported with calcium-type urinary tract calculi, possibly due to inadequate acidification due to deviation of sulfur from sulfate. One patient was a young child, the other asymtomatic until his 20s when he developed recurrent calculi. B_6 seemed helpful over short period of observation. Significance of the biochemical abnormality is unknown and perhaps coincidental.

Cystathioninuria in the range of 160 to 1400 mg per day depending on size of patient and methionine intake. Plasma concentrations range from about 1 to 10 μmole per 100 ml. Normally, cystathionine occurs in the urine and plasma in traces.

Complications
I **Derived:** —
II **Associated:** A variety of serious complications such as thrombocytopenia and heart disease have been reported, although these cannot at present be clearly related to the biochemical defect.

Etiology: Autosomal recessive; McK *21950

Pathogenesis: Apparently includes defect of liver cystathionase needed to bind the coenzyme pyridoxal phosphate.†

Related Facts
I   **Sex Ratio:** M1:F1
II **Risk of Occurrence:** ?
III **Risk of Recurrence for**
   Patient's Sib: 1 in 4 (25%) for each offspring to be affected
   Patient's Child: Not increased unless mate is carrier or homozygote
IV **Age of Detectability:** ?
V   **Prevalence:** About two dozen cases reported although studies for heterozygotes suggest a moderate incidence.

Treatment
I **Primary Prevention:** Genetic counseling
II **Secondary Prevention:** Blood and urine cystathionine concentrations can be decreased to near zero by high doses of vitamin B_6 (pyridoxine hydrochloride), eg 5 to 10 mg/kg in divided doses orally, per day. The significance of this, or desirability, is unknown. Similarly, B_6 administration to pregnant carriers *might* prevent associated defects in the fetus.†
III **Other Therapy:** —

Prognosis: ?

Detection of Carrier: Heterozygotes may have a slightly elevated cystathionine excretion. Frank cystathioninuria can be provoked by administration of L-methionine, 100 mg/kg, in a single oral dose.

†Special Considerations: Problem areas include: the mechanism of B_6 effect, and whether or not the biochemical defect is related to the various disorders described or is coincidental. Patients continue to be reported and discussed who present with some medical problem, while others have no apparent clinical problem - occasionally in the same family. Since this also occurs in other aminoacidurias, the wise approach is to consider this an open question.

In all patients reported in whom it has been tried, except for one Japanese child, administration of high doses of vitamin B_6 has resulted in marked decrease in the aminoaciduria. In vivo and in vitro studies led to the proposal that this could be accounted for by a defective structure of the protein apoenzyme that causes it to bind improperly the coenzyme pyridoxal phosphate. This suggestion remains to be conclusively proved or confirmed.

References:
Frimpter, G.W.: Cystathioninuria. In Nyhan, W.L. (ed.): Heritable Disorders of Amino Acid Metabolism. New York:John Wiley, Inc., 1974, pp. 452-463.
Frimpter, G.W. et al: Cystathioninuria: Management. Am. J. Dis. Child. 113:115, 1967.
Frimpter, G.W. et al: Distribution of sulfur in urine of patients with cystathioninuria before and during administration of pyridoxine. Metabolism 25:355, 1976.
Frimpter, G.W.: Recurrent urinary tract calculi possibly due to inherited cystathioninuria. Aerosp. Med. 44:1300, 1973.
Tada, K. et al: Cystathioninuria not associated with vitamin B_6 dependency: A probably new type of cystathioninuria. Tohoku J. Exp. Med. 95:235, 1968.

Contributor: **George W. Frimpter**

Editor's Computerized Descriptors: CV., GU.

CYSTIC FIBROSIS

Includes: Muco-viscidose-fibrose kystique du pancréas
Zystische Pankreasfibrose
Fibrosis quística
Mucoviscidosis
Cystic fibrosis of pancreas
Pancreatic fibrosis
Fibrocystic disease of pancreas

Excludes: Gluten-induced enteropathy (423)

Minimal Diagnostic Criteria: Quantitative analysis of sweat electrolyte levels with sodium and chloride each exceeding 60mEq/L. The pilocarpine iontophoresis technic for sweat stimulation is the most useful and simple method. It is diagnostic in 98% of the patients especially when combined with characteristic pulmonary disease or pancreatic deficiencies. Examination of digestive fluid for absence of trypsin and increased viscosity is positive in 85% of children.

Clinical Findings: Generalized disorder affecting the exocrine glands of the body with production of abnormal secretions resulting in excessively high sweat electrolytes, pancreatic insufficiency, chronic pulmonary disease and cirrhosis of the liver. Patients (95%) have sweat sodium and chlorides greater than twice normal. (Na 60mEq/L; Cl 60mEq/L). This may lead to heat prostration. Repeated episodes of rectal prolapse (5-10%). Intestinal obstruction (meconium ileus) at birth (5-10%) may have perforation and meconium peritonitis.

Patients (80%) have pancreatic enzyme deficiencies (trypsin, lipase, and amylase) into the GI tract preventing proper digestion and absorption of fats, fat-soluble vitamins and proteins causing malnutrition, failure to thrive, hypoproteinemia with edema. Cirrhosis of the liver secondary to biliary obstruction (1-5%). Portal hypertension and esophageal varices may occur.

Ninety-five percent of patients who survive infancy have pulmonary diseases with hyperinflation, persistent cough, recurrent bronchitis, bronchiolitis, pneumonia, atelectasis, emphysema, fibrosis and destruction of parenchyma. Chronic sinusitis (25%). Nasal polyps develop in 10%. Adult males show lack of spermatogenesis (> 99%).

Complications
I **Derived:** Chronic pulmonary disease. Secondary infection and organ dysfunctions may occur following inspissation and blockage of any collecting system in the body, ie liver, testicle.
II **Associated:** —

Etiology: Autosomal recessive transmission of lethal gene. Gene frequency estimated to be about .016 and heterozygotes represent 3-5% of general Caucasian population in the United States. McK *21970

Pathogenesis: ? Membrane transport defect appears likely.

Related Facts
I **Sex Ratio:** M1:F1
II **Risk of Occurrence:** About 1 in 2000 in U.S.A.; very rare in Negroes and Orientals; most common in Northern Europeans.
III **Risk of Recurrence for**
Patient's Sib: 1 in 4 (25%) for each offspring to be affected
Patient's Child: Homozygote males lack spermatogenesis and females usually die early; therefore, none unless surviving female mates with heterozygote.†
IV **Age of Detectability:** Within 24 hours by sweat electrolyte determination. However, collection of sufficient sweat is difficult until infant is more than one month of age.
V **Prevalence:** Affected males outlive females 6 to 1 by age of 20 years.

Treatment
I **Primary Prevention:** Genetic counseling†
II **Secondary Prevention:** Adequate pancreatic enzyme replacement, adequate salt ingestion, adequate pulmonary therapy, adequate antibiotic therapy.
III **Other Therapy:** Supportive for specific organ system involved.

Prognosis: Average life expectancy of girls is 12 years; of boys, 16 years. This may be improved with meticulous care.

Detection of Carrier: Heterozygote serum factor inhibits action of cilia in explants of rabbit tracheal mucosa but less so than homozygote serum. Metachromatic granules in fibroblasts of skin in both homozygotes and heterozygotes is under study as a test for the latter.

†Special Considerations: Young adults are increasingly being diagnosed as having this condition with apparently reduced expressivity.

References:
Anderson, D. H.: Cystic fibrosis of pancreas. J. Chronic Dis. 7:58, 1958.
Danes, B. S. and Bearn, A. G.: A genetic cell marker in cystic fibrosis of the pancreas. Lancet 1:1061, 1968.
Doershuk, C. F. and Matthews, L. W.: Cystic fibrosis and obstructive pulmonary disease. In Green, M. and Haggerty, R.J. (eds.): Ambulatory Pediatrics. Philadelphia:W.B. Saunders, 1968, p. 707.
Zelkowitz, P. S. and Giammona, S. T.: Cystic fibrosis: Pulmonary studies in children, adolescents and young adults. Am. J. Dis. Child. 117:543, 1969.

Contributor: **Samuel T. Giammona**

Editor's Computerized Descriptors: Nasoph., Sweating, Resp., GI., Liver

CYSTINOSIS

Includes: Cystinose
Cistinosis
Cystine storage disease
Nephropathic cystinosis
Intermediate (late-onset) cystinosis
Benign cystinosis

Excludes: Cystinuria (239)

Minimal Diagnostic Criteria: Refractile bodies seen in the cornea and conjunctiva with a slit lamp by an experienced ophthalmologist, or demonstration of characteristic cystine crystals in either bone marrow, lymph gland, or rectal mucosa biopsy. The biochemical demonstration of increased intracellular cystine is not required for diagnosis.

Clinical Findings: The most characteristic presentation occurs at 6 to 10 months of age, with symptoms related to a deficiency in tubular reabsorption of water, phosphate, sodium, potassium, bicarbonate, glucose, amino acids and other organic acids. The defect in water reabsorption usually accounts for the presenting symptoms of the disease, which are polyuria, polydipsia, and recurrent unexplained fever, probably the result of dehydration. The renal loss of phosphate accounts for the subsequent development of hypophosphatemic rickets, resistant to the usual antirachitic doses of vitamin D. The loss of bicarbonate and potassium results in chronic acidosis and hypokalemia. Affected children show severe growth retardation.

These children also show progressive glomerular damage, which usually progresses to death from uremia within the 1st decade of life. In other families (late-onset cystinosis), attenuated clinical expression permits survival into the 2nd or 3rd decade. In still other families, the kidney is spared and the disorder is benign.

In all 3 types of cystinosis, cystine crystal deposition can be demonstrated in conjunctiva, bone marrow, lymph nodes, and leukocytes. A characteristic retinopathy is observed in patients with nephropathic but not in patients with benign cystinosis. The intracellular cystine content of free (nonprotein) cystine is approximately 100 times normal. The excess cystine appears to be stored in lysosomes. The primary abnormal gene product, leading to cystine accumulation, remains to be identified.

Complications
I **Derived:** Impairment of both renal tubular and glomerular functions.
II **Associated:** Rickets, acidosis, hypokalemia, growth retardation, hypothyroidism and uremia

Etiology: Autosomal recessive; McK *21980, *21990, *22000

Pathogenesis: This is most likely related to the accumulation of cystine, but the exact mechanism causing this is unknown.

Related Facts
I **Sex Ratio:** This should theoretically be 1:1, but in a recent study of 73 children with nephropathic cystinosis, there were 53 males and 20 females.
II **Risk of Occurrence:** ?
III **Risk of Recurrence for**
Patient's Sib: 1 in 4 (25%) for each offspring to be affected
Patient's Child: Zero unless mate is carrier or homozygote
IV **Age of Detectability:** It is possible to diagnose cystinosis in utero by estimating the free-cystine content of cultured amniotic fluid cells. The diagnosis can be made at birth by measuring the leukocyte cystine content. Cystine crystals cannot be demonstrated until 2-4 months of age.
V **Prevalence:** ?

Treatment
I **Primary Prevention:** Genetic counseling
II **Secondary Prevention:** —
III **Other Therapy:** Systematic correction of the renal tubular losses is easily accomplished by fluid, potassium, and alkali replacement, and moderate doses of vitamin D (usually 5000-10,000 units per day). Renal transplantation is now being done for cystinotic children in several centers. Two children have survived 12 years posttransplantation.

Prognosis: Children with nephropathic cystinosis usually die before 10 years of age, unless renal transplantation is performed. Patients with late-onset cystinosis survive for variable lengths of time. Patients with benign cystinosis appear to have a normal life expectancy. The prognosis of children who have had renal transplantation appears to be similar to that of children who have received renal transplants secondary to other causes of renal failure.

Detection of Carrier: Heterozygotes can be detected by a 4 to 5 fold increase in the intracellular content of free cystine in their leukocytes. This measurement, however, is very tedious and cannot be utilized for screening purposes.

Special Considerations: —

References:
Schneider, J. A. et al: Cystinosis and the Fanconi syndrome. In Stanbury, J.B. et al (eds.): Metabolic Basis of Inherited Diseases, 4th. Ed. New York:McGraw Hill. 1978, p. 1660.
Schulman, J.D.:Cystinosis. DHEW Publication no. (NIH) 72-249. Washington:U.S.Government Printing Office, 1973.

Contributor: **Jerry A. Schneider**

Editor's Computerized Descriptors: Eye, Skel., GU.
Also see Section I, Fig. 55

CYSTINURIA

Includes: Cystinurie
Zystinurie
Cistinuria
Cystinuria I, II, III
Cystine-lysine-arginine-ornithinuria
Cystinuria and dibasic aminoaciduria

Excludes: Cystinosis (238)
Familial protein intolerance with defective transport of dibasic
amino acids
Homocystinuria (474)
Hyperdibasic-aminoaciduria (491)
Hypercystinuria (490)

Minimal Diagnostic Criteria: Urinary cyanide-nitroprusside test
yields magenta red color; specific cystine-lysine-arginine-ornithinuria by paper chromatography, paper electrophoresis or column chromatography; normal or decreased plasma concentrations of cystine and dibasic amino acids.

Clinical Findings: Formation of radiopaque cystine calculi in
renal pelvis, ureter or bladder; cystine crystalluria, related to
urinary volume; short stature (statistic correlation only);
markedly increased renal clearance and excretion of cystine, lysine, arginine and ornithine (100%); defective intestinal absorption of cystine, lysine, arginine and ornithine.

Complications
I **Derived:** Renal or ureteral colic, hematuria, dysuria and
urinary tract infections secondary to cystine stone formations; renal insufficiency and uremia secondary to infection,
obstruction and surgical intervention.
II **Associated:** Hyperuricemia; increased incidence of mental
retardation or psychiatric disturbance (?).

Etiology: Autosomal recessive transmission with heterogeneity.
There are at least 3 genotypic variants (Types I, II, III) due to
allelic mutations. Cystinuria also occurs in dogs. McK *22010

Pathogenesis: The mutation affects "carrier protein" (or "reactive site") catalyzing transport of cystine, lysine, arginine and
ornithine in proximal renal tubule and small intestine. Defective
renal tubular reabsorption of cystine produces excessive urinary
excretion, crystalluria and lithiasis due to limited solubility of
cystine in urine (maximum solubility about 300 mg/liter); impaired intestinal absorption of lysine (an essential amino acid)
may explain the observed short stature; dibasic aminoaciduria
has no known clinical significance.

Related Facts
I **Sex Ratio:** M1:F1
II **Risk of Occurrence:** About 1 in 10,000 live births
III **Risk of Recurrence for**
Patient's Sib: 1 in 4 (25%) for each offspring
Patient's Child: 1 in 100
IV **Age of Detectability:** Probably at birth
V **Prevalence:** About 1 in 10,000

Treatment
I **Primary Prevention:** Genetic counseling
II **Secondary Prevention:** High fluid intake; alkalinization of
the urine to increase cystine solubility; oral administration
of D-penicillamine (1-2 gm/24 hr in divided doses†); surgical
removal of renal, ureteral or vesical calculi
III **Other Therapy:** Management of renal insufficiency includes
base replacement, low-protein diet, dialysis.

Prognosis: Life span shortened by more than 10 years in affected
males and less than 10 years in affected females; death due to
renal failure.

Detection of Carrier: Type I heterozygotes detectable only by
studies of intestinal absorption or transport of cystine and dibasic
amino acids. These account for about 2/3 of all carriers. Type II

and Type III heterozygotes excrete increased amounts of cystine
and dibasic amino acids in urine.

†Special Considerations: There is no evidence that the
several different genotypes responsible for cystinuria lead
to clinically different syndromes. Rare cystine calculi may
be formed by Type II or Type III heterozygotes, suggesting
that such individuals should also be encouraged to maintain a high urinary output. Since patients with cystinuria
may form mixed stones and even noncystine stones, all
patients with renal tract calculi should have a nitroprusside test to exclude this disorder. D-penicillamine is effective in prevention and dissolution of stones but also produces a variety of deleterious effects including serum sick-
ness, leukopenia, thrombocytopenia, and a reversible nephrotic syndrome. Also see Citrullinemia: Special Considerations.

References:
Rosenberg, L. E. and Scriver, C. R.: Disorders of amino acid metab-
olism. In Bondy, P.K. and Rosenberg, L.E. (eds.): Diseases of
Metabolism, 7th Ed. Philadelphia:W.B. Saunders, 1974, p. 465.
Scriver, C.R. and Bergeron, M.: Amino acid transport in kidney.
The use of mutation to dissect membrane and transepithelial
transport. In Nyhan, W.L. (ed.): Heritable Disorders of Amino
Acid Metabolism. New York:John Wiley & Son, 1974, p. 515.
Thier, S.O. and Segal, S.: Cystinuria. In Stanbury, J.B. et al (eds.):
The Metabolic Basis of Inherited Disease, 3rd Ed. New York:Mc-
Graw-Hill, 1972, p. 1504.

Contributor: **Leon E. Rosenberg**

Editor's Computerized Descriptors: Skel., GU., Nerve

CYSTS OF SPLEEN

Includes: Kystes spléniques
Milzzysten
Quistes esplénicos
Splenic cysts

Excludes: —

Minimal Diagnostic Criteria: True cysts have a specific type of lining cell other than fibroblasts. For example, true epidermoid cysts contain a lining of stratified squamous epithelium containing prickle cells with intracellular bridges.

Clinical Findings: Classification of splenic cysts (after Fowler). Primary: true cysts with cellular lining, endothelial. Congenital, traumatic, inflammatory either infoliation or dilatation (lymphangiectatic polycystic disease), neoplastic, epidermoid or dermoid (which have no endothelial component), lymphangioma, hemangioma (benign capillary and cavernous), parasitic-echinococcus. Secondary: no cellular lining. Traumatic (blood, serous), degenerative (liquefaction), inflammatory (necrosis, tuberculosis).

Parasitic cysts are probably the most common worldwide but are rare in the United States. In the United States neoplastic cysts are 40% of the total number. Of these, hemangiomas are the most common, dermoids the least common. Twenty percent of cystic neoplasms are epidermoid. The latter are most frequently found in children and young adults and presumably are of congenital origin. The presence of ectodermal tissue in the spleen is unexplained but perhaps due to 1) congenital inclusion of ectodermal tissue, 2) metaplasia of heterotopic endodermal inclusion of the spleen, or less likely, 3) metaplasia of a mesothelial inclusion cyst. Clinical findings are minimal. Vague upper abdominal discomfort; LUQ mass with some abdominal distention as the cyst enlarges. Frequently cysts are completely asymptomatic. The radiographic triad of a normal IVP, inferior displacement of the splenic flexure of the colon and anterior and rightward displacement of the stomach is considered to be almost pathognomonic of a cyst of the spleen. A splenic scan with 198 Au colloid (sequestered in the spleen and liver) shows a large round area of decreased isotope uptake within the spleen. Cysts have also been diagnosed by selective visceral arteriography or by percutaneous splenic cystography. Aspiration of glistening-cholesterol-crystal laden fluid is presumptive evidence of a splenic cyst. Parasitic cysts usually show characteristic calcification.

Complications
I **Derived:** Rupture of the cyst is an extreme rarity.
II **Associated:** —

Etiology: ? Upper abdominal trauma is the only known and most uniformly accepted etiologic factor of secondary splenic cysts.

Pathogenesis: True cysts have a specific type of lining cell other than fibroblasts. Very rare dermoids contain skin appendages and keratinizing epidermis. In secondary cysts the trauma is thought to cause splenic laceration within the capsule, laceration of splenic vessels, hemorrhage, encapsulation of the hematoma, absorption of the blood, fibrous wall formation and persistence of serous fluids (Hoffman).

Related Facts
I **Sex Ratio:** Sex incidence varies in different reports from M3:F2 to M1:F1
II **Risk of Occurrence:** ?
III **Risk of Recurrence for**
   Patient's Sib: ?
   Patient's Child: ?

IV **Age of Detectability:** At any age by radiographic methods described above; two-thirds of cysts are diagnosed during the 2nd and 3rd decades of life.
V **Prevalence:** ?

Treatment
I **Primary Prevention:** —
II **Secondary Prevention:** Treatment is by surgical removal of the spleen.
III **Other Therapy:** —

Prognosis: Excellent with surgery if cyst of spleen is not of malignant origin.

Detection of Carrier: —

Special Considerations: —

References:
Fowler, R.H.: Collective review: Nonparasitic benign cystic tumors of spleen. Int. Abstr. Surg. 96:209, 1953.
Hoffman, E.: Non-parasitic splenic cysts. Am. J. Surg. 93:765, 1957.
McNamara, J.J. et al: Splenic cysts in children. Surgery 64:487, 1968.

Contributor: **Elliot F. Ellis**

Editor's Computerized Descriptors: Spleen, GI.

DARWIN TUBERCLE (MARKER)

Includes: Tubercule de Darwin
Darwinscher Höcker
Punto de Darwin auricular (Marcador)

Excludes: Darwin pointed pinnae (outward pointed projections of ears)
Small enlargement of the ear rim at the Darwin ear point

Minimal Diagnostic Criteria: Tubercle on posterosuperior helix

Clinical Findings: A variable sized tubercle on the posterosuperior helix. An infolded point near the upper lateral rim of the ear. The cartilage is thickened at this point to form a tubercle which can be distinctly seen.

Complications
I   **Derived:** —
II **Associated:** —

Etiology: Autosomal dominant with variable expressivity. Expression varies from a small tubercle to larger infolded point with a series of intermediate forms. Some have the tubercle in only one ear and a few carry the gene without expressing the trait in either ear.

Pathogenesis: —

Related Facts
I   **Sex Ratio:** M50:F45. Evidently sex plays some role in the degree of penetrance of the gene.
II   **Risk of Occurrence:** Finland and England: 1 in 2 live births; Germany: about 1 in 5.
III **Risk of Recurrence for**
    Patient's Sib: 1 in 2 if one parent has the gene; nearly 1 in 1 if both parents have the gene.
    Patient's Child: 1 in 2 if mate does not have the gene; nearly 1 in 1 if mate also has the gene.
IV   **Age of Detectability:** At birth
V   **Prevalence:** Finland about 50%, Germany about 20% and England about 55%

Treatment
I   **Primary Prevention:** Not necessary
II   **Secondary Prevention:** Not needed
III **Other Therapy:** —

Prognosis: Normal for life span, intelligence and function

Detection of Carrier: —

Special Considerations: —

References:
Gates, R.R.: Human Genetics. New York:Macmillan, 1946, vol. I, ch. 13.
McKusick, V. A.: Mendelian Inheritance in Man, 4th Ed. Baltimore: Johns Hopkins Press, 1975, p. 75.
Winchester, A. M.: Genetics; A Survey of the Principles of Heredity, 3rd Ed. Boston: Houghton Mifflin, 1966.

Contributor: A. M. Winchester

Editor's Computerized Descriptor: Ear

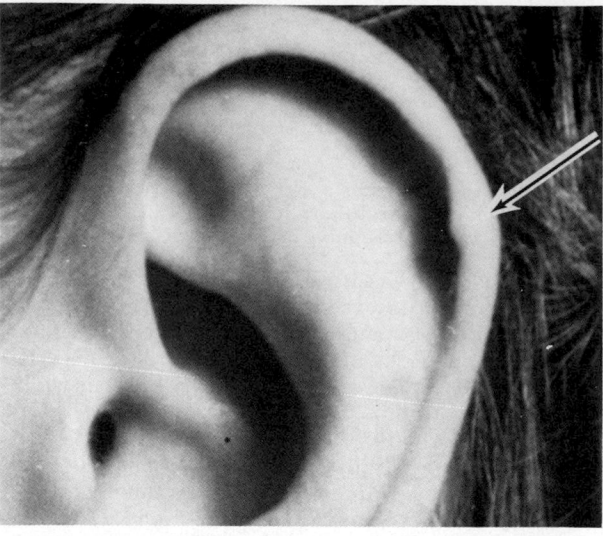

212. Darwin tubercle

DE LANGE SYNDROME

Includes: Syndrome de Cornelia de Lange
Síndrome de de-Lange
Cornelia de Lange syndrome
Typus degenerativus Amstelodamensis

Excludes: —

Minimal Diagnostic Criteria: Physical and mental retardation, hirsutism and synophrys, microcephaly, long or protruding philtrum, anteverted nostrils, small or grossly malformed hands, and webbing of 2nd and 3rd toes.

Clinical Findings: Mental retardation. Growth retardation with low birthweight even at term. Generalized hirsutism, synophrys, long eyelashes. Microcephaly, usually with brachycephaly. Anteverted nostrils, prominent philtrum, thin lips that are turned down at angles of mouth. Limitation of extension of elbows. Single transverse palmar crease, proximally placed thumbs, clinodactyly of 5th finger. Severely malformed upper limbs, ranging from small hands to oligodactyly or phocomelia, and webbing of 2nd and 3rd toes. In addition, neonatal feeding or respiratory problems are often noted. Recurrent respiratory infection, a short neck, low-pitched cry, undescended testes, delayed eruption and wide spacing of teeth are common. Cardiac defects are also common, but hypospadias, cleft palate, recurrent convulsions, herniae and other malformations are less common.

Complications
I   Derived: Neonatal feeding or respiratory difficulties
II Associated: —

Etiology: Unknown in the great majority of cases. Chromosomal abnormalities have been reported in 16 of about 150 patients, but no specific chromosome is involved in all. Familial translocations, giving rise to unbalanced complements with duplication/deficiency states of various chromosomes have been observed.

Pathogenesis: ?

Related Facts
I   Sex Ratio: M1:F1
II   Risk of Occurrence: 1 in > 10,000 live births
III Risk of Recurrence for
    Patient's Sib: Empiric risk of about 4%
    Patient's Child: No children born to affected individuals
IV   Age of Detectability: At birth
V   Prevalence: ?

Treatment
I   Primary Prevention: Genetic counseling
II   Secondary Prevention: None
III Other Therapy: Symptomatic, eg anticonvulsants for those with seizures, tranquilizers for behavioral disorders

Prognosis: Diminished life expectancy; few known patients are adults. Increased susceptibility to infections.

Detection of Carrier: Rarely, recognized by demonstrating a balanced translocation in either parent, or some of the minor clinical features, eg hirsutism and synophrys.

Special Considerations: —

References:
Berg, J.M. et al: The de Lange Syndrome. Oxford: Pergamon Press, 1970.
Falek, A. et al: Familial de Lange syndrome with chromosome abnormalities. Pediatrics 37:92, 1966.
McArthur, R.G. and Edwards, J.H.: De Lange syndrome: Report of 20 cases. Can. Med. Assoc. J. 96:1185, 1967.
Opitz, J.M. et al: The etiology of the Brachmann-de Lange syndrome. In Birth Defects Reprint Series, No. 16, The National Foundation-March of Dimes, 1965, p. 22.

Contributor: **Orlando J. Miller**

Editor's Computerized Descriptors: Vision, Eye, Ear, Face, Oral, Teeth, Nose, Speech, Neck, Skin, Dermatoglyphic, Hair, Skel., Muscle, Resp., CV., GU., Nerve

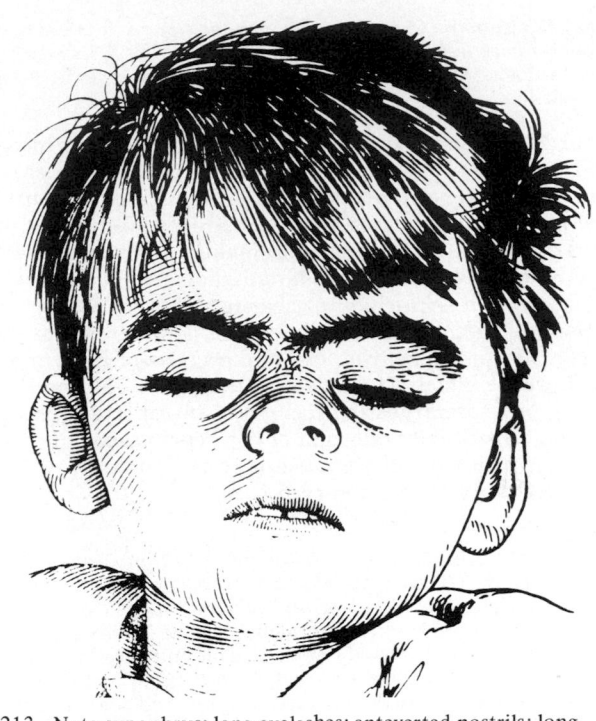

213. Note synophrys; long eyelashes; anteverted nostrils; long philtrum; thin, turned-down lips

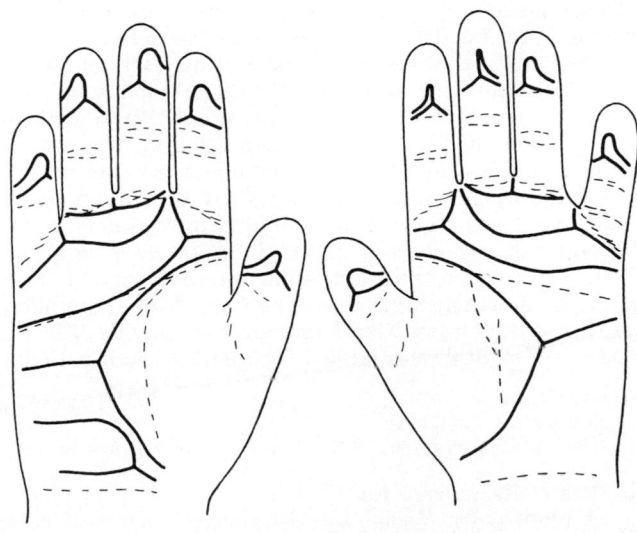

214. Dermatoglyphics in de Lange syndrome

DEAF-MUTISM, SEMILETHAL

Includes: Surdi-mutité semiléthale
Semilethale Form der Taubstummheit
Forma semiletal de sordomudez

Excludes: Autosomal recessive deaf-mutism
Recessive X-linked deaf-mutism
Cardioauditory syndrome (123)

Minimal Diagnostic Criteria: Congenital severe, familial sensorineural deafness with a preponderance of males. The hearing deficit is at least 80 db and there may be small differences between the 2 ears.

Clinical Findings: Congenital deafness often not recognized until after 2 years of age (may be detected in early infancy where newborn screening technics are in use). Very severe hearing loss is suspected from failure to respond to tuning fork testing, noisemakers and speech, with masking when possible. Standard audiometry is confirmatory, showing a sensorineural hearing deficit of at least 80 db. Special audiometry usually cannot be done because of the severity of the hearing loss and because of its symmetry. However, about 11% of the patients are only hard of hearing but special testing has not been reported. Therefore, the possible site of origin of the hearing malfunction is unknown in the individual case prior to demise.
Semilethality is also observed.†

Complications
I   **Derived:** Mental retardation in about 40% of cases
II **Associated:** These patients seldom marry and practically never have children. However, we have not observed visible signs of hypogonadism. Hormonal investigations are missing. The sexual behavior of these deaf-mutes cannot be explained only by the mental retardation in 40% of cases, or by the fear to marry because of their deafness. In some regions, recessive deaf-mutes of another type often marry and have offspring. Strabismus has been observed in 13.5% of these patients.

Etiology: Autosomal recessive, penetrance is total but expressivity is variable. Consanguinity of the patient's parents is found in about 4-10% of cases.

Pathogenesis: The mutism is a consequence of the congenital deafness. The latter is based on the defective development of the inner ear, occurring at an early ontogenic phase. The opinions concerning the anatomopathologic defects are still divergent, but mainly a malformation of the membranous parts of the inner ear is found. The osseous labyrinthine capsule and the middle ear are normal. The vestibular apparatus is seldom involved. In some cases, the defective development of the nerve pathways may be followed up into the gyri of Heschl; in other cases no abnormality is found in the brain. An action of the deaf-mutism gene on the ontogenesis of the brain is all the more likely as this affliction has been found associated with different degrees of mental retardation in about 40% of our patients.

Related Facts
I   **Sex Ratio:** M1.34:F1
II **Risk of Occurrence:** ? Observed only in Eastern Switzerland.
III **Risk of Recurrence for**
    Patient's Sib: Actual, 1 in 17.† Theoretic, 1 in 4 (25%) for each offspring to be affected.
    Patient's Child: Not increased unless mate is carrier or homozygote. To date they seldom marry and very rarely have children.
IV **Age of Detectability:** Usually after 2 years of age except

where newborn hearing screening is available.
V   **Prevalence:** 0.1 to 1% in the examined populations.
    This form of deafness has been observed so far only in the cantons of St. Gallen, Appenzell and Glarus of Eastern Switzerland.

Treatment
I   **Primary Prevention:** Genetic counseling
II **Secondary Prevention:** Hearing aids, auditory training, extensive speech therapy or lip-reading as indicated in the individual case.
III **Other Therapy:** —

Prognosis: Nonprogressive deafness and normal life span. The patients may be integrated into society as far as their mental faculties permit.

Detection of Carrier: —

†Special Considerations: The penetrance of the affliction is total. Its expressivity is variable. Whereas the majority are deaf-mutes, 11% are only hard of hearing. Audiometric differences were also found from one individual to another and from one ear to another. However, these variations in the manifestations of the affliction always lead either to deafness or to definite and early hardness of hearing. Transitional forms with different degrees of hearing impairment, as described in dominant labyrinthine deafness, are not found.

The proportion of afflicted children in a series of brothers and sisters is less than the value for a single recessive inheritance of 25%. The values found varied between 16.29+ 1, 27% and 19.63+ 1, 94%, with the method of Bernstein-Lenz-Hodgben. However, within the afflicted series of brothers and sisters, there was a highly significant difference in the sex ratio between healthy brothers and sisters on the one hand, and the deaf-mute on the other hand ($x^2 = 10.761$). We find too few deaf-mute sisters. This observation may be explained by the hypothesis that the homozygote state of the factor is semilethal, and tends to kill selectively the sex cells with the X-chromosomes, or the female zygotes. The factor might exert its action either in the haplophase or in an early stage of the diplophase. (Sporadic cases of nongenetic or nonrecessive causation may in part account for these findings. Ed.)

References:
Pfändler, U.: Le déficit de sourds-muets dans les fratries atteintes. Arch. Klaus-Stift. Vererb.-Forsch. 38:96, 1963.
Pfändler, U.: Une forme semilétale de la surdimutite récessive dans différentes populations de la Suisse orientale. Bull. Schweiz. Akad. Med. Wiss. 16:255, 1960.
Pfändler, U. and Schnyder, E.: La surdi-mutité récessive dans le Werdenberg (canton de Saint-Gall, Suisse). J. Genet. Hum. 9:158, 1960.
Schwarz, M. and Becker, P. E.: Taubstummheit. In Becker, P.E. (ed.): Humangenetik: Ein kurzes Handbuch in Fünf Bänden. Bd. 4. Stuttgart: Georg Thieme Verlag, 1964, p. 281.

Contributor: **Udo Pfändler**

Editor's Computerized Descriptors: Eye, Hearing, Nerve

DEAFNESS AND ABSENT INCUDO-STAPEDIAL JUNCTION

Includes: Surdité de conduction par malformation des osselets
Durch Ankylose von Hammer und Amboss bedingte Schalleitungsschwerhörigkeit
Sordera de conducción bilateral y ausencia de la articulación yunque-estribo
Bilateral conductive deafness and absent incus-stapes junction

Excludes: Congenital stapes fixation
Occasional small malformations of the middle ear
Hand muscle wasting and sensorineural deafness (450)

Minimal Diagnostic Criteria: Evidence for bilateral conductive deafness and absent incus-stapes junction demonstrated at surgery.

Clinical Findings: This syndrome was discovered in 1962 in a male patient with bilateral conductive deafness, present since birth, normal eardrums and pneumatization. At surgery the following abnormalities were found: the long crus of the incus was curved like a hook; in 1 ear a few fibers of connective tissue extended to the reduced head of the stapes, but in the other ear the stapes head was entirely lacking with no connection between incus and stapes. A similar history of hearing loss was present in 2 brothers.

Histologic examination of the incus shows normal bony tissue and vascularization with no signs of inflammation. Connective tissues take their origin from a marked and fine limited zone in the distal end. Similar surgical findings were present in another child.

Complications
I Derived: —
II Associated: Hypertrophic, thickened ear lobules

Etiology: Autosomal dominant with apparently complete penetrance. The associated trait of thickened ear lobules may be attached to the same dominant genetic factor.

Pathogenesis: Probable failure in the 6th-7th week of fetal life of the rotation and junction of the distal end of the incus with the blastema of the stapes.

Related Facts
I Sex Ratio: M1:F1
II Risk of Occurrence: ?
III Risk of Recurrence for
    Patient's Sib: If parent is affected, 1 in 2 (50%) for each offspring to be affected; otherwise not increased.
    Patient's Child: 1 in 2
IV Age of Detectability: As soon as audiometric testing is possible, the diagnosis may be suspected; strongly suspected if the patient has thickened ear lobules and normal ear drums and confirmed when surgery can be performed.
V Prevalence: ? Only 1 Swiss kindred of 342 members has been reported.

Treatment
I Primary Prevention: Genetic counseling
II Secondary Prevention: Middle ear exploration (tympanotomy). Rotation of the incus to the stapes or prosthesis from the footplate to the malleus.
III Other Therapy: Hearing aid and special seating in school to assure good acquisition of speech, language, and education until corrective surgery can be performed.

Prognosis: Normal for life span and intelligence. Good for function after restored sound conduction.

Detection of Carrier: —

Special Considerations: —

References:

Escher, F. and Hirt, H.: Dominant hereditary conductive deafness through lack of incus-stapes junction. Acta Otolaryngol. (Stockh.) 65:25, 1968.

Contributor: **Franz Escher**

Editor's Computerized Descriptors: Hearing, Ear

DEAFNESS AND ATOPIC DERMATITIS

Includes: Surdité, dermatite atopique
Taubheit und atopische Dermatitis
Sordera y dermatitis atópica
Neural hearing loss and hereditary atopic dermatitis
Atopic dermatitis and neural hearing loss

Excludes: Recessive moderate nonprogressive neural hearing loss

Minimal Diagnostic Criteria: Congenital moderate nonprogressive neural hearing loss followed by atopic dermatitis at about age 10 years.

Clinical Findings: There is a congenital moderate neural hearing loss which may be detected only when the child begins school, and is found in all affected persons. The short increment sensitivity index is positive and the tone decay is negative, suggesting a cochlear hearing loss. Audiograms show a 10-55 db neural hearing loss. Vestibular tests are normal.

All affected persons, at about 10 years of age, also develop an atopic dermatitis with a lichenified erythematous eruption which involves particularly the forearms, elbows, antecubital spaces and sometimes the waist. The popliteal spaces are not involved. There are no other physical or neurologic abnormalities.

Complications
I   Derived: —
II Associated: —

Etiology: Probably autosomal recessive

Pathogenesis: ?

Related Facts
I   **Sex Ratio:** M1:F1
II **Risk of Occurrence:** Very rare
III **Risk of Recurrence for**
    Patient's Sib: 1 in 4 (25%) for each offspring to be affected
    Patient's Child: Not increased unless mate is carrier or homozygote
IV **Age of Detectability:** In early childhood if older sib has complete syndrome, or at about 10 years of age, when neural hearing loss is followed by atopic dermatitis.
V   **Prevalence:** Very rare. Only 3 cases of this disease have been described. These were sibs ranging from 11-14 years of age. With attention to this defect, more cases probably will be found.

Treatment
I   **Primary Prevention:** Genetic counseling
II **Secondary Prevention:** Local therapy for the atopic dermatitis. Hearing aid for the hearing loss
III **Other Therapy:** —

Prognosis: Normal for life span and intelligence

Detection of Carrier: ?

Special Considerations: —

References:
Konigsmark, B.W. et al: Familial neural hearing loss and atopic dermatitis. JAMA 204:953, 1968.

Contributor: **Bruce W. Konigsmark‡**

Editor's Computerized Descriptors: Hearing, Skin

DEAFNESS AND DIABETES

Includes: Surdité, diabète
Taubheit und Diabetes mellitus
Sordera y diabetes
Sensorineural deafness associated with diabetes

Excludes: Perceptive or conductive deafness as a result of infection in the ear of a diabetic

Minimal Diagnostic Criteria: A progressive but subtotal hearing loss involving first high then lower frequencies in a diabetic subject.

Clinical Findings: At present, no test can determine that a hearing loss is caused by diabetes. All clinical investigations in this field are based on statistical analysis in a diabetic population. The hearing has been tested with whispered and spoken words, pure tone audiometry, distorted speech, directional hearing and stapedius reflex changes, but a specific diabetic audiologic pattern has not been established.

Most investigators find a slowly progressing hearing impairment affecting the higher frequencies first and most severely. The hearing loss seldom starts before the age of 30, and it has not been shown to be influenced by the duration or the gravity of the diabetes. In the higher age group diabetes-associated hearing loss may be confused with presbyacusis. In rare cases it may also be confused with progressive hereditary sensorineural deafness.†

Complications
I   **Derived:** Same as those of diabetes generally
II **Associated:** —

Etiology: Genetically determined defect. It is not known whether it is the diabetogenic gene(s), or a gene in some way linked or associated with the diabetogenic gene that is the cause of the hearing loss.†

Pathogenesis: No gross changes observed in the cochlea or auditory nerve. Microscopic changes consist of periodic acid-Schiff positive thickening of the capillaries of the stria vascularis, but it is not known if this per se is the cause of the hearing loss.

The functional hearing loss has a preponderance in the higher frequency area. Deterioration of directional hearing has also been found. As this syndrome is associated with diabetes there is either hypoinsulinemia or a reduced effect of the insulin. In the latter cases, there may be a normo- or even hyperinsulinemia.

Related Facts
I   **Sex Ratio:** M1:F1
II **Risk of Occurrence:** ? (Figures vary between 0-80% in a diabetic population.)
III **Risk of Recurrence for**
    Patient's Sib: ?
    Patient's Child: ?
IV **Age of Detectability:** 30 years or later
V   **Prevalence:** 0-1 in 25,000 in western countries

Treatment
I   **Primary Prevention:** —
II **Secondary Prevention:** Hearing aid and control of diabetes mellitus
III **Other Therapy:** —

Prognosis: Hearing loss will increase with age, but does not lead to complete deafness.

Detection of Carrier: Detection of the diabetic condition plus described hearing loss

†Special Considerations: As the hearing loss in diabetes is not influenced by the duration or the gravity of the diabetes as judged by renal, ocular and neurologic complications, it is unlikely that it is the diabetes per se that leads to hearing deterioration. Instead it may be some additional factor that is in some way linked to the diabetogenic gene(s).

In this connection it is interesting to note the similarities between hearing loss in diabetes and that of presbyacusis and progressive hereditary nerve deafness. In all of these 3 conditions there is a more or less marked genetic component. They all show the same audiologic pattern, similarities in development in time, and histologic changes consisting of periodic acid-Schiff positive thickening of the capillaries of stria vascularis. This could indicate that there are also similarities in the pathogenesis induced by the genetic defect in these conditions.

However, these similarities make it impossible to differentiate clinically between the hearing loss of presbyacusis alone and that associated with diabetes. This problem must be solved before we can come to a clear understanding of the effect of diabetes upon hearing.

References:

Axelsson, A. and Fagerberg, S. E.: Auditory function in diabetes. Acta Otolaryngol. (Stockh.) 66:49, 1968.
Hognestad, S.: Hereditary nerve deafness associated with diabetes. Acta Otolaryngol. (Stockh.) 64:219, 1967.
Jorgensen, M. B.: The inner ear in diabetes mellitus: Histological studies. Arch. Otolaryngol. 74:373, 1961.

Contributor: **Sølve Hognestad**

Editor's Computerized Descriptor: Hearing

DEAFNESS AND EAR PITS

Includes: Surdité, fossettes auriculaires
Taubheit und Ohrgrübchen
Sordera con fóveas auriculares
Preauricular appendages and deafness
Ear pits and external ear malformations with deafness
Deafness with preauricular pits or sinuses
Ear malformations and lateral (or branchial) cervical fistulas and deafness

Excludes: Ear pits (Marker) (329)
Oculo-auriculo-vertebral dysplasia (735)
Mandibulofacial dysostosis (627)
Hemifacial microsomia (457)

Minimal Diagnostic Criteria: Preauricular pits with a conductive, sensorineural or mixed hearing loss which has been present since birth.†

Clinical Findings: The patient may have a normal pinna, a lop-ear deformity, or the ear may be low set. A small pit or sinus is present just in front of the anterior extremity of the helix just superior to the takeoff of the crus helicis. This pit frequently becomes infected, but even in the absence of infection a small amount of fluid may discharge from or can be expressed from the pit. Occasionally the pit communicates with the middle ear, and this can be demonstrated by injecting radiopaque dye and showing the dye in the middle ear by mastoid films or petrous pyramid polytomography. Often the sinus communicates with the external auditory canal. Ear pits may be multiple. They are usually bilateral.

Some patients have typical branchial cleft cysts, sinuses of fistulas in the neck. Preauricular appendages, which may be fleshy, or also contain cartilage, are quite common.

Two types of congenital hearing loss may be seen in this entity and may indeed represent 2 separate clinical syndromes. In some pedigrees, sensorineural hearing loss is noted, in others conductive or mixed. In other pedigrees, however, all types of hearing loss occur. In the cases in which sensorineural hearing loss occurs, other etiologies, such as acoustic trauma and ototoxic drugs, were ruled out. The sensorineural hearing loss may be profound. Exploratory tympanotomy has been done in a few patients with conductive hearing loss and malformed ossicles; specifically absence of the lenticular process of the incus was found. In these instances the air-bone gap on the audiogram will be about 40-60 db, and impedance testing will confirm ossicular discontinuity or fixation, since ossicular fixation is also theoretically possible in these instances. The findings will be distinctly different from those found in middle ear effusions.

Apparently in some pedigrees certain family members show other branchial cleft cysts or sinuses without the ear manifestations.

Complications

I **Derived:** Infection of the preauricular sinus with conductive or mild sensorineural hearing loss: defective speech and language development. With profound sensorineural or severe mixed hearing losses: failure to develop speech and language unless the condition is recognized and early therapy instituted. Psychologic disturbance due to the cosmetic deformity, especially if it is severe.

II **Associated:** Hemifacial microsomia, micrognathia, microtia "occasionally," lateral soft palate fistulas, mandibulofacial dysostosis, narrow external canals, cystathioninuria with brain abnormalities and pituitary disorders. Very rare, colobomata of upper eyelids, epibulbar dermoids, hemivertebrae of the cervical spine, spina bifida (Goldenhar syndrome). Frequency of preauricular pits and appendages approaches 100%.

Etiology: May occur as an autosomal dominant with almost 100% penetrance of branchial fistulas and preauricular pits. The penetrance of hearing loss is reduced, but the degree of its reduction is unknown. Sporadic cases occur and it is possible that some of these are either autosomal recessive or multifactorial. McK *12510

Pathogenesis: ?

Related Facts
I **Sex Ratio:** M1:F<1
II **Risk of Occurrence:** ?
III **Risk of Recurrence for**
  Patient's Sib: When autosomal dominant or autosomal recessive, see Table I AD or AR, respectively.
  Patient's Child: When autosomal dominant or autosomal recessive, see Table I AD or AR, respectively.
IV **Age of Detectability:** At birth, although an associated conductive or mild sensorineural hearing loss may escape detection for some time.
V **Prevalence:** ?

Treatment
I **Primary Prevention:** Genetic counseling
II **Secondary Prevention:** If the preauricular pits become infected, warm compresses and antibiotics are needed. Repeated infections are an indication for surgical excision. Before excising the tract it is important to be sure it does not communicate with the middle ear or ear canal. Failure to do so will leave a deep potential cyst or sinus tract which will become infected, enlarge and conceivably cause cholesteatoma formation with all of its attendant complications. In addition, the fistulous tract may run close to the facial nerve and in excising the tract great care must be taken not to injure the nerve. If there is conductive hearing loss, petrous pyramid polytomography may delineate the middle ear anomaly. Surgical repair of the ossicular abnormality is often possible and may be performed on 1 side at about ages 4-5 years. Repair of the other middle ear may be deferred until adult life, if serviceable hearing is obtained on 1 side. If this is not possible, or if the patient has a sensorineural loss, hearing aids and rehabilitative measures are indicated. Cervical branchial cleft remnants should also be excised, with medical treatment being used as a temporary expedient only in those instances in which infection occurs.
III **Other Therapy:** For concomitant defects when present.

Prognosis: Good for normal life. Fair for restoration to serviceable hearing in instances in which there is a potentially repairable middle ear defect. In mild-to-moderate sensorineural hearing losses, there is a good prognosis for adequate function in school and occupation with hearing aids and aural rehabilitation. In severe, mixed or profound sensorineural hearing losses patients may be limited in speech and oral language but may function well with the use of sign language and lip-reading.

Detection of Carrier: —

†**Special Considerations:** As with any external ear malformation a hearing loss must be considered to be present until proven otherwise.

If the patient should have a tympanic perforation, such a communication might be demonstrated by injecting methylene blue or another harmless colored substance into the sinus opening and watching for its appearance in the middle ear. A bitter substance, such as a local or topical anesthetic, could be instilled through a tiny catheter into the sinus and if the patient tastes it, this might suggest that the substance traversed the middle ear and the eustachian tube into the pharynx.

References:
Fourman, P. and Fourman, J.: Hereditary deafness in family with ear-pits (fistula auris congenita). Br. Med. J. 2:1354, 1955.
Frimpter, G.W. et al: Cystathioninuria. N. Engl. J. Med. 268:333,

1963.
Gorlin, R.J. and Pindborg, J.J.: Syndromes of the Head and Neck. New York:McGraw-Hill, 1964.
McLaurin, J.W. et al: Hereditary branchial anomalies and associated hearing impairment. Laryngoscope 76:1277, 1966.
Wildervanck, L.S.: Hereditary malformations of the ear in three generations. Acta Otolaryngol. (Stockh.) 54:553, 1962.

Contributor: **LaVonne Bergstrom**

Editor's Computerized Descriptors: Eye, Hearing, Ear, Face, Oral, Speech, Neck, Skel.

DEAFNESS AND EPISODIC VERTIGO

Includes: Vertige épisodique avec surdité
Familiärer, periodisch auftretender Schwindel und Hörverlust
Vértigo episódico y sordera familiar
Endolymphatic hydrops
Ménière disease, familial
Vestibular hydrops
Episodic vertigo and hearing loss

Excludes: Acoustic neurinoma
Vestibular neuronitis
Labyrinthitis

Minimal Diagnostic Criteria: Fluctuating hearing loss, episodic vertigo and roaring tinnitus. It is important to emphasize that the vertigo is episodic; that is, usually occurs in attack form and is quite severe and almost always associated with nausea and emesis. The hearing loss is usually fluctuating, although later it may be progressive.

Clinical Findings: Characterized by sensorineural deafness, usually unilateral; episodic true vertigo, often associated with nausea and emesis; tinnitus, usually of a roaring quality; feeling of fullness in ear; occasionally temporal or occipital pain and patient may have cluster or migraine headaches. The attack of dizziness is very often followed by acute anxiety. This entity is familial, as opposed to classic Ménière disease which is not familial.

Complications
I **Derived:** Unsteadiness, vertigo and hearing loss
II **Associated:** Family history of allergy, migraine or cluster headaches, and autonomic dysfunction

Etiology: ? (Probably dominant with reduced penetrance)†

Pathogenesis: The endolymphatic sac of guinea pigs was obstructed and this produced relatively uniform increased volume of endolymph. It is fairly well known that the endolymphatic sac contains a columnar mucosa which is somewhat similar to the renal tubule and the thought is that the endolymphatic sac may play an important role in reabsorption of fluids. Silverstein found increased concentration of certain electrolytes and protein in the endolymphatic sac fluid. Therefore, one of the significant possibilities may be that Ménière disease is a result of inadequate absorption of endolymph. All of the other concepts, specifically those related to autonomic dysfunction and vascular spasm or vascular dilatation, have, in no way, been proved experimentally or clinically.

Related Facts
I   **Sex Ratio:** M?:F?
II **Risk of Occurrence:** ?
III **Risk of Recurrence for**
    Patient's Sib: ?
    Patient's Child: ?
IV **Age of Detectability:** Usually this is a disease which occurs in adults, although several cases have been reported in teenagers. The youngest patient that the author has seen was 14 years of age, in which a true Ménière disease could be identified.
V   **Prevalence:** ?

Treatment
I **Primary Prevention:** —
II **Secondary Prevention:** Various vasodilators have been tried. However, it is important to note that this defect is characterized by exacerbations and remissions and, therefore, it is extremely difficult to document the value of any pharmaceutic agent. It is always important to understand the personality problems and the various anxiety situations that may exist because it has been well documented that stressful situations do seem to precipitate an attack.

Surgery is utilized only in incapacitating vertigo. Labyrinthectomy is used in unilateral Ménière disease where the hearing is almost nonfunctional. Ultrasound labyrinthectomy is used particularly when the hearing on one side seems to be useful because the ultrasound therapy usually can specifically destroy the vestibular labyrinth and spare the cochlea. The use of streptomycin can be used in bilateral Ménière disease where vertigo is again incapacitating. There are many other modifications of surgical procedures that can be used, such as decompressing the endolymphatic sac.

III **Other Therapy:** —

Prognosis: Normal for life span and intelligence. Function depends on severity of the defect.

Detection of Carrier: —

†**Special Considerations:** The factor of heredity in labyrinthine deafness and paroxsymal vertigo has been described by Brown in 1949 and Bernstein in 1965. Brown reported 5 families in which at least 2 members suffered from Ménière disease. Bernstein described 7 families in which more than 1 member had episodic vertigo and hearing loss. Not all of the patients had true Ménière disease. Some may have had vestibular neuronitis, but nevertheless the problem included episodic vertigo and sensorineural hearing loss. Several of these families had a history of allergy and several others had history of migraine headaches.

References:
Bernstein, J. M.: Occurrence of episodic vertigo and hearing loss in families. Ann. Otol. Rhinol. Laryngol. 74:1011, 1965.
Brown, M.R.: The factor of heredity in labyrinthine deafness and paroxysmal vertigo. Ann. Otol. Rhinol. Laryngol. 58:665, 1949.
Kimura, R.S.: Experimental blockage of the endolymphatic duct and sac and its effect on the inner ear of the guinea pig: A study on endolymphatic hydrops. Ann. Otol. Rhinol. Laryngol. 76:664, 1967.
Silverstein, H. and Schuknecht, H. F.: Biochemical studies of inner ear fluid in man; changes in ostosclerosis, Ménière's disease and acoustic neuroma. Arch. Otolaryngol. 84:395, 1966.

Contributor: **Joel M. Bernstein**

Editor's Computerized Descriptors: Hearing, Ear, Nerve

DEAFNESS AND GOITER

Includes: Maladie de Pendred
Taubheit und Struma
Sordera y bocio
Pendred syndrome
Goiter and sensorineural deafness

Excludes: Associations (probably fortuitous) of deafness with other defects of thyroxine synthesis
Associations of deafness with endemic goiter (endemic cretinism)
Iodide transport defect (542)
Defective organification
Defective iodotyrosine coupling
Thyroidal iodotyrosine deiodinase deficiency
Thyroidal and peripheral iodotyrosine deiodinase deficiency
Iodoprotein secretory defect

Minimal Diagnostic Criteria: Perceptive deafness, goiter, and proven discharge of radioiodide with perchlorate or thiocyanate.

Clinical Findings: The sensorineural deafness is congenital or at least of very early onset and probably not progressive. It is perceptive and of profound degree; almost invariably the 2 sides are affected symmetrically. There is variable preservation of hearing in the low tones which occasionally permits appreciation of speech and normal education. However, special education is almost always necessary. Vestibular function is often impaired to a variable extent.

The block in thyroxine synthesis is at the incorporation of iodide into organic form in the thyroglobulin molecule and is detected by demonstrating a discharge of radioiodide from the thyroid gland by perchlorate or thiocyanate. This block is incomplete and of very variable degree and, because of this, the thyroid disorder of Pendred syndrome may take many forms. Thus lifelong euthyroidism is the rule, though hypothyroidism may occur in infancy or following surgical removal of the thyroid. Because of the difficulty in hormone synthesis, hyperplasia of the thyroid gland is usual, though it is of much lesser degree in males than females. Surgery is often unsatisfactory since regrowth of the remnant is common and some affected persons have had 4 or more operations.

In common with other types of goiter associated with defects in thyroxine synthesis, the histologic picture is extremely pleiomorphic and has given rise to suspicions of malignant change, though these are probably unjustified; at any rate, no well-documented cases of metastasis have been reported.

Complications
I **Derived:** Mental and physical retardation may occur in rare cases in whom pronounced hypothyroidism occurs in infancy. Death in infancy may very occasionally be due to respiratory obstruction caused by thyroid enlargement.
II **Associated:** —

Etiology: Autosomal recessive

Pathogenesis: ?

Related Facts
I **Sex Ratio:** M < 1:F1
II **Risk of Occurrence:** 1 in 14,300 births in Great Britain. Occurs in other white populations and also in many other ethnic groups including Japanese, blacks, and populations from India with unknown frequency.
III **Risk of Recurrence for**
Patient's Sib: 1 in 4 except in exceptional circumstances such as when 1 or both parents are affected.
Patient's Child: The reproductive fitness of deaf persons is increasing rapidly and may be 75% or more of normal. Deaf people, however, almost invariably marry within their own group. Several marriages between persons affected with Pendred syndrome have been reported. In such cases the risk is 1 in 1 (100%). In the vast majority of other cases the risk is extremely small, being confined to those who marry heterozygotes, in which case 1 in 2 (50%) of the children will be affected.
IV **Age of Detectability:** Deafness: early infancy (though often not detected until later). The condition could probably be detected at birth if the perchlorate discharge test were applied.
V **Prevalence:** Virtually normal life span hence essentially same as risk of occurrence in a given group.

Treatment
I **Primary Prevention:** Genetic counseling
II **Secondary Prevention:** In cases in which there is pronounced thyroid hyperplasia, prophylactic therapy with exogenous thyroid hormone preparations is effective in obviating the need for surgery and the risk of involved complications.
III **Other Therapy:** Surgery may be necessary for troublesome goiter. There is no therapy for the deafness, only supportive educational measures and the provision of appropriate electronic hearing aids being possible.

Prognosis: Virtually normal life span. There is some risk in the newborn period of suffocation from extremely pronounced thyroid hyperplasia and later in life from surgery of the thyroid gland. In rare cases the complications of gross hypothyroidism may threaten life. There is probably no or minimal risk of malignant neoplasia of the thyroid gland.

Detection of Carrier: ?

Special Considerations: —

References:
Fraser, G.R.: Association of congenital deafness with goiter (Pendred's syndrome); a study of 207 families. Ann. Hum. Genet. 28:201, 1965.
Fraser, G.R. et al: The syndrome of sporadic goitre and congenital deafness. Q.J. Med. 29:279, 1960.

Contributor: **G. R. Fraser**

Editor's Computerized Descriptors: Hearing, Ear, Neck

DEAFNESS AND METAPHYSEAL DYSOSTOSIS

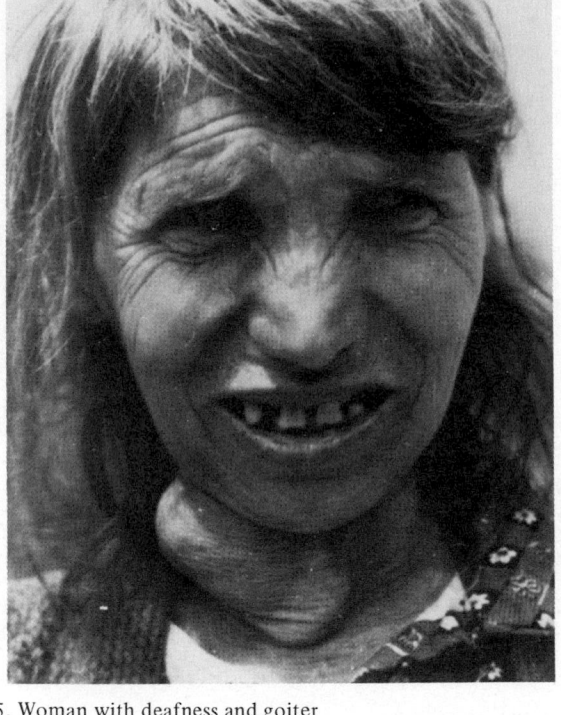

215. Woman with deafness and goiter

Includes: Dysostose métaphysaire, deficience mentale et surdité de conduction
Metaphysäre Chondrodysplasie, geistige Retardierung und Schalleitungs-Schwerhörigkeit
Disostosis metafisaria, retardo mental y sordera de conducción

Excludes: Other disorders associated with metaphyseal dysostosis

Minimal Diagnostic Criteria: Metaphyseal dysostosis and conductive hearing loss.

Clinical Findings: A kindred has been reported in which all 3 sibs were found to have short-limbed dwarfism, metaphyseal dysostosis, conductive hearing loss and mild mental retardation. The parents were 4th cousins. The skeletal disorder can be classified as "metaphyseal dysostosis" since the major lesions consist of widening and fragmentation of the metaphyses of the long bones with relative sparing of the skull, spine and epiphyses. Coxa vara, genua vara, scoliosis or lumbar lordosis were noted. The feet and hands were short and broad and the fingers were loose-jointed. Two sibs were hyperopic and had alternating esotropia. Anterior polar cataract was present in 1 sib. Polytomography revealed bilateral low placement of the ossicles in all 3 sibs. There was a striking upward angulation of the internal auditory canals. Audiologic examination in the 3 boys demonstrated a moderate bilateral conductive hearing deficit.

Complications
I Derived: —
II Associated: —

Etiology: Autosomal recessive

Pathogenesis: ?

Related Facts
I Sex Ratio: M3:F0
II Risk of Occurrence: ?
III Risk of Recurrence for
    Patient's Sib: 1 in 4 (25%) for each offspring to be affected
    Patient's Child: Not increased unless mate is carrier or homozygote
IV Age of Detectability: Early childhood
V Prevalence: ? One reported family with 3 affected sibs

Treatment
I Primary Prevention: Genetic counseling
II Secondary Prevention: Orthopedic therapy and a hearing aid may be useful.
III Other Therapy: —

Prognosis: Probably normal life span

Detection of Carrier: ?

Special Considerations: —

References:
Rimoin, D.L. and McAlister, W.H.: Metaphyseal dysostosis, conductive hearing loss, and mental retardation: A recessively inherited syndrome. In Bergsma, D. (ed.): Part IX. Ear. Birth Defects: Orig. Art. Ser., vol. VII, no. 4. Baltimore: Williams & Wilkins for The National Foundation-March of Dimes, 1971, p. 116.

Contributor: **Cor W.R.J. Cremers**

Editor's Computerized Descriptors: Vision, Eye, Hearing, Ear, Skel.

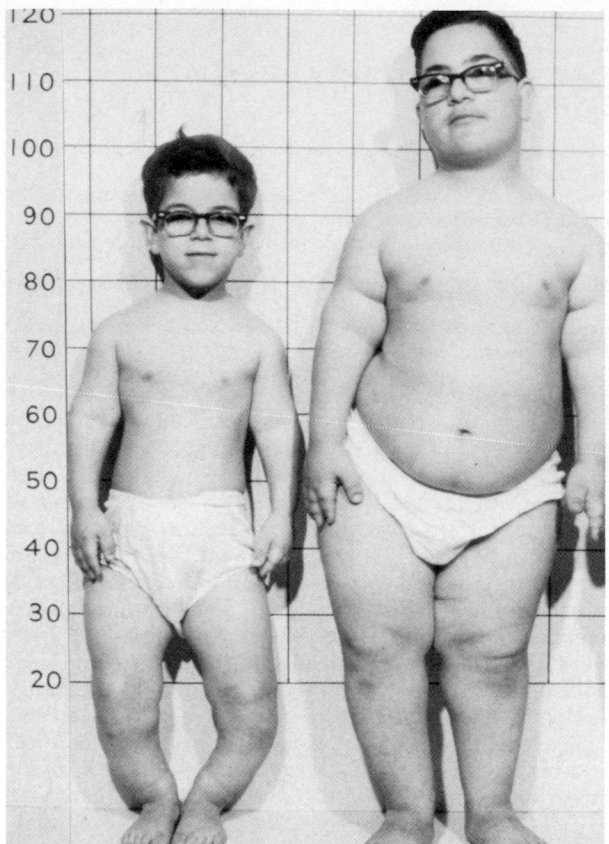

216. Brothers with short stature and skeletal defects secondary to metaphyseal dysostosis

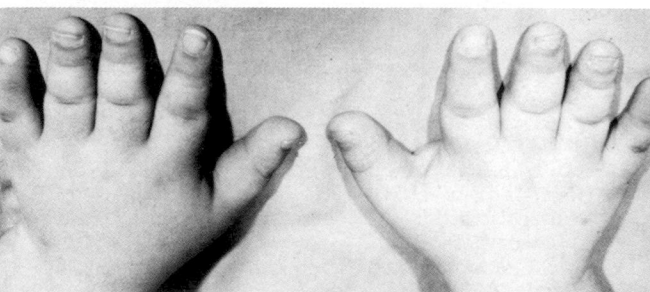

217. Note short, stubby hands with squared-off nails

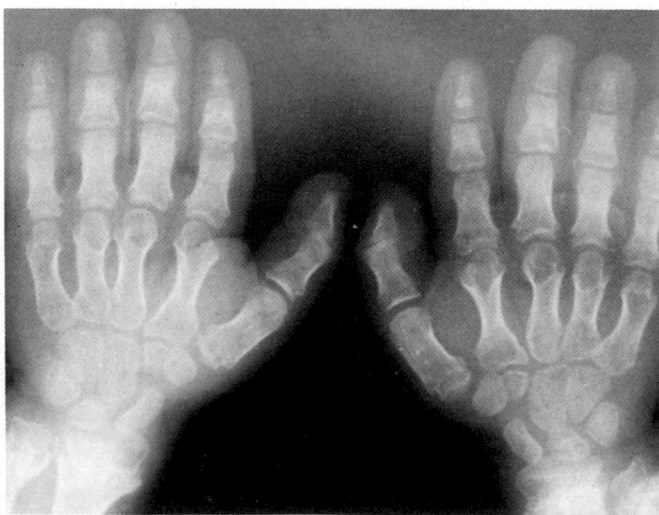

218. Short tubular bones with widened metaphyses; metaphyseal flaring of radius and ulna

DEAFNESS AND MYOPIA

Includes: Surdité cochléaire, myopie et oligophrénie
Innenohrschwerhörigkeit, Myopie und Oligophrenie
Sordera coclear, miopía y oligofrenia
Eldridge syndrome
Recessive myopia and hearing loss
Myopia, cochlear deafness and intellectual impairment
Oligophrenia, cochlear deafness and myopia
Cochlear deafness, myopia and oligophrenia

Excludes: Dominant myopia, hearing loss, peripheral neuropathy and skeletal abnormalities
Usher syndrome (983)
Phytanic acid storage disease (810)
Alström syndrome (41)
Recessive retinal changes, deafness, muscular wasting and mental retardation
Juvenile diabetes mellitus, optic atrophy and deafness (550)
Familial hearing loss, polyneuropathy and optic atrophy
Deafness, myopia, cataract and saddle nose (261)

Minimal Diagnostic Criteria: Cochlear deafness (30-100 db), myopia and intellectual impairment†

Clinical Findings: The natural history of the hearing impairment has not been fully documented but it is probably present at birth and progresses little thereafter. The hearing loss is cochlear in origin. The vestibular function is normal. The eye changes are those of severe myopia diagnosed at 4-6 years of age. EEG and CSF findings provide no consistent evidence of local or diffuse disease of the brain. Nonverbal IQ scores are in the range of 71-82. (Difficulties in the proper evaluation of mental status in the presence of marked sensory deprivation must be recognized.)

Complications
I   **Derived:** —
II **Associated:** †

Etiology: Autosomal recessive

Pathogenesis: Probably an enzyme deficiency

Related Facts
I   **Sex Ratio:** M1:F1
II   **Risk of Occurrence:** ? Higher in some isolated populations, such as Amish communities, because of consanguinity.
III **Risk of Recurrence for**
     Patient's Sib: 1 in 4 (25%) for each offspring to be affected
     Patient's Child: Not increased unless mate is carrier or homozygote
IV   **Age of Detectability:** At birth by newborn hearing tests, (screening or high risk registry) and refraction.
V   **Prevalence:** ?

Treatment
I   **Primary Prevention:** Genetic counseling
II   **Secondary Prevention:** Early detection of hearing and visual loss; early application of hearing aids and corrective lens; early special education.
III **Other Therapy:** —

Prognosis: Normal for life span; function dependent on initial status and subsequent care.†

Detection of Carrier: ?

†Special Considerations: Misdiagnoses such as schizophrenic reaction of childhood type (autism) have been made with resultant delayed onset of special training. Some do have IQ scores in the low normal and can be functional members of society with early diagnosis and training.

References:
Eldridge, R. et al: Cochlear deafness, myopia, and intellectual impairment in an Amish family. Arch. Otolaryngol. 88:49, 1968.
Flynn, P. and Aird, R. B.: A neuroectodermal syndrome of domi-

nant inheritance. J. Neurol. Sci. 2:161, 1965.
Konigsmark, B. W.: Hereditary deafness in man (second of three parts). N. Engl. J. Med. 281:774, 1969.

Contributor: **Lewis N. Neblett**

DEAFNESS AND ONYCHODYSTROPHY

Includes: Surdité avec onycho-dystrophie
Taubheit und Nageldystrophie
Sordera y ónicodistrofia
Nail dystrophy and sensorineural deafness

Excludes: Anonychia, hereditary (66)
Nail-patella syndrome (704)
Pachyonychia congenita (789)

Minimal Diagnostic Criteria: Sensorineural deafness with nail dystrophy

Clinical Findings: Characterized by profound deafness, bilateral, and of sensorineural type, normal or hypoactivity of labyrinth, and the nails of all fingers and toes show dystrophic changes from birth. Strabismus may be found.

Complications
I **Derived:** —
II **Associated:** —

Etiology: Autosomal recessive inheritance, pleiotropic. The parents of the 1 involved family were both 1st cousins on the maternal and 2nd cousins on the paternal side in a family of Jews from Egypt. (Coefficient of consanguinity $F = 0.078$)

Pathogenesis: Ectodermal defect involving ears and nails. Both deafness and dystrophic changes of the nails were found in 2 female sibs, the other members of the family being free of these anomalies. Strabismus was found in both sibs and mother.

Related Facts
I **Sex Ratio:** M1:F1
II **Risk of Occurrence:** Rare
III **Risk of Recurrence for**
   Patient's Sib: 1 in 4 (25%) for each offspring to be affected
   Patient's Child: Not increased unless mate is carrier or homozygote
IV **Age of Detectability:** At birth, although hearing loss may escape immediate notice.
V **Prevalence:** Only 1 family with the syndrome found in the literature.

Treatment
I **Primary Prevention:** Genetic counseling
II **Secondary Prevention:** Habilitation treatment for deafness
III **Other Therapy:** —

Prognosis: Probably normal life span

Detection of Carrier: ?

Special Considerations: —

References:
Cockayne, E. A.: Inherited Abnormalities of Skin and Its Appendages. London:Oxford University Press, 1933, p. 265.
Feinmesser, M. and Zelig, S.: Congenital deafness associated with onychodystrophy. Arch. Otolaryngol. 74:507, 1961.
Goodman, R. M. et al: Hereditary congenital deafness with onychodystrophy. Arch. Otolaryngol. 90:474, 1969.
Roberts, J. A. F.: An Introduction to Medical Genetics, 2nd Ed. London:Oxford University Press, 1959, p. 140.

Contributor: **Moshe Feinmesser**

DEAFNESS AND PROGRESSIVE OPTIC NERVE ATROPHY

Includes: Atrophie optique associée à la surdi-mutité
Opticus-atrophie in Kombination mit Taubheit
Sordera y atrofia del nervio óptico progresiva
Deafness-optic atrophy syndrome

Excludes: Leber optic atrophy (579)
Wolfram syndrome
Deafness-sensorineural, polyneuropathy and optic atrophy (268)
Optico-cochleo-dentate degeneration (759)
Sylvester disease
Syndromes including hearing loss and retinitis pigmentosa

Minimal Diagnostic Criteria: Severe hearing loss in early childhood in association with slowly progressive optic nerve atrophy and the absence of other anomalies or symptoms.

Clinical Findings: 17 cases in 4 families have been described and a Dutch kindred is known by personal communication. Profound bilateral sensorineural hearing loss of 60 to over 90 db, most marked in the midfrequencies, may be present from early childhood. Optic atrophy begins in the 1st decade and progresses very slowly resulting eventually in visual failure in the 2nd-6th decades. In some cases the visual loss was noticed in the 1st decade of life. Funduscopy showed paleness of the optic disk with distinct margins and normal macular reflex and normal retinal periphery. Neurologic examination is normal, except for deafness and optic nerve atrophy. Polytomography of the optic foramina, the chiasmatic region, and the temporal bone is normal. Vestibular function, as tested by electronystagmography, was normal in 2 cases. Color blindness is a common finding.

Complications
I   **Derived:** —
II **Associated:** —

Etiology: Autosomal dominant

Pathogenesis: ?

Related Facts
I   **Sex Ratio:** M1:F1; 17 patients described, 9 males and 8 females.
II **Risk of Occurrence:** ?
III **Risk of Recurrence for**
    Patient's Sib: If parent is affected, 1 in 2 (50%) for each offspring to be affected; otherwise not increased.
    Patient's Child: 1 in 2
IV **Age of Detectability:** Possible in the 1st or 2nd decade of life.
V **Prevalence:** ? Several kindreds have been independently described.

Treatment
I   **Primary Prevention:** Genetic counseling
II **Secondary Prevention:** —
III **Other Therapy:** Because of the severity of the sensorineural hearing loss, special education and hearing aids are necessary.

Prognosis: Probably good for normal life span. Vision decreases progressively to blindness. The hearing loss usually is present in early childhood and probably also progressive.

Detection of Carrier: —

Special Considerations: —

References:
Fraser, G.R.: Deafness with optic atrophy. In The Causes of Profound Deafness in Childhood. Baltimore: The Johns Hopkins Univeristy Press, 1976, p. 145.

Gernet, H.: Hereditäre Opticusatrophie in Kombination mit Taubheit. Ber. Dtsch. Ophthalmol. Ges. 65:545, 1964.
Konigsmark, B.W. et al: Dominant congenital deafness and progressive optic nerve atrophy: Occurrence in four generations of a family. Arch. Ophthalmol. 91:99, 1974.
Konigsmark, B.W. et al: Dominant congenital deafness and progressive optic nerve atrophy. Report of a family through four generations. Acta Genet. Med. Gemellol. (Roma) 23:377, 1974.
Michal, S. et al: Atrophy optique hérédo-familiale dominante associée à la surdi-mutité. Ann. Oculiste (Paris) 201:431, 1968.

Contributor: **Cor W.R.J. Cremers**

Editor's Computerized Descriptors: Vision, Eye, Hearing

DEAFNESS-CONDUCTIVE, AND MALFORMED LOW-SET EARS

Includes: Surdité de conduction-insertion basse des oreilles
Schalleitungsschwerhörigkeit und deformierte, tiefsitzende Ohren
Sordera de conducción y orejas malformadas de implantación baja
Ears, malformed and low-set, with conductive deafness
Conductive deafness with malformed low-set ears

Excludes: Low-set ears as part of other syndromes with multiple
structural abnormalities

Minimal Diagnostic Criteria: Malformed external ears and a
conductive hearing loss in the absence of other major structural
abnormalities are necessary to make the diagnosis.

Clinical Findings: Malformed external ears are found in all cases
with degree of deformity varying from mild cup-shaped deformity
to marked flop-eared deformity. Fifty percent of the affected also
have low-set ears. All affected have a mild-to-moderate hearing
loss. This is always a conductive loss, and is usually worse in the
more affected external ear. Mental retardation is present in 50%
of the affected. Cryptorchism is found in 100% of the males.

Complications
I   **Derived:** Deafness
II   **Associated:** †

Etiology: Autosomal recessive; McK *22130

Pathogenesis: Unknown developmental factors causing structural changes in middle ear bones and external pinna. Pathogenesis of mental retardation also unknown.

Related Facts
I   **Sex Ratio:** M1:F1
II   **Risk of Occurrence:** ?
III   **Risk of Recurrence for**
    Patient's Sib: 1 in 4 (25%) for each offspring to be affected
    Patient's Child: Not increased unless mate is carrier or
      homozygote.
IV   **Age of Detectability:** External ear deformity at birth; deaf-
    ness in infancy.
V   **Prevalence:** ?

Treatment
I   **Primary Prevention:** Genetic counseling
II   **Secondary Prevention:** Some affected may benefit from ear
    surgery.
III   **Other Therapy:** Special education for those mildly retarded
    may be of help. Hearing aids are often useful adjuncts to
    such special education.

Prognosis: Normal for life span

Detection of Carrier: ?

†**Special Considerations:** The description of additional cases will
help to delineate the place (if any) of mental retardation, cryptorchism, and short stature in this syndrome.

References:
Konigsmark, B. W.: Hereditary deafness in man (second of three
    parts). N. Engl. J. Med. 281:713, 1969.
Mengel, M. C. et al: Conductive hearing loss and malformed low-
    set ears, as a possible recessive syndrome. J. Med. Genet. 6:14,
    1969.

Contributor: **Marvin C. Mengel**

Editor's Computerized Descriptors: Hearing, Ear, GU., Nerve

DEAFNESS, DIABETES, PHOTOMYOCLONUS AND NEPHROPATHY

Includes: Photomyoclonie, diabète sucré, surdité de perception,
néphropathie, et encéphalopathie
Photomyoklonus, Diabetes mellitus, Innenohr-Schwerhörigkeit,
Nephropathie, zerebrale Dysfunktion
Fotomioclonus, diabetes mellitus, sordera neurosensorial, ne-
fropatía, y disfunción cerebral.

Excludes: Jakob-Creutzfeld syndrome
Amaurosis
Nephritis and nerve deafness, hereditary (708)

Minimal Diagnostic Criteria: Photomyoclonus, deafness, cerebral dysfunction, diabetes mellitus and nephropathy.

Clinical Findings: Thirteen affected patients in 5 generations of
1 family have been described. Four suffered from the complete
syndrome, the others had only a part of the syndrome. Photomyo-
clonic seizures began about age 20, followed by progressive sensorineural deafness at about age 30-35 and progressive dementia,
cerebellar symptoms, hemiparesis, aphasic and agnosic deficits in
the 4th decade. At this time, diabetes mellitus and low-grade
glomerulo- and pyelonephritis were also diagnosed. Terminally
bizarre myoclonus and bulbar signs were seen. No audiometric
findings were described.

Complications
I   **Derived:** Extreme emaciation and progressive unresponsive-
    ness
II   **Associated:** One patient died from bronchopneumonia.

Etiology: Autosomal dominant

Pathogenesis: In the brain, particularly in the cerebral and cerebellar cortices, generalized neural loss was revealed. Furthermore, the accumulation of abnormal lipids in the brain - most
striking in dentate and inferior olivary nuclei, and in the kidney
suggest a marked lipidosis.

Related Facts
I   **Sex Ratio:** M4:F9 (All 4 patients with complete syndrome
    were female)
II   **Risk of Occurrence:** —
III   **Risk of Recurrence for**
    Patient's Sib: If parent is affected, 1 in 2 (50%) for each
      offspring to be affected; otherwise not increased.
    Patient's Child: 1 in 2
IV   **Age of Detectability:** 3rd-4th decade
V   **Prevalence:** Single reported kindred with multiple affected
    individuals in several generations.

Treatment
I   **Primary Prevention:** Genetic counseling
II   **Secondary Prevention:** Supportive therapy
III   **Other Therapy:** Anticonvulsant medication, tube feeding

Prognosis: Poor

Detection of Carrier: —

Special Considerations: —

References:
Herrman, C., Jr. et al: Hereditary photomyoclonus associated with
    diabetes mellitus, deafness, nephropathy and cerebral dysfunc-
    tion. Neurology 14:212, 1964.

Contributors: **Agnes M. Ickenroth**
                    Cor W.R.J. Cremers

Editor's Computerized Descriptors: Hearing, GU., Nerve

DEAFNESS, DOMINANT LOW-FREQUENCY

Includes: Surdité pour les sons graves
Dominant erblicher Hörverlust niederfrequenter Bereiche
Pérdida de la audición a las frequencias bajas dominante
Hearing loss, familial low-frequency

Excludes: Dominant midfrequency hearing loss
Dominant high-frequency hearing loss

Minimal Diagnostic Criteria: A progressive neural hearing loss by audiometric testing involving low frequencies in the latter half of the 1st or the 2nd decade of life in family with evidence for autosomal dominant inheritance of low-frequency hearing loss.

Clinical Findings: No hearing loss may be noted by affected persons until their 2nd-4th decades of life when they detect a slowly progressive hearing loss. Audiometric testing is necessary to detect affected persons. The hearing loss may be congenital, since the youngest patient tested was 7 years old and had a 25 db low-frequency hearing loss.

Younger-affected persons show hearing loss involving frequencies up to about 2000 Hz. With increasing age the higher frequencies also deteriorate, until finally in old age there is a severe hearing loss involving all frequencies. However, there is moderate individual variation with some affected persons in their middle decades showing a severe hearing loss while some older affected persons have only a moderate loss.

The tone decay test generally is negative suggesting that there is no VIIIth nerve involvement. However, the small increment sensitivity index generally is positive in affected persons, suggesting a cochlear locale for the hearing loss.

Physical, neurologic and laboratory examinations are normal, as is vestibular testing.

Complications
I   **Derived:** —
II **Associated:** —

Etiology: Autosomal dominant

Pathogenesis: ?

Related Facts
I   **Sex Ratio:** M1:F1
II **Risk of Occurrence:** ? †
III **Risk of Recurrence for**
    Patient's Sib: If parent is affected 1 in 2 (50%) for each offspring to be affected; otherwise not increased.
    Patient's Child: 1 in 2
IV **Age of Detectability:** After 5 years of age when audiometric testing can be done.
V **Prevalence:** Too little data available for reasonably accurate estimate. This disease is probably fairly widespread but found only when looked for.

Treatment
I   **Primary Prevention:** Genetic counseling
II **Secondary Prevention:** —
III **Other Therapy:** A hearing aid is indicated when the hearing loss becomes a problem.

Prognosis: Normal for life span and intelligence

Detection of Carrier: —

†Special Considerations: It is quite likely that many patients with familial hearing loss have this disease.

References:
Konigsmark, B.W. et al: Familial low-frequency hearing loss. Laryngoscope 81:759, 1971.

Contributor: **Bruce W. Konigsmark‡**

Editor's Computerized Descriptor: Hearing

DEAFNESS, GOITER AND PERIPHERAL RESISTANCE TO THYROID HORMONE

Includes: Surdité, éphiphyses ponctuées, goitre avec élévation du taux sanguin en hormones thyroïdien
Taubheit-multicentrishche Ossifikation der Epiphysen, hohes eiweissgebundenes Jod
Sordera-epifisis punteadas-bocio y PBI elevado
Goiter with high PBI, deafness and stippled epiphyses
Stippled epiphyses, deafness and goiter with high levels of serum thyroid hormone

Excludes: Neonatal Graves disease
Goitrous cretinism
Congenital epiphysial dysgenesis (dysplasia epiphysialis multiplex, osteochondrodystrophies)

Minimal Diagnostic Criteria: Goiter and thyroid overactivity associated with high levels of free (protein unbound) circulating thyroid hormone in the absence of hyperthyroidism.

Clinical Findings: Goiter, congenital profound sensorineural deafness, birdlike facies, pigeon breast and winged scapulae. Delayed bone age, stippled epiphyses but normal dental development. Clinically euthyroid with normal basal metabolic rate. Elevated level of circulating thyroxine (PBI, BEI and serum thyroxine) in the presence of normal thyroxine-binding capacity of thyroxine-binding globulin (TBG) and prealbumin (TBPA). The thyroxine is the L-isomer. Free thyroxine in blood is elevated. The 24 hour thyroidal[131] I uptake is high (80-50%) and is nonsuppressible with the usual dose of thyroid hormone (thyroxine or triiodothyronine) replacement. Elevated thyroidal iodine release due to the enormous pool size and elevated thyroxine and triiodothyronine degradation rate due to the increase of the extra thyroidal hormonal pool. Normal penetration of thyroxine into liver. Circulating thyrotropin (TSH) levels are normal. The long acting thyroid stimulator (LATS) is absent, as are the thyroglobulin antibodies. Administration of supraphysiologic doses of thyroid hormone fail to suppress the response of TSH to TSH-releasing hormone. Glucocorticoids produce their usual "nonspecific" suppressive effect on TSH. Lymphocytes lack normal receptors for thyroid hormone.

Complications
I   **Derived:** Probably deafness and bony dysgenesis
II **Associated:** Birdlike facies, pigeon breast, winged scapulae, laryngomalacia with stridor in infancy.

Etiology: Behaves as a rare autosomal recessive.

Pathogenesis: It appears to be a congenital metabolic defect associated with variable degrees of tissue response to the action of thyroid hormone, which has been partially compensated by the excess hormone production. Circulating lymphocytes lack the normal, high affinity-low capacity, nuclear thyroid hormone binding "receptor" protein. The latter may represent the biochemical basis for the observed tissue resistance to the hormone.†

Related Facts
I   **Sex Ratio:** M1:F1
II   **Risk of Occurrence:** ?
III **Risk of Recurrence for**
     Patient's Sib: Presumably 1 in 4 (25%) for each offspring to be affected
     Patient's Child: Not increased unless mate is carrier or homozygote.
IV   **Age of Detectability:** Early infancy, by physical examination, bone xrays, and evidence of thyroid hyperactivity with elevated level of circulating thyroid hormone in the presence of euthyroidism.
V   **Prevalence:** ?

Treatment
I   **Primary Prevention:** Genetic counseling
II   **Secondary Prevention:** Special training for deaf-mutism
III **Other Therapy:** —

Prognosis: ? Probably normal life span

Detection of Carrier: ?

†**Special Considerations:** The distinguishing feature of this syndrome is a combination of findings usually associated with hypothyroidism (delayed bone age, stippled epiphyses, congenital deafness and goiter) with blood protein bound thyroxine, free thyroxine and iodine kinetic measurements characteristic of hyperthyroidism. Thyroid clearance of iodide is elevated in the face of normal renal clearance. Plasma iodide and plasma iodide disappearance rates are increased. Thyroid organic iodine content is markedly increased, as is the thyroid iodide secretion rate. Absolute iodine uptake is high. Administration of perchlorate fails to discharge the previously trapped iodine[131]. Administration of thyroxine and triiodothyronine in doses 5-7 fold the normal physiologic amount fails to induce signs of thyrotoxicity, raise the basal metabolic rate, alter body weight, caloric intake, sleeping pulse rate or any other parameter except for an increase in the urinary hydroxyproline excretion from low to normal. Uptake of thyroid hormone and conversion of thyroxine to triiodothyronine by skin fibroblasts grown in culture are normal.

References:
Bernal J. et al: Absent nuclear thyroid hormone receptors and failure of T3-induced TRH suppression in the syndrome of peripheral resistance to thyroid hormone. In Robbins J. and Braverman, L.E. (eds): Thyroid Research, Proc. 7th Int. Thyroid Conf. Amsterdam:Excerpta Medica, 1976, pp. 316-319.
Refetoff, S. et al: Familial syndrome combining deaf-mutism, stippled epiphyses, goiter and abnormally high PBI: Possible target organ refractoriness to thyroid hormone. J. Clin. Endocrinol. 27:279, 1967.
Refetoff, S. et al: Studies on a sibship with apparent hereditary resistance to the intracellular action of thyroid hormone. Metabolism 21:723, 1972.

Contributors: **Loren T. DeWind**
Samuel Refetoff
Leslie J. DeGroot

Editor's Computerized Descriptors: Hearing, Face, Larynx, Neck, Skel., Resp.

DEAFNESS, HYPERPROLINURIA AND ICHTHYOSIS

Includes: Néphropathie, surdité neurosensorielle, hyperprolinurie et ichtyose

Nephropathie, Innenohrschwerhörigkeit, Hyperprolinurie und Ichthyose

Nefropatía, pérdida de la agudeza auditiva neuro-sensorial hiperprolinuria e ictiosis

Excludes: Hyperprolinemia (Marker) (502)

Renal anomalies and hearing loss

Hyperprolinemia and microscopic hematuria

Ichthyosis, strabismus and sensorineural deafness

Minimal Diagnostic Criteria: Hearing loss and ichthyosis with either renal disease or hyperprolinuria or a relative with those conditions.

Clinical Findings: Various combinations of renal disease, hearing loss, ichthyosis and hyperprolinuria were found in 23 of 78 examined members of a kindred. Two of 3 children, born of a consanguineous union of affected parents, showed all elements of the syndrome except hearing loss. In no family members were all symptoms present. Thirteen of 67 tested family members had a sensorineural hearing loss, 8 had a nephropathy, 6 had ichthyosis and 4 had a proline defect. Two of the family members had 3 traits, 5 had 2 traits, 15 had only 1 trait.

The hearing loss is mainly in the frequencies above 4000 cycles/second and is slowly progressive. The degree of hearing loss was > 50 db in persons over 50 years of age and > 30 db in younger people.

Advanced renal disease with chronic renal failure was present in the proband and his younger sister. Six other persons had renal calculi. Histopathologic examination of kidney specimens obtained from the proband showed glomerular and periglomerular sclerosis. The interstitial tissue was infiltrated largely by lymphocytes. The small arteries and arterioles showed variable degrees of medial hypertrophy and subendothelial sclerosis. Electron microscopy showed a thickening of the mesangial basement membrane. Plasma proline levels were elevated in 3 person, and prolinuria was noted in 2 family members.

Complications

I **Derived:** Uremia

II **Associated:** —

Etiology: The evidence suggests an autosomal dominant trait with variable expressivity.

Pathogenesis: ?

Related Facts

I **Sex Ratio:** M13:F10

II **Risk of Occurrence:** ?

III **Risk of Recurrence for**

Patient's Sib: If autosomal dominant and, if parent is affected 1 in 2 (50%) for each offspring to be affected; otherwise not increased.

Patient's Child: If autosomal dominant, 1 in 2

IV **Age of Detectability:** Childhood and adolescence

V **Prevalence:** ?

Treatment

I **Primary Prevention:** Genetic counseling

II **Secondary Prevention:** Treatment of renal calculi and uremia. A hearing aid may be of help.

III **Other Therapy:** —

Prognosis: In absence of uremia, no decrease of life span.

Detection of Carrier: The affected patient is heterozygous for the dominant mutant gene. Close examination of the apparently unaffected individual may reveal minimal expression of the mutant gene.

Special Considerations: —

References:

Goyer, R.A. et al: Hereditary renal disease with neurosensory hearing loss, prolinuria and ichthyosis. Am. J. Med. Sci. 256:166, 1968.

Contributor: **Cor W.R.J. Cremers**

Editor's Computerized Descriptors: Hearing, Skin, GU.

259

DEAFNESS, KERATOPACHYDERMIA AND DIGITAL CONSTRICTIONS

258-500

Includes: Surdité, kératopachydermie, et constrictions digitales
Keratoma hereditarium mutilans
Sordera, queratopaquidermia y constricciones digitales
Vohwinkel syndrome
Mutilating keratoderma
Keratopachydermia, digital constrictions and deafness
Digital constrictions, keratopachydermia and deafness

Excludes: Ainhum
Pseudoainhum
Keratosis palmaris et plantaris with ainhum
Mal de Meleda
High-tone deafness

Minimal Diagnostic Criteria: Palmo-plantar keratoderma, congenital deafness and distal digital constrictions

Clinical Findings: Onset in infancy or early childhood of a diffuse palmo-plantar keratoderma with honeycombed small depressions, starfish-shaped keratoses of the dorsa of hands and feet, and linear keratoses of elbows and knees. Digital band-like constrictions of distal interphalangeal creases develop after age 4-5 years. Patients show congenital high-frequency neural hearing loss and 1 patient is reported with deaf-mutism. Xrays may show constriction of phalangeal bone(s), trophic bony atrophy and regular nodular verrucous soft tissue.

Complications
I **Derived:** Amputation of distal digit(s) because of gangrene or chronic sepsis.
II **Associated:** Diffuse nonscarring alopecia, alopecia areata, ridged dystrophic nails, syndactylia, transient plantar blisters, hyperhidrosis

Etiology: Autosomal dominant McK *12450

Pathogenesis: ?

Related Facts
I **Sex Ratio:** M1:F1
II **Risk of Occurrence:** ?
III **Risk of Recurrence for**
Patient's Sib: If parent is affected, 1 in 2 (50%) for each offspring to be affected; otherwise not increased.
Patient's Child: 1 in 2
IV **Age of Detectability:** Deafness: infancy or early childhood. Keratoderma: infancy or early childhood. Digital constrictions: 4-5 years of age.
V **Prevalence:** ?

Treatment
I **Primary Prevention:** Genetic counseling
II **Secondary Prevention:** 10 - 40% urea solution soaks followed by abrasive filing of hyperkeratosis; 40% salicylic acid plaster with débridement of hyperkeratoses. Excision of keratoses with full thickness skin grafting. Surgical amputation of gangrenous or septic digit(s).
III **Other Therapy:** Specially fitted shoes, avoidance of trauma

Prognosis: Normal for life span and intelligence

Detection of Carrier: —

Special Considerations: —

References:
Gibbs, R. C. and Frank, S. B.: Keratoma hereditaria mutilans (Vohwinkel). Differentiating features of conditions with constriction of digits. Arch. Dermatol. 94:619, 1966.

Contributor: **William C. Gentry, Jr.**

Editor's Computerized Descriptors: Hearing, Skin, Sweating, Hair, Nails, Skel.

DEAFNESS, LOW-TONE

Includes: Surdité pour les basses fréquences
Tiefton-Schwerhörigkeit
Sordera a los tonos bajos
Hearing loss, low-frequency
Low-tone deafness

Excludes: —

Minimal Diagnostic Criteria: This condition is characterized by an upward-sloping pure-tone audiogram with 30 db to 40 db hearing thresholds below 2000 Hz and normal or near-normal thresholds above this level. The disorder presents a symmetric involvement of both ears.

Clinical Findings: Sensorineural hearing loss at low frequencies with normal or near-normal hearing thresholds at higher frequencies and without syndrome identifying associated abnormalities. These children or adults in general recognize the presence of a symmetric bilateral hearing defect among a number of the members of their kindred. The hearing loss is variable in severity and the autosomal dominant mode of inheritance is detected by audiometric testing of as many family members as is possible. Otoneurologic and psychologic evaluations are within normal limits. The low-tone sensorineural component does not appear to progress in severity.

Complications
I   **Derived:** With superimposed acoustic trauma or noise-induced hearing loss in the high frequencies, the audiogram may take on a unique configuration with peaking in the mid-tone range and the previously mild hearing defect may become more clinically noticeable.
II   **Associated:** —

Etiology: Autosomal dominant; McK *12490

Pathogenesis: Audiometric tests suggest a peripheral or cochlear localization of the lesion (ie elevated SISI scores for 250-2000 Hz in affected subjects). Detailed ENT examination, vestibular function testing, and temporal bone xrays have shown no significant abnormalities. It seems likely that the apical cochlear function is defective and that affected patients do not perceive low-frequency sound until the intensity is great enough to stimulate the normal, more proximal portion of the cochlea.

Related Facts
I   **Sex Ratio:** M1:F1
II   **Risk of Occurrence:** ?
III   **Risk of Recurrence for**
     Patient's Sib: If parent is affected 1 in 2 (50%) for each offspring to be affected; otherwise not increased.
     Patient's Child: 1 in 2
IV   **Age of Detectability:** Usually not detected until audiometric screening tests are performed.†
V   **Prevalence:** ? Only 5 recognized kindreds have been reported.

Treatment
I   **Primary Prevention:** Genetic counseling
II   **Secondary Prevention:** Fitting of an adequate wearable hearing aid and remedial program in language, speech and auditory training, when indicated.
III   **Other Therapy:** —

Prognosis: Good with early detection and treatment as outlined. The low-tone hearing loss does not appear to be progressive.

Detection of Carrier: —

†Special Considerations: Affected children and young adults are usually symptomatic but not incapacitated because of the relative sparing of hearing in the speech range. Nevertheless, affected individuals may often experience hearing difficulty in school; this fact emphasizes the importance of recognizing the hereditary nature of the disorder so that hearing loss in other family members may be promptly diagnosed and treated appropriately.

References:
Allen, J.H. et al: (Vanderbilt University Hereditary Deafness Study Group): Dominantly inherited low-frequency hearing loss. Arch. Otolaryngol. 88:242, 1968.

Contributor: **Paul H. Ward**

Editor's Computerized Descriptor: Hearing

DEAFNESS, MYOPIA, CATARACT AND SADDLE NOSE

Includes: Myopie, cataracte, ensellure nasale profonde, hypertélorisme, nanisme, et surdité de perception d'intensité variable

Myopie, Katarakt, Sattelnase, Hypertelorismus, Kleinwuchs, Innenohrschwerhörigkeit

Miopía, catarata, nariz en silla de montar, hipertelorismo, estatura baja y pérdida de la audición neurosensorial de moderada a severa

Marshall syndrome

Abnormal facies, myopia and short stature

Myopia, cataract, saddle nose, hypertelorism, short stature and moderate-to-severe sensorineural hearing loss

Excludes: Oto-oculo-musculo-skeletal syndrome (785)
Facio-oculo-acoustic-renal (FOAR) syndrome

Minimal Diagnostic Criteria: Saddle nose, hypertelorism, high myopia, cataract, and sensorineural hearing loss. The extent of variability is not yet clear.

Clinical Findings: Twenty-one cases of this syndrome have been reported in 5 families. All patients have a severely depressed nasal bridge with anteverted nostrils. Wide-set eyes, myopia, congenital and juvenile cataracts, and a moderate-to-severe sensorineural hearing loss are frequent features of this syndrome. Esotropia, hypertropia, high-arched or cleft palate and retinal detachment have also been noted. The upper incisors protrude in a number of cases. Roentgenologic examinations revealed absent or small nasal bones. The facial appearance is thought to be due to faulty devlopment of the ethmoid bone, which also causes a short anterior cranial fossa. Grossly the saddle-nose deformity becomes less obvious as the patient matures. As infants, the children may "snort" as they breathe, but by 1-2 years of age this upper-airway sound disappears. The degree of myopia is usually > -10 D. In some cases there was a sudden maturation of cataract with glaucoma, necessitating surgery. The moderate-to-severe sensorineural hearing loss is progressive in some cases. By x-ray examination, the internal auditory canals were somewhat narrowed. In 1 case polytomography of the inner ears was normal. In another case vestibular function was normal as assessed by caloric stimulation with ice water.

Complications
I **Derived:** Retinal detachment
II **Associated:** —

Etiology: Autosomal dominant with variable expression

Pathogenesis: ?

Related Facts
I **Sex Ratio:** M1:F1
II **Risk of Occurrence:** ?
III **Risk of Recurrence for**
  Patient's Sib: If parent is affected 1 in 2 (50%) for each offspring to be affected; otherwise not increased.
  Patient's Child: 1 in 2
IV **Age of Detectability:** Early childhood
V **Prevalence:** Several independent pedigrees have been reported.

Treatment
I **Primary Prevention:** Genetic counseling
II **Secondary Prevention:** Surgical treatment of cataract. A hearing aid can be useful in some cases. Special education because of the hearing loss may be necessary.
III **Other Therapy:** —

Prognosis: Probably good for normal life span

Detection of Carrier: —

Special Considerations: —

References:
Keith, C.G. et al: Abnormal facies, myopia, and short stature. Arch. Dis. Child. 47:787, 1972.
Marshall, D.: Ectodermal dysplasia. Report of a kindred with ocular abnormalities and hearing defect. Am. J. Ophthalmol. 45:143, 1958.
O'Donnell, J.J. et al: Generalized osseous abnormalities in the Marshall syndrome. In Bergsma, D. (ed.): Cytogenetics, Environment and Malformation Syndromes. Birth Defects: Orig. Art. Ser., vol. XII, no. 5. New York: Alan R. Liss, Inc. for The National Foundation-March of Dimes, 1976, p. 299.
Ruppert, E.S. et al: Hereditary hearing loss with saddle nose and myopia. Arch. Otolaryngol. 92:95, 1970.
Zellweger, H. et al: The Marshall syndrome: Report of a new family. J. Pediatr. 84:868, 1974.

Contributor: **Cor W.R.J. Cremers**

Editor's Computerized Descriptors: Vision, Eye, Hearing, Oral, Teeth, Nose, Skel., Resp.

DEAFNESS, ONYCHODYSTROPHY AND DIGITAL ANOMALIES

Includes: Onychodysplasie, triphalangie des pouces et des gros orteils, retard mental, épilepsie et surdité de perception
Onychodystrophie, dreigliedrige Daumen und Zehen, geistige Retardierung, Krampfanfälle, angebornene Innenohr-Schwerhörigkeit
Onicodistrofia, pulgares trifálangicos, orejas recortadas y pérdida de la audición neurosensorial
Deafness with onycho-osteo dystrophy and mental retardation (DOOR syndrome)
Onychodystrophy, triphalangeal thumbs and halluces, mental retardation, seizures and congenital sensorineural deafness

Excludes: Onychodystrophy and congenital sensorineural deafness
Onychodystrophy, triphalangeal thumbs and congenital sensorineural deafness (autosomal dominant inheritance)
Onychodystrophy, coniform teeth and sensorineural hearing loss (autosomal dominant inheritance)
Knuckle pads, leukonychia and deafness (558)

Minimal Diagnostic Criteria: Onychodystrophy, triphalangeal thumbs and halluces, mental retardation, seizures, and sensorineural deafness.

Clinical Findings: Three kindreds are reported in which 4 children showed the features of this syndrome. Parental consanguinity was evident in 2 families. Absent or hypoplastic fingernails and toenails were present in 4/4, triphalangeal thumbs and halluces in 4/4, dystrophic terminal phalanges of some or all of the fingers and toes in 4/4. In some patients there were only 2 phalanges in the little fingers, and fusion of the middle and distal phalanges of the 3rd to 5th toes.

Mental retardation was present in 4/4 seizures in 3/4 sensorineural deafness in 4/4. Roentgenograms of the petrous bone were normal in 2/4. Low-set ears were present in 1/4, antimongoloid slant in 1/4. Teeth were yellow in some cases and hypoplastic in one. Dermatoglyphic studies of the finger and toe prints in the 4 cases have shown almost all to be arches. The atd angles were normal. Dermatoglyphics of the parents and the other normal sib were normal in 1 kindred.

Complications
I   Derived: —
II   Associated: —

Etiology: Autosomal recessive

Pathogenesis: ?

Related Facts
I   **Sex Ratio:**   M2:F2
II   **Risk of Occurrence:**   ? Description of the syndrome in 3 families suggests that it may not be exceedingly rare.
III   **Risk of Recurrence for**
    Patient's Sib: 1 in 4 (25%) for each offspring to be affected
    Patient's Child: Not increased unless mate is carrier or homozygote
IV   **Age of Detectability:**   Early childhood
V   **Prevalence:**   ? 3 reported familes with 4 affected individuals. Consanguinity in 2 of 3 reported families suggests this is a moderately rare recessive trait.

Treatment
I   **Primary Prevention:**   Genetic counseling
II   **Secondary Prevention:**   Hearing aid and supportive educational measures.
III   **Other Therapy:**   —

Prognosis: Probably good for normal life span

Detection of Carrier: ?

Special Considerations: —

References:
Cantwell, R.J.: Congenital sensori-neural deafness associated with onycho-osteo dystrophy and mental retardation (D.O.O.R. syndrome). Humangenetik 26:261, 1975.
Qazi, Q.H. and Smithwick, E.M.: Triphalangy of thumbs and great toes. Am. J. Dis. Child. 120:255, 1970.
Walbaum, R. et al: Surdité familiale avec ostéo-onycho-dysplasie, J. Génét. Hum. 18:101, 1970.

Contributor: **Cor W.R.J. Cremers**

Editor's Computerized Descriptors: Eye, Hearing, Ear, Teeth, Dermatoglyphic, Nails, Skel., Nerve

DEAFNESS, PERIPHERAL PULMONARY STENOSES AND BRACHYTELEPHALANGY

Includes: Sténoses pulmonaire multiples, surdité mixte, brachytélé phalangie calcification des cartilages
Periphere Pulmonalstenose, Kombinierte Schwerhörigkeit, Brachytelephalangie, Knorpelverkalkungen
Estenosis pulmonar periférica múltiple, sordera mixta, braquitelefalangia y calcificación de los cartílagos
Multiple peripheral pulmonary stenoses, mixed deafness, brachytelephalangy, calcification of cartilages

Excludes: Familial multiple pulmonary stenoses
Fetal rubella syndrome (384)
Progressive valvular or infundibular pulmonary stenosis, skeletal abnormalities and deafness

Minimal Diagnostic Criteria: Since only 2 sibs with this syndrome have been reported, it is difficult to establish minimal diagnostic criteria. It would seem that calcification of the cartilages, brachytelephalangy, multiple peripheral pulmonary stenoses and mixed or sensorineural deafness must be present.

Clinical Findings: A kindred has been reported in which 2 of 5 sibs had a history of recurrent bronchitis and otitis media. Hearing loss was apparent in both children in the 1st year of life. Both had a mixed hearing loss of 40-70 db; the conductive component was supposedly due to recurrent middle ear infections. Their auricles were large, prominent and tough. Histologic examination of the girl's right auricle showed perichondral and enchondral ossification centers. Abnormal vascular murmurs were detected on routine examinations. Isolated multiple peripheral pulmonary stenoses were diagnosed in both. Pulmonary and aortic valves were intact. There was no evidence of intracardiac lesions. In the girl, the terminal phalanges of both hands were shortened and somewhat malformed, as were the terminal phalanges I-IV on the right, and I, III, IV on the left in the boy. The terminal phalanges of the great toes were similarly malformed in both. In the affected phalanges epiphyseal-metaphyseal fusion was almost complete. Radiographic studies at 8-9 years showed widespread calcification in the cartilages of the nose, larynx including the epiglottis, the trachea, the bronchi and the ribs.

Complications
I **Derived:** Language delay secondary to the hearing loss. Hypertrophy of the right heart.
II **Associated:** —

Etiology: Probably autosomal recessive

Pathogenesis: ?

Related Facts
I **Sex Ratio:** M1:F1
II **Risk of Occurrence:** Probably very rare
III **Risk of Recurrence for**
   Patient's Sib: 1 in 4 (25%) for each sib to be affected
   Patient's Child: Not increased unless mate is carrier or homozygote
IV **Age of Detectability:** First years of life
V **Prevalence:** ? Single reported family with 2 affected sibs

Treatment
I **Primary Prevention:** Genetic counseling
II **Secondary Prevention:** Hearing aid; control of peripheral stenoses
III **Other Therapy:** —

Prognosis: Good for an essentially normal life span

Detection of Carrier: —

Special Considerations: —

References:
Keutel, J. et al: Ein neues autosomal-rezessiv Vererbbares Syndrom. Dtsch. Med. Wochenschr. 96:1676, 1971.
Keutel, J. et al: A new autosomal recessive syndrome: Peripheral pulmonary stenoses, brachytelephalangism, neural hearing loss and abnormal cartilage calcifications/ossifications. In Bergsma D. (ed.): Part XV. Cardiovascular System. Birth Defects: Orig. Art. Ser., vol. VIII, no. 5. Baltimore: Williams & Wilkins for The National Foundation-March of Dimes, 1972, p. 60.

Contributor: **Cor W. R. J. Cremers**

Editor's Computerized Descriptors: Hearing, Ear, Nose, Speech, Skel., Resp., CV.

DEAFNESS, RENAL AND DIGITAL ANOMALIES

Includes: Surdité, anomalies rénales et digitales
Taubheit, renale und digitale Fehlbildungen
Sordera, anomalías renales y digitales
Renal and digital anomalies and deafness
Digital and renal anomalies and deafness

Excludes: Nephritis and nerve deafness, hereditary (708)
Nephrosis, familial (710)
Nephrosis, congenital (709)

Minimal Diagnostic Criteria: Since it is not certain that all 5 boys represent a single entity, it is difficult to establish minimal diagnostic criteria. It would seem that conductive or mixed hearing loss with the typical digital abnormalities must be present with or without renal anomalies or nephrosis.†

Clinical Findings: A kindred has been reported in which 4 of 12 sibs have had renal problems, 3 of 12 a hearing loss and 3 of 12 had similar short distal portions of the great toes and thumbs giving them a bulbous appearance.

Two boys had a conductive hearing loss, a bifid uvula and urinary tract anomalies; one of them had a bladder neck and ureteral obstruction, and the other had a duplication of the renal pelvis and upper ureter on the left. These same 2 boys had a history of allergies but otologic examination showed no evidence of serous otitis media. Middle ear exploration in one case revealed normal ossicles. The 3rd boy with the digital anomalies had a normal uvula, normal urinary tract and a more severe hearing loss, mixed in type. Audiograms on the 3 boys with deafness were abnormal showing varying degrees of conductive or mixed hearing loss. Xrays of the thumbs and great toes showed short, rudimentary distal phalanges with bifurcation at the distal end.

Two other male sibs had clinical and laboratory evidence of nephrosis. One died at almost 5 years of age. Both had normal digits, normal uvula and normal hearing. The mother of these children had hypertension with 2 of her pregnancies. She is otherwise normal.

Complications
I Derived: Language delay secondary to the hearing loss, chronic infection secondary to urinary tract obstruction, nephrosis
II Associated: —

Etiology: Postulated to be either an autosomal recessive or X-linked recessive trait.†

Pathogenesis: ? The authors have speculated that the boys with nephrosis may have an obstructive lesion not detectable by routine radiologic or histologic studies.

Related Facts
I Sex Ratio: All reported cases are males. M1:F0
II Risk of Occurrence: ?
III Risk of Recurrence for
　Patient's Sib: ? If autosomal recessive or X-linked recessive, see Table I AR or X-linked R, respectively.
　Patient's Child: ? If autosomal recessive or X-linked recessive, see Table I AR or X-linked R, respectively.
IV Age of Detectability: At birth by physical examination for digital abnormalities and by audiogram. However routine newborn audiometric screening may miss the conductive hearing loss. IVP and urinalysis necessary to detect renal abnormalities.
V Prevalence: ?

Treatment
I Primary Prevention: Genetic counseling

II Secondary Prevention: Amplification and special training if the hearing loss is severe, corrective surgery for some of the urinary tract abnormalities.
III Other Therapy: Treatment for nephrosis

Prognosis: Varied. It is guarded in cases with nephrosis or more complicated urinary tract abnormalities but probably good in the others.

Detection of Carrier: ? Hypertension during pregnancy may indicate the carrier state in the female.

†Special Considerations: These 5 brothers may have a single entity or they may represent 2 different entities, one characterized by digital abnormalities and hearing loss with urinary tract anomalies, and the other by nephrosis.

References:
Braun, F. C., Jr. and Bayer, J. F.: Familial nephrosis associated with deafness and congenital urinary tract anomalies in siblings. J. Pediatr. 60:33, 1962.

Contributor:　Janet M. Stewart

Editor's Computerized Descriptors: Hearing, Oral, Speech, Skel., GU.

DEAFNESS-SENSORINEURAL, DIVERTICULITIS, AND NEUROPATHY

Includes: Surdité neurosensorielle, diverticulite intestinale et neuropathie

Innenohrschwerhörigkeit, Dünnadarm-Divertikulose, und Neuropathie

Sordera neurosensorial, diverticulitis del intestino delgado y neuropatía

Excludes: Progressive sensorineural deafness and sensory radicular neuropathy

Syndrome of diverticulitis of the small intestine associated with steatorrhea with or without macrocytic anemia

Minimal Diagnostic Criteria: Not yet clear. Sensorineural deafness in childhood, absent gastric motility, small bowel diverticulitis, and progressive sensory neuropathy must be present.

Clinical Findings: A kindred has been reported in which 3 of 6 sibs showed the symptoms of this syndrome. The ages of onset of the progressive bilateral sensorineural deafness were 8, 3, and 9 years, respectively. At 10, 5, and 18 years, respectively, the deafness became total. Histologic examination of the temporal bones in the 1st case showed a type of cochleosaccular degeneration like that seen in the Scheibe type malformation. A history of hearing loss was present on the paternal side in 3 generations but was mild and had a much later onset (40 years or more). Vestibular function was normal in all 3 sibs. Abdominal cramps, vomiting, steatorrhea and hypoalbuminemic edema were present. There was progressive loss of gastric antral motility and multiple diverticula of the ileum and lower jejunum. Inflammation in the diverticula resulted in extensive small bowel ulceration at the mesenteric border diagnosed at autopsy in the 1st patient (age 18), at laparotomy in the 2nd, and is probably present in the 3rd girl. Progressive peripheral neurophathy was seen in all 3 sibs. Histologic examination of the sural nerve showed marked atrophy of the nerve bundles in a thick layer of fibrous tissue. It also showed demyelination of almost all nerve fibers.

Tendon reflexes at knees and ankles were hypoactive or absent. One sib experienced loss of sensation in fingers and toes, and had decreased corneal reflexes. Progressive peripheral sensory loss was noted in the fingertips and below the knees. Bilateral pes cavus was noted in the father and 2 of the affected sibs. Sinus tachycardia was present in all 3 sibs. Acanthosis nigricans developed in the 2 surviving sibs.

Complications
I **Derived:** Steatorrhea and low serum proteins with hypoalbuminemic edema
II **Associated:** —

Etiology: Postulated to be autosomal recessive

Pathogenesis: ?

Related Facts
I **Sex Ratio:** M0:F3
II **Risk of Occurrence:** ? Very rare
III **Risk of Recurrence for**
Patient's Sib: If autosomal recessive, 1 in 4 (25%) for each offspring to be affected
Patient's Child: Not increased unless mate is carrier or homozygote
IV **Age of Detectability:** Childhood or adolescence
V **Prevalence:** Single reported family with 3 affected sibs

Treatment
I **Primary Prevention:** Genetic counseling
II **Secondary Prevention:** Oral antibiotic therapy, medium chain triglyceride diet with methacholine chloride. Improvement of the acanthosis nigricans with topically applied vitamin A acid.
III **Other Therapy:** —

Prognosis: Poor because of the progressive nature of this disorder. One sib died, the 2nd is now bedridden.

Detection of Carrier: —

Special Considerations: —

References:
Groll, A. and Hirschowitz, B.I.: Steatorrhea and familial deafness in two siblings. Clin. Res. 14:47, 1966.

Groll, A. and Hirschowitz, B.I.: Steatorrhea and absent gastric antral motility in three female siblings with familial deafness. Ann. Intern. Med. 68:1147, 1968.

Hirschowitz, B.I. et al: Hereditary nerve deafness in three sisters with absent gastric motility, small bowel diverticulitis and ulceration, and progressive sensory neuropathy. In Bergsma D. (ed.): Part XIII. G.I. Tract Including Liver and Pancreas. Birth Defects: Orig. Art. Ser., vol. VIII, no. 2. Baltimore: Williams & Wilkins for The National Foundation-March of Dimes, 1972, p. 27.

Montes, L.F. et al: Acanthosis nigricans and hypovitaminosis A. Response of topical vitamin A acid. J. Cutan. Pathol. 1:88, 1974.

Contributor: **Cor W.R.J. Cremers**

Editor's Computerized Descriptors: Eye, Hearing, Skin, Skel., CV., GI., Nerve

DEAFNESS-SENSORINEURAL, DYSTONIA AND RETARDATION

Includes: Dystonie, surdité sensorielle, déficit intellectuel inconstant

Dystonie, Schalleitungs-Schwerhörigkeit, möglicherweise geistige Retardierung

Distonía, sordera neurosensorial y posible deterioro intelectual

Excludes: Familial myoclonus, cerebellar ataxia and deafness

Hepatolenticular degeneration (469)

Hyperuricemia, deafness and ataxia (508)

Minimal Diagnostic Criteria: The disease is suspected by the association of sensorineural hearing loss with later appearance of dystonic posturing and progressive deterioration. Mental retardation may be a part of this syndrome.

Clinical Findings: An 8-year-old male presented with deafness, severe dysarthria, striking deterioration of handwriting, occasional bizarre posturing of the head and neck, and hyperactive behavior. The pregnancy, perinatal period, as well as early growth and development, were reportedly normal. Audiometric testing at 2 years confirmed a sensorineural hearing loss. At 7 years his parents noticed increasing distortion of his handwriting as well as dystonic movements of his left hand, and neck. By 9 years he could not walk, was confined to a wheelchair with severe retrocollis in the upright position and was unable to articulate. Although he had a brief period of clinical improvement with L-dopa therapy, he continued to deteriorate and died at 11 years of age.

Although the parents of the proband are clinically normal, the proband's maternal uncle reportedly had hearing loss from age 6, subsequent progressive dystonic posturing, and died in his 20s. The proband's healthy 26-year-old sister has a 6-year-old son who has severe bilateral sensorineural hearing loss, lack of normal language development and severe psychomotor retardation.

Complications
I   **Derived:** Complications are related to the progressive nature of this disorder.
II **Associated:** —

Etiology: Probably X-linked recessive in this single family.†

Pathogenesis: Histopathologic examination of the proband's brain revealed neuronal loss and gliosis in both caudate nuclei, putamen and globus pallidus. Examination of the temporal bone revealed severe degeneration of the sensory epithelium and supporting cells in the basal turn of the cochlea, and absence of the organ of Corti.

Related Facts
I   **Sex Ratio:** M3:F0
II **Risk of Occurrence:** ?
III **Risk of Recurrence for**
     Patient's Sib: See Table I X-linked R
     Patient's Child: See Table I X-linked R. Affected patients unlikely to reproduce.
IV **Age of Detectability:** Onset of hearing loss is evidently present by age 6 with onset of movement disorder soon thereafter.
V   **Prevalence:** There seems to be only 1 reported family with this combination of findings.

Treatment
I   **Primary Prevention:** Genetic counseling
II **Secondary Prevention:** —
III **Other Therapy:** —

Prognosis: Poor

Detection of Carrier: If X-linked, mothers of male probands are obligate carriers. 50% of female sibs would also be expected to carry the mutant gene.

†Special Considerations: It should be noted that torsion dystonia without deafness has been reported in several families, fitting both autosomal dominant and autosomal recessive modes of inheritance.

References:

Eldridge, R.: The torsion dystonias: Literature review and genetic and clinical studies (dystonia musculorum deformans). Neurology (Minneap.) 20:1, 1970.

Scribanu, N. and Kennedy, C.: Familial syndrome with dystonia, neural deafness, and possible intellectual impairment. Clinical course and pathological findings. Adv. Neurol. 14:235, 1976.

Contributors: **Frederick R. Bieber**
                     Walter E. Nance

Editor's Computerized Descriptors: Hearing, Ear, Speech, Nerve

DEAFNESS-SENSORINEURAL, MIDFREQUENCY

Includes: Surdité de perception pour les ondes de fréquence moyenne
Schalleitungsschwerhörigkeit mit vorwiegendem Ausfall mittlerer Frequenzen
Sordera neurosensorial a las frecuencias medias
Hereditary midfrequency nerve loss
"U'-shaped hearing loss
Midfrequency sensorineural deafness

Excludes: Hereditary high-tone deafness
Hand muscle wasting and sensorineural deafness (450)

Minimal Diagnostic Criteria: There must be a hereditary nerve deafness with a loss in the midfrequencies. There is usually good discrimination considering the audiogram. There is no tone decay. The severer losses will show a positive short increment sensitivity index (SISI). No other hereditary defects are found.

Clinical Findings: Midfrequency sensorineural hearing loss is demonstrated by audiometry in members of a family. Several of the affected families show members with hereditary hearing loss, but not all audiometric patterns are "U'-shaped. Some are high-tone, others low-tone, and some flat. The hearing loss reported has been nonprogressive in some families and progressive in others. Other than the hearing impairment, the medical history, physical examination, neurologic and otolaryngologic examinations are negative. Vestibular testing, including caloric examination, is normal. In most of the affected people the hearing loss progressed slowly over the years, paralleling that of presbycusis.

Complications
I   **Derived:** Mild paranoia may develop
II **Associated:** —

Etiology: Possibly autosomal dominant†; McK *12470

Pathogenesis: In most cases a mild-to-moderate hearing loss in early school life is noted. Frequently the hereditary hearing impairment is known in other members of the family. The tone decay tests are usually negative tending to eliminate an 8th nerve lesion. The SISI is positive in most of the individuals with moderate-to-severe hearing loss suggesting a cochlear lesion, probably in the middle turn of the cochlea where the midfrequencies are found. Speech discrimination is remarkably good for the amount of hearing lost in the critical frequencies. In the families with the nonprogressive loss this can be explained by a learning process.

Related Facts
I   **Sex Ratio:** M1:F1 (In 5 families, 36 males: 28 females)
II **Risk of Occurrence:** ?
III **Risk of Recurrence for**
   Patient's Sib: If autosomal dominant and if parent is affected 1 in 2 (50%) for each offspring to be affected; otherwise not increased.
   Patient's Child: If autosomal dominant 1 in 2
IV **Age of Detectability:** In infancy if computerized brain wave response is used; 4-6 years of age if audiometry is employed
V   **Prevalence:** ?

Treatment
I   **Primary Prevention:** Genetic counseling
II **Secondary Prevention:** Hearing aids occasionally needed for socially adequate hearing.
III **Other Therapy:** —

Prognosis: Average life span unaffected, with minimal handicap.

Detection of Carrier: —

†**Special Considerations:** In several families some members showed a "U'-shaped deafness while others showed a high-tone or flat deafness. In some families all showed a "U'-shaped loss. Some families have progressive hearing loss, in others nonprogressive. The kindreds have not been large enough to determine whether we are dealing with 1, 2, or more types of genetic problems.

References:
Konigsmark, B.W. et al: Dominant midfrequency hearing loss. Ann. Otol. Rhinol. Laryngol. 79:42, 1970.
Martensson, B.: Dominant hereditary nerve deafness. Acta Otolaryngol. (Stockh.) 52:270, 1960.
Williams, F. and Roblee, L.A.: Hereditary nerve deafness. Arch. Otolaryngol. 75:69, 1962.

Contributor: **David A. Dolowitz**

Editor's Computerized Descriptor: Hearing

DEAFNESS-SENSORINEURAL, POLYNEUROPATHY AND OPTIC ATROPHY

Includes: Surdité de perception, polynéurite et atrophie optique
Innenohr-Schwerhörigkeit, Polyneuropathie und Opticusatrophie
Sordera neurosensorial, polineuropatía y atrofia óptica
Rosenberg-Chutorian syndrome
Charcot-Marie-Tooth disease with opticoacoustic degeneration
Optic atrophy, nerve deafness and distal neurogenic amyotrophy

Excludes: Phytanic acid storage disease (810)
Wolfram syndrome
Optic atrophy, infantile heredofamilial (755)
Leber optic atrophy (579)
Classic Charcot-Marie-Tooth disease and other spinocerebellar degenerations

Minimal Diagnostic Criteria: Sensorineural deafness, polyneuropathy, optic atrophy.

Clinical Findings: Five patients in 2 families have been described with this symptom complex. In 1 family, 2 brothers and their nephew (son of sister), in another family a brother and sister. Three cases presented in infancy with hearing loss, and 2 at age 8 with hand deformity (ulnar deviation, muscle weakness and wasting). Bilateral optic atrophy, especially temporal sided, resulting in loss of visual acuity beginning with nyctalopia, was seen in 4/5. Bilateral neurogenic hearing loss in 5/5, dysarthria or rhinolalia in 4/5. Gait was deteriorated (broad-based, ataxic) in 4/5. Distal amyotrophy of the upper limbs existed in 4/5 and of the lower limbs in 3/5. Distal sensory impairment was reported in 3/5, peripheral nerve conduction velocity was lowered in 3/5. Muscle biopsy showed features of neurogenic atrophy in 2/5; this was also revealed by EMG in 2/5. Demyelination was seen in sural nerve biopsy in 2/5. Bone deformity, including tarsal bone, chest and spine (scoliosis) occurred in 3/5. All patients had normal intelligence.†

Complications
I **Derived:** The impaired speech may be secondary to deafness. Bone deformities may be due to muscle atrophy.
II **Associated:** Communication handicaps occur, which influence school performance.

Etiology: Autosomal recessive inheritance is likely in the sib pair described by Iwashita et al. Inheritance may be X-linked recessive in the family reported by Rosenberg and Chutorian. Genetic heterogeneity probably exists.†

Pathogenesis: The loss of visual acuity and the hearing loss are caused by optic and acoustic nerve degeneration. The optic atrophy is believed to be due to retrobulbar neuritis. The amyotrophy may be due to motor neuron disease.

Related Facts
I **Sex Ratio:** M4:F1 of the 5 patients described
II **Risk of Occurrence:** ?
III **Risk of Recurrence for**
  Patient's Sib: When autosomal recessive or X-linked recessive, see Table AR or X-linked R, respectively.
  Patient's Child: When autosomal recessive or X-linked recessive, see Table AR or X-linked R, respectively.
IV **Age of Detectability:** In early infancy or youth
V **Prevalence:** ?

Treatment
I **Primary Prevention:** Genetic counseling
II **Secondary Prevention:** —
III **Other Therapy:** A hearing aid may be of help. Special instruction will be needed. Support by cane, braces and special shoes.

Prognosis: Poor for vision and hearing because of the progressive nature of the syndrome.

Detection of Carrier: ?

†Special Considerations: The 2 described families are similar, but not identical. It is difficult to be sure about the exact nosologic classification of this condition.

References:
Iwashita, H. et al: Optic atrophy, neural deafness and distal neurogenic amyotrophy. Arch. Neurol. 22:357, 1970.
Konigsmark, B.W. and Gorlin, R.J.: Optic atrophy, polyneuropathy and sensorineural deafness. In Genetic and Metabolic Deafness. Philadelphia: W.B. Saunders, 1976, p. 108.
Rosenberg, R.N. and Chutorian, A.: Familial optico-acoustic nerve degeneration and polyneuropathy. Neurology 17:827, 1967.

Contributors: **Agnes M. Ickenroth
Cor W.R.J. Cremers**

Editor's Computerized Descriptors: Vision, Eye, Hearing, Speech, Skel., Muscle, Nerve

DEAFNESS-SENSORINEURAL, PROGRESSIVE HIGH-TONE

Includes: Surdité héréditaire progressive pour les tons aigus
Erblicher, progressiver Hörnervlust für hohe Frequenzen
Sordera progresiva hereditaria para las frecuencias elevadas
Hearing loss, hereditary progressive high-tone type
Albrecht syndrome
Progressive high-tone nerve loss

Excludes: U—shaped nonprogressive nerve loss

Minimal Diagnostic Criteria: Progressive high-tone loss of hearing develops in children of families with an affected parent.†

Clinical Findings: During childhood a high-tone hearing loss develops. Recruitment is not demonstrable. Other than slight evidence of tone decay in the high tones there is no evidence of nerve involvement by this method. As the children with the trait become older the hearing impairment spreads, suggesting that the gene has the ability to change the rate of presbycusis.

Complications
I   **Derived:** —
II **Associated:** In one large kindred a parallel finding of nasal septal deviation was reported.

Etiology: Autosomal dominant with complete penetrance

Pathogenesis: ?

Related Facts
I   **Sex Ratio:** M1:F1
II **Risk of Occurrence:** ?
III **Risk of Recurrence for**
   Patient's Sib: If parent is affected 1 in 2 (50%) for each offspring to be affected; otherwise not increased.
   Patient's Child: 1 in 2
IV **Age of Detectability:** As soon as able to take a pure tone audiometric examination, namely 3-6 years of age depending on intelligence.
V   **Prevalence:** ?

Treatment
I   **Primary Prevention:** Genetic counseling
II **Secondary Prevention:** —
III **Other Therapy:** Lip reading or hearing aid in middle age.

Prognosis: Life span not affected - no cases developed total deafness - all could function with a hearing aid or lip reading.

Detection of Carrier: —

†Special Considerations: This condition is well known clinically. There is insufficient fully substantiated autopsy material for pathologic understanding and pathogenesis. The work done clinically shows no recruitment and minimal tone decay which suggests degeneration of the spiral ganglia cells rather than dissolution of the hair cells in the organ of Corti.

References:
Dolowitz, D.A. and Stephens, F.E.: Hereditary nerve deafness. Ann. Otol. Rhinol. Laryngol. 70:851, 1961.
Stephens, F.E. and Dolowitz, D.A.: Hereditary nerve deafness. Am. J. Hum. Genet. 1:37, 1949.

Contributor: David A. Dolowitz

Editor's Computerized Descriptors: Hearing, Nasoph.

DEAFNESS-SENSORINEURAL, RECESSIVE EARLY-ONSET

Includes: Surdité de perception précoce
Frühmanifeste recessive Taubheit
Sordera neural recesiva precoz
Recessive early-onset neural deafness

Excludes: Congenital severe neural deafness
Dominant congenital neural deafness
X-linked congenital neural deafness
X-linked early-onset neural deafness

Minimal Diagnostic Criteria: Severe hearing loss with evidence either by history or by sonogram that some hearing was present during early childhood. Evidence of recessive transmission.

Clinical Findings: During the first several years of life there is some hearing, evidenced by the child learning to speak a few words. Hearing deteriorates until by 5 or 6 years of age there is severe hearing loss. Audiometric testing when the child is 5 years old generally shows a 60-100 db symmetric sensorineural hearing loss. Hearing loss is so severe that no other audiometric tests can be done.
   Caloric vestibular tests show a normal response. Physical and neurologic examinations show no abnormalities except for the hearing loss. Laboratory tests including temporal bone tomograms are normal.

Complications
I   **Derived:** —
II **Associated:** —

Etiology: Autosomal recessive

Pathogenesis: ? †

Related Facts
I   **Sex Ratio:** M1:F1
II **Risk of Occurrence:** Not described in general U. S. population. In Mennonite population of Lancaster, Pa., risk is 1 in 500 live births.
III **Risk of Recurrence for**
   Patient's Sib: 1 in 4 (25%) for each offspring to be affected
   Patient's Child: Not increased unless mate is carrier or homozygote
IV **Age of Detectability:** One or 2 years of age
V   **Prevalence:** 1 in 500 of Mennonite population in Lancaster, Pa.

Treatment
I   **Primary Prevention:** Genetic counseling
II **Secondary Prevention:** The disease should be diagnosed as early as possible and hearing aids used during the period when the child is acquiring speech.
III **Other Therapy:** —

Prognosis: Normal for life span and intelligence

Detection of Carrier: ?

†Special Considerations: The hearing loss is probably due to degeneration, possibly of the hair cells in the organ of Corti as suggested by the following indirect evidence: neurologic examination shows no abnormalities; the vestibular system is also normal, and the inner ear is normal by tomogram.

References:
Mengel, M.C. et al: Recessive early-onset neural deafness. Acta Otolaryngol. (Stockh.) 64:313, 1967.

Contributor: Bruce W. Konigsmark‡

Editor's Computerized Descriptor: Hearing

DEAFNESS-SENSORINEURAL, RECESSIVE PROFOUND

Includes: Surdité sévere récessive neurosensorielle
Rezessive Schalleitungsschwerhörigkeit
Sordera neurosensorial profunda recesiva
Sensorineural deafness, profound
Deafness, severe isolated congenital
Recessive profound sensorineural deafness

Excludes: Progressive deafness
Mild-to-moderate familial deafness
Pre- or neonatally acquired deafness
Deafness occurring with other somatic anomalies or defects

Minimal Diagnostic Criteria: Sensorineural deafness, severe-to-profound. Nonprogressive deafness present at birth or during early months of life. The diagnosis cannot be considered as proved unless a similar deafness is ascertained in at least 1 more family member.

Clinical Findings: The deafness is sensorineural and essentially symmetric bilaterally, present at birth or shortly thereafter and nonprogressive after it becomes manifest. Audiometry shows severe hearing loss, ranging from no response to 80 db average in the speech frequencies. Because of the profundity of the loss, affected persons were in the past placed in manual (signing or finger spelling) programs, and were not trained to speak intelligibly. From this situation arose the term "deaf-mutism", which is a misnomer; none of these people are inherently "mute" except insofar as they have not had oral speech training. It is probable that as many as 45% of this group have no responses to standard audiometry, and the remainder chiefly respond only to the low frequencies: 250, 500 and 1000 Hz. Occasionally there is residual hearing throughout the audiometric range, but severely reduced to levels > 80 db.

Normal vestibular function is usually considered characteristic of this deafness, but some evidence suggests that 35% of this group have no response to rotation tests. Polytomography thus far has not been successful in identifying the pathology of this deafness.

Complications
I   Derived: Defective speech and language development results unless early training is instituted. Emotional problems can occur if the hearing loss is not recognized early and the child is not treated appropriately.
II   Associated: —

Etiology: Autosomal recessive with variable penetrance; several genes are probably involved, and these are capable of variable expression either in the homozygote or heterozygote. No interaction need occur when 2 different recessive genes are involved.

Pathogenesis: No specific histopathology has been identified for this type of deafness, but recessive deafness has been related to the cochleosaccular membranous labyrinth degeneration described by Scheibe. Ormerod suggests that the pathology may resemble that of albino animals with recessive deafness, in which there is attempted maturity of the ear structures, with subsequent degeneration of the scala media. In some, this occurs soon after birth.

Related Facts
I   Sex Ratio: M1:F1
II   Risk of Occurrence: ? Comprises about 22.5% of all deafness
III   Risk of Recurrence for
   Patient's Sib: 1 in 4 (25%) for each offspring to be affected
   Patient's Child: Not increased unless mate is carrier or homozygote for the same recessive gene or genes.
IV   Age of Detectability: When deafness occurs at birth or in the first months of life, it should be identifiable by hearing tests.
V   Prevalence: Phenotype frequency is 1 in 5000 to 1 in 330

Treatment
I   Primary Prevention: Genetic counseling
II   Secondary Prevention: Speech and language dysfunction may be ameliorated by early training in language through auditory or manual learning techniques and oral speech training.
III   Other Therapy: —

Prognosis: Normal for life span; probability is that hearing loss will be stable during life unless other exogenous effects act upon it. The prognosis for speech and language development is fairly good provided that intensive auditory or manual training techniques are instituted before 2 years of age.

Detection of Carrier: Reportedly it may be possible by Bekesy audiometric tests which reveal erratic dips in the audiometric configuration.

Special Considerations: —

References:
Anderson, H. and Wedenberg, E.: Audiometric identification of normal hearing carriers of genes for deafness. Acta Otolaryngol. (Stockh.) 65:535, 1968.
Black, F.O. et al: Congenital Deafness: A New Approach to Early Detection of Deafness Through a High Risk Register. Boulder:- Colorado Ass. University Press, 1971.
Chung, C.S. et al: A note on deafmutism. Ann. Hum. Genet. 23:357, 1959.
Fraser, G.R.: Profound childhood deafness. J. Med. Genet. 1:118, 1964.
Konigsmark, B.W.: Hereditary deafness in man (2nd of 3 parts). N. Engl. J. Med. 281:774, 1969.
Ormerod, F.C.: The pathology of congenital deafness. J. Laryngol. Otol. 74:919, 1960.
Stevenson, A.C. and Cheeseman, E.A.: Hereditary deafmutism, with particular reference to northern Ireland. Ann. Hum. Genet. 20:177, 1956.

Contributor: **Marion P. Downs**

_____

Editor's Computerized Descriptors: Hearing, Speech

DEAFNESS, STREPTOMYCIN-SENSITIVITY

Includes: Surdité causée par la streptomycine
Taubheit durch Streptomycin-Empfindlichkeit
Sordera por sensibilidad a la estreptomicina
Streptomycin-sensitivity deafness

Excludes: Hearing loss due to toxic doses of streptomycin

Minimal Diagnostic Criteria: Normal audiogram and renal function prior to starting streptomycin injections. Significant sensorineural hearing loss after small doses of streptomycin.†

Clinical Findings: Early onset of tinnitus and moderately severe-to-profound hearing loss, usually following small doses of streptomycin sulfate (4-30 gm). Audiometry shows sensorineural hearing loss of 50-100 db. Caloric testing showed either normal responses or directional preponderance. Sibs and parents who did not receive streptomycin had normal audiograms.

Complications
I **Derived:** Vestibular dysfunction
II **Associated:** —

Etiology: Presumed abnormal sensitivity to streptomycin, familial in nature, exact mode of transmission uncertain. The extrinsic causative factor is the chemical streptomycin sulfate. There is some overlap with the reported ototoxic dosage range (for hearing), given as 12-325 gm. However, this wide range may include at the lower end of the spectrum persons who previously had other ototoxic drugs causing subclinical hair cell loss in the inner ear, or initial loss of hair cells subserving high frequencies beyond the reach of conventional audiometry (ie beyond 8000 cps), followed by further hair cell loss due to streptomycin, which loss then became sufficient to cause clinically detectable hearing loss. On the other hand, some of the patients showing hearing loss in the lower dosage ranges may actually be those who demonstrate streptomycin sensitivity.†

Pathogenesis: The deafness and vestibular findings are probably due to destruction of hair cells in the inner ear. Available evidence suggests that initially the 1st row of outer hair cells at the basal turn degenerate and with increasing dosage there is gradual spread of degeneration to all 3 rows of outer hair cells in the basal coil and then progressively to other coils and all rows. Eventually, the inner hair cells also degenerate. The area of hair cell loss is filled in by progressive enlargement of adjacent supporting cells to form a "phalangeal scar," best seen on osmium-stained surface preparations using phase contrast microscopy. Finally, by conventional light microscopy virtually no trace of the organ of Corti can be seen. By electron microscopy, degeneration of neural elements can be seen to lag slightly behind that of the hair cells. The remnants of nerve endings form irregular clumps of dark granules. Later the nerve fibers become rarefied. However, certain nerve fiber bundles seem to be spared.

Related Facts
I **Sex Ratio:** M?:F? Only 1 family has been reported. Four sisters of the family were reported affected. Since the brother and father were not ill, they did not receive streptomycin. The mother also was untreated. Sporadic cases of moderate-to-profound hearing loss have been reported with relatively small doses (12-17 gm at 1 gm/day), but without positive family history. The reports have not specified the sex of all such affected persons.
II **Risk of Occurrence:** ?
III **Risk of Recurrence for**
  Patient's Sib: ?
  Patient's Child: ?

IV **Age of Detectability:** Depends on streptomycin intake
V **Prevalence:** ?

Treatment
I **Primary Prevention:** Avoidance of streptomycin in patients with positive family history of streptomycin sensitivity.
II **Secondary Prevention:** Hearing conservation, ie avoidance of further exposure to ototoxic drugs, avoidance of acoustic trauma and noise exposure and prompt treatment of ear infections.
III **Other Therapy:** Hearing aid, lip-reading and speech training as needed.

Prognosis: Hearing loss is permanent. No effect on life expectancy.

Detection of Carrier: —

†Special Considerations: More studies of affected families are needed to clarify this condition. Pathologic examination of affected ears would be valuable. A search for some genetically determined enzyme deficiency may be fruitful since some hypersensitivity reactions to other drugs have been shown to be on a genetic basis.

References:
Engström, H.H.H. et al: Structural Pattern of the Organ of Corti; a Systematic Mapping of Sensory Cells and Neural Elements. Stockholm: Almqvist & Wiksell, 1966.
Kalow, W.: How genetic factors affect individual drug responses. Hosp. Practice 2:92, 1967.
Pražic, M. et al: Familial sensitivity to streptomycin. J. Laryngol. Otol. 78:1037, 1964.

Contributor: **LaVonne Bergstrom**

***

Editor's Computerized Descriptors: Hearing

272-500

DEAFNESS, TUNE (MARKER)

Includes: Amusie
Incapacidad auditiva para la afinación
Tune deafness (Marker)

Excludes: —

Minimal Diagnostic Criteria: Individuals who are unable to recognize or reproduce (by singing or playing an instrument which is dependent on accurate pitch production) a tune or any series of pitches presented in sequence. These individuals have normal speaking voices, normal hearing and are usually free of neurologic deficits.

Clinical Findings: The affected individual is able to sing only in a monotone and apparently cannot be taught to sing in tune, although usually is able to reproduce the rhythm of the song. Apparently these individuals can be taught to play the piano or other instruments, where ability to distinguish correct pitch is not essential to producing an accurate rendition of the music. Audiometric tests are normal and such individuals often can distinguish differences in pure tone frequencies in isolation, but may be unable to make such discriminations when pitches are presented in groups, as in chords, or in sequence. In fact, cases have been recorded of individuals who had superior pitch discrimination but apparently could not learn the simplest tune. The speaking voice of tune deaf individuals shows all the pitch and modulation characteristics of normal persons. No laryngeal motor abnormalities have been suspected or detected. Appreciation and enjoyment of music may be present, and such individuals may be quite sensitive to the beauties of other forms of art. Often, however, tune deaf persons do not enjoy music.

Complications
I Derived: —
II Associated: —

Etiology: One or more dominant or recessive genes has been proposed. However, the influence of environment has not been disproved. The possibility of fetal or neonatal insult producing a specific learning disability has not been considered, but in the opinion of the author, cannot be ruled out.

Pathogenesis: ? It has been suggested that tune deafness is analogous to dyslexia or that there is some deficit in feedback mechanism, which prevents the individual from imitating a tone or series of tones. There is no information to suggest that neurologic or other learning deficits are more common in the tune deaf than in the general population.

Related Facts
I **Sex Ratio:** ? Possibly M1:F1, although 1 study of school children showed 7% of boys and only 1% of girls to be "monotones." However, this could be culturally determined.
II **Risk of Occurrence:** ?
III **Risk of Recurrence for**
Patient's Sib: ?
Patient's Child: ?
IV **Age of Detectability:** In early childhood or by school years
V **Prevalence:** 1 in 20 of the adult population

Treatment
I **Primary Prevention:** —
II **Secondary Prevention:** There is some evidence that intensive coaching of children aged 3-5 can significantly improve pitch discrimination.
III **Other Therapy:** —

Prognosis: Some tune deaf individuals may outgrow or overcome their deficiency by about age 12. The reason for this is unknown.

Detection of Carrier: —

Special Considerations: —

References:
Cuddy, L.L.: Practice effects in the absolute judgment of pitch. J. Acoust. Soc. Am. 43:1069, 1968.
Deutsch, D.: Music recognition. Psychol. Rev. 76:300, 1969.
Kalmus, H.: Inherited sense defects. Sci. Am. 186:64, 1952.
Shuter, R.: Hereditary and environmental factors in musical ability. Eugen. Rev. 48:149, 1966.

Contributor: **LaVonne Bergstrom**

Editor's Computerized Descriptor: Hearing

DEAFNESS, UNILATERAL INNER EAR

Includes: Surdité de perception (unilatérale)
Einseitige Schallempfindungsschwerhörigkeit
Sordera del oído interno unilateral
Sensorineural unilateral hearing loss
Deafness, congenital unilateral
Unilateral inner ear deafness

Excludes: Deafness and absent incudo-stapedial junction (244)
Syndromes which include unilateral hearing loss
Acquired sensorineural hearing loss
Hand muscle wasting and sensorineural deafness (450)
Deafness-sensorineural, midfrequency (267)

Minimal Diagnostic Criteria: Sensorineural unilateral hearing loss. Polytomographic demonstration of unilateral otic capsule abnormality may be possible.
Positive evidence is difficult without postmortem.†

Clinical Findings: Late recognition is common because of functioning contralateral ear. Unilateral sensorineural hearing loss detectable with audiometric testing. History may be positive or negative for intrauterine disease, (ie viral infection 1st trimester). Family history may be positive or negative for unilateral hearing loss. External ear may be normal or abnormal, (ie associated branchial arch syndrome). Vestibular responses may be normal or abnormal. (Normal caloric responses expected in the Scheibe type abnormality). Petrous pyramid polytomography is abnormal in the Michel and Mondini-Alexander types and is normal in the Siebenmann-Bing and the Scheibe types.

Complications
I **Derived:** Abnormalities of otic capsule have been shown to predispose to otogenic meningitis secondary to otitis media. Possible increase in susceptibility to loss of hearing in contralateral ear.
II **Associated:** —

Etiology: Possibly autosomal dominant

Pathogenesis: Maldevelopment or regression of various components of the inner ear

Related Facts
I **Sex Ratio:** M1:F1
II **Risk of Occurrence:** ?
III **Risk of Recurrence for**
   Patient's Sib: If autosomal dominant and if parent is affected 1 in 2 (50%) for each offspring to be affected; otherwise not increased.
   Patient's Child: If autosomal dominant, 1 in 2
IV **Age of Detectability:** Usually late when using standard hearing testing with careful masking. Possible screening method under laboratory use (PAR technique) not yet tested clinically.
V **Prevalence:** ? Not known for unilateral congenital deafness in general population. Ten percent of severe unilateral deafness related to hereditary factors.

Treatment
I **Primary Prevention:** —
II **Secondary Prevention:** Early monaural screening for hearing defects
III **Other Therapy:** Regular otologic attention to avoid acquired hearing loss in normal contralateral ear. Preferential seating in school.

Prognosis: Normal for life span. Functionally very good unless contralateral ear is affected by other pathology.

Detection of Carrier: —

†Special Considerations: Unilateral congenital deafness is discovered only with difficulty. This disorder may represent an incomplete expression of the more common bilateral congenital deafness. The normal functioning contralateral ear allows adequate speech development. Free field hearing tests would not reveal the abnormality. Late recognition using standard audiometric techniques is usually the case. Some clues for detection would include signs such as inability to use telephone with both ears. This could probably be used as a simple screening test for severe unilateral hearing loss. The most striking histologic feature distinguishing congenital hereditary deafness of the membranous type from congenital-acquired (ie maternal rubella) remains the irregular cochlear duct dilation in the former with normal size or collapse in the latter. Acquired abnormalities of the osseous labyrinth, detectable with polytomography, are rare. Therefore, this radiologic finding, particularly in the absence of a positive history for labyrinthitis or meningitis, would be highly suggestive of a congenital disorder.

References:
Cohn, A.M. et al: Inner ear pathology in unilateral congenital deafness. Ann. Otol. Rhinol. Laryngol. 77:42, 1968.
McConnell, F. and Ward, P. H. (eds.): Deafness in Childhood. Nashville:Vanderbilt University Press, 1967.
Proctor, C. A. and Proctor, B.: Understanding hereditary nerve deafness. Arch. Otolaryngol. 85:23, 1967.

Contributor: **Robert I. Kohut**

Editor's Computerized Descriptors: Hearing, Ear

DEAFNESS, VITILIGO AND MUSCLE WASTING

Includes: Surdité, nanisme, vitiligo, hypotrophie musculaire et achalasie

Taubheit, Kleinwuchs, Vitiligo, Muskelhypotrophie und Achalasie

Sordera, estatura baja, vitíligo, emaciación muscular y acalasia

Sensorineural deafness, short stature, vitiligo, muscle wasting and achalasia

Excludes: Infantile achalasia

Oto-oculo-musculo-skeletal syndrome (785)

Minimal Diagnostic Criteria: Deafness, vitiligo, muscle wasting, achalasia

Clinical Findings: Two children, a boy and a girl, in a family with a consanguineous marriage and sporadic deafness in another part of the family, have been described with the features of this syndrome. The presenting sign was early childhood deafness. In both sibs there was sensorineural hearing loss > 100 db. The achalasia was the cause of frequent vomiting and difficulty in swallowing. Depigmented areas of vitiligo were present on their necks and torsos. Marked muscle wasting was noted in the hands, feet, and legs. Short stature was present only in the boy. Morphologic studies of a biopsy of the boy's anterior tibialis muscle revealed typical groups of small fibers indicative of a neuropathic process. Electromyographic studies performed on both patients were indicative of a neuropathic process with additional evidence of myopathy. Changes in EEG, globulin levels, thymol turbidity test and cephalin-cholesterol flocculation were found. The dermatoglyphics revealed a rare radial loop on R2 of the boy, and R4 on the girl.

Complications

I **Derived:** Failure to thrive and recurrent pneumonia due to achalasia.

II **Associated:** —

Etiology: Probably autosomal recessive

Pathogenesis: —

Related Facts

I **Sex Ratio:** M1:F1 Only 1 boy and 1 girl have been described.

II **Risk of Occurrence:** —

III **Risk of Recurrence for**

Patient's Sib: If autosomal recessive 1 in 4 (25%) for each offspring to be affected.

Patient's Child: If autosomal recessive, not increased unless mate is carrier or homozygote.

IV **Age of Detectability:** Early childhood

V **Prevalence:** 1 reported family with 2 affected sibs

Treatment

I **Primary Prevention:** Genetic counseling

II **Secondary Prevention:** Esophageal dilatation by dilatator or surgical intervention to relieve esophageal obstruction.

III **Other Therapy:** A hearing aid and special education at a school for the deaf.

Prognosis: ?

Detection of Carrier: —

Special Considerations: —

References:

Rozycki, D.L. et al: Autosomal recessive deafness, associated with short stature, vitiligo, muscle wasting and achalasia. Arch. Otolaryngol. 93:194, 1971.

Contributor: **Cor W.R.J. Cremers**

DENS IN DENTE

275-500

Includes: Invagination dentaire

Excludes: Lobodontia (607)

Minimal Diagnostic Criteria: The tooth must show an invagination in enamel or cementum in which there is a direct connection of the outer layer with the inner layer of enamel, or in radicular invaginations of cementum in roentgenograms, or by gross or histologic sections.

Clinical Findings: An invagination of tooth structure, enamel, dentin or cementum, within the crown or root of tooth giving the appearance on roentgenograms of a tooth within a tooth. Teeth affected may be normal, barrel-or peg-shaped. There are no generalized effects.

The teeth affected in order of frequency are:

Maxillary lateral incisors	77%
Maxillary central incisors	6%

Of maxillary incisors only:

Lateral incisor	88%
Central incisor	12%
Unilateral occurrence	40%
Bilateral occurrence	60%

1st, 2nd and 3rd -

maxillary and mandibular molars	5%
Maxillary and mandibular bicuspids	4%
Supernumerary teeth	4%
Maxillary cuspids	3%
Mandibular Incisors	0.4%

The abnormality is found in various degrees:

As a pit in the cingulum of incisors	26.8%
Involving cingulum and pulp chamber	63.9%
Involving cingulum, pulp chamber and root	9.3%
Two or more invaginations in 1 tooth	4.0%

Complications
I **Derived:** Pulpal necrosis or death leading to periapical abscesses, granulomas or cysts. Internal root resorption or pulp stones may also be a sequela of defect.
II **Associated:** Occurs in lobodontia.

Etiology: Essentially unknown. Theories include retardation in growth, constriction due to pressure, an abnormal ingrowth of the tooth, abnormal morphodifferentiation, atavism, trauma, infection, or an invagination of the dental papilla. The condition is possibly a gene(s) mutation resulting in an autosomal dominantly transmitted trait. Hereditary pattern not clear.†

Pathogenesis: Essentially unknown but appears to result from an invagination of dental enamel organ into pulpal space during tooth development.

Related Facts
I **Sex Ratio:** M1:F1
II **Risk of Occurrence:** ?
III **Risk of Recurrence for**
  Patient's Sib: 32%†
  Patient's Child: 43%†
IV **Age of Detectability:** After the coronal portion of the tooth has calcified by radiographs.
V **Prevalence:** In Caucasians, 1 in 77 or 1.31% in a sample of 24,997. Possibly higher in Asians, Indians, and Malaysians. It is rarely seen in Negroes.

Treatment

I **Primary Prevention:** —
II **Secondary Prevention:** Prophylactic dental filling
III **Other Therapy:** Removal of the tooth, possibly root canal treatment

Prognosis: If the defect is treated by means of prophylactic dental filling, a normal life span of the tooth can be expected. If the defect is not treated, a premature loss of the tooth can be expected.

Detection of Carrier: ?

†**Special Considerations:** Risk figures were derived from 26 families wherein 1 member showed the trait. Kindred analysis suggests a dominantly inherited trait with reduced penetrance but is also compatible with a common recessive trait. A definite mode of inheritance has not been determined.

References:
Grahnen, H. et al: Dens invaginatus. I. Clinical, roentgenological, and genetical study of permanent upper lateral incisors. Odontol. Revy. 10:115, 1959.
Hallett, G.E.M.: The incidence, nature and clinical significance of palatal invaginations in the maxillary incisor teeth. Proc. R. Soc. Med. 46:491, 1953.
Oehlers, F.A.C.: Dens invaginatus (dilated composite odontome). I. Variations of the invagination process and associated anterior crown forms. Oral Surg. 10:1204, 1957.

Contributor: **Thomas J. McCarter**

Editor's Computerized Descriptor: Teeth

DENTIN DYSPLASIA, CORONAL

Includes: Dysplasie de la dentine coronaire
Koronare Dentin-Dysplasie
Displasia de la dentina coronaria
Dentin dysplasia, type II
Coronal dentin dysplasia

Excludes: Dentin dysplasia, radicular (278)
Dentino-osseous dysplasia (280)
Dentinogenesis imperfecta† (279)
Osteogenesis imperfecta (777)
Fibrous dysplasia of dentin
Branchio-skeleto-genital syndrome (118)
Pulpal dysplasia† (843)
Calcinosis
Ehlers-Danlos syndrome (338)
Teeth, thistle-shaped pulp chambers (937)
Odontodysplasia (739)

Minimal Diagnostic Criteria: Opalescent primary teeth and normal appearing permanent teeth.

Clinical Findings: Primary teeth are brownish-blue with a translucent opalescent sheen and are identical in appearance to teeth seen in dentinogenesis imperfecta.† Permanent teeth are normal in color, size, and shape. Radiographically, the primary teeth have obliterated pulp chambers and reduced root canals. The permanent teeth have flame-shaped pulp chambers often with a radicular extension and numerous pulp stones. Root formation in permanent teeth is usually normal. Primary teeth abrade rapidly.

Complications
I Derived: —
II Associated: —

Etiology: Autosomal dominant; McK *12542

Pathogenesis: ? The dentin of primary teeth is amorphous resembling a grey granular gelatin with vestiges of tubule formation. The permanent teeth have normal tubular dentin with osteo and tubular denticles in the pulp chamber which is flame-shaped. With age, the pulp chamber becomes obliterated in permanent teeth.

Related Facts
I Sex Ratio: M1:F1
II Risk of Occurrence: ?
III Risk of Recurrence for
    Patient's Sib: If parent is affected, 1 in 2 (50%) for each offspring to be affected; otherwise not increased.
    Patient's Child: 1 in 2
IV Age of Detectability: At 9 to 18 months, upon eruption of primary teeth by visual and radiologic examination.
V Prevalence: ? Rare

Treatment
I Primary Prevention: Genetic counseling
II Secondary Prevention: Crowning of primary teeth. Acid etch restorations.
III Other Therapy: —

Prognosis: Premature loss of teeth may be slightly increased.

Detection of Carrier: —

†Special Considerations: Must be differentiated from dentinogenesis imperfecta in which teeth of both dentitions are opalescent, and from pulpal dysplasia which is associated with growth and developmental retardation.

References:
Giansanti, J.S. and Allen, J.D.: Dentin dysplasia, type II, or dentin dysplasia, coronal type. Oral Surg. 38:911, 1974.
Shields, E.P. et al: A proposed classification for heritable human dentine defects with a description of a new entity. Arch. Oral Biol. 18:543, 1973.

Witkop, C.J., Jr. : Hereditary defects of dentin. Dent. Clin. North Am. 19:25, 1975.

Contributor: **Carl J. Witkop, Jr.**

Editor's Computerized Descriptor: Teeth

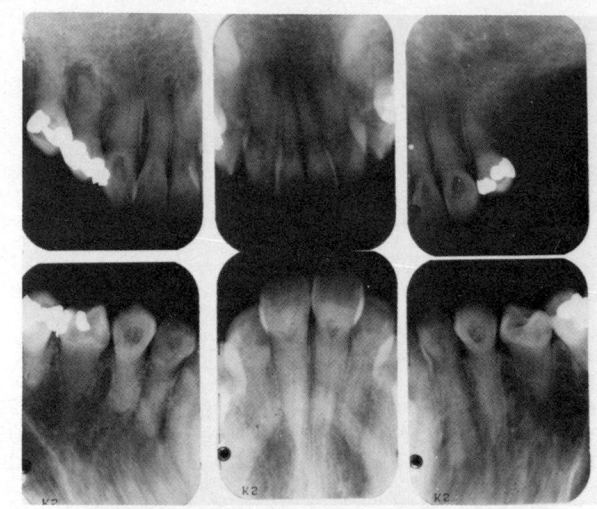

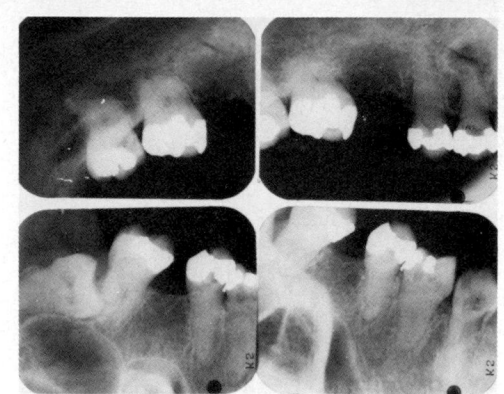

219. Coronal dentin dysplasia

DENTIN DYSPLASIA, RADICULAR

Includes: Dysplasie de la dentine radiculaire
Dentin dysplasie, Typ I
Displasia de la dentina radicular
Rootless teeth
Radicular dentin dysplasia
Dentin dysplasia, type I
Nonopalescent opalescent dentine

Excludes: Dentinogenesis imperfecta (279)
Odontodysplasia (739)
Dentin dysplasia, coronal (277)
Fibrous dysplasia of dentin
Dentino-osseous dysplasia (280)
Branchio-skeleto-genital syndrome (118)
Pulpal dysplasia (843)
Calcinosis
Ehlers-Danlos syndrome (338)
Teeth, thistle-shaped pulp chambers (937)
Osteogenesis imperfecta (777)

Minimal Diagnostic Criteria: Normal colored teeth which by roentgenologic examinations lack pulp chambers or have half-moon shaped pulp chambers and short or abnormal shaped roots.

Clinical Findings: Both dentitions affected. Teeth usually normal in color and contour of crowns, but may have a bluish-brown hue. Teeth are frequently malaligned in arch with a history of drifting. Roentgenographic alterations include absent or half-moon shaped pulp chambers - 100%; short or abnormal shaped roots - 80%; radiolucent areas around roots - 20%. Coronal dentin and enamel histologically normal. Radicular and pulp areas filled with foci of dentin formed in the dental papilla surrounded by dentin formed from the normal root development. The histologic picture resembles a stream flowing around boulders. Vascular channels cap the foci of dentin formed in the papilla. Periapical lesions are radicular cysts. Teeth may exfoliate spontaneously or with minor trauma.†

Complications
I **Derived:** Spontaneous exfoliation of teeth, premature loss of teeth and destruction of jaws by cyst expansion.
II **Associated:** —

Etiology: Autosomal dominant. Five of 22 propositi have had normal parents which may indicate either genetic heterogeneity, lack of penetrance, or high mutation rate. McK *12540

Pathogenesis: A defect in the epithelial root sheath which invades the radicular area and induces mesenchymal cells at many foci to undergo transformation to odontoblasts. These odontoblasts lay down multiple areas of dentin which fuse and become surrounded by a layer of more normal radicular dentin resulting in complete or nearly complete obliteration of pulp chambers and root canals and short abnormal roots. Epithelial rests undergo cystic degeneration forming periapical cysts.

Related Facts
I **Sex Ratio:** M1:F1
II **Risk of Occurrence:** 1 in 50,000 among North American Caucasians
III **Risk of Recurrence for**
Patient's Sib: If parent is affected 1 in 2 (50%) for each offspring to be affected; otherwise not increased.
Patient's Child: 1 in 2
IV **Age of Detectability:** By roentgenologic examination at time of eruption of teeth, 9 to 18 months of age
V **Prevalence:** 1 in 50,000 North American Caucasians

Treatment
I **Primary Prevention:** Genetic counseling
II **Secondary Prevention:** Prosthetic replacement of teeth, extraction, and surgical treatment of cysts
III **Other Therapy:** —

Prognosis: No apparent effect on longevity. Usually complete loss of teeth by 3rd to 4th decade.

Detection of Carrier: —

†Special Considerations: Clinically and histologically identical teeth also occur in dentinoosseous dysplasia and in the branchio-skeleto-genital syndrome.

References:
Bruszt, P.: Sur deux cas de dysplasie dentinaire. Bull. Group. Int. Rech. Sci. Stomatol. 12:107, 1969.
Rushton, M. A.: Anomalies of human dentine. Ann. R. Coll. Surg. Engl. 16:94, 1955.
Sauk, J.J., Jr. et al: An electron optic analysis and explanation for the etiology of dentinal dysplasia. Oral Surg. 33:763, 1972.
Shields, E. D. et al: Heritable defects in dentine; description, differentiation and classification. Arch. Oral Biol. 18:543, 1973.
Witkop, C.J., Jr.: Hereditary defects of dentin. Dent. Clin. North Am. 19:25, 1975.

Contributor: **Carl J. Witkop, Jr.**

Editor's Computerized Descriptor: Teeth

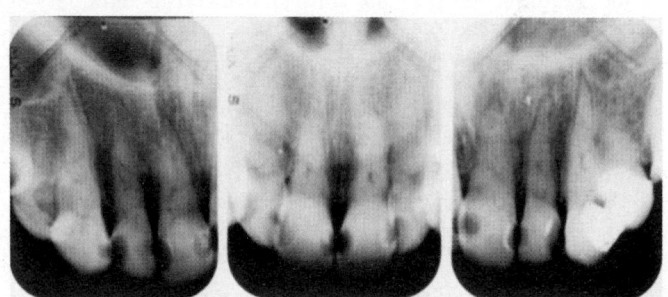
220. Radicular dentin dysplasia

DENTINOGENESIS IMPERFECTA

Includes: Dentinogénèse imparfaite
Opalescent dentin

Excludes: Osteogenesis imperfecta (777)
Odontodysplasia (739)
Branchio-skeleto-genital syndrome (118)
Calcinosis
Ehlers-Danlos syndrome (338)
Pulpal dysplasia (843)
Dentin dysplasia, radicular (278)
Dentin dysplasia, coronal (277)
Fibrous dysplasia of dentin
Dentino-osseous dysplasia (280)

Minimal Diagnostic Criteria: Roentgenologic finding of lack of any pulp chambers in opalescent teeth.†

Clinical Findings: All teeth in both dentitions affected. Teeth bluish-brown to brown in color with opalescent sheen. Crowns are bulbous-shaped. Enamel hypoplastic in about 20%. Enamel fractures and easily abrades. Teeth wear rapidly, and in adults, only roots may remain. Lack of history of repeated fractures and absence of other signs of osteogenesis imperfecta.

Roentgenograms show absence of pulp chambers and root canals. A few may show normal or large chambers or canals as a variation in expressivity.† Short thin roots.

Histologically there are scanty atypical tubules of varying width and length. Interglobular dentin. Lack of scalloping in most cases at dentinoenamel junction. Cell remnants embedded in dentin.

Complications
I **Derived:** Secondary hypoplasia of alveolar process probably from loss of occlusal tooth surface resulting in large gingivae and alveolar ridges. Premature loss of teeth by attrition and pulp exposure and fractures of crown. Occasional periapical cyst formation occurs but less frequently than seen in dentin dysplasia.
II **Associated:** —

Etiology: Autosomal dominant trait of high penetrance, low mutation rate and with variability in expression. Some evidence for linkage with phenylthiocarbamide (PTC) taste ability. McK *12550

Pathogenesis: A defect in odontoblasts which form a defective periodic acid Schiff (PAS) positive matrix. Odontoblasts differentiate and lay down 1-2 mm of fairly normal appearing tubules adjacent to dentinoenamel junction. This layer of odontoblasts degenerates and new layer differentiates from mesenchyme and lays down 1-2 mm of atypical dentin. This process continues until tooth is completely filled. Dentin matrix does not calcify properly, resulting in interglobular type of dentin.

Related Facts
I **Sex Ratio:** M55:F45 Several large studies of over 600 affected persons and their normal sibs have shown a consistent and statistically significant deviation of the expected 1:1 ratio.
II **Risk of Occurrence:** ?
III **Risk of Recurrence for**
    Patient's Sib: If parent is affected, 1 in 2 (50%) for each offspring to be affected; otherwise not increased.
    Patient's Child: 1 in 2†
IV **Age of Detectability:** Upon eruption of teeth at 9-18 months by visual and roentgenologic examination
V **Prevalence:** 1 in 8000 general North American population. Occurs in isolates in higher prevalence. Highest known, Brandywine isolate of Maryland 1 in 15.† Reported nearly exclusively in people of Caucasian ancestry, especially tracing ancestry to Normandy. Unreported in pure Negroes,

Asiatics or Australoid populations.

Treatment
I **Primary Prevention:** Genetic counseling
II **Secondary Prevention:** Crowning usually fails unless teeth are well formed. Children 4-15 years: do NOT extract teeth. Place full denture prosthesis over teeth to maintain alveolar ridge. Adults: full-mouth extraction and prosthetic replacements. Caution! Teeth soft and crush under forcep pressure. Extract by elevation. Recommend treatment at early age as these unsightly teeth affect psychosocial development.
III **Other Therapy:** Alveolectomy may be needed in older children and adults prior to prosthetic replacement.

Prognosis: No decreased longevity in either treated or untreated cases. Early loss of teeth. Risk of alveolar infection. Untreated cases usually develop psychosocial retardation.†

Detection of Carrier: —

†Special Considerations: Genetic heterogeneity may exist in this category. Shields and associates feel that the Brandywine triracial isolate type with an occasional child showing large pulp chambers in primary teeth is a different disease than that found in most families. Studies to date have not shown definitive collagen or glycosaminoglycan differences in the Brandywine type and what these authors term dentinogenesis imperfecta type I (hereditary opalescent dentin).

An occasional variation in the expressivity of this gene is encountered in kindreds of the classic disease. These variants usually affect primary teeth which demonstrate normal-sized or very large pulp chambers (shell teeth). Sections reveal a reduced or absent layer of odontoblasts on the pulpal surface in these instances. Several reports of isolated cases have designated such cases as a separate entity; however, permanent teeth of relatives usually show the classic disease picture. Must be differentiated from dentin dysplasia which usually has a remnant of pulp chamber visible on roentgenologic examination.

Two large studies indicate that there is a significantly increased effective reproductive fitness of 30-35% of affected individuals over their unaffected sibs and the population from which they were derived. Among a triracial isolate, all of the excess was attributable to excess male reproduction and among North American Caucasians to excess female reproduction, possibly indicating psychosocial factors involved with unsightly teeth.

References:
Rushton, M.A.: Anomalies of human dentine; Charles Tomes lecture. Ann. R. Coll. Surg. Engl. 16:94, 1955.
Shields, E.P. et al: A proposed classification for heritable human dentine defects with a description of a new entity. Arch. Oral Biol. 18:543, 1973.
Witkop, C.J., Jr. et al: Medical and dental findings in the Brandywine isolate. Ala. J. Med. Sci. 3:382, 1966.
Witkop, C.J., Jr.: Manifestations of genetic disease in the human pulp. Oral Surg. 32:278, 1971.

Contributor: Carl J. Witkop, Jr.

Editor's Computerized Descriptors: Oral, Teeth
Also see Section I, Fig. 82

DENTINO-OSSEOUS DYSPLASIA

Includes: Dysplasie de la dentition et de l'os
Osseo-dentine Dysplasie
Displasia dentino ósea
Dentin dysplasia with sclerotic bone and skeletal anomalies

Excludes: Dentin dysplasia, radicular† (278)
Dentin dysplasia, coronal† (277)
Dentinogenesis imperfecta (279)
Osteogenesis imperfecta (777)
Fibrous dysplasia of dentin
Branchio-skeleto-genital syndrome† (118)
Pulpal dysplasia (843)
Calcinosis
Ehlers-Danlos syndrome (338)
Teeth, thistle-shaped pulp chambers (937)
Odontodysplasia (739)

Minimal Diagnostic Criteria: Teeth with short roots, obliteration of pulp chambers, and thickened dense cortices of long bones.

Clinical Findings: Both dentitions are affected with dentin dysplasia, radicular type, in which the teeth are of normal color and radiographically show short abnormal roots, lack pulp chambers or have small demilune-shaped pulp chambers and numerous periapical radiolucencies. These latter lesions are areas of granulation tissue. In addition all affected patients have dense thickened cortical layers of bone affecting primarily the long bones, fine trabecular pattern of medullary bone, calcified epiphyseal disks, abnormalities of carpal bones with large sesamoid bones in the hand, exostoses of hand and wrist bones, and medial displacement of thumbs.

Complications
I Derived: Spontaneous exfoliation of teeth.
II Associated: —

Etiology: Autosomal dominant

Pathogenesis: ? Histologically the teeth are identical to those seen in radicular dentin dysplasia with pulpal foci of tubular dentin type denticles surrounded by normal dentin of the radicular sheath. Each denticle is capped by a vascular channel. Epithelial root sheath fragments and invades dental papilla where mesenchymal cells are stimulated to transform into functional odontoblasts, lay down foci of dentin which subsequently become incorporated into the dentin of the developing roots.

Related Facts
I Sex Ratio: M1:F1
II Risk of Occurrence: ?
III Risk of Recurrence for
   Patient's Sib: If parent is affected 1 in 2 (50%) for each offspring to be affected; otherwise not increased
   Patient's Child: 1 in 2
IV Age of Detectability: By radiographic examination, at time of eruption of teeth 9-18 months of age.
V Prevalence: Very rare, 1 large kindred reported.

Treatment
I Primary Prevention: Genetic counseling
II Secondary Prevention: Prosthetic replacement of teeth
III Other Therapy: —

Prognosis: ? Does not appear to decrease longevity. Risk for early loss of teeth.

Detection of Carrier: —

†Special Considerations: Must be differentiated from coronal dentin dysplasia, radicular dentin dysplasia and branchio-skeleto-genital syndrome.

References:

Morris, M.E. and Augsburger, R.H.: Dentine dysplasia with sclerotic bone and skeletal anomalies inherited as an autosomal dominant trait. A new syndrome. Oral Surg. 43(2):267, 1977.

Contributors: **Carl J. Witkop, Jr.**
Merle E. Morris

Editor's Computerized Descriptors: Teeth, Skel.

DERMAL HYPOPLASIA, FOCAL

Includes: Hypoplasie dermique en foyers
Hypoplasia cutis circumscripta
Hipoplasia dérmica focal
Goltz-Gorlin syndrome

Excludes: Poikiloderma congenita
Incontinentia pigmenti (526)
Epidermal nevus syndrome

Minimal Diagnostic Criteria: Dermal hypoplasia with protrusion of fat, areas of underdevelopment and thinness of skin, forming reticular, vermiform, cribriform or sometimes linear streaks.

Clinical Findings: Widespread foci of dermal hypoplasia with herniation of fat and red streaking of the skin (100%). Frequent papillomas of the lips, gums, anus, vulva; sparsity of hair; small stature; asymmetry of face, trunk and limbs; mental retardation, and a variety of cutaneous, skeletal, ocular, oral, dental or soft tissue defects as follows.†

Cutaneous abnormalities: Area of underdevelopment and thinness of skin - reticular, vermiform, cribriform, frequently linear, localized herniations of subcutaneous fat through the attenuated dermis, total absence of the skin from various sites at birth, linear or reticular areas of hyper- or depigmentation of the skin, telangiectasia, papillomas of the lips, gums, base of tongue, circumoral area, anus, vulva, inguinal, axillary and periumbilical skin, an initial inflammatory or desquamative phase, onset with blistering and crusting, urtication or intense reddening of the skin on stroking; lichenoid, follicular hyperkeratotic papules, keratotic lesions on palms and soles, radial folds around the mouth, disorders of sweating (hypo- or hyperhidrosis) especially of palms and soles; scalp hair sparse and brittle, hair totally lacking from small areas of scalp or pubis, localized poliosis; finger and toenails absent, poorly developed, dystrophic, spooned, grooved or depigmented.

Skeletal defects: Small stature, microcrania, rounded skull, pointed chin, thinness and deviation of nasal septum, prognathism, spinal anomalies, kyphosis, scoliosis, fusion and sacralization of vertebrae, spina bifida occulta, anomalies of vertebrae, rudimentary tail, asymmetric development of face, trunk or limbs, absence of part of limb, deformity of bones, anomalies of hands and feet, hypoplasia or absence of digits, polydactyly, claw hand, split hand, syndactyly, fusion of phalanges, camptodactyly, clinodactyly, valgus deformity, generalized osteoporosis.

Ocular anomalies: Anophthalmia, aniridia, wide spacing of eyes, strabismus, nystagmus, heterochromia, blue sclerae, irregularity of pupils, colobomas of iris, choroid, retina, optic nerve, subluxation of lens, microphthalmia, patchy de - or hyperpigmentation of retina, optic atrophy, clouding of cornea or vitreous, ectropion, ptosis, blockage of tear ducts with epiphora.

Oral and dental anomalies: Prognathism, underdevelopment of mandible, overbite, microdontia, dysplasia of teeth, agenesis of teeth, extra incisor, irregular spacing and malocclusion, enamel defects with caries, notching of upper and lower incisors, harelip, high-arched palate, defect in alveolar ridge, median cleft of tongue, double lingual frenulum, hemihypoplasia of tongue, absence of labial sulcus, hypertrophy of gums.

Soft tissue defects: Asymmetry of face, notching or underdevelopment of ala nasi, protrusion and asymmetry of ears, hypoplasia of helix, auricular appendage, combined neurosensory and conductive hearing loss, branchial cleft, mental retardation, thenar and hypothenar hypoplasia, diastasis recti, omphalocele, defect in abdominal muscula-ture, hernia, inguinal, umbilical, rectal prolapse, asymmetry of breast, with lateral displacement of areola, cardiac anomaly (aortic stenosis?) (atrial septal defect with pulmonary hypertension), abnormalities of kidney and ureter, papilloma of stomach wall.

Complications
I **Derived:** Dependent upon associated defects
II **Associated:** Mental retardation, epileptiform seizures

Etiology: Unclear; autosomal dominant or X-linked dominant with lethality in males. McK *30560

Pathogenesis: The preponderance of affected girls and the possibility of increase in miscarriages in mothers, suggests that the syndrome in its fullest expression is lethal in males. The chromosomes of the peripheral blood have been normal in 7 reported cases. The hand anomalies suggest that the abnormal development in this condition occurs before the 8th week of gestation because the digits normally have elongated and separated by that time.

Related Facts
I **Sex Ratio:** M3:F45
II **Risk of Occurrence:** ?
III **Risk of Recurrence for**
  Patient's Sib: No reports of more than 1 case in a sibship, but frequent maternal history of abortions, miscarriages and stillbirths.
  Patient's Child: ?
IV **Age of Detectability:** At birth
V **Prevalence:** Only 48 reported cases

Treatment
I **Primary Prevention:** Genetic counseling
II **Secondary Prevention:** —
III **Other Therapy:** Ocular, dental and orthopedic procedures as indicated

Prognosis: Only risk to life may be from soft tissue defects, especially cardiac and renal. These are uncommon features of this syndrome.

Detection of Carrier: ?

†**Special Considerations:** While some of these children have been mentally retarded, others have been notably intelligent. They may be severely handicapped by skeletal deformities, as well as showing marked cosmetic deformity because of the cutaneous, ocular and skeletal anomalies.

References:
Goltz, R.W. et al: Focal dermal hypoplasia syndrome: A review of the literature and report of two cases. Arch. Dermatol. 101:1, 1970.

Contributor: **Robert Goltz**

Editor's Computerized Descriptors: Eye, Face, Oral, Teeth, Nose, Skin, Sweating, Hair, Nails, Skel. Ear, Nerve , Hearing Muscle, GI., GU.

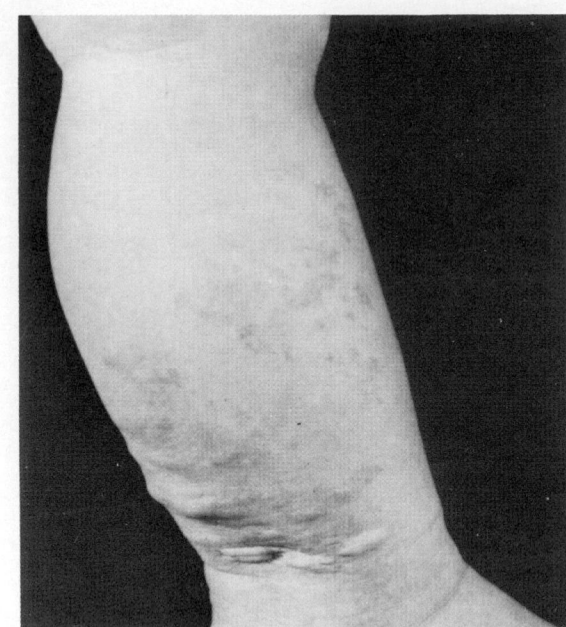

221. Note herniation of subcutaneous fat

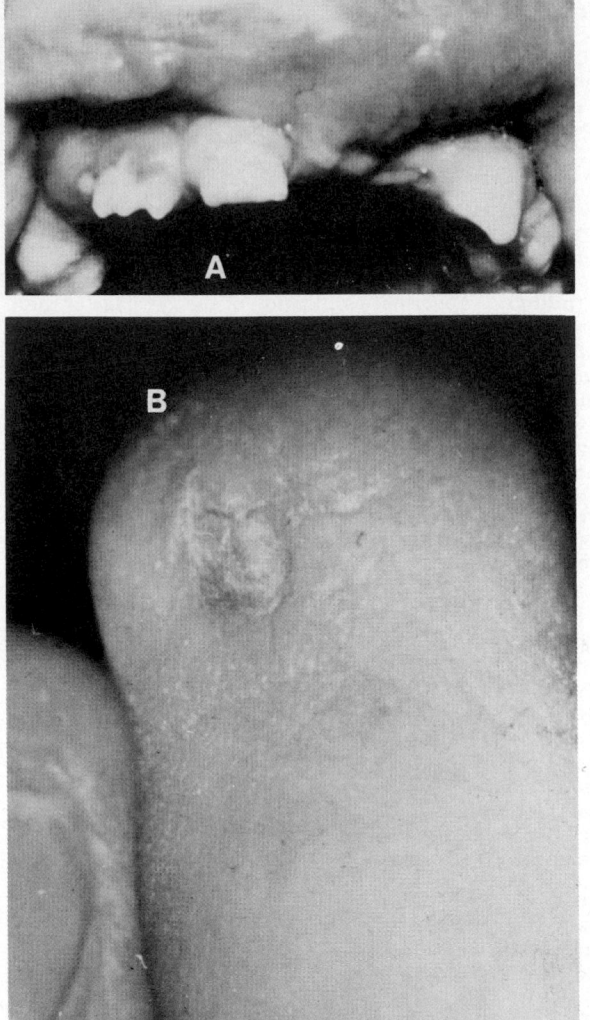

222. A) Irregular shape and spacing of teeth; absent left maxillary central incisor; B) hypoplasia of fingernail

DERMO-CHONDRO-CORNEAL DYSTROPHY OF FRANÇOIS

Includes: Dystrophie dermo-chondro-cornéenne de François
Dystrophia dermato-chondro-cornealis (François)
Distrofia dermo-condro-corneana de François
Cutaneous, cartilaginous and corneal lesions

Excludes: Xanthomatoses
Mucopolysaccharidoses

Minimal Diagnostic Criteria: The triad of cutaneous, cartilaginous and corneal lesions†

Clinical Findings: Abnormal ossification of the cartilage of the hands and feet occurs, leading to marked deformities. Dermal nodules, resembling xanthomata, appear over the dorsal surface of the fingers, posterior surface of the elbows, and on the pinnae. The corneal lesion is characterized by a central epithelial collection of white, irregular opacities causing moderately reduced visual acuity. The stroma, endothelium and periphery of the cornea remain uninvolved.

Complications
I   **Derived:** Reduced visual acuity
II **Associated:** —

Etiology: ? McK *22180

Pathogenesis: ?

Related Facts
I   **Sex Ratio:** ? Too few cases for certainty
II   **Risk of Occurrence:** ?
III **Risk of Recurrence for**
      Patient's Sib: ?
      Patient's Child: ?
IV **Age of Detectability:** —
V   **Prevalence:** Very rare

Treatment
I   **Primary Prevention:** —
II   **Secondary Prevention:** —
III **Other Therapy:** —

Prognosis: ?

Detection of Carrier: —

†**Special Considerations:** François reported 2 sibs (brother and sister) affected with this syndrome in 1949. It is doubtful that any identical cases have subsequently been reported. Jensen, who thought an unusual patient represented this disorder, similarly used the name dermo-chondro-corneal dystrophy. However, the disorder he described actually was rather different in that the corneal lesions resembled pterygia and not epithelial opacities, the skin nodules resembled those of the Urbach-Wiethe syndrome (lipoid proteinosis) and not xanthomata, and the bony changes were mild.

References:
François, J.: Heredity in Ophthalmology. St. Louis:C.V. Mosby, 1961.
François, J.: Dystrophie dermo-chondro-cornéenne familiale. Ann. Oculist (Paris) 182 :409, 1949.
Jensen, V. J.: Dermo-chondro-corneal dystrophy: Report of a case. Acta Ophthalmol. (Kbh.) 36 :71, 1958.

Contributor: **Morton F. Goldberg**

Editor's Computerized Descriptors: Eye, Skin, Skel.

DERMOID CYST OR TERATOMA OF HEAD AND NECK

Includes: Kystes dermoïdes de la tête et du cou
Dermoid Zysten oder Teratome von Kopf und Hals
Quiste dermoide o teratoma de la cabeza y cuello
Dermoids of the head and neck
Monodermoma of head or neck
Bidermoma of head or neck
Tridermoma of head or neck
Embryoma of head or neck
Epignathus
Teratomas of the orbit
Teratoid tumor of head or neck
Hairy cyst on head or neck
Mixed cyst on head or neck
Cervical teratomas
Nasopharyngeal teratomas
Nasal dermoids

Excludes: Other congenital head and neck tumors
Branchial cleft cysts or sinuses (117)
Thyroglossal duct remnant (945)
Lingual thyroids
Inclusion cysts of head or neck lined with squamous epithelium
Preauricular tags and cysts
Salivary gland, mixed tumor (878)

Minimal Diagnostic Criteria: Histopathologic study is necessary to establish the diagnosis.

Clinical Findings: Dermoid cysts or teratomas of the head and neck occur almost exclusively in infants and young children. A review of 103 dermoid cysts of the head and neck revealed the following:

Site	No. of Patients	%
Nose	13	12.6
Orbit	51	49.5
Floor of mouth, submental, submaxillary	24	23.3
Occipital, frontal, lip, neck, soft palate	15	14.6

The signs and symptoms depend upon the size and location of the tumor.

Nasal dermoids are usually detected shortly after birth. A small midline pit or depression on the bridge of the nose with hair protruding from it may be the only abnormality. This pit represents the opening of a sinus tract that may extend between the nasal bones into the cribriform plate or nasal septum. Xrays of the skull and facial bones are essential and injection of the tract with a radiopaque substance before this examination is helpful in establishing the extent of the sinus tract. Nasal obstruction and rhinorrhea may be present.

Teratomas of the orbit are associated with a unilateral exophthalmos and some degree of microphthalmos. The patient with a teratoma is usually born with a mass behind the eye; whereas the dermoid cyst may not become apparent until later in life. Orbital teratomas may extend through defects in the orbit or skull into the anterior cranial fossa, middle cranial fossa, temporal fossa or nasal cavity. Clinical findings will depend upon the size and extensions of the tumor.

Cervical teratomas are rare after age one. Most of these tumors are present at birth with an equal distribution between the 2 sexes. A mass in the neck is the usual presentation. Acute respiratory symptoms of stridor, apnea, and cyanosis result from compression or deviation of the trachea. Dysphagia may arise from esophageal compression. Cystic lymphangioma, congenital goiter, branchial cleft cysts and thyroglossal duct cysts must be considered in the differential diagnosis. These tumors are usually unilateral and quite large, measuring between 5 and 12 cm. The medial border of the tumor may extend across the anterior midline in close relation to the thyroid gland and trachea. They may be solid, multiloculated or cystic. The skin overlying the tumor is movable, the mass may grow to a considerable size causing cosmetic deformities. X-ray examination of the neck mass may reveal areas of calcification within the tumor.

Nasopharyngeal teratomas are present at birth and involve females 6 times as often as males. These tumors may be either pedunculated or sessile. Airway obstruction, cough, rhinorrhea and a nasal or nasopharyngeal tumor are the most common findings. These tumors may be associated with deformities of the skull such as anencephaly, hemicrania or fissures of the palate.

Complications
I   **Derived:**   Airway obstruction, rhinitis and sinusitis, epistaxis, meningitis, cosmetic deformities, exophthalmos, decreased vision, malignant degeneration.
II **Associated:**   The orbital, nasal and nasopharyngeal teratomas may be associated with cranial defects. Cervical teratomas are not associated with these or other defects.

Etiology: ? They are believed to arise from embryonal disturbances of development. A growth disturbance of the primary axis (the notochord and contiguous structures from Hensen node in the early embryo) has been proposed.

Pathogenesis: There is no sharp delineation between dermoid cysts and simple congenital inclusion cysts. As the cyst enlarges and the patient grows, the lesion may migrate away from its primary location. Dermoid cysts may contain a small percentage of mesodermal elements in addition to predominant dermal elements. Teratomas are much more complex tumors and the structure of these tumors varies greatly according to the variety of tissues they contain. Usually they are cystic and the skin-lined cavities contain sebaceous material. The cavities not lined with skin contain mucoid or watery secretions. Skin, hair, bone, cartilage, and teeth may be recognized on gross examination. Microscopically, the tissues within these tumors vary considerably. Skin, hair follicles, sebaceous and sweat glands are common. Respiratory epithelium, intestinal epithelium, nervous tissue, cartilage, bone, and nonstriated muscle are present in varying proportions. Liver, lung, thyroid, and renal tissues are uncommon. Teeth are found in a few tumors. These components are arranged in a chaotic fashion, but closely resemble their normal counterparts. The benign teratoma and dermoid cyst are usually easy to recognize.

Related Facts
I   **Sex Ratio:**   Nasal dermoid: Slight male preponderance
        Orbital dermoid or teratoma: M1:F1
        Cervical dermoid or teratoma: M1:F1
        Nasopharyngeal teratoma: M1:F6
II **Risk of Occurrence:**   ?
III **Risk of Recurrence for**
    Patient's Sib: ?
    Patient's Child: ?
IV **Age of Detectability:**   Nasal: at birth. Orbital dermoid: childhood. Orbital teratoma: at birth. Cervical: at birth. Nasopharyngeal: at birth.
V   **Prevalence:**   ?

Treatment
I   **Primary Prevention:**   —

II **Secondary Prevention:**   Complete surgical excision is required to prevent recurrences and other complications. Combined ophthalmologic, neurosurgical, and otolaryngologic operations may be needed to successfully treat the orbital tumors. Cervical tumors are usually encapsulated with fibrous tissue and this makes complete surgical excision possible.
III **Other Therapy:**   Tracheostomy, an extra-oral feeding route, antibiotics and reconstructive procedures for cosmetic deformities may be necessary.

Prognosis: A normal life span can be expected when the tumor is completely excised. Malignant degeneration is rare.

Detection of Carrier: —

Special Considerations: —

References:
Ariel, I.M. and Pack, G.T.: Cancer and Allied Diseases of Infancy and Childhood. Boston: Little Brown & Co., 1960.
Batsakis, J.G. and Farber, E.R.: Teratomas of the head and neck. E.E.N.T. Dig. 30:67, 1968.
New, G.B. and Erich, J.B.: Dermoid cysts of head and neck. Surg. Gynecol. Obstet. 65:48, 1937.
Willis, R.A.: Teratomas. In Atlas of Tumor Pathology, Section III-fasc. 9:1. Armed Forces Institute of Pathology, Washington, D.C., 1951.

Contributor: **Gerald M. English**

Editor's Computerized Descriptors: Eye, Oral, Nasoph., Nose, Neck, Skel., Resp.

DERMOLIPOMA

Includes: Lipome dermoïde
Dermatolipom
Lipodermoid

Excludes: Lipoma
Orbital and periorbital dermoid cysts (761)

Minimal Diagnostic Criteria: Subconjunctival tumor in upper temporal quadrant and biopsy confirmation

Clinical Findings: Yellowish-white benign congenital tumors made up of cutaneous and fatty elements located subconjunctivally in the upper temporal quadrant between the superior and lateral recti muscles. They may be unilateral or bilateral. There is a tendency for growth after birth.

Complications
I **Derived:** They may enlarge or produce irritation due to piercing hairs.
II **Associated:** 40% of cases of oculoauriculovertebral dysplasia, coloboma, aniridia, microphthalmos, and facial hemiatrophy

Etiology: Possibly autosomal dominant

Pathogenesis: ?

Related Facts
I **Sex Ratio:** M1:F1
II **Risk of Occurrence:** ?
III **Risk of Recurrence for**
   Patient's Sib: When autosomal dominant and if parent is affected, 1 in 2 (50%) for each offspring to be affected; otherwise not increased.
   Patient's Child: 1 in 2 when autosomal dominant
IV **Age of Detectability:** —
V **Prevalence:** ?

Treatment
I **Primary Prevention:** Genetic counseling
II **Secondary Prevention:** —
III **Other Therapy:** Surgical excision if irritation develops or lesion is cosmetically disfiguring.

Prognosis: Excellent, no visual impairment, no threat to life

Detection of Carrier: Affected parent and patient when autosomal dominant

Special Considerations: —

References:
Duke-Elder, S.:System of Ophthalmology, vol. 3, pt. 2. Congenital Deformities. London: Henry Kimpton, 1964, p. 823.

Contributor: **Morton E. Smith**

Editor's Computerized Descriptors: Eye, Face

DEXTROCARDIA, BRONCHIECTASIS AND SINUSITIS SYNDROME

Includes: Syndrome dextro - cardie-bronchiectasies
Dextrokardie-Bronchiektasie-Sinusitis-Syndrom
Síndrome de dextrocardia, bronquiectasias y sinusitis
Kartagener syndrome
Bronchiectasis, sinusitis and dextrocardia

Excludes: Isolated situs inversus
Isolated dextrocardia

Minimal Diagnostic Criteria: This is a clinical diagnosis and can only be considered definite in the isolated patient with no affected relatives if he or she has had thick nasal secretions since infancy, pansinusitis and partial or complete situs inversus.†

Clinical Findings: The affected patients may have all or any combination of these physical features: partial or complete situs inversus, thick nasal secretions from infancy throughout life, pansinusitis from childhood, chronic serous otitis media and bronchiectasis. Many features reflect progressive complications involving the respiratory epithelium that develop at different ages in each patient. Often the situs inversus is unrecognized for many years. Cardiac anomalies may be present, especially if the situs inversus is incomplete.

Complications
I **Derived:** Anosmia, a mild conductive hearing loss, nasal polyps, pneumonia and bronchiectasis
II **Associated:** Asplenia syndrome and cardiac anomalies

Etiology: Autosomal recessive; McK *24440

Pathogenesis: The primary defect in the respiratory epithelium is not known. Apparently, thickened secretions lead to blockage of the paranasal sinuses, eustachian tube, and lobes of the lung and predispose these areas to infection. Slow or absent mucociliary transport in the tracheobronchial tract was found in 2 patients. Immotile spermatozoa have also been observed. The abnormality in both cilia and sperm has been attributed to a lack of normal dynein arms. A transient hypogammaglobulinemia has been documented in 2 children, 1 of whom was simultaneously having recurrent infections. In the same study, the serum immunoglobulins were normal in 8 patients; the 2 youngest patients, ages 3 and 6 years, had persistently low IgA levels. The immunoglobulins in parotid saliva were normal in 8 patients. Possibly serial assays for salivary and serum immunoglobulins (including IgE) on affected infants will reveal transient immunologic abnormalities.

Related Facts
I **Sex Ratio:** M1:F1
II **Risk of Occurrence:** ?
III **Risk of Recurrence for**
   Patient's Sib: 1 in 4 (25%) for each sib
   Patient's Child: Not increased unless mate is carrier or homozygote
IV **Age of Detectability:** Most patients have thick mucoid rhinorrhea and recurrent respiratory infections in the 1st year of life. May be detected in newborn with respiratory distress and atelectasis of left middle lobe.
V **Prevalence:** Rare, but specific data not available

Treatment
I **Primary Prevention:** Genetic counseling†
II **Secondary Prevention:** Otitis media, acute sinusitis and pneumonia should be carefully looked for and vigorously treated. By early treatment of respiratory complications, bronchiectasis may be prevented. A transient low level of serum IgG, if identified, should be treated. Patients with bronchiectasis benefit from the removal of the affected lobes or segments.

III Other Therapy: Long-term treatment of chronic serous otitis, including continuous drainage and ventilation, and use of hearing aid may be warranted.

Prognosis: For life: good, unless the patient has either a severe cardiac anomaly or extensive bronchiectasis. The actual life span is not known, but almost all patients survive to adulthood. For function: pulmonary function tests show that all patients have evidence of ventilatory obstruction, but the severity is quite variable. Mildly affected individuals can engage in vigorous physical activity without difficulty. The patients complain most about the constant rhinorrhea and chronic cough. They are often unaware of their anosmia and mild hearing loss. Infertility may be a problem due to immotile sperm.

Detection of Carrier: —

†Special Considerations: This syndrome includes both developmental structural abnormalities and thick mucoid secretions throughout the entire respiratory epithelium. These seemingly unrelated problems are the pleiotropic effects of a single mutant gene. Numerous family studies have shown a wide phenotypic variability within a sibship. For example, the index patient will have many features of this syndrome, while his brother has only thick nasal secretions and sinusitis and his sister only situs inversus. Yet, all 3 sibs should be considered examples of Kartagener syndrome. Unfortunately, one cannot be certain of this diagnosis if the mildly affected child does not have a more severely affected sib. Obviously, for the purpose of genetic counseling it is equally appropriate to correctly identify the mildly affected child.

References:

Afzelius, B.A.: A human syndrome caused by immotile cilia. Science 193:317, 1976.

Camner, P. et al: Evidence for congenitally nonfunctioning cilia in the tracheobronchia tract in two subjects. Am. Rev. Respir. Dis. 112:807-809, 1975.

Hartline, J.V. and Zelkowitz, P.S.: Kartagener's syndrome in childhood. Am. J. Dis. Child. 121:349-352, 1971.

Holmes, L.B. et al: A reappraisal of Kartagener's syndrome. Am. J. Med. Sci. 255:13-28, 1968.

Contributor: **Lewis B. Holmes**

Editor's Computerized Descriptors: Ear, Nasoph., Resp., CV.

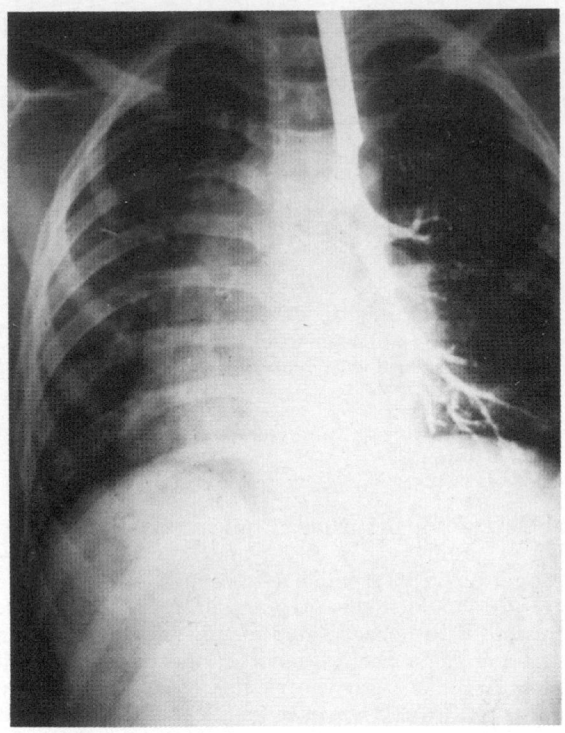

223. Bronchiectasis and dextrocardia

DEXTROPOSITION OF VENTRICULAR SEPTUM AND DOUBLE INLET LEFT VENTRICLE

Includes: Dextroposition du septum ventriculaire
Dextroposition des Kammerseptums-doppelte Einstrombahn des linken Ventrikels
Dextroposición del tabique inter-ventricular y ventrículo izquierdo a doble entrada
Double inlet left ventricle without ventricular inversion
Cor triloculare biatriatum
Holmes heart
Single ventricle with rudimentary outflow chamber
Double inlet left ventricle with ventricular inversion
Univentricular heart

Excludes: Tricuspid valve atresia (968)
Mitral valve atresia (665)
Other forms of functional single ventricle

Minimal Diagnostic Criteria: Clinical evidence of a large left-to-right shunt in a mildly cyanotic infant with electrovectorcardiographic evidence of severe left ventricular hypertrophy should suggest the possibility of double inlet left ventricle with noninversion of the ventricles. Similar clinical findings in the presence of electrovectorcardiographic evidence of right ventricular hypertrophy as evidenced by significant Q waves in lead V_1, plus similar deep Q waves in standard lead III and lead aVF, should suggest the possibility of double inlet left ventricle with inversion of the ventricles. Cardiac catheterization and selective angiocardiography will confirm the exact anatomic situation.

Clinical Findings: Double inlet left ventricle is that cardiac malformation in which both atrioventricular valves open into a large ventricular chamber which morphologically resembles a left ventricle. The mitral valve communicates exclusively with this large left ventricle. The tricuspid valve may also communicate exclusively with the large left ventricle but may override a hypoplastic ventricular septum and open partially into a more or less rudimentary right ventricle. Double inlet left ventricle is usually, but not necessarily, associated with transposition of the great arteries in which case the aorta arises from the rudimentary right ventricle which consists only of a rightward and anteriorly placed infundibular chamber. In the rare instance when the great arteries are normally related (and the ventricles are not inverted), the complex is known as the Holmes heart. The atrial septum is usually intact, although small atrial septal defects may occur. A ventricular septal defect is always present as the route of communication from the large single ventricle to the rudimentary right ventricular infundibular chamber. If the ventricular septal defect is small, there may be functional obstruction to the aorta. Pulmonic or subpulmonic obstruction may also be present, ranging from mild stenosis to complete atresia.

The anatomic complex double inlet left ventricle may also occur in the presence of ventricular inversion. In that condition the large ventricular chamber, which has the internal morphology of a left ventricle and which receives both A-V valves, is located on the right side. The apex of the heart (in situs solitus) usually points to the left, but dextroversion may be present. The pulmonary trunk almost always arises from the main chamber. The left A-V valve (which is morphologically the tricuspid valve) may override the ventricular septum in some cases. The hypoplastic right ventricular infundibular chamber is placed leftward, superiorly and anteriorly and gives origin to the aorta. The

ventricular septum lies in the sagittal plane. As with noninversion, pulmonic or subpulmonic obstruction may be present.

Clinical features are usually those of a large left-to-right shunt with bidirectional intracardiac mixing and are similar for both inversion and noninversion of the ventricles. In the absence of pulmonary stenosis, cyanosis is initially mild. With increased pulmonary vascular resistance, cyanosis will increase. A harsh systolic murmur and systolic thrill are present along the left sternal border and the second sound is single or narrowly split with accentuation of the pulmonic component. A mitral diastolic flow murmur is common and congestive heart failure is frequently present. When pulmonic or subpulmonic obstruction is present, the clinical findings depend upon the degree of obstruction. When mild, the findings may be unchanged. When severe, cyanosis is prominent, the murmurs may be insignificant, and the second sound is single. When obstruction to aortic outflow is present, the clinical picture frequently mimics aortic atresia or severe coarctation of the aorta and survival beyond a few months of life is unlikely.

The electrovectorcardiographic features depend upon whether inversion or noninversion of the ventricles is present. Regardless of the type of single ventricle, there is almost invariably an alteration of the initial cardiac vectors from the anticipated normal. Additional features suggest noninversion from inversion. With noninversion, the ECG and the vectorcardiogram demonstrate marked left ventricular hypertrophy. The mean frontal QRS axis ranges from $+25°$ to $+75°$ and the initial QRS forces are directed leftward and anteriorly, recording little or no Q wave in any of the usual chest leads (V_3R to V_7). The major QRS forces are shifted leftward and posteriorly resulting in rS complexes in lead V_1 and Rs complexes in lead V_6. Left and right atrial enlargement are frequently present. When pulmonic obstruction is present, the ECG is relatively unchanged except that right atrial enlargement is more marked. In the presence of ventricular inversion, the ECG and vectorcardiogram are quite different. As in ventricular inversion with 2 ventricles, the initial QRS forces are directed leftward, superiorly and usually posteriorly, resulting in Q waves in standard lead III, lead aVF and lead V_1. However, the major portion of the QRS forces is directed rightward and anteriorly, indicating anterior chamber hypertrophy, and resulting in qRs complexes in lead V_1 and RS complexes in V_6. The QRS axis in the frontal plane is directed somewhat to the right between 100° and 135°. Cardiac arrhythmias, especially varying degrees of atrioventricular block, are more common in the presence of ventricular inversion. As is the case with noninversion, atrial hypertrophy may be present and when pulmonic obstruction is significant, right atrial enlargement is more marked.

The echocardiographic diagnosis of this disorder requires demonstration that 2 separate atrioventricular valves exist without an intervening ventricular septum. Differential diagnosis of the various forms of single ventricle, as well as some forms of complete atrioventricular canal, is extremely difficult echocardiographically. Nevertheless, the demonstration of the transposed great vessel relationship in the presence of 2 atrioventricular valves and the absence of an intervening ventricular septal echo may suggest a diagnosis of single ventricle. An additional important feature is the identification of a small outflow tract anteriorly located but unrelated to an atrioventricular valve.

Chest roentgenographic findings depend upon the degree of pulmonic obstruction and the position of the right ventricular infundibulum. In the usual case without pulmonic obstruction, there is prominent shunt type vascularity, generalized cardiomegaly, biatrial enlargement and mediastinal findings suggestive of transposition of the great arteries. When pulmonic obstruction is significant, pulmonary arterial vascularity appears normal or decreased, and heart size is normal or slightly enlarged. Chest roentgenograms may suggest the presence of ventricular inversion by the position of the great arteries and the bulge of the infundibular chamber on the left upper border of the cardiac shadow.

Cardiac catheterization demonstrates a lack of significant shunting at the atrial level, based on fully saturated left atrial blood and no significant oxygen increase in the right atrium. Ventricular and peripheral arterial oxygen values show mild desaturation and are about equal. Selective angiocardiography is necessary to demonstrate the precise anatomy. The presence of ventricular inversion is apparent by the position of the infundibular chamber and the orientation of the ventricular septum. The interrelationship of the great arteries is of little value in distinguishing inversion from noninversion. Angiocardiography will demonstrate the presence of 2 independent atrioventricular valves entering a large single ventricle, which communicates with a rudimentary right ventricular infundibular chamber.

Complications
I **Derived:** Persistent cardiac failure and repeated pulmonary infections frequently prove fatal. When pulmonic obstruction is significant, hypoxic complications may occur. Aortic obstruction may result in low cardiac output, poor systemic perfusion and death within the first few months of life.

II **Associated:** —

Etiology: ?

Pathogenesis: Probably due to a failure of alignment of the right portion of the atrioventricular canal with the primitive right ventricle. Thus, the right ventricle does not develop and functions only as an outlet chamber. The reason for the high degree of association of double inlet left ventricle with transposition of the great arteries is unknown.

Related Facts
I **Sex Ratio:** M2:F1
II **Risk of Occurrence:** < 1 in 100 cases of congenital heart defects
III **Risk of Recurrence for**
   Patient's Sib: ?
   Patient's Child: ?
IV **Age of Detectability:** From birth
V **Prevalence:** —

Treatment
I **Primary Prevention:** —
II **Secondary Prevention:** Palliative procedures such as pulmonary artery banding, or systemic-pulmonary artery shunt in the presence of severe pulmonic stenosis, may prolong life.
III **Other Therapy:** As necessary for congestive heart failure and pneumonia.

Prognosis: Poor; survival into adulthood possible with moderate pulmonic obstruction. Most cases die early in life.

Detection of Carrier: Not applicable

Special Considerations: —

References:
De la Cruz, M.V. and Miller, B.L.: Double-inlet left ventricle: Two pathological specimens with comments on the embryology and on its relation to single ventricle. Circulation 37:249, 1968.
Gessner, I.H. et al: The vectorcardiogram in double inlet left ventri-
cle, with and without ventricular inversion. In Hoffman, I. (ed.): Vectorcardiography. Amsterdam: North Holland Publishing Co., 1976.
Goldberg, S.J. et al: Pediatric and Adolescent Echocardiography. Chicago: Year Book Medical Publishers, 1975.
Seward, J. et al: Preoperative and postoperative echocardiographic observations in common ventricle. Circulation (Suppl. II) 52:46, 1975.
Van Praagh, R. et al: Diagnosis of the anatomic types of single or common ventricle. Am. J. Cardiol. 15:345, 1965. (Review)

Contributors: **Ira H. Gessner**
Larry P. Elliott
B. Lynn Miller

Editor's Computerized Descriptors: Resp., CV.

DIABETES INSIPIDUS, VASOPRESSIN-RESISTANT

Includes: Diabète insipide pitresso-résistant
Vasopressin-resistenter Diabetes insipidus
Diabetes insípida nefrogénica
Nephrogenic diabetes insipidus
Vasopressin-resistant diabetes insipidus

Excludes: Vasopressin-responsive diabetes insipidus
Psychogenic polydipsia and polyuria

Minimal Diagnostic Criteria: Hypotonic urine (<300 mOsm/L) with no response to parenteral administration of vasopressin; absence of other proximal or distal tubular abnormalities; exclusion of psychogenic polydipsia, urinary tract obstruction and acute or chronic renal disease.

Clinical Findings: Polyuria and polydipsia (100%); urine osmolality always less than that of serum (<300 mOsm/L) and commonly below 100 mOsm/L.

Complications
I **Derived:** Dehydration if adequate supply of fluid is not available; mental and physical retardation may occur secondary to dehydration.
II **Associated:** —

Etiology: Usually X-linked recessive and occasionally autosomal dominant transmission affecting vasopressin-responsive mechanism in distal tubule and collecting duct.† McK *30480

Pathogenesis: Since vasopressin increases permeability of distal tubule and collecting duct to water, this defect results in inability to concentrate the urine above the osmolality of plasma; severe dehydration will ensue in the absence of sufficient oral or parenteral water replacement.†

Related Facts
I **Sex Ratio:** ? Much more common in males than females
II **Risk of Occurrence:** ?
III **Risk of Recurrence for**
   Patient's Sib: When X-linked recessive or autosomal dominant, see Table I X-linked R or AD, respectively.
   Patient's Child: When X-linked recessive or autosomal dominant, see Table I X-linked R or AD, respectively.
IV **Age of Detectability:** Neonatal†
V **Prevalence:** ?

Treatment
I **Primary Prevention:** Genetic counseling
II **Secondary Prevention:** Adequate water replacement will prevent dehydration; thiazide diuretics reduce urine flow significantly.
III **Other Therapy:** —

Prognosis: Benign if fluid replacement is adequate; episodic dehydration in infancy may impair physical and mental development.

Detection of Carrier: Some mothers and sisters of affected males with X-linked form demonstrate partial impairment of maximum concentrating ability even after parenteral administration of vasopressin.

†Special Considerations: X-linked recessive pattern of inheritance is the rule, but several instances of male-to-male transmission indicate that more than one genetic lesion may result in vasopressin resistance; vasopressin action mediated by adenosine-3', 5'-monophosphate (cyclic AMP) which is formed from ATP by adenyl cyclase; therefore, the genetic defect could involve one of the enzymatic reactions leading to cyclic AMP synthesis as well as an abnormality in distal tubule receptor site for vasopressin; diagnosis difficult to establish in neonates or premature infants who normally demonstrate impaired response to vasopressin; infusion of hypertonic saline may be helpful in distinguishing between true vasopressin resistance and psychogenic polydipsia.

References:
Bode, H. H. and Crawford, J. D.: Nephrogenic diabetes insipidus in North America. The Hopewell hypothesis. N. Engl. J. Med. 280:750, 1969.
Cannon, J. F.: Diabetes insipidus: Clinical and experimental studies with consideration of genetic relationships. Arch. Intern. Med. 96:215, 1955.
Orloff, J. and Burg, M. B.: Vasopressin-resistant diabetes insipidus. In Stanbury, J.B. et al (eds.): The Metabolic Basis of Inherited Disease, 3rd Ed. New York: McGraw-Hill, 1972, p. 1567.
Rosenberg, L. E.: Hereditary diseases with membrane defects. In Dowben, R.M. (ed.): Biological Membranes. Boston: Little, Brown and Co., 1969, p. 255.

Contributor: **Leon E. Rosenberg**

Editor's Computerized Descriptor: GU.

DIAPHRAGM, EVENTRATION

Includes: Éventration diaphragmatique
Zwerchfell-Eventration
Eventración del diafragma
Abnormally high but intact diaphragm arching smoothly from its normal costal attachments
Congenital absence or deficiency of muscle between the pleura and peritoneum
Congenital relaxation of diaphragm
Diaphragm abnormally high

Excludes: Diaphragmatic hernia (289)
Absence of one leaf of diaphragm
Traumatic rupture of diaphragm

Minimal Diagnostic Criteria: Abnormally high but intact diaphragm

Clinical Findings: If diaphragm is only slightly elevated, there may be no symptoms. If diaphragm is markedly elevated, there is limited expansion of the lung and atelectasis on the ipsilateral side. In small infants there may be a dangerous shift of the mediastinum to the contralateral side with further impairment of respiratory function by compression of the lung on the opposite side. Tachypnea is the first symptom which may progress to severe "respiratory fatigue" and death. Congenital absence of muscle in the diaphragm is the least common cause of eventration but usually produces very severe symptoms that are incompatible with life early in the newborn period.

The acquired form of eventration resulting from obstetric delivery may be either temporary or permanent depending on whether the phrenic nerve is merely stretched or irreversibly damaged or avulsed. Symptoms may develop a few days after birth but usually in the neonatal period. If the infant tolerates the restricted expansion of the lungs, a period of observation may be indicated, hoping for spontaneous improvement. If the symptoms persist with progressive fatigue of the infant or if the infant requires extra oxygen or has feeding difficulties due to shortness of breath, a surgical repair should not be delayed.

An AP roentgenogram of the chest shows an elevation of the involved leaf of the diaphragm with a normal position of the opposite leaf. Fluoroscopy shows paradoxical motion of the involved leaf of the diaphragm. On inspiration the involved leaf rises while the uninvolved leaf is depressed and during expiration the reverse occurs. Paradoxical motion also can be demonstrated by a roentgenogram taken in full inspiration and compared to one taken in full expiration.

Complications
I **Derived:** Ipsilateral atelectasis, mediastinal shift, tachypnea
II **Associated:** —

Etiology: ?

Pathogenesis: ? Failure of development of adequate muscular tissue in septum transversum with presence of pleura and peritoneum.

Related Facts
I **Sex Ratio:** M?:F?
II **Risk of Occurrence:** ?
III **Risk of Recurrence for**
 Patient's Sib: ?
 Patient's Child: ?
IV **Age of Detectability:** At birth
V **Prevalence:** ?

Treatment
I **Primary Prevention:** —
II **Secondary Prevention:** Under controlled, intubation anesthesia a thoracotomy is performed on the affected side. A central elipse of the abnormal diaphragm is resected and the defect closed by overlapping the remaining 2 layers using nonabsorbable sutures. The repaired diaphragm after plication should be at the level of a normal diaphragm. A thoracotomy tube is placed on low suction for removal of any serum and protection against the possibility of an unrecognized postoperative pneumothorax.

III **Other Therapy:** —

Prognosis: The prognosis is excellent if surgical plication is performed when needed before the infant has deteriorated from chronic oxygen insufficiency, prolonged atelectasis and associated pneumonia. Follow-ups many years later show the plicated diaphragm remains at a normal level and is relatively fixed, showing little motion with deep inspiration and expiration.

Detection of Carrier: —

Special Considerations: —

References:
Baffles, T. G.: Eventration of the diaphragm. In Mustard, W.T. et al (eds.): Pediatric Surgery. Chicago:Yearbook Medical Publishers, 1969, p. 350.
Bishop, H. C. and Koop, C. E.: Acquired eventration of the diaphragm in infancy. Pediatrics 22:1088, 1958.
Jewett, T. C., Jr. and Thomson, N. B., Jr.: Iatrogenic eventration of the diaphragm in infancy. J. Thorac. Cardiovasc. Surg. 48:861, 1964.

Contributor: **Harry C. Bishop**

Editor's Computerized Descriptors: Muscle, Resp.

DIAPHRAGMATIC HERNIA

Includes: Hernie diaphragmatique congénitale
Angeborene Zwerchfellhernie
Hernia diafragmática congénita
Posterolateral diaphragmatic hernia
Hernia, congenital diaphragmatic
Bochdalek hernia
Anterolateral diaphragmatic hernia
Congenital absence of hemidiaphragm
Retrosternal diaphragmatic hernia
Foramen of Morgagni hernia
Parasternal hernia
Subcostosternal hernia

Excludes: Diaphragm, eventration (288)
Traumatic hernia of diaphragm
Phrenic nerve palsy
Esophageal chalasia (366)
Lax cardia
Congenital short esophagus
Parahiatal hernia
Esophageal stricture
Hiatus hernia (471)

Minimal Diagnostic Criteria: *Posterolateral hernia:* Radiographic demonstration of abdominal viscera in chest with surgical confirmation of posterolateral diaphragmatic defect.

Retrosternal hernia: Radiographic demonstration of abdominal viscera displaced into lower anterior mediastinum.

Clinical Findings: *Posterolateral diaphragmatic hernia:* Severely affected infants present with dyspnea and cyanosis from birth. Symptoms progress with time as swallowed air distends the hollow viscera displaced into the chest and causes further cardiopulmonary compression. Early onset of symptoms and high mortality correlate with the degree of associated pulmonary hypoplasia. Infants with compressed but fully developed lungs have more respiratory reserve and develop symptoms usually after the first 24 hours of life when initial feedings and swallowed air increase the mass lesion in the chest. Hernias through the left leaf of the diaphragm predominate 9:1. Less than one-half of the posterolateral hernias are contained by a hernia sac. Physical findings usually include cyanosis, tracheal shift, lateral displacement of the heart away from the lesion, overexpansion of the affected side with lag in the respiratory cycle, and a scaphoid abdomen. Bowel sounds are seldom audible over the chest of affected newborns. Breath sounds are greatly decreased bilaterally, but more on the affected side. The diagnostic x-ray must include the infant's chest and abdomen to differentiate displaced abdominal viscera from cystic malformations or infectious processes in the lung. Acidosis, arterial hypoxia and hypercarbia are usual laboratory findings in symptomatic infants.

Retrosternal diaphragmatic hernia: Affected infants may present with dyspnea in the first hours of life but more often symptoms are recognized much later in infancy or childhood. These anterior hernias are probably limited in size by the adjacent pericardium and by the usual presence of a containing hernia sac. Right-sided hernias predominate and they are seldom large enough to produce serious symptoms from mass compression in the chest. Symptoms may relate to moderate pulmonary compression or to partial bowel obstruction. Pulmonary hypoplasia is not commonly associated. Diagnosis is often first suspected from routine roentgenograms of the chest.

Complications
I Derived: *Posterolateral hernia:* Preoperative: pneumo-thorax on ipsilateral or more commonly contralateral side of hernia, pneumomediastinum, hypoxia, acidosis and death. Bowel obstruction or volvulus and infarction can occur with late onset of symptoms.

Postoperative: pneumothorax on ipsilateral or contralateral side of repair, bowel obstruction, recurrence of hernia (infrequent), hemorrhage (infrequent), infection (infrequent), progressive cardiopulmonary failure and death (common incidence affected by degree of pulmonary hypoplasia and capacity of abdomen to contain displaced viscera. Tension in abdomen in turn affects function of diaphragm and degree of vena caval compression).

Retrosternal hernia: Preoperative: bowel obstruction, recurrent lung infections. Postoperative: bowel obstruction, recurrence of hernia, hemorrhage, infection (all infrequent).

II Associated: *Posterolateral hernia:* major associated anomalies in 90% if stillborn, 20% if born alive and much lower percentage if infant survives beyond one hour. Anomalies include malformations of CNS, cardiovascular, GU and GI systems.

Retrosternal hernia: associated malformations of cardiovascular, GU and CNS systems are common.

Etiology: ?

Pathogenesis: *Posterolateral hernia:* thought to develop in the 8th to 12th week of fetal life. The formation of the diaphragm, the return of the gut from the yolk stalk and the differentiation of the lung buds all take place at this period. An imbalance in timing is thought to result in thoracic migration of the gut with incomplete closure of the diaphragm and compression of the undeveloped lung buds.

Retrosternal hernia: thought to result from fusion failure of the diaphragm anteriorly or from failure of muscular ingrowth from the cervical myotomes.

Related Facts
I Sex Ratio: Posterolateral hernia, M2:F1. Retrosternal hernia, M?:F?
II Risk of Occurrence: Posterolateral hernia: 1 in 2200 births (0.45 per 1000 total births - England 1962) (0.08 per 1000 live births - Pennsylvania 1962). Retrosternal hernia: ? Probably less than 1 in 1,000,000 live births.
III Risk of Recurrence for
 Patient's Sib: Not increased
 Patient's Child: Not increased
IV Age of Detectability: At birth with chest xray
V Prevalence: ?

Treatment
I Primary Prevention: —
II Secondary Prevention: Surgical repair - Transthoracic or transabdominal reduction of displaced viscera into abdomen with repair of defect in diaphragm. Prosthetic enlargement of abdomen with later staged reconstruction may be required for some complicated posterolateral defects associated with pulmonary hypoplasia.
III Other Therapy: —

Prognosis: Probable normal life span without disability if repair is uncomplicated, pulmonary development is normal and other anomalies do not coexist. Effect of associated pulmonary hypoplasia on life span is unknown.

Detection of Carrier: ?

Special Considerations: —

References:
Butler, N. and Claireaux, A. E.: Congenital diaphragmatic hernia as a cause of perinatal mortality. Lancet 1:659, 1962.
Carter, R.E.B. et al: Hernia and eventration of the diaphragm in childhood. Lancet 1:656, 1962.
Johnson, D. G. et al: Diaphragmatic hernia in infancy: Factors affecting the mortality rate. Surgery 62:1082, 1967.
Whittaker, L.D., Jr. et al: Hernias of the foramen of Bochdalek in children. Mayo Clin. Proc. 43:580, 1968.

DIAPHYSEAL DYSPLASIA

Includes: Dysplasie diaphysaire
Diaphysäre Dysplasie
Displasia diafisiaria
Dysplasia, diaphyseal
Progressive diaphyseal dysplasia
Camurati-Engelmann syndrome
Osteopathia hyperostotica sclerotisans multiplex infantilis
Sclerotic bone disease

Excludes: Hyperostosis corticalis generalisata (497)
Hereditary multiple diaphyseal sclerosis
Hypervitaminosis A
Cortical hyperostosis, infantile (221)
Melorheostosis (641)

Minimal Diagnostic Criteria: Skeletal changes consisting of symmetrically widened, fusiform diaphyses of the long bones with sclerosis of the periosteum and endosteum.†

Clinical Findings: Variable. Some cases are asymptomatic. Characteristically there is: inability to gain weight, often producing a markedly malnourished appearance; wide-based waddling gait; poorly developed muscles, muscle weakness and easy fatigability; aching pains in the limbs or back ranging from minimal to severe; flat, pronated feet; occasionally bowed or knock-knee deformity; increased lumbar lordosis and scoliosis. Puberty is often delayed. Intelligence is normal. The radiographic features include symmetric fusiform enlargement and sclerosis of the diaphyses of the long bones. The cortex is thickened by periosteal and endosteal proliferation of new bone and the area of hyperostosis is usually sharply demarcated from the metaphyses and epiphyses in the growing child. The lesion progresses along the long axis of the long bones both proximally and distally. Eventually no normal trabeculation remains and within the thickened and sclerotic bone there are mottled areas of rarefaction. The base of the skull and frontal areas may be involved; the facial bones, mandible and spine are generally not affected; the ribs, scapulae, pelvis, clavicles, hands and feet are infrequently involved. No consistent abnormalities have been found in routine blood chemistries.

Complications
I **Derived:** Crippling leg pain may incapacitate the individual. Fracture of a long bone is a rare complication.
II **Associated:** —

Etiology: Presumably autosomal dominant. Most reports are of isolated cases. McK *13130

Pathogenesis: ? †

Related Facts
I **Sex Ratio:** M1:F1
II **Risk of Occurrence:** Rare. Less than 30 cases have been reported.
III **Risk of Recurrence for**
    Patient's Sib: If parent is affected 1 in 2 (50%) for each offspring to be affected; otherwise not increased.
    Patient's Child: 1 in 2
IV **Age of Detectability:** The earliest reported case was recognized at the age of 4 months.
V **Prevalence:** ?

Treatment
I **Primary Prevention:** Genetic counseling
II **Secondary Prevention:** Corticosteroids
III **Other Therapy:** —

Prognosis: Life span does not appear to be shortened, though there may be crippling disability. There is some evidence that with cessation of growth there is cessation of progression of the bone lesion.

Detection of Carrier: —

†Special Considerations: In hereditary multiple diaphyseal sclerosis the diaphyseal osteosclerosis and hyperostosis are limited to 1 or more (up to 4) of the long bones, does not seem to be progressive, and muscular development is normal. Because of the associated features muscular dystrophy or poliomyelitis is sometimes diagnosed in these patients.

In diaphyseal dysplasia there appears to be decreased or absent osteoclastic activity and corticosteroids appear to stimulate osteoclasis and decrease lamellar bone deposition.

References:

Clawson, D.K. and Loop, J.W.: Progressive diaphyseal dysplasia (Engelmann's disease). J. Bone Joint Surg. 46:143, 1964.

Rubin, P.: Dynamic Classification of Bone Dysplasias. Chicago: Year Book Medical Publishers, Inc. 1964.

Singleton, E.B. et al: Progressive diaphyseal dysplasia (Engelmann's disease). Radiology 67:233, 1956.

Sparkes, R.S. and Graham, C.B.: Camurati-Engelmann disease. J. Med. Genet. 9:73, 1972.

Contributor: **Charles I. Scott, Jr.**

Editor's Computerized Descriptors: Skel., Muscle

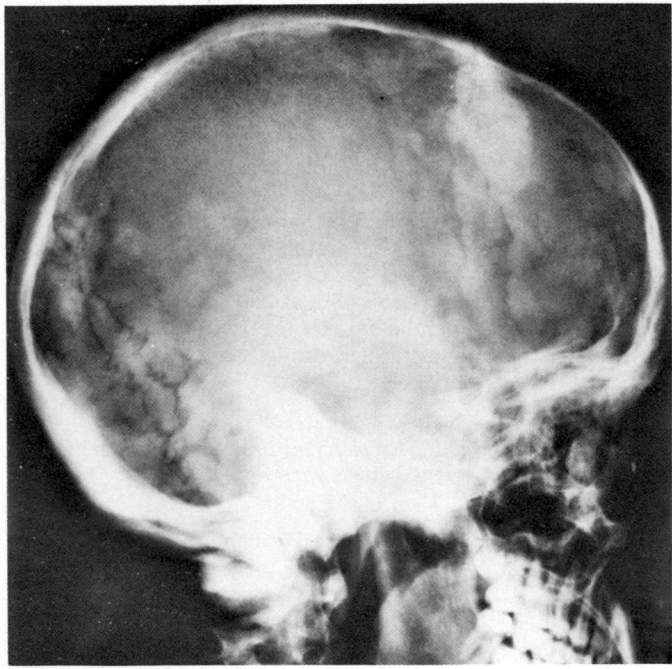

224. Focal sclerosis with more marked thickening in the base than the vault

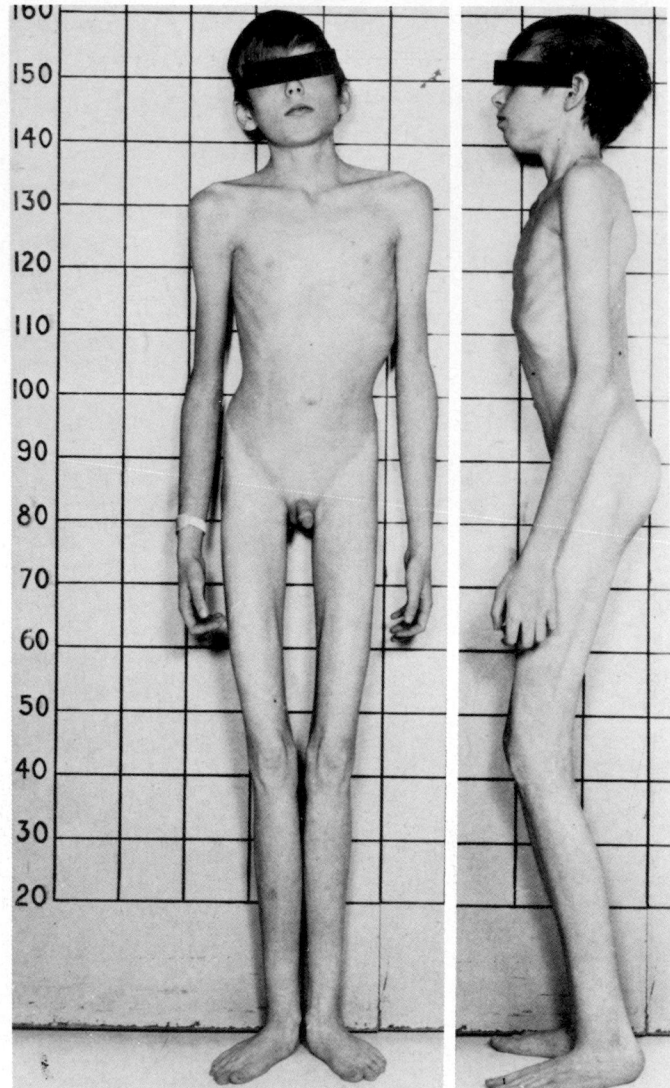

225. Thin body habitus; dorsal scoliosis; flexion deformities at elbows, hips, and knees

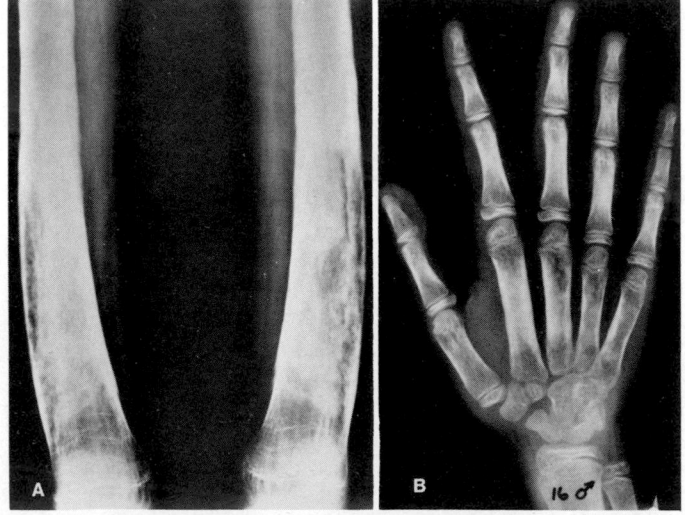

226. A) Swollen diaphyses, particularly in distal portions; irregular cortical thickening; sclerosis; B) wide, poorly modeled metacarpals and phalanges; irregular sclerotic shafts

DIASTEMA, MEDIAN INCISAL (MARKER)

Includes: Diastème des incisives médianes
Diastema der Mittleren Schneidezähne
Diastema de los incisivos medianos (Marcador)
Median incisal diastema

Excludes: Teeth, supernumerary (Marker) (936)

Minimal Diagnostic Criteria: When there exists a natural spacing of 1-3 mm or more between the two central incisors, either in the maxillary dental arch, or in the mandibular dental arch, or in both.

Clinical Findings: A natural spacing of 1-3 mm or more exists between the two central incisors, both in the primary and secondary dentitions. The median diastema is regarded as a normal feature of the primary and mixed dentitions. Only when it persists after the eruption of the secondary canines, is it regarded as being abnormal.

Complications
I **Derived:** —
II **Associated:** Microdontia, macrognathia, peg or missing lateral incisors, midline cysts and supernumerary teeth. Abnormally attached frenum.

Etiology: Essentially unknown. Failure of the frenal attachment to migrate superiorly with relation to the alveolar ridge; McK *12590

Pathogenesis: At birth the frenum is attached to the alveolar ridge with fibers running into the lingual interdental papilla. Normally as the teeth erupt into occlusion and as alveolar bone is deposited, the frenum attachment migrates superiorly with respect to the alveolar ridge. Fibers may persist between the maxillary central incisors and in the V-shaped intermaxillary suture attaching to the outer layer of the periosteum and the connective tissue of the suture, thereby preventing contact between the mesial surfaces of the maxillary central incisors.

Related Facts
I   **Sex Ratio:** M1:F1
II **Risk of Occurrence:** —
III **Risk of Recurrence for**
    Patient's Sib: ?
    Patient's Child: ?
IV **Age of Detectability:** After eruption of anterior teeth by visual examination
V   **Prevalence:** Occurs predominantly between the maxillary central incisors-10 maxillary: 1 mandibular. In 541 patients between ages of 5 and 12 years 51.8% had diastemas.

In deciduous dentition	41.5%
In mixed dentition	61.0%
In permanent dentition	31.5%

Treatment
I   **Primary Prevention:** —
II **Secondary Prevention:** —
III **Other Therapy:** Surgical and orthodontic treatment in severe cases

Prognosis: Very good. Little indication for increased risk of tooth loss. Primarily of concern for esthetic reasons.

Detection of Carrier: —

Special Considerations: —

References:
Jakobsson, S. O.: Diastema mediale: En longitudinell undersökning. Odont. T. 73:127, 1965.
Rao, S. R. and Evans, L. K.: Occurrence of midline diastema in Rochester school children. Unpublished manuscript. 1964.
Taylor, J. E.: Clinical observations relating to normal frenum labii superioris. Am. J. Orthod. 25:646, 1939.

Contributor: **Satish R. Rao**

Editor's Computerized Descriptors: Face, Oral, Teeth

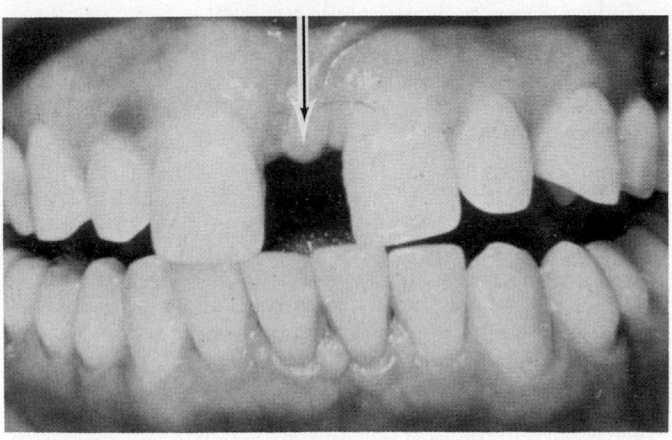

227. Diastema

DIASTEMATOMYELIA

Includes: Diastème de la moëlle (épinière)
Diastematomiélia
Diplomyelia with bony spur
Split notocord syndrome

Excludes: Spinal cord, neurenteric cyst (894)

Minimal Diagnostic Criteria: Clinical and roentgen findings leading to myelography which shows a double column of contrast material surrounding the divided spinal cord with a central dark radiolucent zone of varying extent between the two halves.

Clinical Findings: Most frequent presenting symptoms are gait disturbance with weakness and atrophy of one or both lower limbs. Bladder dysfunction may ensue. Pain in back or legs infrequent. Examination of lower back will show a skin abnormality such as a patch of hair, a cutaneous dimple, hemangioma, or a subcutaneous fat pad (66% of cases). Roentgenographic examination is positive showing spina bifida, scoliosis, or kyphoscoliosis with widening of the interpediculate distances in the region of the spinal cord anomaly. Hemivertebrae or fused vertebrae may also be seen. The finding of a bony spur is not to be expected in every case, because the spur may be fibrous or cartilaginous.

Complications
I **Derived:** Progressive neurologic deficit with bladder dysfunction and upper urinary tract pathology
II **Associated:** Spina bifida distal to the diastematomyelia present > 50%. Scoliosis in nearly all patients (4.9% of scoliosis patients have diastematomyelia).

Etiology: Exact cause not known. May result from hydromyelia in embryo leading to disruption of roof plate and separation of cord lateral masses. Alternately may represent accessory neurenteric canal.

Pathogenesis: During the closure of the neural tube from the primitive neuroectoderm in the 3rd to 4th week of gestation, aberrant mesodermal cells protrude into the neural tissue on its ventral surface instead of becoming arranged around its periphery. All cases reported are below the T-6 level. The spinal cord may be duplicated, but usually has a single dorsal and ventral cell mass with lateral roots and lacks medial roots. Each hemicord is covered with pia, arachnoid and dura. A frequent associated pathologic finding is an enlarged central canal (hydromyelia) cephalad to the diastematomyelia.

Related Facts
I **Sex Ratio:** F > M
II **Risk of Occurrence:** ? Rare
III **Risk of Recurrence for**
    Patient's Sib: ?
    Patient's Child: —
IV **Age of Detectability:** 1-15 years, although an occasional case is diagnosed as an adult
V **Prevalence:** Unusual

Treatment
I **Primary Prevention:** ?
II **Secondary Prevention:** ?
III **Other Therapy:** Surgical removal of the bony spur is indicated if lesion is symptomatic and in all young children when spinal column growth is anticipated to cause later symptoms.

Prognosis: Surgical results are satisfactory in preventing further neurologic loss with the possibility of improving the presurgical status.

Detection of Carrier: ?

Special Considerations: —

References:
Bremer, J. L.: Dorsal intestinal fistula; accessory neurenteric canal; diastematomyelia. Arch. Pathol. 54:132, 1952.
Cohen, J. and Sledge, C. B.: Diastematomyelia. An embryological interpretation with report of a case. Am. J. Dis. Child. 100:257, 1960.
Hendrick, E.B.: On diastematomyelia. In Progress in Neurosurgery. Basel:S. Karger, 1971, pp. 277-288.
Winter, R.B. et al: Diastematomyelia and congenital spine deformities. J. Bone Joint Surg. 56A:27, 1974.

Contributor: **Kenneth Shulman**

Editor's Computerized Descriptors: Skin, Hair, Skel., Muscle, GU., Nerve

DIASTROPHIC DYSPLASIA

Includes: Nanisme diastrophique
Diastrophischer Zwergwuchs
Enanismo diastrófico
Diastrophic dwarfism
Chondrodystrophy with clubfeet
Cherub dwarfs
Dwarfism, diastrophic

Excludes: Arthrogryposis (88)
Achondroplasia with clubfeet

Minimal Diagnostic Criteria: Micromelic short stature, present at birth, with or without hitch-hiker thumbs, symphalangism of the PIP joints, clubfeet, the characteristic swellings of the pinnae or cauliflower deformity.†

Clinical Findings: Marked shortness of stature with micromelia apparent at birth, progressive scoliosis often associated with kyphosis, a characteristic hand deformity with short fingers, synostosis of the proximal interphalangeal (PIP) joints and proximal insertion of the thumb in a hitch-hiker position; with or without hip and knee dislocation on weight bearing and severe bilateral clubfoot deformity. The ears show cystic swellings of the auricles in early infancy which later develop into cauliflower-like deformities with or without calcification and ossifications. Slightly more than 25% of the patients have a cleft palate. Intelligence is normal. On xray the long bones are reduced in length, thick, have broad metaphyses and flattened irregular epiphyses which may be late in mineralizing. The 1st metacarpal is oval or triangular in shape and is set low on the carpus. Other radiographic features include clubfeet, severe, progressive scoliosis, distortion of the pelvic bones, deformed femoral heads, coxa vara with dislocation or subluxation and, at times, calcification or ossification can be demonstrated in the pinnae. In infancy the epiphyses may have a stippled appearance.

Complications
I Derived: Subluxation or dislocation of the hips and knees and secondary degenerative arthritis. Scoliosis may result in marked kyphosis with or without respiratory problems. Failure to correct the clubfoot deformity further complicates ambulation and may be a source of much discomfort.
II Associated: —

Etiology: Autosomal recessive; McK *22260

Pathogenesis: Chondroosseous histopathology is characteristic with focal death of chondrocytes and subsequent cyst formation and intracartilaginous ossification.

Related Facts
I Sex Ratio: M1:F1
II Risk of Occurrence: ?
III Risk of Recurrence for
    Patient's Sib: 1 in 4 (25%) for each offspring to be affected
    Patient's Child: Not increased unless mate is carrier or homozygote
IV Age of Detectability: At birth
V Prevalence: ?

Treatment
I Primary Prevention: Genetic counseling†
II Secondary Prevention: Orthopedic management with the use of surgery, braces, casts and manipulations. Appropriate dental management and surgical closure of the cleft palate when indicated.
III Other Therapy: —

Prognosis: Normal for life span and intelligence. Those with severe kyphoscoliosis are prone to respiratory infections.

Detection of Carrier: ?

†Special Considerations: Because of the different mode of inheritance it is critical for genetic counseling that diastrophic dwarfism be differentiated from achondroplasia. Diastrophics, in comparison to achondroplasts, have normal sized heads and facies, lack trident hand deformities, do not have rhizomelic shortening of the limbs and are not prone to nerve root and cord compression in the lumbar area. Achondroplastic dwarfs lack anomalies of the pinnae, hitch-hiker thumbs and symphalangism, clubfeet, scoliosis and cleft palate. Radiographically the differences are also many and achondroplasia is autosomal dominant.

References:
Langer, L.O., Jr.: Diastrophic dwarfism in early infancy. Am. J. Roentgenol. Radium Ther. Nucl. Med. 93:399, 1965.
Rimoin, D.L. et al: Chrondro-osseous pathology in the chondrodystrophies. Clin. Orthop. 114:137, 1976.
Spranger, J.W. et al: Bone Dysplasias. Philadelphia: W.B. Saunders, 1974.
Walker, B.A. et al: Diastrophic dwarfism. Medicine 51:41, 1972.

Contributor: **Charles I. Scott, Jr.**

Editor's Computerized Descriptors: Ear, Oral, Skel.

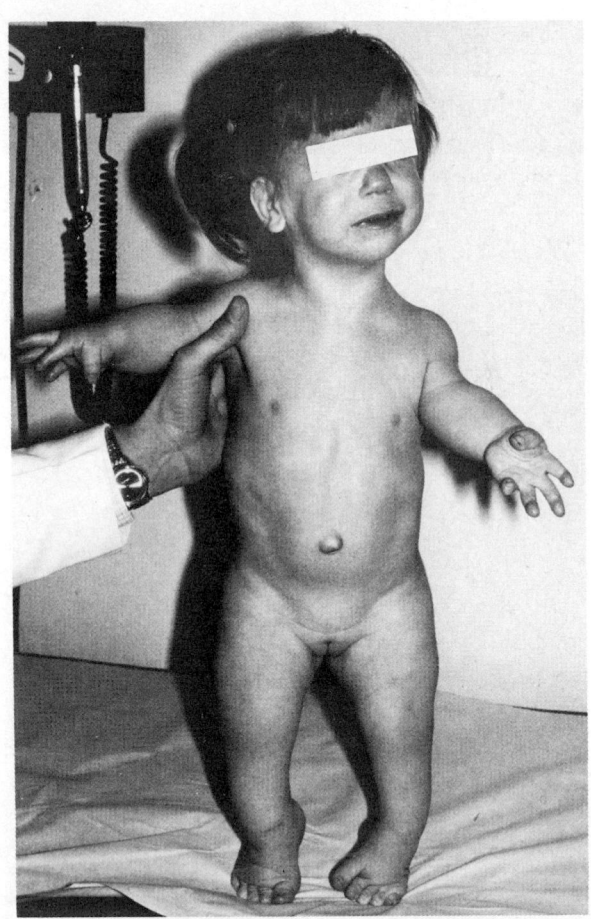

228. Note short limbs, clubfeet, tiptoe stance, and hitch-hiker thumbs

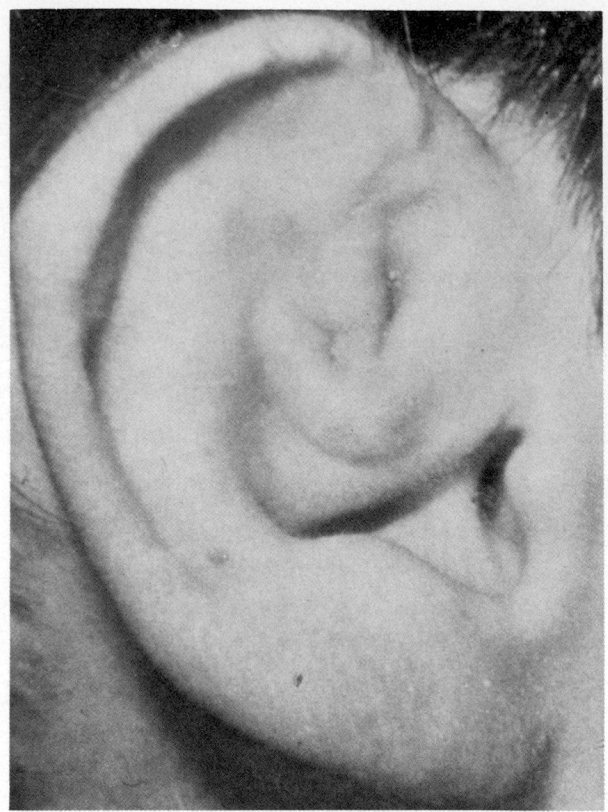

229. Cystic swelling of auricle producing cauliflower ear deformity

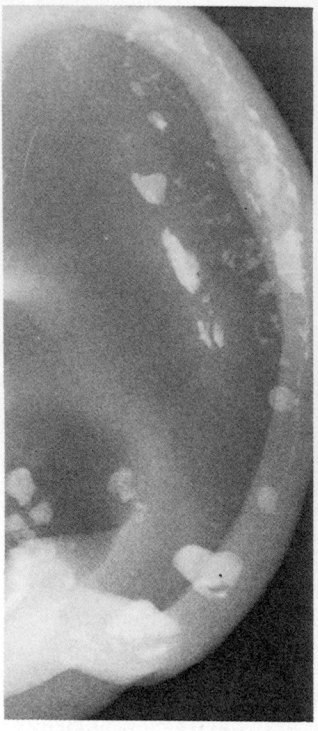

231. Calcification in pinna

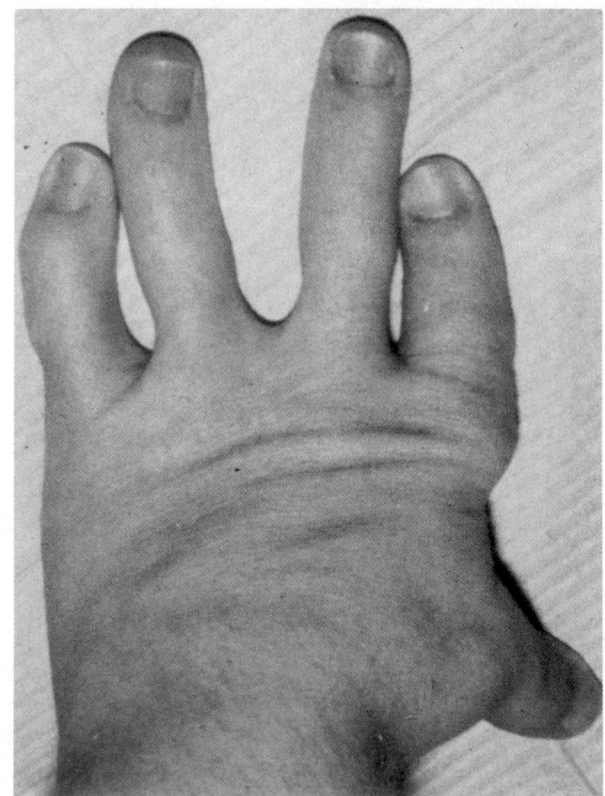

230. Short fingers; proximal thumb (hitch-hiker thumb)

Contributor: **Charles R. Scriver**

DICARBOXYLIC AMINOACIDURIA

Includes: Aminoacidurie dicarboxylique
Dicarboxyaminoacidurie
Aminoaciduria dicarboxílica

Excludes: —

Editor's Computerized Descriptor: GU.

Minimal Diagnostic Criteria: Selective excess of L-glutamate and L-aspartate in urine (dicarboxylicmonoamino acids), identifiable by partition chromatography, electrophoresis or elution chromatography on ion exchange resin columns. The corresponding plasma concentrations are normal. Endogenous renal clearance of both dicarboxylic amino acids is elevated and can exceed creatinine clearance.

Clinical Findings: Incidental finding in 2 infants. A tendency for fasting hypoglycemia, the presence of increased serum ketone bodies and low plasma bicarbonate without a defect in ammoniagenesis, with modest hyperprolinemia (< 1mM; <11.5 md/dl) was observed in Teijema's patient. Similar findings were absent in Melancon's patient.

Complications
I **Derived:** ? Those listed as Associated may be derived.
II **Associated:** Hypoglycemia after mild fasting; ketosis; impaired bicarbonate conservation (probably renal).

Etiology: ? Presumed to be autosomal recessive transmission involving either a defect in selective membrane transport system for dicarboxylicmonoamino acids, or intracellular transamination to keto acids during transepithelial movement.

Pathogenesis: Simple defect in uptake from tubule lumen will not explain C_{glu} and C_{asp} greater than $C_{creatinine}$; therefore impaired intracellular metabolism of amino acid to keto acid with intracellular accumulation and backflux is a possible explanation. Intestinal uptake defect was also suspected in Teijema's proband; pathogenesis (and etiology) of intestinal defect presumably similar to renal defect. †

Related Facts
I **Sex Ratio:** ?
II **Risk of Occurrence:** ?
III **Risk of Recurrence for**
  Patient's Sib: Presumed 1 in 4 (25%) for each offspring to be affected
  Patient's Child: Not increased unless mate is carrier or homozygote
IV **Age of Detectability:** Presumably in newborn period
V **Prevalence:** ?

Treatment
I **Primary Prevention:** Genetic counseling
II **Secondary Prevention:** —
III **Other Therapy:** Frequent feedings of L-glutamine has been demonstrated to prevent hypoglycemia.

Prognosis: ?

Detection of Carrier: Parents of proband have normal urine and plasma amino acid concentration and renal clearance of glutamate and aspartate.

†Special Considerations: Selective dicarboxylicmonoamino aciduria fulfills prediction from Hartnup disorder that there is a separate transepithelial transport system for these anionic amino acids.

References:
Melancon, S.B. et al: Dicarboxylic aminoaciduria: An inborn error of amino acid conservation. J. Pediatr. 91:422, 1977.
Teijema, H.L. et al: Dicarboxylic aminoaciduria: An inborn error of glutamate and aspartate transport with metabolic implications in combination with a hyperprolinemia. Metabolism 23:115, 1974.

DIPLEGIA, SPASTIC

Includes: Diplégie spastique
Spastische Diplegie
Diplegia espástica
Diplegia, infantile spastic
Spastic diplegia, hereditary
Familial spastic diplegia

Excludes: Birth injury
Congenital double hemiplegia
Sjögren-Larsson syndrome

Minimal Diagnostic Criteria: The diagnosis should be considered in an individual with slowly progressive upper motor neuron disease confined to the lower limbs in whom appropriate neurologic and roentgenologic examinations have been negative. A positive family history substantiates the diagnosis.

Clinical Findings: The age of onset of symptoms is variable but most commonly between 2 and 20 years. Patients initially complain of gait disturbances, which may be slowly progressive. An illness which confines the patient to bed may worsen the symptoms, probably secondary to immobility. Characteristically the signs are limited in a symmetric fashion to the lower limbs. Brisk reflexes, increased tone and extensor plantar reflexes are the most common findings. Muscle wasting, weakness, sensory disturbances or sphincter involvement do not occur. Intellect is usually normal. There are no typical roentgenologic or laboratory findings.

Complications
I **Derived:** Deformities such as pes cavus, kyphoscoliosis and contractures of the hips and knees occur
II **Associated:** —

Etiology: Autosomal recessive, but autosomal dominant may occur. McK *27020

Pathogenesis: ? The principal neuropathologic lesions are found in the spinal cord. Demyelination of the corticospinal, spinocerebellar tracts and loss of neurones in the dorsal nuclei of Clarke are the most common findings, and are most prominent in the thoracic and cervical spinal cord. No metabolic or toxic cause has been demonstrated. It is possible that familial spastic diplegia is the result of a very slowly progressive demyelinating disease.

Related Facts
I **Sex Ratio:** M1:F1
II **Risk of Occurrence:** ? Rare
III **Risk of Recurrence for**
  Patient's Sib: If autosomal recessive, or autosomal dominant, see Table I AR or AD, respectively.
  Patient's Child: If autosomal recessive, or autosomal dominant, see Table I AR or AD, respectively.
IV **Age of Detectability:** Variable, usually in 1st decade by physical examination
V **Prevalence:** ? Rare

Treatment
I **Primary Prevention:** Genetic counseling
II **Secondary Prevention:** Physical therapy may be useful. Avoid long periods of immobilization if possible
III **Other Therapy:** None. No drug found to be effective.

Prognosis: Good. Usually only minor incapacity so that patients may lead a full and useful life.

Detection of Carrier: —

Special Considerations: —

References:
Schwarz, G.A. and Liu, C.: Hereditary (familial) spastic paraplegia; further clinical and pathologic observations. Arch. Neurol. Psychiat. 75:144, 1956.
Sjögren, T. and Larsson, T.: Oligophrenia in combination with congenital ichthyosis and spastic disorders. Acta Psychiatr. Scand. 32 (Suppl.) 113:1, 1957.

Contributor: **Robert H. A. Haslam**

Editor's Computerized Descriptor: Nerve

DISTICHIASIS

Includes: Distiquiasis
Distichiasis congenita
Distichiasis congenita vera
Eyelashes, accessory

Excludes: Trichiasis†
Eyelid entropion (372)

Minimal Diagnostic Criteria: Accessory anomalous lashes on posterior edge of the lid margin in addition to the usual normal anterior row of cilia.†

Clinical Findings: An accessory row of lashes on the posterior border of an otherwise normal lid margin. Accessory cilia may vary in number from 3 or 4 to 20. The average number reported is 12 to 15 and they may be present on 1, 2, 3, or all 4 lids. Most commonly, some anomalous cilia are present on all 4 lids. Absence of normal Meibomian glands. Massage of lids produces no secretion from the Meibomian glands. A surprising number of patients have reported little or no irritation. This is probably due to the fact that the anomalous lashes are shorter, thinner and softer than the normal anterior lashes.

Complications
I **Derived:** Conjunctivitis and keratitis from continued conjunctival and corneal irritation by accessory cilia.
II **Associated:** Rarely ectropion or ptosis

Etiology: Autosomal dominant with strong penetrance; McK *12630

Pathogenesis: Probably a heterologous developmental anomaly. May be a sign of atavism in which the cilia are the product of the same anlage but differentiation has failed to take place.

Related Facts
I **Sex Ratio:** M1:F1
II **Risk of Occurrence:** Rare
III **Risk of Recurrence for**
 Patient's Sib: If parent is affected, 1 in 2 (50%) for each offspring to be affected; otherwise not increased.
 Patient's Child: 1 in 2
IV **Age of Detectability:** At birth
V **Prevalence:** Condition is exceedingly rare (about 80 cases have been reported in ophthalmic literature).

Treatment
I **Primary Prevention:** ? Genetic counseling
II **Secondary Prevention:** Resection and plastic repair is best. If only a few lashes, epilation or electrolysis may work.
III **Other Therapy:** —

Prognosis: Good except for ocular discomfort if condition is untreated.

Detection of Carrier: —

†Special Considerations: Because of its rarity the condition is most often confused with trichiasis (anterior row lashes pointing backward). Entropion (ie the whole margin of the lid turned inward) is a less common mistaken diagnosis. All such cases should be examined with good light and high magnification, such as a slit lamp.

References:
Bader, A.: Aplasia congenitalis glandularum Meibomii palpebrae inferioris, von Graefes. Arch. Ophthalmol. 150:411, 1950.
Blatt, N.: Distichiasis congenita vera. Z. Augenheilk. 53:325, 1924.
Pico, G.: Congenital ectropion and distichiasis: Etiologic and hereditary factors; a report of cases and review of literature. Am. J. Ophthalmol. 47:363, 1959.

Contributor: **Sidney A. Fox**

DOUBLE OUTLET RIGHT VENTRICLE WITH ANTERIOR VENTRICULAR SEPTAL DEFECT

Includes: Anomalie des gros vaisseaux (aorte et artère pulmonaire) qui prennent leur origine dans le ventricule droit. Communication inter-ventriculaire antérieure

Doppelte Ausstrombahn des rechten Ventrikels mit anterior gelegenem Ventrikelseptumdefekt

Ventrículo derecho a doble salida con comunicación inter-ventricular anterior

Taussig-Bing syndrome

Origin of both great vessels from right ventricle with subpulmonic ventricular septal defect

Ventricular septal defect with double outlet right ventricle

Excludes: Double outlet right ventricle with posterior ventricular septal defect (298)

Transposition of great vessels (962)

Minimal Diagnostic Criteria: Clinical evidence of cyanosis, cardiomegaly, heart failure, increased pulmonary arterial vascularity and biventricular hypertrophy in an infant who also demonstrates, on plain chest roentgenogram, gross enlargement of the relatively normally situated main pulmonary artery is suggestive of DORV with anterior VSD. The exact anatomic diagnosis depends upon selective angiocardiography.

Clinical Findings: Double outlet right ventricle (DORV) with anterior ventricular septal defect (VSD) is that cardiac malformation in which both the aorta and pulmonary artery arise entirely from the right ventricle. The only outlet from the left ventricle is via a large VSD anterior to or above the crista supraventricularis. This position of the VSD is just inferior to the pulmonary artery. Thus, the pulmonary artery overrides the defect to a varying extent, but arises in otherwise normal fashion from the right ventricular infundibulum. The pulmonary trunk and aorta are normally interrelated externally. However, the aortic valve is displaced to the right and lies higher than normal at about the same level as the pulmonic valve in both the cross-sectional and coronal body planes. Thus, the aortic valve cannot be in continuity with the anterior leaflet of the mitral valve. Right ventricular infundibular obstruction is not seen, but pulmonic valvar stenosis occurs rarely.

Clinical features mimic complete transposition of the great arteries with a VSD. The position of the VSD beneath the pulmonic valve results in selective streaming of left ventricular (oxygenated) blood into the pulmonary artery. The aorta receives primarily right ventricular (desaturated) blood. Thus, the patient is cyanotic from birth, although this may be mild in early infancy. Heart failure, chronic respiratory infections and growth retardation are usually present. A harsh systolic murmur is present at the upper left sternal border but is usually not accompanied by a thrill. The second sound is narrowly split or single and the pulmonic component is accentuated. A diastolic murmur of pulmonic insufficiency is occasionally heard. The ECG shows right axis deviation, right atrial enlargement and biventricular hypertrophy. Plain chest roentgenograms demonstrate markedly increased pulmonary vascularity of a shunt type, a prominent pulmonary artery segment, cardiomegaly involving both ventricles and left atrial enlargement. This is one of the few admixture lesions that is overtly cyanotic with a normally positioned pulmonary artery segment.

Since a great anatomic spectrum exists in this lesion, the echocardiographic differential diagnosis for DORV includes abnormalities in the tetralogy/truncus group as well as those in the transposition group. Identification of septal-aortic override or septal-pulmonic override with mitral semilunar discontinuity is essential for making this diagnosis. It was initially reported that an anterior displacement of the posterior great vessel from the mitral valve was diagnostic of this disorder. However, it has recently been pointed out that great difficulties arise in demonstrating this anterior-posterior displacement. Further, the presence of a subaortic or subpulmonic conus separating this posterior great vessel semilunar valve from the mitral valve is at least as important in delineating these malformations as is the anterior-posterior displacement. Secondary characteristics involving abnormal great vessel orientation may be of use in defining this group. See also Tetralogy of Fallot.

Cardiac catheterization and angiocardiography are necessary to establish the precise anatomy. Significant systemic arterial desaturation is present, and pulmonary artery oxygen saturation exceeds systemic artery saturation. This is in contrast to DORV with a posterior VSD. Catheter position may suggest the abnormal location of the aortic valve. Selective right ventricular angiography will demonstrate denser opacification of the aorta than of the pulmonary artery, while selective left ventricular angiography will demonstrate the VSD and denser opacification of the pulmonary artery than of the aorta. Angiocardiography also demonstrates the abnormal position of the aortic valve and its lack of relation to anterior leaflet of the mitral valve.

Complications
I Derived: Chronic heart failure, frequent respiratory infection, growth failure, and cyanosis may result in early death. With increasing age, pulmonary vascular disease will occur.

II Associated: —

Etiology: Presumably multifactorial inheritance

Pathogenesis: Failure of transfer of the posterior great artery (aorta) to the left ventricle results in DORV. The pathogenesis of the VSD is variable, but apparently is due to faulty development in both the conus septum and the muscular ventricular septum.

Related Facts
I Sex Ratio: M1:F1

II Risk of Occurrence: < 1 in 100 cases of congenital heart disease

III Risk of Recurrence for
Patient's Sib: ?
Patient's Child: ?

IV Age of Detectability: From birth

V Prevalence: ?

Treatment
I Primary Prevention: —

II Secondary Prevention: In infancy, palliative surgery may be necessary. Creation of an atrial septal defect and pulmonary artery banding will increase the amount of intracardiac mixing and thus increase the supply of oxygenated blood to the aorta. The total complex is now amenable to surgical correction by use of the Mustard procedure, originally designed for complete transposition of the great arteries. The atrial portion of the Mustard operation is performed as usual. The VSD is closed by a patch in such a way as to transfer the pulmonary artery to the left ventricle.

III Other Therapy: As necessary for congestive heart failure and pulmonary infection

Prognosis: Overall prognosis is poor with pulmonary arteriolar vascular disease being a common early complication. Survival beyond childhood without surgery is unlikely. With successful corrective surgery, prognosis may be favorable.

Detection of Carrier: —

Special Considerations: —

References:

French, J.W. and Popp, R.L.: The variability of echocardiographic discontinuity in double-outlet right ventricle and truncus arteriosus. Circulation 51:848, 1975.

Neufeld, H.N.: Origin of both great vessels from the right ventricle. In Moss, A.J. and Adams, F.H. (eds.): Heart Disease in Infants, Children and Adolescents. Baltimore: Williams & Wilkins, 1968, p. 577.

Sahn, D.J. et al: Echocardiographic versus anatomic discontinuity. Circulation 53:201, 1976.

Solinger, R. et al: Deductive echocardiographic analysis in infants with congenital heart disease. Circulation 50:1072, 1974.

Van Praagh, R.: What is the Taussig-Bing malformation? Circulation 28:445, 1968.

Contributor: **Ira H. Gessner**

Editor's Computerized Descriptors: Resp., CV.

DOUBLE OUTLET RIGHT VENTRICLE WITH POSTERIOR VENTRICULAR SEPTAL DEFECT

Includes: Anomalie des gros vaisseaux (aorte et artère pulmonaire) qui prennent leur origine dans le ventricule droit. Communication inter-ventriculaire postérieure.
Doppelte Ausstrombahn des rechten Ventrikels mit posterior gelegenem Ventrikelseptumdefekt
Ventrículo derecho a doble salida con comunicación inter-ventricular posterior
Origin of both great vessels from right ventricle with posterior ventricular septal defect

Excludes: Double outlet right ventricle with anterior ventricular septal defect (297)
Tetralogy of Fallot (938)
Transposition of great vessels (962)
Ventricular septal defect (989)

Minimal Diagnostic Criteria: Clinical evidence of a large left-to-right ventricular level shunt with pulmonary hypertension and a superiorly oriented, counterclockwise frontal plane QRS loop should arouse suspicion of DORV with posterior VSD and no pulmonic stenosis. Selective angiography is necessary to establish a correct diagnosis. DORV with posterior VSD and pulmonic stenosis simulates tetralogy of Fallot almost exactly. The presence of marked right atrial enlargement and of atrioventricular conduction delay would suggest DORV with pulmonic stenosis, but selective angiocardiography is necessary to establish the exact anatomy.†

Clinical Findings: Double outlet right ventricle (DORV) with posterior ventricular septal defect (VSD) is that cardiac malformation in which both the aorta and pulmonary artery arise entirely from the right ventricle. The only outlet from the left ventricle is via a large VSD which is posterior in location, ie below the crista supraventricularis. The pulmonary trunk and aorta are normally interrelated externally. However, the aortic valve is displaced to the right and lies higher than normal at about the same level as the pulmonic valve in both the cross-sectional and coronal body planes. The displaced aortic valve results in lack of continuity between the anterior leaflet of the mitral valve and the aortic valve. Obstruction to flow into the pulmonary artery is common, due to right ventricular infundibular hypertrophy. Subaortic obstruction is rarely seen.

Clinical features are related primarily to the degree of pulmonic obstruction. Without pulmonic obstruction, the clinical features closely resemble a large VSD with right ventricular hypertension. Poor growth, frequent respiratory infection and heart failure are present in infancy. A precordial systolic thrill and grade IV/VI harsh systolic murmur along the lower left sternal border, a narrowly split and accentuated second sound, and an apical diastolic murmur of increased mitral valve flow indicate the presence of a large VSD with elevated right ventricular pressure. Cyanosis is usually minimal or absent because the posterior location of the VSD allows left ventricular output to be directed through the VSD towards the aortic valve and thus significant mixing in the right ventricle may not occur. With time, pulmonary arteriolar disease may develop resulting in increased pulmonary vascular resistance. Cyanosis will then become a prominent feature. The ECG demonstrates left atrial enlargement and biventricular hypertrophy. A distinctive ECG feature commonly seen is marked left axis deviation and superior counterclockwise frontal plane QRS forces, similar to that seen in an endocardial cushion defect. Plain chest roentgenograms demonstrate a large pulmonary artery segment, increased pulmonary vascularity of the shunt type, left atrial enlargement and cardiomegaly, findings which are not specific for this malformation. In the presence of significant pulmonic obstruction, the clinical features mimic those of tetralogy of Fallot and indeed may be indistinguishable. Cyanosis is present from early infancy. A left lower parasternal systolic thrill and murmur and a single second sound are found. There is no mitral flow murmur.

The ECG frequently demonstrates right atrial enlargement and always shows right ventricular hypertrophy of the type commonly seen in tetralogy of Fallot. In DORV without pulmonary stenosis, right axis deviation is seen and the QRS forces are directed inferiorly. Delayed atrioventricular conduction time and intraventricular conduction delay are commonly seen. Right atrial enlargement and delayed atrioventricular conduction are unusual in tetralogy of Fallot, providing one of the few distinguishing clinical features between these 2 malformations. Plain chest roentgenograms demonstrate decreased pulmonary arterial vascularity, a prominent aorta, mild cardiomegaly involving the right heart, a small right ventricular outflow tract with absence of a pulmonary artery segment, and no left atrial enlargement, features commonly seen in tetralogy of Fallot as well.

Since a great anatomic spectrum exists in this lesion, the echocardiographic differential diagnosis for DORV includes abnormalities in the tetralogy/truncus group as well as those in the transposition group. Identification of septal-aortic override or septal-pulmonic override with mitral semilunar discontinuity is essential for making this diagnosis. It was initially reported that an anterior displacement of the posterior great vessel from the mitral valve was diagnostic of this disorder. However, it has recently been pointed out that great difficulties arise in demonstrating this anterior-posterior displacement. Further, the presence of a subaortic or subpulmonic conus separating this posterior great vessel semilunar valve from the mitral valve is at least as important in delineating these malformations as is the anterior-posterior displacement. Secondary characteristics involving abnormal great vessel orientation may be of use in defining this group. See also Tetralogy of Fallot.

Cardiac catheterization and selective angiocardiography are necessary to establish the precise anatomic diagnosis. Without pulmonic obstruction, the catheterization findings are those of a large VSD with equal pressures in the left and right ventricles. Mild systemic arterial desaturation is usually seen, although, as mentioned above, streaming of left ventricular blood into the aorta may be so precise that little systemic arterial desaturation is found. Systemic arterial oxygen saturation is significantly greater than pulmonary oxygen saturation. Position of the catheter in the great vessels may suggest the abnormal location of the aortic valve. Selective right and left ventricular angiography will demonstrate the exact anatomic situation, illustrating the lack of continuity of the mitral valve with a semilunar valve, a large posterior VSD and the abnormal location of the aortic valve. In the presence of pulmonic obstruction, the catheterization findings are similar to tetralogy of Fallot. Again, catheter localization of the aortic valve may suggest its abnormal position. Selective right ventricular angiography is necessary to distinguish these 2 malformations, however.

Complications

I   **Derived:**   Without pulmonic stenosis, chronic heart failure, frequent respiratory infections and poor growth occur. Eventual development of pulmonary vascular disease is common. With pulmonic stenosis, hypoxic spells may occur.

II   **Associated:**   —

Etiology: Presumably multifactorial inheritance

Pathogenesis: Failure of transfer of the posterior great artery (aorta) to the left ventricle results in DORV. The conus septum fails to develop properly and a large VSD results. If the conus septum is displaced anteriorly and becomes hypertrophied, infundibular (pulmonic) obstruction results.

Related Facts
I   **Sex Ratio:**   M1:F1
II   **Risk of Occurrence:**   < 1 in 100 cases of congenital heart defects
III   **Risk of Recurrence for**
   Patient's Sib: ?
   Patient's Child: ?
IV   **Age of Detectability:**   From birth
V   **Prevalence:**   ?

Treatment
I   **Primary Prevention:**   —
II   **Secondary Prevention:**   Corrective surgery may be accomplished by construction of a tunnel from the VSD to the root of the aorta. If present, infundibular hypertrophy can be resected. When the aorta is too far removed from the VSD for correction, in the absence of infundibular obstruction, pulmonary artery banding may be performed as a palliative procedure.
III   **Other Therapy:**   As necessary for congestive heart failure and pneumonia.

Prognosis: Poor; survival is enhanced by a moderate degree of pulmonic obstruction.

Detection of Carrier: —

†**Special Considerations:**   DORV may occur in association with the fundamental ventricular abnormality, ventricular inversion. In that instance, since the anatomic right ventricle is located on the left, both great arteries arise from the left-sided right ventricle.

Complete transposition of the great vessels may occur together with DORV. In that situation, the aorta is located to the left and slightly anteriorly arising from the right ventricular infundibulum. The pulmonary artery arises to the right and posterior of the aorta with lack of continuity between the mitral valve and the pulmonic valve. The physiology is similar to the ordinary case of complete transposition of the great vessels with a VSD.

References:
Neufeld, H.N.: Origin of both vessels from the right ventricle. In Moss, A.J. and Adams, F.H. (eds.): Heart Disease in Infants, Children and Adolescents. Baltimore: Williams & Wilkins, 1968, p. 577.

Contributor: **Ira H. Gessner**

Editor's Computerized Descriptors: Resp., CV.

DUBOWITZ SYNDROME

Includes: Syndrome de Dubowitz
Síndrome de Dubowitz

Excludes: Seckel syndrome (881)
Nanocephaly
Fetal alcohol syndrome (379)

Minimal Diagnostic Criteria: Low birthweight, postnatal growth retardation, microcephaly, characteristic facial features.

Clinical Findings: All reported patients have had low birthweight, postnatal growth retardation, and microcephaly. Mental retardation of a mild degree is frequently encountered. The characteristic dysmorphic facial features include: sparse hair, high sloping forehead, flat supraorbital ridges, broad nasal bridge in line with the forehead, telecanthus, ptosis, blepharophimosis with short palpebral fissures, epicanthal folds and micrognathia. The voice is usually high-pitched and hoarse. The lateral portions of the eyebrows may be hypoplastic. Eczema, poor dietary intake, vomiting and chronic diarrhea may occur during the 1st year. Internal abnormalities have not been detected. Hypospadias or cryptorchidism may be encountered in affected males.

Complications
I **Derived:** Shy personality, withdrawal from peers due to short stature.
II **Associated:** Prolapse of rectum due to chronic diarrhea, infection of eczema, failure to thrive, poor school performance.

Etiology: Autosomal recessive; McK *22337

Pathogenesis: ?

Related Facts
I **Sex Ratio:** M1:F1
II **Risk of Occurrence:** ? Probably much more common than the 17 cases would suggest.
III **Risk of Recurrence for**
    Patient's Sib: 1 in 4 (25%) for each offspring to be affected
    Patient's Child: Not increased unless mate is carrier or homozygote
IV **Age of Detectability:** At birth
V **Prevalence:** ?

Treatment
I **Primary Prevention:** Genetic counseling
II **Secondary Prevention:** —
III **Other Therapy:** Surgery for ptosis or ocular abnormality; special education

Prognosis: Probably normal life span

Detection of Carrier: —

Special Considerations: —

References:
Dubowitz, V.: Familial low birthweight dwarfism with an unusual facies and a skin eruption. J. Med. Genet. 2:12, 1965.
Grosse, R. et al: The Dubowitz syndrome. Z. Kinderheilkd. 110:175, 1971.
Majewski, F. et al: A rare type of low birthweight dwarfism: The Dubowitz syndrome. Z. Kinderheilkd. 120:283, 1975.
Opitz, J.M. et al: Studies of malformation syndromes in man XXIV B: The Dubowitz syndrome. Further observations. Z. Kinderheilkd. 116:1, 1973.

Contributor: **R.S. Wilroy, Jr.**

DUODENAL ATRESIA OR STENOSIS

Includes: Atrésie ou sténose duodénale
Duodenalatresie oder-stenose
Atresia o estenosis duodenal

Excludes: Stomach atresia (910)
Duodenal bands
Annular pancreas (62)

Minimal Diagnostic Criteria: Gastric distention usually associated with emesis during the first 24 to 36 hours of life. Characteristic "double bubble" appearance of abdominal roentgenograms with absence of air in remainder of abdomen.

Clinical Findings: The location of the atresia or stenosis is classified as preampullary in approximately 20% and postampullary in approximately 80% of patients. The intestine is shorter than normal in less than 2% of patients. Annular pancreas occurs in approximately 21% and is believed to be a factor producing obstruction in approximately half. Complete interruption of the duodenum with separation of the ends is rare. Approximately 54% of patients are premature by birthweight. Emesis is the first symptom in over 80% of patients and is bile-stained in three-fourths of them. Abdominal distention usually localized to the upper abdomen is seen in over one-third of patients. Meconium is passed in over 52% of patients prior to operation. Jaundice occurs in approximately 37% of patients and occasionally requires exchange transfusion. Plain abdominal roentgenograms with air insufflation of the stomach demonstrate the characteristic "double bubble" appearance for duodenal atresia. Polyhydramnios is present in approximately 45% of mothers. Duodenal stenosis or duodenal diaphragm usually is not recognized until after the first few days of life. Upper GI roentgenograms after barium ingestion is usually necessary to demonstrate this lesion.

Complications
I **Derived:** Intestinal obstruction with emesis and electrolyte depletion. Tracheal aspiration occurs commonly if not relieved.
II **Associated:** Present in approximately 48% of patients. Approximately 30% have chromosome 21 trisomy syndrome. Malrotation of the colon with incomplete intestinal fixation occurs in approximately 22% and congenital heart disease occurs in 20% of the patients. Tracheoesophageal fistula, and renal malformations are slightly less common.

Etiology: ? McK *22340

Pathogenesis: Possible persistence of "solid cord state" of small segment of duodenum during embryonic development. Possible in utero vascular obstruction to segment of duodenum. Possible compression of duodenum by surrounding annular pancreas.

Related Facts
I **Sex Ratio:** M1:F1
II **Risk of Occurrence:** 1 in 10,000 live births with no racial predilection
III **Risk of Recurrence for**
   Patient's Sib: 1 in 10,000
   Patient's Child: 1 in 10,000
IV **Age of Detectability:** As neonate in most patients
V **Prevalence:** ?

Treatment
I **Primary Prevention:** —
II **Secondary Prevention:** Duodenoduodenostomy.†
III **Other Therapy:** Gastrostomy usually recommended

Prognosis: Death from inanition if obstruction is not relieved.

Sixty percent of patients with duodenal atresia, 71% with duodenal diaphragms, and 77% with duodenal stenosis survive. Death is usually attributed to respiratory complications (28%). Late deaths are uncommon.

Detection of Carrier: —

†Special Considerations: Associated malformations frequently complicate postoperative management following duodenoduodenostomy.

References:
Fonkalsrud, E.W. et al: Congenital atresia and stenosis of the duodenum: A review compiled from the members of the Surgical Section of the Academy of Pediatrics. Pediatrics 43:79, 1969.
Lynn, H.B.: Duodenal obstruction. In Mustard, W.T. et al (eds.): Pediatric Surgery. Chicago: Year Book Medical Publishers, 1969, p. 800.

Contributor: **Eric W. Fonkalsrud**

Editor's Computerized Descriptors: CV., GI.

DUPUYTREN CONTRACTURE

Contributor: **Robert A. Norum**

Includes: Contracture de Dupuytren
Dupuytrensche Kontraktur
Palmar fibromatosis
Fibromatosis, palmar

Editor's Computerized Descriptors: Skin, Skel., GU.

Excludes: Camptodactyly

Minimal Diagnostic Criteria: A nodule in the palmar fascia or an interphalangeal band producing a flexion deformity of the PIP joint.

Clinical Findings: Subcutaneous palmar nodules and flexion contractures of the fingers at the proximal interphalangeal (PIP) and metacarpophalangeal joints. Web space contractures draw pairs of digits together. Skin pits are attached to palmar bands. Knuckle pads and the Peyronie fibrous contracture of the penis are sometimes associated. Hand contractures are bilateral in 90%.

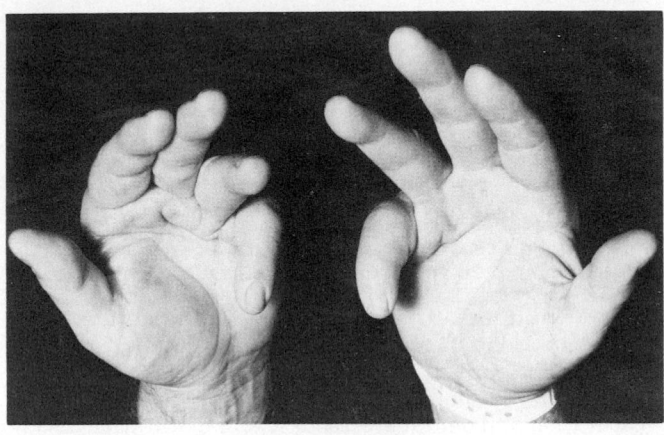

232. Dupuytren contracture

Complications
I **Derived:** Varying loss of function in affected hands
II **Associated:** Knuckle pads are seen in 25% of cases, plantar involvement in 20%, and penile lesions in 3%.

Etiology: Autosomal dominant transmission with variable penetrance is likely, but unproved. Association with epilepsy, alcoholism, pulmonary tuberculosis and chronic invalidism has been suggested but has not been proved.

Pathogenesis: Fibrofatty tissue anterior to the palmar aponeurosis is replaced by centrifugal fibrosis which results in fixation of skin, aponeurosis and skeleton, but not tendons in synovial sheaths. Contracture of newly produced mature collagen results in thickening of nodules and bands and progressively flexes digits at the metacarpophalangeal and PIP joints with hyperextension of the distal interphalangeal joint in advanced stages.

Related Facts
I **Sex Ratio:** Under age 40, M2:F1; over age 40, M1:F1
II **Risk of Occurrence:** ?
III **Risk of Recurrence for**
Patient's Sib: When autosomal dominant and if parent is affected, 1 in 2 (50%) for each offspring to be affected; otherwise not increased
Patient's Child: 1 in 2
IV **Age of Detectability:** Uncommon under age 20
V **Prevalence:** Almost exclusively in people of European descent increasing in frequency from 4% under age 20 years to 20% over age 60.

Treatment
I **Primary Prevention:** Genetic counseling when autosomal dominant
II **Secondary Prevention:** Surgical excision of fibrotic tissue is sometimes indicated†
III **Other Therapy:** —

Prognosis: Normal for life span and intelligence, variable disability in affected hands

Detection of Carrier: —

†**Special Considerations:** About one-third of patients with a strong family history, plantar lesions, knuckle pads, or a penile contracture (Peyronie disease) have recurrence after surgical excision.

References:
Hueston, J. T.: Dupuytren's Contracture. Baltimore: Williams and Wilkins, 1963.
Lygonis, C.: Familiar Dupuytren's contracture. Hereditas 56:142, 1966.
Maza, R.K. and Goodman, R.M.: A family with Dupuytren's contracture. J. Hered. 59:155, 1968.

DWARFISM, LARON

Includes: Nanisme de type Laron
Laron Zwergwuchs
Enanismo de Laron
Familial dwarfism with high plasma immunoreactive human growth hormone (hGH)
Laron dwarfism

Excludes: Growth hormone deficiency, isolated (447)
Panhypopituitarism
Primordial dwarfism
Other causes of proportionate short stature

Minimal Diagnostic Criteria: Proportionate dwarfism with elevated basal plasma hGH; low plasma somatomedin activity; absent response to exogenous hGH administration.

Clinical Findings: Proportionate short stature with growth retardation commencing in early infancy. Normal birthweight and slightly decreased birth length. With growth retardation there are accompanying delays in bone maturation and dental eruption; sexual maturation also is delayed but eventually complete. There may be early delays in motor development. Intelligence usually normal though average IQ may be reduced.

Physically, patients resemble each other closely. Craniofacial disproportion due to maxillary and mandibular hypoplasia results in large appearing head, saddle nose, and "sign of the sunset" eyes. Hair growth may be slow and the hair sparse; the teeth may be discolored and brittle. Hands and feet are relatively small, as apparently are the male genitalia. The truncal obesity and high-pitched voice characteristic of pituitary dwarfs are present. Physically patients cannot be differentiated from those with isolated hGH deficiency, but they are significantly shorter on the average.

Metabolically they are characterized by an elevation of basal immunoreactive hGH levels. However, as in normals, hGH levels are variable and multiple blood samples may have to be analyzed to document elevation. Plasma hGH concentrations rise further in response to provocative stimuli, but fail to be suppressed normally with hyperglycemia. Serum somatomedin levels are low and there is no response to exogenous hGH. Also, there is no sustained response in linear growth with administration of exogenous hGH. Other metabolic parameters show little or no response to hGH administration though variability has been noted. Abnormal glucose metabolism is present with hypersensitivity to insulin, insulinopenia and spontaneous hypoglycemia during infancy and childhood.

Complications
I **Derived:** Spontaneous hypoglycemia of infancy and childhood.
II **Associated:** —

Etiology: Autosomal recessive; McK *26250

Pathogenesis: ? Cannot presently distinguish between the following hypotheses: 1) metabolic defect in somatomedin generation; 2) defective hGH end-organ responsiveness with perhaps an altered hGH receptor site; 3) an abnormal hGH molecule which is immunologically normal but has altered biologic activity.

Related Facts
I **Sex Ratio:** M1:F1 approximately
II **Risk of Occurrence:** ?
III **Risk of Recurrence for**
   Patient's Sib: 1 in 4 (25%) for each offspring to be affected
   Patient's Child: Not increased unless mate is carrier or homozygote

IV **Age of Detectability:** Clinically in early infancy with appearance of growth retardation or hypoglycemia. May be detectable at birth by hGH measurement. However, hGH levels are elvated normally during the first 2-4 weeks of life.
V **Prevalence:** Rare; originally described in oriental Jews but affected individuals in other ethnic groups have been described.

Treatment
I **Primary Prevention:** Genetic counseling
II **Secondary Prevention:** No effective treatment available for short stature.
III **Other Therapy:** Treatment of spontaneous hypoglycemia to prevent CNS damage.

Prognosis: Good for general health; marked dwarfism a certainty.

Detection of Carrier: —

Special Considerations: —

References:
Laron, Z. et al: Pituitary dwarfism with high serum levels of growth hormone. Isr. J. Med. Sci. 4:883, 1968.
Laron, Z. et al: Administration of growth hormone to patients with familial dwarfism with high plasma immunoreactive growth hormone: Measurement of sulfation factor, metabolic and linear growth responses. J. Clin. Endocrinol. Metab. 33:332, 1971.
Rabinowitz, D. and Merimee, T.J.: Isolated human growth hormone deficiency and related disorders. Isr. J. Med. Sci. 9:1601, 1973.

Contributors: **Jonathan Zonana**
David L. Rimoin

Editor's Computerized Descriptors: Eye, Face, Teeth, Nose, Hair, Skel., GU.

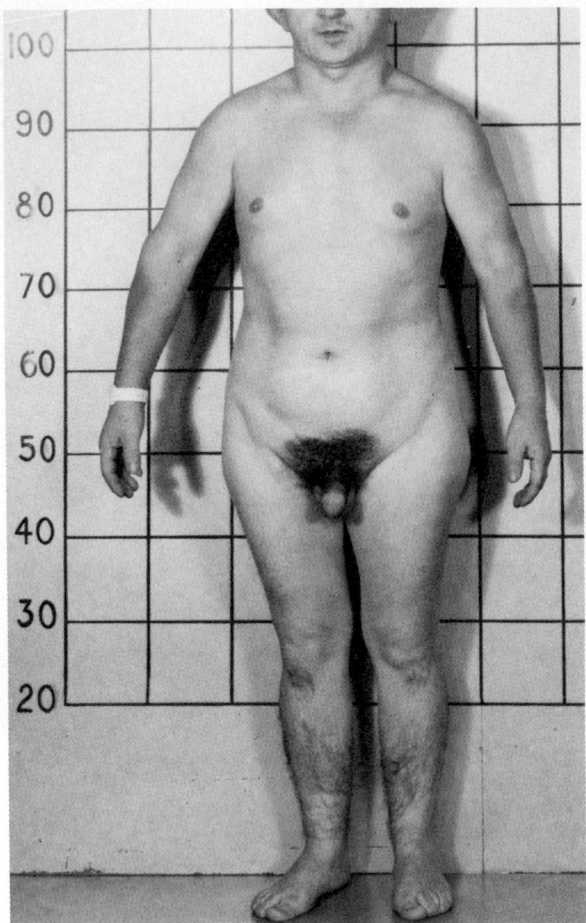

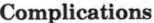

233. Proportionate short stature with high basal levels of hGH, low sulfation factor activity, and peripheral insensitivity to hGH

DWARFISM, PANHYPOPITUITARY

Includes: Nanisme panhypopituaire
Panhypopituitarismus
Enanismo panhipopituitario
Asexual ateleotic dwarfism

Excludes: Congenital absence of the pituitary
Dwarfism, pituitary with abnormal sella turcica (304)
Growth hormone deficiency, isolated† (447)
Dwarfism, Laron (302)

Minimal Diagnostic Criteria: Consistently decreased hGH response to recognized stimuli such as L-dopa, arginine, or insulin-induced hypoglycemia together with evidence of at least one other tropic hormone deficiency: gonadotropins, ACTH or TSH.

Clinical Findings: A deficiency of human growth hormone (hGH) and at least one other pituitary hormone including gonadotropins followed in order of frequency by adrenocorticotropic hormone (ACTH) and thyroid stimulating hormone (TSH) occur in panhypopituitary dwarfism. However, the particular pattern may vary among families and even among affected members of the same family. The clinical findings depend on which pituitary hormone deficiencies are present.

The hGH deficiency results in dwarfism, excess subcutaneous adipose tissue, a high-pitched peculiar voice, soft wrinkled skin, and childlike facies. The growth retardation is not usually evident prior to 6 months of age, and is proportionate although adults retain childlike proportions, ie relatively long trunk and short legs. The deficiency is associated with a marked delay in skeletal bone age. Metabolically the lack of hGH leads to glucose intolerance, decreased lipolysis, a relative insulinopenia and diminished serum somatomedin levels. Gonadotropin deficiency results in complete lack of secondary sexual characteristics. Females demonstrate primary amenorrhea and males, small testes and phallus. When present, ACTH deficiency may contribute to severe hypoglycemic attacks in infancy and childhood. TSH deficiency usually does not result in severe hypothyroidism but may occasionally produce definite signs including slow reflexes, hypometabolism and epiphyseal dysplasia.

Complications
I   **Derived:** Related to particular hormone deficiencies present.
II **Associated:** —

Etiology: Most cases occur sporadically, and the majority are probably not genetic. However, both autosomal recessive and X-linked recessive inheritance patterns have been described; and all 3 forms are clinically and metabolically indistinguishable. McK *26240

Pathogenesis: In most cases a hypothalamic defect is likely, since, in these cases, the pituitary responds to synthetic hypothalamic releasing factors. In the remainder, a structural, degenerative or secretory defect of the pituitary is postulated.

Related Facts
I   **Sex Ratio:** M1:F1 in sporadic and autosomal recessive forms. Only males affected in X-linked recessive form.
II **Risk of Occurrence:** Very low
III **Risk of Recurrence for**
    Patient's Sib: The occurrence in a sporadic family member probably represents a nongenetic case, and the risk of recurrence is negligible. If autosomal or X-linked recessive see Table 1 AR or X-linked R, respectively.
    Patient's Child: If autosomal or X-linked recessive see Table I AR or X-linked R, respectively. Fertility is rare due to gonadotropin deficiency.
IV **Age of Detectability:** Growth retardation is usually not

apparent before 6 months of age, but if suspected, hGH and other hormone deficiencies can be identified at birth.†

V   Prevalence: Very low

Treatment

I   Primary Prevention: Genetic counseling in inherited types.

II   Secondary Prevention: Replacement with hGH and other secondarily deficient hormones, ie thyroxine, cortisone, estrogens, testosterone. In some cases it may be possible to induce fertility by appropriate gonadotropin therapy.

III   Other Therapy: —

Prognosis: Depends upon adequacy of treatment. Relatively normal stature and correction of hormonal deficiency states may result from early diagnosis and appropriate treatment.

Detection of Carrier: —

†Special Considerations: Since patients with isolated growth hormone deficiency usually have delayed puberty, it may be difficult to differentiate panhypopituitary from isolated growth hormone deficient patients in late adolescence. Treatment with growth hormone often stimulates spontaneous puberty in isolated growth hormone deficient patients and may help in this distinction.

References:

Rimoin, D.L. and Schimke, R.N.: Genetic Disorders of the Endocrine Glands. St. Louis: C.V. Mosby, 1971, p. 11.

Rimoin, D.L. Hereditary forms of growth hormone deficiency and resistance. In Bergsma, D. (ed.): Growth Problems and Clinical Advances. Birth Defects: Orig. Art. Ser., vol. XII, no.6. New York: Alan R. Liss, Inc. for The National Foundation-March of Dimes, 1976, p. 15.

Contributors: **William A. Horton**
David L. Rimoin

Editor's Computerized Descriptors: Face, Speech, Skin, Skel., GU.

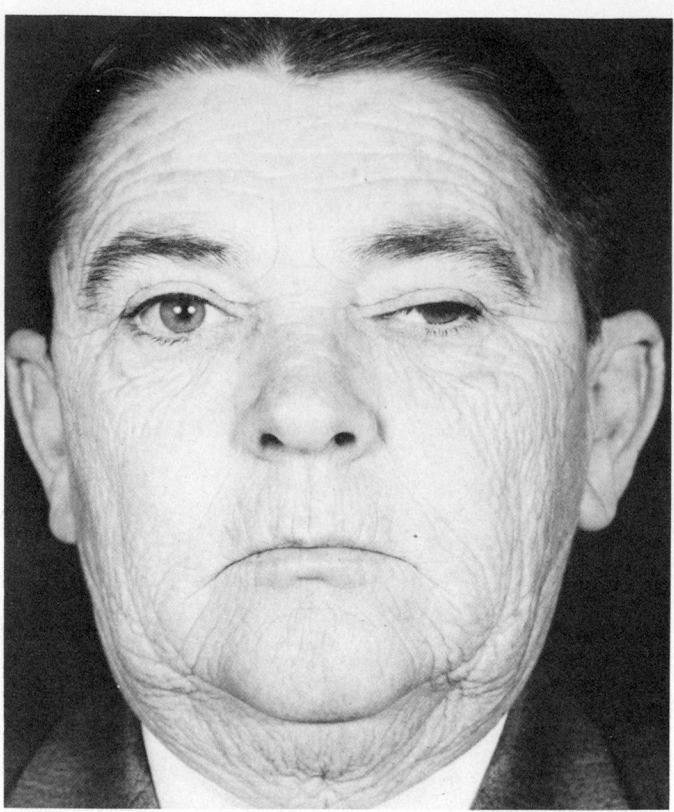

235. Marked wrinkling of face and congenital ptosis in 53-year-old man

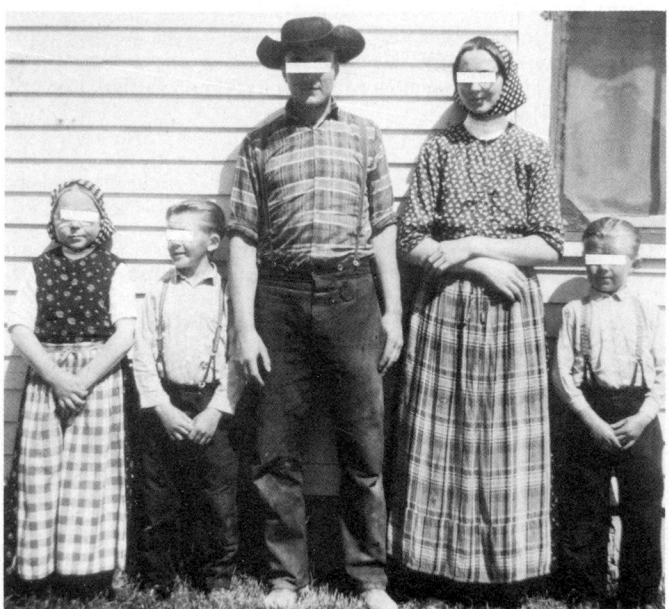

234. Familial panhypopituitarism in a Hutterite sibship. Left to right: female age 31; male, 27; normal brother, 25; normal sister, 24, male, 20

DWARFISM, PITUITARY WITH ABNORMAL SELLA TURCICA

Includes: Nanisme pituitaire avec anomalie de la selle turcique
Familiärer hypophysärer Zwergwuchs mit abnormer sella turcica
Enanismo familiar hipofisario con silla turca anormal

Excludes: Congenital absence of the pituitary
Panhypopituitary dwarfism, familial
Dwarfism, panhypopituitary (303)
Growth hormone deficiency, isolated (447)
Dwarfism, Laron (302)

Minimal Diagnostic Criteria: Characteristically abnormal sella turcica on xray associated with evidence of pituitary insufficiency.†

Clinical Findings: Two female sibs have been reported with severe growth failure, spontaneous hypoglycemia and laboratory evidence of a relative deficiency of human growth hormone (hGH), adrenocorticotropic hormone (ACTH), and thyroid stimulating hormone (TSH). Both had a radiographically abnormal sella turcica located in a morphologically abnormal sphenoid bone. Mental retardation was present in both sibs but may have been due to repeated episodes of hypoglycemia. Gonadotropin status was not known since the oldest sib was only 10 years old.

Complications
I Derived: Related to hormone deficiencies
II Associated: —

Etiology: Probable autosomal recessive inheritance in the 1 family reported.

Pathogenesis: Presumably a defect in the hypothalamic-pituitary axis.

Related Facts
I Sex Ratio: Presumably M1:F1
II Risk of Occurrence: Very low
III Risk of Recurrence for
  Patient's Sib: 1 in 4 (25%) for each offspring to be affected
  Patient's Child: Not increased unless mate is carrier or homozygote
IV Age of Detectability: At birth, if suspected, but growth failure not usually apparent before 6 months.
V Prevalence: Very low

Treatment
I Primary Prevention: Genetic counseling
II Secondary Prevention: Replacement of hGH and secondarily deficient hormones, ie thyroxine, cortisone, estrogen, etc. when needed.
III Other Therapy: —

Prognosis: —

Detection of Carrier: —

†**Special Considerations:** All cases of pituitary dwarfism should have lateral radiographs of the skull to rule out this disorder.

References:
Ferrier, P.E. and Stone, E.F.: Familial pituitary dwarfism associated with an abnormal sella turcica. Pediatrics 43:858, 1969.
Rimoin, D.L. and Schimke, R.N.: Genetic Disorders of the Endocrine Glands. St. Louis: C.V. Mosby, 1971, p. 11.

Contributors: **William A. Horton
David L. Rimoin**

Editor's Computerized Descriptor: Skel.

DWARFISM, SNUB-NOSE

Includes: Nanisme à nez camus
Dominanter Zwergwuchs Typ Levi
Enanismo tipo "nariz aplastada"
Dominantly inherited dwarfism of Levi

Excludes: Other types of low-birthweight dwarfism such as recessively determined hypopituitary dwarfism
Dwarf with lateral asymmetry
Seckel syndrome (881)
Cockayne syndrome (189)

Minimal Diagnostic Criteria: Birthweight is likely to be less than 2.0 kg. Subsequent growth rate will remain below the 3rd percentile for the population under consideration. Snub-nose appearance and stocky build are the rule.†

Clinical Findings: Affected infants are said to be born at full term of low birthweight, but this is not very well documented. Growth rate is consistently slow. Puberty occurs but may be slightly delayed. Skeletal development appears to be normal in most cases. Characteristic appearance includes a stocky build with depressed nasal bridge and brachycephaly. The term "snub-nose" probably is not strictly correct since, while the bridge of the nose is flat, the tip is normal.

Complications
I Derived: —
II Associated: Inguinal hernia, undescended testes

Etiology: Autosomal dominant

Pathogenesis: The pathogenesis of this condition is not known but may involve a defect in secretion of or response to growth hormone or some other factor operative in intrauterine life and responsible for intrauterine growth and the setting of subsequent growth pattern throughout life. A definitive biochemical abnormality has not been found. The only structural defect is gross dwarfism.†

Related Facts
I Sex Ratio: M1:F1
II Risk of Occurrence: ? Rare
III Risk of Recurrence for
  Patient's Sib: If parent is affected 1 in 2 (50%) for each sib; otherwise not increased.
  Patient's Child: 1 in 2. Reproductive fitness (of males at any rate) seems proved from known family histories.
IV Age of Detectability: At birth, but confusion may exist if gestational age is not known; therefore, diagnosis may not be obvious until consistent retardation of growth has been observed from birth.
V Prevalence: ? Rare. Majority of cases have been described in Western Europe.

Treatment
I Primary Prevention: Genetic counseling
II Secondary Prevention: Probably none, but treatment with human growth hormone should be investigated.
III Other Therapy: —

Prognosis: For life: In affected families death in infancy appears relatively common, but other affected individuals have had normal life spans. For intelligence: No effect upon intelligence. For function: None, except that due to small stature. Skeletal abnormalities are absent.

Detection of Carrier: All cases of this dominantly inherited defect are assumed to be heterozygotes.

†**Special Considerations:** This type of dominantly inherited dwarfism does not appear to have been investigated with modern methods and the possibility cannot be excluded that some defect in growth hormone secretion or response is present. However, the consistent statement

that the affected individuals were extremely small at birth is against a defect in secretion of growth hormone as such individuals invariably have a normal birthweight. The morphologically similar snub-nosed dwarfs which have been described as occurring in a recessively determined form may well have been examples of hypopituitary dwarfs with isolated growth hormone deficiency.

References:
Black, J.A.: Low birth-weight dwarfism. Arch. Dis. Child. 36:633, 1961.

Levi, E.: Contributions à la connaissance de la microsomie essentielle hérédo-familiale; distinction de cette forme clinique d'avec les nanismes, les infantilismes et les formes mixtes de ces différentes dystrophies. Nouv. Iconogr. Salpêt. 23:522, 1910.

Warkany, J. et al: Intrauterine growth retardation. Am. J. Dis. Child. 102:249, 1961.

Contributor: John A. Black

Editor's Computerized Descriptors: Nose, Skel., Hernia not CNS, GU.

DYGGVE-MELCHIOR-CLAUSEN SYNDROME

Includes: Syndrome de Dyggve-Melchior-Clausen
Síndrome de Dyggve-Melchior-Clausen

Excludes: Mucopolysaccharidosis IV† (678)
Other mucopolysaccharidoses†
Other spondyloepiphyseal dysplasias

Minimal Diagnostic Criteria: Truncal dwarfism with characteristic radiographic skeletal abnormalities particularly of the vertebral bodies, pelvic and hand bones.

Clinical Findings: Short trunk type of dwarfism, protruding sternum, barrel chest, accentuated spinal curves, restricted joint mobility, waddling gait. Mental retardation in most cases, frequently associated with microcephaly.

Radiographs show characteristic skeletal changes with flat, anteriorly pointed vertebral bodies. In younger patients, the superior and inferior end-plates of the vertebral bodies are notched. Short and broad ilia with defective ossification of their basilar portions and irregularly ossified (lace-like) crests; laterally displaced capital femoral epiphyses; irregular carpal bones, shortened metacarpal bones and phalanges with accessory ossification centers in various metacarpals and phalanges become apparent between the ages of 1 and 13 years.

Complications
I **Derived:** Usual sequelae of marked intellectual impairment.
II **Associated:** —

Etiology: Autosomal recessive; McK *22380

Pathogenesis: ? The association of a skeletal dysplasia with a mental defect in most cases suggests a metabolic disorder affecting mesenchymal and neural cells. An abnormal excretion of carbohydrate-containing substances, possibly glycoproteins, has been found in the urine.†

Related Facts
I **Sex Ratio:** M1:F1
II **Risk of Occurrence:** Rare
III **Risk of Recurrence for**
  Patient's Sib: 1 in 4 (25%) for each offspring to be affected.
  Patient's Child: Not increased unless mate is carrier or homozygote.
IV **Age of Detectability:** Infancy
V **Prevalence:** ?

Treatment
I **Primary Prevention:** Genetic counseling
II **Secondary Prevention:** Appropriate orthopedic measures for patients without mental retardation
III **Other Therapy:** Supportive.

Prognosis: The life expectancy is unknown. The oldest patients with mental retardation are in their 20s; several patients without mental retardation are in their 40s.

Detection of Carrier: ?

†Special Considerations: The Dyggve-Melchior-Clausen syndrome was originally thought to be a mucopolysaccharidosis. Normal urinary excretion of acid mucopolysaccharides and failure to demonstrate mucopolysaccharide storage by microscopic and biochemical means make this improbable. A metabolic error of other complex carbohydrates is not excluded. Most patients are mentally retarded. There are a few isolated and familial cases with the full morphologic manifestation of the condition but normal mentality. It is not clear if this is due to genetic variability or if the Dyggve-Melchior-Clausen phenotype with normal mentality is caused by a different mutation.

References:
Spranger, J. et al: The Dyggve-Melchior-Clausen syndrome. Radiology 114:415, 1975.

Contributor: **Jürgen W. Spranger**

Editor's Computerized Descriptors: Skel. , Nerve

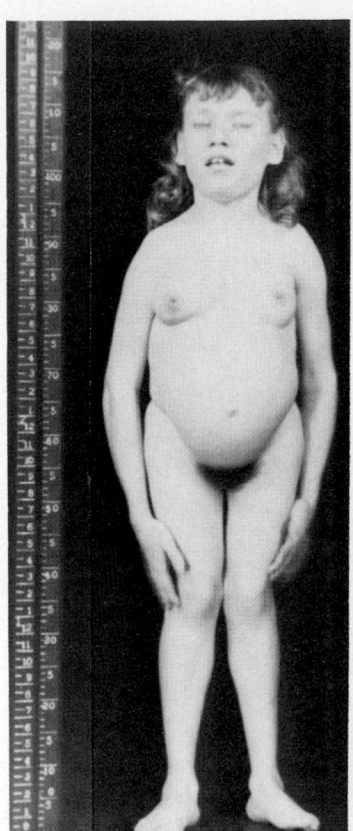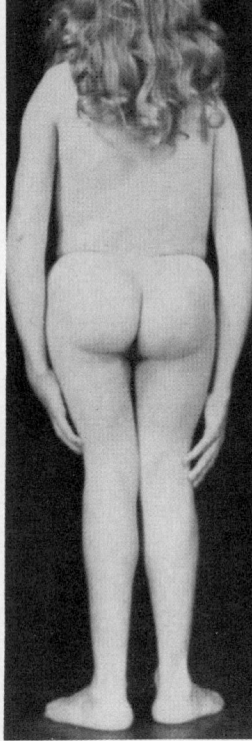

236. Short trunk; lumbar lordosis; marked hip dislocation; relatively long limbs

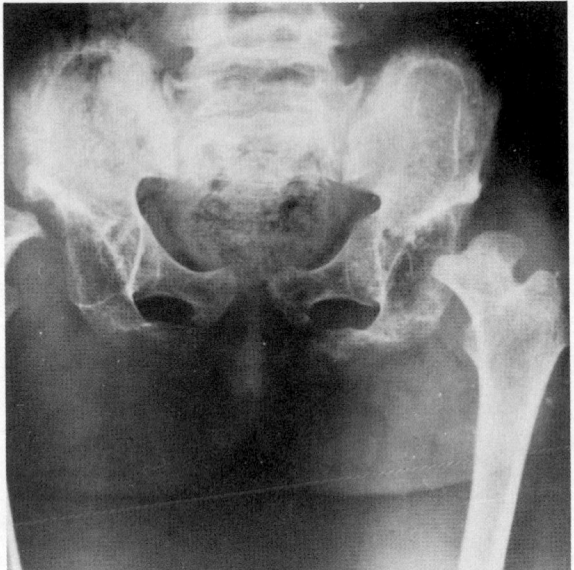

237. Dislocated hips with poorly developed femoral heads, necks, acetabula; increased transverse diameter of pelvic inlet relative to vertical height; lacey appearance of iliac crests

DYSAUTONOMIA

Includes: Disautonomía
Riley-Day syndrome

Excludes: Congenital indifference to pain
Immunodeficiency, common variable (521)

Minimal Diagnostic Criteria: The disease can be suspected on the basis of family history and appearance of swallowing deficits in the newborn. In addition the indifference to pain may be detected at that time.

There is no single diagnostic test. There is an abnormal response to intradermal histamine in which there is a thin red border but no surrounding flare as there is in the normal. Simply scratching the skin does not result in the usual flared response. There are also pharmacologic abnormalities, particularly a hypersensitivity to both cholinergic and adrenergic agents.

Clinical Findings: The process presents as a complex. There are no symptoms or signs which are by themselves pathognomonic of the disease. The constant features include an absence of overflow tears (alacrima), absence of the fungiform papillae of the tongue, vasomotor instability, hypoactive or absent deep tendon reflexes, and relative indifference to pain. In younger children feeding difficulties are very frequent. In addition physical retardation, episodic vomiting, marked emotional instability, scoliosis and disturbances of GI motility are frequent. The most common neurologic feature is the insensitivity to pain.

The incidence of these features is indicated in the following table:

Feature	%
Absence of fungiform papillae	100
Absence of overflow tears	100
Vasomotor disturbance (blotching)	98
Abnormal sweating	97
Episodic fever	92
Incoordination and unsteadiness	90
Swallowing difficulty in infancy	85
Physical retardation	78
Episodic vomiting	67
Breath-holding attacks	66
Marked emotional instability	65
Scoliosis	55
Bowel disturbance	49

Complications

I **Derived:** The complications may come from the insensitivity to pain, scoliosis, or from the GI disturbance, particularly the swallowing deficit. Repeated aspirations and episodes of pneumonia are a common complication. Failure of somatic growth is an integral part of the process; whether it is secondary or primary is not clear.

II **Associated:** —

Etiology: Autosomal recessive and largely confined to Ashkenazi Jews. McK *22390

Pathogenesis: The basic mechanism of the disease is unknown. There are features that suggest that the CNS, both peripheral and autonomic are involved in a defect in neurotransmission. Whether some biochemical abnormality of neuronal maturation or maintenance is at fault has not been clearly established.

Related Facts

I   **Sex Ratio:**   M1:F1
II **Risk of Occurrence:**   ? The disease occurs primarily in Ash-
       kenazi Jewish families.
III **Risk of Recurrence for**
       Patient's Sib: 1 in 4 (25%) for each offspring to be affected
       Patient's Child: Not increased unless mate is carrier or
          homozygote
IV **Age of Detectability:**   The disease can be strongly suspected
       at birth but often the definitive diagnosis is not made until
       later in life.
V   **Prevalence:**   ?

Treatment
I   **Primary Prevention:**   Genetic counseling
II **Secondary Prevention:**   There is no treatment for the dis-
       ease. Complications can be treated particularly in the use of
       antibiotics for repeated episodes of pneumonia.
III **Other Therapy:**   —

Prognosis: The prognosis varies but many cases die in childhood
   or early adult life from the complications of defects in swallowing
   and secondary pneumonia.

Detection of Carrier: ?

Special Considerations: —

References:
   Brunt, P.W. and McKusick, V.A.: Familial dysautonomia. A report
      of genetic and clinical studies, with a review of the literature.
      Medicine 49:343, 1970.
   Riley, C.M.: Familial dysautonomia. Adv. Pediatr. 9:157, 1957.

Contributor: **Guy M. McKhann**

Editor's Computerized Descriptors: Eye, Oral, Nasoph., Skin,
   Nerve , Sweating

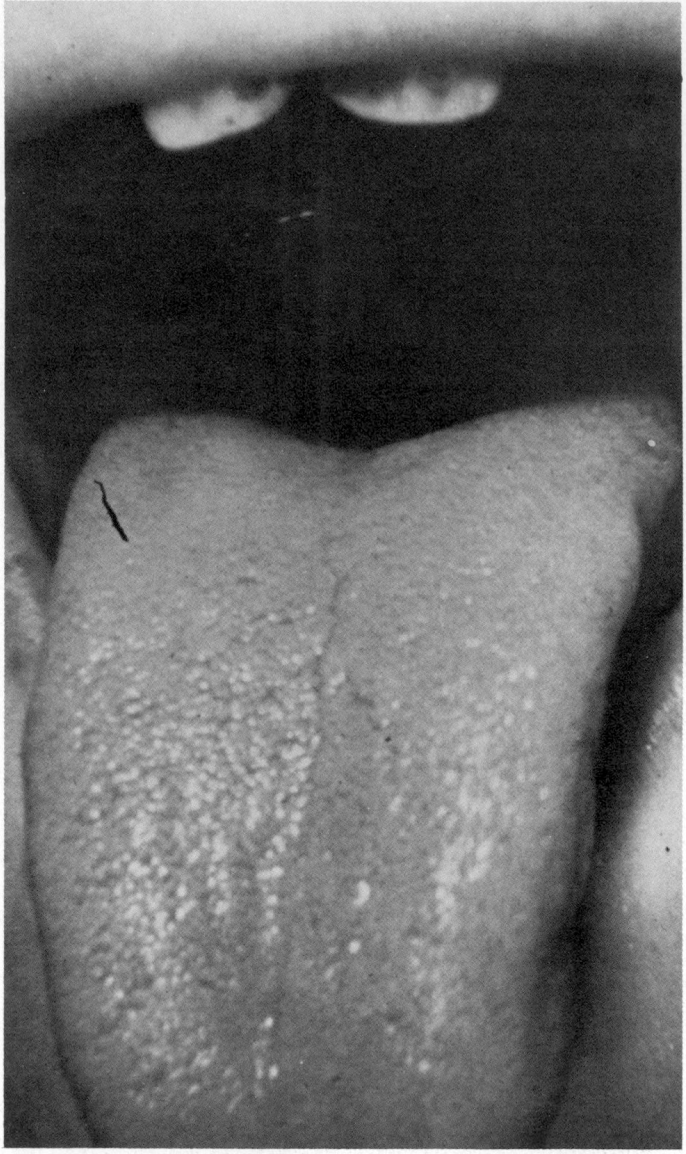

238. Absent fungiform papillae

308
DYSCHONDROSTEOSIS

Includes: Léri dyschondrosteosis
Dyschondrosteose
Discondrostosis
Leri-Weill disease
Mesomelic dwarfism and Madelung deformity
Deformity with mesomelic dwarfism

Excludes: Madelung deformity due to trauma or infection
Other types of mesomelic dwarfism
Turner syndrome (977)

Minimal Diagnostic Criteria: Madelung deformity in a patient with mesomelic short stature.† In a family in which one or more individuals have typical disease, a relative with simple Madelung deformity and normal stature would be considered to be affected.

Clinical Findings: Mild disproportionate short stature with mesomelia of the upper and lower limbs. Usual adult height varies between 137-152 cm. There is a marked modeling deformity of the wrists, with a bayonet-like configuration of the forearm and wrists produced by lateral and dorsal bowing of the radius, most marked distally. The radius is short and thickened. Radiologically, there is a V-shaped deformity of the wrist with slanting at the distal radial contour and dorsal dislocation of the ulna. There is wedging of the carpal bones between the deformed radius and protruding ulna resulting in a triangular configuration with the lunate at the apex. Inconstant features include humeral neck deformities, exostoses of the proximal medial tibia, shortening and thickening of the metacarpals and phalanges, coxa valga, cubitus valgus, lateral subluxation of the patella and osteoarthritis of large joints.

Complications
I **Derived:** Limitation of wrist motion, occasional osteoarthrosis.
II **Associated:** —

Etiology: Autosomal dominant trait, more severe in females. McK *12730

Pathogenesis: ?

Related Facts
I **Sex Ratio:** Relative excess of females
II **Risk of Occurrence:** ? Most common form of mesomelic dwarfism
III **Risk of Recurrence for**
  Patient's Sib: If parent is affected 1 in 2 (50%) for each offspring to be affected; otherwise not increased
  Patient's Child: 1 in 2
IV **Age of Detectability:** Mid to late childhood because of short stature or wrist deformity.
V **Prevalence:** —

Treatment
I **Primary Prevention:** Genetic counseling
II **Secondary Prevention:** Orthopedic surgery for wrist deformity if Madelung deformity is severe.
III **Other Therapy:** —

Prognosis: Normal life span.

Detection of Carrier: —

†**Special Considerations:** There is some controversy as to whether there is a distinct heritable isolated form of Madelung deformity, in the absence of a generalized bone dysplasia. A more severe form of mesomelic dwarfism, similar to mesomelic dysplasia—Langer type, may occur in an individual who is homozygous for the dyschondrosteosis gene.

References:

Felman, A.H. et al: Dyschondrosteose. Am. J. Dis. Child. 120:329, 1970.
Kaitila, I.I. et al: Mesomelic skeletal dysplasias. Clin. Orthop. 114:94, 1976.
Langer, L. O.: Dyschondrosteosis: A hereditable bone dysplasia with characteristic roentgenographic features. Am. J. Roentgenol. Radium Ther. Nucl. Med. 95:178, 1965.

Contributors: **Ralph S. Lachman**
David L. Rimoin

Editor's Computerized Descriptor: Skel.

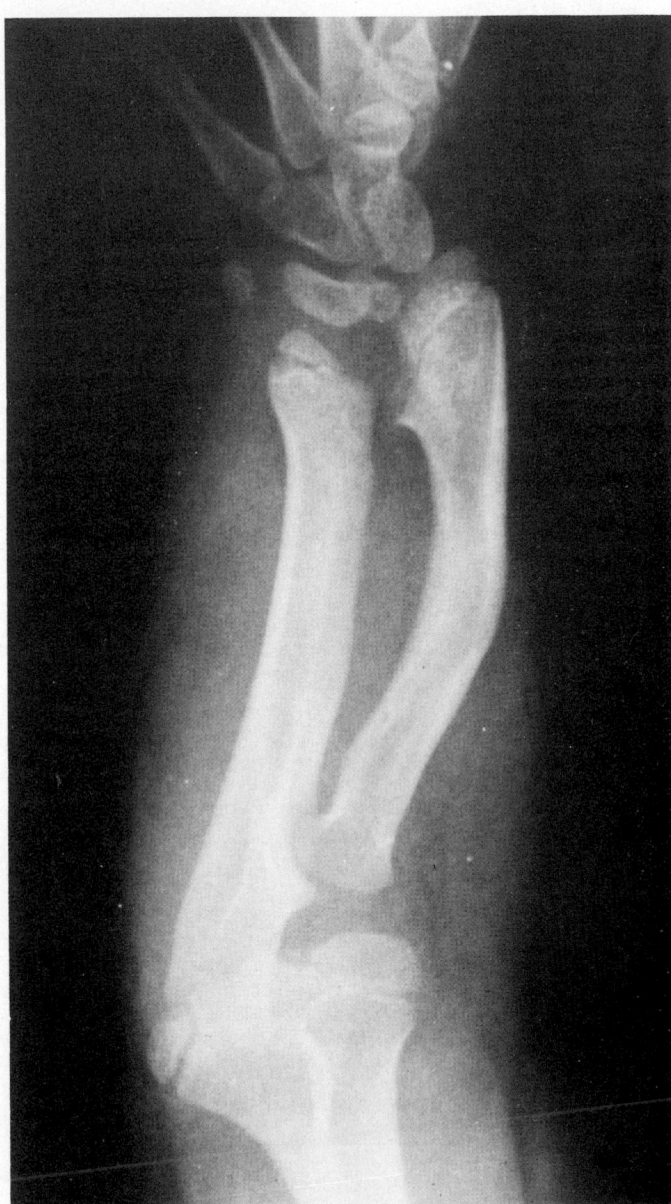

239. Note uneven fusion of distal epiphyses of radius and ulna

DYSCORIA

Includes: Dyscorie
Dyskorie
Discoria
Pupil abnormalities

Excludes: Ocular colobomas (733)
Anisocoria (58)
Polycoria
Corectopia
Pupillary membrane persistence (845)

Minimal Diagnostic Criteria: Abnormality in the shape of the pupil, in the absence of neoplasia or inflammatory processes with synechiae.

Clinical Findings: Abnormally shaped pupils may take the form of a slit (most commonly), hourglass, rectangle or pear. In the absence of malformations of the globe, vision is usually good.

Complications
I   Derived: —
II Associated: Anterior chamber cleavage syndromes

Etiology: Usually autosomal dominant. May also occur sporadically.

Pathogenesis: ? Probably related to abnormal "cleavage" of the anterior chamber during embryonic life

Related Facts
I   Sex Ratio: M1:F1
II   Risk of Occurrence: ?
III Risk of Recurrence for
     Patient's Sib: If parent is affected 1 in 2 (50%) for each offspring to be affected; otherwise not increased.
     Patient's Child: 1 in 2
IV   Age of Detectability: At birth
V   Prevalence: ?

Treatment
I   Primary Prevention: Genetic counseling
II   Secondary Prevention: None indicated in the absence of associated ocular malformations
III Other Therapy: —

Prognosis: Normal for life and intelligence. Good for vision, if independent of associated ocular malformations.

Detection of Carrier: Affected parent and patient when autosomal dominant

Special Considerations: —

References:
Duke-Elder, S.: System of Ophthalmology, vol. 3, part 2. Congenital Deformities. London:Henry Kimpton, 1964.
Henkind, P. et al: Mesodermal dysgenesis of the anterior segment: Rieger's anomaly. Arch. Ophthalmol. 73:810, 1965.
Reese, A. B. and Ellsworth, R. M.: The anterior chamber cleavage syndrome. Arch. Ophthalmol. 75:307, 1966.

Contributor: Morton F. Goldberg

Editor's Computerized Descriptor: Eye

DYSOSTEOSCLEROSIS

Includes: Dysostéosclérose
Dysosteosklerose
Disosteoesclerosis

Excludes: Osteopetrosis†
Pyknodysostosis (846)

Minimal Diagnostic Criteria: Dense osteopetrotic bones with platyspondyly and phalangeal tuft resorption.

Clinical Findings: Short stature with increased bone fragility. Lack of eruption of permanent teeth with enamel hypoplasia. Sclerosis of the base of the skull may lead to optic atrophy, other cranial nerve involvement and upper motor neuron lesions. Radiographic evaluation reveals generalized increased density of the cartilaginous bones including the base of the skull. Platyspondyly and sclerosis of the vertebrae are characteristic features. The metaphyses of long bones are expanded with exaggerated linear growth lines and there is phalangeal tuft resorption.

Complications
I   Derived: Optic atrophy and other cranial nerve involvement, increased predisposition to bone fractures.
II Associated: Progressive mental deterioration and upper motor neurone disease may occur.

Etiology: Autosomal recessive; McK *22430

Pathogenesis: Lack of resorption of calcified cartilage at the growth plate, surrounded by only thin rims of bone. Bone from the orbital roof has been shown to be of a woven nature. The primary defect appears to involve the replacement of calcified cartilage by mature bone.

Related Facts
I   Sex Ratio: —
II   Risk of Occurrence: Very rare
III Risk of Recurrence for
     Patient's Sib: 1 in 4
     Patient's Child: Not increased, unless mate is carrier of homozygote.
IV   Age of Detectability: Early childhood, when xrays are performed for fractures or cranial nerve involvement.
V   Prevalence: —

Treatment
I   Primary Prevention: Genetic counseling
II   Secondary Prevention: Routine treatment of fractures. Repair and capping of teeth, unroofing of the optic canal may be necessary to retard visual loss.
III Other Therapy: —

Prognosis: No adults have yet been reported.

Detection of Carrier: —

†Special Considerations: This disorder may be confused with the more typical forms of osteopetrosis, but can be distinguished by the presence of platyspondyly, radiolucency of the widened submetaphyseal portions of the tubular bones and the absence of hematologic complications.

References:
Leisti J. et al: Dysosteosclerosis. In Bergsma, D. (ed.): Disorders of Connective Tissue. Birth Defects: Orig. Art. Ser., vol. XI, no. 6. Miami: Symposia Specialists for The National Foundation-March of Dimes, 1975, p. 349.
Roy, C. et al: Un nouveau syndrome osseux avec anomalies cutanées et troubles neurologiques. Arch. Fr. Pediatr. 25:983, 1968.
Spranger, J. et al: Die Dysosteosklerose. Fortschr. Rontgenstr. 109:564, 1968.

Contributors: Ralph S. Lachman
David L. Rimoin

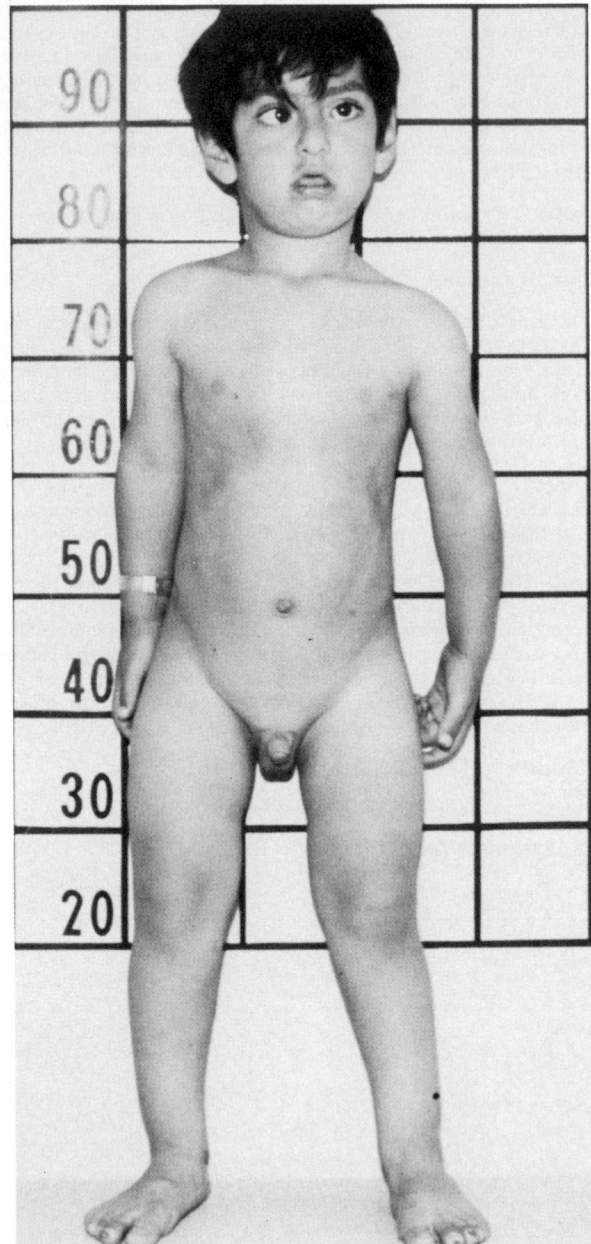

240. Note the disproportionately short limbs and slight bowing of the long bones

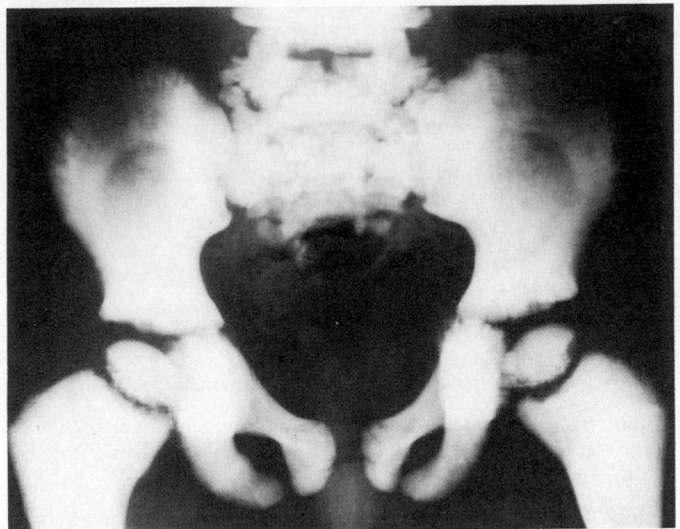

241. Irregularities of iliac crests and acetabular roofs; increased striations extend from these areas

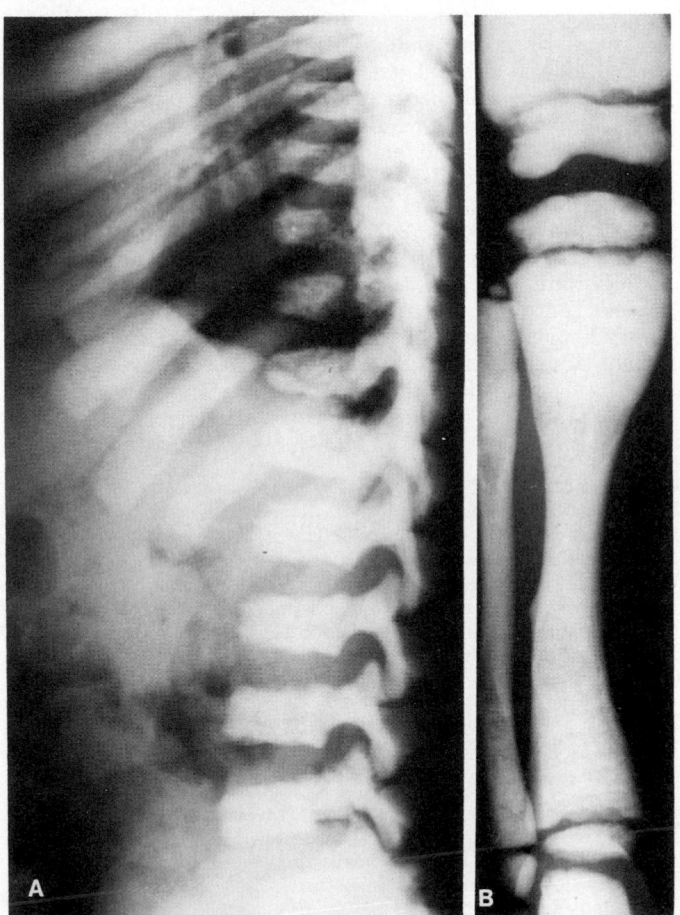

242. A) Note marked sclerosis and platyspondyly; ribs lack normal modeling of distal ends; B) long bones have abnormally molded metaphyses with relatively milder epiphyseal changes; diaphyses show narrowing of marrow cavity

DYSPLASIA EPIPHYSEALIS HEMIMELICA

Includes: Dysplasie épiphysaire hémimélique
Displasia epifisaria hemimélica
Hemimelic skeletal dysplasias
Tarsomegaly
Chondrodystrophie epiphysaire
Benign epiphyseal osteochondroma
Intraarticular osteochondroma of the astragalus
Carpal osteochondroma
Osteochondroma of the distal femoral epiphysis

Excludes: Epiphyseal dysplasia, multiple (358)
Enchondromatosis (345)
Multiple cartilaginous exostoses (685)
Chondrodysplasia punctata, Conradi-Hünermann type (153)

Minimal Diagnostic Criteria: Hemimelic involvement of 1 or more epiphysis or tarsal or carpal bone, with no other affected family member.

Clinical Findings: This is a developmental disorder of childhood in which there is asymmetric cartilaginous overgrowth of 1, or more than 1 epiphysis, or of a tarsal or carpal bone. It is usually limited to the medial or lateral half of a single limb, although the entire epiphysis may at times be involved. The usual presentation is with unilateral swelling about the inner or outer aspects of the ankles or knees, pain, deformity or limitation of motion. The medial side is affected twice as often as the lateral side. Multiple lesions did occur in 2 of 3 cases, but involvement of the upper limbs is rare. Observed frequencies are: the talus, 61.5%; the distal femoral epiphysis, 45.5%; proximal tibial epiphysis, 26.5%; tarsal navicular, 24.5%; medial cuneiform, 17.5%; distal fibular epiphysis, 17.5% and femoral capital epiphysis, 8.8%. The deformities and size of lesions increase with growth of normal bone. The earliest radiographic changes are premature appearance of the osseous centers on the affected side. Thereafter, an irregular radiopacity develops on 1 side of the epiphysis. The lesions appear as irregular, lobulated osseous masses protruding from 1 side of the epiphysis. The final appearance may be similar to an exostosis. There are no characteristic laboratory changes and no known systemic associations.

Complications
I **Derived:** Deformity of the affected bone due to unequal involvement of the epiphysis. The most common deformities are genu valgum or varum and valgus or equinus deformity of the ankle. Pain and limitation of motion may occur at the involved joint. Pain may result from fracture of an exostosis. Occasionally, inequality of limb size, both shortening and lengthening may occur.†
II **Associated:** —

Etiology: ? There is no familial aggregation. The disorder is thought to be an embryopathy of limb bud formation occurring at about the 5th week of fetal development.

Pathogenesis: ? Thought to result from an ectopic focus of proliferating cartilage with subsequent enchondral ossification. Both by gross inspection and microscopically the lesions are indistinguishable from osteocartilaginous exostosis. There are no reports of malignant degeneration.

Related Facts
I **Sex Ratio:** M3:F1
II **Risk of Occurrence:** ?
III **Risk of Recurrence for**
   Patient's Sib: Not thought to be increased
   Patient's Child: Not thought to be increased
IV **Age of Detectability:** May be detected from birth to adult life, with the most frequent ages of detection between 2 and 14 years, by radiographs.
V **Prevalence:** ?

Treatment
I **Primary Prevention:** —
II **Secondary Prevention:** This is a localized deformity in an otherwise normal child and requires early orthopedic correction to avoid deformities of the affected limb. The involved epiphysis should be excised in cases with pain, deformity, unequal limb length or limitation of motion. Recurrence is not known after excision of the involved area. Heel cord lengthening should be performed for the equinus deformity.
III **Other Therapy:** —

Prognosis: Normal for life span and intelligence. Function is also good after early orthopedic correction.

Detection of Carrier: —

†**Special Considerations:** Secondary metaphyseal abnormalities such as bone spurs, or streaking and bowing of the metaphysis as in enchondromatosis may develop. Active growth of lesions may occur in adult life. The exostoses in this condition are distinguished from those in multiple exostoses only by their epiphyseal location and lack of diaphyseal migration.

References:
Kettelkamp, D.B. et al: Dysplasia epiphysealis hemimelica: A report of fifteen cases and review of the literature. J. Bone Joint Surg. 48A:746, 1966.
Rubin, P.: Dynamic Classification of Bone Dysplasias. Chicago: Year Book Medical Publishers, 1964, p. 159.
Theodorou, S. and Lanitis, G.: Dysplasia epiphysialis hemimelica (epiphyseal osteochondromata). Report of two cases and review of the literature. Helv. Paediatr. Acta 23:195, 1968.
Trevor, D.: Tarso-epiphysial aclasis: A congenital error of epiphyseal development. J. Bone Joint Surg. 32B:204, 1950.

Contributor: **Jack R. Lichtenstein**

Editor's Computerized Descriptor: Skel.

EAR, ABSENT TRAGUS

Includes: Absence du tragus
Tragus-Aplasie
Ausencia del trago

Excludes: Microtia-atresia (664)
Atresia alone
Deafness and ear pits (247)
Darwin tubercle (Marker) (241)
Ear lobe pit (Marker) (322)
Ear flare

Minimal Diagnostic Criteria: Absence of tragus of ear†

Clinical Findings: Usually seen only in conditions in which the mandible is also absent or markedly hypoplastic.

Complications
I   **Derived:** —
II **Associated:** Agnathia

Etiology: ?

Pathogenesis: ?

Related Facts
I   **Sex Ratio:** ?
II   **Risk of Occurrence:** Extremely rare
III **Risk of Recurrence for**
     Patient's Sib: ?
     Patient's Child: ?
IV **Age of Detectability:** At birth
V   **Prevalence:** ?

Treatment
I   **Primary Prevention:** —
II   **Secondary Prevention:** If isolated defect, no treatment is needed.
III **Other Therapy:** —

Prognosis: Good for life span, intelligence and function if isolated defect of outer ear, otherwise dependent upon concomitant defects.

Detection of Carrier: —

†Special Considerations: Anomalies of the external ear should suggest the possibility of an anomaly of the middle ear as well. Hearing should be assessed as soon as possible and appropriate therapy instituted. The anatomy of the middle and inner ear should be determined by petrous pyramid polytomography.

References:
Converse, J.M. (ed.): Reconstructive Plastic Surgery. Philadelphia:W.B. Saunders Co., l964, vol. 3.

Contributor: **LaVonne Bergstrom**

Editor's Computerized Descriptors: Ear, Face

EAR, ARTERIOVENOUS FISTULA

Includes: Fistule artério-veineuse de l'oreille externe
Arteriovenöse Fistel des äusseren Ohr
Fístula arteriovenosa del oído externo
Pulsating venous aneurysm of external ear
External ear arteriovenous fistula
Cirsoid aneurysm of external ear
Aneurysm serpentina of external ear
Arteriovenous aneurysm of external ear
External ear aneurysm by anastomosis
Angioma cavernosum of external ear

Excludes: Chondroma of ear
Fibroma of external ear
Lymphangioma of ear
Hemangioma of ear
Nevus flammeus of ear
Dermoid of ear

Minimal Diagnostic Criteria: The history of an enlarged, pinkish to bl...ish, distorted, pulsatile auricle manifesting itself at birth or within the first 2 decades of life plus physical findings of the above signs (perhaps with overlying bruit). Retrograde arteriography may be helpful, but is not essential to the diagnosis.†

Clinical Findings: There is enlargement and distortion of the auricle or a part thereof. This has a pinkish-to-bluish discoloration, often is pulsatile, may have a bruit, and usually involves adjacent portions of cheek, scalp or neck. In 3 of 8 cases, necrosis and hemorrhage occurred from the affected auricle. Ipsilateral increase in facial bone growth has occasionally been observed, usually with the more extensive arteriovenous fistulae. Retrograde arteriography demonstrates increased vascularity of the involved auricle.

Complications
I   **Derived:** Perichondritis of auricle necrosis (ulceration of auricle) in 3 of 8 cases; hemorrhage from auricle in 3 of 8 cases
II   **Associated:** —†

Etiology: ?

Pathogenesis: Normally there are rich anastomoses between the internal carotid and external carotid arteries along the walls of the external auditory meatus. This vascular network along with venous channels differentiates from an embryonal plexus of fine tubules. Most of these channels become obliterated. Congenital arteriovenous fistulae result from failure of obliteration of these embryonal connections. The progressive enlargement of this lesion is apparently due to the ability of arteriovenous fistulae to stimulate the formation of collateral circulation.

Related Facts
I   **Sex Ratio:** M3:F5 (in the 8 cases reported)
II   **Risk of Occurrence:** ?
III **Risk of Recurrence for**
     Patient's Sib: ?
     Patient's Child: ?
IV **Age of Detectability:** From birth through the 2nd decade by means of physical examination
V   **Prevalence:** ?

Treatment
I   **Primary Prevention:** —
II   **Secondary Prevention:** The only successful treatment is complete excision of the involved auricle with plastic or prosthetic reconstruction of the auricle. Attempts at ligation of feeding vessels have been unsuccessful in that some channels are invariably overlooked.
III **Other Therapy:** —

Prognosis: With adequate excision of the lesion, a normal life span can be anticipated. In the untreated patient, death from auricular hemorrhage is possible.

Detection of Carrier: —

†**Special Considerations:** Unlike acquired arteriovenous fistulae occurring in other body regions, there is no related cardiac hypertrophy or failure. This is probably due to the smaller caliber of the arteriovenous communications of the external ear.

References:
Dingman, R.O. and Grabb, W.C.: Congenital arteriovenous fistulae of the external ear. Plast. Reconstr. Surg. 35:620, 1965.

Contributors: **Benjamin C. Leadholm**
LaVonne Bergstrom

Editor's Computerized Descriptors: Ear, Face, Skin

EAR, CUPPED

Includes: Oreille en cupule
Löffelohr
Oreja en copa
Cup ear

Excludes: Microtia-atresia (664)
Atresia alone
Deafness and ear pits (247)
Ear lobe pit (Marker) (322)
Ear flare

Minimal Diagnostic Criteria: Pinna folded forward over external auditory meatus

Clinical Findings: The pinna is cupped forward over the external auditory meatus. The helix is short, extends downward rather than upward and the surface of the ear which normally faces the side of the head is posterolateral or lateral. The ear lobe is also at right angles to the head. The ear appears small, but is actually of normal size. The condition is nearly always bilateral. Hearing is normal.

Complications
I   **Derived:** Psychologic disturbance
II **Associated:** Pierre Robin micrognathia and conductive hearing loss

Etiology: Autosomal dominant with regular penetrance and variable expressivity; McK *12860

Pathogenesis: ? Possible arrest at a fetal stage of development

Related Facts
I   **Sex Ratio:** Ml:Fl
II   **Risk of Occurrence:** ?
III **Risk of Recurrence for**
     Patient's Sib: When autosomal dominant and if parent is affected 1 in 2 (50%) for each offspring to be affected; otherwise not increased.
     Patient's Child: When autosomal dominant 1 in 2
IV   **Age of Detectability:** At birth
V   **Prevalence:** ?

Treatment
I   **Primary Prevention:** Genetic counseling
II   **Secondary Prevention:** Plastic surgical repair may be indicated.
III **Other Therapy:** —

Prognosis: Good for life span, intelligence and function if isolated defect of outer ear, otherwise dependent upon concomitant defects.

Detection of Carrier: —

Special Considerations: —

References:
Converse, J.M. (ed.): Reconstructive Plastic Surgery. Philadelphia:W.B. Saunders Co., 1964, vol. 3
Peterson, D.M. and Schimke, R.N.: Hereditary cup-shaped ears and the Pierre Robin syndrome. J. Med. Genet. 5:52, 1968.
Rogers, B.O.: Microtic, lop, cup and protruding ears: Four directly inheritable deformities. Plast. Reconstr. Surg. 41:208, 1968.

Contributor: **LaVonne Bergstrom**

Editor's Computerized Descriptor: Ear

EAR DYSPLASIAS, INNER

Includes: Dysplasies de l'oreille interne
Dysplasie der Innenohr
Displasias del oído interno
Scheibe cochleosaccular degeneration of inner ear
Mondini-Alexander malformation of inner ear
Bing-Siebenmann dysplasia
Heredodegenerations of inner ear
Abiotrophies of inner ear
Dysgenesis of inner ear
Hypoplasia of inner ear
Inner ear dysplasia

Excludes: Labyrinth aplasia (562)

Minimal Diagnostic Criteria: Severe to profound unilateral or bilateral congenital hearing loss with varying degrees of bony dysplasia of the inner ear detectable by petrous pyramid polytomography. Some types of membranous dysplasia may be inferred from the audiometric pattern or abnormal vestibular testing.

Clinical Findings: Although there is considerable anatomic variation in the inner ear dysplasias, the clinical picture is usually that of moderately severe-to-profound hearing loss. There is considerable evidence from animal studies that 1 type of dysplasia, the cochleosaccular degeneration of Scheibe, may occur in the early neonatal period. By light microscopy, the ears appear normal at birth. Improved techniques for testing hearing in newborn and young infants suggest that a similar phenomenon may occur in some cases of human deafness in which no known exogenous causes of hearing loss can be found. The infant usually babbles and vocalizes normally until about age 6-9 months when his production of vocalization diminishes and changes in pitch. An alert parent may suspect the hearing loss early because of failure to respond to loud, nonvibratory sounds; but often the hearing loss is not suspected or detected until speech and language fail to develop.

Attempts have been made to correlate pathology with audiometric patterns; these have been most successful in cases in which cochleosaccular degeneration occurs. In this entity atrophy of the stria vascularis, degeneration of the organ of Corti and rolling up of the tectorial membrane are constant features which are most marked in the basal turn or the cochlea, in which the higher frequencies are represented. In the apical turn where low frequencies are localized, these structures appear less distorted or may even appear normal. Reissner membrane may be collapsed or the endolymphatic compartment may be dilated. The audiogram often shows residual hearing only in the low frequencies. However, in the Mondini-Alexander malformation audiometric patterns have been quite variable, from profound hearing loss to normal hearing. In this classic malformation the bony cochlea is shorter than the normal 2 1/2 - 2 3/4 turns, and may be only 1 or 1 1/2 turns long. Varying degrees of membranous inner ear malformations are seen. There may be dilatation of the saccule, endolymphatic duct and sac. The bony vestibular labyrinth may show anomalies of the semicircular canals. Varying degrees of hypodevelopment of the acoustic and vestibular ganglia and fibers are seen. The otic capsule may be poorly developed; stapes footplate fixation, other middle ear anomalies or external auditory atresia may be associated.

Petrous pyramid polytomography has shown that at least 11 of 15 possible combinations of inner ear anomalies occur. Therefore, the classic categories need augmentation or revision. These 11 combined anomalies of the inner ear

structures in order of frequency of occurrence, are: (Those that might affect hearing have a # sign.) 1) semicircular canal(s); 2) # cochlea, vestibule and semicircular canal(s); 3) vestibule and semicircular canals; 4) # cochlea, internal meatus, vestibule and semicircular canal(s); 5) # cochlea alone 6) internal meatus only; 7) # cochlea and vestibule; 8) # cochlea and semicircular canal(s); 9) # cochlea and internal meatus; 10) # cochlea, internal meatus and semicircular canals and 11) # internal meatus and semicircular canals.

Diminished vestibular function (caloric tests) is seen in some of these patients but is rarely symptomatic, since it is present from birth or early life.

A membranous cochlear dysplasia associated with nonprogressive high-tone or basin-shaped loss and good speech discrimination was postulated by Alexander in 1927. The literature is confusing as to the precise pathology. Inner ear x-rays are normal.

In the Bing-Siebenmann dysplasia, the bony cochlea and vestibular portions of the inner ear are well formed, but the membranous components of both the inner ear and systems are malformed. Xrays of the inner ear are normal. The organ of Corti consists of a small mound of undifferentiated cells; some remains of the tectorial membrane are present. Reissner membrane is usually collapsed but may be ballooned out so that the cochlear duct is dilated. Aplasia of the membranous vestibular labyrinth may be seen.

It has been shown that the Scheibe and Mondini malformations may be unilateral, and presumably the other malformations may also be unilateral. In these instances, the patient would have normal speech and language development and the unilateral hearing loss might not be discovered until school age or later.

Asymmetry of malformation is not uncommon and the patient may have, for example, a Scheibe malformation of 1 ear and a Mondini malformation of the other. In these instances, the degree or pattern of hearing loss and the x-ray findings may well be different on the 2 sides.

Complications
I Derived: —
II Associated: Scheibe malformation may be found in Waardenburg syndrome, cardioauditory syndrome, chromosome 13-15 trisomy, Usher syndrome, Refsum syndrome, sensory radicular neuropathy, osteitis deformans of Paget, rubella embryopathy.

Mondini-Alexander malformation may be found in Pendred syndrome of deafness and goiter, Klippel-Feil malformation, Wildervanck syndrome, and chromosome 18 trisomy syndrome.

Bing-Siebenmann malformation may be found with mental retardation or retinitis pigmentosa.

Many of these inner ear dysplasias are isolated defects.

Etiology: Unknown, unless associated with a specific genetic syndrome. Varied when part of a syndrome, eg Scheibe malformation usually autosomal recessive, rubella embryopathy is caused by a viral infection.

Pathogenesis: Unknown in humans. Inner ear studies in one 7-week-old embryo aborted because of maternal rubella suggest that Scheibe malformation could occur in utero. Animal studies in the Scheibe malformation show progressive degeneration of a normal-appearing cochlea and saccule.

Pathogenesis of other inner ear dysplasias is unknown, postulated to be an arrest of embryologic development in some instances. However, in other cases the pathology is bizarre and does not correspond with any known normal phase of inner ear development.

Related Facts
I Sex Ratio: ?

II Risk of Occurrence: ?
III Risk of Recurrence for
    Patient's Sib: ?
    Patient's Child: ?
IV Age of Detectability: Bony dysplasias may be diagnosed by petrous pyramid polytomography shortly after birth or as soon as the hearing loss is discovered. Membranous dysplasias cannot be detected except at autopsy, although if associated with a known genetic disease may be inferred as soon as the physical findings of the syndrome are manifest.
V Prevalence: At least 3-4% of profound congenital deafness

Treatment
I Primary Prevention: —
II Secondary Prevention: Hearing aids, auditory and other special training for the hearing handicapped.
III Other Therapy: Hearing conservation, treatment or training as appropriate for associated defects.

Prognosis: Dependent on associated defects for life prognosis. The ability of the hearing-handicapped patient to function in our society is directly related to prompt diagnosis and prompt and vigorous habilitation and training. Most of these individuals have usable residual hearing.

Detection of Carrier: —

Special Considerations: —

References:

Ilies, A.: Pathological changes produced by rubella in a human embryo. Translated and abstracted from Rev. Roum. Embryol. Cytol. 4(2):187, 1967. In Birth Defects Abstracts of Selected Articles, vol. 5, no. 6. 1968.
Lindsay, J.R.: Inner ear pathology in congenital deafness. Otolaryngol. Clin. North Am. 4:249, 1971.
Ormerod, F.C.: The pathology of congenital deafness. J. Laryngol. 74:919, 1960.
Schuknecht, H.F.: Pathology of sensorineural deafness of genetic origin. In McConnell, F. and Ward, P. (eds.): Deafness in Childhood. Nashville:Vanderbilt University Press, 1967, p. 69.
Valvassori, G.E. et al: Inner ear anomalies: Clinical and histopathological considerations. Ann. Otol. Rhinol. Laryngol. 78:929, 1969.

Contributor: **LaVonne Bergstrom**

Editor's Computerized Descriptors: Hearing, Ear, Speech

EAR, ECTOPIC PINNA

Includes: Ectopie du pavillon de l'oreille
Ektopie der Ohrmuschel
Pabellón de la oreja ectópico
Ectopic placement of pinna

Excludes: Microtia-atresia (664)
Atresia alone
Deafness and ear pits (247)
Darwin tubercle (Marker) (241)
Ear lobe pit (Marker) (322)
Ear flare

Minimal Diagnostic Criteria: Normally contoured pinna found in a displaced position without relationship to the external auditory canal, eardrum and middle ear, which are in normal position or normally contoured pinna with associated canal, drum and middle ear all displaced from their usual position.

Clinical Findings: Ectopic placement of the pinna on the head without displacement of the external auditory canal and with normal eardrum and middle ear has been reported in perhaps 2 cases in the literature. In 1 case, there was no evidence of auricular structures or auricular appendages at the normal site, and the opposite pinna was completely normal in form and location. The ectopic ear was also normal in contour except that it seemed attached anteriorly to the forehead and temple by a thick pedicle of tissue. The ear was above its normal position. In other instances, the ear canal and middle ear have been displaced with the pinna.

Complications
I Derived: Malformation of the middle ear and eustachian tube
II Associated: —

Etiology: ?

Pathogenesis: ? Possible intrauterine trauma that led to transplantation of pinna precursor to another area of skull; or amniotic fibrous adhesions that pulled developing pinna into abnormal position.

Related Facts
I Sex Ratio: M?:F?
II Risk of Occurrence: ?
III Risk of Recurrence for
    Patient's Sib: ?
    Patient's Child: ?
IV Age of Detectability: At birth
V Prevalence: ?

Treatment
I Primary Prevention: —
II Secondary Prevention: Plastic surgical repair may be indicated.
    If conductive hearing loss is present, petrous pyramid polytomography should be done to assess the anatomic configuration of the middle ear and if it seems favorable, exploratory tympanotomy and surgical correction should be performed, if feasible. If not feasible, or if unsuccessful, or if the patient has a sensorineural hearing loss, hearing aids should be fitted and aural rehabilitation undertaken.
III Other Therapy: —

Prognosis: Good for life span, intelligence and function if isolated defect of outer ear, otherwise dependent upon concomitant defects.

Detection of Carrier: —

Special Considerations: —

References:

Smith, C.R. et al: Congenital gross displacement of the pinna. Arch. Otolaryngol. 86:49, 1967.

Contributor: **LaVonne Bergstrom**

Editor's Computerized Descriptor: Ear

EAR, EXCHONDROSIS (MARKER)

Includes: Chondromes du pavillon de l'oreille
Ekchondrose des Ohrläppchens
Exocondrosis del pabellón auricular (Marcador)
Exchondrosis of pinna

Excludes: Microtia-atresia (664)
Atresia alone
Deafness and ear pits (247)
Darwin tubercle (Marker) (241)
Ear lobe pit (Marker) (322)
Ear flare

Minimal Diagnostic Criteria: Bump at lower end of posterior surface of ear next to scalp†

Clinical Findings: A cartilaginous bump occurs on the posteromedial surface of the pinna close to its scalp attachment ("posterior ear bump").

Complications
I   **Derived:** —
II **Associated:** —

Etiology: Autosomal dominant; McK *13350

Pathogenesis: ?

Related Facts
I   **Sex Ratio:** M1:F1
II **Risk of Occurrence:** ?
III **Risk of Recurrence for**
    Patient's Sib: If parent is affected 1 in 2 (50%) for each offspring to be affected; otherwise not increased.
    Patient's Child: 1 in 2
IV **Age of Detectability:** At birth
V   **Prevalence:** ?

Treatment
I   **Primary Prevention:** Genetic counseling
II **Secondary Prevention:** Plastic surgical repair may be indicated
III **Other Therapy:** —

Prognosis: Good for life span, intelligence and function if isolated defect of outer ear, otherwise dependent upon concomitant defects.

Detection of Carrier: —

†**Special Considerations:** Anomalies of the external ear should suggest the possibility of an anomaly of the middle ear as well.

References:
Gates, R.R.: Human Genetics. New York: Macmillan, 1946, vol. 1.

Contributor: **LaVonne Bergstrom**

Editor's Computerized Descriptor: Ear

Includes: Exostoses de l'oreille
Gehörgangs-Exostosen
Exostosis auriculares
Multiple compact osteomata
Exostoses of external auditory canal
Ivory exostoses of ear canal
Aural exostoses
Hyperostoses of auditory canal

Excludes: Osteomata of external auditory canal

Minimal Diagnostic Criteria: Small, multiple, bilateral, symmetric, sessile bony masses in the external auditory canals next to the sulcus tympanicus occurring in a child or infant too young for exposure to classic exogenous factors thought to be of importance in etiology of noncongenital exostoses.

Clinical Findings: Exostoses are usually asymptomatic except rarely when they become large enough to obstruct or nearly obstruct the external auditory canal so that cerumen and desquamated canal debris become impacted medial to the exostosis. This may cause a conductive hearing loss or external otitis. In coincidental or secondary suppurative otitis media and tympanic membrane rupture, large exostoses may cause obstruction to drainage and interfere with evaluation and treatment.

On otoscopic examination one sees rounded, sessile, hard, bony nodules protruding from the bony external auditory canal wall near the sulcus tympanicus—these are usually multiple and bilateral. Often the exostoses are on opposing walls of the canal, most commonly the posterior and anterior at the approximate locations of the tympanomastoid and tympanosquamous sutures. The floor of the canal is said to be seldom involved. The skin covering them is usually normal unless self-induced trauma or infection has occurred. Occasionally exostoses of the external auditory canal may be associated with multiple exostoses in other locations, eg the orbit, mandible.

Hyperostoses are similar, but more diffuse, annular or segmented bony thickenings of the external canal. Hyperostosis of other bones of the skull and face may be associated.

There is considerable confusion in distinguishing between exostoses and osteomata of the external auditory canal. Osteomata tend to be unilateral, often pedunculated and usually occur at the junction of bony and cartilaginous canals. Osteomata are generally single but multiple compact osteomata have been described. Osteomas are believed to be rarer than exostoses but more likely to be associated with complications such as infection and hearing loss. As in exostoses and hyperostoses, familial syndromes are known in which osteomata of the external ear canal occur.

Mastoid xrays and petrous pyramid polytomography would be a useful adjunct to physical examination in those cases in which surgery is necessary to determine the extent of involvement, to delineate the course of the facial nerve and to see if concomitant middle or inner ear anomalies or pathology, such as cholesteatoma, are present.

It may be useful to search for generalized bone disease in certain cases. However, no abnormalities of calcium or phosphorus metabolism have been described in aural exostoses per se.

The pathology of the bony tissue in exostoses is felt to be distinct from that of osteomata. Osteomas usually show a thin shell of compact bone over a trabecular, fibrous center, whereas exostoses and hyperostoses are felt to comprise a circumscribed hypertrophy of the periosteal bone.

Complications
I **Derived:** In order of frequency: cerumen impaction, otitis externa, conductive hearing loss, otitis media, cholesteatoma and ossicular disruption. All of these complications are rare. Perforation of the tympanic membrane or damage to the facial nerve could occur as a complication of surgery for exostoses.
II **Associated:** Rarely, exostoses or hyperostoses of other bones

Etiology: ? Possibly multifactorial

Pathogenesis: ?

Related Facts
I **Sex Ratio:** M3:F1
II **Risk of Occurrence:** ? Frequently found in prehistoric Indian skulls, but no ethnic predominance is known in living racial groups. The older literature indicates that this condition comprises some 1 in 270 to 1 in 200 cases of aural disease.
III **Risk of Recurrence for**
   Patient's Sib: ?
   Patient's Child: ?
IV **Age of Detectability:** Not found until symptomatic, or by otoscopy during a routine otolaryngologic examination.
V **Prevalence:** ?

Treatment
I **Primary Prevention:** —
II **Secondary Prevention:** Small exostoses and hyperostoses are best treated with periodic observation and careful aural hygiene (avoidance of self-cleaning or trauma to the ear canal). Keeping water out of the ear is especially important since many otologists feel that water, particularly swimming in cold salt water, may cause or aggravate aural exostoses. Large obstructing exostoses should be removed using an endaural approach, reflecting a tympanomeatal skin flap over the exostoses and removing them with a high-speed drill and dental burrs, followed by the usual postoperative packing and care. Occasionally a postauricular approach may be preferable.
III **Other Therapy:** Tympanoplasty and ossicular reconstruction for those extremely rare cases in which middle ear complications occur. If a cholesteatoma should occur, mastoidectomy of a type dictated by the extent of the pathology would be needed.

Prognosis: Ear function usually normal unless obstruction or infection supervene in which instances conductive hearing loss, tympanic membrane rupture, otitis media, cholesteatoma and ossicular disruption or destruction could occur. Although it is extremely unlikely that this disease would go undetected until cholesteatoma formation, should this occur, it is conceivable that CNS complications of cholesteatoma, such as brain abscess or meningitis, could result and endanger the patient's life.

Detection of Carrier: —

Special Considerations: —

References:
Ballenger, J.J.: Diseases of the Nose, Throat and Ear. Philadelphia:Lea and Febiger, 1969.
Canciullo, R. and Bozzi, A.: Osteomi ed esostosi del condotto uditivo esterno. Otorinolaringol. Ital. 36:294, 1967.
Mawson, S.R.: Diseases of the Ear. Baltimore: Williams & Wilkins, 1963.
Shambaugh, G.E., Jr.: Surgery of the Ear, 2nd Ed. Philadelphia:W.B. Saunders Co., 1967.

Contributor: **LaVonne Bergstrom**

Editor's Computerized Descriptors: Hearing, Ear

EAR, HAIRY

Includes: Hypertrichose des oreilles
Behaarte Ohren
Hipertricosis de las orejas
Hypertrichosis pinnae auris
Hairy pinnae

Excludes: Hairy tragus and meatus acusticus externus in males alone

Minimal Diagnostic Criteria: Hairy ears

Clinical Findings: Up to 1 inch long, coarse hairs growing closely together on the helix of the ears. In the population in India the common site is in the sulcus at the side of ears while in Israeli population and in Malta, hair frequently occurs at the top of the ear.

Complications
I Derived: —
II Associated: In India, 68.9% association with hairy tragus and with higher frequency of baldness. (Frequency of hairy tragus alone 34.6%.) Strong association with age in all populations.

Etiology: Enough data have been accumulated to support the hypothesis that this trait is the only one known to be Y-linked, ie the responsible gene is situated on Y chromosome. High proportion of brothers, fathers and paternal grandfathers of probands are affected at age of expression of the trait. Male relatives from the maternal side are affected only exceptionally, mainly as a coincidence, due to finding a very high frequency of the trait in some populations in India.

Recently the 2-gene hypothesis has been suggested involving 2 nonallelic genes, 1 of which is situated on the nonhomologous part, and the other on homologous part of the Y chromosome (the homologous part of the X chromosome sharing also a corresponding allele). Penetrance is almost complete in older men (above 60 years).

Pathogenesis: ?

Related Facts
I Sex Ratio: M1:F0
II Risk of Occurrence: ?
III Risk of Recurrence for
   Patient's Sib: Almost all male sibs affected at older age
   Patient's Child: Almost all sons of male patients
IV Age of Detectability: Around 20 years of age and later
V Prevalence: The overall mean prevalence in the Indian population is 16.8% (excluding Asian groups of India and the people of the sub-Himalayan region). The higher prevalence was observed in All-Brahmins and All-Kayasthas: 23 to 27%. In West Bengal 60% of males between 70 and 79 years of age were affected. In Israeli population the prevalence in males was only 1.1 to 25.8% depending on age of examined.

Treatment
I Primary Prevention: —
II Secondary Prevention: Cosmetic ?
III Other Therapy: —

Prognosis: Normal for life span, intelligence and function

Detection of Carrier: —

Special Considerations: —

References:
Chakravartti, M.R.: Hairy pinnae in Indian populations. Acta Genet. (Basel) 18:511, 1968.
Dronamraju, K.R.: Hypertrichosis of the pinna of the human ear, Y-linked pedigrees. J. Genet. 57:23, 1960.
Rao, D.C.: Two-gene hypothesis for hairy pinnae of the ear. Acta Genet. Med. Gemellol. (Roma) 19:448, 1969.

Contributor: Jaroslav Červenka

Editor's Computerized Descriptor: Hair
Also see Section I, Fig. 72

EAR LOBE, ABSENT

Includes: Absence du lobe de l'oreille
Aplasie des Ohrläppchens
Ausencia del lóbulo de la oreja

Excludes: Microtia-atresia (664)
Atresia alone
Deafness and ear pits (247)
Darwin tubercle (Marker) (241)
Ear lobe pit (Marker) (322)
Ear flare
Ear lobes attached (323)

Minimal Diagnostic Criteria: Hypoplastic or absent ear lobe†

Clinical Findings: The ear lobe is either absent or hypoplastic. This is often noted in conjunction with syndromes, eg bird-headed dwarfism.

Complications
I **Derived:** —
II **Associated:** Bird-headed dwarfism

Etiology: ?

Pathogenesis: ?

Related Facts
I **Sex Ratio:** Presumed to be M1:F1
II **Risk of Occurrence:** ?
III **Risk of Recurrence for**
    Patient's Sib: —
    Patient's Child: ?
IV **Age of Detectability:** At birth
V **Prevalence:** ? Said to be more frequent in Negroes and Filipinos

Treatment
I **Primary Prevention:** —
II **Secondary Prevention:** If isolated defect no treatment is needed.
III **Other Therapy:** —

Prognosis: Good for life, intelligence and function if isolated defect of outer ear, otherwise dependent upon concomitant defects.

Detection of Carrier: —

†**Special Considerations:** Anomalies of the external ear should suggest the possibility of an anomaly of the middle ear as well. Hearing should be assessed as soon as possible and appropriate therapy instituted.

References:
Smith, D.W.: Recognizable Patterns of Human Malformation: Genetic, Embryologic and Clinical Aspects (Major Problems in Clinical Pediatrics). Philadelphia:W.B. Saunders Co., 1970.

Contributor: **LaVonne Bergstrom**

_____

Editor's Computerized Descriptor: Ear

EAR LOBE, CLEFT

Includes: Fente du lobe de l'oreille
Gespaltenes Ohrläppchen
Lóbulo de la oreja fisurado
Cleft ear lobe

Excludes: Microtia-atresia (664)
Atresia alone
Deafness and ear pits (247)
Darwin tubercle (Marker) (241)
Ear lobe pit (Marker) (322)
Ear flare

Minimal Diagnostic Criteria: Longitudinal cleft of lobule†

Clinical Findings: (Coloboma lobuli). The ear lobe is cleft longitudinally. The cleft may be partial, but usually extends to, but not through, the incisura intertragica. The deformity may be unilateral or bilateral.

Complications
I **Derived:** —
II **Associated:** —

Etiology: ?

Pathogenesis: ?

Related Facts
I **Sex Ratio:** Presumed to be M1:F1
II **Risk of Occurrence:** ?
III **Risk of Recurrence for**
    Patient's Sib: ?
    Patient's Child: ?
IV **Age of Detectability:** At birth
V **Prevalence:** ?

Treatment
I **Primary Prevention:** —
II **Secondary Prevention:** Plastic surgical repair may be indicated.
III **Other Therapy:** —

Prognosis: Good for life span, intelligence and function if isolated defect of outer ear, otherwise dependent upon concomitant defects.

Detection of Carrier: —

†**Special Considerations:** Anomalies of the external ear should suggest the possibility of an anomaly of the middle ear as well.

References:
Converse, J.M. (ed.): Reconstructive Plastic Surgery. Philadelphia: W.B. Saunders Co., 1964, vol. 3.
Rubin, A. (ed.): Handbook of Congenital Malformations. Philadelphia: W.B. Saunders Co., 1967.

Contributor: **LaVonne Bergstrom**

_____

Editor's Computerized Descriptor: Ear

EAR LOBE PIT (MARKER)

Includes: Perforation du pavillon de l'oreille
Ohrläppchen-Fistel
Perforaciones naturales de los pabellones auriculares (Marcador)
Natural earring holes

Excludes: —

Minimal Diagnostic Criteria: Pit in ear lobe

Clinical Findings: Pit about 1 mm deep in ear lobes at about the place where they would normally be pierced for earrings. The holes do not completely penetrate the lobe.

Complications
I **Derived:** —
II **Associated:** —

Etiology: Autosomal dominant with variable expressivity and incomplete penetrance. In about half the cases the pit is in only 1 lobe and in a few cases the gene may be carried without showing pits in either lobe.

Pathogenesis: ?

Related Facts
I **Sex Ratio:** M1:F1
II **Risk of Occurrence:** ? Very rare
III **Risk of Recurrence for**
 Patient's Sib: If parent is affected < 1 in 2 (< 50%) for each offspring to be affected; otherwise not increased
 Patient's Child: < 1 in 2
IV **Age of Detectability:** Young child
V **Prevalence:** ? Very rare

Treatment
I **Primary Prevention:** Not necessary
II **Secondary Prevention:** None needed
III **Other Therapy:** —

Prognosis: Normal for life span, intelligence and function

Detection of Carrier: —

Special Considerations: —

References:
Edmonds, H.W. and Keeler, C.E.: Natural "ear-ring" holes; inherited sinuses of ear lobe. J. Hered. 31:507, 1940.
Winchester, A.M.: Genetics; A Survey of the Principles of Heredity, 3rd Ed. Boston: Houghton Mifflin, 1966, p. 450.

Contributor: **A. M. Winchester**

Editor's Computerized Descriptor: Ear

EAR LOBES, ATTACHED (MARKER)

Includes: Lobes des oreilles attachés
Angewachsen Ohrläppchen
Lóbulos de las orejas pegadas (Marcador)

Excludes: Ear lobe, absent (320)

Minimal Diagnostic Criteria: Attachment of ear lobe

Clinical Findings: Lower part of ear attached directly onto head with no free-hanging lobes. There may be considerable variation in the shape of the lower part of ear.

Complications
I **Derived:** —
II **Associated:** —

Etiology: Overall attachment seems to be recessive to free-hanging ear lobes, but polygenic inheritance affects the angle of attachment.

Pathogenesis: —

Related Facts
I **Sex Ratio:** M1:F1
II **Risk of Occurrence:** About 1 in 7 in Germany
III **Risk of Recurrence for**
 Patient's Sib: About 1 in 4 (25%) when both parents are carriers, about 1 in 2 (50%) when 1 parent shows the trait and the other is a carrier, and close to 1 in 1 (100%) when both parents show the trait.
 Patient's Child: About 1 in 4 (25%) when both parents are carriers, about 1 in 2 (50%) when 1 parent shows the trait and the other is a carrier, and close to 1 in 1 (100%) when both parents show the trait.
IV **Age of Detectability:** At birth
V **Prevalence:** About 15% in Germany

Treatment
I **Primary Prevention:** Not necessary
II **Secondary Prevention:** Not needed
III **Other Therapy:** —

Prognosis: Normal for life span, intelligence and function

Detection of Carrier: —

Special Considerations: —

References:
McKusick, V.A.: Mendelian Inheritance in Man, 4th Ed. Baltimore: Johns Hopkins Press, 1975, p. 88.
Powell, E.F. and Whitney, D.D.: Ear lobe inheritance; unusual 3-generation photographic pedigree-chart. J. Hered. 28:185, 1937.
Winchester, A.M.: Genetics; A Survey of the Principles of Heredity, 3rd Ed. Boston: Houghton Mifflin, 1966.

Contributor: **A. M. Winchester**

Editor's Computerized Descriptor: Ear

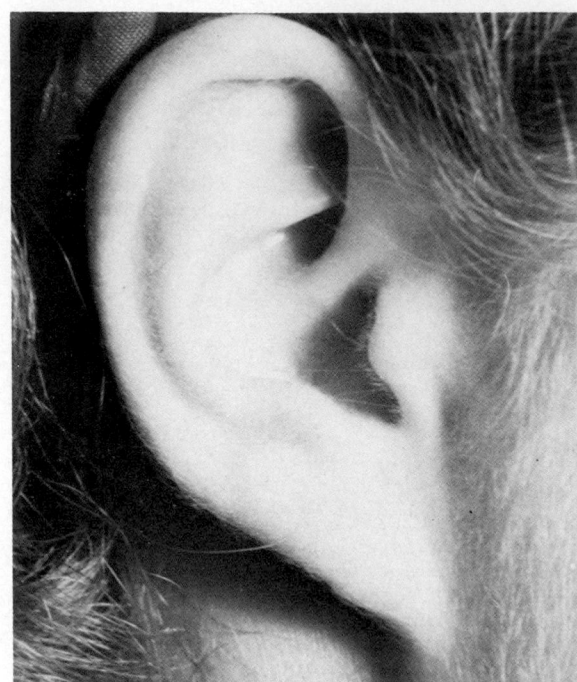

243. Attached ear lobe

EAR LOBES, HYPERTROPHIC THICKENED

Includes: Hypertrophie des lobes de l'oreille
Hypertrophische (fleischige) Ohrläppchen
Lóbulos auriculares engrosados e hipertróficos
Hypertrophic ear lobes

Excludes: Microtia-atresia (664)
Atresia alone
Deafness and ear pits (247)
Darwin tubercle (Marker) (241)
Ear lobe pit (Marker) (322)
Ear flare

Minimal Diagnostic Criteria: Disproportionately large, thick ear lobes†

Clinical Findings: The ear lobe is disproportionately large for the overall size of the ear, is thickened and feels fibrotic in the center of the lobule. All affected persons have an associated conductive hearing loss. The eardrum is normal. At tympanotomy a malformed incus which does not articulate with the stapes is found. Histologic examination of the incus shows a nest of connective tissue fibers at its distal end.

Complications
I   **Derived:** —
II **Associated:** Malformed incus which does not articulate with stapes.

Etiology: Autosomal dominant

Pathogenesis: ?

Related Facts
I   **Sex Ratio:** M1:F1
II   **Risk of Occurrence:** ?
III **Risk of Recurrence for**
    Patient's Sib: If parent is affected 1 in 2 (50%) for each offspring to be affected; otherwise not increased.
    Patient's Child: 1 in 2
IV **Age of Detectability:** At birth, although conductive hearing loss might not be suspected for several years.
V   **Prevalence:** ?

Treatment
I   **Primary Prevention:** Genetic counseling
II **Secondary Prevention:** If isolated defect, no treatment is usually needed.
    If conductive hearing loss is present, petrous pyramid polytomography should be done to assess the anatomic configuration of the middle ear, and, if it seems favorable, exploratory tympanotomy and surgical correction should be performed, if feasible. If not feasible, or, if unsuccessful, or if the patient has a sensorineural hearing loss, hearing aids should be fitted and aural rehabilitation undertaken.
III **Other Therapy:** —

Prognosis: Good for life span, intelligence and function if isolated defect of outer ear, otherwise dependent upon concomitant defects.

Detection of Carrier: —

†Special Considerations: External ear anomalies should also prompt the physician to look for anomalies of other systems and to follow the infant for possible mental retardation. Careful genetic and clinical studies of the family should be carried out if accompanying defects are found.

References:
Konigsmark, B.W.: Hereditary deafness with external-ear abnormalities: A review. Johns Hopkins Med. J. 127:228, 1970.
Wilmot, T.J.: Hereditary conductive deafness due to incus-stapes abnormalities and associated with pinna deformity. J. Laryngol. 84:469, 1970.

EAR, LONG, NARROW, POSTERIORLY ROTATED

Editor's Computerized Descriptors: Hearing, Ear

Includes: Oreilles allongées en rotation postérieure
Langes, schmales, dorsal rotiertes Ohr
Orejas largas, estrechas y con rotación posterior

Excludes: Microtia-atresia (664)
Atresia alone
Deafness and ear pits (247)
Darwin tubercle (Marker) (241)
Ear lobe pit (Marker) (322)
Ear flare

Minimal Diagnostic Criteria: Posterior rotation of ear around axis of external auditory meatus†

Clinical Findings: The ear's configuration is normal except that the ear is somewhat elongated. It may be slightly low set or at the normal height but rotated from the perpendicular more than 10% backward around an axis which goes through both external auditory meati. This may be associated with syndromes such as the broad thumb-hallux syndrome and is suggested in osteogenesis imperfecta. In the latter case, it may be caused by the bulging of the squama of the temporal bone.

Complications
I   **Derived:** —
II **Associated:** Broad thumb-hallux syndrome, osteogenesis imperfecta

Etiology: ?

Pathogenesis: ?

Related Facts
I   **Sex Ratio:** Presumed to be M1:F1
II   **Risk of Occurrence:** ?
III **Risk of Recurrence for**
     Patient's Sib: ?
     Patient's Child: ?
IV   **Age of Detectability:** At birth
V   **Prevalence:** ?

Treatment
I   **Primary Prevention:** —
II   **Secondary Prevention:** If isolated defect, no treatment is usually needed.
III **Other Therapy:** —

Prognosis: Good for life span, intelligence and function if isolated defect of outer ear, otherwise dependent upon concomitant defects.

Detection of Carrier: —

†Special Considerations: Anomalies of the external ear should suggest the possibility of an anomaly of the middle ear as well. Hearing should be assessed as soon as possible and appropriate therapy instituted. The anatomy of the middle and inner ear should be determined by petrous pyramid polytomography. External ear anomalies should also prompt the physician to look for anomalies of other systems, and to follow the infant for possible mental retardation. Careful genetic and clinical studies of the family should be carried out if accompanying defects are found.

References:
Converse, J.M. (ed.): Reconstructive Plastic Surgery. Philadelphia:W.B. Saunders Co., 1964, vol. 3.

Contributor: **LaVonne Bergstrom**

Editor's Computerized Descriptor: Ear

EAR, LOP

Includes: Oreilles flasques
Schlaffe Ohrmuschel
Oreja colgante
Ear, floppy helix of
"Bat ear"

Excludes: Microtia-atresia (664)
Atresia alone
Deafness and ear pits (247)
Darwin tubercle (Marker) (241)
Ear lobe pit (Marker) (322)
Ear flare

Minimal Diagnostic Criteria: Floppy helix, poor development of scapha and anthelix†

Clinical Findings: The concha appears large while the anthelix and scapha are poorly developed so that the ear protrudes, giving a floppy appearance to the helix or the appearance that there is no helix at all. In some instances, the helix droops to a degree sufficient to cover the concha. The condition may be unilateral, but is usually bilateral and fairly symmetric.

Complications
I   **Derived:** Psychologic disturbance due to the deformity
II **Associated:** Reduplicated Darwin tubercle, absence of the lobule, microtia, macrotia, curling or displacement of the ear, facial asymmetry, chromosome 21 trisomy syndrome, occasionally conductive hearing loss.

Etiology: Autosomal dominant in some cases, in others possible arrest at a fetal stage of development. Reason for increased clinical occurrence in males is unknown.

Pathogenesis: ? Rogers has suggested that the lop ear resembles a fetal stage of pinna development, suggesting arrest of development at that stage.

Related Facts
I   **Sex Ratio:** M3:F1
II **Risk of Occurrence:** ?
III **Risk of Recurrence for**
    Patient's Sib: When autosomal dominant and if parent is affected, 1 in 2 (50%) for each offspring to be affected; otherwise not increased.
    Patient's Child: When autosomal dominant 1 in 2
IV **Age of Detectability:** At birth
V   **Prevalence:** 21 in 108,744 pediatric admissions to a hospital

Treatment
I   **Primary Prevention:** Genetic counseling
II **Secondary Prevention:** Plastic surgical repair may be indicated.
    If conductive hearing loss is present, petrous pyramid polytomography should be done to assess the anatomic configuration of the middle ear, and, if it seems favorable, exploratory tympanotomy and surgical correction should be performed, if feasible. If not feasible, or, if unsuccessful, or if the patient has a sensorineural hearing loss, hearing aids should be fitted and aural rehabilitation undertaken.
III **Other Therapy:** —

Prognosis: Good for life span, intelligence and function if isolated defect of outer ear, otherwise dependent upon concomitant defects.

Detection of Carrier: —

†**Special Considerations:** External ear anomalies should also prompt the physician to look for anomalies of other systems and to follow the infant for possible mental retardation. Careful genetic and clinical studies of the family should be carried out if accompanying defects are found.

References:

Converse, J.M. (ed.): Reconstructive Plastic Surgery. Philadelphia:W.B. Saunders, 1964, vol 3.
Konigsmark, B.W.: Hereditary deafness with external-ear abnormalities: A review. Johns Hopkins Med. J. 127:228, 1970.
MacCollum, D.W.: The lop ear. JAMA 110:1427, 1938.
Rogers, B.O.: Microtic, lop, cup and protruding ears: Four directly inheritable deformities. Plast. Reconstr. Surg. 41:208, 1968.

Contributor: **LaVonne Bergstrom**

Editor's Computerized Descriptor: Ear

EAR, LOW-SET

Includes: Insertion basse des oreilles
Tiefsitzende Ohren
Oreja implantada baja
Low-set ear

Excludes: Microtia-atresia (664)
Atresia alone
Deafness and ear pits (247)
Darwin tubercle (Marker) (241)
Ear lobe pit (Marker) (322)
Ear flare

Minimal Diagnostic Criteria: ? Ear set below an arbitrary line drawn between the lateral canthus of the eye and the occipital protuberance. Associated backward rotation of pinna.†

Clinical Findings: By definition an ear is low set when the helix meets the cranium below a line between the outer canthus of the eye and the occipital protuberance. When the head is level the external auditory meatus is normally at about the level of the ala nasi. Low-set ears may be normal in configuration and merely set below the landmarks outlined, with some tendency to backward rotation around an axis passing through both external auditory meati. However, usually low-set ears are also somewhat small with associated minor malformations. The condition is usually bilaterally symmetric.

Complications
I   **Derived:** —
II **Associated:** Seen in many syndromes as well as in otherwise normal individuals. Often the ears are somewhat small and deformed in varying degrees. In some instances conductive hearing loss is associated. Mental retardation present in 50% of Mengel's cases.

Etiology: Probably multifactorial

Pathogenesis: ?

Related Facts
I   **Sex Ratio:** Presumed to be Ml:Fl
II **Risk of Occurrence:** ?
III **Risk of Recurrence for**
    Patient's Sib: ?
    Patient's Child: ?
IV **Age of Detectability:** At birth
V   **Prevalence:** ?

Treatment
I   **Primary Prevention:** —
II **Secondary Prevention:** If isolated defect, no treatment is usually needed. If conductive hearing loss is present, petrous pyramid polytomography should be done to assess the anatomic configuration of the middle ear, and, if it seems favorable, exploratory tympanotomy and surgical correction should be performed, if feasible. If not feasible, or if unsuccessful, or if the patient has a sensorineural hearing loss, hearing aids should be fitted and aural rehabilitation undertaken.
III **Other Therapy:** —

Prognosis: Good for life span, intelligence and function if isolated defect of outer ear, otherwise dependent upon concomitant defects.

Detection of Carrier: —

†Special Considerations: Anomalies of the external ear should suggest the possibility of an anomaly of the middle ear as well. Hearing should be assessed as soon as possible and appropriate therapy instituted. The anatomy of the middle and inner ear should be determined by petrous pyramid polytomography. External ear anomalies should also prompt the physician to look for anomalies of other systems and to follow the infant for possible mental retardation. Careful genetic and clinical studies of the family should be carried out if accompanying defects are found.

References:
Converse, J.M. (ed.): Reconstructive Plastic Surgery. Philadelphia:W.B. Saunders Co., 1964, vol. 3.
Konigsmark, B.W.: Hereditary deafness with external-ear abnormalities: A review. John Hopkins Med. J. 127:228, 1970.
Mengel, M.C. et al: Conductive hearing loss and malformed low-set ears, as a possible recessive syndrome. J. Med. Genet. 6:14, 1969.
Smith, D.W.: Recognizable Patterns of Human Malformation: Genetic, Embryologic and Clinical Aspects (Major Problems in Clinical Pediatrics). Philadelphia:W.B. Saunders, 1970.

Contributor: **LaVonne Bergstrom**

Editor's Computerized Descriptors: Hearing, Ear

EAR, MOZART (MARKER)

Includes: Oreille de Mozart
Mozart-Ohr
Oreja de Mozart (Marcador)
Mozart ear (Marker)

Excludes: Microtia-atresia (664)
Atresia alone
Deafness and ear pits (247)
Darwin tubercle (Marker) (241)
Ear lobe pit (Marker) (322)
Ear flare

Minimal Diagnostic Criteria: Bulging superior margin of pinna due to fusion of crura of the anthelix and the crus helicis.†

Clinical Findings: Said to have been present in the composer, Mozart, and his father. The 2 crura of the anthelix and the crus of the helix are fused, giving a bulging appearance to the cartilaginous framework of the anterosuperior portion of the pinna. The anthelix is also somewhat larger than usual. (None of the usually published portraits of Mozart demonstrate this malformation, although 1 family portrait suggests it.)

Complications
I   Derived: —
II Associated: —

Etiology: Autosomal dominant

Pathogenesis: ?

Related Facts
I   Sex Ratio: Presumed to be Ml:Fl
II   Risk of Occurrence: ?
III Risk of Recurrence for
    Patient's Sib: If parent is affected 1 in 2 (50%) for each offspring to be affected; otherwise not increased.
    Patient's Child: 1 in 2
IV   Age of Detectability: At birth
V   Prevalence: ?

Treatment
I   Primary Prevention: Genetic counseling
II   Secondary Prevention: If isolated defect, no treatment is usually needed.
III Other Therapy: —

Prognosis: Good for life span, intelligence and function if isolated defect of outer ear, otherwise dependent upon concomitant defects.

Detection of Carrier: —

†**Special Considerations:** Anomalies of the external ear should suggest the possibility of an anomaly of the middle ear as well.

References:
Gates, R.R.: Human Genetics. New York: Macmillan Co., 1946, vol. 1.

Contributor: **LaVonne Bergstrom**

Editor's Computerized Descriptor: Ear

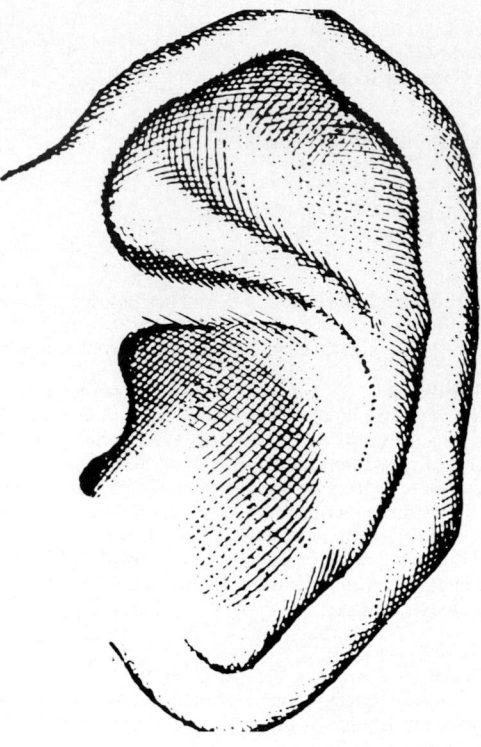

244. Mozart ear

EAR PITS (MARKER)

Includes: Fossettes auriculaires
Ohrgrübchen
Fóveas auriculares (Marcador)
Prehelicine fistula
Preauricular pits
Fistula auris congenita
Congenital sinuses of external ear

Excludes: Deafness and ear pits (247)

Minimal Diagnostic Criteria: A preauricular or anterior helicine pit or sinus in an individual in whom there is a positive family history for the trait.

Clinical Findings: A usually shallow pit, which may be funnel-like or cystic, is located in the descending limb of the helix of the ear or just anterior to it. Occasionally the pit may extend 1 or 2 cm as a sinus tract and rarely may communicate with the middle ear. The trait is unilateral in about 75% of cases and bilateral in about 25% of cases, with right and left sides being involved about equally in unilateral cases. The tracts are lined with squamous or columnar epithelium. If the lining is squamous the usual skin appendages may be present. The pits often discharge a milky substance and are prone to become infected. Occasionally a chronic infection may appear granulomatous.

Complications
I **Derived:** Infection in the sinus
II **Associated:** Branchial fistulas, cleft palate, spina bifida, imperforate anus, renal defects. It is possible that the association of all but branchial fistulas with ear pits is coincidental.

Etiology: Autosomal dominant with incomplete penetrance. One of identical twins may have the trait and not the other.

Pathogenesis: ? It has been theorized that preauricular pits represent abortive accessory ear canals or that they represent areas of failure of fusion of the primitive ear hillocks. However, there is considerable disagreement about this. Both of these theories are somewhat attractive in view of the fact that ear pits are often seen in patients with microtia.

Related Facts
I **Sex Ratio:** One paper indicates M1:F2
II **Risk of Occurrence:** 1 in 50 live births in African tribes, 1 in 500 live births in Europeans
III **Risk of Recurrence for**
   Patient's Sib: Only about 1 in 4 (25%) in dominant pedigrees, because of reduced penetrance.
   Patient's Child: Only about 1 in 4 because of reduced penetrance
IV **Age of Detectability:** At birth
V **Prevalence:** 0.9% among American draftees, 0.2% among white races, 5.2% among American blacks, 4.0 among African blacks, 1 per 1000 in India. "Very prevalent" among the Chinese (exact figures not cited).

Treatment
I **Primary Prevention:** Not necessary
II **Secondary Prevention:** Medical treatment if pits become infected; incision and drainage if an abscess forms; excision of the tract if infection is recurrent or chronic.
III **Other Therapy:** —

Prognosis: Normal for life expectancy, intelligence and function

Detection of Carrier: —

Special Considerations: —

References:
Ewing, M.R.: Congenital sinuses of external ear. J. Laryngol. 61:1823, 1946.
Martins, A.G.: Lateral cervical and preauricular sinuses: Their transmission as dominant characters. Br. Med. J. 1:255, 1961.
Quelprud, T.: Ear pit and its inheritance: Fistula auris congenita, described in 1864, still genetical and embryological puzzle. J. Hered. 31:379, 1940.
Simpkiss, M. and Lowe, A.: Congenital abnormalities in the African newborn. Arch. Dis. Child. 36:404, 1961.
Stiles, K.A.: Inheritance of pitted ear. J. Hered. 36:53, 1945.

Contributor: **LaVonne Bergstrom**

Editor's Computerized Descriptor: Ear

Includes: Anthélix saillant
Ohr, prominente Anthelix
Antihélix auricular prominente
Wildermuth ear

Excludes: Microtia-atresia (664)
Atresia alone
Deafness and ear pits (247)
Darwin tubercle (Marker) (241)
Ear lobe pit (Marker (322)
Ear flare

Minimal Diagnostic Criteria: Prominent anthelix†

Clinical Findings: In this deformity prominence of the anthelix with a very poorly formed helix is seen. It may be present in certain syndromes in which other multiple anomalies may be present, as in chromosome 18q-.

Complications
I **Derived:** —
II **Associated:** May be seen in a number of syndromes, some of which have multiple anomalies. Sensorineural or conductive hearing loss may be present in some instances and probably due to associated middle ear anomalies.

Etiology: ?

Pathogenesis: ?

Related Facts
I **Sex Ratio:** Presumed to be Ml:Fl
II **Risk of Occurrence:** ?
III **Risk of Recurrence for**
  Patient's Sib: ?
  Patient's Child: ?
IV **Age of Detectability:** At birth
V **Prevalence:** ?

Treatment
I **Primary Prevention:** —
II **Secondary Prevention:** If isolated defect, no treatment is usually needed. If conductive hearing loss is present, petrous pyramid polytomography should be done to assess the anatomic configuration of the middle ear, and, if it seems favorable, exploratory tympanotomy and surgical correction should be performed, if feasible. If not feasible, or, if unsuccessful, or if the patient has a sensorineural hearing loss, hearing aids should be fitted and aural rehabilitation undertaken.
III **Other Therapy:** —

Prognosis: Good for life span, intelligence and function if isolated defect of outer ear, otherwise dependent upon concomitant defects.

Detection of Carrier: —

†Special Considerations: Anomalies of the external ear should suggest the possibility of an anomaly of the middle ear as well.

References:
Konigsmark, B.W.: Hereditary deafness with external-ear abnormalities: A review. Johns Hopkins Med. J. 127:228, 1970.
Rubin, A. (ed.): Handbook of Congenital Malformations. Philadelphia:W.B. Saunders, 1967.

Contributor: **LaVonne Bergstrom**

Editor's Computerized Descriptors: Hearing, Ear

Includes: Agénésie partielle de l'oreille avec plicature de l'hélix
Ohr, kleines mit umgeschlagener Helix
Oreja pequeña con hélix doblada
Ear, with folded-down helix (incompletely developed)

Excludes: Microtia-atresia (664)
Atresia alone
Deafness and ear pits (247)
Darwin tubercle (Marker) (241)
Ear lobe pit (Marker (322)
Ear flare

Minimal Diagnostic Criteria: Small ear with helix folded down close to pinna†

Clinical Findings: The ear is small and the helix is folded down close to the pinna in a plane parallel to the top of head. The helix is poorly developed. Congenital absence of the incus-stapes articulation and deformity of incus and stapes may be present causing conductive hearing loss. Similar malformation is part of a number of syndromes.

Complications
I **Derived:** —
II **Associated:** Absence of incus-stapes articulation and deformities of incus and stapes. Chromosome 21 trisomy syndrome.

Etiology: ?

Pathogenesis: ?

Related Facts
I **Sex Ratio:** Presumed to be Ml:Fl
II **Risk of Occurrence:** ?
III **Risk of Recurrence for**
  Patient's Sib: ?
  Patient's Child: ?
IV **Age of Detectability:** At birth
V **Prevalence:** ?

Treatment
I **Primary Prevention:** —
II **Secondary Prevention:** Plastic surgical repair may be indicated.
III **Other Therapy:** —

Prognosis: Good for life span, intelligence and function if isolated defect of outer ear, otherwise dependent upon concomitant defects.

Detection of Carrier: —

†Special Considerations: Anomalies of the external ear should suggest the possibility of an anomaly of the middle ear as well. Hearing should be assessed as soon as possible and appropriate therapy instituted. The anatomy of the middle and inner ear should be determined by petrous pyramid polytomography. External ear anomalies should also prompt the physician to look for anomalies of other systems and to follow the infant for possible mental retardation. Careful genetic and clinical studies of the family should be carried out if accompanying defects are found.

References:
Converse, J.M. (ed.): Reconstructive Plastic Surgery. Philadelphia:W.B. Saunders, 1964, vol. 3.
Konigsmark, B.W.: Hereditary deafness with external-ear abnormalities: A review. Johns Hopkins Med. J. 127:228, 1970.
Rogers, B.O.: Microtic, lop, cup and protruding ears: Four directly inheritable deformities. Plast. Reconstr. Surg. 41:208, 1968.

Contributor: **LaVonne Bergstrom**

Editor's Computerized Descriptors: Hearing, Ear

EBSTEIN ANOMALY

Includes: Maladie d'Ebstein
Ebsteinsche Anomalie
Enfermedad de Ebstein
Ebstein anomaly of tricuspid valve
Tricuspid valve, downward displacement

Excludes: Ebstein anomaly of left atrioventricular valve in cases of ventricular inversion
Other forms of congenital tricuspid valve incompetence

Minimal Diagnostic Criteria: In the acyanotic individual, selective angiocardiography or cardiac catheterization with the intracavitary electrode catheter are necessary to establish a definitive diagnosis. When in a cyanotic individual who has bouts of tachycardia, there is decreased pulmonary vascular markings on chest roentgenograms, an ECG which shows large P waves, a prolonged PR interval and a precordial QRS pattern suggesting RBBB or having no definite criteria for either right or left ventricular hypertrophy, or the type B WPW pattern is present, then the diagnosis of Ebstein anomaly becomes mandatory.

Clinical Findings: The pathology of Ebstein anomaly is extremely variable. The 2 characteristic features are redundancy of valve tissue and adherence of a variable portion of the septal and posterior cusps to the right ventricular wall. Redundancy involves all cusps, although the anterior cusp is always much less affected. The area of adherence may be small, in which case the true origin of the cusps at the atrioventricular annulus is close to the apparent origin; or it may extend all the way down to the ring formed by the parietal band, crista supraventricularis, septal and moderator bands and anterior papillary muscle. That portion of the ventricle between the annulus and the apparent origin of the valve is said to be "atrialized," as it more or less forms a common chamber with the right atrium. The myocardium of the atrialized portion of the right ventricle may be fairly well developed in mild forms of the anomaly. In severe forms it may be fibrous. Both the pathology and pathophysiology are variable. In rare cases of Ebstein anomaly, the valve mechanism may function almost normally. With increasing severity of the anomaly, there is valvar insufficiency or stenosis. In time, right atrial pressure is elevated, the right atrium becomes markedly enlarged and a right-to-left shunt is established through an anatomically patent foramen ovale, or rarely, an atrial septal defect.

The malformation may be so pronounced as to cause intrauterine or neonatal death. Symptoms and signs are commonly present during the 1st month of life, particularly cyanosis, murmurs, congestive heart failure and bouts of tachycardia. Symptoms in the older child and adult are dyspnea on exertion, profound weakness or fatigue, cyanosis, bouts of tachycardia and in the terminal stages, cardiac failure. Auscultation is variable. Often the widely split components of the first sound are followed by a systolic murmur, 2 widely split components of the second sound and frequently a prominent third or fourth sound, producing a "triple" or "quadruple" rhythm. A diastolic murmur may surround either S_3 or S_4, or both.

The ECG either shows a right bundle branch block pattern or the Wolff-Parkinson-White (type B) pattern often with right atrial enlargement and a prolonged PR interval. The vectorcardiogram classically shows P loop changes of right atrial enlargement and slowing of the terminal rightward, superior and anterior QRS forces consistent with RBBB. The radiologic features in infancy are variable ranging from slight to massive cardiac enlargement and often resemble severe pulmonic stenosis with an intact ventricular septum and a right-to-left shunt. In patients of all age groups, certain roentgenographic features are seen: there are varying degrees of right heart enlargement; the pulmonary artery segment is usually inapparent; no left atrial enlargement; the aortic knob is normal or small; pulmonary vascular markings are normal or decreased, and even with chronic congestive heart failure, pleural effusion is not seen.

The echocardiogram shows dilation of the right ventricular cavity and delayed tricuspid closure with respect to mitral diastolic closure. The tricuspid valve excursion is exaggerated and its echo representation is displaced leftward. Many patients have paradoxic septal motion.

Cardiac catheterization, to be diagnostic, must demonstrate that a portion of the right ventricle functions as the right atrium. When, with an intracavitary electrode catheter, right ventricular muscle potentials are recorded in the presence of a right atrial pressure, the diagnosis is established. The hemodynamic findings depend on whether there is tricuspid insufficiency, or stenosis, or both. In cyanotic individuals, the right-to-left shunt is localized to the atrial level. Angiocardiography is best performed in the right ventricle. This outlines clearly the enlarged right atrium, the atrialized right ventricle and the functional right ventricle. The true and apparent annulus divide the inferior margin of the cardiac border in the AP view into 3 distinct compartments.

Complications
I **Derived:** Cerebral abscess, thromboembolic phenomena and organ pathology secondary to chronic congestive failure.
II **Associated:** These most commonly are a ventricular septal defect or pulmonary stenosis or atresia. Extracardiac anomalies are rare.

Etiology: Lithium has been identified as a specific environmental trigger. Multifactorial inheritance.

Pathogenesis: Ebstein anomaly is probably an abnormality of the process of undermining of the embryonic right ventricular myocardium which normally leads to the formation of the tricuspid valve apparatus. In Ebstein anomaly, it remains incomplete and never reaches the annulus. Thus, the normal development of chordae and papillary muscles does not take place, or remains abortive. The relatively normal development of the anterior cusp is probably related to its very early liberation.

Related Facts
I **Sex Ratio:** M1:F1
II **Risk of Occurrence:** Approximately 1 in 200 births with congenital heart disease
III **Risk of Recurrence for**
Patient's Sib: Predicted risk 0.7%; empiric risk 1.1%
Patient's Child: ?
IV **Age of Detectability:** From birth, particularly with selective right ventricular angiocardiography or the intracavitary electrode catheter
V **Prevalence:** 1 in 50,000 to 1 in 20,000 in the pediatric population

Treatment
I **Primary Prevention:** Genetic counseling
II **Secondary Prevention:** Replacement of abnormal tricuspid valve with a prosthesis
III **Other Therapy:** Appropriate drugs or electroshock for bouts of tachycardia. Symptomatic therapy for congestive heart failure. Antibiotic therapy for cerebral abscess.

Prognosis: Variable, depending on the degree of pathologic anatomy and resultant distortion of physiology. Ebstein anomaly may cause neonatal death or be compatible with a normal life span.

Detection of Carrier: —

Special Considerations: —

References:

Goldberg, S.J. et al: Pediatric and Adolescent Echocardiography. Chicago:Year Book Medical Publishers, 1975.

Hernandez, F.A. et al: The intracavitary electrocardiogram in the diagnosis of Ebstein's anomaly. Am. J. Cardiol. 1:181, 1953.

Lundström, N.R.: Echocardiography in the diagnosis of Ebstein's anomaly of the tricuspid valve. Circulation 47:597, 1973.

Schiebler, G.L. et al: Clinical study of twenty-three cases of Ebstein's anomaly of the tricuspid valve. Circulation 19:165, 1959.

Schiebler, G.L. et al: Diseases of the tricuspid valve. In Moss, A.J. and Adams, F.H. (eds.): Heart Disease in Infants, Children, and Adolescents. Baltimore:Williams & Wilkins Co., 1968, p. 492.

Van Mierop, L.H.S. et al: Anomalies of the tricuspid valve resulting in stenosis or incompetence. In Moss, A.J. and Adams, F.H. (eds.): Heart Disease in Infants, Children, and Adolescents, 2nd Ed. Baltimore:Williams & Wilkins Co., 1977.

Contributors: **Gerold L. Schiebler**
L.H.S. Van Mierop

Editor's Computerized Descriptors: Resp., CV.

ECTODERMAL DYSPLASIA, ANHIDROTIC

Includes: Dysplasie ectodermique anhydrotique
Anhidrotische ektodermale Dysplasie
Displasia ectodérmica anhidrótica
Hypohidrotic ectodermal dysplasia
Anhidrosis hypotrichotica
Ectodermal polydysplasia
Christ-Siemens-Touraine syndrome
Hypohidrosis, hypodontia, hypotrichosis syndrome

Excludes: Ectodermal dysplasia, hidrotic (334)

Minimal Diagnostic Criteria: Hypohidrosis, hypodontia, hypotrichosis

Clinical Findings: Hypohidrosis, hypotrichosis, hypodontia to adontia, saddle nose, frontal bossing, pouting lips, periorbital pigment. Hair color lighter than unaffected sibs, eczema, rarely deafness and mental retardation.

Complications
I **Derived:** Inability to control temperature by sweating. Persistent upper respiratory difficulties.
II **Associated:** —

Etiology: X-linked recessive; McK *22490, *30510

Pathogenesis: Absence of eccrine sweat glands in the skin but also absence of mucous glands in the pharynx, larynx, trachea, large and small bronchi and upper esophagus. This leads to the increased susceptibility to infection.

Related Facts
I **Sex Ratio:** M1:F0
II **Risk of Occurrence:** Rare - all races reported.
III **Risk of Recurrence for**
    Patient's Sib: If mother is a carrier, 1 in 2 (50%) for each brother to be affected and 1 in 2 for each sister to be a carrier.
    Patient's Child: 1 in 1 (100%) for carrier daughters; not increased for sons unless wife is a carrier.
IV **Age of Detectability:** Neonatal. High body temperature if hot day.
V **Prevalence:** ?

Treatment
I **Primary Prevention:** Genetic counseling.
II **Secondary Prevention:** Prevent infections by use of vaccines. Removal of any teeth left and replaced with good dentures, plastic surgery. Limited exercise in heat.
III **Other Therapy:** Use of false tears for dryness of eyes.

Prognosis: Fair to good

Detection of Carrier: Mothers may have missing teeth and if given sweat tests may show areas with absence of sweating on trunk.

Special Considerations: —

References:

Kerr, C.B. et al: Gene effect in carriers of anhidrotic ectodermal dysplasia. J. Med. Genet. 3:169, 1966.

Reed, W.B. et al: Clinical spectrum of anhidrotic ectodermal dysplasia. Arch. Dermatol. 102:134, 1970.

Upshaw, B.Y. and Montgomery, H.: Hereditary anhidrotic ectodermal dysplasia: Clinical and pathologic study. Arch. Dermatol. Syph. (Chic.) 60:1170, 1949.

Contributor: **William B. Reed‡**

Editor's Computerized Descriptors: Hearing, Face, Teeth, Nose, Skin, Sweating, Hair, Resp.

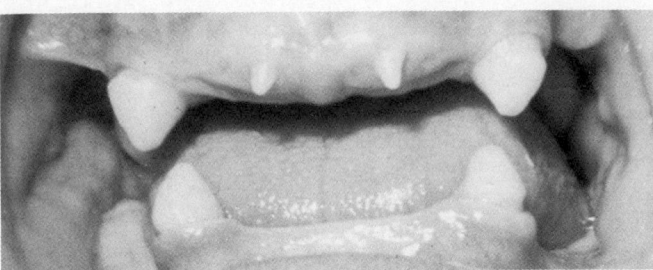

245. Note missing and conical teeth

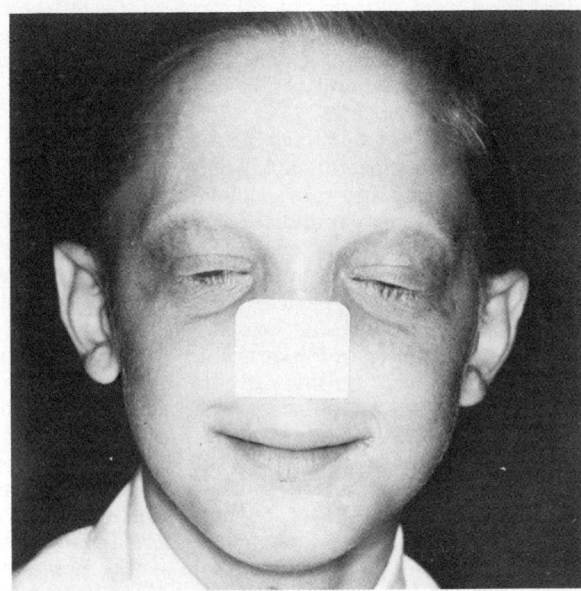

246. Note scanty hair and eyebrows

ECTODERMAL DYSPLASIA, HIDROTIC

Includes: Dysplasie ectodermique hydrotique
Hidrotische ektodermale Dysplasie
Displasia hidrótica ectodérmica
Hereditary ectodermal dystrophy

Excludes: Hidrotic ectodermal dysplasia with deafness
Ectodermal dysplasia, anhidrotic (333)

Minimal Diagnostic Criteria: Variable sparsity of hair and dystrophic nails.

Clinical Findings: Sparse, thin, fragile hair with reduced tensile strength on the head, eyebrows and body. Dystrophic, thick nails with subungual infections. Thick rough skin of palms and soles with brownish pigmentation. Normal sweat glands and teeth. Variable expressivity, especially of hair defect.

Complications
I **Derived:** —
II **Associated:** —

Etiology: Autosomal dominant with complete penetrance; McK *12950

Pathogenesis: Structural defect of keratin resulting from a change in molecular structure involving loss of high molecular weight components of the matrix protein.

Related Facts
I **Sex Ratio:** M1:F1
II **Risk of Occurrence:** Very rare except in certain areas settled by French families carrying the gene, eg near Montreal and New Orleans.
III **Risk of Recurrence for**
 Patient's Sib: If parent is affected, 1 in 2 (50%) for each offspring to be affected; otherwise not increased.
 Patient's Child: 1 in 2 (some evidence of reproductive overcompensation).
IV **Age of Detectability:** Neonatal period
V **Prevalence:** ?

Treatment
I **Primary Prevention:** Genetic counseling
II **Secondary Prevention:** —
III **Other Therapy:** Wigs may be cosmetically and psychologically helpful.

Prognosis: Normal life span

Detection of Carrier: —

Special Considerations: —

References:
Gold, R.J.M. and Kachra, Z.: The molecular defect in hydrotic ectodermal dysplasia. In Brown, A.C. (ed.): The First Human Hair Symposium. New York:Medcom Press, 1974, pp. 260-276.
Williams, M. and Fraser, F. C.: Hydrotic ectodermal dysplasia-Clouston's family revisited. Can. Med. Assoc. J. 96:36, 1967.

Contributor: **F. Clarke Fraser**

Editor's Computerized Descriptors: Skin, Hair, Nails

ECTOPIA CORDIS

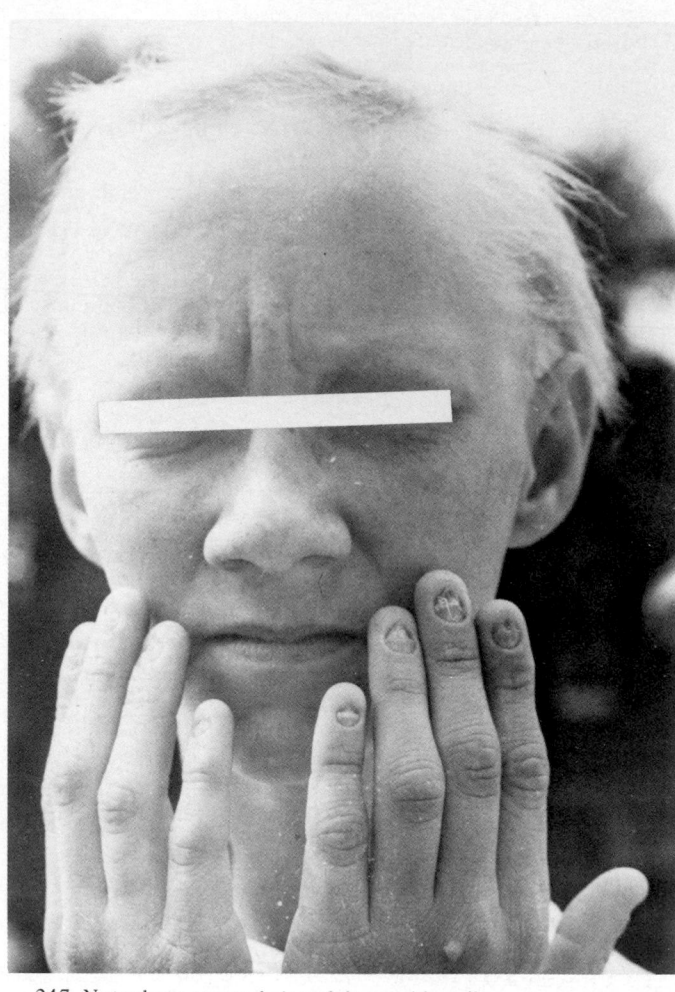

247. Note short, scanty hair and dystrophic nails

Includes: Ectopie cardiaque
Cervical, thoracic (complete or incomplete) and thoracoabdominal ectopia cordis

Excludes: Cardiac malpositions within thorax
Ventricular diverticulum (988)
Pericardium agenesis (805)

Minimal Diagnostic Criteria: Complete or partial thoracic ectopia cordis is apparent on physical examination. The thoracoabdominal type may be suspected if a pulse is apparent in an omphalocele, but angiocardiography may be necessary to demonstrate mild forms. In the rare isolated abdominal variety, the chest film will show an absence of the cardiac shadow, confirming the diagnosis.

Clinical Findings: While several forms of this entity exist, the common pathologic finding in all is partial or complete displacement of the heart from the thorax. This, in nearly all cases, is associated with a midline defect of the anterior body wall at some point.

Various classifications have been proposed based on the location of the displaced heart. There are 2 major clinical forms: the thoracic and thoracoabdominal types. The thoracic type is the most common and accounts for more than two-thirds of the reported cases. The usual anatomic arrangement consists of a completely cleft sternum, absence of the skin and parietal pericardium resulting in total extrophy of the heart with the apex displaced anteriorly and superiorly. Failure of union of the anterior thorax is usually associated with a similar defect in the anterior abdominal wall so that an omphalocele is present. An incomplete variant of the thoracic type exists and is sometimes referred to as the thoracocervical type. The sternum may be united in its inferior portion, but bifid superiorly with the heart being located in the upper thorax and neck. The skin is usually present, though the parietal pericardium may or may not be found. An abdominal defect is not usually present. This form is unusual and represents approximately 5% of the cases. The thoracoabdominal type is the 2nd most common form, comprising 20-25% of the cases. Anatomically, the sternum is usually not fused in its inferior position and this is associated with an anterior defect of the diaphragm and abdominal wall resulting in herniation of the heart inferiorly. Isolated abdominal and true cervical forms are exceedingly rare and are usually associated with other lethal malformations. The physical findings are striking and are usually indicative of the type of ectopia which is present. Diagnosis of the thoracoabdominal type may at times be difficult if there is only minimal herniation. Additional physical findings are largely dependent on the associated heart lesion.

If the diagnosis is not made from physical examination, a chest film may reveal inferior displacement of the heart in the thoracoabdominal type. With minimal herniation, the xray may be normal, though ventricular herniation may cause a slight dextrorotation due to the bilateral symmetry of the diaphragmatic defect. The ECG is of little aid in the diagnosis of ectopia cordis.

Complications

I **Derived:** Cardiac embarrassment from compression or strangulation of cardiovascular structures, death from infection.

II **Associated:** Eighty percent of the complete thoracic and thoracoabdominal forms will have intracardiac anomalies with VSD being the most common. Complex cyanotic lesions have been reported.

Etiology: ?

Pathogenesis: Precise mechanisms are unknown. The complete thoracic form is thought to be secondary to a failure of fusion of the right and left anterior body walls, resulting in a midline defect with cardiac extrophy and omphalocele. Thoracoabdominal ectopia is associated with a failure of development of the septum transversum allowing herniation of the heart through the diaphragm. The true cervical form of ectopia cordis apparently results from a failure of migration of the heart to the thorax from its original position near the mandibular arch.

Related Facts
I   **Sex Ratio:**   M1:F1
II **Risk of Occurrence:**   ? It is a rare lesion with less than 200 cases of all forms reported to date.
III **Risk of Recurrence for**
    Patient's Sib: ?
    Patient's Child: ?
IV **Age of Detectability:**   Thoracic - from birth by physical examination; thoracoabdominal - by physical examination or chest film; angiocardiography may be necessary in some cases.
V   **Prevalence:**   ?

Treatment
I   **Primary Prevention:**   —
II **Secondary Prevention:**   Surgical replacement of the heart in the thorax in a manner which will not lead to cardiac embarrassment.
III **Other Therapy:**   General supportive care of the infant until a definitive surgical procedure can be undertaken.

Prognosis: This depends upon the type of ectopia cordis and the associated malformations. Infants with the complete thoracic form die during the first days of life. Thoracoabdominal forms have been successfully repaired. The incomplete thoracic form is amenable to surgery and offers the best prognosis in that usually there is no associated cardiac malformation. With surgical correction and no associated lesion, a normal life span can be anticipated.

Detection of Carrier: —

Special Considerations: —

References:
Kanagasuntheram, R. and Verzin, J.A.: Ectopia cordis in man. Thorax 17:159, 1962.
Toyama, W.M.: Combined congenital defects of the anterior abdominal wall, sternum, diaphragm, pericardium, and heart: A case report and review of the syndrome. Pediatrics 50:778, 1972.
Van Praagh, R.: Malposition of the heart. In Moss, A.J. and Adams, F.H. (eds.): Heart Disease in Infants, Children, and Adolescents. Baltimore:Williams & Wilkins, 1968, p. 602.

Contributor: **Robert H. Miller**

Editor's Computerized Descriptors: Skel., CV., Muscle

ECTRODACTYLY

Includes: Ectrodactylie
Ektrodactylie
Ectrodactilia
Split-hand deformity
Lobster claw deformity

Excludes: Hanhart syndrome (451)
Brachydactyly (114)
Ring constrictions (874)
Ectrodactyly-ectodermal dysplasia-clefting syndrome (337)
Lacrimo-auriculo-dento-digital (LADD) syndrome

Minimal Diagnostic Criteria: Absence of 1 (central) or more digits.

Clinical Findings: Ectrodactyly refers to a heterogeneous group of hand and foot malformations. The clinical findings range from partial to complete absence of a finger to the cleft hand or foot deformity (absence of the 3rd digit with clefting into the proximal portion of the hand or foot and syndactyly of the remaining digits on each side of the cleft) to monodactyly (absence of all but the 5th digit). Simple absence of a finger usually represents a sporadic event, occurs unilaterally and without foot involvement. The cleft hand/foot and monodactyly malformations appear to reflect different degrees of severity of a common developmental defect and are distinct from the isolated absent finger. This type of anomaly usually occurs bilaterally, foot involvement is frequent and may occur alone, and a positive family history is obtained in about one-half of the cases. Several genetically distinct traits probably manifest this type of anomaly.

Complications
I   **Derived:**   Diminished function related to severity of defect
II **Associated:**   —

Etiology: The sole absence of a digit usually occurs sporadically. Cleft hand/foot and monodactyly deformities often show autosomal dominant transmission with considerable variability in expression. However, pedigrees consistent with autosomal recessive inheritance have been reported.†

Pathogenesis: Presumably suppression of the central and, in more severe cases, also radial rays in the developing limbs.

Related Facts
I   **Sex Ratio:**   M1:F1
II **Risk of Occurrence:**   ? Low
III **Risk of Recurrence for**
    Patient's Sib: Low in general. If parent is affected, 1 in 2 (50%) for each offspring to be affected.
    Patient's Child: Occurrence in a single individual may represent a sporadic event with little risk of recurrence, or a new mutation of an autosomal dominant trait which carries a 1 in 2 (50%) risk for each offspring. Clefting or monodactyly, bilaterality and foot involvement suggest a dominant trait. When autosomal dominant transmission is present, risk is 1 in 2 (50%).
IV **Age of Detectability:**   At birth
V   **Prevalence:**   1.4-8 in 100,000 for cleft hand

Treatment
I   **Primary Prevention:**   Genetic counseling, when autosomal dominant
II **Secondary Prevention:**   Reconstructive surgery when applicable
III **Other Therapy:**   —

Prognosis: Intelligence and life span are normal. Function is dependent on severity of deformity.

Detection of Carrier: —

†**Special Considerations:** Pedigrees consistent with autosomal recessive inheritance (only sibs affected and consanguinity present) have been reported; however, these cases are very rare.

References:

David, T.S: The differential diagnosis of the cleft hand and cleft foot malformations. Hand 6:58, 1974.

Maisels, D.D.: Lobster claw deformities of the hand. Hand 2:79, 1970.

Temtamy, S.A. and McKusick, V.A.: Synopsis of hand malformations with particular emphasis on genetic factors. In Bergsma, D. (ed.): Part III. Limb Malformations, Birth Defects: Orig. Art. Ser., vol. V, no. 3. New York: The National Foundation-March of Dimes, 1969, p. 125.

Contributor: **William A. Horton**

Editor's Computerized Descriptor: Skel.

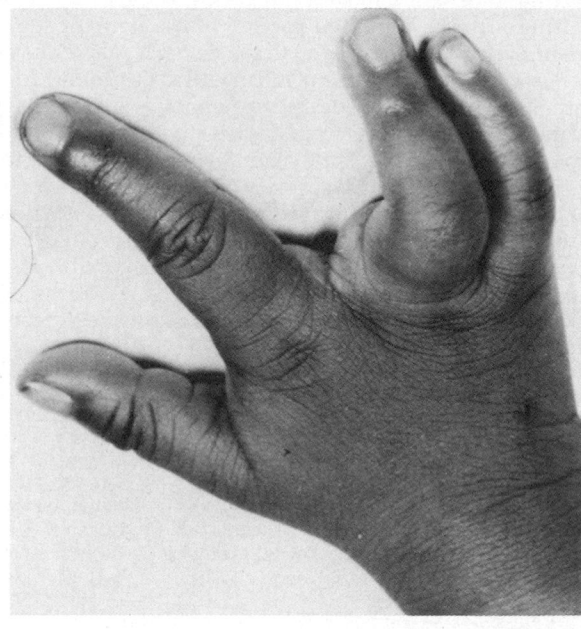

248. Ectrodactyly

ECTRODACTYLY-ECTODERMAL DYSPLASIA-CLEFTING SYNDROME

Includes: Ektrodaktylie-Ektodermale Dysplasie-Spaltsyndrom
Ectrodactilia, displasia ectodérmica y síndrome de acrofisuras
EEC syndrome
Cleft lip-palate with split hand or foot
Split hand or foot with cleft lip

Excludes: Ectrodactyly-cleft palate syndrome (ECP syndrome)†
Rapp-Hodgkin syndrome†
Freire-Maia syndrome†
Roberts syndrome† (875)
Fontaine syndrome†

Minimal Diagnostic Criteria: Abnormalities are facultative and not obligatory. Ectrodactyly is the most commonly occurring feature followed by absent lacrimal puncta and cleft lip-palate in that order.

Clinical Findings: Common features include ectrodactyly of the hands and feet; absent lacrimal puncta; cleft lip-palate; sparse scalp hair, lashes, and eyebrows. Less common features include some degree of soft tissue syndactyly, albinoid alteration of the skin and hair; hypoplastic nails; absent sebaceous glands; numerous pigmented nevi; microcephaly; mental deficiency; conduction deafness; inguinal hernia; absent kidney; hydronephrosis; hydroureter; cryptorchidism; anodontia; oligodontia; enamel hypoplasia; reduced number of meibomian orifices; primary telecanthus.

Complications
I **Derived:** Absent lacrimal puncta are associated with tearing, blepharitis, dacrocystitis, keratoconjunctivitis, and photophobia.
II **Associated:** Xerostomia, deeply furrowed tongue, predisposition to candidiasis.

Etiology: Although most cases have been sporadic, affected sibs with normal parents, and several cases in which the disorder has been transmitted from a parent to one or more children have been reported. The syndrome appears to have autosomal dominant inheritance with incomplete penetrance and variable expressivity, although etiologic heterogeneity with an autosomal recessive form is possible. McK *12990

Pathogenesis: ?

Related Facts
I **Sex Ratio:** M1:F1
II **Risk of Occurrence:** ? Very low
III **Risk of Recurrence for**
  Patient's Sib: When autosomal dominant or autosomal recessive, see Table I AD or AR, respectively.
  Patient's Child: When autosomal dominant or autosomal recessive, see Table I AD or AR, respectively.
IV **Age of Detectability:** At birth by physical examination
V **Prevalence:** ? Rare

Treatment
I **Primary Prevention:** Genetic counseling
II **Secondary Prevention:** Surgical repair of cleft lip-palate. Establish nasolacrimal duct drainage.
III **Other Therapy:** Orthodontic and prosthetic treatment, and speech therapy in some cases.

Prognosis: Good for life span and, in most cases, intelligence; function varies with severity of defects.

Detection of Carrier: —

†**Special Considerations:** The ectrodactyly-ectodermal dysplasia-clefting syndrome should be carefully distinguished from a number of other conditions. The ectrodactyly-cleft palate syndrome is autosomal dominant with incomplete penetrance and variable expressivity. Cleft lip

and absent lacrimal puncta are never seen in this condition. The Rapp-Hodgkin syndrome consists of cleft lip-palate, hypohidrosis, thin wiry hair, and dystrophic nails. Inheritance is autosomal dominant. In the autosomal recessive Freire-Maia syndrome, tetraperomelia is associated with large deformed ears, sparse hair, hypoplastic nipples, oligodontia, conical crown form, hypogonadism, and mental deficiency. In the Roberts syndrome, cleft lip-palate and tetraphocomelia are associated with ocular hypertelorism and enlarged penis or clitoris. Inheritance is autosomal recessive. In the similar or possibly identical pseudothalidomide syndrome, tetraphocomelia and cleft lip-palate are associated with hypoplastic cartilages of the alae and pinnae, facial hemangiomas, and mental deficiency. The autosomal dominant Fontaine syndrome consists of ectrodactyly and syndactyly of the feet, cleft palate (usually submucous), micrognathia, dysplastic ears, and, in some cases, mental deficiency. Isolated ectrodactyly may be inherited as an autosomal dominant and, less commonly, autosomal recessive trait.

References:

Bixler, D. et al: The ectrodactyly-ectodermal dysplasia-clefting (EEC) syndrome. Clin. Genet. 3:43, 1971.

Cohen, M.M., Jr.: Syndromes with cleft lip and palate. J. Oral Surg. (In press.)

Gorlin, R.J. et al: Syndromes of the Head and Neck, 2nd Ed. New York: McGraw-Hill Co., 1976.

Pashayan, H.M. et al: The EEC syndrome. In Bergsma, D. (ed.): Malformation Syndromes. Birth Defects: Orig. Art. Ser., vol. 10, no. 7. Miami: Symposia Specialists for The National Foundation-March of Dimes, 1974, p. 105.

Contributor: **M. Michael Cohen, Jr.**

Editor's Computerized Descriptors: Eye, Hearing, Face, Oral, Teeth, Skin, Hair, Nails, Skel., Hernia not CNS, GU.

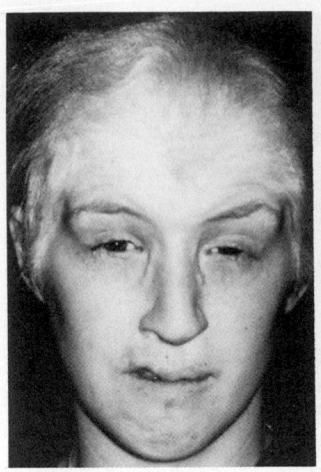
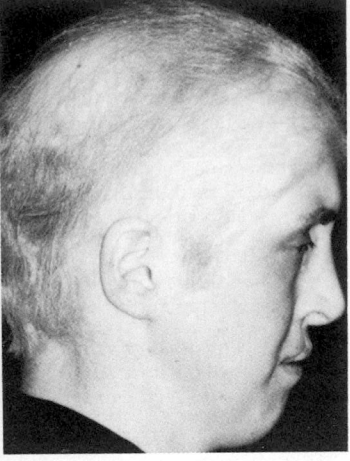

250. Note scanty hair and malar hypoplasia

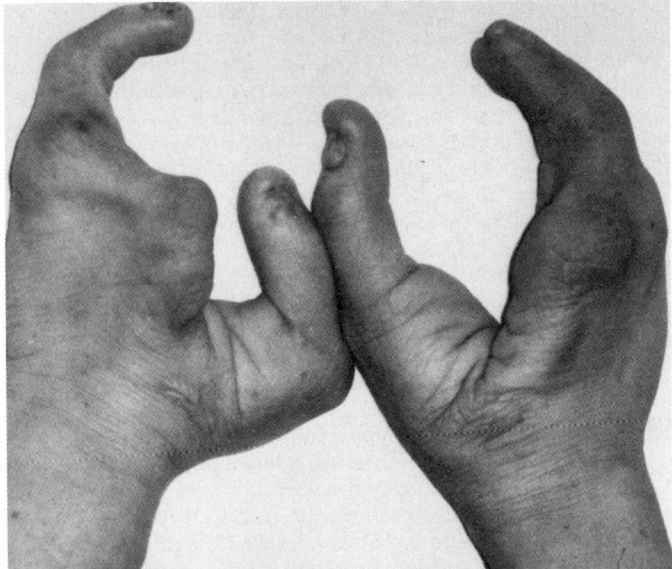

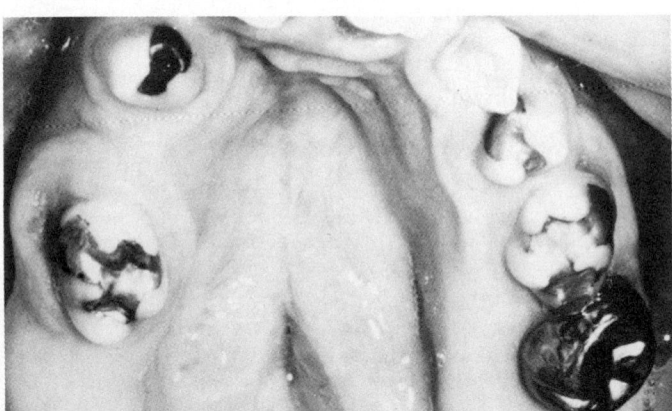

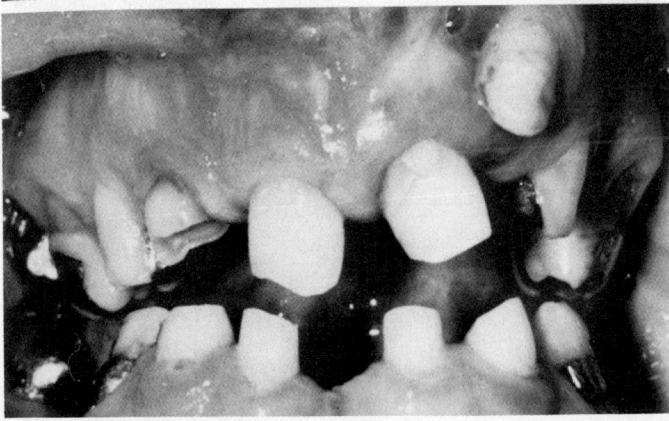

249. Teeth in EEC syndrome

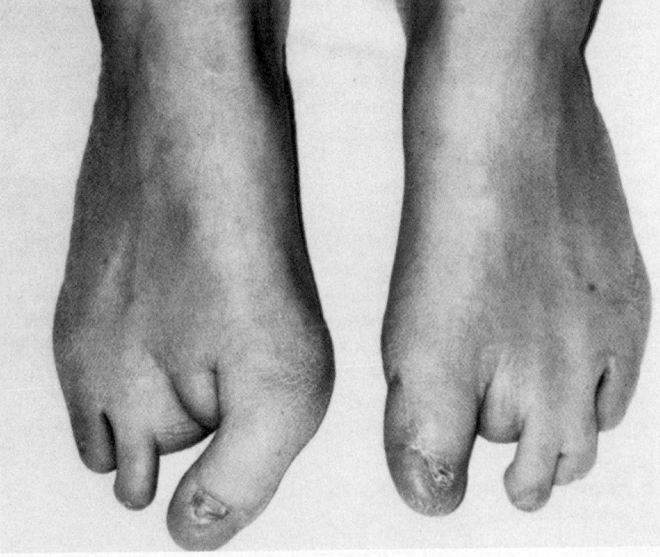

251. Lobster claw configuration of hand and foot

EHLERS-DANLOS SYNDROME

Includes: Syndrome d'Ehlers Danlos
Síndrome de Ehlers-Danlos
Dermatorrhexis cutis hyperelastica
Lysyl hydroxylase deficiency
Hydroxylysine deficient collagen disease
Arthrochalasis multiplex congenita
Procollagen peptidase deficiency

Excludes: Cutis laxa (233)
Larsen syndrome (570)
Congenital ligamentous laxity

Minimal Diagnostic Criteria: Some degree of joint laxity, skin friability and cutaneous hyperextensibiltiy. Biochemical documentation of specific enzyme deficiency in these disorders when it is known.

Clinical Findings: This is a heterogeneous group of connective tissue disorders which share hyperextensibility of joints and skin. At least 7 distinct entities can be recognized on clinical, genetic, and biochemical grounds.

ED-I, the gravis type, is characterized by generalized and severe joint hypermobility. Musculoskeletal deformities, eg pes planus, may occur. Skin hyperextensibility and easy bruising are severe, and increased fragility leads to skin splitting and subsequent "cigarette paper'-like scarring particularly over the forehead, elbows, knees, and shins. Varicose veins occur commonly, as do molluscoid pseudotumors and subcutaneous spheroids. Generalized tissue friability may result in difficulty with wound healing following trauma or surgery as well as premature rupture of fetal membranes.

ED-II, the mitis type, resembles but is milder than ED-I. Joint laxity is often confined to the hands and feet, and cutaneous involvement is minimal. There is a slight tendency toward bruising but little scar formation. Varicose veins are uncommon, and tissue friability is rarely a problem.

ED-III, the benign hypermobility type, shows severe hypermobility of all joints usually without musculoskeletal deformities. Skin changes are minimal.

ED-IV, the arterial, ecchymotic, or Sack type, is the most malignant form due to the tendency toward spontaneous rupture of large and intermediate sized arteries and perforation of the bowel. The skin is very thin and easily bruised, with prominent underlying veins, but stretchability is increased only slightly.

ED-V, the X-linked type, manifests only minimal joint hypermobility in contrast to marked hyperextensibility of the skin. Cutaneous bruisability and fragility are moderately increased.

ED-VI, the ocular type, is characterized by severe scoliosis and ocular fragility in addition to moderate joint and skin involvement. Rupture of the sclera and cornea or retinal detachment often result from minor trauma.

ED-VII, exhibits short stature and extreme generalized joint hypermobility. Subluxations of hips, knees, elbows and feet are common. Infants with this disorder are floppy. There is moderate skin stretchability and bruisability. Abnormal facies including hypertelorism, epicanthal folds and scooped out midfacies may be part of this disorder.

Complications
I   Derived: Depends on particular type
II Associated: —

Etiology: ED-I, II, III-autosomal dominant. "In one case with demonstrated defective synthesis of Type III collagen, there was a partial defect in both parents." (VAM) ED-IV "Evidence for AD in some, AR in others." (VAM) Often sporadic which may represent new dominant mutations. McK *13000
   ED-V - X-linked recessive; McK *30520
   ED-VI, VII - autosomal recessive; McK *22540

Pathogenesis: The friability and hyperextensibility result from defective connective tissue, most likely a collagen abnormality. Specific defects in collagen synthesis have been identified in ED-VI, VII and possibly in ED-IV and V. ED-VI-deficiency of lysyl hydroxylase ED-VII-deficiency of procollagen peptidase ED-IV-diminished synthesis of type III collagen? ED-V-deficiency of lysyl oxidase

Related Facts
I   Sex Ratio: M1:F1 except ED-V, the X-linked form in which only males are affected
II Risk of Occurrence: ?
III Risk of Recurrence for
   Patient's Sib: ED-I, II, III-If parent is affected 1 in 2 (50%) for each offspring to be affected; otherwise not increased
      ED-V-If mother is a carrier 1 in 2 (50%) for each brother to be affected and 1 in 2 (50%) for each sister to be a carrier
      ED-IV-When autosomal dominant or autosomal recessive, see Table I AD or AR, respectively.
      ED-VI,VII-1 in 4 (25%) for each offspring to be affected
   Patient's Child: ED-I, II, III-1 in 2
      ED-IV-When autosomal dominant or autosomal recessive, see Table I AD or I AR, respectively
      ED-V 1 in 1 (100%) for carrier daughters; not increased for sons unless wife is carrier
      ED-VI,VII-Not increased unless mate is carrier or homozygote
IV Age of Detectability: Early childhood
V   Prevalence: ?

Treatment
I   Primary Prevention: Genetic counseling†
II Secondary Prevention: Avoid trauma. Wear protective padding over bony prominences. Meticulous surgical and obstetric care. Repair of superficial lacerations with tape rather than suture. Angiography may be hazardous, particularly in ED-IV.
III Other Therapy: —

Prognosis: Life span is reduced in ED-IV but probably normal in other types. Intelligence is normal.

Detection of Carrier: Not available†

†Special Considerations: Carrier detection may be potentially possible in types VI and VII in which enzyme deficiencies have been identified. Likewise, if amniotic fluid cells express these missing enzymes, prenatal diagnosis would also be potentially available.

References:
Beighton, P. et al: Variants of the Ehlers-Danlos syndrome; clinical, biochemical, hematological, and chromosomal features of 100 patients. Ann. Rheum. Dis. 28:228, 1969.
McKusick, V.A.: Heritable Disorders of Connective Tissue. St. Louis: C.V. Mosby, 1972, p. 292.
McKusick, V.A.: Multiple forms of the Ehlers-Danlos syndrome. Arch.Surg. 109:475, 1974.
McKusick, V.A. and Martin, G.R: Editorial Notes: Molecular defects in collagen. Ann. Intern. Med. 82:585, 1975.

Contributor: William A. Horton

Editor's Computerized Descriptors: Eye, Oral, Skin, Skel., Hernia not CNS, Resp., CV., GI.

ELASTOSIS PERFORANS SERPIGINOSA

Includes: Elastose perforante serpigneuse
Elastoma intrapapillare perforans verruciforme Miescher
Elastosis perforante serpiginosa
Keratosis follicularis serpiginosa
Skin lesions, papular

Excludes: Kyrle disease (561)
Porokeratosis (819)

Minimal Diagnostic Criteria: Ring-like or serpiginous papular skin lesions located over the nape or side of the neck of a young individual. Definite diagnosis is made by histologic examination of the skin lesions.

Clinical Findings: Skin lesions consisting of slightly erythematous or skin colored keratotic papules measuring 2-5 mm. The keratotic papules are arranged at the periphery of a circle or show a serpiginous configuration.

Complications
I   **Derived:**   Development of keloidal scar following surgical manipulation of the skin lesions.
II   **Associated:**   In 26% of the reported cases, elastosis perforans serpiginosa has occurred in association with various heritable disorders such as chromosome 21 trisomy, Ehlers-Danlos syndrome, osteogenesis imperfecta, pseudoxanthoma elasticum and Marfan syndrome. In 2 instances elastosis perforans serpiginosa occurred in patients with Wilson disease during treatment with penicillamine.

Etiology: ?

Pathogenesis: Localized increase of dermal elastic fibers with secondary epidermal and follicular epithelial hyperplasia and transepithelial elimination of the elastic fibers through multiple perforating channels.

Related Facts
I   **Sex Ratio:**   M4:F1
II   **Risk of Occurrence:**   Uncommon
III   **Risk of Recurrence for**
   Patient's Sib: ?
   Patient's Child: ?
IV   **Age of Detectability:**   90% of the patients with elastosis perforans serpiginosa are younger than 30 years of age.
V   **Prevalence:**   Over 120 cases reported

Treatment
I   **Primary Prevention:**   —
II   **Secondary Prevention:**   No effective treatment has been established. Avoidance of surgical manipulation which may result in development of keloidal scar.
III   **Other Therapy:**   —

Prognosis: Normal life expectancy except when complicated by other heritable disorders.

Detection of Carrier: —

Special Considerations: —

References:
Lutz, W.: Keratosis follicularis serpiginosa. Dermatologica 106:318, 1953.
Mehregan, A.H.: Elastosis perforans serpiginosa: A review of the literature and report of 11 cases. Arch. Dermatol. 97:381, 1968.
Mehregan, A.H.: Perforating dermatoses: A clinicopathologic review. Int. J. Dermatol. 16:19, 1977.
Miescher, G.: Elastoma intrapapillare perforans verruciforme. Dermatologica 110:254, 1955.

Contributor: Amir H. Mehregan

_____

Editor's Computerized Descriptor: Skin

ENAMEL AND DENTIN DEFECTS FROM ERYTHROBLASTOSIS FETALIS

Includes: Hypoplasie de l'émail et de la dentine associés à une érythroblastose fétale
Schmelz-dentinverfarbung durch Erythroblastosis Fetalis
Hipoplasia y pigmentación del esmalte y la dentina por eritroblastosis fetal
Rh hump
Enamel shelf
Erythroblastosis fetalis and staining of enamel and dentin
Hemolytic disease of newborn

Excludes: Amelogenesis imperfecta (46)
Enamel and dentin defects from tetracycline (341)
Odontodysplasia (739)

Minimal Diagnostic Criteria: History of parental blood group incompatibilities, and discoloration of primary teeth with or without hypoplasia.

Clinical Findings: Oral: Green, blue or brown intrinsic staining of primary teeth, with or without hypoplastic defects of incisor edges of anterior teeth and midcrown of cuspids, producing ring-like defect ("Rh hump"). General: Infants may be stillborn. Live infants may have: 1) anemia with pallor, 2) icterus, 3) compensatory medullary and extramedullary erythropoiesis, 4) edema (fetal hydrops), 5) manifestations of CNS involvement including convulsions, muscular spasm, opisthotonos, 6) hepatomegaly and splenomegaly. Permanent teeth are unlikely to be affected.

Complications
I   **Derived:**   Psychosocial problems may arise due to unesthetic primary teeth. Dental caries may occur in hypoplastic defects, if present.
II   **Associated:**   Subsequent to dental caries there may be pulpal exposure, periapical infection, granuloma, cyst formation, and loss of teeth, followed by possible drifting of teeth and development of malocclusion.

Etiology: The deposition of hemolyzed blood pigments in developing enamel and dentin produces discoloration; in severe cases hypoplasia due to ameloblastic damage may occur.

Pathogenesis: Anti-Rh or ABO factors produced by maternal antibody system react with fetal Rh or ABO factors to produce a congenital hemolytic anemia.

Related Facts
I   **Sex Ratio:**   M1:F1
II   **Risk of Occurrence:**   Risk of Rh incompatibility is 1 in 200 pregnancies. Postpartum administration of passive Rh immune globulin to Rh- ve mother after birth of Rh+ ve infant has reduced sensitization to 1% or less.
III   **Risk of Recurrence for**
   Patient's Sib: If Rh immune globulin is administered to mother, sensitization is 1% or less; if not administered, risk increases with successive pregnancies.
   Patient's Child: Risk of Rh incompatibility is 1 in 200 pregnancies.
IV   **Age of Detectability:**   Eruption of primary teeth
V   **Prevalence:**   Of "Rh hump" 1 in 2000 children in general population. Prevalence of discolored primary dentition is related to length of icterus - 1 in 10 survivors.

Treatment
I   **Primary Prevention:**   Rh immune globulin is administered to Rh-ve woman within 72 hours following birth of Rh+ve infant, or following induced abortion or miscarriage to prevent Rh immunization.
II   **Secondary Prevention:**   Blood exchanged by pre- or postnatal fetal transfusions. Phototherapy with blue fluorescent bulbs may be of benefit.
III   **Other Therapy:**   Esthetics and function of primary teeth may be restored by complete coverage with crowns.

Prognosis: Treated oral condition: excellent for primary dentition; secondary dentition likely to be unaffected. Untreated oral condition: unesthetic primary teeth may predispose towards childhood psychopathology. Dental caries may occur in hypoplastic defects, if present. Oral condition does not appear to interfere with longevity of patient.

Detection of Carrier: Parental blood grouping and Rh determination will identify the potential to develop this condition in children.

Special Considerations: —

References:
Kotonska, J. et al: The condition of deciduous teeth in children with a history of hematologic disease of newborn. Czas. Stomatol. 26:123, 1973.
McMillan, P. H. and Kashgarian, M.: Relation of human abnormalities of structure and function to abnormalities of the dentition. I. Relation of hypoplasia of enamel to cerebral and ocular disorders. J. Am. Dent. Assoc. 63:38, 1961.
Pollack, W. et al: Prevention of Rh hemolytic disease. Prog. Hematol. 6:121, 1969.

Contributors: **Louise Brearley Messer**
Jay T. Cline
D. H. McKibben, Jr.

Editor's Computerized Descriptors: Teeth, Skin, Spleen, Liver, Nerve

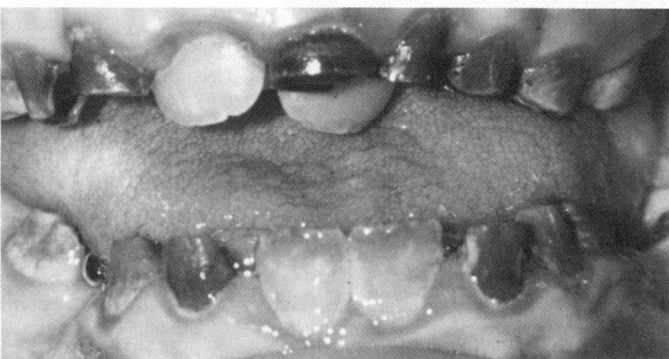

252. Bilirubin staining of teeth

ENAMEL AND DENTIN DEFECTS FROM TETRACYCLINE

Includes: Hypoplasie de l'émail et de la dentine coloration des dents par les tétracyclines
Schmelz-dentinhypoplasie mit Tetrazyklinverfärbung
Hipoplasia del esmalte y la dentina y decoloración por tetraciclinas
Tetracycline discoloration of enamel and dentin

Excludes: Amelogenesis imperfecta (46)
Enamel and dentin defects from erythroblastosis fetalis (340)
Dentinogenesis imperfecta (279)

Minimal Diagnostic Criteria: Yellow, brown or grey discoloration of teeth, distributed in horizontal bands and exhibiting yellow fluorescence under ultraviolet light.

Clinical Findings: Yellow, brown or grey discoloration of enamel and dentin of teeth. Seen most frequently in primary dentition. In severe cases, some enamel of primary molars and cuspids and secondary incisors and molars may be hypoplastic or missing. Incidence is variable, depending upon use of tetracyclines in community in early years of child's life and length of period of administration. Exposure to sunlight may change yellow color to brownish grey. In ultraviolet light affected areas fluoresce pale to bright yellow, although fluorescence may be lost in teeth whose color has changed to brownish grey.

Complications
I Derived: Attrition of the hypoplastic tooth structure
II Associated: Staining of bones

Etiology: Tetracycline administered during the period of tooth calcification. Primary dentition is affected when drug is given during the last 2 months of intrauterine life to 9 months of age. The anterior teeth of the secondary dentition may be affected if administration occurs between birth and 5 years. The degree of involvement depends on total dose. Where this exceeds 100 mg/kg (30-35 mg/kg/day) in first few months of life, discoloration and hypoplasia of enamel of primary dentition can be expected in 90% or more cases. Where drug is given to premature infants shortly after birth, hypoplasia of enamel is more likely to occur.

Involvement of secondary dentition is less common and unlikely with a normal single course of administration but may affect severely the anterior teeth if drug is given over a period of months during the first 5 years of life.

Tetracycline hydrochloride, demethylchlortetracycline and chlortetracycline produce a yellower discoloration than oxytetracycline which causes a paler creamy color. Incidence with long acting new tetracyclines not known.

Pathogenesis: Tetracycline is deposited in developing dentin and enamel.

Related Facts
I Sex Ratio: M1:F1
II Risk of Occurrence: When total dose exceeds 100 mg/kg in the first 12 months, discoloration and hypoplasia of primary dentition occurs in at least 90% of cases. Dose required to produce changes in secondary dentition not known.
III Risk of Recurrence for
Patient's Sib: Not genetic
Patient's Child: Not genetic
IV Age of Detectability: After eruption of teeth
V Prevalence: Variable. Depends upon the use of tetracyclines in the community. Prevalence varies with year and age of children. Has been reported in U.S.A. in children 4-12 years of age, 1 in 24 (urban) and 1 in 71 (rural) in 1964 and 1 in 7 (urban) in 1966.

Treatment

I Primary Prevention: Do not give tetracycline in any form during last 2 months of pregnancy or during first 5 years of life. If tetracycline has to be given during the first 5 years of life, then the shorter the course and the lower the dose the better.

II Secondary Prevention: In general, no treatment. Esthetic crowns may be considered for older children with severe discoloration or hypoplasia of anterior secondary teeth.

III Other Therapy: —

Prognosis: No effect on general health. Teeth may change color and become either darker or lighter with exposure to sunlight. Psychosocial problems may develop in person with severely stained and hypoplastic teeth.

Detection of Carrier: —

Special Considerations: —

References:
Wallman, I. S. and Hilton, H. B.: Teeth pigmented by tetracycline. Lancet 1:827, 1962.
Witkop, C. J., Jr. and Wolf, R. O.: Hypoplasia and intrinsic staining of enamel following tetracycline therapy. JAMA 185:100, 1963.

Contributor: **I. S. Wallman**

Editor's Computerized Descriptor: Teeth
Also see Section I, Fig. 80

ENAMEL, HYPOPLASIA

Includes: Hypoplasie de l'émail
Zahnschmelzhypoplasie
Hipoplasia del esmalte
Mulberry molars
Hutchinson incisors
Intrauterine and neonatal enamel hypoplasia

Excludes: Amelogenesis imperfecta (46)
Enamel and dentin defects from erythroblastosis fetalis (340)
Enamel and dentin defects from tetracycline (341)
Porphyria, erythropoietic (821)

Minimal Diagnostic Criteria: Visual or radiographic evidence of defect in enamel thickness

Clinical Findings: A nonanatomic depression in enamel surface of primary teeth or permanent teeth occurring as a horizontal ring depression or series of pits with or without hypomaturation of enamel.

Complications
I Derived: —
II Associated: A wide variety of associated defects may occur depending upon the etiology of the condition. Sequelae of congenital lues and mental retardation are frequent associated defects.†

Etiology: Hypoplasia of enamel is associated with maternal diabetes, toxemia of pregnancy, prematurity, hypoxia, asphyxia, and congenital syphilis. It occurs in conjunction with motor or sensory brain damage whose etiology may be same factor.

Pathogenesis: Uncertain, except possible direct infection of tooth follicle in congenital syphilis

Related Facts
I Sex Ratio: ?
II Risk of Occurrence: From congenital syphilis: 1 in 3 affected infants; among normal children, unspecified population group: 1 in 11; among brain-damaged children, unspecified population: 1 in 2.
III Risk of Recurrence for
    Patient's Sib: ?
    Patient's Child: ?
IV Age of Detectability: Of primary teeth: 2-5 years by visual, clinical and radiographic examination.
    Of permanent teeth: 6-7 years by visual, clinical and radiographic examination.
V Prevalence: Unspecified population 1 in 3 to 1 in 10; individuals affected with congenital syphilis 1 in 30.

Treatment
I Primary Prevention: Treatment and prevention of maternal infection, toxemia of pregnancy, prematurity, febrile diseases of childhood.
II Secondary Prevention: Crowning of teeth only in severely affected permanent dentition.
III Other Therapy: None indicated

Prognosis: Not a life-threatening condition. Prognosis depends upon associated defects.

Detection of Carrier: Not applicable

†Special Considerations: About half of prenatal and neonatally brain-damaged children have hypoplasia of enamel. Less than 10% of normal children show hypoplasia of enamel and are, as a group, less severely involved.

References:
Grahenén, H. et al: Neonatal asphyxia and mineralisation defects of the primary teeth. Caries Res. 3:301, 1969.
Via, W.F. and Churchill, J.A.: Relationship of enamel hypoplasia to abnormal events of gestation and birth. J. Am. Dent. Assoc. 59:702, 1959.

Contributor: **William F. Via, Jr.**

Editor's Computerized Descriptor: Teeth

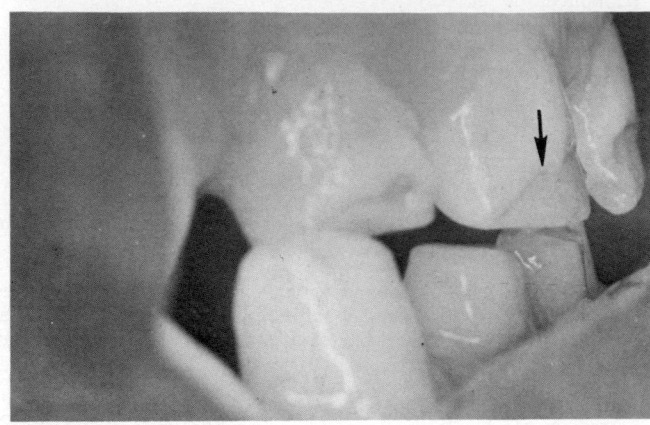

253. Marked enamel hypoplasia

ENCEPHALOCELE

Includes: Enzephalozele
Encefalocele
Cranium bifidum
Cranial meningoencephaloceles

Excludes: Hydrocephaly (481)
Meningocele (642)

Minimal Diagnostic Criteria: A midline mass with underlying bony defect of skull

Clinical Findings: A mass in the midline of the parietal or occipital skull, usually skin covered. Frontal encephaloceles present in the midline (nasion), or in the medial wall of orbit, or as a cystic mass in the nasopharynx. All are present at birth. The infant's neurologic testing is abnormal in those instances of large encephaloceles containing major amounts of brain. The defect in the skull confirmed by xray.

Complications
I **Derived:** If the encephalocele is not skin covered, meningitis may ensue. Improper manipulation of nasal encephaloceles may also lead to meningitis.
II **Associated:** Posterior encephaloceles are associated with abnormalities of the cerebrospinal fluid pathways leading to hydrocephaly in greater than 50% of cases. Two instances of associated myelomeningocele, one lipoma of cauda equina, and the Klippel-Feil anomaly are recorded.

Etiology: ?

Pathogenesis: The basis of the cerebral defect is a failure of closure of the midline with brain protrusion or overgrowth. Many large lesions contain primarily the cranial meninges and cerebrospinal fluid with little brain, suggesting a primary mesodermal failure.

Related Facts
I **Sex Ratio:** M1:F1
II **Risk of Occurrence:** Varies, but probably about 1 in 2000 live births
III **Risk of Recurrence for**
Patient's Sib: CNS anomaly in subsequent sibs (6%)
Patient's Child: ?
IV **Age of Detectability:** At birth
V **Prevalence:** Varies, but highest in Ireland

Treatment
I **Primary Prevention:** ?
II **Secondary Prevention:** Surgical closure as soon after birth as possible, as emergency if encephalocele is open and draining CSF.
III **Other Therapy:** —

Prognosis: Related to presence and amount of brain within sac. Approximately 20% of children will be mentally subnormal or neurologically handicapped. With occipital lesions, successful treatment of the hydrocephaly effects prognosis.

Detection of Carrier: —

Special Considerations: —

References:
Blumenfeld, R. and Skolnick, E. M.: Intranasal encephaloceles. Arch. Otolaryngol. 82:527, 1965.
Dedo, H. H. and Sooy, F. A.: Endaural encephalocele and cerebrospinal fluid otorrhea. Ann. Otol. Rhinol. Laryngol. 79:168, 1970.
Dedo, H. H. and Sooy, F. A.: Endaural brain hernia (encephalocele): Diagnosis and treatment. Laryngoscope 80:1090, 1970.
Lorber, J.: The prognosis of occipital encephalocele. Dev. Med. Child Neurol. (Suppl.) 13:75, 1967.
Mealey, J., Jr. et al: The prognosis of encephaloceles. J. Neurosurg. 32:209, 1970.

Contributor: **Kenneth Shulman**

Editor's Computerized Descriptors: Eye, Nasoph., Skel.

ENCEPHALOPATHY NECROTIZING

Includes: Encéphalopathie nécrosante
Nekrotisierende Enzephalopathie
Encefalopatía necrotizante
Leigh disease
Necrotizing, infantile subacute encephalopathy
Encephalomyelopathy

Excludes: Neuroaxonal dystrophy
Lactic acidosis familial
Wernicke encephalopathy
Neuronal ceroid - lipofuscinoses (713)
Globoid cell sclerosis
Cerebral sclerosis, diffuse

Minimal Diagnostic Criteria: This disease is as yet ill-defined
and may represent several biochemical defects within the pyruvate decarboxylase system. Intermittent symptomatology with
worsening associated with stress is suggestive of the disease. Elevation of serum lactate and pyruvate, a mild persistent acidosis,
elevation of serum and urinary alanine and the presence of an
inhibitor of thiamine triphosphate synthesis are strongly suggestive of the disease. The only definitive diagnostic criteria at
present is neuropathologic.†

Clinical Findings: More than 50 autopsy-proven cases
with variable clinical manifestations have been described.
The disease should be suspected in cases of progressive
neurologic deficit particularly when the progression involves a stepwise loss of function associated with infection.
The classic picture appears to begin in infancy or early
childhood with abnormalities in extraocular movements.
The neurologic symptoms then remain stable or may improve slightly, but again worsen with a 2nd infection. Older
children and adolescents have been reported with a chronic
unremitting course. Intermittent ataxia associated with
stress, but with complete remission has also been reported.
Clinical features vary from case to case, but include: 1)
abnormal eye movements, nystagmus, strabismus, paralysis of upward gaze; 2) sluggish pupils; 3) optic atrophy with
particular involvement of the maculopapular bundle; 4)
bulbar symptoms; 5) cerebellar signs; 6) tremors; 7) ataxia;
8) peripheral neuropathy; 9) pyramidal tract signs; 10) posterior column involvement.

Complications
I **Derived:** Progressive and usually fatal
II **Associated:** —

Etiology: Possibly autosomal recessive; McK *25600

Pathogenesis: ? Pathologically the disease resembles Wernicke encephalopathy (thiamine deficiency). Areas of focal
pathology and vascular proliferation are present in brain-
stem, diencephalon and periaqueductal area with involvement of cerebral and cerebellar hemispheres. There is
demyelination of peripheral nerves. Increasing evidence
suggests that the biochemical defect is in the pyruvate
decarboxylation system, a membrane-bound enzyme-cofac-
tor complex, which involves the enzyme, thiamine, lipoic
acid, CoA and nicotinamide. Several defects in the complex
may be responsible for the variable symptomatology. The
mechanism by which the focal pathology is produced remains unknown, but may be related to the acidosis.

Related Facts
I **Sex Ratio:** M1:F1
II **Risk of Occurrence:** ?
III **Risk of Recurrence for**
   Patient's Sib: Possibly 1 in 4 (25%) for each offspring to be
   affected

Patient's Child: If autosomal recessive, not increased unless mate is carrier or homozygote.

IV Age of Detectability: Considerable variation of onset

V Prevalence: ?

Treatment

I Primary Prevention: Genetic counseling

II Secondary Prevention: Therapy with high doses of thiamine (600-300 mg/d) (3,4) and lipoic acid (4) may have beneficial effects.

III Other Therapy: —

Prognosis: Disease is usually fatal with variable course. Further knowledge of enzymatic defect will permit better definition of disease and its variability and prognosis.

Detection of Carrier: —

†**Special Considerations:** This disease first described in 1951 is doubtless far more common than previously reported. Awareness of the stepwise progression of the intermittent course should lead to heightened suspicion. Hyperalaninemia, hyperalaninuria and elevation of serum lactate and pyruvate serve as preliminary confirmatory data. The value of the test for thiamine triphosphate inhibitor in urine requires further evaluation. It has been suggested that this disease represents another vitamin dependency state, but definitive statements require further biochemical evaluation of the pyruvate decarboxylase complex in this condition.

References:

Cooper, J.R. et al: Experience with phosphoryl-transferase inhibition in subacute necrotizing encephalomyelopathy. N. Engl. J. Med. 283:793, 1970.

Dunn, H. G. and Dolman, C. L.: Necrotizing encephalomyelopathy; report of a case with relapsing polyneuropathy and hyperalaninemia and with manifestations resembling Friedreich's ataxia. Neurology 19:536, 1969.

Hommes, F. A. et al: Leigh's encephalomyelopathy: An inborn error or gluconeogenesis. Arch. Dis. Child. 43:426, 1968.

Lonsdale, D. et al: Intermittent cerebellar ataxia associated with hyperpyruvic acidemia, hyperalaninemia and hyperalaninuria. Pediatrics 43:1025, 1969.

Contributor: **John Mark Freeman**

Editor's Computerized Descriptors: Eye, Nerve

ENCHONDROMATOSIS

Includes: Encondromatosis
Dyschondroplasia
Ollier syndrome
Internal chondromatosis
Multiple enchondromatosis

Excludes: Enchondromatosis and hemangiomas (346)
Multiple cartilaginous exostoses (685)
Osteochondromata
Metachondromatosis (650)

Minimal Diagnostic Criteria: Radiographic evidence of typical enchondromata.

Clinical Findings: Both expansion of the enchondromas and their interference with endochondral ossification produce a wide variety of skeletal deformities affecting primarily tubular bones. Frequent deformities include phalangeal enlargement, asymmetric limb shortening, bowing of long bones, and ulnar deviation of the wrist. Involvement is asymmetric and usually bilateral. Severity ranges from minimal involvement of one limb to marked and generalized deformities. Tumor growth is sporadic through adolescence after which lesions tend to stabilize and may partially regress as cartilage is replaced by mature bone. During adulthood sarcomatous degeneration occurs but is uncommon.

Radiographically the lesions vary from minute foci of incompletely calcified cartilage extending linearly from the growth plate into the metaphysis to large tumorous masses of cartilage producing massive metaphyseal enlargement. Irregular calcifications are found within the tumor. Cortical thinning and disruption often occur in overlying bone and may be associated with abnormal metaphyseal modeling. Radiolucent defects may extend into the shaft of the bone.

Complications

I Derived: Fracture through lesion; chondrosarcoma

II Associated: —

Etiology: All cases appear to be sporadic

Pathogenesis: Enchondromas extending from the growth plate into the metaphysis continue to proliferate causing distortion of the metaphysis and interference with normal endochondral ossification.

Related Facts

I Sex Ratio: M1:F1

II Risk of Occurrence: Very low

III Risk of Recurrence for

Patient's Sib: Very low

Patient's Child: Very low

IV Age of Detectability: At birth

V Prevalence: ?

Treatment

I Primary Prevention: —

II Secondary Prevention: Orthopedic management of deformities; radiographic examination for malignant degeneration if clinically indicated (pain or rapid enlargement in an adult)

III Other Therapy: —

Prognosis: Good

Detection of Carrier: —

Special Considerations: —

References:

Feldman, F.: Cartilaginous lesions of bones and soft tissues. CRC Crit. Rev. Clin. Radiol. Nucl. Med. 4:477, 1974.

Kaufman, H.J.: Enchondromatosis. Semin. Roentgenol. 8:176, 1973.

Manizer, F. et al: The variable manifestations of multiple enchondromatosis. Pediatr. Radiol. 99:377, 1971.

Contributors: **Ralph S. Lachman**
William A. Horton

Editor's Computerized Descriptor: Skel.

ENCHONDROMATOSIS AND HEMANGIOMAS

Includes: Enchondromatose mit Hemangiomen (Maffucci)
Encondromatosis con angiomas
Maffucci syndrome
Hemangiomata and enchondromatosis
Dyschondroplasia and hemangiomatosis (some cases)

Excludes: Hemangiomatosis†
Enchondromatosis† (345)
Angioosteohypertrophy syndrome†
Metachondromatosis† (650)
Dysplasia epiphysealis hemimelia† (311)

Minimal Diagnostic Criteria: Hemangiomas and enchondromas verified by radiologic or pathologic examination.†

Clinical Findings: The cardinal feature of this syndrome is the coexistence of hemangiomas and enchondromas. Superficial or cavernous hemangiomas are usually detected at or shortly after birth. They are usually located on the limbs (97%); however, lingual, umbilical and GI hemangiomas have also been reported. The size of the lesions is not stationary, and they range from a few millimeters to massive clusters, deforming an entire limb. Multiple enchondromata appear in early childhood, and may be clinically heralded by the development of asymmetry of the limbs or face, or by irregular expansion of the small bones of the hands or feet. Radiographic examination typically discloses multiple enchondroma occurring as discrete lesions, or in irregular clusters. With time, massive distortion of a long bone by the enchondromas may occur. Though asymmetry of the enchondral bones of the base of the skull has been observed, these lesions do not appear to produce the massive distortion seen at other sites. There is, for the most part, no correlation between the sites of hemangiomas and enchondromas. Either may be unilateral or bilateral in distribution.

Frequency of Clinical Findings: 1) Enchondromas 100% (bilateral 62%, unilateral 38%); 2) hemangiomas 100% (bilateral 56%, unilateral 44%); 3) sarcomatous degeneration 30%; 4) phlebectasia 25%; 5) phleboliths 43%.

Occasional Clinical Findings: Vitiligo, GI hemangiomas, other malignant tumors 7%, benign tumors 7%, lymphangiomas.

Complications
I **Derived:** Physical handicap due to distortion of limb; malocclusion, if face and jaw are involved. Pathologic fractures, GI bleeding.
II **Associated:** Malignant degeneration of hemangiomas or enchondromas to angiosarcoma or osteosarcoma.

Etiology: ?

Pathogenesis: Two major pathogenetic mechanisms have been proposed. Both the hemangiomas and enchondromas may result from mesodermal dysplasia of the anlagen of vessels and bones in the affected areas. Second, enchondromas may result from failure of resorption of part of the cartilage growth plate of the epiphysis. This failure may be induced by an abnormality of the blood supply to the bone, or by the presence of vascular anomalies, ie hemangiomas within the bone. Careful examination has, on occasion, revealed the coexistence of osseous hemangioma and enchondroma at the same site.

Related Facts
I **Sex Ratio:** M1:F1
II **Risk of Occurrence:** Rare, approximately 100 cases reported.
III **Risk of Recurrence for**
Patient's Sib: No reported familial cases

Patient's Child: No reported familial cases
IV Age of Detectability: Birth or shortly after
V Prevalence: Rare

Treatment
I Primary Prevention: —
II Secondary Prevention: Orthopedic and surgical intervention to minimize deformities. Surveillance for GI lesion and sarcomatous change.
III Other Therapy: Psychosocial support

Prognosis: Patients may live near to normal life span with normal intelligence. Progression of deformities tends to cease by adolescence, though sarcomas may develop later on, and the occurrence of enchondromas may be exacerbated by fractures.

Detection of Carrier: —

†Special Considerations: The accurate recognition of the enchondromatosis and hemangioma syndrome is crucial in view of the increased incidence of malignancy in this disorder. Neither this increased risk nor the degree of deformity seen are encountered in the other entities.

The cornerstone of diagnosis lies in the finding of both enchondromas and hemangiomas. The bony abnormalities of Ollier disease (multiple enchondromatosis) do not differ radiologically or pathologically from those in Maffucci syndrome. The presence of hemangiomas in the latter is the only distinguishing feature between the two. The radiologic finding in Klippel-Trenaunay-Weber is thickening of the bony cortex which is also usually unilateral. There is a clear relationship between the site of hemangioma and bony changes in this as well as the angioosteohypertrophy syndrome.

Hereditary multiple exostoses show misplaced cartilage not to be in the substance of bone, but on its surface, and the protuberances point away from the bone rather than appear to invade its substance.

Metachondromatosis is an entity consisting of both multiple exostoses and enchondroma. There are no associated hemangiomas. Dysplasia epiphysealis hemimelia is an unusual entity consisting of unilateral epiphyseal exostoses, and presents as long bone enlargement and asymmetry of the limbs. There are no associated hemangiomas. The term enchondromatosis is preferable to the less specific dyschondroplasia. It should be noted that early reports use the terms interchangeably.

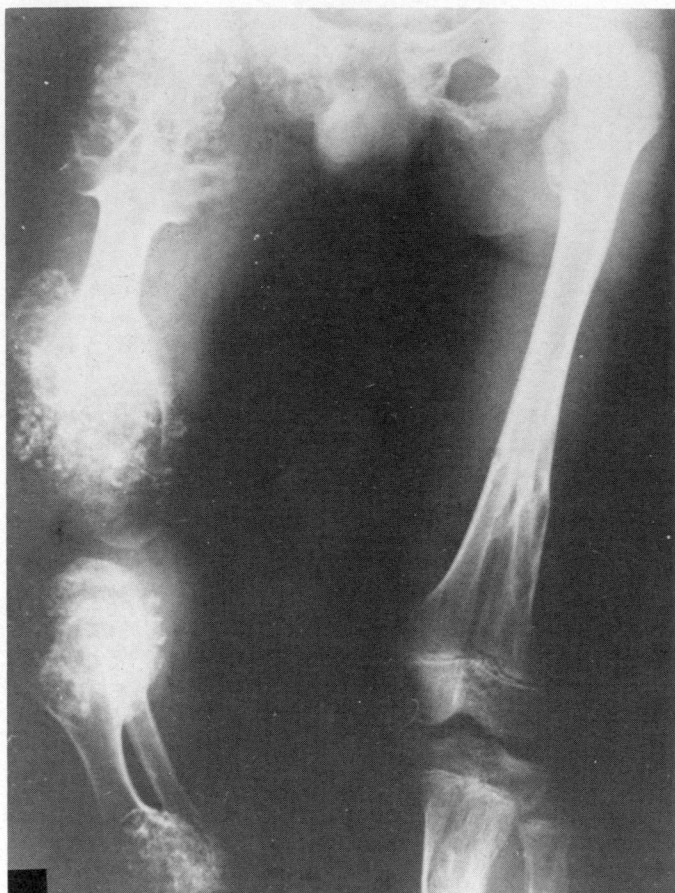

254. Multiple enchondromas

References:
Anderson, I.F.: Maffucci's syndrome - report of a case with review of the literature. S. Afr. Med. J. 39:1066, 1965.
Bean, W.: Dyschondroplasia and hemangiomata. Arch. Int. Med. 95:767, 1955.
Carleton, A. et al: Maffucci's syndrome. Q. J. Med. 11:203, 1942.
Lewis, R.J.: Maffucci's syndrome: Functional and neoplastic significance. J. Bone Joint Surg. (Am.) 7:1465, 1973.

Contributors: **Kathleen Toomey**
David W. Hollister

Editor's Computerized Descriptors: Teeth, Skin, Skel., CV., GI.

ENDOCARDIAL CUSHION DEFECTS

Includes: Défaut des coussins endocardiques
Defekte der Endokardpolster
Defectos de las almohadillas endocárdicas
Endocardial cushion defects, partial type, with interatrial communication
Ostium primum type atrial septal defect, persistent ostium primum
Endocardial cushion defects, partial type, with interventricular communication
Ventricular septal defect of the endocardial cushion defect type
Endocardial cushion defects, partial type, with interatrial and interventricular communication
Endocardial cushion defects, partial type, with left ventricular to right atrial communication
Endocardial cushion defects, partial type, with isolated cleft of the anterior cusp of the mitral valve
Endocardial cushion defects, complete type
Persistent common atrioventricular canal
Atrioventricularis communis

Excludes: Defects at the fossa ovalis
Sinus venosus type atrial septal defects

Minimal Diagnostic Criteria: Clinical findings indicating the presence of an atrial level left-to-right shunt (pulmonary ejection systolic murmur, diastolic tricuspid flow murmur, widely split and fixed components of the second sound at the base), together with an ECG which shows the combination of left axis deviation in the limb leads and mild-to-moderate right ventricular hypertrophy pattern in the precordial leads, and radiographic findings of an atrial level shunt are strongly suggestive of the diagnosis of the partial form of ECD with an atrial level communication. Left ventricular angiogram confirms the diagnosis. Clinical findings suggesting a ventricular level shunt (systolic thrill and loud harsh holosystolic murmur at the lower sternal border, mitral flow murmur) together with an ECG which shows left axis deviation and biventricular hypertrophy, and radiographic findings of a left-to-right shunt beyond the level of the atrioventricular valves suggest the diagnosis of partial form of ECD with interventricular communication. A left ventriculogram confirms the diagnosis. Symptoms in infancy or early childhood of recurrent pneumonitis, dyspnea, feeding difficulties, congestive heart failure, auscultatory findings of a loud, harsh precordial systolic murmur, diastolic flow murmurs (and sometimes also a widely split, fixed second sound at the base), ECG evidence of marked left axis deviation and biventricular enlargement together with radiographs showing moderate-to-marked cardiomegaly, hypervascularity of the lung fields and the absence of left atrial enlargement are strongly suggestive of the diagnosis of complete type of ECD. The left ventricular angiogram is usually diagnostic. In all types of ECD, an apical systolic murmur indicating mitral incompetence is usually, but not invariably, present.

Clinical Findings: Endocardial cushion defects (ECD) comprise a group of pathogenetically related cardiac anomalies thought to be the result of abnormal development of the embryonic atrioventricular endocardial cushions. Pathologic and anatomic features characteristic of endocardial cushion defects and shared by all types to a varying degree are: the aortic cusp of the mitral valve is cleft and its origin is concave, rather than convex towards the atrium as in the normal heart; the ventricular septum has a peculiar "scooped out" appearance; the left ventricular outflow tract is more narrow and elongated than normal; the superoinferior (anteroposterior) diameter of the ventri-

cles is increased at the base. Usually a large, very characteristic interatrial communication, an interventricular communication, or both, is present. The clinical findings in individual cases are determined almost wholly by the type of defect present in the cardiac septum, eg whether there is an intracardiac shunt at the atrial or ventricular level or at both. The cleft mitral valve is usually (but not always) incompetent. The degree of incompetence has a significant, if not dominant, influence on the clinical course.

ECD, partial type with interatrial communication: The interatrial communication is usually quite large and located immediately above the level of the atrioventricular valves. While true atrial septal defects also may be present, the characteristic interatrial communication in ECD corresponds in position to the atrioventricular part of the cardiac septum which is absent in ECD. As compared to a normal heart, the medial portions of the 2 atrioventricular ostia are displaced apically. The atrial septum itself typically is normal and its lower free border, or upper rim of the interatrial communication, corresponds to the line of origin of the anterior mitral cusp of the normal heart. A portion of the ventricular septum of variable size, just below the atrioventricular ostia, is fibrous and contains short chordae tendineae which insert into the medial most portion of the cleft mitral valve.

In cases where the mitral valve is competent, the clinical picture closely resembles that seen in true atrial septal defects (ASD). There is evidence of a large left-to-right shunt at the atrial level with enlargement of the right atrium and the right ventricle and engorgement of the pulmonary arterial tree. Respiratory infections are common, and growth retardation, fatigability and dyspnea are seen more commonly and tend to occur at an earlier age than in cases with true ASD. As in ASD, an ejection type systolic murmur is audible at the left upper sternal border and the second sound at the base is distinctly split, a splitting which varies little or none at all with respiration. A thrill, uncommon in ASD, is present much more often in ECD. Also present along the lower left sternal border is a lower frequency diastolic flow murmur, encompassing S_3 and S_4, which represents relative tricuspid stenosis. In somewhat more than half the cases, a high-pitched, blowing systolic murmur indicating the presence of mitral insufficiency, is present over the apex and transmitted to the axilla. With more severe degrees of valve incompetence, there may be an associated diastolic flow murmur of relative mitral stenosis.

The ECG, with rare exceptions, shows a combination of left axis deviation of -40° to -130°, and a right bundle branch block pattern of right ventricular hypertrophy in the precordial leads. The PR interval is commonly prolonged. The vectorcardiogram characteristically shows a superiorly oriented, counterclockwise inscribed QRS loop in the frontal plane. In cases with significant mitral incompetence, evidence of combined ventricular hypertrophy is found.

Radiographically, the heart tends to be somewhat larger than in patients with ASD. The pulmonary trunk is enlarged and the vascularity is prominent of a shunt type. Left atrial enlargement is absent except in those cases where the atrial communication is small and the mitral insufficiency is moderate to severe.

In contrast to the secundum type of ASD, the echocardiogram shows abnormal thickening of the right ventricular anterior wall and the interventricular septum. In addition, the right ventricular cavity is dilated, as in other types of ASD, and the septal motion may be flat to paradoxical. The mitral valve motion pattern may vary widely from normal to the typical motion pattern of ECD where the valve echocardiographically appears to traverse the septum during diastole.

Cardiac catheterization findings are similar to those found in ASD. An unusually low position of the cardiac catheter as it crosses from right atrium to left atrium may suggest the true nature of the defect. Significant elevation of right ventricular and pulmonary arterial pressures are more common than in ASD. Much more useful in the differentiation between ASD and ECD, however, is angiocardiography. In ASD the left ventricular angiogram is normal; in ECD the left ventriculogram in the frontal plane shows the elongated left ventricular outflow tract ("gooseneck") and the "scooped out" ventricular septum. The long, narrow left ventricular outflow tract is best appreciated during cardiac diastole, whereas during systole the 2 halves of the cleft anterior mitral valve cusp are seen to bulge into the left atrium forming a notch indicating the position of the cleft. Mitral insufficiency, if present, is, of course, readily demonstrated.

ECD, partial type with interventricular communication: The clinical features of this anomaly closely resemble those seen in patients with defects of the basilar portion of the ventricular septum. Mitral incompetence is usually present. Electrocardiographically there is evidence of left ventricular volume overload as in other cases with ventricular septal defects, but the frontal plane axis is typically deviated leftward. In these cases with intact atrial septum, the anterior cusp of the mitral valve, while cleft, originates normally and the "gooseneck" may not be readily apparent on the left ventriculogram.

ECD, partial type with interatrial and interventricular communications: This type is uncommon and the clinical picture resembles that seen in cases where there is a combination of an atrial level and a ventricular level shunt. As in the other types, mitral incompetence is usually present.

ECD, partial type with left ventricular to right atrial shunt: This lesion is extremely uncommon. The clinical, ECG and radiographic findings are similar to those seen in cases with an atrial level shunt, a precordial systolic thrill is almost always present and radiographically the right atrium tends to be more distinctly enlarged. A left ventricular angiogram demonstrates the shunt, but cannot always differentiate it with certainty from cases with a ventricular septal defect and tricuspid valve insufficiency.

ECD, partial type with isolated cleft of the mitral valve: This anomaly is exceedingly rare and is only important when the mitral valve is incompetent. Such cases cannot be differentiated with certainty from other conditions with mitral insufficiency.

ECD, complete type: In this anomaly, the central portion of the cardiac septum is absent and there is a single atrioventricular ostium with free communication between the 4 cardiac chambers. The atrial component of the septal defect is similar to that seen in the partial form with interatrial communication, and the ventricular component of the defect is similar to that seen in the partial form with interventricular communication. In addition to the normal posterior cusp of the mitral valve and the anterior and posterolateral cusps of the tricuspid valve, there is a large anterior cusp which crosses the top of the ventricular septum and inserts on the left side on the anterior papillary muscle of the left ventricle and on the right side on the medial papillary muscle of the right ventricle. In some cases, the cusp is also attached to the top of the ventricular septum. In others, the large anterior cusp may combine with the normal right ventricular anterior tricuspid cusp, in which case the medial papillary muscle is absent. Opposite the large anterior cusp a somewhat smaller, posterior common

cusp inserts, on the left side, onto the posterior left ventricular papillary muscle, and on the right side, usually onto the top of the ventricular septum and sometimes also to a number of small posterior right ventricular papillary muscles.

The common atrioventricular valve may be competent, particularly in very young infants. The complete type of ECD usually causes severe difficulties early in infancy, such as repeated respiratory infections, feeding difficulties, growth retardation, dyspnea and congestive heart failure. Most of the infants die within the first 2 years of life. Cyanosis is rare unless there is an associated obstruction of the right ventricular outflow tract, respiratory infection, heart failure or very high pulmonary vascular resistance. Cardiomegaly develops rapidly after birth. In general, the larger the ventricular component of the defect and the more pronounced the mitral insufficiency, the sicker the child. Extreme degrees of left axis deviation may be seen in the ECG, and marked right ventricular hypertrophy indicating high right ventricular pressures is common. Radiographically, the pulmonary vascularity indicates a large shunt, often with concomitant signs of failure and pneumonia. The heart is usually quite large. Few shunt lesions result in so much cardiomegaly. Signs of left atrial enlargement are usually inapparent except in the presence of significant mitral valve incompetence.

The echocardiogram shows very little to no interventricular septum. The diastolic atrioventricular valve motion is exaggerated and completely crosses the ventricular cavity and in systole the leaflets appear joined at the level of the aortic root. Many patients with the complete defect have pulmonary vascular obstructive disease and the echo of the pulmonary valve is accordingly abnormal, with loss of the "A" dip, flattening of the diastolic slope and a "W" pattern of systolic motion with the early closure occurring in the first one-third of the valve opening trace. In less severe forms of the defect, the valve motion pattern is less exaggerated and more septal representation is noted. Mitral echoes, ordinarily at the plane of the posterior aortic root, can be traced to the anterior border of the left ventricular outflow tract. In most forms of the defect, because of the unusual valve orientation, the E-F slope is difficult to record and generally only the D-E slope is seen in diastole.

Complications

I **Derived:** Congestive heart failure is unusual in infancy and early childhood in the partial form of ECD with an atrial level shunt. It is much more common in those cases where a ventricular level shunt is present, particularly in the complete type of ECD. In these forms, recurrent pneumonitis, growth retardation and dyspnea are also commonly seen. Bacterial endocarditis is uncommon. Increased pulmonary vascular resistance secondary to progressive pulmonary vascular changes tends to develop at a relatively early age, particularly in the complete type of ECD. Right ventricular hypertension is common. Such patients become progressively more cyanotic.

II **Associated:** —

Etiology: Multifactorial inheritance in two-thirds of the cases. Trisomy 21 in one-third of the cases. About 15% of patients with chromosome 21 trisomy have some form of ECD, usually the complete type. ECD, usually the complete type, are also present in the majority of cases of asplenia syndrome and to a lesser extent also in the polysplenia syndrome.

Pathogenesis: ECD are thought to be due to partial or complete failure of fusion of the superior and inferior atrioventricular endocardial cushions. Normally, after fusion, the endocardial cushions bend to form an arc, the convexity of which is toward the atrial side. The atrial septum primum fuses with the high point of the arc, thus dividing it into 2 approximately equal parts. The right half contributes to the ventricular septum, the atrioventricular septum and the medial or septal cusp of the tricuspid valve. The left half of fused cushions plays an important role in the formation of the aortic or anterior cusp of the mitral valve. In ECD, the cushions fuse only in part or not at all, and the arc is usually not formed. The lower border of the atrial septum cannot reach the endocardial cushions and a large interatrial communication remains. In addition, the atrioventricular part of the cardiac septum is not formed. Failure of fusion of the left side of the endocardial cushions explains the cleft in the mitral valve cusp.

Related Facts
I **Sex Ratio:** Ml:Fl
II **Risk of Occurrence:** Approximately 1 in 2500 live births
III **Risk of Recurrence for**
   Patient's Sib: Predicted risk - 2:100; empiric risk - 2.6:100
   Patient's Child: Predicted risk - 2:100; empiric risk - ?
IV **Age of Detectability:** In infancy
V **Prevalence:** 1 in 25,000 of the infant and child population

Treatment
I **Primary Prevention:** —
II **Secondary Prevention:** Banding of the pulmonary trunk has been carried out in individuals with the complete type of ECD and with the partial form with interventricular communication, in an effort to reduce pulmonary blood flow and prevent the development of peripheral vascular changes which result in increased resistance. Results of this procedure have been mediocre, but occasionally, fairly good results have been reported.†
III **Other Therapy:** Children with the more severe forms of ECD usually need vigorous medical therapy for respiratory infections and congestive heart failure in early infancy. Corrective surgery should be carried out as early as possible, even in the more benign forms of the anomaly, particularly if the mitral valve is still competent. Once this valve has become insufficient, the surgical results tend to be mediocre.

Prognosis: The prognosis of the severe forms of the anomaly generally is poor, with most of the infants dying at an early age. The partial form with interatrial communication carries the best prognosis, particularly if the mitral valve is competent. Once mitral insufficiency exists, the prognosis is determined largely by the degree of such insufficiency. Pulmonary vascular changes resulting in high pulmonary vascular resistance tend to occur early in the severe forms of the anomaly.

Detection of Carrier: —

†Special Considerations: Since the prognosis of ECD depends so much on the presence and severity of mitral incompetence, surgery should be carried out as early as is practically feasible, even in mild forms of the anomaly in children who are asymptomatic. It is probably advisable in such cases to simply close the intracardiac communication and not try to repair the cleft in the mitral valve. Such a repair may, in some if not most cases, lead to impaired function of the anterior cusp resulting in turbulence and consequent damage, thereby actually promoting the appearance of mitral insufficiency. Whether or not surgical therapy should be undertaken in children with chromosome 21 trisomy remains an unresolved question and may be other than medical.

References:
Baron, M.G. et al: Endocardial cushion defects: Specific diagnosis by angiocardiography. Am. J. Cardiol. 13:162, 1964.
Edwards, J.E. et al: Persistent common atrioventricular canal. In Edwards, J.E. (ed.): Congenital Heart Disease, Correlation of Pathologic Anatomy and Angiocardiography. Philadelphia:W.B. Saunders Co., 1965, vol. 1 p. 209.
Goldberg, S.J. et al: Pediatric and Adolescent Echocardiography. Chicago: Year Book Medical Publishers, 1975, p. 85.
Keith, J.D. et al: Atrial septal defect. In Heart Disease in Infancy and Childhood, 2nd Ed. New York: Macmillan Co., 1967, p. 392.
Pieroni, D.R. et al: Echocardiography in atrioventricular canal defects: A clinical spectrum. (Abstract) Excerpta Medica, International Congress Series, no. 277, 2nd World Congress on Ultrasonics in Medicine, 1973, p. 12.
Williams, R.G. and Rudd, M.: Echocardiographic features of endocardial cushion defects. Circulation 49:418, 1974.

Contributor: **L.H.S. Van Mierop**

Editor's Computerized Descriptors: Resp., CV.

ENDOCARDIAL FIBROELASTOSIS OF LEFT VENTRICLE

Includes: Fibro-élastose du ventricule gauche
Endokard-Fibroelastose des linken Ventrikels
Fibroelastosis endocárdica del ventrículo izquierdo
Left ventricular subendocardial fibroelastosis
Left ventricular endocardial fibrosis fibroelastosis
Left ventricular primary myocardial hypertrophy with endocardial fibroelastosis
Left ventricular endocardial sclerosis

Excludes: Endocardial fibroelastosis of right ventricle (349)
Endomyocardial fibrosis
Myocarditis
Nonobstructive cardiomyopathy

Minimal Diagnostic Criteria: ECG evidence of extreme left ventricular hypertrophy and T-wave changes, radiographic findings of cardiomegaly with enlargement of the left ventricle and left atrium and hemodynamic and angiographic evidence of altered left ventricular performance with mitral insufficiency. When the above findings occur in a young infant, this diagnosis must be considered.

Clinical Findings: This is a condition wherein the endocardium of the left ventricle is thickened and noncompliant. Symptoms usually occur in the first 12 months of life, infrequently after 1 year of age or before the 1st month. Evidence of cardiac decompensation with rapid onset in a previously healthy infant is the characteristic finding in all clinically recognized cases. With progression, if untreated, the terminal state is peripheral collapse accompanied by greyish cyanosis and feeble pulses. Auscultation of the heart while decompensation is present may reveal only tachycardia and a gallop rhythm. Gross cardiac enlargement is uniformly present. With compensation, a murmur of mitral insufficiency is not uncommonly present and may be clinically obvious in 30-50% of the patients. Most affected infants have accentuated third and fourth heart sounds. The first and second sounds may be normal.

Laboratory Findings: The ECG is considered typical and usually forms the basis of the clinical diagnosis. The principal findings are extreme left ventricular hypertrophy with flattening or inversion of the left precordial T waves. These findings occur in 80-90% of patients. The cardiac radiograms uniformly reveal the heart to be enlarged, particularly the left atrium and ventricle. Evidence of pulmonary venous hypertension or obstruction is invariably present. The functional disorder apparent at cardiac catheterization and angiography is progressive failure of the left ventricle to maintain an adequate contractile state. There is a decrease in left heart output and an increase in left ventricular end systolic, as well as in end diastolic volumes. The result of this alteration is extreme left ventricular dilatation and failure, although a small number of cases, probably less than 10%, may reveal a nondilated left ventricle. This functional disturbance may be due to the altered endocardium which limits contractility or alters metabolism of the myocardium by reducing the oxygen supply to the subendocardial layer. Valvar regurgitation, principally mitral, due to primary involvement, as well as left ventricular dilatation and demonstrable with left ventricular angiography, further adds to the left ventricular work load. Physiologically, left ventricular end diastolic pressure rises and peak dp/dt falls as myocardial contractility is further embarrassed. Myocardial failure ensues. Left atrial pressure rises as does pulmonary venous pressure.

Echocardiography, at present, cannot differentiate this disease from other forms of congestive cardiomyopathy. The left ventricular and septal walls may be abnormally thickened but the endocardial surface may appear normal. The wall motion is poor and the left ventricular cavity is usually dilated with respect to normal. The mitral valve motion is attenuated, and the anterior posterior leaflets are seen together. The anterior leaflet is seemingly displaced posteriorly and does not reach the septum in diastole. The left atrium is dilated to a greater or lesser extent, depending upon the degree of left heart failure or mitral insufficiency.

Pathologic Anatomy: Grossly, the left ventricle is dilated and thickened. The chordae tendineae of the mitral valve are shortened. The endocardium of the left ventricle and, occasionally of the left atrium, is thickened and presents as a glistening, pearly-white lining of the chamber. The mitral valve usually presents a similar appearance. The aortic valve also may be involved. Microscopically, the fundamental pathologic change is the thickened endocardium composed principally of elastic tissue but with an increased amount of collagenous tissue. However, wide variation in the amounts of these elements has been noted to occur. The condition may thus be less specific and more heterogeneous than previously supposed. Myocardial alterations have also been reported with the principal findings being a decrease in the ratio of capillary to myocardial fiber volume. Electron microscopic studies have indicated the composition of the thickened endocardium to be principally fibrin, but this information lacks confirmation by other investigators.

Complications

I   **Derived:** Congestive heart failure with coincident failure to thrive and difficult feeding are the principal complications. The decompensation, often amenable initially to therapy with digitalis preparations, frequently becomes intractable with death occurring in 75% by the end of the 1st year of life. Systemic thromboembolic phenomena represent a serious but little emphasized complication. Emboli from the left ventricle have been reported within all major systemic arterial systems and pulmonary emboli have been reported originating from the right ventricle.

II **Associated:** Associated cardiovascular defects, principally those causing overload of the left ventricle are recognized. Thus, coarctation of the aorta, aortic stenosis and mitral insufficiency are the leading associated abnormalities seen.

Etiology: No specific etiologic agent is known to cause the condition, although a number of agents have been implicated. Originally, the abnormality was thought to be the result of intrauterine infection and was considered a fetal endocarditis. More recently, a number of investigators have reported serologic and cultural evidence for extrauterine or intrauterine infection with Coxsackie as well as other enteroviruses. A relationship to mumps virus has been suggested because of a reportedly high incidence of positive skin tests to mumps antigen in individuals with EFE. However, the initial observation of this relationship has not been regularly reproduced by other investigators.

Evidence of obstruction to the cardiac lymphatics has also been reported further suggesting an inflammatory etiology. A familial incidence is recognized suggesting a hereditary cause. Secondary EFE, occurring with aortic atresia, mitral valvar disease, usually regurgitation, aortic stenosis and aortic coarctation all suggest overload of the left ventricle as a contributing factor. It is not known, however, whether the EFE in these circumstances is identical to that seen with the isolated lesion. Proof of cause is thus singularly lacking in all the aforementioned possibilities.
McK *30530

Pathogenesis: The mode of origin and development of this entity is not known. Whether it develops as a response to one of a number of possible agents over a period of time, or is a basic congenital abnormality of the endocardial surface of the heart, has not been determined. Furthermore, it has not been ascertained whether the lesion is a static one, present as an inherent endocardial defect throughout most of intrauterine and early extrauterine life, or whether if it becomes progressively more severe until it causes left ventricular failure and often death. Thus, if the defect is not progressive, or if progression should be halted, "mild" or subclinical cases might occur. The result would be that the abnormality would be of such a low-grade severity that symptoms might not be produced. Because the lesion is rarely, if ever, accurately diagnosed in an asymptomatic state, and even if entertained in such a state, cannot be definitely proven, the occurrence of sequential structural changes remains conjectural.

Related Facts
I   **Sex Ratio:** MO.6:Fl
II **Risk of Occurrence:** The risk of occurrence, calculated for the general population, is difficult to ascertain. The disease appears to have a higher incidence in colder climates and is less commonly encountered in the tropics. However, a tentative frequency may be arrived at by employing data from several large studies and assuming an overall incidence of congenital heart disease of 10 in 1000 live births. Using this material and the limitations mentioned, EFE may be expected to occur in approximately 1 in 6000 live births. Apparently the incidence of EFE has decreased in the past decade in North America.
III **Risk of Recurrence for**
    Patient's Sib: 3.8%
    Patient's Child: ? Various patterns are identifiable in selected families which include autosomal recessive, autosomal dominant and X-linked recessive. Most cases, however, are sporadic.
IV **Age of Detectability:** Most commonly within the 1st year of life, infrequent before the 1st month and after the 2nd year.
V   **Prevalence:** ?

Treatment
I   **Primary Prevention:** —
II **Secondary Prevention:** —
III **Other Therapy:** Treatment is strictly supportive with efforts to control congestive heart failure. General experience shows that the infant so treated has greater longevity and may survive this disease.

Prognosis: Prognosis depends upon the accuracy of clinical diagnosis. If the criteria previously set forth accurately diagnose EFE, then an estimated 50% or greater of diagnosed and treated patients will survive an indefinite period of time. As soon as the disease produces congestive heart failure, the prognosis without treatment is poor and the infant cannot be expected to survive.

Detection of Carrier: —

Special Considerations: —

References:
Chen, S. et al: Endocardial fibroelastosis: Family studies with special reference to counseling. J. Pediatr. 79:385, 1971.
Goldberg, S.J. et al: Pediatric and Adolescent Echocardiography. Chicago: Year Book Medical Publishers, 1975.
Mitchell, S.C. et al: An epidemiologic assessment of primary endocardial fibroelastosis. Am. J. Cardiol. 18:859, 1966.
Moller, J.H. et al: Endocardial fibroelastosis: A clinical and anatomic study of 47 patients with emphasis on its relationship to mitral insufficiency. Circulation 30:759, 1964.
Sellers, F.J. et al: The diagnosis of primary endocardial fibroelastosis. Circulation 29:49, 1964.
Westwood, M. et al: Heredity in primary endocardial fibroelastosis. Br. Heart J. 37:1077, 1975.

Contributor: **Gordon M. Folger, Jr.**

Editor's Computerized Descriptor: CV.

ENDOCARDIAL FIBROELASTOSIS OF RIGHT VENTRICLE

347-000

Includes: Fibro-élastose du ventricule droit
Endokard-Fibroelastose des rechten Ventrikels
Fibroelastosis endocárdica del ventrículo derecho
Right ventricular subendocardial fibroelastosis
Right ventricular endocardial fibrosis fibroelastosis
Right ventricular primary myocardial hypertrophy with endocardial fibroelastosis

Excludes: Endocardial fibroelastosis of left ventricle (348)
Endomyocardial fibrosis
Endomyocardial sclerosis
Obstructive cardiomyopathy of right ventricle
Myocarditis
Nonobstructive cardiomyopathy

Minimal Diagnostic Criteria: Angiocardiography of the right ventricle demonstrates the small contracted right ventricle.

Clinical Findings: A rare condition of the right ventricle in which the endocardium is thickened and noncompliant. When EFE of the right ventricle occurs as a primary lesion, it may present findings similar to hypoplasia of the right ventricle with cyanosis, evidence of systemic venous engorgement and reduced pulmonary blood flow.

Laboratory Findings: The ECG pattern is similar to that seen with hypoplasia of the right ventricle of other causes. Radiographically the heart is enlarged, the apex tilted up and the pulmonary conus segment is absent. The pulmonary vasculature is reduced. The findings at cardiac catheterization, as with the other laboratory findings, are similar to those seen in pulmonary atresia or extreme stenosis. The right ventricle is diminutive and there is a massive right-to-left shunt at the atrial level.

Pathology: Isolated primary EFE of the right ventricle such as is seen in the left ventricular form is extremely unusual. In this condition, no obstruction to the otherwise normal right ventricle occurs. The gross appearance, however, is identical to the condition as it occurs as a primary lesion of the left ventricle revealing an opaque white endocardium which is thickened on cut section as well as tough and fibrous. The right ventricle, however, is contracted rather than dilated.

Microscopic: The endocardial layer is increased many times its normal thickness with abundance of elastic fibers and an increase in collagenous tissue. The subendocardial-myocardial junction usually shows a few degenerative muscle fibers.

Complications
I **Derived:** Congestive heart failure, right-to-left atrial shunt, hypoxemia and acidosis.
II **Associated:** The condition is nearly always associated with other intracardiac anomalies, principally pulmonary atresia or extreme stenosis with intact ventricular septum.

Etiology: So rare is the primary form of this condition occurring in the right ventricle that no postulations as to its etiology have been made. Familial occurrence in 3 generations has been described.

Pathogenesis: The origin and development of the endocardial fibroelastic thickening is entirely unknown.

Related Facts
I **Sex Ratio:** ?
II **Risk of Occurrence:** ?
III **Risk of Recurrence for**
    Patient's Sib: ?
    Patient's Child: ?

IV **Age of Detectability:** Generally during early infancy, rarely after 2-3 months
V **Prevalence:** ?

Treatment
I **Primary Prevention:** —
II **Secondary Prevention:** Palliative systemic venous to right pulmonary artery anastomosis to improve pulmonary blood flow and reduce right heart work load.
III **Other Therapy:** Symptomatic therapy for congestive heart failure.

Prognosis: Death in early infancy is nearly invariable with survival seldom more than a few months unless a palliative procedure is carried out.

Detection of Carrier: —

Special Considerations: —

References:
Andersen, D.N. and Kelly, J.: Endocardial fibroelastosis; endocardial fibroelastosis associated with congenital malformations of the heart. Pediatrics 18:513, 1956.
Keith, J.D. et al: Pulmonary atresia with normal aortic root. In Heart Disease in Infancy and Childhood, 2nd Ed. New York: Macmillan Co. 1967, p. 818.
Morgan, A.D. et al: Endocardial fibroelastosis of the right ventricle in the newborn: Presenting the clinical picture of the hypoplastic right heart syndrome. Am. J. Cardiol. 18:933, 1966.

Contributor: **Gordon M. Folger, Jr.**

Editor's Computerized Descriptor: CV.

ENDOCRINE NEOPLASIA I, MULTIPLE

Includes: Cancer endocrinien multiple I
Syndrom der multiplen endocrinen Tumoren I
Neoplasia endócrina múltiple tipo I
Multiple endocrine adenomatosis, type I
Wermer syndrome
Zollinger-Ellison syndrome
Forbés-Albright syndrome
Hereditary hyperparathyroidism
MEN I syndrome

Excludes: Endocrine neoplasia II and III, multiple (351, 352)

Minimal Diagnostic Criteria: The presence of any or all of the below tumors (syndromes) in a member of a family in which the various tumors have been found strongly suggests the diagnosis.

Clinical Findings: The age of diagnosis ranges from the 2nd-7th decades of life, rarely in childhood. The presenting symptoms depend upon which endocrine organ is initially involved and whether or not hormonal hypersecretion is clinically significant. More than 1 endocrine gland may be affected simultaneously. Years may elapse between clinical symptoms caused by a single gland dysfunction and that occasioned by others. Affected glands include pituitary, parathyroid, pancreas, adrenal cortex and occasionally thyroid. Bronchial and intestinal carcinoids also have been described.

Pituitary adenomas may give rise to symptoms of acromegaly or the Cushing syndrome if hyperfunctioning. Amenorrhea or galactorrhea or both may be seen (Forbes-Albright syndrome). Headache and visual disturbances secondary to an expanding intrasellar mass are not uncommon.

Parathyroid adenomas are usually multiple; diffuse hyperplasia of all glands may be seen. The parathyroid is the most commonly affected gland in the syndrome(> 80%). Symptoms may be typical of hyperparathyroidism or the elevated blood calcium and parathyroid hormone levels may be discovered only by laboratory screening. Parathyroid carcinoma is rare.

Pancreatic adenomas or adenocarcinomas arise from the islet cells, and symptoms depend on which cell type is involved; ie insulinomas, glucagonomas or gastrinomas. There may be diffuse islet cell hyperplasia or multiple tumor nodules, frequently malignant. Intractable or recurrent peptic ulceration, or both, may result from excess gastrin secretion (Zollinger-Ellison syndrome).

Adrenal cortical hyperplasia or adenomas are not as common, but may be associated with hypercorticism, hyperaldosteronism or with symptoms related to excessive sex steroids. It is questionable as to whether the adrenal is primarily involved or becomes secondarily hypertrophied as a consequence of excess pituitary ACTH secretion or ectopic ACTH secretion from pancreatic or other tumors.

Thyroid involvement is less common and the lesions are not consistent; ie adenomas, thyroiditis and colloid goiter all have been described.

Complications
I **Derived:** Include all those classically associated with hormonal hypersecretion. Ectopic peptide hormone production may be a feature. Carcinoid tumors arising from the bronchi, thymus or upper small intestine may be responsible for excessive secretion of serotonin and the carcinoid syndrome. Pancreatic cholera or the watery diarrhea syndrome has been seen.
II **Associated:** Epithelial thymomas, schwannomas, and multiple benign lipomas have been described.

Etiology: Autosomal dominant disorder with virtually complete penetrance, if the entire age range and variable expressivity are taken into account. McK *13110

Pathogenesis: Suggested defect in neural crest differentiation, but this has been disputed.

Related Facts
I **Sex Ratio:** M1:F1
II **Risk of Occurrence:** Rare
III **Risk of Recurrence for**
   Patient's Sib: If parent affected 1 in 2 (50%) for each offspring to be affected; otherwise not increased, although extensive hormone assays may be necessary to exclude diagnosis even in asymptomatic 1st-degree relatives.
   Patient's Child: 1 in 2
IV **Age of Detectability:** Between 10 and 60 years.
V **Prevalence:** ?

Treatment
I **Primary Prevention:** Genetic counseling, coupled with screening of at-risk relatives with hormone assays (perhaps with discretionary use of provocative or suppressive tests), serum calcium levels and visual field examinations at yearly intervals.
II **Secondary Prevention:** Pituitary lesions may be treated surgically or with appropriate radiotherapy. If hyperparathyroidism or hyperadrenalcorticism develops all parathyroid or adrenal tissue should be removed; the recurrence risk is high. The Zollinger-Ellison syndrome responds to total gastrectomy and rarely metastatic lesions have disappeared on "second look" procedures. Other pancreatic lesions should be treated by surgical excision of the pancreas. Thyroid lesions are usually not malignant and may be managed conservatively. Other miscellaneous tumers—carcinoids, thymomas—should be removed. Lipomas are benign and require no therapy.
III **Other Therapy:** After surgical removal of a gland, hormone replacement therapy is indicated. If the parathyroid glands are totally removed, vitamin D and calcium will be necessary. Nonresectable or metastatic lesions may respond to chemotherapy. Cimetadine has been useful in treatment of gastrin-induced hyperacidity. Prostaglandin inhibitors may be helpful in control of pancreatic cholera.

Prognosis: Good for nonmalignant facet of disease, if symptoms detected early. Poor for pancreatic malignancy, although long-term survivors of Zollinger-Ellison syndrome have been described.

Detection of Carrier: As in Primary Prevention

Special Considerations: —

References:
Schimke, R.N.: Genetics of hormone-producing tumors. Clin. Gastroenterol. 2:661, 1973.
Schimke, R.N.: The multiple endocrine adenoma syndromes. Adv. Intern. Med. 21:294, 1974.

Contributor: **R. Neil Schimke**

Editor's Computerized Descriptors: Vision, Neck, GI., GU.

ENDOCRINE NEOPLASIA II, MULTIPLE

Includes: Cancer endocrinien multiple II
Syndrom der multiplen endocrinen Tumoren II
Neoplasia endócrina múltiple tipo II
Medullary thyroid carcinoma and pheochromocytoma syndrome
Sipple syndrome
Medullary thyroid carcinoma syndrome
Multiple endocrine adenomatosis type II
MEN II syndrome

Excludes: Endocrine neoplasia I and III, multiple (350, 352)
Familial pheochromocytoma
Pheochromocytoma occurring with neurofibromatosis or von Hippel-Lindau syndrome

Minimal Diagnostic Criteria: The presence of pheochromocytoma, medullary thyroid carcinoma, or both, in any member of a family in which others have shown similar lesions suggests the diagnosis. An elevated plasma calcitonin level alone is *not* sufficient for diagnosis since this hormone may be ectopically secreted by lung tumors, pancreatic tumors, and even a sporadic pheochromocytoma.

Clinical Findings: Age of diagnosis is variable but may range from childhood to 7th decade. Patients may present with symptoms related to catecholamine excess, including headache, palpitations, diaphoresis, flushing and either labile or sustained hypertension secondary to pheochromocytoma. The pheochromocytoma may however, be asymptomatic. Pheochromocytomas are bilateral and occasionally, extraadrenal. Malignant degeneration is rare.

Medullary thyroid carcinoma is invariably multifocal, but the nodules may or may not be palpable, and may or may not be detectable by radioactive scanning with radioiodine. Measurements of plasma calcitonin with or without stimulation may be the only means of diagnosis of the asymptomatic patient. The tumor may elaborate ectopic hormones including ACTH. The carcinoid syndrome, as well as the watery diarrhea syndrome, have been seen with these tumors.

Parathyroid hyperplasia or adenomatosis is an additional feature seen frequently. It may be asymptomatic or result in typical symptoms of hyperparathyroidism.

Complications
I **Derived:** Include those associated with catecholamine-induced hypertension: eg cardiac disease, renal damage, strokes and symptoms associated with parathyroid hormone excess. Ectopic hormone production by the medullary carcinoma may lead to a variety of problems depending upon the peptide secreted.
II **Associated:** Gliomas, glioblastomas and meningiomas have been reported. Other tumors and nonmalignant lesions are probably no more common than in the general population.

Etiology: Autosomal dominant disorder with high penetrance and variable expressivity. McK *17140

Pathogenesis: A heritable defect in neural crest differentiation.

Related Facts
I **Sex Ratio:** M1:F1
II **Risk of Occurrence:** ?
III **Risk of Recurrence for**
  Patient's Sib: If parent affected or if 2 sibs affected, 1 in 2 (50%). An apparently sporadic case should not be considered a new mutation until extensive family testing has been undertaken.
  Patient's Child: 1 in 2
IV **Age of Detectability:** Between early childhood and 60 years
V **Prevalence:** ?

Treatment

I **Primary Prevention:** Genetic counseling. Catecholamine assays may reveal pheochromocytoma before hypertension adversely affects the cardiovascular system. Elevated plasma calcitonin levels suggest the presence of thyroid tumors before metastases have developed. Serum calcium and parathyroid hormone levels may be useful in preventing long-term complications of hyperparathyroidism.
II **Secondary Prevention:** Surgical excision of both adrenals if tumors present, since lesions are usually bilateral. Surgical removal of entire thyroid with or without local neck dissection for medullary thyroid tumor. Plasma calcitonin may be useful in determining adequacy of resection and aid in detection of metastases. All parathyroids should be removed if hyperparathyroidism develops to avoid reoperation.
III **Other Therapy:** α and β adrenergic receptor blocking agents may be used if pheochromocytoma is unresectable for whatever reason. Nonresectable thyroid tumors producing ACTH may require adrenalectomy. The watery diarrhea syndrome may respond to prostaglandin synthesis inhibitors. After surgery, appropriate hormone and vitamin replacement is necessary.

Prognosis: Good for pheochromocytoma. Good for medullary thyroid tumor if resected before metastatic disease evident; poor otherwise, although long-lived exceptions have been seen.

Detection of Carrier: As in Primary Prevention

Special Considerations: —

References:
Schimke, R.N.: Familial tumor endocrinopathies. In Bergsma, D.(ed.): Part X. The Endocrine System. Birth Defects; Orig. Art. Ser., vol. VII, no. 6. Baltimore: Williams & Wilkins for The National Foundation-March of Dimes, 1971, p. 55.
Steiner, A.L. et al: Study of a kindred with pheochromocytoma, medullary thyroid carcinoma, hyperparathyroidism and Cushing's disease: Multiple endocrine neoplasm, type 2. Medicine 47:371, 1968.

Contributor: **R. Neil Schimke**

Editor's Computerized Descriptors: Skin, Sweating, CV., GI., Nerve

ENDOCRINE NEOPLASIA III, MULTIPLE

Includes: Cancer endocrinien multiple III
Syndrom der multiplen endocrinen Tumoren III
Neoplasia endócrina múltiple tipo III
Multiple endocrine adenomatosis, type IIb
Pheochromocytoma, medullary thyroid carcinoma and multiple neuroma syndrome
Mucosal neuroma syndrome
MEN III syndrome

Excludes: Endocrine neoplasia I and II, multiple (350, 351)
Other causes of pheochromocytoma and mucosal neuromas
Neurofibromatosis (712)

Minimal Diagnostic Criteria: Not known with certainty since sufficient detailed family studies have not been reported. The facies is virtually pathognomonic of underlying malignancy.

Clinical Findings: The physiognomy is frequently striking and diagnostic. Affected patients may have some or all of the following: neuromas of conjunctiva, nasal, labial and buccal mucosa, tongue and other parts of GI tract including colon with or without megacolon; esthenic habitus; muscular hypotonia; café-au-lait spots or diffuse freckling; large blubbery lips and pseudoprognathism; kyphosis, lordosis, pes cavus, genu valga and generalized joint laxity; absent flare response to intradermal histamine.

Medullary thyroid carcinoma is an apparently invariant feature with all the attendant symptoms (see MEN II syndrome). Prophylactic surgery is probably warranted simply on the basis of the facies; certainly so, if plasma calcitonin is elevated.

Pheochromocytoma is frequently bilateral and may be asymptomatic.

Intestinal symptoms are related to colonic ganglioneuromas (megacolon) or are secondary to excessive prostaglandin or VIP (vasoactive intestinal polypeptide) secreted by the thyroid tumor which may cause diarrhea.

Parathyroid hyperplasia is quite rare.

Complications
I **Derived:** As with MEN II syndrome. Joint laxity may give rise to orthopedic problems. Fluid and electrolyte disturbances result from altered bowel motility. Laryngeal tumor may cause vocal problems. It is conceivable that additional tumors derived from neural crest will be reported. Ectopic hormone production may be less common but in view of the small number of cases reported this may be fortuitous.
II **Associated:** ?

Etiology: Autosomal dominant. Penetrance unknown but probably high. Variable expressivity likely. McK *16230

Pathogenesis: A defect in the differentiation of certain neural crest derivatives.

Related Facts
I **Sex Ratio:** M1:F1
II **Risk of Occurrence:** Probably rarer than MEN I or II
III **Risk of Recurrence for**
　Patient's Sib: 1 in 2 if parent or another sib affected. Sporadic case may be new mutant, but caution must be exercised since penetrance not defined.
　Patient's Child: 1 in 2
IV **Age of Detectability:** As early as infancy and as late as 40 years; conceivably could be detected at birth.
V **Prevalence:** ?

Treatment
I **Primary Prevention:** Genetic counseling; examination of at-risk relatives for neuromas; hormone assays as outlined with MEN II.

II **Secondary Prevention:** Surgical removal of malignant tumors.
III **Other Therapy:** Symptomatic

Prognosis: Depends on tumor type and stage when detected.

Detection of Carrier: Typical facies and physical findings, catecholamine assays, plasma calcitonin levels are all useful in detecting premalignant states.

Special Considerations: —

References:
Khairi, M.R. et al: Mucosal neuromas, pheochromocytoma and medullary thyroid carcinoma: Multiple endocrine neoplasia, type 3. Medicine 54:89, 1975.
Schimke, R.N.: Tumors of the neural crest system. In Mulvihill, J.J. (ed.): Genetics of Human Cancer. New York: Raven Press, 1976, p. 179.

Contributor: **R. Neil Schimke**

Editor's Computerized Descriptors: Face, Oral, Larynx, Skin, Skel., Muscle, Eye, Nose, GI.

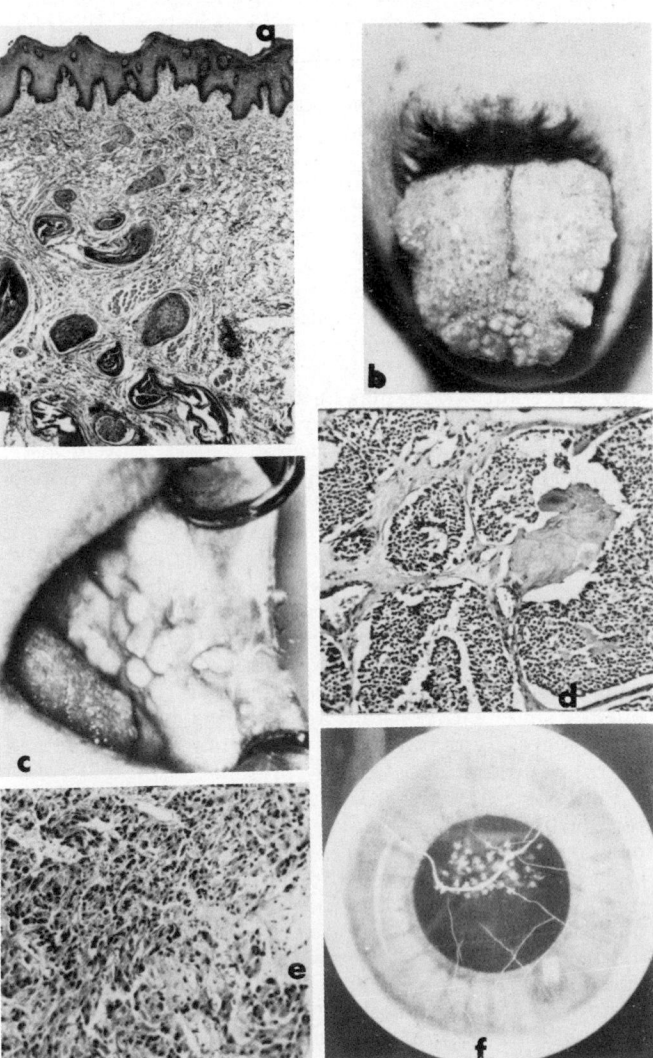

255. A) Photomicrograph of mucosal neuroma; B) nodules of lips and tongue; C) nodules of buccal mucosa; D) medullary carcinoma of thyroid with amyloid production; E) pheochromocytoma; F) thickened corneal nerves

ENDOMYOCARDIAL FIBROSIS OF LEFT VENTRICLE

Includes: Fibrose endomyocardiaque du ventricule gauche
Endomykardfibrose des linken Ventrikels
Fibrosis endomiocárdica del ventrículo izquierdo
Davies disease
Constrictive cardiopathy
African cardiopathy

Excludes: Endomyocardial fibrosis of right ventricle (354)
Endocardial fibroelastosis
Primary myocardial hypertrophy with endocardial fibroelastosis

Minimal Diagnostic Criteria: Hemodynamic data showing malfunction of the left ventricle and angiocardiography demonstrating reduction of myocardial contractility are the principal features. Angiographic demonstration of apical filling defects in the left ventricle, as well as mitral regurgitation, is usually present.

Clinical Findings: Similar to those of endomyocardial fibrosis of the right ventricle.

Cardiomegaly is uncommon as this is a restrictive heart disease. Likewise, displacement of the apical impulse is unusual, and it is rarely prominent or heaving. With pulmonary hypertension secondary to mitral regurgitation and advanced left ventricular disease, an accentuated pulmonary component of the second heart sound may be present. A prominent third heart sound is a constant finding and an opening snap may be detected in one-third to one-half of the cases. A characteristic apical systolic murmur occupying early systole has been reported due to early phase mitral insufficiency with mitral competency occurring in late systole.

Laboratory Findings: Eosinophilia may occur but may be secondary to parasitic infestation. Gamma globulin levels are often elevated. The ECG tracing may be normal and is reportedly rarely helpful. With advanced disease hypertrophy of the left atrium may be seen, and with the development of significant pulmonary hypertension, right atrial hypertrophy and right ventricular hypertrophy develop. Enlargement of the heart is usually present. With pulmonary hypertension, right atrial and ventricular enlargement are usually detectable and left atrial enlargement may be apparent. Pulmonary venous congestion is a frequent finding. Elevation of the left atrial pressure and the left ventricular end diastolic pressure are the usual findings. Pulmonary hypertension is found in nearly 50% of the patients studied but this varies with the degree of left ventricular disease. The left ventricular chamber is frequently small with constant apical filling defects. Contractility is greatly reduced. The left atrium is enlarged and mitral regurgitation is usually present.

Pathologic Anatomy: Grossly, there is a recurring pattern of fibrotic endocardial lesions occurring in 2 areas - one on the posterior wall of the left ventricle involving the endocardium in the area behind the posterior leaflet of the mitral valve, the chordae of the posterior mitral leaflet and a portion of the endocardium of the outflow tract, and one located at the apex of the ventricle tapering toward the endocardium of the septum to terminate at the bases of the posterior papillary muscles. Microscopic findings are the same as EMF of right ventricle.

Complications
I **Derived:** The development of severe pulmonic hypertension secondary to reduced left ventricular compliance and mitral regurgitation is the principal complication. With pulmonary hypertension, right atrial and ventricular dilatation may occur with the possibility of pulmonary embolic phenomena.

Congestive heart failure is a frequent finding and the common cause of death.
II **Associated:** —

Etiology: ? †

Pathogenesis: ? †

Related Facts
I **Sex Ratio:** Ml:Fl
II **Risk of Occurrence:** ?
III **Risk of Recurrence for**
   Patient's Sib: ?
   Patient's Child: ?
IV **Age of Detectability:** Generally early adult life to middle age, rarely in childhood.
V **Prevalence:** ?

Treatment
I **Primary Prevention:** —
II **Secondary Prevention:** —
III **Other Therapy:** Anticongestive measures restore compensation for varying periods of time, but the outcome is uniformly fatal, usually in early middle age.

Prognosis: Poor, with death from the condition occurring uniformly.

Detection of Carrier: —

†**Special Considerations:** For more detailed comment, see Etiology and Pathogenesis of Endomyocardial Fibrosis of Right Ventricle.

References:
Cockshott, W.P.: Angiocardiography of endomyocardial fibrosis. Br. J. Radiol. 38:192, 1965.
Connor, D.H. et al: Endomyocardial fibrosis in Uganda (Davies' disease) I. An epidemiologic, clinical and pathologic study. Am. Heart J. 74:687, 1967.
Connor, D.H. et al: Endomyocardial fibrosis in Uganda (Davies' disease). II. An epidemiologic, clinical and pathologic study. Am. Heart J. 75:107, 1968.
Fowler, J.M. and Somers, K.: Left ventricular endomyocardial fibrosis and mitral incompetence: A new syndrome. Lancet 1:227, 1968.

Contributor: **Gordon M. Folger, Jr.**

Editor's Computerized Descriptors: Resp., CV.

ENDOMYOCARDIAL FIBROSIS OF RIGHT VENTRICLE

Includes: Fibrose endomyocardiaque du ventricule droit
Endomykardfibrose des rechten Ventrikels
Fibrosis endomiocárdica del ventrículo derecho
Davies disease
Constrictive cardiopathy
African cardiopathy

Excludes: Endomyocardial fibrosis of left ventricle (353)
Endocardial fibroelastosis
Primary myocardial hypertrophy with endocardial fibroelastosis

Minimal Diagnostic Criteria: Hemodynamic changes consist principally of evidence for right ventricular dysfunction with elevation of right atrial pressure and right ventricular end diastolic pressures. Cardiac angiography reveals reduction in right ventricular contractility.

Clinical Findings: A disorder of the cardiac connective tissues occurring among native African Negroes, found much less frequently in Negroes from other world areas and rare in non-Negroid populations, in which the ventricular endocardium and subendocardial layers, as well as the supportive tissue of the ventricular wall, are thickened and rendered noncompliant.

Characteristically, evidence of right heart failure occurs insidiously. The involved individual is almost invariably a Negro in the early adult years of life, although children as young as 2 years have been reported to have the condition. Ascites is the most striking feature. Peripheral edema may be present but much less prominent. Hepatosplenomegaly is common with a pulsatile liver frequently present. The cardiac findings consist of enlargement of the heart detectable in 50-60% of patients, a right ventricular lift occurs in approximately half of the patients, an accentuated third heart sound is found in nearly all patients and the murmur of tricuspid insufficiency is found in 15-25% of cases. Pericardial effusion is common, occurring in nearly 50% of reported cases.

Laboratory Findings: Eosinophilia of significance occurs in some individuals but may be secondary to coexisting parasitic infestation. Elevated gamma globulin levels are commonly encountered. The QRS axis is usually normal. QRS voltages are generally normal or decreased with hypertrophy patterns uncommon. Atrial hypertrophy occurs in approximately 50% of individuals and is more often a P mitral configuration or a pattern suggesting hypertrophy of both atria. Less commonly, right atrial enlargement alone is noted. Characteristic or diagnostic ECG patterns have not been reported. Atrial fibrillation occurs at some time in approximately one-third of cases. EMF is restrictive heart disease and gross cardiomegaly is usually due either to enlargement of the right atrium or to the coexistence of a pericardial effusion. Dilatation of the right ventricular infundibular area is, however, a frequent radiographic as well as angiographic finding. Intracardiac calcification may be visualized. Elevation of the right ventricular end diastolic pressure is a constant finding. The right ventricular pressure curve closely resembles that of constrictive pericarditis even though that condition does not coexist. The cardiac output may be normal or reduced. By cardiac angiography, reduced contractility of the right ventricle and a degree of tricuspid insufficiency are common findings. The right ventricular body may appear nearly obliterated with only the dilated infundibular area remaining cavitary.

Pathologic Anatomy: The gross appearance of the heart is that of extreme enlargement of the right atrium, a contracted right ventricle, particularly the apical area with dilatation of the right ventricular outflow area. Significant right ventricular hypertrophy is uncommon. Endocardial fibrosis characteristically is more severe at the apical portion of the right ventricle, usually extending to encase the papillary muscles but sparing the chordae tendineae and the tricuspid valve leaflets. Mural thrombi are often present in the right atrium and may occur in the right ventricle. Calcification in the fibrotic areas occurs occasionally. The microscopic findings are a swollen appearance of the connective tissues of the endocardium and underlying myocardial interstices. The earlier finding that these tissues contain elevated amounts of acid mucopolysaccharide has not been found to be specific for EMF. Distinct increase in cardiac muscle fiber size is recognized. Inflammatory changes are not observed.

Complications
I **Derived:** Congestive heart failure is a uniform finding and the principal cause of death. Pulmonary emboli secondary to thrombi in the right atrium and ventricle are a major complication.
II **Associated:** —

Etiology: No definite etiologic agent has been identified. A number of agents, however, capable of instituting an autoimmune reaction have been considered. Included in these have been infectious agents, toxins and dietary idiosyncracy, none of which have been positively implicated. However, the distribution of the lesion to very specific areas within the heart, and in no other place, and the inability to find immunologically competent cells in areas undergoing change have cast some doubt upon an immunologic origin. Malnutrition has been considered but appears unlikely. Some similarities to rheumatic fever have caused consideration of this disease as the cause of the changes seen, but this, too, is unproven. The disease is seen occasionally in children as young as 2 years, but its clinical onset is more commonly in a young adult.

Pathogenesis: Development of these changes is unknown but is currently thought to be secondary to an autoimmune mechanism, the reaction to an as yet unknown agent.

Related Facts
I **Sex Ratio:** Ml:Fl
II **Risk of Occurrence:** ?
III **Risk of Recurrence for**
    Patient's Sib: ?
    Patient's Child: ?
IV **Age of Detectability:** Generally, early adult life
V **Prevalence:** ?

Treatment
I **Primary Prevention:** —
II **Secondary Prevention:** —
III **Other Therapy:** Anticongestive measures restore compensation for varying periods of time, but it appears that the outcome is uniformly fatal.

Prognosis: Poor, with death from the condition occurring uniformly, usually in the age range from early adulthood to early middle age

Detection of Carrier: —

Special Considerations: —

References:
Cockshott, W.P.: Angiocardiography of endomyocardial fibrosis. Br. J. Radiol. 38:192, 1965.
Connor, D.H. et al: Endomyocardial fibrosis in Uganda (Davies' disease). I. An epidemiologic, clinical and pathologic study. Am.

Heart J. 74:687, 1967.

Connor, D.H. et al: Endomyocardial fibrosis in Uganda (Davies' disease). II. An epidemiologic, clinical and pathologic study. Am. Heart J. 75:107, 1968.

McKinney, B.: Cardiac muscle fiber size in African cardiomyopathies. Am. Heart J. 87:298, 1974.

Somers, K. et al: Clinical features of endomyocardial fibrosis in the right ventricle. Br. Heart. J. 30:309, 1968.

Contributor: **Gordon M. Folger, Jr.**

Editor's Computerized Descriptors: CV. Spleen, Liver

EPIBLEPHARON

Includes: Epiblefarón
Superior epiblepharon
Inferior epiblepharon

Excludes: Eyelid entropion (372)
Blepharochalasis

Minimal Diagnostic Criteria: Horizontal fold of skin on eyelid often exaggerated in downward gaze

Clinical Findings: Both inferior and superior epiblepharon occur. It is a horizontal fold of skin in the tarsal region of the lid. Accessory lid structures are usually normal. The excess skin overhangs the lower portion of the upper lid or overlaps the upper portion of the lower lid. It is most evident near the medial canthi. The overriding of skin may extend to the lid border causing an inturning of the lashes. This is often exaggerated in downward gaze. In early life, this may or may not cause increased lacrimation, photophobia, bulbar conjunctival infection and keratitis. Symptoms are more likely to arise if the condition persists. Infants with epiblepharon characteristically have chubby cheeks, prominent eyes and a narrow interpupillary distance. Epiblepharon is usually bilateral but asymmetric. Inferior epiblepharon tends to disappear with facial growth.

Complications
I   **Derived:** —
II **Associated:**   Paresis of the inferior oblique muscle, eyelid entropion, hypertrophy of the tarsus, and epicanthus

Etiology: For superior epiblepharon autosomal dominant transmission has been demonstrated. Inferior epiblepharon has a familial tendency.

Pathogenesis: It has been postulated that epiblepharon results from incomplete development of the fascial planes, absence of the tarsus, hypertrophy of the marginal portion of the orbicularis, and from anomalous strands of insertions of the vertical recti muscles into the skin of the lids. Superior epiblepharon, in addition to the preceding, has been theorized to result from a Z-shaped kink in the orbicularis fibers or insertion of the levator tendon too close to the lid margin.

Related Facts
I   **Sex Ratio:** M1:F1 probable
II   **Risk of Occurrence:**   Superior epiblepharon is relatively rare, whereas inferior epiblepharon is common, in comparison.
III **Risk of Recurrence for**
     Patient's Sib: For superior epiblepharon: when autosomal dominant and if parent is affected, 1 in 2 (50%) for each offspring to be affected; otherwise not increased
     Patient's Child: For superior epiblepharon: 1 in 2 when autosomal dominant
IV   **Age of Detectability:**   At birth for inferior epiblepharon
V   **Prevalence:**   ?

Treatment
I   **Primary Prevention:**   Genetic counseling when autosomal dominant
II   **Secondary Prevention:**   The overlapping portion of skin may be excised in epiblepharon for either cosmetic purposes or, if repeated keratitis occurs, from inturned lashes. The application of collodion, adhesive, or cellophane tapes from the lower lid to cheek may be of some help to pull the skin fold away from the lid as a temporizing measure. Inferior epiblepharon usually corrects itself spontaneously within the 1st year of life with growth and development of the facial and orbital bone. Its persistence is rare. Irritation of the cornea, if it occurs, is usually temporary and may be less-

ened by the application of a protective ointment. Superior epiblepharon more often requires surgical correction than inferior epiblepharon.

III Other Therapy: —

Prognosis: Excellent for both types

Detection of Carrier: —

Special Considerations: —

References:
Duke-Elder, S.: System of Ophthalmology, vol. 3, part 2. Congenital Deformities. London:Henry Kimpton, 1964, p. 857.
Karlin, D. B.: Congenital entropion, epiblepharon, and antimongoloid obliquity of the palpebral fissure. Am. J. Ophthalmol. 50:487, 1960.
Levitt, J. M.: Epiblepharon and congenital entropion. Am. J. Ophthalmol. 44:112, 1957.
Swan, K. C.: Syndrome of congenital epiblepharon and inferior oblique insufficiency. Am. J. Ophthalmol. 39:130, 1955.

Contributor: **Elsa K. Rahn**

Editor's Computerized Descriptors: Eye, Face

EPICANTHUS

Includes: Epikanthus
Epicanto
Epicanthus supraciliaris
Epicanthus palpebris
Epicanthus tarsalis
Epicanthus inversus
Telecanthus

Excludes: Mongolian fold

Minimal Diagnostic Criteria: No sharp guidelines exist. In many cases the clinical impression is sufficient. Comparison of measurements between inner canthi with normal ranges for the age and racial group are helpful, since mild-to-moderate degrees of epicanthus are normally found in a high percentage of prepubertal Caucasians.†

Clinical Findings: The inner corner of the eye is bridged by an arching fold which extends from the bridge of the nose. The fold frequently covers the inner canthus and curves laterally above and below to fuse with the upper and lower eyelids. The bridge of the nose appears flat and an impression (usually false) of esotropia is created. Telecanthus is a more general term which describes widening of the inner canthal distance for whatever reason.

Complications
I **Derived:** Usually a cosmetic problem. Rarely are the folds wide enough to interfere with nasal field vision.
II **Associated:** Epicanthus with ptosis is associated frequently with esotropia and blepharophimosis and occasionally with epiblepharon, congenital ectropion or entropion, and abnormalities of the caruncle. Simple epicanthus, as the name implies, is inherited as an isolated character. Finally, epicanthus has been described as a component of a wide variety of syndromes. (Epicanthus inversus is a distinct entity associated with ptosis and antimongoloid slant.)

Etiology: Autosomal dominant gene with variable expressivity. (Mongolian fold is an autosomal dominant racial characteristic.) McK *13150

Pathogenesis: There are 3 major theories: excessive skin at the root of the nose; poor development of the bones of the bridge of the nose; and retention of the fetal epicanthal fold normally present in the fetus from the 3rd-6th month.

Related Facts
I **Sex Ratio:** Simple epicanthus: M1:F1; (congenital ptosis with epicanthus: M2:F1)
II **Risk of Occurrence:** Among Caucasians, about 1 in 5 live births
III **Risk of Recurrence for**
Patient's Sib: If parent is affected, 1 in 2 (50%) for each offspring to be affected; otherwise not increased.
Patient's Child: 1 in 2
IV **Age of Detectability:** At birth, but in Caucasians, most disappear by puberty.
V **Prevalence:** Caucasians: 1 in 5 at 1 year; 1 in 33 at 12 years and over. Adult mongoloids: 100 in 143; Negroids: intermediate.

Treatment
I **Primary Prevention:** Genetic counseling
II **Secondary Prevention:** Plastic surgery very rarely indicated to correct loss of nasal field vision.
III **Other Therapy:** —

Prognosis: No complications unless part of a larger syndrome

Detection of Carrier: —

†Special Considerations: It should be reemphasized that simple epicanthus is a variation of normal which usually disappears by puberty in Caucasians (somewhat sooner in females than in males) and therefore should not be operated on prematurely for cosmetic reasons. Furthermore, increased inner canthal distance (as distinct from epicanthus) should lead one to look for other signs of Waardenburg syndrome in order to detect deafness early. More obvious associated defects will lead one to suspect other malformation syndromes such as chromosome 18q-, chromosome 5p-, chromosome 21 trisomy, mucopolysaccharidosis I, oculodentodigital dysplasia, Turner syndrome, pseudo-Turner syndrome.

References:

Christian, J.C. et al: Familial telecanthus with associated congenital anomalies. In Bergsma, D. (ed.): Part II. Malformation Syndromes. Birth Defects: Orig. Art. Ser., vol. V, no. 2. New York: The National Foundation-March of Dimes, 1969, p. 82.

Duke-Elder, S.: System of Ophthalmology, vol. 3, pt. 2. Congenital Deformities. St. Louis: C.V. Mosby Co., 1963, p. 851.

Gellis, S.S. and Feingold, M.: Atlas of Mental Retardation Syndromes: Visual Diagnosis of Facies and Physical Findings. Washington, D.C.: Government Printing Office, 1968.

Johnson, C.C.: Epicanthus. Am. J. Ophthalmol. 66:939, 1968.

Contributor: **Donald R. Bergsma**

Editor's Computerized Descriptor: Eye

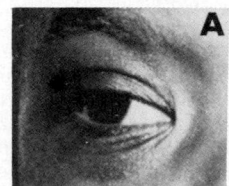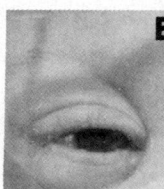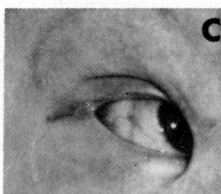

256. Epicanthal fold: A) mild; B) moderate; C) marked

EPIMERASE DEFICIENCY (MARKER)

Includes: Déficit en épimérase
Epimerase-Mangel
Deficiencia de epimerase
Uridine diphosphate galactose 4'-epimerase deficiency

Excludes: Galactokinase deficiency (402)
Galactosemia (403)

Minimal Diagnostic Criteria: Absence or severe deficiency of epimerase from blood cells

Clinical Findings: None in 8 individuals known to be clinically affected

Complications
I **Derived:** —
II **Associated:** —

Etiology: Autosomal recessive; McK *23035

Pathogenesis: —

Related Facts
I **Sex Ratio:** M2:F6
II **Risk of Occurrence:**   ?
III **Risk of Recurrence for**
    Patient's Sib: 1 in 4 for each offspring to be affected
    Patient's Child: Not increased unless mate is carrier or homozygote
IV **Age of Detectability:**   Newborns fed milk have high levels of red blood cell galactose-1-phosphate which may be discovered by bacterial screening test for galactose in blood
V **Prevalence:** ?

Treatment
I **Primary Prevention:** —
II **Secondary Prevention:** —
III **Other Therapy:** —

Prognosis: Normal life span

Detection of Carrier: Erythrocyte epimerase approximately 50% or less of normal

Special Considerations: —

References:

Gitzelmann, R.: Deficiency of uridine diphosphate galactose 4-epimerase in blood cells of an apparently healthy infant: Preliminary communication. Helv. Paediatr. Acta 27:125, 1972.

Gitzelmann, R. and Steinmann, B.: Uridine diphosphate galactose 4-epimerase deficiency: II. Clinical follow-up, biochemical studies and family investigation. Helv. Paediatr. Acta 28:497, 1973.

Mitchell, B. et al: Reversal of UDP-galactose 4-epimerase deficiency of human leukocytes in culture. Proc. Natl. Acad. Sci. USA 72:5026, 1975.

Contributor: **Richard Gitzelmann**

Editor's Computerized Descriptor: —

EPIPHYSEAL DYSPLASIA, MULTIPLE

Includes: Dysplasie polyépiphysaire dominante
Multiple epiphysäre Dysplasie
Displasia epifisaria múltiple
Dysplasia epiphysialis multiplex
Fairbank disease†
Polyosteochondrite (Turpin et Coste)

Excludes: Spondyloepiphyseal dysplasia, tarda (898)
Pseudoachondroplastic dysplasia (828)
Chondrodysplasia punctata
Arthroophthalmopathy (90)
Spondyloepiphyseal dysplasia, congenita (897)

Minimal Diagnostic Criteria: The diagnosis can be made only by roentgenologic study of the epiphysis of the long bones and the hands.

Clinical Findings: Multiple epiphyseal dysplasia manifests itself between the 2nd and 5th years of life with waddling gait or articular limitations. However, the diagnosis of this condition is often late, motivated by discomfort secondary to osteoarthritic changes. Clinically, the limbs appear relatively short but the stature is not much decreased (close to 150 cm in the adult). The shortness of the hand and foot is the most striking. The mobility of the hip joint, sometimes of the shoulder or other articulations, is restricted.

On x-ray examination the epiphysis of the long bones, the carpal and tarsal bones are small, irregular, sometimes fragmented and these changes become progressively more marked. The metaphyses of the long bones are normal in this type but the metacarpals and phalanges are slightly short and their metaphyseal limits are irregular. The vertebral bodies are normal, or sometimes show minimal irregularities of the plates.

Complications
I **Derived:** Osteoarthritic changes appear with advancing age and these are almost constant in the adult, especially in the hip.
II **Associated:** Chondrodysplastic rheumatism is sometimes observed in the adult.

Etiology: Autosomal dominant; McK *13240

Pathogenesis: The appearance of the chondrocytes is similar to pseudoachondroplasia but the alterations are less marked. The swelling of the endoplasmic reticulum, with a sketch of a periodic structure, is visible and suggests an accumulation of an abnormal product. However, unlike pseudoachondroplasia, the proteoglycans of the cartilage seem normal by electrophoretic analysis.

Related Facts
I **Sex Ratio:** M1:F1
II **Risk of Occurrence:** ?
III **Risk of Recurrence for**
 Patient's Sib: If parent is affected, 1 in 2 (50%) for each offspring to be affected; otherwise not increased.
 Patient's Child: 1 in 2
IV **Age of Detectability:** The condition is recognized in childhood by articular limitation or disorder of gait.
V **Prevalence:** ?

Treatment
I **Primary Prevention:** Genetic counseling
II **Secondary Prevention:** —
III **Other Therapy:** Orthopedic surgery of the hip may be indicated (osteotomy of the pelvis, or the collum femoris), sometimes, osteotomy of the leg (correction of genu varum or genu valgum).

Prognosis: Normal life span

Detection of Carrier: —

†Special Considerations: The described type conforms to the Fairbank description but the heterogeneity of the multiple epiphyseal dysplasia is not fully delineated. For example, an autosomal recessive form is probable, and some radiologic difference from the dominant form (flat femoral head, no metaphyseal irregularities of the metacarpals and phalanges) exists. In this form, the chondrocytes contain inclusions probably of lysosomal origin with granular or filamentous material.

References:
Fairbank, H.A.T.: Dysplasia epiphysialis multiplex. Br. J. Surg. 34:225, 1947.
Kahn, M.F. et al: Le rhumatisme chondrodysplasique. Sem. Hop. Paris 46:1938, 1970.
Maroteaux, P. et al: Essai de classification des dysplasies spondylo-épiphysaires. Simep. édit. Lyon, 1968.
Maroteaux, P. et al: Dysplasie poly-épiphysaire probablement récessive autosomique. Apport de l'étude ultrastructurale dans l'isolement de cette forme autonome. Nouv. Presse Med. 4:2169, 1975.

Contributor: **Pierre Maroteaux**

Editor's Computerized Descriptor: Skel.

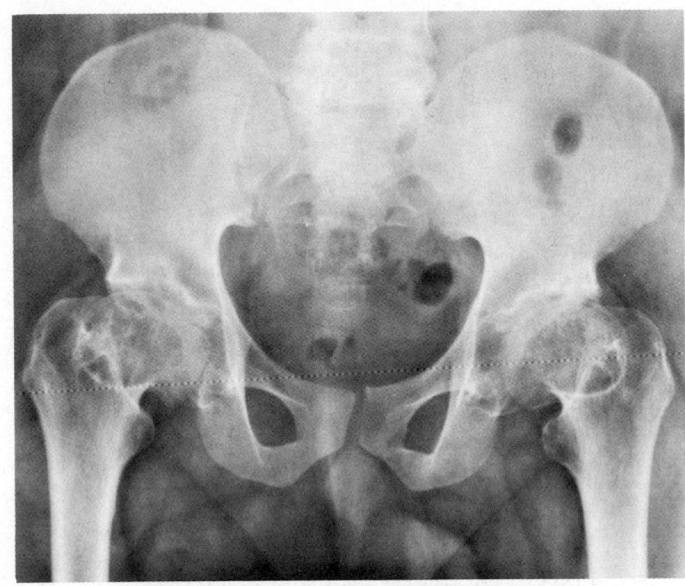

257. Note affected hips and secondary degenerative joint disease

EPITHELIOMA, MULTIPLE SELF-HEALING SQUAMOUS

Includes: Epithélioma multiple à cellules squameuses
Keratoakanthom Typ Ferguson-Smith
Epitelioma escamoso múltiple autocicatrizante
Familial multiple primary self-healing squamous cell epithelioma
Self-healing multiple squamous epithelioma

Excludes: Keratoacanthoma

Minimal Diagnostic Criteria: More than 1 tumor with the histologic appearance of squamous epithelioma. History of self-healing tumors in patient and family members. Characteristic scars.

Clinical Findings: Multiple cutaneous tumors, histologically indistinguishable from well-differentiated squamous epithelioma, affecting principally circumoral region, nose and ears, and less frequently scalp, hands, forearms and legs. Each tumor starts in normal skin as a small papule which enlarges, ulcerates and eventually heals, leaving deep pitted scars with irregular overhanging crenellated borders. Individual tumors last for several months and fresh ones usually appear in numbers rather more than sufficient to balance the healing.

Complications
I **Derived:** Severe trauma resulting from overenthusiastic radiotherapy or surgery
II **Associated:** —

Etiology: Autosomal dominant; McK *13280

Pathogenesis: ? Tumors are thought to arise in pilosebaceous follicles

Related Facts
I **Sex Ratio:** M1:F1
II **Risk of Occurrence:** Very rare
III **Risk of Recurrence for**
  Patient's Sib: If parent is affected, 1 in 2 (50%) for each offspring to be affected; otherwise not increased.
  Patient's Child: 1 in 2
IV **Age of Detectability:** After puberty; 90% of affected men and women have their 1st lesion by 41 and 34 years of age, respectively.
V **Prevalence:** ? 11 families have been reported from Scotland and a similar number from North America and elsewhere.

Treatment
I **Primary Prevention:** Genetic counseling
II **Secondary Prevention:** Individual tumors should be excised as soon as they become apparent. Larger tumors may be excised or curetted.
III **Other Therapy:** Radiotherapy contraindicated

Prognosis: Normal for life span, intelligence and function

Detection of Carrier: —

Special Considerations: —

References:
Currie, A. R. and Smith, J. F.: Multiple primary spontaneous-healing squamous-cell carcinomata of skin. J. Pathol. Bacteriol. 64:827, 1952.
Ferguson-Smith, M.A. et al: Multiple self-healing squamous epithelioma. In Bergsma, D. (ed.): Part XII. Skin, Hair and Nails, Birth Defects: Orig. Art. Ser., vol. VII, no. 8. Baltimore:Williams & Wilkins Co. for The National Foundation- March of Dimes, 1971, p. 157.

Contributor: **Malcolm A. Ferguson-Smith**

Editor's Computerized Descriptor: Skin

EPULIS, CONGENITAL

Includes: Epulis
Épulis congénito
Congenital granular cell tumor
Congenital granular cell myoblastoma
Congenital rhabdomyoma
Myogenic xanthoma
Myoblastic myoma
Myoblastoma
Abrikossoff tumor
Myoepithelial tumor
Nodular myolysis
Granulocellular rhabdomyoma
Granular neuroma
Lipid fibroma
Granular cell neurofibroma
Granular cell perineural fibroblastoma
Granular cell pseudotumor
Lipoid thesaurismosis
Granular cell schwannoma

Excludes: Giant cell granuloma
Giant cell reparative granulomata
Melanotic neuroectodermal tumor of infancy
Eruption cysts
"Fibroma"

Minimal Diagnostic Criteria: A tumor or mass of maxilla or mandible in newborn or neonate having histopathologically distinctive features.

Clinical Findings: The lesion presents congenitally or neonatally as a single, rarely multiple, rounded smooth mass usually of the maxilla or, more rarely, of the mandible, having the color of normal oral mucosa. It is seen more often in females. It has been observed in a 10-week-premature infant.

Complications
I **Derived:** —
II **Associated:** —

Etiology: ?

Pathogenesis: ? The striking histologic similarity noted to exist between congenital epulis and granular cell tumor (granular cell myoblastoma) has led to the assumption that they are identical. This is possibly incorrect. While the histologic features observed in congenital epulis and granular cell tumor are similar, the pathogenesis or cause of the tumors may not be. The 2 conditions have recently been described together in 2 patients.

Related Facts
I **Sex Ratio:** M1:F10
II **Risk of Occurrence:** ?
III **Risk of Recurrence for**
  Patient's Sib: ?
  Patient's Child: ?
IV **Age of Detectability:** At birth, by physical examination and histologic verification
V **Prevalence:** ? Rare

Treatment
I **Primary Prevention:** —
II **Secondary Prevention:** Conservative surgical excision effects cure
III **Other Therapy:** —

Prognosis: Excellent. Recurrence not observed following surgical removal.

Detection of Carrier: —

Special Considerations: —

References:
Carstens, P. H. B.: Ultrastructure of granular cell myoblastoma.

Acta Pathol. Microbiol. Scand. (A)78:685, 1970.

Custer, R. P. and Fust, J. A.: Congenital epulis. Am. J. Clin. Pathol. 22:1044, 1952.

Dixter, C.T. et al: Congenital granular-cell tumor of alveolar ridge and tongue. Report of two cases. Oral Surg. 40:270, 1975.

Fuhr, A.H. and Krogh, H.J.: Congenital epulis of the newborn: Centennial review of the literature and report of a case. J. Oral Surg. 30:30, 1972.

Garancis, J.C. et al: Granular cell myoblastoma. Cancer 25:542, 1970.

Haisken, W. and Langer, E.: Submicroscopic structure of so-called myoblastic myoma (lipid fibroma, granular neuroma). Frankfurt. Z. Pathol. 71:600, 1962.

Hornstein, O. P. and Pape, H. D.: Zur Klinik und Histogenese der sog. Epulis connata. Fortschr. Kiefer Gesichtschir. 14:112, 1970.

Pearse, A. G. E.: The histogenesis of granular cell myoblastoma (? granular-cell perineural fibroblastoma). J. Pathol. Bacteriol. 62:351, 1950.

Vickers, R. A.: Mesenchymal (soft tissue) tumors of the oral region. In Gorlin, R.J. and Goldman, H.M. (eds.): Thoma's Oral Pathology. St. Louis:C.V. Mosby Co., 1970.

Contributor: **Robert A. Vickers**

Editor's Computerized Descriptor: Oral

ERYTHROKERATODERMIA, VARIABLE

Includes: Erythrokeratodermia variabilis Mendes da Costa
Eritroqueratoderma variable
Mendes da Costa syndrome
Keratosis rubra figurata
Erythrokeratoderma figurata variabilis
Erythrokeratoderma progressiva

Excludes: Congenital ichthyosiform erythroderma
Familial annular erythema
Annually recurring erythema
Erythema perstans

Minimal Diagnostic Criteria: Family history of similarly affected individuals having capriciously outlined erythematous patches together with hyperkeratotic plaques not directly related to the erythema. The histologic findings should show a massive laminated hyperkeratosis, acanthosis, and papillomatosis.

Clinical Findings: Capricious, discrete, configurate patches of erythema, extremely variable in size, position, duration and number. Although these are subject to environmental and emotional influence, being relatively transient in nature, some subsequently develop into fixed hyperkeratotic areas. The latter are sharply demarcated, persistent, yellow-brown hyperkeratotic plaques of geographic outline which usually arise on normal skin.

Complications

I Derived: —

II Associated: Atypical forms have been noted in which erythrokeratodermia is associated with neurologic disturbances. Five generations of a French-Canadian kindred exhibited a slowly progressive neurologic defect characterized by depressed deep tendon reflexes, nystagmus, dysarthria, and gait ataxia. There are also isolated reports of erythrokeratodermia occurring with perceptive deafness, psychic, and somatic retardation, and motor dysfunction.

Etiology: In most pedigrees, an autosomal dominant gene of variable expressivity.† McK *13320

Pathogenesis: Approximately one-third of case reports do not mention the presence of erythema. In those cases where it has been noted, it tends to localize to the face, buttocks, and extensor aspect of the limbs.

The hyperkeratotic lesions have a similar distribution. While they usually develop on normal skin, they may occasionally arise from persistent erythrodermic areas. Their tendency is to persist indefinitely, although rarely they may involute spontaneously. The palms and soles show a variable keratoderma. The Koebner phenomenon has been elicited in some of these cases. Autoradiographic studies reveal a normal epidermal proliferation rate indicating this to be a "retention type" of hyperkeratoses. Ultrastructure demonstrates a notable reduction in the number of keratinosomes.

Recent enzyme histochemical studies have demonstrated distinctive findings in 1 pedigree examined. Langerhans cells were absent in the epidermis, while acid phosphatase was found in the stratum corneum in parallel laminated tiers.

Related Facts

I Sex Ratio: M1:F1

II Risk of Occurrence: ? Very rare

III Risk of Recurrence for

Patient's Sib: If parent is affected 1 in 2, (50%) otherwise not increased.

Patient's Child: 1 in 2

IV Age of Detectability: Condition present at birth in some 30% of cases, with majority of remainder noting the onset during the 1st year of life, but onset may be delayed until 3rd year of life or later.

V **Prevalence:** ? Rare. Some 150 cases of variable erythrokeratodermia have been reported, the majority being from Europe. It has occurred in Negroes as well as in Caucasians.

Treatment
I **Primary Prevention:** Genetic counseling
II **Secondary Prevention:** —
III **Other Therapy:** Topical corticosteroids and keratolytics. Vitamin A is of limited benefit.†

Prognosis: The general tendency is for the process to increase in severity until puberty and then remain stationary or show gradual signs of improvement. The general health remains unaffected.

Detection of Carrier: —

†**Special Considerations:** Majority of pedigrees are consistent with an autosomal dominant transmission, but other modes of inheritance cannot be excluded in some families. Thorough examination of the parents, sibs and descendants of an affected individual is important because of the variable expressivity. As this condition is one of cosmetic importance only, only symptomatic therapy is warranted.

References:
Beare, J.M. et al: Atypical erythrokeratoderma with deafness, physical retardation and peripheral neuropathy. Br. J. Dermatol. 87:308, 1972.
Brown, J. and Kierland, R.R.: Erythrokeratoderma variabilis: Report of 3 cases and review of the literature. Arch. Dermatol. 93:194, 1966.
Giroux, J.M. and Barbeau, A.: Erythrokeratodermia with ataxia. Arch. Dermatol. 106:183, 1972.
Noordhoek, F.J.: Over Erythro- et keratodermia variabilis. N.V. Drukerij de Eendracht, Schiedam, W. Germany, 1950.
Schellander, F. and Fritsch, P.: Variable Erythrokeratodermien; Enzymhistochemische und Autoradiographische Untersuchungen an 2 Fällen. Arch. Klin. Exp. Dermatol. 235:241, 1969.
Vandersteen, P.R. and Muller, S.A.: Erythrokeratoderma variabilis: An enzyme histochemical and ultrastructural study. Arch. Dermatol. 103:362, 1971.

Contributor: **Paul R. Vandersteen**

Editor's Computerized Descriptor: Skin

ERYTHROPOIETIC PROTOPORPHYRIA

Includes: Protoporphyrie érythropoiétique
Protoporfiria eritropoyética
Protoporphyria, erythropoietic†

Excludes: Other photosensitizing forms of porphyria
Nonporphyric forms of polymorphic photodermatitis
Lipoid proteinosis (599)

Minimal Diagnostic Criteria: Photosensitivity accompanied by a significantly increased erythrocyte protoporphyrin level. In addition, red cell and normoblast fluorescence should be sought. Fecal protoporphyrin may or may not be increased.

Clinical Findings: Photosensitivity is usually manifested by burning and stinging of skin on exposure to sunlight for periods of minutes up to hours. This may occur through window glass as well as outdoors or through lightweight clothing. The burning may be mild or severe and may persist for days. Most patients also develop erythema and some edema in the affected areas, the latter sometimes persisting for weeks. Occasionally solar urticaria is the main or only manifestation. Vesicles, bullae, and purpura may occur. Scabs and crusts can form on these lesions and heal with superficial scars. Chronic skin lesions are usually mild, especially in patients who live in moderate climates. There may be some thickening and scarring on and around the nose, on the cheeks, and the backs of the hands and fingers. The chronic skin lesions are often more obvious in tropical areas where papular thickening of the skin may produce a "cobblestone" appearance. Absence of lunulae has been observed in some families. Erythrodontia has not been observed in this disease and hirsutism and hyperpigmentation occur only rarely, in contrast to congenital erythropoietic porphyria. Hemolytic anemia occurs only occasionally. It is suspected that there is an increased incidence of gallstones in this disease.

Complications
I **Derived:** Chronic skin lesions and possibly an increased incidence of gallstones
II **Associated:** —

Etiology: Autosomal dominant biochemical defect; McK *17700

Pathogenesis: The specific enzyme defect has not yet been elucidated, but present evidence indicates that excessive protoporphyrin can originate in the liver as well as the bone marrow in this disease.

Related Facts
I **Sex Ratio:** M1:F1
II **Risk of Occurrence:** Exact figures not known, but incidence of disease is much higher than congenital erythropoietic porphyria.
III **Risk of Recurrence for**
Patient's Sib: If parent is affected, 1 in 2 (50%) for each offspring to be affected; otherwise not increased.
Patient's Child: 1 in 2
IV **Age of Detectability:** The disease is detectable by chemical measurement in childhood, but it is not certain at what age the chemical abnormalities are always detectable.
V **Prevalence:** Exact figures not known, but probably 1 in 100,000

Treatment
I **Primary Prevention:** Genetic counseling
II **Secondary Prevention:** Preliminary studies suggest that large doses of β-carotene may be useful (see Mathews-Roth et al 1970). Some success has also been achieved by the topical use of dihydroxyacetone and lawsone in a vanishing cream base (Fusaro and Runge, 1970). Avoidance of sunlight

as much as possible.
III Other Therapy: —

Prognosis: There is no evidence at present to suggest any shortening of life span.

Detection of Carrier: This may be detected as an increase of erythrocyte protoporphyrin or as an increase of fecal protoporphyrin. Both these findings can occur in other disorders and are only specific in detecting carriers of this disease when the findings occur in a family with the disease documented.

†**Special Considerations:** Before this disease was recognized as a type of porphyria it was included in what is now called polymorphic photodermatitis or polymorphic light eruption (which included erythema solare perstans, prurigo aestivale, hydroa aestivale, hydroa vacciniforme, urticaria solaris, eczema solare, etc).

References:
Baer, R.L. et al: Erythropoietic protoporphyria: Photosensitivity patterns in man and laboratory animals. Dermatologica 135:5, 1967.
Fusaro, R.M. and Runge, W.J.: Erythropoietic protoporphyria: IV. Protection from sunlight. Br. Med. J. 1:730, 1970.
Mathews-Roth, M.M. et al: Beta-carotene as a photoprotective agent in erythropoietic protoporphyria. N. Engl. J. Med. 282:1231, 1970.
Reed, W.B. et al: Erythropoietic protoporphyria. JAMA 214:1060, 1970.

Contributor: **Donald P. Tschudy**

Editor's Computerized Descriptor: Skin

ESOPHAGEAL ACHALASIA

Includes: Achalasie oesophagienne
Achalasie
Acalasia esofágica
Cardiospasm
Megaesophagus

Excludes: Stricture of esophagus secondary to reflux
Esophagitis

Minimal Diagnostic Criteria: A large, poorly emptying esophagus without evidence of distal esophagitis or stricture by radiographic and endoscopic examination is diagnostic of achalasia. This is an unusual diagnosis to be made in the young child, but if one follows the rule of investigating persistent respiratory, deglutition or regurgitation complaints by barium swallow examination, it will not be overlooked.

Clinical Findings: Patients with achalasia often present with recurrent pneumonitis, stridor, regurgitation and failure to thrive. The very large, almost constantly filled esophagus may produce symptoms of pressure upon the airway, but most often in the child one finds poor weight gain or even weight loss with the return of undigested food hours or even days after its ingestion. In the young child aspiration pneumonitis may be a problem.

Complications
I Derived: Repeated aspiration pneumonitis, dysphagia or regurgitation with evidences of poor nutrition are less acute but are common presenting complications.
II Associated: —

Etiology: ?

Pathogenesis: This lesion apparently begins at an early age persisting with cardiospasm and leading eventually to secondary changes in the esophagus. Many have proposed abnormalities in the myenteric plexuses and the distal esophagus. A seemingly careful study by Cassella, Brown, Sayre and Ellis demonstrated, by electron microscopy, that the only persistent change in this condition was a Wallerian type degeneration of the vagus nerve. This data was supported experimentally by Long, Neiss, Thal and Truex after high cervical vagotomy in dogs produced a lesion very similar to achalasia. Protracted distal obstruction causes marked muscular hypertrophy of the esophagus. Inherent peristaltic defects which may be present are not helped in any way by this hypertrophy. Long periods of time may be required for resolution of this hypertrophic muscle following relief of the obstruction at the junction.

Related Facts
I Sex Ratio: M?:F?
II Risk of Occurrence: ?
III Risk of Recurrence for
    Patient's Sib: ?
    Patient's Child: ?
IV Age of Detectability: Childhood
V Prevalence: —

Treatment
I Primary Prevention: —
II Secondary Prevention: —
III Other Therapy: —

Prognosis: Of 227 patients treated by Ellis and his coworkers, 82% achieved an excellent or good result, 11% had a fair result and only 7% had a poor result after Heller myotomy. Poor results were considered to be no improvement or worsening of the condition.

Detection of Carrier: —

Special Considerations: —

References:

Cassella, R.R. et al: Achalasia of the esophagus: Pathologic and etiologic considerations. Ann. Surg. 160:474, 1964.

Ellis, F.H., Jr. et al: Esophagomyotomy for esophageal achalasia: Experimental, clinical, and manometric aspects. Ann. Surg. 166:640, 1967.

Long, D.M. et al: The experimental production of cardiospasm in dogs. Surg. Forum 9:408, 1959.

Tachovsky, T.J. et al: The surgical approach to esophageal achalasia in children. J. Pediatr. Surg. 3:226, 1968.

Contributors: **Thomas M. Holder**
Keith W. Ashcraft

Editor's Computerized Descriptors: Resp., GI.

ESOPHAGEAL ATRESIA

Includes: Atrésie oesophagienne
Oesophagusatresie
Atresia esofágica

Excludes: Esophageal atresia and tracheoesophageal fistula (365)
Esophageal stenosis (369)
Tracheoesophageal fistula, isolated

Minimal Diagnostic Criteria: Excessive salivation, regurgitation, obstruction in esophagus as tested by catheter and xray.

Clinical Findings: This defect is first detectable in the immediate neonatal period, usually brought to the attention of the examining physician by an alert nursery nurse. The presence of prematurity and polyhydramnios should suggest to the physician that an appropriate size catheter be passed and xrays taken to rule out the presence of esophageal atresia in the immediate postnatal period.

"Excessive salivation" is noted shortly after birth and is really only apparently excessive because the child cannot swallow his secretions. Regurgitation with feedings are characteristic. If the lesion remains untreated, dehydration or starvation follows.

Children suspected of having this lesion should have a stiff #10 or 12 French catheter passed via nose or mouth into the esophagus. An obstruction met with between 9 and 13 cm from the nares or upper alveolar ridge confirms the presence of atresia. A tube being passed further than this does not exclude atresia since the tube may coil in an atretic proximal esophagus. A portable upright chest xray with the tube in place should be taken in every infant in whom there is any question of esophageal atresia. This will 1) demonstrate the relative length of the upper pouch, 2) confirm the absence of a distal tracheoesophageal fistula, 3) document the status of the lungs, 4) demonstrate abnormalities in cardiac configuration, and 5) show skeletal abnormalities such as hemivertebra. It is helpful to put 1/2 cc of Dionosil into the upper esophagus for clearer identification of the pouch and perhaps demonstration of a fistula from the proximal esophagus to the trachea.

Complications

I   **Derived:** If untreated, the lesion is invariably fatal either through dehydration or starvation.

II **Associated:** Numerous severe congenital anomalies are associated with approximately half of the patients born with esophageal atresia anomalies. In order of frequency, these include congenital heart disease, GI anomalies, GU anomalies, imperforate anus, skeletal deformities, including many arm and hand abnormalities, cleft defects of the face, CNS lesions such as meningoceles or hydrocephaly and chromosome 21 trisomy syndrome. One-third of the patients are premature.

Etiology: Failure of normal development of the esophagus in the 4th embryonic week. Because of the frequency of associated anomalies which are also explainable on the basis of an unknown embryologic insult at approximately the same time, it is felt that this is a random, generalized insult to embryogenesis. The reasons for this insult are completely unknown.

Pathogenesis: Atresia of the esophagus occurs at the end of the 1st month of gestational life. The inability to swallow prevents the fetus participating in the normal turnover of amniotic fluid and may result in polyhydramnios and through this mechanism leads to premature birth. After birth, saliva cannot be swallowed and will be regurgitated through the mouth and nose. Feedings likewise will be taken usually with voracity, only to be returned a few moments later.

Related Facts

I   **Sex Ratio:**   M1:F1
II   **Risk of Occurrence:**   1 in 3000 live births
III   **Risk of Recurrence for**
   Patient's Sib: Not increased
   Patient's Child: Not increased
IV   **Age of Detectability:**   At birth by passage of nasogastric tube
   with chest xray
V   **Prevalence:**   ?

Treatment
I   **Primary Prevention:**   —
II   **Secondary Prevention:**   Establishment of a patent upper GI
   tract. These infants should be detected and treated early
   (preferably 1st day of life) and are best cared for in a pediatric surgical center.
      Preliminary gastrostomy and cervical esophagostomy are
   usually done. Definitive repair with colonic interposition is
   usually done at 1 year of age. Primary anastomosis of esophagus is rarely possible due to distance between upper and
   lower segments.
III   **Other Therapy:**   —

Prognosis: Once surgically corrected, this lesion alone should not
   interfere with the normal life span, but associated anomalies may
   alter the outlook.

Detection of Carrier: —

Special Considerations: —

References:
   Hendren, W.H. and Hale, J.R.: Electromagnetic bougienage to
      lengthen esophageal segments in congenital esophageal atresia.
      N. Engl. J. Med. 293:428, 1975.
   Holder, T.M. and Ashcraft, K.W.: Esophageal atresia and tracheo-
      esophageal fistula. Curr. Probl. Surg., 1966.

Contributors: **Thomas M. Holder**
                  Keith W. Ashcraft

Editor's Computerized Descriptor: GI.

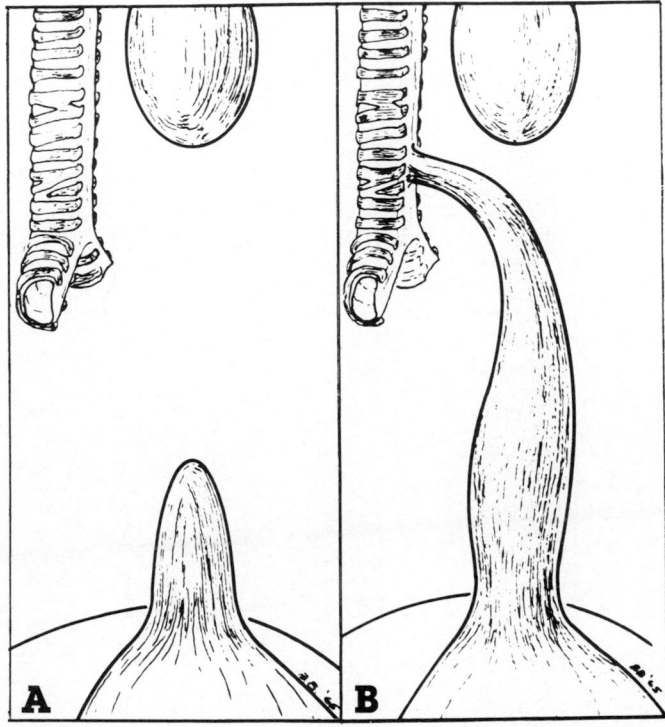

258. A) Esophageal atresia, B) with distal tracheoesophageal fistula

ESOPHAGEAL ATRESIA AND TRACHEOESOPHAGEAL FISTULA

Includes: Atrésie de l'oesophage avec fistule trachéo-oeso-
phagienne
Oesophagusatresie mit tracheo-oesophagealer fistel
Atresia del esófago con fistula traqueoesofágica
Tracheoesophageal fistula and esophageal atresia

Excludes: Laryngeal cleft
Laryngotracheal fissure
Common tracheoesophagus
Esophageal atresia (364)
Tracheoesophageal fistula (960)

Minimal Diagnostic Criteria: Radiographic demonstration of
blind upper esophagus and air in GI tract indicating a lower segment fistula. An upper pouch fistula to the trachea is demonstrated by injection of a small quantity of radiopaque contrast
material under fluoroscopic control.

Clinical Findings: Symptoms are always present from
birth but may not be recognized until the first feedings are
attempted. "Excessive" salivation and regurgitation may
be noted from birth. The salivation is really only apparently excessive because the child cannot swallow his secretions. Coughing, choking and cyanosis are associated with
overflow from a blind esophageal pouch into the trachea.
Tracheoesophageal fistula (TEF) communication may exist
between the distal esophageal segment > 85%, the proximal esophageal pouch < 1%, or between both segments <
1%.
   Acid reflux of gastric content through a distal segment
TEF combines with overflow of saliva and feedings from
the upper pouch to produce progressive chemical and bacterial aspiration pneumonia. Symptoms of tachypnea,
cyanosis and dyspnea progress to eventual collapse and
death. Gaseous distention of the GI tract is associated with
a patent fistula between the trachea and the lower esophageal segment. This may not be appreciated without a
radiograph. Absence of air in the GI tract does not exclude
the uncommon fistulous communication between trachea
and proximal esophageal pouch or the less common situation where a distal segment fistula is occluded with a
mucus plug. The failure of a catheter to pass from the nose
or mouth into the stomach raises initial suspicion of esophageal atresia. The presence or absence of associated TEF
requires radiographic study. The most common variety
with proximal blind esophageal pouch and distal TEF is
confirmed by a lateral radiograph demonstrating a coiled
catheter in the proximal esophageal segment and air in the
GI tract.
   Fistulae from the upper pouch of the trachea are frequently missed. Careful instillation of contrast media under fluoroscopic control is the best way to avoid spillover of
the material into the trachea yet demonstrate a fistula, if
present.

Complications
I   **Derived:**   *Before corrective surgery:* Repeated contamination
      of the airway with ingested liquids and regurgitated gastric
      contents leads to varying degrees of pneumonitis. The infant
      forces air through the tracheoesophageal fistula into the
      stomach when crying, which makes regurgitation easier.
      The gastric distention also elevates the diaphragm and inter-
      feres with respiratory activity in the early neonatal period.
         After surgical treatment: Recurrence of isolated TEF; leak
      from tracheal or esophageal closure leading to mediastinitis,
      unrecognized pneumothorax, recurrent laryngeal nerve in-
      jury causing laryngeal obstruction, esophageal stenosis and
      tracheal stenosis. Gastroesophageal reflux of some degree is

present following repair of esophageal atresia in almost all cases. When severe, it may result in aspiration, apneic episodes or esophagitis and stricture.

II **Associated:** Over half (58%) have associated defects including: cardiac, GI, GU, musculoskeletal, CNS, facial and other anomalies, or imperforate anus.

Etiology: Failure of normal development and division of the tracheobronchial tree in the 4th embryonic week. Because of the frequency of associated anomalies which are also explainable on the basis of an unknown embryologic insult at approximately the same time, it is felt that this is a random, generalized insult to embryogenesis. The reasons for this insult are completely unknown. TEF with esophageal atresia has been reported in sibs and in one member of twins; only on 6 occasions has there been a report of both twins being affected by this disorder.

Pathogenesis: Atresia of the esophagus and tracheoesophageal fistula occurs at the end of the 1st month of gestational life. The inability to swallow effectively prevents the fetus participating in the normal turnover of amniotic fluid and may result in polyhydramnios and, through this mechanism, to premature birth. After birth, saliva cannot be properly swallowed and will be regurgitated through the mouth and nose. Feedings, likewise, will be taken with voracity, only to be returned a few moments later. There may be a communication between the upper esophageal pouch and the trachea which will allow saliva to be constantly discharged into the airway, resulting in bacterial pneumonitis. More frequently, there is a communication between the distal esophagus and the airway, allowing for gastric acid to be regurgitated into the airway, resulting in a severe chemical pneumonitis. The latter probably becomes rapidly infected. With crying in the neonatal period, the intratracheal pressure is raised and air passes freely down the distal tracheoesophageal fistula into the stomach. The stomach distends and, depending upon the child's position, allows for easy regurgitation of gastric acid up into the airway. A 2nd feature is the distention of the stomach interfering with the normal diaphragmatic motion in the newborn and thus creating respiratory insufficiency.

Related Facts
I   **Sex Ratio:**   M1:F1
II **Risk of Occurrence:**   1 in 3000 live births
III **Risk of Recurrence for**
     Patient's Sib: Not increased
     Patient's Child: Not increased
IV **Age of Detectability:**   At birth or after liquid feeding
V   **Prevalence:**   ?

Treatment
I   **Primary Prevention:**   —
II **Secondary Prevention:**   Surgical division of fistula with closure of tracheal defect and primary or staged reconstruction of esophageal atresia.†
III **Other Therapy:**   —

Prognosis: Probably normal life span without disability, if repair of isolated fistula is uncomplicated and other anomalies do not coexist. Abnormalities of lower esophageal motility may persist indefinitely. Prognosis then depends upon severity of disorder and degree of gastroesophageal reflux or aspiration.

Detection of Carrier: —

†**Special Considerations:** In the surgically corrected child with esophageal atresia and TEF there are occasional late anastomotic strictures of the esophagus which produce dysphagia. The presence of a mechanical obstruction can be determined by a contrast radiographic study to demonstrate the esophagus. There is evidence to suggest that even in the absence of organic stricture, an inherent neuromuscular defect may exist below the level of the

anastomosis or the tracheoesophageal fistula which will interfere with normal swallowing. This may be a troublesome complication, but is not likely to cause nutritional difficulties.

References:
Haight, C.: Congenital esophageal atresia and tracheoesophageal fistula. In Benson, C.D. et al (eds.): Pediatric Surgery. Chicago: Year Book Medical Publishers, 1962, vol. 1, p. 266.
Holder, T. M. and Ashcraft, K. W.: Esophageal atresia and tracheoesophageal fistula. Curr. Probl. Surg., 1, 1966.

Contributors: **Dale G. Johnson**
                     Thomas M. Holder

Editor's Computerized Descriptors: Resp., GI.

ESOPHAGEAL CHALASIA

Includes: Reflux oesophagien
Chalasie
Calasia esofágica
Gastroesophageal reflux without radiographically or surgically de-
monstrable hiatus hernia

Excludes: Hiatus hernia (471)

Minimal Diagnostic Criteria: Chalasia may be assumed if by
esophagram there is a relaxed cardiac sphincter with easy gastroesophageal reflux and if hiatus hernia is excluded. The demonstration of actual herniation of the stomach above the diaphragm
is often very difficult. Persistence of vomiting, failure to thrive,
unexplained anemia, or respiratory distress due to regurgitation
or aspiration should prompt barium studies of the esophagus.

Clinical Findings: Chalasia and gastroesophageal reflux is
a common condition among newborns and is usually self-
limiting. Persistent easy regurgitation or even vomiting of
a mildly projectile nature after feedings is aggravated by
lying down, being handled or by crying. Respiratory distress may occur due to laryngospasm or aspiration may
lead to pneumonitis. This may be severe in either case and
even life-threatening. Propping the infant upright in a
chalasia chair coupled with thickened feedings and a
period of rest after feedings will generally obviate the reflux and control symptoms to a large degree until such time
as the cardiac sphincter mechanism begins to function normally and the reflux ceases to become a problem.

Complications
I **Derived:** Although chalasia is generally self-limiting, rarely
peptic esophagitis may lead to stricture formation requiring
operative relief. The pulmonary aspiration and laryngos-
pasm may be most severe and the cause of greatest morbidity.

II **Associated:** —

Etiology: ? An immaturity or a neuromuscular imbalance of the
sphincter mechanism at the gastroesophageal junction is believed
to be present.

Pathogenesis: Since there is no effective sphincter "mechanism"
at the gastroesophageal junction in these children, any activity
which increases intraabdominal pressure relative to the intrathoracic pressure will result in reflux. With a full stomach, normal
inspiratory activity may result in regurgitation of liquid content
up into the esophagus and aspiration may be possible. Also in the
prone or supine position the stomach will empty into the esophagus quite readily because of gravity.

Related Facts
I **Sex Ratio:** M1:F1
II **Risk of Occurrence:** ?
III **Risk of Recurrence for**
   Patient's Sib: ?
   Patient's Child: ?
IV **Age of Detectability:** Neonatal period
V **Prevalence:** ?

Treatment
I **Primary Prevention:** —
II **Secondary Prevention:** A chalasia chair at a 60° upright
position at all times day and night and avoidance of stimulation of the child immediately after feeding will tend to overcome the symptoms. Severe acute or chronic sequelae of
gastroesophageal reflux are becoming more regularly recognized. These complications are usually respiratory and may
be manifested by recurrent croup-like symptoms, aspiration
pneumonitis and even sudden infant death. Fundoplication
is recommended for complicated cases where positional
therapy has been ineffective.

III **Other Therapy:** —

Prognosis: The large majority will respond to nonoperative management, and the prognosis is excellent in most cases.

Detection of Carrier: —

Special Considerations: —

References:
Botha, G. S. M.: The Gastro-Esophageal Junction: Clinical Applications to Oesophageal and Gastric Surgery. Boston: Little, Brown
and Co., 1962, p.341.
Randolph, J.G. et al: Surgical treatment of gastroesophageal reflux
in infants. Ann. Surg. 180:479, 1974.

Contributors: **Thomas M. Holder**
Keith W. Ashcraft

Editor's Computerized Descriptors: Resp., GI.

ESOPHAGEAL DIVERTICULUM

Includes: Diverticule de l'oesophage
Oesophagusdivertikel
Divertículo del esófago
Pharyngoesophageal diverticulum
True esophageal diverticulum

Excludes: Pulsion or tension esophageal diverticula
Esophageal duplication (368)

Minimal Diagnostic Criteria: Dysphagia, regurgitation and barium contrast study of the esophagus.†

Clinical Findings: These usually produce symptoms at a very early age either of esophageal obstruction or aspiration or obstruction of airway. Regurgitated food may be old and is unchanged by gastric acid. There may be a mass lesion visible in the neck if the diverticulum is high, or by chest xray if it is low. The obstructive symptoms at the thoracic inlet may be severe and are notably intermittent. Since the lesion makes aspiration easy, pneumonitis may be the prominent presenting feature. Barium swallow oftentimes will show contrast material in a pouch, or external pressure upon an esophagus if the pouch should be filled with food.

Complications
I **Derived:** Aspiration is the most prominent threat, complete airway obstruction with asphyxiation may occur. Starvation is a late inexcusable complication.
II **Associated:** —

Etiology: ?

Pathogenesis: A true diverticulum is generally located in the upper one-third of the esophagus and contains mucosa, submucosa and muscular coats thus differentiating it from an acquired pulsion diverticulum. Obstruction secondary to a filled diverticulum produces the symptoms which call attention to the malformation.

Related Facts
I **Sex Ratio:** M?:F?
II **Risk of Occurrence:** ?
III **Risk of Recurrence for**
  Patient's Sib: ?
  Patient's Child: ?
IV **Age of Detectability:** Early neonatal period
V **Prevalence:** Very rare

Treatment
I **Primary Prevention:** —
II **Secondary Prevention:** Surgical excision is the only treatment of lasting benefit.
III **Other Therapy:** —

Prognosis: The prognosis is excellent once surgical treatment has been carried out.†

Detection of Carrier: —

†**Special Considerations:** These are extremely rare lesions but may be fatal by the mechanism of airway obstruction before they have been diagnosed.

References:
Haight, C.: The esophagus. In Benson, C.D. et al (eds.): Pediatric Surgery. Chicago: Year Book Medical Publishers, 1962, vol. 1, p. 266.

Contributors: **Thomas M. Holder**
Keith W. Ashcraft

Editor's Computerized Descriptors: Resp., GI.

ESOPHAGEAL DUPLICATION

Includes: Duplication de l'oesophage
Duplikation des Oesophagus
Duplicación del esófago
Esophageal cyst

Excludes: Esophageal diverticulum (367)
Bronchogenic cysts

Minimal Diagnostic Criteria: Mass lesion in the posterior mediastinum seen on barium contrast xray to be in continuity with the musculature of the esophagus.

Clinical Findings: Dysphagia is the single most common symptom of esophageal duplication. Respiratory distress, either as a result of partial obstruction of the esophagus by the extrinsic pressure created by this mass or by actual pressure upon the trachea, may also be the presenting complaint. Occasionally ulceration will result in bleeding as the presenting feature. A number of these lesions are incidental findings on chest xrays, and on very careful questioning absolutely no symptoms can be elicited referable to the lesion. A duplication is generally found in the older child or adult and will appear on xray as a posterior, usually well-rounded, mediastinal mass. A smooth filling defect in the esophagus on barium study suggests extrinsic pressure.

Complications
I **Derived:** Regurgitation of food, persistent respiratory problems, failure to thrive. Anemia may ensue if bleeding is a symptom.
II **Associated:** —

Etiology: ?

Pathogenesis: It is suspected that vacuoles develop in the thickened endoderm of the primitive foregut, and this may persist as a cystic duplication. Proof for this theory is lacking, but support is gained from the fact that a common muscular wall is shared by the true esophagus and by the duplicated segment. These lesions grow with the child, and most are separate, although rarely there may be a small communication with the esophageal lumen. They are oftentimes filled with a thin fluid and gradually enlarge. The lining may occasionally bear respiratory epithelium. Most are squamous lined, and all are located within the muscle of the esophageal wall.

Related Facts
I **Sex Ratio:** M1:F1
II **Risk of Occurrence:** ?
III **Risk of Recurrence for**
  Patient's Sib: ?
  Patient's Child: ?
IV **Age of Detectability:** Infancy to adulthood
V **Prevalence:** ?

Treatment
I **Primary Prevention:** —
II **Secondary Prevention:** Surgical removal
III **Other Therapy:** —

Prognosis: Complete recovery following surgical removal is to be expected.

Detection of Carrier: —

Special Considerations: —

References:
Gross R.E.: Surgery of Infancy and Childhood. Philadelphia: W.B. Saunders, 1953.

Holder, T.M.: The esophagus and stomach. In Walters, W. (ed.): Lewis-Walters Practice of Surgery. Hagerstown: W.F. Prior, 1965.

Contributors: **Thomas M. Holder**
Keith W. Ashcraft

Editor's Computerized Descriptors: Resp., GI.

ESOPHAGEAL STENOSIS

Includes: Sténose de l'oesophage
Oesophagusstenose
Estenosis del esófago
Congenital esophageal stricture
Esophageal web or veil
Congenital diaphragm of esophagus

Excludes: Upper esophageal web of Plummer-Vinson syndrome
Lower esophageal lesions such as Schatzke ring
Strictures secondary to reflux esophagitis
Esophageal lesions, acquired

Minimal Diagnostic Criteria: Neonatal dysphagia and regurgitation barium study are evidence for esophageal stricture. Acquired lesions in distal third of esophagus must be ruled out. There are children with hiatus hernia known to have had severe esophageal strictures in the 1st week or 2 of life. The strictures are presumed by most to be acquired lesions secondary to a hiatus hernia.

Clinical Findings: Dysphagia beginning in the immediate neonatal period is a necessity for the diagnosis of congenital esophageal stenosis. It may be more severe at one time than another and will obviously become more troublesome with the addition of semisolids and solids to the diet. Regurgitation of unchanged food is characteristic of this lesion. Aspiration pneumonitis is certainly not an infrequent finding because the reflex epiglottic closure mechanisms in the newborn infant are probably immature and fail to prevent aspiration with regurgitation. Barium swallow shows a narrowing or web characteristically in the middle third just below the tracheal bifurcation with proximal dilatation being very frequent.

Complications
I   **Derived:** Failure to thrive is the most common complication of this lesion. Aspiration may occur. Too often the early regurgitation or difficulty with swallowing is passed off as "normal" in the newborn infant, and thus complete radiographic investigation may not be carried out until failure to gain weight is noticed. Very occasionally a bolus of solid food which would normally pass will lodge causing an acute obstruction, as will small foreign bodies, but generally the patient who presents in this way is older than a neonate.
II   **Associated:** —

Etiology: ?

Pathogenesis: It has been postulated that most of these lesions of a congenital stenotic nature occur at the point where the esophagus gives origin to the tracheobronchial tree, ie the bifurcation of the trachea, and the same point where esophageal atresia occurs. Esophageal stenosis is unusual, but the documented ones consist of a firm, fibrous ring or web of mucosa only varying in length. The obstruction results in dilatation proximal to the stenosis with subsequent hypertrophy of the muscle.

Related Facts
I   **Sex Ratio:** M1:F1
II   **Risk of Occurrence:** ?
III   **Risk of Recurrence for**
      Patient's Sib: ?
      Patient's Child: ?
IV   **Age of Detectability:** Usually neonatal
V   **Prevalence:** ?

Treatment
I   **Primary Prevention:** —
II   **Secondary Prevention:** Dilatations will normally suffice. Some children will require resection with esophagostomy, and some with longer strictures may even require esophageal substitution procedures.

III **Other Therapy:** None is needed if the obstruction is relieved.

Prognosis: The prognosis is excellent once the condition is relieved.

Detection of Carrier: —

Special Considerations: —

References:
Gross, R. E.: Surgery of Infancy and Childhood. Philadelphia: W.B. Saunders, 1953.
Holder, T. M.: The esophagus and stomach. In Walters, W. (ed.): Lewis-Walters Practice of Surgery. Hagerstown: W.F. Prior, 1965.

Contributors: **Thomas M. Holder**
Keith W. Ashcraft

Editor's Computerized Descriptors: Resp., GI.

EUSTACHIAN TUBE DEFECTS

Includes: Anomalies de la trompe d'eustache
Fehlbildungen der Eustachischen Röhre
Defectos de la trompa de eustaquio
Eustachian tube atresia
Congenital defects of eustachian tube
Eustachian tube cysts
Eustachian tube tumors

Excludes: Functional defects secondary to cleft palate
Carcinoma and other acquired tumors of the nasopharynx

Minimal Diagnostic Criteria: Intractable serous or chronic otitis media with conductive hearing loss and evidence of a congenital defect of the 1st, 2nd or 3rd branchial arch.

Clinical Findings: Congenital defects of the eustachian tube are evident primarily by intractable serous otitis media or chronic otitis media with perforation or cholesteatoma. A cyst or tumor may be seen in the nasopharynx or protympanum. If found in association with absence of tympanic portion of the temporal bone, an external canal bony atresia plate will be seen. Audiometric findings consist of a conductive hearing loss.

Complications
I **Derived:** Tympanic membrane perforation with hearing loss. Middle ear cholesteatoma secondary to perforation or severe retraction.
II **Associated:** Eustachian tube abnormalities frequently seen with brachycephaly, where a short straight infantile tube is found; and in dolichocephaly, in which there is a marked narrowing and angulation of the isthmus, with an easily obstructed lumen.

Etiology: ?

Pathogenesis: These lesions are rare and diversified.†

Related Facts
I **Sex Ratio:** M?:F?
II **Risk of Occurrence:** ? Very rare
III **Risk of Recurrence for**
  Patient's Sib: ?
  Patient's Child: ?
IV **Age of Detectability:** Audiometric and otologic examination may reveal hearing loss with serous otitis within the first 6 months of life.
V **Prevalence:** ? Very rare

Treatment
I **Primary Prevention:** —
II **Secondary Prevention:** Permanent artificial middle ear ventilation is necessary to prevent serous otitis and retraction cholesteatoma.
III **Other Therapy:** —

Prognosis: Good unless abnormality is due to neoplasm. Prognosis poor for adequate ear function unless artificial middle ear ventilation is provided.

Detection of Carrier: —

†**Special Considerations:** There is an extreme paucity of histopathologic material concerning defects of the eustachian tube. 1) Reported congenital neoplasms of the eustachian tube are extremely rare, but include 2 dysontogenic dermoids. 2) Branchial cyst of arch III origin has been reported as a mass below the floor of the eustachian tube with obstruction. 3) Bony defects of development have been associated with external canal atresia and defects of the tympanic cavity. 4) Multiple temporal bones have been examined histologically by Schuknecht and no eustachian tube abnormalities found in cases of: chondrodystrophy, meatal atresia, cretinism, craniofacial dysostosis, mucopolysac-

charidosis I, osteogenesis imperfecta, phocomelia, rubella embryopathy, Paget disease, otosclerosis, renal rickets, osteomalacia, or temporal bone fractures.

References:
Krukover, I. cited in Weltzer, P.: Anatomy and physiology of the ear. Arch. Otolaryngol. 7:167, 1928.
Proctor, B.: Embryology and anatomy of the eustachian tube. Arch. Otolaryngol. 86:503, 1967.
Schuknecht, H.F. and Kerr, A.G.: Pathology of the eustachian tube. Arch. Otolaryngol. 86:497, 1967.

Contributor: Daniel R. Miller

Editor's Computerized Descriptors: Hearing, Ear, Nasoph., Skel.

EYELID ECTROPION, CONGENITAL

Includes: Ectropion congénital
Angeborene Lid-Ektropie
Ectropión congénito de los párpados
Congenital ectropion of conjunctiva
Congenital ectropion of lids

Excludes: Total eversion of upper lids

Minimal Diagnostic Criteria: A space exists not only between the lid margin and the globe, but also the lids do not appose each other when closed.

Clinical Findings: The lid margins are everted exposing the palpebral conjunctiva. Ectropion is more common in the lower than the upper lids because the tarsal plates of the latter are stronger and because the effects of gravity predispose to eversion of the lower but not the upper lids.†

Complications
I   **Derived:** Ectropion of the lower lid leads to pooling of tears and epiphoria. If associated with lagophthalmos (poor closure of eyelids secondary to defective orbicularis muscle), exposure keratitis may result.
II **Associated:** Ptosis, strabismus, lagophthalmos, absence of lacrimal puncta, madarosis, distichiasis (double rows of eyelashes), euryblepharon (long lid fissures), blepharophimosis (short lid fissures) and hypoplasia of the tarsal plates and meibomian glands. Ectropion has been reported in association with chromosome 21 trisomy and with abnormal chromosome 1.

Etiology: Unknown since cases are rare and usually sporadic. A few kindreds with this syndrome are compatible with autosomal dominant inheritance.

Pathogenesis: ?

Related Facts
I   **Sex Ratio:** M?:F?
II   **Risk of Occurrence:** Unknown specifically but rare
III **Risk of Recurrence for**
     Patient's Sib: When autosomal dominant, 1 in 2 (50%) for each offspring to be affected.
     Patient's Child: When autosomal dominant, 1 in 2
IV   **Age of Detectability:** At birth
V   **Prevalence:** ?

Treatment
I   **Primary Prevention:** Genetic counseling when autosomal dominant
II   **Secondary Prevention:** Plastic eyelid surgery
III **Other Therapy:** Prevention of exposure keratitis

Prognosis: Usually nonprogressive except for threat of exposure keratitis

Detection of Carrier: —

†Special Considerations: Ectropion may occur secondarily to microphthalmos, buphthalmos and orbitopalpebral cysts as well as to a number of congenital diseases which cause shrinkage of skin of the lids; eg ichthyosis, keratosis follicularis, spinulosa decalvans, erythroderma ichthyosiforme congenitum, xeroderma pigmentosum and lamellar exfoliation of the newborn. Total eversion of the upper lids in otherwise normal newborns is thought to be secondary to birth trauma. The lids are edematous and the conjunctiva chemotic. Eversion disappears as the swelling resolves in 2 or 3 weeks. The corneas must meanwhile be protected.

References:
Duke-Elder, S.: System of Ophthalmology. vol. 3, pt. 2. Congenital

Deformities. St. Louis: C.V. Mosby Co., 1963, p. 864.

Johnson, C.C. and McGowan, B.L.: Persistent congenital ectropion of all four eyelids with megaloblepharon. Am. J. Ophthalmol. 67:252, 1969.

Mortada, A.: Lamella exfoliation of the newborn and ectropion of the eyelids. Ophthalmologica (Basel) 152:68, 1966.

Waardenburg, P.J. et al: Genetics and Ophthalmology. Oxford: Blackwell Scientific Publications, Ltd., 1961 vol. 1. p. 235.

Contributor: Donald R. Bergsma

Editor's Computerized Descriptor: Eye

EYELID ENTROPION

Includes: Entropion
Entropion des Augenlids
Entropión del párpado
Congenital entropion of lid

Excludes: Entropion of iris
Secondary entropion
Epiblepharon (355)

Minimal Diagnostic Criteria: Inversion of tarsus

Clinical Findings: The tarsus of the eyelid is inverted or turned inward toward the globe with resultant rubbing of the lashes against the cornea. It usually affects the lower lid and is more often bilateral than unilateral. It may be found as an isolated phenomenon or in association with other anomalies, especially epicanthus and epiblepharon. The latter has been postulated to cause, in some instances, entropion. In the presence of anomalies of the globe, such as microphthalmia or anophthalmia, both upper and lower lids may be secondarily inverted.

Complications
I   **Derived:**   Keratitis and traumatic pannus are seen from trauma of the lashes rubbing against the cornea.
II   **Associated:**   Epicanthus, epiblepharon, antimongoloid obliquity of the palpebral fissures, anophthalmia, microphthalmia, polytrichia, bone defects of skull and clubfeet

Etiology: Autosomal dominant transmission has been reported.

Pathogenesis: Defective development of the tarsal plate, hypertrophy of the tarsus, hypertrophy of the palpebral portion of the orbicularis muscle, and attachments of the orbicularis and inferior rectus muscles into the skin of the lid have all been implicated as possible factors in the pathogenesis of entropion.

In combination with epiblepharon, the excess fold of skin may cause backward pressure on the ciliary margin with inward turning of the lid.

Lack of support to the lid margins in the presence of small or absent globes may result in the inward turning from a mechanical defect.

Related Facts
I   **Sex Ratio:**   M1:F1
II   **Risk of Occurrence:**   Rare
III   **Risk of Recurrence for**
   Patient's Sib: When autosomal dominant and if parent is affected, 1 in 2 (50%) for each offspring to be affected; otherwise not increased.
   Patient's Child: 1 in 2, when autosomal dominant
IV   **Age of Detectability:**   At birth
V   **Prevalence:**   Rare

Treatment
I   **Primary Prevention:**   Genetic counseling
II   **Secondary Prevention:**   Surgical repair is usually necessary in entropion. The type of procedure is dependent upon the area and extent of involvement and associated complications.
III   **Other Therapy:**   —

Prognosis: Good

Detection of Carrier: Affected parent and patient when autosomal dominant

Special Considerations: —

References:
Bacskulin, J. and Bacskulin, E.: Beitrag zur Klinik und Therapie des kongenitalen Entropiums. Ophthalmologica 151:555, 1966.
Hiles, D.A. and Wilder, L.W.: Congenital entropion of the upper lids. J. Pediatr. Ophthalmol. 6:157, 1969.

Contributor: Elsa K. Rahn

FABRY DISEASE

Includes: Maladie de Fabry
Mb. Fabry
Enfermedad de Fabry
Angiokeratoma corporis diffusum universale
Glycolipid lipidosis
Di- and trihexosyl ceramide lipidosis
Fabry-Anderson disease
Hereditary dystopic lipidosis
Ruiter-Pompen-Wyers syndrome

Excludes: Angiokeratoma Mibelli
Hereditary hemorrhagic telangiectasia
Rheumatic fever
Erythromelalgia

Minimal Diagnostic Criteria: Hemizygotes can be diagnosed by a history of acroparesthesia and the presence of the characteristic skin lesions and corneal opacities. Heterozygotes may be asymptomatic or manifest attenuated symptoms, particularly corneal lesions. Birefringent lipid can be observed histologically in biopsied tissues, bone marrow macrophages, or urinary sediment. All cases should be confirmed biochemically by the demonstration of increased levels of trihexosyl ceramide in urinary sediment, plasma, or cultured fibroblasts, or by deficient α-galactosidase A activity in plasma, isolated leukocytes, tears or cultured fibroblasts.†

Clinical Findings: *Hemizygous males* usually have the onset of the disease during childhood or adolescence. It is characterized by periodic, excruciating acroparesthesia which may become more frequent and severe with age. These painful episodes may last several days and are associated with a low grade fever and an elevation of the erythrocyte sedimentation rate; these symptoms have frequently led to the misdiagnosis of rheumatic fever. During the 2nd and 3rd decades of life, these recurrent episodes may become progressively more painful and debilitating. The cutaneous vascular lesions, angiokeratoma, usually appear during childhood and progressively increase in number with age. Characteristically, they are most dense between the umbilicus and knees and do not blanch with pressure. Variants without these lesions have also been reported. Ocular manifestations include aneurysmal dilation and tortuosity of conjunctival and retinal vessels and corneal opacities. The opacities are characterized by diffuse haziness or whorled streaks in the corneal epithelium and must be observed by slit-lamp microscopy. With increasing age, the major symptoms result from involvement of the renal-cardiovascular system. Early in the course of the disease, casts, red cells, and lipid inclusions with characteristic birefringent "Maltese crosses" appear in the urinary sediment. Proteinuria, isothenuria, and gradual deterioration of renal function and development of azotemia occur in the 2nd to 4th decade of life. Cardiovascular findings in late maturity may include hypertension, left ventricular hypertrophy, myocardial ischemia or infarction, and cerebral vascular disease. Nausea, vomiting, diarrhea, and abdominal or flank pain are common GI symptoms. Hypohydrosis is a common feature; other less frequent symptoms include massive edema of the legs, and dyspnea. Musculoskeletal system findings include a permanent deformity of the distal interphalangeal joint of the fingers, osteoporosis of dorsal vertebrae, and avascular necrosis of the head of femur and talus. These patients have a mild hypochromic microcytic anemia, presumably due to decreased red cell survival. Many hemizygotes appear to have growth retardation or delayed puberty. Affected individuals may complain of fatigue and weakness and may be incapacitated for prolonged periods of time. Death most often results from uremia or vascular disease of the heart or brain during the 4th decade of life.

Heterozygous females may be asymptomatic or may, in attenuated form, manifest many of the same symptoms as the hemizygous males. Skin lesions and corneal opacities are present in the majority of these carriers of the Fabry gene. The clinical course and prognosis are more favorable in heterozygotes than hemizygotes and a reasonable longevity may be expected. With age, however, most heterozygotes become more symptomatic and death usually results from renal or cardiac insufficiency. Rare heterozygous females as severely affected as hemizygous males have been described.

Complications
I   **Derived:** Renal insufficiency leading to uremia, cardiovascular involvement.
II **Associated:** Seizures, subacute bacterial endocarditis, chronic bronchitis.

Etiology: X-linked transmission with complete penetrance and variable clinical expressivity in hemizygous males. Expressivity in heterozygous females ranges from usually asymptomatic individuals to rare females with severe manifestations of the disease.† McK *30150

Pathogenesis: Fabry disease is characterized by the systemic accumulation of the glycosphingolipids, trihexosyl and digalactosyl ceramide, particularly in the cardiovascular-renal system. The anatomic and physiologic alterations in this disorder result from the unique tissue distribution of the deposited glycosphingolipids. The progressive onset of the clinical manifestations suggests that, as the deposition of glycosphingolipid at a particular site reaches "threshold level" the resultant clinical or functional symptom becomes manifest. The primary metabolic defect is the defective activity of the lysosomal hydrolase, α-galactosidase A, which normally catabolizes the accumulated glycosphingolipids. Tetrahexosyl ceramide, released from senescent erythrocytes, is the metabolic precursor of trihexosyl ceramide and is the major erythrocyte glycosphingolipid. It has been postulated that the defective enzymatic activity results in the accumulation of trihexosyl ceramide in tissues and particularly in the plasma. Accumulated plasma trihexosyl ceramide presumably gains access to the endothelial and adjacent epithelial cells of the glomerulus and to endothelial and adjacent perithelial cells of blood vessels throughout the body; these vascular sites are the most involved areas of glycosphingolipid deposition in this disease.

Related Facts
I   **Sex Ratio:** M1:F(rare). Disease manifestations usually limited to males.
II **Risk of Occurrence:** ? estimate: approximately 1/40,000
III **Risk of Recurrence for**
    Patient's Sib: If mother is a carrier, 1 in 2 (50%) for each brother to be affected and 1 in 2 for each sister to be a carrier.
    Patient's Child: For hemizygous patients, all daughters will be carriers, all sons will be normal. For heterozygous patients, 1 in 2 (50%) daughters will be carriers of the gene, 1 in 2 (50%) sons will be affected.
IV **Age of Detectability:** Antenatal, as well as postnatal, diagnosis of hemizygotes can be accomplished by demonstration of the enzymatic deficiency. Screening of suspected individuals can be done in the first days of life by determining the α-galactosidase A activity in plasma or tears.
V   **Prevalence:** Of the over 200 cases reported, most have oc-

curred in Caucasians of Western European extraction; however, Oriental, Negro, Egyptian, and Latin American patients have been described. The disease has not been reported in American Indians.

Treatment
I   **Primary Prevention:** Genetic counseling
II **Secondary Prevention:** Heterozygote identification and antenatal detection. Enzyme replacement therapy may be feasible in the future. Kidney transplantation in appropriate individuals.
III **Other Therapy:** Painful Fabry crises may be relieved and prevented by low-maintenance doses of diphenylhydantoin or carbamazepine. Treatment of renal, cardiovascular, pulmonary and musculoskeletal problems remains symptomatic at present.

Prognosis: Average reported life span of affected males is 41 years. Asymptomatic heterozygotes generally have a normal life span; however, symptomatic heterozygotes have been reported to expire in the 4th and 5th decades of life.

Detection of Carrier: Heterozygotes for Fabry disease can be biochemically identified by their intermediate levels of 1) increased trihexosyl ceramide in urinary sediment or cultured fibroblasts, or 2) α-galactosidase A activity in plasma, leukocytes, tears or cultured fibroblasts.

†Special Considerations: Hemizygotic variants without the classic skin lesions have been reported. Interfamilial variation in the clinical manifestations suggests multiple mutant alleles at the X-linked locus for this disorder. Enzyme replacement therapy is experimental at present; further experience will determine its therapeutic effectiveness.

References:
Desnick, R.J. et al: Fabry's disease: Enzymatic diagnosis of hemizygotes and heterozygotes. Alpha-galactosidase activities in plasma, serum, leukocytes and urine. J. Lab. Clin. Med. 81:157, 1973.
Desnick, R.J. et al: Towards enzyme therapy for lysosomal storage diseases. Physiol. Rev. 56:57, 1976.
Desnick, R.J. et al: Fabry's disease. In Stanbury, J.B. et al (eds.): The Metabolic Basis of Inherited Disease, 4th Ed. New York: McGraw-Hill, 1976.
Johnson, D.L. et al: Fabry disease: Diagnosis of hemizygotes and heterozygotes by α-galactosidase A activity in tears. Clin. Chim. Acta 63:81, 1975.
Lockman, L.A. et al: Relief of the painful crises of Fabry's disease by diphenylhydantoin. Neurology (Minneap.) 23:871, 1973.

Contributor: **Robert J. Desnick**

Editor's Computerized Descriptors: Eye, Skin, Skel., GU., Nerve, GI., Muscle
Also see Section I, Fig. 92

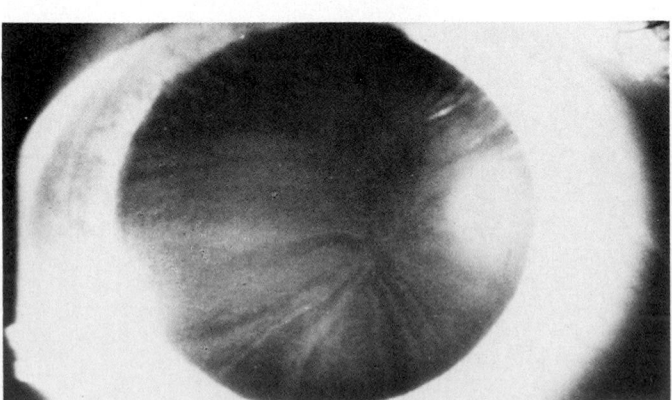

259. Cornea verticillata

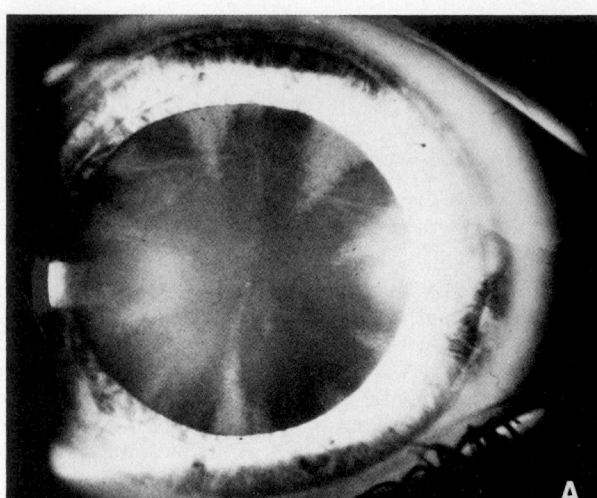

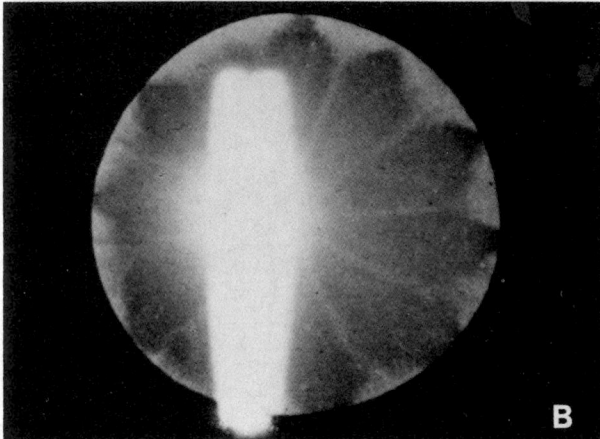

260. A) Wedge-shaped anterior opacities of the lens; B) posterior spoke-like opacities of the lens

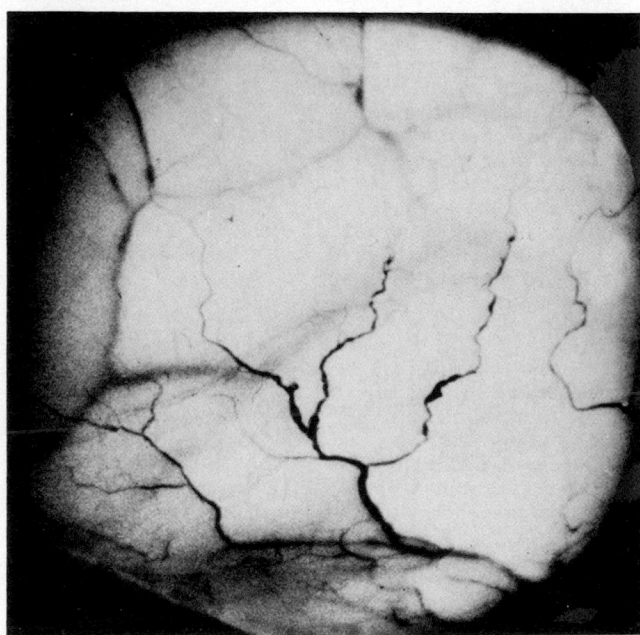

261. Tortuosity and irregularity in caliber of conjuctival vessels in Fabry disease

FACIAL CLEFT, LATERAL

Includes: Fissure latérale
Laterale Gesichtsspalte
Fisura facial lateral
Macrostomia
Cleft, facial lateral

Excludes: Facial cleft, oblique (375)

Minimal Diagnostic Criteria: Lateral facial cleft extending from either corner of the mouth.

Clinical Findings: Facial cleft extending from the corners of the mouth laterally. May be unilateral or bilateral.

Complications
I   **Derived:** —
II **Associated:** One case each of grooves above ears, dorsal sinus of nose, auricular deformity, preauricular appendages, syndactyly one hand.

Etiology: ?

Pathogenesis: ? As maxillary and mandibular processes are not separated during embryogenesis and hence do not fuse, defect is probably secondary to rupture along developmental furrow between the maxillary and mandibular processes during embryogenesis.

Related Facts
I   **Sex Ratio:** M2:F3 (5 cases)
II   **Risk of Occurrence:** ? 1 in 100 cleft lips are lateral cleft.
III **Risk of Recurrence for**
      Patient's Sib: ?
      Patient's Child: ?
IV   **Age of Detectability:** At birth by visual examination
V   **Prevalence:** ?

Treatment
I   **Primary Prevention:** —
II   **Secondary Prevention:** Operative closure of cleft, Z-plasty.
III **Other Therapy:** Repair other associated congenital anomalies.

Prognosis: Normal life span

Detection of Carrier: —

Special Considerations: —

References:
Blackfield, H. M. and Wilde, N. J.: Lateral facial clefts. Plast. Reconstr. Surg. 6:68, 1950.
Grabb, W. C.: The first and second branchial arch syndrome. Plast. Reconstr. Surg. 36:485, 1965.
May H.: Transverse facial clefts and their repair. Plast. Reconstr. Surg. 29:240, 1962.
Pitanguy, I. and Franco, T.: Nonoperated facial fissures in adults. Plast. Reconstr. Surg. 39:569, 1967.
Stark, R. B. and Saunders, D. E.: The first branchial syndrome. Plast. Reconstr. Surg. 29:229, 1962.

Contributors: **Harry M. Blackfield**
John Q. Owsley, Jr.
Stephen H. Miller

Editor's Computerized Descriptors: Ear, Face, Skel.

FACIAL CLEFT, OBLIQUE

Includes: Fissure oblique de la face
Schräge Gesichtsspalte
Fisura facial oblicua
Cleft, facial oblique
Meloschisis

Excludes: Other types of facial clefting, although they may be associated with the basic defect

Minimal Diagnostic Criteria: Oblique facial clefting

Clinical Findings: Oblique facial clefts are variable in pattern and extent. Involvement may be unilateral or bilateral. In some cases the nostril may be involved. In other cases the cleft may skirt the ala. Clefting may be superficial or may involve the underlying bone. When clefting involves the orbital margin, the eyelid usually fails to develop, leaving the eye globe exposed. Alar clefts or colobomas may represent incomplete forms of the condition.

Complications
I   **Derived:** —
II **Associated:** Almost always include cleft lip, cleft palate, or lateral facial clefting and, in some cases, hydrocephaly, encephalocele, structural abnormalities of the eye, arthrogryposis, talipes, adactyly, GU anomalies

Etiology: ?

Pathogenesis: ? †

Related Facts
I   **Sex Ratio:** Probably M1:F1
II   **Risk of Occurrence:** ?
III **Risk of Recurrence for**
     Patient's Sib: ?
     Patient's Child: ?
IV   **Age of Detectability:** At birth by physical examination
V   **Prevalence:** 1 in 1300 cases of orofacial clefting

Treatment
I   **Primary Prevention:** ?
II   **Secondary Prevention:** Surgical correction
III **Other Therapy:** —

Prognosis: Depends on the nature of the associated anomalies and on the extent of facial clefting.

Detection of Carrier: —

†**Special Considerations:** Oblique clefts are variable in pattern and most frequently do not follow the epithelial grooves of facial development. Therefore, embryologic explanations based on facial development do not explain many cases.

References:
Gorlin, R. J. and Goldman, H. M. (eds.): Thoma's Oral Pathology, 6th Ed. St. Louis:C.V. Mosby, 1976, vol. 1, p. 47.
Gorlin, R.J. et al: Syndromes of the Head and Neck, 2nd Ed. New York:McGraw-Hill, 1976.

Contributor: **M. Michael Cohen, Jr.**

Editor's Computerized Descriptors: Eye, Face, Oral, Nose, Skel., GU., Nerve

FACIAL DIPLEGIA, CONGENITAL

Includes: Diplégie faciale congénitale
Diplegia facial congénita
Möbius syndrome
Nuclear hypoplasia congenital (6th and 7th cranial nerves)
Facial diplegia (6th and 7th cranial nerves)

Excludes: Congenital muscular dystrophy

Minimal Diagnostic Criteria: A nonprogressive, congenital syndrome characterized by paralysis of the 6th and 7th cranial nerves.

Clinical Findings: The outstanding finding is facial paralysis, which is usually bilateral. When the paralysis is incomplete, the lower face and platysma tend to be spared. The weakness may cause difficulty in feeding in the neonatal period. There may be drooling of saliva, lodging of food in the cheeks and indistinct speech at a later age. The facies is mask-like. Approximately 75% of the patients have paralysis of the lateral rectus muscle. The abducens paralysis tends to be bilateral and complete. External ophthalmoplegia has been reported in 25%.

Paralysis and hypoplasia of the tongue, as well as weakness of the palate, are occasionally noted.

There are no diagnostic laboratory tests. The pneumoencephalogram may reveal enlarged basal cisterns.

Complications
I   **Derived:** An infant may fail to thrive because of difficulty in feeding secondary to weakness of the facial muscles. Corneal and conjunctival ulceration may result due to incomplete closure of the lids. Bulbar paralysis may result in aspiration of secretions producing bronchopneumonia.
II **Associated:** Mental retardation of a moderate degree has been recorded in 10% of the cases. Bilateral talipes equinovarus, hypoplasia or absence of the pectoralis muscle, congenital amputations, syndactyly, brachydactyly, ear lobe deformities and deafness may occur.

Etiology: Autosomal dominant transmission occurs. However, frequency of consanguineous marriages is a feature of many reported patients. McK *15790

Pathogenesis: ? Nuclear hypoplasia accounting for the cranial nerve paralysis has been documented in a few well-studied cases. Electromyographic studies tend to verify a supranuclear or nuclear cause for the palsies noted on examination.

Related Facts
I   **Sex Ratio:** M1:F1
II   **Risk of Occurrence:** ?
III **Risk of Recurrence for**
     Patient's Sib: When autosomal dominant or autosomal recessive, see Table I AD or AR, respectively.
     Patient's Child: When autosomal dominant or autosomal recessive, see Table I AD or AR, respectively.
IV   **Age of Detectability:** At birth by physical examination
V   **Prevalence:** ?

Treatment
I   **Primary Prevention:** Genetic counseling
II   **Secondary Prevention:** A special diet may be helpful to prevent aspiration. Very occasionally tube feeding may be necessary in the neonatal period to overcome poor suck and maintain nutrition.
III **Other Therapy:** Early recognition and treatment of associated malformations or complications such as corneal ulceration.

Prognosis: Good if complications can be avoided. Compatible with a normal life span.

Detection of Carrier: —

Special Considerations: —

References:
Henderson, J.L.: Congenital facial diplegia syndrome: Clinical features, pathology and aetiology; review of 61 cases. Brain 62:381, 1939.

Contributor: **Robert H. A. Haslam**

Editor's Computerized Descriptors: Eye, Hearing, Ear, Face, Oral, Speech, Skel., Muscle, GI., Nerve

FACIAL PALSY, CONGENITAL

Includes: Paralysie faciale congénitale
Angeborene Fazialisparese
Parálisis facial congénita
Congenital unilateral facial palsy
Congenital bilateral facial palsy
Nuclear facial palsy
Familial congenital peripheral facial paralysis
Congenital partial facial palsy

Excludes: Facial palsy, late-onset (378)
Facial palsy due to birth trauma or misapplication of forceps
Agenesis of facial musculature
Congenital facial palsy which is part of syndromes, eg Möbius syndrome and Melkersson-Rosenthal syndrome
Sporadic cases of Bell palsy

Minimal Diagnostic Criteria: Bilateral (occasionally unilateral) peripheral palsy present from birth and not caused by trauma. Electrodiagnostic tests will show denervation as differentiated from muscular agenesis. Petrous pyramid polytomography may show middle ear anomalies or an aberrant course of the facial nerve canal.†

Clinical Findings: Peripheral facial palsy is present at birth and is usually bilateral. Some pedigrees have been described in which each affected member was involved unilaterally and on the same side. History and physical findings are negative for birth trauma and, unlike most cases due to obstetric forceps pressure, no degree of recovery has been reported. In most instances no other neurologic deficits can be found, although in some families scattered members have shown associated homolateral ptosis or nystagmus or strabismus. In some instances associated congenital conductive hearing loss due to middle ear malformations has been reported, but these appeared to be sporadic.

Various laboratory tests may be helpful in differential diagnosis, prognosis and in determining whether therapy might be beneficial in some instances. However, for therapy to have optimum results, evaluation should be carried out at about 7-14 days of age. Four tests have been found useful: the facial nerve excitability test, the strength-duration or intensity-duration test (recorded graphically), electromyography, and facial muscle biopsy in selected cases. A newer test, stapedius reflex testing with the acoustic bridge, may help establish site of lesion but needs to be combined with audiometric examination so that the level of hearing and type of hearing loss (if one exists) may be documented.

The facial nerve-excitability test is most useful in unilateral cases where the response between the normal and abnormal side can be compared. In neurapraxia (physiologic or conductive block), there will be no difference in excitability between the normal and abnormal nerve. In partial denervation, the involved nerve will require more intensity of stimulation to evoke a response. In both of these instances, recovery can be anticipated and a good prognosis given but confirmation should be obtained using strength-duration testing. This test is of no value if performed before the 14th day *after onset of paralysis*. However, the time of onset of paralysis in congenital cases is unknown. Therefore, it might be worthwhile trying the test before the 14th day of life.

In total denervation no response to facial nerve-excitability stimulation is seen. Accordingly, this test is useful for both unilateral and bilateral facial weakness. Strength-duration curves are confirmatory.

Facial nerve-excitability and strength-duration tests are best carried out in the infant under light general anesthesia which can then be deepened for definitive surgery, should this prove advisable. Electromyography and stapedius testing should be done without anesthetic, although sedation may be required. In the absence of muscle potentials of any kind, specific muscle biopsy might be advisable in some instances to rule out absence of muscle fibers.

The stapedius reflex will be absent in lesions proximal to the takeoff of the main trunk of the facial nerve as it descends through the mastoid. If hearing loss is also present, it is needful to measure acoustic impedance to see if an associated anomaly of the middle ear ossicles may exist.

Instances of partial facial palsy have been reported in which only the lower half of the face was paralyzed. The stapedius reflex was also impaired but taste and lacrimation were unimpaired. This was believed to be a partial nuclear lesion, not cortical.

Petrous pyramid polytomography may delineate the anatomy of the facial nerve canal in the temporal bone and is a useful adjunct to diagnosis and therapy. It should be remembered, however, that the facial nerve may not be in the fallopian canal.

Complications
I **Derived:** Corneal drying and ulceration could occur if the eye is unable to be closed sufficiently. Most patients, however, have an adequate Bell phenomenon. Eventually, denervated muscles undergo atrophy and fibrosis, and if the defect is unilateral, pulling of the opposite facial muscles will make the asymmetry even more noticeable. Bilateral involvement of the buccinator muscles may make feeding of the newborn infant very difficult but children and adults compensate for this.

II **Associated:** Middle ear anomalies, usually of 2nd branchial arch origin but sometimes involving 1st arch structures, may be associated without mandibulofacial anomalies. Associated deficits of other cranial nerves have been reported in scattered patients. Isolated absence or abnormality of the ramus mandibularus of the facial nerve associated with cardiac defects has been reported but this appears to be a separate entity.

Etiology: Autosomal dominant with high penetrance. In congenital unilateral facial palsy, partial agenesis of the motor nucleus of the 7th cranial nerve has been found at autopsy. If hypoplasia of the facial nerve is found combined with middle ear anomalies, some cause for branchial arch malformation may exist. Thalidomide ingestion by the mother during pregnancy may cause facial nerve agenesis.

Pathogenesis: The pathogenesis is unknown except that in instances of bony compression of the facial nerve within the temporal bone, it is believed the blood supply to the nerve is compromised. Wide variations in the anatomy of the facial nerve and the fallopian canal are known to occur. Hypoplasia and "hyperplasia" of the nerve have been reported. The facial nerve lies encased in a bony canal which may be abnormally narrow and compress the nerve. Narrowing at the stylomastoid foramen has been reported. Secondary edema may cause further decrease of the blood supply with death of the nerve fibers. There is some experimental evidence that ischemia of the facial nerve causes paralysis.

Related Facts
I **Sex Ratio:** M1:F1
II **Risk of Occurrence:** ?
III **Risk of Recurrence for**
   Patient's Sib: If parent is affected 1 in 2 (50%) for each offspring to be affected; otherwise not increased.
   Patient's Child: 1 in 2
IV **Age of Detectability:** At birth. In unilateral cases the facial

asymmetry is obvious. Bilateral cases may go unrecognized for a prolonged time. Detection is by physical examination and confirmation is by electrodiagnostic testing.
V **Prevalence:** ?

Treatment
I **Primary Prevention:** Genetic counseling
II **Secondary Prevention:** Surgical decompression of the facial nerve in the temporal bone may be useful in early cases. This technique has so seldom been used in such ideal cases that its success cannot be assessed.

Later, plastic and reconstructive procedures, such as fascial slings and reinnervation of the facial musculature using other nearby motor nerves, might be done. Reinnervation of already atrophic or fibrotic muscles is hopeless, and electromyography should be done before attempting any such procedure.†

III **Other Therapy:** If the patient has inadequate eye closure, tarsorrhaphy should be performed and the patient might be given safety glasses as additional protection.

Tube feeding, gavage or feeding with a syringe may be necessary in the bilaterally-affected infant who cannot suck. Cervical esophagotomy or gastrostomy might be indicated in extreme cases.

Surgical correction of associated middle ear anomalies which have caused conductive hearing loss may be feasible. In inoperable cases a hearing aid should be prescribed if the hearing loss is bilateral.

Prognosis: Normal for life span and intelligence. For function: without therapy, no recovery may be anticipated. With therapy, variable degrees of recovery may be possible.†

Detection of Carrier: —

†**Special Considerations:** Those physicians caring for these infants need to be aware that a more sophisticated approach to the problem than mere observation is now available. Facial paralysis is a major disability and every attempt should be made to diagnose and, if possible, treat it early.

Middle ear anomalies may be present in some instances, causing a maximum conductive hearing loss. Audiometry should be done early to rule out this possibility and appropriate habilitation begun.

In many cases the etiology or pathogenesis remain unknown because either a "wait-and-see" or a hopeless attitude is taken by parents or physician. Very few patients have electrodiagnostic studies made shortly after birth and even fewer patients have surgical exploration and decompression of the facial nerve as it courses through the temporal bone.

References:
McHugh, H.E. et al: Facial paralysis and muscle agenesis in the newborn. Arch. Otolaryngol. 89:131, 1969.
Rubin, A.: Handbook of Congenital Malformations. Philadelphia:W.B. Saunders Co., 1967.
Skyberg, D. and van der Hagen, C.B.: Congenital hereditary unilateral facial palsy in four generations. Acta Paediatr. Scand. (Suppl.) 159:77, 1965.

Contributor: **LaVonne Bergstrom**

Editor's Computerized Descriptors: Eye, Hearing, Face, Skel., Nerve

FACIAL PALSY, LATE-ONSET

Includes: Paralysie faciale à début tardif
Spätmanifeste Fazialisparese
Parálisis facial de comienzo tardío
Single or recurrent episodes of Bell palsy

Excludes: Facial palsy, congenital (377)
Melkersson-Rosenthal syndrome
Sporadic cases of Bell palsy

Minimal Diagnostic Criteria: Typical peripheral facial palsy not present at birth, often recurrent; occurring in a family or kindred.†

Clinical Findings: Inability to move the ipsilateral muscles of the face or close the eye. Decreased salivary secretion of the submaxillary gland, decreased tearing of the eye, diminished or absent stapedius reflex or impaired taste sensation on the ipsilateral side may be present.

Affected persons may show 1 or repeated episodes of peripheral facial palsy. Family history reveals an increased incidence of Bell palsy among family members over more than 1 generation. One survey found such an incidence to be 9 times greater in the families of patients with Bell palsy as compared to the families of control patients. The same study showed that the episodes of Bell palsy in families could not be associated with exogenous factors, such as viral outbreaks, although in 1 family several members had repeated episodes of facial palsy associated with upper respiratory and ear infections. Disorders such as diabetes or hypertension do not seem to be associated with an increased incidence of familial Bell palsy.

There seems to be some tendency for episodes of Bell palsy to recur on the same side, suggesting an anatomic variation as a factor in etiology. Usually the palsy recovers spontaneously. However, in some instances nerve excitability may be lost; and in those instances the nerve would not be expected to recover without treatment. Pain, when it occurs, is a poor prognostic sign and also suggests the need for urgent surgical intervention. Jepson reported the following findings for facial nerve lesions at different levels:

Regional Diagnosis	Taste	Lacrimation	Stapedius Reflex
Nuclear	+	+	-
Suprageniculate	±	-	-
Transgeniculate	-	-	-
Suprastapedial	-	+	-
Infrastapedial	-	+	+
Infrachordal	+	+	+

Complications

I Derived: The nerve may fail to recover causing permanent paralysis. This may occur in 10-25% of cases. There is some evidence that less recovery occurs after repeated episodes of facial palsy. Corneal drying and ulceration may occur if there is inadequate eye closure.

II Associated: —

Etiology: Autosomal dominant with reduced penetrance. There may be patients with autosomal recessive inheritance. (Hypersensitivity to cold or to horse serum has been associated with increased susceptibility to facial paralysis in experimental animals.)

Pathogenesis: ? A patient was described who had Bell palsy prior to dying of a ruptured aneurysm and had blanching, localized areas of constriction or edema of the facial nerve. Facial nerve was surrounded by and contained dilated and engorged veins and venules. Myelin sheath and axis cylinder had degenerated both proximal and distal to this geniculate ganglion. The neural sheaths were empty and swollen. The greater superficial petrosal nerve was degenerated. Some of the ganglion cells of the geniculate ganglion stained paler than on the normal side; some cells were pyknotic. The facial nerve nucleus was normal.

Related Facts

I   Sex Ratio: M1:F1
II Risk of Occurrence: ?
III Risk of Recurrence for
  Patient's Sib: When autosomal dominant or autosomal recessive, see Table I AD 85% or AR, respectively.
  Patient's Child: When autosomal dominant or autosomal recessive, see Table I AD 85% or AR, respectively.
IV Age of Detectability: When it first occurs, usually in adults.
V   Prevalence: ?

Treatment

I   Primary Prevention: Genetic counseling
II Secondary Prevention: If nerve excitability remains equal to that of the normal side, a conduction block exists. Testing should be done twice daily for up to 2 weeks to be certain denervation is not occurring. Probably no therapy is needed in these cases but if the palsy persists more than a few weeks, massage, local heat and electrical stimulation of the facial muscles to minimize atrophy and fibrosis may be beneficial.

If denervation occurs and if other neurologic deficits or a systemic cause are not present, immediate surgical decompression of the nerve throughout its course in the temporal bone seems to be of benefit. This should be done as soon as denervation becomes apparent. However, it may be of some benefit even after a prolonged period of denervation. In late cases, anastomosis of the facial nerve with another nerve, excision of an involved segment and grafting have been proposed. To minimize deformity, fascial slings may be created to support the sagging paralyzed side of the face.

If coverage of the eye is inadequate, temporary or permanent tarsorrhaphy should be done.†

III Other Therapy: Other medical treatments have been proposed. These include the administration of steroids, vasodilating drugs and stellate ganglion block. However, their efficacy seems to approximate the spontaneous recovery rate.

Prognosis: Normal for life span and intelligence. Spontaneous recovery of nerve function occurs in 75-90% of cases. In some cases recovery is partial, resulting in synkinesis or only partial movement.

Detection of Carrier: —

†Special Considerations: Careful electrodiagnostic testing and neurologic examination of patients are essential for accurate diagnosis and rational therapy. An expectant attitude is not sufficient.

References:
Alter, M.: Familial aggregation of Bell's palsy. Arch. Neurol. 8:557, 1963.
DeSanto, L.W. and Schubert, H.A.: Bell's palsy: Ten cases in a family. Arch. Otolaryngol. 89:700, 1969.
Fowler, E.P., Jr.: The pathologic findings in a case of facial paralysis. Trans. Am. Acad. Ophthalmol. Otolaryngol. 67:187, 1963.
McGovern, F.H.: A review of the experimental aspects of Bell's palsy. Laryngoscope. 78:324, 1968.
Sullivan, J.A. et al: Management of Bell's palsy. Arch. Otolaryngol. 89:144, 1969.

Contributor: **LaVonne Bergstrom**

Editor's Computerized Descriptors: Eye, Nerve, Face

FETAL ALCOHOL SYNDROME

Teratology 12:1, 1975.

Contributor: **Kenneth Lyons Jones**

Includes: Syndrome d'imprégnation alcoolique de foetus
Embryofetales Alkohol Syndrom
Síndrome fetal por alcohol

Editor's Computerized Descriptors: Eye, Dermatoglyphic, Skel., CV., Nerve

Excludes: —

Minimal Diagnostic Criteria: Prenatal-onset growth deficiency; microcephaly; mental retardation; short palpebral fissures in a child born to a severe chronic alcoholic mother.

Clinical Findings: Prenatal-onset growth deficiency with birth length more severely affected than birthweight; postnatal linear growth rate 65% of normal, and average postnatal rate of weight gain 40% of normal; mental retardation (average IQ 63); microcephaly; short palpebral fissures; variable joint anomalies consisting of congenital hip dislocations, inability to extend metacarpal-phalangeal joints; altered palmar crease patterns; cardiac defects, (primarily ventricular septal defect); fine motor dysfunction (weak grasp, poor eye-hand coordination, tremulousness in the newborn period). This disorder has been seen only in offspring of severe chronic alcoholic mothers. The effects on the offspring of less severe maternal alcohol consumption are unknown.

Complications
I   Derived: —
II Associated: —

Etiology: The similarity in this pattern of malformations suggests a singular etiology most likely related to chronic maternal alcoholism. Ethanol itself is the most likely possibility. However, one of its breakdown products such as acetaldehyde has not been ruled out. Other possibilities include the indirect effects of maternal undernutrition or deficiency of a specific nutrient or vitamin.

Pathogenesis: —

Related Facts
I   Sex Ratio: M1:F1
II Risk of Occurrence: Available evidence suggests that the fetal alcohol syndrome occurs in approximately one-third of infants born to severe chronic alcoholic mothers. This figure is derived from evaluation of 23 children born to chronic alcoholic women ascertained from the Perinatal Collaborative Study of the National Institute·of Neurologic Disease and Stroke.
III Risk of Recurrence for
   Patient's Sib: Documentation in some cases of normal, older sibs of affected children born prior to the onset of maternal alcoholism suggests that recurrence risk might be related to control of maternal alcoholism.
   Patient's Child: None
IV Age of Detectability: At birth
V   Prevalence: ?

Treatment
I   Primary Prevention: Avoidance of pregnancy in severe chronic alcoholic women.
II Secondary Prevention: Corrective as appropriate
III Other Therapy: —

Prognosis: Life span reduced in relation to degree of cardiac or brain defect. Mild-to-moderate mental retardation in all cases.

Detection of Carrier: —

Special Considerations: —

References:
Jones, K.L. et al: Pattern of malformation in offspring of chronic alcoholic mothers. Lancet 1:1267, 1973.
Jones, K.L. and Smith, D.W.: The fetal alcohol syndrome.

FETAL AMINOPTERIN SYNDROME

Includes: Embryopathies et foetopathies dues à l'aminophtérine
Intrauteriner Aminopterin Schaden
Lesión fetal por aminopterina
Fetal damage from 4-amino-pteroyl-glutamic acid
Aminopterin damage in utero

Excludes: —

Minimal Diagnostic Criteria: Documentation of mother using aminopterin during pregnancy plus differential diagnosis.

Clinical Findings: Aminopterin given to a woman in the first trimester of pregnancy can cause depression of fetal hematopoiesis, necrosis of the liver or adrenals or fetal death. In an older fetus the drug may induce congenital malformations such as hydrocephaly, meningoencephalocele or harelip and cleft palate. If the fetus lives to near term, anencephaly, partial craniostenosis, particularly cranial dysplasia (lack of ossification of the cranial bones), have been observed. Facial anomalies, posterior cleft palate, clubhands and clubfeet also occur. In case of survival the disease picture can improve and ossification of the skull bones progresses slowly. Shortening of the forearms and coxa vara deformity of the hips may persist. There may be mental retardation.

Complications
I **Derived:** —
II **Associated:** —

Etiology: Aminopterin during pregnancy. Dose range in reported cases varied from 6 to 12 mg over 2-5 day period.

Pathogenesis: ?

Related Facts
I **Sex Ratio:** Ml:Fl
II **Risk of Occurrence:** Not genetic
III **Risk of Recurrence for**
    Patient's Sib: Not genetic
    Patient's Child: Not genetic
IV **Age of Detectability:** At birth or early infancy
V **Prevalence:** ?

Treatment
I **Primary Prevention:** Avoidance of aminopterin during pregnancy
II **Secondary Prevention:** —
III **Other Therapy:** —

Prognosis: Varies with kind and severity of defects present

Detection of Carrier: —

Special Considerations: —

References:
Howard, M.J. and Rudd, N.L.: The natural history of aminopterin-induced embryopathy. In Bergsma, D. and Lowry, R.B. (eds.): Natural History of Specific Birth Defects. Birth Defects: Orig. Art. Ser., vol. XIII, no. 3C. New York: Alan R. Liss for The National Foundation-March of Dimes, 1977, p. 85.
Meltzer, H.J.: Congenital anomalies due to attempted abortion with 4-amino-pteroylglutamic acid. JAMA 161:1253, 1956.
Shaw, E.B. and Steinbach, H.L.: Aminopterin-induced fetal malformation; survival of infant after attempted abortion. Am. J. Dis. Child. 115:477, 1968.
Shaw, E.B.: Fetal damage due to maternal aminopterin ingestion. Am. J. Dis. Child. 124:93, 1972.
Thiersch, J.B.: Therapeutic abortions with folic acid antagonist, 4-aminopteroylglutamic acid (4-amino P.G.A.) administered by oral route. Am. J. Obstet. Gynecol. 63:1298, 1952.
Warkany, J. et al: Attempted abortion with aminopterin (4-amino-pteroylglutamic acid); malformations of the child. Am. J. Dis. Child. 97:274, 1959.
Warkany, J.: Aminopterin and methotrexate folic acid deficiency. Teratology 17:353-358, 1978.

Contributor: **Josef Warkany**

Editor's Computerized Descriptors: Face, Oral, Skel., Nerve

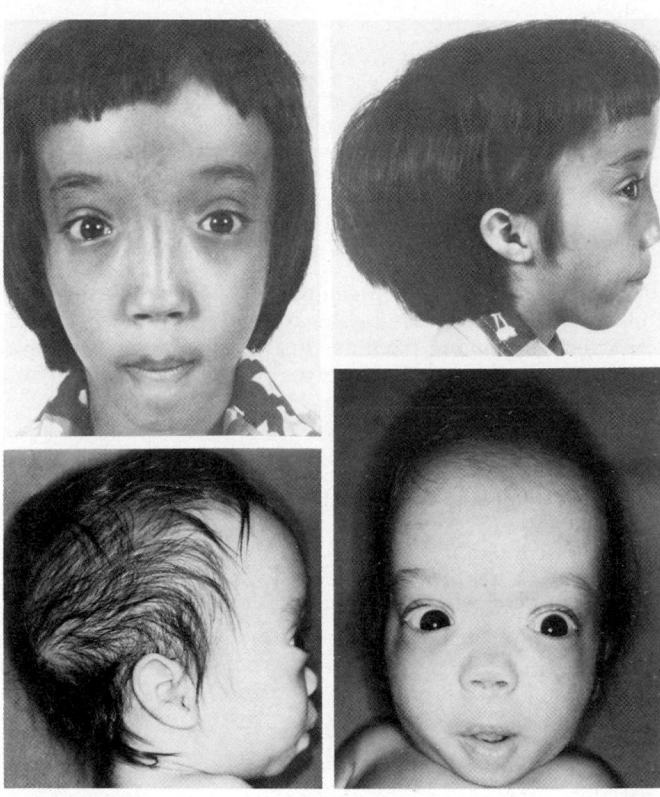

262. Note facial features including broad frontonasal bridge, hypertelorism, and micrognathia

FETAL CYTOMEGALOVIRUS SYNDROME

Includes: Maladie des inclusions cytomégaliques
Zytomegalie
Infección por citomegalovirus
Salivary gland virus infection
Congenital cytomegalic inclusion disease
Cytomegalovirus infection
Cytomegalovirus in utero

Excludes: —

Minimal Diagnostic Criteria: Intrauterine growth retardation associated with hepatosplenomegaly, purpura, jaundice, erythroblastemia and thrombocytopenia in the neonatal period should lead to strong suspicion of cytomegalovirus infection. Intracranial calcifications and microcephaly with or without generalized systemic disease may be caused by this agent. Infection beyond the neonatal period may result in an infectious mononucleosis-like syndrome, isolated hepatomegaly or severe pulmonary infection in immunologically altered hosts.†

Clinical Findings: Cytomegalovirus, when transmitted in utero to the conceptus may be associated with a spectrum of infection ranging from asymptomatic viruria to severe systemic disease which involves the brain, lungs, liver, spleen, bone marrow.

Manifestations with frequencies of over 50% include:

Hepatosplenomegaly	90%
Thrombocytopenia or petechia	70%
Jaundice	60%
Hemolytic anemia	55%

Manifestations with frequencies of less than 50% include:

Microcephaly	40%
Intrauterine growth retardation	35%
Cerebral calcifications	25%
Metaphysitis	25%
Pneumonia	25%
Chorioretinitis	5%
Hydrocephaly	rare
Congenital ascites	rare
Seizures	?

Complications

I **Derived:** When infection with cytomegalovirus is mild, there may be no permanent sequelae. If the disease is clinically detectable at birth, approximately 80% of infants have sequelae related to the CNS. These include varying degrees of mental retardation, spasticity, hyperactivity and convulsive seizures. Microcephaly may be present at birth but may not become apparent until 18 months of age. Hepatosplenomegaly is the most common manifestation at birth and may persist up to 4 years. Despite extensive involvement of the liver at the time of infection, chronic liver problems are rare. The major histologic findings on liver biopsies with clinical and chemical evidence of liver dysfunction include varying degrees of portal fibrosis, hepatitis with giant cells, and cholangitis.

In one series, 5 of 18 infants had structural abnormalities of derivatives of the 1st embryonic arch which included high-arched palate and micrognathia, facial weakness, deafness and cleft of hard and soft palate.

II **Associated:** Microgyria, porencephaly, hypoplasia of cerebellar hemisphere, absence of olfactory bulbs and tracts, hearing loss with inner ear involvement, pulmonary valvular stenosis, mitral stenosis, atrial septal defect.

Etiology: Caused by human specific cytomegalovirus. Organism can be cultured in vitro only in human fibroblast cells. Fine structure of a particle from culture material reveals a capsomere-like herpes simplex virus. The nucleoprotein is DNA. Cytomegaloviruses are species specific and infect man, monkeys and rodents.

Pathogenesis: Infection usually takes place in utero in the 3rd or 4th month of gestation by transplacental transmission. The mother is usually asymptomatic. Cytomegalovirus multiplies within cells and destroys them. Cytomegalovirus causes a disseminated necrotizing, calcifying encephalitis. Infection may be acquired in the early postnatal period via transfusion of whole fresh blood.†

Related Facts
I   **Sex Ratio:** M1:F1
II **Risk of Occurrence:** 1 in 3500 live births
III **Risk of Recurrence for**
    Patient's Sib: Second intrauterine infection not documented
    Patient's Child: —
IV **Age of Detectability:** Newborn, by isolation of virus or serology †
V   **Prevalence:** ?

Treatment
I   **Primary Prevention:** ?
II **Secondary Prevention:** ?
III **Other Therapy:** Isolated reports suggest thymidine analogs floxuridine or idoxuridine may be helpful. 9-D-Arabinofuranosyladenine has been effective in vitro against cytomegalovirus. No clinical trials have been reported.

Prognosis: Infants with severe infection usually die in the newborn period as a result of cerebral involvement. Severely infected infants who survive the newborn period and who are severely retarded have expired with superimposed infections. Other infants with severe infection in the newborn period who have survived have had seizures, may be spastic or mentally retarded. Infants with mild disease at birth may develop within normal limits.

Detection of Carrier: Cytomegalovirus infection in pregnant woman, who is usually asymptomatic.

†Special Considerations: There are no clinical stigmata that can differentiate this in utero infection from that of rubella, toxoplasmosis or syphilis. Cerebral calcifications may be periventricular but may also be flat disseminated calcifications, just as occurs in toxoplasmosis. Chorioretinitis occurs much less frequently than with toxoplasmosis, is usually peripheral but may also be macular. Microcephaly without systemic disease may be caused by cytomegalovirus.

Although a variety of tests are available to aid in the diagnosis of congenital cytomegalovirus infection, isolation of the organism remains the most reliable method but is also cumbersome. For technical reasons, many laboratories rely on less specific tests. Characteristic inclusion cells are only seen in 30% of cases and other types of cells may be easily confused with true cytomegalic cells. It should be remembered that although serum macroglobulins are usually elevated, infants with mild infection may have normal IgM levels. Serologic tests are diagnostic if elevated after 6 months of life when endogenous antibody production accounts for the majority of measured antibody. This test does not distinguish congenital from postnatal acquired infection in older infants. Recently, a simple fluorescent test to demonstrate macroglobulin specific antibodies has been developed for cytomegalic inclusion disease. The test is simple yet reliable in diagnosing congenital infection in the very young infant but is not available in every laboratory.

References:
Hanshaw, J. B.: Congenital and acquired cytomegalovirus infection. Pediatr. Clin. North Am. 13:279, 1966.

McCracken, G.H. Jr. et al: Congenital cytomegalic inclusion disease. Am. J. Dis. Child. 117:522, 1969.

Weller, T. H. and Hanshaw, J. B.: Virologic and clinical observations on cytomegalic inclusion disease. N. Engl. J. Med. 266:1233, 1962.

Contributor: **Henry R. Shinefield**

Editor's Computerized Descriptors: Vision, Eye, Hearing, Face, Oral, Skin, Skel., Resp., CV., Spleen, Liver, Nerve

FETAL HYDANTOIN SYNDROME

Includes: Embryopathie due à l'hydantoïne
Fetales Hydantoin-Syndrom
Síndrome hidantoínico fetal
Dilantin syndrome
Fetal damage from hydantoin anticonvulsants

Excludes: Fetal damage from other anticonvulsants
Coffin Siris syndrome
Noonan syndrome (720)

Minimal Diagnostic Criteria: The diagnosis may be considered in any infant exposed prenatally to hydantoin anticonvulsants and who manifests several of the features cited below.

Clinical Findings: Major manifestations which characterize children exposed prenatally to hydantoin anticonvulsants include abnormalities of growth such as pre- and postnatal growth deficiency, microcephaly and abnormalities of performance such as developmental delays or mental retardation. These children also have dysmorphic craniofacial features commonly including short nose with broad depressed bridge and inner epicanthic folds, mild hypertelorism, ptosis of the eyelid, strabismus, wide mouth and metopic sutural ridging. Less commonly short neck with mild webbing and cleft lip or palate may occur. Limb anomalies include hypoplasia of nails and distal phalanges with an increased frequency of low arch digital dermal ridge patterns, and finger-like thumb.

Complications
I   **Derived:**   Failure to thrive in infancy. Mild-to-moderate mental retardation may be present in 60% or more of children seriously affected physically.
II   **Associated:**   Cardiac anomalies, GU or CNS anomalies, serious limb reduction defects, or diaphragmatic hernia.

Etiology: Maternal treatment with an hydantoin anticonvulsant (diphenylhydantoin, mephenytoin, ethotoin) during early pregnancy. A specific sensitive period of fetal development has not been defined.

Pathogenesis: —

Related Facts
I   **Sex Ratio:**   M1:F1
II   **Risk of Occurrence:**   The full pattern of abnormalities recognizable as the fetal hydantoin syndrome is now estimated to occur in at least 10% of exposed infants. However, an additional 30% may show some abnormalities consistent with the prenatal effects of hydantoins. The full syndrome has only been seen in infants whose prenatal drug exposures included an hydantoin. The relative contribution of possible genetic and other factors affecting hydantoin metabolism is unclear at present.
III   **Risk of Recurrence for**
   Patient's Sib: As under Risk of Occurrence
   Patient's Child: None, unless patient is a female and is treated with an hydantoin anticonvulsant during her pregnancy.
IV   **Age of Detectability:**   At birth or early infancy
V   **Prevalence:**   Estimates of the frequency of hydantoin therapy of mothers during pregnancy vary but may be approximately 1/500 pregnancies (0.2%). This would suggest that at least 1 in 5000 children may have this condition.

Treatment
I   **Primary Prevention:**   Avoidance of hydantoin anticonvulsants during pregnancy. Women with seizure disorders should be informed of the nature and magnitude of risks to the fetus arising from hydantoin therapy prior to considering a pregnancy.
II   **Secondary Prevention:**   Surgical correction of major defects

may be necessary. In mildly affected children, nail abnormalities may improve with time. Effective remedies for deficiencies of growth and performance have not been demonstrated.

III Other Therapy: —

Prognosis: Dependent upon severity of involvement

Detection of Carrier: Not applicable

Special Considerations: —

References:
Fedrick, J.: Epilepsy and pregnancy: A report from the Oxford record linkage study. Br. Med. J. 2:442, 1973.
Hanson, J.W. and Smith, D.W.: The fetal hydantoin syndrome. J. Pediatr. 87:285, 1975.
Hanson, J.W. et al: Risks to the offspring of women treated with hydantoin anticonvulsants, with emphasis on the fetal hydantoin syndrome. J. Pediatr. 89:662, 1975.
Hill, R.M. et al: Infants exposed in utero to antiepileptic drugs. Am. J. Dis. Child. 127:645, 1974.
Monson, R.R. et al: Diphenylhydantoin and selected congenital malformations. N. Engl. J. Med. 289:1049, 1973.

Contributor: **James W. Hanson**

Editor's Computerized Descriptors: Eye, Face, Oral, Nose, Skin, Dermatoglyphic, Nails, Skel., Muscle, CV., Nerve

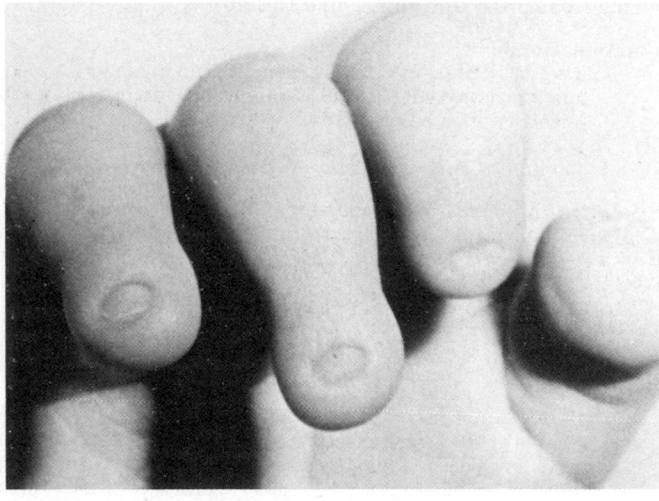

263. Distal hypoplasia of fingers and nails

383

FETAL RADIATION SYNDROME 380-500

Includes: Embryopathie due à la radioactivité
Strahlenembryopathie
Embriopatía por radiación
Radiation teratogenesis
Leukemogenesis
Radiation embryopathy

Excludes: Effects of radiation prior to conception

Minimal Diagnostic Criteria: Radiation embryopathy has no pathognomonic features. The influence of radiation exposure can be demonstrated only by showing that rates for specific disorders significantly exceed normal expectation. The best biologic dosimeter in man to date is the presence of complex cytogenetic abnormalities detectable in peripheral blood. Such abnormalities were found in 39% of persons 20 years after exposure in utero (maternal dose = 100 rad or more), as compared with 2% of controls. Chromosomal aberrations were found even in the leukocytes of persons exposed in utero during the 1st trimester.

Clinical Findings: Mental retardation and head circumference 3 or more SD below the average for age and sex; also growth retardation. In less severe cases there may be normal intelligence with head circumference 2-3 SD below the average for age and sex. No other anomalies in man have been shown to be radiation-induced but fetal wastage may occur 7 times more often than usual following heavy radiation exposures during pregnancy.

Radiation in sufficient dose during intrauterine life may be leukemogenic but present evidence is based only on small (diagnostic) exposures. Reports of an excess of leukemia and all other neoplasms of childhood following such exposures during pregnancy may not represent a direct causal effect; ie diagnostic radiation may merely be an indicator (concomitant) of the real reason for the excessive cancer occurrence.

Among the Japanese exposed in utero to the atomic bomb, no excess of deaths occurred through 20 years of age. The possibility that intrauterine radiation exposure may result in diminished fertility or sterility cannot yet be evaluated. Radiation nephropathy has been observed in a child whose mother received massive radiotherapy early in pregnancy for Hodgkin disease.

Complications
I Derived: Unexceptional, except that there may be fear of radiation effects among parents of exposed children with no abnormalities.
II Associated: As under Clinical Findings.

Etiology: The sources of radiation in sufficient dose to produce embryopathy may be radiologic equipment or nuclear weapons. There may be interaction with other environmental agents.

Pathogenesis: Unknown, except for the possible influence of somatic mutations, as suggested by the presence of cytogenetic abnormalities.

Related Facts
I Sex Ratio: M1:F1
II Risk of Occurrence: Among women who were within 1200 meters of the Hiroshima hypocenter and who had last menstruated 7 - 15 weeks before, 11 delivered liveborn children, 8 of whom had small head circumferences and mental retardation. At further distances there was a dose-response relationship. The frequency of leukemia was about 1 in 60 during the first 12 years following exposure of survivors who had been within 1000 meters of the Hiroshima hypocenter (all ages, but none were in utero at the time).
III Risk of Recurrence for
Patient's Sib: †

IV **Age of Detectability:** Small head size is detectable at birth, and mental retardation is recognizable during the 1st year of life.

V **Prevalence:** These disorders have been observed only after therapeutic or heavy accidental radiation exposure.

Treatment

I **Primary Prevention:** Avoidance of large radiation exposures during early pregnancy, including the interval following menstruation when pregnancy is likely to be unsuspected. Therapeutic abortion should *not* be recommended following diagnostic abdominal radiation, since the increased risk, if any, to the fetus is extremely small.

II **Secondary Prevention:** Persons with radiation-induced anomalies should avoid additional radiation exposures which may be incompletely additive with regard to leukemogenesis among other late effects.

III **Other Therapy:** —

Prognosis: Retardation of intelligence may be minimal to severe. On the basis of animal experimentation, shortening of life span may occur and fertility may be impaired.

Detection of Carrier: There are no carriers.

†**Special Considerations:** The radiation effects noted to date in man are somatic, not genetic.

References:
Bloom, A.D. et al: Cytogenetics of the in utero exposed to Hiroshima and Nagasaki. Lancet 2:10, 1968.
Miller, R. W.: Effects of ionizing radiation from the atomic bomb on Japanese children. Pediatrics 41:257, 1968.
Wood, J. W. et al: In utero exposure to the Hiroshima atomic bomb: An evaluation of head size and mental retardation: 20 years later. Pediatrics 39:385, 1967.
Wood, J. W. et al: Mental retardation in children exposed in utero to the atomic bombs in Hiroshima and Nagasaki. Am. J. Public Health 57:1381, 1967.
Wood, J.W. et al: The growth and development of children exposed in utero to the atomic bombs in Hiroshima and Nagasaki. Am. J. Public Health 57:1374, 1967.

Contributor: **Robert W. Miller**

Editor's Computerized Descriptors: Skel., Nerve

FETAL RUBELLA SYNDROME

Includes: Rubéole congénitale
Rötelnembryopathie
Rubella malformation syndrome
Expanded rubella syndrome
Gregg syndrome
Congenital rubella

Excludes: Microcephaly (659)

Minimal Diagnostic Criteria: Congenital rubella should be suspected in any child with one or more of the typical defects described below, especially when a history of rubella during pregnancy can be obtained. The presence of retinopathy is most helpful in patients with unexplained congenital deafness. The diagnosis may be confirmed by isolation of rubella virus from a pharyngeal swab, cerebrospinal fluid, cataractous lens or other tissue. The presence in the serum of a newborn infant of specific rubella IgM antibody or persistence of any rubella antibody after 8-12 months of age (in the absence of postnatal rubella) is also diagnostic. The rubella hemagglutination inhibition (HI) antibody test is the most sensitive, convenient, economical and reliable of the antibody tests.

Clinical Findings: Fetal infection with rubella virus may cause spontaneous abortion, stillbirth or a variety of birth defects occurring singly or in combination. Transient neonatal manifestations include low birthweight, hepatosplenomegaly, purpura, bulging unusually large anterior fontanel and metopic suture, corneal clouding, and jaundice. Laboratory studies during this period may also reveal thrombocytopenia, hemolytic or hypoplastic anemia, hepatitis, radiographic lesions in the metaphyseal portions of the long bones, pleocytosis and elevated protein levels in the cerebrospinal fluid, elevated serum IgM (and less frequently IgA) and persistence of rubella virus in many organs. Pneumonia, meningitis, encephalitis, and rarely, intermittent rash may develop during infancy.

Permanent stigmata include sensorineural deafness which may be bilateral or unilateral, mild to profound; congenital heart disease, almost always patent ductus arteriosus with or without pulmonary artery or valvular stenosis, septal defect or aortic arch abnormalities; cataract, unilateral or bilateral, with or without microphthalmia; retinopathy; glaucoma; and high myopia. Encephalitis may lead to varying degrees of psychomotor retardation with intellectual or motor impairment, including typical spastic cerebral palsy.†

Complications

I **Derived:** Deafness (usually sensorineural, rarely conductive), language delay, blindness or low vision, congestive heart failure, mental retardation, cerebral palsy and emotional disturbances.

II **Associated:** Inguinal hernia, abnormal incidence of certain dermatoglyphic patterns, skin dimpling and pigmented macular skin lesions.

Etiology: Rubella virus is a moderate-sized, pleomorphic, ether-sensitive RNA-containing virus which has been placed tentatively in the paramyxovirus group.

Pathogenesis: In postnatal rubella infection, viremia occurs for as long as 1 week before onset of the rash. Viremia also occurs in subclinical rubella. When a pregnant woman develops rubella before the 16th gestational week, placental infection following maternal viremia may lead to fetal viremia and disseminated fetal infection involving virtually every organ. Rubella virus infection of human fetal tissue inhibits mitosis, and elicits an inflammatory response in certain organs. Anomalies result from varying degrees of undergrowth or hypoplasia, inflammatory responses and their sequelae. Changes in the inner ear eg are confined to the endolymphatic spaces of the cochlea and saccule. Cataract, glaucoma, sensorineural hearing loss and neurologic impairment may progress after birth as a consequence of the continued virus infection.

Related Facts
I **Sex Ratio:** M1:F1
II **Risk of Occurrence:** Depends on prevalence of rubella in the community; may exceed 1 in 100 live births during epidemic years or less than 1 in 10,000 live births during immediate postepidemic years.
III **Risk of Recurrence for**
   Patient's Sib: None
   Patient's Child: None
IV **Age of Detectability:** At birth or infancy if rubella virus is isolated from an infected child. Antibody studies on cord blood may be diagnostic. Hearing loss eg may be detected early by alert parents, nurse or pediatrician. However, in some cases clinical stigmata alone may not be detectable for months or rarely, several years.
V **Prevalence:** ?

Treatment
I **Primary Prevention:** Rubella vaccination of all children. Human immunoglobulin (gamma globulin) but effectiveness is questionable.
II **Secondary Prevention:** Some of the neonatal manifestations of congenital rubella are self-limited and resolve spontaneously eg thrombocytopenic purpura, hepatitis, bone lesions and hemolytic anemia. Therapy for specific defects requires the services of a variety of specialists. Ideally, a multidisciplinary team should provide the coordinated care necessary for the multihandicapped child. No variation from established procedures is required, (eg early congestive heart failure is justification for cardiac catheterization, angiocardiography and surgical correction of a patent ductus arteriosus during infancy). Surgery for bilateral cataracts should usually be delayed until 6-12 months of age. Congenital glaucoma requires immediate surgery. Amplification and auditory training are indicated as soon as significant hearing loss is determined. Specialists in rehabilitation medicine, and education of the handicapped, should be an integral part of the treatment team.
III **Other Therapy:** None

Prognosis: Varies critically with the timing of the maternal infection. For multihandicapped infants, especially those with neonatal thrombocytopenic purpura, the mortality rate is high. A death rate of 35% was observed during the 1st year of life in 1 group of 58 infants with purpura. The overall mortality for infants with manifestations of congenital rubella detected during the 1st year of life is 10-20%. For those who survive infancy, most may anticipate normal life span. The exceptions are those severely retarded nonambulatory children who require institutional care. When provided early with intensive treatment and special education, many multihandicapped children may make reasonable socio-economic adjustments. The usual causes of death during early infancy are congestive heart failure, sepsis and general debility.†

Detection of Carrier: Rubella infection in pregnant women

†Special Considerations: The infant with congenital rubella may shed virus in pharyngeal secretions, urine, stool and tears for months after birth, hence he must be considered contagious to all susceptible persons with whom he may have direct contact. Virus shedding is uncommon

(< 10%) after age 1 year and has not been reported after 2 years of age.

Children with congenital rubella may appear clinically normal at birth and during early infancy. All infants whose mothers are suspected of having had rubella during pregnancy should be studied for laboratory and clinical signs. Any positive finding warrants regular evaluation during infancy and early childhood with special emphasis on detection of ocular, audiologic and neurologic defects. Cardiac lesions are less likely to be overlooked.

Sensory deprivation from auditory or ocular defects compounds any intellectual deficit associated with the sequelae of congenital rubella encephalitis. Early efforts at habilitation and education should include intensive family counseling and stimulation designed to "reach" the intact senses.

Premature labeling of a child with congenital rubella as "suitable for custodial care" should be avoided. Because of the chronic virus infection and the sensory deficits, some infants exhibit a degree of psychomotor retardation which does not accurately reflect their potential for learning. A trial in a multidisciplinary diagnostic teaching program, geared to multihandicapped preschool children, may provide helpful information on a child's ability to learn.

References:
Cooper, L. Z. and Krugman, S.: The rubella problem. In Dowling, H.F. (ed.): Disease-a-Month. Chicago:Year Book Medical Publishers, Inc., 1969.
Desmond, M.M. et al: Congenital rubella encephalitis: Course and early sequelae. J. Pediatr. 71:311, 1967.
Krugman, S.: Rubella symposium. Am. J. Dis. Child. 110:345, 1965.

Contributors: **Louis Z. Cooper**
Saul Krugman

Editor's Computerized Descriptors: Vision, Eye, Hearing, Skin, Skel., Resp., CV., Spleen, Liver, Nerve
Also see Section I, Figs. 28, 76

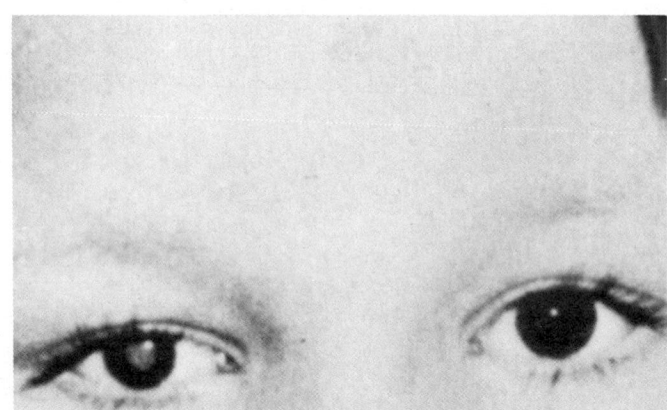
264. Congenital rubella cataract and microphthalmia OD

FETAL SYPHILIS SYNDROME

Includes: Angeborene Lues
Sífilis congénita
Treponema pallidum in utero
Syphilis, congenital

Excludes: —

Minimal Diagnostic Criteria: With newly acquired, untreated disease in the pregnant mother, the newborn infant should be considered to be infected. If syphilis was acquired by the mother but was not treated in the 2 years prior to the present delivery, the infant should be carefully observed. Clinical diagnosis in newborns may be difficult. In some cases, there is no clinical or laboratory evidence of infection at the time of birth but these will appear in the early months of life. Most rapid means of diagnosis of congenital syphilis is by dark-field examination of moist skin lesions or mucopurulent drainage from the nares if these are present or by careful serologic testing.†

Clinical Findings: Since Treponema pallidum can invade and variably damage almost any organ system to any degree, congenital syphilis is generally characterized by protean manifestations.

Early characteristic lesions are similar to those of secondary syphilis in the adult. The most distinctive are as follows: maculopapular, bullous, vesicular, eczematous or annular cutaneous lesions. Distribution is significant; involvements may be generalized but can include localized lesions in the circumoral and anogenital regions, palms and soles. Flat condylomata can occur in the perianal region. Mucus patches and fissures may occur on lips or perianal region. Purulent and hemorrhagic rhinitis (snuffles) are due to involvement of nasal mucosa. Osseous lesions may be clinically silent and demonstrable only on roentgenograms. Osteochondritis commonly may involve the long bones and occasionally the small bones of hands and feet (dactylitis). Diffuse periostitis can develop but usually occurs well after osteochondritis. CNS involvements are frequent, dangerous and often clinically inapparent early in the infection. For these reasons, spinal fluid examinations should be performed in all infants with suspected infection. Typical positive findings are those of meningeal inflammation. Hematopoietic system-anemia (frequent); hepatosplenomegaly and jaundice (frequent); lung - pneumonia alba (uncommon except in severe disease); kidney-albuminuria; occasionally nephrotic syndrome.

Late manifestations include lesions which occur in early childhood and are thought to be caused by hypersensitivity: interstitial keratitis and gummatous degenerations of various organs. Scarring from early lesions causes typical stigmata. Later in life, these classically include: saddle nose, saber shin, Hutchinson teeth, mulberry molars and other dental anomalies; a multitude of CNS abnormalities including vestibular dysfunction and sensorineural deafness and, occasionally, aortic valvulitis.

Complications
I **Derived:** Mental retardation
II **Associated:** —

Etiology: Infection of a human fetus by Treponema pallidum between the 20th week of gestation and birth

Pathogenesis: Infection may result in abortion, stillbirth, delivery of symptomatic infant or a neonate who appears normal but develops signs of infection in the early months of life.

Related Facts

I **Sex Ratio:** M1:F1
II **Risk of Occurrence:** ? Frequency increasing
III **Risk of Recurrence for**
    Patient's Sib: ? Dependent upon effective treatment of infected mother and her possible reinfection
    Patient's Child: None
IV **Age of Detectability:** At birth or early infancy, by dark-field examination or serology
V **Prevalence:** ? Frequency increasing

Treatment
I **Primary Prevention:** Prompt treatment and reporting of all cases of early or latent syphilis.
II **Secondary Prevention:** Experience has shown that the Treponema pallidum still retains a high sensitivity to penicillin and application of this drug has been successful in cures. Therefore, penicillin is the drug of choice in the treatment of congenital syphilis.

Careful diagnosis and adequate treatment of the mother will cure active infection in utero, providing the fetus has been exposed to the medication for a sufficient period of time prior to delivery. Care should be taken to employ drugs that are proven to cross the placenta (penicillin and erythromycin; because of its adverse effects on the fetus, tetracycline should be avoided, if possible). Residual effects, caused by tissue damage to the fetus before treatment, may be present at delivery and result in stigmata later in life.

Children under 2 years may be treated with benthazine penicillin G, 50,000 units/kg body wt, given as a single dose; or procaine penicillin G with 20% aluminum monostearate (PAM), 100,000 units/kg body wt, given in 3 divided doses at 3-day intervals; or aqueous procaine penicillin, 100,000 units/kg body wt, given in 10 daily doses of 10,000 units/kg body wt. The latter treatment schedule should be employed if laboratory evidence of CNS involvement is present at delivery.
III **Other Therapy:** Therapy for deafness due to late congenital syphilis should not only include appropriate doses of penicillin but also corticosteroids.

Prognosis: Dependent upon degree of tissue involvement and promptness of effective therapy

Detection of Carrier: Early or latent syphilitic infection in pregnant women

†**Special Considerations:** The interpretation of positive serology in cord or neonatal sera for the purpose of diagnosing congenital syphilis is frequently complicated by the presence of both nontreponemal or treponemal maternal antibodies which can be transferred to the fetus in both infected and uninfected pregnancies. Antibodies transferred from maternal to fetal sera during pregnancy are contained in the G fraction of the serum immunoglobulins. Maternal VDRL antibodies usually disappear during the first 3 or 4 months following delivery, while maternal antibodies reactive in the fluorescent treponemal antibody test (FTA-ABS) may be detectable for as long as 6 months. In some cases of congenital syphilis, antibody production can be initiated in utero. Fetally produced antibodies are contained in the M globulin fractions of cord or neonatal sera collected from infected neonates. The following serologic findings in the infant strongly suggest intrauterine antibody production and, hence, active infections: levels of treponemal or nontreponemal antibodies 4-fold above those in the maternal sera; a rapid increase in titers of syphilis antibodies in the 1st week of life; demonstration of M treponemal or nontreponemal antibodies. This can be rapidly detected in the M-FTA-ABS test.

Under most circumstances, treatment should be deferred until the diagnosis of congenital syphilis is confirmed either by the demonstration of Treponema pallidum or by serologic methods. However, early and adequate treatment of infants with congenital syphilis is imperative in order to avoid CNS damage. The following therapeutic guidelines are helpful when confirmation of infection cannot be readily obtained.

Treatment should be immediately instituted and completed with the following: 1) any clinical evidence of infection in infants with positive syphilis serology; 2) history or serologic evidence of newly acquired infection by the mother during the course of the pregnancy; 3) if a suspected infant must be treated for any other reason, therapy should be adequate to cure syphilis.

References:
Brown, W. J. and Moore, M. B., Jr.: Congenital syphilis in the United States. Clin. Pediatr. (Phila.) 2:220, 1963.
Curtis, A. C. and Philpott, O. S.: Prenatal syphilis. Med. Clin. North Am. 48:707, 1964.
Harris, W. D. and Cave, V. G.: Congenital syphilis in the newborn; diagnosis and treatment. JAMA 194:1312, 1965.
Kampmeier, R. H.: Syphilis: The same old disease. South. Med. J. 53:2, 1965. (Editorial)
Scotti, A. T. and Logan, L.: A specific IgM antibody test in neonatal syphilis. J. Pediatr. 73:242, 1968.
Tuffanelli, D.L. et al: Fluorescent treponemal-antibody absorption tests: Studies of false-positive reactions to tests for syphilis. N. Engl. J. Med. 276:258, 1967.

Contributors: **Charles A. Alford, Jr.**
John Simpson

Editor's Computerized Descriptors: Eye, Hearing, Ear, Teeth, Nasoph., Nose, Skin, Skel., Resp., CV., Spleen, Liver, GU., Nerve

FETAL THALIDOMIDE SYNDROME

Includes: Embryopathie causée par le thalidomide
Thalidomid-Embryopathie
Embriopatía por talidomida

Excludes: Similar limb or other developmental defects not causally related to thalidomide

Minimal Diagnostic Criteria: Maternal ingestion of 1 tablet (100 mg) of thalidomide at the critical stage of embryonic development (4 - 6 weeks) and resulting developmental defects.

Clinical Findings: May affect the development of almost any organ; however, the most obvious finding is reduction deformities of the limbs ranging from hypoplasia of 1 or more digits to total absence of all limbs. The association of phocomelia, hearing loss, nasal hemangioma, duodenal stenosis and other defects, sometimes is described as thalidomide syndrome.

Complications
I **Derived:** Deafness, blindness, congenital defects of the heart, kidney, GI tract and other organs. Severely involved fetuses may be stillborn.
II **Associated:** —

Etiology: Maternally ingested thalidomide at critical stage of embryonic development (4 - 6 weeks).

Pathogenesis: —

Related Facts
I **Sex Ratio:** M1:F1
II **Risk of Occurrence:** †
III **Risk of Recurrence for**
    Patient's Sib: None
    Patient's Child: None
IV **Age of Detectability:** At birth
V **Prevalence:** Highest where thalidomide was most used. An iatrogenic epidemic 1959-1962. Smaller number of similar defects of unknown etiology occurred prior to and following withdrawal of thalidomide.†

Treatment
I **Primary Prevention:** Avoidance of thalidomide in early pregnancy
II **Secondary Prevention:** Corrective as appropriate. Prostheses as indicated.
III **Other Therapy:** Supportive care dependent on defect

Prognosis: Normal life span if only limbs are involved. Life span reduced in relation to type and degree of heart, kidney or other organ defects.

Detection of Carrier: —

†**Special Considerations:** Thalidomide (DL-α-phthalimidoglutarimide) (Thalidomide, Contergan, Distavol, Kevadon) was synthesized in 1956 in the laboratories of Chimie Grunenthal Gm Btl, Stolberg, Germany. It was first listed in the German registry of approved drugs in 1957 and was prescribed for its sedative effect. In 1960-1961, several reports of peripheral neuritis as a thalidomide side effect were published. In 1961 and 1962, MacBride, Weicker and Lenz separately directed attention to the increased incidence of reduction deformities of the limbs and maternal ingestion of thalidomide. The drug was withdrawn from the world market in early 1962 and the incidence of limb deformities returned to the pre-thalidomide level. On a world-wide basis, probably 10,000 neonates had thalidomide embryopathy.

References:
Lenz, W.: Kindliche Missbildungen nach Medikament-Einnahme während der Gravidität? Dtsch. Med. Wochenschr. 86:2555,

1961.

McBride, W. G.: Thalidomide and congenital abnormalities. Lancet 2:1358, 1961.

Swinyard, C. A. (ed.): Limb Development and Deformity: Problems of Evaluation and Rehabilitation. Springfield:Charles C Thomas Co., 1969.

Contributor: **Chester A. Swinyard**

Editor's Computerized Descriptors: Vision, Hearing, Nose, Skel., CV., GI., GU.

FETAL TOXOPLASMOSIS SYNDROME

Includes: Toxoplasmose congénitale
Angeborene Toxoplasmose
Toxoplasmosis, infantile
Chorioretinitis, toxoplasmic

Excludes: Fetal rubella syndrome (384)
Fetal cytomegalovirus syndrome (381)
Erythroblastosis fetalis

Minimal Diagnostic Criteria: High-titered toxoplasma antibodies in the serum of both the mother and infant are suggestive, but must be interpreted with caution because latent acquired toxoplasmosis is frequent in the obstetric age group (30%) and these antibodies are transmitted to the infant. In uninfected infants passively acquired transplacental antibodies will fall in titer about 50% per month. In infected infants the titer will be maintained, and may fluctuate for a few months before rising, reflecting antibody production by the infant. A fluorescent antibody test showing elevated IgM globulins (20mg%) and specific toxoplasma IgM antibodies in the IFA test supports the diagnosis in a young infant. Specific diagnosis may be made by isolating the parasite from spinal or ventricular fluid, biopsy tissue or autopsy material, by intraperitoneal inoculation of mice.

Clinical Findings: Infection of the fetus by toxoplasma (T.) gondii leads to signs and symptoms covering a wide spectrum from stillborn infants to essentially healthy, but infected children. Prematurity is frequent but birthweight is usually within the normal range for the gestation period. The most common findings are those reflecting involvement of the CNS, including hydrocephaly or microcephaly, unilateral or bilateral retinochoroiditis with microphthalmia and other abnormalities secondary to diffuse encephalomyelitis such as convulsions, psychomotor disturbances and cerebral calcifications. Spinal and ventricular fluid is often xanthochromic with mononuclear pleocytosis and elevated protein. Systemic signs include fever, hepatomegaly, jaundice, splenomegaly, pneumonitis, carditis and a maculopapular skin rash.

Children who appear healthy at birth may show evidence later in life of CNS disease such as mental retardation, seizures, or recurrent episodes of retinochoroiditis.

Complications

I   **Derived:** In survivors of severe disease, mental retardation over 80%, convulsions or other neurologic abnormalities in about 80%, sight is impaired in over half and deafness has been reported in over 10%. When only ocular manifestations are observed in infancy, the retinochoroiditis may recur and continue to blindness or to secondary glaucoma requiring enucleation.

The complications which may follow subclinical infection have not been studied. Mental retardation, cerebral calcifications, convulsions, deafness, retinochoroiditis and other neurologic manifestations have been observed in older children in whom the infection was not suspected in infancy. Retinochoroiditis with onset in adult life may be due to congenital T. gondii which was clinically undetectable at birth.

II **Associated:** —

Etiology: Transplacental transmission of T. gondii to the fetus from a mother initially infected during pregnancy.

Pathogenesis: Spread of T. gondii from mother to fetus via the placenta; proliferation of T. gondii leading to necrosis in many fetal tissues, especially the brain.

Related Facts

I Sex Ratio: M1:F1

II Risk of Occurrence: (Based on few studies at present) 1 in 500 in low-income Negro populations in Birmingham, Ala. 1 in 1350 in New York Hospital, mixed ethnic populations.

III Risk of Recurrence for
Patient's Sib: No proven risk
Patient's Child: No proven risk

IV Age of Detectability: (Closely associated with clinical severity). The infection in stillborn and fatal cases can be diagnosed at autopsy, by visualization or isolation of the parasite; in newborns by clinically characteristic disease and by isolation of T. gondii from spinal or ventricular fluid or biopsied tissue and by high-titered antibodies in mother and infant including toxoplasma specific IgM antibodies in the infant; in infants age 4-8 months. The clinical diagnosis is confirmed by a comparison of toxoplasma antibody titers in mother and infant with a high titer maintained by the infant because in the infected infant, the titer remains high whereas in the uninfected, the titer will have fallen about 50% per month; in older ages the diagnosis is frequently made by positive toxoplasma antibody tests on the child, but the older the patient is the less confidence can be placed in these positive tests because of the possibility of acquired infection after birth.

V Prevalence: ? Possibly about 1 in 1000

Treatment

I Primary Prevention: Avoiding the sources of infection before and during pregnancy: a) ingestion of rare meat and b) exposure to cat feces or soil potentially contaminated by them. Cats that hunt or are fed raw meat are potential vectors and excrete oocysts for 1-2 weeks after the infectious meal. One to 3 days after *Toxoplasma* oocysts are excreted in cat feces, they become infective. They remain infective in water or moist soil for weeks and months. In recent studies oocyst survival has been shown for over a year. Drying and heat kill them. Precautions should include feeding cats only canned or dried foods, removing cat feces from "litterpans" daily (before the oocysts have sporulated), and using plastic gloves when handling cat-contaminated litterpans and work gloves when handling soil. c) Children's sandboxes should be covered when not in use. d) The children of mothers with remote infection are protected. e) No vaccine is at present available.

II Secondary Prevention: Detection of recently acquired toxoplasmosis in gravid patients by clinical evidence and serologic testing. When detected early enough, therapeutic abortion has been used. Chemotherapy with sulfadiazine and pyrimethamine is of questionable value. It should be used only in the second half of pregnancy together with Leucovorin. In the first trimester these drugs should be avoided because of their teratogenic effect.

III Other Therapy: Identify the infants with clinically inapparent infections and treat them, hopefully, to prevent the development of clinical involvement of the CNS or retina. Prompt treatment of infants with sulfadiazine and pyrimethamine is recommended but is seldom of value because treatment cannot reverse the damage due to necrosis.

Prognosis: Estimates are based on few studies. Death in 7%; survival with severe damage (mental retardation, etc) in 8%; survival with ocular damage in 25%; survival with an unknown portion showing sequelae from an infection that was subclinical in infancy in 60%.

Detection of Carrier: Not applicable. A chronically infected carrier mother is immune and will not infect her infant in utero.

Special Considerations: —

References:
Alford, C.A. et al: Subclinical central nervous system disease of neonates. A prospective study of infants born with increased levels of IgM. J. Pediatr. 75:1167, 1969.
Desmonts, G. et al: Le toxoplasme, la mere et l'enfant. Arch. Fr. Pediatr. 22:1183, 1965.
Frenkel, J. K.: Toxoplasmosis. Mechanisms of infection, laboratory diagnosis and management. Curr. Top. Pathol. 54:28, 1971.
Kimball, A.C. et al: Congenital toxoplasmosis: A prospective study of 4,048 obstetric patients. Am. J. Obstet. Gynecol. 111:211, 1971.

Contributors: **B. H. Kean**
Anne C. Kimball

Editor's Computerized Descriptors: Vision, Eye, Hearing, Skin, Skel., Resp., CV., Spleen, Liver, Nerve
Also see Section I, Figs. 25, 26

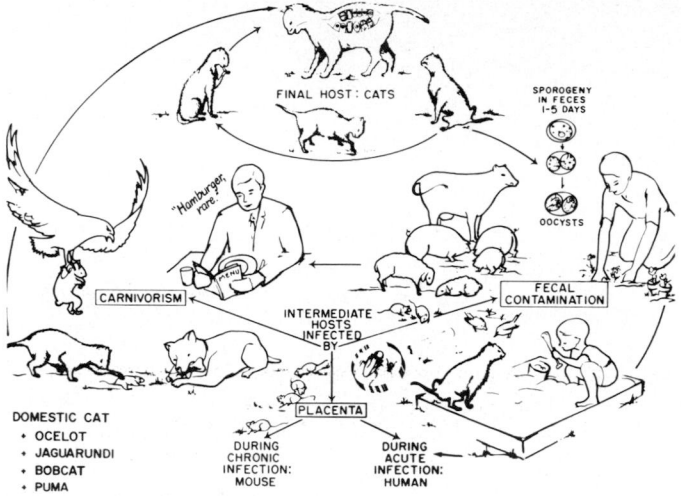

265. Postulated epidemiology of toxoplasmosis transmission

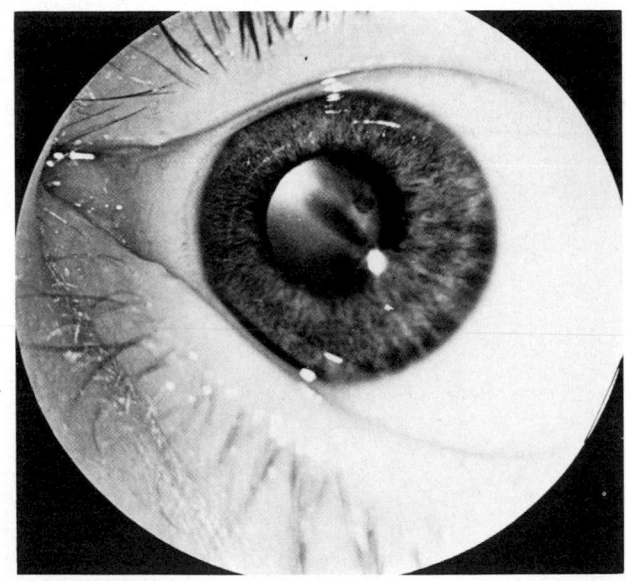

266. Note inflammatory membrane behind lens

FETAL TRIMETHADIONE SYNDROME

Includes: Embryopathie due à le triméthadione
Fetales Trimethadion-Syndrom
Síndrome de la trimetadiona fetal
Tridione syndrome
Paradione syndrome
Fetal damage from oxazolidine anticonvulsants

Excludes: Fetal damage from other anticonvulsants

Minimal Diagnostic Criteria: The diagnosis may be considered in any child exposed prenatally to oxazolidine anticonvulsants, who also manifests several of the features below. There is some variability in the manifestations in individual patients.

Clinical Findings: Common abnormalities which characterize children exposed prenatally to oxazolidine anticonvulsants include prenatal onset growth deficiency, mental deficiency, dysmorphic craniofacial features, and cardiac defects. The craniofacies displays mild brachycephaly with midfacial hypoplasia, short nose with broad depressed nasal bridge and epicanthic folds, synophrys with "V'-shaped eyebrows; low-set posteriorly rotated ears with a poorly developed, cupped or overlapping helix; mild micrognathia, broad lateral palatine ridges, and irregular dentition. The most frequent cardiac defects are septal defects and tetralogy of Fallot. Affected children also frequently have minor genital anomalies including hypospadias or clitoral enlargement.

Less commonly, these children have microcephaly, strabismus, ptosis, visual and hearing deficits, facial hemangiomas, scoliosis, transposition of the great vessels, hypoplastic heart, pyloric stenosis, renal anomalies, umbilical and inguinal herniae, dislocated hips, ambiguous genitalia, and single palmar creases.

Complications
I   **Derived:** Growth deficiency, speech disorders, visual and hearing deficits, mental deficiency.
II **Associated:** —

Etiology: Maternal treatment with an oxazolidine anticonvulsant (trimethadione, paramethadione) during pregnancy.†

Pathogenesis: ?

Related Facts
I   **Sex Ratio:** M1:F1
II **Risk of Occurrence:** Current epidemiologic data is inadequate to provide an accurate risk estimate among exposed infants. However, case reports suggest that trimethadione may be a potent teratogen.
III **Risk of Recurrence for**
    Patient's Sib: None unless an oxazolidine anticonvulsant is taken during pregnancy.
    Patient's Child: None unless an oxazolidine anticonvulsant is taken during pregnancy.
IV **Age of Detectability:** At birth or early infancy
V   **Prevalence:** Rare. Oxazolidine anticonvulsants are uncommonly employed during childbearing years.

Treatment
I   **Primary Prevention:** Avoidance of oxazolidine anticonvulsants during pregnancy. Women with seizure disorders should be informed of the nature of risks to the fetus arising from oxazolidine therapy prior to considering a pregnancy.
II **Secondary Prevention:** Surgical correction of major defects may be necessary. Effective remedies for deficiencies of growth and performance have not been demonstrated. Speech therapy may be of value in some cases.
III **Other Therapy:** Early childhood stimulation and appropriate educational placement may be of benefit.

Prognosis: Mental deficiency and serious cardiac defects give many cases a poor prognosis.

Detection of Carrier: —

†**Special Considerations:** Trimethadione and paramethadione are no longer regarded as the drugs of choice in any seizure disorder and should only be utilized when other safer agents are ineffective. Furthermore, the types of seizure disorders for which these agents are most effective are rare in women of childbearing age. Thus, there is seldom an indication for using this dangerous class of drugs in a potentially pregnant woman. Unfortunately, the safety for the fetus of alternative drugs is not clearly established at the present time.

References:
German, J. et al: Trimethadione and human teratogenesis. Teratology 3:349, 1970.
Zackai, E.H. et al: The fetal trimethadione syndrome. J. Pediatr. 87:280, 1975.

Contributor: **James W. Hanson**

Editor's Computerized Descriptors: Vision, Eye, Hearing, Ear, Face, Teeth, Nose, Speech, Skin, Hair, Skel., Hernia not CNS, CV., GI., GU., Nerve

FETAL WARFARIN SYNDROME

Includes: Embryopathie due à la warfarine
Cumarin-Embryopathie
Embriopatía por warfarina
Vitamin K-antagonist embryopathy
Coumadin embryopathy
Oral anticoagulant embryopathy
Warfarin embryopathy

Excludes: Chondrodysplasia punctata, rhizomelic type (154)
Chondrodysplasia punctata, Conradi-Hünermann type (153)

Minimal Diagnostic Criteria: Documented history of maternal ingestion of vitamin K-antagonist anticoagulant in therapeutic doses during the 1st trimester of pregnancy in association with 1 or more common malformations, ie hypoplastic nose, stippled epiphyses, eye abnormality.

Clinical Findings: Maternal vitamin K-antagonist therapy during the 1st trimester results in a recognizable complex of abnormalities in some newborns. Summary of 11 affected cases: 1) hypoplastic nose with underdeveloped nasal cartilage resulting in an upturned appearance (100%) (also choanal stenosis-2/11, respiratory distress-5/11) 2) bony abnormalities primarily stippling of epiphyses, particularly in the lumbosacral and cervical vertebrae, trochanters of femurs, and calcaneus (90%) (also broad short hands-5/11, short distal phalanges-4/11, skull abnormality-3/11) 3) ophthalmologic abnormalities (45%) (blindness-3/11, optic atrophy-2/11, hypertelorism-2/11, cataract-1/11, microphthalmia-1/11, prominent eyes with small eyelids-1/11) 4) mental retardation (36%) (all of the retarded children have additional problems: 3 are blind, 1 with occipital meningomyelocele and hydrocephaly, and the 4th has deafness and seizures) 5) intrauterine growth retardation (27%) 6) neck anomalies (27%) Other features seen-hypotonia, poorly developed ears, seizures, occipital meningomyelocele with hydrocephaly, posterior cleft of cervical vertebrae, short neck, persistent truncus arteriosus, severely short long bones, large tongue, hypertrophied clitoris, single umbilical artery. Two cases have multiple severe malformations.

Vitamin K-antagonist therapy with onset during the 2nd or 3rd trimester is not associated with the above but may result in an increased number of stillbirths and abortions. In addition, among living children CNS malformations may be observed with an increased frequency.

Complications
I   **Derived:** Infants may have bleeding problems at birth, if mother is still on anticoagulants.
II **Associated:** —

Etiology: Teratogenic effect of vitamin K-antagonist anticoagulant drugs during the 1st trimester. Malformations may be time-specific.

Pathogenesis: Not known whether malformations are due to hemorrhage with secondary scarring, a direct effect of drugs on tissue, or a deficiency of vitamin K in tissue.

Related Facts
I   **Sex Ratio:** M1:F1
II **Risk of Occurrence:** Not all women taking oral anticoagulants during the 1st trimester have affected children. At least half of reported cases of maternal coumadin use in the 1st trimester are said to be normal. Less than half of all affected cases are seriously affected. Thus, the risk of a child being seriously affected would apppear to be less than 25%.
III **Risk of Recurrence for**
    Patient's Sib: ? Depends on whether mother is still taking the drug.
    Patient's Child: None
IV **Age of Detectability:** At birth (stippled bones seen on xray may be gone by 1 year of age so radiographs should be taken at birth)
V   **Prevalence:** Rare

Treatment
I   **Primary Prevention:** Maternal use of heparin during 1st trimester, if anticoagulation is required.
II **Secondary Prevention:** —
III **Other Therapy:** —

Prognosis: Varies with severity of defects. Most infants have shown cosmetic improvement of nose with growth. Stippling of long bones is usually no longer evident by 1 year of age.

Detection of Carrier: —

Special Considerations: —

References:
Becker, M.H. et al: Chondrodysplasia punctata. Is maternal warfarin therapy a factor? Am. J. Dis. Child. 129:356, 1975.
Hall, J.G.: Embryopathy associated with oral anticoagulant therapy. In Bergsma, D. (ed.): Cytogenetics, Environment and Malformation Syndromes. Birth Defects: Orig. Art. Ser., vol. XII, no. 5. New York: Alan R. Liss for The National Foundation-March of Dimes, 1976, p. 33.
Pettifor, J. M. and Benson, R.: Congenital malformations associated with the administration of oral anticoagulants during pregnancy. J. Pediatr. 86:459, 1975.
Shaul, W.L. et al: Chondrodysplasia punctata and maternal warfarin use during pregnancy. Am. J. Dis. Child. 129:360, 1975.
Shaul, W.L. and Hall, J.G.: Multiple congenital anomalies associated with oral anticoagulants. Am. J. Obstet. Gynecol. 127:191, 1977.
Warkany, J. and Bofinger, M.: Coumadin and congenital malformations. J. Med. Hyg. 33:1454, 1975.

Contributor: **Judith G. Hall**

Editor's Computerized Descriptors: Vision, Eye, Hearing, Ear, Oral, Nasoph., Nose, Neck, Skel., CV., GU., Nerve , Resp.

FIBROUS DYSPLASIA, MONOSTOTIC

387-500

Includes: Dysplasie fibreuse monostotique
Fibrose Dysplasie
Displasia fibrosa monostótica
Jaffe-Lichtenstein disease

Excludes: Fibrous dysplasia, polyostotic (391)
Unicameral bone cyst
Aneurysmal bone cyst
Ossifying fibroma

Minimal Diagnostic Criteria: This disorder may be suspected on radiologic grounds, but the diagnosis can only be made by biopsy and histologic confirmation.†

Clinical Findings: This disease is characterized by a solitary pseudocystic lesion of bone which usually develops during childhood or adolescence. The individual lesion is identical to that found in polyostotic fibrous dysplasia, but it is isolated to 1 area and is not associated with extraskeletal manifestations. The lesions are most common in the craniofacial bones, ribs, vertebrae, and long bones. The craniofacial lesions can produce deformities secondary to the presence of a mass, or difficulty in chewing because of maxillary enlargement. Lesions in the ribs are usually discovered incidentally on routine chest xrays. Involvement of the vertebrae may produce low back pain. Those lesions affecting the long bones usually present as a mass. The earliest radiologic changes are loss of density in the site where bone is being replaced by fibrous tissue. Later the whole shaft may exhibit a ground-glass appearance with expansion of the medullary cavity and internal atrophy of the cortical walls. Diagnosis can only be made on microscopic confirmation of the typical lesion consisting of whorls of fibrous tissue with interspersed islands of bony trabeculae and calcified cartilage.

Complications
I **Derived:** —
II **Associated:** —

Etiology: ?

Pathogenesis: ?

Related Facts
I **Sex Ratio:** M1:F1
II **Risk of Occurrence:** ?
III **Risk of Recurrence for**
    Patient's Sib: ? (All cases have been sporadic)
    Patient's Child: ?
IV **Age of Detectability:** Can be detected in early childhood by skeletal xrays.
V **Prevalence:** ?

Treatment
I **Primary Prevention:** —
II **Secondary Prevention:** Orthopedic procedures such as curettage of the lesion and packing with bone chips
III **Other Therapy:** —

Prognosis: Normal for life span. Lesions may progressively increase in size. Regrowth has often occurred following curettage, which has apparently been incomplete.

Detection of Carrier: —

†Special Considerations: The term "Jaffe-Lichtenstein syndrome" should be restricted to those cases of fibrous dysplasia which are monostotic. The polyostotic form of the disease is often associated with endocrine and skin manifestations and probably represents a completely distinct entity. This disorder may appear identical radiographically to unicameral bone cysts, aneurysmal bone cysts and ossifying fibromas. The diagnosis can only be confirmed upon histologic examination of biopsied tissue.

References:
Harris, W.H. et al: The natural history of fibrous dysplasia. J. Bone Joint Surg. 44A:207, 1962.
Jaffe, H.L. and Lichtenstein, L.: Non-osteogenic fibroma of bone. Am. J. Pathol. 18:205, 1942.

Contributors: **David L. Rimoin**
David W. Hollister

Editor's Computerized Descriptors: Face, Oral, Skel.

FIBROUS DYSPLASIA, POLYOSTOTIC

Includes: Dysplasie fibreuse polyostotique
Polyostotische Fibrose Dysplasie
Displasia fibrosa polióstica
Polyostotic fibrous dysplasia, skin pigmentation and sexual precocity
McCune-Albright syndrome

Excludes: Fibrous dysplasia, monostotic (390)
Neurofibromatosis (712)
Hyperparathyroidism

Minimal Diagnostic Criteria: Diagnosis of this disorder can be made by the classic radiographic appearance of polyostotic fibrous dysplasia, with or without the associated skin or endocrine anomalies. Neither the skin lesions nor sexual precocity are required to make a diagnosis.†

Clinical Findings: The classic triad of this syndrome consists of polyostotic fibrous dysplasia, skin pigmentation and sexual precocity. It is now obvious, however, that in some individuals the skeletal disorder can occur alone or with only 1 of the cutaneous or endocrine components. The bone disorder consists of patchy areas of rarefaction with a pseudocystic appearance. The lesions may be disseminated throughout the skeleton, and are most frequently found in the lower limbs, less frequently in the upper limbs, and rarely in the skull. The skull may be involved, however, by a sclerotic overgrowth of bone at the base, which may be so dense that the sella cannot be visualized. Deforming overgrowth of the skull, jaw, or facial bones may occur. The skeletal lesions result in frequent fractures, deformity, and leg length discrepancy. In 1 series, 70% of the patients presented with a limp, leg fracture, or limb pain; 60% had leg length discrepancy; 85% had experienced at least 1 fracture; and 40% had experienced 3 or more fractures. Serum alkaline phosphatase levels are elevated in about 1/3 of the patients. The lesions may progress by extension, increasing deformity, or by the appearance of new lesions. There is no evidence for a change in the frequency of fractures with puberty. Fracture healing is not delayed. The skeletal lesions consist of poorly differentiated fibrous tissue with fibrous bone trabeculae interspersed; in some specimens multiple islands of cartilage have been found. Sarcomatous degeneration in an area of fibrous dysplasia has been described on 2 occasions.

The skin lesions consist of brown nonelevated patches of pigmentation with an irregular outline. They are frequently present at birth. Distribution is often unilateral and segmental and they may overlie areas of bone involvement.

The sexual precocity occurs primarily in females, but several affected males have been described with precocious puberty. Approximately 50% of females with polyostotic fibrous dysplasia have sexual precocity. It usually first presents as abnormal vaginal bleeding which may occur as early as 3 months of age. In contrast to most types of sexual precocity, the vaginal bleeding, which is usually scanty and irregular, precedes the breast development and sexual hair growth by as much as 7 years. The ovaries have been found to contain follicles in various stages of development, sometimes with large follicular cysts. There is no evidence of ovulation or corpus luteum formation. Urinary gonadotropins are usually low to absent, but high peaks of urinary LH have been detected. Urinary estrogen, 17-hydroxycorticoid and 17-ketosteroid concentrations have been elevated in some patients. At the regular time of puberty, ovulation and regular periods occur, and fertility is not impaired. Affected males usually do not have sexual abnormalities, but precocious puberty has been described in a few males, 1 of whom had active spermatogenesis. Advanced skeletal and accelerated growth in childhood may occur in patients with sexual precocity. Adult height, however, is usually normal or somewhat decreased. Diffuse or nodular thyroid enlargement is frequent, and mild hyperthyroidism is also common; parathyroid hyperplasia has been described in several patients.

Skeletal xrays reveal hypo- or hypersclerotic cysts which may be scattered throughout the skeleton. They are not bilaterally symmetric, and may have a segmental distribution. They have a ground-glass appearance due to a myriad of thin calcified trabeculae. There is variability in the overlying cortical thickness, and the periosteal surface is smooth. Other disorders, such as unicameral bone cysts, aneurysmal bone cysts, and nonossified fibromata may appear similar radiographically. Involvement of the entire bone from epiphyseal plate to epiphyseal plate and the increased density of the base of the skull, however, are not found in these other disorders. The skeletal lesions may result in bending or bowing of the affected bones, the classic deformity being the "shepherd's crook" malformation of the femoral neck.

Complications
I   **Derived:** The skeletal lesions may result in multiple fractures, leg length discrepancy, bowing of the limbs, a waddling gait, and persistent pain. The sclerotic lesions of the base of the skull may result in obliteration of the nasal sinuses, facial asymmetry, and rarely may impinge upon the optic nerves resulting in optic atrophy. Sarcomatous degeneration of the bony lesions has been described in 2 patients. The multiple fractures may result in partial-to-complete disability, and multiple fractures of the ribs may predispose to pneumonia.
II **Associated:** —

Etiology: ?

Pathogenesis: ?

Related Facts
I   **Sex Ratio:** Approximately M1:F1 (For the skeletal disorder)
II   **Risk of Occurrence:** ?
III **Risk of Recurrence for**
    Patient's Sib: ? (All cases to date have been sporadic, including discordant identical twins.)
    Patient's Child: ?
IV **Age of Detectability:** The disease may be detected at birth by the pigmented skin lesions; in infancy or childhood by sexual precocity; or in childhood or adolescence by the deformities, fractures, or leg length discrepancy resulting from the fibrous dysplasia of bone.
V   **Prevalence:** ?

Treatment
I   **Primary Prevention:** —
II **Secondary Prevention:** Orthopedic surgical correction for progressive deformity, nonunion of fractures, femoral shaft fractures in adults or persistent pain. Medroxyprogesterone may be used for sexual precocity.
III **Other Therapy:** —

Prognosis: The life span is apparently normal. When the fibrous dysplasia is extensive early in life, the progression of the disorder is marked and the prognosis is poor.

Detection of Carrier: —

†**Special Considerations:** The association of polyostotic fibrous dysplasia, sexual precocity, and skin pigmentation has been known as the McCune-Albright syndrome. It is apparent, however, that the polyostotic fibrous dysplasia is the only invariable

feature of this disorder, and it may occur alone or in conjunction with only 1 of the associated anomalies. Polyostotic fibrous dysplasia with or without the associated skin and endocrine manifestations should be considered as a unified syndrome.

References:
Alexander, F.W.: Polyostotic fibrous dysplasia with raised steroid excretion. Arch. Dis. Child. 46:91, 1971.
Benedict, P.H.: Endocrine features in Albright's syndrome (fibrous dysplasia of bone). Metabolism 11:30, 1962.
Harris, W.H. et al: The natural history of fibrous dysplasia. J. Bone Joint Surg. 44A:207, 1962.

Contributors: **David L. Rimoin**
                    David W. Hollister

Editor's Computerized Descriptors: Face, Skin, Skel., GU.

FIBULA DYSPLASIA AND BRACHYDACTYLY

Includes: Dysplasie du péroné et brachydactylie
Fibula-Dysplasie mit Brachydaktylie
Displasia del peroné y braquidactilia
Brachydactyly and fibula dysplasia

Excludes: Other types of brachydactyly

Minimal Diagnostic Criteria: Fibula dysplasia with brachydactyly†

Clinical Findings: Characterized by shortening of metacarpals, small carpals and short middle phalanx of index fingers causing brachydactyly with radial deviation. Both reported cases had almost complete absence of the fibula bilaterally. There was tibiotarsal dislocation and brachydactyly of the toes which were deviated laterally.

Complications
I **Derived:** Orthopedic complications result from the bony deformities, especially in the legs.
II **Associated:** —

Etiology: Autosomal recessive inheritance is likely because the patients were sibs and the parents were 1st cousins.

Pathogenesis: ?

Related Facts
I **Sex Ratio:** M1:F1
II **Risk of Occurrence:** ?
III **Risk of Recurrence for**
    Patient's Sib: Presumably 1 in 4 (25%) for each offspring to be affected
    Patient's Child: Not increased unless mate is carrier or homozygote.
IV **Age of Detectability:** Infancy
V **Prevalence:** ?

Treatment
I **Primary Prevention:** If autosomal recessive, genetic counseling
II **Secondary Prevention:** Appropriate orthopedic procedures to feet and hands
III **Other Therapy:** —

Prognosis: Normal for life span and intelligence with variable function

Detection of Carrier: ?

†Special Considerations: The chief distinction between this condition and other types of brachydactyly (types AI-5 and B-E) is the fibula dysplasia.

References:
Grebe, H.: Chondrodysplasie. Rome Int. Greg. Mendel., 1955, p. 300.

Contributor: **David C. Siggers**

Editor's Computerized Descriptor: Skel.

Includes: Absence de dermatoglyphes
Fehlen von Fingerbeerenmustern
Ausencia de huellas dactilares
Absent fingerprints

Excludes: Keratosis palmaris et plantaris
Hypoplasia of dermal ridges

Minimal Diagnostic Criteria: Complete absence of finger, palm, and toeprint dermatoglyphics from birth.

Clinical Findings: Complete absence of dermatoglyphics (finger, palm, and toeprints) from birth. Of 16 affected members in 4 generations, all had congenital milia which lasted for about 6 months and absent ridge formation. Bilateral webbing of the toes and bilateral flexion contractures of the fingers or the toes were present in all members either alone or in combination. No other evidence of an ectodermal defect was present. Their intelligence, physical findings, including teeth and fingernails, patterns of illness, and the like were not remarkable.

Complications
I **Derived:** Painful fissures and discomfort of the palms and soles during hot or cold weather.
II **Associated:** —

Etiology: Autosomal dominant; McK *13600

Pathogenesis: Highly speculative. It has been suggested that the family carries a genetic factor for a congenital epidermolytic process. This would be severe enough to lead to massive sloughing and would involve only the volar surfaces. If this process occurred, the new skin would lack ridges and the contractures would be induced by the fetal reparative activities.

Related Facts
I **Sex Ratio:** M1:F1
II **Risk of Occurrence:** ?
III **Risk of Recurrence for**
 Patient's Sib: If parent is affected 1 in 2 (50%) for each offspring to be affected; otherwise not increased
 Patient's Child: < 1 in 2
IV **Age of Detectability:** At birth
V **Prevalence:** Only 1 kindred has been reported to date.

Treatment
I **Primary Prevention:** Genetic counseling
II **Secondary Prevention:** —
III **Other Therapy:** —

Prognosis: Normal life span

Detection of Carrier: —

Special Considerations: —

References:
Baird, H.W.: Absence of fingerprints in four generations. Lancet 2:1250, 1968.
Baird, H.W.: Kindred showing congenital absence of the dermal ridges (fingerprints) and associated anomalies. J. Pediatr. 64:621, 1964.

Contributor: **Henry W. Baird**

Editor's Computerized Descriptors: Skin, Dermatoglyphic, Skel.

Includes: Dysplasie frontométaphysaire
Frontometaphysäre Dysplasie
Displasia frontometafisaria

Excludes: Osteodysplasty (775)
Craniometaphyseal dysplasia (228)
Pyle disease (847)
Other craniotubular dysplasias

Minimal Diagnostic Criteria: Peculiar facial appearance, dental abnormalities, multiple joint contractures, skeletal dysplasia with metaphyseal modeling defects of the tubular bones, calvarial hyperostosis, abnormal pelvic appearance.

Clinical Findings: Peculiar face with prominent supraorbital ridges (in most patients); a small pointed chin, micrognathia; high-arched palate, malaligned, small teeth, unerupted or congenitally missing teeth. Relatively short trunk with a straight thoracic spine or thoracic lordosis, scoliosis; pectus excavatum or carinatum, winging of the scapulae; relatively long hands and feet, multiple joint contractures of the large and small joints.

Radiographs reveal diffuse hyperostosis of the calvaria, most prominently in the frontal region, underdeveloped paranasal sinuses, micrognathia, multiple dental abnormalities; abnormalities of the cervical spine, dorsally flattened vertebral bodies; irregular contours of the ribs; flared iliac wings with abnormally constricted lower portions of the ilia and constricted pelvic outlet; small capital femoral epiphyses; coxa valga, metaphyseal flaring and tortuosity of the shafts of the long tubular bones; small carpal bones with pronounced underdevelopment of the proximal row; extended lack of metaphyseal modeling of the short tubular bones.

Complications
I **Derived:** Progression of joint contractures, joint pain, muscular hypotrophy, hammer toe, progressive thickening of the cranial vault; combined sensorineural and conductive hearing loss; psychologic problems due to facial appearance.
II **Associated:** Impaired vision due to congenital esotropia and secondary amblyopia; hyperopia; bifid uvula, recurrent respiratory and middle ear infections; cardiac defects.

Etiology: Autosomal dominant.† There may also be an X-limited form.

Pathogenesis: ?

Related Facts
I **Sex Ratio:** M1:F1
II **Risk of Occurrence:** ?
III **Risk of Recurrence for**
 Patient's Sib: If parent is affected 1 in 2 (50%); otherwise not increased.
 Patient's Child: 1 in 2
IV **Age of Detectability:** Early infancy (joint contractures). Skeletal changes in young children.
V **Prevalence:** ?

Treatment
I **Primary Prevention:** Genetic counseling
II **Secondary Prevention:** —
III **Other Therapy:** Appropriate for orthopedic, dental and hearing problems. Surgical removal of the frontal torus has been recommended for cosmetic reasons.

Prognosis: Psychomotor development and life expectancy are normal in most patients. The complications listed above may interfere with the patient's physical and social performance.

Detection of Carrier: Skeletal radiographs may detect abnormal bone modeling or cranial hyperostosis in otherwise unaffected relatives.

†**Special Considerations:** The similar clinical and radiographic findings suggest that osteodysplasty and frontometaphyseal dysplasia are the same condition. There are, however, subtle differences in the appearance of the vertebral bodies and hand bones of reported cases. Further observations are needed to show whether these differences are consistent or if they are variable manifestations of the same mutation.

References:
Gorlin, R. J. and Cohen, M.M.: Frontometaphyseal dysplasia. Am. J. Dis. Child. 118:487, 1969.
Holt, J.F. et al: Frontometaphyseal dysplasia. Radiol. Clin. North Am. 10:225, 1972.

Contributor: **Jürgen W. Spranger**

Editor's Computerized Descriptors: Vision, Eye, Hearing, Face, Oral, Teeth, Skel.

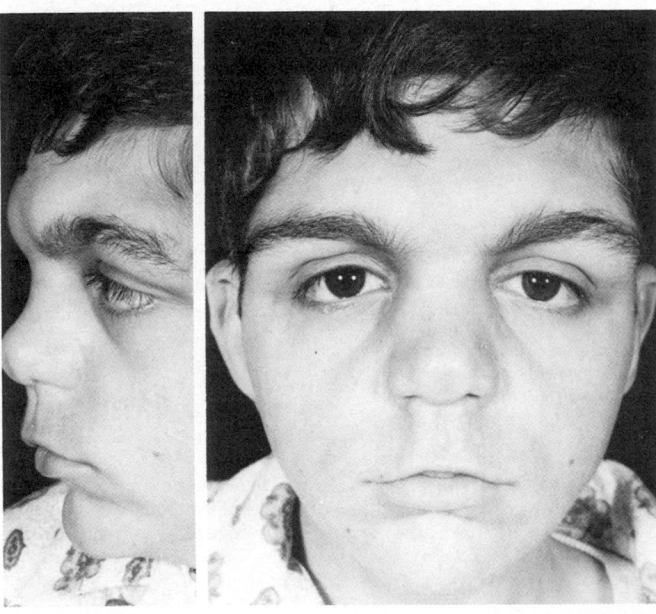

267. Note broad nasal bridge, thickened nares, prominent supra-orbital ridge, and small pointed chin

FRUCTOSE-1-PHOSPHATE ALDOLASE DEFICIENCY

Includes: Déficit en fructose-1-phosphate aldolase
Fruktose-1-Phosphat-Aldolase Mangel
Deficiencia de fructosa-1-fosfato aldolasa
Fructosemia
Fructose intolerance

Excludes: Galactose and fructose intolerance
Fructosuria (Marker) (397)
Fructose-1, 6-diphosphatase deficiency (396)

Minimal Diagnostic Criteria: An IV fructose tolerance test with 3 gm of fructose per m^2 in children and 0.25 gm of fructose per kg in adults leads to a sustained fall in blood glucose, hypoglycemic symptoms and hypophosphatemia. Blood glucose and inorganic serum phosphorus must be determined in 15 minute intervals up to 120 minutes. A fall of blood glucose of more than 40% from the initial value lasting for 1/2 hour or longer proves the diagnosis of fructose intolerance. This diagnosis is confirmed by the measurement of the ratio of the hepatic aldolase activities to fructose-1,6-diphosphate and fructose-1-phosphate respectively, which is above 5.0 (normal ratio 1.4).†

Clinical Findings: The major symptoms are: failure to thrive 100%, vomiting 100%, hepatomegaly 100%, jaundice 100% and seizures caused by hypoglycemia 100%. The acute syndrome after fructose ingestion consists of nausea, vomiting, all signs and symptoms of hypoglycemia and fructosuria. Hypoglucosemia develops rapidly after fructose intake and reaches its lowest values after 30-60 minutes. Children demonstrate symptoms faster than adults. At the same time the level of serum inorganic phosphorus falls in a sustained manner. After massive doses of fructose, hyperbilirubinemia and a rise of serum levels of hepatic enzymes (eg sorbitol dehydrogenase and glutamate-pyruvate-transhydrogenase) may be seen. Transient aminoaciduria of the "hepatic type" may occur. The chronic syndrome is seen only in babies during infancy. It is caused by prolonged intake of fructose, most often in the form of saccharose (table sugar or sucrose) and fruit juices.

Fructosuria is present after fructose intake. Later fibrosis and cirrhosis of the liver may develop together with ascites and edema. If the condition is not recognized in due time, the babies may die in a cachectic state. Tubular acidosis has been described. The teeth of older children and of adult patients with fructose intolerance regularly are free from dental caries. All patients from the age of 6 months onward develop a strong aversion to all food stuffs which are sweet and contain fructose and they thus protect themselves from getting ill.

Complications
I **Derived:** If fructose ingestion continues, cachexia, liver failure and dehydration result.
II **Associated:** —

Etiology: Autosomal recessive deficiency of fructose-1-phosphate aldolase in liver, kidney and mucosa of small bowel; McK *22960

Pathogenesis: Since fructose-1-phosphate aldolase is needed only for the metabolism of fructose, patients with fructose intolerance are perfectly healthy as long as no fructose is ingested. Fructokinase is present in normal amounts and fructose is phosphorylated primarily by the liver to fructose-1-phosphate which accumulates intracellularly. Fructose-1-phosphate blocks glycogenolysis and gluconeogenesis leading to hypoglucosemia. Fructose-1-

phosphate impedes the action of phosphorylase and thus the formation of glucose-1-phosphate from glycogen. On the other hand, fructose-1-phosphate appears to inhibit the formation of fructose-1,6-diphosphate aldolase which is also present in the liver. Hepatocellular damage is also believed to be caused by the accumulation of fructose-1-phosphate.

Related Facts
I   **Sex Ratio:**   M1:F1
II **Risk of Occurrence:**   ?
III **Risk of Recurrence for**
    Patient's Sib: 1 in 4 (25%) for each offspring to be affected
    Patient's Child: Not increased, unless mate is carrier or homozygote
IV **Age of Detectability:**   At birth, by fructose tolerance test or enzyme determination in liver biopsy
V   **Prevalence:**   ?

Treatment
I   **Primary Prevention:**   Genetic counseling
II **Secondary Prevention:**   All fructose-containing food stuffs must be completely avoided. Hypoglycemic attacks caused by the ingestion of fructose may be relieved instantaneously by the IV administration of glucose. There is no specific treatment for hepatocellular damage in fructose intolerance with the exception of complete avoidance of any fructose-containing food stuffs.
III **Other Therapy:**   —

Prognosis: The prognosis is very bad when the condition is not recognized. The earlier fructose is started and continued, the faster the condition deteriorates. Babies with fructose intolerance who were persistently fed fructose died between 2 and 6 months of age. The cause of death is cachexia, liver failure and dehydration. Death due to hypoglycemia has not been described. No residual brain damage was found in any surviving child or adult with fructose intolerance.

Hepatocellular damage is usually reversible when the children are taken off fructose. Children recover fully and life span is normal.

Detection of Carrier: The heterozygous carriers of fructose intolerance are not detectable clinically with the use of fructose tolerance tests. An intermediate ratio of hepatic fructose-1-phosphate to fructose-1,6-diphosphate aldolase activity between normal subjects and patients with fructose intolerance is to be expected, but has not yet been proven.

†**Special Considerations:**   Fructose intolerance is not the same as fructosuria, another anomaly of fructose metabolism characterized by a lack of fructokinase. Another disorder of fructose metabolism distinct from fructose intolerance is fructose and galactose intolerance. Two sisters displayed severe hypoglycemic attacks after fructose as well as galactose ingestion, accompanied by hyperinsulinism which is not present in fructose intolerance. Nausea and vomiting, typical for fructose intolerance, were absent in these 2 cases, neither of whom developed a distaste toward sweet food stuffs.

References:
Black, J. A. and Simpson, K.: Fructose intolerance. Br. Med. J. 4:138, 1967.
Froesch, E. R.: Essential fructosuria and hereditary fructose intolerance. In Stanbury, J.B. et al (eds.): The Metabolic Basis of Inherited Disease, 3rd Ed. New York:McGraw-Hill, 1972, p. 131.
Mass, R. E. et al: The association of hereditary fructose intolerance and renal tubular acidosis. Am. J. Med. Sci. 251:516, 1966.

Contributor: **E. R. Froesch**

Editor's Computerized Descriptors: Nose, Skin, GI., Liver, GU., Nerve

FRUCTOSE-1,6-DIPHOSPHATASE DEFICIENCY

Includes: Déficit en fructose-1,6-diphosphatase hépatique
Fruktose-1,6-Diphosphatasemangel
Deficiencia de fructosa-1,6-difosfatasa
Hepatic fructose-1,6-diphosphatase deficiency

Excludes: Fructose-1-phosphate adolase deficiency (395)
Pyruvate carboxylase deficiency with lactic acidemia (850)
Myopathy with lactic acidemia (697)
Glycogenosis, type I† (425)
Glycogenosis, type III† (426)

Minimal Diagnostic Criteria: Absence or severe deficiency of hepatic fructose-1,6-diphosphatase. Hypoglycemia and lactic acidosis with fasting.

Clinical Findings: This inborn error of hepatic gluconeogenesis presents in the immediate neonatal period with acute episodes of hyperventilation, convulsions, coma, lactic acidosis, hypoglycemia, ketosis, and hyperalaninemia. Later, these symptoms occur in the fasting state and are often provoked by febrile infections. Peculiar EEG patterns during the acute episodes have been reported. During the asymptomatic intervals, mild hepatomegaly (fatty infiltration), muscle hypotonia and hyperventilation may be marked. There is normal psychomotor development.

Blood glucose is reduced after fasting and may fall below 10-20 mg/dl. Lactate is usually elevated and after fasting may be > 200 mg/dl. The lactate falls rapidly with correction of the hypoglycemia. Alanine may be elevated, especially during acidosis. Glucagon fails to raise blood glucose after prolonged fasting but postprandially it raises blood glucose to normal.

Complications
I   **Derived:**   —
II **Associated:**   —

Etiology: Autosomal recessive; McK *22970

Pathogenesis: In this defect of hepatic gluconeogenesis, blood glucose cannot be maintained after depletion of liver glycogen stores. Prolonged fasting is poorly tolerated. Mild fructose and sorbitol intolerance exists and is caused by the inhibition of hepatic glycogenolysis by certain phosphate esters.

Related Facts
I   **Sex Ratio:**   M4:F10
II **Risk of Occurrence:**   ?
III **Risk of Recurrence for**
    Patient's Sib: 1 in 4 (25%) for each offspring to be affected.
    Patient's Child: Not increased unless mate is carrier or homozygote.
IV **Age of Detectability:**   Any age
V   **Prevalence:**   ?

Treatment
I   **Primary Prevention:**   Genetic counseling
II **Secondary Prevention:**   Avoidance of prolonged fasting, especially during febrile infections. Restriction of dietary fructose and sorbitol, reduction of proteins and fats. As weight reduction is difficult to achieve, caloric intake may have to be closely watched in order to prevent obesity. Prompt correction of hypoglycemia and acidosis.
    Caution: The infusion of sorbitol for suspected brain edema has been lethal in 1 child!
III **Other Therapy:**   Treatment with folic acid has been suggested but remains to be proved beneficial.

Prognosis: Acute episodes are life-threatening. Growth, psychomotor and intellectual development seem unimpaired if acute episodes can be prevented.

Detection of Carrier: In the 3 parents examined, the activity of hepatic frutose-1,6-diphosphatase was reduced to approximately 1/2 of the normal or less.

†**Special Considerations:** This disorder may be difficult to distinguish initially from glycogen storage disease especially type I, but also type III. The blood lactate levels should distinguish it from type III, and the response to glucagon following an adequate carbohydrate intake should distinguish it from type I. Increased glycogen storage may be found in the liver of these patients.

References:

Baerlocher, K. et al: Infantile lactic acidosis due to hereditary fructose 1,6-diphosphatase deficiency. Helv. Paediatr. Acta 26:489, 1971.

Baker, L. and Winegrad, A.I.: Fasting hypoglycaemia and metabolic acidosis associated with deficiency of hepatic fructose-1,6-diphosphatase activity. Lancet 2:13, 1970.

Gitzelmann, R. et al: Hereditäre Störungen im Fruktose-und Galaktosestoffwechsel. Monatsschr. Kinderheilkd. 121:174, 1973.

Greene, H.L. et al: "Ketotic Hypoglycemia" due to hepatic fructose-1,6-diphosphatase deficiency: Treatment with folic acid. Am. J. Dis. Child. 124:415, 1972.

Hülsmann, W.C. and Fernandes, J.: A child with lactacidemia and fructose diphosphatase deficiency in the liver. Pediatr. Res. 5:633, 1971.

Retbi, J.-M et al: Acidose lactique et hypoglycémie à début néonatal par déficit congénital en fructose-1,6-diphosphatase hépatique. Arch. Fr. Pediatr. 32:367, 1975.

Contributor: **Richard Gitzelmann**

Editor's Computerized Descriptors: Resp., Nerve, Muscle

FRUCTOSURIA (MARKER)

Includes: Fruktosurie
Essential fructosuria

Excludes: Fructose-1-phosphate aldolase deficiency (395)

Minimal Diagnostic Criteria: The reducing sugar in the urine must be identified as fructose.† Blood fructose levels after oral administration of fructose (1 gm per kg body weight) are markedly increased (above 25 mg per 100 ml), and levels remain high 4 hours later. Following an oral fructose load, fructose appears rapidly in the urine. Glucose and galactose metabolism are normal.

Clinical Findings: Individuals are normal except for the presence of a reducing sugar in the urine (positive Benedict, positive Fehling, positive Nylander qualitative tests); negative glucose-oxidase (Testape or Clinistix). It is important as a differential for diabetes mellitus.

Complications
I **Derived:** —
II **Associated:** —

Etiology: Autosomal recessive deficiency of fructokinase; McK *22980

Pathogenesis: Fructose is excreted in the urine because of a lack of hepatic fructokinase which normally catalyzes the conversion of fructose to fructose 1-phosphate.

Related Facts
I **Sex Ratio:** M1:F1
II **Risk of Occurrence:** ?
III **Risk of Recurrence for**
  Patient's Sib: 1 in 4 (25%) for each offspring to be affected
  Patient's Child: Not increased, unless mate is carrier or homozygote
IV **Age of Detectability:** Any age, dependent upon diet, if urine examined for reducing sugar (fructose).
V **Prevalence:** 1 in 130,000 of general population; 18 of 50 cases have occurred in Jews.

Treatment
I **Primary Prevention:** Genetic counseling
II **Secondary Prevention:** Eliminate fructose from diet. Insulin is usually without effect.
III **Other Therapy:** —

Prognosis: Excellent

Detection of Carrier: ?

†**Special Considerations:** Fructose is fermentable by yeast, yields a positive Selivanoff reaction and is levorotatory. Its identity is confirmed by paper chromatographic techniques.

References:

Froesch, E. R.: Essential fructosuria and hereditary fructose intolerance. In Stanbury, J.B. et al (eds.): The Metabolic Basis of Inherited Disease, 3rd Ed. New York:McGraw-Hill, 1972, p. 131.

Laron, Z.: Essential benign fructosuria. Arch. Dis. Child. 36:273, 1961.

Lasker, M.: Essential fructosuria. Hum. Biol. 13:51, 1941.

Schapira, F. et al: La lésion enzymatique de la fructosuria bénigne. Enzym. Biol. Clin. 1:170, 1961-62.

Contributor: **Maurice D. Kogut**

Editor's Computerized Descriptor: —

FUCOSIDOSIS

Includes: Fukosidose
"Mucopolysaccharidosis F"

Excludes: Mucopolysaccharidoses
Mucolipidoses I, II, III, and IV
G_{M2}-gangliosidosis with hexosaminidase A deficiency (434)
G_{M2}-gangliosidosis with hexosaminidase A and B deficiency (433)
Mannosidosis
Aspartylglucosaminuria
Fabry disease (373)

Minimal Diagnostic Criteria: In deteriorating nervous system diseases of young children, proof of involvement with this syndrome, after general review of features, involves demonstration (leukocytes, cultured skin fibroblasts) of absent α-L-fucosidase activity and increased tissue levels of fucose-containing polysaccharides and sphingolipids. Plasma is convenient for screening, but a small percentage of normal individuals have no detectable activity. Localized deficiencies limited to cultured fibroblasts have been encountered while normal activity was preserved in leukocytes and plasma. The significance of these findings is unknown.

Clinical Findings: At least 20 patients have now been identified. A great deal of clinical heterogeneity is apparent, but 2 main groups can be delineated. In Type 1, corresponding to the original disease description, the children make fair progress in the 1st year of life, but then have progressive cerebral degeneration, with weakness and hypotonia followed by the picture of spastic quadriplegia. They have thick skin, with abundant sweating and cardiomegaly. Seizures are not frequent. Of note is a markedly increased sodium and chloride level in sweat (3-9x N), and a progressive impairment of gallbladder function. Spinal fluid is normal and urinary mucopolysaccharides are not increased, but a number of fucose-containing oligosaccharides and glycopeptides have been detected. Faint corneal cloudiness may be present. There is a brachycephalic skull, with frontal bulging, and lumbar kyphosis with hypoplasia and beaking of L-2 and L-3. The special features of the illness are an accumulation of fucose-containing neutral polysaccharides in vacuolated lymphocytes, skin, liver and other tissues (intracellular), an increase of fucose-containing lipids in liver and brain and an absence of α-L-fucosidase in tissue assays.†

In Type 2, the children present with delayed psychomotor development. Angiokeratomas, similar to those of Fabry disease, may appear around age 5 years. Neurologic symptoms include spasticity, contractures, peripheral neuropathy and amyotrophy. There is no visceromegaly. Skeletal abnormalities are discrete, resembling those of Mucopolysaccharidosis III.

Complications
I   **Derived:** Chronic recurrent respiratory infection is a problem, as well as the easy dehydration and electrolyte depletion from sweat losses. In these children there is progressive weight loss, as well as signs of myocarditis.
II **Associated:** Thickened skin, muscle contractures.

Etiology: Autosomal recessive; deficiency of α-L-fucosidase has been found in liver, lung, kidney, brain, skin fibroblasts, leukocytes and serum. McK *23000

Pathogenesis: A gradual increase in the levels of fucose-containing polysaccharides and glycolipids is noted in most tissues, including brain, apparently correlating with the above-mentioned deficiency of tissue fucosidase. Changes are notable also in the muco-secreting glands, skin and lymphocytes. The white matter of the brain shows demyelination and gliosis. Electron microscopic studies of the liver cells have revealed cytoplasmic vacuoles surrounded by a single membrane, containing granular inclusion and lamellar bodies. Similar lamellar bodies, with a larger periodicity, are also seen in mitochondria.†

Related Facts
I   **Sex Ratio:**   M1:F1
II   **Risk of Occurrence:**   ?
III **Risk of Recurrence for**
     Patient's Sib: 1 in 4 (25%) for each offspring to be affected
     Patient's Child: Not increased unless mate is carrier or homozygote
IV   **Age of Detectability:**   Prenatal diagnosis has been attempted. One affected fetus was mistaken for a heterozygote.
V   **Prevalence:**   ?

Treatment
I   **Primary Prevention:**   Genetic counseling
II   **Secondary Prevention:**   Attention to hydration needs
III **Other Therapy:**   Use of antibiotics

Prognosis: Death has occurred at around 5 years of age in Type 1. Survival to adulthood can be expected in Type 2 (the oldest patient on record is now 24 years).

Detection of Carrier: Most heterozygotes have intermediate α-L-fucosidase activity in cultured skin fibroblasts or leukocytes. Overlap between heterozygously involved individuals and normals occasionally occurs. Until a statistically significant number of obligatory heterozygotes has been studied, individuals with equivocal activities are best considered at risk.

†**Special Considerations:** Fucose is known to be part of glycoproteins and sphingolipids with blood group activity (A, B, H, and Lewis), and also of uromucoid, a urinary glycoprotein. From the generalized involvement of tissues in the present condition, it can be inferred that fucose-containing compounds represent a common cell constituent which might contribute to its biochemical individualization.

At least 6 α-L-fucosidase isozymes are known. All of them are barely detectable in both types of fucosidosis. Attempts to relate the clinical expression to the Lewis blood types have not been conclusive.

References:
Borrone, C. et al: Fucosidosis. J. Pediatr. 84:727, 1974.
Brill, P.W.: Roentgenographic findings in Fucosidosis Type 2. Am. J. Roentgenol. Radium Ther. Nucl. Med. 124:75, 1975.
Durand, P. et al: Fucosidosis. J. Pediatr. 75:665, 1969.
Humbel, R. and Collart, M.: Oligosaccharides in urine of patients with glycoprotein storage diseases. Clin. Chim. Acta 60:143, 1975.
Philippart, M.: Glycolipids. Adv. Exp. Med. Biol., 25:231, 1972.

Contributor: **Michel Philippart**

Editor's Computerized Descriptors: Eye, Face, Skin, Sweating, Skel., Muscle, CV., Liver, Nerve

FUNDUS ALBIPUNCTATUS

Includes: Fundus albipunctatus cum hemeralopia
Fundo albino puntato

Excludes: Progressive albipunctate dystrophy
Retinitis punctata albescens
Uyemura syndrome
Vitamin A deficiency †
Oxalate retinopathy †
Fleck retina of Kandori

Minimal Diagnostic Criteria: Typical fundus findings with night-blindness that becomes normal with time and a normal ERG after appropriate adaptation.

Clinical Findings: Multiple yellow-white dots, sparing the macula, are seen deep in the retina and are associated with congenital stationary nightblindness. The dots are most dense in the posterior pole and are more scattered towards the periphery. The size of the spots has been described as that of a second order arteriole, and they are fairly uniform. The retinal vessels and the optic disk remain normal.

Visual functions are well preserved; acuity is normal, color vision is normal and visual fields are full.

Dark adaptometry shows a marked delay in both cone and rod function so that the normal cone threshold, usually achieved at 10 minutes after a standard bleach, is delayed for up to 1 hour and the final rod threshold may not be achieved for 3 hours with a normal of 30 minutes. Electroretinography parallels the course of adaptation so that a normal ERG is recordable after appropriate adaptation but only a cone-dominated ERG is seen if done in a routine fashion. The EOG has a reduced light rise but this, too, becomes normal after prolonged dark adaptation. Kinetic studies of pigment regeneration show marked delays in both rods and cones.

Complications
I   Derived: —
II Associated: —

Etiology: Autosomal recessive

Pathogenesis: All evidence points to a defect in rate of pigment regeneration with a disturbance in the receptor outer segment-pigment epithelial complex. No histologic examinations have yet been reported.

Related Facts
I   Sex Ratio: M1:F1
II Risk of Occurrence: Rare
III Risk of Recurrence for
    Patient's Sib: 1 in 4 (25%) for each offspring to be affected
    Patient's Child: Not markedly increased unless mate is carrier or homozygote
IV Age of Detectability: 1st decade of life
V   Prevalence: ?

Treatment
I   Primary Prevention: Genetic counseling
II Secondary Prevention: —
III Other Therapy: Night vision pocketscope

Prognosis: Normal life span

Detection of Carrier: —

†Special Considerations: The appearance of white dots in the fundus has been reported in vitamin A deficiency and generalized oxalosis. However, these abnormalities have not been seen in fundus albipunctatus patients.

References:

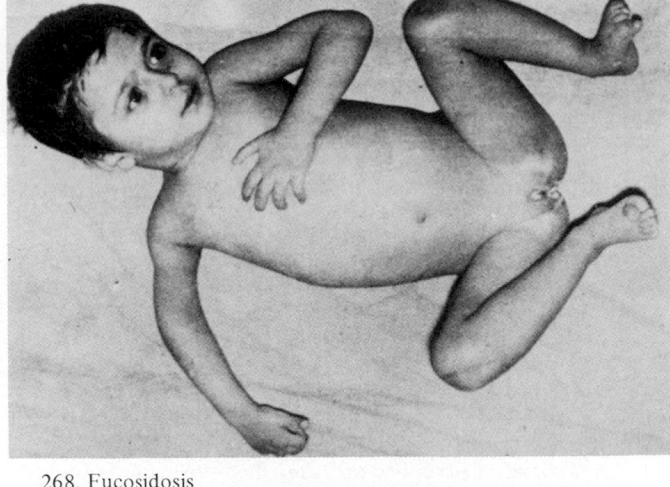

268. Fucosidosis

Carr, R.E.: Congenital stationary nightblindness. Trans. Am. Ophthalmol. Soc. 72:448, 1974.

Carr, R.E. et al: Fluorescein angiography and vitamin A and oxalate levels in fundus albipunctatus. Am. J. Ophthalmol. 82:549, 1976.

Franceschetti, A. et al: Chorioretinal Heredodegenerations. Springfield: Charles C Thomas, 1974.

Contributor: **Mitchel L. Wolf**

Editor's Computerized Descriptor: Eye

FUNDUS FLAVIMACULATUS

Includes: Dystrophie maculaire ponctuée
Fundus flavimaculatus with macular degeneration
Macular degeneration and fundus flavimaculatus
Stargardt disease

Excludes: Fundus albipunctatus (399)
Ocular drusen (734)
Fleck retina of Kandori

Minimal Diagnostic Criteria: Characteristic ophthalmoscopic appearance

Clinical Findings: The term "fundus flavimaculatus" was coined in 1963 by Franceschetti to describe a picture of yellow-white flecks in the deeper retinal layer of the posterior pole of the retina. The lesions vary in size, shape, opaqueness, and density, and occasionally have some surrounding brownish pigmentation. The peripheral lesions are usually asymptomatic but central visual loss occurs if the flecks are present in the foveal area.

An associated atrophic macular degeneration is present in the majority of patients and visual loss may antedate observable pathology. The macular lesion is, for all practical purposes, identical with that described by Stargardt in 1909, and, in the past few years, many authors have equated Stargardt disease with that form of fundus flavimaculatus associated with macular degeneration.

The ophthalmoscopic picture in the periphery changes as new flecks appear and old flecks coalesce or become faint. Fluorescein angiography demonstrates the opaque nature of fresh flecks as well as pigment epithelial defects corresponding to resorbed flecks. Since the disease is characterized by coalescence and resorption of flecks, an end-stage picture of widespread pigment epithelial and choriocapillaris atrophy may be part of this syndrome.

Psychophysical and electrophysiologic abnormalities have been reported and are more likely to be found when the disease is severe. Dark adaptation is often prolonged, the EOG may be abnormal, and the ERG is affected when there is marked peripheral involvement. That is, most patients with the disease have macular degeneration without evidence of diffuse cone abnormality but some display signs of severe rod and cone disease in addition to macular degeneration. Whether the limited form progresses to diffuse form is a matter of debate. The macular degeneration in the limited form of the disease is progressive.

Complications
I   **Derived:**   Macular degeneration; in some cases widespread retinal degeneration
II **Associated:**   —

Etiology: Autosomal recessive inheritance most often, but dominant pedigrees occur. McK *23010

Pathogenesis: Histologic studies show altered morphologic characteristics of pigment epithelium consisting of 1) a displacement of the nucleus from the base of the pigment epithelial cell towards the center or inner surface; 2) a peculiar line of condensation of pigment granules in the center or near the inner surface of the cell, frequently at the level of the displaced nucleus; 3) accumulation of an acid mucopolysaccharide largely within the inner half of the cell in circumscribed areas; and 4) great variations in the size of cells.

Related Facts
I   **Sex Ratio:**   M1:F1
II   **Risk of Occurrence:**   ?
III **Risk of Recurrence for**
      Patient's Sib: When autosomal dominant or autosomal

recessive, see Table I AD or AR, respectively.

Patient's Child: When autosomal dominant or autosomal recessive, see Table I AD or AR, respectively. Minimal in autosomal recessive pedigrees.

IV Age of Detectability: Visual symptoms usually occur between 10 and 30 years.

V Prevalence: ?

Treatment

I Primary Prevention: Genetic counseling

II Secondary Prevention: —

III Other Therapy: —

Prognosis: Normal life span with frequent impairment of central vision

Detection of Carrier: —

Special Considerations: —

References:

Ernest, J.T. and Krill, A.E.: Fluorescein studies in fundus flavimaculatus and drusen. Am. J. Ophthalmol. 62:1, 1966.

Fishman, G.: Fundus flavimaculatus. Arch. Ophthalmol. 94:2061, 1976.

Hadden, O.B. and Gass, J.D.M. Fundus flavimaculatus and Stargardt's disease. Am. J. Ophthalmol. 82:527, 1976.

Irvine, A.R. and Wergeland, F.L.: Stargardt's hereditary progressive macular degeneration. Br. J. Ophthalmol. 56:817, 1972.

Klein, D.: Genetic approach to the nosology of retinal disorders. In Bergsma, D. (ed.): Part VIII. Eye. Birth Defects: Orig. Art. Ser., vol. VII, no. 3. Baltimore: Williams & Wilkins for The National Foundation-March of Dimes, 1971, p. 52.

Klien, B.A. and Krill, A.E.: Fundus flavimaculatus; clinical, functional and histopathologic observations. Am. J. Ophthalmol. 64:3, 1967.

Contributors: **Mitchel L. Wolf**
Donald R. Bergsma
Alex E. Krill‡

Editor's Computerized Descriptors: Vision, Eye

G SYNDROME

Includes: Syndrome G
Sindrome G
Hypospadias-dysphagia syndrome
Opitz-Frias syndrome

Excludes: Aarskog syndrome (1)

Minimal Diagnostic Criteria: Characteristic appearance, unusual type of hypospadias, dysphagia and hoarse voice. Some heterozygotes may have no manifestations at all, 1 apparently affected male only had the characteristic facies; some heterozygotes only have stridor ("wheezers").†

Clinical Findings: Range from congenital lethal severity, or neonatal lethality with multiple congenital anomalies, to a less severe form predominantly with functional swallowing problems - which, if managed properly, may allow survival - to very mild forms with minimal or no functional impairment, usually ascertained on family studies. Most of the severely affected patients are males, though 1 neonatally lethally affected infant was a female. The facial appearance is characteristic: hypertelorism with relatively flattened bridge of nose, prominence of parietal eminences and occiput with relatively dolichocephalic skull and large anterior fontanels, relatively narrow, slit-like palpebral fissures with slight mongoloid or antimongoloid slant, epicanthic folds with or without an accessory fold following the upper lid partly to the outer canthus, strabismus, anteversion of nostrils, philtrum relatively flat and inapparent, with relatively severe micrognathia. Voice and cry are hoarse; usually no other external anomalies are evident except for hypospadias and occasional imperforate anus with rectourethral fistula. The hypospadias is unusual - it ranges in severity from mild coronal to perineoscrotal degrees, with chordee at times pulling tip of glans to anterior edge of anus. Labioscrotal folds may be incompletely fused but testes are usually descended; the 2 halves of the scrotum may be incompletely descended and cover the phallus. An occasional patient may have a cleft lip and cleft palate.

The combination of characteristic facies and genital defects with hoarse or stridulous cry is diagnostic and should immediately lead the clinician to search for the potentially fatal esophageal functional defect which leads to repeated aspiration. In severe cases the infant sucks eagerly but chokes, coughs and becomes cyanotic, develops respiratory distress, increase in stridor, aspiration pneumonia, patchy atelectasis and emphysema, and in chronic cases bronchiectasis. Cinefluoroscopic studies should be done with a water soluble contrast medium; they usually show severely disordered esophageal motion with some or much of the bolus entering the trachea, and much gastroesophageal reflux which may be designated "hiatus hernia" and lead to surgical repair. In severe cases the functional defects may have additional anatomic bases - laryngeal cleft with hypoplasia of epiglottis, vocal cords and larynx, and high bifurcation of trachea, hypoplasia of 1 lung, duodenal stricture. The functional defect usually requires surgery (gastrostomy; in extreme cases ligation of the esophagus with cervical esophagostomy). Survivors mature in their swallowing capacity in a few months to a year to the point where they can eat a normal diet, but continue to choke and aspirate if forced to drink fluids rapidly. They continue to have a relatively hoarse voice and stridor which leads family members to call such individuals and other heterozygotes "wheezers" and which frequently leads to a false diagnosis of respiratory allergy and asthma.

Not all survivors are of normal intelligence; the surviving male of the family had an IQ of 93 at 7 years with an apparently organic learning problem (midline brain defect affecting corpus callosum?); the patient of Frias and Rosenbloom, and all 4 patients of van Biervliet and van Heuvel were mildly retarded. Survivors generally show normal growth of height, weight, and CNS, and have an unusually cheerful personality.

Autopsy may show the above-mentioned anomalies plus CHD: anomalous venous return to the heart, midline position of the heart, with patency of foramen ovale and ductus arteriosus, unlobed lungs, bifid renal pelvis with double ureter, Meckel diverticulum and absence of gallbladder, short or bifid uvula, bifid tip of tongue. Dermatoglyphics are probably normal.

Complications
I **Derived:** Aspiration, pneumonia, death. Respiratory insufficiency in cases of unilateral pulmonary hypoplasia?
II **Associated:** Mental retardation

Etiology: Most likely an autosomal dominant mutation with some male sex-limitation; male-to-male transmission has been suggested but remains unconfirmed; X-linked inheritance has not been ruled out and could account for apparently greater heterogeneity of clinical manifestations in females than in males.

Pathogenesis: The clinical manifestations suggest that this mutation acts primarily on midline organs and structures, less effectively on paramedian structures.

Related Facts
I **Sex Ratio:** Severe dysphagia-hypospadias complex confined to males, though some females may have more or less severe pulmonary manifestations.
II **Risk of Occurrence:** ?
III **Risk of Recurrence for**
    Patient's Sib: If autosomal dominant, see Table I AD (keep in mind possibility of male sex limitation and new mutation, but examine parents minutely before giving negligibly small recurrence risk); if X-linked incompletely recessive, see Table 1 X-linked R.
    Patient's Child: See Table 1
IV **Age of Detectability:** Any age, including neonatal, by physical examination
V **Prevalence:** ?

Treatment
I **Primary Prevention:** Genetic counseling
II **Secondary Prevention:** Any child suspected at birth of having the G syndrome should be fed only water; fluoroesophagraphy should be performed with a contrast medium least harmful to the lungs. If a swallowing defect is demonstrated, a feeding jejunostomy should should be established immediately. If the patient survives to 1 year of age the esophagus can probably be reanastomosed.
III **Other Therapy:** Supportive pediatric care to supplement surgical management. Hypospadias repair is indicated if the patient survives past infancy.

Prognosis: In cases of severe dysphagia, death is usually due to aspiration and inanition. In successfully treated cases prognosis for life, growth and reproduction is presumably normal, although some individuals may be mildly mentally retarded.

Detection of Carrier: Most heterozygotes appear to be relatively healthy persons-some have lifelong stridor. Any suspected carrier (close relative of proband and presence of stridor) should have a chest film to rule out pulmonary anomalies.

†**Special Considerations:** Patients with Aarskog syndrome are short of stature and have a facial appearance similar to patients with the G syndrome. However, dysphagia and pulmonary difficulties have not been observed in that syndrome.

References:
Coburn, T.P.: G syndrome. Am. J. Dis. Child. 120:466, 1970.

Frias, J.L. and Rosenbloom, A.L.: Two new familial cases of the G syndrome. In Bergsma, D. (ed.): Malformation Syndromes. Birth Defects: Orig. Art. Ser., vol. XI, no. 2. Amsterdam: Excerpta Medica for The National Foundation-March of Dimes, 1975, p. 54.
Gilbert, E.F. et al: The pathologic anatomy of the G syndrome. Z. Kinderheilkd. 111:290, 1972.
Kasner, J. et al: Studies of malformation syndromes VID: The G syndrome. Further observations. Z. Kinderheilkd. 118:81, 1974.
Little, J.R. and Opitz, J.M.: The G syndrome. (Letter to the editor) Am. J. Dis. Child. 121:505, 1971.
Opitz, J. M. et al: The G syndrome of multiple congenital anomalies. In Bergsma, D. (ed.): Part II Malformation Syndromes. Birth Defects: Orig. Art. Ser., vol. V, no. 2 White Plains:The National Foundation-March of Dimes, 1969, p. 95.
Pedersen, I.L. et al: The G syndrome; a four generation family study. Hum. Hered. 26:66, 1976.
van Biervliet, J.P.G.M. and van Heuvel, J.O.: Familial occurrence of the
syndrome. Clin. Genet. 7:238, 1975.

Contributor: John M. Opitz

Editor's Computerized Descriptors: Eye, Face, Oral, Nasoph., Nose, Larynx, Speech, Skel., Resp., CV., GI., GU., Nerve

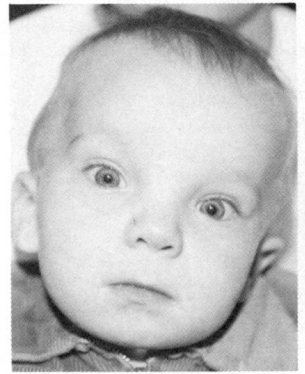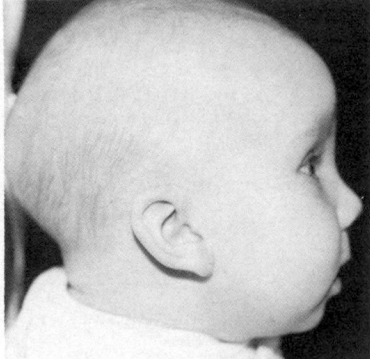

269. Note prominent parietal and occipital skull, posterior rotation of ears, sparse eyebrows, and anteverted nares

GALACTOKINASE DEFICIENCY

Includes: Déficit en galactokinase
Galaktokinasemangel
Deficiencia en galactoquinasa
Agalactokinase

Excludes: Galactosemia (403)

Minimal Diagnostic Criteria: Absence of erythrocyte galactokinase

Clinical Findings: Nuclear and/or zonular cataracts in early infancy, hypergalactosemia, galactose-galactitol-glucose diabetes.

Complications
I   **Derived:** Nuclear and/or zonular cataracts. A peculiar type of polyneuropathy observed in an adult patient who refused treatment may represent a complication of untreated galactokinase deficiency of long standing.
II   **Associated:**   —

Etiology: Autosomal recessive transmission of galactokinase deficiency; McK *23020

Pathogenesis: Inability to metabolize galactose normally with resulting accumulation of galactitol in the intra- and extra- cellular fluids. Galactitol accumulation in the lens causes osmotic swelling, electrolyte imbalance, protein denaturation and thus the formation of "sugar" cataract.

Related Facts
I   **Sex Ratio:** M1:F2 (only approx. 20 patients are known)
II   **Risk of Occurrence:** ? Galactokinase deficiency was originally reported in 3 gypsy families but has since been discovered in various other ethnic groups.
III   **Risk of Recurrence for**
    Patient's Sib: 1 in 4 (25%) for each offspring to be affected
    Patient's Child: Not increased unless mate is carrier or homozygote
IV   **Age of Detectability:** Any age. Newborns fed milk have hypergalactosemia which can be discovered in the routine newborn screening program (microbiologic or enzymatic assay of galactose in dried blood spots), and galactosuria (testing for reducing substances in urine).
V   **Prevalence:** ? 1:100,000 or less.

Treatment
I   **Primary Prevention:** Genetic counseling
II   **Secondary Prevention:** Exclusion of milk, milk products, and other sources of galactose from the diet prevents formation of cataracts. Early cataracts are reversible under galactose exclusion diet.
III   **Other Therapy:** Surgical removal of cataracts. Diet should be established prior to operation as it may help in the prevention of recurring cataracts.

Prognosis: Normal life span. Recurring cataracts after surgical removal of cataract may require discission.

Detection of Carrier: Red blood cell galactokinase approximately 50% of normal

Special Considerations: —

References:
Gitzelmann, R.: Deficiency of erythrocyte galactokinase in a patient with galactose diabetes. Lancet 2:670, 1965.
Gitzelmann, R.: Hereditary galactokinase deficiency: A newly recognized cause of juvenile cataracts. Pediatr. Res. 1:14, 1967.
Gitzelmann R. et al: Galactose metabolism in a patient with hereditary galactokinase deficiency. Eur. J. Clin. Invest. 4:79, 1974.

Contributor: **Richard Gitzelmann**

Editor's Computerized Descriptor: Eye

GALACTOSEMIA

Includes: Galaktosämie
Galactose-1-phosphate uridyl transferase deficiency
Galactosemia-Duarte and Negro variants

Excludes: Galactokinase deficiency (402)

Minimal Diagnostic Criteria: Diagnosis depends upon demonstrating the absence of galactose-1-phosphate uridyl transferase activity in red cells.

Clinical Findings: The infant affected with galactosemia usually appears normal at birth; the symptoms do not develop until milk feedings are given. Excluding patients diagnosed at birth, the findings in 43 symptomatic patients revealed that most had hepatomegaly 90%, jaundice 78%, anorexia and weight loss 54%. Frequently found were: cataracts 42%, vomiting 37%, abdominal distention 20% and lethargy 16%. Ascites, splenomegaly and dark urine were each found in 14%. Bulging anterior fontanel was present in 9%; pallor, cyanosis, diarrhea and mental retardation (moderate or severe) were each present in 7%. Hemorrhagic phenomena were found in 5%; generalized edema, cholelithiasis, acholic stools, dysuria and frequency were each present in 2%.

One of the earliest signs is jaundice which appears at 4 - 10 days of age and which may last for more than 6 weeks. Lethargy and hypotonia are frequent. Food may be refused, vomiting is common, and diarrhea appears occasionally. The clinical course of some infants is fulminant, and in these patients death may occur early from infection, inanition or hepatic failure. The diagnosis of overwhelming sepsis is often suggested by clinical manifestations.

Galactosemia may vary in severity, but the symptoms in the majority of the cases reported have been severe. In a small number of milder cases, the diagnosis may be overlooked for weeks or months. Digestive difficulties, retarded physical and mental development, hepatic enlargement, cataracts and perhaps intolerance to milk should suggest the possibility of galactosemia.

Mature cataracts are usually a late manifestation of the disease. Untreated children who survive beyond the first weeks usually manifest signs of mental retardation which may be moderate or severe. Specific neurologic abnormalities are usually absent.

Complications
I   **Derived:** Overwhelming infection is the most common complication in infancy, and it often results in death, if untreated. Additional complications include hypoglycemia, convulsions, gallstones and gangrene of the limbs secondary to septicemia.
II   **Associated:**   —

Etiology: Autosomal recessive. Presently available evidence suggests a structural change affecting the reactive site of the enzyme.† McK *23040

Pathogenesis: The absence of galactose-1-phosphate uridyl transferase causes galactose, galactose-1-phosphate and galactitol to accumulate. It has been shown that galactose-1-phosphate may be inhibitory to certain enzyme systems. In galactokinase deficiency, galactose-1-phosphate does not accumulate but galactitol does, and nuclear cataracts also occur. Therefore, it is assumed that the cataract of galactosemia results from galactitol accumulation and that galactose-1-phosphate is responsible for the other clinical manifestations. Bilirubin retention may be a result of injury to hepatic cells by metabolites of galactose. Mild hemolysis may be a contributing factor, but the anemia usually accompanying the disease is unexplained.

Transferase activity was reported present during the rapid growth phase of fibroblasts derived from skin of galactosemia patients. The normal transferase and the Duarte variant can be demonstrated in gel electrophoresis, but this is not possible for the galactosemia homozygote due to absent or very low activity.†

Related Facts
I **Sex Ratio:** M1:F1
II **Risk of Occurrence:** ?
III **Risk of Recurrence for**
  Patient's Sib: 1 in 4 (25%) for each offspring to be affected
  Patient's Child: Not increased unless mate is carrier or homozygote.
IV **Age of Detectability:** At birth by absence of enzyme in erythrocytes
V **Prevalence:** Uncertain; a recent estimate is 1 in 40,000. Galactosemia appears to be generally distributed.

Treatment
I **Primary Prevention:** Genetic counseling
II **Secondary Prevention:** Early exclusion of milk and milk products from the diet prevents appearance of the clinical manifestations of the disease. Later institution of treatment results in reversal of symptomatology except for matured cataracts and mental retardation. A number of milk substitutes are available, including casein hydrolysates and soy bean products. Fortunately, exogenous galactose is dispensable. Galactolipids and other essential galactose-containing compounds are provided endogenously from UDPG via reversal of the epimerase system. Consequently, normal physical growth and maturation are possible.
III **Other Therapy:** Appropriate therapy must be undertaken to control infection, correct fluid and electrolyte imbalance and manage bleeding manifestations. Emotional aspects of long-term dietary therapy may require attention.

Prognosis: With untreated galactosemia patients' mortality is high in the first few months of life. The untreated patients who survive usually develop nuclear cataracts and mental retardation. Long-term studies are not yet available, but the life span of the treated galactosemic individual should be similar to that of the general population.

Detection of Carrier: The heterozygote has about 50% of normal galactose-1-phosphate uridyl transferase activity in erythrocytes and is usually asymptomatic.

†Special Considerations: Beutler reported a transferase deficiency (the Duarte variant) different from that commonly described. In the families studied, homozygotes had about half the normal erythrocyte enzyme activity and that for heterozygotes averaged about 75% of normal. Homozygotes for this defect are asymptomatic. Pedigree analysis has suggested that the gene for the Duarte variant is an allele of the galactosemia gene.

References:
Donnell, G. N. et al: Galactosemia. Biochem. Med. 1:29, 1967.
Segal, S.: Disorders of galactose metabolism. In Stanbury, J.B. et al (eds): The Metabolic Basis of Inherited Disease, 4th Ed. New York:McGraw-Hill, l978, p. 160.
Woolf, L. I.: Inherited metabolic disorders: Galactosemia. In Sobotka, H. and Steward, C.P. (eds.): Advances in Clinical Chemistry. New York:Academic Press, 1962, vol. 5.

Contributors: **George N. Donnell**
William R. Bergren

Editor's Computerized Descriptors: Eye, Skin, Skel., Muscle, Resp., Spleen, GI., Liver, Nerve, GU.

GALLBLADDER ANOMALIES

Includes: Anomalies de la vésicule biliaire
Gallenblasen-Fehlbildungen
Anomalías de la vesícula biliar
Absence of gallbladder
Duplication of gallbladder
Diverticulum of gallbladder
Bilobed gallbladder
Ectopic gallbladder
Cystic artery anomalies
Floating gallbladder

Excludes: Cholesterolosis
Cholecystitis
Cholelithiasis
Hydrops of gallbladder
Choledochal cyst (149)

Minimal Diagnostic Criteria: Usually asymptomatic. Rarely diagnosis of duplication is made by xray when 2 rows of stones are observed. "Floating" gallbladder causes sudden right-upper quadrant pain, nausea and vomiting if torsion occurs.

Clinical Findings: *Congenital absence of gallbladder* (gallbladder agenesis): A rare occurrence as an isolated entity and has no known sequelae. Approximately in 1 of every 5 cases of biliary atresia, the gallbladder is completely absent.

Duplication of gallbladder (double gallbladder): The 2nd gallbladder may be alongside the normal organ or may reside in an unusual location, eg in the left lobe of the liver. The duplication is usually the same size as the normal organ. It commonly has a separate cystic duct which empties independently into the common bile duct, and rarely, empties into a common "Y"-shaped cystic duct. There are no characteristic symptoms or signs to make it obvious with diagnosis usually achieved at operation or as an autopsy finding. Rarely, diagnosis is made by xray, observing 2 rows of stones on cholecystogram.

Bilobed gallbladder (bifid, partially divided gallbladder): This is a very rare defect in which 2 cavities join into a single cystic duct. Two clinical types are noted; those with an internal septum dividing them or a truly paired fundic variety. These are usually asymptomatic.

Diverticulum of gallbladder: A diverticulum can be located anywhere along the free surface of the organ from neck to fundus. Rarely, stones may form in a narrow-necked diverticulum due to stasis.

'Floating" gallbladder: This anomaly refers to a gallbladder that hangs from a long mesentery which attaches either to the entire organ, or more rarely, the neck and cystic duct only, letting the fundus hang free. Torsion may complicate the latter type with subsequent infarction (rare in childhood). These instances are characterized by right-upper quadrant pain, nausea, and vomiting.

Anomalous location or ectopic gallbladder: There are 3 specific types each rarely observed; intrahepatic, left-sided, and retrodisplaced. The intrahepatic variety is of surgical significance because of the difficulty encountered during cholecystectomy for cholelithiasis and cholecystitis. The incidence of gallstone formation is considered to be quite high in cases of intrahepatic gallbladder.

Anomalies of the cystic artery: The cystic artery arises from the right hepatic artery in 75% of cases, the common hepatic artery in 15% and the left hepatic artery in 10%. In 25% of cases a double cystic artery is observed.

Complications
I **Derived:** —

II Associated: —

Etiology: ?

Pathogenesis: ?

Related Facts
I Sex Ratio: M?:F?
II Risk of Occurrence: Very rare except for gallbladder agenesis which occurs in 1 in 3300 live births and duplication of gallbladder 1 in 4000 live births.
III Risk of Recurrence for
Patient's Sib: ?
Patient's Child: ?
IV Age of Detectability: ?
V Prevalence: ?

Treatment
I Primary Prevention: —
II Secondary Prevention: —
III Other Therapy: —

Prognosis: Normal life span

Detection of Carrier: —

Special Considerations: —

References:
Flannery, M.G. and Caster, M.P.: Congenital abnormalities of the gallbladder. Surg. Gynecol. Obstet. 103:439, 1956.
Gross, R.E.: Congenital anomalies of the gallbladder: Review of 148 cases with report of a double gallbladder. Arch. Surg. 32:131, 1936.

Contributors: **Jay L. Grosfeld**
H. William Clatworthy, Jr.

Editor's Computerized Descriptors: CV., GI.

GASTROSCHISIS

Includes: Gastrosquisis

Excludes: Omphalocele (748)

Minimal Diagnostic Criteria: Presence of lateral abdominal wall defect with eviscerated bowel. Umbilicus intact.

Clinical Findings: Viscera exposed and eviscerated from abdomen through defect generally to the right and lateral to umbilical orifice. Umbilicus normally closed. Viscera may be covered by thick green-brown exudate obscuring details of bowel wall. Intestines seem foreshortened. Anomalies of bowel may be obscured by edema of bowel and exudate. Defect in abdominal wall generally small, 3-5 cm.

Complications
I Derived: Intestinal obstruction due to angulation of gut, adhesions or atresia secondary to vascular impairment of bowel wall.
II Associated: Malrotation of intestine

Etiology: ?

Pathogenesis: Failure in development of part of lateral embryonic fold of abdominal wall may result in defect to side, generally right, of normally formed umbilicus.

Related Facts
I Sex Ratio: M?:F?
II Risk of Occurrence: 1 in 20,000 to 1 in 30,000 live births
III Risk of Recurrence for
Patient's Sib: ?
Patient's Child: —
IV Age of Detectability: At birth
V Prevalence: ?

Treatment
I Primary Prevention: None known
II Secondary Prevention: Return of viscera to abdominal cavity surgically.† Where abdominal cavity is too small one must use silastic sheeting as temporary covering with serial removal for reconstitution of abdominal wall.
III Other Therapy: —

Prognosis: With staged repair and support, mortality has dropped to 20-30% in most series.

Detection of Carrier: —

†Special Considerations: Related atresias of gut must be searched for and repaired. Establishment of GI function is slow. Babies generally must be supported with central venous feeding (hyperalimentation) during staged repairs.

References:
Cordero, L. et al: Staged repair of gastroschisis with silastic sheeting. Surgery. 65:4, 1969.
Rickham, P.P.: Exomphalos and gastroschisis. In Rickham, P.P. and Johnston, J.H. (eds.) Neonatal Surgery. New York: Appleton-Century-Crofts, 1969, p. 254.

Contributor: **Lawrence K. Pickett**

Editor's Computerized Descriptors: Hernia not CNS, GI.

GAUCHER DISEASE

Includes: Maladie de Gaucher
Mb. Gaucher
Enfermedad de Gaucher
Cerebroside lipidosis
Cerebrosidosis
Glucocerebrosidosis

Excludes: Niemann-Pick disease (717)
G_{M1}-gangliosidosis, type 1 (431)
Sea-blue histiocytosis
Other sphingolipidoses

Minimal Diagnostic Criteria: The infantile patient presents a characteristic appearance of neurologic abnormalities plus visceromegaly. In the chronic form obscure splenomegaly, or skeletal difficulties, suggest the diagnosis.

Gaucher cells (large histiocytic elements, with a "wrinkled-appearing" cytoplasm) can usually be demonstrated on the initial marrow examination. In a few reports they have been identified sparsely in the marrow of obligatory heterozygotes. Rarely, cells of somewhat similar appearance may be found in the marrow of patients with chronic leukemia or hemolytic anemia.

An elevated level of tartrate-resistant acid phosphatase in the serum is generally viewed as critical to the support of the diagnosis.

Ultimately, it must be demonstrated that there is an increase in glucocerebrosides in the involved tissues or in the plasma, or a deficiency of β-glucosidase in the tissues or the circulating white blood cells.

Clinical Findings: In the so-called *Acute* or *Infantile* form of Gaucher disease, the child presents a picture of "pseudobulbar palsy," with strabismus, difficulty in swallowing, laryngeal spasm, a common position of comfort with the head extended (resembling opisthotonus), and developmental retardation. Simultaneously there is significant enlargement of the liver and spleen. There are troubling episodes of aspiration, with chronic bronchopneumonia and increasing debility. Most such infants die by 6-12 months of age; in a few (? "*Subacute*" type) the neurologic handicaps may be milder in the early months, and survival may be possible until 2 years or so of age. Another group of patients who also have nervous system involvement, have been labeled the *Juvenile* type. They show a gradually increasing dementia during middle to late childhood, often with behavioral changes, seizures, extrapyramidal and cerebellar signs, and difficulties from pulmonary disease. Organomegaly is mild. Some aspects of this infrequent clinical picture remain obscure, and the diagnosis should be made with caution. (It is seen more frequently in certain areas in Sweden.)

By far the most common type of Gaucher disease is the *Chronic* or *Adult* form, probably representing 90% of the total. In spite of the "adult" designation, the 1st symptoms may appear as early as 1 year of age. The presenting clinical features are abdominal enlargement (from the notable increase in spleen and liver size) and orthopedic difficulties. Symptoms in the bones and joints (pain, pathologic fractures, aseptic necrosis) result from the handicaps of a greatly expanded medullary cavity volume, and xrays show tubulation failure and areas of dissolution in the long bones and vertebrae. Yellow patches on the sclerae ("pingueculae") are seen in about a quarter of the adults and abnormal pigmentation of the face, neck, hands, or shins may occur.

Complications

I Derived: In time the marrow-suppressing effects of the continuing splenomegaly produce a lowering of all formed blood elements. When the thrombocytopenia reaches critical levels, various hemorrhagic symptoms appear, including easy bruising and epistaxis. The effects of the hepatic involvement appear to be unimportant and portal hypertension is almost unknown. Splenic rupture has been rarely reported. As mentioned, skeletal complications are common, with fractures of the femoral neck and the vertebral bodies most important, plus the secondary development of aseptic necrosis of the femoral head. In the infantile patient, pneumonia occurs plus the effects of increasing cerebral handicap.

II Associated: Immunoglobulin abnormalities have been reported rarely

Etiology: Autosomal recessive in each form of Gaucher disease. McK *23080 (In 2 families only, there has been evidence of dominant transmission of the chronic form.) There are no genetic interrelationships among the various forms of the disease.

A reduction in the levels of β-glucosidase has been found at many sites (liver, spleen, white blood cells, etc).

There is also a consistent increase in acid phosphatase activity, histochemically demonstrable in the cytoplasm of the Gaucher cells, with excretion producing an elevation in the serum level of tartrate-resistant acid phosphatase.

Pathogenesis: The tissue deficiency of β-glucosidase, which seems to be the cerebroside-cleaving enzyme, correlates well with the cytoplasmic accumulation in histiocytes of glycolipid which cannot be catabolized. There are 2 theories about the actual origin of the cellular cerebroside augmentation. The traditional view would be that it arises from local, in situ synthesis preeminently, and it has been demonstrated that isolated normal spleen or liver slices are capable of normal cerebroside biosynthesis. Another hypothesis views the major source of stockpiled glycolipid as arising from the normal breakdown of white and red blood cells, the engulfed products of which are then blocked from further catabolism. The majority of the material in the visceral cells is of the usual gluco- form. The mechanism of the cerebral handicap in the infantile form is not well understood, but it is of interest to note that some neurones (eg in the thalamus) show mild distention with PAS-positive material. It has not been possible to formulate a satisfactory explanation for the role of the greatly increased amount of the special "Gaucher acid phosphatase" in the final disease picture, but its origin does appear to be directly from tissues rich in Gaucher cells.

Related Facts
I Sex Ratio: M1:F1
II Risk of Occurrence: Gaucher disease is uncommon but not rare. About 350 patients have been reported.
III Risk of Recurrence for
    Patient's Sib: 1 in 4 (25%) for each offspring to be affected
    Patient's Child: Not increased unless mate is carrier or homozygote
IV Age of Detectability: Prenatal diagnosis possible in cell culture from amniotic fluid. For patients with infantile Gaucher disease, stiffness and irritability commonly begin by 2-3 months of age, organomegaly by 3-6 months, and respiratory distress by 3 months or soon after. In the chronic form, enlargement of the liver and spleen may on occasion be detected as early as 1 year of age.
V Prevalence: About two-thirds of the patients with chronic Gaucher disease are of Ashkenazi Jewish ancestry, where the carrier rate apparently approximates that for Tay-Sachs disease.

Treatment
I Primary Prevention: Genetic counseling
II Secondary Prevention: Splenectomy provides useful permanent control of the hemorrhagic symptoms, but should

only be pursued when there are serious clinical issues in this area. Informed conservative orthopedic supervision can keep the skeletal complications to a minimum. Simple immobilization is required for the acute pain episodes. Eventual "total hip replacement" operations may be necessary for management of the late effects in adult life.

III Other Therapy: Individuals and families need considerable general support and reassurance. Trials of "enzyme replacement therapy" are of experimental relevance only at this time.

Prognosis: There is only a 1-2 year survival in the infantile form. For the chronically-involved patient of the usual sort, however, there should be no shortening of normal life expectancy.

Detection of Carrier: Heterozygote identification by β-glucosidase analysis on white blood cells or cultured fibroblasts is possible.

Special Considerations: —

References:
Crocker, A. C. and Landing, B. H.: Phosphatase studies in Gaucher's disease. Metabolism 9:341, 1960.
Fredrickson, D.S. and Sloan, H.R.: Glucosyl ceramide lipidoses: Gaucher's disease. In Stanbury, J.B. et al (eds.): The Metabolic Basis of Inherited Disease, 3rd Ed. New York:McGraw-Hill, 1972, p. 730.
Matoth, Y. and Fried, K.: Chronic Gaucher's disease; clinical observations on 34 patients. Isr. J. Med. Sci. 1:521, 1965.
Schettler, G. and Kahlke, W.: Gaucher's disease. In Schettler, G. (ed.): Lipids and Lipidoses. New York:Springer Verlag, 1967, p. 260.

Contributor: **Michel Philippart**

Editor's Computerized Descriptors: Eye, Nasoph., Larynx, Skin, Skel., Muscle, Resp., Spleen, GI., Liver, Nerve

GINGIVAL FIBROMATOSIS

Includes: Fibromatose gingivale
Fibromatosis gingivae

Excludes: Gingival fibromatosis and hypertrichosis (410)
Symmetric gingival fibromatosis
Gingival fibromatosis and digital anomalies (409)
Gingival fibromatosis and multiple hyaline fibromas (411)
Gingival fibromatosis, Cowden type (412)
Gingival fibromatosis, depigmentation, and microphthalmia (413)
Gingival dystrophy
Dilantin and other causes of gingival enlargement

Minimal Diagnostic Criteria: Hard, firm, noninflammatory enlargement of all of the gingivae. All of the gingivae usually involved at some stage in this disease. Early at the initiation of the enlargement, only a portion of the gingivae around erupting teeth may be involved or after surgical removal, recurrences may initially be localized. Local gingival fibromatosis has been observed in sibs and relatives in what appears to be a recessive form of the disease. Symmetric gingival fibromatosis usually involves only the molar area bilaterally, has its onset after 12 years of age, is generally less firm than gingival fibromatosis and is nonfamilial in most reported examples.†

Clinical Findings: Generalized gingival enlargement involves all of the gingivae in both jaws. The gums are hard, firm and of normal color and have a normal or accentuated stippling resembling an orange peel. The gums may be smooth or partially lobulated around the necks of teeth. All teeth may be completely covered by the tissue, but more frequently the crowns are partly exposed. In untreated cases the gingivae may reach enormous size and protrude from mouth. Radiographically, the teeth may undergo root resorption within the gingiva.

Complications
I Derived: Interference with tooth eruption and exfoliation. Difficulties in chewing, swallowing, speech and respiration. Drooling with secondary ulceration of extruded gingivae and lips. Gingival infection and dentigerous cysts develop around unerupted teeth.
II Associated: None. There is no statistically higher risk for oligophrenia or epilepsy in cases with only gingival fibromatosis. However, when accompanied by *hypertrichosis* the risk for these defects is considerable.

Etiology: Autosomal dominant. Approximately 80% of reported cases are familial and 20% reported as isolated cases or familial history not investigated.

Pathogenesis: Initiating event not fully understood but gingival enlargement is intimately associated with the presence of erupted teeth. As either the primary teeth, the secondary teeth or both begin to erupt there is a progressive enlargement of the gingivae. In nearly all cases, extraction of the teeth causes a regression and disappearance of the gingival lesion. Histologically, the tissue is composed of dense mature hyperplastic and hypertrophic collagen bundles in the lamina propria and submucosa. Evidence for inflammatory elements is absent or scanty foci of chronic inflammatory infiltrate are found between bundles of connective tissue or localized to secondarily traumatized or infected areas. The condition has been compared to a keloid as an overresponse of gingival connective tissue to the trauma of tooth eruption and erupted teeth.

Related Facts
I Sex Ratio: M1:F1
II Risk of Occurrence: Rare
III Risk of Recurrence for
Patient's Sib: If parent is affected 1 in 2 (50%) for each

offspring to be affected; otherwise not increased.
Patient's Child: 1 in 2. Recessive forms known.

IV Age of Detectability: At time of eruption of teeth. Approximately 50% begin at the eruption of primary teeth 6 months to 3 years and 50% at the time of eruption of the permanent teeth 5 to 12 years. Those that have their onset during eruption of the primary teeth also have involvement of the permanent dentition.

V Prevalence: ? Rare

Treatment
I Primary Prevention: Genetic counseling

II Secondary Prevention: Conservative treatment should be tried first consisting of gingivectomy followed by good oral hygiene. Many cases tend to recur. These refractive cases can be treated by extraction of all teeth and gingivectomy.

III Other Therapy: Prosthetic replacement of teeth.

Prognosis: Good. Normal life span.

Detection of Carrier: —

†**Special Considerations:** Genetic heterogeneity exists in this category. Dilantin, lesions of the diencephalon, certain blood and endocrine disorders may have generalized gingival enlargement which follows the onset of these conditions. Has been reported in Caucasians and American Negroes.

References:
Jorgenson, R.J. and Cocker, M.E.: Variation in the inheritance and expression of gingival fibromatosis. J. Periodontol. 45:472, 1974.

Rushton, M. A.: Hereditary or idiopathic hyperplasia of the gums. Dent. Practit. 7:136, 1957.

Witkop, C. J., Jr.: Heterogeneity in gingival fibromatosis. In Bergsma, D. (ed.): Part XI. Orofacial Structures. Birth Defects: Orig. Art. Ser., vol. VII, no. 7. Baltimore: Williams and Wilkins Co. for The National Foundation - March of Dimes, 1971, p. 210.

Contributor: **Carl J. Witkop, Jr.**

Editor's Computerized Descriptors: Oral, Teeth
Also see Section I, Fig. 89

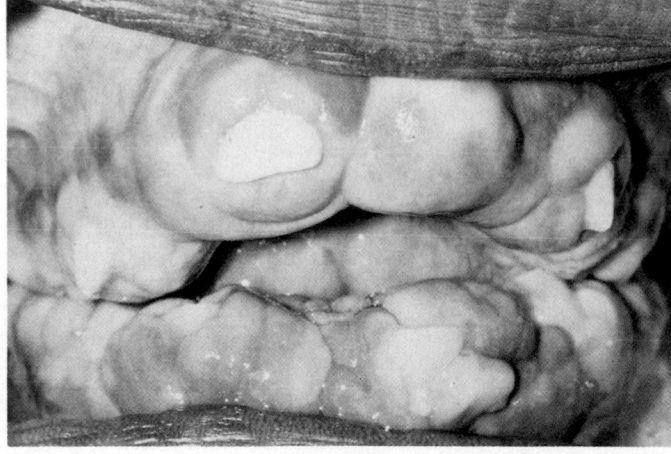

270. Marked gingival hypertrophy secondary to fibromatosis

GINGIVAL FIBROMATOSIS AND CORNEAL DYSTROPHY

Includes: Fibromatose gingivale, anomalie de l'éruption dentaire et dystrophie cornéenne

Fibromatosis gingivae, gestörter Zahndurchbruch und Hornhautdystrophie

Fibromatosis gingival, alteración de la erupción dentaria y distrofia corneana

Corneal opacities and gingival fibromatosis

Rutherfurd syndrome

Disturbed eruption of teeth, corneal dystrophy and gingival fibromatosis

Corneal dystrophy, disturbed eruption of teeth and gingival fibromatosis

Gingival fibromatosis, disturbed eruption of teeth and corneal dystrophy

Excludes: Gingival fibromatosis (407)

Gingival fibromatosis and hypertrichosis (410)

Symmetric gingival fibromatosis

Gingival fibromatosis and digital anomalies (409)

Gingival fibromatosis and multiple hyaline fibromas (411)

Gingival fibromatosis, Cowden type (412)

Gingival fibromatosis, depigmentation and microphthalmia (413)

Minimal Diagnostic Criteria: The presence of gingival fibromatosis and curtain-like corneal opacities affecting the upper half of the eye.

Clinical Findings: Generalized dense fibrotic enlarged gingivae cover the teeth which fail to erupt. Both primary and secondary teeth may be embedded within the fibrotic gums during the period of mixed dentition with root resorption of the primary teeth occurring within the gums. A few teeth of either dentition may erupt and be visible in the mouth and are frequently hypoplastic being peg- or cone-shaped. Curtain-like corneal opacities involve the superior portion of each cornea; the lower portion of the eye is usually spared. Complete visual loss due to vascularization of cornea occurs in the 5th decade.

Complications
I Derived: Tooth fragments from incomplete exfoliation may remain within the gingivae. Dentigerous cysts and gingival infections. Loss of vision.

II Associated: Possibly oligophrenia. Two affected kindred members were also mentally retarded. Skull asymmetry and undescended testes noted in one infant.

Etiology: Autosomal dominant; McK *18090

Pathogenesis: Essentially unknown. Dense fibrotic gingivae are present in infancy and primary teeth fail to erupt. The secondary dentition fails to appear but by radiographs full primary dentition undergoing root resorption may be present. Corneal opacities involving the upper portion of the eye vascularize with age.

Related Facts
I Sex Ratio: M1:F1

II Risk of Occurrence: ? Very rare

III Risk of Recurrence for
Patient's Sib: If parent is affected, 1 in 2 (50%) for each offspring to be affected; otherwise not increased.
Patient's Child: 1 in 2

IV Age of Detectability: Early infancy by clinically noting gingival fibromatosis and corneal opacities.

V Prevalence: ? Very rare. Has been reported in only one English kindred by 1971.

Treatment
I Primary Prevention: Genetic counseling

II Secondary Prevention: Gingivectomy, surgical removal of cysts

III Other Therapy: —

Prognosis: Good except for visual defect. Probably does not affect longevity significantly. Patients have survived to 6th decade.

Detection of Carrier: —

Special Considerations: —

References:
Houston, I. B. and Shotts, N.: Rutherfurd's syndrome; a familial oculodental disorder. Acta Paediatr. Scand. 55:233, 1966.
Rutherfurd, M. E.: Three generations of inherited dental defect. Br. Med. J. 2:9, 1931.
Witkop, C. J., Jr.: Heterogeneity in gingival fibromatosis. In Bergsma, D. (ed.): Part XI. Orofacial Structures. Birth Defects: Orig. Art. Ser., vol. VII, no. 7. Baltimore:Williams and Wilkins Co. for The National Foundation - March of Dimes, 1971, p. 210.

Contributor: **Carl J. Witkop, Jr.**

Editor's Computerized Descriptors: Vision, Eye, Oral, Teeth
Also see Section I, Fig. 89

GINGIVAL FIBROMATOSIS AND DIGITAL ANOMALIES

Includes: Fibromatose gingivale-anomalies des doigts, des oreilles et du nez avec hépatosplénomégalie
Fibromatosis gingivae mit Fehlbildungen von Fingern, Ohr, Nase und Hepatosplenomegalie
Fibromatosis gingival y anomalías auriculares y nasales con hepatoesplenomelia
Phalangeal hypoplasia and gingival fibromatosis
Digital, ear, nose anomalies, gingival fibromatosis, and hepatosplenomegaly
Ear, nose, digital anomalies, gingival fibromatosis, and hepatosplenomegaly
Nose, ear, digital anomalies, gingival fibromatosis, and hepatosplenomegaly
Hepatosplenomegaly, gingival fibromatosis, digital, ear, and nose anomalies
Gingival fibromatosis, digital, ear, nose anomalies and hepatosplenomegaly

Excludes: Gingival fibromatosis (407)
Symmetric gingival fibromatosis
Gingival fibromatosis and hypertrichosis (410)
Gingival fibromatosis and multiple hyaline fibromas (411)
Gingival fibromatosis and corneal dystrophy (408)
Gingival fibromatosis, Cowden type (412)
Gingival fibromatosis, depigmentation and microphthalmia (413)
Other causes of gingival enlargement

Minimal Diagnostic Criteria: Gingival fibromatosis in a patient with clinical or radiographic evidence of hypoplasia of terminal phalanges and nails

Clinical Findings: At birth, there is absence or dysplasia of toe and fingernails with clubbed or tree frog-like fingers and toes with radiographic evidence of hypoplasia of terminal phalangeal bones. Gingival fibromatosis is noted at the time of eruption of primary teeth. Hyperextensibility of the metacarpophalangeal joints, soft bulky cartilage in nose and ears. Hepatosplenomegaly occurs in over half of the affected patients.†

Complications
I **Derived:** Massive overgrowth of gingiva has resulted in malocclusion, salivation with secondary lesions at commissures of lips, defects of mastication, speech and swallowing, exfoliation of teeth, secondary infections of gingivae, protrusion of lips with xerostomia. Hepatosplenomegaly has led to misdiagnosis of anemia and tumor.
II **Associated:** One patient had giant oral melanotic nevus of palate and buccal mucosa.

Etiology: Autosomal dominant in most cases reported. No affected parent in 2 carefully examined patients and their parents. Chromosomes found to be normal.

Pathogenesis: Essentially unknown

Related Facts
I **Sex Ratio:** M1:F1
II **Risk of Occurrence:** ? Very rare†
III **Risk of Recurrence for**
     Patient's Sib: If parent is affected, 1 in 2 (50%) for each offspring to be affected; otherwise not increased.
     Patient's Child: 1 in 2
IV **Age of Detectability:** Early infancy by clinical and radiographic examination of terminal phalanges and noting nose and ear defects. All signs of syndrome may not be present until eruption of teeth at 2 - 3 years of age.
V **Prevalence:** ? Very rare, less than 20 cases reported

Treatment
I **Primary Prevention:** Genetic counseling
II **Secondary Prevention:** Good oral hygiene delays onset and reduces severity of gingival lesions. Excision of gingival tissue with pressure packs and good oral hygiene. May recur

despite treatment.

III Other Therapy: ?

Prognosis: Fair to good. Not known if hepatosplenomegaly contributes to decreased longevity. Persons with trait have survived to 6th decade.

Detection of Carrier: —

†Special Considerations: Has been reported in persons of East Indian ancestry from India and West Indies most frequently, but also known in isolated cases in Caucasians. No cases among Mongoloids, Capoids, Australoids or Congoids reported.

References:
Laband, P.F. et al: Hereditary gingival fibromatosis: Report of an affected family with associated splenomegaly and skeletal and soft tissue abnormalities. Oral Surg. 17:339, 1964.
Läwen, (Königsberg): Chirurgische Demonstrationen. Demonstration von Bildern eines Falles von Elephantiasis gingivae (diffuse Zahnfleischfibromatose, Gingivitis hypertrophica, diffuse fibromatose Entartung der Gingiva) bei einem 15 jahrigen Jungen. Zentralbl. Chir. 56:626, 1929.
Witkop, C. J., Jr.: Heterogeneity in gingival fibromatosis. In Bergsma, D. (ed.): Part XI. Orofacial Structures. Birth Defects : Orig. Art. Ser., vol. VII, no. 7. Baltimore:Williams and Wilkins for The National Foundation-March of Dimes, 1971, p.210.

Contributor: Carl J. Witkop, Jr.

Editor's Computerized Descriptors: Ear, Oral, Nose, Nails, Skel., Spleen, Liver , Teeth
Also see Section I, Fig. 89

GINGIVAL FIBROMATOSIS AND HYPERTRICHOSIS

Includes: Fibromatose gingivale avec hypertrichose
Fibromatosis gingivae mit Hypertrichose
Fibromatosis gingival con hipertricosis
Hirsutism and gingival enlargement
Hair, excessive and gingival enlargement

Excludes: Gingival fibromatosis and digital anomalies (409)
Gingival fibromatosis and multiple hyaline fibromas (411)
Gingival fibromatosis and corneal dystrophy (408)
Gingival fibromatosis, Cowden type (412)
Gingival fibromatosis, depigmentation and microphthalmia (413)
Symmetric gingival fibromatosis
Other causes of gingival hyperplasia

Minimal Diagnostic Criteria: Gingival enlargement in patient with hirsutism

Clinical Findings: Usually hypertrichosis is noted first. Within the first 2 years after birth, child develops excessive hair on head, face and body which tends to be black even in blond families. Enlargement of the gingiva is usually noted when teeth fail to appear on schedule. The patient has a slowly progressive firm fibrotic enlargement of gums which are covered with normal appearing mucosa, often showing normal "orange peel" stippling which in untreated cases may fill oral cavity and protrude from mouth. A few teeth may erupt only to be recovered by the expanding gingival tissue or the teeth may exfoliate prematurely. About one-half of children also have epileptic attacks or oligophrenia.†

Complications
I **Derived:** Interference with chewing, respiration and speech. Failure of eruption or exfoliation of teeth. Periodontal abscesses. Xerostomia and dribbling of saliva from mouth. Trauma to tongue and body secondary to epileptic seizures.
II **Associated:** Patients with gingival fibromatosis and hypertrichosis have a·high risk for epilepsy and oligophrenia in contrast to those patients with gingival fibromatosis without hirsutism who do not. About one-half (22/52) reported cases have had either oligophrenia or epilepsy or both.

Etiology: Most cases are autosomal dominant. Approximately one-fourth of the reported cases (12/52) have been sporadic with no family history. Question if recessive form exists.† McK *13540

Pathogenesis: Essentially unknown. Gingival overgrowth with proliferation and hypertrophy of collagen fibers develops about the time of eruption of primary teeth.

Related Facts
I   **Sex Ratio:** M1:F1
II **Risk of Occurrence:** ? Rare
III **Risk of Recurrence for**
      Patient's Sib: If parent is affected, 1 in 2 (50%) for each offspring to be affected; otherwise not increased.†
      Patient's Child: 1 in 2†
IV **Age of Detectability:** Nearly all cases noted before 2 years of age. Most diagnosed before 1 year of age.
V   **Prevalence:** ? Rare (less than 60 cases reported by 1970).

Treatment
I   **Primary Prevention:** Genetic counseling
II **Secondary Prevention:** Surgical excision with pressure dressings should be tried first. Many patients have recurrence. Extraction of teeth and gingivectomy usually prevent the recurrence of the gingival lesions except in very rare instances. Dilantin or other epileptic controlling therapy. Depilatory treatment for hirsutism.
III **Other Therapy:** Full denture prosthesis, special education if oligophrenia is present.

Prognosis: Fair, data on longevity not available. For gingival fibromatosis, excellent with adequate treatment; for epilepsy, fair with therapy; for oligophrenia, poor.

Detection of Carrier: †

†Special Considerations: All reported cases have been in Caucasians. One Filipino case. A recessive form may exist as several families have had sibs but not parents affected. It is in these nonfamilial cases where oligophrenia and epilepsy occur most frequently. It is not known if this is really a different entity from gingival fibromatosis with hypertrichosis and fibroadenomas of breasts as this may resemble gingival fibromatosis, hypertrichosis and fibroadenomas of breasts, especially before the age of onset of the breast lesions in a girl showing few of the signs associated with fibroadenoma syndrome. See Byars and Sarnat (1944) and Byars and Jurkiewicz (1961) under latter entry. Family history and associated defects important in distinguishing the two conditions.

References:

Byars, L. T. and Sarnat, B. G.: Congenital macrogingivae (fibromatosis gingivae) and hypertrichosis. Surgery 15:964, 1944.

Jorgenson, R.J. and Cocker, M.E.: Variation in the inheritance and expression of gingival fibromatosis. J. Periodontol. 45:472, 1974.

Witkop, C. J., Jr.: Heterogeneity in gingival fibromatosis. In Bergsma, D. (ed.): Part XI. Orafacial Structures. Birth Defects: Orig. Art. Ser., vol. VII, no. 7. Baltimore: Williams and Wilkins, Co. for The National Foundation - March of Dimes, 1971, p. 210.

Contributor: **Carl J. Witkop, Jr.**

Editor's Computerized Descriptors: Oral, Teeth, Hair, Nerve

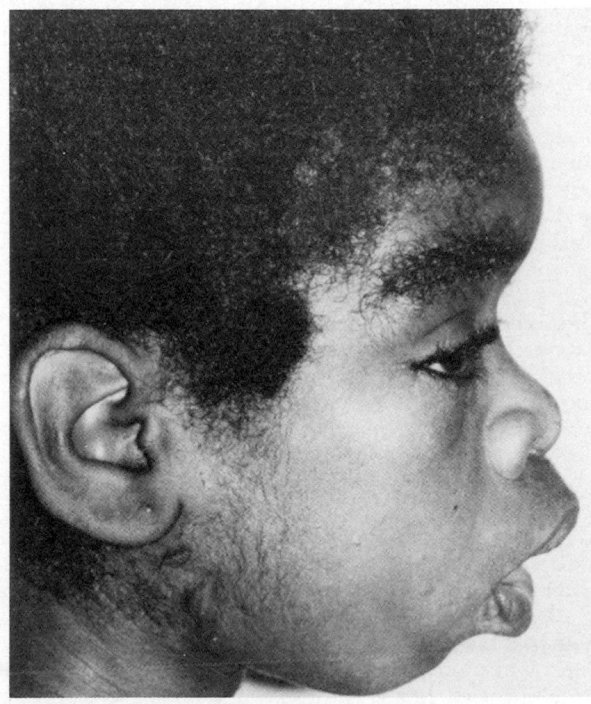

271. Note hypertrichosis; lip protrusion secondary to gingival fibromatosis

GINGIVAL FIBROMATOSIS AND MULTIPLE HYALINE FIBROMAS

Includes: Fibromatose gingivale et fibromes hyalines multiples
Fibromatosis gingivae mit multiplen hyalinen Fibromen
Fibromatosis gingival con fibromas hialinos múltiples
Murray syndrome
Fibromatosis hyalinica multiplex juvenilis
Hyaline fibromas and gingival fibromatosis
Juvenile hyaline fibromatosis

Excludes: Gingival fibromatosis (407)
Symmetric gingival fibromatosis
Gingival fibromatosis and digital anomalies (409)
Gingival fibromatosis and corneal dystrophy (408)
Gingival fibromatosis and hypertrichosis (410)
Gingival fibromatosis, Cowden type (412)
Gingival fibromatosis, depigmentation and microphthalmia (413)
Cylindromas of scalp (235)

Minimal Diagnostic Criteria: Gingival fibromatosis and multiple hyaline fibromata. Histologic criteria may be needed for definitive diagnosis.†

Clinical Findings: Gingival enlargement may be present at birth or develops during the first 2 years of life. All of the gingivae are involved with a hard, firm, slowly enlarging lesion. In early childhood, sub- and periungual growths appear and slowly enlarge. Multiple firm, painless, elastic nodules adherent to the overlying skin develop by coalescence and growth of white miliary nodules. These slowly enlarge and may reach orange-sized pendulous tumors. Tumors usually appear first on the head, face, shoulders and digits. Those involving the trunk, back, thighs, and legs usually develop later in childhood. The scalp tumors resemble turban tumors. There have been no café-au-lait spots, hypertrichosis, epilepsy, neurofibromata, hemangiomas, osteochondromata, dermoids, juvenile aponeurotic fibromata, keloids or oligophrenia in the cases reported. Radiographic survey may show destructive long bone lesions. Common laboratory tests have been normal.

Complications
I **Derived:** Malocclusion, interference with speech, local irritation depending on site of tumor involvement
II **Associated:** Flexural contractures of limbs noted in some cases.

Etiology: Autosomal recessive

Pathogenesis: Slowly enlarging gingivae are ascribable to deposits of PAS-positive amorphous substance in the lamina propria without inflammatory infiltrates. Tumors are composed of a hyaline homogenous amorphous, acidophilic, PAS-positive, ground substance in which are embedded abundant blood vessels and ovoid-to-spindle-shaped cells forming minute streaks. Between cells are fine silver staining fibers. The sections have the appearance of pseudocartilage but only minute amounts of hyaluronic acid are found on electrophoresis of tumor extracts. True cartilage, elastic, or nervous tissue has not been observed in tumors.

Related Facts
I **Sex Ratio:** M1:F1
II **Risk of Occurrence:** Very rare
III **Risk of Recurrence for**
    Patient's Sib: 1 in 4 (25%) for each offspring to be affected
    Patient's Child: Not increased unless mate is carrier or homozygote
IV **Age of Detectability:** Perinatal to 2 years of age
V **Prevalence:** ? Very rare, reported in Europeans and Japanese.

Treatment

I Primary Prevention: Genetic counseling

II Secondary Prevention: Extraction of teeth and gingivectomy. Surgical removal of tumors has met with variable success; several have recurred at surgical site.

III Other Therapy: Prosthetic replacement of teeth

Prognosis: Not a sufficient number of cases to give definite statement. However, one case has survived to 6th decade of life. Surgical excision of tumors has met with only partial success as tumors tend to recur.

Detection of Carrier: ?

†Special Considerations: The original cases were described by Murray in 1871 and were thought by later investigators to be examples of neurofibromatosis. Neurofibromatosis can affect gingivae but the neurofibromata are usually localized and do not involve all of the gums as is seen in this disease. Ungual fibromata may occur in both conditions. Tuberous sclerosis may have nodular tumors of the face and nose in addition to a generalized pebbly appearing lesion of the gums. The nodules in tuberous sclerosis usually do not reach the size seen in this disease and the histologic picture is different. Osteochondromatoses of the Ollier and Maffucci types can be differentiated from this disease by the occurrence in the former diseases of hemangiomas and true cartilage and osseous containing tumors.

References:

Drescher, E. et al: Juvenile fibromatosis in siblings (fibromatosis hyalinica multiplex juvenilis). J. Pediatr. Surg. 2:427, 1967.

Kitano, Y.: Juvenile hyalin fibromatosis. Arch. Dermatol. 112:86, 1976.

Whitfield, A. and Robinson, A. H.: A further report on the remarkable series of cases of molluscum fibrosum in children (communicated to the Society by Dr. John Murray in 1873). Med. - chir. Trans. (London) 86:293, 1903.

Witkop, C. J., Jr.: Heterogeneity in gingival fibromatosis. In Bergsma, D. (ed.): Part XI. Orofacial Structures. Birth Defects: Orig. Art. Ser., vol. VII, no. 7. Baltimore: Williams and Wilkins for The National Foundation-March of Dimes, 1971, p. 210.

Contributors: **Carl J. Witkop, Jr.**
Edward Drescher‡
Yukio Kitano

Editor's Computerized Descriptors: Oral, Skin, Nails, Skel. Also see Section I, Fig. 89

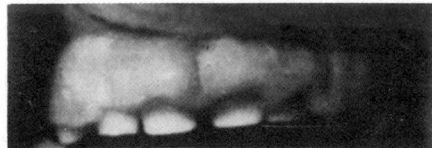

272. Gingival hypertrophy

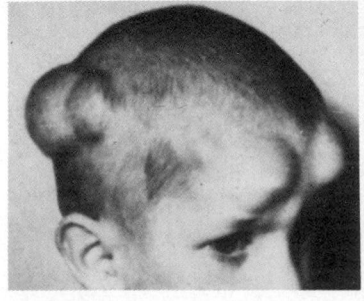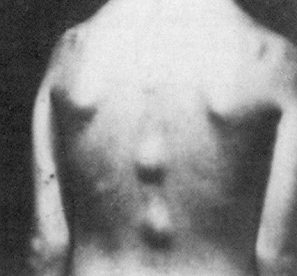

273. Multiple hyaline fibromas

GINGIVAL FIBROMATOSIS, COWDEN TYPE

Includes: Fibromatose gingivale hypertrychose et fibroadénomes mammaires
Fibromatosis gingivae, Hypertrichose und Fibroadenome der Mammae
Fibromatosis gingival, hipertricosis y fibroadenomas mamarios
Cowden disease
Hypertrichosis, gingival fibromatosis and fibroadenomas of breasts
Breast fibroadenomas, hypertrichosis and gingival fibromatosis
Multiple hamartoma syndrome
Gingival fibromatosis, hypertrichosis and fibroadenomas of breasts

Excludes: Gingival fibromatosis (407)
Gingival fibromatosis and hypertrichosis (410)
Symmetric gingival fibromatosis
Gingival fibromatosis and digital anomalies (409)
Gingival fibromatosis and multiple hyaline fibromas (411)
Gingival fibromatosis and corneal dystrophy (408)
Gingival fibromatosis, depigmentation and microphthalmia (413)

Minimal Diagnostic Criteria: Mucosal and cutaneous papillomatosis and fibromatosis, fibrocystic breast disease in the female.

Clinical Findings: The most constant findings have been gingival fibromatosis appearing from birth to 1 year of age, hypertrichosis appearing from birth to 5 years of age and massive "virginal" bilateral enlargement of breasts after puberty. Breast enlargement seems to coincide with a "precipitating" event such as first menarche, or breast development may be normal for a time with enlargement occurring later, in some at the time of first pregnancy. Initial growth is rapid, the breasts may double in size within a few months with a later slowing rate of enlargement so that 2 years have elapsed in some instances before the breasts reach a size sufficiently great to cause the patient to seek medical attention. In other examples, enlargement has been so rapid that within an 8-month-span the breasts hung to a level of the pubes. The breast lesions are giant fibroadenomas which undergo early malignant degeneration. At birth the hair may be coarse and black, the child frequently being the only black-haired child in the sibship. Hypertrichosis involves trunk, face, arms and legs and may increase at menarche. Axillary and pubic hair have a normal female distribution. There are usually no other indications of endocrine or gonadal dysfunction such as menstrual abnormalities, changes in features, voice, size of feet or hands, striae pigmentation, loss of libido or urinary symptoms. Gingival enlargement may be accompanied by hyperkeratosis or parakeratosis of the overlying epithelium or a generalized hyperkeratotic papillomatosis of lips, oral and pharyngeal mucosa. Mild mental retardation in about 50%.

Patients described under the term Cowden disease or multiple hamartoma syndrome have extensive facial tricholemmomas, and mucosal papillomatosis and fibromatosis. Verrucous lesions appear throughout the oral cavity, about all facial orifices, on the extensor surfaces of the limbs, and punctate keratoderma may be seen on palmar and plantar surfaces. All affected women have fibrocystic breast disease which may become malignant. Precocious breast hypertrophy has been seen in only 2 females. Gynecomastia occurred in 1 male. Thyroid adenoma and goiter, thyroiditis, thyroid hypofunction and thyroid carcinoma occur more frequently in women. Gynecologic abnormalities include menstrual irregularity, miscarriage, stillbirth, uterine fibroid tumors and ovarian cyst. The GI tract may be involved with polyposis of the stomach, colon and rectum, submucosal neuroma, leiomyoma, diverticulae and perirectal abscess. Carcinoma of the colon has developed in one patient. Skeletal abnormalities are diverse and include adenoid facies, mandibular hypoplasia, high-arched palate, pectus excavatum, scoliosis and bone cysts.

Complications
I   **Derived:** Malignant degeneration of breast lesions, lordosis, rupture of breast cysts, difficulties in speech, mastication, swallowing and respiration, dentigerous cysts, retained tooth fragments within gingivae.
II **Associated:** Thyroid adenoma, goiter and carcinoma; uterine fibroids, ovarian cyst, miscarriage and stillbirth; benign and malignant GI tumors; cutaneous neuromas, hemangiomas, lipomas, and carcinoma of the endometrium and ovaries.

Etiology: ? Some cases may have no family history, whereas evidence for autosomal dominant inheritance pattern has been noted in families with Cowden disease. McK *15835

Pathogenesis: Initial precipitating event is unknown. Children are born with coarse, black hair and are frequently the only black-haired children in the sibship. Gingival enlargement may be present at birth or noted by one year of age. Hirsutism may be congenital or develop as late as 4 to 5 years. Breast enlargement occurs after puberty at time of first menses or later and may occur at first pregnancy. Gingival lesions are composed of thick dense bundles of mature collagen bands in submucosa and lamina propria. The overlying epithelium is hyperkeratotic. Verrucous papillary growths arise about facial orifices, on the oral mucosa and on glabrous skin surfaces. Breast lesions have features of fibrocystic disease or giant fibroadenomas. Ductal carcinomas have been found in some cases. Thyroid tumors with histologic changes indistinguishable from carcinoma are reported. Chromosomal structure and numbers have been normal in 3 patients. An autosomal dominant inheritance pattern with variable expressivity has been proposed for Cowden disease. Electron microscopic examinations of warty cutaneous lesions do not demonstrate viral particles.

Related Facts
I   **Sex Ratio:** M8:F9
II **Risk of Occurrence:** ? Rare
III **Risk of Recurrence for**
      Patient's Sib: ?
      Patient's Child: ? 50%
IV **Age of Detectability:** For full syndrome, puberty to young adult. For gingival fibromatosis and hirsutism, birth to 4 years.†
V   **Prevalence:** ? Rare

Treatment
I   **Primary Prevention:** ?
II **Secondary Prevention:** Surgical removal of excess gingival tissue but it often recurs. If lesion recurs, extraction of all teeth, then gingivectomy. Surgical removal of malignant tumors of breast, thyroid or GI tract if they arise.
III **Other Therapy:** Full dentures. Depilatories. Plastic repair of breasts. Special education for those with oligophrenia.

Prognosis: Good with early surgical removal of breast adenomas. Fair if malignant transformation has occurred.

Detection of Carrier: —

†**Special Considerations:** It is not known if this condition is really a different entity from gingival fibromatosis and hypertrichosis. Of 40 familial cases (M22:F18) with gingival fibromatosis and hypertrichosis, none have been reported with breast lesions. At least 12 isolated cases of gingival

fibromatosis and hypertrichosis have been reported (M4:F8) which in all respects resemble this entry prior to the time breast lesions occur. It is not known if these cases are simply gingival fibromatosis, hypertrichosis and fibroadenomas of the breast at an age prior to the age of onset of the breast lesions. One such case did eventually develop giant fibroadenomas of the breast.

Some of the isolated cases of gingival fibromatosis and hypertrichosis are male; one male with Cowden disease had gynecomastia. Further, gingival fibromatosis alone has been reported in familial form (M44:F58) and in isolated cases not associated with Dilantin therapy (M15:F12). In none of these reports is virginal enlargement of breasts associated. It is not certain whether patients with only gingival fibromatosis might later develop changes in the other organ systems affected in Cowden disease. However, in both the familial and isolated cases with only gingival fibromatosis none of the other signs and symptoms reported in Cowden disease were present.

References:
Byars, L. T. and Jurkiewicz, M.: Congenital macrogingivae and hypertrichosis with subsequent giant fibroadenomas of the breasts. Plast. Reconstr. Surg. 27:608, 1961.
Gentry, W.C., Jr., et al: The multiple hamartoma syndrome (Cowden's disease). Arch. Dermatol. 109:521, 1974.
Lloyd, K. M., 2nd, and Dennis, M.: Cowden's disease. A possible new symptom complex with multiple system involvement. Ann. Intern. Med. 58:136, 1963.
Witkop, C. J., Jr.: Heterogeneity in gingival fibromatosis. In Bergsma, D. (ed.): Part XI. Orofacial Structures. Birth Defects: Orig. Art. Ser., vol. VII, no. 7. Baltimore:Williams and Wilkins Co. for The National Foundation - March of Dimes, 1971, p. 210.

Contributors: **Carl J. Witkop, Jr.**
William C. Gentry, Jr.

Editor's Computerized Descriptors: Face, Oral, Teeth, Nasoph., Skin, Hair, Skel., GI., GU.
Also see Section I, Fig. 89

GINGIVAL FIBROMATOSIS, DEPIGMENTATION AND MICROPHTHALMIA

Includes: Fibromatose gingivale depigmentation microphthalmie, oligophrénie et athétose
Fibromatosis gingivae, Pigmentmangel, Mikrophthalmie, Oligophrenie und Athetose
Fibromatosis gingival con depigmentación, microftalmia, oligofrenia y atetosis
Depigmentation, gingival fibromatosis, microphthalmia, oligophrenia and athetosis
Microphthalmia, gingival fibromatosis, depigmentation, oligophrenia and athetosis
Oligophrenia, gingival fibromatosis, depigmentation, microphthalmia, and athetosis
Athetosis, gingival fibromatosis, depigmentation, microphthalmia, and oligophrenia
Gingival fibromatosis, depigmentation, microphthalmia, oligophrenia and athetosis

Excludes: Gingival fibromatosis (407)
Gingival fibromatosis and hypertrichosis (410)
Symmetric gingival fibromatosis
Gingival fibromatosis and digital anomalies (409)
Gingival fibromatosis and multiple hyaline fibromas (411)
Gingival fibromatosis and corneal dystrophy (408)
Gingival fibromatosis, Cowden type (412)

Minimal Diagnostic Criteria: Gingival fibromatosis in a patient with depigmentation, microphthalmia, oligophrenia and athetosis. No available information on the absence of one or more of these signs as possible variations in expressivity in this syndrome because all patients have shown all of these signs.

Clinical Findings: Gingival fibromatosis and high-arched palate constricted in the bicuspid region are found in conjunction with severe oligophrenia in children with athetosis, depigmentation and microphthalmia. Children are depigmented at birth and have small eyes, with coarse, jerky horizontal nystagmus and dense diffused, generalized corneal opacities which become heavily vascularized with spastic ectropion and injected palpebral conjunctivae. Head size is normal. By 3 months of age random athetoid movements, constant sucking sounds and weak high-pitched cry are noted and developmental parameters such as head holding, sitting and walking are not reached. Hyperextension of head, flexion contractures of limbs, shoulders and hips develop in late infancy. All deep tendon reflexes symmetrically exaggerated with plantar responses extensor bilaterally. Grasp and sucking reflexes retained into childhood. No clonus is elicited. Depigmentation of all of the skin and hair is present and hair shaft is thin. Hair bulbs show a decreased number of melanocytes with clumps of melanosomes within melanocyte cytoplasm. The hair bulb tyrosine test is weakly positive showing tyrosinase is present but melanocytes are seen arranged in a pinion gear fashion within the hair bulbs. Limited clinical and laboratory investigations have been done in this disease. The following tests were found normal: routine blood, urine, electroencephalogram, urine chromatography, fasting serum phenylalanine and tyrosine, cerebrospinal fluid glucose, protein, cells, lactic dehydrogenase and karyotype. One child had steep, basilar angle compatible with compensated hydrocephaly on skull radiographs.

Complications
I   **Derived:** Erythrodermia on even brief exposure to sunlight. Generalized sequelae of severe oligophrenia with institutionalization, growth and weight retardation, flexion contractures, underdeveloped secondary sex characteristics.

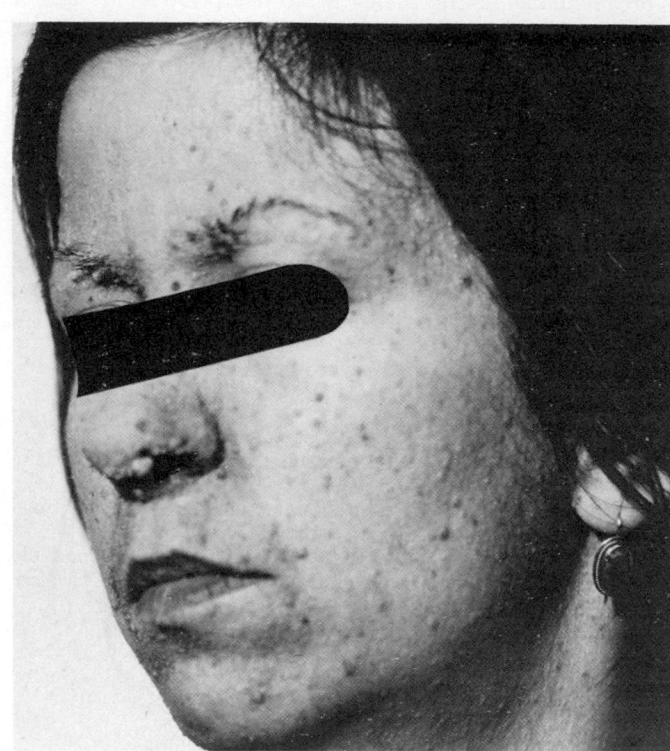

274. Typical facies of patient with Cowden disease

II Associated: —

Etiology: Autosomal recessive

Pathogenesis: ?

Related Facts
I **Sex Ratio:** M1:F1 (postulated, too few cases)
II **Risk of Occurrence:** Very rare
III **Risk of Recurrence for**
    Patient's Sib: 1 in 4 (25%) for each offspring to be affected
    Patient's Child: Patients do not reproduce.
IV **Age of Detectability:** Neonatal to early infancy by physical
    examination
V **Prevalence:** Very rare; one family reported by 1971.

Treatment
I **Primary Prevention:** Genetic counseling
II **Secondary Prevention:** ?
III **Other Therapy:** Nursing care, institutionalization

Prognosis: Reduced life span. Three children died by age 10 years.
One living less than 10 years of age. Essentially no data. Lethal
without intensive care.

Detection of Carrier: —

Special Considerations: —

References:
Cross, H.E. et al: A new oculocerebral syndrome with hypopigmen-
tation. J. Pediatr. 70:398, 1967.
Witkop, C.J., Jr. et al: Classification of albinism in man. In Bergs-
ma, D. (ed.): Part XII. Skin, Hair and Nails. Birth Defects: Orig.
Art. Ser., vol. VII, no. 8. Baltimore: Williams and Wilkins for The
National Foundation - March of Dimes, 1971, p. 13.
Witkop, C.J., Jr. et al: Oculocutaneous albinism. In Nyhan, N.L.
(ed.): Heritable Disorders of Amino Acid Metabolism - Patterns
of Genetic Variation and Expression. New York:John Wiley &
Sons, 1974.

Contributors: **Carl J. Witkop, Jr.**
                  Harold E. Cross

Editor's Computerized Descriptors: Eye, Face, Oral, Speech,
Skin, Hair, Skel., Nerve
Also see Section I, Fig. 89

GLAUCOMA, CONGENITAL

Includes: Glaucome congénital
Angeborene Glaukom
Glaucoma congénito
Congenital buphthalmos
Glaucoma, infantile

Excludes: Primary open angle glaucoma
Angle closure glaucoma
Secondary glaucoma
Goniodysgenesis (439)
"Juvenile" glaucoma
Aniridia (57)

Minimal Diagnostic Criteria: Elevated intraocular pressure or
corneal enlargement, ruptures in Descemet membrane, corneal
edema†

Clinical Findings: This relatively rare form of glaucoma is diagnosed within the 1st year of life in 80% of cases. The early clinical
signs include lacrimation, photophobia, blepharospasm, corneal
clouding (edema), corneal enlargement, ruptures in Descemet
membrane, cupping and atrophy of the optic disks. The globe
eventually becomes enlarged.† It is bilateral in 75% of cases and
more common in males. Examination under anesthesia confirms
the above findings plus increased intraocular pressure with poor
outflow facilities.

Complications
I **Derived:** Enlargement of globe, visual loss, postoperative
    complications
II **Associated:** Aniridia, cataracts, pyloric stenosis, deafness,
    mental retardation, cardiac anomalies, Marfan syndrome,
    Pierre-Robin syndrome, homocystinuria, Axenfeld syn-
    drome, Lowe syndrome, spherophakia, persistent hyper-
    plastic primary vitreous, Sturge-Weber syndrome, neurofi-
    bromatosis, trisomy D, trisomy F, rubella, and Rubinstein-
    Taybi syndrome.†

Etiology: Autosomal recessive with sporadic cases more common;
McK *23130

Pathogenesis: May be due to failure of the normal cleavage process of the iris from the angle structures with remaining underdeveloped mesodermal tissue blocking the outflow channels or to
persistence of a thin "cellophane'-like membrane over the
trabecular meshwork, or a combination of above.

Related Facts
I **Sex Ratio:** M3:F1
II **Risk of Occurrence:** 1:10,000 births
III **Risk of Recurrence for**
    Patient's Sib: When autosomal recessive, 1 in 4 (25%) for
    each offspring to be affected.
    Patient's Child: When autosomal recessive, not increased
    unless mate is carrier or homozygote.
IV **Age of Detectability:** 60% in 1st 6 months, 80% in 1st year
V **Prevalence:** The incidence varies between .03-.08% of oph-
    thalmic patients.

Treatment
I **Primary Prevention:** Genetic counseling when autosomal
    recessive
II **Secondary Prevention:** Medical treatment virtually ineffec-
    tive. Surgery should be performed as early as possible and
    the procedure of choice is goniotomy.
III **Other Therapy:** Other surgical procedures often resorted to
    when repeated goniotomies fail.

Prognosis: If the pressure is elevated at birth, there is less chance
of cure than if the symptoms appear after the 2nd month. Surgery
can be successful in salvaging the eye in 80% of the latter cases.
Vision may be poor, however, due to amblyopia and damaged
optic nerve. Although spontaneous remissions have been reported, most infants go blind unless successful surgery is per-

formed.

Detection of Carrier: —

†**Special Considerations:** The differential diagnosis includes congenital megalocornea, trauma with resultant corneal haze, rubella keratitis or metabolic diseases causing corneal haze. Unilateral congenital glaucoma may be associated with Sturge-Weber syndrome or neurofibromatosis.

References:

Haas, J.: Principles and problems of therapy in congenital glaucoma. Invest. Ophthalmol. 7:140, 1968.

Hetherington, J., Jr. and Shaffer, R.N.: Tonometry and tonography in congenital glaucoma. Invest. Ophthalmol. 7:134, 1968.

Jerndal, T.: Varieties of congenital glaucoma. Acta Ophthalmol. (Kbh.) 46:153, 1968.

Kass, M. et al: Chronic topical corticosteroid use simulating congenital glaucoma. J. Pediatr. 81:1175, 1972.

Kolker, A. and Hetherington, J. (eds.): Becker and Shaffer's Diagnosis and Therapy of the Glaucomas. 4th Ed. St. Louis: C.V. Mosby, 1976.

Kwitko, M.L.: Congenital glaucoma: A clinical study. Can. J. Ophthalmol. 2:91, 1967.

Richardson, K.T. and Shaffer, R.N.: Optic-nerve cupping in congenital glaucoma. Am. J. Ophthalmol. 62:507, 1966.

Richardson, K.T., Jr. et al: Long-term functional results in infantile glaucoma. Trans. Am. Acad. Ophthalmol. Otolaryngol. 71:833, 1967.

Sears, M.L.: Congenital glaucoma in neonatal rubella. Br. J. Ophthalmol. 51:744, 1967.

Shaffer, R.N.: Genetics and the congenital glaucomas. Am. J. Ophthalmol. 60:981, 1965.

Shaffer, R.N. and Weiss, D.I.: Congenital and Pediatric Glaucoma. St. Louis: C.V. Mosby, 1970.

Worst, J.G.: Congenital glaucoma: Remarks on the aspect of chamber angle, ontogenetic and pathogenetic background, and mode of action of goniotomy. Invest. Ophthalmol. 7:127, 1968.

Contributor: **Morton E. Smith**

Editor's Computerized Descriptors: Vision, Eye
Also see Section I, Figs. 39, 68

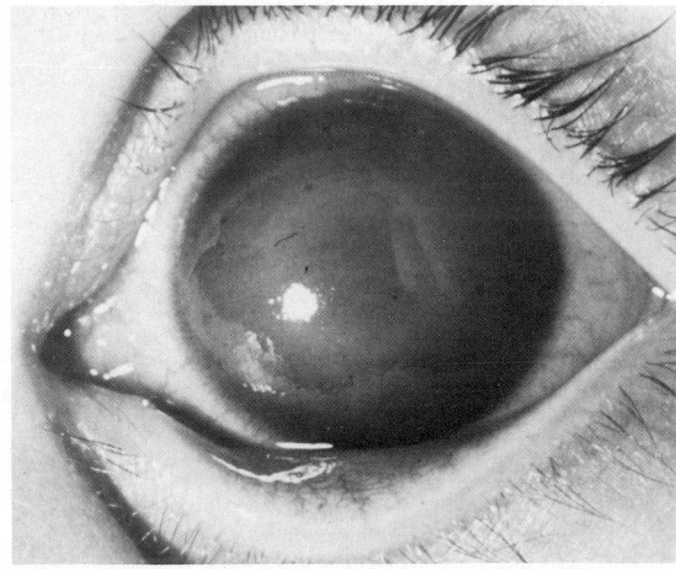

275. Congenital glaucoma

GLOBOID CELL LEUKODYSTROPHY

Includes: Sclérose cérébrale à cellules globoïdes
Mb. Krabbe
Esclerosis a células globoides
Cerebral sclerosis - diffuse Krabbe type
Krabbe disease

Excludes: Metachromatic leukodystrophies (651)
Sudanophilic leukodystrophy
Pelizaeus-Merzbacher syndrome (803)
Brain, spongy degeneration (115)
Other leukodystrophies of nervous system
Other degenerative diseases of nervous system

Minimal Diagnostic Criteria: The diagnosis can be suspected on the basis of the clinical history and is aided by a positive family history. The spinal fluid protein is usually elevated and there is said to be an increase in albumin and in α-2 globulin and a reduction of β-1 globulin and gamma globulin fractions of CSF. The peripheral nervous system is also involved and peripheral nerve conduction velocities are delayed.

The diagnosis can be confirmed by biochemical studies which can be carried out on leukocytes, skin fibroblasts, on somatic organs or brain. Biochemical defect is in an acid hydrolase of lysosomal origin, cerebroside β-galactosidase. The affected individuals have less than 10% of control levels of activity of this enzyme.

Clinical Findings: This is a disease of infants and young children with clinical onset around 4-6 months of age. The children usually appear to be irritable and are often thought to have GI disturbances. By 6-8 months of age it is apparent that the child is making no developmental progress and there is progressive deterioration and loss of any motor skills which may have developed. By 9-12 months of age the child feeds poorly, stops using his limbs in any meaningful way, will be quite spastic and will appear to be blind and deaf and unresponsive to all incoming stimuli. With increasing age convulsions become common and are quite refractory to anticonvulsant therapy. The patient may have unexplained temperature elevation and death is usually from aspiration pneumonia.

Complications
I **Derived:** Feeding disorders, seizures and aspiration pneumonia
II **Associated:** —

Etiology: The condition is autosomal recessive with the biochemical defect being absence or deficiency of cerebroside β-galactosidase. The defect is generalized and can be detected in somatic organs, brain, leukocytes and skin fibroblasts. (There is a similar disease in the cairn terrier with a similar enzymatic defect.) McK *24520

Pathogenesis: There is widespread severe demyelination, a loss of oligodendroglia and the presence of multinucleated giant cells (globoid cells) in the white matter of the CNS. Biochemically there is a marked decrease in the concentration of sulfatide and a relative preservation in the concentration of cerebroside. In the peripheral nervous system there is segmental demyelination. These changes are secondary to a biochemical defect, the deficiency or absence of cerebroside β-galactosidase.

Related Facts
I   **Sex Ratio:** M1:F1
II **Risk of Occurrence:** ?
III **Risk of Recurrence for**
     Patient's Sib: 1 in 4 (25%) for each offspring to be affected
     Patient's Child: (Condition is lethal in early childhood.)

IV Age of Detectability: The condition can be diagnosed at birth using leukocytes or fibroblasts for the assay of β-galactosidase. It is conceivable that the condition can be diagnosed in utero using amnionic cells. It is also possible, by these means, to detect the heterozygote carrier.

V Prevalence: ?

Treatment
I Primary Prevention: Genetic counseling
II Secondary Prevention: There are no known agents which will alter the course of the disease.
III Other Therapy: Supportive measures to minimize aspiration

Prognosis: Death occurs within 6-24 months after onset of disease.

Detection of Carrier: The heterozygote can be determined by enzymatic assay of leukocytes or fibroblasts for cerebroside β-galactosidase.

Special Considerations: —

References:
Farrell, D.F. et al: Globoid cell (Krabbe's) leukodystrophy: Heterozygote detection in cultured skin fibroblasts. Am. J. Hum. Genet. 25:604, 1973.
Suzuki, Y. and Suzuki, K.: Krabbe's globoid cell leukodystrophy: Deficiency of galacto-cerebrosidase in serum, leukocytes, and fibroblasts. Science 171:73, 1971.

Contributor: **Guy M. McKhann**

Editor's Computerized Descriptors: Vision, Hearing, Nerve

GLOMUS TUMORS, MULTIPLE

Includes: Tumeurs glomiques multiples
Multiple glomus Tumoren
Tumores múltiples de los glomus
Glomangiomas
Multiple glomus tumors

Excludes: Solitary glomus tumor
Solitary glomangioma

Minimal Diagnostic Criteria: Positive diagnosis by biopsy. The characteristic histopathologic features are endothelial-lined dilated vascular spaces which are surrounded by one or more layers of the oval glomus tumor (smooth muscle) cells.

Clinical Findings: Multiple flesh-colored to blue nodules in the skin, 0.3 to 3.0 cm in diameter. They may occasionally involve deeper structures such as bone. The lesions are usually regional but may be generalized. The lesions are soft, movable, sometimes tender. No changes are ordinarily seen in the overlying epidermis.

Complications
I Derived: —
II Associated: †

Etiology: ? But an autosomal dominant pattern of inheritance has been seen in several families. McK *13800

Pathogenesis: Several authors have considered these tumors to be a benign hyperplasia of the normal cutaneous arteriovenous anastomosis. The average age of development of the regional type is 29 years and that of the generalized type 40 years. One-third of all cases appear before age 20. Some cases have been apparent at birth.

Related Facts
I Sex Ratio: Males affected slightly more than females.
II Risk of Occurrence: Very rare
III Risk of Recurrence for
  Patient's Sib: When autosomal dominant and if parent is affected, 1 in 2 (50%) for each offspring to be affected; otherwise not increased.
  Patient's Child: When autosomal dominant, 1 in 2
IV Age of Detectability: Average age 29 years for the regional type, 40 years for the generalized type
V Prevalence: Less than 50 cases in medical literature

Treatment
I Primary Prevention: Genetic counseling
II Secondary Prevention: Surgical excision of the lesion
III Other Therapy: —

Prognosis: Normal for life span and intelligence. Functional disability may result from pain or rarely, deformity of the limb. The lesions have no malignant potential.

Detection of Carrier: ?

†Special Considerations: A case has been reported with deformities of the affected limb consisting of hypoplasia with precocious closure of the epiphyses and bradymetacarpia. Another case had some atrophy of the affected limb and (by arteriography) many abnormal ballooning blood vessels at the end of arteries and arteriovenous anastomoses corresponding to tumors.

References:
Goodman, T.F., Jr. and Abele, D.C.: Multiple glomus tumors: A clinical and electron microscopic study. Arch. Dermatol. 103:11, 1971.
Gordon, B. and Hyman, A.B.: Multiple nontender glomus tumors: Report of a case with 33 lesions. Arch. Dermatol. 83:640, 1961.
Sluiter, J.T. and Postma, C.: Multiple glomus tumors of the skin. Acta Derm. Venereol. (Stockh.) 39:98, 1959.

Contributors: **Thomas F. Goodman, Jr.**
Donald C. Abele

Editor's Computerized Descriptors: Skin, Muscle,

GLOSSITIS, MEDIAN RHOMBOID

Includes: Glossite rhomboide médiane
Mediane rhomboide Glossitis
Glositis mediana romboidea
Median rhomboid, glossitis

Excludes: Lingual tonsil
Lingual thyroid
Central papillary atrophy
Tongue, geographic (954)

Minimal Diagnostic Criteria: A history or observation of persistent ovoid area free of papillae in midline immediately anterior to V formed by circumvallate papillae, which, in children, may increase in size, but no more rapidly than the tongue as a whole.

Clinical Findings: An ovoid or rhomboid nodular, fissured or smooth, red mass or zone situated in the midline of the dorsum of the tongue, just anterior to the V formed by the circumvallate papillae. It is usually somewhat elevated. No association with other birth defects has been suggested.

Microscopically, the epithelium tends to be noncornified and may be unusually thin or may show acanthosis with elongated rete ridges. A chronic inflammatory infiltrate of varying intensity is usually present, but it should be borne in mind that biopsy sampling may be biased in favor of symptom-producing (ie inflamed) lesions. There is no abnormality in the position or amount of underlying skeletal muscle.

Complications
I **Derived:** Food and detritus accumulation in fissures may lead to chronic inflammation, which may have painful episodes. Frequency data are not available, but inflammation appears to be relatively common and tenderness or pain relatively uncommon.
II **Associated:** —

Etiology: ?

Pathogenesis: Thought to be failure of the lateral lingual tubercules to completely overgrow the tuberculum impar during the development of the tongue, resulting in a zone of nonpapillated mucosa. Some workers have described a smooth-surfaced lesion, somewhat anterior to the usual location that is inflammatory and often regresses with treatment. This seems to be a separate entity — central papillary atrophy.

Related Facts
I **Sex Ratio:** Some reports indicate a preponderance of males and others show an equal sex distribution.
II **Risk of Occurrence:** The incidence has not been observed, but it is probably nearly identical to the prevalence.
III **Risk of Recurrence for**
    Patient's Sib: ?
    Patient's Child: ?
IV **Age of Detectability:** At birth, by direct examination of the posterior dorsum of the tongue. Theoretically, it should also be detectable in aborted fetuses 7 to 8 weeks and older. However, it may be more difficult to detect in young children due to small size and relative lack of color distinction from surrounding lingual mucosa.
V **Prevalence:** 1 in 384 (Caucasian); 1 in 660 (Negro)

Treatment
I **Primary Prevention:** —
II **Secondary Prevention:** —
III **Other Therapy:** None indicated except as follows: hygienic measures, such as brushing or lavage of fissures, if chronic inflammation and tenderness are present to an annoying degree; partial or total excision if diagnosis is uncertain, if lesion appears to be enlarging, if hygienic measures fail to relieve tenderness, or if the patient has an intractable fear

that the lesion is cancerous.

Prognosis: Excellent. Does not appear to reduce longevity.

Detection of Carrier: ?

Special Considerations: —

References:
Farman, A.G. et al: Central papillary atrophy of the tongue. Oral Surg. 43:48, 1977.
Halperin, V. et al: Occurrence of Fordyce spots, benign migratory glossitis, median rhomboid glossitis and fissured tongue in 2,478 dental patients. Oral Surg. 6:1072, 1953.
Richardson, E. R.: Incidence of geographic tongue and median rhomboid glossitis in 3,319 Negro college students. Oral Surg. 26:623, 1968.

Contributor: **Robert S. Redman**

Editor's Computerized Descriptor: Oral

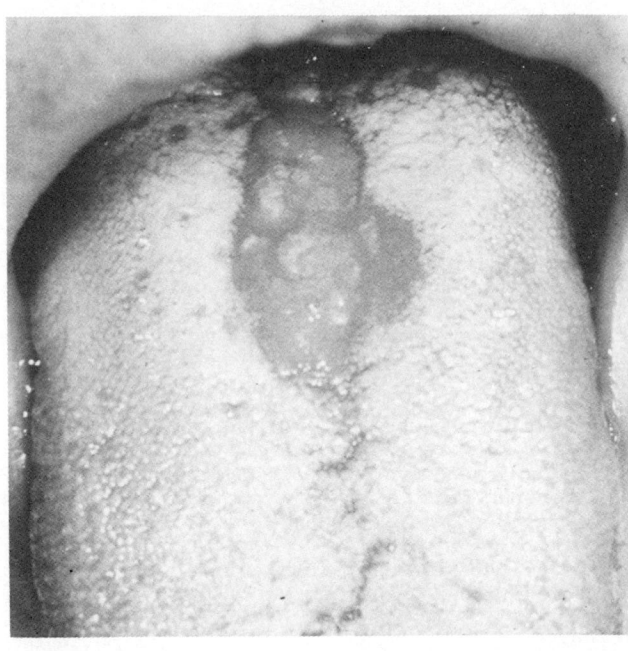

276. Rhomboid glossitis

GLUCOGLYCINURIA (MARKER)

Includes: Glucoglycinurie
Glukoglyzinurie
Glucoglicinuria (Marcador)

Excludes: Renal glucosuria
Hyperglycinemia
Cystic fibrosis (237)

Minimal Diagnostic Criteria: Glucosuria associated with reduced "venous" plasma threshold and normal T_m (Reubi type B renal glucosuria).
Renal hyperglycinuria, Cgly > 8.6 ml/min /1.73M^2. No other evidence of renal tubular dysfunction.

Clinical Findings: Fourteen members in a Swiss pedigree of 45 members exhibited isolated glucosuria and hyperglycinuria. All but the 9 1/2 year-old male proband were healthy; the latter presented with a clinical condition compatible with cystic fibrosis. Investigations indicated that the glucosuria was the result of reduced tubular reabsorption; the plasma threshold for glucosuria was reduced (79mg%), whereas the T_m glucose was normal (386 mg /min /1.73M^2); a load: T_m ratio of 4 was achieved. Hyperglycinuria was less well-studied, but it was clearly documented when the plasma concentration of glycine was normal. No other disturbance of renal function was discovered. Intestinal transport was not investigated.

Complications
I   **Derived:** —
II **Associated:** —

Etiology: Probably autosomal dominant defect of renal tubule

Pathogenesis: Deficiency of tubular absorptive mechanism(s) for both glucose and glycine.†

Related Facts
I   **Sex Ratio:** M9:F5, in one pedigree
II **Risk of Occurrence:** ?
III **Risk of Recurrence for**
    Patient's Sib: If parent is affected, probably 1 in 2 (50%) for each offspring to be affected; otherwise not increased.
    Patient's Child: 1 in 2
IV **Age of Detectability:** Early infancy probably
V   **Prevalence:** ?

Treatment
I   **Primary Prevention:** Genetic counseling
II **Secondary Prevention:** —
III **Other Therapy:** —

Prognosis: Normal life span; apparently harmless trait as described

Detection of Carrier: Trait so far identified only in carriers.

†**Special Considerations:** Reubi type B glucosuria describes reduced affinity (increased Km value) of transport system for glucose, assuming Michaelis kinetics for its uptake. This type of glucosuria is one predictable mode of expression for a mutant genotype affecting glucose transport. However, this type of glucosuria should not necessarily be associated with impaired glycine transport since the 2 molecules do not share a common mode of transport. An immediate interpretation of the data presented by the Swiss pedigree, which is compatible with current thinking about "transport" genotypes and phenotypes, is not apparent.
Glucoglycinuria has been described, accompanied by a phosphate transport defect (Scriver, C.R. et al: Pediatrics

34:357, 1964); in the latter case, the transport defect was clearly of the "low-T_m" type.

Numerous causes of isolated hyperglycinuria exist, all of which are distinguished from the Swiss trait.

References:

Käser, H. et al: Glucoglycinuria: A new familial syndrome. J. Pediatr. 61:386, 1962.

Reubi, F.: Physiopathologie et diagnostic diabète rénal. Rev. franç. Étud. clin. biol. 1:575, 1956.

Wyngaarden, J.B. and Segal, S.: The hyperglycinurias. In Stanbury, J.B. et al (eds.): The Metabolic Basis of Inherited Disease. 2nd Ed. New York: McGraw-Hill, 1966, p. 341.

Contributor: **Charles R. Scriver**

Editor's Computerized Descriptor: GU.

GLUCOSE-GALACTOSE MALABSORPTION

Includes: Malabsorption du glucose et du galactose
Glukose-Galaktose-Malabsorption
Malabsorción del glucosa-galactosa
Intestinal monosaccharide intolerance
Galactose-glucose malabsorption

Excludes: Disaccharidase deficiency
Disaccharide intolerance
Renal glycosuria (Marker) (861)

Minimal Diagnostic Criteria: Specific monosaccharide intolerance for glucose and galactose; osmotic diarrhea associated with flat oral glucose tolerance test; intermittent glycosuria when euglycemic; demonstration of defect in uptake of glucose or galactose by jejunal mucosa; absence of disaccharidase deficiency.

Clinical Findings: Severe diarrhea in neonatal period (nearly 100%). Intolerance to formulae containing glucose or galactose in any form. Amelioration of symptoms when fed fructose as carbohydrate source (100%). Large amounts of glucose and galactose in feces (100%).

Complications
I **Derived:** Severe dehydration and shock secondary to diarrhea; failure to thrive if undiagnosed and not treated with fructose-containing formulae.
II **Associated:** —

Etiology: Autosomal recessive transmission affecting specific glucose-galactose "carrier protein" in small intestine and kidney. McK *23160

Pathogenesis: Intestinal transport defect leads to osmotic diarrhea and dehydration when glucose or galactose are ingested; failure to thrive produced by diarrheal episodes, inanition and dehydration; renal tubular defect of no apparent clinical significance.†

Related Facts
I **Sex Ratio:** M1:F1
II **Risk of Occurrence:** ?
III **Risk of Recurrence for**
    Patient's Sib: 1 in 4 (25%) for each offspring to be affected
    Patient's Child: Increased if mate is carrier or homozygote; magnitude of risk undefined pending data on risk of occurrence.
IV **Age of Detectability:** Soon after birth
V **Prevalence:** Less than 20 cases reported

Treatment
I **Primary Prevention:** Genetic counseling
II **Secondary Prevention:** Removal of glucose or galactose-containing foodstuffs from the diet.
III **Other Therapy:** Oral or parenteral fluid replacement for dehydration

Prognosis: Early demise if untreated; no shortening of life span if glucose and galactose are avoided; symptoms seem to ameliorate with age.

Detection of Carrier: Reduced uptake of glucose by jejunal mucosa demonstrable in both parents of 1 affected child.

†Special Considerations: Intestinal transport and absorption of glucose is completely defective whereas renal tubular reabsorption of glucose is only modestly impaired, thus demonstrating that at least 2 systems mediate glucose reabsorption in renal tubule in contrast to single mechanism in the intestine; normal affinity but reduced capacity for intestinal glucose transport in jejunal mucosa of obligate heterozygotes implies that mutation affects number of carrier molecules.

References:

Elsas, L.J., Jr. et al: Renal and intestinal hexose transport in familial glucose-galactose malabsorption. J. Clin. Invest. 49:576, 1970.

Meeuwisse, G.W. and Dahlqvist, A.: Glucose-galactose malabsorption: A study with biopsy of the small intestinal mucosa. Acta Paediatr. (Uppsala) 57:273, 1968.

Schneider, A.J. et al: Glucose-galactose malabsorption: Report of a case with autoradiographic studies of a mucosal biopsy. N. Engl. J. Med. 274:305, 1966.

Stirling, C.E. et al: Quantitative radioautography of sugar transport in intestinal biopsies from normal humans and a patient with glucose-galactose malabsorption. J. Clin Invest. 51:438, 1972.

Contributor: **Leon E. Rosenberg**

Editor's Computerized Descriptor: GI.

GLUCOSE-6-PHOSPHATE DEHYDROGENASE DEFICIENCY

Includes: Déficit en glucose-6-phosphate déhydrogénase
Glukose-6-phosphat Dehydrogenase-Mangel
Deficiencia en glucosa-6-fosfato dehidrogenasa
Congenital nonspherocytic hemolytic anemia associated with G6PD deficiency
Primaquine sensitive anemia
Favism
G6PD deficiency
Dehydrogenase deficiency, glucose-6-phosphate

Excludes: Other causes of congenital nonspherocytic hemolytic anemia
Drug-induced hemolysis not associated with deficient G6PD

Minimal Diagnostic Criteria: Quantitative assay of erythrocyte G6PD. Several screening tests are also available.†

Clinical Findings: Clinical findings in a specific patient are a function of: 1) The molecular variant of G6PD present in that patient. 2) The presence of other, as yet undefined genetic abnormalities which may interact with G6PD deficiency (eg favism). 3) Environmental factors- in particular, the presence of oxidant drugs and chemicals.

In general, the defect is characterized by one or more of the following:

Episodic hemolysis following ingestion of an oxidant drug (eg primaquine), exposure to certain chemicals (eg naphthalene), or during either viral or bacterial infections. Two or 3 days after exposure to a hemolytic agent hemolysis ensues with hemoglobinuria, jaundice, increasing anemia, reticulocytosis and occasionally even prostration, abdominal and back pain, and death. Heinz bodies may be found within the red cells during the early phases of hemolysis but not later. Despite continued presence of the hemolytic agent, recovery may ensue and a stage of compensated hemolysis be reached, characterized by normal hemoglobin levels but evidence of shortened erythrocyte survival.

Chronic unremitting hemolysis present from birth (congenital nonsperocytic hemolytic anemia), hyperbilirubinemia, anemia, reticulocytosis, and splenomegaly. Hemolysis in these patients may be exacerbated by exposure to hemolytic agents.

Favism; some, but not all, patients with the Mediterranean variant of G6PD undergo episodes of severe hemolysis following ingestion of fava beans or inhalation of fava bean pollen. Favism has also been noted in South China, but not in patients with the African (A-) G6PD variant.

Neonatal hyperbilirubinemia occurs frequently in Oriental (China, Thailand) and Mediterranean (Greece, Italy, Israel) G6PD-deficient infants. Full-term American Negroes with G6PD deficiency are not more susceptible than normal to hyperbilirubinemia but premature infants are. In Greece, other undefined genetic factors may act in concert with G6PD deficiency to produce hyperbilirubinemia in as many as 43% of G6PD-deficient infants.

Complications
I   **Derived:** The expected sequelae of chronic jaundice or anemia may occur (eg gallstones, congestive heart failure).
II **Associated:** Abnormal glucose tolerance tests have been reported.

Etiology: X-linked recessive; McK *30590

Pathogenesis: Deficiency of G6PD leads to diminished generation of NADPH, an essential reducing agent in the erythrocyte, and renders the cell incapable of converting

GSSG to GSH. Devoid of its endogenous reducing power the cell becomes susceptible to both exogenous (eg drugs) and endogenous (eg H_2O_2) oxidants which may attack membrane, hemoglobin or enzyme S-H groups; may oxidize hemoglobin or enzyme S-H groups; may oxidize hemoglobin to methemoglobin; or may peroxidate membrane lipids. One consequence of the oxidative attack upon hemoglobin is the formation of intraerythrocytic Heinz bodies which represent aggregates of denatured hemoglobin. Removal of such inclusion bodies by the spleen may result in loss of cell membrane and partial cell fragmentation. The ultimate cause of hemolysis is not known but is thought to be the consequence of membrane injury either as a result of Heinz body formation or following a direct oxidative assault on structural components essential for membrane integrity.

Related Facts

I **Sex Ratio:** M > F Severe phenotypic expression of deficiency almost always in males or in homozygous females, who are numerically far less frequent than affected males. Heterozygous females demonstrate variable, intermediate levels of enzyme deficiency and are usually clinically normal.

II **Risk of Occurrence:**
(For males)

American Negroes	10-14%
Ashkenazic Jews	0.4%
Sephardic Jews	
Kurdish	53%
Iraq	24%
Iran	15%
Yemen	5%
Arabs	14-8%
Sardinians	4-30%
Greeks	0.7-12.5%
Chinese	5.5%
Filipinos	13%

III **Risk of Recurrence for**
Patient's Sib: If mother is a carrier, 1 in 2 (50%) for each brother to be affected and 1 in 2 for each sister to be a carrier.
Patient's Child: 1 in 1 (100%) for each daughter to be a carrier; not increased for sons unless wife is a carrier.
IV **Age of Detectability:** At birth (assay of erythrocyte G6PD)
V **Prevalence:** See Risk of Occurrence†

Treatment

I **Primary Prevention:** Genetic counseling
II **Secondary Prevention:** Avoidance of agents capable of inducing hemolysis. These include:
Antimalarials-(primaquine, pamaquine, pentaquine, plasmoquine, quinocide, atabrine, quinine**).
Sulfonamides-(sulfanilamide, N^2 acetylsulfanilamide, sulfacetamide, sulfamethoxypyridazine, salicylazosulfapyridine, sulfisoxazole, sulfapyridine).
Nitrofurans-(nitrofurantoin, furazolidone, furaltadone, nitrofurazone).
Antipyretics and analgesics-(acetylsalicylic acid, acetanilide, acetophenetidin, antipyrine**, aminopyrine**, p-aminosalicylic acid).
Sulfones-
Others-(simercapriol, methylene blue, naphthalene, phenylhydrazine, probenecid, vitamin K (large doses of water soluble analogs), chloramphenicol**, quinidine**, fava beans**, chloroquine, nalidixic acid, orinase.
**These agents produce hemolysis in Caucasians but apparently not in Negroes.
III **Other Therapy:** Supportive blood transfusions when necessary for acute hemolytic anemia. Cholecystectomy if gallstones ensue. Splenectomy usually of little or no benefit in G6PD-deficient patients with chronic congenital nonspherocytic hemolytic anemia.

Prognosis: Most affected males will survive into adulthood and

normal longevity is common. However, in one survey of American Negroes, the incidence of G6PD deficiency was 12% in males but declines to 8% in those over 40 suggesting an unfavorable influence of G6PD deficiency on mortality. Heterozygous females appear to have a normal life expectancy.

Detection of Carrier: Heterozygous, carrier females are usually free of clinical manifestations of G6PD deficiency (but hemolysis may ensue in some following exposure to hemolytic agents) and identification therefore depends upon quantitative assay of the erythrocyte enzyme. In individual carriers, enzyme activity may range from the low levels found in hemizygous males to levels indistinguishable from normal. Special tests are available to aid in identification of the latter group.

†**Special Considerations:** More than 150 molecular variants of human G6PD have been described. Their differentiation has been on the basis of electrophoresis, pH maximal activity, substrate kinetics, and utilization of alternate substrates. Normally Caucasians have the B+ isoenzyme, identified by its electrophoretic migration, as do approximately 70% of American Negroes. 18% of Negroes have the A+ isoenzyme which is structurally distinguished from the B+ by a single amino acid substitution of aspartic acid for asparagine. G6PD-deficient American Negro males have a different A isoenzyme (A-), so named because its electrophoretic migration is identical to the A+ isoenzyme. The activity of the A- enzyme may be normal in reticulocytes but it declines rapidly as the cell ages. Thus the older erythrocytes are particularly liable to hemolysis. Caucasians with G6PD deficiency may have a B isoenzyme (B-) or one of the many other variants mentioned. Even reticulocytes from these patients are deficient in G6PD activity. Hemolysis upon exposure to an oxidant is, therefore, often more severe in this group.

Other tissues (WBC, lens, liver, skin, platelets) may demonstrate deficient G6PD activity (WBC G6PD is normal in G6PD-deficient Negroes, however).

References:
Beutler, E.: Abnormalities of the hexose monophosphate shunt. Semin. Hematol. 8:311, 1971.
Beutler, E. and Yoshida, A.: Human glucose-6-phosphate dehydrogenase variants: A supplementary tabulation. Ann. Hum. Genet. 37:151, 1973.
Piomelli, S.: G6PD deficiency and related disorders of the pentose pathway. In Nathan, D. G. and Oski, F. A. (eds.): Hematology of Infancy and Childhood, Philadelphia:W. B. Saunders Co., 1974, p. 346.
Yoshida, A. et al: Human glucose-6-phosphate dehydrogenase variants. Bull. WHO 45:243, 1971.

Contributors: **William C. Mentzer, Jr.**
Louis K. Diamond

Editor's Computerized Descriptors: CV., Spleen, GI.

GLUTARIC ACIDURIA

Includes: Acidurie glutarique
Glutar-Acidurie
Aciduria glutárica

Excludes: —

Minimal Diagnostic Criteria: Elevated concentrations of glutaric and β-hydroxy-glutaric acids in urine.

Clinical Findings: Patients appear normal at birth but episodes of hypotonia, vomiting and metabolic acidemia appear in the 1st year of life. The chronic picture is dominated by dystonic posturing, involuntary movements, and usually mental retardation.

Urinary excretion of glutaric acid may be in excess of 1 gm/day. This compound is normally found in urine only in ketosis, and even then in amounts less than 0.1 mg/mg creatinine. β-hydroxy-glutaric and occasionally glutaconic acids are also found in the urine. Glutaric acid concentrations are also elevated in serum, CSF, and in tissues.

Complications
I **Derived:** Death, mental retardation, choreoathetosis
II **Associated:** —

Etiology: Autosomal recessive

Pathogenesis: Deficient activity of glutaryl-CoA dehydrogenase. Accumulation of 5-carbon dicarboxylic acids may impair synthesis of γ-aminobutyric acid (GABA) in the brain.

Related Facts
I **Sex Ratio:** M1:F1
II **Risk of Occurrence:** ?
III **Risk of Recurrence for**
   Patient's Sib: 1 in 4 (25%) for each offspring to be affected
   Patient's Child: Not increased unless mate is carrier or homozygote. Most patients do not survive to childbearing age.
IV **Age of Detectability:** Presumably at birth, by demonstration of glutaric aciduria or by enzyme assay in peripheral leukocytes. Detection in utero may be possible by enzyme assay in cultured amniotic cells.
V **Prevalence:** ?

Treatment
I **Primary Prevention:** Genetic counseling
II **Secondary Prevention:** The usefulness of dietary restriction of glutarigenic amino acids (lysine, hydroxylysine, tryptophan) is unknown.
III **Other Therapy:** Treatment of acute episodes of acidosis and dehydration with fluids and bicarbonate.

Prognosis: Most patients are retarded and incapacitated by the movement disorder. Death may be common during acute episodes.

Detection of Carrier: Demonstration of reduced activity (about 25% of normal) of glutaryl-CoA dehydrogenase in peripheral leukocytes.

Special Considerations: —

References:
Goodman, S.I. et al: Glutaric aciduria; a 'new' disorder of amino acid metabolism. Biochem. Med. 12:12, 1975.
Goodman, S.I. and Kohlhoff, J.G.: Glutaric aciduria; inherited deficiency of glutaryl-CoA dehydrogenase activity. Biochem. Med. 13:138, 1975.
Stokke, O. et al: Glutaric aciduria; presence of glutaconic and β-hydroxyglutaric acids in urine. Biochem. Med. 12:386, 1975.
Stokke, O. et al: Inhibition of brain glutamate decarboxylase by glutarate, glutaconate, and β-hydroxyglutarate: Explanation of the symptoms of glutaric aciduria? Clin. Chim. Acta 66:411, 1976.

Contributor: **Stephen I. Goodman**

GLUTATHIONURIA

Includes: Glutathionurie
Glutathionmangel
Glutationuria
Gamma-glutamyl transpeptidase deficiency
Glutathionase deficiency

Excludes: —

Minimal Diagnostic Criteria: Marked increase in excretion of urinary glutathione, increased plasma glutathione concentrations, and normal concentration of erythrocyte glutathione. A severe reduction of the activity of gamma-glutamyl transpeptidase has been demonstrated in serum, urine, leukocytes, and cultured skin fibroblasts.

Clinical Findings: Two or possibly 3 patients with this disorder have been described. One was an adult male with mild mental retardation and no other clinical abnormalities. Another was a 22-year-old female who spends most of her time in an institution for the retarded. This individual had episodes of colic and vomiting as an infant. She walked and was toilet trained at a normal time but speech was slow, and tantrums were prominent from age 3 to 5. Her IQ was in the low 60s on several testings. At age 12, behavioral problems became more severe and an EEG showed mild generalized dysrhythmia. Severe behavioral abnormalities continued, including several instances of self-inflicted injury, suicidal threats, and attacks on hospital staff and other patients. Physical examination was normal. A 3rd patient who may have this disorder was briefly described by O'Daly; attempts to obtain further information or confirmation of diagnosis on this patient, described as "a child suffering from a psychiatric disorder," have been unsuccessful.

Complications
I **Derived:** The few patients described have had some abnormality in mental function. Whether this is a consequence of the enzyme defect or a coincidental finding is presently unknown.
II **Associated:** —

Etiology: Possibly autosomal recessive

Pathogenesis: Generalized deficiency of gamma-glutamyl transpeptidase.

Related Facts
I **Sex Ratio:** Possibly M1:F1
II **Risk of Occurrence:** ?
III **Risk of Recurrence for**
  Patient's Sib: If autosomal recessive, 1 in 4 (25%) for each offspring to be affected.
  Patient's Child: ? None of the patients is known to have children.
IV **Age of Detectability:** Presumably at birth by enzyme assay of peripheral leukocytes or demonstration of glutathionuria. Since gamma-glutamyl transpeptidase is present in normal cultured amniotic fluid cells, antenatal diagnosis of this disorder might be possible.
V **Prevalence:** ?

Treatment
I **Primary Prevention:** Genetic counseling; possibly antenatal diagnosis. The possibility that glutathionuria is usually a harmless disorder must be considered.
II **Secondary Prevention:** —
III **Other Therapy:** —

Prognosis: ?

Detection of Carrier: —

Special Considerations: —

References:
Goodman, S.I. et al: Serum gamma-glutamyl transpeptidase deficiency. Lancet 1:243, 1971.
O'Daly, S.: An abnormal sulphydryl compound in urine. Ir. J. Med. Sci. 7:578, 1968.
Schulman, J.D. et al: Glutathionuria: Inborn error of metabolism due to tissue deficiency of gamma-glutamyl transpeptidase. Biochem. Biophys. Res. Commun. 65:68, 1975.

Contributors: **Stephen I. Goodman**
A.D. Patrick
Joseph D. Schulman

Editor's Computerized Descriptors: Speech, GI., Nerve

GLUTEN-INDUCED ENTEROPATHY

Includes: Maladie coéliaque
Gluten-induzierte Enteropathie
Enteropatía causada por el gluten
Celiac sprue
Celiac disease

Excludes: Other types of intestinal malabsorption

Minimal Diagnostic Criteria: Flattened jejunal mucosa found on jejunal biopsy. Restoration of normal growth and remission of symptoms on exclusion of all gluten from the diet.

Clinical Findings: Failure to thrive. The passage of loose, pale, bulky, greasy and foul-smelling stools. Irritability.

Biochemical studies may show raised fecal fat (in the presence of normal fecal nitrogen) abnormal xylose absorption, abnormal fat and glucose tolerance tests.

Biopsy of the jejunal mucosa shows a flattened mucosa with a loss of microvilli, and increased depth of crypts.

Retarded bone age.

Onset usually in late infancy or early childhood, but may be in adult life.

Complications
I **Derived:** Small stature. Secondary nutritional deficiencies, including deficiencies of vitamin D, folic acid, and iron.
II **Associated:** Increased risk of lymphoma and GI carcinomas. About 75% of patients with dermatitis herpetiformis have histologic features of celiac disease, which respond to a gluten-free diet.
   Possibly increased risk of diabetes mellitus, autoimmune thyroiditis and diffuse interstitial lung disease.

Etiology: A dominant gene, making those who carry it liable to develop the disease, is probably very closely linked to the HLA-B locus; but other unknown factors, genetic or environmental, influence its expression. The association is usually with the HLA-B8 antigen (present in about 25% of Caucasians, but in 85% of those with celiac disease).

Pathogenesis: Toxicity has been observed in a fraction of molecular weight approximately 3000, prepared by enzymatic degradation of gliadin.

The mechanism may be immunologic, or secondary to a mucosal enzyme defect.

Disturbances in both cellular and humoral immune mechanisms have been observed, but have not been firmly implicated in pathogenesis.

Related Facts
I **Sex Ratio:** M1.0:F1.5 (approx.)
II **Risk of Occurrence:** Wide racial variation, probably due to both genetic and environmental (eg variations in wheat consumption) factors. About 1 in 2000 live births in most populations of North European derivation, but higher in Ireland and Scotland.
III **Risk of Recurrence for**
   Patient's Sib: About 3% for clinical disease, but for subclinical disease with abnormal biopsy about 10%.
   Patient's Child: About 3% for clinical disease, but for subclinical disease with abnormal biopsy about 10%.
IV **Age of Detectability:** In infancy when gluten-containing grains are added to the diet.
V **Prevalence:** About 1 in 2000

Treatment
I **Primary Prevention:** Genetic counseling
II **Secondary Prevention:** Gluten-free diet is dramatically effective and permits first accelerated and then normal growth.†
III **Other Therapy:** Usually none required

Prognosis: Normal life span in most cases, if treated, but increased risk of malignancy may persist despite a gluten-free diet.

However, the gluten-free diet should probably be lifelong since recovery from the primary injurious effect of gluten does not appear to take place.

Detection of Carrier: Relatives of patients may be found to have abnormal jejunal mucosa without symptoms and with steatorrhea.

†**Special Considerations:** Some 30% of adult patients with a flat jejunal mucosa and steatorrhea do not respond to a gluten-free diet. At present these cases are best regarded as a distinct group.

References:
Anderson, C.M. et al: Coeliac disease: Some still controversial aspects. Arch. Dis. Child. 47:292, 1972.
European Soc. for Paediatric Gastroenterology: Diagnostic criteria in coeliac disease. Acta Paediatr. Scand. 59:461, 1970.
Hekkens, W.T.J.M. and Pena, A.S. (eds.): Proc. of 2nd International Coeliac Symposium. Leiden:Stenfert-Kroese, 1974.
Management of coeliac disease. Br. Med. J. 21:April 1973.
Mann, J.G. et al: The subtle and variable expressions of gluten-induced enteropathy. Am. J. Med. 48:357, 1970.
Townley, R.R. and Barnes, G.L.: Intestinal biopsy in childhood. Arch. Dis. Child. 48:480, 1973.
Young, W.F. and Pringle, E.M.: 110 children with coeliac disease. Arch. Dis. Child. 46:421, 1971.

Contributors: **Cedric O. Carter**
                     Nicholas R. Dennis

Editor's Computerized Descriptors: Skel., GI.

GLYCOGEN SYNTHETASE DEFICIENCY

Includes: Déficit en glycogène synthétase
Glykogen-Synthetase-Mangel
Deficiencia de glucógeno-sintetasa
Aglycogenosis
Glycogen deficiency syndrome with visceral fatty metamorphosis

Excludes: Glycogenoses

Minimal Diagnostic Criteria: Fasting hypoglycemia, extremely low hepatic glycogen stores (<0.5 gm/100 gm wet weight), very low glycogen synthetase activity (uridine diphosphoglucose (UDPG)-glycogen transglucosylase activity).

Clinical Findings: Lethargy, somnolence, unconsciousness, coma, convulsions, sweating, poor feeding, poor weight gain, tachycardia, hepatomegaly, microcephaly, delayed motor development, mental retardation. Laboratory findings include: low blood glucose (fasting), ketosis, metabolic acidosis, negative response to glucagon when fasting, low urinary catecholamines when hypoglycemic.

Complications
I Derived: Delayed motor development, mental retardation, microcephaly
II Associated: —

Etiology: Probably autosomal recessive with complete penetrance and variable expressivity of glycogen synthetase deficiency.†
McK *24060

Pathogenesis: Affected patients have very low (or no) glycogen stores and are unable to release glucose from liver to blood (in amounts coincident with peripheral utilization). Gluconeogenesis is also impaired, but mechanism is unclear. Fasting hypoglycemia leads to acute and chronic neurologic symptoms and signs.

Related Facts
I Sex Ratio: M2:F1 Only 6 patients described
II Risk of Occurrence: ? Very rare
III Risk of Recurrence for
  Patient's Sib: Probably 1 in 4 (25%) for each offspring to be affected
  Patient's Child: Probably not increased unless mate is carrier or homozygote
IV Age of Detectability: Newborn period by biochemical methods
V Prevalence: ? Very rare

Treatment
I Primary Prevention: Genetic counseling
II Secondary Prevention: Frequent or continuous carbohydrate feedings to prevent fasting hypoglycemia, ketosis, and metabolic acidosis.
III Other Therapy: —

Prognosis: For life: without treatment—grave; with treatment: guarded and variable (depending on severity of metabolic defect(s). For normal development: guarded (even with treatment).

Detection of Carrier: ?

†Special Considerations: Two sibships have been reported along with several isolated patients. In the 1st sibship, glycogen synthetase was deficient, while in the 2nd other enzyme activities in addition to glycogen synthetase were absent or low (hepatic phosphorylase, muscle phosphorylase, muscle UDPG pyrophosphorylase and muscle phosphoglucomutase). It would appear that aglycogenosis may represent a group of diseases, rather than a single defect.

References:
Dykes, J.R.W. and Spencer-Peet, J.: Hepatic glycogen synthetase deficiency: Further studies on a family. Arch. Dis. Child. 47:558, 1972.
Lewis, G.M. et al: Infantile hypoglycaemia due to inherited deficiency of glycogen synthetase in liver. Arch. Dis. Child. 38:40, 1963.
Parr, J. et al: Symptomatic hypoglycemia, visceral fatty metamorphosis, and aglycogenosis in an infant lacking glycogen synthetase and phosphorylase. Pediatrics 35:770, 1965.

Contributor: **Thomas M. Teree**

Editor's Computerized Descriptors: Skel., CV., GI., Liver, Nerve

GLYCOGENOSIS, TYPE I

Includes: Glycogenose, type I
Glykogenose, Typ I
Glucogenosis, tipo I
Glycogen storage disease, type I
von Gierke disease

Excludes: Hepatomegaly of a wide variety of etiologies
Hypoglycemia of other causes
All other glycogenoses

Minimal Diagnostic Criteria: An infant or child with a fasting blood lactate over 30 mg%, a low fasting blood glucose, unresponsive to glucagon, with poor growth and a very large liver probably has type I glycogenosis. The definitive diagnosis rests on the demonstration of the absence of glucose-6-phosphatase in the liver.

Clinical Findings: In the neonatal period hypoglycemic seizures or hepatomegaly may be the cardinal finding. As feedings become less frequent or infections supervene, hypoglycemia and ketoacidosis will be seen. Delayed growth becomes apparent by 1 year of age. Difficulty handling simple respiratory infections becomes a problem. At about 2 years of age nose bleeds usually begin, often in association with URI. Motor development is usually somewhat delayed. As the child grows older, he becomes better able to tolerate hypoglycemia. Xanthoma develops in about 10% of patients. The physical examination reveals a short, cherub-faced individual with protuberant abdomen. The liver, but not the spleen, is very large. Muscular tone is usually relatively poor. These individuals have high blood lactates, low fasting blood glucose which fails to rise with glucagon or epinepherine, high blood lipids, high uric acid and increased number of platelets.

Complications
I   **Derived:** Death from rapidly evolving ketoacidosis precipitated by infection in the early years, "dwarfism", gout after puberty, hepatomata.
II   **Associated:** —

Etiology: Autosomal recessive biochemical defect; McK *23220

Pathogenesis: Absence of glucose-6-phosphatase in the liver, kidney and intestinal mucosa

Related Facts
I   **Sex Ratio:** Approximately M1:F1
II   **Risk of Occurrence:** Estimated 1 in 400,000 live births in Sweden. Approximately the same in the U.S.A.
III   **Risk of Recurrence for**
    Patient's Sib: 1 in 4 (25%) for each offspring to be affected
    Patient's Child: Not increased unless mate is carrier or homozygote
IV   **Age of Detectability:** At birth
V   **Prevalence:** ? Rare

Treatment
I   **Primary Prevention:** Genetic counseling
II   **Secondary Prevention:** Frequent (every 3 to 4 hours) high carbohydrate feedings
III   **Other Therapy:** Use of an alkalinizing agent (eg Polycitra [R]) during periods of stress to prevent ketoacidosis. Allopurinol is useful in controlling the uric acid level after puberty. Frequent carbohydrate feedings during the day combined with constant nasogastric infusion of glucose at night correct the secondary metabolic aberrations and permit growth.

Prognosis: Death within the first 2 years with ketoacidosis is less frequent today. Death with hepatomata at 8-10 years of age or later is reported. Death in the 3rd decade with gouty nephritis is reported. Insufficient data is available on the course of the condition in adulthood.

Detection of Carrier: One report described detection of the heterozygote by determining the level of glucose-6-phosphatase by peroral intestinal biopsy.

Special Considerations: —

References:
Greene, H.L. et al: Nocturnal intragastric feeding for Type I glycogen-storage disease. N. Engl. J. Med. 294:423, 1976.
Moses, S.W. and Gutman, A.: Inborn errors of glycogen metabolism. Adv. Pediatr. 19:95, 1971.

Contributor: **James B. Sidbury, Jr.**

Editor's Computerized Descriptors: Face, Nasoph., Skin, Skel., Muscle, GI., Liver, Nerve

GLYCOGENOSIS, TYPE III

Includes: Glycogenose, type III
Glykogenose, Typ III
Glucogenosis, tipo III
Glycogen storage disease, type III
Forbes disease

Excludes: All other glycogenoses
Hepatomegaly of a variety of etiologies
Hypoglycemia of other causes

Minimal Diagnostic Criteria: The plasma lactate is normal. The demonstration of a failure of blood glucose to rise in response to glucagon administration in the fasting state which then responds postprandially is a useful screening procedure. The definitive diagnosis can be made only by the determination of amylo-1,6-glucosidase and amylo-1,4→1,4-glucantransferase in liver and muscle.

Clinical Findings: This type glycogenosis is rarely symptomatic in the neonatal period. There is a much wider spectrum of severity in type III than is seen in type I. The course for the first 4-6 years may be clinically indistinguishable from type I. There may be the short stature, the hypoglycemia with failure to respond to glucagon, hyperlipemia, episodes of ketoacidosis, poor handling of infections, epistaxis and massive hepatomegaly. They do not show the high fasting blood lactate levels, and hypoglycemia is rarely severe. Physical examination may show the cherub-faced, dwarfed individual with a markedly protuberant abdomen due to massive hepatomegaly. Other individuals may have virtually no difficulty and they are detected only because of the protuberant abdomen and hepatomegaly. At least 1 patient was detected in adulthood because of symptomatic myopathy. These individuals tend to become asymptomatic around puberty and the liver decreases progressively in size.

Complications
I **Derived:** Hypoglycemia may be symptomatic in the first 5 years of life with stress or fasting. Myopathy has been reported in older patients.
II **Associated:** —

Etiology: Appears to be an autosomal recessive biochemical defect. McK *23240

Pathogenesis: An absence or deficiency of amylo-1,6-glucosidase and amylo-1,4→1,4-glucantransferase. Both may be absent from liver and muscle or one of several permutations of distribution.

Related Facts
I **Sex Ratio:** Approximately M1:F1
II **Risk of Occurrence:** ?
III **Risk of Recurrence for**
  Patient's Sib: 1 in 4 (25%) for each offspring to be affected
  Patient's Child: Not increased unless mate is carrier or homozygote
IV **Age of Detectability:** At birth
V **Prevalence:** ?

Treatment
I **Primary Prevention:** Genetic counseling
II **Secondary Prevention:** High protein diet
III **Other Therapy:** Treatment of hypoglycemia and ketoacidosis symptomatically when it occurs.

Prognosis: Normal life expectancy anticipated

Detection of Carrier: ?

Special Considerations: —

References:

Moses, S.W. and Gutman, A.: Inborn errors of glycogen metabolism. Adv. Pediatr. 19:95, 1972.
Van Hoof, F. and Hers, H.G.: The subgroups of type III glycogenosis. Eur. J. Biochem. 2:265, 1967.

Contributor: **James B. Sidbury, Jr.**

Editor's Computerized Descriptors: Face, Nasoph., Skel., GI., Liver

GLYCOGENOSIS, TYPE VI

Includes: Glycogenose, type VI
Glykogenose, Typ VI
Glucogenosis, tipo VI
Glycogen storage disease, type VI

Excludes: Other hepatic glycogenoses
Hepatomegaly of a variety of etiologies

Minimal Diagnostic Criteria: Low leukocyte phosphorylase activity is helpful but a liver biopsy with assay of liver glycogen content and phosphorylase activity is definitive.

Clinical Findings: This type of glycogen storage disease has been confused by the inclusion of type IX patients and those otherwise not classifiable. This has understandably muddied accurate clinical description. Present data indicate these patients have very large livers, moderate intermittent hypoglycemia, growth retardation, and other symptoms very similar to type I. The range of the clinical spectrum is not yet clear.

Complications
I   **Derived:** Episodes of hypoglycemia
II **Associated:** —

Etiology: Autosomal recessive biochemical defect; McK *23270

Pathogenesis: Decrease in liver phosphorylase activity

Related Facts
I   **Sex Ratio:** M1:F1
II **Risk of Occurrence:** ?
III **Risk of Recurrence for**
   Patient's Sib: 1 in 4 (25%) for each offspring to be affected
   Patient's Child: Not increased unless mate is carrier or homozygote
IV **Age of Detectability:** Presumably at birth
V   **Prevalence:** ?

Treatment
I   **Primary Prevention:** Genetic counseling
II **Secondary Prevention:** None needed
III **Other Therapy:** —

Prognosis: Inadequate information available.

Detection of Carrier: ?

Special Considerations: —

References:
—

Contributor: **James B. Sidbury, Jr.**

Editor's Computerized Descriptor: Liver

GLYCOGENOSIS, TYPE VII

Includes: Glycogenose, type VII
Glykogenose, Typ VII
Glucogenosis, tipo VII
Glycogen storage disease, type VII

Excludes: Glycogenosis, types II, IV and V (11, 116, 698)
Idiopathic myoglobinuria
Muscular dystrophy
Other myopathies
Neurogenic muscle disease

Minimal Diagnostic Criteria: The anoxic exercise test is a useful screening test but the diagnosis requires the demonstration of abnormally low levels of phosphofructokinase activity in the muscle. The erythrocytes show diminished (approximately 50% of normal) activity of the enzyme also.

Clinical Findings: Muscle cramps induced by exercise from school age. Severe exercise may be associated with nausea, abdominal pain, severe crampy muscle pains followed in a few hours by myoglobinuria. By limitation of exertion may lead relatively normal life. Physical examination normal in resting state. Serum creatine phosphokinase and aldolase elevated. No rise in blood lactate when the forearm was subjected to an anoxic exercise test and muscular contracture of forearm muscles developed during test.

Complications
I   **Derived:** No permanent disability has been found to date. All of the individuals reported were relatively young (< 40 years of age). Recurrent attacks might be expected in time to result in muscle atrophy.
II **Associated:** —

Etiology: Appears to be an autosomal recessive biochemical defect; McK *23280

Pathogenesis: Deficiency of the muscle form of phosphofructokinase

Related Facts
I   **Sex Ratio:** Approximately M1:F1
II **Risk of Occurrence:** ? Reported in only 2 families; 1 Japanese, 1 Jewish
III **Risk of Recurrence for**
   Patient's Sib: 1 in 4 (25%) for each offspring to be affected
   Patient's Child: Not increased unless mate is carrier or homozygote
IV **Age of Detectability:** Presumably at birth but the 1st symptoms are reported about the time of beginning school.
V   **Prevalence:** ? Reported in only 2 families

Treatment
I   **Primary Prevention:** Genetic counseling
II **Secondary Prevention:** Avoidance of vigorous or sudden bursts of activity. These individuals can handle moderate, paced activity without symptoms.
III **Other Therapy:** Vocational guidance toward sedentary employment.

Prognosis: Normal for life span and intelligence

Detection of Carrier: Erythrocyte phosphofructokinase activity intermediate between normal and homozygote. Muscle enzyme activity determination in 2 obligatory heterozygotes showed 1 to have a normal activity level and the other to be intermediate.

Special Considerations: —

References:
Howell, R.R.: The glycogen storage diseases. In Stanbury, J.B. et al (eds.): The Metabolic Basis of Inherited Disease. 4th Ed. New York: McGraw-Hill, 1977.
Layzer, R.B. et al: Muscle phosphofructokinase deficiency. Arch. Neurol. 17:512, 1967.

Tarui, S. et al: Enzymatic basis for the coexistence of myopathy and hemolytic disease in inherited muscle phosphofructokinase deficiency. Biochem. Biophys. Res. Commun. 34:77, 1969.

Tarui, S. et al: Phosphofructokinase deficiency in skeletal muscle. A new type of glycogenosis. Biochem. Biophys. Res. Commun. 19:517, 1965.

Contributor: **James B. Sidbury, Jr.**

Editor's Computerized Descriptors: Muscle, GI.

429   **426-500**

GLYCOGENOSIS, TYPE VIII

Includes: Glycogenose, type VIII
Glykogenose, Typ VIII
Glucogenosis, tipo VIII
Glycogen storage disease, type VIII

Excludes: Glycogenosis, types II, IV and V (11, 116, 698)
Idiopathic myoglobinuria
Muscular dystrophy
Other myopathies
Neurogenic muscle disease

Minimal Diagnostic Criteria: The anoxic exercise test is a useful screening test, but the definitive diagnosis requires the demonstration of diminished lactate production by muscle homogenate when glucose-1-phosphate or glucose-6-phosphate is added as substrate, but normal lactate production when fructose-6-phosphate or fructose-1, 6-diphosphate are added. The activity of phosphohexoisomerase was normal.

Clinical Findings: Muscle pain, stiffness and fatigability after exercise, later onset, ie 35 years of age. The symptoms occurred a few hours after moderately heavy exercise and they were prominent during rest or at the end of the day. The symptoms were relieved by rest for several days. Myoglobinuria may occur after heavy exercise. The physical examination showed no abnormality; specifically no weakness nor atrophy. The creatine phosphokinase was elevated. There was no blood lactate rise when the forearm was subjected to anoxic exercise, nor, however, was there any associated muscle contracture. The lactate response was reported to be normal after an oral fructose load.

Complications
I   **Derived:**   The condition appears to be progressive and interferes with the individual's ability to do physically active work.
II   **Associated:**   —

Etiology: ? Presumed to be a genetically determined biochemical defect.

Pathogenesis: The implication of the findings is that there is an inhibitor of phosphohexoisomerase present in the muscle of these individuals.

Related Facts
I   **Sex Ratio:**   M?:F? Only report describes 2 brothers.
II   **Risk of Occurrence:**   ? Reported in 2 Japanese brothers
III **Risk of Recurrence for**
     Patient's Sib: ? (Presuming recessive transmission) 1 in 4 (25%) for each offspring to be affected
     Patient's Child: Not increased unless mate is carrier or homozygote
IV   **Age of Detectability:**   35 years or older
V   **Prevalence:**   ?

Treatment
I   **Primary Prevention:**   —
II   **Secondary Prevention:**   Avoidance of excessive physical activity. It is reported that fructose administered orally prevented the occurrence of symptoms.
III **Other Therapy:**   —

Prognosis: ? Inadequate information to project a prognosis

Detection of Carrier: No attempts were apparently made to identify the heterozygous state.

Special Considerations: —

References:
Howell, R.R.: The glycogen storage diseases. In Stanbury, J.B. et al (eds.): The Metabolic Basis of Inherited Disease. 4th Ed. New

482

York: McGraw-Hill, 1977.
Satoyoshi, E. and Kowa, H.: A new myopathy due to glycolytic abnormalities. Trans. Am. Neurol. Assoc. 90:46, 1965.

Contributor: **James B. Sidbury, Jr.**

_____

Editor's Computerized Descriptor: Muscle

GLYCOGENOSIS, TYPE IX

Includes: Glycogenose, type IX
Glykogenose, Typ IX
Glucogenosis, tipo IX
Glycogen storage disease, type IX

Excludes: Other hepatic glycogenoses
Hepatomegaly of a variety of etiologies

Minimal Diagnostic Criteria: Hepatomegaly. Low leukocyte phosphorylase in affected male, mother and 50% of female sibs.† Demonstration of decreased liver phosphorylase kinase activity is definitive.

Clinical Findings: A mild disease in males. No symptoms in infancy other than hepatomegaly. Mild degree of muscular weakness. The serum transaminases are elevated as in other glycogenoses. Hypoglycemia is minimal, fasting lactate may be slightly elevated, serum lipids elevated and serum uric acid may be elevated.

Complications
I   **Derived:**   Mild muscular weakness, fatigability.
II   **Associated:** —

Etiology: X-linked enzymatic defect

Pathogenesis: Deficiency of phosphorylase kinase in liver, not muscle.

Related Facts
I   **Sex Ratio:**   M1:F0
II   **Risk of Occurrence:**   ?
III **Risk of Recurrence for**
     Patient's Sib: If mother is a carrier 1 in 2 (50%) for each
   •   brother to be affected and 1 in 2 (50%) for each sister to be a carrier
     Patient's Child: 1 in 1 (100%) for carrier daughters; not increased for sons unless wife is a carrier.
IV **Age of Detectability:**   Presumably at birth
V   **Prevalence:**   ?

Treatment
I   **Primary Prevention:**   Genetic counseling
II   **Secondary Prevention:**   None needed
III **Other Therapy:** —

Prognosis: Good. Liver diminishes in size at puberty.

Detection of Carrier: With assay of the enzyme activity in leukocytes

†Special Considerations: The female carrier has an enlarged liver for the first few years of life. Usually normal by 6 years.

References:
Huijing, F.: Glycogen storage disease type VIa: Low phosphorylase kinase activity caused by a low enzyme - substrate affinity. Biochem. Biophys. Acta 206:199, 1970.
Sidbury, J.B.: The glycogenoses. In Gardner, L.I. (ed.) Endocrine and Genetic Diseases of Childhood. Philadelphia: W.B. Saunders, 1976.

Contributor: **James B. Sidbury, Jr.**

_____

Editor's Computerized Descriptors: Muscle, Liver

G~M1~-GANGLIOSIDOSIS, TYPE 1

Includes: Gangliosidose-type I
G_{M1} Gangliosidose, Typ I
Gangliosidosis G_{M1} tipo I
Generalized gangliosidosis, type 1
Familial neurovisceral lipidosis
Cerebral G_{M1}-gangliosidosis

Excludes: Mucopolysaccharidoses
G_{M2}-gangliosidosis with hexosaminidase A deficiency (434)
Niemann-Pick disease (717)
G_{M1}-gangliosidosis, type 2 (432)
Fucosidosis (398)
Mucolipidoses

Minimal Diagnostic Criteria: This diagnosis should be considered in a retarded infant with visceromegaly who has the characteristic bone changes and facies. Further support would be given by the vacuolized lymphocytes and marrow cells, and renal biopsy if available. Urinary mucopolysaccharide levels are normal. Diagnosis rests with demonstration of the G_{M1}-ganglioside increase in brain and ganglioside and mucopolysaccharide increases in the viscera, plus the deficiency of β-galactosidase activity in brain, liver, cultured skin fibroblasts, leukocytes, or urine.†

Clinical Findings: These infants demonstrate early and severe retardation of mental and motor development, and all have shown an unusual facial appearance with flat nose, full forehead and impression of wide-spaced eyes. Characteristic are changes in the long bones by xray (first periosteal cloaking, then architectural modifications similar to those in Hurler disease), hypoplasia or beaking of the vertebral bodies, enlargement of the liver (and, less notably, the spleen), gingival hyperplasia, generalized edema, glomerular epithelial cytoplasmic vacuolization, foam cells in the marrow, and vacuolization of circulating lymphocytes. Cherry-red macular changes have been seen in a half of the patients. All children have an increase in G_{M1}-ganglioside in brain and viscera, and a deficiency of β-galactosidase in tissues and body fluids.

Complications
I   **Derived:** Growth and nutritional failure, increasing nervous system compromise, control of infection, seizures. Death is accompanied by recurrent bronchopneumonia.
II   **Associated:** Cataracts have been found in 1 patient.

Etiology: Autosomal recessive inheritance. The fundamental defect is felt to be a deficiency of lysosomal β-galactosidase in brain and other organs. McK *23050

Pathogenesis: β-galactosidase is known to be involved in the cleavage of galactose from ganglioside, galactose-containing mucopolysaccharides, and glycoproteins. Hence, a deficiency of this enzyme would constitute a reasonable basis for accumulation of these substrates in the tissue. It is probable that the neuronal gangliosidosis is responsible for the cumulative cerebral handicaps, the skeletal mucopolysaccharidosis is the setting for the bony deformities, and both elements contribute to the visceral histiocytosis with organomegaly.

Related Facts
I   **Sex Ratio:** M1:F1
II   **Risk of Occurrence:** ?
III   **Risk of Recurrence for**
    Patient's Sib: 1 in 4 (25%) for each offspring to be affected
    Patient's Child: Homozygotes die in early infancy or early childhood.
IV   **Age of Detectability:** Prenatal diagnosis has been accomplished. At birth, would depend on the vigor with which specific signs are sought in new infants; clinical evidence is present by several months of age.
V   **Prevalence:** Low. There are more than 50 patients on record,

but many others undoubtedly exist in unclassified categories in other studies. No increased gene frequency has been identified with any particular ethnic group, except for a suspicion of increased frequency on Malta.

Treatment
I   **Primary Prevention:** Genetic counseling
II   **Secondary Prevention:** —
III   **Other Therapy:** The supportive treatment would be that for any of the debilitating, brain-handicapping sphingolipidosis disorders.

Prognosis: Most patients with this disease have expired by 2 years of age (with exceptional children reaching up to 4 years).

Detection of Carrier: Identification of heterozygously involved individuals is possible by assay of β-galactosidase activity in leukocytes and cultured fibroblasts from skin biopsy.

†Special Considerations: It is only in the recent years that the really critical progress has been made in the establishment of the phenotypic classification for unusual children formerly viewed as "atypically" involved in inborn error syndromes bearing partial relationship to Hurler syndrome, Niemann-Pick and Tay-Sachs diseases. Now 6 or more syndromes have been recorded in this area (the 2 types of gangliosidosis, I-cell disease, fucosidosis, lipomucopolysaccharidosis, metachromatic leukodystrophy variant, etc), with the definitive studies dependent on careful analysis of tissue glycolipids and polysaccharides, plus enzyme assays. β-galactosidase abnormalities are common to several of these diseases, but thus far the deficiency has been most extreme in generalized gangliosidosis. Experience in the clinical diagnosis of the syndromes will grow now, if coordinated with well-controlled laboratory support.

References:
Landing, B.H. et al: Familial neurovisceral lipidosis. Am. J. Dis Child. 108:503, 1964.
O'Brien, J.S.: The gangliosidoses. In Standbury, J.B. et al (eds.): The Metabolic Basis of Inherited Disease, 4th Ed. New York:McGraw-Hill, 1978, p. 841.
O'Brien, J.S.: Generalized gangliosidosis: A review. J. Pediatr. 75:167, 1969.
O'Brien, J.S et al: Generalized gangliosidosis; another inborn error of ganglioside metabolism? Am. J. Dis. Child. 109:338, 1965.
Okada, S. and O'Brien, J.S.: Generalized gangliosidosis: Beta-galactosidase deficiency. Science 160:1002, 1968.

Contributor: **John S. O'Brien**

Editor's Computerized Descriptors: Eye, Face, Oral, Nose, Skin, Skel., Spleen, Liver, Nerve

G$_{M1}$-GANGLIOSIDOSIS, TYPE 2

Includes: Gangliosidose-type II
G$_{M1}$ Gangliosidose, Typ II
Gangliosidosis G$_{M1}$ tipo 2
Late infantile systemic lipidosis
G$_{M1}$-gangliosidosis of late onset without bony deformities

Excludes: Neuronal ceroid-lipofuscinoses (713)
G$_{M1}$-gangliosidosis, type 1 (431)
Juvenile lipidosis
Other sphingolipidoses

Minimal Diagnostic Criteria: Clinical suspicion for this syndrome is raised by the finding of an infant who shows spasticity and ataxia late in the 1st year of life, with subsequent further deterioration. Support would be given by identification of marrow foam cells or neuronal lipidosis. Diagnosis depends on chemical studies - increased G$_{M1}$-ganglioside in brain and deficient β-galactosidase in tissues, leukocytes or urine.

Clinical Findings: Children with this diagnosis begin to show mental and motor retardation by 6-12 months of age, with progressive spasticity, ataxia, weakness and then rigidity, seizures and dementia. They expire by 3 to 10 years of age (rarely later). The fundi are generally normal and the viscera are not enlarged. Foam cells are often found in the marrow, but the bones are normal or mildly dysplastic by xray, as is the face. Vacuolated cells in the liver, spleen and glomeruli are notable in some of the patients and lipidosis of the central and autonomic nervous system neurones is general. As in the generalized gangliosidosis syndrome, G$_{M1}$-ganglioside accumulates in the brain and a keratan-sulfate-like polysaccharide in the liver. β-galactosidase activity is deficient in the brain, liver, leukocytes and cultured fibroblasts. Urinary mucopolysaccharide levels have varied, with occasional elevations.†

Complications
I Derived: The clinical problems are found as expected in a deteriorating cerebral condition, including in this instance special difficulties in the management of seizures.
II Associated: —

Etiology: Autosomal recessive inheritance. The basic defect is thought to be the β-galactosidase deficiency. Analysis of total enzyme, and its electrophoretic components, has not to date allowed any specific differentiation from the β-galactosidase deficiency of G$_{M1}$-gangliosidosis type 1. McK *23060

Pathogenesis: The enzyme deficiency presumably accounts for the neuronal handicap, which, in turn, lies behind the neurologic deterioration. The visceral changes are moderate but of the same basic origin.

Related Facts
I Sex Ratio: M1:F1
II Risk of Occurrence: ? Low
III Risk of Recurrence for
    Patient's Sib: 1 in 4 (25%) for each offspring to be affected
    Patient's Child: Homozygotes have all died in childhood.
IV Age of Detectability: The basic enzyme defect would be identifiable in cultured fetal cells from amniocentesis or in the infant at any time after birth.
V Prevalence: Low (about 20 patients identified to date), with no special predilection in any particular ethnic group.

Treatment
I Primary Prevention: Genetic counseling
II Secondary Prevention: —
III Other Therapy: Assistance to the family in the dilemma of a child with degenerative CNS disease.

Prognosis: Most patients die in early or middle childhood, but survival has been noted up to 20 years.

Detection of Carrier: β-galactosidase assay of the circulating leukocytes has been abnormal in the parents of involved children.

†Special Considerations: It is worthy of comment that children with this disease bear considerable resemblance to the clinical picture of so-called "late infantile amaurotic idiocy" (Jansky-Bielschowsky), although marrow foam cells are lacking and macular pigmentation is prominent in the latter condition. It is possible that some patients with G$_{M1}$-gangliosidosis, type 2, have been listed in earlier reports as examples of Jansky-Bielschowsky disease. The definitive examination obviously involves the enzyme assay.

References:
Derry, D.M. et al: Late infantile systemic lipidosis; major monosialogangliosidosis delineation of two types. Neurology (Minneap.) 18:340, 1968.
O'Brien, J.S.: Generalized gangliosidosis. In Standbury, J.B. et al (eds.): The Metabolic Basis of Inherited Disease, 4th Ed. New York:McGraw-Hill, 1978, p. 841.
O'Brien, J.S.: Generalized gangliosidosis. In Bergsma D. (ed.): Part IV. Skeletal Dysplasias. Birth Defects: Orig. Art. Ser., vol. V, no. 4. New York:The National Foundation- March of Dimes, 1969, p. 190.
Suzuki, K. et al: Morphological, histochemical and biochemical studies on a case of systemic late infantile lipidosis (generalized gangliosidosis). J. Neuropathol. Exp. Neurol. 27:15, 1968.
Wolfe, L.S. et al: GM1-gangliosidosis without chondrodystrophy or visceromegaly. Neurology (Minneap.) 20:23, 1970,

Contributor: **John S. O'Brien**

Editor's Computerized Descriptors: Muscle, Nerve

G$_{M2}$-GANGLIOSIDOSIS WITH HEXOSAMINIDASE A AND B DEFICIENCY

Includes: Gangliosidose G$_{M2}$ avec déficit en hexosaminidase A et B
G$_{M2}$ Gangliosidose mit Hexosaminidase-A und B Mangel
Gangliosidosis G$_{M2}$ con deficiencia de hexosaminidasa A y B
Sandhoff disease
Systemic G$_{M2}$-gangliosidosis

Excludes: G$_{M2}$-gangliosidosis with hexosaminidase A deficiency (434)

Minimal Diagnostic Criteria: Clinical findings below plus A and B deficiency of hexosaminidase activity in serum or tissues†

Clinical Findings: Psychomotor retardation evident by 6 months or perhaps earlier, with cherry-red macula, hepatosplenomegaly, nystagmus, and diffuse EEG abnormality. Later progression includes failure to attain milestones with appearance of seizures, myoclonic jerks, exaggerated startle response, and finally spastic tetraparesis, blindness, and loss of contact with environment, with death by 2-3 years.

Complications
I **Derived:** Relentlessly progressive and ultimately fatal disease usually terminating with bulbar incompetence and resulting pneumonitis.
II **Associated:** —

Etiology: Presumably autosomal recessive; McK *26880

Pathogenesis: Lack of A hexosaminidase enzyme activity resulting in failure of normal ganglioside catabolism and concomitant accumulation of G$_{M2}$-ganglioside (Tay-Sachs ganglioside) in brain as well as the sphingolipid globoside or aminoglycolipid, a normal constituent of visceral tissues. Both compounds have an amino sugar (hexosamine) as the terminal sugar.

Related Facts
I **Sex Ratio:** M?:F? Too few cases exist to estimate sex ratio
II **Risk of Occurrence:** ?
III **Risk of Recurrence for**
    Patient's Sib: If autosomal recessive 1 in 4 (25%) for each offspring to be affected
    Patient's Child: (Patients die early.)
IV **Age of Detectability:** Prenatally by amniocentesis or as early as clinically suspected
V **Prevalence:** —

Treatment
I **Primary Prevention:** Genetic counseling
II **Secondary Prevention:** ?
III **Other Therapy:** Supportive

Prognosis: Relentless progression to death

Detection of Carrier: Enzyme determination of serum, white blood cells, or skin fibroblasts

†**Special Considerations:** Where the clinical presentation contains features of classic Tay-Sachs disease, plus visceromegaly one must consider this variant.

References:
Sandhoff, K. et al: Deficient hexosaminidase activity in an exceptional case of Tay-Sachs disease with additional storage of kidney globoside in visceral organs. Pathol. Eur. 3:278, 1968.

Contributor: **Guy M. McKhann**

Editor's Computerized Descriptors: Vision, Eye, Spleen, Liver, Nerve

G$_{M2}$-GANGLIOSIDOSIS WITH HEXOSAMINIDASE A DEFICIENCY

Includes: Gangliosidose G$_{M2}$ avec déficit en hexosaminidase A
G$_{M2}$-Gangliosidose mit Hexosaminidase-A-Mangel
Gangliosidosis G$_{M2}$ con deficiencia de hexosaminidasa A
Tay-Sachs disease

Excludes: G$_{M2}$-Gangliosidosis with hexosaminidase A and B deficiency (433)
Ceroidlipofuscinoses
G$_{M1}$-gangliosidoses and leukodystrophies

Minimal Diagnostic Criteria: The clinical picture is quite distinctive and the appearance of psychomotor delay and a cherry-red spot strongly suggest a neuronal storage disease. The disease occurs primarily in Ashkenazi Jews. The disease can be established by finding a deficiency of hexosaminidase A in serum or tissues.†

Clinical Findings: The clinical picture is characterized by psychomotor retardation and deterioration, blindness, the appearance of a cherry-red spot in the macula and the persistence of exaggerated response to sounds. The psychomotor retardation is evident from 4-6 months of age when the child fails to develop normal milestones. In addition, the child is quite apathetic and unresponsive to a number of exogenous stimuli. It is rare for a case of Tay-Sachs disease to reach the stage of sitting without support or to crawl. There is hypotonia, and poor head control is often an early sign.

The blindness is noted toward the latter part of the 1st year in life and there is often a dissociation between the child's responses to auditory stimuli, which may be exaggerated, and his response to visual stimuli. The exaggerated response to sound may initially look like a Moro reflex but can be an exaggerated jerk of the arms and legs to any sound stimulus.

Seizures are a later manifestation which may be quite refractory to any convulsant medication. EEG abnormalities appear toward the end of the 1st year of life and will develop into paroxysmal discharges which decrease as the child reaches a more advanced form of the disease.

As the disease progresses the child reaches a vegetative state being quite hypotonic with exaggerated reflexes. The exaggerated response to sound diminishes and the child often develops megalencephaly. Death usually occurs by age 2 but a few children have lived to age 3 or 4.

Complications
I **Derived:** The disease is relentlessly progressive and ultimately fatal. Death is usually associated with aspiration pneumonia.
II **Associated:** —

Etiology: The basic defect in the disease is the failure of the degradation of G$_{M2}$-ganglioside. The enzymatic defect is the deficiency of hexosaminidase A. This defect is inherited as an autosomal recessive with a high gene frequency in Ashkenazi Jews. McK *27280

Pathogenesis: G$_{M2}$-gangliosidosis is a failure of the degradation of G$_{M2}$-ganglioside and a subsequent storage of this ganglioside in neurons throughout the body. The neurons become ballooned out and accumulate within them G$_{M2}$-gangliosides complexed with other lipids which are identifiable by electron microscopy as membranous cytoplasmic bodies. Some neurons, such as granular cells of the cerebellum, apparently cannot accumulate this particular lipid and degenerate quite early in the course of the disease.

There is no accumulation of ganglioside in other organs. However, the metabolic defect is present in other tissues.

The disease can be diagnosed in utero by demonstration of the enzymatic defect in amniotic cells as well as at birth from examination of serum or skin fibroblasts. In addition, the heterozygote can be determined by skin fibroblasts or other tissue.

Related Facts
I **Sex Ratio:** M1:F1
II **Risk of Occurrence:** For Ashkenazi Jewish families the incidence is 1 in 3600 live births. (The gene frequency in Ashkenazi families is 1 in 30. In Sephardic Jews the carrier rate is 1 in 250 and in non-Jews it is 1 in 300.)
III **Risk of Recurrence for**
    Patient's Sib: 1 in 4 (25%) for each offspring to be affected
    Patient's Child: The condition is lethal in early childhood.
IV **Age of Detectability:** By clinical grounds 4-6 months.
V **Prevalence:** Very low because of early death

Treatment
I **Primary Prevention:** Genetic counseling
II **Secondary Prevention:** There is no proven therapy at present
III **Other Therapy:** —

Prognosis: The disease is progressive and death occurs by 3-4 years of age.

Detection of Carrier: The heterozygote can be detected by enzymatic assay of serum or skin fibroblasts. Carriers usually have 40-60% of the activity of control patients.

†**Special Considerations:** There is confusion in the literature about later life forms of Tay-Sachs disease. It is our recommendation that Tay-Sachs disease be restricted to the G_{M2}-gangliosidosis in which the defect is deficiency of hexosaminidase A, and the clinical characteristics as described in this report.

References:
O'Brien, J.S. et al: Tay-Sachs disease. Detection of heterozygotes and homozygotes by serum hexosaminidase assay. N. Engl. J. Med. 283:15, 1970.
O'Brien, J.S.: Ganglioside-storage diseases. N. Engl. J. Med. 284:893, 1971.
O'Brien, J.S. et al: Tay-Sachs disease: Prenatal diagnosis. Science. 172:61, 1971.

Contributor: **Guy M. McKhann**

Editor's Computerized Descriptors: Eye, Muscle, Nerve, Vision
Also see Section I, Fig. 24

GOITER, GOITROGEN-INDUCED

Includes: Crétinisme acquis
  Chemisch induzierte Struma
  Bocio causado por bociógenos
  Congenital goiter
  Iodide goiter
  Propylthiouracil (PTU) goiter
  Goitrogen-induced goiter

Excludes: Thyroid dysgenesis (946)
  Goitrous cretinism
  Endemic goiter
  Congenital enzymatic goiter

Minimal Diagnostic Criteria: Goiter, history of maternal ingestion of PTU or iodides

Clinical Findings: Goiter, hypothyroidism may or may not occur, hyperbilirubinemia may occur with hypothyroidism, PBI high with iodide goiter and low with PTU goiter.

Complications
I **Derived:** Theoretically mental retardation can result but is seldom observed. Occasionally large goiters may produce respiratory distress and asphyxia due to tracheal compression.
II **Associated:** —

Etiology: Maternal ingestion of propylthiouracil or iodide in excess. Chronic intake of cough mixture containing K1 is a frequent source of iodide excess to fetus.

Pathogenesis: Fetal thyroid uptake of iodide transferred across the placenta starts at approximately the 12th week of gestation. Apparently excess iodide in the fetal thyroid inhibits synthesis and release of thyroid hormone; this in turn stimulates pituitary thyrotropic hormone and is followed by hypertrophy of the thyroid gland.

Related Facts
I **Sex Ratio:** M1:F1
II **Risk of Occurrence:** ?
III **Risk of Recurrence for**
    Patient's Sib: Not genetic
    Patient's Child: Not genetic
IV **Age of Detectability:** At birth
V **Prevalence:** ?

Treatment
I **Primary Prevention:** Administration of reduced amounts of goitrogen in pregnancy. Mothers who are taking antithyroid drugs or iodides, which are secreted in milk, should not nurse their babies.
II **Secondary Prevention:** Administration of thyroid hormone during pregnancy in large amounts which may cross the placenta and prevent the iatrogenic goiter. When goiter is present, desiccated thyroid-grain-1-per day should be given to infant until goiter regresses.
III **Other Therapy:** —

Prognosis: Good. Condition is not life-jeopardizing.

Detection of Carrier: Not applicable

Special Considerations: —

References:
Bernhard, W.G. et al: Congenital goiter: Report of a fatal case with postmortem findings. Arch. Pathol. 60:635, 1955.
Burrow, G.N.: Neonatal goiter after maternal propylthiouracil therapy. J. Clin. Endocrinol. 25:403, 1965.
Crawford, J.D.: Symposium on endocrinology; goiters in childhood. Pediatrics 17:437, 1956.
Murray, I.P., and Stewart, R.D.: Iodide goitre. Lancet 1:922, 1967.
Wolff, J.: Iodide goiter and the pharmocologic effects of excess iodide. Am. J. Med. 47:101, 1969.

GONADAL DYSGENESIS, XX TYPE

Includes: Dysgénésie ovarienne
Familiäre Ovarialdysgenesie
Disgenesia ovárica familiar
Familial ovarian dysgenesis
Ovarian dysgenesis, familial
XX form of pure gonadal dysgenesis
XX Gonadal dysgenesis

Excludes: Gonadal dysgenesis, XY type (437)
Turner syndrome (977)
Chromosome 45,X/46,XY mosaicism (173)

Minimal Diagnostic Criteria: Streak gonads in 46,XX individual with female external genitalia and normal müllerian development. Fibrous streaks should be demonstrated by laparoscopy or laparotomy or deduced on the basis of elevated gonadotropin levels. A monosomic (45,X) cell line should be excluded.

Clinical Findings: Individuals with gonadal dysgenesis may have an apparently normal female (46,XX) chromosomal complement with female external genitalia. Their external genitalia and their streak gonads are indistinguishable from individuals who have gonadal dysgenesis and a 45,X chromosomal complement. The endocrine features and the lack of secondary sexual development are similar to other individuals with streak gonads. Estrogen levels are decreased; FSH and LH levels are increased. Müllerian derivatives remain infantile yet well differentiated. Most individuals with XX gonadal dysgenesis are normal in stature. Only a few XX gonadal dysgenesis patients have features of the Turner stigmata, and in many of these undetected 45,X/46,XX mosaicism may be suspected.

The diagnosis is applied only to individuals whose gonads either consist of bilateral streak gonads or show endocrine evidence of ovarian failure (elevated FSH and LH levels). However, in at least 2 families one 46,XX sib had bilateral streak gonads, whereas another had primary amenorrhea and extreme ovarian hypoplasia with a few follicles. These observations suggest that oocytes may develop in some individuals who carry the abnormal allele.

Complications
I **Derived:** Hypogonadism; infertility
II **Associated:** Neurosensory deafness†

Etiology: An autosomal recessive gene. Among some 130 cases are 14 familial aggregates. In each aggregate, sibs were the only relatives affected, and in 3 families parents were consanguineous. McK *23330

Pathogenesis: No data have proved informative. 45,X cells are unlikely to be present yet undetected in available tissues, although monosomy limited to germ cells cannot be excluded.

Related Facts
I **Sex Ratio:** M0:F1
II **Risk of Occurrence:** ?
III **Risk of Recurrence for**
    Patient's Sib: 1 in 4 for 46,XX sibs; 1 in 8 for all sibs
    Patient's Child: All patients are infertile
IV **Age of Detectability:** At puberty because of primary amenorrhea
V **Prevalence:** ? but rare. Approximately 130 cases have been reported; however, the disorder occurs in about 20% of individuals with primary amenorrhea.

Treatment
I **Primary Prevention:** Genetic counseling
II **Secondary Prevention:** Treatment of hypogonadism by administration of estrogens. Assessment for auditory deficits.
III **Other Therapy:** —

Prognosis: Probably normal life span

Detection of Carrier: ?

†**Special Considerations:** In the 1st edition of this Compendium XX gonadal dysgenesis was divided into forms associated with a) normal or tall stature, and b) short stature. Recent analysis by this reviewer suggests no evidence for bimodality with respect to stature. On the other hand, in 4 families and in 2 sporadic cases individuals have had both XX gonadal dysgenesis and neurosensory deafness. Possible explanations for the coexistence of these anomalies include genetic heterogeneity or pleiotropy for the gene causing XX gonadal dysgenesis. In addition, in 3 other families, each apparently unique, 46,XX females with gonadal dysgenesis had a specific pattern of somatic abnormalities, none associated with the Turner stigmata; in each family the anomalies were different and in each an allele different from XX gonadal dysgenesis can be suspected (see Simpson, 1978).

References:
Boczkowski, K.: Pure gonadal dysgenesis and ovarian dysplasia in sisters. Am. J. Obstet. Gynecol. 106:626, 1970.
Inhorn, S.L. and Opitz, J.M.: Abnormalities of sex development. In Bloodworth, J.M.B. (ed.): Endocrine Pathology. Baltimore: Williams & Wilkins, 1968. p. 529.
Simpson, J.L.: Gonadal dysgenesis and sex chromosomal abnormalities: Phenotypic-karyotypic correlations. In Porter, I.H. (ed.): Genetic Mechanisms of Sex Determination. New York: Academic Press, 1978.
Simpson, J.L. et al: Gonadal dysgenesis in individuals with apparently normal chromosomal complements: Tabulation of cases and compilation of genetic data. In Bergsma, D (ed.): Part X, The Endocrine System. Birth Defects: Orig. Art. Ser. vol. VII, no. 6. Baltimore: Williams & Wilkins for The National Foundation-March of Dimes, 1971, p 215.
Simpson, J.L.: Disorders of Sexual Differentiation: Etiology and Clinical Delineation. New York: Academic Press, 1976.

Contributor: **Joe Leigh Simpson**

Editor's Computerized Descriptors: Hearing, GU.

GONADAL DYSGENESIS, XY TYPE

Includes: Syndrome de Swyer
Síndrome de Swyer
Swyer syndrome
Pure testicular dysgenesis
XY form of pure gonadal dysgenesis
XY Gonadal dysgenesis

Excludes: Chromosome 45,X/46,XY mosaicism (173)
Gonadal dysgenesis, XX type (436)
Turner syndrome (977)
Agonadia (29)
Androgen insensitivity syndrome, complete (49)

Minimal Diagnostic Criteria: Streak gonads in a 46,XY individual with female external genitalia and normal müllerian derivatives. The diagnosis may properly be applied to 46,XY individuals who have normal female external genitalia or minimal clitoral hypertrophy and either gonadoblastomas or dysgerminomas.

Clinical Findings: Individuals with a normal male (46,XY) chromosomal complement may show bilateral streak gonads, female external genitalia and müllerian derivatives (uterus and fallopian tubes). No somatic abnormalities are present. The streak gonads in these individuals are usually histologically indistinguishable from the gonads of individuals with a 45,X complement. As result of lack of gonadal development, these individuals do not menstruate, and fail to develop breasts or pubic and axillary hair. Their external genitalia are female, yet sexually infantile. The uterus and fallopian tubes are likewise small yet well differentiated. Estrogen and testosterone levels are decreased; gonadotropin levels are increased. In XY gonadal dysgenesis the streak gonads may undergo neoplastic transformation to dysgerminomas or gonadoblastomas. Approximately 20-30% of reported XY gonadal dysgenesis patients have such a tumor, which may or may not be associated with virilization or feminization.

Complications
I **Derived:** Effects of hypogonadism; infertility. Gonadal neoplasia is associated with 20-30% of individuals with XY gonadal dysgenesis. Feminization or masculinization may occur as result of these tumors.
II **Associated:** None. If features of the Turner stigmata are present, undetected monosomic (45,X) cells should be suspected.

Etiology: XY gonadal dysgenesis results from an X-linked recessive or male-limited autosomal dominant gene. There are at least 15 familial aggregates. These include 1 set of concordantly affected monozygotic twins, 11 families with multiple affected sibs of nonconsanguineous parents, 1 family compatible with several modes of inheritance, and 3 families in which the trait segregated in the manner expected of an X-linked recessive or male-limited autosomal dominant gene.†

Pathogenesis: Extensive investigations indicate that 45,X cells are unlikely to be present; however, monosomy limited to germ cells cannot be excluded. Suppression of H-Y antigen is an attractive hypothesis.

Related Facts
I **Sex Ratio:** M1:F0
II **Risk of Occurrence:** ?
III **Risk of Recurrence for**
   Patient's Sib: 1 in 2 for 46,XY sibs; 1 in 4 for all sibs. Other 46,XY individuals in the maternal kindred may be at risk, eg 1st cousins and uncles.
   Patient's Child: All patients are infertile.
IV **Age of Detectability:** Usually at puberty because of primary amenorrhea. A few patients may be detected before puberty

if other relatives are affected or if gonadoblastomas or dysgerminomas produce feminization, virilization or pelvic pain.

V Prevalence: ? About 130 cases have been reported.

Treatment

I Primary Prevention: Genetic counseling

II Secondary Prevention: Treatment of hypogonadism by administration of estrogen; removal of gonadal streaks to prevent neoplastic transformation. Following diagnosis, gonadal extirpation should be performed without delay.

III Other Therapy: —

Prognosis: Probably normal life span, although gonadal streaks could undergo malignant transformation. Infertility.

Detection of Carrier: No information

†Special Considerations: In at least 3 other families at least one 46,XY sib had XY gonadal dysgenesis, whereas another sib had genital ambiguity, bilateral testes and müllerian derivatives (uterus and fallopian tubes). Possible explanations include 1) undetected 45,X cells in several family members (familial mosaicism), thus explaining the presence of a uterus (see 45,X/46,XY mosaicism), 2) the gene controlling XY gonadal dysgenesis is capable of varied expressivity, or 3) a gene different from that producing XY gonadal dysgenesis is capable of varied expressivity.

References:

Espiner, E.A. et al: Familial syndrome of streak gonads and normal male karyotype in five phenotypic females. N. Engl. J. Med. 283:6, 1970.

Scully, R.E.: Gonadoblastoma. A review of 74 cases. Cancer 25:1340, 1970.

Simpson, J.L. et al: Gonadal dysgenesis in individuals with apparently normal chromosomal complements: Tabulation of cases and compilation of genetic data. Part X. The Endocrine System. Birth Defects: Orig. Art. Ser. vol. VII, no. 6 . Baltimore: Williams & Wilkins for The National Foundation-March of Dimes, 1971, p. 215.

Simpson, J.L.: Disorders of Sexual Differentiation: Etiology and Clinical Delineation. New York: Academic Press, 1976.

Simpson, J.L.: Gonadal dysgenesis and sex chromosome abnormalities: Phenotypic-karyotypic correlations. In Porter, I.H. (ed.): Genetic Mechanisms of Sex Determination. New York:Academic Press, 1978.

Contributor: **Joe Leigh Simpson**

Editor's Computerized Descriptors: Hair, GU.

GONADOTROPIN DEFICIENCY, ISOLATED

Includes: Déficit isolé en gonadotropine
Isolierter Gonadotropin-Mangel
Deficiencia aislada de gonadotropina
Fertile eunuch syndrome
Isolated LH deficiency
Isolated FSH deficiency

Excludes: Panhypopituitary dwarfism, familial
Kallmann syndrome

Minimal Diagnostic Criteria: Deficiency of FSH or LH associated with otherwise normal pituitary function.

Clinical Findings: In the isolated gonadotropin deficiency (IGD) syndrome, the absence of pituitary gonadotropins results in failure of normal sexual maturation, infertility, and complete lack of secondary sexual characteristics in both sexes. Specifically, males have small testes which may be cryptorchid, prepubertal genitalia with an unrugated scrotum and small penis, absent beard, scant axillary and pubic hair with a female escutcheon, high voice and eunuchoid habitus. Females share the habitus, reduced axillary and pubic hair and also manifest primary amenorrhea, infantile uterus and ovaries, and lack of breast development. Most patients with IGD have low circulating levels of follicle stimulating hormone (FSH) and lutenizing hormone (LH) and do not show a gonadotropin response to clomiphene citrate ingestion or lutenizing hormone releasing factor (LRF) infusion. (Some patients do, however, exhibit an LRF response).

A few patients with otherwise typical IGD have low LH levels but normal spermatogenesis and FSH levels. These patients have been termed fertile eunuchs and appear to have an isolated deficiency of LH. At least some may have a diminished FSH response to clomiphene citrate; this has been interpreted as a "reduced FSH reserve." Hence, many authors feel that the fertile eunuch is only a clinical variant of the IGD syndrome. In addition, at least 1 female has been described with primary amenorrhea, poor sexual development, low FSH, but high LH. It is not clear if this represents a separate syndrome of isolated FSH deficiency or is a clinical variant of the IGD syndrome.

Complications

I Derived: See Clinical Findings

II Associated: —

Etiology: The vast majority of cases are sporadic, but autosomal recessive inheritance is recognized. Also, X-linked recessive or sex-limited autosomal dominant inheritance has been described in 1 family. McK *22720

Pathogenesis: Most cases probably represent a hypothalamic defect in LRF release, but pituitary defects have also been postulated. The pathogenesis is likely heterogeneous.

Related Facts

I Sex Ratio: M1:F1 (except in 1 family where only males were affected).

II Risk of Occurrence: Very low

III Risk of Recurrence for
    Patient's Sib: Generally very low, but may be as high as 25%
    Patient's Child: Negligible

IV Age of Detectability: Usually during mid-adolescence when anticipated puberty fails to occur.†

V Prevalence: Very low

Treatment

I Primary Prevention: Genetic counseling

II Secondary Prevention: Replacement of secondarily deficient hormones, ie testosterone, estrogen, will result in development of secondary sexual characteristics. Treatment with a combination of human menopausal gonadotropins (HMG) and human chorionic gonadotropins (HCG) will also produce secondary sexual development and often fertility as well.

III Other Therapy: —

Prognosis: Appropriate treatment results in relatively normal life.

Detection of Carrier: —

†**Special Considerations:** During adolescence it may be difficult to differentiate IGD from constitutional delay. Administration of LRF will often help to distinguish these 2 disorders since patients with constitutional delay usually show some rise in gonadotropins, whereas those with IGD usually do not.

References:
Rabinowitz, D. and Spitz, I.M.: Isolated gonadotropin deficiency and related disorders. Isr. J. Med. Sci. 11:1011, 1975.
Rimoin, D.L. and Schimke, R.N.: Genetic Disorders of the Endocrine Gland. St. Louis: C.V. Mosby, 1971, p. 11.
Spitz, I.M. et al: Isolated gonadotropin deficiency, a heterogeneous syndrome. N. Engl. J. Med. 290:10, 1974.

Contributors: **William A. Horton**
David L. Rimoin

Editor's Computerized Descriptors: Speech, Hair, GU.

GONIODYSGENESIS

Includes: Goniodisgenesis
Iridocorneal mesodermal dysgenesis
Mesoectodermal dysgenesis of iris and cornea
Rieger syndrome
Posterior embryotoxon
Mesoectodermal dysgenesis of anterior segment
Axenfeld anomaly
Dysgenesis mesostromal
Hypodontia-mesoectodermal dysgenesis of iris and cornea
Posterior marginal dysplasia of cornea
Anterior chamber cleavage syndrome
Peter anomaly
Congenital anterior staphyloma
Iridogoniodysgenesis

Excludes: Essential iris atrophy
Polycoria
Glaucoma, congenital (414)

Minimal Diagnostic Criteria: The least severe form is merely the presence of posterior embryotoxon.

Clinical Findings: This congenital defect represents a mesodermal dysplasia of the anterior ocular segment. It may present as any one of several forms depending upon the severity of the dysplasia; hence the confusion of the appropriate term to apply. Goniodysgenesis is suggested as the most useful term.

Posterior embryotoxon is the mildest form in which there is an unusual prominence and forward displacement of the Schwalbe line, which stands out like an encircling glass rod inside the limbus. This can easily be seen by external inspection or slit-lamp examination and it is estimated to be present to some degree in 15% of individuals. When dense bands of iris tissue extend and attach to this posterior embryotoxon, it is referred to as the Axenfeld anomaly.

Rieger anomaly is the term used when there is hypoplasia of the iris stroma with adhesions of stroma to the posterior embryotoxon. Rieger syndrome is the term used when the findings of Rieger anomaly are associated with other defects such as missing or cone-shaped teeth and hypoplasia of the maxilla. Complications such as glaucoma and cataracts are more common with this more severe form of goniodysgenesis.

Peter anomaly is the term most frequently used when the mesodermal dysgenesis of the anterior ocular segment includes a central corneal stromal opacity with a defect in the posterior stroma and the Descemet membrane.

Congenital anterior staphyloma is a severe degree of the entity in which there is disorganization of the anterior chamber with a staphylomatous opaque cornea. These eyes usually have severe glaucoma and eventually become phthisical.

Complications
I **Derived:** Glaucoma, cataracts, subluxated or dislocated lenses, opacification of cornea, phthisis bulbi.
II **Associated:** Dental anomalies in Rieger syndrome, myotonic dystrophy, mental retardation and myopathies have been reported.

Etiology: Autosomal dominant in many cases with extreme variability in its expression. One member of a family may have a severe form whereas only minimal signs will be present in another family member. Some cases are associated with chromosomal aberrations, eg deletion of the short arm of 4 and syndrome 18q. McK *18050

Pathogenesis: Presumed to be a developmental aberration of the mesodermal and possibly ectodermal germ layers of the anterior ocular segment.

Related Facts
I **Sex Ratio:** M1:F1
II **Risk of Occurrence:** ? Rare
III **Risk of Recurrence for**
Patient's Sib: <1 in 2 (<50%) for each offspring to be affected in the autosomal dominant cases
Patient's Child: <1 in 2
IV **Age of Detectability:** At birth
V **Prevalence:** ? Rare

Treatment
I **Primary Prevention:** Genetic counseling when autosomal dominant
II **Secondary Prevention:** Control of glaucoma, cataract extraction, corneal transplant, enucleation to relieve pain or cosmesis.
III **Other Therapy:** —

Prognosis: Normal for life span and intelligence; poor for vision

Detection of Carrier: —

Special Considerations: —

References:
Alkemade, P.P.H.: Dysgenesis Mesodermalis of the Iris and Cornea. Springfield: Charles C Thomas, 1969, p. 95.
François, J.: Affections of the cornea. In Heredity in Ophthalmology. St. Louis: C.V. Mosby, 1961, p. 290.
Henkind, P. et al: Mesodermal dysgenesis of the anterior segment: Rieger's anomaly. Arch. Ophthalmol. 73:810, 1965.
Ing, M.R.: Bilateral anterior staphylomata. J. Pediatr. Ophthalmol. 4:22, 1967.
Mills, D.W.: Mesodermal dysgenesis of the anterior segment of the eye. Can. J. Opthalmol. 2:279, 1967.
Nakanasighi, I. and Brown, S.: The histopathology and ultrastructure of congenital central corneal opacity (Peter's anomaly). Am. J. Ophthalmol. 72:801, 1971.
Reese, A.B. and Ellsworth, R.M.: The anterior chamber cleavage syndrome. Arch. Ophthalmol. 75:307, 1966.
Waring, G.O. et al: Anterior chamber cleavage syndrome. A stepladder classification. Surv. Ophthalmol. 20:3, 1975.

Contributor: **Morton E. Smith**

Editor's Computerized Descriptors: Eye, Face, Teeth

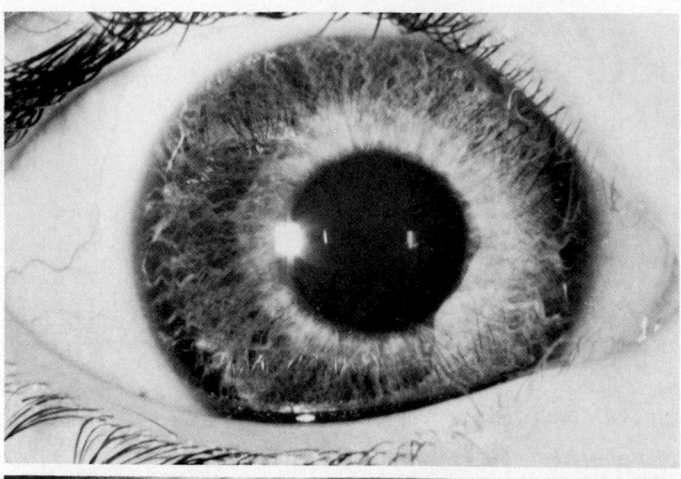

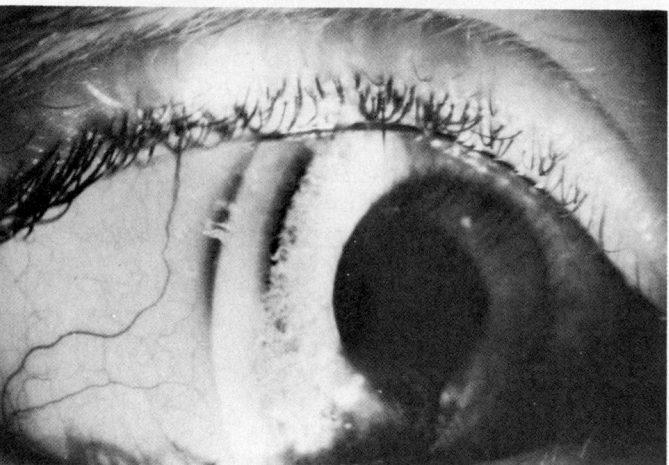

277. Slit-lamp examination of cornea demonstrates hypoplasia of anterior stromal leaf of cornea, trabecular iris adhesions, anterior displacement, and thickening of Schwalbe ring

GORLIN-CHAUDHRY-MOSS SYNDROME

Includes: Syndrome de Gorlin-Chaudhry-Moss
Síndrome de Gorlin-Chaudhry-Moss

Excludes: —

Minimal Diagnostic Criteria: Only 2 known cases as described below.

Clinical Findings: The only 2 known cases are sisters issuing from a nonconsanguineous marriage. Both had mild growth and mental retardation, midfacial flattening, painful ulceration of the skin near the metatarsal arch, hypertrichosis, umbilical hernia, mild microphthalmia, hypodontia, patent ductus arteriosus and hypoplasia of the labia majora. Both girls were brachycephalic due to premature closure of the coronal sutures.

Complications
I   **Derived:** —
II **Associated:** —

Etiology: Possibly autosomal recessive

Pathogenesis: ?

Related Facts
I   **Sex Ratio:** M?:F?
II   **Risk of Occurrence:** ?
III **Risk of Recurrence for**
     Patient's Sib: If autosomal recessive, 1 in 4 (25%) for each sib
     Patient's Child: Not increased unless mate is heterozygote or homozygote.
IV **Age of Detectability:** At birth
V   **Prevalence:** ?

Treatment
I   **Primary Prevention:** Genetic counseling
II **Secondary Prevention:** ?
III **Other Therapy:** ?

Prognosis: For life: ? For intelligence: mild deficit probable. For function: ?

Detection of Carrier: —

Special Considerations: —

References:
Gorlin, R.J. et al: Craniofacial dysostosis, patent ductus arteriosus, hypertrichosis, hypoplasia of labia majora, dental and eye anomalies-a new syndrome? J.Pediatr. 56:778, 1960.

Contributor: **Robert J. Gorlin**

Editor's Computerized Descriptors: Eye, Face, Teeth, Skin, Hair, Skel., Hernia not CNS, CV., GU., Nerve

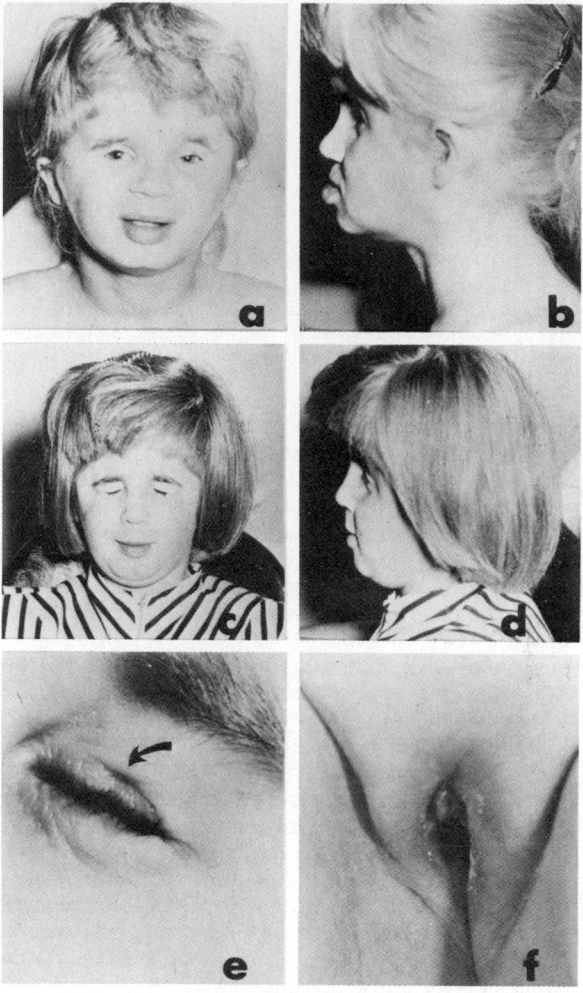

278. A & B) Note pronounced maxillary hypoplasia and low-set frontal hairline; C & D) milder maxillary hypoplasia, antimongoloid obliquity and hypertrichosis; E) notched defect of upper eyelid; F) hypoplastic labia majora with gaping fourchette

Includes: Goutte
Gicht
Gota
Primary familial hyperuricemia
Partial deficiencies of hypoxanthine guanine phosphoribosyl transferase
Hyperuricemia, primary

Excludes: Secondary hyperuricemia

Minimal Diagnostic Criteria: Uric acid concentrations in plasma of patients with gout are over 6 mg/100ml. However, a certain number of normal individuals have concentrations as high as 7 mg/100 ml. In the absence of impaired renal function, patients with gout seldom have concentrations higher than 8 to 12 mg/100 ml. These values reflect the concentrations of supersaturated solutions of sodium urate in plasma.

Clinical Findings: Primary gout refers to a heterogeneous group of conditions for which the diagnostic hallmark is hyperuricemia. With time, hyperuricemic individuals develop recurrent attacks of acute arthritis. Hematuria, crystalluria, urinary tract stones and progressive nephropathy also occur regularly. Urate is deposited in tophi in soft tissues, especially around the joints and in cartilage. Chronic gout leads to deformities of the limbs and destruction of bone.

Some patients with gout have an increased rate of uric acid synthesis. This usually is true of patients presenting with clinical manifestations of hyperuricemia in childhood as well as of a certain proportion of adults with gout. A large number of adults appear to have hyperuricemia on the basis of diminished renal elimination of uric acid. Among those with increased rates of purine synthesis, some have been shown to have partial deficiencies of the enzyme hypoxanthine guanine phosphoribosyl transferase, which is completely deficient in the Lesch-Nyhan syndrome. Initial distinction among these conditions can be made by quantitating the excretion of uric acid in the urine. Another subgroup of patients with overproduction of purine de novo has been shown to have an abnormality in the enzyme phosphoribosyl pyrophosphate (PRPP) synthetase. This is an interesting disorder in that the patients have more activity than normal. An adult with overproduction gout generally excretes over 600 mg per day.

Complications
I   **Derived:**   cf Clinical Findings; renal failure
II   **Associated:**   Obesity, hypertensive cardiovascular disease, diabetes.

Etiology: Gout is clearly multifactorial and probably polygenic. In a small number of patients there is a single gene defect and the primary site of gene action is in the activity of the enzyme hypoxanthine guanine phosphoribosyl transferase or in that of PRPP synthetase. In either case there is increased synthesis of uric acid. There are other patients with increased rates of uric acid synthesis in whom the site of the defect has not been established. In others with gout it is apparent that the transport of urate in the renal tubule is abnormal. Genetic control of uric acid concentrations in normal individuals is almost certainly polygenic and these influences are present in hyperuricemias as well. It seems likely that a number of the diseases we know as gout will ultimately be found to be determined by single gene defects. Some of these may be transmitted as autosomal dominants, and some as autosomal recessives. Hypoxanthine guanine phosphoribosyl transferase activity

is determined by genes on the X chromosome; deficiency of this enzyme is transmitted as an X-linked recessive character. McK *30800

Pathogenesis: cf Etiology. Most of the clinical manifestations of gout can be readily correlated with the occurrence of supersaturated solutions of urate in body fluids and consequent precipitation in tissues. The acute inflammatory reaction in the joint has been correlated with the physicochemical characteristics of the crystal encountered there, a needle-like crystal which is engulfed by leukocytes in the inflammatory process.

Related Facts
I   **Sex Ratio:**   M95:F5 in large series. The hypoxanthine guanine phosphoribosyl transferase deficiency disease has not been seen in the female.
II   **Risk of Occurrence:**   ? cf V Prevalence
III **Risk of Recurrence for**
     Patient's Sib: Hyperuricemia has been found in 25-72% of relatives of gouty patients. With hypoxanthine guanine phosphoribosyl transferase deficiency, (HGPTD), see Table I X-linked R; without HGPTD see Table I AR.
     Patient's Child: With HGPTD see Table I X-linked R; without HGPTD see Table I AR.
IV   **Age of Detectability:**   The time of onset of hyperuricemia in individuals ultimately having clinical gout is quite variable. Clinical manifestations are rare before the menopause in the female.
V   **Prevalence:**   1 in 500 to 1 in 330 in the United States and Europe. Higher among inhabitants of the Philippine and Marianas Islands. In the Maori of New Zealand, 1 in 12 men.

Treatment
I   **Primary Prevention:**   Genetic counseling
II   **Secondary Prevention:**   Hyperuricemia can be controlled in many patients using uricosuric agents, such as probenecid, salicylates or sulfinpyrazone. Allopurinol, the xanthine oxidase inhibitor, hydroxypyrazolo (3,4-D) pyrimidine is more uniformly effective even in patients otherwise difficult to control. It is the drug of choice in patients excreting large amounts of urate and may be the drug of choice in patients needing treatment for hyperuricemia. Control of hyperuricemia in this way will prevent nephropathy and stones, and prevent or resolve tophi. The number of attacks of acute arthritis in treated patients appears to be decreasing.
III **Other Therapy:**   Colchicine is the drug of choice in the treatment of acute gouty arthritis. Phenylbutazone, indomethacin and adrenal steroids are also effective.

Prognosis: Progressive nephropathy may be lethal. Early prevention of nephropathy should lead to a normal life span.

Detection of Carrier: —

Special Considerations: —

References:
Becker, M.A. et al: Gout with purine overproduction due to increased phosphoribosyl pyrophosphate synthetase activity. Am. J. Med. 55:232, 1973.
Gutman, A. B. (ed.): Proceedings of Conference on Gout and Purine Metabolism. Arthritis Rheum. 8:591, 1965.
Kelley, W.N. et al: A specific enzyme defect in gout associated with overproduction of uric acid. Proc. Natl. Acad. Sci. USA 57:1735, 1967.
Wyngaarden, J.B.: Gout. In Stanbury, J.B. et al (eds.): The Metabolic Basis of Inherited Disease. New York:McGraw-Hill, 1972, p. 889.

Contributor: **William L. Nyhan**

Editor's Computerized Descriptors: Skel., GU.

GRANULOMATOUS DISEASE OF FEMALES, CHRONIC

Includes: Maladie granulomatéine chronique observée chez les femmes
Chronische Granulomatose beim weiblichen Geschlecht
Granulomatosis crónica de las mujeres
Fatal granulomatous disease of females
Lipochrome histiocytosis of females

Excludes: Granulomatous disease of males, chronic (443)
Job syndrome†

Minimal Diagnostic Criteria: In both females and males in vitro demonstration of intracellular bactericidal deficiency when neutrophils are challenged with *Staphylococcus aureus* and inability of latex-stimulated neutrophils to reduce tetrazolium salts. Bactericidal capacity for *Streptococcus fecalis* is normal.

Clinical Findings: The clinical, radiologic and histopathologic features of chronic granulomatous disease (CGD) of females cannot be distinguished from the classic disease in males. Similarly, immunoglobulin levels are often elevated but other immunologic analysis is normal.

Lipochrome histiocytosis, described in 3 sisters, differs from CGD in that arthritis is a feature and granulomas are not present. All have survived into adult life. The susceptibility to bacterial infection is identical.

Complications
I **Derived:** Disability and eventual death result from uncontrolled infections.
II **Associated:** —

Etiology: Lipochrome histiocytosis is familial with no known molecular abnormality. CGD of females is presumed to be autosomal recessive. A deficiency of leukocyte glutathione peroxidase has been reported in several female children with CGD. An affected brother of one of them has been found to have glutathione peroxidase deficiency.†

Pathogenesis: Engulfment of bacteria is normal but catalase-positive bacteria including many of low pathogenicity are not killed. Persisting viable intracellular bacteria are protected from antibiotics which may lead to disseminated chronic infection with granuloma formation.

Related Facts
I **Sex Ratio:** ? At least one family known with an affected sister and brother.
II **Risk of Occurrence:** ? About 15% of known cases of CGD are girls.
III **Risk of Recurrence for**
Patient's Sib: 1 in 4 (25%) if autosomal recessive.
Patient's Child: If autosomal recessive, not increased unless mate is carrier or homozygote.
IV **Age of Detectability:** Earliest age not established
V **Prevalence:** Rare

Treatment
I **Primary Prevention:** Genetic counseling
II **Secondary Prevention:** Prompt recognition of new infections and intensive prolonged therapy with appropriate antibiotics and surgical drainage as required. Regular pulmonary therapy helps lessen pulmonary complications.
III **Other Therapy:** Use of continuous antibiotic therapy is debated.

Prognosis: The disease has been uniformly fatal in the past with an average life span of 7-8 years with CGD and 35 years with lipochrome histiocytosis.

Detection of Carrier: Undetectable by the standard tests. In one female with CGD, both parents had intermediate glutathione peroxidase values. In another family, the parents had normal values.

†Special Considerations: Job syndrome is clinically distinct with recurrent cold staphylococcal abscesses and severe atopic dermatitis. Hyperimmunoglobulinemia E and defective neutrophil chemotaxis have been described but the leukocyte defects typical of CGD are absent.

CGD females who have been tested are not lacking neutrophil Kx antigen.

References:
Azimi, P. et al: Chronic granulomatous disease in three female siblings. JAMA 206:2865, 1968.
Holmes, B. et al: Chronic granulomatous disease in females. N. Engl. J. Med. 283:217, 1970.
Malawista, S.E. and Gifford, R.H.: Chronic granulomatous disease of childhood (CGD) with leukocyte glutathione peroxidase (LGP) deficiency in a brother and sister: A likely autosomal recessive inheritance. Clin. Res. 23:416A, 1975.
Marsh, W.L. et al: Chronic granulomatous disease and the Kell blood groups. Br. J. Haematol. 29:247, 1975.
Quie, P. G. et al: Defective polymorphonuclear-leukocyte function and chronic granulomatous disease in two female children. N. Engl. J. Med. 278:967, 1968.
Rodey, G. E. et al: Leukocyte function in lipochrome histiocytosis. Am. J. Med. 49:322, 1970.
White, L. R. et al: Leukocytes in Job's syndrome. Lancet 1:630, 1969.

Contributor: **Elizabeth M. Smithwick**

Editor's Computerized Descriptors: Skin, Spleen, GU. Eye, Oral, Nasoph., Skel., CV., Lymphatic, Liver, Resp., GI.

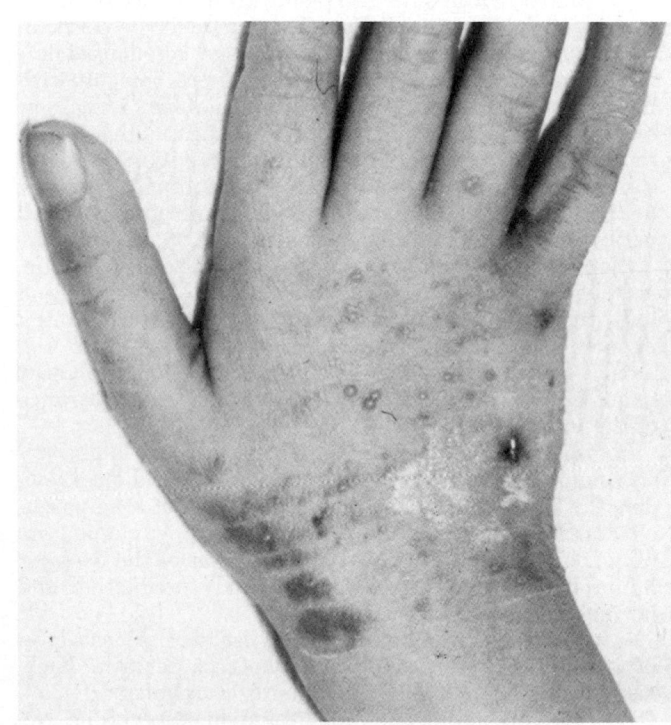

279. Hand lesions in chronic granulomatous disease

GRANULOMATOUS DISEASE OF MALES, CHRONIC

Includes: Maladie granulomateuse chronique atteignant les garçons
Chronische Granulomatose beim männlichen Geschlecht
Enfermedad granulomatosa crónica del varón
Fatal granulomatous disease of males
Chronic granulomatous disease of childhood
Chronic familial granulomatosis
Progressive septic granulomatous disease
Congenital dysphagocytosis
Pigmented lipid histiocytosis

Excludes: Granulomatous disease of females, chronic (442)
Specific granulomatous disease (acid-fast, mycotic etc)
Chédiak-Higashi syndrome (143)
Job syndrome

Minimal Diagnostic Criteria: Male sex. Neutrophils capable in vitro of ingesting organisms but selectively fail to kill catalase-positive bacteria, eg staphylococci; catalase-negative bacteria, eg streptococci are killed normally. Demonstration of an associated defect in leukocyte oxidative metabolism, eg inability of latex-stimulated neutrophils to reduce colorless tetrazolium salts to a blue color.

Clinical Findings: This disease is characterized clinically by recurrent, severe suppurative infections, usually with low-grade pathogens, and histopathologically by granuloma formation.

Onset of disease typically occurs in early infancy. Common clinical features, in decreasing order of incidence, include: marked lymphadenopathy, particularly cervical, and often requiring incision and drainage; eczematoid dermatitis; destructive pulmonary disease; hepatomegaly with liver abscesses; splenomegaly; unexplained fever; osteomyelitis which frequently involves the small bones of the hands and feet; rhinitis and conjunctivitis; ulcerative stomatitis; persistent diarrhea, on occasion with steatorrhea and vitamin B_{12} malabsorption; perianal abscesses; and pericarditis. Healing progresses slowly.

Biopsy and autopsy material demonstrate characteristic, although nonspecific, granulomas at sites of infection and infiltration of visceral organs with histiocytes containing pigmented lipid material. This chromolipoid "ceroid" pigment, presumed to be a secondary phenomenon, is present in quantities sufficient to cause a yellow-brown appearance of the unstained tissue.†

Common laboratory findings are neutrophilic leukocytosis, anemia, elevated sedimentation rate and radiologic evidence of pulmonary disease, eg infiltration of lung parenchyma, hilar adenopathy, encapsulated pneumonia. Immunologic studies usually show elevation of the 3 major immunoglobulins with normal antibody production and normal cell-mediated immunity.

Infectious agents most frequently isolated are catalase-positive bacteria, including Staphylococci, Serratia, Klebsiella-Aerobacter, Pseudomonas, enteric organisms (E. coli, Proteus, Salmonella), and fungi (Candida, Aspergillus, Nocardia).

Complications
I **Derived:** Severe infections leading to disabling sequelae and a decreased life span.
II **Associated:** Potential transfusion hazard in patients with the McLeod or K_0 phenotype. Transfusions will result in antibody formation to Kell antigens present on red cells of virtually all blood donors.†

Etiology: In the predominant form, almost certainly X-linked recessive; mothers and sisters can be identified as carriers. Autosomal recessive transmission is suggested when the disease occurs in sibs of both sexes, or when the carrier state cannot be identified in the family of an affected male. Some of the latter may be due to a new somatic mutation of the X chromosome.

Pathogenesis: Neutrophils and monocytes ingest bacteria and fungi but cannot kill certain organisms effectively. Following particle ingestion, leukocytes manifest many abnormalities of oxidative metabolism, including defective generation of hydrogen peroxide and superoxide radicals which appear critical for bactericidal activity. Bacteria producing hydrogen peroxide are killed almost normally. Prolonged retention of material resulting from defective intracellular kill and digestion leads to granuloma formation. The basic underlying defect is debated and may indeed be different in various forms of the disease.†

Related Facts
I **Sex Ratio:** M1:F0 in X-linked recessive.
II **Risk of Occurrence:** Estimated at 1 in 1,000,000 to 1 in 100,000 live births
III **Risk of Recurrence for**
  Patient's Sib: If mother is a carrier, 1 in 2 (50%) for each brother to be affected and 1 in 2 for each sister to be a carrier.
  Patient's Child: Patients usually die very early. (Theoretically, 1 in 1 (100%) for carrier daughters; not increased for sons unless wife is a carrier.)
IV **Age of Detectability:** Affected males have been detected as early as 2 days of age.
V **Prevalence:** High lethality in childhood, therefore extremely rare in the general population.

Treatment
I **Primary Prevention:** Genetic counseling
II **Secondary Prevention:** Prompt recognition of infection with identification of organism and aggressive prolonged therapy with appropriate antibiotics; surgical drainage as necessary. Attention to regular pulmonary therapy helps to lessen pulmonary complications.
III **Other Therapy:** Use of continuous antibiotic therapy is debated.

Prognosis: In its classic form, the disease has been uniformly fatal and as many as one-third of the children die before 7 years of age. Life span ranges from several months to young adulthood; the oldest survivor is not known. The disease has generally been more severe in males than in females but greater clinical variability is now recognized.

Detection of Carrier: The majority of obligate heterozygote carriers of X-linked disease have been identified on the basis of an intermediate defect in neutrophil bactericidal ability and reduction of NBT. The defect has been shown in carriers tested as early as 4 years of age. However, there are limitations in the identification of all potential carriers, both in the classic X-linked form with early onset and in those families where the diagnosis is made later. Efforts to detect heterozygote carriers among family members of older affected males have often been unsuccessful with currently available tests.†

†Special Considerations: Lipochrome histiocytosis is not restricted to this disease. Ceroid is also found in Niemann-Pick disease, Gaucher disease, Wolman disease and various xanthomatous lesions.

Some boys with X-linked disease have the very rare McLeod red cell phenotype. The antigen Kx, related to the Kell blood group system and present on neutrophils and monocytes of normals, has been found to be lacking on leukocytes from males with X-linked disease. This membrane abnormality may be related to the impaired bactericidal activity.

It has been reported that leukocytes from affected males have an abnormality of NADH oxidase, of NADPH oxidase and of G6PD; the exact defect remains to be confirmed.

Patients have been described with low to undetectable G6PD in their leukocytes and a functional defect almost identical to chronic granulomatous disease.

Carriers are not unusually susceptible to infection but a lupus-like illness has been described in several carrier mothers.

References:
Baehner, R.L.: The growth and development of our understanding of chronic granulomatous disease. In Bellanti, J.A. and Dayton, D.H. (eds.): The Phagocytic Cell in Host Resistance. New York:Raven Press, 1975, p. 173.
Baehner, R.L. and Nathan, D.G.: Quantitative nitroblue tetrazolium test in chronic granulomatous disease. N. Engl. J. Med. 278:971, 1968.
Johnston, R.B. and Baehner, R.L.: Chronic granulomatous disease: Correlation between pathogenesis and clinical findings. Pediatrics 48:730, 1971.
Landing, B. H. and Shirkey, H. S.: A syndrome of recurrent infection and infiltration of viscera by pigmented lipid histiocytes. Pediatrics 20:431, 1957.
Marsh, W.L. et al: Antigens of the Kell blood group system on neutrophils and monocytes: Their relation to chronic granulomatous disease. J. Pediatr. 87:1117, 1975.
Repine, J.E. et al: Spectrum of function of neutrophils from carriers of sex-linked chronic granulomatous disease. J. Pediatr. 87:901, 1975.

Contributor: **Elizabeth M. Smithwick**

Editor's Computerized Descriptors: Eye, Oral, Nasoph., Skin, Skel., Resp., Lymphatic, Liver, GU. CV., Spleen, GI.

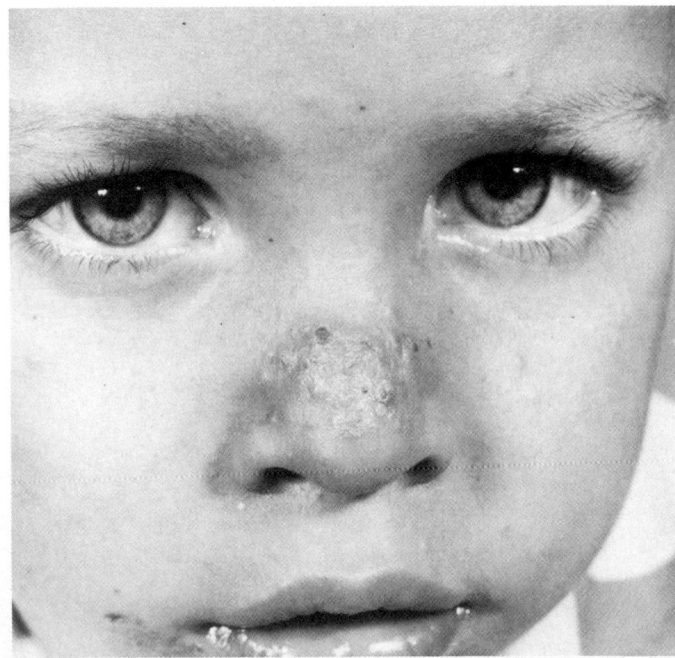

280. Pustular miliaria in chronic granulomatous disease

GRANULOSIS RUBRA NASI

Includes: Nose, red skin and papules on

Excludes: Rosacea
Lupus vulgaris
Lupus erythematosus

Minimal Diagnostic Criteria: Excess sweating and redness of nose

Clinical Findings: Marked sweating confined to the nose, occasionally surrounding areas of the face also involved, redness of the nose with papules, rarely numerous small vesicles. There are no reports of associated palmar or solar hyperhidrosis, or of associated excessive perspiration elsewhere on the body. No unique laboratory or roentgenographic findings. The histologic changes consist of hyperemia of the superficial cutis, perivascular infiltrates of neutrophilic leukocytes, plasma cells and histiocytes. There is no evidence of destruction of sweat glands or their ducts; however, varying degrees of ductal dilatation is observed.

Complications
I   Derived: —
II Associated: —

Etiology: Autosomal dominant

Pathogenesis: ? It is felt this entity represents a vasomotor disorder. (Local sepsis, eg tuberculosis, and chemical contact allergies have been considered.)

Related Facts
I   Sex Ratio: ?
II   Risk of Occurrence: ?
III Risk of Recurrence for
     Patient's Sib: If parent is affected 1 in 2 (50%) for each offspring to be affected; otherwise not increased.
     Patient's Child: 1 in 2
IV   Age of Detectability: ?
V   Prevalence: ?

Treatment
I   Primary Prevention: Genetic counseling
II   Secondary Prevention: —
III Other Therapy: —

Prognosis: Normal for life expectancy, intelligence and function. Condition usually clears at puberty, rarely persists into adulthood.

Detection of Carrier: —

Special Considerations: —

References:
Binazzi, M.: Ulteriori relievi su di una osservazione di granulosis rubra nasi ereditaria. Rass. Dermatol. Sif. 11:23, 1958.
Cockayne, E.A.: Inherited Abnormalities of the Skin and Its Appendages. London:Humphrey Milford, 1933.
Hellier, F.F.: Granulosis rubra nasi in mother and daughter. Br. Med. J. 2:1068, 1937.

Contributor: **Kent F. Jacobs**

Editor's Computerized Descriptors: Nose, Skin, Sweating

GREBE SYNDROME

Editor's Computerized Descriptor: Skel.

Includes: Syndrome de Grebe
Síndrome de Grebe
Grebe disease
Grebe chondrodysplasia

Excludes: Achondrogenesis, Langer-Saldino type (8)
Achondrogenesis, Parenti-Fraccaro type (9)

Minimal Diagnostic Criteria: Dwarfism due almost entirely to pronounced shortening of the long bones. These changes are extreme in the digits and polydactyly may be present. Xrays show aplasias and hypoplasias of the limb bones.

Clinical Findings: Short stature due to short limbs. Short upper limbs with progressive shortening from proximal to distal segments. The hands and fingers may be extremely short and the fingers resemble toes. Polydactyly is frequent and the limbs tend to be obese. Shortening of the lower limbs is more severe than the upper limbs. The feet are short, broad and in valgus position. Rudimentary toes may be present. The trunk, head and intelligence are normal. X-ray abnormalities are confined to the limbs which show variable aplasia or hypoplasia of all bony elements; the changes are more severe from proximal to distal.

Complications
I **Derived:** —
II **Associated:** —

Etiology: Autosomal recessive

Pathogenesis: ?

Related Facts
I **Sex Ratio:** M1:F1
II **Risk of Occurrence:** Extremely rare
III **Risk of Recurrence for**
 Patient's Sib: 1 in 4 (25%) for each offspring to be affected
 Patient's Child: Not increased unless mate is carrier or homozygote
IV **Age of Detectability:** At birth
V **Prevalence:** Extremely rare; 47 of 56 reported cases occurred in an inbred Brazilian population described by Quelce-Salgado.†

Treatment
I **Primary Prevention:** Genetic counseling
II **Secondary Prevention:** —
III **Other Therapy:** Orthopedic care as indicated.

Prognosis: According to Quelce-Salgado many of the affected Brazilians in his study were stillborn or died in infancy. Survival to adulthood was illustrated in a case reported by Scott.

Detection of Carrier: ?

†Special Considerations: Since Grebe first reported this condition, rarely has it been described except for the large number of cases in a highly inbred population of Brazilians. This disorder has inappropriately been included as a type of achondrogenesis. Grebe syndrome is a distinct chondrodysplasia affecting only the limbs and is rarely associated with early infant deaths.

References:
Freire-Maia, N. and Lenz, W.D.: Discussion. In Bergsma, D. (ed.): Part IV. Skeletal Dysplasias. Birth Defects:Orig. Art. Ser., vol. V, no. 4. New York:The National Foundation-March of Dimes, 1969, p. 14.
Grebe, H.: Die Achondrogenesis. Ein einfach rezessives Erbmerkmal. Folia Hered. Path. 2:23, 1952.
Quelce-Salgado, A.: A rare genetic syndrome. Lancet 1:1430, 1968.
Romeo, G. et al: Heterogeneity of nonlethal severe short-limbed dwarfism. J. Pediatr. 91:918, 1977.

Contributor: **Charles I. Scott, Jr.**

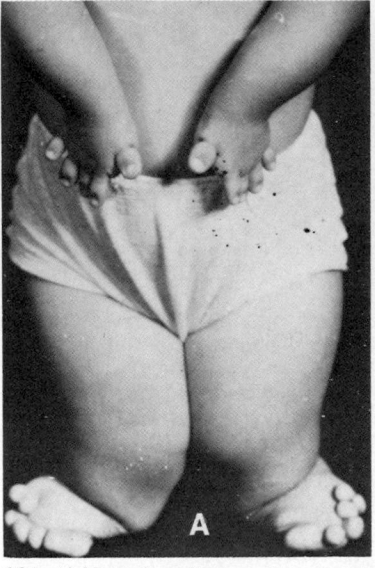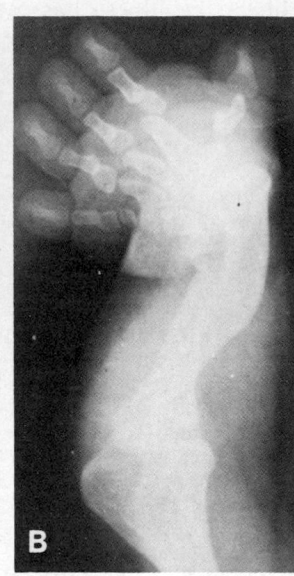

281. A) Note short limbs and postaxial polydactyly of feet;
B) markedly bowed and short radius and hypoplastic ulna

GROUP-SPECIFIC COMPONENT (MARKER)

Includes: Protéines de groupe
Gruppenspezifische Eiweisskomponente
Componente del grupo específico Gc (Marcador)
Group-specific protein
Gc

Excludes: —

Minimal Diagnostic Criteria: The group-specific component is an α_2-globulin of human serum

Clinical Findings: The group-specific component is an α_2-globulin of human serum with genetically determined variations. The different genetic types can be distinguished by electrophoretic procedures including immunoelectrophoresis on agar-gel, starch- and polyacrylamide-gel electrophoresis. The 3 common Gc types are designated Gc 1-1, Gc 2-1, and Gc 2-2, and are determined by a pair of autosomal alleles, Gc^1 and Gc^2. Gc 1-1 has the electrophoretic mobility of a fast α_2-globulin; it is electrophoretically heterogeneous and consists of 2 separable components. Gc 2-2 migrates as a slow α_2-globulin and appears to be homogeneous electrophoretically. Individuals heterozygous for this trait (Gc 2-1) have the products of both alleles in their serum; by electrophoretic procedures 3 components can be disclosed.

Gc has a molecular weight of 50,000 and a sedimentation rate of 4.1 S. It contains 3.3% carbohydrates and is devoid of sialic acid and lipids. The group-specific component is composed of different structural subunits, supposedly 2 polypeptide chains of a molecular weight of 25,000. The structural differences between the various genetic types have not been identified, but may reside in single amino acid substitutions as suggested by the presently available peptide mapping date.

The group-specific component has the capacity to bind vitamin D and serves presumably as the transport protein for this substance in the blood circulation. The serum concentration in healthy individuals is approximately 40 mg/100 ml. There are slight but significant differences in the concentrations among the different genetic types: persons with Gc 1-1 have on the average higher levels than individuals with Gc 2-1; persons with Gc 2-1 have higher concentrations than individuals with Gc 2-2. Gc is increased in sera of pregnant women. Since the group-specific component is synthesized in the liver, patients with severe liver diseases tend to have, therefore, very low Gc serum levels. The Gc is also present in plasma, cerebrospinal fluid, ascites fluid and normal urine. The group-specific component has been identified in subhuman primates; homologous proteins are presumably also present in all other mammals.

The practical application of the Gc system is at present restricted to the use as an additional genetic marker in studies of human populations, in twin diagnosis, and in cases of disputed paternity.

Complications
I **Derived:** —
II **Associated:** —

Etiology: Autosomal codominant; McK *13920

Pathogenesis: —

Related Facts
I **Sex Ratio:** M1:F1
II **Risk of Occurrence:** Each child has Gc^1 or Gc^2
III **Risk of Recurrence for**

Patient's Sib: If a parent has Gc^1, 1 in 2 for Gc^1; if a parent has Gc^2, 1 in 2 for Gc^2.
Patient's Child: If a parent has Gc^1, 1 in 2 for Gc^1; if a parent has Gc^2, 1 in 2 for Gc^2.
IV **Age of Detectability:** Infancy
V **Prevalence:** Gc^1 and Gc^2 appear to have a worldwide distribution: both alleles have been disclosed in every population examined. In most populations, Gc^1 is more common than Gc^2, the frequency of the latter varies from 0.011 in an Australian aborigine tribe from Cundeelee in the Western Desert to 0.385 in a population of Finns from the island of Kokar. In some South American Indian tribes, however, Gc^2 is more common than Gc^1. Most Caucasian and Asian populations have Gc^2 frequencies between 0.20 and 0.30, Negro populations have lower Gc^2 frequencies between 0.03 and 0.11. The mechanisms responsible for the observed differences in allelic distribution are not known. A number of rare genetic variants in the Gc system have been discovered which include the faster migrating Gc Aborigine, Gc Darmstadt, Gc Wien, Gc Japanese and Gc Opava, the slower migrating Gc Bangkok and Gc Z, and the variants Gc Chippewa and Gc Norway. The structural loci for the group-specific component and for albumin are genetically linked.

Treatment
I **Primary Prevention:** —
II **Secondary Prevention:** —
III **Other Therapy:** —

Prognosis: —

Detection of Carrier: —

Special Considerations: —

References:
Cleve, H.: The variants of the group-specific component. A review of their distribution in human populations. Isr. J. Med. Sci. 9:1133, 1973.
Cleve, H. and Bearn, A. G.: The group-specific component of serum; genetic and chemical considerations. Prog. Med. Genet. 2:64, 1962.
Daiger, S.P. et al: Group-specific component proteins bind vitamin D and 25-hydroxy-vitamin D. Proc. Natl. Acad. Sci. USA 72:2076, 1975.
Hirschfeld, J.: The Gc-system; immuno-electrophoretic studies of normal human sera with special reference to a new genetically determined serum system (Gc). Prog. Allergy 6:155, 1962.

Contributor: **Hartwig Cleve**

Editor's Computerized Descriptor: —

GROWTH HORMONE DEFICIENCY, ISOLATED

Includes: Déficit isolé en hormone de croissance
Isolierter Wachtumshormon-Mangel
Deficiencia aislada de hormona de crecimiento
Sexual ateleotic dwarfism

Excludes: Congenital absence of pituitary
Panhypopituitary dwarfism, familial
Dwarfism, panhypopituitary† (303)
Dwarfism, pituitary with abnormal sella turcica (304)
Dwarfism, Laron (302)

Minimal Diagnostic Criteria: Evidence of hGH deficiency (poor response to recognized hGH stimuli, ie L-dopa, arginine infusion, insulin-induced hypoglycemia) in the absence of other pituitary hormone deficiencies.†

Clinical Findings: Isolated growth hormone deficiency (IGHD) refers to a heterogeneous group of disorders which differ clinically, biochemically and genetically. The most common, IGHD, type I, is characterized by proportionate dwarfism, excessive subcutaneous adipose tissue, particularly of the trunk, soft wrinkled skin, round doll-like facies and a peculiar high-pitched voice. Birth length and weight are normal but hypoglycemic episodes may be a problem during infancy. Growth retardation begins at birth, but usually is not apparent before 6 months of age. Skeletal bone age is mildly retarded. Normal sexual development occurs but often is delayed until the late teens or early 20s; and patients are fertile. Metabolic abnormalities include glucose intolerance unassociated with ketosis or diabetic vascular complications, insulinopenia following glucose ingestion or arginine infusion, prolonged hypoglycemia following insulin infusion and diminished lipolysis. Human growth hormone (hGH) replacement results in correction of these abnormalities.

IGHD, type II, a rarer and less well-defined form, differs from IGHD, type I, in that patients lack the wrinkled skin and peculiar voice and tend to be somewhat more obese. Although they have glucose intolerance and decreased lipolysis, they demonstrate an increased rather than a decreased insulin response to glucose ingestion or arginine infusion and a relative resistance to insulin infusion. Furthermore, these metabolic abnormalities may not be corrected with hGH treatment. Hence, these patients show a relative resistance to the metabolic effects of both insulin and hGH. Probably IGHD, type II is a heterogeneous disorder, as patients have been described with different combinations of metabolic abnormalities.

Several other IGHD variants have been described, but are primarily single family reports. One form, referred to as type A, differs from IGHD, type I, by more severe dwarfism and the appearance of high concentrations of hGH antibodies following hGH treatment.

Complications
I   **Derived:** See Clinical Findings
II **Associated:** —

Etiology: IGHD, type 1: Almost all families show autosomal recessive inheritance, but autosomal dominant inheritance may occur rarely in patients with this constellation of metabolic abnormalities. McK *26240
IGHD, type II: Most cases are sporadic, but autosomal dominant inheritance has been recognized.
Type A: Autosomal recessive inheritance pattern.

Pathogenesis: A variety of defects in the hypothalamic-pituitary axis has been postulated, all of which could ultimately lead to isolated growth hormone deficiency. Somatotropic cells have been identified in the pituitaries of several autopsied cases of IGHD, type I, suggesting a primary hypothalamic defect.

Related Facts
I   **Sex Ratio:** M1:F1
II   **Risk of Occurrence:** ? Low
III **Risk of Recurrence for**
     Patient's Sib: IGHD type I: When autosomal dominant or autosomal recessive, see Table I AD or AR, respectively.
     IGHD, type II: Negligible, unless parent is affected then 1 in 2 (50%) for each offspring to be affected; otherwise not increased.
     Type A: 1 in 4 (25%) for each offspring to be affected.
     Patient's Child: IGHD, type I: When autosomal dominant or autosomal recessive, see Table I AD or AR, respectively.
     IGHD, type II: 1 in 2
     Type A: Not increased unless mate is carrier or homozygote.
IV   **Age of Detectability:** At birth, but usually not suspected before 6 months of age.
V   **Prevalence:** Very low

Treatment
I   **Primary Prevention:** Genetic counseling
II   **Secondary Prevention:** Replacement with hGH as early as possible. Pregnant females with the disorder need cesarean section since children, whether affected or unaffected, will be of normal size at birth.
III **Other Therapy:** —

Prognosis: —

Detection of Carrier: —

†Special Considerations: Since patients with IGHD usually have late puberty, it may be difficult to differentiate them from those with panhypopituitarism during late adolescence. Treatment with hGH often stimulates spontaneous puberty in IGHD patients and may be helpful in distinguishing these patients.

References:
Rimoin, D.L. and Schimke, R.N.: Genetic Disorders of the Endocrine Glands. St. Louis: C.V. Mosby, 1971, p. 11.
Rimoin, D.L.: Hereditary forms of growth hormone deficiency and resistance. In Bergsma, D. (ed.): Growth Problems and Clinical Advances. Birth Defects: Orig. Art. Ser., vol. XII, no. 6. New York: Alan R. Liss, Inc. for the National Foundation-March of Dimes, 1976, p. 15.

Contributors: **William A. Horton**
                    David L. Rimoin

Editor's Computerized Descriptors: Face, Speech, Skin, Skel., GU.

GUSTATORY SWEATING

282. A & B) Phenotype of isolated deficiency of hGH, type I;
C) normal daughter of B

Includes: Sudation gustative
 Sialorrhoea hereditaria
 Sudación asociada a la gustación
 Auriculotemporal syndrome
 Frey syndrome
 Sweating, gustatory

Excludes: Posttraumatic and postoperative gustatory sweating
 Postencephalitic gustatory sweating
 Parotid duct fistula
 Syringomyelia gustatory sweating

Minimal Diagnostic Criteria: A lifelong history of facial and neck sweating, with or without flushing, during or after eating obtained from a person who has no medically or surgically induced neurologic deficits. A strong positive family history is usually present.

Clinical Findings: At the time of or just after eating or drinking, perspiration of the face and neck is noted. The face and neck areas may show associated flushing. No increase of sweating or flushing is noted in other areas of the body. The symptoms appear with any food or beverage, but there are no symptoms or findings to suggest specific food allergy. There is no history of trauma or surgery in the area, nor of encephalitis or neurologic deficits. Generally the symptoms have been lifelong or date from infancy; often a family history can be obtained.

Complications
I   **Derived:** Social embarrassment or in extreme cases withdrawal from social contacts might occur.
II **Associated:** —

Etiology: Appears to be autosomal dominant.

Pathogenesis: ?

Related Facts
I   **Sex Ratio:** M > 1:F1 in the cases reported, but the total incidence reported is so low that it is impossible to say whether this is a true difference.†
II **Risk of Occurrence:** ? The known cases have been in American Negroes as reported by Mailander; and 3 generations of Zuni Indians with the syndrome have been studied by Jacobs. However, there is no reason to believe that other ethnic groups might not also be affected.†
III **Risk of Recurrence for**
    Patient's Sib: If parent is affected, 1 in 2 (50%) for each offspring to be affected; otherwise not increased.
    Patient's Child: 1 in 2
IV **Age of Detectability:** Infancy
V   **Prevalence:** ?

Treatment
I   **Primary Prevention:** Genetic counseling
II **Secondary Prevention:** Intratympanic section of Jacobsen nerve might be successful in interrupting the efferent innervation to the parotid gland. This is postulated on the theory that aberrant autonomic innervation occurs. It is thought that the sweat glands and blood vessels of the skin are innervated by parasympathetic rather than sympathetic fibers. A topical preparation, such as 3% scopalamine cream, may be useful in instances where the sweating is not profuse. In mild cases simple assurance to the patient that he does not have a serious or life-threatening disorder may be sufficient. Intracranial section of the 9th cranial nerve is not justified for this benign disease. X-ray therapy of the skin would require near-cancerocidal doses to destroy the sweat glands and also is not indicated.
III **Other Therapy:** —

Prognosis: Good for normal life span. Total function of the patient is limited only if he tends to withdraw from society.

Detection of Carrier: —

†**Special Considerations:** As pointed out by Mailander, the incidence of this disorder may be higher than reported, since affected individuals may tend to deny the symptoms or withdraw from society. Also, in both ethnic groups in which this condition has been described there is a tendency to ignore such physical complaints or at least not to bring them to medical attention. Often this is an incidental finding when the patient is receiving medical care for an unrelated problem. An erroneous diagnosis of parotid fistula or neuropsychiatric disease is often made and proper therapy not instituted.

References:
Mailander, J.C.: Hereditary gustatory sweating. JAMA 201:203, 1967.

Contributors: **Kent F. Jacobs**
LaVonne Bergstrom

Editor's Computerized Descriptor: Sweating

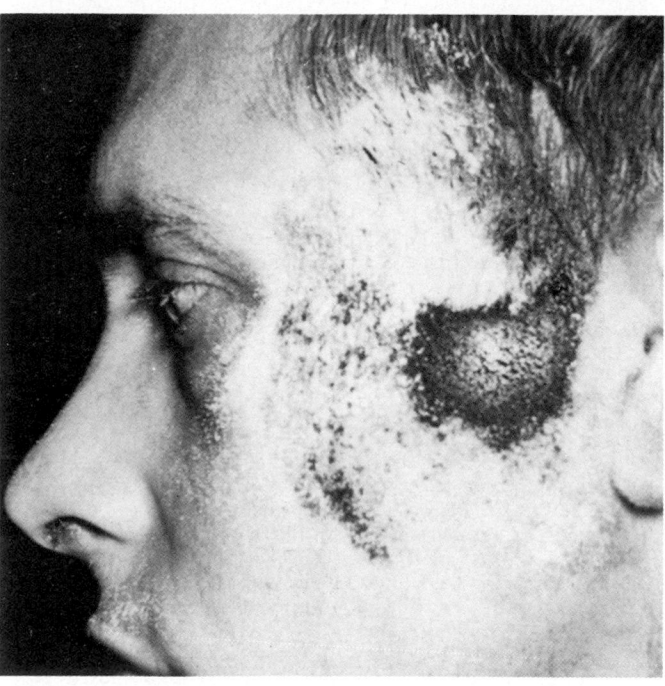

283. Gustatory sweating

GYRATE ATROPHY

Includes: Atrophie gyrée de la chorio-rétine
Atrophia gyrata choroideae et retinae
Atrofia girata
Ornithuria with retinal degeneration

Excludes: Tapetochoroidal dystrophy (925)
Choroidal sclerosis
Myopic choroidosis

Minimal Diagnostic Criteria: Typical retinal findings and elevated plasma ornithine.

Clinical Findings: Gyrate atrophy is an autosomal recessive degeneration of retina and choroid which begins in the 1st decade of life with the development of sharply demarcated atrophic areas in the equatorial region. These foci merge to form scalloped plaques which eventually involve most of the eyegrounds. The choriocapillaris disappears except in the macula and the far periphery and a velvety pigment with glistening granules is seen in these areas. This pigment blocks fluorescein dye as opposed to the end-stage situation in choroideremia where the dye is seen. The disk remains pink but the retinal vessels gradually narrow.

All those affected are myopic. Dark adaptation is impaired early and the nightblindness is progressive. Visual fields correspond to the fundus changes with a broadening ring scotoma leaving only a small central island. Acquired tritanopia is often present. Central acuity is maintained intact into the 4th decade but eventually severe impairment occurs. Cataracts are frequent and are the complicated type. ERGs are usually unrecordable and the EOG is severely impaired.

Recent studies have demonstrated a marked elevation in plasma ornithine, 10-20 times normal, with a corresponding overflow ornithuria.

Complications
I **Derived:** Cataract, myopia
II **Associated:** Adler anomaly of leukocytes in some patients

Etiology: Autosomal recessive; McK * 22990

Pathogenesis: The role of elevated ornithine is unclear as hyperornithemia when part of other generalized biochemical disorders is compatible with a normal fundus and electrophysiology.

Related Facts
I **Sex Ratio:** M1:F1
II **Risk of Occurrence:** —
III **Risk of Recurrence for**
Patient's Sib: 1 in 4 (25%) for each offspring to be affected
Patient's Child: Not markedly increased unless mate is carrier or homozygote
IV **Age of Detectability:** 1st decade
V **Prevalence:** —

Treatment
I **Primary Prevention:** Genetic counseling
II **Secondary Prevention:** —
III **Other Therapy:** —

Prognosis: Normal life span with eventual severe visual loss.

Detection of Carrier: The eye examination is normal. However, mildly elevated ornithine levels have been reported and significantly abnormal ornithine loading tests are present.

Special Considerations: —

References:
Berson, E.L. et al: Plasma amino acids in hereditary retinal disease: Ornithine, lysine, and taurine. Br. J. Ophthalmol. 60:142,

1976.

Franceschetti, A. et al: Chorioretinal Heredodegenerations. Springfield: Charles C Thomas, 1974.

Takki, K.: Gyrate atrophy of the choroid and retina associated with hyperornithenaemia. Br. J. Ophthalmol. 58:3, 1974.

Takki, K. and Simell, O. Genetic aspects in gyrate atrophy of the choroid and retina with hyperornithenaemia. Br. J. Ophthalmol. 58:907, 1974.

Contributor: **Mitchel L. Wolf**

Editor's Computerized Descriptors: Vision, Eye

HAND MUSCLE WASTING AND SENSORINEURAL DEAFNESS

Includes: Anomalies des mains-surdité de perception
Hand Fehlbildung und Innenohrschwerhörigkeit
Anomalías de las manos y sordera neuro-sensorial
Deafness, sensorineural and hand muscle wasting

Excludes: Proximal symphalangism
Hand anomaly associated with dwarfism

Minimal Diagnostic Criteria: Congenital flexion contractures and atrophy of thenar, hypothenar and interosseous muscles in a patient with congenital sensorineural hearing loss and normal joints by radiography.†

Clinical Findings: The patients manifest familial congenital bilateral or unilateral sensorineural hearing losses of varying degrees. A congenital hand abnormality is seen in both normal-hearing and deaf patients. There are congenital flexion contractures of the digits and wasting of the thenar, hypothenar and interosseous muscles which are nonprogressive. Flexion creases over the interphalangeal joints are absent. Active and passive flexion and extension of the fingers is limited. Some of the fingers may show ulnar deviation. There may be muscle weakness, most marked in the distribution of the ulnar nerve. There is no pain; there are no other neurologic deficits; nerve conduction studies and electromyography are normal. Dermatoglyphics show a striking vertical orientation of the palmar digital lines. Xrays in both adults and children show normal joints. Petrous pyramid polytomography, electronystagmography and various laboratory tests (CBC, urinalysis, serum electrolytes, BUN, blood glucose, serum glutamic oxalic transaminase, aldolase, CPK, urine and plasma amino acid screening, urine mucopolysaccharide screening, ECG and karyotype) are normal.

Complications
I   **Derived:** Failure to acquire speech and language in a patient with profound hearing loss. Articulation errors and poor school progress in patients with lesser degrees of hearing loss.
II **Associated:** Limitation of motion of other joints has been seen. These include the wrist, toes, forearm pronation and supination, elbow extension.

Etiology: Autosomal dominant with complete penetrance but variable expressivity

Pathogenesis: ?

Related Facts
I   **Sex Ratio:**   M1:F1
II   **Risk of Occurrence:**   ?
III **Risk of Recurrence for**
     Patient's Sib: If parent is affected, 1 in 2 (50%) for each offspring to be affected; otherwise not increased.
     Patient's Child: 1 in 2
IV   **Age of Detectability:** The hand abnormality is detectable at birth and if bilateral, the hearing loss may be detected at birth also, unless the loss is mild. A unilateral loss may escape detection for years.
V   **Prevalence:**   ?

Treatment
I   **Primary Prevention:**   Genetic counseling
II   **Secondary Prevention:** Hearing loss, if significant, should be treated by the use of auditory habilitation with hearing aids and special speech training. Less severe losses may be managed by preferential seating in school, lip-reading training and the use of hearing conservation (regular otologic and audiologic checkups, avoidance of acoustic trauma and oto-

toxic drugs). Mumps immunization might be desirable in susceptible patients with unilateral hearing loss. Physical therapy may be of benefit in patients with more severe contractures.

III Other Therapy: —

Prognosis: Normal for life expectancy and intelligence. There is some evidence to suggest that the inner ears in these patients may be more susceptible to injury from febrile illnesses.

Detection of Carrier: —

†Special Considerations: An infant with the characteristic hand abnormality should have audiometric evaluation and periodic follow-up to rule out hearing loss. The hearing loss is the only potential serious disability, as the hand abnormality seems not to hinder patients in their daily activities and occupations.

References:
Stewart, J.M. and Bergstrom, L.: Familial hand abnormality and sensori-neural deafness: New syndrome. J. Pediatr. 78:102, 1971.

Contributors: **Janet M. Stewart**
              LaVonne Bergstrom

Editor's Computerized Descriptors: Hearing, Speech, Dermatoglyphic, Muscle

HANHART SYNDROME

Includes: Syndrome de Hanhart
Síndrome de Hanhart
Aglossia-adactylia syndrome
Hypoglossia-hypodactylia syndrome
Ankyloglossum superior syndrome
Glossopalatine ankylosis syndrome
Aglossia congenita
Peromelia and micrognathia

Excludes: Ectrodactyly (336)
Acheiropody
Oro-facio-digital syndromes (770, 771)
Charlie M. syndrome†
Poland-Möbius syndrome†
Ring constrictions (874)
Cleft lip-lateral synechiae syndrome†

Minimal Diagnostic Criteria: Absence of distal portions of the limbs to variable degrees in conjunction with (usually severe) micrognathia or microglossia.

Clinical Findings: Absence of distal portions of the limbs, including complete or partial adactyly, acheiria/apodia or absence of legs, arms, forearms and thighs. Characteristically, the severity varies in different limbs. The feet are almost always affected. Micrognathia and microglossia are present, may be severe and associated with cleft palate, synechiae, syngnathia, oligodontia and microstomia. Congenital unilateral or bilateral cranial nerve palsies may occur.† A few patients have been mentally retarded, one had an imperforate anus.

Complications
I   **Derived:** Physical limitations due to limb defects; speech and hearing deficit; neonatal respiratory and feeding difficulties.
II **Associated:** Breech presentation

Etiology: ? McK *26130

Pathogenesis: Malformation with developmental field defect in distal limbs and orofacial region of incomplete rather than abnormal development. Bersu et al have postulated that the defect may result from deficient mesodermal proliferation in the embryonal "Ektodermring," beginning about the 4th week of development.

Related Facts
I   **Sex Ratio:** M1:F1
II   **Risk of Occurrence:** Small
III **Risk of Recurrence for**
       Patient's Sib: Small
       Patient's Child: ?
IV   **Age of Detectability:** At birth
V   **Prevalence:** At least 1 in 500,000

Treatment
I   **Primary Prevention:** —
II   **Secondary Prevention:** Neonatal respiratory and nutritional care
III **Other Therapy:** Constructive orofacial surgery, limb and dental prostheses, speech habilitation

Prognosis: Increased neonatal death rate, with insufficiently explained cause in some instances. Other patients have an apparently normal life span. Intelligence is normal in almost all patients and their personality often delightful.

Detection of Carrier: —

†Special Considerations: Traditionally, patients with cranial nerve palsy have been diagnosed as having the Möbius syndrome. These include a) patients with limb defects of the "Hanhart type," b) patients with symbrachydactyly (usually in upper limbs only) or pectoralis muscle hypoplasia of the "Poland type," c) patients with other, and d) patients with no associated anomalies. We suggest distinguishing the following conditions not on the basis of presence or absence of cranial nerve palsy, but on the basis of the associated anomalies: 1) the Hanhart syndrome (with and without cranial nerve palsy), 2) the Poland-Möbius syndrome (complete or incomplete combination of symbrachydactyly, chest defect, cranial nerve palsy), 3) the cleft palate/lateral synechiae syndrome, 4) isolated cranial nerve palsy (autosomal dominant), 5) the Charlie M. syndrome, and 6) others. Of further importance is that the orofacial and acral abnormalities (the "Kettner anomaly") in the Hanhart syndrome and the symbrachydactyly and chest defect (the "Poland anomaly") in the Poland-Möbius syndrome represent nonspecific developmental field defects which may occur in other genetic or nongenetic syndromes.

References:

Bersu, E.T. et al: Studies of malformation syndromes in man XXXXIA: Anatomical studies in the Hanhart syndrome-a pathogenetic hypothesis. Eur. J. Pediatr. 122:1, 1976.

Gorlin, R.J. et al: Syndromes of the Head and Neck. 2nd Ed. New York: McGraw-Hill, 1976, p. 571.

Herrmann, J. et al: Studies of malformation syndromes of man XXXXIB: Nosologic studies in the Hanhart and the Möbius syndromes. Eur. J. Pediatr. 122:19, 1976.

Contributor: **Jürgen Herrmann**

Editor's Computerized Descriptors: Eye, Hearing, Face, Oral, Teeth, Skel., Resp., Nerve

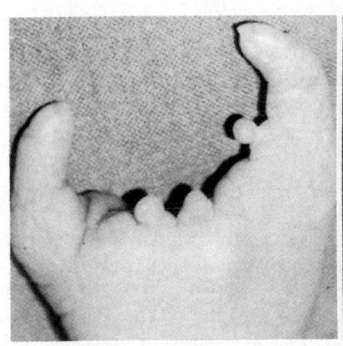 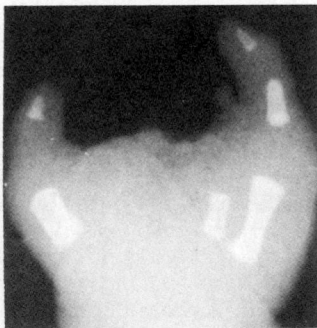

284. Crab-type deformity of hand

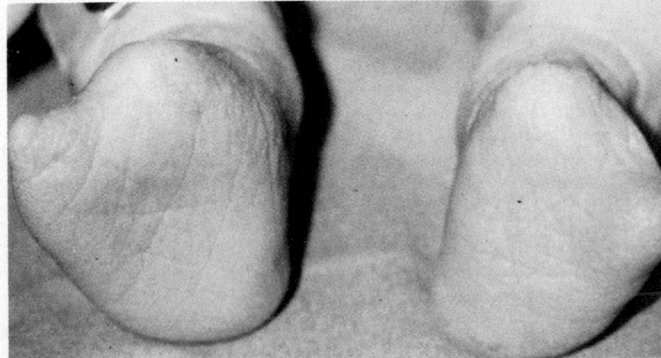

285. Loss of anterior one-third of foot

HAPTOGLOBIN (MARKER)

Includes: Haptoglobine
Haptoglobina (Marcador)
Hemoglobin-binding α_2 globulins
Hemoglobin-binding β_2 globulins

Excludes: Heme-binding protein (hemopexin)

Minimal Diagnostic Criteria: Measurement of hemoglobulin-binding capacity and electrophoretic determination of phenotype.

Clinical Findings: Haptoglobin (Hp) levels in plasma (expressed as the hemoglobin-binding capacity) normally vary over a wide range of about 30-180 mg%, although the level is fairly constant in any given healthy individual. Men have generally higher levels than women, and this may be due to a hormonal effect. Newborn infants usually have little or no demonstrable haptoglobin and adult levels are reached at about 1 year. In conditions associated with inflammatory reactions, neoplasia or severe stress, the Hp level is usually increased, sometimes exceeding 1000 mg%. Conversely, in hemolytic states, Hp is either decreased or absent, unless the hemolysis is entirely extravascular. Hp is also decreased in severe liver disease, presumably because synthesis of Hp occurs in that organ. Measurements of Hp are of some value in following the course of liver disease and in determining the presence of increased intravascular hemolysis. However, hypohaptoglobinemia can occur in apparently normal subjects, including about 1% of white subjects, 10% of black children and about 4% of black adults; therefore, decreased or absent Hp must be evaluated with caution.

The common electrophoretic phenotypes are Hp 1-1, 2-2 and 2-1 representing homo- and heterozygosity for 2 codominant alleles, Hp^1 and Hp^2. Although there is considerable heterogeneity in the geographic distribution of these genes, there is no convincing evidence available for an association between Hp genetic type and disease.

Complications
I **Derived:** —
II **Associated:** —

Etiology: Autosomal dominant transmission of each allele; McK *14010, *14020

Pathogenesis: —

Related Facts
I **Sex Ratio:** M1:F1
II **Risk of Occurrence:** ?
III **Risk of Recurrence for**
    Patient's Sib: If parent has allele Hp^1 or Hp^2, 1 in 2 (50%) for that allele for each offspring
    Patient's Child: 1 in 2
IV **Age of Detectability:** —
V **Prevalence:** ?

Treatment
I **Primary Prevention:** —
II **Secondary Prevention:** —
III **Other Therapy:** —

Prognosis: Normal life span

Detection of Carrier: The haptoglobin phenotype is determined by performing electrophoresis in starch gel or acrylamide gel on serum to which hemoglobin has been added in excess of the binding capacity. The three common types have a characteristic appearance. About 10% of blacks have a quantitatively altered Hp 2-1 type called Hp 2-1 (Mod), in which there is a shift in concentration of Hp 2-1 components toward the fastest moving bands. The inheritance of this phenotype is consistent with the existence of a third allele, Hp^{2M}. However, the possibility of a genetic event such as regulator gene mutation cannot be entirely ruled out.

Special Considerations: —

References:
Black, J.A. and Dixon, G.H.: Amino acid sequence of alpha chains of human haptoglobins. Nature 218:736, 1968.
Giblett, E.R.: Genetic Markers in Human Blood. Oxford:Blackwell Scientific Ltd., 1969.
Javid, J.: Human serum haptoglobins: A brief review. Semin. Hematol. 4:35, 1967.

Contributor: **Eloise R. Giblett**

Editor's Computerized Descriptor: —

HARTNUP DISORDER

Includes: Maladie de Hartnup
Hartnupsche Krankheit
Enfermedad de Hartnup

Excludes: Pellagra

Minimal Diagnostic Criteria: Specific hyper-α-aminoaciduria, involving neutral and ring-structured amino acids, but excluding dicarboxylic and dibasic amino acids, the imino acids, and glycine. Feces contains excess of same group of amino acids, which appear in excess in the urine. For another form of trait, intestinal defect is absent (presumably a different mutation).

Clinical Findings: May be asymptomatic. Usually discovered in patients with intermittent psychiatric disorder, or mild mental retardation. Photosensitivity of exposed areas of skin occurs after sufficient UV dosage. Intermittency of clinical manifestations is characteristic. Conditioning factors, if they exist, have not been fully clarified, but marginal nutrition is suspected to be important in precipitating symptoms. Impaired nicotinic acid nutrition is implicated particularly.
  Plasma levels of tryptophan metabolites are slightly depressed. The same amino acids are affected by the intestinal and renal tubular transport defects.

Complications
I **Derived:** Pellagra-like symptoms related to impaired endogenous synthesis of nicotinic acid, under marginal nutritional intake. Intermittent and reversible "psychosis" may occur.
II **Associated:** —

Etiology: Autosomal recessive; McK *23450

Pathogenesis: Deficiency of group-specific membrane transport system for certain aliphatic and ring-structured neutral α-amino acids. Transport of oligopeptides involving the same amino acids is normal.
  Biochemical characteristics include: specific hyper-α-aminoaciduria (it excludes the dibasic amino acids, the dicarboxylic amino acids, the imino acids, and glycine); and high clearance (renal) mechanism for the aminoaciduria. Urine also contains excessive amounts of tryptophan derivatives, such as indoxyl sulfate, indole-3-acetic acid, and indolylacetyl glutamine, which are of intestinal origin, secondary to impaired intestinal absorption of tryptophan, and can be suppressed with neomycin.

Related Facts
I **Sex Ratio:** Ml:Fl (approximate)
II **Risk of Occurrence:** About 1 in 14,500 live births (Massachussetts survey)
III **Risk of Recurrence for**
  Patient's Sib: 1 in 4 (25%) for each offspring to be affected
  Patient's Child: Not increased unless mate is carrier or homozygote.
IV **Age of Detectability:** In newborn
V **Prevalence:** Since many cases are asymptomatic the "disease" prevalence is lower than the "trait" occurrence.†

Treatment
I **Primary Prevention:** Genetic counseling
II **Secondary Prevention:** Good protein nutrition; nicotinic acid supplements to offset proposed deficiency in endogenous synthesis of coenzyme and prevent pellagra-like symptoms.
III **Other Therapy:** —

Prognosis: Normal life span

Detection of Carrier: No identifying characteristics under usual prevailing conditions. Renal T_m should be lower than normal for amino acids whose transport is affected by trait.

†**Special Considerations:** Symptomatic trait is world-wide, but it

is very infrequently found in North America, where high standard of nutrition may offset features of trait likely to precipitate symptoms.

References:

Jepson, J.B.: Hartnup disease. In Stanbury, J.B. et al (eds.): The Metabolic Basis of Inherited Disease, 4th Ed. New York:McGraw-Hill, 1978, p. 1563.

Milne, M.D. et al: The metabolic disorder in Hartnup disease. Q. J. Med. 29:407, 1960.

Scriver, C. R.: Hartnup disease: A genetic modification of intestinal and renal transport of certain neutral alpha-amino acids. N. Engl. J. Med. 273:530, 1965.

Contributor: **Charles R. Scriver**

Editor's Computerized Descriptors: Skin, Nerve

HEART BLOCK, CONGENITAL COMPLETE

Includes: Bloc cardiaque complet d'origine congénitale
Angeborener kompletter atrioventrikulärer Block
Bloqueo aurículo-ventricular completo congénito
Complete atrioventricular (A-V) block
Third degree atrioventricular block
Congenital complete sinoatrial block
Congenital complete heart block

Excludes: Acquired complete atrioventricular block
Other forms of atrioventricular dissociation such as acceleration of the AV junctional pacemaker during acute rheumatic fever, digitalis intoxication or following open heart operations

Minimal Diagnostic Criteria: A slow heart rate, changing intensity of the first heart sound, and "cannon waves" in the jugular pulse should suggest the diagnosis. It is established, however, with the ECG. The presence or absence of additional cardiac malformations often requires cardiac catheterization and angiocardiography.

Clinical Findings: There may be a complete anatomic interruption of the electrical conduction pathway which normally connects the atria and the ventricles. Congenital complete heart block (CHB) is present at birth but, in the majority of cases, the diagnosis is not made until early infancy or during childhood. In these children, it is difficult to distinguish whether the heart block is congenital or acquired. The criteria for congenital CHB are: 1) an abnormally slow heart rate at an early age; 2) early documentation by ECG of the dissociation between atrial and ventricular excitation, and 3) the absence of other causes for A-V block eg diphtheritic or viral myocarditis.

Congenital CHB may occur as a single anomaly or with associated congenital cardiac defects. In CHB slow fetal, infant or childhood heart rate between 30 and 80 beats per minute at rest is the most striking sign. Bounding pulses are often found. Pulse pressures range from 35 to 100 mm Hg. "Cannon waves" (expression of atrial contraction against the closed A-V valves during ventricular systole) may be seen as irregular bounding venous pressure pulses in the neck veins, more often noted in older children. Upon auscultation, variation of intensity of the first heart sound is almost always present. The second sound is usually normal in intensity and splits conventionally with respiration. Third and fourth heart sounds may be present, and may summate intermittently to an especially loud diastolic filling sound. A systolic ejection type murmur, grade II-III/VI, over the left midsternal border is the rule. This murmur is due to the large stroke volume. Additionally, an apical middiastolic flow murmur is often present. Cases without any murmur have also been reported. Most of the children are asymptomatic even at exercise. Some develop dyspnea and fatigue during exertion.

In the group with an associated malformation of the heart, the clinical symptoms and signs are modified by and may be predominantly those of the defect (cyanosis, signs of large shunts and cardiac failure may be present). The coincidence of CHB with congenital heart disease jeopardizes the hemodynamic compensation.

The ECG in complete A-V block shows independent atrial and ventricular rhythms with a slower ventricular than atrial rate. Both rhythms are usually stable. The atria are under the control of the sinus node and beat a normal rate for age (85 beats per minute in the older child at rest) and commonly show a sinus arrhythmia phasic variation. The ventricles beat at about 30-80 beats per minute, often approximately half the atrial rate. In most cases the ventricular rate increases in response to physical exertion, at times to 150% of the resting rate. P waves may be tall and broad, suggesting right and left atrial enlargement, or an ectopic pacemaker in the atria. Atrial fibrillation may also occur. The QRS complex is usually of normal duration indicating an origin of excitation proximal to the bifurcation of the bundle of His. Prolongation of the QRS complex (more than 0.10 msec) suggests a lower ventricular pacemaker; and there is some evidence that these cases are more prone to Adams-Stokes attacks. Right and left bundle branch block patterns have been described, as well as signs of left or biventricular hypertrophy. The QRS axis is in the normal range for age with a slight tendency to left axis deviation. In cases with congenital heart disease and complete A-V block, the ECG may be modified according to the type of malformation; however CHB may be associated with an abnormal sequence of activation (due primarily to the site of initiation of the ventricular beat) making the ECG contours not truly representative of hypertrophy, etc. Complete sinoatrial block, a rare form of CHB, may be suspected when there is no evidence of atrial activity on the ECG and the ventricular rate is slow.

Roentgenologically, in the absence of associated problems, the heart may be normal in size but in most cases there is cardiomegaly with evidence of left ventricular enlargement, and a minor degree of pulmonary venous obstruction as a result of elevated left atrial pressure. In cases with cardiac malformations, the roentgenologic findings vary with the hemodynamics of that particular lesion.

Cardiac catheterization in CHB without associated heart disease usually reveals a mild right ventricular and pulmonary arterial systolic hypertension, a mild elevation of left atrial mean, and left ventricular and aortic systolic pressures. Cardiac output is usually normal in spite of the slow heart rate: this is accomplished by increasing the stroke volume 50 to 100%. When there are associated heart disorders, the hemodynamic and angiocardiographic findings reflect both defects. An electrophysiologic study recording the His bundle potential with an electrode catheter can demonstrate the level of A-V block whether at the head of the A-V node or lower within the ventricles. Atrial pacing can confirm a presumptive diagnosis of sinoatrial block by showing capture and A-V conduction.

The echocardiogram in A-V block shows varying amplitudes and timing of the mitral valve A wave (which follows atrial systole) depending upon the relationship of the ECG P wave to the QRS complex. The cardiac cavity dimensions vary in size and may exceed normal. Fetal echocardiography may be the earliest sign of CHB in showing the consistently slow fetal heart rate.

Complications
I **Derived:** Adams-Stokes attacks (ventricular asystole or fibrillation) are the most serious complication. According to the length of the ventricular standstill and the interruption of the peripheral circulation, the attacks may be lethal (if the heart does not start to beat again) or may result in dizziness, unconsciousness and convulsions. In a large series, the incidence of this complication in all cases (with and without associated congenital heart disease) is about 10%. Heart failure is a major problem in the neonate with a slow ventricular rate or when congenital heart defects are present.
II **Associated:** Most common is inversion of the ventricles with transposition (corrected transposition of the great arteries) with a ventricular septal defect. Other abnoralities (ASD, VSD, PDA, single ventricle or endocardial fibroelastosis) may be found. The overall incidence of associated heart defects is more than 50%.

Etiology: The familial form is most often autosomal recessive,

although there are reports of autosomal dominant families. Multifactorial inheritance and in utero myocarditis may also be considered. McK *23470

Pathogenesis: Discontinuity of the A-V conduction system may result from underdevelopment (or abnormal resorption) of components or from abnormal development of the central fibrous body. In cases where there is no anatomic interruption of the conduction pathway, functional blockage of the electrical excitation is assumed.

Related Facts
I **Sex Ratio:** M1.8:F1
II **Risk of Occurrence:** 1 in 20,000 live births
III **Risk of Recurrence for**
  Patient's Sib: 2.5% in sporadic occurrence, may be 50% in familial occurrence
  Patient's Child: 2.5% sporadic; high, familial
IV **Age of Detectability:** Before birth
V **Prevalence:** ?

Treatment
I **Primary Prevention:** Genetic counseling in the familial form
II **Secondary Prevention:** Implantation of an artificial electronic pacemaker should be considered in those cases: a) with the first definite Adams-Stokes attack, even mild, eg dizziness, since even the first Adams-Stokes episode may occasionally be fatal; b) in a neonate with a slow ventricular rate (40 or less) and a fast atrial rate (140 or greater) or with signs of congestive heart failure; c) for intractable congestive heart failure, more likely when there is an associated cardiac defect. Temporary pacemaker therapy is advisable for most patients with complete heart block who are to undergo general anesthesia for any operative procedure including implantation of a pacemaker. Isoproterenol may be used intravenously in the interim preparatory to establishing pacemaker control. Questionable is longterm therapy with isoproterenol.
III **Other Therapy:** Digitalis is indicated in congestive heart failure. Isoproterenol may be helpful.

Prognosis: In the majority of cases (those without congenital heart disease and presenting after the first few months of life) the outlook is good. An adequate response of ventricular rate to exercise is a favorable sign. Widening of the QRS complex, compared to that on a previous ECG, indicates deterioration. The familial occurrence of congenital complete A-V block seems to be associated with a greater likelihood of Adams-Stokes attacks and a high mortality. If congenital heart disease is present, the prognosis is poor. Causes of death in these cases is mainly congestive heart failure. The wider application of pacemaker therapy may improve the outlook in these individuals.

Detection of Carrier: Not applicable

Special Considerations: —

References:
Crittenden, I.H. et al: Familial congenital heart block. Am. J. Dis Child. 108:104, 1964.
Genrey, J. et al: Permanent implantation of pacemakers in infants, children and adolescents: Long-term follow-up. Circulation 53:243, 1976.
Gochberg, S.H.: Congenital heart block. Am. J. Obstet Gynecol. 88:238, 1964.
Goldberg, S.J. et al: Pediatric and Adolescent Echocardiography. Chicago: Year Book Medical Publishers, 1975.
Lev, M.: The pathology of complete atrioventricular block. Prog. Cardiovasc. Dis. VI:315, 1964.
Michaelsson, M. and Engle, M.A.: Congenital complete heart block: An international study of the natural history. Cardiovasc. Clin. 4:85, 1972.

Contributors: B. Lynn Miller
Henry J. L. Marriott

Editor's Computerized Descriptor: CV.

HEART-HAND SYNDROME

Includes: Syndrome cardiomélique
Kardiomeler Syndrom
Síndrome cardiomélico
Atriodigital dysplasia
Cardiac limb syndrome
Holt-Oram syndrome
Upper limb cardiovascular syndrome
Heart upper limb syndrome
Cardiomelic syndrome

Excludes: Radial defects (853)
Thrombocytopenia with absent radius (941)
Fanconi anemia
Chondroectodermal dysplasia (156)
Autosomal trisomies
Vater association (987)

Minimal Diagnostic Criteria: Thumb anomaly (triphalangism, hypoplasia or absence) with congenital heart disease.

Clinical Findings: Congenital heart disease, usually secundum atrial septal defect (ASD), and skeletal anomalies of the upper limb, usually thumb hypoplasia, triphalangism or absence; upper limb phocomelia occasionally occurs. The 1st metacarpal has both a proximal and a distal epiphyseal ossification center and the carpal bones may be either absent or increased in number. The triphalangeal thumb is usually in the same plane as the fingers. The radius, ulna, and humerus may be abnormal; inability to supinate and pronate the hand is common. The scapulae and clavicles may also be anomalous and the pectoralis major absent; pectus excavatum has been reported. The lower limbs are not affected.

The cardiac anomaly is ASD in over two-thirds of the cases; other congenital heart defects reported include the following: patent ductus arteriosus, coarctation of the aorta, ventricular septal defect (VSD), transposition of the great vessels, single coronary artery and prolapsed mitral valve. ECG may show a prolonged P-R interval; atrial arrythmias occur. Occasionally either the cardiac or upper limb anomalies occur alone. Families have been reported where VSD occurs consistently as the cardiac anomaly; this may indicate genetic heterogeneity in the heart-hand syndrome.

Complications
I **Derived:** Lack of opposition of the thumb
II **Associated:** —

Etiology: Autosomal dominant with variable expression; McK *14290

Pathogenesis: ? Similar skeletal and cardiac abnormalities are seen as a result of thalidomide embryopathy, the critical time being the 4th and 5th weeks of pregnancy. It is likely that in this syndrome the abnormal gene is active at this same stage in embryogenesis.

Related Facts
I **Sex Ratio:** M1:F1
II **Risk of Occurrence:** Uncommon
III **Risk of Recurrence for**
    Patient's Sib: 1 in 2 (50%) if parent affected; otherwise not increased.
    Patient's Child: 1 in 2
IV **Age of Detectability:** Infancy
V **Prevalence:** Uncommon, but cases have been reported from many different populations and in both Caucasians and Negroes.

Treatment

I **Primary Prevention:** Genetic counseling
II **Secondary Prevention:** Appropriate operative treatment for congenital heart disease and for skeletal anomalies.
III **Other Therapy:** —

Prognosis: Normal for intelligence. Life span and function depend upon cardiac and bone anomalies.

Detection of Carrier: —

Special Considerations: —

References:

Holt, M. and Oram, S.: Familial heart disease with skeletal malformations. Br. Heart J. 22:236, 1960.
Kaufman, R.L. et al: Variable expression of Holt-Oram syndrome. Am. J. Dis. Child. 127:21, 1974.
Lewis, K.B. et al: The upper limb cardiovascular syndrome. An autosomal dominant genetic effect on embryogenesis. JAMA 193:1080, 1965.
Poznanski, A.K. et al: Skeletal manifestations of the Holt-Oram syndrome. Radiology 94:45, 1970.

Contributor: **David C. Siggers**

Editor's Computerized Descriptors: Skel., Muscle, CV.

HEMANGIOMA AND THROMBOCYTOPENIA SYNDROME

Includes: Syndrome de thrombocytopénie avec hémangiome
Kasabach-Merritt Syndrom
Sindrome de hemangioma y trombocitopenia
All vascular tumors (malignant and benign) of hemangioid cell derivation associated with sudden spontaneous hemorrhage
Thrombocytopenia and hemangioma syndrome

Excludes: Hemangiomas with rapid growth, ulceration, without spontaneous hemorrhage

Minimal Diagnostic Criteria: Hemangioma (small or large) with associated systemic hemorrhagic symptoms.†

Clinical Findings: Characterized by normal appearing hemangioma suddenly increasing in size 100%, associated thrombocytopenia 100%, petechiae and ecchymoses 75%, marked decrease in hemoglobin and erythrocyte levels 75%, hypofibrinogenemia, decreased prothrombin.

Complications

I **Derived:** Death through hemorrhage in 21% of reported cases, platelet sequestration within the capillary bed of the hemangioma.
II **Associated:** —

Etiology: ?

Pathogenesis: ? Associated fibrinogen depletion in some cases. Isoagglutinins are not likely.

Related Facts

I **Sex Ratio:** M1:F1
II **Risk of Occurrence:** 1 in 500 reported hemangiomas in teaching hospital files
III **Risk of Recurrence for**
  Patient's Sib: ?
  Patient's Child: ?
IV **Age of Detectability:** Birth through 73 years, median age 5 weeks. Detected primarily through platelet counts.
V **Prevalence:** 1 in 500 cases of hemangiomas. Hemangiomas alone occur in 1 in 12 infants under 1 year of age.

Treatment

I **Primary Prevention:** —
II **Secondary Prevention:** Irradiation, surgical extirpation of tumor if feasible, splenectomy, systemic steroids
III **Other Therapy:** Heparinization when fibrinogen is decreased, whole blood transfusions

Prognosis: Mortality rate 21%; median age at death 5 weeks; preceding statistics for treated cases only; untreated statistics unknown; usual cause of death is hemorrhage.

Detection of Carrier: —

†Special Considerations: The size or the type of the vascular tumor in no way determines the possible development of this syndrome.

References:

Kasabach, H.H. and Merritt, K.K.: Capillary hemangioma with extensive purpura: Report of a case. Am. J. Dis. Child. 59:1063, 1940.
Shim, W.K.: Hemangiomas of infancy complicated by thrombocytopenia. Am. J. Surg. 116:896, 1968.
Wilson, C.J. and Haggard, M.E.: Giant vascular tumors and thrombocytopenia. Arch. Dermatol. 81:432, 1960.

Contributor: **Charles J. Wilson**

Editor's Computerized Descriptors: Skin, CV
Also see Section I, Fig. 100

HEMIFACIAL MICROSOMIA

Includes: Hypoplasie faciale unilatérale avec microsomie
Hemifaziale Mikrosomie
Microsomía hemifacial
Facial hypoplasia unilateral
Otomandibular dysostosis
First arch syndrome

Excludes: Oculo-auriculo-vertebral dysplasia (735)
Mandibulofacial dysostosis (627)
Hemifacial atrophy

Minimal Diagnostic Criteria: Unilateral ear abnormalities and hypoplasia of the mandibular condyle and ramus.

Clinical Findings: The abnormalities are unilateral. Ear: aplasia, hypoplasia and a variety of other malformations of the pinna - 100%. The external canal may be absent or the opening covered by skin. Preauricular skin tags - 95%. Eye abnormalities: lower palpebral fissure on the affected side, microphthalmia, cysts, iris and choroid colobomas and strabismus. Facial muscles are hypoplastic giving the impression of macrostomia or if macrostomia is present, it appears larger. Malocclusion is present on the affected side - 90%. Hypoplasia of the maxilla and mandible - 95%. Pulmonary agenesis on the affected side has been reported.

Complications
I **Derived:** Decreased hearing and malocclusion on the affected side
II **Associated:** —

Etiology: ?

Pathogenesis: Possibly results from a vascular abnormality during embryogenesis.

Related Facts
I **Sex Ratio:** M1:F1
II **Risk of Occurrence:** ?
III **Risk of Recurrence for**
   Patient's Sib: Probably essentially zero
   Patient's Child: Probably essentially zero
IV **Age of Detectability:** At birth by clinical examination
V **Prevalence:** ?

Treatment
I **Primary Prevention:** —
II **Secondary Prevention:** —
III **Other Therapy:** The ear and mandibular abnormalities may be repaired by plastic surgery and dental care may prevent the malocclusion.

Prognosis: Excellent. Normal life span.

Detection of Carrier: —

Special Considerations: —

References:
François, J. and Haustrate, L.: Anomalies colobomateuses du globe oculaire et syndrome du premier arch. Ann. Oculist. (Paris) 187:340, 1954.
Gorlin, R. J. and Pindborg, J. J.: Syndromes of the Head and Neck. New York:McGraw-Hill, 1964.
Kazajian, V. H.: Congenital absence of the ramus of the mandible. Am. J. Orthod. 26:175, 1940.
Ross, R.B.: Lateral facial dysplasia. In Bergsma, D. (ed.): Morphogenesis and Malformation of Face and Brain. Birth Defects: Orig. Art. Ser., vol XI, no. 7. New York:Alan Liss, Inc. for The National Foundation-March of Dimes, 1975, p. 51.

Contributor: **Murray Feingold**

Editor's Computerized Descriptors: Eye, Hearing, Ear, Face, Teeth, Muscle, Resp.

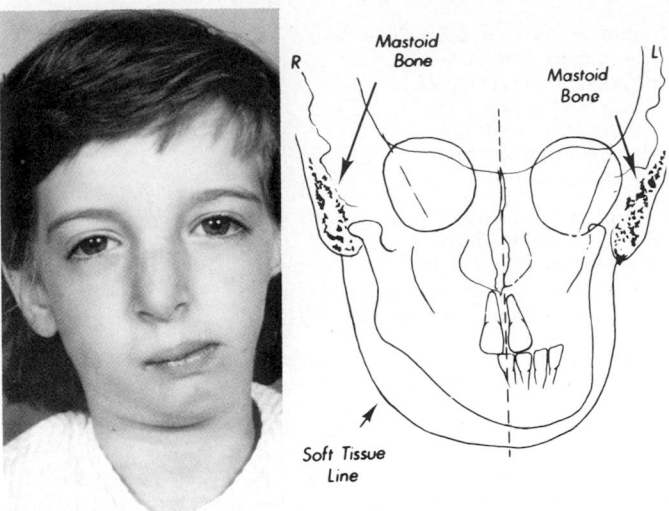

286. Full face and graphic illustration exhibit facial asymmetry with external ear and contiguous with anatomic anomalies

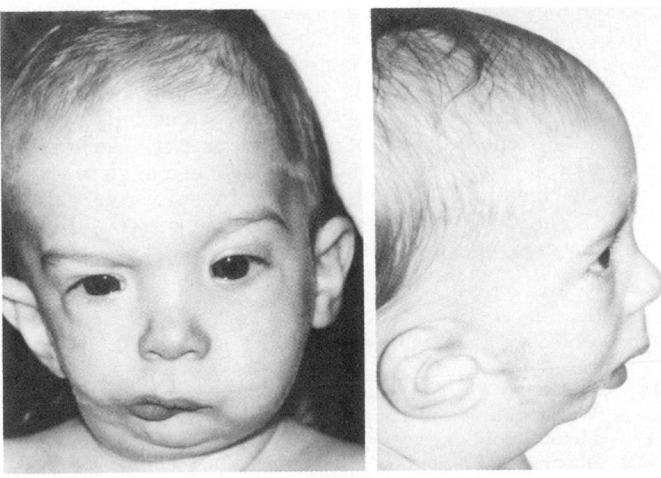

287. Note facial asymmetry secondary to hemifacial microsomia

HEMIHYPERTROPHY

Includes: Hémi-hypertrophie
Hemihipertrofia
Isolated hemihypertrophy
Congenital asymmetry
Unilateral hypertrophy
Hemifacial hypertrophy
Hemigigantism

Excludes: Congenital hemiatrophy
Silver syndrome (887)
Neurofibromatosis (712)
Underlying vascular anomalies
Beckwith-Wiedemann syndrome (104)

Minimal Diagnostic Criteria: Diagnosis is made from evidence of gross body asymmetry (total or partial) which is easily perceptible on external examination. Mild forms of asymmetry are very common, often go unnoticed and are normal variations.†

Clinical Findings: Hemihypertrophy varies considerably in the severity and extent of involvement. External examination may show enlargement of an entire side (total hemihypertrophy) or specific regions of the body (partial or segmental), and occasionally different anatomic areas on both sides of the body (crossed). The hemihypertrophy may affect not only the visible portions of the body (skin, soft tissue and musculoskeletal system), but also the internal organs of the enlarged side. There are no specific laboratory abnormalities and roentgenologic examination may show advanced bone age in the hypertrophied limbs and enlarged viscera (eg kidney on IVP). Approximately 20-30% of the reported cases of hemihypertrophy have hamartomatous lesions (eg pigmented nevi, hemangiomas) or various congenital defects, especially mental retardation and GU anomalies. There is an increased susceptibility to childhood neoplasms of the kidney, adrenal cortex and liver.

Complications
I   **Derived:** Leg-length discrepancy often leads to difficulty in locomotion.
II **Associated:** Predisposition to childhood cancers including Wilms tumor, adrenocortical neoplasms and hepatoblastoma. Medullary sponge kidney and other GU defects may impair renal function. Internal hamartomatous growths can cause liver failure and hemangiomas may rupture.

Etiology: Seven cases have been reported among sibs or successive generations in the maternal line. In addition, 7 other cases have been reported with a variety of chromosomal abnormalities in blood leukocytes or skin fibroblasts (different forms of mosaicism and in one case a pair of elongated No. 16 chromosomes). Most cases studied have had no familial aggregation, chromosomal defect or unusual environmental exposures. It seems likely that the origins of hemihypertrophy are heterogeneous: genic, chromosomal and other factors which are as yet unknown.

Pathogenesis: The nature of hemihypertrophy suggests origins in the very early stages of embryogenesis. The histopathology shows cellular hyperplasia rather than cellular hypertrophy. No metabolic or endocrine defect has been described.

Related Facts
I   **Sex Ratio:** M1:F1
II   **Risk of Occurrence:** 1 in 14,300 births followed to age 6, as reported from the registry of malformations in Birmingham, England.
III **Risk of Recurrence for**
     Patient's Sib: No reliable data, but scattered case reports suggest a slightly increased risk.
     Patient's Child: Possibly slightly increased risk among offspring of affected mothers.

IV **Age of Detectability:** Ordinarily, soon after birth, but severity of asymmetry may increase or diminish with advancing age.
V   **Prevalence:** Uncommon, specific figures not available

Treatment
I   **Primary Prevention:** —
II   **Secondary Prevention:** Orthopedic procedures, such as epiphysiodesis for leg-length asymmetry. Surgical procedures for correction of associated congenital and hamartomatous defects; careful follow-up with periodic examinations through age 6 for early detection of abdominal neoplasia and surgical intervention in appropriate cases.
III **Other Therapy:** —

Prognosis: Average life span, though not affected by hemihypertrophy itself, seems diminished by associated defects such as neoplasia, renal anomalies and hamartomas. Mental retardation occurs in some cases. Limb asymmetry may interfere to some extent with function, and renal anomalies may produce problems.

Detection of Carrier: —

†Special Considerations: Diagnosis from clinical evidence of gross asymmetry between two sides of the body. The condition should be distinguished from 1) hemiatrophy, which shows unilaterally subnormal development, muscle weakness or neurologic deficit; 2) hemihypertrophy secondary to hemangiomatous, lymphangiomatous, or lipomatous malformations; 3) hemihypertrophy associated with primary neurocutaneous disorders or multiple-defect syndromes in which body asymmetry is only one of several major anomalies (eg Silver syndrome and Beckwith-Wiedemann syndrome). Hemihypertrophy shares with the neurocutaneous syndromes and the Beckwith-Wiedemann syndrome a susceptibility to hamartomatous growths and neoplasms, but the origins of hemihypertrophy are much less clearly genetic. One-third of the cases with childhood neoplasms had tumors in a side which was externally unaffected by hemihypertrophy, suggesting that the oncogenic stimulus does not necessarily lateralize to the larger side. Components of this malformation - neoplasia syndrome may be spread over the family tree, as suggested by Meadows et al, reporting a woman with congenital hemihypertrophy who had 3 children with Wilms tumor and a 4th with a urinary tract defect.

References:
Fraumeni, J.F., Jr. et al: Wilms' tumor and congenital hemihypertrophy: Report of five new cases and review of literature. Pediatrics 40:886, 1967.
Meadows, A.T. et al: Wilms' tumor in 3 children of a woman with congenital hemihypertrophy. N. Engl. J. Med. 291:23, 1974.
Pfister, R.C. et al: Congenital asymmetry (hemihypertrophy) and abdominal disease. Radiology 116:686, 1975.
Ringrose, R.E. et al: Hemihypertrophy. Pediatrics 36:434, 1965.

Contributor: **Joseph F. Fraumeni, Jr.**

Editor's Computerized Descriptors: Skel., Skin, CV., GU.

HEMIMELIA AND SCALP-SKULL DEFECTS

Includes: Hemimelie
Absence defect of limbs, scalp and skull
Scalp-skull and limbs, absence defect of

Excludes: Localized absence of skin (608)

Minimal Diagnostic Criteria: Bony abnormalities in hands or feet with scalp and skull defects.†

Clinical Findings: Denuded ulcerated area or areas on the vertex of the scalp present at birth, a bony defect of the skull underlying the scalp defect. The skull and scalp defects usually heal spontaneously in the 1st few months, but in a minority of cases plastic surgery has been required. The limb abnormalities are variable in severity, the fingers and toes may be absent or short and the metacarpals may also be absent. The most severely affected individuals had absent lower limbs below the midcalf and absent fingers. Adams and Oliver (1945) described 8 probable cases in 3 generations of a pedigree.

Complications
I Derived: —
II Associated: —

Etiology: Probably autosomal dominant

Pathogenesis: ?

Related Facts
I   Sex Ratio: M1:F1
II Risk of Occurrence: ? Very uncommon
III Risk of Recurrence for
     Patient's Sib: If autosomal dominant and if 1 parent is affected 1 in 2 (50%) for each offspring to be affected; otherwise not increased
     Patient's Child: 1 in 2
IV Age of Detectability: At birth
V   Prevalence: ?

Treatment
I   Primary Prevention: Genetic counseling when autosomal dominant
II Secondary Prevention: Plastic surgery to scalp if required and appropriate prostheses for limbs
III Other Therapy: —

Prognosis: Normal for life span and intelligence. Variable for function

Detection of Carrier: —

†**Special Considerations:** The skull and scalp defects resemble aplasia cutis congenita which has been reported in families with apparently recessive inheritance.

References:
Adams, F.H. and Oliver, C.D.: Hereditary deformities in man due to arrested development. J. Hered. 36:3, 1945.
Hodgman, J.E. et al: Congenital scalp defects in twin sisters. Am. J. Dis. Child. 110:293, 1965.

Contributor: David C. Siggers

***

Editor's Computerized Descriptors: Skin, Skel.

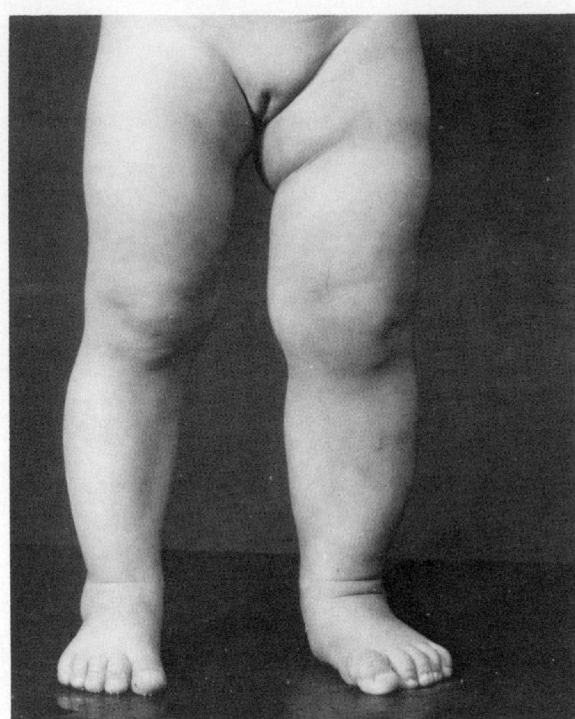

288. Note enlargement of left lower limb

HEMOCHROMATOSIS, IDIOPATHIC

Includes: Hémochromatose, idiopathique
Hämochromatose
Neonatal hemochromatosis
Juvenile hemochromatosis
Adult hemochromatosis
Bronze diabetes
Congenital pigmentary cirrhosis
Iron retention

Excludes: Hemochromatosis acquired from transfusion or high iron diet

Minimal Diagnostic Criteria: Proof of large iron overload is requisite. The desferrioxamine urinary iron excretion test is preferred. Either values over 8 mg/24h or values steadily increasing at 2 or 3 year intervals and associated with normal erythrocyte output and survival while on a normal diet are required.†
Familial involvement, though not prerequisite, is an important support for the diagnosis.

Clinical Findings: After a silent asymptomatic progressive loading of about 15 gm of iron at a rate of 1-5 mg a day, the clinical disease generally becomes evident in the 4th decade (often later and with reduced frequency in females). The clinical onset may be with diabetes mellitus (50%) or one or several of the following:

General weakness	45%
Loss of libido	15%
Variously localized pains mainly hepatalagia	30%
Metallic grey hue or banal bronze tan	90%
(The latter has been usually overlooked)	

Ultimately diabetes mellitus occurs in 60-80% of patients with hemochromatosis and 70% of these become insulin dependent. Endocrine deficiencies are in most instances dependent on pituitary insufficiency, mainly gonadotropic (FSH < 5 mouse units, low 17-ketosteroid urinary output), rarely adrenotropic or thyrotropic. Liver hypertrophic cirrhosis is regularly found, but portal hypertension is uncommon, as is liver cellular failure; functional hepatic tests remain within normal limits for a fairly long period. Cardiac involvement is frequently restricted to ECG findings: low voltage, flattening or inversion of T waves, and partial blocks. Articular pain with or without radiologic chondrocalcinosis is not uncommon.

Hemochromatosis is rarely noted before the age of 35 (90% occur after 35) but it may appear at any age. In early onset cases the rate of iron overloading is faster and the disease is more acute, but involves basically the same organ impairments and the same genetic transmission. The greatest difference is the outstanding severity of the cardiac involvement in children, for which there is no adequate explanation. This is frequently associated with congestive acute asystole. The hormonal involvement is also altered by the age at onset. Primary infantilism is associated with early onset, regressive infantilism with onset at puberty and secondary gonadal atrophy in young men after a period of normal sexual life.

Complications
I **Derived:** Nonspecific cellular insufficiencies ultimately resulting from the siderosclerosis of the various organs including the usual complications of diabetes (when associated with hemochromatosis†), ketonemic or hypoglycemic coma, thought to be due to variations in sensitivity to insulin, and late degenerative sequelae whose frequency is now considered to be comparable to that observed in late onset diabetes, since there is increased longevity of patients with

hemochromatosis. Liver failure (edema, ascites, jaundice) and cirrhosis, with rare visceral hemorrhage due to portal hypertension. Cardiac damage, various types of dysrhythmia (ventricular extrasystoles, paroxysmal auricular or supraventricular tachycardia), acute bouts of pseudopericarditis with prognosis much better than that of terminal congestive failure with biventricular dilatation and anasarca.

II **Associated:** Diabetes mellitus resulting from the coexistence in affected individuals of a familial predisposition to diabetes†, and a low insulin output due to pancreatic siderosclerosis. Hepatoma or cholangioma occurring with even higher frequency than in other types of cirrhosis, independent of correct depletion therapy.

Etiology: Genetically determined autosomal recessive defect. The mutant gene has been hypothesized to be one of the genes involved in the diabetic constitution.

Pathogenesis: The one known constant consequence is progressive iron overloading eventually leading to organ damage presumably through siderosclerosis.

Related Facts
I **Sex Ratio:** M1:F 0.1-0.2 This difference is due to iron loss in females (10-20 gm/lifetime).
II **Risk of Occurrence:** ?
III **Risk of Recurrence for**
    Patient's Sib: 1 in 4, see Table I AR.
    Patient's Child: None, see Table I AR, unless mated to an occasional heterozygous carrier.
IV **Age of Detectability:** Usually around the age of 40 when decompensation occurs. In the sibship of an index case, theoretically the disease may be detected quite early through demonstration of an iron overload which steadily increases at yearly intervals.
V **Prevalence:** ? Rare, but worldwide, with a tendency to be infrequent in areas of prevailing iron deficiency and to concentrate where consanguinity is more common.

Treatment
I **Primary Prevention:** Genetic counseling
II **Secondary Prevention:** Removal of excess body iron through phlebotomies at weekly intervals progressively restores normal color to the skin, liver size and function, frequently improves cardiac condition, usually prevents enhancement of endocrine deficiencies, rarely reduces insulin requirements, and has generally little influence on articular involvement. Once returned to normal, a few venesections a year prevent resumption of iron overload. Desferrioxamine injections are a useful adjuvant, and the sole possible treatment when venesections are contraindicated. Preventive venesection therapy, when started in the latent phase, prevents the organic injuries characteristic of the decompensation period. Corticosteroids and alcoholic beverages should be avoided.
III **Other Therapy:** Supportive treatment for existing organ damage; oral hypoglycemic drugs and insulin in 70% of associated diabetes; testosterone for impotence; usual management of liver cirrhosis with rare indications for portocaval anastomosis.

Prognosis: Altogether different in early and late onset of the disease. It is worse the younger the patient is at clinical onset. Overall life expectancy after diagnosis, initially rather short, was extended to about 5 years after the insulin era, and needs to be reexamined now that sufficient time has elapsed since the introduction of venesection therapy. This is especially true when early diagnosis is achieved in the asymptomatic phase through family studies. Major causes of death may be summarized as: cardiac failure 30%, hepatic coma 15%, hematemeses 15%, hepatoma 15%, diabetic coma 5%.

Detection of Carrier: 25% of heterozygous carriers of the mutant gene have slightly abnormal iron stores, rarely exceeding 3 gm, when on a normal diet. They may be detected by the finding of serum iron and unsaturated iron-binding capacity (UIBC) abnormalities. They may be differentiated from homozygotes by a post desferrioxamine injection with subsequent urinary excretion of iron much less than 4 mg. They tend to be stable with time.

†**Special Considerations:** Ascertainment of a large enough iron overload using desferrioxamine is basic to the differentiation of patients with the disease (homozygotes) from healthy carriers of the mutant gene (heterozygotes). For this purpose neither histology, nor plasma iron study are adequate. Histologic quantitation of iron is frequently misleading, this being particularly the case when the size of the liver is not taken into account. Impressive amounts of iron have been found on the smear coexistent with as little as 2-3 gm of iron excess. Serum iron and UIBC similarly, have proved to be misleading. Their maximum possible alterations are restricted by the actual quantity of circulating transferrin. They are reached at a level of iron overload well below the upper limit found in heterozygotes.

The utilization of histology and the findings in the plasma as criteria for the diagnosis of the disease have contributed greatly to erroneous conclusion of dominant inheritance in idiopathic hemochromatosis.

A study of 72 patients with hemochromatosis designed to reexamine the influence of iron overload on the appearance of diabetes in this disease revealed no compulsory relationship between iron overload and diabetes.

HLA A$_3$ is found in 78.4% of these patients as opposed to 27.0% in controls, HLA B$_{14}$ in 25.5% as opposed to 3.4% in controls.

References:

Balcerzak, S.P. et al: Diabetes mellitus and idiopathic hemochromatosis. Am. J. Med. Sci. 255:53, 1968.

Pollycove, M.: Hemochromatosis. In Stanbury, J.B. et al (eds.): The Metabolic Basis of Inherited Disease, 3rd Ed. New York: McGraw-Hill, 1972, p. 1051.

Saddi, R. and Feingold, J.: Idiopathic haemochromatosis and diabetes mellitus. 1) Rev. Franc. Étud. Clin. Biol. 14:252, 1969. 2) Clin. Genet. 5:242, 1974.

Saddi, R. and Feingold, J.: Idiopathic haemochromatosis: An autosomal recessive disease. 1) Rev. Franc. Étud. Clin. Biol. 14:238, 1969. 2) Clin. Genet. 5:234, 1974.

Saddi, R. and Feingold, J.: Idiopathic haemochromatosis: A genetic approach to the prognosis for children born in hemochromatosic families. In Barltrop, D. and Burland, W.L. (eds.): Glaxo Symposium on Mineral Metabolism in Pediatrics. Oxford: Blackwell Scientific, 1969, p. 153.

Contributors: **Raymond Saddi**
Georges Schapira

Editor's Computerized Descriptors: Skin, Skel., Muscle, CV., GI., Liver, GU., Nerve

HEMOPHILIA A

Includes: Hémophilie A
Hämophilie A
Hemofilia A
AHG deficiency
Factor VIII deficiency
Classic hemophilia
AHF deficiency

Excludes: Von Willebrand disease (996)
Hemophilia B (462)
Plasma thromboplastin antecedent (PTA) deficiency

Minimal Diagnostic Criteria: Assay of Factor VIII activity below 30% of normal. Most severe cases are below 1%. Assay of Factor VIII antigen is normal.

Clinical Findings: Hemorrhage into the tissues after slight or painless injury is often the earliest sign as an infant begins to stand or move about. Ecchymoses are more common than petechiae. The initial manifestation may also be bleeding following a surgical procedure, such as circumcision. Also, uncontrolled bleeding into a bruise, from a torn frenulum of the tongue, or after loss of a deciduous tooth may be the first warning that the child is a "bleeder." Hemorrhage into joints is frequent and can be crippling to severe hemophiliacs (Factor VIII levels less than 1%). On the other hand, milder variants do exist and such individuals may have no bleeding trouble until severe trauma occurs or a serious operation is undertaken.

Complications
I **Derived:** Hemorrhage in and around joints will often lead to permanent limitation of motion, particularly if replacement therapy with Factor VIII-containing blood products is not promptly instituted. Hemorrhages compromising vital areas such as the brain, pharynx, trachea or oropharynx are dangerous, and were often fatal before specific replacement therapy was available and used freely.
II **Associated:** Transfusion-induced hepatitis. 10-20% of patients develop inhibitors to Factor VIII making them unresponsive to therapy.

Etiology: X-linked recessive transmission of decreased Factor VIII activity, through production of an abnormal inactive protein. McK *30670

Pathogenesis: Hemophilia A results from the production of a structurally and functionally abnormal Factor VIII rather than from decreased production of the normal protein. This is inferred from the presence in hemophilic plasma of a protein that reacts with antibodies against purified Factor VIII.

Related Facts
I **Sex Ratio:** M1:F0
II **Risk of Occurrence:** 1 in 2500 live male births
III **Risk of Recurrence for**
   Patient's Sib: If mother is a carrier 1 in 2 (50%) for each brother to be affected and 1 in 2 for each sister to be a carrier.
   Patient's Child: 1 in 1 (100%) for each daughter to be a carrier; not increased for sons unless wife is a carrier.
IV **Age of Detectability:** At birth (Factor VIII does not cross the placenta).
V **Prevalence:** Unknown, but less than the frequency at birth, because risk of death in all age groups is considerably higher than in the unaffected population.

Treatment
I **Primary Prevention:** Genetic counseling
II **Secondary Prevention:** Patients at particularly high risk from trauma or with a clustering of recent hemorrhagic episodes can be protected with regular prophylactic therapy

either daily, every second day or as infrequently as twice a week. The concentrates now available are only effective intravenously. Short-term prophylactic therapy is recommended prior to, and following, surgical and dental procedures. Aspirin often prolongs the bleeding time substantially and should be avoided.

III Other Therapy: Hemorrhagic episodes are treated with a concentrate of Factor VIII obtained from human plasma. Fresh frozen plasma or lyophilized plasma may be used when no concentrate is available. Duration of treatment, interval between treatments and dosage depend on the location and extent of the bleeding as well as on the level of the patient's Factor VIII. These variables are discussed in detail in the references. The average half-life of Factor VIII is about 12 hours. Replacement therapy over a period of days, therefore, requires administration of Factor VIII at 12- or 24- hour intervals. Responsiveness to Factor VIII concentrate can be checked by determining whether a prolonged partial thromboplastin time is corrected.

Most hemorrhagic episodes can be managed without hospitalization. About 10% of patients develop an inhibitor to Factor VIII at some time in the course of their disease, apparently unrelated to the number of treatments previously administered. This results in decreased responsiveness to replacement therapy with human Factor VIII.

Prognosis: The introduction of replacement therapy, with Factor VIII concentrates used more regularly and earlier in the disease, has resulted in a dramatic prolongation of useful and relatively unrestricted, active life.

Detection of Carrier: Female carriers are usually asymptomatic. Their Factor VIII activity is, on the average, intermediate between that of normal and affected individuals. Serial assays of Factor VIII activity in a single individual can vary considerably; occasionally, the status of a prospective carrier is in doubt even after a number of determinations. The ratio of Factor VIII activity to the amount of cross-reacting material to Factor VIII (material reacting with antibodies to purified Factor VIII) will identify a female carrier in about 80% of cases.

Special Considerations: —

References:
Abildgaard, C.F.: Current concepts in the management of hemophilia. Semin. Hematol. 12:223, 1975.
Brinkhous, K.M. and Hemker, H.C. (eds.): Handbook of Hemophilia. Amsterdam: Excerpta Medica, 1975.

Contributors: **Marion A. Koerper**
Louis K. Diamond

Editor's Computerized Descriptor: Skin

HEMOPHILIA B

Includes: Hémophilie B
Hämophilie B
Hemofilia B
Factor IX deficiency
Plasma thromboplastin component (PTC) deficiency
Christmas disease factor deficiency

Excludes: Hemophilia A (461)
Plasma thromboplastin antecedent (PTA) deficiency
Deficiencies of other specific plasma factors

Minimal Diagnostic Criteria: Assay of Factor IX of less than 30% of normal activity. Most clinically recognized cases have less than 5% of normal activity.

Clinical Findings: Manifestations are similar to those of hemophilia A (Factor VIII deficiency), though often somewhat milder. Spontaneous bleeding is rare in patients with more than 1% of normal Factor IX activity and those with over 2% are only mildly affected.

Complications
I Derived: Hemorrhage in and around joints will often lead to permanent limitation of motion, particularly if replacement therapy with Factor IX-containing blood products is not promptly instituted. Hemorrhage compromising vital areas such as the brain or the trachea or oropharynx are dangerous, and were often fatal before specific replacement therapy was available and used freely.
II Associated: Hepatitis due to transfusions of blood products. Inhibitors to Factor IX decrease responsiveness to Factor IX therapy in 10% of patients.

Etiology: X-linked inheritance; McK *30690

Pathogenesis: Some cases of hemophilia B result from production of a structurally or functionally abnormal protein while others result from decreased production of Factor IX.

Related Facts
I Sex Ratio: M1:F0
II Risk of Occurrence: 1 in > 2500 live male births
III Risk of Recurrence for
  Patient's Sib: If mother is a carrier 1 in 2 (50%) for each brother to be affected and 1 in 2 for each sister to be a carrier
  Patient's Child: 1 in 1 (100%) for each daughter to be a carrier; not increased for sons unless wife is a carrier
IV Age of Detectability: At birth (Factor IX does not cross the placenta) for severe cases but not for mild cases since Factor IX level is normally low in the neonate.
V Prevalence: Unknown, but less than the frequency at birth, because risk of death in all age groups is considerably higher than in the unaffected populations.

Treatment
I Primary Prevention: Genetic counseling
II Secondary Prevention: A concentrate of Factors II, VII, IX and X facilitates short-term prophylactic therapy prior to, and following, surgical and dental procedures. Continued prophylactic therapy is possible with administration of concentrate as infrequently as twice a week.
III Other Therapy: Hemorrhagic episodes are treated with a concentrate of Factors II, VII, IX and X obtained from human plasma. Fresh frozen plasma may be used when no concentrate is available. Duration of treatment, interval between treatments, and dosage depend on the location and extent of bleeding (see references). After administration of a dose of concentrate, there is an early phase of rapid disappearance of activity from the bloodstream with a T 1/2 averaging about 5 hours followed after about 22 hours by a slower rate of disappearance with a T 1/2 of about 30 hours. Thus therapeutic levels of Factor IX activity can be maintained with single injections every one or 2 days. Inhibitors

to Factor IX may develop at some time in the course of the disease in about 10% of patients. The result is decreased responsiveness to replacement therapy.

Prognosis: The introduction of replacement therapy with a concentrate of Factors II, VII, IX and X has led to a decreased incidence of chronic damage to joints and to a marked prolongation of useful and active life.

Detection of Carrier: Female carriers are usually asymptomatic. Their Factor IX activity is generally intermediate between that of normal and affected individuals. Serial assays in a single individual can vary considerably; occasionally the status of a prospective carrier remains in doubt even after several determinations.

Special Considerations: —

References:
Abildgaard, C.F.: Current concepts in the management of Hemophilia. Semin. Hematol. 12:223, 1975.
Biggs, R. and Macfarlane, R. G. (eds.): Treatment of Haemophilia and Other Coagulation Disorders. 2nd Ed. Philadelphia:F.A. Davis, 1976.
Brinkhous, K.M. and Hemker, H.C. (eds.): Handbook of Hemophilia. Amsterdam: Excerpta Medica, 1975.

Contributors: **Marion A. Koerper**
Louis K. Diamond

Editor's Computerized Descriptor: Skin

HEPATIC AGENESIS   458-500

463

Includes: Agénésie hépatique
Leberaplasie
Agenesia hepática
Absence of liver

Excludes: Biliary atresia (110)

Minimal Diagnostic Criteria: Complete absence of liver

Clinical Findings: Agenesis of the liver is incompatible with life. This finding has been reported in stillborn fetuses usually in association with other severe anomalies.

Complications
I   **Derived:** —
II   **Associated:** —

Etiology: Failure of development of hepatic bud from foregut; cause unknown.

Pathogenesis: ?

Related Facts
I   **Sex Ratio:** M?:F?
II   **Risk of Occurrence:** ?
III   **Risk of Recurrence for**
     Patient's Sib: ?
     Patient's Child: ?
IV   **Age of Detectability:** In stillborn
V   **Prevalence:** ?

Treatment
I   **Primary Prevention:** —
II   **Secondary Prevention:** Not possible
III   **Other Therapy:** Not possible

Prognosis: Incompatible with life

Detection of Carrier: —

Special Considerations: —

References:
—

Contributors: **Jay L. Grosfeld**
H. William Clatworthy, Jr.

Editor's Computerized Descriptor: Liver

HEPATIC ARTERIAL ANOMALIES

Includes: Anomalies artérielles hépatiques
Anomalien der a. hepatica
Anomaliás de las arterias hepáticas
Aberrant hepatic arterial supply

Excludes: Hepatic venous anomalies (468)
Hepatic hemangiomatosis (466)

Minimal Diagnostic Criteria: Direct visualization either by angiography or at operation.

Clinical Findings: The common hepatic artery arises from the celiac axis and bifurcates into a right and left hepatic artery in the great majority of cases. The right hepatic artery divides into anterior and posterior segmental branches and the left hepatic into the medial and lateral branches to supply their appropriate lobes and segments.

    In 17% of people, the right hepatic artery arises in an aberrant fashion from the superior mesenteric artery. In from 14-23% of cases, the left hepatic artery originates directly from the left gastric artery. The recognition of these aberrant vessels is of great importance during the performance of hepatobiliary or gastric operations.

Complications
I   **Derived:** —
II **Associated:** Injury during operation

Etiology: ?

Pathogenesis: ?

Related Facts
I   **Sex Ratio:** M?:F?
II   **Risk of Occurrence:** ?
III **Risk of Recurrence for**
     Patient's Sib: ?
     Patient's Child: ?
IV **Age of Detectability:** ?
V   **Prevalence:** ?

Treatment
I   **Primary Prevention:** —
II   **Secondary Prevention:** —
III **Other Therapy:** —

Prognosis: ?

Detection of Carrier: —

Special Considerations: —

References:
Michels, N.: The hepatic, cystic and retroduodenal arteries and their relation to the biliary ducts. Ann. Surg. 133:503, 1951.
Michels, N.: Blood Supply and the Anatomy of the Upper Abdominal Organs. Philadelphia:J.B. Lippincott, 1955.

Contributors: **Jay L. Grosfeld**
                H. William Clatworthy, Jr.

Editor's Computerized Descriptor: CV.

HEPATIC CYST, SOLITARY

Includes: Kyste hépatique solitaire
Solitäre Leberzyste
Quiste hepático solitario
Nonparasitic hepatic cyst
Hepatic cyst, unilocular
Liver cyst, solitary but multilocular

Excludes: Liver, hamartoma (604)
Liver, polycystic disease (605)
Parasitic cysts
Choledochal cyst (149)

Minimal Diagnostic Criteria: Mass in right-upper quadrant makes solitary hepatic cyst a possible diagnosis.†

Clinical Findings: Solitary hepatic cysts are unilocular (90%) or multilocular (10%), and are usually located in the anteroinferior margin of the right lobe. While most of these cysts are slow growing and asymptomatic, pain and the presence of a mass are not uncommon findings. Pain may be due to distention of the liver capsule, resulting from torsion of a pedunculated cyst, or hemorrhage into the cyst.†

Complications
I   **Derived:** Torsion of pedunculated tumor, hemorrhage, infection, and rarely, portal hypertension.
II **Associated:** Strangulation due to torsion of a pedunculated lesion, rupture and hemorrhage into the abdominal cavity, and rarely, development of portal hypertension with bleeding varices.

Etiology: True etiology is unknown; however, it is thought that these cysts arise from aberrant bile ducts obstructed by congenital malformation.

Pathogenesis: The solitary hepatic cyst is noncalcific, lined with an inner layer of cuboidal epithelial cells or a dense fibrous layer. The outer layer often contains portions of bile duct remnants. The cyst has low internal tension and fluid that contains albumin, cholesterol, mucin, and epithelial elements. Infection, hemorrhage into and torsion of the cysts may occur.

Related Facts
I   **Sex Ratio:** M1:F4
II   **Risk of Occurrence:** ?
III **Risk of Recurrence for**
     Patient's Sib: ?
     Patient's Child: ?
IV **Age of Detectability:** The majority of these cysts are asymptomatic and usually do not present until the 4th or 5th decade or are incidental findings at necropsy studies.
V   **Prevalence:** ? 1 in 1000 "autopsy material"

Treatment
I   **Primary Prevention:** —
II   **Secondary Prevention:** Simple excision of the cyst is the treatment of choice when possible, with internal drainage as an alternate. Under certain conditions, hepatic lobectomy may be required. Marsupialization should be avoided because of the prolonged and persistent drainage.
III **Other Therapy:** —

Prognosis: Good. Many remain asymptomatic throughout life and are noted only as an autopsy finding. Others are usually amenable to up-to-date operative extirpation. Overall mortality rate due to the cyst is 2.4-5.0%.

Detection of Carrier: —

†Special Considerations: Solitary hepatic cysts (nonparasitic) are rarely observed in childhood where the presence of a mass requires investigation and subsequent diagnosis. Although often asymptomatic throughout life, the cyst is potentially dangerous.

References:

Clark, D.D. et al: Solitary hepatic cysts. Surgery 61:687, 1967.

Henson, S.W., Jr. et al: Benign tumors of the liver. III. Solitary cysts. Surg. Gynecol. Obstet. 103:607, 1956.

Longmire, W.P., Jr.: Hepatic surgery: Trauma, tumors and cysts. Ann. Surg. 161:1, 1965.

Contributors: **Jay L. Grosfeld**
H. William Clatworthy, Jr.

Editor's Computerized Descriptor: Liver

HEPATIC HEMANGIOMATOSIS

Includes: Hémangiomatose hépatique
Hämangiomatose der Leber
Hemangiomatosis hepática
Hepatic infantile hemangioendothelioma
Diffuse capillary or cavernous hemangioma of liver

Excludes: Liver, hamartoma (604)
Solitary hepatic hemangioma

Minimal Diagnostic Criteria: Consider hepatic hemangiomatosis in any infant in the first 6 months of life with hepatomegaly, congestive heart failure, and cutaneous hemangiomas. Confirm with hepatic scintiscan and celiac angiogram.†

Clinical Findings: Hepatic hemangiomatosis of infancy usually presents with the triad of progressive hepatomegaly (100%), congestive heart failure (93%), and multiple cutaneous hemangiomas (86%). These lesions attain their maximum growth rate in the first 6 months of life. Due to their immense size, they may trap platelets causing thrombocytopenia, produce arteriovenous shunting leading to cardiac failure, or may cause symptoms by compressing adjacent viscera. Hepatic hemangiomatosis is a diffuse process usually involving the entire organ. A wide pulse pressure, bounding peripheral pulses, and a systolic bruit and thrill over the liver can usually be observed. Jaundice is rare and ascites has not been observed. Dilutional anemia may be noted as a result of compensatory expansion of plasma volume. Flat-plate and erect abdominal xrays may show an enlarged liver shadow. Hepatic scintiscan will show a large filling defect. Celiac angiogram shows a characteristic arteriovenous blush within the liver with a large celiac axis and hepatic artery. A decrease in the circumference of the abdominal aorta beyond the celiac axis consistent with the diversion of blood flow through the liver is also seen.

Complications
I **Derived:** Thrombocytopenia due to platelet trapping, congestive heart failure due to arteriovenous shunting, hemorrhage due to rupture of hemangioma.
II **Associated:**   Multiple cutaneous hemangiomas

Etiology: These tumors represent a congenital vascular malformation composed of endothelial-lined channels of capillary size and are very cellular. Capillary hemangiomas usually involve the skin, but may be of multicentric origin which helps explain occurrence in the liver.

Pathogenesis: The pathophysiology of hepatic hemangiomatosis includes a wide-open conduit between the hepatic artery and veins. The A-V fistula increases the venous return to the heart, and raises the cardiac output with subsequent increase in right atrial pressure as congestive failure occurs. The severity of the symptoms corresponds to the natural history of the tumor and its growth pattern.

Related Facts
I **Sex Ratio:** M1:F2
II **Risk of Occurrence:**   ?
III **Risk of Recurrence for**
     Patient's Sib: ?
     Patient's Child: ?
IV **Age of Detectability:**   Usually within the first 6 months of life
V **Prevalence:**   ?

Treatment
I **Primary Prevention:** —
II **Secondary Prevention:** Corticosteroid therapy, radiation, and hepatic-artery ligation have all been employed with

some degree of success. Steroids are also useful if thrombocytopenia is present.†

III Other Therapy: Digitalis derivatives and diuretics alone do not improve most infants in failure because of the large A-V shunts.

Prognosis: Mortality is greater than 90% if diuretics or digitalis alone are employed. In all fatal cases, death occurs within 6 months of birth during the rapid growth of the lesion and prior to spontaneous involution.†

Detection of Carrier: —

†Special Considerations: The triad of hepatomegaly, cutaneous hemangiomas, and congestive heart failure in the absence of congenital heart disease strongly suggests the diagnosis. Congestive heart failure develops within 6 weeks of birth in 50% of cases. The failure of digitalis and diuretics in the past makes other avenues of therapy a most important consideration. Since the liver is diffusely involved by hemangioendothelioma, hepatic lobectomy is also an ineffective form of treatment.

Steroids have caused noticeable regression of hemangioma within 2 weeks of therapy. Although the mechanism of steroid therapy is unknown, it is suggested that the rapidly proliferating endothelium in the hemangioma is sensitive to circulating steroids.

Although radiotherapy is a somewhat controversial method of therapy, occasional reports of its effectiveness have been recorded.

Hepatic-artery ligation has been successfully employed when accomplished proximal to the collateral branches so that obliteration of all arterial inflow is prevented.

All of these adjuncts to therapy hopefully are employed to "buy time" until spontaneous involution and shrinkage of the tumor occurs.

References:
DeLorimier, A.A. et al: Hepatic-artery ligation for hepatic hemangiomatosis. N. Engl. J. Med. 277:333, 1967.

Fost, N.C. and Esterly, N.B.: Successful treatment of juvenile hemangiomas with prednisone. J. Pediatr. 72:351, 1968.

Goldberg, S.J. and Fonkalsrud, E.W.: Successful treatment of hepatic hemangioma with corticosteroids. JAMA 208:2473, 1969.

Contributors: **Jay L. Grosfeld**
H. William Clatworthy, Jr.

Editor's Computerized Descriptors: Skin, CV., Liver

HEPATIC LOBES, ACCESSORY

Includes: Lobes hépatiques accessoires
Akzessorisch Leberlappen
Lóbulos hepáticos accesorios
Hepatic lobes anomalous
Accessory hepatic lobes

Excludes: —

Minimal Diagnostic Criteria: Evidence of additional hepatic lobe

Clinical Findings: The lobes of the liver may vary in size and shape with either one being absent, or there may be more than 2. The Reidel lobe is a tongue-like downward projection of liver tissue from the right lobe. This may resemble a large or mobile right kidney and rarely causes concern as a possible hepatic neoplasm.

Accessory lobes are not uncommonly seen in cases of anterior abdominal wall defects (ie omphalocele) where liver tissue may project through the defect.

Complications
I   Derived: —
II Associated: Omphalocele

Etiology: ?

Pathogenesis: ?

Related Facts
I   Sex Ratio: M?:F?
II Risk of Occurrence: ?
III Risk of Recurrence for
     Patient's Sib: ?
     Patient's Child: ?
IV Age of Detectability: ?
V   Prevalence: ?

Treatment
I   Primary Prevention: —
II Secondary Prevention: —
III Other Therapy: —

Prognosis: ?

Detection of Carrier: —

Special Considerations: —

References: —

Contributors: **Jay L. Grosfeld**
H. William Clatworthy, Jr.

Editor's Computerized Descriptors: Hernia not CNS, GI., Liver

HEPATIC VENOUS ANOMALIES

Includes: Anomalie de la veine hépatique
Fehlbildungen der v. hepatica
Anomalía venosa hepática
Preduodenal portal vein
Anterior duodenal portal vein
Portal-vein atresia
Cavernous transformation of portal vein
Total anomalous hepatic venous return

Excludes: Hepatic arterial anomalies (464)
Hepatic hemangiomatosis (466)

Minimal Diagnostic Criteria: See Clinical Findings by type of anomaly.

Clinical Findings: *Preduodenal portal vein* is a rare congenital anomaly that occurs when the embryonic caudal branch persists between 2 primitive vitelline veins while the middle and cephalic branches atrophy placing the portal vein anterior to the pancreas and duodenum. Preduodenal portal vein is of surgical significance since it may readily cause difficulties in operations involving the duodenum and biliary tract. Its presence should be observed and care taken not to divide it inadvertently.

Portal-vein atresia: Excessive obliteration of the fetal umbilical vein and ductus venosus may lead to involvement of the portal vein resulting in atresia or stenosis. The atresia may involve the whole extent of the vein or may be localized to the portion just proximal to its division into its 2 main branches in the porta hepatis.

Cavernous transformation of portal vein: Controversy exists whether this anomaly represented by spongy trabeculated venous lakes involving the portal vein is an angiomatous tumor or a result of portal vein thrombosis with recanalization and compensatory enlargement of collateral capillaries and veins. This is frequently associated with portal hypertension, splenomegaly, and bleeding esophageal varices.

Other hepatic vein anomalies: Rarely, the portal vein may enter directly into the vena cava by-passing the liver or may enter directly into the right atrium. Duplication of the portal vein has been seen, but is quite rare.

In certain cases of total anomalous hepatic venous return, the pulmonary veins may drain directly into the portal vein or the ductus venosus. The pulmonary plexus drains into a common channel closely associated with the esophagus, and pierces the diaphragm entering the portal venous system. Eighty-three percent of these cases occur in male infants.

Complications
I   **Derived:** —
II **Associated:** Biliary atresia, situs inversus, complete bowel rotation, dextrocardia, and most frequently, duodenal atresia or stenosis are associated with preduodenal portal vein. Portal hypertension, splenomegaly, and rarely, variceal hemorrhage may be associated with portal-vein atresia or cavernous transformation of portal vein.

Etiology: ?

Pathogenesis: ?

Related Facts
I   **Sex Ratio:** M?:F?
II **Risk of Occurrence:** ?
III **Risk of Recurrence for**
    Patient's Sib: ?
    Patient's Child: ?
IV **Age of Detectability:** ?

V   **Prevalence:** ?

Treatment
I   **Primary Prevention:** ?
II **Secondary Prevention:** ?
III **Other Therapy:** ?

Prognosis: ?

Detection of Carrier: —

Special Considerations: —

References:
Boles, E.T., Jr. et al: Preduodenal portal vein. Pediatrics 28:805, 1961.
Marks, C.: Developmental basis of the portal venous system. Am. J. Surg. 117:671, 1969.

Contributors: **Jay L. Grosfeld**
H. William Clatworthy, Jr.

———————————

Editor's Computerized Descriptors: CV., Spleen, GI., Liver

HEPATOLENTICULAR DEGENERATION

Includes: Dégénérescence hépato-lenticulaire
Hepatolentikuläre Degeneration
Degeneración hepatolenticular
Wilson disease
Hypoceruloplasminemia
Progressive lenticular degeneration
Ceruloplasmin deficiency
Copper retention
Inherited copper toxicosis

Excludes: Cerebro-hepato-renal syndrome (139)

Minimal Diagnostic Criteria: In an asymptomatic patient, a persistently lowered serum concentration of ceruloplasmin (< 20 mg%) and elevation of the hepatic concentration of copper (> 250 mcgs/g dry liver) are required. Transient deficiency of ceruloplasmin occurs in the normal neonate and in patients with sprue, malabsorption, protein-losing enteropathy, nephrotic syndrome, or severe malnutrition, such as kwashiorkor. Transient, or prolonged, deficiency of ceruloplasmin occurs in about 10% of heterozygous carriers of the disorder. About 2% of patients exhibit a normal concentration of ceruloplasmin (> 20 mg%). Elevation of the hepatic concentration of copper also occurs in the neonatal state and in biliary atresia or biliary cirrhosis. In the last two, however, the concentration of serum ceruloplasm is almost invariably normal.

With neurologic signs and symptoms, the presence of Kayser-Fleischer rings is invariable. The absence of these rings, confirmed by a trained observer using a slit lamp, rules out the diagnosis in such a symptomatic individual.

Clinical Findings: Before the age of 5 or 6 years the patient is almost invariably asymptomatic. Between this age and the 5th decade clinical manifestations occur. Most patients, however, become affected in late childhood or adolescence. The onset is most often apparent as dysfunction of the liver or the CNS, but not infrequently the kidney is involved.

Hepatitis, clinically indistinguishable from the viral disease, or findings of portal obstruction, such as GI hemorrhage or ascites, may appear and disappear with no apparent residua. Hemolytic anemia accompanied by jaundice, may herald the onset.

Neurologic involvement, insidiously appearing, may at first take the form of open-mouthedness, drooling, and dysarthria. Later, or without these, intention or resting tremors, rigidity and difficulty in using arms and legs may supervene. Rarely, convulsions may occur.

Neurotic, psychotic or behavioral disturbances are not infrequent.

Occasionally Kayser-Fleischer rings are discovered incidentally. Abdominal pain, amenorrhea, or thrombocytopenia, leukopenia, or anemia, the last three generally resulting from hypersplenism, may first be seen. Evidence of renal glomerular or tubular dysfunction has indicated the onset in a very few patients.

It is common for the 24 hour urinary copper excretion to exceed 100 mcgs and for the free copper in serum to exceed 10 mcgs%. Other chemical findings - such as hypoalbuminemia, aminoaciduria or hypouricemia - reflect hepatic or renal dysfunction and are, therefore, not often found in patients who are asymptomatic or only minimally ill.

Histologic examination of a liver biopsy may reveal increased fat, pigmentation, and active or inactive cirrhosis.

Complications

I **Derived:** Most commonly any of the consequences of hepatic parenchymal or circulatory dysfunction. Other possible complications are implicit in the clinical findings given above.
II **Associated:** —

Etiology: Autosomal recessive; McK *27790

Pathogenesis: Defective regulation of copper balance, which is accompanied by persistent hypoceruloplasminemia, leads to a net positive copper balance possibly due to decreased biliary excretion of this metal. The excess copper, deposited in liver, brain and eyes—as well as in almost every other organ and tissue in the body—results in damage and the characteristic pathologic findings.

Related Facts
I **Sex Ratio:** M1:F1
II **Risk of Occurrence:** 1 in 200,000 (approximate) live births in the general world population
III **Risk of Recurrence for**
  Patient's Sib: 1 in 4 (25%) for each offspring to be affected
  Patient's Child: Not increased unless mate is a carrier or homozygote
IV **Age of Detectability:** From 6 months on
V **Prevalence:** About 1 in 200,000 in the general world population

Treatment
I **Primary Prevention:** Genetic counseling
II **Secondary Prevention:** Individuals with a persistent deficiency of ceruloplasmin and an elevated hepatic copper concentration, with or without histologic damage, should receive lifelong decopperizing therapy. This consists of the administration of about 1 gm of D-penicillamine (Cuprimine R) daily in 4 divided doses on an empty stomach together with pyridoxine, 25 mgs/daily. Avoidance of foods rich in copper (liver, mushrooms, chocolate, nuts, and shellfish) is possibly of additional value. Periodic analyses of a 24-hour collection of urine for copper should be made so that the dose of penicillamine can be adjusted to keep the daily output of copper close to 1.0 mg or more. Penicillamine may induce various forms of toxicity, some fatal.†
  Treatment of the clinically affected individual is the same as prophylaxis except that the improvement of clinical manifestations, or the lack of it, may also serve as a guide to dosage of penicillamine.
III **Other Therapy:** Physical, speech and psychotherapy are occasionally very helpful. Nonspecific treatment of liver disease is useful as indicated.

Prognosis: Based on observations in individual patients for close to 20 years, it may be possible to delay indefinitely the onset of clinical disease by continued prophylactic treatment.
  Clinical improvement can generally be expected with treatment. Neurologic improvement is most frequent and marked; and improvement in hepatic disturbance and of the psychiatric disorders also occurs. Discontinuance of therapy is generally followed by a relapse, hepatic or neurologic, within 1-3 months.

Detection of Carrier: Heterozygous individuals are clinically normal though roughly 10% may show moderate decrease in serum ceruloplasmin concentration and moderate increase of hepatic copper concentration (to about 100 mcgs/g of dry liver).
  Various abnormalities in the metabolism of administered radioactive ^{64}Cu have been used to detect the carrier state.
  Unfortunately even the best of these tests leaves a fair number of individuals unclassified with respect to their heterozygosity or homozygosity.

†**Special Considerations:** Surgery in treated patients must be undertaken with awareness of the effects of penicillamine on wound-healing.

References:
Bergsma, D. (ed.): Wilson's Disease. Birth Defects: Orig. Art. Ser., vol. IV, no. 2. New York:The National Foundation-March of Dimes, 1968.

Scheinberg, I.H. and Sternlieb, I.: Wilson's disease. Annu. Rev. Med. 16:119, 1965.

Sternlieb, I. et al: Detection of heterozygous carrier of Wilson's disease gene. J. Clin. Invest. 40:707, 1961.

Sternlieb, I. and Scheinberg, I. H.: Penicillamine therapy for hepatolenticular degeneration. JAMA 189:748, 1964.

Sternlieb, I.: Prevention of Wilson's disease in asymptomatic patients. N. Engl. J. Med. 278:352, 1968.

Tauxe, W.N. et al: Radiocopper studies in patients with Wilson's disease and their relatives. Am. J. Med. 41:375, 1966.

Walshe, J.M.: Wilson's disease: A review. In Peisach, J. et al (eds.): Biochemistry of Copper. New York:Academic Press, 1966, p. 475.

Contributor: **I. Herbert Scheinberg**

Editor's Computerized Descriptors: Eye, Face, Oral, Speech, GI., Liver, GU., Nerve
Also see Section I, Figs. 57, 58

HERRMANN-OPITZ ARTHROGRYPOSIS SYNDROME

Includes: Síndrome de artrogriposis de Herrmann-Opitz
VSR syndrome

Excludes: Other arthrogryposis syndromes

Minimal Diagnostic Criteria: Appropriate skeletal findings in multiple areas (craniofacial, skeleton, limbs, vertebrae) and congenital joint contractures.

Clinical Findings: The syndrome represents a generalized bone dysplasia manifested by congenital joint contractures. The 3 reported affected persons showed: shortness of stature, mesomelic shortness of upper limbs, rhizomelic shortness of lower limbs, craniofacial dysostosis (with trigonocephaly, prominent zygomatic bones, broad maxillary and mandibular bones and cleft palate), costovertebral anomalies (inluding scoliosis, sagittal cleft of vertebral bodies, broad ribs) and flexion contractures at the elbow, wrist, finger and ankle joints. Intelligence was normal.

Complications
I   **Derived:**   Limitation of movements including intrauterine activity; cutaneous dimples and dislocations at contracted joints; abnormal flexion creases; respiratory infections due to decreased mobility of chest.
II   **Associated:**   Postterm delivery; inguinal hernia

Etiology: Apparently autosomal dominant

Pathogenesis: Many of the clinical manifestations can be related to a primary skeletal abnormality (of unknown type) of a generalized nature.

Related Facts
I   **Sex Ratio:**   Presumably M1:F1
II   **Risk of Occurrence:**   Small
III   **Risk of Recurrence for**
   Patient's Sib: If parent is affected 1 in 2 (50%) for each offspring to be affected; otherwise not increased
   Patient's Child: 1 in 2
IV   **Age of Detectability:**   At birth. Prenatal diagnosis is perhaps possible, but has not been attempted.
V   **Prevalence:**   Apparently rare

Treatment
I   **Primary Prevention:**   Genetic counseling
II   **Secondary Prevention:**   Intensive orthopedic treatment including multiple surgical procedures to correct contractures; cleft palate repair.
III   **Other Therapy:**   Supportive care for neonatal feeding and respiratory infections.

Prognosis: Good. Adequate recovery of joint mobility is possible.

Detection of Carrier: —

Special Considerations: —

References:
Herrmann, J. and Opitz, J.M.: The VSR syndrome. In Bergsma, D. (ed.): Skeletal Dysplasias, Birth Defects: Orig. Art. Ser., vol. X, no. 9. Miami: Symposia Specialists for The National Foundation-March of Dimes, 1974, p. 227.

Contributor: **Jürgen Herrmann**

Editor's Computerized Descriptors: Face, Oral, Skin, Skel., Resp.

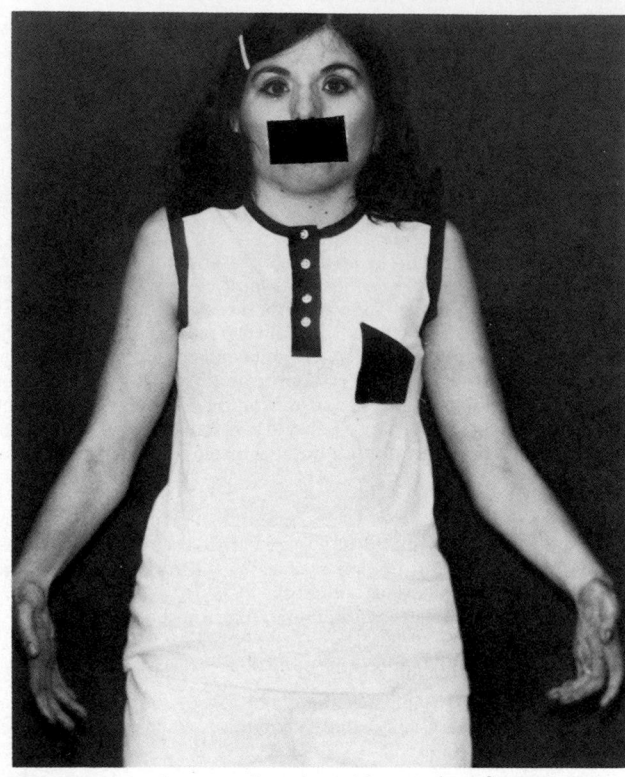

289. Note broad zygomatic and nasal bones; short forearms; arthrogryposis of shoulder, elbow, and finger joints with secondary muscular atrophy

HIATUS HERNIA

Includes: Hernie hiatale
Hiatushernie
Hernia hiatal
Esophageal hiatus hernia
Diaphragmatic esophageal hiatus hernia
Most instances of "short esophagus"
Most children with distal esophageal webs or strictures
Most persistent gastroesophageal reflux

Excludes: Self-limited reflux of chalasia and the very rare congenitally short esophagus

Minimal Diagnostic Criteria: Persistent vomiting beyond 4 weeks of age associated with failure to thrive would suggest pathology at the gastroesophageal junction. While it may be difficult to demonstrate gastroesophageal reflux radiographically in some children, it is much more difficult to demonstrate actual herniation of the stomach above the diaphragm, and this is the only absolute diagnostic criteria.

Clinical Findings: Persistent regurgitation or vomiting immediately after feeding, especially upon assuming the supine position is characteristic of hiatus hernia with gastroesophageal reflux. After the age of 1 month, this symptom requires further investigation. Recurrent pneumonitis believed due to aspiration, weight loss or failure to thrive, unexplained anemia, or the finding of esophageal stricture due to peptic esophagitis, all suggest the presence of hiatus hernia with gastroesophageal reflux.

Complications
I   **Derived:** Because of the frequent and easy vomiting of food, failure to thrive or actual weight loss is probably the most prominent complication. Aspiration pneumonitis is a frequent problem which calls the attention of the physician to the possibility of hiatus hernia and reflux. The sequelae of reflux esophagitis, bleeding and stricture formation, often are the first clues to the malformation. In the very young child the pain associated with esophagitis may go unnoticed until stricture formation has occurred. GI bleeding may similarly be of such a slow nature as to be barely detectable, particularly if the child is on an iron preparation.
II **Associated:** Cahill, Aberdeen and Waterston suggest there are commonly associated anomalies with hiatus hernia - mental retardation, pyloric stenosis and contortion of the neck being the most common. Leape and Holder do not feel there are any particular associated malformations.

Etiology: Unknown, although presumably laxity in the esophageal hiatus along with laxity in the phrenoesophageal membrane lead to displacement of the gastroesophageal junction above the diaphragm and therefore reflux.

Pathogenesis: A structural defect exists at the esophageal hiatus. Because of the sling arrangement of the 2 arms of the right crus, their contraction with inspiration serves as a "pinchcock" mechanism to prevent reflux during the period of negative intrathoracic pressure. The angle of His has been suggested by some to be of significance in maintaining integrity of the gastroesophageal junction and prevention of reflux, although this mechanism certainly is controversial. The role of the phrenoesophageal ligament in keeping the gastroesophageal junction below the diaphragm is likewise a matter of controversy. It has been shown, however, that in the presence of herniation of the stomach up into the chest, the phrenoesophageal ligament serves as a means of opening the gastroesophageal junction thereby producing easy reflux. This is, of course, related to the presence of the physiologic sphincter at the distal end of the esophagus and thus its placement up into the chest favors reflux.

Related Facts

I   Sex Ratio: M1:F1
II Risk of Occurrence: ?
III Risk of Recurrence for
        Patient's Sib: ?
        Patient's Child: ?
IV Age of Detectability: After about 1 month of age
V   Prevalence: —

Treatment
I   Primary Prevention: —
II Secondary Prevention: Reestablishment of the gastroeso-phageal junction below the diaphragm by one means or an-other, thereby enhancing the action of the physiologic distal esophageal sphincter, aided by the constantly positive in-traabdominal pressure. The restoration of the angle of His by fundoplication procedures is probably of value. Only a small proportion of patients with esophageal hiatus hernia come to operation. Most can be treated satisfactorily with thickened feedings and positioning in a "chalasia chair" fol-lowing eating until such time as gastroesophageal reflux subsides spontaneously. Many feel congenital hiatus hernia will resolve as does the umbilical hernia, and thus preven-tion of complications during this time is the aim of treat-ment. These children should be followed closely. If a hernia is demonstrated and there is evidence of esophagitis, the hernia should be repaired. Lack of response to nonoperative therapy and failure to gain are also indications for repair.†
III Other Therapy: —

Prognosis: The prognosis for unoperated patients is difficult to predict. In our series of 35 patients with gastroesophageal reflux treated over a 3-year period by fundoplication, only 1 has had recurrence of reflux.

Detection of Carrier: —

†Special Considerations: While some people have felt that hiatus hernia in childhood is not a congenital anomaly but is associated with a congenitally short esophagus, this, in all probability, is not the case. That a congenitally short esophagus does exist has been demonstrated by Barrett, but it is extremely rare, and most of the short esophagi associated with hiatus hernia are due to cicatricial shorten-ing from reflux esophagitis. Muscle spasm from esophagitis also will accentuate any tendency toward shortening of the esophagus.

Perhaps the respiratory complications of gastroeso-phageal reflux associated with hiatus hernia are the most feared of complications. Sudden death may follow laryngos-pasm due to reflux, or chronic respiratory disorders may produce long-term disability. With the excellent outlook of fundoplication in the child and the low morbidity of surgi-cal repair more emphasis is being placed upon early correc-tion and prevention of long-term or fatal complications.

References:
Belsey, R.: The pulmonary complications of oesophageal disease. Br. J. Dis. Chest 54:342, 1960.
Cahill, J.L. et al: Results of surgical treatment of esophageal hiatal hernia in infancy and childhood. Surgery 66:596, 1969.

Contributors: **Thomas M. Holder**
Keith W. Ashcraft

Editor's Computerized Descriptors: Resp., GI.

HISTIDINEMIA

Includes: Histidinémie
Histidinämie
Histidine metabolism disturbance
Disturbance of histidine metabolism

Excludes: Histidinuria of pregnancy
Phenylketonuria (808)

Minimal Diagnostic Criteria: Minimal biochemical findings should consist of persistent histidinemia with values above 6 mg/100 ml.

Clinical Findings: Emotional instability, tremor of hands, behavioral disturbances, scholastic failure, mild degree of retardation and speech impairment are relatively common. A gross degree of mental retardation is uncommon. The biochemical aberrations can also be found in otherwise healthy looking people. Laboratory findings include: posi-tive urinary tests with ferric chloride or Phenistix. In-creased concentration of histidine in plasma; values are generally above 6 mg/100 ml. Increased urinary output of histidine exceeding twice that of normal for comparable age.

Exaggerated response to an orally administered loading dose of 150 mg L-histidine per kg of body weight. The plasma peak at about 2 hours after ingestion of the dose should rise to values, about or generally above 15 mg/100 ml. The return to the baseline is generally delayed beyond the normal 6 hours after the administration of the dose.

Absence of histidase activity in the liver and also in the stratum corneum. Additional laboratory findings are: a) persistently low glutamic acid and high α-alanine in biologic fluids, and b) the presence of imidazolepyruvic, imidazolelactic and imidazoleacetic acids in the urine of the patients as shown by paper chromatography.

Complications
I   Derived: Scholastic failure, emotional and behavior prob-lems, speech impairment, mild or moderate degree of mental retardation.†
II Associated: —

Etiology: Autosomal recessive enzyme defect. Heterogeneity ex-ists.† McK *23580

Pathogenesis: The lack of histidase activity causes histidine to be pushed through the subsidiary pathway of transamination or deaminization to form imidazolepyruvic acid. The latter may then be reduced to imidazolelactic acid or converted to imidazoleacetic acid by decarboxylation. Imidazolepyruvic acid, similar to the products of many subsidiary pathways, appears in abundance in urine.†

Related Facts
I   Sex Ratio: M1:F2 (not yet explained)
II Risk of Occurrence: ?
III Risk of Recurrence for
        Patient's Sib: 1 in 4 (25%) for each offspring to be affected
        Patient's Child: Not increased, unless mate is carrier or homozygote
IV Age of Detectability: First week of life by blood histidine test or a histidase test of stratum corneum. Screening of the newborns for histidinemia is required by law in New York State since 1974.
V   Prevalence: ? 1 in 12,000 births, similar to phenylketonuria.

Treatment
I   Primary Prevention: Genetic counseling
II Secondary Prevention: Dietary treatment is in experimen-tal stages.
III Other Therapy: —

Prognosis: Normal life span

Detection of Carrier: LaDu's enzymic technique carried out on stratum corneum will identify the heterozygote. Stratum corneum can be conveniently obtained from the cuticles, the heel of the foot and the toes. Administration of a loading dose of 150 mg/kg of histidine may also help to identify the carrier.

†**Special Considerations:** The relationship of biochemical anomaly to speech or mental retardation has not been clarified.

References:
Auerback, V.H. et al: Histidinemia: Direct demonstration of absent histidine activity in liver and further observations on the histidinemia disorder. In Nyhan, W.L. (ed.): Amino Acid Metabolism and Genetic Variation. New York:McGraw-Hill, 1967, p. 145.

Ghadimi, H: Histidinemia: Emerging clinical picture. In Nyhan, W.L. (ed.): Heritable Disorders of Amino Acid Metabolism: Patterns of Clinical Expression and Genetic Variation. New York:John Wiley & Sons, 1974, p. 265

Zannoni, V. G. and LaDu, B. N.: Determination of histidine, alphadeaminase in human stratum corneum and its absence in histidinaemia. Biochem. J. 88:160, 1963.

Contributor: **H. Ghadimi**

Editor's Computerized Descriptors: Speech, Nerve

HOLOPROSENCEPHALY

Includes: Holoprosencéphalie
Holoprosenzephalie
Holoprosencefalia
Arhinencephaly

Excludes: Lip, median cleft of upper (595)

Minimal Diagnostic Criteria: Bilateral cleft lip, hypotelorism and psychomotor retardation strongly suggest the diagnosis. Absence of the philtrum is helpful. The demonstration of diffuse posterior transillumination or pneumocephalic evidence of prosencephalic disorganization establishes the diagnosis.†

Clinical Findings: Bilateral cleft lip, usually with absent philtrum. Hypotelorism with interorbital ridge distance <1.0 cm. Severe psychomotor retardation and seizures. Wide temperature fluctuations. Increased posterior transillumination is common. Pneumoencephalogram shows variable malformations of the prosencephalon, from absence of the corpus callosum to a large single fused ventricle. Those patients with holoprosencephaly due to 13-15 trisomy have associated polydactyly or syndactyly, colobomas, severe cardiac and GI defects.

Complications
I **Derived:** Six patients have been reported with autopsy or in vivo evidence of ACTH - adrenal axis failure. Two patients have had pitressin-responsive diabetes insipidus. No cases of thyrotropin or growth hormone deficiency have been recognized.
II **Associated:** Those patients with 13-15 trisomy have the extracranial anomalies of that syndrome.

Etiology: Approximately half of the reported cases where data are available are due to chromosome 13-15 trisomy. The etiology of the rest of the cases is unknown. Six instances of familial occurrence have been reported, but no demonstrable mode of genetic transmission has been proven. McK *23610

Pathogenesis: The basis of the cerebral defect in this disorder is a failure of evagination of the secondary telencephalic vesicles and a failure of cleavage of the prosencephalon. This results in an absence of the olfactory bulbs. However, the remainder of the formations of the rhinencephalon are present but hypoplastic. Since the differentiation of the forebrain and face is induced by the precordial mesoderm, the severity of the anomalies of the face and brain usually, but not always, correlate.

Related Facts
I **Sex Ratio:** M1:F2 in reported cases
II **Risk of Occurrence:** ?
III **Risk of Recurrence for**
   Patient's Sib: ?
   Patient's Child: ?
IV **Age of Detectability:** At birth by inspection
V **Prevalence:** ?

Treatment
I **Primary Prevention:** ?
II **Secondary Prevention:** ?
III **Other Therapy:** Treatment of seizures. Detection and treatment of hormonal deficiencies.

Prognosis: Most patients have died before 6 months of age. Survival beyond 1 year is rare.

Detection of Carrier: ?

†**Special Considerations:** The clinical picture of holoprosencephaly can be viewed as part of a spectrum of facial anomalies including cyclopia, ethmocephaly and cebocephaly. They all share similar cerebral malformations.

The patient with holoprosencephaly due to chromosome 13-15 trisomy can usually be identified before karyotype analysis because of the extracephalic malformations which are rarely found in patients with holoprosencephaly and normal chromosomes.

References:
Cohen, M.M., Jr.: Holoprosencephaly revisited. Am. J. Dis. Child. 127:597, 1974.
DeMyer, W. et al: The face predicts the brain: Diagnostic significance of median facial anomalies for holoprosencephaly (arhinencephaly). Pediatrics 34:256, 1964.
Godeano, D. et al: Familial holoprosencephaly with median cleft lip. J. Genet. Hum. 21:223, 1973.
Hintz, R.L. et al: Familial holoprosencephaly with endocrine dysgenesis. J. Pediatr. 72:81, 1968.

Contributor: **Raymond L. Hintz**

Editor's Computerized Descriptors: Eye, Face, Nerve

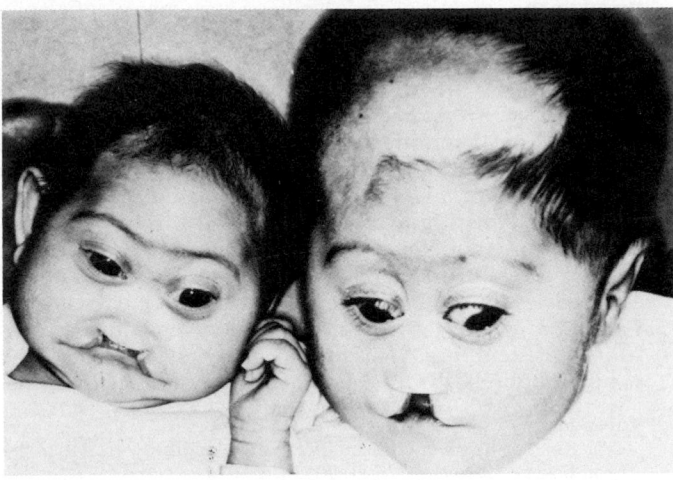

290. Note premaxillary agenesis and ocular hypotelorism

HOMOCYSTINURIA

Includes: Homozystinurie
Homocistinuria
Cystathionine synthase deficiency

Excludes: —

Minimal Diagnostic Criteria: Persistent urinary excretion of homocystine, with elevated plasma concentrations of homocystine and methionine.†

Clinical Findings: Almost all untreated patients have abnormalities of the skeletal system that are detectable visually or roentgenologically. These include genu valgum, pes cavus, pectus excavatum or carinatum, scoliosis, kyphosis, dolichostenomelia, and crowding and irregular alignment of the teeth. Osteoporosis is common, and fractures are frequent. Restricted mobility of joints may occur.

Ectopia lentis is present in the great majority of patients who survive into the 2nd decade. This leads to such complications as myopia, optic atrophy, retinal detachment, and glaucoma.

The cardinal circulatory feature is thrombosis. Occlusion of the coronary, carotid and renal arteries, lesser arteries and veins, and generalized venous thrombosis, may cause hemiplegia, renal hypertension or early death.

Half to two-thirds of untreated patients have some degree of mental retardation usually of mild or moderate degree. A malar flush or livido reticularis may be present but abnormalities of the skin are frequently absent.

The roentgenologic findings are those expected for the characteristic skeletal abnormalities. The EEG usually shows an abnormal pattern, particularly in patients who have suffered cerebrovascular thromboses.

Biochemical studies show elevations in plasma concentrations of methionine, homocysteine, homocystine, and the mixed disulfide of cysteine and homocysteine. Fasting plasma methionine concentrations in untreated patients range from 5 to 100 times the upper limit of normal (30 μ moles/ml), while concentrations of homocystine (undetectable in normal plasma) range from 50 to 200 μmoles/ml. Plasma cystine concentrations are markedly decreased.†

Homocysteine, homocystine, and the mixed disulfide of cysteine and homocysteine are routinely present in the urine. The daily excretion of homocystine in the urine may exceed 1 mM (268 mg). In addition, smaller amounts of methionine, and of a number of unusual amino acids derived from homocysteine (including S-adenosylhomocysteine, 5-amino-4-imidazolecarboxamide-5'-S-homocysteinylriboside, α-hydroxy-γ-mercaptobutyrate-homocysteine disulfide, and homolanthionine) are present in the urine.†

Genetic heterogeneity is indicated by the fact that about half of all patients respond to large doses of pyridoxine (B$_6$) with marked decreases in concentrations of homocystine in body fluids, while biochemical abnormalities are unchanged by pyridoxine therapy in the remainder of patients.

Complications
I   **Derived:** Mental retardation in one-half to two-thirds of cases; skeletal malformations and progressive ectopia lentis in almost all cases; intravascular thromboses, from minor to lethal, occurring at any time from infancy to the 5th decade of life.
II **Associated:** —

Etiology: Autosomal recessive. There is more than one genetic variant.† McK *23620

Pathogenesis: Deficiency of cystathionine synthase in liver, brain or cultured fibroblasts, cultured lymphocytes.

Related Facts

I Sex Ratio: M1:F1

II Risk of Occurrence: Much lower than that for phenylketonuria

III Risk of Recurrence for
  Patient's Sib: 1 in 4 (25%) for each offspring to be affected
  Patient's Child: Not increased unless mate is carrier or homozygote

IV Age of Detectability: Can be detected within 48 to 96 hours of birth by identification of homocystine in urine, or by measurement of elevated methionine concentration in blood.

V Prevalence: Uncertain for North American and European populations, but probably less than 1 in 100,000 population. Prevalence higher in Ireland, and among persons of Irish ancestry.

Treatment

I Primary Prevention: Genetic counseling

II Secondary Prevention: The approximately 50% of patients who have the B6- responsive form of cystathionine synthase deficiency should be treated with pyridoxine in amounts (up to 1000 mg orally per day) which minimize homocystine levels in plasma. This treatment, started early in infancy, and continued indefinitely, can prevent all manifestations of the disease. Patients whose disorder fails to respond to pyridoxine, should be placed on a low methionine diet with supplemental L-cystine. If started in infancy and pursued vigorously, this diet is effective in minimizing the skeletal malformations and eye changes, and in preventing mental retardation. If started later in childhood, the same treatment is valuable in preventing intravascular thromboses.†

III Other Therapy: Trauma and unnecessary surgery should be carefully avoided to decrease the likelihood of thromboses. Dipyridamole and aspirin may be helpful in preventing the platelet aggregations that lead to intravascular thromboses.

Prognosis: Life span markedly reduced due to thrombotic episodes in untreated patients. Life span should be normal in B6-responsive patients, due to the ease of this form of treatment. Life span will probably be reduced in B6-unresponsive patients, since the low methionine diet is difficult to continue indefinitely, and rarely succeeds in reducing plasma homocysteine and homocystine to the normal undetectable levels.

Detection of Carrier: Assay of cystathionine synthase in biopsy specimens of liver obtained from obligate heterozygotes shows enzyme activity about one-half that found in normal subjects. The enzyme can also be assayed in cultured fibroblasts and in phytohemagglutinin-stimulated short-term lymphocyte cultures. Heterozygosity can usually be determined by either of these tissue culture enzyme assays, but there is some overlap between heterozygotes and normal controls.

†Special Considerations: The diagnosis of homocystinuria due to cystathionine synthase deficiency is suggested by a positive cyanide-nitroprusside screening test on urine, or by the finding of an elevated methionine concentration in plasma on unidimensional paper chromatographic screening of blood or serum. Since the cyanide-nitroprusside screening test is also positive in urine of patients with cystinuria and urine of heterozygotes for cystinuria, two-dimensional paper chromatography for amino acids is required on urine specimens that react positively to this test. Detection of homocystine in urine, or the finding of elevated methionine in screening tests of blood, should be followed by automatic amino acid chromatography of fasting plasma. If the methionine concentration is elevated in plasma, and homocystine is present, the diagnosis of homocystinuria due to cystathionine synthase deficiency is established. Repeated careful measurement of

homocystine concentrations in plasma on the amino acid analyzer is essential for monitoring the response of patients to treatment with either pyridoxine or a low methionine diet.

Since homocystinuria may mimic the skeletal features of the Marfan syndrome, and since about 5% of patients with nontraumatic dislocation of the lenses have homocystinuria, the disorder should be searched for in all patients with apparent Marfan syndrome or with dislocated lenses. Additionally, homocystinuria should be ruled out in all infants and children with unexplained thrombotic disease.

In addition to cystathionine synthase deficiency, 3 other genetically determined conditions may give rise to the excretion of homocystine in urine and to the appearance of this amino acid in plasma. In each of these conditions, the remethylation of homocysteine to methionine is impaired. This remethylation pathway fails if 1) there is a defect in the formation of the coenzymatically active vitamin B_{12} derivative methyl-B_{12} from hydroxy-B_{12}, 2) a failure of transport of the vitamin B_{12}-intrinsic factor complex through the intestinal wall, or 3) an enzymatic deficiency of $N^{5,10}$-methylenetetrahydrofolate reductase leading to failure of the normal conversion of $N^{5,10}$-methylenetetrahydrofolate to N^5-methyltetrahydrofolate. Each of these genetic disorders is rarer than cystathionine synthase deficiency. Clinical manifestations do not include dislocated ocular lenses, and skeletal abnormalities and a thromboembolic tendency are mild or absent. Each of the 3 disorders is easily distinguished biochemically from cystathionine synthase deficiency by the presence of normal or decreased levels of methionine in plasma, rather than the elevated levels always present in classic homocystinuria. Treatment with a low methionine diet is harmful and contraindicated in the 3 disorders involving failure of the remethylation pathway from homocysteine to methionine.

References:
Harker, L.A. et al: Homocystinemia: Vascular injury and arterial thrombosis. N. Engl. J. Med. 291:537, 1974.
Mudd, S.H.: Homocystinuria and homocysteine metabolism: Selected aspects. In Nyhan, W.L. (ed.): Heritable Disorders of Amino Acid Metabolism. New York:John Wiley & Sons, 1974, p. 429.
Perry, T.L.: Homocystinuria. In Nyhan, W.L. (ed.): Heritable Disorders of Amino Acid Metabolism. New York:John Wiley & Sons, 1974, p. 395.

Contributor: **Thomas L. Perry**

Editor's Computerized Descriptors: Vision, Eye, Teeth, Skin, Skel., CV., GU., Nerve
Also see Section I, Fig. 61

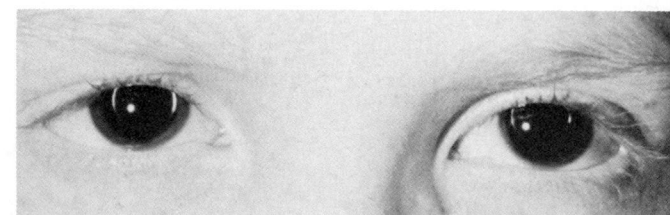

291. Note lens dislocation

HORNER SYNDROME

Includes: Syndrome de Horner
Síndrome de Horner
Congenital Horner syndrome
Oculopupillary syndrome
Oculosympathetic syndrome
Miosis and partial ptosis

Excludes: Acquired Horner syndrome

Minimal Diagnostic Criteria: Miosis and partial ptosis of the affected side

Clinical Findings: The symptom-complex includes on the affected side: miosis, partial ptosis of the upper lid, anhidrosis. The first two components are the most constant. Heterochromia iridis may be a part of the syndrome when the onset occurred before birth or within the first 2 years of life. The findings depend upon the site of interruption of the sympathetic nervous system between the hypothalamus and the orbit. Langham and Weinstein have proposed that pre- and postcervical ganglionic lesions in man can be differentiated by the presence or absence of supersensitivity of the affected eye to adrenergic amines applied topically. The absence of supersensitivity appears to be indicative of a preganglionic lesion of the sympathetic tract. In post-ganglionic lesions, sympathetic denervation supersensitivity of the pupil is due to the inability of the presynaptic endings to reabsorb catecholamines. The pupillary reaction to light and accommodation are maintained but may be diminished.

Complications
I **Derived:** Alteration of tear secretion on the affected side, cataract formation, increase in the amplitude of accommodation, and glaucoma
II **Associated:** Facial hemiatrophy

Etiology: Autosomal dominant. May result from birth trauma, infection or neoplastic lesion. McK *14300

Pathogenesis: Any interruption of the autonomic nervous system from the hypothalamus to the orbit

Related Facts
I **Sex Ratio:** Ml:Fl
II **Risk of Occurrence:** Rare
III **Risk of Recurrence for**
Patient's Sib: When autosomal dominant and if parent is affected, 1 in 2 (50%) for each offspring to be affected; otherwise not increased.
Patient's Child: When autosomal dominant, 1 in 2
IV **Age of Detectability:** At birth
V **Prevalence:** Rare

Treatment
I **Primary Prevention:** Genetic counseling
II **Secondary Prevention:** —
III **Other Therapy:** Early removal of neoplasm if present

Prognosis: Dependent upon associated findings. Early surgical removal of a neoplasm may be lifesaving.

Detection of Carrier: Affected parent and patient

Special Considerations: —

References:
Giles, C. L. and Henderson, J. W.: Horner's syndrome: An analysis of 216 cases. Am. J. Ophthalmol. 46:289, 1958.
Korczyn, A.D.: Denervation supersensitivity in Horner's syndrome. Ophthalmologica 170:313-319, 1975.
Langham, M. E. and Weinstein, G. W.: Horner's syndrome: Ocular supersensitivity to adrenergic amines. Arch. Ophthalmol. 78:462, 1967.
Weinstein, G. W. and Langham, M. E.: Horner's syndrome and glaucoma: Report of a case. Arch. Ophthalmol. 82:483, 1969.

Contributor: **Elsa K. Rahn**

Editor's Computerized Descriptor: Eye

HUMAN ALLOTYPES (MARKERS)

Includes: Allotypes chez l'homme
Menschliche Allotypen
Alotipos humanos (Marcadores)
Gamma globulin (Gm) antigen
Inv antigen type
Gm antigen type

Excludes: —

Minimal Diagnostic Criteria: The presence of Inv (Km), Gm or A2m antigens

Clinical Findings: No clinical symptoms are attributable to the presence or absence of Gm or Inv allotypes, but the Am allotypes may be associated with transfusion reactions.
The Gm antigens are found upon the heavy chains of IgG and the Am antigens are found on the heavy chains of IgA2. The Inv(Km) antigens are found upon the kappa light chains of the immunoglobulin molecules. Because IgG readily crosses the placenta, an individual's Gm and Inv types cannot ordinarily be determined before 6 months of age. IgA on the other hand does not cross the placenta, hence typing may be done in infants.†

Complications
I   **Derived:** —
II **Associated:** —

Etiology: These are normal antigens transmitted as autosomal codominant alleles.†

Pathogenesis: Anti-IgA antibodies may occur as the result of transfusion or of the injection of Ig, possibly also as the result of immunization across the placenta, because of a placental rupture.

Related Facts
I   **Sex Ratio:** M1:F1
II **Risk of Occurrence:** These normal antigens are present in all races but with different frequencies.
III **Risk of Recurrence for**
    Patient's Sib: As for codominant alleles
    Patient's Child: As for codominant alleles
IV **Age of Detectability:** After 6 months of age
V   **Prevalence:** Worldwide distribution

Treatment
I   **Primary Prevention:** —
II **Secondary Prevention:** —
III **Other Therapy:** —

Prognosis: Normal life span

Detection of Carrier: —

†**Special Considerations:** The antigens are inherited in different complexes (haplotypes) in each of the several races of man. Accordingly, they are extensively used for human population studies. They may also, in the hands of experts and with caution, be used for paternity testing and for identification of individuals.

References:
Giblett, E.R.: Genetic markers in the human blood. Oxford: Blackwell Scientific Pub. Ltd., 1969.
Grubb, R.: The genetic markers of human immunoglobulins. New York: Springer-Verlag, 1970.
Steinberg, A.G.: Globulin polymorphisms in man. Annu. Rev. Genet. 3:25, 1969.

Contributor: **Arthur G. Steinberg**

Editor's Computerized Descriptor: —

HUMERORADIAL SYNOSTOSIS

Includes: Synostose huméro-radiale
Humeroradiale Synostose
Sinostosis húmeroradial

Excludes: Radioulnar synostosis (854)
Acrocephalosyndactyly (14)

Minimal Diagnostic Criteria: Radiographic evidence of fusion of humerus and radius

Clinical Findings: Severely reduced or absent flexion and extension at the elbow with radiographic evidence of fusion between the humerus and radius on one or both sides establishes the diagnosis. A number of other abnormalities such as microcephaly, occipital meningocele, coloboma, and microphthalmia have each been found in one case. Although 2 sons of second cousins once removed had elbow abnormalities, both patients had several other abnormalities for which they were not concordant, casting doubt on the conclusion that they had the same genetic syndrome. Humeroradial synostosis may be associated with a number of distinct syndromes of diverse etiology.

Complications
I   **Derived:** Absent motion of elbow
II **Associated:** Not yet certain, see Clinical Findings.

Etiology: Possibly autosomal recessive; McK *23640

Pathogenesis: ?

Related Facts
I   **Sex Ratio:** M1:F1
II **Risk of Occurrence:** Rare
III **Risk of Recurrence for**
    Patient's Sib: ?
    Patient's Child: ?
IV **Age of Detectability:** At birth, by examination and xray
V   **Prevalence:** Rare

Treatment
I   **Primary Prevention:** ?
II **Secondary Prevention:** ?
III **Other Therapy:** —

Prognosis: ? Probably normal for life span depending on associated abnormalities

Detection of Carrier: —

Special Considerations: —

References:
Bagnasco, F.M.: Congenital symmetrical humeroradial synostosis. NY State J. Med. 74:549, 1974.
Keutel, J. et al: Eine wahrscheinlich autosomal recessiv vererbte Skelettmissbildung mit humeroradialsynostose. Humangenetik 9:43, 1970.
Say, B. et al: Humeroradial synostosis, a case report. Humangenetik 19:341, 1973.

Contributor: **Robert A. Norum**

Editor's Computerized Descriptor: Skel.

HUNTINGTON CHOREA

Includes: Chorée de Huntington
Chorea Huntington
Corea de Huntington
Progressive chorea

Excludes: Sydenham chorea
Familial paroxysmal choreal athetosis
Torsion dystonia (957)
Hepatolenticular degeneration (469)
Hallervorden-Spatz syndrome

Minimal Diagnostic Criteria: The age of onset, the progressive chorea and dementia are strongly suggestive of the diagnosis. However, the diagnosis cannot be established unless a positive family history is obtained. There is no specific diagnostic test. However, on pneumoencephalography the atrophy of the caudate may be demonstrable particularly in advanced cases.

Clinical Findings: The cardinal features are chorea and dementia. The choreiform movements are rapid and involve the limbs, trunk and face. The movements are constantly changing and are brought on or exaggerated by attempts at voluntary movement. They are not stereotyped. At times the movements are slower and twisting and some patients have postural deformities suggestive of torsion dystonia.

The gait is clumsy and the patient often makes a shuffling, writhing, twisting movement of the body and arms as he attempts to walk. The speech is likely to be indistinct and the tongue and palate are involved in movement abnormalities.

The dementia appears independently of the movement disorders and in some families dementia is the prominent symptom. In others the dementia appears months or years after the movement disorder has been present. Psychiatric symptoms often are a 1st manifestation of the dementia and emotional instability and paranoia may be the 1st signs of the disturbance in mentation.

The course is inexorably progressive with the disease lasting 10-20 years. The age of onset is usually between ages 35 and 40. However, there are a few cases in childhood and a few cases that first appear after the age of 50 or 60.

There is a form in which the movement disorder is more one of rigidity, similar to what one sees in parkinsonism. This form is more likely to occur in younger children. Some patients with this form subsequently develop the choreic manifestations as the disease progresses.

It should be noted that children often present with mental retardation, seizures and difficulties in speech. The movement disorder is less prominent and a diagnosis in childhood may be dependent on obtaining a family history compatible with autosomal dominant inheritance.

Complications
I **Derived:** In the advanced cases there are complications associated with being bedridden such as ulcerations of skin, pneumonia and urinary tract infections.
II **Associated:** —

Etiology: Autosomal dominant; McK *14310

Pathogenesis: The biochemical defect underlying this disease has not been elucidated. Pathologically, the brunt of the disease is on the basal ganglia and cerebral cortex. The caudate becomes shrunken and demyelinated and has a marked gliosis with a loss of neurons, particularly small ganglion cells. The cerebral cortex may show damage with atrophy and loss of neurons, particularly in the 3rd and 5th layers.

Related Facts

I **Sex Ratio:** M1:F1
II **Risk of Occurrence:** ?
III **Risk of Recurrence for**
Patient's Sib: If parent is affected 1 in 2 (50%) for each offspring to be affected; otherwise not increased
Patient's Child: 1 in 2
IV **Age of Detectability:** Usually 35 and 40 years, rarely in childhood or after 50 years of age. There is no diagnostic test for the disease in patients prior to the appearance of neurologic or psychiatric symptoms.
V **Prevalence:** About 1 in 18,000 as reported in England and Minnesota; 1 in 20,000 in Switzerland; 1 in 25,000 in Michigan but only 1 in 333,000 in Japan.

Treatment
I **Primary Prevention:** Genetic counseling (limited by usual late onset)
II **Secondary Prevention:** There is no satisfactory treatment for this disease. Diazepam has been used to decrease the rigidity and perhaps alter the movement disorder. However, there is nothing that can stop the inexorable progression.
III **Other Therapy:** Supportive measures may prevent some of the longer terms of complications particularly in the bedridden patient.

Prognosis: Inexorable progression with death during 2nd decade following onset.

Detection of Carrier: —

Special Considerations: —

References:
Chandler, J.H. et al: Huntington's chorea in Michigan. Neurology 10:148, 1960.
Vessie, P.R.: On the transmission of Huntington's chorea for 300 years—the Bures family group. J. Nerv. Ment. Dis. 76:553, 1932.

Contributor: **Guy M. McKhann**

Editor's Computerized Descriptors: Speech, Skel., Nerve

HYALOIDEORETINAL DEGENERATION OF WAGNER

Includes: Dégénération hyaloide de la rétine
Hyaloideo-retinale Degeneration von Wagner
Degeneración hialoidea retineana de Wagner
Favre microfibrillary vitreoretinal dystrophy

Excludes: Retinoschisis (871)
Hyaloideotapetoretinal degeneration of the Favre-Goldman type
Pigmented paravenous degeneration

Minimal Diagnostic Criteria: An autosomal dominant vitreoretinal degeneration showing most of the above features.

Clinical Findings: The prominent features of this disease may include: 1) liquefaction and destruction of the vitreous body which may even give the appearance of being almost optically empty on the slit lamp, 2) partial or even total detachment of the vitreous body with thickening of the posterior hyaloid membrane which may have a fenestrated aspect, 3) greyish-white nonvascularized filaments or membranes which often have holes of various sizes and are usually preretinal or retinal in location and generally in the equatorial region, 4) retinal pigmentation particularly in the inferior temporal peripheral retina and often perivascular and in some cases completely ensheathing the vessels, 5) depigmentation of the posterior eyegrounds or in the periphery, 6) sheathing of the peripheral vessels, 7) numerous small shiny white intraretinal spots, 8) major and minor cysts sometimes with a defect in the anterior wall located in the peripheral retina. Retinoschisis is frequently noted in the inferior temporal retina, and 9) localized or diffuse choroidal atrophy especially around the optic disk.

Most patients have moderate myopic astigmatism. Retinal detachment is a frequent complication. Lenticular opacities are common beyond the age of 10. These opacities start as whitish, punctate and streaked densities in the posterior cortex. By the 3rd or 4th decade there is often rapid progression possibly to the extent of necessitating cataract extraction which may be quite difficult because of the liquefied vitreous. Glaucoma is common in patients beyond the age of 30 years and may be associated with iris atrophy and membranous abnormalities of the angle. Functionally, the visual acuity is normal unless reduced by ocular complications; color vision is normal; dark-adaptation is normal; ERG is subnormal; visual fields often show nasal or concentric narrowing. Annular scotomas have been observed in a number of cases. A detachment may affect most of the above parameters.

Complications
I   **Derived:** Cataracts, retinal detachment, glaucoma
II **Associated:** Epicanthus, broad sunken nasal bridge, receding chin, cleft palate, genu valgum, hyperextensible joints, chondrodysplasia. However, those patients with the clefting syndromes may have a distinct disease.

Etiology: Autosomal dominant with almost 100% penetrance; McK *14320

Pathogenesis: It is likely that this condition represents a fairly widespread disturbance of mesodermal development. The occurrence of vitreal and retinal changes, anomalies of the chamber angles, atrophy of the iris, together with cleft palate, genu valgum and facial deformity support this notion. Histologic examination of several eyes has been reported. The preretinal membrane visible in the ophthalmoscope, which is avascular, departs from the equatorial area and extends forward, merging into the hyaloid membrane. The retina, on histologic examination, has shown cystic degeneration, irregular areas of atrophy, and peripheral perivascular accumulations of pigment. The retinal vessels often have thickened walls and the choroid is atrophic.

Related Facts
I   **Sex Ratio:** M1:F1
II   **Risk of Occurrence:** ?
III **Risk of Recurrence for**
     Patient's Sib: If parent is affected, 1 in 2 (50%) for each offspring to be affected; otherwise not increased.
     Patient's Child: 1 in 2
IV   **Age of Detectability:** Generally diagnosed in the 1st decade
V   **Prevalence:** ?

Treatment
I   **Primary Prevention:** Genetic counseling
II   **Secondary Prevention:** —
III **Other Therapy:** Essentially the management of complications. Cataract extraction deferred as long as possible since complications may be anticipated owing to the liquefied vitreous. Superficial diathermy prior to cataract extraction has been advised. When retinoschisis is present, many authors consider that surgical intervention does not carry a good prognosis but, as shown in senile retinoschisis, segmental photocoagulation may cause a disappearance of the abnormality. When a detachment exists, it should be treated first and then a coexisting retinoschisis should be photocoagulated. The glaucoma in these individuals runs a benign course and is relatively easy to treat medically.

Prognosis: Normal life span

Detection of Carrier: —

Special Considerations: —

References:
Alexander, R.L. and Shea, M.: Wagner's disease. Arch. Ophthalmol. 74:310, 1965.
Böhringer, H.R. et al: Zur Klinik und Pathologie der Degeneration hyaloideo-retinalis hereditaria (Wagner). Ophthalmologica 139:330, 1960.
Deutman, A.F.: Vitreoretinal dystrophies. In Krill, A.E. and Archer, D.B. (eds.): Krill's Hereditary and Choroidal Diseases. vol II. Clinical Characteristics. Hagerstown:Harper & Row, 1977.
Brandsen, E.: Hereditary hyaloideo-retinal degeneration (Wagner) in a Danish family. Acta. Ophthalmol. (Kbh.) 44:223 1966.
Hirose, T. et al: Wagner's hereditary vitreoretinal degeneration and retinal detachment. Arch. Ophthalmol. 89:176, 1973.
Klein, D.: Genetic approach to the nosology of retinal disorders. In Bergsma, D. (ed.): Part VIII. Eye. Birth Defects: Orig. Art. Ser., vol. VII, no. 3. Baltimore: Williams & Wilkins for The National Foundation-March of Dimes, 1971, p. 52.

Contributors: **Alex E. Krill‡**
                   Mitchel L. Wolf
                   Donald R. Bergsma

Editor's Computerized Descriptors: Vision, Eye

HYDRANENCEPHALY

Includes: Hydranencéphalie
Hydranenzephalie
Hidranencefalía
Schizencephaly with head enlargement

Excludes: Anencephaly (52)
Hydrocephaly (481)

Minimal Diagnostic Criteria: Diagnosis suggested by transillumination, but since this can occur in extreme hydrocephaly, angiogram or air study becomes diagnostic, showing no cerebral cortex. Angiogram may demonstrate occlusion of the carotid arteries as they enter the cranium.

Clinical Findings: An enlarged head at birth with large fontanel. Skull vault is thin. Neurologic function may be assessed as "normal" with preservation of Moro reflex, rooting and sucking. Poor temperature control, increasing blindness and loss of electrical activity on EEG may be present. Optic fundi show pale disks but optic nerve is present. Normal pupillary light reflex. Head transilluminates. On fontanel tap, cerebrospinal fluid obtained immediately upon puncture of dura. A condition in which the cerebral cortex is absent though skull or cranial meninges are intact. Thalami present. Choroid plexus present. Brain stem and optic nerves intact.

Complications
I   **Derived:**   Progressive head enlargement due to failure of CSF absorption
II   **Associated:**   —

Etiology: ?

Pathogenesis: Evidence is accumulating that hydranencephaly is due to an early fetal obstruction of the carotid vessels as they enter the cranial vault with secondary degeneration of developing cerebral hemispheres. Those structures supplied by the basilar artery are spared including the basal portions of the temporal and occipital lobes, the hippocampi and basal nuclei, brain stem and cerebellum. Hydranencephaly differs from extreme porencephaly by the former's symmetry and absence of ependymal lining of large cystic cavities.

Related Facts
I   **Sex Ratio:**   ?
II   **Risk of Occurrence:**   Rare
III   **Risk of Recurrence for**
   Patient's Sib: ?
   Patient's Child: ?
IV   **Age of Detectability:**   At birth
V   **Prevalence:**   Rare

Treatment
I   **Primary Prevention:**   —
II   **Secondary Prevention:**   Rarely a survivor is reported after shunt operation.
III   **Other Therapy:**   —

Prognosis: Most infants die by age 4 months.

Detection of Carrier: ?

Special Considerations: —

References:
Hamby W.B. et al: Hydranencephaly: Clinical diagnosis; presentation of 7 cases. Pediatrics 6:371, 1950.
Lorber, J.: Hydranencephaly with normal development. Dev. Med. Child. Neurol. 7:628, 1965.

Contributor: Kenneth Shulman

HYDROCEPHALY

Includes: Hydrocéphalie
Hydrozephalie
Hidrocefalía
Hydrocephalus
Stenosis of aqueduct of Sylvius
Dandy-Walker syndrome
Atresia of foramina of Luschka and Magendie
All varieties of extra- and intraventricular congenital obstructive hydrocephaly

Excludes: Acquired hydrocephaly due to tumor, infection
Subarachnoid hemorrhage
Hydranencephaly (480)
Myelomeningocele (693)
Encephalocele (343)
Achondroplasia (10)
Mucopolysaccharidosis I-H (674)

Minimal Diagnostic Criteria: Ventricular dilatation on air study. The various types of hydrocephaly have characteristic air studies.

Clinical Findings: An enlarged head either present at birth (30%) or detected during the first 3 months of life (50%); distended scalp veins; a large tense fontanel; "sunsetting" of pupils. The cerebrospinal fluid is normal as is the EEG. If the cortical mantle is extremely thin (1 cm), transillumination is positive. Pneumoencephalogram, or ventriculogram, shows enlarged ventricles with obstruction of air either within or outside the ventricle.

Complications
I **Derived:** Mental retardation if untreated
II **Associated:** Myelomeningocele, spina bifida cystica, encephalocele, Klippel-Feil syndrome

Etiology: Genetically heterogeneous - autosomal recessive for many cases including patients with atresia of foramina of Luschka and Magendie; X-linked recessive for congenital stenosis of aqueduct of Sylvius; in such instances the aqueduct in its entire length, but most stenotic at inferior portion without ependymitis or gliosis. Holmes et al believe that the syndrome of X-linked hydrocephalus comprises manifestations that are neither obligatory nor pathognomonic and that the entire syndrome represents a genetically nonspecific set of secondary manifestations due to congenital obstructive hydrocephalus. MIM *30000

Pathogenesis: All hydrocephaly is obstructive in that a normal amount of CSF is produced, but cannot be absorbed because of obstruction in the CSF pathways. Intraventricular obstruction occurs at the aqueduct of Sylvius or outlets of 4th ventricle. As fluid accumulates within the ventricle under increased pressure, the ependymal lining is disrupted allowing CSF to pass into the periventricular white matter causing myelin and axonal loss. The ventricles gradually increase in size attendant upon such loss of white matter resulting ultimately in a thin mantle of brain containing chiefly cerebral gray matter.

Related Facts
I **Sex Ratio:** M1:F < 1 in aqueduct stenosis only
II **Risk of Occurrence:** 1 in 2000 live births
III **Risk of Recurrence for**
Patient's Sib: When autosomal recessive see Table 1 AR; when X-linked see Table I X-linked R.
Patient's Child: When autosomal recessive see Table 1 AR; when X-linked see Table I X-linked R.
If hydrocephalic sib or maternal male relative, there is a 25% recurrence rate for each pregnancy and a 50% recurrence rate for each male pregnancy.
IV **Age of Detectability:** At birth: 30%; by first year: 80%
V **Prevalence:** ?

Treatment
I **Primary Prevention:** Genetic counseling
II **Secondary Prevention:** Surgical by-pass (shunt) carrying fluid from head into the vascular system, peritoneum, etc.†
III **Other Therapy:** —

Prognosis: With shunt treatment, 80% of children reach 5 years of age, and 80% of survivors are normal or educable.

Detection of Carrier: ?

†Special Considerations: The acquired varieties of hydrocephaly, ie tumor, infection, subarachnoid hemorrhage or cyst, require direct surgical approach to the obstructing lesion.

References:
Gregory, G.A.: Continuous positive airway pressure and hydrocephalus. Lancet 2:911, 1973.
Holmes, L.B. et al: X-linked aqueductal stenosis. Clinical and neuropathological findings in two families. Pediatrics 51:697, 1973.
Johnson, R. T. and Johnson, K. P.: Hydrocephalus following viral infection: The pathology of aqueductal stenosis developing after experimental mumps virus infection. J. Neuropathol. Exp. Neurol. 27:591, 1968.
Shulman, K.: Workshop in Hydrocephalus. Philadelphia: University of Pennsylvania Press, 1966.
Vert, P. et al: Continuous positive airway pressure and hydrocephalus. Lancet 2:319, 1973.

Contributor: **Kenneth Shulman**

Editor's Computerized Descriptors: Eye, Skin, Skel., Nerve

HYDROXYPROLINEMIA (MARKER)

Includes: Hydroxyprolinémie
Hydroxyprolinämie
Hidroxiprolinemia

Excludes: Disorders of bound hydroxyproline metabolism

Minimal Diagnostic Criteria: Free hydroxyproline concentration in plasma 20-40 times above normal concentration of < 0.01 μmoles/ml. Free hydroxyproline excretion in urine is increased, but other amino acids are normal unless plasma concentration of hydroxyproline exceeds about 0.75 μmoles/ml; at this concentration, proline and glycine will be excreted. Bound hydroxyproline excretion is normal.†

Clinical Findings: A biochemical phenotype. No proven association with clinical disease. Condition reported in 4 probands; consanguinity present in 2 of the 4 pedigrees.

Complications
I   **Derived:** —
II **Associated:** Possibly mental retardation

Etiology: Probably autosomal recessive enzyme defect; McK *23700

Pathogenesis: "Hydroxyproline oxidase" deficiency†

Related Facts
I   **Sex Ratio:** M1:F1
II   **Risk of Occurrence:** Probably very rare
III **Risk of Recurrence for**
     Patient's Sib: Probably 1 in 4 (25%) for each offspring to have the trait.
     Patient's Child: Not increased unless mate is carrier or homozygote
IV   **Age of Detectability:** Presumably detectable in newborn
V   **Prevalence:** Probably very rare

Treatment
I   **Primary Prevention:** —
II   **Secondary Prevention:** None. Protein (gelatin) restriction of no use. Ascorbic acid depletion does not alter hydroxyprolinemia.
III **Other Therapy:** —

Prognosis: ?

Detection of Carrier: ?

†**Special Considerations:** Source of *free* hydroxyproline is apparently normal collagen turnover. Collagen breakdown not abnormal and excretion pattern of bound hydroxyproline is normal. Enzymes controlling metabolism of free hydroxyproline in mammalian tissue proven to be independent of those controlling L-proline biosynthesis and degradation.

References:
Efron, M.L. et al: Hydroxyprolinemia. II. A rare metabolic disease due to a deficiency of the enzyme "hydroxyproline oxidase". N. Engl. J. Med. 272:1299, 1965.
Pelkonen, R. and Kivirikko, K.I.: Hydroxyprolinemia. N. Engl. J. Med. 283:451, 1970.
Scriver, C.R.: Disorders of proline and hydroxyproline metabolism. In Stanbury, J.B. et al (eds.): The Metabolic Basis of Inherited Disease, 4th Ed. New York:McGraw-Hill, 1976.

Contributor: **Charles R. Scriver**

Editor's Computerized Descriptor: —

HYMEN, IMPERFORATE

Includes: Imperforation de l'hymen
Hymen imperforatus
Himen imperforado
Some causes of hydrometrocolpos
Imperforate hymen

Excludes: Müllerian aplasia (682)
Vaginal atresia† (984)
All forms of female pseudohermaphroditism
All forms of male pseudohermaphroditism

Minimal Diagnostic Criteria: Nonpatent hymen in a female (46,XX) with otherwise normal external and internal genitalia.

Clinical Findings: In imperforate hymen the central portion of the hymen fails to develop its usual orifice. The external genitalia, vagina, cervix, uterus, fallopian tubes and ovaries are otherwise normal for females. No somatic anomalies are present.
  As result of absence of the hymenal orifice, mucus or blood may accumulate and, hence, prevent outflow of menstrual fluid. Examination may reveal a bulging hymen, but usually no other abnormalities. Secondary sex development is otherwise normal.

Complications
I   **Derived:** Hydrocolpos or hydrometrocolpos
II **Associated:** Usually none, although theoretically retention of blood could predispose to infection. Distention of uterus could occur theoretically but seems rare.

Etiology: ? In 1 family 3 sibs were affected, but heritable tendencies have not been observed frequently. Not all cases are necessarily congenital; perhaps some occasionally result from inflammatory causes.

Pathogenesis: Most investigators believe that the hymen arises from the urogenital sinus at the site at which the sinovaginal bulbs invaginate to form the caudal portion of the vagina; however, others believe that the hymen is a remnant of the urogenital membrane. Irrespective of origin, the hymen is ordinarily perforated after formation. Absence of perforation produces an imperforate hymen. Alternatively, postnatal inflammatory causes could sometimes lead to occlusion of a previously patent hymen.

Related Facts
I   **Sex Ratio:** F1:M0
II   **Risk of Occurrence:** ? But relatively rare.
III **Risk of Recurrence for**
     Patient's Sib: ? But apparently low.
     Patient's Child: ? But apparently low.
IV   **Age of Detectability:** Usually at puberty because of hydrometrocolpos. Occasionally at birth because of hydrocolpos.
V   **Prevalence:** ? But relatively rare.

Treatment
I   **Primary Prevention:** Cruciform incisions in central portion of hymen.
II   **Secondary Prevention:** —
III **Other Therapy:** —

Prognosis: Normal life span; normal fertility.

Detection of Carrier: —

†**Special Considerations:** Imperforate hymen should be distinguished from vaginal atresia. In the latter the lower portion of the vagina fails to form, and the nonpatent portion is too thick for simple incision.

References:
Jones, H.W., Jr. and Scott, W.M.: Hermaphroditism, Genital Anomalies, and Related Endocrine Disorders, 2nd Ed. Baltimore: Williams & Wilkins, 1971.
McIlroy, D.M. and Ward, I.V.: Three cases of imperforate hymen occurring in one family. Proc. R. Soc. Med. 23:633, 1930.

Contributor: Joe Leigh Simpson

Editor's Computerized Descriptor: GU.

Includes: Hyperaldostéronisme familial suppressible par les glucocorticoïdes
Familiärer Glukokortikoid-supprimierbarer Hyperaldosteronismus
Hiperaldosteronismo
Nontumorous primary aldosteronism

Excludes: Hypertensive forms of congenital adrenal hyperplasia a) 17-hydroxylase deficiency b) 11-hydroxylase deficiency
Primary hyperaldosteronism (Conn syndrome)

Minimal Diagnostic Criteria: These must include hypokalemic alkalosis, hypertension, and hyperaldosteronism which suppress with glucocorticoids in the absence of a known enzyme block in adrenal steroid synthesis.

Clinical Findings: This is a familial disease characterized by hypertension, hypokalemic alkalosis, elevated aldosterone and suppressed renin. Polyuria has been reported. No specific enzyme defect has been identified from analysis of plasma and urinary steroids. Deficiency of 17-hydroxylase is readily excluded by finding normal or intermittently elevated 17-ketosteroids and 17-ketogenic steroids in urine, and 11-hydroxylase deficiency is excluded by the lack of significant quantities of deoxycorticosterone (DOC) and 11-deoxycortisol (Compound-S). Growth and sexual development are normal and reproductive capacity is unimpaired. Patients may present late in life with hypertension as the major finding.

Complications
I   **Derived:** Persistent hypertension may lead to renovascular changes and poor suppression of elevated blood pressure by glucocorticoids. The sequelae of hypokalemia may also be present.
II **Associated:** —

Etiology: This is a familial disease. Limited studies suggest an autosomal dominant or X-linked dominant form of inheritance.

Pathogenesis: The hypertension, hypokalemia and low renin are due to the known effects of aldosterone. Suppressibility by glucocorticoids implies an enzyme defect but none has been hitherto identified.

Related Facts
I   **Sex Ratio:** M1:F1
II   **Risk of Occurrence:** Rare
III **Risk of Recurrence for**
     Patient's Sib: 1 in 2 (50%) if autosomal dominant and if parent affected; negligible if autosomal dominant fresh mutation; 1 in 2 (50%) for both sexes if X-linked dominant and if mother affected; 100% for sisters and zero for brothers if proband a girl, if X-linked dominant, and father affected.
     Patient's Child: 1 in 2 (50%) if autosomal dominant; 1 in 2 for both sexes if X-linked dominant and proband a female; 100% for daughters and zero for sons if X-linked dominant and proband a male.
IV   **Age of Detectability:** May be detected from childhood to adult life.
V   **Prevalence:** ?

Treatment
I   **Primary Prevention:** After the index case is identified, genetic counseling and screening for affected individuals can be performed.
II   **Secondary Prevention:** Treatment with glucocorticoids such as dexamethasone or prednisone reverses all the clinical findings. Several weeks of therapy may be required for reversal of hypertension. Spironolactone may be required in long-standing cases.

III Other Therapy: —

Prognosis: Prognosis is excellent if treated before irreversible renovascular hypertension occurs.

Detection of Carrier: —

Special Considerations: —

References:
Giebink, G.S. et al: A kindred with familial glucocorticoid-suppressible aldosteronism. J. Clin. Endocrinol. Metab. 36:715, 1973.

Contributor: **Mark A. Sperling**

Editor's Computerized Descriptor: CV.

HYPERAMMONEMIA

Includes: Hyperammonémie
Hyperammonämie
Hiperamonemia
Ornithinemia†
Carbamyl phosphate synthetase deficiency†
Ornithine transcarbamylase deficiency

Excludes: Lysine intolerance
Hyperglycinemia
Citrullinemia (174)
Argininemia (86)
Argininosuccinic aciduria (87)
Hyperdibasic-aminoaciduria (491)

Minimal Diagnostic Criteria: Elevated blood ammonia levels, especially after high-protein containing meals. Diagnosis made by liver or intestinal biopsy or peripheral leukocytes with decrease of ornithine transcarbamylase (OTC) with or without decreased carbamyl phosphate synthetase. Urinary glutamine and orotic acid are elevated.

Clinical Findings: At least 20 families have now been described. Most patients are detected before 4 years of age, and, like others with urea cycle defects and ammonia intoxication, have mental and physical retardation, protein intolerance, raised plasma levels of ammonia, glutamine, ornithine, orotic acid, and sometimes alanine. Urinary ammonia and pyrimidine metabolites are increased. Vomiting, lethargy, and coma are associated with elevated plasma ammonia levels. Later, spasticity and cerebral atrophy occur. Almost all the reported children are girls. Four boys with a similar syndrome are considered to be variants, with a milder disease. Eight other boys died in the first 10 days of life. One male neonate, sib of a girl with hyperammonemia, was controlled for 54 days with exchange transfusions, peritoneal dialysis, and essential amino acid supplements with excess aspartate and arginine.

Complications
I **Derived:** Mental retardation, agitation, seizures, stupor, cortical atrophy
II **Associated:** —

Etiology: X-linked dominant; McK *31125, also see *23720, *23730.

Pathogenesis: Defect of liver ornithine transcarbamylase or of liver carbamyl phosphate synthetase.

Related Facts
I **Sex Ratio:** Probably M1:F1. Most males die in early infancy with complete absence of OTC. A few males with variant forms have lived longer. Living females are heterozygous and have partial OTC deficiency.
II **Risk of Occurrence:** Rare
III **Risk of Recurrence for**
　Patient's Sib: If mother is a carrier 1 in 2 (50%). Probably lethal in boys; varying severity of disease in girls.
　Patient's Child: Males have died early; females died early or were X-linked dominant carriers.
IV **Age of Detectability:** At birth
V **Prevalence:** Uncommon

Treatment
I **Primary Prevention:** Genetic counseling
II **Secondary Prevention:** Low-protein, high-carbohydrate diet, and monitor blood ammonia.
III **Other Therapy:** Various agents have been utilized to decrease ammonia intoxication with partial success. These include exchange transfusions, dialysis, mixtures of pyrrolidone carboxylate and arginine, guanidinosuccinate, keto analogs of essential amino acids, and others.

Prognosis: With good monitoring of ammonia levels in heterozygotes, probably reasonably good both for life and mental development. In homozygous boys, prognosis is poor.

Detection of Carrier: Female carriers may be symptomatic or asymptomatic. Levels of OTC are decreased in white cells and liver.

†Special Considerations: A 21-year-old woman and a 1 1/2-year-old boy have been described with mental retardation, seizures, irritability, and abnormal EEG. Both had elevated blood levels of ammonia and ornithine and excreted excessive homocitrulline. Chemical abnormalities decreased when protein intake was decreased, and diet was supplemented with lysine. A defect in ornithine transport into the mitochondria has been suggested.

Six related subjects with similar chemical and clinical findings also developed bleeding tendencies in infancy. They were found to have decreased carbamyl phosphate synthetase I activity and abnormal hepatic mitochondria.

In a study of 22 patients in 15 families with gyrate atrophy of the choroid and retina, plasma levels of ornithine were increased 10- to 20-fold. No other clinical abnormalities were found (Takki).

Three patients have been described with carbamyl phosphate synthetase deficiency. Symptoms were similar to those with other causes of ammonemia and decreased with reduced protein intake. In 1 family, a girl was hospitalized at 20 days of age because of poor feeding, lethargy and convulsions. She was fed a low-protein diet and improved but died at 7 months. Her sister and brother had died at 4 weeks of age following similar symptoms.

In another family with carbamyl phosphate synthetase deficiency, a male infant fed poorly, developed hypertonia, and died at 75 hours. A 13-year-old mentally retarded girl was given keto analogs of essential amino acids with decrease in blood ammonia and decrease in seizures.

References:
Bachman, C.: Urea cycle. In Nyhan, W.L. (ed.): Heritable Disorders of Amino Acid Metabolism. New York: Wiley, 1974, chap. 18.

Batshaw, M. et al: Treatment of carbamyl phosphate synthetase deficiency with keto analogues of essential amino acids. N. Engl. J. Med. 292:1085, 1975.

Fell, V. et al: Ornithinemia, hyperammonemia, and homocitrullinuria. Am. J. Dis. Child. 127:752, 1974.

Gatfield, P.D. et al: Hyperornithinemia, hyperammonemia and homocitrullinuria associated with decreased carbamyl phosphate synthetase I activity. Pediatr. Res. 9:488, 1975.

Gelehrter, T.D. and Snodgrass, P.J.: Lethal neonatal deficiency of carbamyl phosphate synthetase. N. Engl. J. Med. 290:430, 1974.

Hommes, F.A. et al: Carbamyl-phosphate synthetase deficiency in an infant with severe cerebral damage. Arch. Dis. Child. 44:688, 1969.

Shih, V.E. et al; Hyperornithinemia, hyperammonemia, and homocitrullinuria. Am. J. Dis. Child. 117:83, 1969.

Snyderman, S.E. et al: The therapy of hyperammonemia due to ornithine transcarbamylase deficiency in a male infant. Pediatrics 56:65, 1975.

Takki, K.: Gyrate atrophy of the choroid and retina associated with hyperornithinemia. Doctoral Thesis. Department of Ophthalmology and the Children's Hospital, University of Helsinki, Finland, 1975.

Contributor: **Lewis A. Barness**

Editor's Computerized Descriptor: Nerve

HYPERBETA-ALANINEMIA

Includes: Hyper-bêta-alaninémie
Hyperbetaalaninämie
Hiper-beta-alaninemia

Excludes: Carnosinemia† (126)

Minimal Diagnostic Criteria: Persistent elevation of β-alanine in plasma above the normal level of 0.014 μmoles/ml. Excessive urinary excretion of β-alanine, βAIB, and taurine. Presence of GABA in urine. Normal carnosine concentration in urine and plasma, but excessive in tissues.†

Clinical Findings: Symptoms included postnatal onset of somnolence, hypotonia, depressed reflexes, and intermittent seizures which could not be controlled by the usual anticonvulsant medications. This fatal condition identified so far in one infant. Fetal movements were thought to have been diminished. Two other pregnancies of the mother resulted in premature stillbirths in the 3rd trimester. β-alanine was present in excessive amounts in plasma, CSF, and urine; the latter also contained β-aminoisobutyric acid and taurine in excessive amounts, directly proportional to the concentration of β-alanine. Gamma-aminobutyric acid (GABA) was also present in urine, plasma and CSF, independent of the β-alanine concentration. GABA concentration in postmortem brain tissue was greatly increased. Brain and muscle contained β-alanine and carnosine in excess at postmortem.†

Complications
I **Derived:** Seizures and inhibition of CNS function
II **Associated:** —

Etiology: Probably autosomal recessive transmission of enzyme defect

Pathogenesis: ? Deficiency of β-alanine transaminase suspected†

Related Facts
I **Sex Ratio:** ?
II **Risk of Occurrence:** ? Rare
III **Risk of Recurrence for**
 Patient's Sib: When autosomal recessive, 1 in 4 (25%) for each offspring to be affected
 Patient's Child: Not increased unless mate is carrier or homozygote
IV **Age of Detectability:** Clinically in early newborn period; biochemical defect also presumably present at this time.
V **Prevalence:** ? Rare

Treatment
I **Primary Prevention:** Genetic counseling
II **Secondary Prevention:** Large doses of pyridoxine may bring about biochemical and eventual clinical improvement, and this therapy should be attempted as early as possible in any future patient.
III **Other Therapy:** —

Prognosis: Apparently fatal, or likely to cause severe retardation in surviving patients.

Detection of Carrier: ?

†Special Considerations: Mechanism of hyper-β-aminoaciduria is combined overflow and competition, analagous to origin of iminoglycinuria in hyperprolinemia. The condition is of particular interest because of evidence - for a membrane transport system with preference for β-amino compounds; for a significant metabolic pool of free β-alanine in man; that the bound β-alanine pool (carnosine) in man is equilibrated with the free pool; that impaired β-alanine metabolism in this case influences GABA metabolism; that carnosine and β-alanine in excess in brain interferes with cerebral function.

References:

Scriver, C. R. et al: Hyper-beta-alaninemia associated with beta-aminoaciduria and gamma-aminobutyricaciduria, somnolence and seizures. N. Engl. J. Med. 274:635, 1966.

Contributor: **Charles R. Scriver**

Editor's Computerized Descriptor: Nerve

HYPERBILIRUBINEMIA I (MARKER)

Includes: Hyperbilirubinémie
Hyperbilirubinämie
Hiperbilirubinemia (Marcador)
Hyperbilirubinemia unconjugated
Constitutional hepatic dysfunction
Jaundice chronic benign
Gilbert disease

Excludes: "Shunt" hyperbilirubinemia
Compensated hemolytic states
Chronic unconjugated hyperbilirubinemia after viral hepatitis

Minimal Diagnostic Criteria: Chronic unconjugated hyperbilirubinemia with serum bilirubin concentrations of 1.5-5.0 mg% in absence of hepatic or splenic enlargement or signs of hemolysis.†

Clinical Findings: Icteric sclerae and mucous membranes with serum unconjugated bilirubin concentrations fluctuating between 1.5 to 5.0 mg%.
Conventional hematologic and liver function tests, hepatic morphologic examinations including electron microscopy, and examinations of pigment composition of bile are normal.

Complications
I   **Derived:** —
II **Associated:** ?†

Etiology: Autosomal dominant; McK *14350

Pathogenesis: Impaired transfer of bilirubin and other organic anions from plasma into liver cells is postulated as well as alterations in glucuronyl transferase activity.

Related Facts
I   **Sex Ratio:** M1:F1
II   **Risk of Occurrence:** ? Rare
III **Risk of Recurrence for**
    Patient's Sib: If parent is affected, 1 in 2 (50%) for each offspring to be affected; otherwise not increased.
    Patient's Child: 1 in 2
IV **Age of Detectability:** Approximately at end of first month of life by persistent mild unconjugated hyperbilirubinemia.
V   **Prevalence:** Relatively common. Over 300 patients in literature.

Treatment
I   **Primary Prevention:** Genetic counseling
II   **Secondary Prevention:** None
III **Other Therapy:** Phenobarbitol administration ameliorates hyperbilirubinemia. Exposure to light also reduces hyperbilirubinemia.

Prognosis: Excellent. This is solely a cosmetic disorder.

Detection of Carrier: —

†Special Considerations: A relatively high frequency of mild unconjugated hyperbilirubinemia has been observed in families with Type II hepatic glucuronyl transferase deficiency although the significance of this association is uncertain. Mutant Southdown sheep in the United States have hyperbilirubinemia and photosensitivity.

References:

Arias, I. M.: Chronic unconjugated hyperbilirubinemia without overt signs of hemolysis in adolescents and adults. J. Clin. Invest. 41:2233, 1962.

Foulk, W.T. et al: Constitutional hepatic dysfunction (Gilbert's disease): Its natural history and related syndromes. Medicine (Baltimore) 28:25, 1959.

Powell, L.W. et al: Idiopathic unconjugated hyperbilirubinemia (Gilbert's syndrome): A study of 42 families. N. Engl. J. Med. 277:1108, 1967.

Smith, P.M. et al: Studies on the familial incidence and clinical history of patients with chronic unconjugated hyperbilirubinemia. Gut 8:449, 1967.

Contributor: **Irwin M. Arias**

Editor's Computerized Descriptors: Eye, Oral

HYPERCHOLESTEREMIA

Includes: Hypercholestérolémie
Hypercholesterinämie
Hipercolesteremia
Hyperlipoproteinemia II
Fredrickson type II hyperlipoproteinemia
Hyperbetalipoproteinemia
Hypercholesteremic xanthomatosis
Hyperlipidemia II

Excludes: Hyperprebeta-lipoproteinemia (500)
Other beta- and prebeta-lipoproteinemias

Minimal Diagnostic Criteria: Diagnosis in the (relatively infrequent) homozygous individual is based on his early xanthomata, the massive serum cholesterol increase, and the positive family history of similar but milder disease.

For the heterozygously involved patient, the presence of a clear serum with a continued increase in cholesterol level over the age-related norms, without other explanation for the hypercholesteremia, suggests this type of intrinsic disease. Family history abnormalities are usually evident, and support to the diagnosis is given by the characteristic xanthomas, corneal changes, and coronary disease. Demonstration of the betalipoprotein increase is a valuable correlation.

Clinical Findings: In the *heterozygously* involved patient, xanthomatous lesions appear in the tendons and on the eyelids (xanthelasmata) in the 3rd-4th decades of life, with evidence of coronary heart disease occurring simultaneously or somewhat later. The knuckles and the Achilles tendons are the most common sites for the nodules. Premature corneal arcus may also be found. Peripheral vascular disease is not conspicuous. Characteristically the serum is clear, with triglyceride levels often normal, cholesterol level 300-500 mg%, and phospholipids mildly increased. Postheparin lipolytic activity is normal. On serum electrophoresis, a sharp increased band of betalipoprotein is seen, with prebeta normal or slightly increased. Glucose tolerance tests are normal.

The *homozygously* involved individual (both of whose parents are heterozygotes) develops conspicuous cutaneous xanthomas (becoming tuberous) in the 1st decade, as well as prominent tendinous lesions and early corneal arcus. His coronary or valvular atheromata usually produce fatal cardiac disease by the age of 20 years. In this instance the serum cholesterol levels vary from 600-1200 mg%, with moderate phospholipid increases as well.

Complications
I **Derived:** Cardiovascular disease. Xanthomata may be mechanically troubling.
II **Associated:** Hyperuricemia in certain pedigrees. Cholecystitis or cholelithiasis may have an increased incidence. Migratory arthritis is sometimes noted.

Etiology: Autosomal dominant. The molecular mechanism appears to be a defective cell surface receptor which normally binds low density lipoprotein. Normal binding results in a) inhibition of biosynthesis of 3-hydroxy-3-methylglutaryl coenzyme A reductase, which is the rate-controlling enzyme in cholesterol biosynthesis, and b) degradation of low density lipoprotein. Thus, homozygously involved individuals, and to a lesser extent heterozygous persons exhibit both overproduction and impaired removal of betalipoprotein.

Pathogenesis: By present understanding the prolonged presence of increased serum betalipoprotein levels is thought to lead to direct lipid deposition (primarily as cholesterol esters) in the arterial walls, tendons, and subcutaneous tissue, with the attendant consequences of atheromatosis and xanthomatosis.

Related Facts
I   **Sex Ratio:** M1:F1
II   **Risk of Occurrence:** About 1-2 per 1000 in the general population. Heterozygotes are commonly found in hospital practice.
III   **Risk of Recurrence for**
   Patient's Sib: In families exhibiting the complete clinical picture and if the proband is homozygously affected, his sibs have a 1 in 2 risk for having heterozygous involvement and a 1 in 4 risk for homozygous disease-the parents must be affected by this schema. If the patient is heterozygously involved, then his parents also must have 1 member affected, and the sibs have a 1 in 2 risk; if 2 parents are affected, then the sib risk is 1 in 2 for heterozygosity and 1 in 4 for homozygosity.
   Patient's Child: 1 in 2 at risk if the proband is heterozygously involved, but 100% for at least heterozygosity if the proband is a homozygote. (The reproductive fitness of heterozygotes is normal.)
IV   **Age of Detectability:** For homozygous involvement: very early (? cord blood at birth). The presence of the heterozygous state may also be detected at birth but sometimes requires some years of feeding and several samples during childhood for ascertainment.
V   **Prevalence:** Relatively frequent; no special population or ethnic group has been identified for increased occurrence.

Treatment
I   **Primary Prevention:** Genetic counseling
II   **Secondary Prevention:** Serum cholesterol levels in heterozygously-involved individuals are usually partially moderated by control of excessive body weight and employment of a diet which restricts dairy and animal fats (with substitution of unsaturated vegetable and fish fats). Useful further management is achieved by chemotherapy, although reports from various centers differ on the value of different drugs. Cholestyramine and nicotinic acid have been partially effective. Ileal by-pass surgery can be considered in special instances.
III   **Other Therapy:** Special cardiac management

Prognosis: The mortality is determined by the cardiovascular involvement. In homozygotes, expiration is by young adult life. Heterozygously-involved males usually have premature coronary disease of a critical type; females may be later in developing these symptoms.

Detection of Carrier: In this circumstance of dominant inheritance the "carrier" is clinically involved; early identification of increased serum cholesterol or betalipoprotein levels is possible (see above).

Special Considerations: —

References:
Brown, M.S. and Goldstein, J.L.: Familial hypercholesterolemia: Genetic, biochemical and pathophysiologic considerations. Adv. Intern. Med. 20:273, 1975.
Fredrickson, D.S. et al: Fat transport in lipoproteins—an integrated approach to mechanisms and disorders. N. Engl. J. Med. 276:34, 1967.
Galbraith, A. and Hatch, F.T.: A system of proportioned fat diets for clinical use. Am. J. Clin. Nutr. 16:480, 1965.
Goldstein, J.L. and Brown, M.S.: Hyperlipidemia in coronary heart disease: A biochemical genetic approach. J. Lab. Clin. Med. 85:15, 1975.
Lees, R.S. and Wilson, D.E.: The treatment of hyperlipidemia. N. Engl. J. Med. 284:186, 1971.
Nevin, N.C. and Slack, J.: Hyperlipidaemic xanthomatosis. II. Mode of inheritance in 55 families with essential hyperlipidaemia and xanthomatosis. J. Med. Genet. 5:9, 1968.
Nikkilä, E.A. and Aro, A.: Family study of serum lipids and lipoproteins in coronary heart disease. Lancet 1:954, 1973.

Contributors: **Frederick T. Hatch**
Robert S. Lees

Editor's Computerized Descriptors: Eye, Skin, Skel., CV.

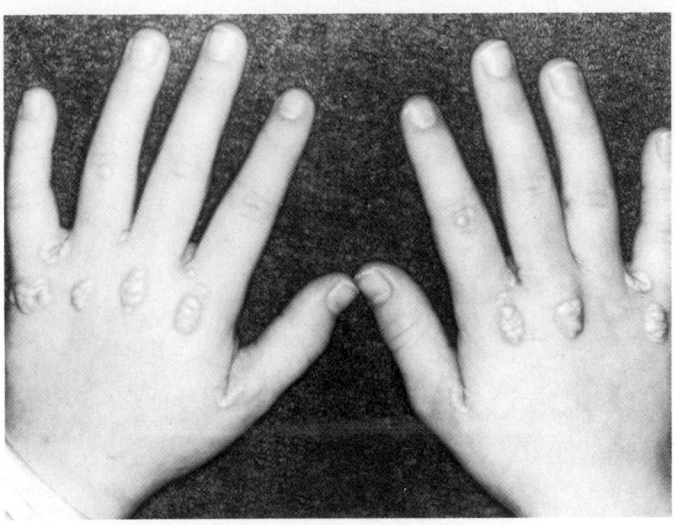

292. Xanthomata

HYPERCHYLOMICRONEMIA

Includes: Hyperchylomicronémie
Fett-induzierte Hyperlipämie
Hiperquilomicronemia
Hyperlipoproteinemia I
Fredrickson type I hyperlipoproteinemia
Idiopathic familial hyperlipemia
Exogenous hypertriglyceridemia
Familial deficiency of postheparin lipolytic activity
Fat-induced hyperlipemia
Hyperlipidemia I
Bürger-Grütz syndrome

Excludes: Hyperprebeta-lipoproteinemia and hyperchylomicronemia (501)
Hyperprebeta-lipoproteinemia (500)

Minimal Diagnostic Criteria: There is grossly lipemic serum and a heavy chylomicron band in lipoprotein electrophoresis, except after strict limitation of dietary fat. Proof of diagnosis requires demonstration of a) relationship of the lipemia to dietary fat intake, and b) deficiency of plasma postheparin lipolytic activity ("clearing factor"). Specific assays for differentiating lipoprotein lipase from hepatic lipase (not deficient in this syndrome) are available.

The glucose tolerance test is normal, and electrophoretic beta- and prebetalipoproteins are not increased.

Clinical Findings: Not infrequently this syndrome is first detected by the accidental finding of grossly lactescent or creamy serum in blood specimens drawn for other purposes. Involved patients are clinically well except for the occasional occurrence of abdominal pain attacks ("crises") of obscure origin, with prostration, vomiting, and spasm of the abdominal wall (self-limited), and the intermittent development of crops of eruptive cutaneous xanthomata. The latter typically appear as small yellow or orange papules in groups on the buttocks, face, limbs, and palate. Tendinous, tuberous and palmar xanthomata are absent, as are corneal arcus lesions and cardiovascular complications. Lipemia retinalis is usually evident, and moderate inconstant enlargement of the liver and spleen may occur. The serum is conspicuously creamy, with a discrete separation of a white layer ("creaming") on standing. The vast bulk of the increased total serum lipid level is triglyceride, with minor increases in cholesterol and phospholipids.

Complications
I   **Derived:**   Skin xanthoma formation may be sufficiently objectionable to the patient to provide motivation for the adoption of a dietary program. Foam cells may be found in the bone marrow (and in the liver and spleen), but no clinical difficulties derive from this secondary phenomenon.
II   **Associated:**   Pancreatitis has been proved to cause the attacks of abdominal pain in many instances.

Etiology: Autosomal recessive. The basic defect appears to be in the lipoprotein lipase enzyme system, which is essential for the normal clearing of ingested fat in the form of chylomicrons from the plasma. McK *23860

Pathogenesis: The delay in clearance of chylomicrons derived from dietary fat leads to a massive elevation of serum triglycerides (and to a minor degree of cholesterol). The foam cell accumulations in marrow and viscera, and the eruptive xanthomata, probably reflect a responsive reticuloendothelial cell uptake of excess lipid.

Related Facts
I   **Sex Ratio:**   M1:F1
II   **Risk of Occurrence:**   Low
III   **Risk of Recurrence for**
Patient's Sib: 1 in 4 (25%) for each offspring to be affected

Patient's Child: Not increased unless mate is carrier or homozygote
IV   **Age of Detectability:**   A few days after birth by plasma postheparin lipolytic activity testing.
V   **Prevalence:**   Probably low. No definite predilection is known for any population or ethnic group. Phenocopies can occur in alcoholism with secondary pancreatitis.

Treatment
I   **Primary Prevention:**   Genetic counseling
II   **Secondary Prevention:**   Modification of the hyperchylomicronemia per se can be accomplished by restriction of dietary fat of all types to less than 25 gm per day. At this level the serum lipids are still not normal, but abdominal pain attacks are eliminated and eruptive xanthomata controlled.

Medium-chain triglyceride substitution for some dietary fat is helpful for temporary use, but may not be safe for long-term therapy. Heparin treatment is not effective. Unnecessary surgery during the episodes of abdominal pain must be prevented.
III   **Other Therapy:**   —

Prognosis: By current concepts, a normal life span is to be anticipated. Reassurance is usually needed because of the automatic alarm induced by the appearance of the patient's serum.

Detection of Carrier: Mild serum triglyceride elevations have occasionally been reported for heterozygotes, but this is of dubious significance. More pertinent, parents and sibs of patients have postheparin lipolytic activity results in the lower quartile of the normal distribution.

Special Considerations: —

References:
Fredrickson, D.S. and Levy, R.I.: Familial hyperlipoproteinemia. In Stanbury, J.B. et al (eds.): The Metabolic Basis of Inherited Disease, 3rd Ed. New York:McGraw-Hill, 1972, p. 545.
Havel, R.J. and Gordon, R.S., Jr.: Idiopathic hyperlipemia; metabolic studies in an affected family. J. Clin. Invest. 39:1777, 1960.
Huttunen, J.K. et al: Effect of fasting on two postheparin plasma triglyceride lipases and triglyceride removal in obese subjects. Eur. J. Clin. Invest. 5:435, 1975.
Reissell, P.K. et al: Treatment of hypertriglyceridemia. Am. J. Clin. Nutr. 19:84, 1966.

Contributor: **Frederick T. Hatch**

Editor's Computerized Descriptors: Skin, Spleen, GI., Liver

HYPERCYSTINURIA (MARKER)

Includes: Hypercystinurie
Hyperzystinurie
Hipercistinuria (Marcador)
Cystinuria without dibasic aminoaciduria

Excludes: Cystinuria (239)
Cystinosis (238)
Homocystinuria (474)

Minimal Diagnostic Criteria: Positive urinary cyanide-nitroprusside test; distinctly increased renal clearance of cystine but not of lysine, arginine or ornithine.

Clinical Findings: Probably none; disorder has been described in only 1 family to date.†

Complications
I   **Derived:** —
II **Associated:** Hypocalcemia and tetany reported in 1 of 2 affected sibs.

Etiology: ? By analogy with cystinuria, presumed to be autosomal recessive transmission involving cystine-specific carrier protein in renal tubule.

Pathogenesis: Transport defect for cystine leads to increased renal clearance and excretion; urinary tract calculi not described to date.

Related Facts
I   **Sex Ratio:** ?
II   **Risk of Occurrence:** ?
III **Risk of Recurrence for**
    Patient's Sib: Presumed 1 in 4 (25%) for each offspring to be affected
    Patient's Child: Not increased unless mate is carrier or homozygote.
IV **Age of Detectability:** ?
V   **Prevalence:** ?

Treatment
I   **Primary Prevention:** Genetic counseling
II   **Secondary Prevention:** —
III **Other Therapy:** —

Prognosis: Probably normal life span

Detection of Carrier: No method known; parents of affected children excreted normal amounts of cystine in the urine.

†**Special Considerations:** Biochemical abnormality significant because it adds considerable evidence in vivo for a tubular transport system for cystine unshared with the dibasic amino acids; no data available concerning intestinal transport of cystine.

References:
Brodehl, J. et al: Isolierter Defekt der tubulären, Cystin-Rückresorption in einer Familie mit idiopathischem Hypoparathyroidismus. Klin. Wochenschr. 45:38, 1967.
Rosenberg, L.E. and Scriver, C.R.: Disorders of amino acid metabolism. In Bondy, P.K. and Rosenberg, L.E. (eds.): Diseases of Metabolism, 7th Ed. Philadelphia:W.B. Saunders Co., 1974, p. 465.

Contributor: **Leon E. Rosenberg**

Editor's Computerized Descriptor: —

HYPERDIBASIC-AMINOACIDURIA

Includes: Amino-acidurie-hyperdibasique
Vermehrte Ausscheidung dibasischer Aminosäuren
Hiper-dibásico-aminoaciduria
Protein intolerance (probably)
Lysinuric protein intolerance
Congenital lysinuria
Hyperlysinuria with hyperammonemia

Excludes: Cystinuria (239)

Minimal Diagnostic Criteria: Normal cystine concentration in urine of < 60 mg/gm creatinine and selective increase in excretion of lysine, ornithine and arginine. Concentration of dibasic amino acids in plasma is normal, or lower than normal. Thus renal clearance is elevated and net tubular absorption is decreased. Excretion rates of dibasic amino acids in subjects with the dominant trait resemble those of the Type III cystinuric trait. An in vivo intestinal transport defect for lysine is present in "Canadian" and "Finnish" probands. Cystine transport is normal in the dominant Canadian trait.

Clinical Findings: One French-Canadian pedigree described in which a dominantly inherited trait appeared in 13 members in 2 generations. All affected subjects had excessive urinary excretion of "dibasic" amino acids without hypercystinuria. No clinical symptoms were directly associated with the presence of the trait.

Twenty-one Finnish patients (probands and sibs) with renal hyperdibasicaminoaciduria and with protein intolerance have been described. Condition characterized by failure to thrive, diarrhea, and vomiting in the infant fed cow's milk, and later by severe aversion to protein-rich food. The patients show growth retardation, enlargement of the liver and often of the spleen. Symptoms associated with hyperammonemia are provoked by protein intake or by loading with alanine; symptoms can be improved by reduction of protein in the diet, and by arginine supplementation. Patients are homozygous; heterozygotes for the trait are symptom free. A mentally retarded patient reported from the U.S.A. (Kihara et al) with severe hyperdibasicaminoaciduria and without hyperammonemia or protein intolerance is probably the homozygous form of the "Canadian" trait. The parents of this patient have moderate hyperdibasicaminoaciduria. Three additional probands (unreported) probably with the homozygous "Canadian" form have been observed in Finland.

Two patients have been studied in Japan and one in the United States whose clinical and laboratory findings closely resembled those of the Finnish trait.

An in vivo intestinal transport defect for lysine is present in all the traits. Intestinal cystine transport has been studied only in the French-Canadian trait; it was found to be normal.

Complications
I   **Derived:** Impaired growth, osteoporosis, and muscular hypotonia in patients with protein intolerance. Increased protein intake causes periods of stupor and, if continuous, probably mental retardation through hyperammonemia.
II **Associated:** —

Etiology: Autosomal recessive defect in "Finnish" and "Canadian" traits. Original finding in Canadian pedigree was expressed dominantly; heterozygotes for lysinuric protein intolerance have less obvious expression of the mutant allele. Therefore, 2 different alleles proposed for "Canadian" and "Finnish" types of hyperdibasicaminoaciduria. McK *22270

Pathogenesis: Deficiency of membrane transport system shared by "dibasic" amino acids, but excluding cystine.†

Related Facts

I **Sex Ratio:** M1:F1 (approximate)

II **Risk of Occurrence:** Approximately 1 in 60,000 live births per lysinuric protein intolerance in Finland. Rarer elsewhere.

III **Risk of Recurrence for**

Patient's Sib: If autosomal recessive or autosomal dominant, see Table I AR or AD, respectively.

Patient's Child: If autosomal recessive or autosomal dominant, see Table I AR or AD, respectively.

IV **Age of Detectability:** In early life theoretically, and diagnosis in infancy has been made frequently.

V **Prevalence:** ? Rare

Treatment

I **Primary Prevention:** Genetic counseling

II **Secondary Prevention:** Protein intake < 1.2 - 1.5 g/kg/day in the lysinuric protein intolerance. L-arginine supplement, 0.5 - 1.0 g/meal considered beneficial. No treatment indicated in "Canadian" form.

III **Other Therapy:** —

Prognosis: Probably normal life span

Detection of Carrier: Modest hyperdibasicaminoaciduria characterizes carrier of the "Canadian" (without protein intolerance) phenotype. Finnish (with protein intolerance) heterozygotes have normal or only slightly increased dibasic amino excretion.

†**Special Considerations:** Two types of hyperdibasicaminoaciduria appear to exist. In the first ("Canadian") type, dibasic amino acid transport is defective in the renal tubule and in the intestine, but not in the liver. In the second ("Finnish") type, the defect is shared by the liver, and failure of the urea cycle, hyperammonemia, and protein intolerance are added to the picture, because the liver becomes deficient in the urea cycle intermediates arginine and ornithine. The alleles are also expressed differently in quantitative and qualitative terms in the heterozygotes for the 2 traits.

References:

Kihara, H. et al: Hyperdibasicaminoaciduria in a mentally retarded homozygote with a peculiar response to phenothiazines. Pediatrics 51:223, 1973.

Oyanagi, K. et al: Congenital lysinuria: A new inherited transport disorder of dibasic amino acids. J. Pediatr. 77:259, 1970.

Simell, O. et al: Lysinuric protein intolerance. Am. J. Med. 50.000, 1975.

Whelan, D. T. and Scriver, C. R.: Hyperdibasicaminoaciduria: An inherited disorder of amino acid transport. Pediatr. Res. 2:523, 1968.

Contributors: **Charles R. Scriver**
Olli G. Simell

Editor's Computerized Descriptors: Skel., Muscle, Spleen, GI., Liver

HYPERGLYCINEMIA, NONKETOTIC

Includes: Hyperglycinémie sans cétose
Nicht-ketotische Form der Hyperglyzinämie
Hiperglicinemia no cetónica
Hyperglycinemia with hypooxaluria
Idiopathic hyperglycinemia
Hereditary hyperglycinemia
Nonketotic hyperglycinemia

Excludes: Glycinuria without hyperglycinemia
Glucoglycinuria (418)
Propionic acidemia (826)

Minimal Diagnostic Criteria: Increased concentrations of glycine in the blood without recurrent ketoacidosis. Propionic acidemia should probably be excluded for we have seen a patient with propionic acidemia who presented repeatedly with severe illness and hyperglycinemia but no ketosis.

Clinical Findings: Onset of lethargy within the first days of life and convulsions at 3 days to 6 weeks. The 3 patients described in detail developed severe mental retardation. Two had irritability and microcephaly. One was markedly hypertonic and hyperreflexic, another was hypotonic and hyperreflexic. Porencephaly and ventricular dilatation were seen on pneumoencephalography. The EEG was abnormal.

Plasma concentrations of glycine are distinctly elevated but tend to be considerably lower than in ketotic hyperglycinemia. A range of 5 to 11 mg/100 ml has been reported. Concentrations of glycine in the cerebrospinal fluid are elevated. Urinary excretion of oxalate appears not to be a consistent characteristic of the disease. Only one of the patients reported has had neutropenia. This observation may relate to the lower concentrations of glycine than in ketotic hyperglycinemia.

Complications

I **Derived:** Those of severe convulsive disorder and mental retardation

II **Associated:** —

Etiology: Probably autosomal recessive

Pathogenesis: A defect has been found in vivo that is consistent with a lack in an enzyme catalyzing the conversion of glycine to CO_2 and hydroxymethyltetrahydrofolic acid. Studies in vitro have revealed evidence of a similar defect in the cleavage of glycine.

Related Facts

I **Sex Ratio:** Probably M1:F1 (all 3 documented patients have been males)

II **Risk of Occurrence:** Very rare

III **Risk of Recurrence for**

Patient's Sib: Probably 1 in 4 (25%) for each offspring to be affected

Patient's Child: Probably not increased unless mate is carrier or homozygote

IV **Age of Detectability:** Presumably it should be detectable within days of birth by quantitative assay of the plasma concentration of glycine.

V **Prevalence:** Very rare

Treatment

I **Primary Prevention:** Genetic counseling

II **Secondary Prevention:** ?

III **Other Therapy:** Anticonvulsant medications

Prognosis: Generally grave. Most patients have died in infancy. Three patients reported are alive and have severe mental retardation.

Detection of Carrier: Not available.

Special Considerations: —

References:
Ando, T. et al: Metabolism of glycine in the nonketotic hyperglycinemia. Pediatr. Res. 2:254, 1968.
DeGroot, C.J. et al: Nonketotic hyperglycinemia: An in vitro study of the glycine-serine conversion in liver of three patients and the effect of dietary methionine. Pediatr. Res. 4:238, 1970.
Gerritsen, T. et al: A new type of idiopathic hyperglycinemia with hypooxaluria. Pediatrics 36:822, 1965.
Rampini, S. et al: Klinisches Bild und Bestimmung von Glyoxylsäure und Oxalsäure im Urin bei je einem Patienten mit der acidotischen und der nicht-acidotischen Form. Helv. Paediatr. Acta 22: 135, 1967.
Tada, K. et al: Hyperglycinemia: A defect in glycine cleavage reaction. Tohoku J. Exp. Med. 98:289, 1969.
Wadlington, W. B. et al: Hyperglycinemia and propionyl CoA carboxylase deficiency and episodic severe illness without consistent ketosis. J. Pediatr. 86:707, 1975.
Ziter F.A. et al: The clinical findings in a patient with nonketotic hyperglycinemia. Pediatr. Res. 2:250, 1968.

Contributor: **William L. Nyhan**

Editor's Computerized Descriptors: Skel., Muscle, Nerve

HYPERHIDROSIS, PREMATURE HAIR GREYING AND PREMOLAR APLASIA

Includes: Syndrome hyperhidrose-blanchîment précoce des cheveux-aplasie des prémolaires
Syndrom von Hyperhydrose, vorzeitig ergrautem Haar und Aplasie der Prämolaren
Hiperhidrosis, encanecimiento prematuro y aplasia de los premolares
Böök syndrome
Premolar aplasia, hyperhidrosis and canities
Hair greying, premolar aplasia and hyperhidrosis

Excludes: Ectodermal dysplasia, anhidrotic (333)
Hypodontia and nail dysgenesis (511)
Werner syndrome (998)

Minimal Diagnostic Criteria: For single cases the presence of all three signs must be required. Otherwise diagnosis is aided by etiology and distribution of signs in affected family members.

Clinical Findings: (Based on 18 clinically examined patients from one pedigree.)
Premolar aplasia, confirmed in 17 patients (15 by x-ray films and inconclusive in one due to unknown number of extractions). Lacking all 8 premolars 9/17. Lacking from 1-5 premolars 8/17.
Hyperhidrosis occurred in 67% of the patients and was not seen in other members of the family.
Premature hair greying (canities prematura) occurred in all patients. Age of onset was from 6-10 years for 39%, from 11-20 years for 50% and from 21-23 years for 11%.

Complications
I   **Derived:** Persistence of primary teeth until adult age in the premolar region and frequently backward dislocation of canines.
II **Associated:** —

Etiology: Autosomal dominant; McK *11230

Pathogenesis: ?

Related Facts
I   **Sex Ratio:** M1:F1
II **Risk of Occurrence:** ?
III **Risk of Recurrence for**
    Patient's Sib: If parent is affected 1 in 2 (50%) for each offspring to be affected; otherwise not increased.
    Patient's Child: 1 in 2
IV **Age of Detectability:** See Clinical Findings.
V   **Prevalence:** ?

Treatment
I   **Primary Prevention:** Genetic counseling
II **Secondary Prevention:** —
III **Other Therapy:** Dental prosthesis and orthodontic treatment

Prognosis: Excellent with no significant consequences for the patient's health or life expectancy.

Detection of Carrier: Evidently complete penetrance in respect of premolar aplasia and premature hair greying in all heterozygotes

Special Considerations: —

References:
Böök, J. A.: Clinical and genetical studies of hypodontia. I. Premolar aplasia, hyperhidrosis and canities prematura: A new hereditary syndrome in man. Am. J. Hum. Genet. 2:240, 1950.

Contributor: **Jan A. Böök**

Editor's Computerized Descriptors: Teeth, Sweating, Hair

HYPERKERATOSIS PALMOPLANTARIS AND PERIODONTOCLASIA

Contributor: **Heddie O. Sedano**

Editor's Computerized Descriptors: Eye, Oral, Teeth, Skin

Includes: Hyperkeratose palmoplantaire et périodontoclasie
Keratosis palmoplantaris und Periodontoklasie
Queratosis palmoplantar y periodontoclasia
Parodontopathia acroectodermalis
Papillon-Lefèvre syndrome
Periodontoclasia and hyperkeratosis palmoplantaris

Excludes: Werner syndrome (998)
Pachyonychia congenita (789)
All other keratosis palmoplantaris

Minimal Diagnostic Criteria: Hyperkeratosis of palms and soles. Periodontoclasia of both dentitions.

Clinical Findings: Hyperkeratosis of palms and soles. Severe periodontal destruction (periodontoclasia) of both primary and secondary dentition with consequent shedding of all teeth. Severe gingivostomatitis. Occasional ectopic calcification of the tentorium and choroid.

Complications
I   **Derived:**   Regional adenopathy
II   **Associated:**   —

Etiology: Autosomal recessive

Pathogenesis: ?

Related Facts
I   **Sex Ratio:**   M1:F1
II   **Risk of Occurrence:**   —
III   **Risk of Recurrence for**
    Patient's Sib: 1 in 4 (25%) for each offspring to be affected
    Patient's Child: Not increased unless mate is carrier or homozygote.
IV   **Age of Detectability:**   It can be suspected at birth because of redness or hyperkeratosis palmoplantaris; positive diagnosis cannot be established until dental involvement, age 4 - 5 years.
V   **Prevalence:**   Approximately 1 in 1,000,000 general population

Treatment
I   **Primary Prevention:**   Genetic counseling
II   **Secondary Prevention:**   Extraction of teeth and dental prosthesis. There is no known treatment for hyperkeratosis.
III   **Other Therapy:**   —

Prognosis: By age 5 - 6 years all of the primary teeth are lost. By age 13 - 14 all of the secondary teeth are lost. However, general health is not impaired.

Detection of Carrier: ?

Special Considerations: —

References:
Bach, J.N. and Levan, N.E.: Papillon-Lefèvre syndrome. Arch. Dermatol. 97:154, 1968.
Giansanti, J.S. et al: Palmar-plantar hyperkeratosis and concomitant periodontal destruction (Papillon-Lefèvre syndrome). Oral Surg. 36:40, 1973.
Gorlin, R.J. et al: The syndrome of palmar-plantar hyperkeratosis and premature periodontal destruction of the teeth: A clinical and genetic analysis of the Papillon-Lefèvre syndrome. J. Pediatr. 65:895, 1964.
Jansen, L. H.: Le caractère héréditaire de l'hyperkératose palmoplantaire avec paradentose (Papillon-Lefèvre). J. Genet. Hum. 5:216, 1956.
Papillon, M. M. and Lefèvre, P.: Deux cas de kératodermie palmaire et plantaire symétrique familiale (maladie de Meleda) chez le frère et la soeur. Coexistence dans le deux cas d'altérations dentaires graves. Bull. Soc. Franc. Derm. Syph. 31:82, 1924.

HYPERLIPOPROTEINEMIA III

Includes: Hyperlipoprotéinémie type III
Hyperlipoproteinämie III
Hiperlipoproteinemia tipo III
Fredrickson type III hyperlipoproteinemia
"Broad beta" syndrome
Hyperlipidemia III

Excludes: Hypercholesteremia (488)

Minimal Diagnostic Criteria: On regular diet, lipoprotein findings as below. Lipoprotein with beta mobility is present in the supernatant fraction after ultracentrifugation of serum for 18 hours. Very low density lipoprotein shows increased ratio of cholesterol to triglyceride.

Clinical Findings: This condition is rarely diagnosed before the 4th decade.

The serum is opalescent or creamy, the range for cholesterol is 400-600 mg% and triglycerides 175-1500. By electrophoresis, chylomicrons are usually absent, betalipoprotein increased, prebetalipoprotein normal or increased and α-1-lipoprotein normal or decreased. The postheparin lipolytic activity is normal but glucose tolerance is abnormal in 40%.

Xanthomata, tendinous or tuberous, may appear after age 25, with planar deposits in palmar creases and fingertips. Xanthelasmata and corneal arcus occur. Both coronary disease and peripheral vascular disease are usual in males over 45 years and in females over 55 years. Abdominal pain and hepatosplenomegaly are not found in hyperlipoproteinemia type III.

Complications
I   **Derived:** Coronary disease, peripheral vascular insufficiency, xanthomas
II **Associated:** Diabetes, hyperuricemia common

Etiology: Inheritable, but mode of genetic transmission unclear. Both overproduction and a block in clearance of very low density lipoprotein have been proposed. Arginine-rich apolipoprotein often elevated. McK *14450

Pathogenesis: The increased low-density lipoprotein evidently has a tendency for deposition in the arterial walls (and xanthomata).

Related Facts
I   **Sex Ratio:** M1:F1
II **Risk of Occurrence:** ? Infrequent
III **Risk of Recurrence for**
  Patient's Sib: 1 in 4 (25%) for each offspring to be affected; 11 of 68 sibs were involved.
  Patient's Child: Not increased unless mate is carrier or homozygote
IV **Age of Detectability:** Reported patients have been in 40-60 year age range with a few in the 2nd and 3rd decades.
V   **Prevalence:** Delayed expression may mask identification. Phenocopies occur by diabetes and lupus erythematosus.

Treatment
I   **Primary Prevention:** None
II **Secondary Prevention:** Weight reduction, reduced intake of saturated fats and cholesterol, balanced with moderate carbohydrates. Clofibrate and nicotinic acid may be useful.
III **Other Therapy:** —

Prognosis: Affected by coronary and peripheral vascular disease (better than for hypercholesteremia). Reproductive fitness is normal.

Detection of Carrier: Heterozygotes often have a type IV pattern of hyperlipoproteinemia.

Special Considerations: —

References:
Fredrickson, D.S. et al: Fat transport in lipoproteins—an integrated approach to mechanisms and disorders. N. Engl. J. Med. 276:34, 1967.
Fredrickson, D.S. et al: Type III hyperlipoproteinemia: An analysis of two contemporary definitions. Ann. Intern. Med. 82:150, 1975.
Hazzard, W.R. et al: Broad-beta disease (Type III hyperlipoproteinemia) in a large kindred; evidence for a monogenic mechanism. Ann. Intern. Med. 82:141, 1975.
Morganroth, J. et al: The biochemical, clinical, and genetic features of Type III hyperlipoproteinemia. Ann. Intern. Med. 82:158, 1975.
Stern, M.P. et al: Acquired Type III hyperlipoproteinemia; report of three cases associated with systemic lupus erythematosus and diabetic ketoacidosis. Arch. Intern. Med. 130:817, 1972.

Contributors: **Frederick T. Hatch**
Robert I. Levy
Gerald M. Reaven

Editor's Computerized Descriptors: Eye, Skin , CV.

HYPERLIPOPROTEINEMIA, COMBINED

Includes: Hyperlipidémie combinée
Kombinierte Hyperlipoproteinämie
Hiperlipoproteinemia combinada
Combined hyperlipidemia
Familial combined hyperlipoproteinemia
Combined hyperlipoproteinemia

Excludes: Hypercholesteremia (488)
Hyperprebeta-lipoproteinemia (500)
Hyperlipoproteinemia III (495)

Minimal Diagnostic Criteria: Diagnosis is based upon plasma lipid or lipoprotein elevations, absence of xanthomas, and absence of isolated elevations of cholesterol and low density lipoprotein among relatives.

Clinical Findings: A heritable disorder in which serum cholesterol and triglyceride levels both are elevated. Low density and very low density lipoprotein concentrations also are elevated but, in contrast to those in hyperlipoproteinemia III, are of normal electrophoretic mobility. The condition quite frequently is identified among young to middle-aged survivors of myocardial infarction. Therefore, it is associated with coronary atherosclerosis. Other clinical characteristics include impaired glucose tolerance, obesity and hyperuricemia; xanthomas are absent. Lipoprotein lipase levels are normal.

Complications
I **Derived:** Coronary heart disease.
II **Associated:** Mild diabetes, hyperuricemia.

Etiology: Genetic analysis suggests possible autosomal dominant inheritance.

Pathogenesis: Tentatively, the defect, of unknown nature, involves metabolism of triglycerides with secondary elevation of serum cholesterol. The elevated lipoprotein levels presumably enhance lipid deposition in artery walls (atherosclerosis).

Related Facts
I **Sex Ratio:** M1:F1
II **Risk of Occurrence:** Approximately 1-2 per 1000.
III **Risk of Recurrence for**
     Patient's Sib: Approximately 1 in 2 show some lipid abnormality.
     Patient's Child: About 1 in 3
IV **Age of Detectability:** Lipid abnormalities detectable in childhood but may not conform to described phenotype.
V **Prevalence:** Uncertain. Phenocopies by overnutrition and possibly other causes.

Treatment
I **Primary Prevention:** Genetic counseling, if familial basis established.
II **Secondary Prevention:** Weight reduction, reduced intake of saturated fats and cholesterol. Clofibrate or nicotinic acid may be helpful.
III **Other Therapy:** —

Prognosis: Death probably by coronary heart disease in 4th-6th decades.

Detection of Carrier: —

Special Considerations: —

References:
Glueck, C.J. et al: Familial combined hyperlipoproteinemia: Studies in 91 adults and 95 children from 33 kindreds. Metabolism 22:1403, 1973.
Goldstein, J.L. et al: Hyperlipidemia in coronary heart disease: Genetic analysis of lipid levels in 176 families and delineation of a new inherited disorder, combined hyperlipidemia. J. Clin. Invest. 52:1544, 1973.
Rose, H.G. et al: Inheritance of combined hyperlipoproteinemia: Evidence for a new lipoprotein phenotype. Am. J. Med. 54:148, 1973.

Contributor: **Frederick T. Hatch**

Editor's Computerized Descriptors: Skin, CV.

HYPEROSTOSIS CORTICALIS GENERALISATA

Includes: Hyperostose corticale généralisée
Hiperostosis cortical generalizada
Van Buchem syndrome
Hyperostose endostale

Excludes: Hypertrophic osteoarthropathy
Pachydermoperiostosis (788)

Minimal Diagnostic Criteria: The diagnosis can only be made by roentgenologic study of the skull and long bones. The regular thickening of the diaphyseal cortex without increased diameter is characteristic with prominence of the mandible and thickening of the skull.

Clinical Findings: Thickening and widening of the chin can be observed in the adolescent and becomes very striking in the adult patient. A thickened clavicle also may be palpable in adolescents but the hands and feet have normal dimensions. Patients have no unusual movements. Often the disease is detected during routine x-ray examination which reveals symmetric thickening of the diaphyseal cortex of the long bones without increased diameter. The base and roof of the skull are thicker but all sinuses are pneumatized. The prominence and thickening of the mandible are typical. The spinal processes of the vertebrae are sclerotic as are vertebral bodies, but to a lesser degree. In affected children hyperostosis of the skull and diaphyseal cortex are present but the mandibular changes are not yet characteristic. The serum alkaline phosphatase concentration is often elevated.†

Complications
I   **Derived:** The osteosclerosis of the base of the skull often causes compression of cranial nerves. Paralysis of the facial nerve and perceptive deafness are especially frequent. Spontaneous fractures and anemia do not occur.
II   **Associated:** —

Etiology: Autosomal recessive†; McK *23910

Pathogenesis: In 2 of Van Buchem's patients, the plasma calcitonin was markedly elevated, but normal in 2 other patients. No conclusion is possible relative to the action of calcitonin to the pathogenesis of hyperostosis corticalis.

Related Facts
I   **Sex Ratio:** M1:F1
II   **Risk of Occurrence:** ?
III **Risk of Recurrence for**
     Patient's Sib: 1 in 4 (25%) for each sib to be affected
     Patient's Child: Not increased unless mate is carrier or homozygote
IV   **Age of Detectability:** The condition may be recognized in childhood but most often the disease is detected in the adult.
V   **Prevalence:** ?

Treatment
I   **Primary Prevention:** Genetic counseling
II   **Secondary Prevention:** Surgical decompression may be attempted for cranial nerve involvement
III **Other Therapy:** Supportive

Prognosis: Life expectancy is apparently normal

Detection of Carrier: —

†**Special Considerations:** Another form of hyperostosis corticalis generalisata, first described by Worth and Wollin seems to be inherited as an autosomal dominant trait. In this form, the deformity of the mandible is mild and a torus palatinus is often present. Xrays show an identical involvement of the skull and long bones and sclerosis of the pelvis and vertebrae. The serum alkaline phosphatase concentration is normal.

Kenny and Caffey have described another dominant syndrome: congenital stenosis of medullary spaces in tubular bone. In this syndrome, the diaphyses are reduced in width and the marrow cavity is filiform.

References:
Kenny, F.M. and Linarelli, L.: Dwarfism and cortical thickening of tubular bones. Transient hypocalcemia in a mother and son. Am. J. Dis. Child. 111:201, 1966.
Maroteaux, P. et al: L'hyperostose corticale généralisée à transmission dominante (type Worth). Arch. Fr. Pediatr. 28:685, 1971.
Van Buchem, F.S. et al: Hyperostosis corticalis generalisata. Report of seven cases. Am. J. Med. 33:387, 1962.
Van Buchem, F.S.: The pathogenesis of hyperostosis corticalis generalisata and calcitonin. Proc. Kon. Ned. Akad. Wet. (Biol. Med.) 73:243, 1970.
Worth, H.M. and Wollin, D.G.: Hyperostosis corticalis generalisata congenita. J. Can. Assoc. Radiol. 17:67, 1966.

Contributor: Pierre Maroteaux

Editor's Computerized Descriptors: Eye, Hearing, Face, Skel., Nerve

HYPEROSTOSIS FRONTALIS INTERNA

Includes: Hyperostose frontale interne
Hiperostosis frontal interna
Hyperostosis calvariae interna
Morgagni-Stewart-Morel syndrome
Metabolic craniopathy
Endostosis cranii

Excludes: Leontiasis oseii
Paget disease

Minimal Diagnostic Criteria: Radiographic evidence of hyperostosis of the inner table of the frontal bone.†

Clinical Findings: Hyperostosis of the inner table of the cranium confined primarily to the frontal or frontal-parietal areas. This anomaly has been reported in association with a variety of endocrine and neuropsychiatric disturbances such as obesity, virilization, gonadal disturbances, headache, epilepsy, psychosis, etc occurring primarily in middle-aged and elderly women. There is some question as to whether this variable constellation of abnormalities represents a true syndrome or is merely coincidental. Radiographs reveal a bony proliferation of the inner table of the skull, with or without involvement of the diploë, confined primarily to the frontal bone. The outer table of the calvarium is uninvolved.

Complications
I   **Derived:** There is some controversy as to whether this endostosis can result in headache and endocrine imbalance or whether it is simply an incidental finding in middle-aged women and produces no symptoms.
II **Associated:** —

Etiology: The occurrence of this anomaly in multiple generations of several families suggests dominant inheritance, either sex-limited autosomal or X-linked transmission.

Pathogenesis: ?

Related Facts
I   **Sex Ratio:** M1:F9
II   **Risk of Occurrence.** ?
III **Risk of Recurrence for**
      Patient's Sib: ?
      Patient's Child: ?
IV   **Age of Detectability:** Usually found in middle-aged females but it has been reported occasionally in adolescence.
V   **Prevalence:** ? High in 47, XXX females

Treatment
I   **Primary Prevention:** —
II   **Secondary Prevention:** —
III **Other Therapy:** —

Prognosis: Normal life span

Detection of Carrier: —

†Special Considerations: There is some doubt as to whether hyperostosis frontalis interna is more than a common benign anatomic peculiarity found in up to 12% of normal women. This lesion has been described in association with myotonic dystrophy, Crouzon disease and a variety of other disorders. It must be distinguished from leontiasis oseii, Paget disease and the congenital anemias. Increased serum alkaline phosphatase levels have been found in about one-half of a group of affected females.

References:
Gegick, C.G. et al: Hyperostosis frontalis interna and hyperphosphatasemia. Ann. Intern. Med. 79:71, 1973.
Kunkle, E.C.: Hyperostosis of skull. JAMA 178:533, 1961.
Moore, S.: Hyperostosis Cranii. Springfield: Charles C Thomas, 1955.
Perou, M.L.: Cranial Hyperostosis, Hyperostosis Cranii or H.C. Springfield: Charles C Thomas, 1964.

Contributor: **David L. Rimoin**

Editor's Computerized Descriptors: Skel., Nerve

HYPERPARATHYROIDISM, NEONATAL FAMILIAL

Includes: Hyperparathyrodoïdie néo-natale familiale
Angeborener, familiärer Hyperparathyreoidismus
Hiperparatiroidismo neonatal familiar
Hereditary parathyroid hyperplasia
Neonatal familial primary hyperparathyroidism
Congenital hyperparathyroidism

Excludes: Congenital hyperparathyroidism secondary to maternal hypoparathyroidism
Endocrine neoplasia, multiple (350, 351, 352)

Minimal Diagnostic Criteria: Hypercalcemia with elevated serum immunoreactive parathyroid hormone level. X-ray evidence of skeletal demineralization is a characteristic finding.

Clinical Findings: Common symptoms in the early weeks of life in the afflicted infants include poor feeding, constipation, respiratory difficulty, failure to thrive, unexplained anemia, hepatomegaly, splenomegaly, seizures, polydypsia, polyuria, and hypotonia. In spite of generalized hypotonia, tendon reflexes may be exaggerated. Extreme hypercalcemia is commmon with peak serum calcium concentrations ranging between 15 and 30 mg/dl. Hypophosphatemia, hypercalcinuria, hyperphosphaturia, and aminoaciduria have been noted in most infants when appropriate measurements have been made. Skeletal roentgenograms reveal demineralization, subperiosteal resorption, and pathologic fractures. Serum alkaline phosphatase values are usually within normal range despite clear evidence of bone involvement. Renal calcinosis is a common finding.

Complications
I **Derived:** Skeletal demineralization with pathologic fractures; renal calcinosis.
II **Associated:** Failure to thrive; hypotonia

Etiology: Possibly 2 distinct patterns of inheritance: autosomal recessive and autosomal dominant. There have been 16 reported cases of infantile hereditary parathyroid hyperplasia. The familial occurrence has been documented and consanguinity has been noted in 2 cases. McK *23920

Pathogenesis: The pathogenesis of parathyroid chief cell hyperplasia observed in this disorder is unknown.

Related Facts
I **Sex Ratio:** M1:F1
II **Risk of Occurrence:** ?
III **Risk of Recurrence for**
   Patient's Sib: When autosomal dominant or autosomal recessive, see Table I AD or AR, respectively.
   Patient's Child: When autosomal dominant or autosomal recessive, see Table I AD or AR, respectively.
IV **Age of Detectability:** In most infants the condition was diagnosed by the age of 4 months.
V **Prevalence:** ?

Treatment
I **Primary Prevention:** Genetic counseling
II **Secondary Prevention:** Neonatal familial hyperparathyroidism is considered a surgical emergency requiring parathyroidectomy. Since recurrence has been observed in 2 infants following subtotal parathyroidectomy the treatment of choice may be total parathyroidectomy.
III **Other Therapy:** Measures to combat hypercalcemia may be needed prior to surgery. Postoperative treatment of hypoparathyroidism requires vitamin D therapy and calcium supplements.

Prognosis: If untreated, the disease progresses and death occurs in the early months of life. Of 5 infants who were subjected to parathyroidectomy, 4 survived, and 1 died 13 days postoperatively.

Detection of Carrier: —

Special Considerations: —

References:
Goldbloom, R.B. et al: Hereditary parathyroid hyperplasia; A surgical emergency of early infancy. Pediatrics 49:514, 1972.
Hillman, D.A. et al: Neonatal familial primary hyperparathyroidism. N. Engl. J. Med. 270:483, 1964.
Spiegel, A.M. et al: Neonatal primary hyperparathyroidsim with autosomal dominant inheritance. J. Pediatr. 90:269, 1977.

Contributors: **David W. Gardner**
                    Constantine S. Anast

Editor's Computerized Descriptors: Skel., Muscle, Resp., Spleen, GI., Liver, GU., Nerve

HYPERPREBETA-LIPOPROTEINEMIA

Includes: Hyperbêta-lipoprotéinémie
Kohlenhydrat-induzierte Hyperlipämie
Hiperprebeta-lipoproteinemia
Hyperlipoproteinemia IV
Fredrickson type IV hyperlipoproteinemia
Carbohydrate-induced hyperlipemia
Endogenous hypertriglyceridemia
Hyperlipidemia IV

Excludes: Hyperchylomicronemia (489)

Minimal Diagnostic Criteria: On regular diet, lipoprotein findings as below. First-degree relatives may have similar findings, but no relatives have Types I, III, or V patterns.

Clinical Findings: This condition is usually identified in young adults. The serum is opalescent or creamy, the range for cholesterol is 200-1000 mg% and triglycerides 200-3000. By electrophoresis, chylomicrons are absent, betalipoprotein moderately decreased, prebetalipoprotein greatly increased and α-1-lipoprotein moderately decreased. The postheparin lipolytic activity is usually normal but glucose tolerance is abnormal in 90%.

Eruptive xanthomata occasionally occur on the buttocks, arms or legs. Xanthelasmata and corneal arcus are not present. Peripheral vascular disease may be present. Coronary disease is frequent but occurs later than in hypercholesteremia. Hepatosplenomegaly is occasionally found but abdominal pain does not occur.

Complications
I **Derived:** Coronary disease
II **Associated:** Relationship to diabetes confusing

Etiology: ? Possibly autosomal dominant. There is an apparent sensitivity to increased intake of calories or carbohydrate.

Pathogenesis: There is an impaired insulin regulation of serum glucose, with overproduction and possibly defective clearing of triglyceride. Excessive carbohydrate intake can induce chylomicronemia.

Related Facts
I **Sex Ratio:** M1:F1
II **Risk of Occurrence:** 2-3 per 1000
III **Risk of Recurrence for**
    Patient's Sib: 1 in 2 for adult sibs
    Patient's Child: Expressed in childhood only when both parents affected
IV **Age of Detectability:** Young adults
V **Prevalence:** Difficult to determine (phenocopies by diabetes, alcoholism, nephrosis, overnutrition)

Treatment
I **Primary Prevention:** —
II **Secondary Prevention:** Weight reduction, low carbohydrate diet, emphasis on polyunsaturated fats. Clofibrate, nicotinic acid, or neomycin may be helpful.
III **Other Therapy:** —

Prognosis: Death probably by coronary disease (but not early)

Detection of Carrier: —

Special Considerations: —

References:
Ahrens, E.J., Jr. et al: Carbohydrate-induced and fat-induced lipemia. Trans. Assoc. Am. Physicians 74:134, 1961.
Bierman, E.L. and Porte, D., Jr.: Carbohydrate intolerance and lipemia. Ann. Intern. Med. 68:926, 1968.
Brunzell, J.D. et al: Evidence for a common, saturable triglyceride removal mechanism for chylomicrons and very low density lipoproteins in man. J. Clin. Invest. 52:1578, 1973.
Fredrickson, D.S. and Levy, R.I.: Familial hyperlipoproteinemia. In Stanbury, J.B. et al (eds.): The Metabolic Basis of Inherited Disease, 3rd Ed. New York:McGraw Hill, 1972, p. 545.
Olefasky, J.M. et al: Reappraisal of the role of insulin in hypertriglyceridemia. Am. J. Med. 57:551, 1974.
Reissell, P.K. et al: Treatment of hypertriglyceridemia. Am. J. Clin. Nutr. 19:84, 1966.

Contributors: **Frederick T. Hatch**
                 Gerald M. Reaven

Editor's Computerized Descriptors: Skin, Spleen, CV.

HYPERPREBETA-LIPOPROTEINEMIA AND HYPERCHYLOMICRONEMIA

Includes: Hyperbêtalipoprotéinémie avec hyperchylomicronémie
Hyperlipämie Typ V n. Fredrickson
Hiperprebeta-lipoproteinemia e hiperquilomicronemia
Hyperlipoproteinemia V
Fredrickson type V hyperlipoproteinemia
Hyperlipidemia V

Excludes: Hyperprebeta-lipoproteinemia (500)
Hyperchylomicronemia (489)

Minimal Diagnostic Criteria: On regular diet, lipoprotein findings as below. Same or hyperpre-β-lipoproteinemia pattern in parents or adult sibs.

Clinical Findings: This condition is usually detected in the 30-40-year age group, rarely earlier. The serum is creamy. The range of cholesterol is 180-550 mg% and triglycerides 750-3700. By electrophoresis, chylomicrons are present, β-lipoprotein normal or decreased, prebetalipoprotein is increased with trailing, and alpha-1-lipoprotein is normal or decreased. The postheparin lipolytic activity has a low normal level and glucose tolerance is usually abnormal.

Eruptive xanthomata frequently occur on the buttocks, arms or legs. Xanthelasmata and corneal arcus are not found. Peripheral vascular disease has not been reported. Coronary disease is frequent but less significant. Abdominal pain may be present and severe, and hepatosplenomegaly is commonly found.

Complications
I **Derived:** Coronary disease, abdominal pain
II **Associated:** —

Etiology: ? One element may be homozygosity for hyperpre-β-lipoproteinemia. There is an apparent sensitivity to increased intake of both fat and carbohydrate. Possible double mutation, one being that for hyperpre-β-lipoproteinemia.

Pathogenesis: Possibly carbohydrate sensitivity is most basic; and saturation of subnormal triglyceride clearing mechanism. Restricted carbohydrate intake may eliminate chylomicronemia leaving only hyperpreβlipoproteinemia.

Related Facts
I **Sex Ratio:** M?:F? both sexes reported
II **Risk of Occurrence:** Rare
III **Risk of Recurrence for**
  Patient's Sib: ? Some relatives have hyperpre-β-lipoproteinemia or this condition.
  Patient's Child: ? Some relatives have hyperpre-β-lipoproteinemia
IV **Age of Detectability:** 3rd-4th decade usually, ? earlier
V **Prevalence:** Rare. Phenocopies by alcoholism, insulinopenic diabetes, nephrosis, and pancreatitis.

Treatment
I **Primary Prevention:** —
II **Secondary Prevention:** Weight reduction, diet moderate in both fat (polyunsaturated) and carbohydrate, high in protein. Clofibrate or nicotinic acid may be helpful.
III **Other Therapy:** —

Prognosis: ? Probably limited by coronary disease.

Detection of Carrier: ? Some heterozygotes simulate patients with hyperpre-β-lipoproteinemia.

Special Considerations: —

References:
Brunzell, J.D. et al: Evidence for a common, saturable, triglyceride removal mechanism for chylomicrons and very low density lipo-proteins in man. J. Clin. Invest. 52:1578, 1973.
Fredrickson, D.S. and Levy, R.I.: Familial hyperlipoproteinemia. In Stanbury, J.B. et al (eds.): The Metabolic Basis of Inherited Disease, 3rd Ed. New York:McGraw-Hill, 1972, p. 545.
Greenberger, N.J. et al: Pancreatitis and hyperlipemia; a study of serum lipid alterations in 25 patients with acute pancreatitis. Medicine 45:161, 1966.

Contributors: **Frederick T. Hatch**
Gerald M. Reaven

Editor's Computerized Descriptors: Skin, Spleen, Liver, CV.

HYPERPROLINEMIA (MARKER)

Includes: Hyperprolinémie
Hyperprolinämie
Hiperprolinemia (Marcador)
Hyperprolinemia type I
Hyperprolinemia type II†

Excludes: —

Minimal Diagnostic Criteria: *Type I:* Persistent elevation of plasma proline concentration above 5 mg/100 dl. Hyperaminoaciduria comprising proline (overflow), and glycine and hydroxyproline (competition) found when plasma proline concentration exceeds 8 mg/100 dl about 0.70 μmole/ml. *Type II:* Same as type I, except proline concentration usually much higher (20-40 mg/100 dl). Urine contains δ'-pyrroline-5-carboxylic acid (PC) and δ'-pyrroline-3-hydroxy-5-carboxylate† the corresponding metabolite of hydroxyproline, as well as proline, glycine and hydroxyproline.

Clinical Findings: A biochemical phenotype. No proven association with clinical disease, although identified frequently in pedigrees containing renal disease or convulsive disorders. The occurrence of subjects in such pedigrees with disease, but no hyperprolinemia, and the converse, and clearcut examples of independent modes of inheritance of the familial disease trait and of hyperprolinemia, support the belief that hyperprolinemia and disease traits are probably incidentally associated.

Complications
I **Derived:** —
II **Associated:** Possibly convulsive disorders, renal disease

Etiology: Autosomal recessive for both types. The possibility of associated genes at different loci has not been ruled out to account for associated renal and CNS disease. McK *23950, *23951

Pathogenesis: With requisite confidence: Type I proline oxidase deficiency. Type II δ'-pyrroline-5-carboxylic acid dehydrogenase deficiency; detectable in fibroblasts cultured from skin biopsy and in leukocytes. Relationship to convulsive disorders and renal disease is unknown.

Related Facts
I **Sex Ratio:** M1:F1
II **Risk of Occurrence:** <1 in 20,000 live births
III **Risk of Recurrence for**
    Patient's Sib: 1 in 4 (25%) for each offspring to be affected
    Patient's Child: Not increased unless mate is carrier or homozygote
IV **Age of Detectability:** Presumably detectable in newborn
V **Prevalence:** < 1 in 20,000

Treatment
I **Primary Prevention:** Not necessary
II **Secondary Prevention:** None. No effective way to restrict proline accumulation. No proven benefit from such attempts.
III **Other Therapy:** —

Prognosis: Apparently benign trait

Detection of Carrier: No consistent finding known; some Type 1 heterozygotes manifest modest hyperprolinemia. Type II heterozygotes do not have hyperprolinemia.

†**Special Considerations:** Trait identified in Caucasians of Europe and North America, and also in the North American Indian. Two enzyme defects can cause the same trait, but PC-dehydrogenase deficiency is associated with greater hyperprolinemia than that caused by proline oxidase deficiency. The latter enzyme may be shared in hydroxyproline metabolism and account for evidence for impaired oxidation of the second imino acid in type II hyperprolinemia.
Complex hyperaminoaciduria (proline, glycine and hydroxyproline) is of combined prerenal and renal origin. It does not appear unless plasma proline is sufficiently elevated (> 8 mg/100 dl). Identification of trait by detection of hyperaminoaciduria requires discrimination from renal iminoglycinuria.

References:
Efron, M. L.: Familial hyperprolinemia: Report of a second case, associated with congenital renal malformations, hereditary hematuria and mild mental retardation, with demonstration of an enzyme defect. N. Engl. J. Med. 272 :1243, 1965.

Schafer, I. A. et al: Familial hyperprolinemia, cerebral dysfunction and renal anomalies occurring in a family with hereditary nephropathy and deafness, N. Engl. J. Med. 267 :51, 1962.

Scriver, C.R.: Disorders of proline and hydroxyproline metabolism. In Stanbury, J.B. et al (eds.): The Metabolic Basis of Inherited Disease, 4th Ed. New York:McGraw-Hill Book Co.,1976, p. 336.

Valle, D.L. et al: Type II hyperprolinemia: Absence of δ'-pyrroline-5-carboxylic acid dehydrogenase activity. Science 185:1053, 1974.

Contributor: **Charles R. Scriver**

Editor's Computerized Descriptor: —

HYPERSARCOSINEMIA

Includes: Hypersarcosinémie
Hypersarkosinämie
Hipersarcosinemia

Excludes: —

Minimal Diagnostic Criteria: Increased sarcosine blood levels; high sarcosine excretion in the urine.

Clinical Findings: Relationship to disease is unknown. Seven patients with hypersarcosinemia have been described. No consistent clinical syndrome has been identified. The 2 original patients had subnormal intelligence. Dysphagia and hepatosplenomegaly may be related.

The 2 original patients had increased levels of sarcosine in the blood 1.4-5.6 mg% as compared with 0-0.2 for controls. Urinary sarcosine excretion was 77-168 mg/24 hr in the less-than-one-year-old patients, and 474-703 mg/24 hr in the 6-year-old.

Complications
I **Derived:** —
II **Associated:** —

Etiology: Probably autosomal recessive of enzyme defect

Pathogenesis: Deficiency of sarosine dehydrogenase in the liver. Relationship to disease unknown.

Related Facts
I **Sex Ratio:** M1:F1 probable
II **Risk of Occurrence:** Extremely low
III **Risk of Recurrence for**
  Patient's Sib: Probably 1 in 4 (25%) for each offspring to be affected
  Patient's Child: Not increased unless mate is carrier or homozygote
IV **Age of Detectability:** Before age 3 months by urine analysis
V **Prevalence:** Extremely rare

Treatment
I **Primary Prevention:** Genetic counseling
II **Secondary Prevention:** ?
III **Other Therapy:** —

Prognosis: Normal life span

Detection of Carrier: Oral tolerance test with sarcosine or dimethylglycine (DMG) (100 mg/kg body weight). In carriers excretion of sarcosine in the urine of more than 100 mg/8 hrs after sarcosine load or more than 15 mg/8 hrs after DMG load identifies carrier state.

Special Considerations: —

References:
Gerritsen, T. and Waisman, H. A.: Hypersarcosinemia: An inborn error of metabolism. N. Engl. J. Med. 275 :66, 1966.
Gerritsen, T.: Sarcosine dehydrogenase deficiency, the enzyme defect in hypersarcosinemia. Helv. Paediatr. Acta 27:33, 1972
Hagge, W. et al: Hypersarcosinemia. (Abstract) Pediatr. Res. 1:409, 1967
Tippett,P. and Danks, D.M.: The clinical and biochemical findings in three cases of hypersarcosinemia and one case of transient hypersarcosinuria with folic acid deficiency. Helv. Paediatr. Acta 29:261, 1974

Contributor: Theo Gerritsen

Editor's Computerized Descriptors: Liver, Nerve

HYPERTELORISM

Includes: Hypertélorisme
Hypertelorismus
Hipertelorismo
Euryopia
Ocular hypertelorism
Greig syndrome

Excludes: Pseudohypertelorism (usually secondary to epicanthus or telecanthus)

Minimal Diagnostic Criteria: Increased interpupillary or interorbital distance for the patient's age, sex and race. Normal means and standard deviation are being developed. (See Christian and Jöhr references.) Telecanthus often accompanies hypertelorism, but one should not be misled by the clinical impression of hypertelorism frequently produced by telecanthus in the presence of normal ocular separation.

Clinical Findings: Increased interorbital distance with increased interpupillary distance can be found as a primary defect or secondary to other developmental malformations of the cranium and face. Typically, the nasal bridge is broad and often depressed and the forehead prominent. Exotropia frequently occurs, making measurement of the interpupillary distance difficult. (It can be accomplished, however, by alternate fixation on a common point.) Usually mentality is not affected. The condition is usually bilaterally symmetric.

Complications
I **Derived:** Occasionally, narrowing of the optic canals produces optic atrophy. Frequently the wide-set orbits lead to exotropia.
II **Associated:** Abnormal dentition, acrocyanosis, arched palate, enlarged terminal phalanges, rudimentary clavicles, syndactyly and undescended testes.

Etiology: ? Most primary hypertelorism occurs sporadically, although families with apparent autosomal dominant or recessive inheritance have been described. Secondary hypertelorism has been described as part of many syndromes: acrocephalosyndactyly, cerebral gigantism, cerebrohepatorenal syndrome, chondrodystrophia calcificans congenita, chromosome 4p-, chromosome 5p-, craniofacial dysostosis, familial metaphyseal dysplasia, mucopolysaccharidosis I, hydrocephaly, infantile hypercalcemia, Kleeblattschädel, median cleft face, nevoid basal cell carcinoma, orofaciodigital syndrome, otopalatodigital syndrome, chromosome 18q-, and others. McK *14540

Pathogenesis: ? Disproportionate growth, embryonic fixation and secondary effects of other malformations are implicated in some cases.

Related Facts
I **Sex Ratio:** ?
II **Risk of Occurrence:** ?
III **Risk of Recurrence for**
  Patient's Sib: When autosomal dominant or autosomal recessive, see Table I AD or AR, respectively.
  Patient's Child: When autosomal dominant or autosomal recessive, see Table I AD or AR, respectively.
IV **Age of Detectability:** Variable. Usually in infancy or early childhood.
V **Prevalence:** ?

Treatment
I **Primary Prevention:** Genetic counseling
II **Secondary Prevention:** Extraocular muscle surgery to reduce strabismus
III **Other Therapy:** Plastic surgery to decrease associated surface malformations

Prognosis: Primary hypertelorism is usually associated with a normal life span. Secondary hypertelorism is dictated by the primary cause.

Detection of Carrier: —

Special Considerations: —

References:
Christian, J.C. et al: Familial telecanthus with associated congenital anomalies. In Bergsma, D. (ed.): Part II. Malformation Syndromes. Birth Defects: Orig. Art. Ser., New York:The National Foundation-March of Dimes, vol. V, no. 2, 1969, p. 82.
Duke-Elder, S.: System of Ophthalmology, vol. 3, pt. 2. Congenital Defects, St. Louis: C.V. Mosby, Co., 1963, p. 1053.
Gellis, S.S. and Feingold, M.: Atlas of Mental Retardation Syndromes: Visual Diagnosis of Facies and Physical Findings. Washington,D.C.: U.S. Government Printing Office, 1968.
Jöhr, P.: Valeurs moyennes et limites normales en fonction de l'âge, le quelques mésures de la tête et de la regien orbitaire. J. Génét. Hum. 2:247, 1953.

Contributor: Donald R. Bergsma

Editor's Computerized Descriptors: Eye, Nose

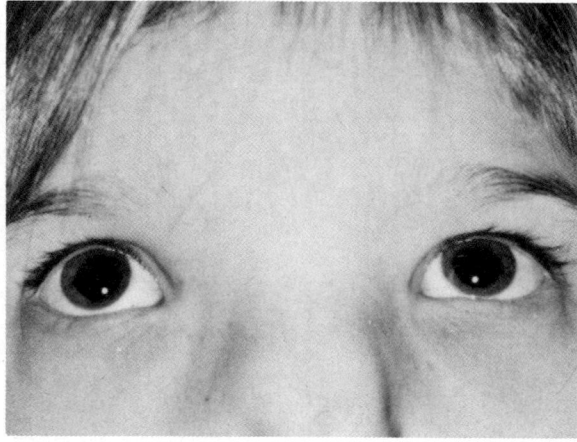

293. Ocular hypertelorism

Includes: Syndrome hypertélorisme-hypospadias
Hypertelorismus-Hypospadie-Syndrom
Síndrome de hipertelorismo e hipospadias
BBB syndrome
Familial telecanthus with associated anomalies
Hypospadias-hypertelorism syndrome
Telecanthus-hypospadias syndrome
Telecanthus with associated abnormalities

Excludes: Isolated hypospadias
Waardenburg syndrome (997)

Minimal Diagnostic Criteria: A male with widely spaced inner canthi and hypospadias or one of these findings and a family history of other affected individuals. A female with telecanthus and affected male relatives.†

Clinical Findings: A total of 26 affected males have been reported. The following clinical findings have been recorded: wide-spaced inner canthi (telecanthus or apparent hypertelorism) 96%, hypospadias 96%, cranial asymmetry (plagiocephaly) 60%, mental retardation 50%, strabismus 42%, cryptorchidism 35%, cleft lip and palate 23% and urinary tract abnormalities 19%. Other findings have been ear anomalies, congenital heart defects, multiple lipomata, flame nevi, imperforate anus, bifid uvula, epicanthal folds, diastasis recti and umbilical or inguinal herniae.

The affected males have come from 16 families and telecanthic females have been found in all but 3 reported families. Females have been reported to have telecanthus and no other findings. The telecanthus has been of variable degree and one obligate carrier female had an inner canthal distance within the normal range.

Complications
I **Derived:** Urinary tract infections; amblyopia ex anopsia
II **Associated:** Not yet discernible

Etiology: A dominant trait with no documented case of male-to-male transmission

Pathogenesis: The most striking findings are midline defects, particularly of the craniofacial skeleton and the genital tubercle. Like-sexed twinning and midline clefts of the face previously have been reported associated in families. The present syndrome seems to be associated with twinning more than can be expected by chance alone. Three affected individuals have been twins (2 pairs concordant and 1 pair discordant for the trait). Therefore, there may be a pathogenic relationship between the process of twinning and this syndrome.

Related Facts
I **Sex Ratio:** M1:F1 (M26:F25 among observed cases)
II **Risk of Occurrence:** ? The 26 reported in 16 families have come from only 4 medical centers suggesting that the syndrome is not widely diagnosed.
III **Risk of Recurrence for**
  Patient's Sib: If autosomal dominant and if parent is affected, 1 in 2 (50%) for each offspring to be affected; otherwise not increased.
  Patient's Child: 1 in 2 if autosomal dominant.
IV **Age of Detectability:** At birth by physical examination
V **Prevalence:** ?

Treatment
I **Primary Prevention:** Genetic counseling
II **Secondary Prevention:** —
III **Other Therapy:** Repair of hypospadias and cleft palate, and appropriate therapy for associated birth defects.

Prognosis: Five affected males have died in infancy; no affected females are known to have died from the syndrome. Mental retardation occurred in 50% of affected males; no known mental retardation in the affected females. In general, the associated congenital anomalies are surgically correctable.

Detection of Carrier: Finding of isolated telecanthus in female.

†Special Considerations: The name hypertelorism-hypospadias syndrome was chosen because it reflects the clinically most evident and common findings in the affected males; however, not all affected individuals with wide-spaced inner canthi (telecanthus) have increased distance between the bony orbits (hypertelorism).

Before more definite conclusions can be drawn about the spectrum of the clinical syndrome and pathogenic factors, there is a great need for further patient documentation and study.

References:
Christian, J.C. et al: Familial telecanthus with associated congenital anomalies. In Bergsma, D. (ed.): Part II. Malformation Syndromes. Birth Defects: Orig. Art. Ser., vol. V, no. 2. New York:- The National Foundation-March of Dimes, 1969, p. 82.
Michaelis, E. and Mortier, N.: Association of hypertelorism and hypospadias-the BBB syndrome. Helv. Paediatr. Acta 27:575, 1972.
Opitz, J.M. et al: The BBB syndrome-familial telecanthus with associated congenital anomalies. In Malformation Syndromes, op. cit., p. 86.
Summitt, R.L. and Wilroy, R.S., Jr.: Further studies of the telecanthus-hypospadias syndrome. (Abstract) Pediatr. Res. 8:442, 1974.

Contributor: **Joe C. Christian**

Editor's Computerized Descriptors: Eye, Face, Oral, Skin, Skel., Muscle, Hernia not CNS, CV., GU., Nerve

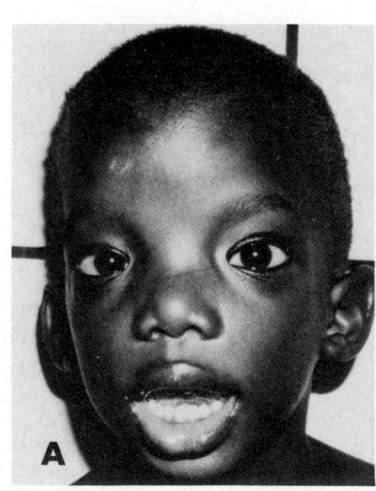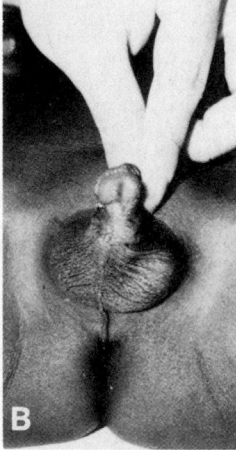

294. A) Hypertelorism, epicanthic folds, and esotropia; B) glandular hypospadias

HYPERTELORISM, MICROTIA, FACIAL CLEFTING AND CONDUCTIVE DEAFNESS

Includes: Hypertélorisme, microtie et la fissure de la lèvre et du palais
Hypertelorismus, Microtie und Lippe und Gaumenspalten
Hipertelorismo, microtia, hendidura facial y sordera de conducción
Microtia, facial clefting, hypertelorism
Bixler syndrome
HMC syndrome

Excludes: Oto-palato-digital syndrome (786)
Median cleft face syndrome (635)

Minimal Diagnostic Criteria: Hypertelorism, microtia and cleft lip and palate

Clinical Findings: Five patients in 3 families, among them a pair of identical twins, have been described with features of this syndrome. Hypertelorism is present in all 5, microtia with meatal atresia is present in all 5, unilateral cleft lip and palate in 4, microcephaly in 2/5, syndactyly of 2nd and 3rd toes in 4/5, shortening of the 5th finger in 4/5, mandibular arch hypoplasia in 5/5, flattened angle of mandible in 5/5, broad nasal tip in 3/5, bifid nose in 1/5, microstomia in 3/5, bilateral thenar hypoplasia in 4/5, ectopic kidneys in 3/5, congenital heart anomalies in 3/5, vertebral anomalies in 4/5. Reduced body weight and size are present in 5/5. In 2 cases polytomographic examination revealed hypoplasia of the auditory ossicles and normal vestibula, cochlea, semicircular canals and internal auditory canals bilaterally. Congenital heart and vertebral anomalies are seen in several family members.

Complications
I   Derived: Because of cleft palate there are, in the early years, problems with feeding and aspiration. Speech defects may be present later. The frequency of recurrent nasal and paranasal infections is higher.
II Associated: Mental retardation

Etiology: Autosomal recessive and autosomal dominant inheritance have been proposed, though the presence of this syndrome in 2 of 4 sibs with normal parents strongly suggests the former.

Pathogenesis: ?

Related Facts
I   Sex Ratio: M3:F2
II Risk of Occurrence: ?
III Risk of Recurrence for
    Patient's Sib: When autosomal recessive or autosomal dominant, see Table I AR or AD, respectively.
    Patient's Child: When autosomal recessive or autosomal dominant, see Table I AR or AD, respectively.
IV Age of Detectability: At birth
V   Prevalence: ? 3 reported families with 5 affected individuals.

Treatment
I   Primary Prevention: Genetic counseling
II Secondary Prevention: Reconstructive surgery of the external auditory canal and auricle. Plastic surgery to repair cleft lip and palate.
III Other Therapy: Hearing aid and special training because of this hearing loss. Orthodontic treatment and speech therapy in cases of cleft palate.

Prognosis: Probably normal life span

Detection of Carrier: ?

Special Considerations: —

References:
Bixler, D. et al: Hypertelorism, microtia and facial clefting. A

newly described inherited syndrome. Am. J. Dis. Child. 118:495, 1969.

Ionasescu, V. and Roberts, R.J.: Variant of Bixler syndrome. J. Genet. Hum. 22:133,1974.

Schweckendiek, W. et al: H.M.C. syndrome in identical twins. Hum. Genet. 33:315, 1976.

Contributors: **Agnes M. Ickenroth**
Cor W.R.J. Cremers

Editor's Computerized Descriptors: Eye, Hearing, Ear, Face, Oral, Nasoph., Nose, Speech, Skin, Skel., CV., GI., GU.

HYPERTRICHOSIS LANUGINOSA

Includes: Hypertrichose congénitale-hirsutisme
Hipertricosis lanuginosa
Congenital hypertrichosis lanuginosa
Hypertrichosis universalis congenita
Edentate hypertrichosis
Hypertrichosis of the dog-man

Excludes: Acquired hypertrichosis or hirsutism associated with endocrine disturbance
Senility or metabolic disorders, such as porphyria and the mucopolysaccharidoses
Gingival fibromatosis and hypertrichosis (410)
Localized hypertrichosis either sporadic or associated with nevi and spina bifida
Hypertrichosis cubiti
Other forms of familial localized hypertrichosis

Minimal Diagnostic Criteria: Generalized hairiness in excess of the amount usually present in persons of the same sex, age, and race.

Clinical Findings: Excessive growth of hair on all parts of the body except the palms, soles, and mucous membranes. The teeth may be abnormal but there are no systemic ramifications. The undue hairiness is usually present at birth, and increases during infancy. It may partially resolve during later childhood.

Complications
I   **Derived:** Psychosocial problems due to the unusual appearance of the patient
II **Associated:** —

Etiology: Autosomal dominant. There is probably a high degree of penetrance but expression is variable. McK *14570

Pathogenesis: ? It is possible that the hair follicles are unduly responsive, or that a biosynthetic defect exists in one of the hormones which controls nonsexual hair growth.

Related Facts
I   **Sex Ratio:** M1:F1
II   **Risk of Occurrence:** Remote
III **Risk of Recurrence for**
      Patient's Sib: If parent is affected, 1 in 2 (50%) for each offspring to be affected; otherwise not increased.
      Patient's Child: 1 in 2
IV   **Age of Detectability:** At birth
V   **Prevalence:** Very rare. Less than 40 cases in the world literature. Reported in Britain, Europe, U.S.A., Canary Isles, Burma and East Africa.

Treatment
I   **Primary Prevention:** Genetic counseling
II   **Secondary Prevention:** Removal of unsightly hair with shaving, depilatory applications, diathermy or radiation. Camouflage by bleaching or makeup.†
III **Other Therapy:** —

Prognosis: Normal for life span, intelligence and function

Detection of Carrier: —

†Special Considerations: The undue hairiness poses serious cosmetic problems especially to females. Apart from variable abnormalities in the teeth, the condition is harmless. In the past, several affected individuals were well-known circus exhibitionists. (Jo-Jo, the Human Skye Terrier; Shwe-Maong, the dog-faced man of Burma, his affected daughter Maphoon and her son Moung Phoset.)

References:
Beighton, P.: Congenital hypertrichosis lanuginosa. Arch. Dermatol. 101:669, 1970.
Danforth, C. H.: Studies on hair; with special reference to hypertrichosis. Arch. Dermatol. Syph. (Chic.) 12:380, 1925.

Felgenhauer, W. R.: Hypertrichosis lanuginosa universalis. J. Genet. Hum. 17:1, 1969.

Contributor: **Peter Beighton**

Editor's Computerized Descriptor: Hair

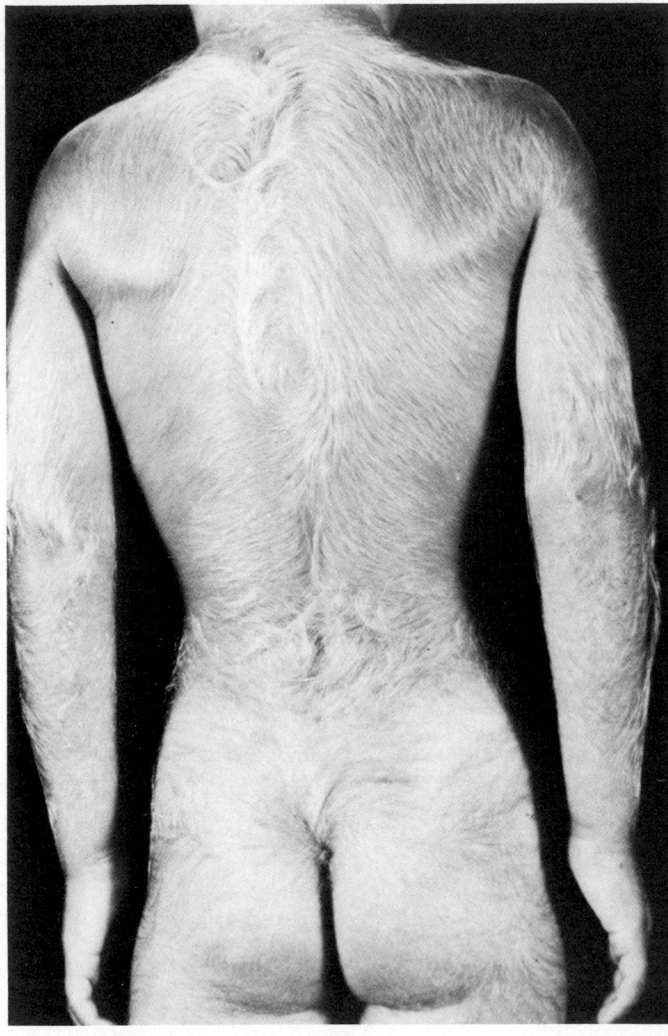

295. Congenital hypertrichosis universalis

HYPERURICEMIA, DEAFNESS AND ATAXIA

Includes: Syndrome hyperuricémie-surdité - ataxie
Hyperuricämie-Schwerhörigkeit-Ataxie
Hiperuricemia-sordera y ataxia
Deafness, sensorineural, ataxia and hyperuricemia

Excludes: Lesch-Nyhan syndrome (588)
Gout (441)
Lipodystrophy and neurologic defect

Minimal Diagnostic Criteria: Hyperuricemia† prior to onset of renal dysfunction (ie primary hyperuricemia), normal hypoxanthine-guanine phosphoribosyltranferase in the erythrocytes, onset in adolescence of progressive spinocerebellar ataxia and sensorineural hearing loss, still later onset of renal dysfunction.

Clinical Findings: Onset of elevated blood uric acid level in late childhood or at puberty. In adolescence or early adult life, progressive spinocerebellar ataxia and sensorineural hearing loss begin. Later, renal disease, slurred speech and occasionally gout occur. Apparently all hyperuricemic individuals with this syndrome develop ataxia and hearing loss. Two adult females with the syndrome have also developed cervicodorsal fat pad ("buffalo hump") without Cushing syndrome and with normal steroid levels. Muscle wasting and weakness are inconstant features. One member of a family studied has developed cardiomyopathy. There is no mental retardation or self-mutilation.

Audiograms show a high-frequency sensorineural loss in the younger affected members, a sloping sensorineural loss in early adult life; and the most severely affected individual has virtually complete loss of hearing. A highly positive SISI is found on special testing, indicating cochlear involvement rather than neural or central involvement. Electronystagmography shows changes consistent with a vestibular lesion central to the labyrinth. Petrous pyramid tomography is normal.

Standard renal function tests are normal in the younger affected members, abnormal in older members. IV pyelography is normal. Erythrocyte hypoxanthine-guanine phosphoribosyltransferase levels are normal. Muscle biopsies of affected members with muscle weakness are consistent with a neurogenic myopathy.

Complications
I   Derived: Nephrolithiasis
II Associated: Congestive heart failure secondary to cardiomyopathy

Etiology: This would seem to be of autosomal dominant inheritance. The hyperuricemia appears to be primary since it antedates the renal dysfunction, but the cause of the hyperuricemia is unknown. Whether the hyperuricemia causes the deafness and ataxia or whether they are merely associated defects is unknown.

Pathogenesis: Muscle biopsy microscopic changes show denervating disease of the long-standing chronic type. No enzyme deficiencies were demonstrated including erythrocyte hypoxanthine-guanine phosphoribosyltransferase. Muscle enzymes were normal. No hormonal effects were demonstrated in 1 adult female with cervicodorsal fat pad.

Related Facts
I   Sex Ratio: M1:F1, although kindred studied contains fewer postadolescent females than males.
II Risk of Occurrence: ? Thus far only described in 1 large Mexican-American kindred living in Pueblo, Colorado.
III Risk of Recurrence for
   Patient's Sib: —
   Patient's Child: —

IV Age of Detectability: Adolescence by blood uric acid, clinical evaluation and audiometry
V Prevalence: ?

Treatment
I Primary Prevention: Genetic counseling
II Secondary Prevention: Allopurinol will reduce blood uric acid levels and, therefore, should prevent gout and nephrolithiasis. However, it has had no retarding or beneficial effects on the deafness, ataxia, muscle weakness or wasting.
III Other Therapy: Hearing aids and speech training. Treatment for congestive heart failure secondary to cardiomyopathy.

Prognosis: Progression of hearing loss, ataxia, muscle weakness and probably of renal disease. Whether or not life span will be shortened remains to be seen.

Detection of Carrier: Family history and uric acid levels are the only means presently available for detection in preclinical cases.

†Special Considerations: Normal Values Serum Uric Acid (Uricase Method) (mgm/100 cc)

Adult and postpubertal males	7.0 or less
Males age 12-18	6.5 or less
Females	6.5 or less
Adolescent females	6.0 or less
Postmenopausal females	7.0 or less
Children	5.5 or less

(Premature infants may have transient renal insufficiency during which time the uric acid may rise temporarily to higher levels.)

References:
Kelley, W.N. et al: A specific enzyme defect in gout assoicated with overproduction of uric acid. Proc. Natl. Acad. Sci. USA 57:1735, 1967.
Rosenberg, A.L. and Bartholomew, B.: Gout and uric acid. Bull. Rheum. Dis. 19:543, 1969.
Rosenberg, A.L. et al: Hyperuricemia and neurologic deficits: A family study. N. Engl. J. Med. 282:992, 1970.

Contributor: **LaVonne Bergstrom**

Editor's Computerized Descriptors: Hearing, Speech, Skin, Skel., Muscle, CV., GU., Nerve

HYPERVALINEMIA

Includes: Hypervalinémie
Hypervalinämie
Hipervalinemia

Excludes: —

Minimal Diagnostic Criteria: Hypervalinemia (10 mg%) and an increased excretion of valine in the urine, in the absence of a ketoaciduria. The other branched-chain amino acids, leucine and isoleucine, are normal.
The specific enzymatic defect is demonstrable in the peripheral leukocyte.

Clinical Findings: Only one patient has been described so far. Therefore, it is not certain whether the clinical findings are coincidental or secondary to the metabolic defect. The effects of a low-valine diet suggest that at least some of the findings are caused directly or indirectly by the hypervalinemia. The patient was a hyperkinetic Japanese child, now 5 years old, mentally and physically retarded. Poor feeding and vomiting were prominent early in infancy.

Complications
I Derived: Probably vomiting, hyperkinesia, mental and physical retardation
II Associated: —

Etiology: Probably autosomal recessive; McK *27710

Pathogenesis: Inability to degrade valine at the first metabolic step (transaminase). This is proximal to the block in maple syrup urine disease.

Related Facts
I Sex Ratio: M1:F1 probable
II Risk of Occurrence: Very rare
III Risk of Recurrence for
Patient's Sib: Probably 1 in 4 (25%) for each offspring to be affected
Patient's Child: Probably not increased unless mate is carrier or homozygote
IV Age of Detectability: ?
V Prevalence: Very rare

Treatment
I Primary Prevention: Genetic counseling
II Secondary Prevention: A low-valine diet was instituted for a brief period of time with lowering of blood valine level, cessation of vomiting, weight gain and reduction in hyperkinesia.
III Other Therapy: —

Prognosis: ?

Detection of Carrier: This has not been conclusively demonstrated to be an inherited disease.

Special Considerations: —

References:
Dancis, J. et al: Hypervalinemia: A defect in valine transamination. Pediatrics 39:813, 1967.
Wada, Y.: Idiopathic hypervalinemia: Valine alpha-keto-acids in blood following an oral dose of valine. Tohoku J. Exp. Med. 87:322, 1965.
Wada, Y. et al: Idiopathic hypervalinemia: Probably a new entity of inborn error of valine metabolism. Tohoku J. Exp. Med. 81:46, 1963.

Contributor: **Joseph Dancis**

Editor's Computerized Descriptors: GI., Nerve

HYPOCHONDROPLASIA

Includes: Hypochondroplasie
Hipocondroplasia

Excludes: Other forms of short-limb dwarfism
Achondroplasia (10)

Minimal Diagnostic Criteria: Mild-to-moderate short-limb dwarfism with combination of clinical and radiographic features listed below.†

Clinical Findings: Both children and adults have small stature with disproportionately short limbs. Hands and feet are short and broad. The relative shortening of the limbs may be mild. Limitation of motion at elbow common. No trident hand deformity. Fibulae are disproportionately long, and mild bowleg and heel varus deformities may be present. Head is normal sized, tends to be brachycephalic with prominent forehead. No depression of nasal bridge or other facial abnormality. Adult height 46 1/2 to 58 in.

Radiographic findings include shortened ilia which may be somewhat square but usually have some flaring of iliac crests. The sacrosciatic notches are not reduced in width. The sacrum usually articulates low in relation to the iliac crests. The pelvic changes are less marked than in achondroplasia and may be within normal limits (frontal projection). The interpediculate distance is the same or narrows from L1 to L5 (frontal projection). These abnormalities are not as marked as in achondroplasia and are usually not present in infants and young children. In most older children and adults, the backs of the lumbar bodies have a concave configuration, less marked than that in achondroplasia. Pedicles are usually short (lateral projection).

Limbs are short, so visual impression is that of mildly widened diaphyses and mildly flared metaphyses. Sites of muscle attachments are prominent. Ulnae are relatively short with a bulbous enlargement of radial aspect of distal ulnar epiphysis and prominence of ulnar styloid. Square configuration of proximal tibial epiphysis and flare of adjacent metaphysis. Fibulae are disproportionately long. In early childhood, there may be shallow V-shaped indentation of distal femoral metaphysis-not as marked as in achondroplasia. This is not a diagnostic finding as a similar change occurs in other short-limb dwarf conditions. (All limb findings in frontal projection.) The skull is normal. No abnormal laboratory findings.

Complications
I Derived: Chronic serous otitis media. Rootlet irritation in some older individuals might be expected because of small bony dimensions in lower lumbar spine.

II Associated: —

Etiology: Autosomal dominant

Pathogenesis: Relatively slow enchondral bone growth with normal membranous ossification.

Related Facts
I Sex Ratio: M1:F1
II Risk of Occurrence: ?
III Risk of Recurrence for
  Patient's Sib: If parent is affected, 1 in 2 (50%) for each offspring to be affected; otherwise not increased.
  Patient's Child: 1 in 2 if mate unaffected
IV Age of Detectability: Although mean birth length is decreased, unless expected, the mild-to-moderate short stature may not be noticed until 3-4 years of age.
V Prevalence: ? †

Treatment
I Primary Prevention: Genetic counseling
II Secondary Prevention: —
III Other Therapy: Cesarean section necessary for delivery in most pregnant hypochondroplasts.

Prognosis: Normal life span

Detection of Carrier: —

†Special Considerations: Hypochondroplasia is a recently recognized entity. The diagnosis of hypochondroplasia cannot be established in sporadic cases until midchildhood. Before this age, height may be in lower range of normal and radiographic changes likewise may be within normal limits. At age 5-6 years, and in the older individual, the physical appearance and radiographic changes are qualitatively similar to those of achondroplasia but deviate from normal to a lesser degree. There is considerable variability in the severity of changes in hypochondroplasia so that in the severely involved hypochondroplastic, the differential diagnostic consideration is achondroplasia, and, in the mildly involved hypochondroplastic the differential diagnostic consideration is the small normal person. Individuals with the changes of both achondroplasia and hypochondroplasia have not been seen in the same family. Thus, it does not appear to represent mild achondroplasia, although severely affected hypochondroplasts have been so diagnosed in the past. It is not an exceedingly rare condition in the experience of physicians aware of its existence. However, too few cases have been reported to estimate its true frequency. It has been postulated that hypochondroplasia may represent an allelic mutation to achondroplasia. In mild cases, the disproportion may not be readily apparent without performing anthropometric measurements and many cases have been considered at first to be proportionate and have received unnecessary endocrine evaluations.

References:
Beals, R.K.: Hypochondroplasia: A report of five kindreds. J. Bone Joint Surg. 51A:728, 1969.
Kozlowski, K. and Zychowicz, C.: Hypochondroplasie. Fortschr. Röntgenstr. 100:529, 1964.
Rimoin, D.L.: The chondrodystrophies. Adv. Hum. Genet. 5:1, 1975.
Walker, B.A. et al: Hypochondroplasia. Am. J. Dis. Child. 122:95, 1971.

Contributors: **David L. Rimoin**
Leonard O. Langer, Jr.

Editor's Computerized Descriptor: Skel.

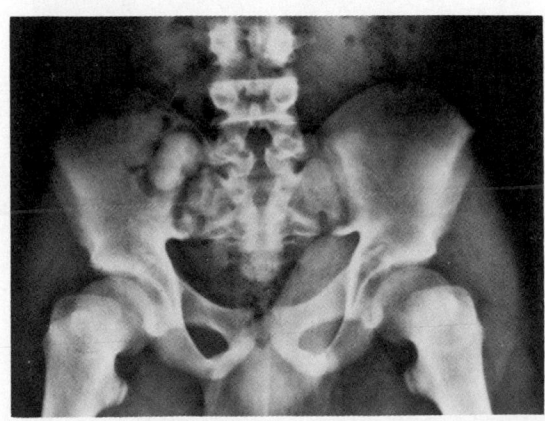

296. Lumbar spine tapers from top to bottom. Note narrow spinal canal and sacrum with posterior midline cleft; small greater sciatic notches

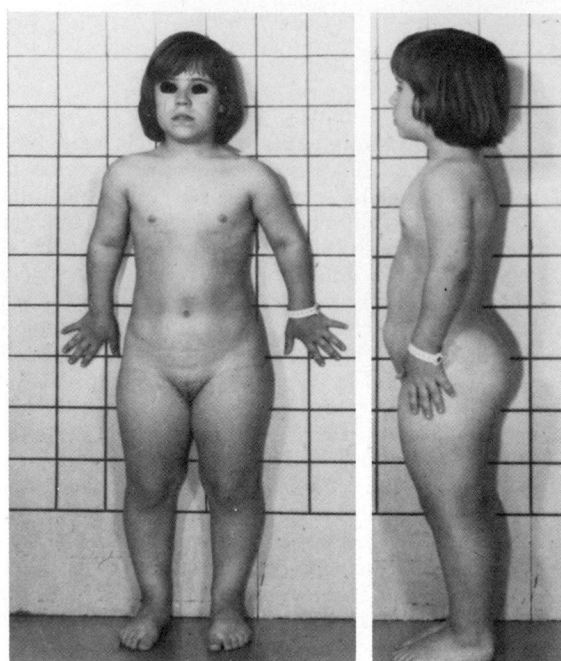

297. Note short stature, disproportionately short limbs, normal head, and limitation of elbow extension

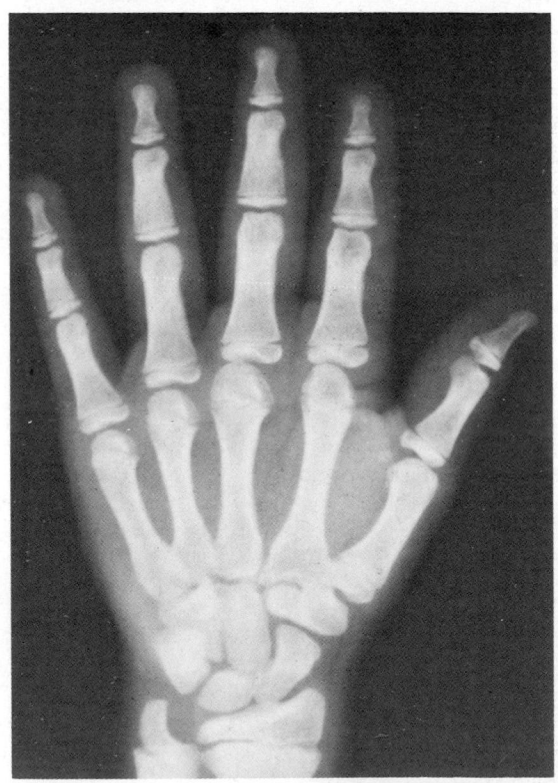

298. Note generalized shortening of bones; long and curved styloid ulna

HYPODONTIA AND NAIL DYSGENESIS

Includes: Hypodontie avec dysgénésie des ongles
Hypodontie und Nageldysgenesie
Hipodoncia con disgenesia de las uñas
Tooth and nail syndrome
Nail dysgenesis and hypodontia

Excludes: Ectodermal dysplasia, anhidrotic (333)
Ectodermal dysplasia, ungual type
Chondroectodermal dysplasia (156)

Minimal Diagnostic Criteria: Congenitally missing teeth and history of slow growth of nails.†

Clinical Findings: Children have congenitally missing teeth (from one to seldom more than 20) and a retardation in growth of nails best seen from birth to 3 years of age without other signs of anhidrotic ectodermal dysplasia. Nails are small, thin and often spoon-shaped. Older children and adults frequently have normal fingernails but small spoon-shaped toenails.

Congenitally missing teeth	100%
Hypoplasia of toe or fingernals	100%
Fine hair	50%
Eversion of lips	20%

Complications
I   **Derived:** Possible loss of vertical face dimension due to loss of teeth resulting in eversion of lips.
II **Associated:** —

Etiology: Autosomal dominant with variable expressivity; McK *18950

Pathogenesis: Essentially unknown. Gene probably acts on specialized ectodermal cells involved in dental lamina and anlage of nails. Nails may be absent at birth or not require cutting until age 2-3 years. Primary and permanent teeth, or only permanent teeth, may be missing. About half of patients have fine hair.

Related Facts
I   **Sex Ratio:** M1:F1
II   **Risk of Occurrence:**   ?
III **Risk of Recurrence for**
      Patient's Sib: If parent is affected 1 in 2 (50%) for each offspring to be affected; otherwise not increased.
      Patient's Child: 1 in 2
IV   **Age of Detectability:** May suspect disorder at birth when physical examination reveals absence of one or more toe or fingernails. Detection usually occurs at 4-5 years with absence of teeth, and history or findings of absent or hypoplastic nails, or after 7 to 15 years with absence of permanent teeth, and history or findings of hypoplastic nails.
V   **Prevalence:** ? Probably fairly common. 1 to 2 in 10,000 as over 10 kindreds collected in 1 year. Occurs in high frequency among Dutch Mennonites of Canada.

Treatment
I   **Primary Prevention:** Genetic counseling
II   **Secondary Prevention:**   ?
III **Other Therapy:** Dental restoration

Prognosis: No reduced longevity or fitness noted in kindreds examined.

Detection of Carrier: —

†**Special Considerations:** It is one cause of congenitally missing teeth that should be differentiated from the X-linked and autosomal recessive forms of anhidrotic or hypohidrotic ectodermal dysplasia wherein missing teeth are common and the unguinal form common in French Canadians but without missing teeth. Hypoplasia of nails frequently noted in retrospect by history of mother not trimming nails until child is 18 to 24 months of age. Toenails are usually more severely affected than fingernails.

References:
Hudson, C.D. and Witkop, C.J., Jr.: Autosomal dominant hypodontia with nail dysgenesis. Report of twenty-nine cases in six families. Oral Surg. 39:409, 1975.
Witkop, C.J., Jr.: Genetic disease of the oral cavity. In Tiecke, R.W. (ed.): Oral Pathology. New York:McGraw-Hill, 1965, p. 786.

Contributors: **Carl J. Witkop, Jr.**
Carolyn D. Hudson

Editor's Computerized Descriptors: Face, Teeth, Hair, Nails

HYPOGLYCEMIA, FAMILIAL NEONATAL

Includes: Hypoglycémie néo-natale
Neugeborenen Hypoglykämie
Hipoglicemia neonatal
Infantile hypoglycemosis, familial
Leucine-sensitive hypoglycemia of infancy, familial
Severe, recurrent, or persistent neonatal and infantile hypoglycemia, familial

Excludes: Early transitional neonatal hypoglycemia
Secondary transient neonatal hypoglycemia
Classic transient hypoglycemia of infants who are small for gestational age
Hormone deficiencies of hypothalamus, pituitary, adrenal cortex, glucagon(?), epinephrine(?)
Hyperinsulinism associated with Beckwith-Wiedemann syndrome, islet cell insulinoma, islet cell hyperplasia or nesidioblastosis
Hereditary defects in carbohydrate metabolism due to hepatic glycogenosis, galactosemia, hepatic glycogen synthetase deficiency, fructose 1,6 diphosphatase deficiency, fructose-1-phosphate aldolase deficiency
Hereditary defects in amino or organic acid metabolism due to maple syrup urine disease, tyrosinosis, methylmalonic acidemia, propionic acidemia
Hereditary defects in urea synthesis and other hyperammonemic states
Idiopathic spontaneous hypoglycemosis
Familial endocrine adenomatosis

Minimal Diagnostic Criteria: Onset of symptomatic and documented hypoglycemia during infancy or early childhood. Family history of similar disease in sibs or close relatives. Persistently low blood glucose levels. Leucine sensitivity present in most when tested in infancy. Absence of pancreatic pathology such as islet cell adenoma, although a variety of degrees of islet cell hyperplasia and absence of alpha cells has been reported.† Gross malformations of the CNS have not been reported but varying degrees of functional brain impairment are common when onset is early. Spontaneous improvement is very common after 1 to 7 years of active hypoglycemia. Adults are free of spontaneous hypoglycemia.

Clinical Findings:

Convulsions	98%
Onset in 1st year of life	98%
Drowsiness, limpness, staring	98%
Positive history in close relatives	98-100%
Strabismus, alternating type	80%
Delayed mental development if onset before 6 months	51-80%
Prolonged unconsciousness if onset after 6 months uncommon	10-20%

Laboratory Findings Include:	
Absence of ketosis	100%
Normal pituitary adrenocortical function	100%
Absence of nonglucose sugars from blood and urine	100%
Normal serum and urine amino acid patterns	100%
Normal blood ammonia and liver function tests	100%
Normal response to glucagon or epinephrine	100%
Low blood glucose during seizures	100%

Low fasting blood glucose	95%
Abnormal serum glucose: insulin ratios when glucose is low	100%
Hypoglycemic response to tolbutamide	80-?%
Hypoglycemic response to L-leucine during active phase	65%

Complications

I **Derived:** Mental retardation in 51 to 80% if onset is in the first 6 months of life, and 10 to 20% if onset is after the first 6 months of life. Persistent tendency to convulsions, not associated with hypoglycemia and with frequency similar to that for mental retardation cited above. Strabismus, the alternating type, is very common during active hypoglycemia and occasionally persists. Ataxia from cerebellar dysfunction may be present during active phase but is rarely permanent. Spasticity similarly present early and tends to improve with age, but may remain permanently.

II **Associated:** —

Etiology: Appearance of 2nd generation cases in 1 large kindred suggests autosomal dominant inheritance pattern with incomplete penetrance. Autosomal recessive inheritance is possible in some cases. McK *24080

Pathogenesis: Nearly all appear to have leucine-induced hyperinsulinism when appropriately studied. The findings of beta cell hyperplasia, absence of alpha cells and no pancreatic pathology causes uncertainty regarding the primary role of the pancreas. The universal tendency to outgrow the disease further clouds pathogenesis.

Related Facts

I **Sex Ratio:** Probably M1:F1
II **Risk of Occurrence:** Extremely rare, only reports are in whites of Northern European background.
III **Risk of Recurrence for**
  Patient's Sib: If autosomal dominant or recessive, see Table I AD or I AR, respectively.
  Patient's Child: If autosomal dominant or recessive, see Table I AD or I AR, respectively.
IV **Age of Detectability:** From birth to 2 years of age by plasma glucose determinations paired with serum insulin.
V **Prevalence:** Extremely rare, only 8 families reported.

Treatment

I **Primary Prevention:** Genetic counseling
II **Secondary Prevention:** A diet high in carbohydrate with frequent feeding. Minimal adequate protein intake, drug therapy with ACTH, corticosteroids, diazoxide[R], or zinc glucagon and partial pancreatectomy. Surgery for squint.
III **Other Therapy:** Anticonvulsant drugs and appropriate supportive measures for mild mental retardation and neuromotor handicaps such as special teaching and physical therapy.

Prognosis: No evidence that life span is shortened even if untreated. Mental retardation is a complication.

Detection of Carrier: ?

†**Special Considerations:** Except for functioning islet cell adenoma, other causes of persistent hypoglycemia can be ruled out by appropriate studies. When an infant has no family history of hypoglycemia (such as when the 1st child affected in a family is studied) but otherwise fulfills all criteria, surgical exploration of the pancreas and partial pancreatectomy is necessary for diagnosis. There is no other certain method of ruling out an islet cell adenoma. When other members of the family have neonatal hypoglycemia, the decision to do pancreatic surgery must be based on other considerations. Islet cell adenomata can be familial when associated with endocrine adenomatosis, but if other affected family members did not have adenomata the decision to do surgery would be based only on a need for therapy by partial pancreatectomy. The reported changes of pancreatic histology other than adenoma do not correlate with clinical responses to surgery. Improvement of a temporary nature can be expected whether or not islet pathology is found. Occasionally the improvement is prolonged in such cases.

References:
Cochrane, W.A.: Idiopathic infantile hypoglycemia and leucine sensitivity. Metabolism 9:386, 1960.
Sauls, H.S.: Hypoglycemia in childhood. In Kelley, V. (ed.): Metabolic, Endocrine and Genetic Disorders of Childhood. Hagerstown: Harper and Row, 1974, p. 703.
Ulstrom, R.A.: Idiopathic spontaneous hypoglycemia. In Linevek, F. (ed.): Erbliche Stoffwechselkrankheiten. Munich: Urban and Schwarzenberg, 1962, p. 225.

Contributor: **Robert A. Ulstrom**

Editor's Computerized Descriptors: Eye, Nerve

HYPOGLYCEMIA, LEUCINE-INDUCED

Includes: Hypoglycémie induit par la leucine
Leuzin-induzierte Hypoglykämie
Hipoglicemia inducida por la leucina
Leucine-sensitive hypoglycemia
Leucine-induced hypoglycemia

Excludes: Hypoglycemia, familial neonatal (512)

Minimal Diagnostic Criteria: Leucine tolerance test - dose - 150 mg (L-leucine)/kg p.o. or 75 mg/kg IV. Response - blood sugar decrease of 50% or more from fasting level within 1 hour of giving L-leucine. Initial fasting blood sugar should be above 40 mg%.†

Clinical Findings: Pallor, cyanotic episodes, lethargy, poor feeding, apnea, twitching, convulsions, hypoglycemia accentuated or induced by high-protein feeding- (blood glucose below 40 mg% on 2 or more occasions), strabismus.

Complications
I **Derived:** Mental and developmental retardation in approximately 75% of cases
II **Associated:** —

Etiology: Possibly autosomal recessive sensitivity to L-leucine, L-isoleucine and α-ketoisocaproic acid. McK *24080

Pathogenesis: L-leucine stimulates insulin release from pancreatic B cells in sensitive patients. L-leucine also inhibits hepatic gluconeogenesis in tissue slices. Microscopic hyperplasia of pancreatic islet B cells has been found in some patients.

Related Facts
I **Sex Ratio:** M1.5:F1
II **Risk of Occurrence:** ?
III **Risk of Recurrence for**
    Patient's Sib: Possibly 1 in 4 (25%) for each offspring to be affected
    Patient's Child: Not increased unless mate is carrier or homozygote
IV **Age of Detectability:** At birth by leucine tolerance test
V **Prevalence:** Rare; 50+ patients in English literature

Treatment
I **Primary Prevention:** Genetic counseling
II **Secondary Prevention:** Low leucine diet with postprandial glucose supplementation. Long acting epinephrine. Diazoxide - if above fail to keep blood glucose levels in normal range - side effects include neutropenia, hirsutism, elevated uric acid levels.
III **Other Therapy:** Anticonvulsant drugs

Prognosis: Poor for normal development. Good for life. Leucine sensitivity seems to subside in some children and tends to improve spontaneously by 4-6 years of age. Death, when untreated, is secondary to hypoglycemic convulsions.

Detection of Carrier: ?

†Special Considerations: Leucine sensitivity type of hypoglycemia was first described in 1956 in a child whose hypoglycemia was made worse by high-protein feedings. It has been postulated that from 25-33% of all cases of "idiopathic hypoglycemia" are leucine-sensitive. In order to make the diagnosis, one's index of suspicion for hypoglycemia must be high and if hypoglycemia is found then one must rule out the leucine-sensitive type. This is done by a leucine tolerance test. This is performed after as long a fast as is tolerated by the patient. When performing a leucine tolerance test, a syringe of 50% glucose and of glucagon should be by the bedside so that if the patient has symptoms associated with the hypoglycemia caused by the leucine stimulus, the study can be promptly terminated. A decrease in blood glucose of 50% or more from fasting in the first hour is diagnostic of leucine-sensitive type of hypoglycemia.

References:
Cochrane, W.A. et al: Familial hypoglycemia precipitated by amino acids. J. Clin. Invest. 35:411, 1956.
Cornblath, M. and Schwartz, R.: Disorders of carbohydrate metabolism in infancy. In Major Problems in Clinical Pediatrics. Philadelphia:W.B. Saunders, 1966, vol. 3.
Fajans, S. S.: Leucine-induced hypoglycemia. N. Engl. J. Med. 272:1224, 1965.
Griese, G. G. and Wenzel, F. J.: Leucine-sensitive hypoglycemia treated with long-acting epinephrine. Pediatrics 35:709, 1965.
Roth, H. and Segal, S.: The dietary management of leucine-sensitive hypoglycemia, with report of a case. Pediatrics 34:831, 1964.

Contributors: **Samuel S. Obenshain**
Robert Schwartz

Editor's Computerized Descriptors: Eye, Resp., GI., Nerve

HYPOMAGNESEMIA, PRIMARY

Includes: Hypomagnesémie essentielle
Primäre Hypomagnesiämie
Hipomagnesemia primaria
Familial hypomagnesemia
Primary infantile hypomagnesemia
Neonatal hypomagnesemia with selective malabsorption of magnesium
Primary hypomagnesemia with secondary hypocalcemia

Excludes: Hypomagnesemia associated with GI and renal disorders, including renal tubular defect in reabsorption of magnesium
Transient hypomagnesemia of the newborn

Minimal Diagnostic Criteria: Hypomagnesemia usually with secondary hypocalcemia; exclusion of other disorders including transient neonatal hypomagnesemia, GI and renal disorders.

Clinical Findings: Tetany and convulsions in early weeks of life associated with hypomagnesemia and hypocalcemia. Serum inorganic phosphate normal or somewhat increased. Hypoalbuminemia, anasarca and diarrhea are occasional findings. Hypocalcemia and symptoms are resistant to calcium and vitamin D therapy but respond well to magnesium treatment.

Complications
I **Derived:** Convulsions, tetany, hypocalcemia, diarrhea, hypoalbuminemia
II **Associated:** Possible psychomotor retardation

Etiology: ? Possibly X-linked recessive. 12 or 13 reported cases have been males. Brothers have been affected in 2 families.

Pathogenesis: Isolated defect in intestinal transport of magnesium. Hypocalcemia due to impaired secretion of parathyroid hormone or impaired end-organ responsiveness to parathyroid hormone each of which may result from magnesium deficiency. Magnesium repletion corrects these abnormalities. Hypoalbuminemia has variously been attributed to impaired synthesis of albumin and to protein-losing enteropathy induced by magnesium deficiency.

Related Facts
I **Sex Ratio:** M12:F1
II **Risk of Occurrence:** Rare
III **Risk of Recurrence for**
  Patient's Sib: If mother is a carrier 1 in 2 (50%) for each brother to be affected and 1 in 2 (50%) for each sister to be a carrier, if X-linked recessive.
  Patient's Child: 1 in 1 (100%) for carrier daughters; not increased for sons unless wife is a carrier, if X-linked recessive.
IV **Age of Detectability:** Usually during first few months of life.
V **Prevalence:** ?

Treatment
I **Primary Prevention:** Genetic counseling
II **Secondary Prevention:** Early recognition of affected infants and treatment with magnesium supplements
III **Other Therapy:** —

Prognosis: Death may occur in untreated infants during early months of life. Life span probably not affected with early and continuous treatment.

Detection of Carrier: ?

Special Considerations: —

References:
Anast, C.S. et al: Impaired release of parathyroid hormone in magnesium deficiency. Clin. Endocrinol. Metabol. 42:707, 1976.
Lombeck, I. et al: Primary hypomagnesemia. Z. Kinderheilkd. 118:249, 1975.
Paunier, L. et al: Primary hypomagnesemia with secondary hypocalcemia in an infant. Pediatrics 41:385, 1968.

Suh, S.M. et al: Pathogenesis of hypocalcemia in primary hypomagnesemia: Normal end-organ responsiveness to parathyroid hormone, impaired parathyroid gland function. J. Clin. Invest. 52:153, 1973.
Vainsel, M. et al: Tetany due to hypomagnesaemia with secondary hypocalcaemia. Arch. Dis. Child. 45:254, 1970.
Woodard, J.C. et al: Primary hypomagnesemia with secondary hypocalcemia, diarrhea and insensitivity to parathyroid hormone. Am. J. Dig. Dis. 17:612, 1972.

Contributors: **Constantine S. Anast**
David W. Gardner

Editor's Computerized Descriptor: Nerve

HYPOPARATHYROIDISM, X-LINKED INFANTILE

Includes: Hypoparathyroïde infantile liée au sexe
X-Chromosomaler infantiler Hypoparathyreoidismus
Hipoparatiroidismo infantil ligado al X
X-linked neonatal hypoparathyroidism

Excludes: Thymic agenesis (943)
Juvenile and adult onset idiopathic hypoparathyroidism

Minimal Diagnostic Criteria: Hypocalcemia and hyperphosphatemia in the presence of low or undetectable serum immunoreactive parathyroid hormone level. Similar chemical findings may be observed in neonatal hypocalcemic tetany, but in contrast to idiopathic hypoparathyroidism, the chemical and clinical abnormalities in neonatal tetany are transient. Other hypocalcemic disorders, including renal insufficiency and pseudohypoparathyroidism, are characterized by elevated serum immunoreactive parathyroid hormone levels.

Clinical Findings: Convulsive seizures and increased neuromuscular irritability with signs and symptoms of tetany or its equivalent are prominent features of infantile hypoparathyroidism. The symptoms include muscle rigidity, laryngeal stridor, and carpopedal spasm. Hyperreflexia is common and Chvostek and Trousseau signs frequently are positive. Diarrhea may be present and is secondary to hyperexcitability of gut muscles induced by hypocalcemia. Ocular manifestations include photophobia, blepharospasm, conjunctivitis, keratitis, corneal ulcerations, and lens opacity. Dental abnormalities, including aplasia or hypoplasia of teeth, may occur if hypoparathyroidism develops during the time that the teeth are being formed. Skeletal x-ray films usually reveal no significant changes from normal. Symmetric calcification of the cerebral basal ganglia may be observed. In some children there may be signs of increased intracranial pressure; the underlying cause of this manifestation is poorly understood.

Complications
I **Derived:** Tetany, convulsions, diarrhea, cataracts and other eye manifestations. Possible impaired intellectual ability in the presence of hypocalcemia which may improve with correction of serum calcium.
II **Associated:** —

Etiology: X-linked recessive; McK *30770

Pathogenesis: ?

Related Facts
I **Sex Ratio:** M1:F0
II **Risk of Occurrence:** ?
III **Risk of Recurrence for**
    Patient's Sib: If mother is a carrier, 1 in 2 (50%) for each brother to be affected and 1 in 2 for each sister to be a carrier.
    Patient's Child: 1 in 1 (100%) for carrier daughters: not increased for sons unless wife is a carrier.
IV **Age of Detectability:** During 1st year of life.
V **Prevalence:** ?

Treatment
I **Primary Prevention:** Genetic counseling
II **Secondary Prevention:** Pharmacologic doses of vitamin D or dihydrotachysterol. Recent studies in older subjects with hypoparathyroidism suggest that 1-α-hydroxyvitamin D_3 or 1, 25-dihydroxyvitamin D_3 may be the treatment of choice, since there is impaired conversion of 25-hydroxy D_3 to 1, 25-hydroxy D_3 in hypoparathyroidism.
III **Other Therapy:** IV calcium therapy is indicated in the presence of hypocalcemic tetany or convulsions.

Prognosis: If untreated, convulsions and death may occur. With adequate treatment, the prognosis for life is good.

Detection of Carrier: ?

Special Considerations: —

References:
Anast, C.: Disorders of the parathyroids. In Kelley, V.A. (ed.): Metabolic, Endocrine and Genetic Disorders of Children. Hagerstown: Harper & Row, 1974, p. 531.
Klein, R. and Haddow, J.: Hypoparathyroidism. In Gardner, L.I. (ed.): Endocrine and Genetic Diseases of Childhood and Adolescence, 2nd Ed. Philadelphia: W.B. Saunders Co., 1975, p. 408.
Peden, V.H.: True idiopathic hypoparathyroidism as a sex-linked recessive trait. Am. J. Hum. Genet. 12:323, 1960.

Contributors: **Constantine S. Anast**
                   David W. Gardner

Editor's Computerized Descriptors: Eye, Teeth, Neck, Resp., GI., Nerve

HYPOPHOSPHATASIA

Includes: Hypophosphatasie
Hipofosfatasia
Pseudohypophosphatasia

Excludes: —

Minimal Diagnostic Criteria: 1) Low alkaline phosphatase activity (total and bone fraction) in plasma (serum) at saturating concentration of substrate (16 mM); or reduced activity at lower substrate concentration (4 mM) in pseudohypophosphatasia which has normal total activity at the high concentration (16 mM) of substrate; 2) phosphoethanolaminuria; 3) histochemical evidence of low alkaline phosphatase activity in bone.

Clinical Findings: Expression of major phenotype (inadequate mature bone formation) varies from intrauterine death to modest handicap in childhood and adulthood.

Those affected with the severe congenital form may be stillborn or die from early respiratory insufficiency. Infantile cases suffer early failure to thrive, hypotonia and irritability, severe nonrachitic skeletal deformity, and hypercalcemia. Spontaneous improvement has been observed in infancy. In the intermediate form, bone changes are less severe and premature loss of deciduous teeth is characteristic. In general, skeletal findings are variable and include: craniosynostosis, bowed lower limbs with overlying cutaneous dimpling, a small thorax with short ribs and rachitic rosary deformity. Gait may be awkward. "Poker-spine" and shortness of stature in childhood and adulthood may occur. In the mild form phosphoethanolaminuria occurs alone or with bone signs (pseudofracture and pathologic fractures) in adult life.

X-ray examination may show decreased mineralization of skull, delayed closure of fontanels and irregularly decreased metaphyseal mineralization. Nephrocalcinosis may be present.

Complications

I **Derived:** Fractures and deformity; increased intracranial pressure (from craniostenosis); sequelae of chronic hypercalcemia.

II **Associated:** Secondary to craniostenosis if untreated.

Etiology: Autosomal recessive transmission (with modulators?); probably more than 1 allele (eg pseudohypophosphatasia). Phenotypic variation within sibships suggests that severe and moderate forms may (not) be necessarily different allelic forms.

Pathogenesis: The exact mutant gene product has not been identified. Its cardinal effects are: inadequate calcification of osteoid tissue; "prerenal" phosphoethanolaminuria secondary to saturation of β-amino acid transport system by high filtered load of phosphoethanolamine. Cleavage of several organic phosphate esters is impaired in the presence of reduced total activity of alkaline phosphatase, or of an apparently altered affinity of the phosphatase for its substrate in pseudohypophosphatasia.

Related Facts

I **Sex Ratio:** M1:F1

II **Risk of Occurrence:** Rare, true frequency not determined.

III **Risk of Recurrence for**
Patient's Sib: 1 in 4 (25%) for each offspring to be affected.
Patient's Child: —

IV **Age of Detectability:** At birth or prenatally†

V **Prevalence:** ?

Treatment

I **Primary Prevention:** Genetic counseling

II **Secondary Prevention:** Prenatal diagnosis

III **Other Therapy:** No generally accepted therapy; hypercalcemia should be avoided (low calcium diet, steroids). Early surgical correction of craniosynostosis recommended. Evaluation of any treatment difficult because of unpredictable and spontaneous improvement of clinical course in some patients with severe phenotype.

Prognosis: Variable from intrauterine death to nearly symptomless course.

Detection of Carrier: About 60% of carriers can be recognized from elevation of urine and plasma phosphoethanolamine concentration. Liver disease, scurvy and hypothyroidism are also associated with elevated phosphoethanolaminuria. Depressed plasma alkaline phosphatase activity is a less reliable index, unless bone fraction is specified.

†Special Considerations: Intrauterine diagnosis of greatly reduced alkaline phosphatase activity in amniocytes from homozygotes is now possible. Long-chain triglycerides stimulate intestinal alkaline phosphatase activity and cause plasma enzyme activity to rise; this response is intact in patients indicating that intestinal alkaline phosphatase is present in hypophosphatasia.

References:

Bartter, F.C.: Hypophosphatasia. In Stanbury, J.B. et al (eds.): The Metabolic Basis of Inherited Disease. 3rd Ed. New York: McGraw-Hill, 1972, p. 1295.

Rasmussen, K.: Phosphorylethanolaminuria and hypophosphatasia. Dan. Med. Bull. 15:1, 1968.

Rattenbury, J.M. et al: Letter. Prenatal diagnosis of hypophosphatasia. Lancet 1:306, 1976.

Scriver, C.R. and Cameron, D.: Pseudohypophosphatasia. N. Engl. J. Med. 251:604, 1969.

Smith, D.W.: Recognizable Patterns of Human Malformation. 2nd Ed. Philadelphia: W.B. Saunders, 1976, p. 218.

Warshaw, J.B. et al: Serum alkaline phosphatase in hypophosphatasia. J. Clin. Invest. 50:2137, 1971.

Contributors: **Charles R. Scriver**
Donald Fraser

Editor's Computerized Descriptors: Teeth, Skel., Resp., Muscle, Nerve

HYPOPHOSPHATEMIA

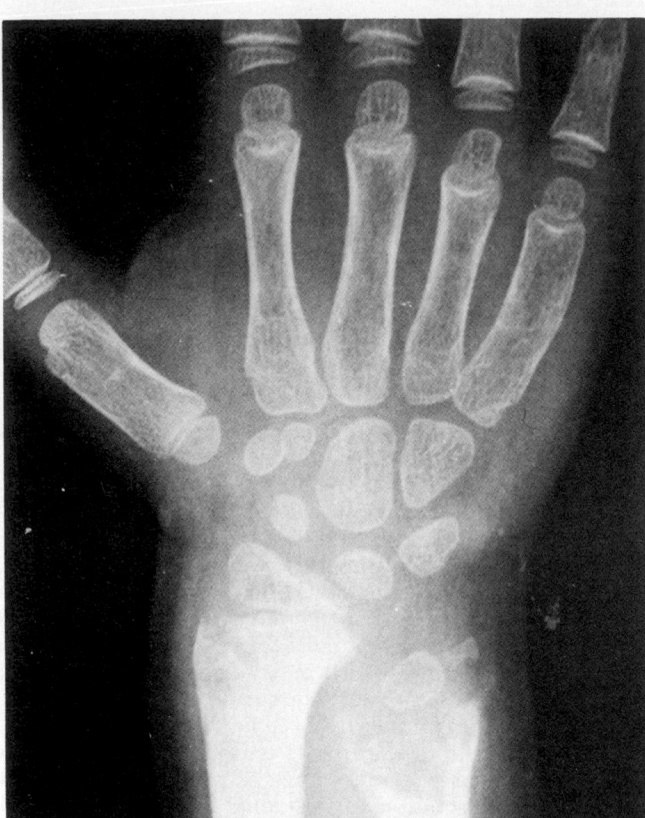

299. Coarse bony trabecular pattern in carpals, metacarpals and phalanges. Irregular ossification of distal radius and ulna, and deep cup-shaped defect of distal ulna with island of coarsely trabeculated bone

Includes: Hypophosphatémie
Hypophosphatämie
Hipofosfatemia
Vitamin D-resistant rickets
Familial hypophosphatemia (X-linked)

Excludes: Hypophosphatemic rickets with glycinuria, glucosuria
Acidosis

Minimal Diagnostic Criteria: A low concentration of inorganic phosphate in the plasma or serum in a fasting subject; exclusion of other possible causes; failure to repair hypophosphatemia or the active rickets with amounts of vitamin D that would cure vitamin D-deficiency rickets. Normal iPTH in serum.†

Clinical Findings: Carriers of the gene have hypophosphatemia or depressed phosphate T_m. Males have hypophosphatemia (low serum inorganic phosphorus) with active, "vitamin D-resistant" rickets in childhood, and short stature. Females have a range of abnormalities from asymptomatic hypophosphatemia, with no other clinical or chemical abnormalities - to florid rickets and shortened stature.

The hypophosphatemia is detectable immediately after birth, evidence of rickets appears later. There is no response to the usual (physiologic) amounts of vitamin D. The serum alkaline phosphatase is elevated when active rickets or osteomalacia is present. Serum calcium is usually normal or low-normal. Serum immunoreactive PTH (iPTH) is normal or minimally elevated in untreated patients.

Associated x-ray findings include: typical changes of active rickets in childhood and of osteomalacia in the adult; and coarsened trabeculation of long bones.

Complications
I **Derived:** Rachitic deformities and shortened stature; particularly of lower limbs in childhood; limitation of motion at large joints (hips, knees, elbows) in adults, due to bony overgrowth at tendinous insertions. Acquired dolichocephalic skull.

II **Associated:** —

Etiology: X-linked dominant. Sporadic cases fulfilling biochemical and clinical criteria may represent new mutations with a general frequency of 1 in 200,000 per X-linked gene per generation. McK *30780

Pathogenesis: Recent evidence indicates that affected persons have an abnormal transepithelial system for reclamation of phosphate in kidney. "Negative reabsorption" of phosphate can even occur at elevated levels of serum phosphate, suggesting that the transport defect permits excessive phosphate backflux at the luminal membrane. Evidence exists both for and against a coexistent deficiency of transepithelial absorption of phosphate in the intestine. Phosphate entry into erythrocytes is not impaired by the X-linked allele.

Related Facts
I **Sex Ratio:** M1:F1.7
II **Risk of Occurrence:** ?
III **Risk of Recurrence for**
   Patient's Sib: If carrier parent is female, 1 in 2 (50%) that each sib will be affected. If carrier parent is male, 1 in 1 (100%) that each sister will be a carrier; risk not increased for brothers.
   Patient's Child: If patient is female, 1 in 2 (50%) for each offspring to be affected; if patient is male, 1 in 1 (100%) for daughters and not increased for sons.
IV **Age of Detectability:** Usually under 1 year
V **Prevalence:** ?

Treatment

I **Primary Prevention:** Genetic counseling

II **Secondary Prevention:** Early recognition of affected infant particularly in affected families. Early, continuous and carefully monitored treatment with supplemental intake of inorganic phosphate (1-4 g per day every 4 hr x 5); supportive vitamin D to prevent hypocalcemia.

III **Other Therapy:** Corrective orthopedic surgery for existing limb deformities.

Prognosis: Life span probably not affected. Early and continuous adequate phosphate treatment throughout the growth period can prevent deformities and impairment of linear growth.

Detection of Carrier: Low value (> 2SD below age specific mean value) for fasting (morning) serum inorganic phosphorus will identify majority of carriers: measurement of Tm_{Pi} recommended in critical equivocal subjects.

†**Special Considerations:** In all patients with hypophosphatemia and rickets, other multifactorial causes should be excluded, (eg Fanconi renal tubular syndrome). There are rare instances of isolated renal glycosuria or glycinuria associated with what appears otherwise to be simple hypophosphatemic rickets; these may represent different genetic disorders or may be simple chance association of findings.

References:

Arnaud, C. et al: Serum parathyroid hormone in X-linked hypophosphatemia. Science 173:845, 1971.

Glorieux, F. and Scriver, C.R.: Loss of a PTH-sensitive component of phosphate transport in X-linked hypophosphatemia. Science 175:997, 1972.

Glorieux, F. et al: Use of phosphate and vitamin D to prevent dwarfism and rickets in X-linked hypophosphatemia. N. Engl. J. Med. 287:481, 1972.

Contributor: **Charles R. Scriver**

Editor's Computerized Descriptor: Skel.

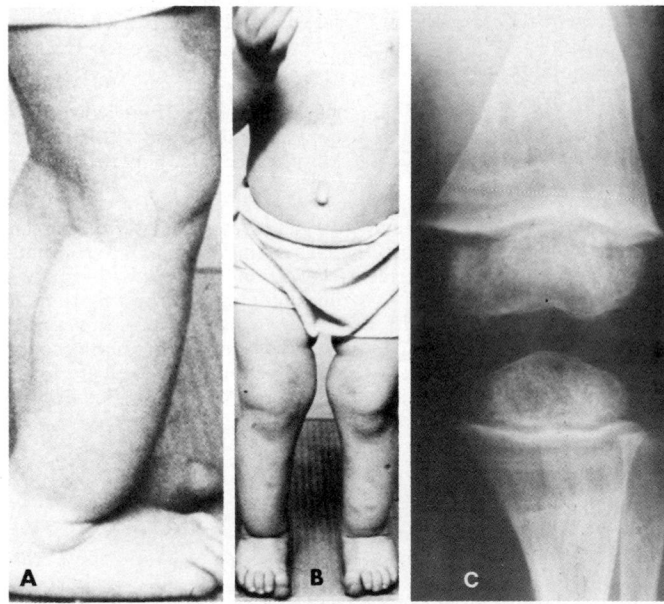

300. A & B) At age 3, note marked anterior bowing of lower 3rd of tibias, with minimal lateral bowing; C) radiograph prior to vitamin D therapy

HYPOSPADIAS

Includes: Hypospadie
Hipospadias
Hypospadias with or without chordee

Excludes: Dystopia of the meatus
Curvature of the penis
Penoscrotal transposition
Scrotal bipartition
Congenital urethral fistula
True hermaphroditism (971)
Chromosome 45,X/46,XY mosaicism (173)

Minimal Diagnostic Criteria: The presence of a urethral meatus at a location other than the tip of the glans penis in an otherwise normal boy and deficiency in redundancy of the foreskin on the ventral aspect of the penis.

Clinical Findings: The hypospadic boy is readily recognized by physical examination. The foreskin of the penis is normally redundant on the dorsal aspect, but on the ventral aspect of the penis there is only a single covering layer of the foreskin. The urethral meatus is not at the tip of the glans penis. In approximately half of the cases, there is associated chordee, which is the downward curvature of the glans penis with resultant penile deformity. This chordee causes the patient to void in the direction of his feet, rather than forward; it also results in painful erection in later life.

It is important to separate out cases of intersexuality from the large group of hypospadic boys. The child who is a pseudohermaphrodite or a true hermaphrodite often presents a more severe degree of hypospadias. In these cases, chromosomal analysis and, occasionally, gonadal biopsy and laparotomy will clarify the situation.

Hypospadias can usefully be classified by location of the meatus into 1st degree (60%)-at the coronal sulcus, 2nd degree (15%)-along the shaft of the penis, 3rd degree (20%)-at the level of the scrotum, and 4th degree (5%)-in the perineum.†

Complications

I **Derived:** Perhaps the most significant complication of hypospadias is urethral meatal stenosis, which is not infrequent, although precise occurrence figures are not available. Obstructive uropathy with progressive azotemia and eventual renal failure may occur.

II **Associated:** The inability to impregnate can complicate untreated hypospadias with chordee. The deformed penis is very painful when erect and the deformity per se can preclude vaginal intromission. Both of these factors can hamper normal sexual activity and lead to a status of functional sterility.†

Etiology: ?

Pathogenesis: ?

Related Facts

I **Sex Ratio:** M10,000:F1
II **Risk of Occurrence:** 1 in 186 live births (McIntosh)
III **Risk of Recurrence for**
   Patient's Sib: —12% (Sorenson)
   Patient's Child: Unknown, but hypospadias does occur in families with variable modes of inheritance.
IV **Age of Detectability:** At birth
V **Prevalence:** ?

Treatment

I **Primary Prevention:** —
II **Secondary Prevention:** Surgery to correct the hypospadias deformity.†
III **Other Therapy:** —

Prognosis: The prognosis for hypospadias is generally good. Uncomplicated hypospadias is almost always successfully operated upon. There is no shortening of the life expectancy, and the affected individual functions quite normally. Neither should there be any difficulty with procreation, except in the most unusual of circumstances, or patients with coincident cryptorchidism.

Detection of Carrier: —

†Special Considerations: There are many other system anomalies associated with hypospadias. In a series of 489 hypospadic patients, Kennedy found nongenitourinary tract malformations as follows: neuromuscular 6.3%, GI 2.8%, cardiovascular 3.0%, respiratory 1.0%, ENT 1.0%, eye 0.8%, and GU tract anomalies as follows: cryptorchidism 10.2%, bifid scrotum 6.3%, pseudohermaphrodite 2.8%, bladder neck obstruction 2.0%, hydrocele 0.1%, microcephaly 1.0%, true hermaphroditism 0.6%, renal ectopia 0.4%, horseshoe kidney 0.4%, others 3.0%.

The primary therapeutic approach is surgical. The objectives of surgery are to straighten the penis to allow the child to void into the bowl while standing up, and to permit impregnation. Both these goals are achieved by positioning the urethral meatus at the tip of the glans penis. This also presents a cosmetically more acceptable penis. This surgery should be undertaken at age 2-4, so that repair is completed by school age.

If chordee is present, the penis needs to be straightened and then the defect in urethral length is corrected. There are also instances of hypospadias without chordee in which the urethral length and appearance of the penis can be improved by urologic surgery. Fistulas requiring additional surgery may occur following hypospadias repair in about 10-15% of cases.

The series of Smythe and Forsythe also emphasizes the need to investigate outlet obstructive anomalies, which occurred in 13.3% of their patients.

Hypospadias occurs in females, although the number of reported cases is quite small. The anomaly is a defect of the inferior wall of the urethra and the superior wall of the vagina, such that the girl urinates from a recessed meatus.

Hypospadias is also found in the following syndromes: Smith-Lemli-Opitz, Silver-Russell, pterygium syndrome, Lenz microphthalmia, G syndrome and hypertelorism with hypospadias. The latter is an autosomal dominant syndrome which is restricted to the male.

Chromosomal abnormalities are frequently associated with hypospadias. These include the Down syndrome and the 4p- syndrome. In the latter, all described cases have hypospadias. The sex chromosome abnormalities associated with hypospadias are Klinefelter syndrome (47,XXY), gonadal dysgenesis (47,XYY), true hermaphroditism and states of intersexuality.

References:

Antolak, S.J., Jr. et al: Female hypospadias. J. Urol. 102:640, 1969.

Campbell, M.F.: Textbook of Urology. Philadelphia: W.B. Saunders, 1970.

Juberg, R.C. et al: Chromosome studies in patients with hypospadias. Pediatrics 43:578, 1969.

Kennedy, P.A., Jr.: Hypospadias: A twenty year review of 489 cases. J. Urol. 85:814, 1961.

McIntosh, R. et al: The incidence of congenital malformations: A study of 5,964 pregnancies. Pediatrics 14:505, 1954.

Smythe, B.T. and Forsythe, I.W.: Hypospadias and associated anomalies of the genitourinary tract. J. Urol. 82:109, 1959.

Contributors: **David T. Mininberg**
                    Nesrin Bingol
                    Edward Wasserman

Editor's Computerized Descriptor: GU.

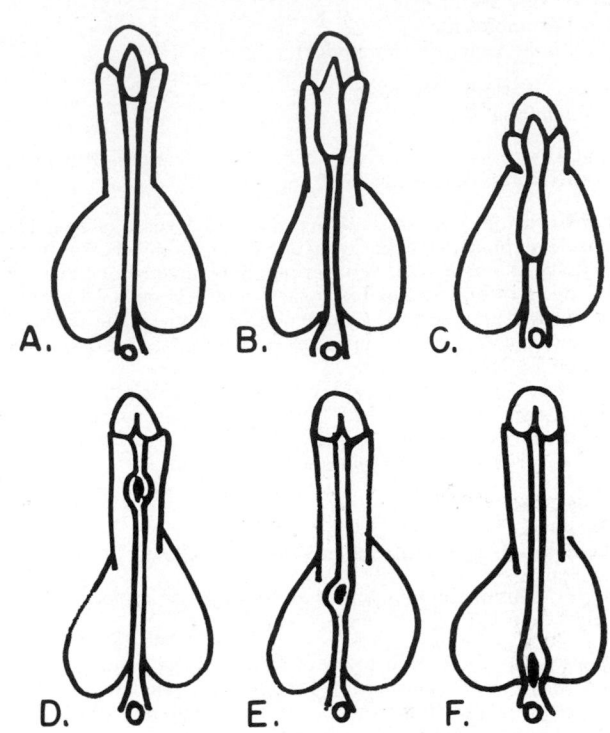

301. Schematic hypospadias: A) glandular; B & C) peniglandular; D) penile; E) scrotal; F) perineal

IMIDAZOLE AMINOACIDURIA (MARKER)

514-500

Includes: Imidazolurie
Imidazol-Aminoazidurie
Imidazol aminoaciduria (Marcador)

Excludes: Histidinemia (472)
Carnosinemia (126)

Minimal Diagnostic Criteria: Frequent elevations of urinary carnosine and anserine above 20 mg/24 hr.

Clinical Findings: Onset is between 5 and 8 years of age. The imidazole aminoaciduria has been documented in 9 of 20 patients with juvenile amaurotic retardation (Spielmeyer-Vogt disease; see Neuronal Ceroid - Lipofuscinoses) and in 6 out of 8 normal individuals examined in the immediate kinship of the patients. The imidazole aminoaciduria includes carnosine, anserine, histidine, and 1-methyl histidine.

The excretion of the imidazoles varies from time to time in the same patient and ranges from 20-100 mg/day of carnosine and anserine (normal values: 5-7 and 2-3 mg/day, respectively). The plasma levels of these compounds were normal.

Complications
I   Derived: —
II   Associated: Juvenile amaurotic retardation†

Etiology: Dominant genetically determined transport or biochemical defect (?)

Pathogenesis: The high urinary excretion of the imidazole compounds with normal plasma levels suggests a renal abnormality in the clearance of these substances rather than a specific enzymatic block. Biochemical studies however, indicate that there may be an increased conversion of histidine to carnosine and anserine with a concomitant decrease in the catabolism of histidine.

Related Facts
I   **Sex Ratio:** M1:F1 probable
II   **Risk of Occurrence:** ?
III **Risk of Recurrence for**
     Patient's Sib: ?
     Patient's Child: ?
IV   **Age of Detectability:** Early childhood by amino acid chromatography of the urine
V   **Prevalence:** ?

Treatment
I   **Primary Prevention:** —
II   **Secondary Prevention:** —
III **Other Therapy:** —

Prognosis: Early death, if associated with juvenile amaurotic retardation

Detection of Carrier: —

†Special Considerations: Found in association with several birth defects, especially in patients with juvenile amaurotic retardation and, significantly, also in relatives of such patients.

In selected populations imidazole aminoaciduria was found in 9 of 20 examined with the neurologic disease, and in 6 of 8 in the immediate kinships examined who had no sign of the neurologic disease. Most kindreds of Spielmeyer-Vogt disease subsequently examined have not had imidazole aminoaciduria. Together the data suggest that the chemical marker may be unrelated to the clinical disease.

References:
Bessman, S. P. and Baldwin, R.: Imidazole aminoaciduria in cerebromacular degeneration. Science 135:789, 1962.
Levenson, J. et al: Carnosine excretion in juvenile amaurotic idiocy. Lancet 2:756, 1964.
Tocci, P. M. and Bessman, S. P.: Histidine peptiduria. In Nyhan, W.L. (ed.): Amino Acid Metabolism and Genetic Variation. New York:McGraw-Hill, 1967, p. 161.

Contributor: **Paul M. Tocci**

Editor's Computerized Descriptor: Nerve

IMINOGLYCINURIA (MARKER)

Includes: Iminoglycénurie
Iminoglyzinurie
Iminoglicinuria (Marcador)
Renal iminoglycinuria
Hyperglycinuria of DeVries et al

Excludes: Hyperprolinemia (Marker) (502)
Iminoglycinuria of normal newborn

Minimal Diagnostic Criteria: Homozygote: Normal plasma concentration of proline, hydroxyproline and glycine. Presence of large amounts of imino acids and glycine in urine of any patient older than 6 months. Heterozygote: Glycinuria exceeding 160 μ moles/g total urinary nitrogen, or renal clearance exceeding 8.6 ml/min/$1.73M^2$ in one type of heterozygote; the other (silent) type has normal glycine excretion.

Clinical Findings: No proven disease occurs with the trait. Its occasional association with seizures, or mental retardation, is probably fortuitous. Numerous healthy children and adults have now been recognized with selective impairment of cellular transport of proline, hydroxyproline and glycine. Plasma levels of affected amino acids are normal. In homozygote, net renal tubular reabsorption of proline, hydroxyproline and glycine is about 80, 80, and 60%, respectively, of normal. An intestinal transport defect restricted to the iminoglycine group of amino acids has also been identified in some, but not in all pedigrees. Most heterozygotes have abnormal endogenous glycine absorption (hence DeVries' description of dominantly inherited hyperglycinuria). Evidence for "silent" heterozygotes exists.† On this basis, and on apparent evidence for heteroallelic homozygotes in some pedigrees, it is assumed that more than one mutant genotype determines the renal iminoglycinuric trait.

Complications
I **Derived:** —
II **Associated:** —

Etiology: Autosomal recessive transmission

Pathogenesis: Deficiency of high capacity, low affinity, group-specific membrane transport system (protein or permease) common to proline, hydroxyproline and glycine

Related Facts
I **Sex Ratio:** M1:F1 (approximate)
II **Risk of Occurrence:** About 1 in 17,000 live births for homozygous trait. 100% for *normal* transient trait at birth, and during first few months of life
III **Risk of Recurrence for**
  Patient's Sib: 1 in 4 (25%) for each offspring to be affected
  Patient's Child: Not increased unless mate is carrier or homozygote.
IV **Age of Detectability:** At birth
V **Prevalence:** 1 in 17,000 based on newborn surveys

Treatment
I **Primary Prevention:** Genetic counseling
II **Secondary Prevention:** —
III **Other Therapy:** Care for associated illnesses (if any)

Prognosis: Normal life span

Detection of Carrier: Hyperglycinuria in most heterozygotes

†**Special Considerations:** Renal iminoglycinuria is normally present in human newborn. "Maturation" of transport system occurs in early infancy, and renal tubular conservation of imino acids and glycine should have approached adult values by 6th month of life.

One pedigree (Family A, Scriver, 1968) contained a patient whose phenotype corresponded to the homozygous form of the trait. The father was a proven heterozygote. The mother did not have hyperglycinuria. Thus, she was apparently a "silent" obligate heterozygote. This suggests the presence of two different mutant alleles at the same locus for the trait (later confirmed in other pedigrees).

Other evidence for more than one genotype rests in the demonstration of an intestinal transport defect in some homozygotes, and the failure to identify this feature in other homozygotes.

References:
Rosenberg, L.E. et al: II. Familial iminoglycinuria: An inborn error of renal tubular transport. N. Engl. J. Med. 278:1407, 1968.
Scriver, C.R.: Familial iminoglycinuria. In Stanbury, J.B. et al (eds.): The Metabolic Basis of Inherited Disease, 3rd Ed. New York:McGraw-Hill, 1972, p. 1520.
Scriver, C.R.: Renal tubular transport of proline, hydroxyproline and glycine: 3. Genetic basis for more than one mode of uptake in human kidney. J. Clin. Invest. 47:823, 1968.
Whelan, D.T. and Scriver, C.R.: Cystathioninuria and renal iminoglycinuria in a pedigree. A perspective on counselling. N. Engl. J. Med. 278:924, 1968.

Contributor: **Charles R. Scriver**

Editor's Computerized Descriptor: —

IMMUNODEFICIENCY, COMMON VARIABLE

Includes: Déficit immunologique tardif (acquis)
Spätmanifester Immunkörpermangel
Deficiencia inmunológica tardía
Dysgammaglobulinemia
Hypogammaglobulinemia†
Acquired agammaglobulinemia
Common variable immunodeficiency
Late-occurring immunologic deficiency

Excludes: Agammaglobulinemia, X-linked infantile (27)
Immunodeficiency, X-linked severe combined (524)
Immunodeficiency, severe combined (522)
Immunodeficiencies with thymoma

Minimal Diagnostic Criteria: Hypogammaglobulinemia, low levels of all or some of the immunoglobulins, deficient immunologic functions which are not secondary to myeloma, lymphatic leukemia, or Hodgkin disease or immunosuppressive treatment, or associated with thymoma.

Clinical Findings: Increased susceptibility to infections, hypogammaglobulinemia and immunologic deficiencies, deficiency of some immunoglobulins but not others (40%), rheumatoid disease (30%), dermatomyositis and other autoimmune diseases (10%), intestinal malabsorption and sprue-like state (40-50%), and pernicious anemia (5%). Immunologic function is impaired and deficiencies include both cell-mediated and humoral immune deficiencies. Quantitative immunoglobulin defects variable from time to time in same patient and from patient to patient in same family.

Complications
I **Derived:** Frequent GI malignancy (10%), lymphoreticular malignancy (15%), pneumonias (100%), chronic sinopulmonary disease (90+ %), meningitis (50%), bronchiectasis (40-50%), rheumatoid disease (30%), and mesenchymal diseases (15%), extreme hypertrophy of lymph nodes and spleen (20%), diarrheal states including malabsorption, giardiasis and other parasites and bacterial overgrowth.
II **Associated:** —

Etiology: Abiotrophic, sometimes clearly transmitted as autosomal recessive; occasionally transmitted as autosomal dominant. McK *24050

Pathogenesis: Progressive loss of immunologic function due often to genetically determined failure of plasma cell production and deficiency of function of small lymphocytes, including deficiency of immunoglobulins IgG, IgA, IgM, IgD, or IgE. Often cells which suppress immune responses may participate in some deficiency of both cell-mediated and humoral immunities.

Related Facts
I **Sex Ratio:** M1:F1
II **Risk of Occurrence:** ?
III **Risk of Recurrence for**
   Patient's Sib: When autosomal recessive or autosomal dominant, see Table I AR or AD, respectively.
   Patient's Child: When autosomal recessive or autosomal dominant, see Table I AR or AD, respectively.
IV **Age of Detectability:** After 2 years of age to adult life
V **Prevalence:** ?

Treatment
I **Primary Prevention:** Genetic counseling
II **Secondary Prevention:** Gamma globulin therapy 0.6 cc/kg/d. Plasma therapy from selected donor every 3 to 4 weeks may be helpful.
III **Other Therapy:** Specific antibiotic treatment of intercurrent infection, prophylactic antibiotics may be required.

Prognosis: Even with replacement therapy, the risk of malignancy, progressive sinopulmonary infection and mesenchymal disease is high. Prognosis must be guarded.

Detection of Carrier: —

†**Special Considerations:** Although in some instances the late-occurring immunologic deficiency is clearly an inherited birth defect, its late occurrence stamps it as an abiotropism. Included in this category are those diseases previously termed primary immunologic deficiencies of adults, acquired agammaglobulinemia, acquired hypogammaglobulinemia, late-occurring agammaglobulinemia and hypogammaglobulinemia, dysgammaglobulinemia, and sporadic agammaglobulinemia and hypogammaglobulinemia. Members of both sexes may be involved. This grouping may include several separate diseases which will be distinguishable from one another.

References:
Wollheim, F. A.: Primary "acquired" hypogammaglobulinemia: Genetic defect or acquired disease? In Bergsma, D. and Good, R.A. (eds.): Immunologic Deficiency Diseases of Man. Birth Defects: Orig. Art. Ser., vol. IV, no. 1. White Plains:The National Foundation-March of Dimes, 1968, p. 311.

Contributor: **Robert A. Good**

Editor's Computerized Descriptors: Nasoph., Resp., Lymphatic, Spleen

IMMUNODEFICIENCY, SEVERE COMBINED

Includes: Agammaglobulinémie lymphopénique
Lymphopenische Agammaglobulinämie, Autosomal-rezessive Form
Agamaglobulinemia linfopénica autosómica recesiva
Lymphopenic agammaglobulinemia, autosomal recessive
Swiss-type agammaglobulinemia, autosomal recessive
Nonplasmatic autosomal recessive thymic alymphoplasia or alymphocytosis
Autosomal recessive primary or essential lymphocytothesis
Autosomal recessive hereditary lymphocytoplasmic dysgenesis
Severe dual system immunodeficiency

Excludes: Immunodeficiency, X-linked severe combined (524)
Agammaglobulinemia, X-linked infantile (27)
Thymic agenesis (943)
Late occurring lymphopenic agammaglobulinemia $\pm$ thymoma

Minimal Diagnostic Criteria: Although severe combined immunodeficiency comprises a spectrum of disorders, certain immunologic and pathologic features are almost uniformly seen and help to establish the diagnosis. A family history of severe combined immunodeficiency should alert to the possibility of this diagnosis. Infants with recurrent or chronic infections of the respiratory tract, skin, or GI system should be suspect for combined immunodeficiency. Disseminated BCG-osis or disseminated vaccinia in an infant strongly suggests the possibility of this disorder. Lymphopenia is not an invariable feature of the disease but is significant, if present. Low or undetectable levels of immunoglobulins, particularly IgM and IgA, are also not invariably present but if detected suggest severe deficiency of the humoral immune system. Lack of development of isohemagglutinins and failure to elicit antibody responses following immunization with DPT or typhoid antigens are constant features of this disorder. Early failure to develop antibody to such challenges occurs in up to 20% of normal newborns, but is significantly abnormal in infancy. Profound deficiencies of thymus-dependent immunity are documented by absence of or profound deficiencies in lymphoproliferative responses to mitogens, particularly PHA, and to allogenic cell stimuli, failure to develop a positive skin test following sensitization with DNCB, and inability to reject allogenic skin grafts. Lymph nodes are difficult to detect, but when biopsied reveal the pathologic features described below. Thymus biopsy by the supersternal route is being used with increasing frequency. The thymus, when found, has the architecture detailed below.

Clinical Findings: Clinical: Affected children usually appear normal at birth and begin to grow normally. Within weeks to months patients usually present with infections of skin and mucosal surfaces, such as oral moniliasis, gastroenteritis, diarrhea, malabsorption syndrome; bacterial or fungal infections of the skin, bronchitis and pneumonia. Lymph nodes draining areas of superficial infection may be conspicuously absent on palpation; and generalized skin eruption, either eczematoid or morbilliform, may be present. Tonsils and adenoids are absent.

Occasionally acute fulminating sepsis occurs. Progressive deterioration ensues over weeks to months with no real control of infection by standard anti-infectious and supportive therapy. In the absence of immunologic reconstitution, affected children, once they have developed infections, are never truly well. Age at death rarely exceeds one year. The usual bacterial infectious agents of this age group usually give way, under antibiotic therapy, to resistant, ubiquitous organisms of generally low pathogenicity. Frequently encountered are: monilial infection of respiratory or GI tract, coliform or micrococcal enteritis, pseudomonas or pneumocystis carinii pneumonia. Measles, cytomegalovirus, and varicella may cause disseminated giant cell inclusion body virus infection and fatal pneumonia. Adenovirus has been reported to cause similar disease. Disseminated BCG-osis, disseminated progressive vaccinia or vaccinia gangrenosum regularly follow immunization with these agents. Progressive disseminated infection from these or other attenuated vaccines in an infant with no other explanation of cause is strongly suggestive of severe combined immunologic deficiency disease. Fatal acute graft-vs-host disease (GVHD) may follow the administration of viable allogenic white cells in blood transfusions. A chronic form of GVHD with scaling erythroderma, diarrhea, malabsorption, and adenopathy due to maternal-fetal or intrauterine transfusion has been reported.

Laboratory Findings: Severe combined immunodeficiency occurs in 2 major forms which can be differentiated by the presence of normal or deficient levels of adenosine deaminase (ADA) in the red cells and lymphocytes. The deficiency in ADA may be only apparent in that an inhibitor of this enzyme has recently been described in some patients with this form of disease. Immunologic features of the 2 disorders are very similar. Absolute lymphocyte counts are generally $< 1500/mm^3$ and frequently $< 1000/mm^3.$ However, lymphopenia is not a necessary feature of this disease. Small lymphocytes usually represent a low percentage of the total number of lymphocytes in the peripheral blood. The classification of these lymphocytes by surface markers reveals abnormally low numbers of T lymphocytes as characterized by the capacity to spontaneously rosette with sheep red cells. Similarly, Ig-bearing lymphocytes are usually, although not always, reduced in number. Immunoglobulin levels are generally markedly abnormal. Normal levels of IgG, derived transplacentally from the mother, may persist for the first 3 months of life. IgM and IgA are usually very low or undetectable. Similarly salivary immunoglobulins are usually undetectable. In variants of this disorder, immunoglobulins may be detected at low normal concentrations; however, in all forms of the disease, antibody responses to antigenic challenges such as diphtheria, tetanus, pertussis or typhoid vaccines are conspicuously absent. Isoagglutinins, except as derived from maternal sources, are not detectable. Skin sensitivity cannot be induced to dinitrochlorobenzene (DNCB) or other exogenous skin sensitizing agents. Skin reactivity to Candida albicans remains negative following documented infection with this organism. Rejection of allogenic skin grafts is either markedly delayed or does not occur. In vitro lymphoproliferative responses to the mitogens phytohemagglutinin (PHA) or concanavalin A are either very low or not detectable. Responses to allogenic stimulation with mitomycin-treated heterologous lymphocytes are usually, though not invariably, markedly deficient. The lymphocytes cannot be induced by mitogen, antigen or allogenic cell stimulation to produce lymphokines. Total serum complement levels may be normal but in many of these patients levels of C1q and C8 are significantly decreased.

Pathologic Alterations: Thymus pathology differs in patients with and without ADA deficiency. The thymus in the enzyme-deficient patient is abnormally small but reveals evidence of some differentiation of a normal thymic vasculature and suggests thymic atrophy. By contrast, in the patients with normal levels of ADA the thymus is vestigial usually weighing 2 gm or less. It is usually found high in the thorax or in the neck. The thymus is morphologically embryonal and devoid of lymphoid infiltration, Hassal corpuscles or a normal vasculature. Corticomedullary organization is absent. The tissue consists of reticulum cells and epithelial cells with few if any lymphocytes. In each disorder the lymph nodes, when found, are strikingly devoid of lymphocytic infiltration. The normal lymph node architecture does not develop. The patients who have complicating chronic or acute GVHD may have lymph nodes with marked disorganization of the normal lymphoid architecture. Germinal centers are absent and the node consists predominantly of whorls of reticulum cells, occasional lymphocytes, and some eosinophils. Additional pathologic features include the absence of lymphoid cell aggregates or plasma cells in the lamina propria of the small intestine and appendix. Plasma cells are similarly lacking in the bone marrow. Peyer patches may not be evident on gross inspection of the ilium and appendix.

Complications
I **Derived:** The infections which have invariably been a cause of death in patients with this disease may be regarded as a complication of exposure to organisms against which the patient with primary immunologic deficiency cannot manifest a normal response.
II **Associated:** —

Etiology: Autosomal recessive transmission of defective gene.† Population data suggest that this may in fact be a final common path for a number of independent genetic entities. As similar degrees of developmental arrest affect both the thymic-dependent and independent lymphoid systems, it is reasonable to suppose that the gene defects reside in the lymphoid stem cell line rather than in one of the traffic organs such as the thymus through which lymphoid progenitors migrate. McK *20250

Pathogenesis: The basic defect in severe combined immunodeficiency without ADA deficiency is presumed to consist of homozygous absence or abnormality of a gene product essential for the development and differentiation of lymphoid stem cells. In the absence of trafficking by competent lymphoid stem cells, the thymus never undergoes transformation from its embryonic epithelial form to normal lymphoid morphology. Early thymic development may occur in the ADA-deficient form. At biopsy, the small thymus appears atrophic. In either form, peripheral lymphoid tissues are not populated. Both the cellular-delayed hypersensitivity and humoral circulating antibody systems fail to function.

Related Facts
I **Sex Ratio:** M1:F1
II **Risk of Occurrence:** About 2 per million live births in outbred population and 1 per 10,000 in 1st cousin matings. These figures are based on an estimated gene frequency of about 1.5×10^{-3} calculated from population data for Western Europe and North America.
III **Risk of Recurrence for**
   Patient's Sib: 1 in 4 (25%) for each offspring to be affected.
   Patient's Child: Affected persons die early.
IV **Age of Detectability:** In neonatal period if appropriate examinations are done.
V **Prevalence:** Prevalence equals risk of occurrence for the age group under about 4 months. Thereafter, it falls to near zero by 2 years as affected children almost invariably fail to survive to this age.

Treatment
I **Primary Prevention:** Genetic counseling
II **Secondary Prevention:** Experience to date suggests that the disease may be totally correctable by replacement of the missing tissue-functional lymphoid stem cells from the bone marrow of a histocompatible donor. Histocompatibility at the HLA-D locus, demonstrated by failure of a prospective donor's lymphocytes to respond to MLC against the patient's

lymphocytes, is critical to successful engraftment without lethal GVHD. Using this criterion, successful reconstitution of immune function with related, non-sib donors and even unrelated donors has been achieved. Laboratory evidence of immunologic reconstitution has been documented with unmatched marrow cells but, in such instances, the immunologically competent cells of the graft become sensitized and then reject their host. Reconstitution of T-cell function with fetal thymus and of both T- and B-cell function with fetal liver have been reported in patients with multiple variants of this disease, including the ADA-deficient form. In one form of SCID with ADA deficiency, significant though transient increments in T-cell function have followed transfusion of normal ADA+ red cells.
III **Other Therapy:** Unreconstituted patients are at constant risk of life-threatening infection; and, if definitive therapy is possible, they should be afforded every feasible benefit of protective isolation prior to satisfactory completion of grafting. Equipment and procedures have been developed for the germ-free cesarean delivery of high-risk infants, for total body decontamination of individuals who already have a bacterial flora (in the absence of gross infection with significant tissue damage), and for maintenance in a totally germ-free environment. Patients with defective delayed hypersensitivity are also unable to eliminate foreign immunologically competent cells encountered in blood or platelet-concentrate transfusions, and fatal GVHD has been reported following transfusion of blood as old as 19 days. As 1500 r of x-irradiation effectively destroys the reproductive potential of circulating lymphoid cells without interfering with either red cells or platelet function, it is recommended that transfusion packs for patients with confirmed or suspected diagnoses including defective delayed hypersensitivity be irradiated with 1500 r prior to administration. Exogenous gamma globulin has not been found to improve survival statistics in this disease.

Prognosis: Average duration of life approximately 6 months. Range: 1 month to about 2 years. Usual cause of death: chronic progressive infection with organisms of generally low pathogenicity.

Detection of Carrier: For patients with normal ADA, definitive identification presently possible only through production of affected offspring. The parents of patients with the ADA-deficient form may be detected by subnormal levels of ADA in the red cells and leukocytes. Prenatal diagnosis of affected offspring by enzyme levels in cultured amniotic fibroblasts is also possible in the ADA-deficient form.

†Special Considerations: The failure of induction of mitotic activity in peripheral leukocytes by PHA or heterologous tissue antigens, whether measured as deficient blast transformation, uptake of labeled DNA precursors or appearance of metaphase chromosome patterns, is a reflection of the absence of circulating cells which can be induced to enter mitosis by these agents, particularly the immunocompetent T lymphocyte. Chromosome karyotypes from such patients, when desired, may be obtained from either skin (fibroblast culture) or bone marrow (mitoses in granulocyte precursors). The more severe forms of X-linked lymphopenic agammaglobulinemia may be clinically and pathologically indistinguishable from the autosomal recessive disease; and, in the not frequently encountered isolated case in a small outbred sibship, differentiation cannot be made on a pedigree basis either. Assignment of hereditary pattern is inconsequential for the management of the patient, as it is the same for both syndromes, though the clinical course is usually slightly more acute in the autosomal recessive form and satisfactory immunologic reconstitution has been accomplished as of the date of writing only in the X-linked form. A difference occurs in the genetic counseling of possible carrier females. However, carriers of the autosomal recessive disease can reduce the probability of occurrence to about .005 per child simply by the avoidance of inbreeding, while carriers of the X-linked form can expect 1 in 2 sons to be affected regardless of their choice of a marital partner. Lymph nodes for diagnostic biopsy are ideally taken about 1 week after stimulation by low doses of typhoid-paratyphoid vaccine or other antigens to the area of drainage, ie an inguinal node stimulated by antigen administration to the corresponding thigh.

References:
Bergsma, D. (ed.): Immunodeficiency in Man and Animals, Birth Defects: Orig. Art. Ser., vol. XI, no. 1. Sunderland, MA: Sinauer Assoc., Inc. for The National Foundation-March of Dimes, 1975.
Buckley, R.H. et al: Correction of severe combined immunodeficiency by fetal liver cells. N. Engl. J. Med. 294:1076, 1976.
Dupont, B. et al: Transplantation of immunocompetent cells. In Brent, L. and Holbrow, J. (eds.): Progress in Immunology II. Clinical Aspects II. New York: American Elsevier Publishing, 1974, vol. V, p. 203.
Fudenberg, H. et al: Primary immunodeficiencies: Report of a W.H.O. Committee. Pediatrics 47:927, 1971.
Hoyer, J.R. et al: Lymphopenic forms of congenital immunologic deficiency diseases. Medicine (Baltimore) 47:201, 1968.
Meuwissen, H.J. et al: Combined immunodeficiency associated with adenosine deaminase deficiency. J. Pediatr. 86:169, 1975.
Polmar, S.H. et al: Restoration of in vitro lymphocyte responses with exogenous adenosine deaminase in a patient with severe combined immunodeficiency. Lancet 2:743, 1975.

Contributor: **Richard J. O'Reilly**

Editor's Computerized Descriptors: Oral, Nasoph., Skin, Resp., Lymphatic, Thymus, GI.

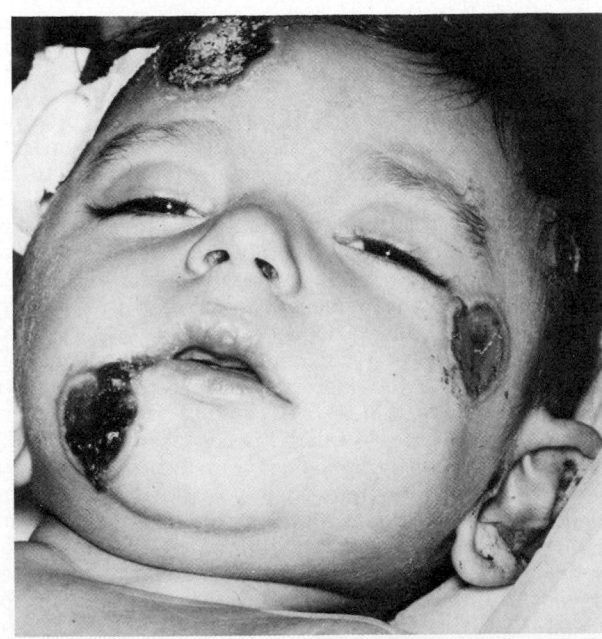

302. Progressive vaccinia. Note secondary lesions of face demonstrating characteristic extension, central necrosis and lack of inflammation

IMMUNODEFICIENCY WITH WISKOTT-ALDRICH SYNDROME

Includes: Syndrome de Wiskott-Aldrich
Ekzem-Thrombozytopenie-Diarrhoe-Syndrom
Síndrome de eczema, trombocitopenia y diarrea infecciosa
Wiskott-Aldrich syndrome
Eczema, thrombocytopenia, diarrhea, and infection syndrome

Excludes: Thrombocytopenia with absent radius (941)

Minimal Diagnostic Criteria: Thrombocytopenia, defective epinephrine or ADP-induced platelet aggregation, absent isohemagglutinins, failure to produce antibody in response to polysaccharide antigens, male.†

Clinical Findings: Thrombocytopenia 100%, eczema 100%, absent isohemagglutinins 100%, draining ears, lymphoid malignancy, high IgA, low IgM, normal-to-high IgG. These patterns probably present late in disease, but immunoglobulin levels can be normal early (before 2 years of age). Susceptibility to infection; frequent death from generalized herpes simplex infection.

Complications
I **Derived:** Lymphoid malignancy
II **Associated:** Autoimmune disorders, particularly hemolytic anemia.

Etiology: Usually X-linked recessive. A constant feature is the inability to form antibodies to certain polysaccharide antigens. Since the ability to form other antibodies is unaltered, the basic defect seems to be one of processing or recognition of this particular class of antigens. The relationship of this defect to thrombocytopenia is unclear.† The platelets are morphologically small. Epinephrine ADP and collagen-induced platelet aggregation is abnormal. Platelet hexokinase and glycogen levels are low, and energy metabolism defective. McK *30100

Pathogenesis: Thrombocytopenia is present from birth and bloody diarrhea usually occurs before the 6th month of life. Later in the course of the disease (by 1 - 2 years), the characteristic immunoglobulin pattern of elevated IgA and decreased IgM is seen. Hypercatabolism of immunoglobulin has been documented. Deficiency of cellular immunities to varying degrees also occurs as the disease progresses and is associated with morphologic changes in the thymic-dependent areas of lymphoid tissue. The high tendency to develop malignancy as a terminal event is postulated to be related to the role of immune deficits in tumorigenesis.

Related Facts
I **Sex Ratio:** M1:F0
II **Risk of Occurrence:** ?
III **Risk of Recurrence for**
   Patient's Sib: If mother is a carrier, 1 in 2 (50%) for each brother to be affected and 1 in 2 for each sister to be a carrier.
   Patient's Child: 1 in 1 (100%) for carrier daughters; not increased for sons unless wife is a carrier. (Reproductive fitness minimal because of early death).
IV **Age of Detectability:** With positive family history should be possible in newborn period; if none, should be possible at 12 months if history suggestive and patient fails to respond to challenge with polysaccharide antigen. Diagnosis suggested earlier by abnormalities in platelet function.
V **Prevalence:** ?

Treatment
I **Primary Prevention:** Genetic counseling
II **Secondary Prevention:** —
III **Other Therapy:** Blood transfusions, platelet transfusions as needed. Bone marrow transplantation reported successful in 3 cases. Transfer factor has been variably reported to be beneficial, particularly in reducing incidence of recurrent

infection.

Prognosis: Average life span treated - ? Average life span untreated - to adolescence or early adulthood. Usual cause of death: overwhelming infection from herpes, Pneumocystis carinii pneumonia, lymphoid malignancy, hemorrhage.

Detection of Carrier: Not yet feasible

†Special Considerations: A few isolated reports of X-linked thrombocytopenia with immunoglobulin alterations similar to those found in this syndrome and with immunoglobulin alterations and absent isohemagglutinins in some but not all have been described. Some of the 1st-degree relatives (female as well as male) have shown immunoglobulin level alterations or absent isohemagglutinins. The relationship of this X-linked syndrome to the so-called eczema, thrombocytopenia, diarrhea, and infection syndrome is unknown.

References:

Bach, F. H. et al: Bone marrow transplantation in a patient with the Wiskott-Aldrich syndrome. Lancet 2:1364, 1968.
Baldini, M.G.: Nature of the platelet defect in the Wiskott-Aldrich syndrome. Ann. N.Y. Acad. Sci. 201:437, 1972.
Blaese, R.M. et al: The Wiskott-Aldrich syndrome: A disorder with a possible defect in antigen processing or recognition. Lancet 1:1056, 1968.
Cooper, M.D. et al: Wiskott-Aldrich syndrome: An immunologic deficiency disease involving the efferent limb of immunity. Am. J. Med. 44:499, 1968.
Levin, A.S. et al: Wiskott-Aldrich syndrome. A genetically determined cellular immunologic deficiency: Clinical and laboratory responses to therapy with transfer factor. Proc. Natl. Acad. Sci. USA 67:821, 1970.

Contributors: **Richard Hong**
Richard J. O'Reilly

Editor's Computerized Descriptors: Ear, Skin, Lymphatic

IMMUNODEFICIENCY, X-LINKED SEVERE COMBINED

Includes: Déficit immunologique lymphopénique lié au sexe
Geschlechtsgebundener lymphopenischer Immunkörpermangel
Deficiencia inmunológica linfopénica ligada al sexo
Thymic alymphoplasia
Gitlin form of alymphopenic immunologic deficiency
Immunodeficiency, X-linked severe dual system
X-linked recessive lymphopenic agammaglobulinemia
X-linked lymphopenic immunologic deficiency
Primary essential lymphopenia (X-linked)
Congenital thymic dysplasia
Alymphocytosis
Lymphocytophisis
X-linked thymic epithelial hypoplasia
Swiss type agammaglobulinemia, X-linked
X-linked recessive form of lymphopenic hypogammaglobulinemia
X-linked severe dual system immunodeficiency

Excludes: Agammaglobulinemia, X-linked infantile (27)
Thymic agenesis (943)
Reticular dysgenesis
Immunodeficiency, severe combined (522)
Thymoma and agammaglobulinemia syndrome (944)
Immunodeficiency with Wiskott-Aldrich syndrome (523)

Minimal Diagnostic Criteria: Male infant with recurrent severe infections, absent or low isohemagglutinins, absent or low immunoglobulins, positive Schick test following DPT immunization, no response to DNFB skin test after sensitization or inability to reject an allogeneic skin graft of lymphocytes following PHA stimulation. Secondarily, lateral x-ray views of oropharynx and retrosternum reveal absence of adenoid and thymic shadows, respectively. Without a positive family history of previous male infant deaths, X-linked recessive lymphopenic immunologic deficiency disease may not be distinguishable from autosomal recessive lymphopenic agammaglobulinemia.†

Clinical Findings: Recurrent severe infections in a male child of pneumonia, meningitis, otitis, pyoderma, moniliasis, sepsis or diarrhea, eczema, undue susceptibility to common viral diseases (eg varicella, rubeola), progressive vaccinia following smallpox vaccination, fatal generalized BCG reactions, absence of lymph nodes, small or absent tonsils, poor growth, furuncles, family history of male infant deaths, absent isohemagglutinins, positive Schick test following DPT immunization, absent-to-low levels of serum immunoglobulins (IgM, IgG and IgA), lymphopenia (variable), markedly reduced proportion of E-rosetting T lymphocytes, negative skin tests to candida, trichophyton and PPD, negative skin test to DNFB 2 weeks after sensitization, poor-to-absent lymphoblast transformation following phytohemagglutinin stimulation, poor skin graft rejection, inability to form antibody following typhoid immunization, retrosternal radiolucency on lateral chest xray, absent thymic shadow on mediastinal CO_2 insufflation, absent adenoid shadow on lateral xray, lymph node biopsy before and after antigenic stimulation shows lack of architectural differentiation into cortex and medulla, absent germinal centers, sparse lymphoid elements and absent plasma cells. The bone marrow singularly lacks plasma cells.

Complications
I   **Derived:** Pneumonitis invariably occurs in these patients, the most common organisms which prove fatal are pseudomonas, enterobacteriaceae, cytomegalovirus, pneumocystis carinii and rubeola virus. Deaths from varicella pneumonia have also been reported. Other infectious complications include meningitis, sepsis, chronic otitis

media, moniliasis and furunculosis. Chronic diarrhea and malabsorption secondary to fungal or parasitic infections may contribute to marked failure to thrive. Vaccination with any live virus can lead to uncontrollable reactions. Fatal reactions have also been reported following BCG vaccination. Fatal graft-versus-host reactions following fresh whole blood transfusions are among the most common causes of death in these infants who lack the ability to reject incompatible lymphocytes. Graft-versus-host disease occurs 7-25 days after transfusion beginning with a coarse, maculopapular rash over the entire body, followed by diarrhea, hemolytic anemia, hepatosplenomegaly, progressive hepatitis, fever, pancytopenia and death. A chronic form of GVHD, marked by scaling erythroderma, histiocytic infiltration in the nodes, and chronic diarrhea may develop secondary to maternal-fetal transfusion or intrauterine transfusion for erythroblastosis fetalis.

II **Associated:** Malabsorption syndrome and lymphosarcoma. These are all extremely rare since patients with X-linked lymphopenic immunologic deficiency usually die before 2 years of age.

Etiology: Genetically determined defect in immune system, inherited in an X-linked recessive manner. McK *30040

Pathogenesis: Because both thymic-dependent (delayed hypersensitivity) and thymic-independent (circulating antibodies) systems are involved in this disease, an abnormality of the immunologic stem cell line has been postulated. During the 1st few months of life, these infants are partially protected by placentally transferred circulating antibodies. In the ensuing months, the immunoglobulin level falls as no new antibodies are being synthesized and, for unknown reasons, the number of circulating lymphocytes - especially the small lymphocytes - decreases. With the failure of both immunologic systems, recurrent infections follow. The danger of fatal GVHD secondary to fresh whole blood transfusions is a constant feature of the disease. On postmortem examination, both gross and microscopic abnormalities are found in the thymus, lymph nodes, spleen and GI tract. These consist mainly of marked depletion of all lymphoid elements, especially lymphocytes and plasma cells.

Related Facts
I **Sex Ratio:** M1:F0
II **Risk of Occurrence:** 1 in 1,000,000. The recorded incidence of the X-linked recessive form of lymphopenic agammaglobulinemia has been higher in the United States than in Europe. The autosomal recessive (Swiss) type of lymphopenic agammaglobulinemia is more commonly seen in Europe.
III **Risk of Recurrence for**
 Patient's Sib: If mother is a carrier, 1 in 2 (50%) for each brother to be affected and 1 in 2 for each sister to be a carrier.
 Patient's Child: 1 in 1 (100%) for carrier daughters; not increased for sons unless wife is a carrier. (Patients die very early.)
IV **Age of Detectability:** The diagnosis can be made shortly after birth by lymph node biopsy, low or absent lymphocyte responses to PHA, inability to reject skin grafts or to form antibody following antigenic stimulation (eg typhoid antigen), absent isohemagglutinins and quantitative low or absent immunoglobulins. A positive family history should increase the index of suspicion.
V **Prevalence:** Less than 1 in 1,000,000 under 1 year of age. Seldom seen above 2 years of age.

Treatment
I **Primary Prevention:** Genetic counseling
II **Secondary Prevention:** Recent experience indicates that reconstitution of the immunologic capacity of these patients is possible by implantation of immunologically competent lymphocytes or a stem cell source from a donor who is histocompatible at the HLA locus, particularly the D locus as detected by mutual nonresponsiveness in mixed leukocyte culture. Allogenic fetal liver cell transplants may also provide partial or complete reconstitution without lethal GVHD.
III **Other Therapy:** For a number of years, gamma globulin replacement therapy and antibiotics, when necessary, have been used to support these patients. Although this regimen, coupled with good pulmonary hygiene, has probably prolonged the life span of these infants, few have survived beyond the 2nd birthday.

Blood transfusion: Whenever whole blood transfusion becomes necessary in the treatment of these patients, care must be taken to minimize the number of viable histoincompatible lymphocytes in the transfusate in order to prevent GVHD from occurring. This can be accomplished by utilizing buffy-coat poor blood irradiated with 1500r.

Prognosis: Poor. With the exception of patients in whom the immunologic system was reconstituted by bone marrow transplantation from a histocompatible sib, both treated and untreated patients have died before 2 years of age of overwhelming infections. In contrast, patients with autosomal recessive lymphopenic agammaglobulinemia die during the first 9 months of life.

Detection of Carrier: —

†**Special Considerations:** Patients with X-linked recessive lymphopenic immunologic deficiency do not always manifest as severe a lymphopenia as do those infants with the autosomal recessive (Swiss) type of lymphopenic agammaglobulinemia. Lymphopenia is also occasionally missed when the total lymphocyte count alone is followed. Lymphopenia in these patients refers primarily to decreased numbers of circulating small lymphocytes. The X-linked and autosomal recessive forms can be differentiated on histologic examination of lymphoid tissues, the former group showing generally less severe depletion of lymphoid elements. Occasionally, normal lymphocyte counts are observed in these patients until relatively late in the course of their disease.

References:
Buckley, R.H. et al: Correction of severe combined immunodeficiency by fetal liver cells. N. Engl. J. Med. 294:1076, 1976.
Dupont, B. et al: Transplantation of immunocompetent cells. In Brent, L. and Holbrow, J. (eds.): Progress in Immunology II. Clinical Aspects II. New York: American Elsevier Publishing Co., 1974, vol. V, p. 203.
Gatti, R.A. et al: Immunological reconstitution of sex-linked lymphopenic immunological deficiency. Lancet 2:1366, 1968.
Gitlin, D. and Craig, J.M.: The thymus and other lymphoid tissues in congenital agammaglobulinemia. I. Thymic alymphoplasia and lymphocytic hypoplasia and their relation to infection. Pediatrics 32:517, 1963.

Contributors: **Richard A. Gatti**
Richard J. O'Reilly

Editor's Computerized Descriptors: Nasoph., Skin, Lymphatic, GI., Nerve

IMMUNOGLOBULIN A DEFICIENCY

Includes: Déficit en immunoglobuline A
IgA-Mangel
Deficiencia en inmunoglobulina A
Isolated IgA deficiency
Dysgammaglobulinemia type IV

Excludes: Ataxia-telangiectasia (94)
Immunodeficiency, severe combined (522)
Immunodeficiency, X-linked severe combined (524)

Minimal Diagnostic Criteria: IgA in serum < 3 SD below mean for age. IgA in secretions usually also is low; a few cases with IgA present in secretion.

Clinical Findings: None specific except those of associated defects when these are present.†

Complications
I **Derived:** Increased susceptibility to respiratory infection and GI disease.
II **Associated:** A number of defects are present, but whether they are commonly associated epiphenomena or derivative consequences is unknown. The following have been described: arthritis 26 cases, SLE 10 cases, thyroiditis 8 cases, pernicious anemia 6 cases, sprue syndrome 8 cases, hepatic cirrhosis 15 cases, "lupoid" hepatitis 5 cases, dermatomyositis 3 cases, pulmonary hemosiderosis 5 cases, idiopathic Addison disease 2 cases, Sjögren disease 2 cases, Coombs positive hemolytic anemia 2 cases, regional enteritis 1 case, ulcerative colitis 1 case, ITP 1 case, mental retardation 3 cases, epilepsy (before treatment) 5 cases. Cancers of epithelial origin (gastric or pulmonary) may have an increased incidence. A large family with IgA deficiency and correlated early onset COPD has been reported.

Etiology: Occurs constantly as a part of congenital agammaglobulinemia syndromes, or unassociated with other immunologic defects. A familial autosomal form has been described. No definite chromosomal abnormality has been identified. Since IgA-bearing lymphocytes are in most, if not all cases, normal in numbers, this may reflect the presence of an abnormality or suppression of cellular differentiation leading to an inability to secrete IgA, rather than a lack of a gene controlling the constant region of the α chain. This is compatible with the finding that the deficiency has been found to include both IgA_1 and IgA_2 subclasses in studied cases.

Drug-induced IgA deficiency reported in phenytoin (Dilantin) treated patients with epilepsy. The number of IgA-bearing B lymphocytes is normal.

Pathogenesis: Perhaps related to local antibody deficiency but many people with isolated IgA deficiency seem perfectly normal. Relation to associated diseases entirely unclear.

Related Facts
I **Sex Ratio:** M1:F2
II **Risk of Occurrence:** 1 in 600 live births. Higher in selected groups ("collagen diseases").
III **Risk of Recurrence for**
  Patient's Sib: ?
  Patient's Child: ?
IV **Age of Detectability:** 1 year of age for certain by immunoquantitation.
V **Prevalence:** 1 in 600 of normal population; higher in those with collagen diseases.

Treatment
I **Primary Prevention:** —
II **Secondary Prevention:** Supportive measures for chronic sinusitis, avoidance of gluten in sprue when sensitivity is shown.

III **Other Therapy:** Fresh plasma infusions in sprue and chronic respiratory infection may be of benefit, but severe anaphylactic transfusion reactions have occurred in patients lacking IgA and having anti-IgA. If blood transfusions are required, washed, packed cells are indicated.

Prognosis: Is that of the associated disease; in many cases compatible with normal longevity.

Detection of Carrier: ?

†**Special Considerations:** Other laboratory findings: 60% have anti-IgA antibodies; not all of these can be explained as due to prior plasma, or gammaglobulin therapy. Increased IgG or IgM frequently found. Antimilk antibodies (hemagglutinating or precipitating) are found in 50% and antibovidae antibodies in 40%. Secretory component levels are usually normal.

References:
Amman, A. and Hong, R.: Selective IgA deficiency: Presentation of 30 cases and a review of the literature. Medicine 50:223, 1971.
Goldberg, L. S. and Fudenberg, H. H.: Selective absence of IgA: A family study. J. Lab. Clin. Med. 72:204, 1968.
Hobbs, J. R.: Immune imbalance in dysgammaglobulinemia type IV. Lancet 1:110, 1968.
Kersey, J.H. et al: Immunodeficiency and cancer. Adv. Cancer Res. 18:211, 1973.
Lawton, A.R. et al: IgA determinants on B-lymphocytes in patients with deficiency of circulating IgA. J. Lab. Clin. Med. 80:26, 1972.
Seager, J. et al: IgA deficiency, epilepsy, and phenytoin treatment. Lancet 2:632, 1975.
Van Loghem, E.: Familial occurrence of isolated IgA deficiency associated with antibodies to IgA. Evidence against a structural gene defect. Eur. J. Immunol. 4:57, 1974.
Vjas, G. and Fudenberg, H.H.: $Am(1)_1$ the first genetic marker of human immunoglobulin A. Proc. Natl. Acad. Sci. USA 64:1211, 1969.

Contributors: **Robert A. Good**
Charlotte Cunningham-Rundles

Editor's Computerized Descriptors: Resp., GI., Liver

INCONTINENTIA PIGMENTI

Includes: Bloch-Sulzberger syndrome
Incontinentia pigmenti achromians

Excludes: Naegeli syndrome (703)

Minimal Diagnostic Criteria: Skin lesions, with or without alopecia, tooth anomalies.

Clinical Findings: Characterized at birth or neonatal period by inflammation and bullae in females. The lesions are arranged in linear fashion and may come and go. They are then replaced by hypertrophic verrucous bands. Then a bizarre pattern of spattered or band-like hyperpigmentation appears mostly on the trunk but also on the scalp and limbs. The hyperpigmentation slowly fades and is about gone by the 3rd decade. Not in every case is the typical hyperpigmentation preceded by inflammation and blisters. Alopecia of scalp, dental, ocular, and osseous anomalies, deformities of ears, small stature, neurologic changes and occasionally mental retardation occur. In incontinentia pigmenti achromians, band-like depigmentation occurs.

Complications
I   **Derived:** Convulsions, retrolental fibroplasia, supernumerary tragi, extra ribs, hemivertebrae
II   **Associated:** —

Etiology: Probably X-linked dominant with lethality in the male; McK *30830

Pathogenesis: ?

Related Facts
I   **Sex Ratio:** The disorder occurs clinically almost exclusively in females.
II   **Risk of Occurrence:** Rare
III   **Risk of Recurrence for**
   Patient's Sib: If affected patient is female, 1 in 2 (50%) for each female sib to be affected. If affected patient is male, risk for each affected sister is 1:2 (50%) and not increased for brothers.
   Patient's Child: If mother is affected, 1:2 (50%) of female offspring is affected; 1 in 2 males dies in utero; the remaining male is normal.
IV   **Age of Detectability:** —
V   **Prevalence:** —

Treatment
I   **Primary Prevention:** Genetic counseling
II   **Secondary Prevention:** Determination of sex of fetus by amniocentesis is not helpful.
III   **Other Therapy:** —

Prognosis: Normal life span. Some patients are mentally retarded. Disability may result from neurologic, ocular, osseous and other changes. Reproductive fitness somewhat impaired by major defects.

Detection of Carrier: —

Special Considerations: —

References:
Bloch, B.: Eigentümliche, bisher nicht beschriebene, Pigmentaffektion (incontinentia pigmenti). Schweiz. Med. Wochenschr. 7:404, 1926.
Carney, R.G.: Incontinentia pigmenti: Report of 5 cases and review of literature. Arch. Dermatol. Syph. 64:126, 1951.
Carney, R.G. and Carney, R.G., Jr.: Incontinentia pigmenti. Arch. Dermatol. 102:157, 1970.
Carney, R.G., Jr.: Incontinentia pigmenti, a world statistical analysis. Arch. Dermatol. 112:535, 1976.
Curth, H.O. and Warburton, D.: The genetics of incontinentia pig-
menti. Arch. Dermatol. 92:229, 1965.
Hamada, T. et al: Incontinentia pigmenti achromians (Ito). Arch. Dermatol. 96:673, 1967.
Sulzberger, M.B.: Über eine bisher nicht beschriebene congenitale Pigmentanomalie (incontinentia pigmenti). Arch. Dermatol. Syph. (Berl.) 154:19, 1928.

Contributor: **Helen Ollendorff Curth**

Editor's Computerized Descriptors: Eye, Ear, Teeth, Skin, Hair, Skel., Nerve

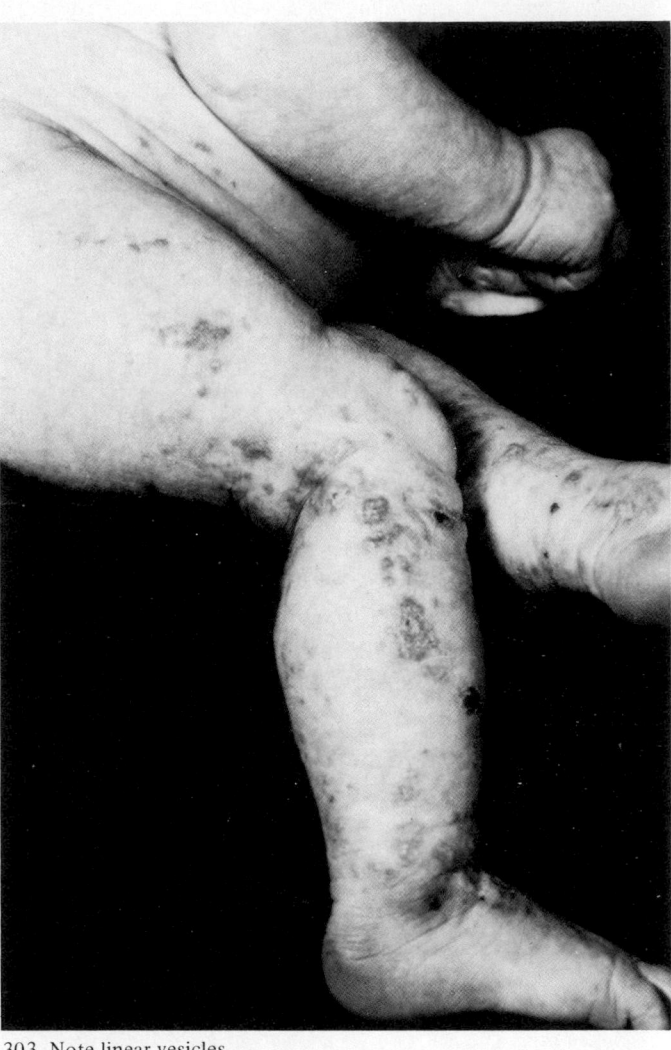

303. Note linear vesicles

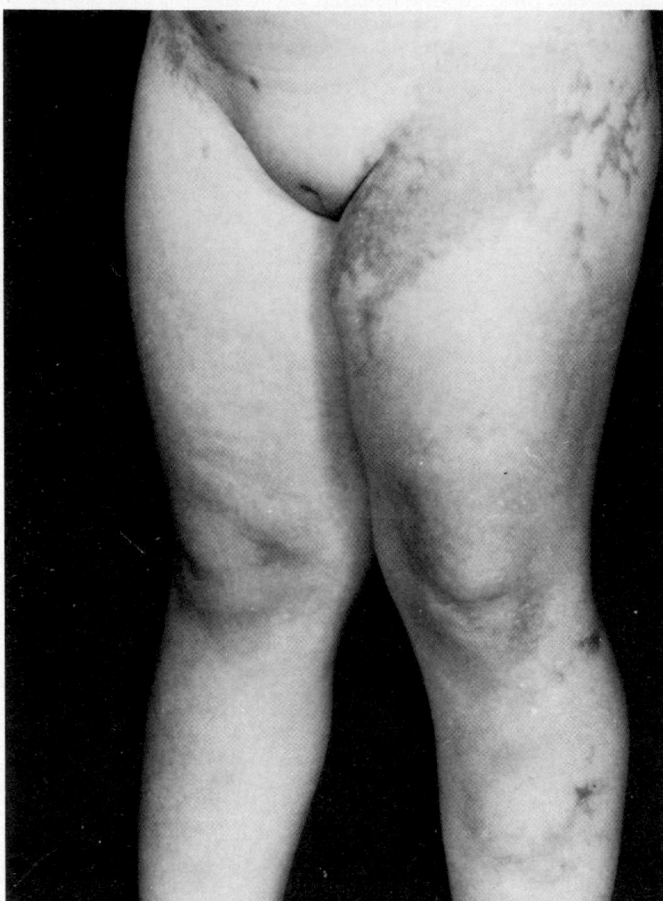

304. Note spattered hyperpigmentation

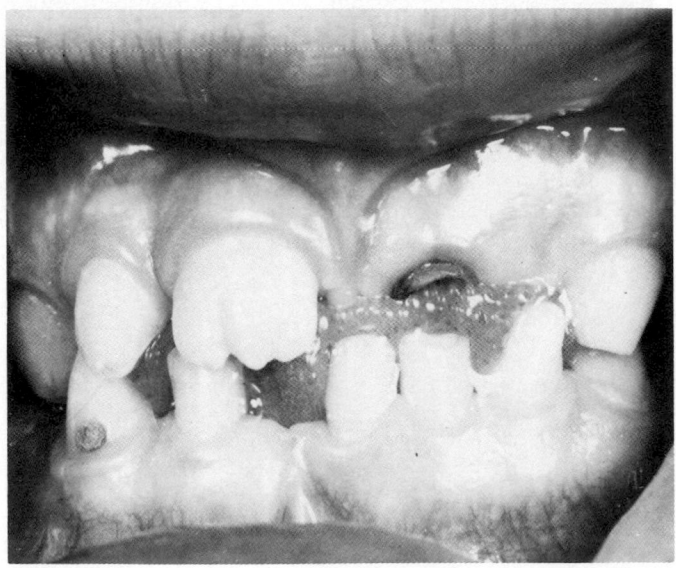

305. Dysplastic and conical teeth secondary to incontinentia pigmenti

INDEPENDENT ORIGIN OF IPSILATERAL VERTEBRAL ARTERY

Includes: Origine anormale de l'artère vertébrale
Direkter Abgang der a. vertebralis aus der Aorta
Origen anormal de la arteria vertebral
Ipsilateral vertebral artery directly from aortic arch rather than from subclavian artery

Excludes: Other abnormal origin of vertebral artery

Minimal Diagnostic Criteria: Selective aortic arch aortography

Clinical Findings: This anomaly is found incidentally and is asymptomatic. The anomaly was found in 6% of patients. There are no cases described with symptomatology that could be attributed to this type of malformation. However, it is important to look for it (during a radiologic contrast examination) particularly when the vertebral artery is not filled from the usual position.
The recognition of this abnormal vessel may become very important if it is associated with other anomalies of the aortic arch that are to be repaired surgically, such as hypoplastic arch syndrome and aortic coarctation. The possibility of resecting it with the involved portion of the aortic arch is very real.

Complications
I   Derived: —
II   Associated: —

Etiology: ?

Pathogenesis: Normally, the first portion of the vertebral artery is derived from the precostal longitudinal anastomoses between the cervical intersegmental arteries, the remainder from the postcostal longitudinal anastomoses. In abnormal origin of the vertebral artery from the aorta, the first part of the vessel is derived from a more anteriorly located channel.

Related Facts
I   Sex Ratio: ?
II   Risk of Occurrence: ?
III Risk of Recurrence for
        Patient's Sib: ?
        Patient's Child: ?
IV   Age of Detectability: At any age by arch aortography
V   Prevalence: ?

Treatment
I   Primary Prevention: —
II   Secondary Prevention: —
III Other Therapy: —

Prognosis: Excellent; should have a normal life span.

Detection of Carrier: —

Special Considerations: —

References:
Bosniak, M.A.: An analysis of some anatomic-roentgenologic aspects of the brachiocephalic vessels. Am. J. Roentgenol. Radium Ther. Nucl. Med. 91:1222, 1964.
Liechty, J.D. et al: Variations pertaining to the aortic arches and their branches. Q. Bull. Northw. Univ. Med. Sch. 31:136, 1957.
Sutton, D. and Davies, E.R.: Arch aortography and cerebrovascular insufficiency. Clin. Radiol. 17:330, 1966.

Contributors: **Juan R. Guerrero
Charles E. Mullins
Dan G. McNamara**

Editor's Computerized Descriptor: CV.

INFERIOR VENA CAVA, ABSENT HEPATIC SEGMENT

Includes: Absence du segment hépatique de la veine cave inférieure
Fehlendes hepatisches Segment der Vena cava inferior
Ausencia del segmento hepático de la vena cava inferior
Infrahepatic interruption of inferior vena cava
Absent inferior vena cava
Azygos continuation of inferior vena cava
Absent hepatic segment of inferior vena cava

Excludes: —

Minimal Diagnostic Criteria: The roentgenologic findings mentioned below, patients suspected of polysplenia, venous angiography.

Clinical Findings: In this condition the inferior vena cava (IVC) is absent between the renal veins and the hepatic veins and the systemic venous drainage from below the interruption is via an enlarged azygos vein to the superior vena cava. Less often, the hemiazygos vein is the alternative venous pathway and empties into a persistent left superior vena cava.

The anomaly by itself does not alter hemodynamics and is not responsible for symptomatology. It may be identified on xray by absence of the inferior vena caval density at the cardiophrenic angle in the lateral view. The collateral route of flow to the right SVC by the azygos vein creates a large rounded density seen in the right lung field just above the SVC-RA junction. This anomaly is almost invariably present when the roentgenogram shows the stomach in a malposed position. In other words, if the thoracic contents are in their usual position (situs solitus) and the stomach is right-sided, or if the thoracic contents indicate situs inversus and the stomach is left-sided, absent hepatic segment of the IVC is present until proven otherwise.

It may occur as an isolated anomaly, but usually there are associated cardiovascular defects. It is particularly common as part of the polysplenia syndrome.

Complications
I **Derived:** Inadvertent ligation of the azygos vein may lead to death. During cardiopulmonary bypass, the surgeon must recognize and deal with the altered systemic venous drainage.
II **Associated:** Multiple spleens, abnormal cardiac situs, isolated abdominal situs inversus

Etiology: ?

Pathogenesis: The anomaly is due to hypoplasia or aplasia of the anastomosis which normally develops between right subcardinal and proximal vitelline venous systems (renal and posthepatic segments of the IVC).

Related Facts
I **Sex Ratio:** Probably M1:F1
II **Risk of Occurrence:** Approximately 1 in 100 patients with congenital heart disease
III **Risk of Recurrence for**
   Patient's Sib: ?
   Patient's Child: ?
IV **Age of Detectability:** From birth by selective angiography
V **Prevalence:** ?

Treatment
I **Primary Prevention:** —
II **Secondary Prevention:** —
III **Other Therapy:** —

Prognosis: In the rare situation where there are no associated cardiac anomalies longevity is normal. Interruption of the IVC with azygos continuation does not influence the prognosis of other conditions.

Detection of Carrier: —

Special Considerations: —

References:
Anderson, R.C. et al: Anomalous inferior vena cava with azygos continuation (infrahepatic interruption of the inferior vena cava): Report of 15 new cases. J. Pediatr. 59:370, 1961.
Lucas, R.V., Jr. and Schmidt, R.E.: Anomalous venous connection, pulmonary and systemic. In Moss, A.J. and Adams, F.H. (eds.): Heart Disease in Infants, Children, and Adolescents. Baltimore: Williams and Wilkins, 1968, p. 720.

Contributor: **Russell V. Lucas, Jr.**

Editor's Computerized Descriptors: Resp., CV., GI.

INGUINAL HERNIA

Includes: Hernie inguinale
Leistenbruch
Hernia inguinal
Hernia, inguinal direct or indirect
Hydrocele
Communicating hydrocele
Sliding hernia
Incarcerated hernia
Strangulated hernia

Excludes: Femoral hernia
Ventral hernia
Varicocele

Minimal Diagnostic Criteria: Presence or history of mass in groin on straining or at rest. Thickened cord structures with history of mass. Persistent hydrocele in child over 1 year of age. Palpation of inguinal ring is invalid in children for detection of hernia. Irreducible mass in inguinal region of infant or child with no symptoms probably is hydrocele of the spermatic cord. Irreducible mass in inguinal canal of female infant or child without symptoms probably represents sliding hernia containing an ovary. Hydrocele of the canal of Nuck also presents as asymptomatic mass in female infant. Differential diagnosis must be made at operation.

Clinical Findings: Presence of mass in groin or scrotum in males and groin in females. Mass may be intermittent and more evident on straining, crying, etc or constant in case of hydrocele with or without herniated viscera. Discomfort and distress may be evident in older children. Intestinal obstruction may be evident with hernia difficult to reduce, ie incarceration. In the absence of a mass there may be "thickened" cord structures or a "silk glove" sensation on palpation of the cord structures at the level of the pubic spine. Persistent hydrocele in children over 1 year of age generally signifies presence of hernia. A hydrocele present in a toddler or infant at the end of the day but absent in the morning should be considered a communicating hydrocele or congenital hernia.

Complications
I **Derived:** Intestinal obstruction may result from incarceration. Strangulation or ischemic change in bowel wall due to incarceration may result in intestinal perforation, shock, peritonitis and death if not treated promptly. Testicular atrophy may result from incarceration with resultant ischemia of testis. Ovarian atrophy may result from incarceration with ischemia of ovary.
II **Associated:** Undescended testis. Herniae more frequent in premature infants.

Etiology: ?

Pathogenesis: Most inguinal herniae in children are indirect herniae. Less than 1% are direct. The indirect hernia is the result of a failure of obliteration of the processus vaginalis, a projection of the peritoneal cavity into the inguinal canal and scrotum. The processus vaginalis obliterates itself except around testis where it becomes the tunica vaginalis. Proximal obliteration of the processus may leave a potential space for fluid collection and hydrocele formation. Hydrocele may be of tunica vaginalis or of cord with no testicular component. Hydroceles are very common in 1st months of life as processus vaginalis is obliterating. If hydrocele persists after 1 year of age a hernia is present 95% of the time. A sudden appearance of a hydrocele of the cord is generally followed at an unspeci-

fied period of time by a clinically evident hernia. Infants and children present with clinical evidence of bilateral herniae 30% of the time. Right herniae are 3-4 times more common than left presentations.

Related Facts
I **Sex Ratio:** M9:F1
II **Risk of Occurrence:** ?
III **Risk of Recurrence for**
Patient's Sib: ?
Patient's Child: ?
IV **Age of Detectability:** Any age from birth through infancy and childhood
V **Prevalence:** 1 in 100 children under 12 years of age will have herniae. (Newcastle, England Study)

Treatment
I **Primary Prevention:** —
II **Secondary Prevention:** When noted, sac should be dissected from cord structures up to internal inguinal ring and excised. Anatomic repair of groin structures is all that is necessary. Hydroceles should be treated just as herniae with removal of residual processus vaginalis down to but not necessarily including tunica vaginalis. When associated with undescended testis, orchidopexy should be carried out at time of herniorrhaphy. When incarceration presents, and has been present for less than 12 hours and there is no evidence of bowel ischemia, attempts should be made at reduction via sedation, ice bag and gentle continuous pressure upward (taxis). Immediate operation should follow failure of reduction. If reduction is accomplished, repair should be delayed 24-48 hours to allow edema of tissues to subside.†
III **Other Therapy:** —

Prognosis: Normal life expectancy with exceedingly rare recurrence

Detection of Carrier: —

†Special Considerations: In infants, particularly, if a hernia is symptomatic on 1 side, other side may harbor asymptomatic patent processus vaginalis. Not all patients with patent processus vaginalis will develop herniae. Though patent processus vaginalis is very frequent on the uninvolved side, most series where only symptomatic herniae are repaired, have only 2-6% of patients return for a hernia on the other side. Enthusiasm for exploration of the uninvolved side is waning.

Direct inguinal hernia is very rare, probably 1% of cases or less. Repair is similar to adult or acquired direct hernia with so-called Cooper ligament repair.

The sliding hernia should be repaired with inversion of the sac by a purse string suture. Care in ligation of the sac in all females should be exercised to prevent injury to the fallopian tube in the neck of the sac.

In bilateral herniae in an infant with external female genitalia with 1 or 2 palpable gonads in the canal, the gonads should be visualized and biopsied if abnormal. True intersex with ovotestis or testicular feminization syndrome may be discovered very early in 0.1-0.5% of cases.

References:
Potts, W.J.: Inguinal hernia in infants. Pediatrics 1:772, 1948.
Swenson, O.: Diagnosis and treatment of inguinal hernia. Pediatrics 34:412, 1964.

Contributor: **Lawrence K. Pickett**

Editor's Computerized Descriptors: GI., GU.

INTERNAL CAROTID ARTERY ANEURYSM OF MIDDLE EAR

Includes: Anévrisme de l'oreille moyenne
Aneurysma der a. carotis im Bereich des Mittelohrs
Aneurisma de la carótida interna del oído medio
Aneurysm of middle ear
Middle ear aneurysm of internal carotid artery
Carotid artery aneurysm

Excludes: Arteriovenous aneurysm of internal carotid artery
Chemodectoma of middle ear (145)
Posttraumatic carotid artery aneurysm in middle ear
Aneurysm of the lateral dural sinus

Minimal Diagnostic Criteria: Aneurysm of middle ear demonstrated by carotid angiography

Clinical Findings: The patient may present with spontaneous bleeding from the ear or profuse bleeding after mild trauma. There may be a history of or symptoms suggesting acute suppurative ear disease or chronic adhesive otitis, and profuse, pulsatile, bright red bleeding follows attempted myringotomy. The patient may complain of pulsatile tinnitus, deafness, vertigo or facial nerve weakness. CNS symptoms, headache, vomiting, convulsions and cranial nerve palsies may be seen with extensive aneurysms. The patient may have had previous mastoidectomy associated with severe intraoperative bleeding from the middle ear. In some cases there may be associated bleeding from the nose.

Physical examination may show a red bulge and visible pulsation behind the tympanic membrane. Pneumatic otoscopy under operating microscope magnification may show blanching with pressure. Often a bruit can be heard over the skull or over the carotid artery system in the neck. Facial paresis or palsy may be present as well as nystagmus. Caloric examination might demonstrate asymmetric response or absent response to stimuli on the involved side. Conductive, sensorineural or mixed hearing loss is often present, and complete hearing loss may occur.

Clinical examination usually does not reveal the true nature of the problem which, however, becomes evident on carotid angiography. Angiography is diagnostic and delineates the extent of the aneurysm and rules out multiple aneurysms, since their incidence in all intracranial aneurysm patients is 13-25%.

Complications
I   **Derived:** Anemia, shock, hypoxemia and death from hemorrhage; facial or vestibular paresis or palsy; hearing loss; bone erosion; CNS symptoms, eg seizures, coma and cranial nerve palsies.
II **Associated:** Strabismus was reported in only 1 case. In another, a large anomalous trigeminal or auditory artery and a rudimentary vertebral artery were found in association with absence of the opposite carotid artery system.

Etiology: ?

Pathogenesis: This is a type of the berry aneurysm seen elsewhere intracranially, possibly caused by a developmental deficiency in the medial layer of arteries or weaknesses in the wall where embryonic capillary plexuses opened. However, there is considerable disagreement about both of these concepts.

Related Facts
I   **Sex Ratio:** Probably M1:F1 (only 8 cases)
II **Risk of Occurrence:** ?
III **Risk of Recurrence for**
     Patient's Sib: ?
     Patient's Child: ?

IV **Age of Detectability:** Variable. Detected when aural bleeding occurs, but it would be possible to suspect the diagnosis in a patient who presents with a feeling of stuffiness in the ear, pulsatile tinnitus, hearing loss, vertigo or facial weakness. The presence of a pulsatile middle ear mass in a child is especially suspicious.
V   **Prevalence:** ?

Treatment
I   **Primary Prevention:** —
II **Secondary Prevention:** Ligation of the homolateral common carotid artery may be effective. However, surgical exposure of the middle ear via a tympanotomy approach, mastoidectomy approach or temporal bone resection approach with control of the carotid artery in the neck may be necessary. Resection or clipping of the aneurysm can then be accomplished. Cryoprobe therapy is not effective. Ligation of the internal carotid artery may be necessary; in about 25% of patients various motor, sensory and speech deficits or even death may ensue.
III **Other Therapy:** Tight packing of the external auditory canal or mastoid cavity (if there is one) with hemostatic gauze or sponge material or ordinary dry strip packing, digital compression of the carotid artery in the neck, blood transfusions and other supportive measures may be needed for management of acute hemorrhage prior to definitive diagnosis and therapy.†

Prognosis: Death may result from exsanguinating hemorrhage. This occurred in 2 of the 8 reported cases, as compared to a mortality rate of 44-55% in other intracranial aneurysms. Complete hearing loss may occur secondary to bone erosion from the aneurysm, from tight emergency aural packing or from necessary definitive surgery. Less frequently, facial paresis or palsy, vestibular loss and CNS damage occur.

The likelihood of rebleeding is high in patients in whom only emergency tamponade is performed; but rebleeding has not been reported after definitive surgery.

Detection of Carrier: —

†Special Considerations: Patients who present with profuse aural bleeding should be controlled by emergency and supportive measures and then given definitive diagnostic measures and definitive therapy promptly, as the likelihood of rebleeding is high.

References:
Allen, G.W.: Angiography in otolaryngology. Laryngoscope 77:1909, 1967.
Anderson, W.A.D.: Synopsis of Pathology, 5th Ed. St. Louis:C.V. Mosby Co., 1960, vol. 1.
Conley, J. and Hildyard, V.: Aneurysm of the internal carotid artery presenting in the middle ear. Arch. Otolaryngol. 90:35, 1969.
Ehni, G. and Barrett, J.H.: Hemorrhage from the ear due to an aneurysm of the internal carotid artery. N. Engl. J. Med. 262:1323, 1960.
Grinker, R.R. and Sahs, A.L.: Neurology, 6th Ed. Springfield; Charles C Thomas, 1966.
Stallings, J.O. and McCabe, B.F.: Congenital middle ear aneurysm of internal carotid. Arch. Otolaryngol. 90:39, 1969.

Contributors: **LaVonne Bergstrom**
Victor H. Hildyard

Editor's Computerized Descriptors: Eye, Hearing, Ear, CV., Nerve

INTESTINAL ATRESIA OR STENOSIS

Includes: Atrésie ou sténose intestinale
Dünndarmatresie (-stenose)
Estenosis o atresia intestinal
Ileal atresia or stenosis
Jejunal atresia or stenosis

Excludes: Duodenal atresia or stenosis (300)
Cystic fibrosis with meconium ileus
Colon aganglionosis (192)
Gastroschisis (405)
Omphalocele (748)

Minimal Diagnostic Criteria: Intestinal obstruction with x-ray confirmation

Clinical Findings: Intestinal obstruction of the newborn with abdominal distention, vomiting and obstipation. Stenosis may become clinically apparent later in infancy with constipation or diarrhea (secondary to alterations in intestinal flora in obstructed segment) the paramount symptom. Atresia occurs in the jejunum (50%), the ileum (43%) and in both jejunum and ileum, ie multiple points of atresia (7%).

Complete or partial occlusion of the lumen of the jejunum or ileum presents in the gross form as either 1) an internal "diaphragm" (19%), 2) constriction of the muscular layers and obliteration of the lumen resulting in a "cord-like" structure connecting the proximal and distal segments (31%), or 3) complete separation of the proximal and distal ends with defect in the mesentery (45%). Stenosis is relatively uncommon, accounting for 4% of these anomalies distal to the duodenum.

Complications
I **Derived:** .a) Meconium peritonitis: evidence of intrauterine (sterile) peritonitis with no demonstrable intestinal perforation at the time of birth (12%). b) Intestinal perforation: perforation of the proximal, dilated, intestinal segment apparent at birth (5%). c) Volvulus with infarction: infarction of the proximal atretic segment resulting from volvulus and ischemia without perforation (2%).
II **Associated:** a) Incomplete rotation of colon: (9%), b) Cardiovascular anomalies (2%), c) Omphalocele-gastroschisis (2%), d) Chromosome 21 trisomy syndrome (1%), e) Esophageal atresia (1%), f) Intestinal duplication (1%), g) Colon aganglionosis (1%), h) Skeletal abnormalities (.5%), i) Urinary tract anomalies (.2%), j) CNS abnormalities (.2%), k) Pulmonary anomalies (.1%), l) Meckel diverticulum (.1%).

Etiology: Atresia is secondary to other intestinal or abdominal birth defects (25%). Etiology in the remainder is unknown.

Pathogenesis: Intrauterine intestinal ischemia resulting from interference with mesenteric blood supply. This occurs as a result of a variety of factors in the final one-third of pregnancy. All forms of intestinal atresia and of stenosis have been produced in experimental animals (dog, sheep, and rabbit) by various forms of mesenteric vascular occlusion.†

Related Facts
I **Sex Ratio:** M1:F1
II **Risk of Occurrence:** 1 in 330 live births in Great Britain and U.S.A., 1 in 400 live births in Denmark.
III **Risk of Recurrence for**
Patient's Sib: If atresia is secondary to meconium ileus or to total colon aganglionosis, the incidence in sibs and children is high. The risk in other forms of atresia is relatively low.
Patient's Child: Same
IV **Age of Detectability:** Symptoms and signs of intestinal obstruction secondary to atresia are recognized at birth or during the initial week of life. Stenosis may be detected in childhood or even in adulthood.
V **Prevalence:** ?

Treatment
I **Primary Prevention:** —
II **Secondary Prevention:** Surgical correction of intestinal defect with restoration of continuity.†
III **Other Therapy:** Recognition of the basic primary defects, ie meconium ileus, aganglionosis, etc.

Prognosis: Normal life span, except when associated with meconium ileus when it is reduced by pulmonary, late intestinal, hepatic and other problems associated with this disease state.

Detection of Carrier: —

†**Special Considerations:** Intestinal atresia or stenosis is regarded as always "secondary" to some other intrauterine disease process which results in mesenteric vascular occlusion. In approximately 25% of the instances of atresia this responsible factor is another recognized disease state, ie meconium ileus, colon aganglionosis, gastroschisis, etc. In the others, however, only evidence for intrauterine intestinal infarction is present, ie mesenteric scars, granulomas adjacent to the intestinal defect, and histologic changes in the segments and the mesentery which suggest prior infarction. It is believed that vascular insufficiency exists in the intestinal segments which are immediately proximal and immediately distal to the atresia. The most significant advance in therapy has been the recognition that a wide resection of the (apparently uninvolved) proximal and distal jejunal segments (in jejunal atresia) results in improved intestinal motility following resection and an increased survival in the neonatal period. It has not been demonstrated that this is true in ileal atresia.

References:
DeLorimier, A.A. et al: Congenital atresia and stenosis of the jejunum and ileum. Surgery 65:819, 1969.
Louw, J.H.: Resection and end-to-end anastomosis in the management of atresia and stenosis of the small bowel. Surgery 62:940, 1967.
Nixon, H.H.: Intestinal obstruction in the newborn. Arch. Dis. Child. 30:13, 1955.

Contributor: **Daniel M. Hays**

Editor's Computerized Descriptors: CV., GI.

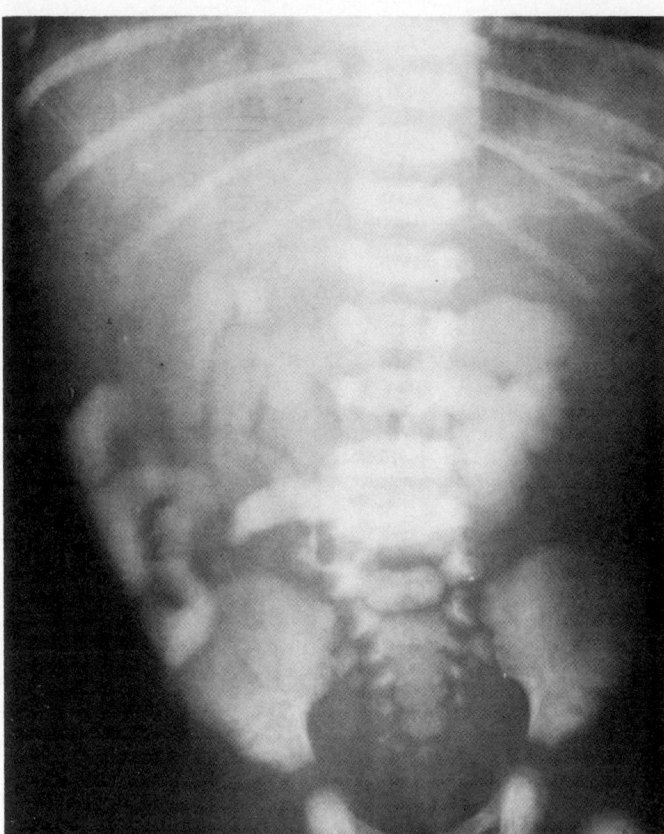

306. Abdomen in recumbent position. Note Levine tube in stomach; no air distal to stomach; multiple opacities with a calcium density in midabdomen

INTESTINAL DUPLICATION

Includes: Duplication intestinale
Intestinale Duplikation
Duplicación intestinal
Enteric cyst
Enterogenous cyst
Enterocystoma
Duodenal duplication
Jejunal duplication
Ileal duplication

Excludes: Esophageal duplication (368)
Stomach duplication (912)
Colon duplication (194)
True intestinal diverticula
Mesenteric cysts (645)
Omental cyst

Minimal Diagnostic Criteria: Intestinal dysfunction and mass demonstrated by xrays. Thoracic skeletal defects associated with duodenal or upper jejunal duplication lead to diagnosis in one-quarter of these cases.

Clinical Findings: Intestinal dysfunction or partial obstruction with nausea, vomiting, distention, crampy pain, commonly a mass, and occasionally with local impairment of arterial or venous circulation causing acute symptoms and inflammation. Rarely ulceration and hemorrhage occur when bowel communication exists. Xrays show mass with distortion of bowel lumen occasionally with air in duplication.

Complications
I   **Derived:**   Slow development of symptoms correlates with increasing mass with more acute symptomatology due to erosion, hemorrhage, perforation, or strangulation of the involved segment. Duodenal duplication may have common duct obstruction and rarely compromised pancreatic drainage due to the mass. Rarely the mass may initiate a volvulus.
II **Associated:**   Congenital abnormalities of cardiovascular, skeletal, and urogenital systems and thoracic skeletal defects. Carcinoma has been reported in a duplication.

Etiology: ? Probably due to intrauterine local vascular accident. Abnormal vacuolization with diverticular formation or longitudinal coalescence in bowel during embryonic solid stage can explain longitudinal duplication.

Pathogenesis: Duplication commonly is between mesenteric leaves but it may be beside the main bowel tube. Mesentery may be split with separate leaves to duplicate the intestine. Duplicate contains all intestinal layers with one or more muscular coats and with a mucosal lining which is that of the parent segment or is often gastric in type. Contents are clear, colorless, generally mucoid, and with vascular compromise, necrosis may be present.

Related Facts
I   **Sex Ratio:**   M1:F1
II   **Risk of Occurrence:**   Rare
III **Risk of Recurrence for**
        Patient's Sib: ?
        Patient's Child: ?
IV   **Age of Detectability:**   Generally infancy and childhood
V   **Prevalence:**   ?

Treatment
I   **Primary Prevention:**   —
II   **Secondary Prevention:**   —
III **Other Therapy:**   Treatment is surgical. For duodenal type with side-to-side anastomosis or cyst-jejunostomy. Jejunal and ileal duplications surgically excised with resection of parent enteric tube with its common blood supply; only rarely duplication will be dissected from mesentery as in mesenteric or omental cysts.

Prognosis: —

Detection of Carrier: —

Special Considerations: —

References:
  Bermer, J. L.: Diverticula and duplications of the intestinal tract. Arch. Pathol. 38:132, 1944.
  Gross, R. E.: Duplications of the alimentary tract. In Gross, R.E. (ed.): The Surgery of Infancy and Childhood: Its Principles and Techniques. Philadelphia:W.B. Saunders Co., 1953.
  Hudson, H. W., Jr.: Giant diverticula or reduplication of the intestinal tract. N. Engl. J. Med. 213:1123, 1935.
  Inouye, W.Y. et al: Duodenal duplication; case report and literature review. Ann. Surg. 162:910, 1965.
  Mellish, R. W. and Koop, C. E.: Clinical manifestations of duplication of the bowel. Pediatrics 27:397, 1961.
  Mustard, W.T. et al (eds.): Pediatric Surgery, 2nd Ed. Chicago: Year Book Medical Publishers, 1969, p. 834.

Contributor: **Newlin Hastings**

Editor's Computerized Descriptors: Skel., CV., GI., GU.

INTESTINAL ENTEROKINASE DEFICIENCY

Includes: Déficit en enterokinase
Intestinaler Enterokinasemangel
Deficiencia de enteroquinasa intestinal
Primary enterokinase deficiency

Excludes: Trypsinogen deficiency (973)
Generalized pancreatic exocrine insufficiency
Secondary enterokinase deficiency

Minimal Diagnostic Criteria: Normal small bowel histology with decreased enterokinase activity is diagnostic of primary enterokinase deficiency.†

Clinical Findings: Patients present from early infancy with diarrhea (100%) and failure to thrive (100%). They will be found to excrete large amounts of fecal nitrogen. As a result of a negative nitrogen balance, hypoproteinemia and edema are usually apparent. Malnutrition may also result in failure of synthesis of pancreatic lipase and amylase as well as intestinal disaccharidases and result in generalized malabsorption of all nutrients. Steatorrhea and carbohydrate intolerance are clinically evident in this circumstance.

Complications
I   **Derived:** Protein malabsorption; malnutrition; failure to thrive (poor weight gain and short stature); hypoproteinemia; generalized pancreatic exocrine dysfunction secondary to malnutrition; intestinal disaccharidase deficiency secondary to malnutrition; and generalized malabsorption.
II **Associated:** Short stature

Etiology: The finding of this abnormality in 2 sibs, the offspring of unaffected parents, suggests that it is an inherited disease. The mode of transmission is unknown, but may be autosomal recessive. McK *22620

Pathogenesis: The pancreatic peptidases, trypsin, chymotrypsin, carboxypeptidase and elastase, are secreted as proenzymes that require activation within the intestinal lumen. The peptidopeptidase of intestinal origin that initiates pancreatic propeptidase activation is enterokinase. In the absence of enterokinase, the rate of conversion of trypsinogen to trypsin is subnormal resulting in concentrations of trypsin that are inadequate for protein hydrolysis including activation of chymotrypsinogen, procarboxypeptidase and proelastase. Lipase and amylase are secreted as functional enzymes not requiring activation. They are of normal activity in the patient with enterokinase deficiency.

Related Facts
I   **Sex Ratio:** M1:F1
II   **Risk of Occurrence:**   ?
III **Risk of Recurrence for**
       Patient's Sib: ? Has occurred in 2 sibs
       Patient's Child: ?
IV   **Age of Detectability:** Early infancy
V   **Prevalence:**   ? 6 cases have been reported

Treatment
I   **Primary Prevention:** —
II   **Secondary Prevention:** Orally administered enterokinase or pancreatic extract normalizes intestinal function.
III **Other Therapy:** —

Prognosis: Excellent. Most patients have continued short stature, apparently from early severe malnutrition.

Detection of Carrier: —

†Special Considerations: Study of pancreatic exocrine function is also diagnostic. In baseline-and secretin-stimulated samples of duodenal aspirate, trypsinogen levels will be normal but trypsin will be of low or absent activity. Trypsinogen may be activated to trypsin by incubation with enterokinase or trypsin (16-hour incubation at 4° C results in activation in some patients). The patient's duodenal fluid will have normal tryptic activity after incubation.

Histologic exam should also be performed since some patients with abnormal small bowel mucosa will have low levels of enterokinase activity.

The malnourished patient may have subnormal secretion of all pancreatic enzymes. Therefore, it is necessary to attain a state of adequate nutrition before pancreatic function studies are completed.

References:
Follett, G.F. and MacDonald, T.H.: Intestinal enterokinase deficiency. Acta Paediatr. Scand. 65:653, 1976.
Haworth, J.C. et al: Intestinal enterokinase deficiency. Arch. Dis. Child. 50:277, 1975.
Tarlow, M.J. et al: Intestinal enterokinase deficiency. Arch. Dis. Child. 45:651, 1970.

Contributor: **Peter F. Whitington**

Editor's Computerized Descriptor: GI.

INTESTINAL LYMPHANGIECTASIA

Includes: Lymphangiectasie intestinale
Intestinale Lymphangiektasie
Linfangiectasia intestinal
Protein-losing enteropathy with dilated intestinal lymphatics

Excludes: Lymphedema I (614)
Lymphedema II (615)
Protein-losing enteropathy without dilated lymphatic channels
Protein-losing enteropathy with dilated intestinal lymphatics secondary to congestive heart failure
Whipple syndrome
Mesenteric neoplasms

Minimal Diagnostic Criteria: Dilated lymphatic channels of the small bowel as demonstrated by peroral biopsy or laparotomy is the hallmark morphologic lesion of this disorder and is required for its diagnosis.

The direct demonstration of GI protein loss, hypoalbuminemia, hypogammaglobulinemia, lymphocytopenia and generalized edema are also important diagnostic features present in virtually all patients. Direct demonstration of excessive GI protein loss using intravenously administered radiolabeled macromolecules such as ^{51}Cr labeled serum proteins, ^{59}Fe dextran, ^{95}Nb albumin, or ^{131}I PVP should be performed to differentiate this syndrome from disorders where the hypoproteinemia is secondary to decreased protein synthesis or accelerated endogenous protein catabolism.

Other causes of protein-losing enteropathy with disorders of intestinal lymphatic channels, such as severe congestive heart failure, Whipple syndrome or mesenteric malignancy, should be looked for and excluded.†

Clinical Findings: The patients with intestinal lymphangiectasia have a generalized disorder of development of lymphatic channels with grossly dilated lymphatic vessels in the lamina propria of the small bowel demonstrable in all cases. The patients have edema which may be asymmetric (15%) and which may involve the macula, producing reversible blindness (7%). Chylous effusion is present at the onset or develops during the course of the disease in 45% of the patients. All patients have significant excessive loss of serum proteins into the GI tract through the disordered lymphatic channels. They have hypoalbuminemia (100%) and a marked reduction of IgG (97%). A significant but less marked reduction in the concentration of fibrinogen (30%), transferrin (50%), IgM (40%), and IgA (70%) is noted in many patients.

GI symptoms are usually mild, but may on occasion be entirely absent or severe. Diarrhea and steatorrhea (mild 60%, severe 20%), vomiting (15%), and abdominal pain (15%) are present in these patients. Carbohydrate absorption tests - including glucose, xylose and lactose tolerance tests - are within normal limits in most of the patients studied. Roentgenograms of the GI tract are completely negative in 20% of the patients, show mild mucosal edema of the small bowel in 70% of the patients, and show significant segmentation and puddling of the barium in the remaining 10% of the patients. On biopsy of the small bowel, the hallmark morphologic lesion of the disease is revealed. It is a dilatation of the lymphatic vessels of the lamina propria. Hypocalcemic tetany is present in 12% of the patients and is most common in those patients with steatorrhea. It is thought to be associated with malabsorption or loss of calcium into the GI tract. Lymphocytopenia (mean lymphocyte count 700 compared to 2400 in controls), secondary to the loss of lymphocytes into the bowel, is present in over 90% of the patients. As a consequence of this lymphocytopenia, 83% of the patients show skin anergy and are unable to manifest delayed hypersensitivity responses (tuberculin-type responses), and are unable to reject skin grafts from unrelated donors.

Less frequent findings include anemia and reduction in the serum concentration of fat soluble vitamins and B$_{12}$. Growth retardation (linear growth below 3rd%) is present in the majority of children with onset of edema and diarrhea within the first 5 years of life. It may be extreme in those patients with associated severe malabsorption.

Complications
I Derived: Tuberculous infections and reticuloendothelial malignancies develop in 3-5% of the cases, possibly due to the lymphocytopenia and inability to make cellular immune responses.

Chronic respiratory diseases (5-10%) associated with the disorder of delayed hypersensitivity and with abnormalities of lymphatics of the lungs.

Intestinal obstruction due to adhesions occur especially in those patients with chylous ascites.

Deficiency of fat-soluble vitamins, including vitamin K (20%) may cause hypoprothrombinemia.

II Associated: Congenital glaucoma (3 in 75 cases). Peliosis hepatis (2 cases). Charcot-Marie-Tooth syndrome (2 cases). Tetralogy of Fallot (1 case).

Etiology: ? The fact that 7 families have been reported with normal parents but with 2-4 affected sibs of both sexes suggests an autosomal recessive mode of inheritance in some cases. The majority of cases (over 75%) are, however, sporadic.

Pathogenesis: The basic defect appears to be a generalized disorder in lymphatic channel development with the most obvious disorder affecting small bowel lymphatics. As a consequence serum proteins, lymphocytes, as well as lipids, iron, copper and calcium are lost into the GI lumen. Hypoproteinemia results when the rate of protein loss and catabolism exceeds the body's capacity to synthesize the protein. The edema and effusions are due both to the extreme hypoproteinemia and the generalized disorder of lymphatic channels. The abnormalities in in vivo cellular (tuberculin-type) responses and the increased incidence in tuberculosis and reticuloendothelial neoplasms appear to be secondary to the lymphocytopenia that results from the loss of lymphocytes into the GI tract.

The hypocalcemia and malabsorption are due to an abnormality of absorption from the bowel, as well as loss of fat and calcium by direct loss of lymph into the bowel.

Related Facts
I Sex Ratio: M1:F1.34
II Risk of Occurrence: No reliable occurrence figures are available. Approximately 100 cases are known. Cases have been reported in Negro, Oriental and Caucasian races.
III Risk of Recurrence for
Patient's Sib: Not well-defined. Most cases, approximately 75%, are sporadic; however, 7 families with 2-4 affected sibs have been reported. Although there are unaffected sibs in these families, the rates of affected to unaffected sibs are not known.
Patient's Child: One case of lymphedema in an offspring of the proband has been reported. Otherwise, there are no reports of an affected individual in 2 generations. The patients have frequently reproduced, although those patients with chylous ascites and vitamin deficiency may have reduced fertility.
IV Age of Detectability: Generalized edema, chylous effusions, asymmetric edema, diarrhea, or hypocalcemia may be the presenting symptom and is first detected at birth or in the first few weeks of life in 25% of the patients. In the remaining patients, the age of onset ranges to young adult life with

a mean age of onset of 10 years.
V Prevalence: Specific figures are not available.

Treatment
I Primary Prevention: —
II Secondary Prevention: A very low-fat diet or a diet in which medium chain triglycerides are used in lieu of long chain triglycerides has been effective in significantly decreasing the hypoproteinemia, GI protein loss, edema and diarrhea in approximately 50% of the patients. Such therapy has been of value in increasing the growth rate in children. In 5-10% of the cases, resection of a localized area of intestinal lymphangiectasia results in amelioration of the symptoms.
III Other Therapy: Diuretics are useful in reducing edema and effusions as well as in reversing blindness in the cases with macular edema. Other therapy such as surgical relief of intestinal obstruction or ligation of thoracic duct in patients with isolated chylothorax may be indicated.

Prognosis: For life: In general, life expectancy is somewhat shortened. In infancy, death may be related to extreme malabsorption, intestinal obstruction, or infections, especially in debilitated patients. Many cases, especially those with late onset, may be stable over periods from 2 to more than 40 years.

For intelligence: No effect upon intelligence

For function: Approximately 30% of the patients are unable to work because of extreme fatigue and weakness associated with the hypoproteinemia.

Detection of Carrier: No means known

†Special Considerations: It should be emphasized that the primary features of this disorder, including edema, excessive GI protein loss, lymphocytopenia and dilated lymphatics of the small intestine, may be seen in patients with Whipple syndrome, mesenteric tumors, or cardiac disorders, especially constrictive pericarditis. Significant care should be taken to rule out congestive failure in all patients with a tentative diagnosis of intestinal lymphangiectasia. The disorders of lymphocyte and protein metabolism are completely reversible in such patients when successful surgical or medical therapy of the cardiac disease is possible. In addition, it should be noted that patients with intestinal lymphangiectasia have skin anergy and thus skin tests, such as the tuberculin skin test, cannot be used in the diagnosis of such chronic infectious disorders.

References:
Jeffries, G.H. et al: Low-fat diet in intestinal lymphangiectasia: Its effect on albumin metabolism. N. Engl. J. Med. 270:761, 1964.
Waldmann, T. A.: Protein-losing enteropathy. Gastroenterology 50:422, 1966.
Waldmann, T.A. et al: The role of the gastrointestinal system in "idiopathic hypoproteinemia." Gastroenterology 41:197, 1961.

Contributor: **Thomas A. Waldmann**

Editor's Computerized Descriptors: Eye, Skin, Lymphatic, GI.

INTESTINAL POLYPOSIS I & II

Includes: Polypose colique
Polyposis coli
Poliposis del colon
Colon polyposis
Polyposis I & II, intestinal
Familial polyposis coli
Peutz-Jeghers syndrome

Excludes: Intestinal polyposis III (536)

Minimal Diagnostic Criteria: *Polyposis I:* polyps in colon
Polyposis II: polyps in jejunum

Clinical Findings: The most common presenting findings are increased frequency of stools and rectal bleeding. Mucoid discharge may accompany the bleeding and some children have a history of pain or prolapse or tenesmus (about 50%). Digital examination of the rectum reveals innumerable polyps. The extent of polypoid involvement is ascertained by proctoscopic examination and air-contrast barium enema examination.

The distribution of polyps with familial polyposis I is limited to the colon, but involvement of any part of the GI tract may be seen in polyposis II with the jejunum consistently involved.

Microscopically polyps are true adenomatous polyps, either sessile or pedunculated, and vary in size from 1 mm to several centimeters in diameter.

Polyposis I: The polyps are usually limited to the colon, may be very numerous and may develop very early (youngest patient 13 mos; under 13 yrs 6.6% have polyps; 95% affected by age 21 yrs). Carcinoma may develop early and in untreated patients malignant change is almost certain with increasing age, especially in the rectosigmoid.

Polyposis II: The polyps may occur throughout the GI tract but jejunal polyps are regularly present. Melanoplakia may be found on the lips, buccal mucosa and the digits. Carcinoma of intestinal polyps is rare. Ovarian tumors occur.

Complications
I **Derived:** *Polyposis I:* Bloody diarrhea, inanition and carcinoma of the colon (children under 13 years of age 6.6%, adults 100% of untreated patients).
Polyposis II: Intussusception
II **Associated:** *Polyposis I:* -
Polyposis II: Ovarian tumor

Etiology: Single dominant pleiotropic gene with variable penetrance for both types; McK *17510, *17520

Pathogenesis: *Polyposis I:* Carcinoma is most common in the rectosigmoid, particularly when there is an increased concentration of polyps there, but it is not known whether the development of cancer is also genetically linked and, therefore, independent of polyp formation or represents carcinomatous change within an enlarging polyp.
Polyposis II: Carcinoma of polyps rare, but prone to granulosa cell tumor of ovary

Related Facts
I **Sex Ratio:** M1:F1
II **Risk of Occurrence:** ? Estimates vary from 1 in 8300 to 1 in 29,000 live births
III **Risk of Recurrence for**
Patient's Sib: If parent is affected, 1 in 2 (50%) for each offspring to be affected; otherwise not increased.
Patient's Child: 1 in 2
IV **Age of Detectability:** Varies, from 13 months to adulthood
V **Prevalence:** ?

Treatment
I **Primary Prevention:** Genetic counseling
II **Secondary Prevention:** For polyposis I total colectomy with ileostomy or subtotal colectomy and ileoproctostomy as soon as the diagnosis is made. The remaining rectal polyps following ileoproctostomy may undergo spontaneous regression; others must be fulgurated and rectum kept free of polyps on biannual examination.
III **Other Therapy:** —

Prognosis: Carcinoma of the colon will develop in all untreated patients with polyposis I with average age of death from cancer at 41.5 years. Incidence of malignancy in the terminal rectal segment following ileoproctostomy is between 4 and 16%.

Detection of Carrier: —

Special Considerations: —

References:
Abramson, D. J.: Multiple polyposis in children: A review and report of case in a six-year-old child who had associated nephrosis and asthma. Surgery 61:288, 1967.
McKusick, V. A.: Genetic factors in intestinal polyposis. JAMA 182:271, 1962.

Contributor: **Robert J. Touloukian**

Editor's Computerized Descriptors: Oral, Skin, GI., GU.

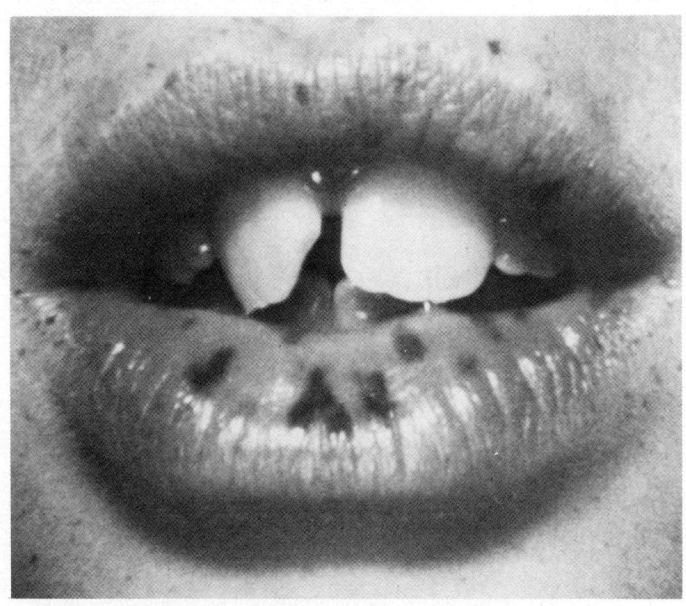

307. Lip pigmentation in intestinal polyposis II

INTESTINAL POLYPOSIS III

Includes: Syndrome de Gardner
Síndrome de Gardner
Polyposis III, intestinal
Gardner syndrome

Excludes: Intestinal polyposis I & II (535)

Minimal Diagnostic Criteria: The presence of any of the lesions cited in clinical findings in patients with a family history, especially of intestinal polyposis (usually present if looked for).†

Clinical Findings: Multiple osteomas of the facial bones (frontal, ethmoid, spheroid, maxilla, mandible, and zygoma); epidermoid or sebaceous cysts, and desmoids or fibromas of the skin; and multiple polyposis of the large bowel. Multiple cystic odontomas have also been described. The intestinal polyps frequently undergo malignant degeneration. Diagnosis is usually made by intestinal symptoms (bleeding, etc) due to polyps. The youngest age reported for the intestinal polyps is 4 years (asymptomatic - discovered as result of family history). The osteomas and odontomas are frequently incidental findings or become manifest in the 2nd or 3rd decade. Osteomas also occur in the long bones.

    The desmoids, fibromas, fibrosarcomas, and lipomas may occur in areas of previous skin incisions or arise de novo on the chest, back, scalp or upper limbs. Epidermoid or sebaceous cysts may occur in any of the usual locations.

Complications
I **Derived:** Intestinal obstruction or bleeding from polyps. Malignant change in the adenomatous polyps is a serious complication.
II **Associated:** ? Torus palatinus may be part of the syndrome, but occurs in 20-25% of the normal population.

Etiology: Autosomal dominant with moderate penetrance and variable expressivity; McK *17530

Pathogenesis: ?

Related Facts
I **Sex Ratio:** M1:F1
II **Risk of Occurrence:** ? Thought to be higher than apparent because some findings (osteomas) are not routinely looked for, and others (sebaceous cysts) are very common in normal population and, hence, unreported.
III **Risk of Recurrence for**
    Patient's Sib: If parent is affected, < 1 in 2 (< 50%) for each offspring to be affected; otherwise not increased.
    Patient's Child: < 1 in 2
IV **Age of Detectability:** Early childhood by sigmoidoscopy and barium enema
V **Prevalence:** ?

Treatment
I **Primary Prevention:** Genetic counseling
II **Secondary Prevention:** May require total colectomy where multiple intestinal polyps are found because of high frequency of malignancy. Other lesions, epidermoid cysts, desmoids, or fibromas, should be excised. Desmoids or fibromas may also be malignant.
III **Other Therapy:** —

Prognosis: Good, if no malignancy in intestinal adenomas or connective tissue tumors. Poor, if malignancy is present.

Detection of Carrier: —

†**Special Considerations:** Family members need thorough periodic examinations, including sigmoidoscopy and barium enema (where indicated) as the adenomatous polyps or other soft tissue tumors may appear at any age. Because of the propensity

for malignancy, lesions should be excised. Differential diagnosis between desmoids and fibrosarcomas may be very difficult. No laboratory tests have yielded any information on these patients. Skeletal x-ray survey is indicated in family members, including skull, facial bones and mandible series.

References:
Gorlin, R.J. and Chaudhry, A.P.: Multiple osteomatosis, fibromas, lipomas, fibrosarcomas of the skin and mesentery, epidermoid inclusion cysts of the skin, leiomyomas and multiple intestinal polyposis. N. Engl. J. Med. 263:1151, 1960.
Jones, E.L. and Cornell, W.P.: Gardner's syndrome; review of the literature and report on a family. Arch. Surg. 92:287, 1966.

Contributor: **Raymond P. Wood, II**

Editor's Computerized Descriptors: Face, Oral, Skin, Skel., GI., GU.

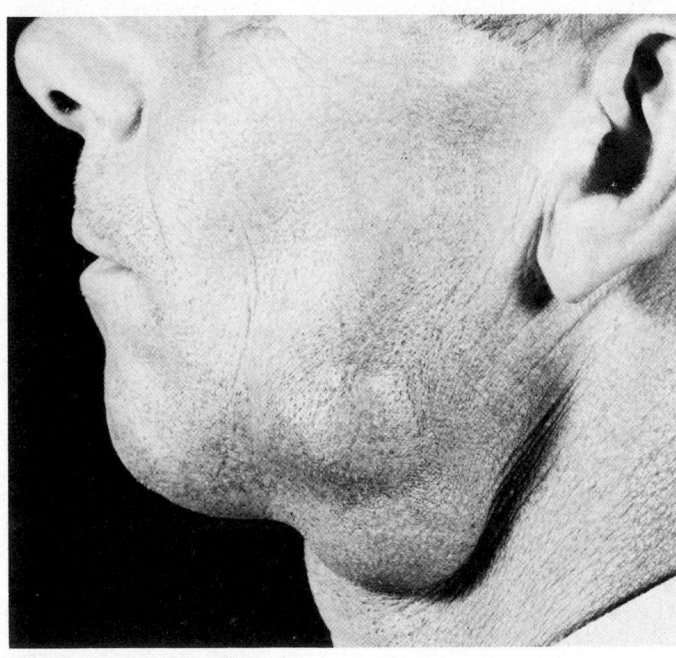

308. Osteoma of mandible

INTESTINAL ROTATION, INCOMPLETE

Includes: Rotation intestinale incompléte
Malrotation
Rotación intestinal incompleta
Intestinal malrotation
Malrotation of midgut
Nonrotation of midgut

Excludes: Intestinal atresia or stenosis (531)
Duodenal atresia or stenosis (300)

Minimal Diagnostic Criteria: Clinical findings as listed below plus typical roentgenographic findings.

Clinical Findings: Bile-stained emesis, malabsorption of fats and recurrent abdominal pain. The patient with this anatomic abnormality usually is presented to the physician in 1 of the following 3 ways:

1) Sudden onset of bile-stained emesis with complete intestinal obstruction. (This is indicative of volvulus of the midgut.)†

2) Recurrent vomiting with symptom free intervals. (This is indicative of partial obstruction of the duodenum due to the Ladd bands.)

3) Malabsorption of fats. (This is due to lymphatic obstruction of the small bowel mesentery.)

Any patient who has abnormal fat content of the stools or who has recurrent vomiting should have a complete radiographic intestinal study to prove or disprove malrotation of the midgut. Patients have been treated for "psychogenic" vomiting or malabsorptive disorders to no avail and only have alleviation of their symptoms by surgical therapy.

Complications
I **Derived:** Midgut volvulus. The incompletely rotated midgut is on a narrow mesenteric pedicle which allows and encourages volvulus resulting in vascular impairment, bowel necrosis and death unless timely therapy (surgical) is instituted.
II **Associated:** Malabsorption of fats with malnutrition.

Etiology: ?

Pathogenesis: During embryonic development, the intestine grows at a more rapid rate than does the celomic cavity. Part of the intestine develops in the base of the umbilical cord, and in the normal sequence of events returns to the celomic cavity and simultaneously rotates in a counter clockwise direction around the superior mesenteric pedicle. Eventually the cecum and right colon are fixed to the posterior parietes by the Toldt fusion fascia. If the rotation does not proceed to completion, fixation of the right colon does not occur and the entire intestine is on a narrowed pedicle.

Related Facts
I **Sex Ratio:** M1:F1
II **Risk of Occurrence:** ?
III **Risk of Recurrence for**
Patient's Sib: ?
Patient's Child: ?
IV **Age of Detectability:** Over one-half of the patients become symptomatic within the first 10 days of life and three-quarters within the 1st month of life. The remainder can remain asymptomatic or become symptomatic at any age.
V **Prevalence:** ?

Treatment
I **Primary Prevention:** ?
II **Secondary Prevention:** ?
III **Other Therapy:** The only effective therapy for this anomaly is surgical correction of the abnormally narrow mesenteric base by lysis of Ladd bands which traverse from the distal small bowel mesentery to the right posterior abdominal wall lateral to the duodenum. If volvulus is present detorsion is accomplished prior to the lysis of Ladd bands.

Prognosis: If the patient is operated upon prior to vascular impairment of the small bowel, the prognosis is excellent both short- and long-term.

Detection of Carrier: —

†Special Considerations: If an infant feeds well during the early hours or days of life and has the sudden onset of bile-stained emesis, midgut volvulus secondary to malrotation should be ruled out on an emergency basis. Observation without appropriate x-ray studies may allow the infant to progress to complete bowel necrosis before therapy is instituted.

References:
Gross, R.E.: The Surgery of Infancy and Childhood: Its Principles and Techniques. Philadelphia:W.B. Saunders Co., 1953, p. 192.
Snyder, W.H., Jr. and Chaffin, L.: Malrotation of the intestine. In Mustard, W.T. et al (eds.): Pediatric Surgery, 2nd Ed. Chicago:-Year Book Medical Publishers, 1969, vol. 2, p. 808.

Contributor: **Morton M. Woolley**

Editor's Computerized Descriptor: GI.

INTRAEPITHELIAL DYSKERATOSIS

Includes: Dyskératose intra-épithéliale
Intraepitheliale Dyskeratose
Disqueratosis intraepitelial
Dyskeratosis, intraepithelial

Excludes: Dermal hypoplasia, focal (281)
Dyskeratosis congenita
Focal epithelial hyperplasia of oral mucosa
Mucosa, white folded dysplasia (681)
Leukoedema
Pachyonychia congenita (789)
Leukoplakia

Minimal Diagnostic Criteria: Perilimbal gelatinous plaques on a hyperemic bulbar conjunctiva with white shaggy lesions of oral mucosa. Diagnosis made on Papanicoleau stained smear with compatible history or tissue section.†

Clinical Findings: White soft shaggy lesions of oral mucosa. Gelatinous perilimbal plaques of bulbar conjunctiva with a hyperemic base which have a vernal exacerbation and autumnal remission leading to temporary blindness in summer in about one-fourth of cases. Vascularization of cornea with loss of vision is terminal result in persons in 5th to 6th decade. Occasional involvement of conjunctiva of lid with white plaques. Roentgenologic findings are normal. Exfoliative cytologic smears of oral and eye lesions stained with Papanicoleau stain are characterized by 2 types of cells: elongated waxy orangeophilic cells (resembling the grains of keratosis follicularis) and a cell-within-cell body consisting of a central abnormal cell and a normal appearing surrounding epithelial cell. Central cell is dyskeratotic, orangeophilic with abnormal nucleus. The surrounding cell appears normal but with an excentric nucleus and refractile hyaline membrane separating normal cells from the central cell. Histologic characteristics show a thickened stratum spinosum containing many dyskeratotic waxy appearing cells with elongated nuclei and cell-within-cell dyskeratotic bodies. No basal lacuni or inflammation in the lamina propria other than dilated vessels.

Complications
I **Derived:** Temporary blindness in about one-fourth of cases in summer. Vascularization of cornea in late adulthood with loss of vision.
II **Associated:** —

Etiology: A gene mutation resulting in an autosomal dominantly transmitted trait with 97% penetrance and moderate variation in expressivity. The severity of manifestation of the eye lesion depending on response to unknown environmental factors such that there is a vernal exacerbation and autumnal remission. McK *12760

Pathogenesis: Primary protein defect is unknown. However, by analogy with the fact that identical cellular lesions can be produced experimentally in man by use of agents affecting nucleic acid integrity (X-radiation, methotrexate, 5 fluorouracil) the gene defect appears to result in nucleic acid damage to epithelial cell nuclei. These damaged cells are then surrounded by normal epithelial cells and exfoliated. Electron microscopic features show degenerated cell surrounded by a more normal appearing epithelial cell. Included cell shows dense bundles of tonofibrils and nuclear fragments.

Related Facts
I **Sex Ratio:** M1:F1
II **Risk of Occurrence:** Very rare, only 3 kindreds known
III **Risk of Recurrence for**
   Patient's Sib: If parent is affected, 1 in 2 (50%) for each

offspring to be affected; otherwise not increased
   Patient's Child: 1 in 2
IV **Age of Detectability:** By visual examination most cases detected by one year of age. Confirmed by exfoliative cytology or biopsy.
V **Prevalence:** Very rare. Only 3 large kindreds known. In Haliwa Indians of North Carolina 1 in 52.

Treatment
I **Primary Prevention:** Genetic counseling
II **Secondary Prevention:** †
III **Other Therapy:** Avoidance of sunlight and dust reduces the severity of eye lesions.

Prognosis: No reduced longevity. Lesion does not appear to predispose to neoplastic change. Blindness from vascularization of cornea in 5th to 6th decade in about 50%.

Detection of Carrier: —

†**Special Considerations:** Must be differentiated from white folded dysplasia of mucosa, especially if such patients also have pterygia, and histologically from keratosis follicularis which shows basilar clefting absent in benign intraepithelial dyskeratosis. Cortisone eye drops temporarily reduce the hyperemia of conjunctivae but do not alter the basic lesion.

References: Sadeghi, E.M. and Witkop, C.J.,Jr.: **Ultrastructural study of hereditary benign intraepithelial dyskeratosis. Oral Surg. 44:567, 1977.**
Von Sallmann, L. and Paton, D.: Hereditary benign intraepithelial dyskeratosis. I. Ocular manifestations. Arch. Ophthalmol. 63:421, 1960.
Witkop, C. J., Jr.: Epithelial intracellular bodies associated with hereditary dyskeratoses and cancer therapy. In Proc. 1st Int. Cong. Exfoliative Cytology, Vienna, 1961. Philadelphia:J.B. Lippincott, 1962, p.259.
Witkop, C.J., Jr. et al: Hereditary benign intraepithelial dyskeratosis. II. Oral manifestations and hereditary transmission. Arch. Pathol. 70:696, 1960.

Contributor: **Carl J. Witkop, Jr.**

Editor's Computerized Descriptors: Vision, Eye, Oral

INTRAOSSEOUS FIBROUS SWELLING OF JAWS

Includes: Gonflement fibreux des maxillaires
Cherubismus
Tumefacción fibrosa intraósea mandibular
Cherubism

Excludes: Giant cell tumor of jaws
Giant cell (reparative) granuloma of jaws
Fibrous dysplasia of jaws
Pseudohypoparathyroidism (830)
Infantile cortical hyperostosis of jaws
Basal cell nevus syndrome (101)
Dentigerous keratocysts
Odontogenic keratocysts

Minimal Diagnostic Criteria: Clinical swellings at angles of mandible with roentgenographic evidence of bilateral, radiolucent lesions in molar-angle region. Biopsy should be performed to establish diagnosis because facial swelling and roentgenographic evidence of cystic appearing lesions can occur at angles of mandible in basal cell nevus syndrome and from bilateral dentigerous or odontogenic keratocysts.

Clinical Findings: Exaggerated chubbiness of face, especially over angles of mandible. In more severe cases there may be extensive maxillary swelling with involvement of orbital floor causing upward displacement of globe and exposure of scleral rims. In extreme cases the swellings may result in a grotesque facial deformity. Swellings are due to expansion of mandible and maxilla. Roentgenologically the lesions are bilaterally symmetric, radiolucent and usually multilocular in character. Alkaline phosphatase may be slightly elevated. Other laboratory studies generally within normal limits. In several reports lesions have been noted in other bones (rib, humerus, femur). These appear to be incidental findings and may not be related to cherubism. In some cases, the submandibular and cervical lymph nodes have been enlarged 50%. Bilateral symmetric involvement of mandibular molar region, angle of mandible or ascending ramus of mandible 100%. Involvement of entire mandible - frequency unknown probably less than 25%. Bilateral symmetric involvement of posterior maxillary (tuberosity) area 60%. Involvement of entire maxilla - frequency unknown probably less· than 20%. There is apparently a considerable range in extent of involvement in cherubism. While bilateral lesions at the angles of the mandible are necessary for the diagnosis and represent the consistent feature of the disease, cases are known where children first presented with unilateral swellings but developed bilateral involvement while under observation. Expansion of the posterior maxillary region (tuberosity) represents the mildest maxillary involvement and is present in about two-thirds of cases. In the more severe examples, the entire maxilla and mandible may be involved. The affected child is normal at birth and swellings may become apparent between 1 and 8 years of age. The natural history of this disease is not well understood and treatment is not standardized. Some instances regress without treatment in early adult life while in others the deformity remains or is slowly progressive. No instances of malignant change are known.

Complications
I **Derived:** In severe cases there may be a grotesque deformity and difficulty with mastication, swallowing, respiration or speech and visual distortions such as diplopia. Tumor may displace teeth.
II **Associated:** Several reports of asymptomatic, isolated lesions in other bones. In most cases these have not been studied histologically and the relation of such lesions to cherubism is uncertain. Several cases have had multiple warty nevi or multiple café-au-lait spots.

Etiology: Autosomal dominant with variable expressivity and possibly reduced penetrance in females (50-70%). Isolated cases may be due to new mutations. In many instances 1 parent will have only a history of prominent facial swellings or roentgenographic evidence of abnormal bone pattern in mandible, but is not overtly affected at the time of examination. Some lesions may heal spontaneously. McK *11840

Pathogenesis: Mode of development unknown. Grossly the lesion is soft-to-fibrous in character and appears whitish to reddish in color. Microscopically, it is composed of fibroblasts, polyhedral mononuclear cells and varying numbers of multinucleated giant cells. The tissue closely resembles that of the giant cell granuloma (benign giant cell tumor) of the jaws. Some authorities consider that cherubism is microscopically indistinguishable from giant cell granuloma while others believe the microscopic features of cherubism are distinctive and diagnostic. (This contributor subscribes to the former view.) Lesions continue to enlarge until about time of puberty when they often but not always regress and in some patients small lesions completely heal with only slight enlargement of bones as the end-result.

Related Facts
I **Sex Ratio:** Probably essentially M1:F1. Reported cases show male predominance (actual M2:F1) but male-to-male transmission rules out X-linkage.
II **Risk of Occurrence:** ?
III **Risk of Recurrence for**
     Patient's Sib: If parent is affected, 1 in 2 (50%) for each offspring to be affected; otherwise not increased.
     Patient's Child: 1 in 2
IV **Age of Detectability:** Facial swelling usually becomes noticeable between age 2-4 years. In less severe cases swelling may not be apparent until age 6 or 7 years. In a few instances swellings have been apparent by age 1.
V **Prevalence:** ? Rare, less than 70 documented cases by 1970.

Treatment
I **Primary Prevention:** Genetic counseling
II **Secondary Prevention:** Management not standardized. Some cases have apparently shown regression and considerable improvement in early adult life. In others the deformity has continued and even slowly progressed. Conservative surgical curettage performed early has given good results in some cases and poor results in others. A more radical surgical approach has been advocated for extensive lesions. Others have suggested delay of therapy until late adolescence or early adult life and then perform operative reduction of the expanded bone. Radiation therapy has given poor results and is contraindicated due to the possible sequelae of osteoradionecrosis and induction of sarcoma.
III **Other Therapy:** Prosthetic replacement of teeth

Prognosis: Good as far as life expectancy is concerned. Facial swellings may cause varying degrees of cosmetic and psychologic disability.

Detection of Carrier: —

Special Considerations: —

References:
Anderson, D. E. and McClendon, J. L.: Cherubism- hereditary fibrous dysplasia of the jaws. I. Genetic considerations. Oral Surg. 15 :(Suppl. 2) 5, 1962.
Hamner, J. E., III and Ketcham, A. S.: Cherubism: An analysis of treatment. Cancer 23 :1133, 1969.

Contributor: **Charles A. Waldron**

INVERSION OF VENTRICLES WITH TRANSPOSITION OF GREAT ARTERIES

Includes: Inversion des ventricules avec transposition des gros vaisseaux
Inversion der Ventrikel mit Transposition der grossen Gefässe
Inversión ventricular con transposición de los grandes vasos
Inverted transposition
Corrected transposition of great vessels or arteries
L-transposition with situs solitus
Great arteries, inversion of ventricles with transposition of

Excludes: Transposition of great vessels (962)
Common ventricle with noninversion
Common ventricle with inversion of infundibulum (corrected transposition with rudimentary ventricle or single ventricle with congenitally corrected transposition)
Dextrocardia with situs inversus and L-transposition
Transposition complexes with asplenia or polysplenia
Inversion of ventricles without transposition of great arteries (541)

Minimal Diagnostic Criteria: The clinical findings plus selective ventriculography are essential to the diagnosis.

Clinical Findings: In inverted transposition with situs solitus, systemic venous blood enters a normally located right atrium and passes through a morphologic mitral valve into a morphologic left ventricle. The pulmonary artery arises from this venous ventricle dorsally and medially to its normal location. As is normal in the morphologic left ventricle, the A-V valve is in continuity with the semilunar valve. The pulmonary veins empty into a normal left atrium. The blood passes through a morphologic tricuspid valve, often abnormal, into a morphologic right ventricle. The left-sided A-V valve is separated from the semilunar (aortic) valve by a crista supraventricularis as is expected in the morphologic right ventricle. The aortic valve takes the position usually occupied by the pulmonary valve. The anterior and leftward located aorta gives rise to a coronary artery pattern, which is the mirror image of normal. Although the pulmonary artery arises medially and posteriorly from the venous ventricle and the aorta arises anteriorly and laterally from the arterial ventricle, in the absence of any associated anomalies, the flow of blood follows a normal route. Thus, though anatomically abnormal, the hearts of these patients may be hemodynamically normal. In the very rare instance of inverted transposition with situs inversus, all the above anatomy is mirror image. In those rare individuals with inverted transposition without any associated cardiac malformations, symptoms are usually absent. However, since the conduction system below the A-V node is also inverted and portions of it are thought to be longer and thus more prone to injury, these patients may have varying degrees of A-V block and sequelae such as an Adams-Stokes attack.

Physical examination in uncomplicated cases is of limited value. The second heart sound at the left base may be palpable and much louder than normal. Closure of the aortic valve, which in this anomaly is situated close to the anterior chest wall, is responsible for this apparently accentuated sound. In the large majority of individuals with inverted transposition, other cardiovascular malformations are present. Lesions of the left A-V valve (morphologic tricuspid valve) are so frequent that they can almost be considered a basic part of this entity. Such lesions, particularly when associated with an Ebstein-type malformation, usually cause insufficiency. Rarely, stenosis and atresia are present. Ventricular septal defect and valvar pulmonic stenosis are other commonly associated lesions.

Less commonly, atrial septal defects, subpulmonic stenosis and patent ductus arteriosus are reported. Rarely, coarctation of the aorta or aortic valve anomalies causing stenosis or regurgitation coexist. In individuals with inverted transposition and one or more of the associated defects, symptoms and physical findings depend primarily on the associated defect. The incidence of A-V block is so high that inverted transposition must be suspected whenever congenital heart disease and arrhythmias coexist. Seventy-five percent of patients with associated defects have symptoms in the 1st month of life. With survival to adulthood, decreased exercise tolerance, arrhythmias and cardiac failure are the primary clinical manifestations.

Roentgenographically, when situs solitus with dextroversion is present, inverted transposition exists in 80% of the cases. Other findings include a narrow cardiac pedicle, absence of a discrete pulmonary artery knob, and a smooth and sloping left upper border caused by the lateral and anterior position of the aorta. Left atrial enlargement exists when left A-V valve insufficiency or a large left-to-right shunt are present. Without associated defects, or with minimal "left A-V valve insufficiency," chest roentgenograms may be relatively normal. However, since associated defects are very common, cardiomegaly and increased pulmonary vascularity are often noted.

The ECG commonly shows various conduction disturbances, such as prolonged PR interval, complete heart block, Wolff-Parkinson-White syndrome or atrial fibrillation. The P wave is abnormal in greater than 90% of the cases revealing left, right or biatrial enlargement. The Q wave in lead V_6 is almost always absent, whereas an initial Q wave is present in V_1 in about 60% of the cases. The QRS duration is prolonged in approximately one-third of the cases. Cardiac catheterization and selective angiocardiography provide data to confirm this anomaly and any associated defects. Complete heart block or repeated bouts of paroxysmal atrial tachycardia often occur during catheterization.

Complications
I **Derived:** The spectrum of complications is as varied as the associated cardiac defects and is directly related to them. Left A-V valve (mitral) insufficiency is common. Progression of conduction defects to complete heart block occurs with ensuing decrease of cardiac function leading to intractable failure and terminal pulmonary edema. Recurrent pulmonary infections are often associated with chronic failure. Subacute bacterial endocarditis occurs, usually when inverted transposition is associated with a ventricular septal defect or pulmonary stenosis.

II **Associated:** —

Etiology: Presumably multifactorial inheritance

Pathogenesis: Inversion of the ventricles with transposition of the great vessels is due to a single embryologic error-inversion (abnormal rotation) of the bulboventricular loop.

Related Facts
I **Sex Ratio:** M2.6:F1
II **Risk of Occurrence:** Approximately 1 in 16,000
III **Risk of Recurrence for**
    Patient's Sib: Probably less than 2%
    Patient's Child: ?
IV **Age of Detectability:** From birth by selective ventriculography
V **Prevalence:** Approximately 1 in 16,000 in the pediatric population

Treatment
I **Primary Prevention:** —
II **Secondary Prevention:** Though technically more difficult because of the course of the coronary arteries and the frequent development of serious arrhythmias, surgical repair of these associated lesions should be attempted when indicated on the basis of symptoms and the pathophysiology.
III **Other Therapy:** Therapy for congestive heart failure, pneumonia and subacute bacterial endocarditis when indicated. In long-standing cases of complete A-V block, isoproterenol is temporarily useful in accelerating the idioventricular pacemaker, but pacemakers are eventually required in most instances.

Prognosis: Some patients with inverted transposition without any other associated cardiovascular anomaly do have a normal life span. Yet, other patients who have no associated defects can develop arrhythmias with varying degrees of A-V block leading to decreased cardiac function and ensuing cardiac failure. The prognosis in general is serious because of the very high incidence of associated cardiac lesions. More than half of the patients die from congestive heart failure. Arrhythmias and pulmonary infections are responsible for other deaths. Approximately 60% die within the 1st year of life or by late adolescence from congestive heart failure. The prognosis for children with any cardiac anomaly and inverted transposition is poorer than the same anomaly alone.

Detection of Carrier: —

Special Considerations: —

References:
Elliott, L.P. et al: Coronary arterial patterns in transposition complexes: Anatomic and angiocardiographic studies. Am. J. Cardiol. 17:362, 1966.
Schiebler, G.L. et al: Congenital corrected transposition of the great vessels: A study of 33 cases. Pediatrics 27:(Suppl.)5:849, 1961.
Van Mierop, L.H. and Wiglesworth, F.W.: Pathogenesis of transposition complexes. III. True transposition of the great vessels. Am. J. Cardiol. 12:233, 1963.

Contributor: **Gerold L. Schiebler**

Editor's Computerized Descriptor: CV.

INVERSION OF VENTRICLES WITHOUT TRANSPOSITION OF GREAT ARTERIES

Includes: Inversion des ventricules sans transposition des gros vaisseaux
Inversion der Ventrikel ohne Transposition der grossen Gefässe
Inversión ventricular sin transposición de los grandes vasos
Inversion of ventricles without reversal of arterial trunks
Isolated ventricular inversion
Ventricular inversion without transposition of great arteries

Excludes: Inversion of ventricles with transposition of great arteries (540)

Minimal Diagnostic Criteria: Selective arterial and venous ventriculography are essential to the anatomic confirmation of this entity.

Clinical Findings: The atria, ventricles and their atrioventricular valves are identical to those described for inversion of the ventricles with transposition of the great vessels. Systemic venous blood enters a normally located right atrium and passes through a morphologic mitral valve into a morphologic left ventricle. The aorta, however, arises posteriorly and to the right of the pulmonary artery from the right-sided morphologic left ventricle. The pulmonary veins empty into a normally located left atrium. Blood passes through a morphologic tricuspid valve into a morphologic right ventricle from which the pulmonary trunk arises anteriorly and to the left of the aorta. The right coronary artery arises above the right lateral aortic valve sinus and gives rise to the anterior descending coronary artery. The left coronary artery arises above the left aortic valve sinus and gives rise to the left marginal artery and distal circumflex coronary artery. As in essentially all forms of inversion with 2 ventricles, the coronary artery pattern is inverted. From the side, the great vessels do not appear transposed because the aorta is posterior to the pulmonary trunk. In the frontal view, the aorta lies to the left of the pulmonary trunk, and its ascending portion may be convex to the left. Thus, anatomically, the great vessels are not considered transposed because the anterior leaflet of the mitral valve is in continuity with aortic valve tissue.

As the hemodynamics are the same as in complete transposition of the great arteries, patients having this entity have similar signs and symptoms. In other words, the aorta arises from the venous ventricle and the pulmonary trunk arises from the arterial ventricle. Maintenance of life depends primarily on the associated defects. With only a patent foramen ovale or small atrial septal defect, cyanosis is apparent at birth, and congestive heart failure and poor weight gain occur early in life. A soft systolic murmur, grade 2/6 or less, is heard and the second heart sound is single. If a large ventricular septal defect (VSD) is also present, allowing good mixing of the arterial and venous streams and also an increased pulmonary blood flow, cyanosis is minimal; but congestive heart failure, repeated respiratory infections and poor weight gain are commonly seen. Such patients have a loud systolic murmur and thrill along the lower left sternal border and a diastolic flow murmur over the midprecordium and apex.

The ideal set of associated anomalies is a large VSD and an appropriate degree of pulmonary stenosis. The VSD allows excellent mixing at the ventricular level, and the pulmonary stenosis prevents volume overload of the heart and congestive heart failure. Such patients have a normal sized heart, a single component of S_2 and a harsh systolic murmur along the left sternal border. These patients have mild-to-moderate cyanosis at rest, increasing with activity.

With age, cyanosis gradually increases, exercise tolerance decreases and clubbing develops. Besides VSD and various types of right ventricular outflow tract obstruction, patent ductus arteriosus and right aortic arch have been observed.

Analysis of the electrovectorcardiogram shows that the initial QRS forces are directed abnormally to the left and slightly anteriorly. The QRS loop shows slowing of ventricular depolarization, but the pattern of the intraventricular block is not classic right or left heart block. This QRS loop is so inscribed as to record either a QR or R complex in the right precordial leads. This QR pattern, in itself, always suggests inversion of the ventricles. The axis varies from mild right axis deviation to mild left axis deviation.

The echocardiographic demonstration of a right-sided mitral valve and a left-sided tricuspid valve in the presence of ventricular inversion is extremely difficult. Single-crystal findings have appeared unreliable although it has been reported that tricuspid valves can be identified by their lack of semilunar continuity and mitral valves by the presence of semilunar continuity. This is an extremely difficult differential to achieve. High resolution real-time cross-sectional echocardiographic systems can differentiate the morphology of tricuspid and mitral valves as well as their relationship to the atrioventricular septum for the determination of the ventricular situs. The abnormal orientation of ventricles as well as the ventricular septum in this disorder sometimes makes the M-mode differential diagnosis between these disorders and forms of single ventricle extremely difficult.

Chest roentgenograms are identical to cases with double inlet left ventricle with inversion and transposition. With large communications between the 2 circulations, the pulmonary vascularity is prominent and of the shunt type. In the presence of a severe degree of obstruction to pulmonary blood flow, pulmonary vascularity is diminished.

Cardiac catheterization provides data similar to that obtained in cases of complete transposition of the great arteries. Ventricular angiocardiography is identical to that described for inversion of the ventricles. The diagnosis is based upon the site of origin of the great vessels and the relationship of the right AV valve with aortic valvar tissue. In the AP view, the aorta appears transposed in that it arises to the left of the pulmonary trunk. In the lateral view, however, the great vessels appear normally related. The aorta arises posterior to the pulmonary trunk and there is a fibrous continuity between the anterior leaflet of the right-sided bicuspid AV valve and the aortic valve. The pulmonary trunk arises from the right ventricular infundibulum. The pulmonary valve is superior and anterior to the aortic valve. Associated intracardiac or extracardiac anomalies will be defined in the conventional manner. Another important angiocardiographic finding is the anterior descending coronary artery arising from the right coronary artery as is typical in all cases with the basic ventricular arrangement of inversion of the ventricles with or without transposition of the great arteries.

Complications
I **Derived:** Congestive heart failure, recurrent respiratory infections, growth failure are the common complications in infancy. In older individuals, polycythemia and its sequelae are the rule.

II **Associated:** —

Etiology: ?

Pathogenesis: Inversion of the ventricles without transposition of the great arteries is due to 2 embryologic errors - inversion of the bulboventricular loop and that pathologic abnormality which, occurring with a normally developing loop, will result in transposition of the great arteries.

Related Facts
I **Sex Ratio:** ?
II **Risk of Occurrence:** ?
III **Risk of Recurrence for**
   Patient's Sib: ?
   Patient's Child: ?
IV **Age of Detectability:** From birth, by selective ventriculography
V **Prevalence:** Less than 10 cases known to authors

Treatment
I **Primary Prevention:** —
II **Secondary Prevention:** Palliative surgery in infancy varies with the hemodynamic state. With marked increased pulmonary blood flow, pulmonary artery banding and creation of an atrial septal defect are advised. In those patients with inadequate mixing, a balloon catheter atrial septostomy or Blalock-Hanlon procedure is advisable. With severe right ventricular outflow tract obstruction, a shunt procedure may be indicated. Corrective surgery using the Mustard procedure and correcting the associated defects is feasible.
III **Other Therapy:** Therapy for congestive heart failure and upper respiratory infections.

Prognosis: Depends on the associated defects. Best prognosis is when a large VSD and moderate pulmonic stenosis are present. Because of the paucity of cases reported or recognized, no further statements can be made in regard to morbidity, mortality or life expectancy.

Detection of Carrier: —

Special Considerations: —

References:
Henry, W.L. et al: Evaluation of atrial ventricular valve morphology in congenital heart disease by real-time cross-sectional echocardiography. Circulation 52 (Suppl. II): 120, 1975.
Solinger, R. et al: Deductive echocardiographic analysis in infants with congenital heart disease. Circulation 50:1072, 1974.
Van Mierop, L.H.S.: In Netter, F.H. (ed.): Ciba Collection of Medical Illustrations. The Heart. Summit, New Jersey: Ciba Publishing Co., 1969. vol. 5, p. 118.
Van Praagh, R. and Van Praagh, S.: Isolated ventricular inversion: A consideration of the morphogenesis, definition and diagnosis of nontransposed and transposed great arteries. Am. J. Cardiol. 17:395, 1966.

Contributors: **Larry P. Elliott**
Gerold L. Schiebler
L. H. S. Van Mierop

Editor's Computerized Descriptors: Resp., CV.

IODIDE TRANSPORT DEFECT

Includes: Anomalie du transport de l'iode
Störung des Jod-Transports
Defecto del transporte del yodo
Iodide trapping defect
Hypothyroidism, congenital
Goiter, familial
Partial iodide transport defect

Excludes: Thyrotropin (TSH) unresponsiveness (948)
Thyroid dysgenesis (946)
Other types of thyroid dyshormonogenesis
Goiter, goitrogen-induced (435)

Minimal Diagnostic Criteria: Congenital hypothyroidism, or compensated hypothyroidism; an absent or very reduced RAI uptake in the presence of normal or increased serum TSH levels, and low salivary to plasma iodide ratio. Known goitrogens must be absent from the diet.

Clinical Findings: All patients have been hypothyroid usually presenting during infancy with developmental, growth and skeletal retardation. Other stigmata of congenital hypothyroidism such as lethargy, constipation, macroglossia, dry skin, umbilical hernia and cretinoid facies are present. Goiter may be present at birth but usually appears in early childhood. Laboratory findings include a low serum thryoxine with a low radioactive iodine (RAI) uptake with no increase after exogenous thyrotropin (TSH) administration. Defective iodide concentrating ability can be demonstrated in the salivary glands and gastric mucosa as well. Thyroid pathology reveals glandular hyperplasia with a low iodine content, and defective in vitro iodide uptake as well.†

Complications
I **Derived:** Congenital hypothyroidism with mental and physical retardation.
II **Associated:** Occasionally mechanical airway obstruction secondary to a large goiter.

Etiology: Autosomal recessive †

Pathogenesis: The transport defect may be due either to an altered postulated membrane iodide receptor or carrier, or an altered energy supply to this active transport system.

Related Facts
I **Sex Ratio:** M1:F1
II **Risk of Occurrence:** Rare
III **Risk of Recurrence for**
   Patient's Sib: 1 in 4 (25%) for each offspring to be affected.
   Patient's Child: Not increased unless mate is carrier or homozygote.
IV **Age of Detectability:** Clinical symptoms of congenital hypothyroidism are usually apparent during the 1st half year of life. Occasionally goiter is present at birth. Serum thyroxine or TSH screening may be diagnostic at birth.
V **Prevalence:** Rare. However, since the defect can be treated with a high iodide intake, the defect may not be apparent in areas of high dietary iodide intake.

Treatment
I **Primary Prevention:** Genetic counseling
II **Secondary Prevention:** Early replacement therapy with thyroxine to prevent hypothyroidism. Iodide therapy also has been successfully utilized.
III **Other Therapy:** Surgical removal of goiter if airway obstruction is present. Educational programs for the problem of mental retardation.

Prognosis: Prevention of mental retardation is dependent on early treatment in infancy.

Detection of Carrier: ? No defect of iodide concentrating ability has been demonstrable in obligate heterozygotes.

†**Special Considerations:** Heterogeneity in the iodide transport defect exists. Three patients with a defect in thyroidal iodide transport but with some residual concentrating ability of their salivary glands and gastric mucosa have been described. Clinically, they are congenitally hypothyroid, and the defect in these cases also appears to be transmitted as an autosomal recessive trait. Whether they represent a different mutation at the same gene locus involved in the complete defect, or a separate basic defect of iodide transport is unknown.

References:

Medeivos-Neto, G.A. et al: Partial defect of iodide trapping mechanism in two siblings with congenital goiter and hypothyroidism. J. Clin. Endocrinol. Metab. 35:370, 1972.

Stanbury, J.B. and Chapman, E.M.: Congenital hypothyroidism with goiter. Absence of an iodide-concentrating mechanism. Lancet 1:1162, 1960.

Stanbury, J.B.: Inborn errors of the thyroid. In Steinberg, A.G. and Bearn, A.G. (eds.): Progress in Medical Genetics. New York: Grune & Stratton, 1974, vol. X, p. 55.

Contributor: **Jonathan Zonana**

Editor's Computerized Descriptors: Face, Oral, Neck, Skel., Hernia not CNS, Skin, Nerve

IODOTYROSINE DEIODINASE DEFICIENCY

Includes: Anomalie de la deshalogénation des iodotyrosines
Jodthyrosin-Dejodinase-Mangel
Deficiencia de iodotirosina deiodonasa
Iodotyrosine dehalogenase deficiency
Hypothyroidism, congenital
Goiter, familial
Partial iodotyrosine deiodinase deficiency
Peripheral iodotyrosine deiodinase deficiency
Thyroidal deiodination deficiency

Excludes: Other types of thyroid dyshormonogenesis
Goitrogen-or iodide-induced goiter
Thyroid dysgenesis (946)

Minimal Diagnostic Criteria: Congenital hypothyroidsim, or compensated hypothyroidism with a rapid and high thyroid uptake and turnover of radioiodine; no deiodination of injected labeled MIT or DIT; and probably MIT and DIT and their derivatives in abnormally high concentration in plasma and urine.

Clinical Findings: Patients with the complete form of iodotyrosine deiodinase deficiency, presumably homozygous for the trait, have the typical clinical appearance of congenital hypothyroidism with impairment of intellect and somatic retardation. Other signs and symptoms include lethargy, hypotonia, macroglossia, dry skin, umbilical hernia and cretinoid facies. There is a variable age of onset in the development of goiter which may be present at birth but usually develops during childhood. Clinical laboratory findings are a low serum thyroxine, with a rapid and high uptake and turnover of radioactive iodine. Moniodotyrosine (MIT) and diiodotyrosine (DIT) and their derivatives are probably present in abnormally high concentrations in the plasma and urine. Exogenous IV administration of MIT or DIT results in their excretion unchanged in the urine indicating a deficient peripheral deiodination of these compounds as well. Thyroid biopsy reveals glandular hyperplasia, and the absence of in vitro deiodination of MIT and DIT.

Some presumedly heterozygous relatives of these patients, especially females, have goiters but are euthyroid. They display a partial impairment in peripheral deiodination when given exogenous DIT intravenously.†

Complications
I **Derived:** Congenital hypothyroidism with resultant mental and growth retardation.
II **Associated:** Occasionally airway obstruction due to an enlarged goiter.

Etiology: Autosomal recessive. Homozygous state manifesting congenital hypothyroidism; heterozygotes, especially females, may manifest euthyroid goiter.† McK *27480

Pathogenesis: The iodotyrosine deiodinase enzyme is not involved in the direct synthesis of T_4 or T_3, but functions as a salvage mechanism for iodide recovery from thyroglobulin bound MIT and DIT not utilized in synthesis. A defect in this enzyme results in continued loss of iodinated precursors and depletion of available iodine stores with resultant hypothyroidism. Consistent with this is the observation that replacement therapy with a large excess of iodide can reestablish a euthyroid state.

Related Facts
I **Sex Ratio:** M1:F1
II **Risk of Occurrence:** ? Since iodide therapy can ameliorate the disorder, it may not be clinically apparent in areas with a high dietary iodide intake.
III **Risk of Recurrence for**
Patient's Sib: 1 in 4 (25%) for homozygous hypothyroid state and 1 in 2 (50%) for heterozygous state.

Patient's Child: Very low for homozygous state-100% for heterozygous state

IV **Age of Detectability:** Symptoms of congenital hypothyroidism usually are apparent during the 1st half year of life, occasionally with goiter. Serum thyroxine or TSH screening could detect this at birth.

V **Prevalence:** ?

Treatment
I **Primary Prevention:** Genetic counseling
II **Secondary Prevention:** Early replacement therapy with thyroxine to prevent congenital hypothyroidism. Iodide treatment has been successful although large doses are necessary.
III **Other Therapy:** Surgical removal of a goiter may be necessary due to pressure symptoms. Educational programs for the problem of mental retardation.

Prognosis: Good with early treatment of hypothyroidism. Poor mental development, if treated late.

Detection of Carrier: IV radioiodine-labeled diiodotyrosine (DIT) test may distinguish the heterozygous state.

†Special Considerations: Heterogeneity of iodotyrosine deiodinase defects has become apparent. Patients have been described with a partial deiodination deficiency, a deficient thyroidal deiodination with normal peripheral deiodination, as well as a peripheral defect with a normal thyroidal iodotyrosine deiodinase activity. Clinically, these patients usually have been euthyroid with goiter. The genetic etiology of each of these types is unclear. They may represent other mutations at the same locus, or at a different locus, perhaps affecting different tissue isoenzymes or enzyme subunits.

References:
Stanbury, J.B. Familial goiter. In Stanbury, J.B. et al(eds.): The Metabolic Basis of Inherited Disease, 4th Ed. New York: McGraw-Hill, 1978, p. 206.
Stanbury, J.B.: Inborn errors of the thyroid. In Steinberg, A.G. and Bearn, A.G. (eds.): Progress in Medical Genetics. New York: Grune & Stratton, 1974, vol. X, p. 55.

Contributor: **Jonathan Zonana**

Editor's Computerized Descriptors: Face, Oral, Neck, Skin, Skel., Muscle, Hernia not CNS, Resp., Nerve

IRIS COLOBOMA AND ANAL ATRESIA SYNDROME

Includes: Syndrome colobome-atrésie anale
Katzenaugen-Syndrom
Síndrome de coloboma y atresia anal
Cat eye syndrome
Anal atresia and iris coloboma

Excludes: Other causes of coloboma or anal atresia

Minimal Diagnostic Criteria: Iris coloboma, anal atresia (usually with rectovaginal or rectoperineal fistula), preauricular tags.

Clinical Findings: Iris coloboma, usually bilateral, and sometimes coloboma of the choroid and microphthalmia. The patients may exhibit a peculiar facies with a depressed nasal bridge, hypertelorism, epicanthus, downward slanting of palpebral fissures and micrognathia. Deformities of the ears are frequently associated with preauricular cutaneous tags, dimples or fistulae. Anal (and rectal) atresia with rectovaginal or rectoperineal fistula is common. Malformations of the kidneys, such as horseshoe kidney or agenesis, and hydronephrosis and cysticoureteral reflux have been noted. Rib anomalies, hemivertebrae and hip dislocation may be associated. Cardiovascular abnormalities comprise septum defects or total anomalous pulmonary venous return as well as tetralogy of Fallot. Dermatoglyphics may be unusual. A 4-finger line is frequently seen. Two-thirds of the patients are mentally retarded.

Complications
I **Derived:** Cardiovascular failure, infections of the urinary tract, hydronephrosis, glaucoma, cataract
II **Associated:** —

Etiology: Probably due to a chromosomal imbalance. An additional small extra chromosome generally with mosaicism has been found in more than 30 cases. This chromosome is satellited even on both arms: it otherwise resembles an acrocentric chromosome, the long arm of which is deleted. Morphologic variability, differences in heterochromatic staining and fluorescence as well as in the replication pattern suggest heterogeneity. Its origin and constitution have not been elucidated. The extra chromosome may be transmitted through 2 generations.†

Pathogenesis: ?

Related Facts
I **Sex Ratio:** M15:F18 in 33 patients with a chromosomal abnormality
II **Risk of Occurrence:** Probably rare
III **Risk of Recurrence for**
  Patient's Sib: Increased
  Patient's Child: Increased
IV **Age of Detectability:** At birth
V **Prevalence:** Rare

Treatment
I **Primary Prevention:** ?
II **Secondary Prevention:** —
III **Other Therapy:** Corrective surgery

Prognosis: Life span depends upon cardiovascular and renal functions. Various degrees of mental deficiency.

Detection of Carrier: By cytogenetic studies

†Special Considerations: In a few cases, no chromosomal aberration was found. Occurrence in 2 sisters and in a male infant of related parents suggests homozygosity of a rare autosomal recessive gene which imitates the phenotype of a specific partial trisomy. From a number of observations of single features of cat eye syndrome and various additional extra chromosomes, one could speculate that this syndrome represents either a selected association of anomalies or the complete phenotype of a partial trisomy.

References:

Franklin, R.C. and Parslow, M.I.: The cat eye syndrome. Review and two further cases occurring in female siblings with normal chromosomes. Acta Paediatr. Scand. 61:581-586, 1972.

Kunze, J. et al: Cat eye syndrome. Humangenetik 26:271-289, 1972.

Contributor: **R. A. Pfeiffer**

Editor's Computerized Descriptors: Eye, Ear, Oral, Skel., CV., GI., Liver, GU., Face, Nose, Nerve

Also see Section I, Fig. 47

---

545   **540-500**
ISOLATED MECONIUM ILEUS

Includes: Ileus meconial
Mekoniumileus, isoliert
Íleo meconial aislado
Meconium ileus, isolated

Excludes: Cystic fibrosis (237)

Minimal Diagnostic Criteria: Intestinal obstruction in a child with no evidence of cystic fibrosis but films and operative findings consistent with inspissated meconium.

Clinical Findings: Twelve patients have been described initially. Rickham estimates that 25% of cases of meconium obstruction are not associated with mucoviscidosis.

Complications
I   **Derived:**   Intestinal obstruction, perforation and meconium peritonitis
II **Associated:** —

Etiology: ?

Pathogenesis: Unknown but presumed to be abnormal form of meconium; no cases studied to date.

Related Facts
I   **Sex Ratio:**   M1:F1
II   **Risk of Occurrence:**   Estimated 1 in 8000
III **Risk of Recurrence for**
     Patient's Sib: ?
     Patient's Child: ?
IV   **Age of Detectability:**   Newborn by x-ray and physical examination
V   **Prevalence:**   25% of cases identified as meconium ileus

Treatment
I   **Primary Prevention:** —
II   **Secondary Prevention:**   Gastrografin enemas or surgery with N-acetylcystine irrigations
III **Other Therapy:**   Resection of bowel for perforation with some type of exteriorization.

Prognosis: Excellent

Detection of Carrier: —

Special Considerations: —

References:

Rickham, P.P.: Progress in Pediatric Surgery. Baltimore: University Park Press, 1971, Vol. II, p. 73.

Rickham, P.P. et al: Neonatal meconium obstruction in the absence of mucoviscidosis. Am. J. Surg. 109:173, 1965.

Contributors: **Lawrence K. Pickett**
Stephen L. Gans

Editor's Computerized Descriptor: GI.

ISOLATION OF SUBCLAVIAN ARTERY FROM AORTA

Includes: Séparation de l'artère sous-clavière et de l'aorte
Anomaler Ursprung der A. subclavia
Aislamiento de la arteria subclavia de la aorta
Isolation of subclavian artery types I, II and III
Congenital atresia of the subclavian artery
Congenital "subclavian steal" syndrome
Subclavian artery, isolation from aorta

Excludes: Traumatic or atherosclerotic occlusion at origin of subclavian artery
Surgical division of subclavian artery with anastomosis of proximal portion to pulmonary artery branch (Blalock-Taussig operation)

Minimal Diagnostic Criteria: Among cases with a left aortic arch, this lesion must be suspected in any patient with diminished pulsations in the right arm. This is especially true in those with coarctation of the aorta or roentgen signs of aberrant right subclavian artery.

In patients with a right aortic arch, roentgen signs of this vessel anomaly plus diminished pulsations in the left arm suggest this condition. Correlation of additional roentgen findings (presence or absence of an aberrant left subclavian artery and left carotid artery pulsations) allows the observer to differentiate each of the three major types.

Definitive diagnosis is based on selective thoracic aortography.

Clinical Findings: With this anomaly, the subclavian artery is completely isolated from the aorta. There may be either a right or left aortic arch. The contralateral subclavian is always the one isolated from the aorta, ie right aortic arch with isolated left subclavian artery. In all cases, the "atretic" proximal portion of the subclavian probably had its origin as part of the ductus arteriosus. The normally higher systemic arterial perfusion pressure prevents pulmonary to subclavian flow even before the ductus arteriosus closes. The distal subclavian artery flow is via collaterals about the neck and shoulder. The vertebral artery contributes a large amount of this collateral and, when the vertebral to subclavian artery flow reaches a critical amount, symptoms of basilar insufficiency will occur because of the blood shunted from the basilar artery into the subclavian. Of the cases reported in English literature, the majority had a right aortic arch. Of these, approximately one-half had tetralogy of Fallot. Other congenital anomalies included some type of aortic abnormality such as coarctation of the aorta, cervical aortic arch and supravalvar aortic stenosis. Among reported cases with a right aortic arch, only a few have been diagnosed during life. Of the cases with a left aortic arch, they almost invariably had an associated coarctation of the aorta.

The main clinical findings would be that of the underlying congenital heart defect, together with a delayed and diminished pulse, plus a lowered blood pressure in the affected arm. Those cases which survive into late childhood or beyond may have the "subclavian steal" syndrome- basilar artery insufficiency or unilateral upper limb numbness or weakness. The vascular syndrome with right arch may occur in one of three forms. In the first type, the left subclavian artery has become isolated from the aortic arch and is connected to the left pulmonary artery by way of a ductus arteriosus. In the second type, an atretic aberrant left subclavian artery originates from a retroesophageal diverticulum. A vascular ring is present. In a third type with right aortic arch, the brachiocephalic vessels display the usual branching pattern, however the first major artery, the innominate artery, is atretic. Thus, the proximal portions of the left common carotid and left subclavian arteries are also atretic.

Thoracic roentgenograms with barium swallow correlated with left peripheral artery pulses enable the observer to distinguish each major type. Obviously, all types with right arch show the usual roentgenologic signs of the right aortic arch. With either isolation of the left subclavian artery (Type I) or atresia of the innominate artery (Type III), there is absence of a retroesophageal indentation on the barium-filled esophagus. With an aberrant, yet atretic, left subclavian artery (Type II), the aortic diverticulum or site of origin of the left subclavian artery produces a wide concave impression caused by the aortic diverticulum on the posterior aspect of the barium-filled esophagus. This, together with diminished pulsation in the left arm, indicates either atresia or severe stenosis of the left subclavian artery at its origin from the diverticulum. The presence of an aortic diverticulum means that there is an ipsilateral ductus or ligament and also a vascular ring (usually "loose" or nonobstructive) is present.

In patients with right aortic arch, diminished pulsation in the left arm and absence of a retroesophageal compression, additional attention should be given to carotid pulsations. In isolation of the left subclavian artery, the pulsations in both carotids, right arm and both legs will be equal. In the type with atresia of the innominate artery, the amplitude of pulsation in the left carotid will be diminished as well. Definitive diagnosis is made with selective aortography.

Complications
I **Derived:** "Subclavian steal" syndrome developing sometime after childhood. Blalock-Taussig operations on the involved side are unsuccessful because of the low flow and pressure in the isolated subclavian plus the subclavian artery may already communicate with the pulmonary artery.
II **Associated:** Tetralogy of Fallot, coarctation of the aorta.

Etiology: ?

Pathogenesis: Believed due to resorption of the aortic arch both distally and proximally to the isolated subclavian artery. Then, in the fetus, the only communication between the heart and the subclavian artery is the persistent patent ductus arteriosus. The opposite aortic arch develops normally.

Related Facts
I **Sex Ratio:** M1:F1
II **Risk of Occurrence:** Exceedingly rare
III **Risk of Recurrence for**
   Patient's Sib: ? No known case of an affected relative
   Patient's Child: ? No known case of an affected offspring
IV **Age of Detectability:** From birth by aortography
V **Prevalence:** ? Exceedingly rare; unknown number of asymptomatic adults.

Treatment
I **Primary Prevention:** —
II **Secondary Prevention:** If an associated congenital heart defect is present, this should be treated in the usual recommended manner, realizing ipsilateral Blalock-Taussig operations are not beneficial in this condition. Otherwise, an isolated subclavian artery deserves no treatment unless "subclavian steal" symptoms are present, in which case the treatment would be ligating the vertebral artery or conceivably inserting an aorta to subclavian artery graft.
III **Other Therapy:** —

Prognosis: Entirely dependent upon associated congenital heart defect.

Detection of Carrier: —

Special Considerations: —

References:

Lansing, A. M. and Murphy, J.: Origin of the left subclavian artery from the pulmonary artery with congenital subclavian steal: Surgical implications in cyanotic patients. Ann. Thorac. Surg. 5:146, 1968.

Stewart, J.R. et al: An Atlas of Vascular Rings and Related Malformations of the Aortic Arch System. Springfield:Charles C Thomas, 1964.

Victorica, B.E. et al: Right aortic arch associated with contralateral congenital subclavian steal syndrome. Am. J. Roentgenol. Radium Ther. Nucl. Med. 108:582, 1970.

Contributors: **Thomas A. Vargo**
Charles E. Mullins
Dan G. McNamara

Editor's Computerized Descriptor: CV.

ISOVALERICACIDEMIA

Includes: Acidémie isovalérique
Isovaleriazidämie
Sweaty feet syndrome

Excludes: —

Minimal Diagnostic Criteria: Extreme elevations of serum isovaleric acid during acute attacks, with more modest elevations during apparent compensation. Urinary excretion of excesses of isovaleric acid and isovalerylglycine. Reduction in the capacity to degrade isovaleric acid is demonstrable in peripheral leukocyte and in skin fibroblast.

Clinical Findings: Onset is usually acute during the first weeks of life with vomiting, acidosis and rapidly progressive neurologic signs. A characteristic "sweaty feet" odor may be noted. Death has occurred within a few weeks in over half the cases. The survivors experience intermittent acute attacks of vomiting, acidosis, ataxia, tremors, progressing to lethargy and coma. Leukopenia, anemia and thrombocytopenia may complicate the acute episode. Mental retardation is common with an IQ in the range of 50 - 80. There appears to be variability in the severity of the disease.†

Complications

I **Derived:** The characteristic disagreeable odor, and periodic attacks of acidosis and coma are clearly related to the metabolic defect.

II **Associated:** It is not as certain that the mental retardation is so related, though it seems likely.

Etiology: Probably autosomal recessive; McK *24350

Pathogenesis: Inability to degrade leucine. The defective enzyme is probably isovaleryl-CoA dehydrogenase, though it has not been conclusively demonstrated. This is one step below the block in maple syrup urine disease, involving the conversion of isovaleric acid to β-methylcrotonic acid.

Related Facts

I **Sex Ratio:** M1:F1

II **Risk of Occurrence:** Very rare

III **Risk of Recurrence for**
Patient's Sib: Probably 1 in 4 (25%) for each offspring to be affected
Patient's Child: Not increased, unless mate is carrier or homozygote

IV **Age of Detectability:** Enzyme defect should be demonstrable at birth. Onset of symptoms may be in newborn period or delayed for many months.

V **Prevalence:** Very rare

Treatment

I **Primary Prevention:** Genetic counseling; antepartum diagnosis should be possible.

II **Secondary Prevention:** Infusions of glucose solutions are usually adequate for acute attacks. Long-range treatment attempts to achieve biochemical normality with dietary control. This should be individualized, using low protein diets, and if necessary, restricted leucine intake.

III **Other Therapy:** —

Prognosis: Appears to be influenced by severity of disease, age of diagnosis and institution of treatment. Normal physical and mental growth are possible.

Detection of Carrier: ?

†**Special Considerations:** There is no aminoacidemia, aminoaciduria or ketoaciduria, so that the usual screening procedures are not informative. The distinctive odor should alert the clinician. Gas phase chromatography is the definitive approach to the diagnosis of isovalericacidemia. Screening of the urine for isovalerylglycine is the most convenient and reliable approach to screening.

References:

Ando, T. and Nyhan, W. L.: A simple screening method for detecting isovaleric acidemia. Clin. Chem. 16:420, 1970.
Efron, M. L.: Isovaleric acidemia. Am. J. Dis. Child. 113:74, 1967.
Levy, H.L. et al: Isovaleric acidemia. Results of family study and dietary treatment. Pediatrics 52:83, 1973.
Shih, V.E. et al: Diagnosis of isovaleric acidemia in cultured fibroblasts. Clin. Chim. Acta 48:437, 1973.

Contributor: **Joseph Dancis**

—————————————

Editor's Computerized Descriptors: GI., Nerve

JAW-WINKING SYNDROME

Includes: Mâchoires à clignotement
Maxillopalpebrale Synkinese
Sincinesia máxilo-palpebral
Marcus Gunn phenomenon
Maxillopalpebral synkinesis
Hereditary palpebromaxillary synergy
Synkinetic ptosis
Pterygoid-levator synkinesis

Excludes: Winking-jaw phenomenon of Wartenberg
Reversed Marcus Gunn phenomenon

Minimal Diagnostic Criteria: Retraction of the upper lid upon movement of the jaw

Clinical Findings: The classic Marcus Gunn syndrome, which is the most common, consists of unilateral ptosis at rest with elevation of the apparently paretic upper lid to a level higher than that of the other eye upon opening the mouth. Usually if the jaw is deviated to the affected side the ptosis increases, but if deviated to the opposite side maximal retraction occurs. Typically the ptosis recurs if the mouth is held open. Affected individuals habitually open the mouth when looking upwards. The phenomenon occurs more frequently on the left than the right. It rarely occurs bilaterally. Multiple variations of the classic syndrome have been described. Examples are retraction only with side-to-side motion of the jaw, or with masseter function, or with inspiration, or with eye movements.

Complications
I **Derived:** Basically cosmetic
II **Associated:** None, except for occasional associated anomalous movements of the extraocular muscles resulting in strabismus

Etiology: Unknown save for those families in which an irregular autosomal dominant inheritance pattern exists. Multiple occurrences in the sibship of only 1 generation may represent autosomal recessive inheritance.

Pathogenesis: The pathogenesis has not been definitely established and many theories have been set forth. Anomalous connections or a reflex arc between the nuclei of the external pterygoid muscle (mesencephalic root C_5) and the levator palpebris (C_3) have been postulated. Antidromic nerve impulses and spread of stimulus rather than direct connection between nuclei also have been implicated.

Related Facts
I **Sex Ratio:** M1+:F1
II **Risk of Occurrence:** ? It has been estimated as the cause of 2% of congenital ptosis.
III **Risk of Recurrence for**
  Patient's Sib: When autosomal dominant and parent is affected, < 1 in 2 (< 50%) for each offspring to be affected; otherwise not increased.
  Patient's Child: < 1 in 2
IV **Age of Detectability:** Soon after birth, since the phenomenon is most noticeable during sucking.
V **Prevalence:** ?

Treatment
I **Primary Prevention:** —
II **Secondary Prevention:** Usually unwarranted. Some success has occurred with section of the motor root of the trigeminal nerve. More experience is available for the procedure of sectioning the levator muscle and using a fascial sling to the orbicularis to produce voluntary lid control.
III **Other Therapy:** —

Prognosis: The condition usually grows slowly less noticeable with age.

Detection of Carrier: —

Special Considerations: —

References:

Beard, C.: Ptosis. St. Louis: C.V. Mosby, 1969, pp. 34, 44, 47-48, 102, 104, 188.

Duke-Elder, S.: System of Ophthalmology, vol. 3, pt. 2. Congenital Deformities, St. Louis:C.V. Mosby Co., 1963, p. 900.

Falls, H.F. et al: Three cases of Marcus Gunn phenomenon in two generations. Am. J. Ophthalmol. 32:53, 1949.

Kuder, G.G. and Laws, H.W.: Hereditary Marcus Gunn phenomenon. Can. J. Ophthalmol. 3:97, 1968.

Walsh, F.B. and Hoyt, W.F.: Clinical Neuroophthalmology, 3rd Ed. Baltimore: Williams & Wilkins, 1969, vol. 1, p. 309.

Contributor: **Donald R. Bergsma**

Editor's Computerized Descriptors: Eye, Face

JUVENILE DIABETES MELLITUS

Includes: Diabète sucré juvénile
Juveniler Diabetes mellitus
Diabetes mellitus juvenil
Labile diabetes mellitus
Ketosis-prone diabetes mellitus

Excludes: Maturity onset diabetes mellitus
Diabetes mellitus secondary to pituitary or adrenocortical abnormalities or to pancreatectomy
Juvenile diabetes mellitus, optic atrophy and deafness (550)
Renal glycosuria (Marker) (861)

Minimal Diagnostic Criteria: A decreased glucose tolerance and no increase in plasma immunoreactive insulin are essential for the diagnosis of diabetes mellitus. In association with the above symptoms and in the absence of obvious endocrinopathy an abnormal increase in blood sugar plus glycosuria can usually be considered diagnostic.

Clinical Findings: The juvenile form of diabetes mellitus, in contrast to the maturity onset or adult form of the disease, is characterized by rapid onset, episodes of hypoglycemia, proneness to ketoacidosis, an almost absolute requirement for insulin and the lack of obesity as an associated finding. The natural history of the illness in children is characterized by 4 stages. The first, beginning with conception, may be termed prediabetes. The only recognized abnormalities that may exist during this period are in the level of insulin activity and the presence of insulin antagonists in the serum. The 2nd stage, subclinical diabetes, is a period during which stress resulting from illness, surgery, trauma or emotional upheavals will produce a detectable abnormality in carbohydrate metabolism. In this stage carbohydrate metabolism appears to be normal during intervening periods. The 2nd stage may last for several months to many years. The 3rd stage, latent diabetes, is usually brief in children and is defined as a period when the glucose tolerance is abnormal, but fasting blood sugars are within the normal range. The 4th stage is overt diabetes, when insulin treatment is required. During the first few weeks of this stage the insulin requirement will approximate 2 units/kg body wt/day. This abruptly drops after 2 to 6 weeks to a requirement of less than 1/2 unit/kg body wt/day. This low level of requirement will last for 2 to 24 months and during this period ketoacidosis and hypoglycemia are rare, and responsiveness to sulfonylurea compounds is usually present. At the end of this period the total diabetic state ensues and is present the remainder of the individual's life. The insulin requirement will average approximately 1 unit/kg body wt/day and will increase with periods of illness, inactivity and at adolescence.

Symptoms occur with the following frequency ranges:

Polyuria	75-80%
Polydipsia	70-80%
Weight loss or failure to gain weight	50-60%
Lassitude and malaise	40-50%
Polyphagia	40-50%
Nocturia	35-40%
Abdominal pain	10-15%
Hyperventilation	5-10%

Laboratory Findings Include:	
Abnormal glucose tolerance	100%
Glycosuria ultimately	100%
Initial glycosuria	60-80%
Ketosis with ketonuria, initially	20-25%

Metabolic acidosis	15-20%
Hypoglycemia	< 5%

Complications
I **Derived:** Ketoacidosis, coma, hypoglycemia
II **Associated:** Vascular changes in many organs, most notably in the eyes and kidneys. The onset of these changes is generally accepted to occur with clinical significance 5 to 15 years after adolescence and without regard to the duration of the disease in the preadolescent.

Etiology: Probably polygenic; resembles autosomal recessive. Occurs in dogs and mice.

Pathogenesis: A relative or absolute insulin deficiency alters glucose transport. Several insulin antagonists have been identified. The sequence which yields arteriolar and capillary wall changes or microscopic nephrosclerosis is unknown.

Related Facts
I **Sex Ratio:** M1:F1 in children; M1:F2 in older patients
II **Risk of Occurrence:** 1 in 25 to 1 in 40 for all diabetes with onset at any age; 1 in 600 to 1 in 1000 will develop diabetes prior to age 15.
III **Risk of Recurrence for**
  Patient's Sib: 1 in 4 (25%) for each offspring to be affected
  Patient's Child: Not increased unless mate is carrier or homozygote (gene frequency is high).
IV **Age of Detectability:** Rarely prior to one year of age
V **Prevalence:** 1 in 59 diagnosed patients for all diabetes, including all ages

Treatment
I **Primary Prevention:** Genetic counseling
II **Secondary Prevention:** Insulin
III **Other Therapy:** Dietary restrictions, varying from minimal concern for excessive carbohydrate to carefully prescribed diets, are considered useful in management. The extent of restriction depends on the philosophic view of the physician. Support in behavioral and social areas is of greatest consequence in the successful management of children with diabetes mellitus. More emphasis is required in these areas than in any other aspect of the illness.

Prognosis: If untreated, death in approximately 6 months. With appropriate treatment there is a 75 to 95% mortality in 45 years.

Detection of Carrier: Studies in progress on use of steroid stressed glucose tolerance test.

Special Considerations: —

References:
Drash, A.: Diabetes mellitus in childhood: A review. J. Pediatr. 78:919, 1971.
Jackson, R. et al: The definition of chemical diabetes in children. Metabolism 22:229, 1973.
Kohrman, A.F. and Weil, W.B.: Juvenile diabetes mellitus. Adv. Pediatr. 18:123, 1971.
Rosenbloom, A.L.: The natural history of diabetes mellitus. Public Health Rev. 2:115, 1973.
Weil, W.B.: Juvenile diabetes mellitus. N. Engl. J. Med. 278:829, 1968.
Weil, W.B.: Diabetes mellitus in children. In Barnett, H. (ed.): Pediatrics, 16th Ed. New York: Appleton-Century-Crofts, 1976.

Contributor: **William B. Weil, Jr.**

Editor's Computerized Descriptors: Eye, Resp., GU.

550 **545-500**
JUVENILE DIABETES MELLITUS, OPTIC ATROPHY AND DEAFNESS

Includes: Diabète sucré juvénile avec atrophie optique et surdité
Juveniler Diabetes mellitus, Optikusatrophie und Taubheit
Diabetes mellitus juvenil, atrofia óptica y sordera
Diabetes insipidus and optic atrophy
Recessive optic atrophy, hearing loss and juvenile diabetes
Diabetes mellitus and optic atrophy
Optic atrophy, juvenile diabetes and deafness

Excludes: Laurence-Moon-Biedl syndrome (578)
Friedreich ataxia and the condition described by Alström, Hallgren, Nilsson and Åsander (1959).

Minimal Diagnostic Criteria: Juvenile diabetes mellitus and optic atrophy†

Clinical Findings: Diabetes mellitus and optic atrophy both tend to be of childhood onset, though either may occur first. The optic atrophy is usually bilateral and symmetric and leads to rapid deterioration of vision. Cataracts also have been reported. In one variant of this syndrome, an unusual type of sideroblastic anemia may be present. The EEG is usually abnormal and the CSF fluid protein level may be raised. Deafness is not an invariable accompaniment, but when it occurs it is bilateral, perceptive, progressive, and of mild-to-moderate degree. It tends to affect the high tones more than the low. Typically it is not sufficiently severe to necessitate special education.
  Other components of the syndrome include diabetes insipidus in several cases, retinal pigmentary degeneration and evidence of more widespread neurologic involvement.

Complications
I **Derived:** Those of juvenile diabetes mellitus and severe optic atrophy (ie visual handicap leading to blindness)
II **Associated:** —

Etiology: Homozygosity for a gene with pleiotropic effects and perhaps also more than 1 locus may be involved. Autosomal recessive type transmission occurs. McK *22230

Pathogenesis: ?

Related Facts
I **Sex Ratio:** M1:F1 (There is some suggestion that associated diabetes insipidus occurs preferentially in females.)
II **Risk of Occurrence:** 1 in 100,000 births or less (Montreal)
III **Risk of Recurrence for**
  Patient's Sib: When autosomal recessive, 1 in 4 (25%) for each offspring to be affected
  Patient's Child: When autosomal recessive, not increased unless mate is carrier or homozygote. (With heterozygote mate it is 1 in 2 but such heterozygotes are rare in the general population. The reproductive fitness of affected individuals is, of course, much reduced both on account of juvenile diabetes mellitus and of the visual handicap consequent to the optic atrophy. No example of a documented case having offspring has been recorded.)
IV **Age of Detectability:** Very variable since the diagnosis cannot be made until both diabetes mellitus and optic atrophy are present.
V **Prevalence:** Approaching risk of occurrence as prognosis of condition improves and expectation of life increases.

Treatment
I **Primary Prevention:** Genetic counseling
II **Secondary Prevention:** —
III **Other Therapy:** As for other forms of juvenile diabetes mellitus

Prognosis: Unknown but probably similar to other forms of juvenile diabetes mellitus.

Detection of Carrier: ?

†**Special Considerations:** It has been suggested that heterozygotes may be affected by juvenile diabetes mellitus without other features of the syndrome.

References:
Fraser, F.C. and Gunn, T.: Diabetes mellitus, diabetes insipidus, and optic atrophy. An autosomal recessive syndrome? J. Med. Genet. 14:190, 1977.
Järnerot, G.: Diabetes mellitus with optic atrophy—thalassemia-like sideroblastic anemia and weak isoagglutinins—a new genetic syndrome? Acta Med. Scand. 193:359, 1973.
Rose, F.C. et al: The association of juvenile diabetes mellitus and optic atrophy: Clinical and genetical aspects. Q. J. Med. 35:385, 1966.

Contributor: **G. R. Fraser**

Editor's Computerized Descriptors: Vision, Eye, Hearing, Nerve

KELOID

Includes: Chéloïde
Queloide
Spontaneous keloids
Traumatic keloids
Cicatricial keloids

Excludes: Hypertrophic scars

Minimal Diagnostic Criteria: Firm, smooth papule or plaque

Clinical Findings: A raised, firm, smooth, pink or flesh-colored papule or plaque on the skin. Rarely tender or painful.

Complications
I   **Derived:** —
II   **Associated:** Common in Turner syndrome

Etiology: Autosomal dominant. Keloids may develop following injury to the skin, such as mechanical trauma, burns, inflammation, tension, vaccination.

Pathogenesis: ?

Related Facts
I   **Sex Ratio:** M1:F2
II   **Risk of Occurrence:** ?
III **Risk of Recurrence for**
      Patient's Sib: If parent is affected 1 in 2 (50%) for each offspring to be affected; otherwise not increased.
      Patient's Child: 1 in 2
IV   **Age of Detectability:** Most common in the 2nd and 3rd decade. Rare in infancy and old age.
V   **Prevalence:** 1 in 1100 in England
                1 in 400 in Breslau, Germany
                1 in 625 in the United States
                1 in 14 in Swiss children under the age of 10
                1 in 8 in Swiss children 10-15 years of age
                1 in 6 in the Congo

Treatment
I   **Primary Prevention:** Genetic counseling
II   **Secondary Prevention:** Avoidance of elective surgery in those patients predisposed to form keloids. Therapy, mainly for cosmetic purposes, is often of limited help. Treatment modalities include excision, irradiation, and local injection of corticosteroid drugs. Some keloids improve or resolve spontaneously after a period of time.
III **Other Therapy:** —

Prognosis: Normal for life span, intelligence and function

Detection of Carrier: —

Special Considerations: —

References:
Bloom, D.: Heredity of keloids; review of literature and report of family with multiple keloids in 5 generations. N.Y. State J. Med. 56:511, 1956.
Ketchum, L.D.: Hypertrophic scars and keloids. Clin. Plast. Surg. 4:301, 1977.
Koonin, A.J.: The aetiology of keloids: A review of the literature and a new hypothesis. S. Afr. Med. J. 38:913, 1964.

Contributor: **James L. Barrett**

Editor's Computerized Descriptor: Skin

KERATOCONUS

Includes: Kératocone
Keratokonus
Queratocono
Conical cornea
Cornea, conical

Excludes: Lenticonus (585)

Minimal Diagnostic Criteria: Asymmetric myopic astigmatism with any of the physical signs cited below or with a positive family history for full-blown keratoconus, conical cornea per se.

Clinical Findings: Noninflammatory, progressive ectasia of the central cornea results in myopic astigmatism, conical projection of the corneal apex, a surrounding ring of iron-containing pigment (Fleischer ring), protrusion of the lower lid by the conical cornea on downward gaze (Munson sign), vertical stretch marks in the posterior stroma, and ruptures in the Descemet and Bowman membranes. Abnormal reflexes are seen with the keratoscope, retinoscope, ophthalmoscope, or ophthalmometer (keratometer). Occasionally, acute ectasia, caused by sudden rupture of Descemet membrane and the endothelium, occurs allowing aqueous to penetrate and cause total opacification of the stroma. The corneal thinning is usually bilateral but asymmetric, and begins at about puberty. There are variable stages of remission and exacerbation.

Complications
I **Derived:** Acute ectasia, reduced visual acuity
II **Associated:** Marfan syndrome, chromosome 21 trisomy, pigmentary retinopathy, amaurosis congenita of Leber, atopic dermatitis, vernal keratopathy, and other disorders.

Etiology: May be either autosomal recessive or autosomal dominant.

Pathogenesis: ? Possibly related to degenerative processes in the basement membrane of the corneal basal epithelium or in Bowman membrane, or possibly to abnormalities in the stromal collagen itself. G-6-PDH deficiency has been reported in the corneal epithelium.

Related Facts
I **Sex Ratio:** M4:F6
II **Risk of Occurrence:** ?
III **Risk of Recurrence for**
   Patient's Sib: When autosomal recessive or autosomal dominant, see Table I AR or AD, respectively.
   Patient's Child: When autosomal recessive or autosomal dominant, see Table I AR or AD, respectively.
IV **Age of Detectability:** —
V **Prevalence:** High incidence of acute ectasia in chromosome 21 trisomy and in amaurosis congenita of Leber

Treatment
I **Primary Prevention:** Genetic counseling
II **Secondary Prevention:** —
III **Other Therapy:** Pressure patch for acute ectasia, contact lens for early cases with irregular astigmatism, penetrating keratoplasty in advanced cases

Prognosis: Variable; good for keratoplasty

Detection of Carrier: Refraction reveals asymmetric myopic astigmatism in affected family members.

Special Considerations: —

References:
Cullen, J. F. and Butler, H. G.: Mongolism (Down's syndrome) and keratoconus. Br. J. Ophthalmol. 47:321, 1963.
Duke-Elder, S.: System of Ophthalmology, vol. 8, part 2. Diseases of the Outer Eye. London:Henry Kimpton, 1965.
Goldberg, M. F.: A review of selected inherited corneal dystrophies associated with systemic diseases. In Bergsma, D. (ed.): Part VIII. Eye. Birth Defects: Orig. Art. Ser., vol. VII, no. 3. Baltimore:Williams and Wilkins Co., for The National Foundation-March of Dimes, 1971, p. 13.
Hammerstein, W.: Zur Genetik des Keratoconus. Albrecht von Graefes Arch. Klin. Exp. Ophthalmol. 190:293, 1974.
Karel, I.: Keratoconus in congenital diffuse tapetoretinal degeneration. Ophthalmologica (Basel) 155:8, 1968.
Kim, J.O. and Hassard, D.T.R.: On the enzymology of the cornea. Can. J. Opthalmol. 8:151, 1973.

Contributors: **Morton F. Goldberg**
                      Joel Sugar

Editor's Computerized Descriptors: Vision, Eye
Also see Section I, Fig. 49

KERATOPATHY, BAND-SHAPED

Includes: Kératopathie en bande
Bandförmige Keratopathie
Queratopatía en bandas
Band keratitis
Band-shaped keratopathy

Excludes: Vogt limbal girdle
Calcareous degeneration of Axenfeld

Minimal Diagnostic Criteria: White material in Bowman membrane occupying the interpalpebral space and having characteristic lacunae.

Clinical Findings: Slow, progressive development of a white band in Bowman membrane, beginning near the limbus in the interpalpebral space and extending centrally. Rarely, the band begins centrally and extends horizontally to the peripheral cornea. There is usually a clear space between the ends of the band and the limbus. Small, dark, pathognomonic clear spaces or lacunae are present. Corneal sensation is usually intact. Irritative episodes do not occur unless calcified plaques erode the overlying epithelium. If the band occupies the visual axis, acuity can be diminished.

Complications
I **Derived:** Epithelial erosions, decreased visual acuity
II **Associated:** †

Etiology: May be autosomal recessive; heterogeneity exists.†
McK *21750

Pathogenesis: Speculative as follows: supersaturation of the interpalpebral cornea with calcium salts, due to evaporation of water in this location, or loss of carbon dioxide to the atmosphere in the interpalpebral location with consequent elevation of the pH and precipitation of calcium salts, or massage of calcium salts to the interpalpebral area by the lids.

Related Facts
I **Sex Ratio:** M1:F1
II **Risk of Occurrence:** ?
III **Risk of Recurrence for**
Patient's Sib: When autosomal recessive, 1 in 4 (25%) for each offspring to be affected.
Patient's Child: Not increased unless mate is carrier or homozygote.
IV **Age of Detectability:** Two forms exist. One with onset of corneal changes in infancy, the other with no changes until old age.
V **Prevalence:** ?

Treatment
I **Primary Prevention:** Genetic counseling, prevention of congenital syphilis, corneal trauma or hypercalcemia†
II **Secondary Prevention:** Treatment of primary ocular disease and of hypercalcemia, chelation of corneal calcium with topically applied EDTA which is successful in removing corneal calcium.
III **Other Therapy:** —

Prognosis: Depends upon underlying systemic or local disease.

Detection of Carrier: —

†**Special Considerations:** Band keratopathy may develop secondary to a variety of conditions, including: 1) Secondary to ocular disease eg juvenile iridocyclitis and rheumatoid arthritis (Still disease), Norrie disease, uveitis in adults, syphilitic interstitial keratitis, longstanding glaucoma. 2) Secondary to chronic corneal trauma, eg exogenous irritants. 3) Secondary to hypercalcemia, regardless of its etiology, or hypophosphatasia. 4) Secondary to gout (rare). 5) "Familial" cases of primary band keratopathy a) juvenile, b) senile. (X-linked recessive band keratopathy, as reported by Duke-Elder and Leigh (see References) is, in reality, Norrie disease with secondary corneal calcification.

References:
Duke-Elder, S. and Leigh, A.G.: System of Ophthalomology, vol. 8, part 2. Diseases of the Outer Eye. London:Henry Kimpton, 1965.
Fishman, R.S. and Sunderman, F.W.: Band keratopathy in gout. Arch. Ophthalmol. 75:367, 1966.
Goldberg, M.F.: A review of selected inherited corneal dystrophies associated with systemic diseases. In Bergsma, D. (ed.): Part VIII. Eye. Birth Defects: Orig. Art. Ser., vol. VII, no. 3. Baltimore: Williams and Wilkins Co., for The National Foundation-March of Dimes, 1971, p. 13.
Lessel, S. and Norton, E.W.: Band keratopathy and conjunctival calcification in hypophosphatasia. Arch. Ophthalmol. 71:497, 1964.
Streiff, E.B. and Zwahlen, P.: Une famille avec degenerescence en bandelette de la cornee. Ophthalmologica 111:129, 1946.
Wagener, H.P.: The ocular manifestations of hypercalcemia. Am. J. Med. Sci. 231:218, 1956.
Warburg, M. Norrie's disease: A congenital progressive oculo-acoustico-cerebral degeneration. Acta Ophthalmol. (Suppl.) (Kbh.) 89:1, 1966.

Contributors: **Morton F. Goldberg**
Joel Sugar

Editor's Computerized Descriptor: Eye

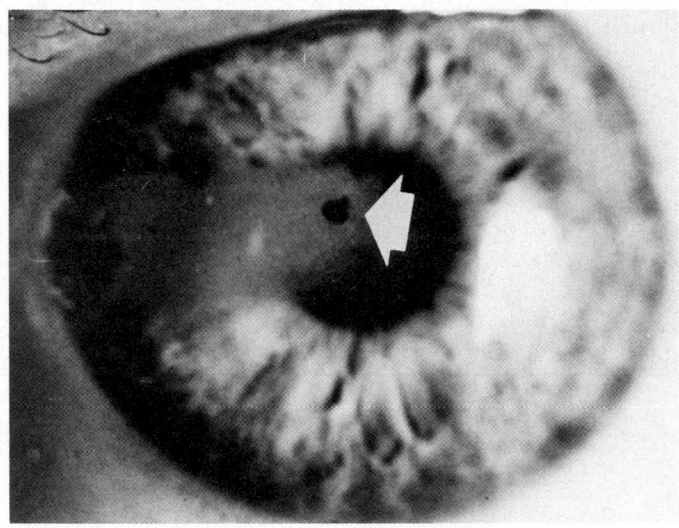

309. Note clear fenestration in white haze (arrow)

KGB SYNDROME

Includes: Síndrome de Herrmann-Pallister-Tiddy-Opitz tipo KGB Short stature, characteristic facies, mental retardation, macrodontia and skeletal anomalies

Excludes: Other malformation-mental retardation syndromes

Minimal Diagnostic Criteria: Rounded face, bow-shaped narrow lips, macrodontia and broad eyebrows in a short, mentally retarded person combined with radiographic abnormalities of ribs, vertebrae, hips and hands.

Clinical Findings: Based on 7 cases from 3 families this syndrome is recognized as showing great variability in expression. Findings in the majority of patients include shortness of stature (below 3rd%), moderate mental retardation, biparietal prominence, brachycephaly, round face, telecanthus, broad eyebrows, short alveolar ridges, macrodontia, cervical ribs, abnormal vertebrae, short femoral necks, short tubular bones in hands, delayed bone age, syndactyly of toes 2-3, palmar distal axial triradius and simian crease. The EEG was abnormal in 2 cases investigated. Other significant low-frequency findings include pectus excavatum, hip dysplasia, hexadactyly, and hearing deficit.

Complications
I **Derived:** Deformities and pain secondary to skeletal manifestations. Crowding and noneruption of teeth.
II **Associated:** —

Etiology: Apparently autosomal dominant

Pathogenesis: ? Many of the manifestations seem related to skeletal defects.

Related Facts
I   **Sex Ratio:** Probably M1:F1
II   **Risk of Occurrence:** Small
III **Risk of Recurrence for**
     Patient's Sib: 1 in 2 (50%) if parent is affected, presumably negligible if parent is not affected.
     Patient's Child: 1 in 2
IV   **Age of Detectability:** At birth
V   **Prevalence:** ?

Treatment
I   **Primary Prevention:** Genetic counseling
II   **Secondary Prevention:** Supportive and symptomatic, including especially a) orthopedic surgery for spine or hip problems, b) dental care, c) hearing aid and speech therapy.
III **Other Therapy:** —

Prognosis: Apparently good for life span; dependent on degree of mental retardation and skeletal manifestations.

Detection of Carrier: —

Special Considerations: —

References:
Herrmann, J. et al: The KGB syndrome-a syndrome of short stature, characteristic facies, mental retardation, macrodontia and skeletal abnormalities. In Bergsma, D. (ed.): New Chromosomal and Malformation Syndromes. Birth Defects: Orig. Art. Ser., vol. XI, no. 5. Miami: Symposia Specialists for The National Foundation-March of Dimes, 1975, p. 7.

Contributor: Jürgen Herrmann

Editor's Computerized Descriptors: Eye, Hearing, Face, Teeth, Dermatoglyphic, Hair, Skel., Nerve

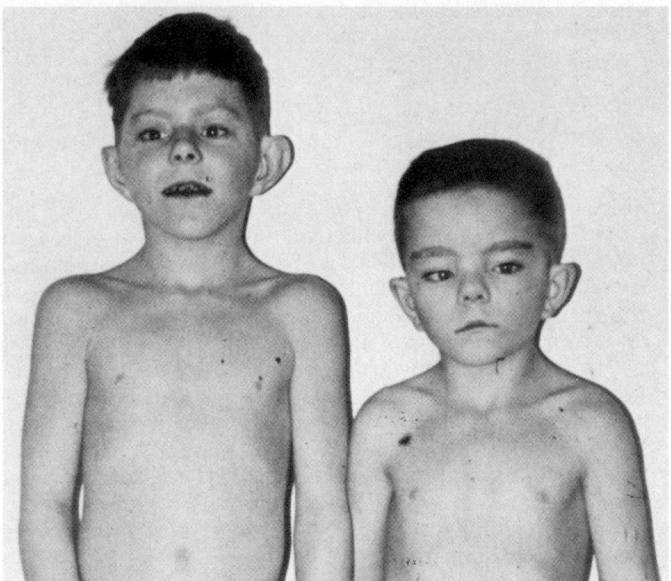

310. Note pectus excavatum and typical facial appearance

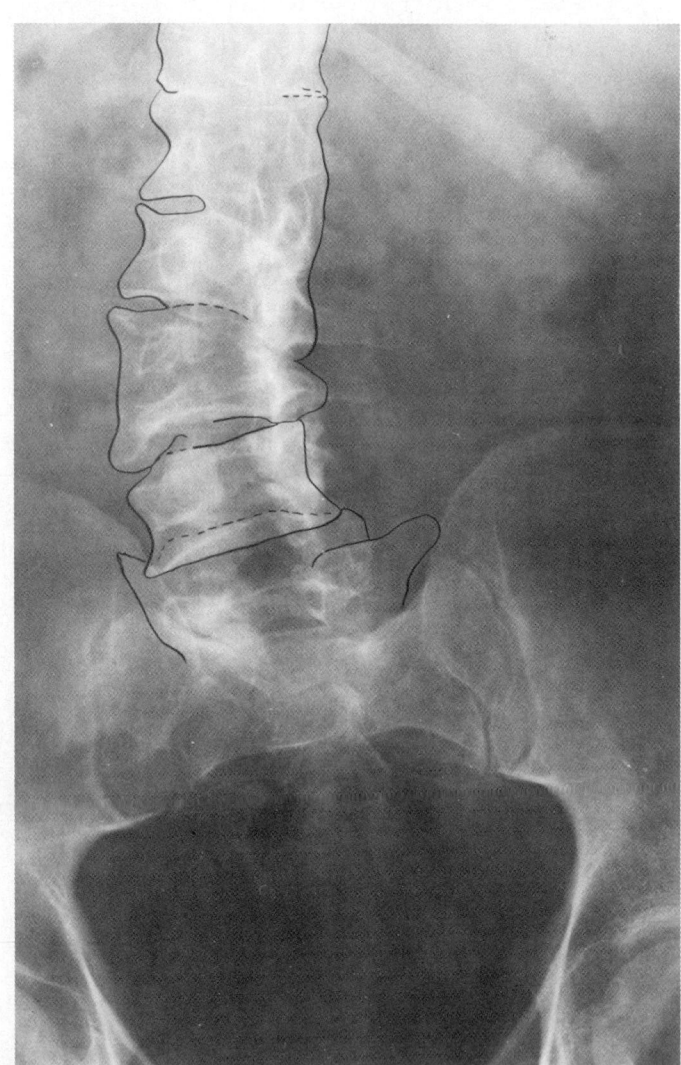

311. Note block vertebrae T12-L2; deformed and partially collapsed L3-L5 vertebral bodies; short femoral necks

fism. Arch. Dis. child. 46:656, 1971.

KLEEBLATTSCHÄDEL ANOMALY

Contributor: **Judith G. Hall**

Includes: Crâne en feuille de trèfle
Deformidad craneana tri-lobulada
Cloverleaf skull syndrome

Editor's Computerized Descriptors: Eye, Ear, Face, Nose, Skel.

Excludes: —

Minimal Diagnostic Criteria: Intrauterine craniosynostosis with a trilobar skull configuration.

Clinical Findings: Trilobed skull deformity at birth results from intrauterine fusion of cranial sutures. Increased intracranial pressure leads to bulging in some areas and craniolacunar pattern (Lückenschädel) in other areas of the cranium. Facial malformations include high forehead, severe proptosis or exophthalmos, beaked nose, midfacial hypoplasia and downward displacement of ears. These abnormalities can be seen as a) an isolated finding; b) associated with other minor localized malformations (vertebral anomaly, elbow or knee ankylosis, hand and foot syndactyly); c) associated with a generalized chondrodystrophy similar to thanatophoric dysplasia; or d) in families with inherited craniosynostosis (Crouzon, Apert, Carpenter, Pfeiffer syndromes).†

Complications
I Derived: Most severely affected individuals are stillborn or die in infancy. Eyes are severely exophthalmic and corneas are exposed to trauma. If patients survive, increased intracranial pressure leads to CNS complications and severe mental retardation.
II Associated: —

Etiology: When associated with thanatophoric dysplasia, appears to be transmitted as an autosomal recessive trait. When associated with an inherited craniosynostosis syndrome, it may occur in other affected individuals. If isolated or associated with minor anomalies, it appears to be sporadic with unknown etiology.

Pathogenesis: Abnormal cranial bone growth is thought to cause premature fusion of sutures. Subsequent brain growth results in bulging in areas of least resistance.

Related Facts
I Sex Ratio: M1:F1
II Risk of Occurrence: Rare
III Risk of Recurrence for
   Patient's Sib: Not increased if isolated defect.
   Patient's Child: Not increased if isolated defect.
IV Age of Detectability: At birth or prenatally
V Prevalence: Rare

Treatment
I Primary Prevention: Genetic counseling
II Secondary Prevention: Prenatal diagnosis in familial cases. Neurosurgery for craniosynostosis in mild cases.
III Other Therapy: —

Prognosis: Poor in severe cases.

Detection of Carrier: —

†Special Considerations: Kleeblattschädel anomalad appears to be a morphologic feature seen in numerous disorders. The skull is quite variable in shape, size, and evolution depending on which sutures are affected and at what stage in development they fuse.

References:
Cohen, M.M.: The Kleeblattschädel phenomenon: Sign or syndrome? Am. J. Dis. Child. 124:944, 1972.
Iannaccone, G. et al: The so-called "Cloverleaf Skull Syndrome." Pediatr. Radiol. 2:175, 1974.
Partington, M.W. et al: Cloverleaf skull and thanatophoric dwar-

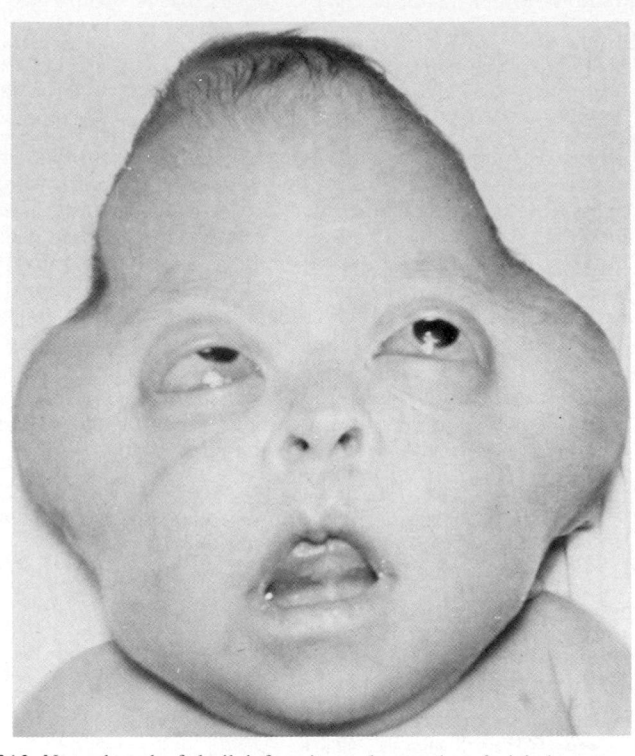

312. Note cloverleaf skull deformity and secondary facial changes

KLINEFELTER SYNDROME

Includes: Syndrome de Klinefelter
Síndrome de Klinefelter
True Klinefelter syndrome
Seminiferous tubule dysgenesis
Primary micro-orchidism

Excludes: All other forms of male hypogonadism
Del Castillo syndrome
Gonadotropin deficiency, isolated (438)

Minimal Diagnostic Criteria: X-chromatin positive male with normal male genitalia, small, firm testes and karyotypic abnormality (most commonly 47,XXY).†

Clinical Findings: Most affected individuals appear grossly normal and the diagnosis is usually not suspected during the examination of neonates or infants except when the testes are found to be significantly smaller than normal. However, multiple minor anomalies are common in the Klinefelter syndrome. Brachycephalic skull configuration, at times with low nuchal hairline, minor defects of differentiation of auricles, clinodactyly of 5th fingers at times with only 1 flexion crease on that finger, simian creases and other variations of palmar crease patterns, decreased total ridge count of fingertip dermatoglyphic patterns, increased incidence of hypothenar patterns with distal axial palmar triradius. Radioulnar synostosis occurs with increased incidence in this syndrome. In individuals with more complex sex chromosome aneuploidy (48,XXXY; 49,XXXXY; 49,XXXYY, etc) multiple somatic anomalies and mental retardation are common.

Pubertal hypogonadism usually leads to tall stature (on the average 10 cm taller than XY males), disturbed body proportions (ie lower body segment > upper body segment, but span ≤ height), deficient maturation of male secondary sexual characteristics, more or less pronounced gynecomastia in some one-half of cases, later disturbances of sexual function (complete infertility, impotence, lack of libido), osteoporosis, and frequent truncal obesity. Average intelligence is reduced, some 15% are definitely mentally retarded. About 1% of all males with an IQ of 90 or less are X-chromatin positive. Personality and character trait disturbances, emotional and behavioral troubles, alcoholism, minor criminality and outright psychosis occur commonly in this syndrome. The true frequency of such manifestations is unknown since patients with these problems are ascertained more frequently than those without. Neurologic abnormalities (seizures, tremor, neuromuscular disorders) have also been reported.

Neonatally and in childhood the number of spermatogonia is less than in control males of the same age. At and after puberty progressive sclerosis and hyalinization of seminiferous tubules leads to loss of germinal tissue with consequent secondary clumping ("nodular hyperplasia") of Leydig cells which are ultimately also lost in a process of progressive fibrosis and atrophy. This process is associated with diminished excretion of 17-ketosteroids and increasing levels of urinary gonadotropins which ultimately reach castrate levels.

Complications
I   **Derived:** Psychologic and psychiatric complications of a person with less than normal IQ, hypogonadism, and impotence. Vertebral collapse due to osteoporosis.
II   **Associated:** —

Etiology: Gonosomal aneuploidy with or without mosaicism: 47,XXY; 46,XY/47,XXY and 46,XX/47,XXY types are the most frequent. More complex forms of gonosomal aneuploidy are rare to very rare. Meiotic nondisjunction in either parent results in aneuploidy while mitotic nondisjunction after fertilization results in mosaicism. The XXY form occurs in the tortoise shell male cat and in mouse, pig and dog.

Pathogenesis: Pathogenesis of seminiferous tubule dysgenesis is unknown. Eunuchoidism and other manifestations of hypogonadism presumably due to progressive testicular sclerosis with loss of germinal and endocrine tissue.

About 2/3 of 47,XXY cases are of the $X^M X^M Y$ type, 1/3 are $X^M X^P Y$.† In the former class, increased maternal age supports the hypothesis of maternal meiotic nondisjunction; maternal age is not increased in the mosaic or $X^M X^P Y$ cases.

Related Facts
I   **Sex Ratio:**   M1:F0
II   **Risk of Occurrence:**   Buccal smear survey: incidence of males with X-chromatin: 1 in 590 live-born males (1 in 1250 to 1 in 1100 live-born infants). Neonatal chromosome surveys: approximately 1 in 500 live-born males.
III   **Risk of Recurrence for**
   Patient's Sib: Presumably not significantly increased
   Patient's Child: Only 4 fertile 46,XY/47,XXY mosaics are known; 1 child was a 47,XXY male, all other offspring were presumably normal. All 47,XXY patients are infertile.
IV   **Age of Detectability:**   Prenatally by examination of fetal cells, at birth by buccal smear, small testes; later on the basis of clinical findings.
V   **Prevalence:**   Presumably around 1 in 1000, primarily in the general Caucasian populations.
   In institutions for the mentally retarded around 1 in 100 male inmates.
   Among populations of infertile men: 1 in 77 to 1 in 24 of all infertile men; 1 in 9 to 1 in 5 for men with high grades of infertility (ie azoospermia or sperm count less than 1 x 10^6 per ml).
   Among men in psychiatric institutions: 1 in 169

Treatment
I   **Primary Prevention:**   —
II   **Secondary Prevention:**   Diagnosis by amniocentesis. Treatment of hypogonadism, supportive psychotherapy for emotional complications.
III   **Other Therapy:**   As indicated

Prognosis: Life span presumably normal

Detection of Carrier: —

†**Special Considerations:**   The patients with more complex gonosomal aneuploidy (48,XXXY; 49,XXXXY; 48,XXYY; 49,XXXYY, etc) are usually ascertained on the basis of mental retardation, generally with multiple anomalies. 47,XYY individuals are not to be considered as having the Klinefelter syndrome. Rarely do patients with a condition essentially indistinguishable from the Klinefelter syndrome have a presumed 46,XX constitution.

Note: X^M equals maternally derived X chromosomes, and X^P equals paternally derived X chromosomes.

References:
Inhorn, S.L. and Opitz, J.M.: Abnormalities of sex development. In Bloodworth, J.M.B., Jr. (ed.): Endocrine Pathology. Baltimore: Williams & Wilkins, 1968, p. 580.
Nielsen, J.: Klinefelter's syndrome and the XYY syndrome. Acta Psychiatr. Scand. (Suppl.) 45:209, 1, 1969.
Overzier, C.: The so-called true Klinefelter syndrome. In Overzier, C. (ed.): Intersexuality. New York: Academic Press, 1963, p. 277.
Zuppinger, K. et al: Klinefelter's syndrome; a clinical and cytogenetic study in 24 cases. Acta Endocrinol. (Kbh.) 54:(Suppl.) 113:5, 1967.

Contributor: **John M. Opitz**

Editor's Computerized Descriptors: Dermatoglyphic, Hair,

KNIEST DYSPLASIA

Includes: Syndrome de Kniest
Kniest-Syndrom
Síndrome de Kniest
Metatropic dysplasia, type II
Pseudometatropic dwarfism
Swiss-cheese cartilage syndrome

Excludes: Metatropic dysplasia† (656)
Spondyloepiphyseal dysplasia
Mucopolysaccharidosis IV (678)

Minimal Diagnostic Criteria: Disproportionate dwarfism with typical x-ray changes in the skeleton, frequently myopia and typical flat facies. Characteristic chondroosseous histopathology may be used to verify the diagnosis.

Clinical Findings: Disproportionate dwarfism and kyphoscoliosis associated with flat facies and prominent eyes, cleft palate, hearing loss, myopia, and limited joint motion. The skeletal abnormalities are recognizable at birth with shortening and deformity of the limbs and stiff joints. Marked lumbar lordosis and kyphoscoliosis develop in childhood resulting in disproportionate shortening of the trunk. Walking is delayed and difficult. The long bones are short and bowed and the joints appear enlarged. There is limitation of joint motion with pain, stiffness and flexion contractures of the major joints. The flexion contractures in the hips produce a characteristic stance. The fingers appear long and knobby, and flexion is limited resulting in an inability to form a fist. The face is flat and dish-shaped with prominent wide-set eyes, flat nasal bridge and a broad mouth. There is severe myopia which frequently leads to retinal detachment. Umbilical and inguinal herniae are common. Cleft palate may lead to chronic otitis media and both conductive and neurosensory hearing loss are common. Recurrent respiratory distress with tracheomalacia may occur in infancy. Motor milestones and speech development may be delayed, but intelligence usually is normal.

The characteristic radiographic abnormalities during the newborn period include dumbbell-shaped femora, hypoplastic pelvic bones, vertical clefts of the vertebrae, and platyspondyly.† In infancy and childhood one sees a dessert-cup shaped pelvis, increased soft tissue densities around the joints, enlarged epiphyses, cloud-like calcifications near the epiphyseal plates, and flat elongated vertebral bodies with cloud-like calcifications. The bones of the hands are osteoporotic and show delay in formation of epiphyses; soft tissue swelling occurs near the joints. There are fragmented accessory ossification centers and joint spaces are narrowed. The femoral heads show a marked delay in ossification and may not appear until mid-childhood. In adult life, there is rhizomelic short stature but the cloud calcifications disappear after epiphyseal fusion. Hands show a bulbous enlargement of the ends of the short tubular bones, short thumb tufts, and a flat and squared appearance of the metacarpal-phalangeal joints.

Complications
I **Derived:** Myopia may lead to retinal detachment. Shortened and deformed bones and limitation of joint motion may lead to severe orthopedic complications. Cleft palate may lead to speech impairment and chronic otitis media.
II **Associated:** —

Etiology: Probable autosomal dominant trait; McK *15655

Pathogenesis: The chondroosseous histopathology is abnormal and distinctive. Resting cartilage contains large cells, a loosely woven matrix with irregular staining, and many "holes" which

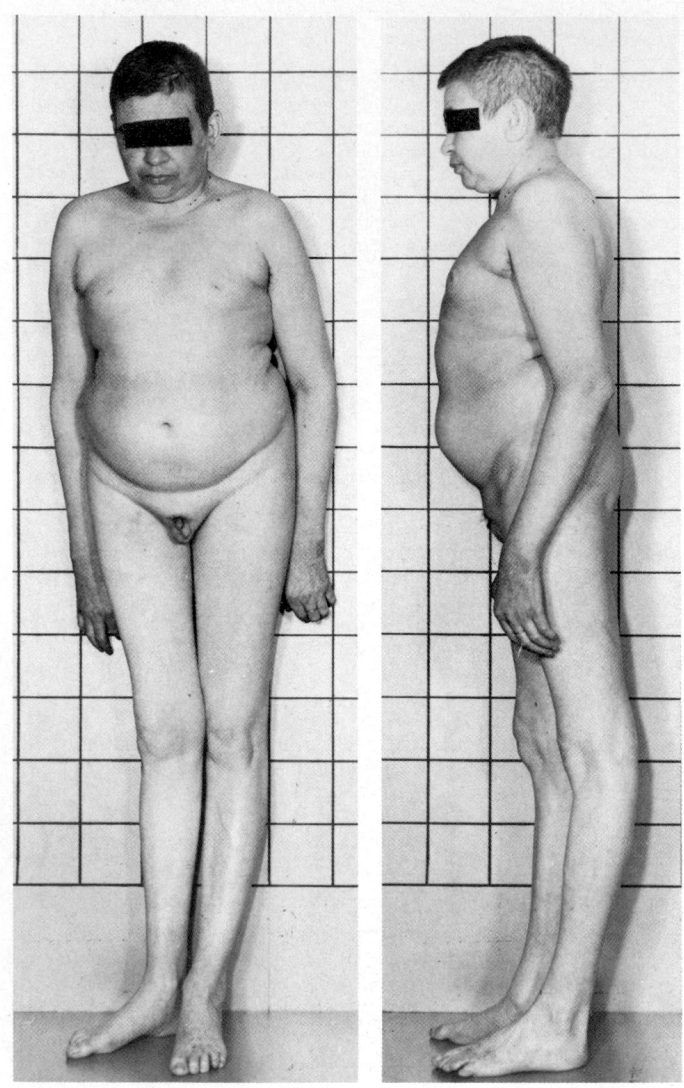

313. Note truncal obesity

have been likened to "swiss-cheese cartilage." The growth plate contains hypercellular cartilage with ballooned chondrocytes and sparse matrix. Ultrastructural studies have revealed chondrocytes filled with dilated cisterna of endoplasmic reticulum. Increased urinary excretion of keratosulfate has been described in several patients.

Related Facts

I **Sex Ratio:** M1:F1
II **Risk of Occurrence:** ?
III **Risk of Recurrence for**
  Patient's Sib: If parent is affected 1 in 2 (50%) for each offspring to be affected; otherwise not increased.
  Patient's Child: 1 in 2
IV **Age of Detectability:** Newborn period because of abnormal appearing limbs with bulbous metaphyses and distinctive skeletal x-ray changes.
V **Prevalence:** ?

Treatment

I **Primary Prevention:** Genetic counseling
II **Secondary Prevention:** Orthopedic surgery for joint contractures, kyphoscoliosis, and epiphyseal dysplasia; repair of cleft palate, frequent regular ophthalmologic examinations for detection and prevention of retinal detachment.
III **Other Therapy:** —

Prognosis: Apparently normal for life.

Detection of Carrier: ?

†**Special Considerations:** This condition had been confused with metatropic dwarfism in the past because of the similar dumbbell appearance of the long bones in the newborn. These 2 disorders can be readily distinguished on the basis of skeletal radiographs and clinical features.

References:

Lachman, R.S. et al: The Kniest syndrome. Am. J. Roentgenol. Radium Ther. Nucl. Med. 123:805, 1975.
Maroteaux, P. and Spranger, J.: La maladie de Kniest. Arch. Fr. Pediatr. 30:735, 1973.
Rimoin, D.L. et al: Metatropic dwarfism, the Kniest syndrome, and the pseudoachondroplastic dysplasias. Clin. Orthop. 114:70. 1976.

Contributors: **Ralph S. Lachman**
David L. Rimoin

Editor's Computerized Descriptors: Vision, Eye, Hearing, Face, Oral, Teeth, Nose, Skel., Hernia not CNS, Resp.

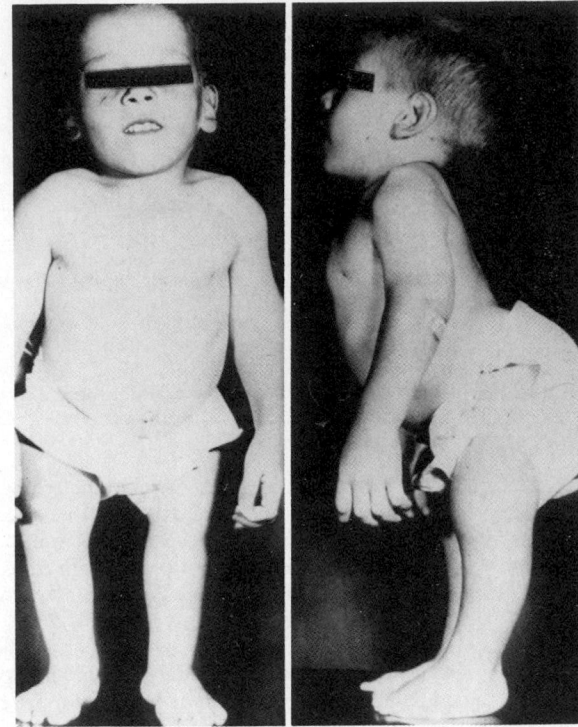

314. Note round facies; shortening of trunk and limbs. Pelvis and trunk are bent forward, secondary to flexion contractures of the hip

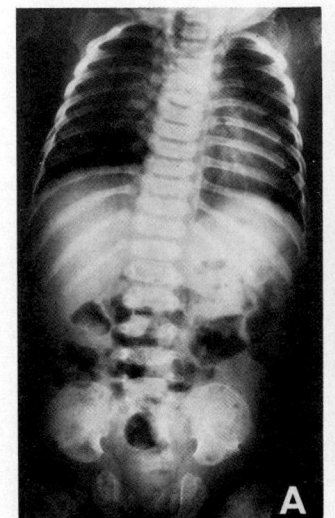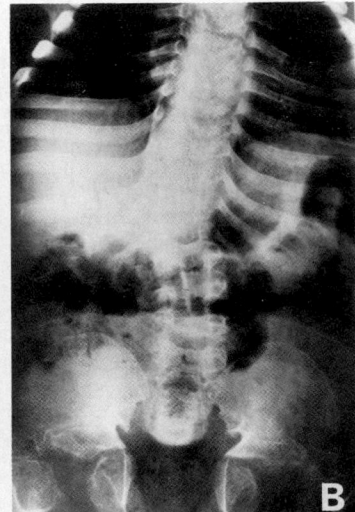

315. Note generalized platyspondyly, broad thoracic cage, and decreased intercostal distances; B) moderately severe thoracolumbar scoliosis; decreased vertical diameter of ilia

KNUCKLE PADS, LEUKONYCHIA AND DEAFNESS

Includes: Kératose palmaire-leuconychie-surdité
Knöchelpolster, leukonychie und Taubheit
Queratosis palmar, leuconiquia y sordera
Bart-Pumphrey syndrome
Leukonychia, knuckle pads and deafness
Deafness, knuckle pads and leukonychia

Excludes: Dominantly inherited sensorineural hearing loss without appropriate cutaneous findings
Knuckle pads without deafness
Leukonychia without deafness

Minimal Diagnostic Criteria: Sensorineural deafness and total leukonychia (nails need not be dead white) when there is a family history of deafness and knuckle pads.

Clinical Findings: Characterized by sensorineural deafness, detection of which may require audiometric studies, apparently 100%; conductive loss present in some cases; increased whiteness of finger and toenails seen in all cases studied, apparently 100%; knuckle pads are usually found; keratoderma palmare et plantare may be a feature.

The hearing loss and knuckle pads are first observed in infancy or early childhood. Leukonychia probably begins in early childhood. Hearing loss has apparently been progressive in some cases. All patients have sensorineural loss, with the defect in the cochlea. Some patients have a superimposed conductive loss which may or may not be associated with structural abnormalities of the middle ear. Keratoderma palmare et plantare has been seen only in adults with the syndrome.

Complications
I   **Derived:** —
II **Associated:** —

Etiology: Autosomal dominant transmission with complete penetrance, but variable expressivity; McK *14920

Pathogenesis: ?

Related Facts
I   **Sex Ratio:** M1:F1
II   **Risk of Occurrence:** ? Very uncommon
III **Risk of Recurrence for**
  Patient's Sib: If parent is affected, 1 in 2 (50%) for each offspring to be affected; otherwise not increased.
  Patient's Child: 1 in 2. Reproductive fitness unimpaired.
IV   **Age of Detectability:** With positive family history, audiometry might establish diagnosis in infancy or early childhood.
V   **Prevalence:** Probably rare. One pedigree has been reported. An isolated case with all the features of the syndrome has also been reported; other members of the family had various abnormalities, but none had the syndrome of knuckle pads, leukonychia and deafness.

Treatment
I   **Primary Prevention:** Genetic counseling
II   **Secondary Prevention:** —
III **Other Therapy:** That appropriate for the degree of hearing loss, including hearing aid and speech therapy, if indicated.

Prognosis: Normal life span and intelligence

Detection of Carrier: —

Special Considerations: —

References:
Bart, R. S. and Pumphrey, R. E.: Knuckle pads, leukonychia and deafness: A dominantly inherited syndrome. N. Engl. J. Med. 276:202, 1967.
Konigsmark, B. W.: Hereditary deafness in man. N. Engl. J. Med. 281:713, 1969.

Contributor: **Robert S. Bart**

Editor's Computerized Descriptors: Hearing, Skin, Nails

KOILONYCHIA

Includes: Coelonychie
Koilonychie
Coiloniquia
Hereditary koilonychia
Spoon nails

Excludes: Secondary koilonychia

Minimal Diagnostic Criteria: Concavity of the fingernails. Toenails are commonly concave in normal children hence unimportant unless fingernails are involved. The great majority of isolated cases of koilonychia are not hereditary but rather traumatic or secondary to a large number of medical disorders.

Clinical Findings: Concave nail shape with everted edges, commonly thin nail. Thumb almost always affected, toenails in over 50%. Not all nails are involved in each patient. Occasionally, a wide fissure is seen in the center of the nail in addition to spooning. Rarely associated with monilethrix, palmar hyperkeratosis, steatocystoma multiplex, and nail-patella syndrome.

Complications
I **Derived:** —
II **Associated:** —

Etiology: Autosomal dominant with a high degree of penetrance. Variable expressivity in degree of nail involvement. McK *14930

Pathogenesis: ?

Related Facts
I **Sex Ratio:** M1:F1
II **Risk of Occurrence:** Rare
III **Risk of Recurrence for**
  Patient's Sib: When autosomal dominant and if parent is affected, 1 in 2 (50%) for each offspring to be affected; otherwise not increased.
  Patient's Child: When autosomal dominant, 1 in 2
IV **Age of Detectability:** At birth or early childhood
V **Prevalence:** Rare

Treatment
I **Primary Prevention:** Genetic counseling when autosomal dominant
II **Secondary Prevention:** Occasionally a deformed toenail that causes discomfort is permanently destroyed surgically.
III **Other Therapy:** —

Prognosis: Normal for life span, intelligence and function

Detection of Carrier: —

Special Considerations: —

References:
Bergeron, J. R. and Stone, O. J.: Koilonychia: A report of familial spoon nails. Arch. Dermatol. 95:351, 1967.
Hellier, F. F.: Hereditary koilonychia. Br. J. Dermatol. 62:213, 1950.
Stone, O. J. and Maberry, J. D.: Spoon nails and clubbing: Review and possible structural mechanisms. Tex. St. J. Med. 61:620, 1965.

Contributor: **Orville J. Stone**

Editor's Computerized Descriptor: Nails

KUSKOKWIM SYNDROME

Includes: Syndrome de la rivière Kuskokwim
Síndrome de Kuskokwim

Excludes: Arthrogryposis (88)

Minimal Diagnostic Criteria: Multiple joint contractures predominantly affecting the knees and ankles, with atrophy or compensatory hypertrophy of associated muscle groups, normal intelligence and evidence of a recessive mode of inheritance.†

Clinical Findings: The chief findings are multiple joint contractures affecting the knees and ankles, with atrophy or compensatory hypertrophy of associated muscle groups. Gait is accomplished on the knees or by a duck-like waddle. Flexion contractures are also found at the elbows. Pigmented nevi and diminished corneal reflexes have been noted in several patients. Intellectual function is not impaired. General laboratory studies, electromyography and muscle biopsies fail to show abnormalities. X-ray features include hypoplasia of the 1st or 2nd lumbar vertebral body, progressive elongation of the pedicles of the 5th lumbar vertebra producing spondylolisthesis, osteolytic areas in the outer clavicle and proximal humerus in children and hypoplasia of the patella associated with knee contractures.

Complications
I **Derived:** The patella, normally placed at birth, migrates proximally through attenuation and elongation of the patella tendon. Equinus and planovalgus foot deformities commonly occur.
II **Associated:** —

Etiology: Thought to be autosomal recessive; McK *20820

Pathogenesis: ? †

Related Facts
I **Sex Ratio:** M1:F1
II **Risk of Occurrence:** ?
III **Risk of Recurrence for**
  Patient's Sib: 1 in 4 (25%) for each offspring to be affected
  Patient's Child: Not increased unless mate is carrier or homozygote
IV **Age of Detectability:** At birth
V **Prevalence:** ? 17 cases have been reported, all in Eskimos in the Kuskokwim River delta of Southwestern Alaska.

Treatment
I **Primary Prevention:** Genetic counseling
II **Secondary Prevention:** Orthopedic measures with use of surgery, casting, bracing and passive manipulation
III **Other Therapy:** —

Prognosis: Normal for life span and intelligence. Function variable.

Detection of Carrier: ?

†Special Considerations: This syndrome is differentiated from arthrogryposis multiplex congenita by the mode of inheritance, lack of laboratory evidence of abnormality of the muscles about affected joints and certain radiographic abnormalities. In the Kuskokwim syndrome abnormal muscle attachment, involving predominantly the tendons of extensor muscles which are under constant strain, is believed to be the primary problem.

References:
Petajan, J.H. et al: Arthrogryposis syndrome (Kuskokwim disease) in the Eskimo. JAMA 209:1481, 1969.
Wright, D.G. and Aase, J.: The Kuskokwim syndrome: An inherited form of arthrogryposis in the Alaskan Eskimo. In Bergsma, D. (ed.): Part III. Limb Malformations. Birth Defects: Orig. Art. Ser., vol. V, no. 4. New York: The National Foundation-March of Dimes, 1969, p. 91.

Contributor: **Charles I. Scott, Jr.**

Editor's Computerized Descriptors: Skin, Skel., Muscle

KYRLE DISEASE

Includes: Maladie de Kyrle
Enfermedad de Kyrle
Hyperkeratosis follicularis et parafollicularis in cutem penetrans
Hyperkeratosis penetrans

Excludes: Reactive perforating collagenosis
Elastosis perforans serpiginosa (339)
Perforating folliculitis

Minimal Diagnostic Criteria: A keratotic plug fills an epithelial invagination. Parakeratosis is in parts of the plug. Basophilic cellular debris not staining with elastic tissue stains is with the plug. Abnormal (parakeratotic) keratinization of all the epidermal cells including the basal cells is present in at least 1 region deep to the plug. In these foci, epidermal disruption usually occurs resulting in the presence of keratinized cells in the dermis accompanied by a granulomatous reaction. Serial histologic sections may be necessary to confirm the diagnosis.

Clinical Findings: Characterized by chronic, scattered, generalized papular eruptions with hyperkeratotic cone-shaped plugs that may be plaque-like, but do not involve the mucosae, palmar or plantar surfaces. Tend to be on the extensor surfaces and involve the legs most often.†

Complications
I Derived: —
II Associated: Error in glucose metabolism, hepatic insufficiency, congestive heart failure, albuminuria.

Etiology: ?†

Pathogenesis: The basic defect is focal parakeratotic keratinization through all layers of the epidermis that results in keratin-dermal contact. When this occurs a granulomatous reaction may ensue.†

Related Facts
I **Sex Ratio:** M2:F3
II **Risk of Occurrence:** Rare
III **Risk of Recurrence for**
      Patient's Sib: ?
      Patient's Child: ?
IV **Age of Detectability:** After 20th year by clinical observation.
V **Prevalence:** Rare

Treatment
I **Primary Prevention:** —
II **Secondary Prevention:** —
III **Other Therapy:** —

Prognosis: Good for life span and function. May be poor esthetically.

Detection of Carrier: —

†Special Considerations: Genodermatosis is not confirmed and only presupposed on the basis of some sibs reported with the disorder. No generation order has been reported. Perforating folliculitis has been proposed for a common acute, follicular eruption similar to Kyrle disease. In this disorder the foreign body is fractured hair shaft while in Kyrle disease keratin from parakeratinization is the foreign body. There most likely is an idiopathic and acquired form; however, the pathogenesis common to both is the chronic parakeratinization of the epidermal cells which may or may not be follicular.

References:
Carter, V.H. and Constantine, V.S.: Kyrle's disease: I. Clinical findings in 5 cases and review of literature. Arch. Dermatol. 97:624, 1968.
Constantine, V.S. and Carter, V.H.: Kyrle's disease: II. Histopathologic findings in 5 cases and review of literature. Arch. Dermatol. 97:633, 1968.
Tappeiner, J. et al: Morbus Kyrle. Hautarzt 20:296, 1969.

Contributor: **Vernon H. Carter**

Editor's Computerized Descriptor: Skin

LABYRINTH APLASIA

Includes: Aplasie labyrinthique
Aplasie der labyrinths
Aplasia del laberinto
Agenesis of inner ear
Michel malformation of inner ear
Inner ear, aplasia

Excludes: Partial aplasias or dysplasias of the inner ear, eg Mondini and Scheibe malformations
Total obliteration of the inner ear caused by new bone formation following suppurative labyrinthitis

Minimal Diagnostic Criteria: Total absence of hearing and vestibular response, either unilateral or bilateral, and xrays which show absence of inner ear structure and internal auditory meatus.

Clinical Findings: Labyrinthine aplasia is a developmental anomaly which occurs as a result of dysplasia of the petrous bone. The degree of hearing loss may not be suspected until the child or infant fails to respond to sound after an adequate trial with powerful hearing aids. The pinna, external canal and tympanic membrane are nearly always normal, and facial nerve function is usually intact. Vestibular symptoms are usually absent, but caloric examination shows no peripheral vestibular response.

If the deformity is unilateral and involves only the inner ear the hearing loss may go undetected for a number of years, since the child uses his normal ear to acquire speech and language. The total hearing loss may only be found after school screening audiometry shows a hearing loss which is confirmed by further testing.

Aplasia of the inner ear may be suggested by absence of bony inner ear cavities and the internal auditory meatus on standard mastoid films. It is confirmed by petrous pyramid polytomography which also shows a normal middle ear and external canal.

At autopsy the petrous bone may show aplasia or hypoplasia. Aplasia is very rare. At times there may be spaces in the bony labyrinth which do not, however, resemble in any way inner ear structures. In Michel's original case the stapes and stapedius tendon were also absent.†

Complications
I **Derived:** Inability to acquire speech and language through the auditory route, even with amplification, if the defect is bilateral.
II **Associated:** Absence of stapes and stapedius tendon. Mental retardation is said by Ormerod to occur "often." However, some of the retardation may have been secondary to total hearing deficit.

Etiology: Unknown except in those cases of maternal ingestion of thalidomide during pregnancy.

Pathogenesis: ?

Related Facts
I **Sex Ratio:** ?
II **Risk of Occurrence:** ?
III **Risk of Recurrence for**
 Patient's Sib: ?
 Patient's Child: ?
IV **Age of Detectability:** Potentially in infancy by petrous pyramid polytomography.
V **Prevalence:** Thought to occur in about 1% of congenitally deaf children who have severe to profound sensorineural hearing loss (Ormerod).

Treatment
I **Primary Prevention:** —
II **Secondary Prevention:** Unilateral: hearing conservation to

prevent injury to the normal ear. Bilateral: prompt institution of methods other than auditory for language acquisition.

III Other Therapy: —

Prognosis: Normal for life span. With advancing age and related changes in the central vestibular system or with acquired visual problems, eg cataracts of old age, some symptomatic vestibular problems, possibly disabling, might occur if defect is bilateral.

Detection of Carrier: Not applicable

†Special Considerations: The patient may show no response to sound at all if the malformation is bilateral. Behavioral audiometry, play conditioning, reflex responses, evoked response audiometry, and psychogalvanometric skin response audiometry all fail to elicit valid hearing responses. Tactile responses to low frequencies presented by bone conduction may be falsely interpreted as true hearing responses.

Apparent lack of response to amplified sound is an indication for petrous pyramid polytomography. Absence of the inner ear will then indicate that training should be redirected into manual and visual methods as early as possible so that acquisition of language and its dependent skills, reading and writing, may be optimum.

In the few instances in which the mother ingested thalidomide during early pregnancy the external ear, canal and facial nerve all may be abnormal or absent. In thalidomide ears there has been absence of the internal auditory canal, inner ear, facial, and VIII cranial nerves.

References:
Ormerod, F.C.: The pathology of congenital deafness. J. Laryngol. 74:919, 1960.
Schuknecht, H.F.: Pathology of sensorineural deafness of genetic origin. In McConnell, F. and Wards, P.H. (eds.): Deafness in Childhood. Nashville: Vanderbilt University Press, 1967, p. 69.
Valvassori, E.E. et al: Inner ear anomalies: Clinical and histopathological considerations. Ann. Otol. Rhinol. Laryngol. 78:929, 1969.

Contributor: **LaVonne Bergstrom**

Editor's Computerized Descriptors: Hearing, Ear, Speech, Skel.

563
558-500
LACRIMAL CANALICULUS ATRESIA

Includes: Atrésie des canaux lacrymaux
Tränengangsatresie
Atresia del canalículo lacrimal
Atresia of canaliculus and punctum
Absence of lacrimal canaliculus, complete or incomplete

Excludes: Congenital impatency of nasolacrimal ducts

Minimal Diagnostic Criteria: See anatomic considerations below.

Clinical Findings: Absence of the punctum invariably occurs in the absence of the canaliculus, whereas atresia of the punctum may occur with intact canaliculus. The patient presents with epiphora (tearing) if both canaliculi on 1 side are missing, and also if only the upper is present. Presence of the lower punctum and canaliculus usually is sufficient to prevent tearing. Absence of the total lacrimal passage is frequently secondary to gross malformations such as cyclopia, arrhinencephaly or cryptophthalmos. Absence of the punctum and canaliculus may be secondary to a coloboma of the eyelid.

Complications
I   Derived: Epiphora. The incidence of dacryocystitis is increased.
II Associated: —

Etiology: Usually secondary to an autosomal dominant gene with variable penetrance and expression. Some cases are secondary to gross malformations. Some sporadic cases are thought to be secondary to amniotic bands.

Pathogenesis: Lack of or incomplete outbudding of the superior end of the ectodermal core which sinks into the mesoderm at the facial fissure.

Related Facts
I   Sex Ratio: ? But no deviation from M1:F1 is reported.
II Risk of Occurrence: ? But absence of punctum and canaliculus is considered rare whereas atresia of punctum is considered relatively common.
III Risk of Recurrence for
    Patient's Sib: When autosomal dominant and parent is affected, < 1 in 2 (< 50%) for each offspring to be affected; otherwise not increased.
    Patient's Child: < 1 in 2
IV Age of Detectability: At birth
V   Prevalence: ?

Treatment
I   Primary Prevention: Genetic counseling
II Secondary Prevention: Insertion of silastic tubing to create an endothelized channel meets with variable success. If an atretic punctum is present, probing may establish a channel to the canaliculus.
III Other Therapy: Topical and, if necessary, systemic antibiotics and hot compresses if inflammation occurs.

Prognosis: Normal life span, if isolated; prognosis of gross malformation, if secondary. Repeated inflammation can be expected if it once occurs.

Detection of Carrier: Affected parent and patient

Special Considerations: —

References:
Duke-Elder, S.: System of Ophthalmology. vol. 3, pt. 2. Congenital Deformities. St Louis: C.V. Mosby, 1963. p. 923.
Waardenburg, P.J. et al: Genetics and Ophthalmology. Oxford: Blackwell Scientific Publications, 1961, vol. 1, p. 293.
Werb, A.: The management of canalicular occlusion. Trans. Ophthalmol. Soc. NZ 28:41, 1976.

Contributor: **Donald R. Bergsma**

LACRIMAL GLAND, ECTOPIC

Includes: Ectopie des glandes lacrymales
Ektopie der Tränendrüse
Glándula lacrimal ectópica
Aberrant lacrimal gland
Congenital dislocation of lacrimal gland

Excludes: Prolapse of normal lacrimal gland

Minimal Diagnostic Criteria: As indicated under Clinical Findings, histologic examination to rule out neoplasm

Clinical Findings: Ectopic lacrimal gland tissue is most often seen under the palpebral or bulbar conjunctiva, particularly in the lateral half of the globe. Differentiation from a true neoplasm is of practical importance. Ectopic lacrimal gland has also been described in the uveal tract and in the orbit.

Complications
I **Derived:** There may be spread of the tissue onto the cornea with visual impairment. It may lie on the lateral rectus giving rise to a strabismus.
II **Associated:** Blepharochalasis, coloboma of the lids

Etiology: ?

Pathogenesis: ?

Related Facts
I **Sex Ratio:** M1:F1
II **Risk of Occurrence:** ? Rare
III **Risk of Recurrence for**
Patient's Sib: ?
Patient's Child: ?
IV **Age of Detectability:** At birth
V **Prevalence:** ? Rare

Treatment
I **Primary Prevention:** —
II **Secondary Prevention:** —
III **Other Therapy:** Surgical removal for cosmetic purposes and histologic confirmation

Prognosis: Good, no visual impairment or threat to life unless neoplasm is present.

Detection of Carrier: —

Special Considerations: —

References:
Dallachy, R.: Ectopic lacrimal glandular tissue within the eyeball. Br. J. Ophthalmol. 45:808, 1961.
Duke-Elder, S.: System of Ophthalmology. vol. 3, pt. 2. Congenital Deformities. London: Henry Kimpton, 1964.
Green, W.R. and Zimmerman, L.E.: Ectopic lacrimal gland tissue: Report of 8 cases with orbital involvement. Arch. Ophthalmol. 78:318, 1967.

Contributor: **Morton E. Smith**

Editor's Computerized Descriptor: Eye

Includes: Fistule des voies lacrymales
Tränensackfistel
Fístula del saco lacrimal
Lacrimal passage ectasia
Fistula of lacrimal sac

Excludes: Puncta and canaliculi, supernumerary (844)
Lacrimal sac fistula secondary to trauma

Minimal Diagnostic Criteria: Opening from lacrimal passage to skin

Clinical Findings: Simple lacrimal fistula presents a small opening on the upper nasal aspect of the cheek through which tear fluid drains. Larger ectasia of the lacrimal passage is often part of a facial cleft accompanied by other malformations such as colobomata of the lids, cleft lip or palate, dermoids, deformed auricles, defects in the orbital bones with encephalocele, etc.

Complications
I **Derived:** Dacryocystitis (often the presenting problem)
II **Associated:** See Clinical Findings.

Etiology: ?

Pathogenesis: There are 2 major theories: persistence of the embryonic facial cleft between the nasal and maxillary processes, and trauma caused by amniotic bands.

Related Facts
I **Sex Ratio:** ?
II **Risk of Occurrence:** ? But rare. Highest estimate is 1 in 4000 live births.
III **Risk of Recurrence for**
Patient's Sib: ? Familial grouping has seldom been reported.
Patient's Child: ?
IV **Age of Detectability:** At birth
V **Prevalence:** ? But rare

Treatment
I **Primary Prevention:** —
II **Secondary Prevention:** Excision of the fistulous tract, probing or dacryocystorhinostomy if lacrimal passage to nose is blocked.
III **Other Therapy:** Topical antibiotics and hot compresses if inflammation occurs.

Prognosis: Normal life span unless part of larger syndrome. Repeated inflammation can be expected if it once occurs.

Detection of Carrier: ?

Special Considerations: —

References:
Bacskulin, J. and Bacskulin, E.: Klinik und Therapie der kongenitalen Tränensackfisteln. Folia Ophthalmol. Jap. 17:1026, 1966.
Duke-Elder, S.: System of Ophthalmology, vol. 3, pt. 2. Congenital Deformities. St. Louis: C.V. Mosby, 1963, p. 924.
Masi, A.: Congenital fistula of the lacrimal sac. Arch. Ophthalmol 81:701, 1969.

Contributor: **Donald R. Bergsma**

Editor's Computerized Descriptors: Eye, Skin

Includes: Déficit congénital en lactase
Angeborener Laktasemangel
Deficiencia congénita en lactasa
Early-onset alactasia
Hereditary lactase deficiency (insufficiency)
Congenital alactasia

Excludes: Acquired and secondary lactase deficiency
Lactase deficiency, primary (567)
Lactose intolerance (569)
Sucrase-isomaltase deficiency (920)
Glucose-galactose malabsorption (419)
Monosaccharide intolerance

Minimal Diagnostic Criteria: Fermentative diarrhea from birth with lactose ingestion, absent with other carbohydrates. Deliberate feeding of measured dose of lactose yields flat serum glucose curve, abdominal discomfort, explosive stool of pH below 5.0 with reducing sugars. These findings do not occur on feeding glucose, galactose or sucrose. If one is certain that the condition is hereditary, these criteria may suffice if the patient's condition precludes peroral biopsy. In all other instances it is essential to demonstrate normal intestinal histology with decreased or absent lactase activity.†

Clinical Findings: Symptoms of fermentative diarrhea (100%) and failure to thrive (100%) begin with initial ingestion of lactose (in human or cow's milk) at birth. Infants almost always have abdominal distention, suffer crampy abdominal pain and vomit sporadically. They usually appear to be very hungry, despite diarrhea, unless the debilitating effects of secondary dehydration, acidosis and inanition supervene. Diarrhea clears as soon as lactose is removed from the diet.

The stool is fluid and quite frothy from contained gas as it is passed, usually explosively. The pH of fresh stool is always below 5.0 if lactose has been ingested; such stool usually contains reducing sugars which can be identified as one or more of the following: lactose, glucose and galactose. Lactosuria occurs in about a third of the patients. Ingestion of a standard dose of lactose (1.5-2.0 gm/kg or 45-60 gm/m^2) is always associated with a flat 3 hour "tolerance curve" for serum glucose; the test dose almost universally produces clinical discomfort and explosive diarrhea during the 3 hour observation period. Accordingly, the oral loading test should be performed in a diarrhea-free period.

Peroral biopsy specimen of the upper small intestinal mucosa is histologically normal, but contains decreased β glycosidase (lactase) activity when this is compared with the activity of the maltose, sucrose or isomaltose digesting enzymes, or when assayed in relation to unit weight of tissue, or to protein content of the tissue.

Complications
I **Derived:** Dehydration, electrolyte and acid-base disturbance in almost 100% of cases.
II **Associated:** Failure to thrive, or death, in all cases if correct diagnosis is not made or treatment instituted early enough.

Etiology: Possibly autosomal recessive

Pathogenesis: Ingested lactose is not hydrolyzed to the component monosaccharides in the upper small intestine as in normal individuals and therefore passes undigested to the colon. Here the disaccharide is hydrolyzed and fermented and resultant mixture contains 2 and 3 carbon volatile acids, glucose and galactose, and often some undigested lactose. The increase in osmolarity of the colonic contents induces net flux of water into the lumen. A combination of the irritant effect of excessive fermentation, increased colonic gas and distention of the bowel walls by the increase in fluid results in explosive passage of the loose stool.

Related Facts
I **Sex Ratio:** M1:F1 probable (from 19 cases described)
II **Risk of Occurrence:** ?
III **Risk of Recurrence for**
 Patient's Sib: Probably 1 in 4 (25%) for each offspring to be affected
 Patient's Child: Not increased unless mate is carrier or homozygote
IV **Age of Detectability:** At birth, by lactose loading test and assay of enzymes in intestinal mucosal biopsy specimen
V **Prevalence:** ?

Treatment
I **Primary Prevention:** Genetic counseling
II **Secondary Prevention:** Avoidance of lactose in the diet. This includes all forms of mammalian milk and milk products. Small amounts of milk solids in foods may be tolerated by some patients.
III **Other Therapy:** Fluid and electrolyte support may be necessitated during the diarrhea activity which results from upsets with lactose ingestion.

Prognosis: Current indications are for normal life span if patient is diagnosed and treated early. If not recognized in infancy, patients may die of severe inanition and electrolyte disturbances.

Detection of Carrier: Lactase activity has not been investigated in heterozygotes.

†Special Considerations: The condition must be distinguished from 2 closely allied conditions: 1) Durant first described, and others also reported, infants with diarrhea on ingestion of lactose. These patients additionally displayed excessive vomiting, lactosemia, lactosuria, other urinary sugars, aminoaciduria or renal acidosis. Lactase activity was not studied in these patients and the outcomes varied from clearance of the intolerance to lactose to death in infancy. (See Lactose Intolerance). 2) Infants may develop transitory lactose intolerance in the course of acute diarrhea of presumed infectious origin. These infants also display lactosemia and lactosuria. Although confirmatory biopsy is not available in all cases, it is assumed that the defect in lactose absorption is secondary to temporary mucosal damage and secondary loss of enzyme activity which returns to normal after a number of weeks or months on a lactose-free diet.

It is generally difficult to differentiate congenital lactase deficiency from secondary defects in the young infant. However, lactosemia, lactosuria, presence of other urinary sugars, histologically abnormal intestinal mucosal specimens and development of tolerance to lactose after a period of its withdrawal from the diet all point away from the diagnosis of congenital lactase deficiency. (See also Special Considerations for Primary Lactase Deficiency).

References:
Davidson, M.: Disaccharide intolerance. Pediatr. Clin. North Am. 14:93, 1967.
Holzel, A.: Development of intestinal enzyme systems and its relation to diarrhoea. Pediatr. Clin. North Am. 12:635, 1965.
Levin, B. et al: Congenital lactose malabsorption. Arch. Dis. Child. 45:173, 1970.
Prader, A. and Auricchio, S.: Defects of intestinal disaccharide absorption. Annu. Rev. Med. 16:345, 1965.

Contributor: **Murray Davidson**

Editor's Computerized Descriptor: GI.

LACTASE DEFICIENCY, PRIMARY

Includes: Déficit primaire en lactase
Primärer Laktasemangel
Deficiencia primaria de lactasa
Late-onset alactasia
Adult lactase deficiency
Adult lactose intolerance
Noncongenital isolated lactase deficiency (insufficiency)
Racial lactase deficiency
Primary lactase deficiency

Excludes: Acquired and secondary lactase deficiency
Lactose intolerance (569)
Monosaccharide intolerance
Sucrase-isomaltase deficiency (920)
Lactase deficiency, congenital (566)

Minimal Diagnostic Criteria: Patients must have a history of normal tolerance to mammalian milk in infancy with development of clinical intolerance to lactose-containing foods in later childhood or adult life. The discomfort, bloating and fermentative diarrhea which occur with lactose ingestion should be absent with other carbohydrates. Ingestion of a standard dose of lactose (15-20 gm/kg or 45-60 gm/m^2) is always associated with a flat 3-hour "tolerance curve" for serum glucose; in some reports the clinical discomfort and explosive diarrhea, usually associated with the test among children with congenital lactase deficiency, was not observed at these doses among adults with primary lactase deficiency. However, feeding of 100 gm/m^2 produces symptoms more uniformly. The loose stools are pH below 5.0 and contain any or all of lactose, glucose and galactose. These findings do not occur on feeding glucose, galactose or sucrose.

Peroral biopsy is necessary to distinguish patients from those with secondary forms of insufficiency. Peroral biopsy specimen of the upper small intestinal mucosa is histologically normal, but contains decreased β-glycosidase (lactase) activity when this is compared with the activity of the maltose, sucrose or isomaltose digesting enzymes, or when assayed in relation to unit weight of tissue or to protein content of the tissue.†

Clinical Findings: Ingestion of milk or other lactose-containing foods usually causes abdominal bloating, cramping and sometimes diarrhea. The difficulty is absent in infants and appears in childhood or in adult life. Individuals with primary lactase deficiency are frequently asymptomatic, if it is their normal pattern not to ingest significant quantities of milk and milk products.

The syndrome has been reported from a number of laboratories to occur in Caucasian adults, as an explanation for "milk allergy." In the United States the adult deficiency is reported with increased frequency among Blacks and Orientals.†

Complications
I **Derived:** While dehydration, electrolyte and acid base disturbances, plus failure to thrive are theoretically possible in individuals with primary lactase deficiency (similar to those of individuals with congenital lactase deficiency) these are not reported. A combination of larger body size, less dependence on milk as an important dietary constituent, and less total diminution of lactase activity than in patients affected with congenital lactase deficiency may account for the differences in incidence of these complications.
II **Associated:** —

Etiology: Probably autosomal dominant

Pathogenesis: It seems likely that individuals with primary lactase deficiency have normal lactase activity at birth, although this has not been proved. Gradual reduction in production of this enzyme with aging ultimately reduces lactase activity below a threshold level. From this time on, ingested lactose is not hydrolyzed to the component monosaccharides in the upper small intestine, as in normal individuals, and passes undigested to the colon. In this organ the disaccharide is hydrolyzed and fermented and the resultant mixture contains 2 and 3 carbon volatile acids, glucose and galactose, and often some undigested lactose. The increase in osmolality of the colonic contents induces net flux of water to the lumen. A combination of the irritant effect of the excessive fermentation, increased colonic gas and distention of the bowel wall by the increase in fluid, results in explosive passage of the loose stool.

Related Facts
I   **Sex Ratio:**   M1:F1 probable
II **Risk of Occurrence:**   ? generally; more than 50% of American Blacks.
III **Risk of Recurrence for**
    Patient's Sib: Probably 50-100% for each offspring to be affected
    Patient's Child: Probably 50-100%. If mate is carrier or homozygote probability is 100%.
IV **Age of Detectability:**   In late childhood or adult life, by lactose loading test and assay of enzymes in intestinal mucosal biopsy specimen
V   **Prevalence:**   Cook has demonstrated an increased incidence among the Baganda children and adults in neighboring Bantu tribes of Uganda. Other Ugandan tribes, the Rwanda and Ankole, most of whom have an Hamitic ancestry, have much higher levels of lactase. Kretchmer similarly reports deficiency among the Yoruba, Hausa, and Ibo while the Fulani are lactose tolerant among the tribes of Nigeria. Since the unions of Yoruba and Europeans produce offspring who are approximately 50% nondigesters of lactose, he concludes that the allele is dominant. Nondigesters are virtually 100% of pure Greenland Eskimos. The increased incidence of deficiency among Blacks and Orientals in the United States also suggests a genetic etiology. Ferguson and Maxwell report a Caucasian sibship in which 2 of 6 children demonstrated hypolactasia. The parents were normal. These latter data raise a question with respect to dominance of the allele, but may be explained by variable penetrance.

Treatment
I   **Primary Prevention:** —
II **Secondary Prevention:**   Avoidance of lactose in the diet. This includes all forms of mammalian milk and milk products. Small amounts of milk solids in foods may be tolerated by some patients. Patients and their physicians should be aware of the common use of lactose as the major component of most medicinal pills.
III **Other Therapy:**   Fluid and electrolyte support may be necessitated during the diarrheal activity which results from upsets with lactose ingestion.

Prognosis: Excellent for life and freedom from morbidity if lactose is avoided in the diet.

Detection of Carrier: ?

†**Special Considerations:**   The condition may be a variant of congenital lactase deficiency. It has been postulated that 3 alleles may occupy the locus which controls lactase production, with the normal gene dominant, the others being recessive.

Secondary lactase deficiency may be differentiated from the primary defect by 4 distinguishing criteria: 1) Mucosal biopsy specimens from patients with primary lactase deficiency are normal on histologic examination but are distorted in accordance with the appropriate underlying condition among patients with secondary lactase deficiency. 2) In primary lactase deficiency, reduction of lactase activity in mucosal specimens is isolated, while in secondary deficiencies there is loss of activity of all disaccharidases. With ingestion of lactose, both groups would demonstrate flat serum glucose curves and GI intolerance. 3) However, lactosemia, lactosuria and presence of other urinary sugars are reported only with secondary deficiencies. 4) Development of tolerance to lactose after a period of its withdrawal from the diet, or after treatment for an underlying malabsorptive condition, precludes the diagnosis of primary lactase deficiency.

References:
Bayless, T. M. and Rosensweig, N. S.: A racial difference in incidence of lactase deficiency: A survey of milk intolerance and lactase deficiency in healthy adult males. JAMA 197:968, 1966.
Chung, M. H. and McGill, D. B.: Lactase deficiency in Orientals. Gastroenterology 54:255, 1968.
Cook, G. C. and Kajubi, S. K.: Tribal incidence of lactase deficiency in Uganda. Lancet 1:725, 1966.
Dahlqvist, A. and Lindquist, B.: Lactose intolerance and protein malnutrition. Acta Paediatr. Scand. 60:488, 1971.
Ferguson, A. and Maxwell, J. D.: Genetic aetiology of lactose intolerance. Lancet 2:188, 1967.
Kretchmer, N.: Memorial lecture: Lactose and lactase - a historical perspective. Gastroenterology 61:805, 1971.
Ransome-Kuti, O. et al: A genetic study of lactose digestion in Nigerian families. Gastroenterology 68:431, 1975.

Contributor: **Murray Davidson**

Editor's Computerized Descriptor: GI.

LACTATE DEHYDROGENASE ISOZYMES

Includes: Lactate déshydrogénase
Laktat Dehydrogenase
Lactato deshidrogenasa
Nicotinamide adenine dinucleotide and oxidoreductase

Excludes: —

Minimal Diagnostic Criteria: Relatively simple electrophoretic techniques are available for determining the isozyme composition of tissues and body fluids. In normal serum, LDH isozymes are present in the following proportions: LDH-2 > LDH-1 > LDH-3 > LDH-4 > LDH-5. A variety of diseases exhibit unique changes in serum isozyme patterns. LDH-1 is markedly increased in myocardial infarction, and LDH-5 in infectious hepatitis.

Analysis of tissue isozyme patterns may also have diagnostic application. In chickens and humans a form of muscular dystrophy is associated with a failure of development of the adult isozyme pattern. Whether this abnormality is a primary or secondary event is unknown. These findings suggest that isozymic analyses may be helpful in determining at what period of development a metabolic abnormality occurs.†

Clinical Findings: Abnormal elevation or depression of lactate dehydrogenase isozymes are associated with certain disease states but are not proved causes thereof.† Lactate dehydrogenase (LDH) is an enzyme of the Embden-Myerhoff pathway which catalyzes the interconversion of pyruvate and lactate. Nicotinamide adenine dinucleotide (NAD) is a specific cofactor, NAD being formed during the reduction of pyruvate and nicotinamide adenine dehydrogenase (NADH) during the oxidation of lactate.

LDH exists in multiple molecular forms (isozymes) in the somatic and gametic tissues of many mammalian and avian species. Five molecular forms of LDH are present in human somatic tissues: LDH-1, LDH-2, LDH-3, LDH-4 and LDH-5. The type and amount of the molecular forms vary for each tissue. In adult human heart and kidney, the major forms are LDH-1, LDH-2 and LDH-3, whereas in adult human muscle and liver the dominant form is LDH-5. Multiple forms of LDH may exist in single cells. Thus hemolysates of thoroughly washed erythrocytes exhibit 3 isozymes, LDH-1, LDH-2 and LDH-3. A 6th isozymic form of LDH (LDH-X) appears in testis at the time of puberty. LDH-X is the predominant form of LDH in sperm.

The relative distribution of isozymes in each human tissue changes during development. In heart, for example, the pattern exhibited by adults is not attained until 3 years of age. In testis, the adult complement of isozymes appears at the time of puberty. Thus each tissue exhibits a unique profile of isozyme development.

Complications
I   **Derived:** —
II **Associated:** Myocardial infarction, infectious hepatitis, hemolytic disorders, meningitis and muscular dystrophy

Etiology: Autosomal dominant transmission of isozymes. Discovery of polypeptide A and B variants in human and animal tissues, together with appropriate genetic studies, showed that the synthesis of A and B polypeptides is controlled by 2 separate nonallelic genes. Observations on pigeon testes have shown that the synthesis of the LDH-X subunit (C) is controlled by a 3rd genetic locus in the pigeon. The total complement of LDH isozymes can be explained on the basis of the activity of genes at 3 loci, A, B

and C, each being responsible for the synthesis of a corresponding polypeptide. The C locus, in contrast to the other loci, is not activated until pubescence in the male and remains inactive in the female.

Pathogenesis: —

Related Facts
I   **Sex Ratio:** For LDH-1, -2, -3, -4 and -5 M1:F1; for LDH-X M1:F0
II   **Risk of Occurrence:** Normally present
III **Risk of Recurrence for**
    Patient's Sib: 1 in 2 (50%) for each offspring for each appropriate LDH
    Patient's Child: 1 in 2
IV **Age of Detectability:** Adult isozyme pattern in heart at age 3 and LDH-X in testis at puberty
V   **Prevalence:** Each isozyme normally present at proper age and in appropriate tissue

Treatment
I   **Primary Prevention:** Not applicable
II   **Secondary Prevention:** Not applicable
III **Other Therapy:** —

Prognosis: Normal life span

Detection of Carrier: —

†Special Considerations: Molecular forms of lactate dehydrogenase (LDH) in heart and kidney are to a large extent different from those in muscle and liver. Each tissue exhibits characteristic changes of the isozyme patterns during development, and in at least one tissue, the testis, an entirely new isozyme appears at the time of puberty. Isozymic analysis of tissues and body fluids may aid in diagnosing certain diseases - myocardial infarction, infectious hepatitis, hemolytic disorders, meningitis, etc. Also further studies on the molecular heterogeneity of LDH, as well as other enzymes, will increase our understanding of the biochemical processes that accompany growth and development.

References:
Markert, C. L.: Epigenetic control of specific protein synthesis in differentiating cells. In Locke, M. (ed.): Cytodifferentiation and Macromolecular Synthesis. New York:Academic Press, 1963, p. 65.
Wroblewski, F. and Gregory, K. K.: Lactic dehydrogenase isozymes and their distribution in normal tissues and plasma and in disease states. Ann. N. Y. Acad. Sci. 94:912, 1961.
Zinkham, W. H.: Lactate dehydrogenase isozymes of testis and sperm: Biological and biochemical properties and genetic control. Ann. N. Y. Acad. Sci. 151:598, 1968.
Zinkham, W. H. et al: Isozymes: Biological and clinical significance. Pediatrics 37:120, 1966.

Contributor: **William H. Zinkham**

Editor's Computerized Descriptors: Muscle, Liver, CV.

LACTOSE INTOLERANCE

Includes: Intolérance au lactose
Laktoseintoleranz
Intolerancia a la lactosa

Excludes: Monosaccharide malabsorption
Sucrase-isomaltase deficiency (920)
Acquired or symptomatic disaccharidase deficiency syndromes
  due to celiac disease
Protein malnutrition (kwashiorkor)
Lactase deficiency, congenital (566)

Minimal Diagnostic Criteria: The lactose intolerance can
be studied with blood sugar curves after lactose oral loading tests (2 gm/kg/body wt or 50 gm/m^2 body surface area,
dissolved in water). The oral loading tests must be performed in a diarrhea-free period, that is, after eliminating
the lactose from the food. The values which do not exceed
20 mg above fasting level are rather indicative of an impaired lactose digestion. As a consequence of such loading,
diarrhea is present. By contrast, ingestion of the 2 monosaccharides, glucose and galactose, which constitute the
lactose (1 gm/kg/body wt), does not lead to diarrhea, does
not cause pH and lactic acid changes in the feces, and is
followed by a normal increase of blood glucose. The direct
assay of lactase activities in a peroral suction biopsy of the
intestinal mucosa is the method for confirming the diagnosis. Absence of lactase activity in the presence of other
disaccharidases can be considered very important proof.

Lactase activity is usually reduced to near zero but less
than 5 units of lactase per gm of protein in a mucosal biopsy
may be regarded as lactase deficiency, whereas over 10
units per gm is considered normal. A single biopsy may be
misleading.

Follow-up study must demonstrate that the defect is permanent; a diagnosis of lactose intolerance could be dis-
carded, if a regressive evolution and an early reappearance
of intestinal lactase activity after withdrawal of lactose
from the diet, is noted.

Clinical Findings: Fermentative diarrhea from the 1st days of
life in a milk-fed baby (100%); followed, if severe, by dehydration
and failure to thrive (94%) and if prolonged, by malnutrition;
sometimes associated with abdominal distention, cramping pain,
flatulence and rarely with vomiting.

Fecal pH below 6 and sometimes closer to 5 (100%), large quantities of low molecular weight organic acids and more than 1 mg
of lactic acid in random samples of 1 gm dried feces (90%); lactose
or glucose plus galactose are excreted in the feces (53%); in about
34% of patients there was a discrete lactosuria (often > 500
mg/100 cc); steatorrhea is unusual but it may occur.

Complications
I   **Derived:** A few patients manifest possible lesions of the intes-
    tinal mucosa, malabsorption of fat monosaccharides and also
    xylose; rarely, a complicating atrophy of the intestinal
    mucosa followed by severe manifestations and malnutrition
    may occur.
II **Associated:** —

Etiology: Possibly autosomal recessive transmission. (See Special
Considerations for Primary Lactase Deficiency.)

Pathogenesis: The symptoms from lactase 1 deficiency
only appear after ingestion of lactose. Deficient hydrolysis
of lactose leads to the retention of sugar in the gut, with an
increase in osmotic pressure and a compensatory influx of
water in the intestinal lumen.

That, and bacterial fermentation resulting in the formation of abnormal quantities of short-chain fatty acids and
especially of lactic acid, cause the evacuation of frequent,
frothy, sour-smelling stools. There may be a slight increase
in the passage of unhydrolyzed lactose into blood and this
is reflected by an increase in excretion of lactose in urine.

In any case, however, it is justified to distinguish between 2 types of "congenital lactose intolerance" because
of the absence or the presence of lactosuria. Lactosuria is
a feature which is related to the amount of lactose in the
gut and to possible lesions of the intestinal mucosa.†

Related Facts
I   **Sex Ratio:** M1:F1
II   **Risk of Occurrence:** ?
III **Risk of Recurrence for**
       Patient's Sib: —
       Patient's Child: —
IV   **Age of Detectability:** First week of life by lactose tolerance
       tests and in vitro assay of mucosal disaccharidase activity
V   **Prevalence:** ?

Treatment
I   **Primary Prevention:** —
II   **Secondary Prevention:** Exclusion of lactose from the diet
       results in a prompt cessation of all symptoms; a too-early
       resumption of milk feeding may end in the reappearance of
       all symptoms. Most patients are able to tolerate small
       amounts of lactose.
III **Other Therapy:** Replacing milk by a lactose-free soya prepa-
       ration with added sucrose or dextri-maltose. Other milk
       preparations and synthetic milk without lactose are known.
       An alternative treatment is to give lactase by mouth with
       each milk feeding or better, first to incubate with lactase in
       order to split the nonabsorbable lactose into absorbable
       monosaccharides glucose and galactose.

Prognosis: Its severity depends on the amount of lactose
ingested, the amount of intestinal lactase, and the presence
of secondary lesions of intestinal mucosa. A severe form
carries a poor prognosis since 12 of the 21 patients reported
died; 14 of the 21 cases treated with a proper diet showed
clinical improvement, although 5 of them subsequently
died. The other case has a more benign course and appears
to respond rapidly to therapy.

Follow-up studies are scarce, but seem to indicate that
surviving patients have normal carbohydrate absorption as
well as negative disaccharide excretion after 2 years of age.
The prognosis in acquired lactose intolerance is excellent
as long as lactose is omitted from the diet.

Detection of Carrier: ?

†**Special Considerations:** Intestinal lactase 1 deficiency or
absence. It is known that 2 distinct mucosal enzymes have
lactase activity. The lactase 1 is the enzyme that hydrolyzes
lactose and cellobiose in the intestine. This enzyme is
located in the brush-border. Lactase 2 which is present,
either soluble in the cytoplasm or in lysosomes, accounts
for a small fraction of the total lactase activity and hydrolyzes hetero-β-galactosides. The absence for a long time of
lactase 1 activity supports the finding that the condition
may be an inborn error. An argument favoring the existence of congenital lactase deficiency is the occurrence of
the disease in sibs, as shown in some families. Secondary
lactase deficiency to gastroenteric infections or disturbances occurs more frequently. All or most disaccharidases
may be reduced subsequent to intestinal and other disease.
As a rule, lactase is the first enzyme to disappear and the
last to return on recovery.

References:
Durand, P. (ed.): Disorders Due to Intestinal Defective Carbohydrate Digestion and Absorption. New York:Grune and Stratton, 1964.

Frézal, J. and Rey, J.: Inborn errors of digestive enzymes. Proc. 3rd Int. Congr. Hum. Genet., Chicago, 1966. Baltimore:Johns Hopkins Press, 1967, p. 153.

Holzel, A.: Sugar malabsorption due to deficiencies of disaccharidase activities and of monosaccharide transport. Arch. Dis. Child. 42:341, 1967.

Contributor: **Paolo Durand**

Editor's Computerized Descriptor: GI.

LARSEN SYNDROME

Includes: Syndrome de Larsen
Síndrome de Larsen
Multiple congenital dislocations with unusual facies and skeletal abnormalities

Excludes: Arthrogryposis (88)

Minimal Diagnostic Criteria: Flat facies with depressed nasal bridge and prominent forehead; dislocations of multiple major joints and cylindrical, nontapering fingers.†

Clinical Findings: Congenital joint dislocations, usually bilaterally, involving the elbows, hips and knees (typically anterior dislocation of the tibia on the femur); subluxation of the shoulders; cylindrical fingers; broad, spatulate thumbs; short metacarpals; short nails; equinovarus or valgus feet; unusual facies characterized by a prominent or bossed forehead, flat and depressed nasal bridge and wide-set eyes. In addition to radiographic demonstration of the foregoing malformations, a number of skeletal anomalies may be demonstrated; a juxtacalcaneal accessory ossification center and abnormalities of vertebral segmentation especially in the upper thoracic and cervical spine.

Complications
I   **Derived:** In early infancy decreased rigidity of the cartilage of the rib cage, epiglottis, arytenoid, and possibly trachea may cause respiratory difficulties. One child died of respiratory complications following general anesthesia.
II **Associated:** Congenital heart disease and cleft palate without cleft lip are occasionally reported.

Etiology: Genetic heterogeneity is present with both autosomal dominant and autosomal recessive modes of transmission being recognized. Differentiation between the 2 forms may be difficult. McK *24560

Pathogenesis: ? The basic defect may be the mesenchymal connective tissue.

Related Facts
I   **Sex Ratio:** M1:F1
II **Risk of Occurrence:** Very rare
III **Risk of Recurrence for**
    Patient's Sib: When autosomal recessive or autosomal dominant, see Table I AR or AD, respectively.
    Patient's Child: When autosomal recessive or autosomal dominant, see Table I AR or AD, respectively.
IV **Age of Detectability:** At birth by physical examination
V   **Prevalence:** ?

Treatment
I   **Primary Prevention:** Genetic counseling
II **Secondary Prevention:** Early, intensive and continued orthopedic care
III **Other Therapy:** In cases with cleft palate, speech therapy and plastic surgery

Prognosis: Inadequate long-term data. Physically handicapped to a variable degree depending on nature and extent of patient's condition and results of orthopedic surgery.

Detection of Carrier: —

†**Special Considerations:** Cases of Larsen syndrome have been reported under other names primarily centering on the striking knee deformities: genu recurvatum; congenital hyperextension and subluxation of the knee. In arthrogryposis multiplex congenita, the facies is not unusual, the fingers taper normally, muscle mass is usually reduced and it is usually nongenetic in etiology.

References:

Gorlin, R.J. and Pindborg, J.J.: Syndromes of the Head and Neck. New York: McGraw-Hill, 1964.

Harris, R. and Cullen, C.H.: Autosomal dominant inheritance in Larsen's syndrome. Clin. Genet. 2:87, 1971.

Larsen, L.J. et al: Multiple congenital dislocations associated with characteristic facial abnormality. J. Pediatr. 37:574, 1950.

Latta, R.J. et al: Larsen's syndrome: A skeletal dysplasia with multiple joint dislocations and unusual facies. J. Pediatr. 78:291, 1971.

Steel, H.H. and Kohl, H.: Multiple congenital dislocations associated with other skeletal anomalies (Larsen's syndrome) in three siblings. J. Bone Joint Surg. 54A:75, 1972.

Contributor: **Charles I. Scott, Jr.**

Editor's Computerized Descriptors: Eye, Face, Oral, Nose, Nails, Skel., Resp., CV.

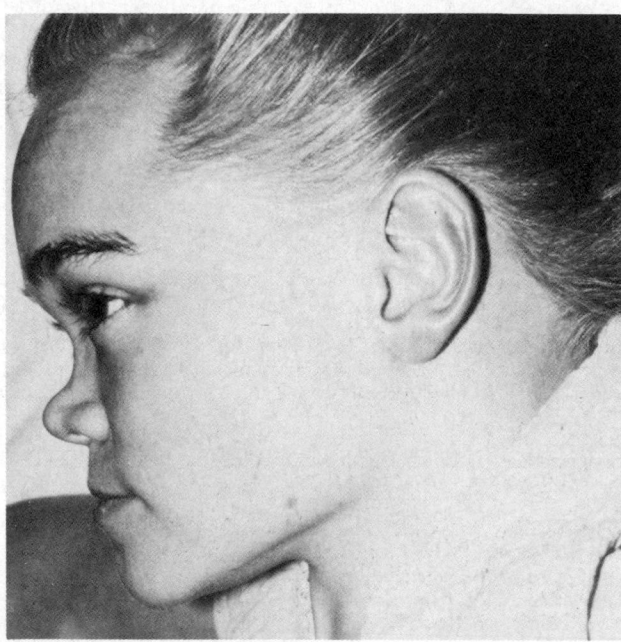

316. Profile showing depressed nasal bridge

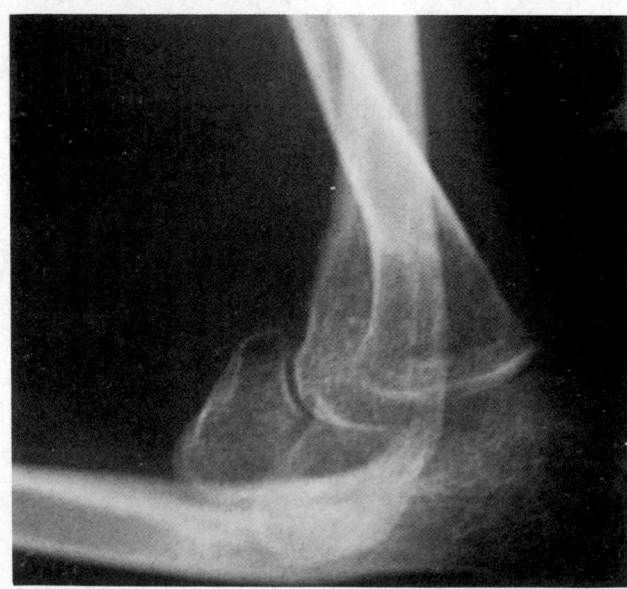

317. Right elbow, lateral view. Note joint dislocation, underdeveloped bones; accessory ulnar ossicle

LARYNGEAL ATRESIA

Includes: Atrésie laryngée
Kehlkopfatresie
Atresia laríngea
Congenital partial atresia of larynx
Stenosis at the conus elasticus
Glottic atresia
Congenital laryngeal atresia
Atresia of larynx types I, II and III

Excludes: Laryngomalacia (576)
Laryngocele (575)
Laryngeal cysts (572)
Tracheoesophageal fistula (960)
Subglottic stenosis (919)
Laryngeal web (574)

Minimal Diagnostic Criteria: Asphyxia neonatorum or stridor at birth with complete or partial laryngeal obstruction

Clinical Findings: Incompatible with life unless it is recognized immediately at birth and steps are taken at once to establish an airway. When the obstruction is incomplete, the signs and symptoms are related to the functioning diameter of the stenosed lumen. Marked respiratory effort without air exchange or stridor at birth, with or without cyanosis, depending on the severity of the stenosis, is the first sign of laryngeal obstruction.

Direct laryngoscopy will reveal a complete or partial membranous occlusion of the larynx. Smith and Bain distinguish 3 types of atresia:

Type I supraglottic and infraglottic parts are atretic
Type II atresia is infraglottic
Type III atresia is glottic

Complications
I **Derived:** Neonatal death is extremely high with complete laryngeal atresia. In mild cases (ie stenosis or partial atresia) recurrent episodes of "croup" and repeated superimposed respiratory infections simulating laryngotracheobronchitis are common. Complications associated with tracheostomy in the newborn must also be considered.
II **Associated:** About half the cases reported in the literature had other potentially fatal malformations. Malformations include the CNS (hydrocephaly, malformations of the aqueduct); alimentary system (esophageal atresia, bronchoesophageal fistula, tracheoesophageal fistula and atresia); urogenital system (hypoplasia of kidney, hydroureter, urethral atresia, vesicovaginal fistula, bicornuate uterus) and skeletal system (varus deformity of feet, partial absence of cervical vertebrae, absence of radius, syndactyly).

Etiology: ? The various types of atresia are the result of arrest of development.

Pathogenesis: ?

Related Facts
I **Sex Ratio:** ? Probably M1:F1
II **Risk of Occurrence:** ? †
III **Risk of Recurrence for**
Patient's Sib: ?
Patient's Child: ?
IV **Age of Detectability:** At birth
V **Prevalence:** ?

Treatment
I **Primary Prevention:** —
II **Secondary Prevention:** Establishment of immediate diagnosis and provision of immediate airway (ie tracheostomy)
III **Other Therapy:** Treatment of secondary infections and stridor

Prognosis: The vast majority of newborns with complete laryngeal atresia die because the condition is not recognized and not treated immediately or because of other fatal anomalies. If the child survives the neonatal period, with proper surgical and medical treatment he will have a normal life span unless beset by serious associated malformations.

Detection of Carrier: —

†Special Considerations: There is little doubt that atresia of the larynx is closely related to laryngeal webs, not only in its presenting signs and pathologic findings, but also in its mode of genesis. Most authors feel that the condition has not been recognized in many infants and, as webs are not uncommon, it is safe to assume that atresia too is no rarity. Baker and Savetsky believe that heredity is a factor in "congenital partial atresia of the larynx" (study includes laryngeal webs and other types of laryngeal stenosis) as was demonstrated in a mother and her 2 children, all of whom had this entity.

References:
Baker, D.C., Jr. and Savetsky, L.: Congenital partial atresia of the larynx. Laryngoscope 78:616, 1966.
Holinger, P.H. and Brown, W.: Congenital webs, cysts, laryngoceles and other anomalies of the larynx. Ann. Otol. Rhinol. Laryngol. 76:744, 1967.
Holinger, P.H. et al: Pediatric laryngology. Otolaryngol. Clin. North Am. 3(2):625, 1970.
Jackson, C.: Anomalies of the larynx. In Maloney, W.H. (ed.): Otolaryngology. Hagerstown: Harper & Row, 1969, vol. 4.
Smith, I.I. and Bain, A.D.: Congenital atresia of the larynx. Ann. Otol. Rhinol. Laryngol. 74:338, 1965.

Contributor: **Lewis N. Neblett**

Editor's Computerized Descriptors: Larynx, Resp.

LARYNGEAL CYSTS

Includes: Kystes laryngés
Kehlkopfzysten
Quistes laríngeos
Congenital cysts of larynx
Glottic cysts

Excludes: Laryngocele (575)
Mucosal retention cysts
Thyroglossal duct remnant (945)

Minimal Diagnostic Criteria: Infant with stridor, dyspnea and a hoarse or absent cry. Lateral neck xray suggestive of laryngeal mass. Identification of cyst overhanging glottis, in false cord, aryepiglottic fold, or arytenoids: by direct laryngoscopy.

Clinical Findings: Hoarseness, muffled cry, stridor, suprasternal and epigastric retractions; dyspnea and cyanosis in varying degrees of severity may increase to complete aphonia and total respiratory obstruction. Cysts may enlarge to affect deglutition. Lateral xrays of the neck reveal round shadow with loss of the normal laryngeal outlines.

Complications
I **Derived:** Respiratory obstruction necessitating tracheotomy. Dysphagia may increase to complete inability to take oral feedings.
II **Associated:** Funnel chest may develop due to prolonged epigastric indrawing.

Etiology: ?

Pathogenesis: Most congenital cysts are confined to the immediate neighborhood of the ventricular appendix. They probably are the result of simple disturbances in fetal development. From the point of view of embryology congenital laryngeal cysts are considered as secondary malformations formed during the development of the Morgagni ventricle.

Congenital cysts and laryngoceles have a similar development, but cysts do not communicate with the interior of the larynx. Laryngoceles admittedly become clinically perceptible only when swollen by air forced into them, or when filled with a collection of fluid; thus congenital laryngoceles and cysts are often indistinguishable from each other. Glottic cysts have their origin in the true and false cords. Laryngoceles, however, originate from the ventricle. Some consider that these cysts arise from the mesodermal tissue of the branchial arches, whereas others suggest that they arise from cells that participate in the formation of the appendix of the laryngeal ventricle and name them dysontogenic laryngeal cysts of appendicular origin.

Related Facts
I **Sex Ratio:** M1:F4
II **Risk of Occurrence:** Rare
III **Risk of Recurrence for**
Patient's Sib: ?
Patient's Child: ?
IV **Age of Detectability:** From birth onward as symptoms progress to necessitate laryngeal examination, usually before 6 months of age.
V **Prevalence:** ?

Treatment
I **Primary Prevention:** —
II **Secondary Prevention:** Tracheotomy; aspiration or removal of the cysts or lateral pharyngotomy or thyrotomy for exposure and removal of the cyst.
III **Other Therapy:** —

Prognosis: Normal for life span. Defect is life threatening only if the cyst produces total obstruction to respiration or deglutition, or becomes infected.

Detection of Carrier: —

Special Considerations: —

References:
Holinger, P.H.: Clinical aspects of congenital anomalies of the larynx, trachea, bronchi and oesophagus. J. Laryngol. Otol. 75:1, 1961.
Holinger, P.H. and Steinmann, E.P.: Congenital cysts of larynx. Pract. Oto-Rhinol-Laryngol. (Basel) 9:Fasc. 3:129, 1947.
New, G.B. and Erich, J.B.: Congenital cysts of the larynx: Report of case. Arch. Otolaryngol. 30:943, 1939.

Contributor: **Paul H. Holinger**

Editor's Computerized Descriptors: Larynx, Speech, Resp.

LARYNGEAL VENTRICLE, PROLAPSE

Includes: Prolapsus du ventricule laryngée
Prolaps des Kehlkopfdeckels
Prolapso del ventrículo laríngeo
Eversion of sacculus
Eversion of ventricle
Prolapse of laryngeal ventricle

Excludes: Laryngocele (575)
Hyperplasia of larynx
Chronic laryngitis
Laryngeal polyp
Reinke edema

Minimal Diagnostic Criteria: Direct laryngoscopic examination, manipulation of the mass to determine its site of origin, and biopsy to establish its histopathologic characteristics are necessary to establish the diagnosis.

Clinical Findings: When a mass of prolapsed tissue extends onto the true vocal cords an irritating, nonproductive cough and intermittent hoarseness are the usual symptoms. The degree of hoarseness varies depending on the size of the mass. Pain is rare and airway obstruction becomes a problem only after the mass reaches a size that occludes the glottic airway.

Idiopathic or true eversion of the ventricular mucosa is rare because this tissue is normally firmly attached to underlying structures. An associated disease that contributes to the development of saccular eversion should always be suspected. Eversion of the sacculus has been detected in persons from the 2nd to the 6th decades of life and is more common in men than in women. In one third of reported cases the lesion was bilateral, with the remainder divided nearly equally between the right and left sides of the larynx.

Examination reveals a smooth, pear-shaped, pale red mass protruding from the ventricle onto the true vocal cord. This mass moves freely when palpated during direct laryngoscopy and can usually be pushed back into the ventricle. It should not be difficult to determine that the mass originates from the ventricle and not from the vocal cords. Aspiration during direct laryngoscopy may be required to distinguish this lesion from a cyst and biopsies should be made to rule out possibility of a neoplasm.

Complications
I **Derived:** Neoplasms, recurrent airway obstruction.
II **Associated:** —

Etiology: ? Infections of the larynx, cysts of the false vocal cord, aryepiglottic fold and ventricle, neoplasms of the larynx, chronic cough from pulmonary disease and external laryngeal trauma have all been implicated. No known familial incidence exists.

Pathogenesis: Eversion of the sacculus, or appendix of the ventricle, or a portion of the ventricular mucosa produces a mass that lies upon the true vocal cord. The prolapsed sacculus is lined with ciliated pseudostratified columnar epithelium resting on an intact basement membrane.

Related Facts
I **Sex Ratio:** M5:F1
II **Risk of Occurrence:** ?
III **Risk of Recurrence for**
    Patient's Sib: ?
    Patient's Child: ?
IV **Age of Detectability:** Usually during early adulthood by indirect mirror examination of the larynx.
V **Prevalence:** ?

Treatment

I Primary Prevention: —

II Secondary Prevention: Surgical excision during direct laryngoscopy. Appropriate treatment of associated diseases.

III Other Therapy: Tracheostomy may be required when airway obstruction occurs.

Prognosis: The prognosis is good when the mass is completely excised; however, any underlying disease may require more extensive therapy. In these patients the prognosis will depend on the success or failure of treatment for these disorders.

Detection of Carrier: —

Special Considerations: —

References:
Freedman, A. O.: Diseases of the ventricle of Morgagni; with special references to pyocele of congenital air sac of ventricle. Arch. Otolaryngol. 28:329, 1938.

MacKenzie, J. N.: Prolapse of the laryngeal ventricles with illustrative cases. Med. News. 40:567, 1882.

Moore, I.: So-called prolapse of the laryngeal ventricle, and eversion of the sacculus. J. Laryngol. 37:265, 1922.

Contributor: **Gerald M. English**

Editor's Computerized Descriptors: Larynx, Speech, Resp.

LARYNGEAL WEB

Includes: Palmure laryngée
Kehlkopfmembran
Membrana laríngea
Glottic web
Subglottic web
Supraglottic web

Excludes: Laryngeal atresia (571)
Subglottic stenosis (919)

Minimal Diagnostic Criteria: Diagnosis is based on the presence of a membranous web in the supraglottic, glottic or subglottic larynx.

Clinical Findings: A laryngeal web or other laryngeal anomaly must be considered in a newborn with evidence of upper airway obstruction or dysphonia. In adults and older children, hoarseness or dyspnea on exertion may be due to a laryngeal web. The diagnosis is made by direct laryngoscopy or by indirect laryngoscopy in those who are old enough to cooperate. The location of laryngeal webs and their frequency are as follows: supraglottic 12.5%, glottic 79.0% and subglottic 8.5%.

Most commonly the webs are greyish-white and glistening in appearance; however they may be greyish-yellow, pink, or hyperemic. Some of the reported webs have consisted of only a thin translucent membrane, but they usually are thin posteriorly and thicker (up to 1.5 cm) anteriorly. In order of frequency, extent of the webs has been as follows: anterior two-thirds, anterior one-half, anterior one-third, anterior one-fourth, anterior three-fourths, anterior four-fifths and, finally, almost total occlusion of the airway.

Histologically, the superior surface of the web is lined by squamous epithelium, which may show thickening. The inferior surface is covered by normal mucous membrane. The thickened anterior portion of the web contains dense fibrous tissue, mucous glands and striated muscle fibers.

The severity of the symptoms is dependent upon the extent of the web. In infants, the most common signs in the order of their frequency are: aphonia, inspiratory and expiratory stridor, difficulty in feeding and attacks of dyspnea. The most common symptoms in older children and adults are: hoarseness, dyspnea on exertion or dyspnea with respiratory tract infections, a weak, high-pitched voice or easy tiring of the voice. Subglottic and supraglottic webs, when symptomatic, cause dyspnea which is constant or present with exertion, depending upon the severity of the airway occlusion.

Complications

I Derived: Significant obstruction of the airway, which fortunately is uncommon. The most common problem has been dysphonia.

II Associated: In the largest series reported, 11.3% of the cases were associated with other anomalies. The associated anomalies have been: coloboma of the eye, nictitating membrane of the eye, ptosis of eyelids, bifid uvula and soft palate, adherent lingual frenulum, talipomanus (clubhands), syndactyly, stenosis of ureter, imperforate anus and supernumerary breasts.

Etiology: ?

Pathogenesis: Differentiation of the larynx occurs between the 4th and 10th weeks of gestation. In the development of the larynx there is epithelial fusion between the 2 sides which is thought to dissolve at about the 10th week. A laryngeal web is thought to be the result of inadequate dissolution of the connection between the

2 sides of the developing larynx.

Related Facts

I **Sex Ratio:** M1:F1, possibly a slight female predominance (55 female: 45 male)

II **Risk of Occurrence:** ? Estimated as 1 in 100,000.

III **Risk of Recurrence for**
  Patient's Sib: ? Probably no increased risk unless there is a positive family history of the anomaly.
  Patient's Child: ?

IV **Age of Detectability:** At birth by direct laryngoscopy

V **Prevalence:** ? Estimated as 1 in 100,000. No known ethnic or geographic prevalence.

Treatment

I **Primary Prevention:** —

II **Secondary Prevention:** Treatment of a web is dependent upon its thickness, extent, and location. A small web of the supraglottic or subglottic larynx which causes no respiratory distress does not require treatment. Some glottic webs, which do not cause respiratory distress may be treated because of vocal disturbances. Thin webs may respond to simple tearing with the bronchoscope, with a dilator, or with laryngeal forceps. Tearing of the web must be performed with caution to avoid injuring the vocal cords. Thicker laryngeal webs require surgical division of the web followed by insertion of a sheet of metal or other material between the edges of the web to prevent recurrence. The inserted plate or keel is anchored to the skin or the thyroid cartilage and is left in place for about 6 weeks. Any patient with an extensive membranous web which does not respond to simple tearing requires tracheotomy.

III **Other Therapy:** —

Prognosis: A severe web can cause death due to upper airway obstruction at the time of birth, if untreated. A large web which does not cause respiratory distress alone may contribute to a patient's death when combined with pulmonary or other respiratory tract disease. When treated, laryngeal web should not affect the patient's life span.

Detection of Carrier: —

Special Considerations: —

References:

Holinger, P.H. et al: Congenital anomalies of the larynx. Ann. Otol. Rhinol. Laryngol. 63:581, 1954.

McHugh, H.E. and Loch, W.E.: Congenital webs of the larynx. Laryngoscope 52:43, 1942.

McNaught, R.C.: Surgical correction of anterior web of the larynx. Laryngoscope 60:264, 1950.

Contributor: **Raymond O. Smith, Jr.**

___

Editor's Computerized Descriptors: Larynx, Speech, Resp.

LARYNGOCELE

Includes: Laryngozele
Laringocele
Laryngoceles; internal, external or combined
Laryngeal hernia
Laryngeal pouch
Laryngeal aerocele
Diverticulum of larynx
Ventricular cyst of larynx
Laryngeal mucocele
Laryngeal pyocele

Excludes: Laryngeal ventricle, prolapse (573)
Laryngeal cysts (572)

Minimal Diagnostic Criteria: Ventricular cystic mass or neck mass over the thyrohyoid membrane. Direct visualization by endoscopy is required to establish the diagnosis and rule out a coexistent disease.

Clinical Findings: A cyst-like mass is present in the neck and laryngeal ventricle. The external component may enlarge with straining and decrease with rest. It may collapse with gentle pressure. This lesion arises as a saccular dilatation of the saccus or appendix of the laryngeal ventricle or the sinus of Morgagni. There is a herniation of mucosa from the ventricle upward and lateral to the false vocal cord. This cystic mass may remain within the interior of the larynx or pass through the thyrohyoid membrane at the perforation site of the neurovascular bundle (superior laryngeal nerve and vessels). This gives rise to the classification of laryngoceles as: internal, external or combined. They have also been classified by their content as: aerocele, pyocele or mucocele.

The laryngeal appendix is larger in Caucasians than in other racial groups. In other primates it may extend into the neck across the chest and into the axilla. In the orangutan a structure similar to a laryngocele is thought to be an air reservoir for use during climbing and phonation.

The clinical symptoms vary with the extent and location of the lesion. The patient's voice may be normal, hoarse or aphonic. There is often a cystic swelling of the neck between the hyoid bone and the thyroid cartilage. Compression of the mass may produce gurgling and hissing in the throat (Bryce sign). The mass may also increase with straining and decrease with rest. Dysphagia and aspiration often develop with large lesions. Airway obstruction and asphyxiation are potential dangers. Small laryngoceles may be entirely asymptomatic.

Complications

I **Derived:** Infection, aspiration, obstruction, carcinoma of larynx

II **Associated:** —

Etiology: Many factors are implicated in the development of this lesion. Increased intraglottic pressure caused by coughing, singing, glass blowing, weight lifting and wind instrument playing are associated with this condition. A weakness or deficiency of the thyrohyoid membrane, herniation of the laryngeal ventricle, and an enlarged, weak-walled saccus have been suggested as factors in the development of this lesion.

Pathogenesis: Increased intraluminal laryngeal pressure in persons with congenitally large ventricular appendices are the major considerations in this disease. The laryngeal appendix becomes dilated with an increase in intraluminal pressure from straining, coughing, glass blowing, wind instrument playing and singing. This dilated saccus then expands up into the false cord, the aryepiglottic fold, or both, and passes into the neck through the perforation of the neurovascular bundle in the thyrohyoid ligament. These cysts are lined with ciliated respiratory epithelium containing mucous secreting glands. Varying degrees of inflammatory reaction will be present in the wall of the cyst.

Related Facts
I   Sex Ratio: M1:F1
II   Risk of Occurrence: ?
III Risk of Recurrence for
     Patient's Sib: ?
     Patient's Child: ?
IV Age of Detectability: ?
V   Prevalence: 183 cases reported through 1968.

Treatment
I   Primary Prevention: —
II   Secondary Prevention: One-stage surgical excision of the lesion through an external incision in any patient with a symptomatic laryngocele. Treatment of infections with antibiotics. Incision and drainage only are to be avoided; however, where acute infection occurs this may become necessary.
III Other Therapy: Tracheostomy when airway obstruction or aspiration are problems

Prognosis: Good for normal life span, intelligence and function when adequately treated.

Detection of Carrier: —

Special Considerations: —

References:
Ballenger, J. J.: Diseases of Nose, Throat and Ear. Philadelphia: Lea and Febiger, 1969, p. 308.
English, G. M. and DeBlanc, G. B.: Laryngocele: A case presenting with acute airway obstruction. Laryngoscope 78:386, 1968.
Fredrickson, J. M. and Ward, P. H.: Laryngocele ventricularis. Arch. Otolaryngol. 76:568, 1962.
Holinger, P. H. and Steinmann, E. P.: Congenital cysts of larynx. Pract. Oto-Rhino-Laryngol. 9:Fasc. 3:129, 1947.
Macfie, D. D.: Asymptomatic laryngoceles in wind-instrument bandsmen. Arch. Otolaryngol. 83:270, 1966.

Contributor: **Gerald M. English**

Editor's Computerized Descriptors: Larynx, Speech, Neck, Resp.

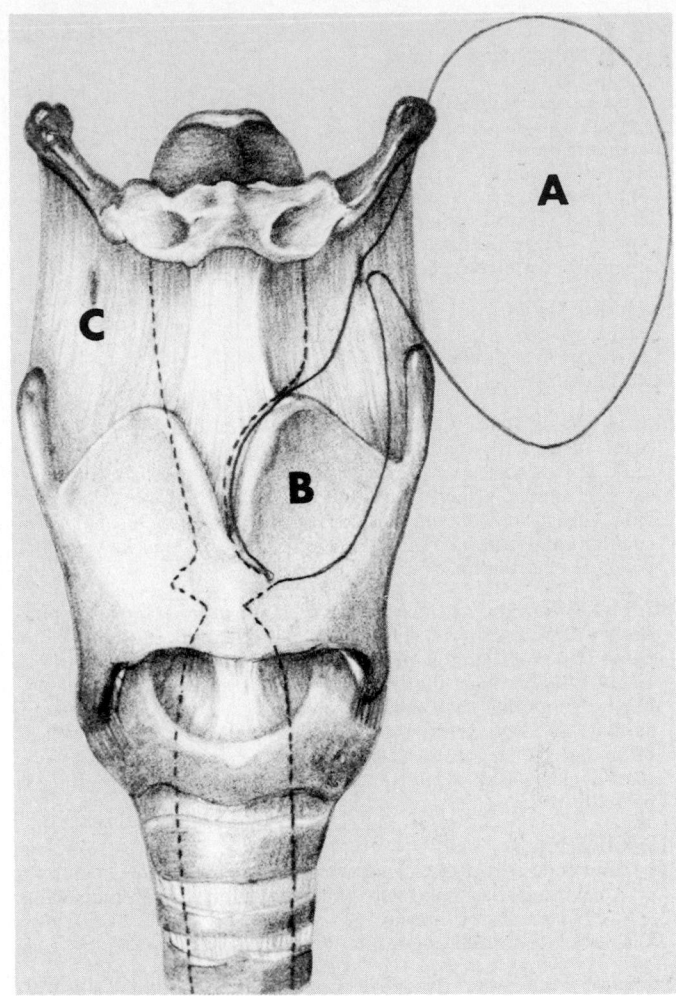

318. Laryngocele within larynx. External component (A) is connected with internal component (B) through thyrohyoid membrane at perforation of neurovascular bundle (C)

LARYNGOMALACIA

Includes: Laryngomalacie
Laryngomalazie
Laringomalacia
Congenital croup
Congenital stridor
Laryngeal stridor, congenital
Larynx, congenital flaccid
Congenital laryngeal chondromalacia

Excludes: Croup
Specific croup
Laryngismus stridulous
Laryngeal atresia (571)

Minimal Diagnostic Criteria: Persistent stuttering inspiratory respirations with episodes of cyanosis especially during feeding; neck, chest and esophageal xrays negative for possible thyroglossal duct cyst, tracheal compression, mediastinal mass, vascular ring. Direct laryngoscopy shows fluttering arytenoids, curled or tubular epiglottis and demonstrates absence of other laryngeal or tracheal obstruction.†

Clinical Findings: Stridorous, noisy, inspiratory crowing respirations with intermittent episodes of hypoxia and cyanosis, accompanied by indrawing at the suprasternal notch and epigastrium. Usually begins shortly after birth and increases in severity, lasting 6-18 months, then gradually subsides. Direct laryngoscopy shows flaccidity of all supraglottic structures; the epiglottis is often curled or tubular and soft, as are the arytenoids and aryepiglottic folds, which all flutter during inspiration. Cord motility is normal.

Complications
I   **Derived:** Failure to gain weight in severe cases. Pectus excavatum associated with the constant epigastric indrawing. Hypoxia and cyanosis.
II **Associated:** Micrognathia, macroglossia.

Etiology: One report describes postmortem findings of 3 sibs with congenital stridor. A 4th sib was normal.

Pathogenesis: Exaggerated or persistent infantile features of the larynx, tubular longitudinal folding of the epiglottis; inward rolling of the arytenoids and aryepiglottic folds have been recorded as postmortem findings. Histologically, edema and a slight increase in the lymphatic and polymorphonuclear cellular elements of the submucosa were found. Kelemen describes cartilages found to be about one-half the thickness of control specimens, which seems especially significant.

Related Facts
I   **Sex Ratio:** M2:F1
II **Risk of Occurrence:** ?
III **Risk of Recurrence for**
    Patient's Sib: ?
    Patient's Child: ?
IV **Age of Detectability:** 1-6 months by direct laryngoscopy
V   **Prevalence:** Most common of congenital laryngeal anomalies, constituting 650 of a series of 866 laryngeal anomalies.

Treatment
I   **Primary Prevention:** —
II **Secondary Prevention:** Interrupt feeding frequently to assist breathing; place infant in position of least obstruction. Tracheotomy only in severe involvement.
III **Other Therapy:** —

Prognosis: Normal for life span, intelligence and function

Detection of Carrier: —

†Special Considerations: Stridor is the auditory evidence of upper airway obstruction; therefore, laryngomalacia must be differentiated from all other causes of stridor in infants. Direct laryngoscopy usually shows a curled and flaccid epiglottis with soft, edematous-appearing arytenoids that are drawn into the glottis with a fluttering appearance with each inspiration. The symptom is exaggerated when the infant is on its back and decreases in severity when the infant lies on its abdomen. The noise is increased with total relaxation, as during sleep, or with vigorous crying. Bronchoscopy often shows an associated, similar tracheo-and bronchomalacia.

References:
Finlay, H.V.L.: Familial congenital stridor. Arch. Dis. Child. 24:219, 1949.
Holinger, P.H. and Brown, W.T.: Congenital webs, cysts, laryngoceles and other anomalies of the larynx. Ann. Otol. Rhinol. Laryngol. 76:744, 1967.
Kelemen, G.: Congenital laryngeal stridor. Arch. Otolaryngol. 58:245, 1953.
Schwartz, L.: Congenital laryngeal stridor (inspiratory laryngeal collapse): New theory as to its underlying cause and desirability of a change in terminology. Arch. Otolaryngol. 39:403, 1944.

Contributor: **Paul H. Holinger**

Editor's Computerized Descriptors: Larynx, Skel., Resp.

LARYNGO-TRACHEO-ESOPHAGEAL CLEFT

Editor's Computerized Descriptors: Larynx, Speech, Resp., GI.

Includes: Fistule laryngo-trachéo-oesophagienne
Laryngo-tracheo-ösophageale Spalte
Fisura laringo-tráqueo-esofágica
Cleft larynx, posterior
Congenital posterior cleft of larynx and trachea with persistent esophagotrachea

Excludes: Tracheoesophageal fistula (960)

Minimal Diagnostic Criteria: Direct visualization of the defect by endoscopy is required to establish the diagnosis.

Clinical Findings: This defect in the posterior wall of the larynx and trachea produces a common communication with the esophagus. The clinical symptoms vary somewhat with the extent of the defect but in all cases they demonstrate respiratory difficulties with feedings. Voice quality is abnormal, varying from hoarseness to aphonia. Inspiratory stridor may be present. Except for the abnormal voice, symptoms are similar to those of tracheoesophageal fistula.

Complications
I   **Derived:**   Repeated aspiration of feeding results in respiratory distress and pneumonitis. This complication has frequently been fatal. Feeding problems result in nutritional deficiency.
II   **Associated:**   —

Etiology: ?

Pathogenesis: Laryngotracheoesophageal cleft develops from an arrest in the rostral advancement of the tracheoesophageal septum and failure of dorsal fusion of the cricoid cartilage. This defect occurs at about the 35th gestational day, which is approximately 10 days prior to fusion of the cricoid cartilage.

Related Facts
I   **Sex Ratio:**   M1:F1
II   **Risk of Occurrence:**   Rare
III   **Risk of Recurrence for**
     Patient's Sib: Two sets of cases have occurred in sibs.
     Patient's Child: ?
IV   **Age of Detectability:**   Immediately after birth
V   **Prevalence:**   Rare, only 31 cases have been reported. Four clefts, however, were found in a series of 2000 consecutive autopsies at a pediatric hospital.

Treatment
I   **Primary Prevention:**   —
II   **Secondary Prevention:**   Surgical closure of the defect has been successful in 5 cases where the cleft was limited to the cervical area.
III   **Other Therapy:**   —

Prognosis: Normal for life span, intelligence and function, if surgery is successful.

Detection of Carrier: —

Special Considerations: —

References:
Blumberg, J.B. et al: Laryngotracheoesophageal cleft, the embryologic implications: Review of the literature. Surgery 57:599, 1965.
Delahunty, J. E. and Cherry, J.: Congenital laryngeal cleft. Ann. Otol. Rhinol. Laryngol. 78:96, 1969.
Imbrie, J. D. and Doyle, P. J.: Laryngotracheoesophageal cleft. Report of a case and review of the literature. Laryngoscope 79:1252, 1969.

Contributors: **Patrick J. Doyle**
                    Donald Imbrie

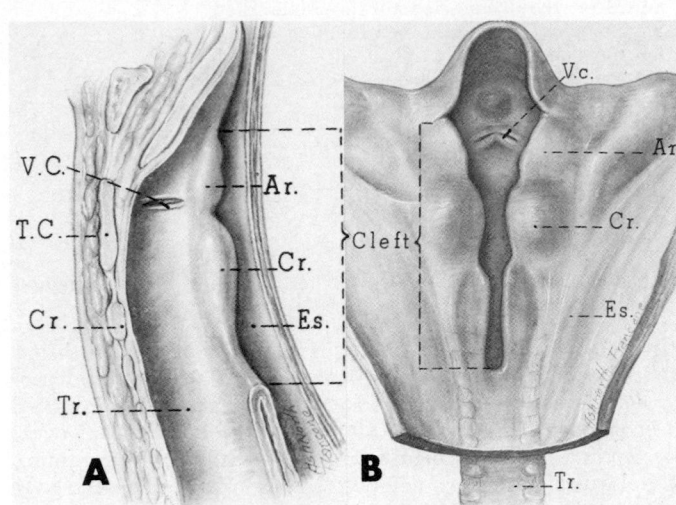

319. A) Lateral and B) PA views of cleft. V.C. = vocal cords; T.C. = thyroid cartilage; Cr. = cricoid; Tr. = trachea; Ar.= arytenoids; Es. = esophagus

LAURENCE-MOON-BIEDL SYNDROME

Includes: Syndrome de Laurence-Moon-Biedl
Síndrome de Laurence-Moon-Biedl
Laurence-Moon syndrome
Laurence-Moon-Biedl-Bardet syndrome
Bardet-Biedl syndrome

Excludes: Alström syndrome† (41)
Prader-Willi syndrome† (823)
Biemond II syndrome†
Usher syndrome† (983)
Acrocephalopolysyndactyly† (13)

Minimal Diagnostic Criteria: Obesity, hypogonadism, mental retardation and characteristic ocular and digital findings.

Clinical Findings: The 5 cardinal signs of this condition are retinal pigmentary degeneration, obesity, genital hypoplasia, mental retardation and polydactyly. When these occur together the diagnosis is straightforward.† However, incomplete and atypical forms of the disorder are common. Relatives of affected persons have been noted to have only 1 or 2 features characteristic of the syndrome.
The relative frequency of these signs are:

ocular signs	93%
obesity	91%
mental defect	86%
digital anomaly	75%
hypogonadism	66%

Pigmentary retinal degeneration occurs in 90% of those affected with loss of central and peripheral vision as well as pigmentary changes in the fundus. Findings typical of retinitis pigmentosa are found in 15% of patients with this condition. The age of onset of degenerative retinal changes is variable but approximately 75% of those who have pigmentary changes are blind by age 20 and 87% by age 30 years. Generally, there is loss of central vision followed by peripheral loss. Nightblindness may be the presenting visual sign. Electroretinography shows the pattern of tapetoretinal degeneration.

Generally the obesity in LMB has its onset in infancy or early childhood and progresses with age. Distribution of adipose tissue is generalized with prominence on the trunk and proximal limbs.

Some degree of mental retardation is found in 86% of patients with this condition. Associated neurologic disorders include seizures, spinocerebellar and extrapyramidal disorders. Structural brain abnormalities such as atrophic or enlarged gyri, hydrocephalus, asymmetric cerebral hemispheres, and thinning and absence of corpus callosum have been reported. Characteristic neuropathologic changes have not been described. EEG abnormalities are frequently present with poorly organized background and diffuse dysrhythmias. Less frequent neurologic defects include hypotonia, hyporeflexia, hyperreflexia and cranial nerve paralysis.

Digital anomalies include syndactyly with or without polydactyly which is postaxial and may occur on any or all limbs. Short and broad fingers and toes may occur. When polydactyly is absent, x-ray examination may show digital malformations, usually of the 5th digit. Other skeletal defects include microcephaly, brachycephaly and oxycephaly, enlargement of parietal foramina and hyperostosis frontalis.

Hypogenitalism is not always present but is more frequently diagnosed in males. Delayed or incomplete pubertal development occurs as well as a wide variety of genital defects including small phallus, bifid scrotum, hypospadias and cryptorchidism. About half of affected females have some indication of hypogonadism, such as delayed puberty, vaginal atresia, double uterus and vaginal septum. Both primary germinal hypoplasia and hypogonadotropic hypogonadism are described.

Endocrine disturbances are not frequent but include diabetes insipidus, tall and short stature, and rarely, abnormal glucose tolerance. Renal abnormalities are frequent and include renal dysplasia, cystic kidneys, glomerulonephritis, pyelonephritis, nephrosclerosis, hydroureter, hydronephrosis, fetal lobulations and persistent urogenital sinus.

Congenital cardiovascular defects are common and highly varied. No one congenital heart lesion is characteristically present. Acquired left ventricular hypertrophy or systemic hypertension may be present. Other associated defects include: anal atresia, microstomia, cleft lip and palate, progressive nerve deafness, hypertrichosis, congenital cystic dilatation of the bile duct and webbed neck.

Complications
I **Derived:** Left ventricular hypertrophy associated with renal disease, systemic hypertension, azotemia, uremia, renal failure, blindness.
II **Associated:** —

Etiology: Generally this is thought to result from an autosomal recessive gene. Genetic heterogeneity is likely in this condition. Irregular dominant and multifactorial inheritance have been suggested by some authors. McK *20990, *24580

Pathogenesis: ?

Related Facts
I **Sex Ratio:** M1:F1 Probably
II **Risk of Occurrence:** Rare
III **Risk of Recurrence for**
Patient's Sib: If autosomal recessive, 1 in 4 (25%) for each offspring to be affected
Patient's Child: If autosomal recessive, not increased unless mate is carrier or homozygote.
IV **Age of Detectability:** Childhood or adolescence
V **Prevalence:** 1 in 175,000 in Switzerland

Treatment
I **Primary Prevention:** Genetic counseling
II **Secondary Prevention:** Supportive. Early diagnosis of congenital heart disease and renal disease may affect mortality.
III **Other Therapy:** Reading aids if needed.

Prognosis: Normal life span if no cardiac or renal abnormalities. If these are present, then prognosis depends upon severity of associated complications.

Detection of Carrier: —

†Special Considerations: Diagnosis may be difficult in incomplete, abortive and atypical forms. Careful examination of family members in these cases may help distinguish this condition from exclusion syndromes.

References:
Bauman, M.L. and Hogan, G.R.: Laurence-Moon-Biedl syndrome. Am. J. Dis. Child. 126:119, 1973.
Bergsma, D. and Brown, K.S.: Assessment of ophthalmologic, endocrinologic and genetic findings in the Bardet-Biedl syndrome. In Bergsma, D.(ed.): Malformation Syndromes. Birth Defects: Orig. Art. Ser., vol. XI, no. 2. Amsterdam: Excerpta Medica for The National Foundation-March of Dimes, 1975, p. 132.
Berson, E.L. et al: Progressive cone-rod degeneration. Arch. Ophthalmol. 80:68, 1968.
Hurley, R.M. et al: The renal lesion of the Laurence-Moon-Biedl syndrome. J. Pediatr. 87:206, 1975.

Klein, D. and Ammann, F. The syndrome of Laurence-Moon-Bardet-Biedl and allied diseases in Switzerland. J. Neurol. Sci. 9:479, 1969.

Nadjmi, B. et al: Laurence-Moon-Biedl syndrome. Am. J. Dis. Child. 117:352, 1939.

Contributor: **Marylou Buyse**

Editor's Computerized Descriptors: Vision, Eye, Hearing, Face, Oral, Skin, Hair, Skel., CV., GI., GU., Nerve

LEBER OPTIC ATROPHY

Includes: Atrophie optique de Leber
Lebersche Opticusatrophie
Atrofia óptica de Leber

Excludes: Optic atrophy, infantile heredofamilial (755)

Minimal Diagnostic Criteria: Central visual loss, optic atrophy.

Clinical Findings: There is sudden loss of central vision occurring in the 2nd and 3rd decades of life. The loss of central vision, which is usually bilateral, progresses rapidly. Elevation of the optic disk and swelling of nerve fiber bundles may be observed. Headaches may accompany the onset of visual loss. Progressive atrophy ensues, leaving a flat pale disk. The visual fields show large dense central scotomas.

Complications
I **Derived:** —
II **Associated:** Rare cerebellar and pyramidal tract signs

Etiology: The disorder with male preponderance, has been considered X-linked recessive, but does not conform to rigid mendelian rules. There is absence of transmission through males, and passage occurs from the female to most of her offspring. The exact etiology remains obscure. Theories include: an infective agent, especially a slow virus; failure to detoxify cyanide; and opticochiasmatic arachnoidal adhesions.†

Pathogenesis: —

Related Facts
I **Sex Ratio:** ?
II **Risk of Occurrence:** ?
III **Risk of Recurrence for**
  Patient's Sib: If X-linked recessive, and mother is a carrier, 1 in 2 (50%) for each brother to be affected and 1 in 2 (50%) for each sister to be a carrier.
  Patient's Child: If X-linked recessive, 1 in 1 (100%) for carrier daughters; not increased for sons unless wife is a carrier.
IV **Age of Detectability:** Typically in the late teens to middle 20s, but the range is from 5-65.
V **Prevalence:** —

Treatment
I **Primary Prevention:** —
II **Secondary Prevention:** —
III **Other Therapy:** Unconfirmed approaches include the use of hydroxocobalamin, and lysis of opticochiasmatic arachnoidal adhesions.

Prognosis: Progressive visual loss

Detection of Carrier: —

†**Special Considerations:** The genetic etiology of this condition is not yet established. Genetic heterogeneity and the excess incidence in males may well add to the difficulty of determining the mode of genetic transmission.

References:
Glazer, J.: Heredofamilial disorders of the optic nerve. In Goldberg, M. (ed.): Genetic and Metabolic Eye Disease. Boston: Little, Brown and Co., 1974.

Seedorff, T.: Leber's disease V. Acta Ophthalmol. (Kbh) 48:186. 1970.

Contributor: **Morton E. Smith**

Editor's Computerized Descriptors: Vision, Eye, Nerve

LECITHIN:CHOLESTEROL ACYL TRANSFERASE DEFICIENCY

Includes: Déficit en lecithine - cholestérol acyl transférase
Lecithin-Cholesterin-Acyl-Transferase Mangel
Lecitina: deficiencia de colesterol acil transferasa
LCAT deficiency
Familial plasma cholesteryl ester deficiency

Excludes: Cholesteryl ester storage disease (151)
Analphalipoproteinemia (48)
Wolman disease (1003)

Minimal Diagnostic Criteria: Presence of corneal opacities, anemia and proteinuria associated with hyperlipemia and reduced levels of plasma cholesterol esters and elevated plasma unesterified cholesterol. All patients have very low (or absent) levels of activity of the enzyme "plasma lecithin:cholesterol acyl transferase" (LCAT).

Clinical Findings: Markedly reduced levels of plasma cholesterol esters and increased levels of unesterified cholesterol are invariable; plasma lecithin is usually elevated and plasma lysolecithin is usually depressed. Six of the 7 known cases have been hyperlipemic. No pre-β-or α-lipoproteins can be detected by paper electrophoresis; the very low density lipoproteins migrate in the β position instead of the usual pre-β position; most of the high density lipoproteins migrate in the α_2 position instead of the usual α_1 position. Very high antistreptolysin titers were found in all of the patients with sheep erythrocytes, but not with rabbit erythrocytes. Corneal opacities, proteinuria and normochromic anemia are constant features; target cells were present in the blood of all patients. Foam cells may be found in the bone marrow (50%) and in the kidney (3 of 3). Two of the 7 patients developed total renal failure. There are no neurologic symptoms.

Complications
I **Derived:** Progressive renal failure; possibly accelerated atherosclerosis.
II **Associated:** —

Etiology: Autosomal recessive mode of transmission. The homozygote apparently cannot make the enzyme (or the normal enzyme) plasma lecithin:cholesterol acyl transferase. McK *24590

Pathogenesis: The sequence of events that causes the development of clinical symptoms is not clear. It has been suggested that plasma LCAT deficiency prevents the maintenance of the normal balance between cholesterol and cholesterol esters in cell (plasma) membranes. Unesterified cholesterol may, therefore, accumulate in the cell membrane and interfere with cellular function; erythrocytes from patients do contain increased amounts of cholesterol and lecithin.

Related Facts
I **Sex Ratio:** M2:F5 in the 7 known cases
II **Risk of Occurrence:** ? All patients were Scandinavian thus far
III **Risk of Recurrence for**
   Patient's Sib: 1 in 4 (25%) for each offspring to be affected
   Patient's Child: Not increased unless mate is carrier or homozygote (Probands do survive to childbearing age and have offspring.)
IV **Age of Detectability:** Probably at birth by plasma enzyme determination
V **Prevalence:** < 1 in 100,000

Treatment
I **Primary Prevention:** Genetic counseling
II **Secondary Prevention:** Frequent transfusions of plasma provide the enzyme LCAT and may be able to prevent the progression of the disease.

III **Other Therapy:** Renal dialysis in the event of kidney failure

Prognosis: Guarded: one of 7 patients has died from renal failure; a 2nd has no kidney function. All patients surviving have marked proteinuria.

Detection of Carrier: ?

Special Considerations: —

References:
Glomset, J.A.: The plasma lecithin:cholesterol acyltransferase reaction. J. Lipid Res. 9:155, 1968.
Norum, K.R. and Gjone, E.: Familial serum-cholesterol esterification failure: A new inborn error of metabolism. Biochim. Biophys. Acta (Amst.) 144:698, 1967.
Norum, K.R. et al: Familial lecithin: Cholesterol acyl transferase deficiency. In Standbury, J.B. et al (eds): The Metabolic Basis of Inherited Disease, 3rd Ed. New York:McGraw-Hill, 1972, p. 531.

Contributor: **Howard R. Sloan**

Editor's Computerized Descriptors: Eye, GU.

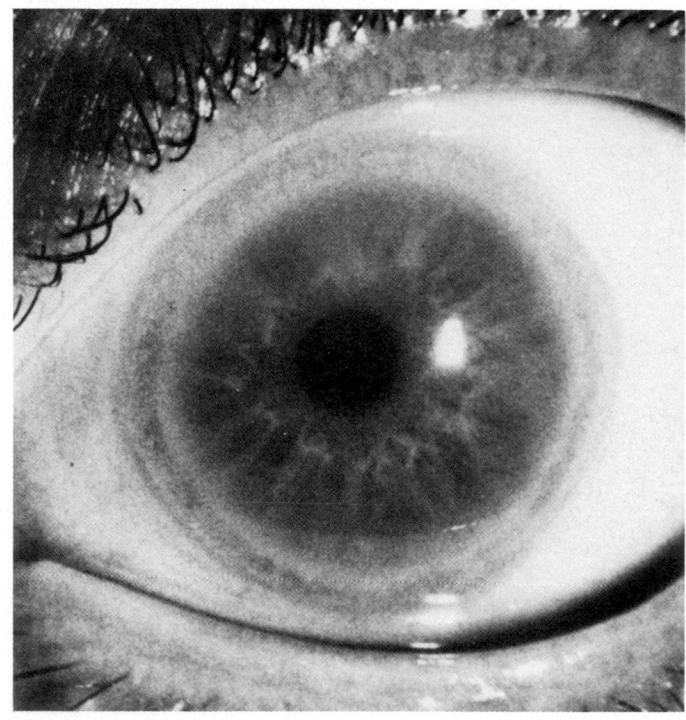

320. Corneal cloudiness

LEFT VENTRICLE, DOUBLE OUTLET

Includes: Ventricule gauche à double issue
Ursprung beider grosser Arterien aus dem linken Ventrikel
Ventrículo izquierdo a doble salida
Double outlet left ventricle with intact ventricular septum and atresia of right ventricular infundibulum
Double outlet left ventricle with ventricular septal defect
Double outlet left ventricle with ventricular septal defect and pulmonary stenosis

Excludes: Single or common ventricle with both great vessels arising from a common left or primitive ventricle
Double outlet right ventricle with ventricular inversion.

Minimal Diagnostic Criteria: Origin of both pulmonary artery and aorta entirely or predominantly above the left ventricle. May have various associated cardiac defects; VSD, pulmonary stenosis, right ventricular infundibular atresia, tricuspid valve stenosis, atresia or straddling.

Clinical Findings: This rare anomaly occurs when both pulmonary artery and the aorta arise entirely or predominantly above the morphologically left ventricle. Both semilunar valves may have fibrous continuity with the mitral valve. The right ventricle may be normally formed, but may be hypoplastic with infundibular atresia. Atria and viscera are usually in solitus arrangement, with concordant relation of atria and ventricles. The semilunar valves may be in the same coronal plane, or the aortic valve level may be anterior or posterior to the pulmonary valve level. The aorta has usually been to the right of the pulmonary trunk. The ventricular septal defect (VSD) may be subaortic or subpulmonic in location or confluent with both great vessels.

The presence or absence of pulmonary stenosis largely determines the clinical course. Cyanosis is prominent with significant pulmonary stenosis and VSD, and the clinical picture may be indistinguishable from that of tetralogy of Fallot. Clinical signs in this group include a prominent ejection systolic murmur due to pulmonary stenosis, and an accentuated single second heart sound at the base. ECGs show right axis deviation and right ventricular hypertrophy. Chest roentgenograms show slight cardiac enlargement and decreased pulmonary vascular markings.

In contrast, patients with VSD but without pulmonary stenosis are relatively acyanotic initially and present with congestive cardiac failure. Pulmonary artery hypertension with increased pulmonary blood flow is clinically evident. The precordium is hyperactive, and the second heart sound split with pulmonary closure accentuation. A pansystolic murmur is present at the lower left sternal border with sometimes a prominent mid-diastolic flow murmur. ECG shows combined ventricular hypertrophy. The chest roentgenogram shows a large heart with increased pulmonary vascularity; findings which may suggest the diagnosis of transposition of the great arteries with VSD.

Hemodynamic data from the published cases showed a systolic pressure gradient at the pulmonary or subpulmonary valve level in 4 cases; right ventricular infundibular atresia was present in 1 patient, and no obstruction was present in the remaining 2. Right ventricular hypertension was present in all patients. In the infant with an intact ventricular septum, the right ventricular peak systolic pressure was greater than the systemic level. The observation of almost identical oxygen saturations in the aorta, pulmonary artery and left ventricle in a cyanotic patient suspected clinically as having tetralogy of Fallot, seems to be an important clue to the diagnosis of double outlet left ventricle with pulmonary stenosis.

Selective biplane angiography with injections into both the right and left ventricle establishes the diagnosis by demonstrating both vessels arising predominantly to the left of the septum above the morphologically left ventricle, and establishes the presence or absence of pulmonary or subpulmonary stenosis, the presence or absence of a VSD, and the status of the atrio-ventricular valves.

At surgery, external inspection of the position of the great arteries has not been helpful in suggesting the diagnosis of double outlet left ventricle, since the great arteries may be similar in appearance to that seen in patients with tetralogy of Fallot, or they may be malposed in a manner similar to that noted in complete transposition of the great arteries or double outlet right ventricle. However, careful analysis of arterioventricular connections during cardiopulmonary bypass can establish the diagnosis.

Complications
I   **Derived:** —
II **Associated:** —

Etiology: ?

Pathogenesis: Van Praagh postulated abnormal conal growth resulting in essentially no conal tissue beneath both the great vessels, which leaves them in a side-by-side position above the left ventricle with both semilunar valves in fibrous continuity with the mitral valve. Anderson emphasized rather an absorptive process involving both the right and left ventricular conus.

Related Facts
I   **Sex Ratio:** In cases in which sex is known, predominantly male
II **Risk of Occurrence:** ? Very rare
III **Risk of Recurrence for**
    Patient's Sib: ?
    Patient's Child: ?
IV **Age of Detectability:** From birth
V   **Prevalence:** Rare. (Van Praagh and Weinberg have recently reviewed 35 well-documented cases based upon personal examinations and the literature.)

Treatment
I   **Primary Prevention:** ?
II **Secondary Prevention:** Surgical:
    Palliative surgery: A) systemic-pulmonary artery shunt for cyanotic infants with diminished pulmonary blood flow; B) pulmonary artery banding for acyanotic infants with markedly increased pulmonary blood flow.
    Corrective surgery for both groups: A) intraventricular diversion of blood from right ventricle to pulmonary artery with patch repair of VSD; B) radical reconstruction with pericardial tunnel or extracardiac valve-bearing conduit from right ventricle to pulmonary artery and patch closure of VSD; C) Fontan-type precedure when coexistent tricuspid atresia.
III **Other Therapy:** —

Prognosis: Following intracardiac repair patients reported alive and improved.

Detection of Carrier: —

Special Considerations: —

References:
Anderson, R.H. et al: Double outlet left ventricle. Br. Heart J. 36:554, 1974.
Bharati, S. et al: Morphologic spectrum of double outlet left ventricle and its surgical significance. Circulation 56:43, 1977.
Kerr, A.R. et al: Double-outlet left ventricle with ventricular septal defect and pulmonary stenosis: Report of surgical repair. Am. Heart J. 81:688, 1971.
Pacifico, A.D. et al: Surgical treatment of double-outlet left ventri-

cle. Circulation III-47 & 48: III-19-III-23, 1973.

Paul, M.H., et al: Double-outlet left ventricle with an intact ventricular septum. Circulation 41:129, 1970.
Van Mierop, L.H.S. and Wiglesworth, F.W.: Pathogenesis of transposition complexes. II. Anomalies due to faulty transfer of the posterior pulmonary artery. Am. J. Cardiol. 12:226, 1962.
Van Praagh, R. and Weinberg, P.M.: Double outlet left ventricle. In Moss, A.J. and Adams, F.H. (eds.): Heart Disease in Infants, Children, and Adolescents. Baltimore: Williams & Wilkins, chapt. 22. (In press)

Contributors: **Kalim U. Aziz**
Milton H. Paul

Editor's Computerized Descriptors: Resp., CV.

LEFT VENTRICLE, SINGLE PAPILLARY MUSCLE

Includes: Muscle papillaire unique du ventricule gauche
Singulärer Papillarmuskel des linken Ventrikels
Músculo papilar único del ventrículo izquierdo
Parachute mitral valve

Excludes: Other anatomic forms of congenital mitral stenosis

Minimal Diagnostic Criteria: While obstruction at the mitral valve may be diagnosed at cardiac catheterization, a parachute deformity can only be suspected. The demonstration of a single, large papillary muscle on a left ventriculogram supports the diagnosis. The diagnosis cannot be made with certainty, however, except by direct visualization.

Clinical Findings: In its pure form, this entity consists of a mitral valve with normal leaflets and commissures. The chordae tendineae, however, are thickened, shortened and converge into a single or nearly single papillary muscle, much as the shrouds of a parachute, hence the descriptive name. While the leaflets and commissures are normal, the short, thickened chordae tendineae with their single point of insertion may severely compromise the effective mitral valve orifice as blood must flow through the interchordal spaces. In addition, the normal mobility of the leaflets is lacking because of the thickened chordae. The clinical manifestations, then, are those of mitral stenosis.

The actual symptomatology is quite variable and dependent on the presence, or absence, of associated lesions. In general, however, symptoms lead to a diagnosis of congenital heart disease early in life. Dyspnea, congestive heart failure and pulmonary infections are common presenting complaints. Right ventricular hypertrophy can usually be detected on physical examination. A systolic murmur at the apex and accentuated first and second sounds are frequent auscultatory findings. The classic diastolic murmur of mitral stenosis is variable. If a diastolic murmur is present, it may be secondary to increased flow from an associated left-to-right shunt lesion. However, if the murmur has a presystolic accentuation, anatomic mitral valve obstruction should be suspected. Unlike acquired mitral stenosis, the opening snap is an infrequent finding. Either an associated obstructive lesion or congestive heart failure may mask the characteristic murmur.

The chest film may show pulmonary venous obstruction and an enlarged heart with discrete left atrial enlargement. The cardiogram will reflect right-sided enlargement and left atrial enlargement. It cannot be overemphasized, however, that the characteristic physical and laboratory findings may be masked by coexisting lesions.

Coexisting left heart lesions have been stressed in most case reports. These include supravalvar stenosing ring of the mitral valve, aortic stenosis, subaortic stenosis and coarctation of the aorta. Additionally, fibroelastotic changes in the left heart are not uncommon. In at least 3 cases, however, right ventricular outflow tract obstruction, either at the pulmonic valve or below, has been reported.

The echocardiographic features of this anomaly reflect both its anatomy and physiology. The mitral valve motion pattern is reduced in velocity and amplitude, similar to the pattern seen in mitral stenosis (see Mitral Valve Stenosis). The left ventricular cavity has greater than normal papillary muscle echoes.

Cardiac catheterization data usually will show elevated pulmonary artery and pulmonary arterial wedge pressures secondary to obstruction; however, a simultaneous comparison of left atrial pressure with left ventricular diastolic pressure is mandatory to confirm a pressure difference across the valve. As with the clinical findings, catheterization data may be misleading because of associated defects.†

Complications
I **Derived:** Frequent pulmonary infections, growth failure and death from congestive heart failure.
II **Associated:** —

Etiology: ?

Pathogenesis: ?

Related Facts
I **Sex Ratio:** M?:F?
II **Risk of Occurrence:** ?
III **Risk of Recurrence for**
  Patient's Sib: ?
  Patient's Child: ?
IV **Age of Detectability:** In the neonatal period, by selective left ventricular angiocardiography.
V **Prevalence:** ?

Treatment
I **Primary Prevention:** —
II **Secondary Prevention:** Operative intervention to relieve severe obstruction of flow through the mitral valve. This particular form of congenital mitral stenosis is apparently most successfully dealt with by valve replacement.†
III **Other Therapy:** Symptomatic therapy for congestive heart failure and respiratory infections.

Prognosis: This depends on the associated lesions. Most patients are severely symptomatic and die in early childhood. Recently, several successful valve replacements have been reported in children in whom the associated cardiac lesions were not severe. The long-term prognosis for the operated children is not known.

Detection of Carrier: —

†**Special Considerations:** Congenital mitral stenosis is a very rare lesion. The parachute deformity of the mitral valve is only one form. Undoubtedly there are reported cases of congenital mitral stenosis which include this deformity. Its frequency as a cause of hemodynamic abnormality is not now known. Its significance is related to the inability to correct this lesion with conservative valvotomy. Thus, a decision for the necessity of surgical intervention must include the probability of mitral valve replacement.

References:
Glancy, D.L. et al: Parachute mitral valve. Further observations and associated lesions. Am. J. Cardiol. 27:309, 1971.
Hastreiter, A.R.: Endocardial fibroelastosis. In Moss, A.J. and Adams, F.H. (eds.): Heart Disease in Infants, Children, and Adolescents. Baltimore: Williams & Wilkins, 1968, p. 760.
Shone, J.D. et al: The developmental complex of "parachute mitral valve," supravalvular ring of left atrium, subaortic stenosis and coarctation of aorta. Am. J. Cardiol. 11:714, 1963.
Simon, A.L. et al: The angiographic features of a case of parachute mitral valve. Am. Heart J. 77:809, 1969.
Terzaki, A.K. et al: Successful surgical treatment for "parachute mitral valve" complex: Report of 2 cases. J. Thorac. Cardiovasc. Surg. 56:1, 1968.
Williams, D.E. et al: Cross-sectional echocardiographic localization of the sites of left ventricular outflow tract obstruction. Am. J. Cardiol. 37(2):250, 1976.

Contributor: **Robert H. Miller**

Editor's Computerized Descriptor: CV.

LENS AND PUPIL, ECTOPIC

Includes: Ectopie du cristallin et de la pupille
Ectopia del cristalino y de la pupila
Congenital ectopic lens and pupil
Ectopia lentis et pupillae

Excludes: Lens, ectopic (584)

Minimal Diagnostic Criteria: Dislocation of the pupil and lens

Clinical Findings: Incomplete dislocation (subluxation) of both lenses with ectopic pupils is present at birth. Usually the lenses and pupils are displaced in opposite directions with the lenses most frequently displaced inferiorly. The direction may vary, however, and rare patients exhibit considerable asymmetry in the 2 eyes. The pupil is often oval or slit-shaped. Vision is often reduced and monocular diplopia may be present. Aphakic vision is sometimes seen.

Complications
I **Derived:** Aphakia, glaucoma, retinal detachment
II **Associated:** —

Etiology: Autosomal recessive

Pathogenesis: ?

Related Facts
I **Sex Ratio:** M1:F1
II **Risk of Occurrence:** ?
III **Risk of Recurrence for**
  Patient's Sib: 1 in 4 (25%) for each offspring to be affected
  Patient's Child: Not increased unless mate is carrier or homozygote
IV **Age of Detectability:** At birth
V **Prevalence:** Rare

Treatment
I **Primary Prevention:** Genetic counseling
II **Secondary Prevention:** Optical iridectomy or lens extraction may rarely be needed.
III **Other Therapy:** —

Prognosis: Normal life span, ocular prognosis dependent upon degree of defect

Detection of Carrier: —

Special Considerations: —

References:
Diethelm, W.: Über Ectopia Lentis ohne Arachnodaktylie und ihre Beziehungen zur ectopia Lentis et Pupillae. Ophthalmologica 114:16, 1947.
Franceschetti, A.: Ectopia Lentis et Pupillae congenita als rezessives Erbleiden und ihre Manifestierung durch Konsanguinität. Klin. Monatsbl. Augenheilkd. 78:351, 1927.

Contributor: **Harold E. Cross**

Editor's Computerized Descriptors: Vision, Eye

LENS, ECTOPIC

Includes: Luxation congénitale du cristallin
Angeborene Linsenektopie
Luxación congénita del cristalino
Dislocation of ocular lens
Subluxation of lens
Congenital ectopia lentis

Excludes: Marfan syndrome (630)
Spherophakia-brachymorphia syndrome (893)
Homocystinuria (474)
Sulfite oxidase deficiency (921)
Lens and pupil, ectopic (583)

Minimal Diagnostic Criteria: Dilated slit-lamp biomicroscopy may be needed to identify minimal dislocation.

Clinical Findings: The isolated abnormality of incomplete dislocation (subluxation) of the lens may be present at birth or occur later. The patient may have no symptoms or may complain of poor vision and monocular diplopia. Physical signs include iridodonesis, irregularly deep anterior chambers and uncorrected poor visual acuity in some cases. Bilateral dislocation is the rule.

Complications
I   **Derived:** Glaucoma, cataract, detached retina
II **Associated:** Cataract, myopia, astigmatism, aniridia, persistent pupillary membrane, colobomas

Etiology: Autosomal dominant. Most likely, heterogeneity exists with at least two recognizable disorders: simple ectopia lentis as a congenital, usually benign abnormality, and spontaneous late subluxation which is usually detected after the 3rd decade of life and often complicated by glaucoma. McK *12960

Pathogenesis: Structural defect of lens zonules which may relate to persistence of the vascular tunic of the lens.

Related Facts
I   **Sex Ratio:** M1:F1
II   **Risk of Occurrence:** ?
III **Risk of Recurrence for**
     Patient's Sib: If parent is affected, 1 in 2 (50%) for each offspring to be affected, otherwise not increased.
     Patient's Child: 1 in 2
IV   **Age of Detectability:** Usually at birth
V   **Prevalence:** Rare

Treatment
I   **Primary Prevention:** Genetic counseling
II   **Secondary Prevention:** —
III **Other Therapy:** Optical iridectomy; cataract extraction when indicated

Prognosis: Normal life span, ocular prognosis guarded

Detection of Carrier: —

Special Considerations: —

References:
Duke-Elder, S.: System of Ophthalmology, vol. 3, part 2. Congenital Deformities. London:Henry Kimpton, 1964.
François, J.: Congenital Cataracts. Netherlands: C.C Thomas, 1963, p. 72.
Stevenson, R. E.: Ectopia lentis et pupillae. In Bergsma, D. (ed.): Part VIII. Eye. Birth Defects: Orig. Art. Ser., vol. VII, no. 3. Baltimore:Williams and Wilkins for The National Foundation-March of Dimes, 1971, p. 173.

Contributor: **Harold E. Cross**

Editor's Computerized Descriptors: Vision, Eye

LENTICONUS

Includes: Lenticone
Lenticono
Lentiglobus

Excludes: Keratoconus (552)
Megalocornea (637)

Minimal Diagnostic Criteria: Slit-lamp evidence of protruded lens surface

Clinical Findings: Protrusion of the anterior or posterior surface of the lens occurs in either a conical (conus) or a spherical (globus) shape. The anterior variety usually presents as bilateral localized thickenings of the anterior lens cortex. The central lens is highly myopic but may be clear. Although probably present at birth, the youngest described patient was 4 years old. The deformity may be progressive leading to further diminution of vision.
An oil globule appearance is characteristic of the posterior variety. Central high myopia is also found. On slit-lamp examination there is a ring reflex. This condition is usually unilateral. Visual acuity is poor.

Complications
I   **Derived:** Anterior polar cataracts may develop in anterior lenticonus.
II **Associated:** Posterior polar lens opacities are common (80%) concomitant features of posterior lentiglobus. Other associations include uveal colobomas, microphthalmos, lens colobomas, oxycephaly, deafness, hypertelorism and Alport syndrome. Associated defects are rare in anterior lenticonus, although it has been reported with rubella embryopathy and a variety of forms of congenital cataract.

Etiology: ?

Pathogenesis: Delayed separation of the lens vesicle from the surface epithelium in anterior lenticonus, and posterior hyaloid artery persistence with a weak posterior capsule or overgrowth of lens fibers in posterior lentiglobus have been suggested to be the mechanisms responsible for the defects.

Related Facts
I   **Sex Ratio:** Lenticonus M > :F; Lentiglobus M2:F3
II   **Risk of Occurrence:** ?
III **Risk of Recurrence for**
     Patient's Sib: ?
     Patient's Child: ?
IV   **Age of Detectability:** At 4 years, probably earlier
V   **Prevalence:** Unknown, but anterior lenticonus is rarer than posterior lentiglobus

Treatment
I   **Primary Prevention:** —
II   **Secondary Prevention:** —
III **Other Therapy:** Lens extraction where indicated

Prognosis: Life span normal; visual prognosis variable

Detection of Carrier: —

Special Considerations: —

References:
Duke-Elder, S.: System of Ophthalmology, vol. 3, part 2. Congenital Deformities. London:Henry Kimpton, 1964, p. 696.

Contributor: **Harold E. Cross**

Editor's Computerized Descriptors: Vision, Eye

LENTIGINES SYNDROME, MULTIPLE

Includes: Lentiginose profuse ou diffuse
Syndrom der multiplen Lentigines
Síndrome de lentigos múltiples
Leopard syndrome
Cardiocutaneous syndrome
Multiple lentigines syndrome

Excludes: Noonan syndrome (720)

Minimal Diagnostic Criteria: A combination of most or all of the below findings should be present for the diagnosis. Some patients have all of the findings except lentigines.

Clinical Findings: The syndrome consists of multiple lentigines (ca 80%); ECG abnormalities of the S_1, S_2, S_3 type indicative of aberrant interventricular conduction (ca 95%); ocular hypertelorism (ca 75%); pulmonary stenosis, either valvular or infundibular (ca 95%); abnormalities of the genitalia, such as cryptorchidism, development and descent of only one testicle, hypospadias (ca 50% of affected males); retardation of growth (ca 90%); sensorineural deafness (ca 15%); winging of the scapulae (ca 50%); and mild pterygium colli (ca 35%).

Other findings include triangular face with biparietal bossing and eyelid ptosis. Various other cardiac findings have included hypertrophic cardiomyopathy, aortic valvular dysplasia, heart block, and atrial septal defect.

Complications
I **Derived:** Sterility, if cryptorchidism is bilateral
II **Associated:** Not yet discernible

Etiology: Autosomal dominant transmission of mutant gene with high penetrance and variable expressivity; McK *15110

Pathogenesis: ?

Related Facts
I **Sex Ratio:** M1:F1
II **Risk of Occurrence:** ?
III **Risk of Recurrence for**
  Patient's Sib: 1 in 2 if a parent is affected, negligible if it can be determined with certainty that neither parent is affected.
  Patient's Child: 1 in 2 regardless of the sex of the next child and regardless of the sex of the affected parent. An affected person need not manifest lentigines and, hence, may escape detection. Affected males may have a somewhat reduced reproductive fitness due to cryptorchidism.
IV **Age of Detectability:** Four to 5 years of age since lentigines usually become abundant by this time. Possibly earlier if there is involved sib.
V **Prevalence:** ?

Treatment
I **Primary Prevention:** Genetic counseling
II **Secondary Prevention:** Surgical correction of cryptorchidism and of cardiac lesion
III **Other Therapy:** —

Prognosis: For life: Good, since pulmonary stenosis is rarely seriously disabling in affected persons. For intelligence: No intellectual deficit and essentially normal for function, unless hampered by deafness or pulmonary stenosis.

Detection of Carrier: Detailed examination will usually allow detection of affected individuals who do not have lentigines.

Special Considerations: —

References:
Gorlin, R.J. et al: Multiple lentigines syndrome. Am. J. Dis Child. 117:562, 1969.
Gorlin, R.J. et al: The Leopard (multiple lentigines) syndrome revisited. In Bergsma, D. (ed.): Part IX. Ear. Birth Defects: Orig. Art. Ser., vol. VII, no. 4. Baltimore: The Williams and Wilkins Co., for The National Foundation - March of Dimes, 1971, p. 110.
Polani, P.E. and Moynahan, E.J.: Progressive cardiopathic lentigines. Q. J. Med. 41:205, 1972.

Contributor: **Robert J. Gorlin**

Editor's Computerized Descriptors: Eye, Hearing, Skin, Skel., CV., GU.

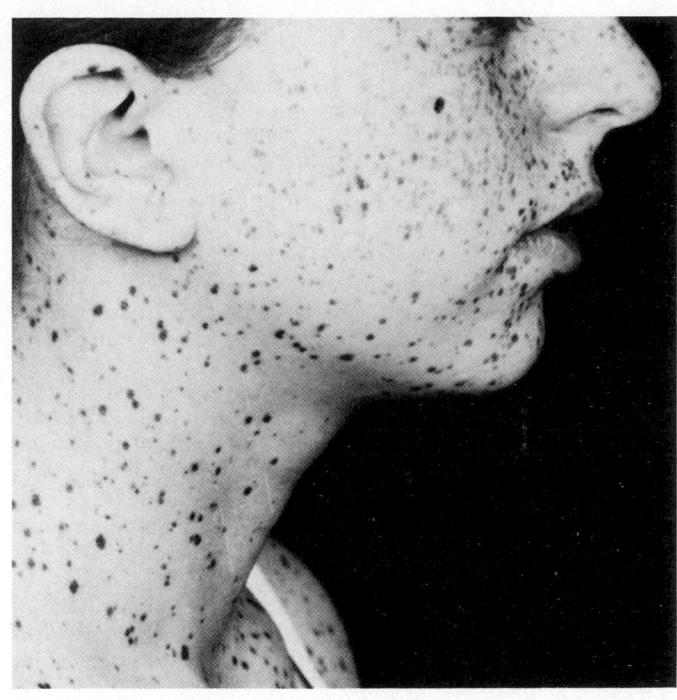

321. Multiple lentigines

LEPRECHAUNISM

Includes: Lépréchaunisme
Leprechaunismus
Leprechaunismo
Donohue syndrome

Excludes: Cockayne syndrome (189)
Chromosome 8 trisomy syndrome (157)

Minimal Diagnostic Criteria: Because of the fact that a diagnosis of leprechaunism must be made primarily upon the basis of clinical findings, only arbitrary minimal diagnostic criteria can be proposed. A presumptive clinical diagnosis of leprechaunism may be made if the patient exhibits malignant failure to thrive, elfin facies with thick lips, large low-set ears, hirsutism, prominent breasts and external genitalia. The clinical diagnosis is supported by the demonstration of abnormal carbohydrate metabolism with increased hepatic glycogen, hepatic siderosis, hyperplasia of the endocrine pancreas, and by ovarian cystic changes.

Clinical Findings: Findings here will be based on a review of 15 cases of leprechaunism, 11 females and 4 males. Approximately 20 cases have been reported; however, 5 are so atypical as to raise serious doubts concerning their validity. Leprechaunism becomes apparent in early infancy and is usually fatal in the early months of life, 11 of the 15 known cases having died at 21 days to 24 months of age. Some investigators suggest that death in infancy is necessary for the diagnosis of leprechaunism. Leprechaunism is characterized by grotesque elfin facies with a flat nasal bridge and flaring nostrils (15/15); thick lips (9/15); large, low-set ears (14/15); hirsutism (11/15); breast enlargement (11/15 including 2 males); prominent clitoris and labia minora in 10 of 11 females and a large penis in all males; deficiency of subcutaneous tissue leading to the presence of excessive folding of the skin, particularly that of the limbs (12/14); motor and mental retardation (10/10); and severe failure to thrive leading to extreme marasmus (14/14) and death in the early months of life (11/15).

Other less frequently noted features include microcephaly, hypertelorism, high or narrowly arched palate, cardiac murmur, umbilical and inguinal herniae or diastasis recti, cryptorchidism, poor muscle tone, unusally large hands and feet, and delayed skeletal maturation. Poley has suggested that cholestatic jaundice, observed in several cases, be considered a feature of leprechaunism.

Complications
I   **Derived:** Susceptibility to infection, early death
II   **Associated:** —

Etiology: Probably autosomal recessive mutant allele; McK *24620

Pathogenesis: ? †

Related Facts
I   **Sex Ratio:** M1:F3
II   **Risk of Occurrence:** Rare
III **Risk of Recurrence for**
     Patient's Sib: Maximum risk of 1 in 4 if an autosomal recessive mutant allele is operative.
     Patient's Child: Probably a lethal condition with "O" reproductive fitness
IV   **Age of Detectability:** In early infancy
V   **Prevalence:** ?

Treatment
I   **Primary Prevention:** Genetic counseling
II   **Secondary Prevention:** —
III **Other Therapy:** Various complications, particularly infections, should be treated as indicated. Utilization of gastros-

tomy feedings has been of temporary benefit in some cases.

Prognosis: Eleven of 15 reported cases have died before 2 years of age. All cases have demonstrated severe motor-mental defect and progressive marasmus.

Detection of Carrier: —

†**Special Considerations:** The occurrence of 2 affected sibs in each of 2 reported sibships, the possibility of multiple affected sibs in 3 other reported families, parental consanguinity in at least 2 families, and the uniform occurrence of normal parents of affected infants suggest that leprechaunism is produced by an autosomal recessive mutant allele in the homozygous state. No causative chromosome abnormality has been reported.

If this condition is produced by an autosomal recessive mutant allele, the primary effect of the mutation has thus far escaped elucidation. Several bits of evidence suggest a metabolic-endocrine aberration in individual patients, but none is uniformly present. A frequently reported abnormality is that involving regulation of carbohydrate metabolism. Such an abnormality is suggested by the occurrence of hypoglycemia, hyperinsulinism, a decreased blood sugar response to adrenalin and glucagon, an exaggerated response to insulin, and hyperplasia and increased numbers of pancreatic islets of Langerhans with evidence that the hyperplasia is due to an increased number of β cells. Enlargement of the external genitalia, maturation of seminiferous tubules in the testicles of affected males, cystic ovaries and histologic changes in the thyroid gland have all suggested excessive stimulation by trophic hormones, and in 1 case this was supported by the presence of an increased number of pituitary basophils. However, the pituitary gland has been normal in other cases.

Leprechaunism constitutes, at best, a formal genesis syndrome; ie a phenotype shared completely or in part by several individuals to the extent that the similarities must be based on a common dysmorphogenetic process. This, however, does not necessarily specify that the same etiology is operative in every case. The absence of a definable common metabolic alteration in affected cases leaves open the possibility that this phenotype could represent a heterogeneous group of coincidentally phenotypically similar but etiologically unrelated patients. Many of the common phenotypic features could be secondary to marasmus whatever the cause. The fact that a similar phenotype can be acquired and is reversible is demonstrated by the case of Hopwood and associates. Some cases reported in the literature as leprechaunism have been excluded from this review, because their phenotypes seemed distinctly different. Such an exclusion is to some extent arbitrary. In the opinion of this contributor, leprechaunism and the Cockayne syndrome are clearly different entities.

References:
Dekaban, A.: Metabolic and chromosomal studies in Leprechaunism. Arch. Dis. Child. 40:632, 1965.
der Kaloustian,V.M. et al: Leprechaunism. A report of two new cases. Am. J. Dis. Child. 122:442, 1971.
Donohue, W.L. and Uchida, I.: Leprechaunism: Euphuism for a rare familial disorder. J. Pediatr. 45:505, 1954.
Gamstorp, I.: Donohue's syndrome-leprechaunism-Cockayne's syndrome. Eur. Neurol. 7:26, 1972.
Hopwood, N.J. and Powell, G.F.: Emotional deprivation. Report of a case with features of leprechaunism. Am. J. Dis. Child. 127:892, 1974.
Kálló, A. et al: Leprechaunism (Donohue's syndrome). J. Pediatr. 66:372, 1965.
Ordway, N.K. and Stout, L.C.: Intrauterine growth retardation, jaundice, and hypoglycemia in a neonate. J. Pediatr. 83:867,

1973.

Rogers, D.R.: Leprechaunism (Donohue's syndrome). A possible case, with emphasis on changes in the adenohypophysis. Am. J. Clin. Pathol. 45:614, 1966.

Summitt, R.L. and Favara, B.E.: Leprechaunism (Donohue's syndrome): Case report. J. Pediatr. 74:601, 1969.

Uematsu, K. et al: Leprechaunism (Donohue's syndrome)-Two autopsy cases. Acta. Pathol. Jph. 24:309, 1974.

Contributor: **Robert L. Summitt**

Editor's Computerized Descriptors: Eye, Ear, Face, Nose, Skin, Hair, Skel., Muscle, Hernia not CNS, CV., Liver, GU., Nerve

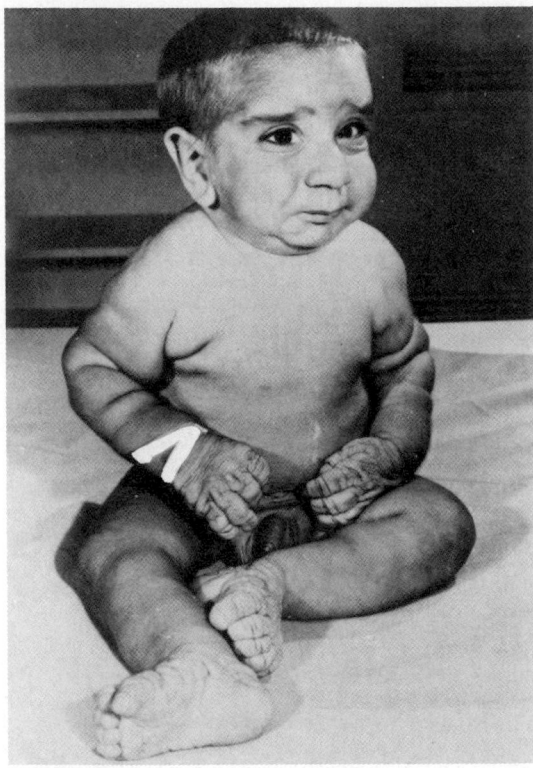

322. Note large hands and feet with marked redundancy and wrinkling of overlying skin

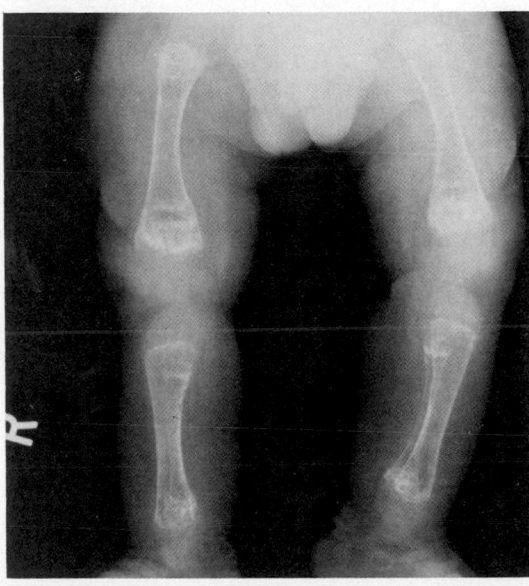

323. Failure in epiphyseal and linear growth of long bones

LESCH-NYHAN SYNDROME

Includes: Syndrome de Lesch-Nyhan
Síndrome de Lesch-Nyhan
X-linked primary hyperuricemia
Hypoxanthine guanine phosphoribosyl transferase deficiency
Disorder of uric acid metabolism and central nervous system function

Excludes: Gout (441)

Minimal Diagnostic Criteria: Most patients with complete absence of hypoxanthine guanine phosphoribosyl transferase activity will be found to have the complete picture including hyperuricemia (cf Gout) and evidence of cerebral dysfunction such as choreoathetosis, cerebral palsy, mental retardation and self-mutilation.

Clinical Findings: Patients appear normal at birth but develop progressive choreoathetosis and spastic cerebral palsy. Mental retardation and motor defect are such that these patients do not walk and few can sit without assistance. They are characterized by bizarre aggressive behavior whose most prominent manifestation is self-mutilation, usually by biting. In addition to these features relevant to the nervous system, these patients have all the clinical findings of gout, including hyperuricemia, hematuria, crystalluria, urinary tract stones, nephropathy, tophi, and acute arthritis. Mild anemia is common and megaloblasts are occasionally seen in the marrow.

Complications
I **Derived:** Nephropathy; renal failure; athetoid dysphagia is extreme and vomiting is prominent; thus these patients are hard to feed. They may die of inanition or aspiration and pneumonia, as well as of renal failure.
II **Associated:** —

Etiology: X-linked recessive transmission; McK *30800

Pathogenesis: Absence of hypoxanthine guanine phosphoribosyl transferase activity. The manner in which this leads to the cerebral manifestations of the disease is unknown.

Related Facts
I **Sex Ratio:** M1:F0
II **Risk of Occurrence:** ?
III **Risk of Recurrence for**
    Patient's Sib: If mother is a carrier, 1 in 2 (50%) for each brother to be affected and 1 in 2 for each sister to be a carrier.
    Patient's Child: 1 in 1 (100%) for carrier daughters; not increased for sons unless wife is a carrier. No patient with this disease has reproduced. It is not likely that one will.
IV **Age of Detectability:** At birth; it is now possible to detect prior to birth by assay of the enzyme in cultured cells obtained by amniocentesis.
V **Prevalence:** ?

Treatment
I **Primary Prevention:** Genetic counseling
II **Secondary Prevention:** See Treatment for Gout. Allopurinol is excellent therapy for the management of hyperuricemia. It will prevent all of those manifestations of this disease that are direct consequences of elevated concentrations of uric acid. It does not prevent or alleviate the cerebral manifestations.
III **Other Therapy:** Appropriate binding of hands and elbows to prevent mutilation of hands.

Prognosis: In the absence of allopurinol most patients have died under 5 years of age. A few long survivors have lived to 20 years.

Detection of Carrier: Culture of fibroblasts from the skin and cloning have yielded two populations of cells from the maternal heterozygote. One population has normal enzyme activity and the other is completely deficient like the patient's. This identifies the carrier and is consistent with the Lyon hypothesis. Hair follicles are also largely clonal and they are the most practical method for the detection of the heterozygote by analysis of the enzyme activity in hair roots. The blood cannot be used for this purpose as the blood of the maternal carrier of this disease is always normal.

Special Considerations: —

References:

Bland, J.: Proceedings of the Seminars on the Lesch-Nyhan syndrome. Fed. Proc. 27:1019, 1968.

Francke, U. et al: Detection of heterozygous carriers of the Lesch-Nyhan syndrome by electrophoresis of hair root lysates. J. Pediatr. 82:472, 1973.

Gartler, S.M. et al: Lesch-Nyhan syndrome: Rapid detection of heterozygotes by use of hair follicles. Science 172:572, 1971.

Lesch, M. and Nyhan, W.L.: A familial disorder of uric acid metabolism and central nervous system function. Am. J. Med. 36:561, 1964.

Migeon, B.R. et al: X-linked hypoxanthine-guanine phosphoribosyl transferase deficiency: Heterozygote has two clonal populations. Science 160:425, 1968.

Nyhan, W.L.: The Lesch-Nyhan syndrome. Annu. Rev. Med. 24:41, 1973.

Nyhan, W.L. et al: Hemizygous expression of glucose-6-phosphate dehydrogenase in erythrocytes of heterozygotes for the Lesch-Nyhan syndrome. Proc. Natl. Acad. Sci. USA. 65:214, 1970.

Contributor: **William L. Nyhan**

Editor's Computerized Descriptors: Skel., GU., Nerve

LEUKONYCHIA

Includes: Leuconychie
Leukonychie
Leuconiquia
Leukonychia partialis, striata, and totalis

Excludes: Leukonychia, punctate

Minimal Diagnostic Criteria: White discoloration of nail

Clinical Findings: A whitish discoloration of the nails either as a single, broad, or transverse band, one or more narrow bands, a large white area, or a completely white nail. Either the fingers, toes, or both may be involved. The nails are not brittle or frayed. The thickness of the nails appears average and no grooves or other irregularities are observed.

Complications
I Derived: —
II Associated: Reported association with leukotrichia, total alopecia, extensive vitiligo, and multiple cyst formation.

Etiology: Autosomal dominant for leukonychia totalis; McK *15160

Pathogenesis: Two major theories advocate that the white color is due to opacity of the nail plate. One theory holds that abnormal keratinization of the nail plate is sufficient to cause the opacity; while the other postulates that air must be present within the nail plate.

Related Facts
I Sex Ratio: M1:F1.5 ?
II Risk of Occurrence: ?
III Risk of Recurrence for
  Patient's Sib: For leukonychia totalis, if parent is affected 1 in 2 (50%) for each offspring to be affected; otherwise not increased.
  Patient's Child: 1 in 2
IV Age of Detectability: At birth
V Prevalence: ?

Treatment
I Primary Prevention: Genetic counseling
II Secondary Prevention: —
III Other Therapy: —

Prognosis: Normal life span

Detection of Carrier: —

Special Considerations: —

References:

Albright, S. D., 3d. and Wheeler, C. E., Jr.: Leukonychia: Total and partial leukonychia in a single family with a review of the literature. Arch. Dermatol. 90:392, 1964.

Medansky, R. S. and Fox, J. M.: Hereditary leukonychia totalis. Arch. Dermatol. 82:412, 1960.

Contributor: **Roland S. Medansky**

Editor's Computerized Descriptor: Nails

LIDDLE SYNDROME

Includes: Syndrome de Liddle
Síndrome de Liddle
Potassium-losing nephropathy with low aldosterone

Excludes: All forms of hypokalemic alkalosis, renal potassium loss and hyperaldosteronism

Minimal Diagnostic Criteria: Potassium-losing nephritis with subnormal-to-low aldosterone secretion.

Clinical Findings: This syndrome is characterized by hypokalemic alkalosis, hypertension, and renal potassium wasting of as much as 80 mEq of K+ daily. Growth is unaffected. Polydipsia and polyuria, and an inability to concentrate urine are also present. In contrast to expectations, aldosterone secretion is low and does not increase with sodium deprivation even when potassium stores are repleted. Neither spironolactone which blocks the renal tubular effects of aldosterone, nor a drug (SU9055) blocking aldosterone biosynthesis, modifies the renal loss of electrolytes. Renin levels are normal or high, which is different from the situation in hyperaldosteronism where renin levels are low. There is a satisfactory renal response to ammonium chloride, acetezolamide and exogenous aldosterone, and renal function appears normal apart from the potassium loss. Triamterene, which blocks renal tubular exchange of potassium for sodium is effective, correcting the high blood pressure, hypokalemic alkalosis, and increasing sodium excretion.

Complications
I **Derived:** The complications are related to the degree of hypokalemia. However, the original report concerned a 16-year-old girl, and the disease thus appears compatible with life.
II **Associated:** —

Etiology: This is a familial defect probably with autosomal dominant inheritance.

Pathogenesis: The pathogenesis is not entirely understood but probably affects membrane transport of potassium at the renal tubular level.

Related Facts
I **Sex Ratio:** M1:F1
II **Risk of Occurrence:** ?
III **Risk of Recurrence for**
 Patient's Sib: If parent is affected 1 in 2 (50%) for each offspring to be affected; otherwise not increased.
 Patient's Child: 1 in 2
IV **Age of Detectability:** Birth onwards
V **Prevalence:** ?

Treatment
I **Primary Prevention:** Genetic counseling
II **Secondary Prevention:** Triamterene is effective in correcting blood pressure, potassium loss and alkalosis. This therapy should be maintained since the clinical findings return on discontinuation of treatment.
III **Other Therapy:** —

Prognosis: The prognosis appears normal for life span if treated.

Detection of Carrier: —

Special Considerations: —

References:
Aarskog, D. et al: Hypertension and hypokalemic alkalosis associated with underproduction of aldosterone. Pediatrics 39:884, 1967.
Liddle, C.W. et al: A familial renal disorder simulating primary aldosteronism but with negligible aldosterone secretion. In Baulieu, E.E. and Robel, P. (eds.): Aldosterone, A Symposium. Oxford: Blackwell Scientific Publications, 1964, p. 352.
Milora, B. et al: A familial syndrome resembling primary aldosteronism but with subnormal aldosterone secretion. Clin. Res. 16:199, 1968.

Contributor: **Mark A. Sperling**

Editor's Computerized Descriptor: GU.

LIMBAL DERMOID

Includes: Dermoide du limbe
Epibulbäres Dermoid
Dermoide limbal
Dermoid of the cornea
Conjunctival dermoid
Epibulbar dermoid

Excludes: Dermolipoma (284)
Orbital and periorbital dermoid cysts (761)

Minimal Diagnostic Criteria: Solid tumor usually at limbus

Clinical Findings: This is a pink white solid tumor which usually occurs at the limbus. It usually remains stationary but rarely may encroach upon the cornea or actually invade the globe.

Complications
I **Derived:** Invasion of the globe with secondary glaucoma; astigmatism
II **Associated:** Mandibulofacial dysostosis; Goldenhar syndrome; auricular appendages

Etiology: ?

Pathogenesis: ?

Related Facts
I **Sex Ratio:** M?:F?
II **Risk of Occurrence:** ? Rare
III **Risk of Recurrence for**
    Patient's Sib: ?
    Patient's Child: ?
IV **Age of Detectability:** At birth
V **Prevalence:** ? Rare

Treatment
I **Primary Prevention:** —
II **Secondary Prevention:** Excision
III **Other Therapy:** —

Prognosis: Excellent for life span, intelligence and for function, if excised early

Detection of Carrier: —

Special Considerations: —

References:
Duke-Elder, S.: System of Ophthalmology, vol. 3, pt 2. Congenital Deformities. St. Louis: C.V. Mosby, 1964, p. 535.
Schultz, G. et al: Ocular dermoids and auricular appendages. Am. J. Ophthalmol. 63:938, 1967.
Schulze, R.: Limbal dermoid tumor with intraocular extension. Arch. Ophthalmol. 75:803, 1966.

Contributor: **Morton E. Smith**

Editor's Computerized Descriptors: Vision, Eye

LIMB-OTO-CARDIAC SYNDROME

Includes: L'association phocomélie-ectrodactylie, malformations des oreilles avec surdité, arythmie sinusale
Hypoplasie der oberen Extremitäten, Ohrfehlbildungen mit Taubheit, und kardialer arrythmie
Hipoplasia de las extremidades superiores, arritmia cardíaca, oído externo malformado y sordera de conducción

Excludes: Heart-hand syndrome (455)
Fetal thalidomide syndrome (386)

Minimal Diagnostic Criteria: Hypoplasia of upper limbs, cardiac arrhythmia, malformed external ear, unilateral conduction deafness.

Clinical Findings: Hypoplasia of the upper limbs, sinus arrhythmia, malformed external ears and profound unilateral conduction deafness have been reported in a father and son. The malformation of the upper limbs is characterized by the absence of the radius, hypoplasia of the humerus, and the absence of 2 metacarpals and 2 or 3 fingers on each side. The malformation of the middle ear was characterized by the absence of the incus and stapes and an aplasia of the oval window.†

Complications
I **Derived:** —
II **Associated:** —

Etiology: Autosomal dominant inheritance is suggested.

Pathogenesis: ?

Related Facts
I **Sex Ratio:** M2:F0
II **Risk of Occurrence:** ?
III **Risk of Recurrence for**
    Patient's Sib: ?
    Patient's Child: ?
IV **Age of Detectability:** At birth
V **Prevalence:** Very rare. 1 reported family with 2 affected males, a father and son.

Treatment
I **Primary Prevention:** Genetic counseling
II **Secondary Prevention:** —
III **Other Therapy:** Surgery?†

Prognosis: Probably normal life span; intelligence is normal.

Detection of Carrier: —

†Special Considerations: Because of the absence of the oval window, reconstructive middle ear surgery was impossible in these cases.

References:
Stoll, C. et al: L'association phocomélie-ectrodactylie, malformations des oreilles avec surdité, arythmie sinusale. Arch. Fr. Pediatr. 31:669, 1974.

Contributors: **Agnes M. Ickenroth
Cor W.R.J. Cremers**

Editor's Computerized Descriptors: Hearing, Ear, Skel., CV.

LINEAR NEVUS SEBACEOUS SYNDROME

Includes: Syndrome de naevus sébacé
Syndrom des Lineären Naevus sebaceus
Síndrome de nevus sebáceos lineares
New neurocutaneous syndrome
Multiple choristomas, convulsions and mental retardation
Nevus sebaceous of Jadassohn
Nevi, linear sebaceous

Excludes: Other phakomatosis disorders
Tuberous sclerosis (975)
Sturge-Weber syndrome (915)
Neurofibromatosis (712)

Minimal Diagnostic Criteria: Mental retardation, seizures, linear sebaceous nevi on the face, and multiple nevi are the most common abnormalities.

Clinical Findings: The clinical findings, based upon reports of 7 cases, include multiple congenital anomalies involving the skin, eyes, brain, and cardiovascular system. Multiple sebaceous nevi are present on the face, scalp, palatine mucosa, neck and body. Characteristically, 1 nevus extends from the forehead to the tip of the nose. Affected children have been mentally retarded and have seizures. Hydrocephaly has been demonstrated radiographically. Failure to thrive with poor growth and development has been seen in most cases. Severe involvement of the eyes has been described with nystagmus, scarification and vascularization of the cornea, slanting palpebral fissures, choroidal coloboma, corectopia, lipodermoids, and blindness. The nasal bridge may be depressed, the teeth hypoplastic and the palatine mucosa thickened, secondary to the presence of nevi. One reported case had coarctation of the aorta and in another case, diffuse bony changes were seen similar to those found in rickets.†

Complications
I **Derived:** Secondary infections may lead to death. Failure to thrive.
II **Associated:** —

Etiology: ?

Pathogenesis: ?

Related Facts
I **Sex Ratio:** 3 males and 4 females have been completely described.
II **Risk of Occurrence:** ?
III **Risk of Recurrence for**
  Patient's Sib: ?
  Patient's Child: ?
IV **Age of Detectability:** At birth by clinical examination
V **Prevalence:** ? The condition has been described in Caucasian, Negro and Mongolian races.

Treatment
I **Primary Prevention:** —
II **Secondary Prevention:** Anticonvulsant medication
III **Other Therapy:** Supportive, custodial care may be necessary.

Prognosis: For life: One reported case died at 8 years of age. Four others range up to 12 years. Uniform profound mental retardation is the overwhelming limiting factor and is aggravated by severe convulsive seizures.

Detection of Carrier: ?

†Special Considerations: Since so few cases have been reported, it is not yet possible clearly to delineate this syndrome. Biopsy of skin and conjunctival lesions has been helpful in establishing this diagnosis. This syndrome might overlap in some of the clinical findings with other phakomatoses. Some of the affected children have been severely affected with anomalies of many systems while others have had only seizures, mental retardation and linear sebaceous nevi.

Laboratory findings: EEGs have all been abnormal due to seizure activity. One case (Herbst) revealed a typical hypsarrythmic pattern. ECG may be abnormal due to cardiac involvement. One case was found to have a renal tubular defect with loss of amino acids but not glucose, phosphorus or potassium. Chromosomal studies have revealed no abnormality.

Biopsy of skin and conjunctival lesions has demonstrated multiple choristomas and hamartomas with hyperplastic sebaceous glands, atypical apocrine glands and immature hair follicles. The finding of sebaceous glands, hair follicles and sweat glands in the conjunctiva is quite rare.

X-ray findings: 1 case demonstrated asymmetry of the skull, deformity of the left sphenoid bone, depressed and widened sella turcica and coarctation of the aorta with hypoplasia of the aorta. Pneumoencephalograms have revealed hydrocephaly. Another case had generalized osteomalacia with rickets, swollen soft tissues, lytic defects in the ribs and malformed clavicles.

References:
Berg, J.M. and Crome, L.: A possible case of atypical tuberous sclerosis. J. Ment. Defic. Res. 4:24, 1960.
Bianchine, J.W.: The nevus sebaceous of Jadassohn. Am. J. Dis. Child. 120:223, 1970.
Feuerstein, R.C. and Mims, L.C.: Linear nevus sebaceus with convulsions and mental retardation. Am. J. Dis. Child. 104:675, 1962.
Herbst, B. and Cohen, M.E.: Linear nevus sebaceus. Arch. Neurol. 24:317, 1971.
Marden, P.M. and Venters, H.D., Jr.: A new neurocutaneous syndrome. Am. J. Dis. Child. 112:79, 1966.
Monahan, R.H. et al: Multiple choristomas, convulsions, and mental retardation as a new neurocutaneous syndrome. Am. J. Ophthalmol. (Suppl.) 64:529, 1967.
Sugarman, G.I. and Reed, W.B.: Two unusual neurocutaneous disorders with facial cutaneous signs. Arch. Neurol. 21:242, 1969.

Contributor: **Philip M. Marden**

Editor's Computerized Descriptors: Vision, Eye, Oral, Teeth, Nose, Skin, Skel., CV., Nerve

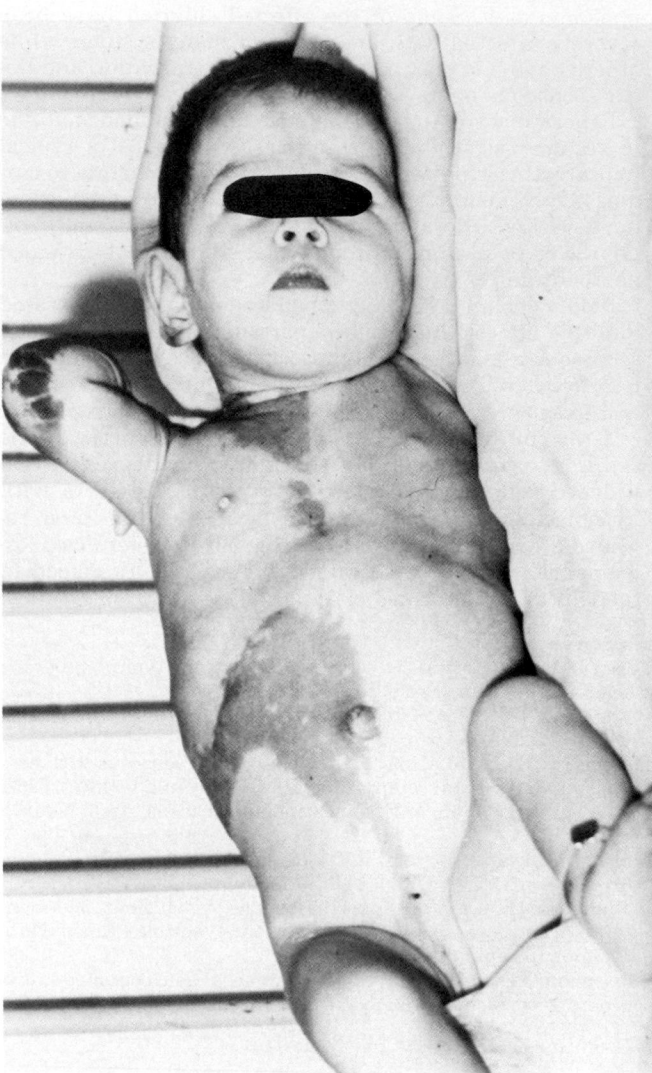

324. Note asymmetry and linear distribution of skin lesion

LIP, DOUBLE

Includes: Duplicité labiale
Doppellippe
Labio doble

Excludes: Blepharochalasis, double lip and nontoxic thyroid enlargement (111)

Minimal Diagnostic Criteria: The appearance of 2 vermilion borders of the upper lip when smiling in a patient without blepharochalasis and nontoxic thyroid enlargement.

Clinical Findings: The vermilion border of the lip is divided into 2 parts by a transverse furrow so that the inner portion of the lip, the pars villosa, sags below the outer portion, the pars glabrosa. When the lip is drawn tightly across the teeth in smiling, it gives the impression of 2 vermilion margins of the lip. In most cases only the upper lip is involved but occasionally the lower lip may also be affected.

Complications
I **Derived:** None. May be of cosmetic concern to patient.
II **Associated:** May occur as 1 sign of the triad of Ascher syndrome (double lip, blepharochalasis and nontoxic thyroid enlargement).

Etiology: ? May be genetic. Has been observed in sibs.

Pathogenesis: Opinion that defect is ascribable to displacement of fibers of orbicularis oris associated with a herniation of submucosa due to hypertrophy of the glandular and submucous tissues.

Related Facts
I **Sex Ratio:** M1:F1
II **Risk of Occurrence:** ? Rare
III **Risk of Recurrence for**
Patient's Sib: ?
Patient's Child: ?
IV **Age of Detectability:** Infancy
V **Prevalence:** Chileans 1 in 480; Caucasians (Utah) 1 in 200.

Treatment
I **Primary Prevention:** —
II **Secondary Prevention:** Surgical repair with pressure dressings
III **Other Therapy:** —

Prognosis: Excellent. Is of cosmetic concern only. General health is not impaired.

Detection of Carrier: —

Special Considerations: —

References:
Guerrero-Santos, J. and Altamirano, J.T.: The use of W-plasty for the correction of double lip deformity. Plast. Reconstr. Surg. 39:478, 1967.
Witkop, C.J., Jr.: The face and oral structures. In Rubin, A. (ed.): Handbook of Congenital Malformations. Philadelphia:W.B. Saunders Co., 1967, p. 103.

Contributor: **M. Michael Cohen, Sr.**

Editor's Computerized Descriptor: Face

LIP, MEDIAN CLEFT OF UPPER

Includes: Fissure médiane de là levre supérieure
Mittlere Unterlippenspalte
Fisura mediana del labio superior
True median cleft
Median cleft of upper lip

Excludes: Oro-facio-digital syndrome I (770)
Oro-facio-digital syndrome II (771)
Holoprosencephaly with premaxillary agenesis

Minimal Diagnostic Criteria: True median clefting of the upper lip

Clinical Findings: Midline clefting of the upper lip†

Complications
I   **Derived:** —
II **Associated:** Bifid nose, ocular hypertelorism, widow's peak, notching or coloboma of nose.

Etiology: ?

Pathogenesis: Midline mesenchymal filling defect with persistent infranasal furrow.

Related Facts
I   **Sex Ratio:** M1:F1, probably
II   **Risk of Occurrence:** Very rare
III **Risk of Recurrence for**
     Patient's Sib: ?
     Patient's Child: ?
IV   **Age of Detectability:** At birth, by physical examination
V   **Prevalence:** Very rare

Treatment
I   **Primary Prevention:** ?
II   **Secondary Prevention:** Surgical correction of defect
III **Other Therapy:** —

Prognosis: Excellent for life

Detection of Carrier: —

†**Special Considerations:** It is important to distinguish true median clefting from median pseudoclefts. True median clefting occurs as an isolated defect or as part of frontonasal dysplasia. Median pseudoclefting is found in those cases of holoprosencephaly which are associated with premaxillary agenesis and also in cases of orofaciodigital syndrome I which is associated with a hyperplastic frenum.

References:
Gorlin, R.J. and Goldman, H.M. (eds.): Thoma's Oral Pathology. 6th Ed. St. Louis: C.V. Mosby, 1970, vol. 1, p. 48.
Gorlin, R.J. and Pindborg, J.J.: Syndromes of the Head and Neck. New York: McGraw-Hill, 1964.

Contributor: **M. Michael Cohen, Jr.**

Editor's Computerized Descriptor : Face

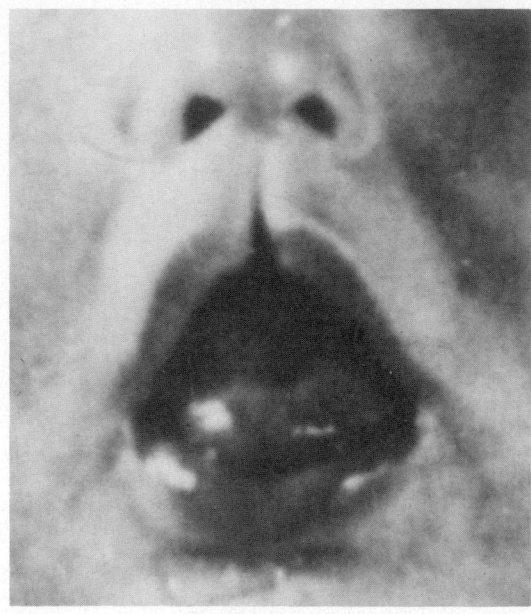

325. Midline cleft of upper lip

LIP PITS OR MOUNDS (MARKER)

Includes: Fossettes labiales
Lippengrübchen
Fóveas o montículos labiales (Marcador)
Commissural lip pits (isolated trait)
Paramedian pits of lower lip (isolated trait)†
Pits of upper lip

Excludes: Cleft lip or palate and lip pits or mounds (177)
Popliteal pterygium syndrome (818)
Oro-facio-digital syndrome I (770)
Cleft lip or palate and filiform fusion of eyelids (176)

Minimal Diagnostic Criteria: Presence of pits on the vermilion border of lips

Clinical Findings: *Commissural lip pits* are small openings or fistulas on the lip vermilion portion located in lip angles. They are either bilateral or unilateral. The pits do not cause any discomfort or esthetic problems.

Paramedian pits of lower lip are usually bilateral or occasionally unilateral fistulas located lateral to the midline on the vermilion border of the lower lip. The openings may be minute, but occur in the center of a mound of lip tissue, or may be fistulas 10 to 15 deep excreting mucous. Rarely, a single centrally located pit.

Pits of upper lip are exceedingly rare and are usually unilateral openings on the vermilion border.

Complications
I **Derived:** Rarely infection
II **Associated:** Commissural lip pits are associated with aural sinuses (auricular pits) in 3.8%. Paramedian lip pits are associated with cleft lip/palate syndromes, particularly cleft lip or palate and lip pits, cleft lip or palate and filiform fusion of eyelids, and popliteal pterygium syndrome. Pits of upper lip are associated with cysts in line of fusion of premaxilla and maxillary processes.

Etiology: *Commissural lip pits:* no genetic study has been published but there are reports of familial occurrence suggesting autosomal dominant transmission. (Father and son, mother and 2 sons, father and 2 daughters, mother and son and daughter and transmission through 3 generations.)

Paramedian lip pits: have been reported in kindreds showing autosomal dominant transmission and with no known relative showing cleft lip/palate. However, data are still insufficient to say with certainty whether this occurs as an isolated trait or whether it is always part of the cleft lip or palate and lip pits syndromes.

Pits of upper lip: probably nongenetic origin

Pathogenesis: *Commissural lip pits* originate from epithelial rests in the line of the embryonal furrow between maxillary and mandibular processes.

Paramedian lip pits originate as vestigial remnants of the "lateral sulci" appearing in the embryonic mandible at the 7.5 to 12.5 mm long stage.

Pits of upper lip due to failure of complete fusion of premaxilla and maxillary processes.

Related Facts
I **Sex Ratio:** *Commissural lip pits:* M1:F1 in Caucasians, American Negroes and North American Indians (Chippewa)
Paramedian lip pits: M1:F1 in Caucasians
Pits of upper lip: ? Very rare
II **Risk of Occurrence:** ?
III **Risk of Recurrence for**
Patient's Sib: *Commissural lip pits:* ? †
Paramedian lip pits: Not known for isolated trait
Patient's Child: *Commissural lip pits:* ? †
Paramedian lip pits: Not known for isolated trait
IV **Age of Detectability:** At birth
V **Prevalence:** *Commissural lip pits:* Caucasians: 1 in 500 to 1 in 83; American Negroes: 1 in 48; North American Indians (Chippewa): 1 in 110
Paramedian lip pits: ?

Treatment
I **Primary Prevention:** —
II **Secondary Prevention:** *Commissural lip pits-* no treatment necessary. *Paramedian lip pits-* plastic surgery. *Pits of upper lip-* surgical excision.
III **Other Therapy:** —

Prognosis: Normal for life span and intelligence when isolated trait

Detection of Carrier: ?

†Special Considerations: While kindreds are known wherein individuals have had only paramedian lip pits in general, these are not extensive kindreds. Kindreds more fully documented have individuals with clefts of lip and palate. For this reason, individuals or families with paramedian pits should elicit a high degree of suspicion that they also have high risk for clefts of lip or palate.

References:
Baker, W. R.: Pits of the lip commissures in Caucasoid males. Oral Surg. 21:56, 1966.
Červenka, J. et al: The syndrome of pits of the lower lip and cleft lip and/or palate: Genetic considerations. Am. J. Hum. Genet. 19:416, 1967.
Everett, F. G. and Wescott, W. B.: Commissural lip pits. Oral Surg. 14:202, 1961.
Fenner, von W. and v. der Leyen, U. -E.: Über die kongenitale Oberlippenfistel. Dtsch. Zahnaerztl. Z. 24:963, 1969.

Contributor: **Jaroslav Červenka**

Editor's Computerized Descriptors: Ear, Face, Oral

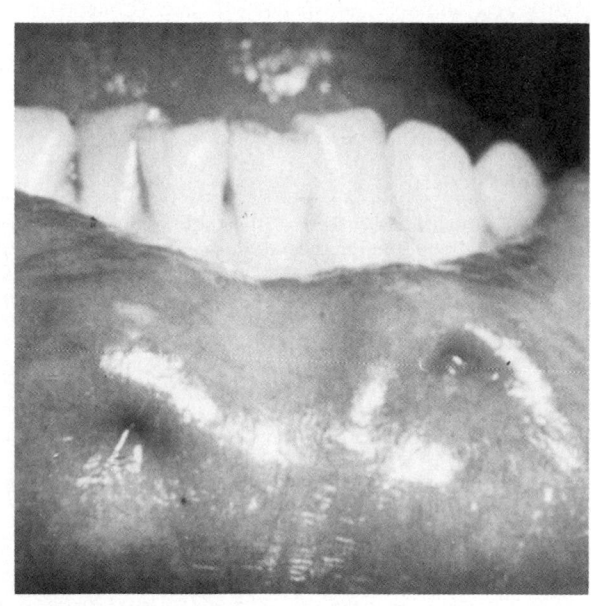

326. Lower lip pits

LIPASE DEFICIENCY, CONGENITAL ISOLATED

Includes: Déficit congénital isolé en lipase
Angeborener isolierter Lipasemangel
Deficiéncia congénita aislada de lipasa
Congenital pancreatic lipase deficiency
Congenital isolated lipase deficiency

Excludes: Co-lipase deficiency
Generalized pancreatic exocrine insufficiency

Minimal Diagnostic Criteria: Basal-and-secretin-stimulated pancreatic juices obtained by peroral duodenal intubation are found to contain normal activities of peptidases and amylase but to be deficient in lipase. Lipase assays are reliable only if performed by experienced investigators. Reproducibility is marginal and incubation conditions are critical.

Co-lipase is necessary for optimal function of lipase in the conditions present in the intestinal lumen. In vivo, co-lipase deficiency could masquerade as lipase deficiency.

Clinical Findings: Steatorrhea is the only significant clinical finding. All patients have had the onset of oily, slightly foul stools in early infancy. The oil separates from the bulk movement and will solidify at room temperature. Soiling of clothing with oil is common.

Normal growth and development is the rule. Abdominal distention is unusual.

Complications
I **Derived:** Steatorrhea
II **Associated:** —

Etiology: The mode of transmission is unknown but the pattern strongly suggests an autosomal recessive mutant allele. McK *24660

Pathogenesis: Pancreatic lipase is essential for optimal fat absorption. Hydrolysis of triglycerides to α-fatty acids and β-monoglycerides occurs at the surface of emulsified fat globules by the action of pancreatic lipase in the presence of bile salts and co-lipase. In the absence of lipase, limited hydrolysis occurs as a result of the action of gastric lipolytic activity and pancreatic esterase. The coefficient of fat absorption in the lipase deficient patient is 50-80%.

Related Facts
I **Sex Ratio:** M3:F1 (4 cases in which sex reported)
II **Risk of Occurrence:** ?
III **Risk of Recurrence for**
Patient's Sib: 1 in 4 (25%) for each offspring to be affected, if autosomal recessive.
Patient's Child: If autosomal recessive, not increased unless mate is carrier or homozygote.
IV **Age of Detectability:** Infancy
V **Prevalence:** ?; 7 cases have been reported.

Treatment
I **Primary Prevention:** Genetic counseling of parents of an affected individual.
II **Secondary Prevention:** Treatment with orally administered pancreatic enzyme replacement improves fat absorption but does not usually normalize function. Dietary fat restriction is necessary to abolish steatorrhea. Medium chain triglycerides may be used as a fat substitute when needed for nutrition in the infant.
III **Other Therapy:** —

Prognosis: Excellent

Detection of Carrier: —

Special Considerations: —

References:
Muller, D.P.R. et al: Studies on the mechanism of fat absorption in congenital isolated lipase deficeincy (Abstr.). Gut 16:838, 1975.
Sheldon, W.: Congenital pancreatic lipase deficiency. Arch. Dis. Child. 39:268, 1964.

Contributor: Peter F. Whitington

Editor's Computerized Descriptor: GI.

LIPOGRANULOMATOSIS

Includes: Lipogranulomatose
Farber disease
Disseminated lipogranulomatosis

Excludes: Histiocytoses
Rheumatoid arthritis
Lipoid dermatoarthritis
Sarcoid arthritis

Minimal Diagnostic Criteria: The hallmark of this syndrome has been the presence of discrete lumpy masses over the wrists and ankles, shown on biopsy to involve a proliferation of histiocytes, lymphocytes, fibroblasts, etc.

Mild evidence is usually available of local foam cell formation, positive for glycolipid histochemical reactions in the granulomas, plus comparable chemical changes in the liver, kidney, and other solid organs.

For the typical, infancy-involved patient, there are also signs of CNS disease (distended neurones on biopsy or autopsy, occasionally even with macular changes).

Clinical Findings: A total of 14 children to date have been identified with this syndrome. Eleven of them have had a rapidly progressive, debilitating course, with death before their 2nd birthday. The principal findings have been early onset of hoarseness, noisy respirations, restriction of joint movements, fleshy subcutaneous masses on the dorsal surfaces of the wrists and ankles, slowed development, irritability and chronic nutritional failure. The other three children had long-standing difficulties from arthropathy, granulomatous masses arising from synovium, tendon sheaths, or subcutaneous connective tissue, and skin nodules or other texture changes. One of these, a boy of 17, is in generally good condition; another boy died at 16 years of age in a cachectic state. This latter group has been spared evident CNS involvement.

Complications
I **Derived:** The affected infants have shown severe progressive joint swelling and restriction, gradual cerebral failure, and recurrent pulmonary infections. In the typical situation trials of corticosteroid therapy have added to growth failure, osteoporosis, and proclivity for infections.
II **Associated:** Subcutaneous nodules in locations other than in relation to joints have been seen in infants. Zetterström's older patient also showed more indurated skin problems, including diffuse flesh-colored papular eruptions and xanthoma-like growths on the face and hands.

Etiology: The syndrome has major characteristics of an inborn error of metabolism, and can be presumed to have autosomal recessive genetic transmission. Multiplex involvement is known in 1 sibship, and no occurrence has been seen in more than 1 generation. McK *22800

The identification by Moser's group of an acid ceramidase deficiency in the tissues of 4 patients strongly suggests that this is the basic enzymopathy.

Pathogenesis: Various degrees of increase in ceramide level, sometimes quite striking, have been found in kidney, liver, brain, spleen, and subcutaneous nodules from Farber disease patients, correlating with foam cell formation and acid ceramidase deficiency in these sites. It is postulated that this situation then is one of a lysosomal storage disease, where some other milder sphingolipid alterations could also be occurring secondarily. Other manifestations remain puzzling, particularly the periarticular and cutaneous granulomata which show mainly a reactive and infiltrative picture resembling to some extent histiocytoses or extreme rheumatoid phenomena. It has been pointed out by North et al that in children sarcoid can produce arthropathy and masses of considerable similarity to those in lipogranulomatosis, although no direct relationship is implied.

Related Facts
I **Sex Ratio:** Probably M1:F1 (M5:F9 in children reported to date)
II **Risk of Occurrence:** Very low. Two of the 13 involved families have been of Azore Portuguese origin, but the syndrome is unknown on the Portuguese mainland. The other cases show a wide distribution of origins, without evidence for a selective gene frequency alteration.
III **Risk of Recurrence for**
Patient's Sib: 1 in 4 (25%) for each offspring to be affected
Patient's Child: Not increased unless mate is carrier or homozygote. Patients usually die before maturity.
IV **Age of Detectability:** Clinical expression is evident within the first few months of life for the infant patients; joint swellings may not be detected until 2 or 3 years of life in the others.
V **Prevalence:** ?

Treatment
I **Primary Prevention:** Genetic counseling
II **Secondary Prevention:** —
III **Other Therapy:** Therapy has not been shown to be of fundamental value. Specifically, corticosteroid therapy has not been of benefit, nor has radiotherapy to masses or altered joints. In a single patient, some suggestion was recorded that oral alkylating agent treatment (chlorambucil) may have retarded the joint or periarticular changes.

Prognosis: Ten infant patients have died, all before 2 years of age. One child, as mentioned, is now 17 years of age, without signs of CNS involvement, and one died at 16 years of age (pathologic examination of the brain normal).

Detection of Carrier: ?

Special Considerations: —

References:
Crocker, A.C. et al: The "lipogranulomatosis" syndrome; review, with report of patient showing milder involvement. In Aronson, S.M. and Volk, B.W. (eds.): Inborn Disorders of Sphingolipid Metabolism. Oxford:Pergamon Press, 1967, p. 485.
Dulaney, J. et al: The biochemical defect in Farber's disease. In Volk, B.W. and Schneck, L. (eds.): Current Trends in Sphingolipidoses and Allied Disorders. New York:Plenum Press, 1976, p. 403.
Farber, S. et al: Lipogranulomatosis: A new lipo-glyco-protein storage disease. J. Mt. Sinai Hosp. 24:816, 1957.
North, A. F. et al: Sarcoid arthritis in children. Am. J. Med. 48:449, 1970.
Samuelsson, K. and Zetterström, R.: Ceramides in a patient with lipogranulomatosis (Farber's disease) with chronic course. Scand. J. Clin. Lab. Invest. 27:393, 1971.

Contributor: **Allen C. Crocker**

Editor's Computerized Descriptors: Speech, Skin, Skel., Resp.

LIPOID PROTEINOSIS

Includes: Protéinose lipoidique
Lipoidproteinose
Proteinosis lipodea
Urbach-Wiethe syndrome
Hyalinosis cutis et mucosae
Lipoglycoproteinosis

Excludes: —

Minimal Diagnostic Criteria: Characteristic clinical findings usually sufficient. Biopsy of skin is confirmatory.†

Clinical Findings: Deposits of an abnormal chemical substance into skin and oropharyngeal mucosa produce most of the clinical findings, arranged here in approximate order of frequency: marked hoarseness (and chronic or acute laryngeal obstruction); thickening of tongue and lips; short frenulum of tongue; papules, flesh-colored, 1-3 mm diameter, dome-shaped or flat-topped and sometimes verrucous, on the margins of eyelids, axillae, gluteal cleft, scrotum and dorsal hands; thickened, rough and infiltrated plaques or areas of skin over the elbows, knees, and to a lesser extent, the hands; prominent pock-like scarring of face and upper trunk; relative sparseness of hair; yellowish or "waxy" appearance of facial skin; slow-healing posttraumatic ulcers, especially at elbows, knees and legs; epilepsy (perhaps 20%). May be related to a characteristic calcification in the hippocampal gyri of the temporal lobes; faulty dentition with no characteristic pattern.

Complications
I **Derived:** Death from acute laryngeal obstruction
II **Associated:** Need for tracheostomy for acute or chronic laryngeal obstruction; slow-healing skin ulcers.

Etiology: Probably autosomal recessive. Expressivity is variable, yet affected individuals usually show sufficient presence of almost all facets of the disorder that they seem amazingly to resemble each other. McK *24710

Pathogenesis: A complex glycolipoprotein is deposited around small blood vessels, starting in utero in some if not in all cases, since some affected individuals are hoarse at birth. Many organs have been shown to receive the deposit, although there are "favorite" areas, for no known reason. The deposition tends to increase until early adult life and then remains fairly stable. In some cases the lipid-staining characteristics of the deposit are not found, suggesting a loose binding. No similar abnormal substance has been found in the blood of patients, nor are other studies of blood lipids or proteins consistently abnormal. Instances of such abnormalities are probably coincidental. The clinical symptoms are dependent upon the quantity of the abnormal substance which may happen to accumulate and thus disturb function or appearance at the site of deposition.

Related Facts
I   **Sex Ratio:** M1:F1
II **Risk of Occurrence:** Rare
III **Risk of Recurrence for**
    Patient's Sib: Probably 1 in 4 (25%) for each offspring to be affected
    Patient's Child: Probably not increased unless mate is carrier or homozygote
IV **Age of Detectability:** At birth, if baby is hoarse or cutaneous lesions are present. Otherwise anytime in childhood or early adult life that manifestations become observable.
V   **Prevalence:** Extremely low but probably slightly greater in South Africa.

Treatment

I   **Primary Prevention:** Genetic counseling
II **Secondary Prevention:** Prophylactic tracheostomy if any important degree of laryngeal obstruction. Papules may be scraped or excised from vocal cords to provide some increased vocal power. Symptomatic management of epilepsy.
III **Other Therapy:** —

Prognosis: Generally excellent for life unless acute or chronic laryngeal complications intervene, but little prospect for any improvement in cosmetic effect of cutaneous or mucocutaneous lesions or dysfunctional effect of laryngeal or cerebral lesions.

Detection of Carrier: ?

†**Special Considerations:** Biopsy specimens should be fixed in formalin and frozen sections requested for fat stains.

References:
Burnett, J. W. and Marcy, S. M.: Lipoid proteinosis. Am. J. Dis. Child. 105:81, 1963.
Caplan, R. M.: Lipoid proteinosis: A review including some new observations. Univ. Mich. Med. Bull. 28:365, 1962.
Caplan, R. M.: Visceral involvement in lipoid proteinosis. Arch. Dermatol. 95:149, 1967.
Gordon, H. et al: Lipoid proteinosis. In Bergsma, D. (ed.): Part XII. Skin, Hair and Nails. Birth Defects: Orig. Art. Ser., vol. VII, no. 8. Baltimore: Williams & Wilkins Co., for The National Foundation - March of Dimes, 1971, p. 164.
Hofer, P.A. and Bergenholtz, A.: Oral manifestations in Urbach-Wiethe disease. Odont. Revy 26:39, 1975.

Contributor: **Richard M. Caplan**

Editor's Computerized Descriptors: Face, Oral, Larynx, Speech, Skin, Resp., Hair

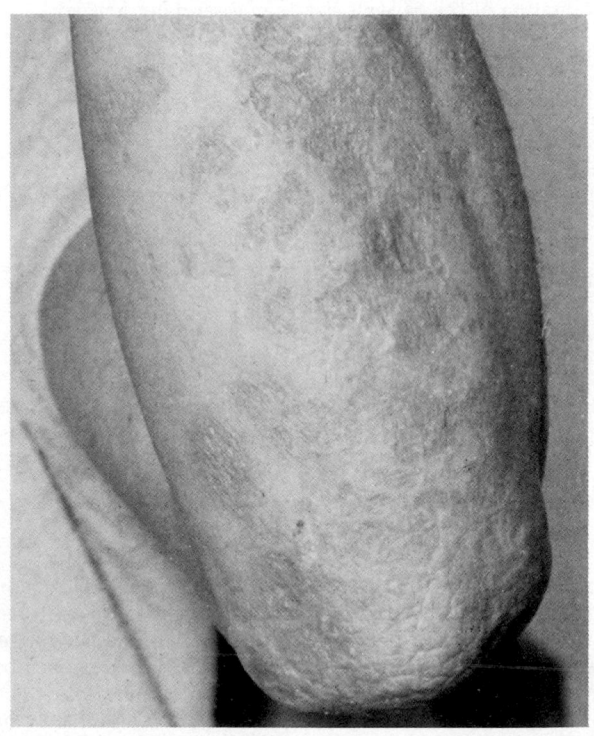

327. Large atrophic scars

LIPOMAS, FAMILIAL SYMMETRIC

Includes: Lipomes symétriques familiaux
Familiäre symmetrischelipome
Lipomatosis simétrica familiar
Multiple symmetric lipomatosis
Hereditary multiple lipomata
Multiple circumscribed lipomas

Excludes: Benign diffuse symmetric lipomatosis
Multiple lipomas
Adiposis dolorosa

Minimal Diagnostic Criteria: Presence of multiple lipomas in typical locations and a familial history of such tumors.†

Clinical Findings: Multiple, nontender, subcutaneous lipomas under 5 cm in diameter. Generally located on trunk, arms and thighs in a symmetric manner. No constitutional abnormalities are present.

Complications
I **Derived:** Nerve compression producing pain or rarely paralysis and fat necrosis from trauma.
II **Associated:** Multiple telangiectases, neurofibromatosis, tylosis of palms and soles, Gardner syndrome (rarely has lipomas).

Etiology: Probably autosomal dominant with complete penetrance in males; McK *15190

Pathogenesis: The lipomas may gradually increase in number as early as puberty, but more commonly erupt during the 3rd or 4th decade occasionally accompanied by pain or tenderness. A period of stability is reached with cessation of pain. Rarely spontaneous regression occurs. The relationship of lipomas to neurofibromas has been raised, but this has not been substantiated. Laboratory evaluation of the patients has been essentially normal.

Related Facts
I **Sex Ratio:** M4:F1
II **Risk of Occurrence:** ?
III **Risk of Recurrence for**
   Patient's Sib: 1 in 2 (50%) for affected brothers; may be detected in sisters.
   Patient's Child: 1 in 2 for affected sons; may be detected in daughters.
IV **Age of Detectability:** Adolescence to 5th decade
V **Prevalence:** ? Not rare, more frequent than is generally thought.

Treatment
I **Primary Prevention:** Genetic counseling
II **Secondary Prevention:** —
III **Other Therapy:** Excision if lipomas are greater than 5 cm in size, if pain or ulceration is prominent. Liposarcomas are very rare complication.

Prognosis: Normal for life span and intelligence

Detection of Carrier: —

†**Special Considerations:** Familial symmetric lipomas must be differentiated from similar conditions such as benign diffuse symmetric lipomatosis which usually presents as massive fat deposits in a horse-collar distribution around the neck or occasionally diffusely on upper trunk. Occasionally patients have multiple lipomas spread randomly over the body in an asymmetric manner and without familial history. Adiposis dolorosa (Dercum disease) occurs predominantly in menopausal women and is characterized by a lumpy accumulation of fat on the thighs and abdomen. Often these patients complain of severe pain or tenderness in these fatty accumulations.

References:

Das Gupta, T.K.: Tumors and tumor-like conditions of the adipose tissue. In Ravitch, M.M. et al (eds.): Current Problems in Surgery. Chicago: Year Book Medical Publishers, 1970.
Muller, R.: Observation sur la transmission hereditaire de la lipomatose circonscribe multiple. Dermatologica 103:253, 1951.
Osment, L.S.: Cutaneous lipomatosis. Surg. Gynecol. Obstet. 127:129, 1968.

Contributor: **E. George Thorne**

Editor's Computerized Descriptor: Skin

LIPOMATOSIS OF FACE AND NECK

Contributor: **LaVonne Bergstrom**

Editor's Computerized Descriptors: Skin, Skel., Resp.

Includes: Lipomatose de la face et du cou
Lipomatose von Gesicht und Hals
Lipomatosis de la cara y del cuello
Adenolipomatosis
Cervical lipomatosis, familial benign
Benign symmetric lipomatosis
Face, diffuse symmetric lipomatosis of

Excludes: Generalized multiple lipomatosis
Neurofibromatosis (712)
Parotitis, punctate (799)

Minimal Diagnostic Criteria: Symmetric masses in the head and neck region which are clinically and pathologically identical to lipoma.†

Clinical Findings: Symmetric fatty growths may involve the neck, parotid area, occipital area and, in some instances, the neck and axilla. When the neck, axillary and orbital regions are affected it has been called adenolipomatosis, although lymph nodes are not involved. Telangiectasis and hypertrophy of bone or muscle may accompany the fatty growths. This disorder may be confused with neurofibromatosis. Some cases have shown an elevated blood cholesterol. Onset is usually in adulthood. In most cases the masses are painless. They remain quiescent for many years but may suddenly enlarge. The major disabilities are cosmetic and respiratory obstruction from lipoma in the neck.

Complications
I **Derived:** Upper respiratory obstruction
II **Associated:** —

Etiology: Probably autosomal dominant

Pathogenesis: —

Related Facts
I **Sex Ratio:** M < 1:F1
II **Risk of Occurrence:** ?
III **Risk of Recurrence for**
    Patient's Sib: When autosomal dominant, if parent is affected, 1 in 2 (50%) for each offspring to be affected; otherwise not increased.
    Patient's Child: 1 in 2
IV **Age of Detectability:** When tumors become clinically evident
V **Prevalence:** Very rare

Treatment
I **Primary Prevention:** Genetic counseling
II **Secondary Prevention:** Surgical removal is the only effective treatment to obtain tissue for diagnosis, to improve appearance, to relieve airway obstruction.
III **Other Therapy:** —

Prognosis: Normal for life span

Detection of Carrier: —

†**Special Considerations:** This is probably only one manifestation of several varieties of hereditary fatty tumors which can involve almost any area of the body. At present it is not certain that those confined to the face and neck are a separate entity. It may occur as a sporadic phenomenon.

References:
McKusick, V.A.: Familial benign cervical lipomatosis. In Medical Genetics, 1961. J. Chronic Dis. 15:417, 1962.
Pack, G.T. and Ariel, I.M.: Tumors of adipose tissue. In Tumors of the Soft Somatic Tissues; a Clinical Treatise. New York:Hoeber-Harper, 1958, p. 343.

LIPOMENINGOCELE

Includes: Lipomeningozelen
Intraspinal lipomas
Cauda equina lipoma
Spinal dysraphism syndrome
Lumbosacral lipoma

Excludes: Dermal sinus tract
Myelomeningocele (693)

Minimal Diagnostic Criteria: Mass on back with spina bifida and widening of interpedicular distances. Myelogram will show widened subarachnoid space with filling defect of lipoma at termination of spinal cord.

Clinical Findings: Skin covered mass in lumbosacral region noted at birth. May have angioma or hair tuft associated. Normal neurologic function for legs and sphincters or minor deficits. Spina bifida on xrays. As child grows, scoliosis and neurologic loss may occur as with diastematomyelia.

Complications
I **Derived:** Progressive neurologic and sphincter loss, progressive orthopedic deformity
II **Associated:** Minor dysraphic changes in spinal cord, ie enlarged central canal

Etiology: ?

Pathogenesis: Displaced or heterotopic adipose tissue

Related Facts
I **Sex Ratio:** F > M
II **Risk of Occurrence:** ?
III **Risk of Recurrence for**
  Patient's Sib: ?
  Patient's Child: ?
IV **Age of Detectability:** At birth
V **Prevalence:** ?

Treatment
I **Primary Prevention:** —
II **Secondary Prevention:** Exploration and excision of lipomatous tissue particularly that bridging skin mass to cord so that spinal cord may ascend with growth. Neurologic loss can be stabilized by surgery and may possibly be prevented by earlier surgery.
III **Other Therapy:** —

Prognosis: Good

Detection of Carrier: ?

Special Considerations: —

References:
Dubowitz, V. et al: Lipoma of the cauda equina. Arch. Dis. Child. 40:207, 1965.
James, C.C.M. and Lassman, L.: Spinal Dysraphism. London: Butterworth, 1972, p. 98.

Contributor: **Kenneth Shulman**

Editor's Computerized Descriptors: Skel., Nerve

LISSENCEPHALY SYNDROME

Includes: Lissencéphalie
Lissenzephalie
Síndrome de lisencefalía

Excludes: —

Minimal Diagnostic Criteria: Microcephaly, characteristic appearance, characteristic clinical course, with or without associated hepatosplenomegaly and prolonged neonatal jaundice, urinary tract infections and other anomalies.†

Clinical Findings: Prenatal indication of possible abnormality (polyhydramnios) in half the cases; intrauterine growth may be reduced; subsequent severe failure to thrive with height and weight falling below 3rd percentile. Congenital microcephaly in all cases - considerable ventricular dilation represents hydrocephaly ex vacuo. In severe, "typical" cases the appearance is striking and diagnostic: forehead is high and may be narrow, particularly in the temporal area; occiput is prominent. Slight downward slanting of palpebral fissures and anteversion of nostrils. Circumlimbal clouding of corneas may be present, ears are slightly posteriorly rotated and show minor anomalies of differentiation. Micrognathia is common. Hirsutism may be extensive. Remarkable ability to fold skin of forehead into many wrinkles is a striking feature of the syndrome and the lips may have a "carp-mouth" appearance.

Polydactyly (to date unilateral-preaxial in 1 case, site? in another case), camptodactyly, simian creases, incomplete cutaneous syndactyly of the 2nd and 3rd toes and a short perineal body may be seen. Affected males have had cryptorchidism and indicated inguinal herniae. Congenital heart disease (5/9 patients), agenesis of 1 kidney and duodenal atresia have been seen.

Neonatally frequent cyanosis and apneic spells, and feeble cry. Initial hypotonia; early, usually severe feeding difficulties (gavage feedings, gastrostomy may be required) and failure to thrive. Initial paucity of movements gradually replaced by onset of seizures and signs of decerebration with spells of rigidity and opisthotonus. Psychomotor maturation does not occur, patients show few responses to stimuli but may be intermittently severely hyperactive.

One-third of patients have had hepatosplenomegaly with severe and prolonged neonatal jaundice (bile stasis ?); some patients have urinary tract infections.

EEG abnormalities are nonspecific at first and then develop into a more or less typical hypsarrhythmic pattern. The suspected CNS defect can be confirmed by air studies. At autopsy the brain shows essentially no sulci and gyri and a severe arrest of development of gray matter associated in 2 cases, with a Dandy-Walker like dilation of the 4th ventricle and hypoplasia of midline portions of the cerebellum.

Complications
I **Derived:** This is a condition invariably fatal in infancy or childhood; seizures are generally refractory to ordinary anticonvulsant drugs, ACTH or adrenocortical steroids.
II **Associated:** —

Etiology: Presumed to be due to the homozygous state of an uncommon autosomal recessive gene. McK *24720

Pathogenesis: ?

Related Facts
I **Sex Ratio:** Presumably M1:F1
II **Risk of Occurrence:** ? Rare
III **Risk of Recurrence for**

Patient's Sib: Presumably 1 in 4 (25%) for each sib
Patient's Child: Homozygotes are not viable
IV **Age of Detectability:** At birth by physical examination, confirmed by course and pneumoencephalogram or CAT scan
V **Prevalence:** ? Rare

Treatment
I **Primary Prevention:** Genetic counseling after birth of 1st affected child
II **Secondary Prevention:** Possible correction of duodenal atresia; if present, treatment of congestive heart failure. Discontinuation of treatment only after consultation with parents and only after CNS diagnosis of lissencephaly is established and confirmed by course and EEG pattern.
III **Other Therapy:** Supportive until death

Prognosis: Condition is invariably fatal in infancy or childhood.

Detection of Carrier: —

†**Special Considerations:** Lissencephaly per se is an etiologically nonspecific brain malformation and may occur without other associated malformations and possibly, in more or less complete form in other syndromes. Conversely, it is quite conceivable that lissencephaly is not an obligatory part of "the" lissencephaly syndrome, but that other CNS defects may occur in that syndrome. Under such circumstances a diagnosis of "the" lissencephaly syndrome can be made only if an affected sib had lissencephaly.

References:
Dieker, H. et al: The lissencephaly syndrome. In Bergsma, D. (ed.): Part II. Malformation Syndromes. Birth Defects: Orig. Art. Ser., vol V, no. 2. White Plains:The National Foundation-March of Dimes, 1969, p. 53.

Contributor: **John M. Opitz**

Editor's Computerized Descriptors: Eye, Ear, Face, Nose, Skin, Dermatoglyphic, Hair, Skel., Muscle, Hernia not CNS, CV., Spleen, GI., Liver, GU., Nerve

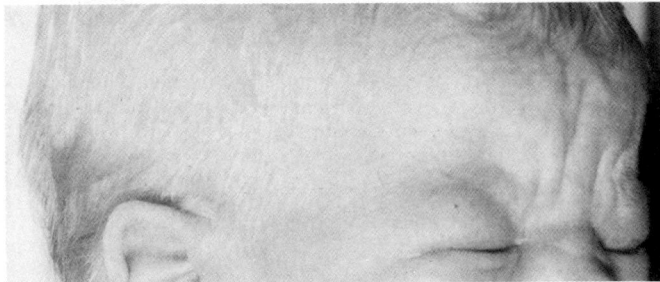

328. Note wrinkled forehead

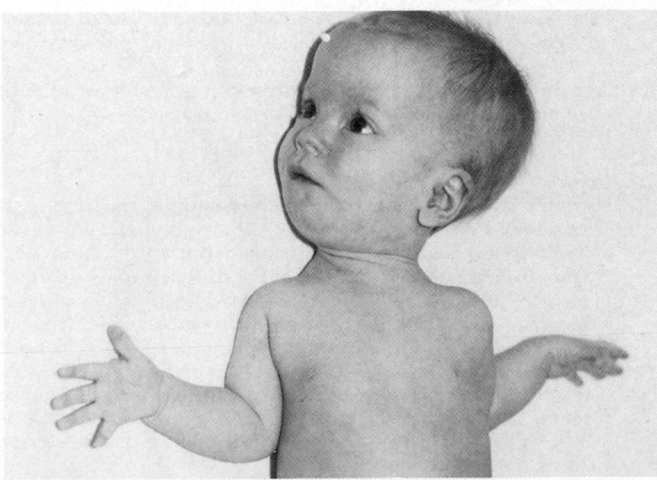

329. Seven-month-old with lissencephaly

LIVER HAMARTOMA

Includes: Hamartome hépatique
Leber-Hamartom
Hamartoma del hígado
Mesenchymal hamartoma of liver
Cystic hamartoma of liver
Hepatic hamartoma
Hamartoma of liver

Excludes: Hepatic hemangiomatosis (466)
Hepatic cyst, solitary (465)
Hepatic nodular hyperplasia
Hepatic adenoma

Minimal Diagnostic Criteria: Large asymptomatic right-upper quadrant mass in an infant. Actual histologic evaluation is necessary for final diagnosis.†

Clinical Findings: Mesenchymal hamartoma of the liver is a rare benign tumor of infancy that is usually asymptomatic except for the presence of a mass. Most are located in the right lobe of the liver with one-third of the cases on a pedicle. These tumors may be exceptionally large and occupy much of the peritoneal cavity.†

Complications
I **Derived:** Respiratory embarrassment from diaphragmatic elevation due to large mass, rarely torsion of tumor on pedicle.
II **Associated:** —

Etiology: The tumor is composed of collagenous tissue thought to arise from primitive mesenchyme and small cystic areas with distorted hepatic tissue components.

Pathogenesis: Grossly the lesion appears as a reddish-brown firm elastic tumor that is solitary and spherical. They are quite large, weighing between 1500-3060 gm. There are 2 types; one in which loose collagenous fibrous stroma predominate, the other in which multiple small cysts predominate. The cyst walls may be of bile duct or lymphangiomatous origin. Smaller cysts have a single layer of lining cells while larger cysts are usually devoid of lining cells.

Related Facts
I **Sex Ratio:** M?:F?
II **Risk of Occurrence:** ?
III **Risk of Recurrence for**
Patient's Sib: ?
Patient's Child: ?
IV **Age of Detectability:** Usually detected within the first 2 years of life
V **Prevalence:** ?

Treatment
I **Primary Prevention:** —
II **Secondary Prevention:** The therapy of choice for mesenchymal hamartoma of the liver is surgical resection. This is simple, if a pedicle is present (1/3 of cases), since it is not necessary to resect beyond the tumor into normal liver when diagnosis can be established at the time of operation. When such distinction cannot be made, hepatic lobectomy is indicated.
III **Other Therapy:** —

Prognosis: Excellent when resection is possible

Detection of Carrier: —

†**Special Considerations:** Mesenchymal hamartoma of the liver is an interesting congenital lesion that only recently has been appreciated as an entity. This lesion should be differentiated from hemangiomatosis (which is a more diffuse lesion with skin components and heart failure) and from solitary cysts and polycystic disease of the liver. It is important to separate this entity from true hepatic adeno-

mas and focal nodular hyperplasia. True hepatic adenomas are very rare and consist of normal-appearing or atypical liver cells arranged in cords and occasionally forming bile ducts. Portal triads and central veins are absent. Hepatic adenomas are usually solitary and occur in otherwise normal livers. Focal nodular hyperplasia is a "tumor-like" condition that is seen with regeneration following liver injury. The cause of this disorder is unknown, however, some type of injury to the liver and interference with and diminution of the blood supply has been suggested. There is a strikingly similar gross appearance of many of these tumors and conditions so that differentiation by appearance alone is quite unreliable and careful microscopic analysis is important.

References:

Edmondson, H.A.: Differential diagnosis of tumors and tumor-like lesions of the liver in infancy and childhood. Am. J. Dis. Child. 91:168, 1956.

Ishida, M. et al: Mesenchymal hamartoma of the liver. Ann. Surg. 164:175, 1966.

Contributors: **Jay L. Grosfeld**
H. William Clatworthy, Jr.

Editor's Computerized Descriptors: GI., Liver

LIVER, POLYCYSTIC DISEASE

Includes: Maladie polykystique du foie
Zystenleber
Enfermedad poliquística del hígado
Polycystic disease of kidneys with liver involvement
Hepatic cysts, multiple
Liver cysts, multiple

Excludes: Hepatic cyst, solitary (465)
Liver hamartoma (604)
Parasitic cysts
Fibrocystic disease of liver
Choledochal cyst (149)

Minimal Diagnostic Criteria: A positive family history of polycystic, renal, or hepatic disease should lead one to investigate the patient. The final diagnosis depends on visualization of multiple cysts.

Clinical Findings: Polycystic disease of the liver is a generalized familial condition frequently associated with polycystic disease of the kidneys (60%), and of other organs such as the lung and pancreas. The lesion presents as a multinodular mass with the liver being filled at all depths and levels with multiple cysts. Painful distention of the liver capsule and portal hypertension are problems rarely encountered. Hepatic angiography and scintiscan are helpful diagnostic aids. The majority of cases are asymptomatic.

Complications
I   **Derived:** Pain from distention of liver capsule by the cysts, or torsion, portal hypertension due to partial obstruction from compression of splanchnic inflow, which may lead to splenomegaly and hemorrhage from esophageal varices.
II **Associated:** Rarely, the cyst may become secondarily infected.

Etiology: Familial disorder that appears to be transmitted in 2 ways. The form that is symptomatic in adults is inherited as an autosomal dominant (common), while the form of the disease symptomatic in infancy (rare) is inherited as an autosomal recessive. Although the etiology is obscure, it is presumably due to retention of fluid in aberrant ducts. McK *17390, *26320

Pathogenesis: The cyst wall is under low tension. The contents (either clear or slightly yellow) are sterile, and similar to serum in electrolyte and enzyme content. The cysts are lined with a cuboidal epithelium similar to primitive bile ducts.

Related Facts
I   **Sex Ratio:** M1:F1
II   **Risk of Occurrence:** ?
III **Risk of Recurrence for**
      Patient's Sib: When (late-onset) autosomal dominant, see Table I AD; when (early-onset) autosomal recessive, see Table I AR.
      Patient's Child: When (late-onset) autosomal dominant, see Table I AD; when (early-onset) autosomal recessive, see Table I AR.
IV   **Age of Detectability:** When autosomal recessive, in infancy; when autosomal dominant in late adulthood.
V   **Prevalence:** ?

Treatment
I   **Primary Prevention:** Genetic counseling
II   **Secondary Prevention:** In cases of symptomatic polycystic liver disease, excisional or resectional therapy is impractical and often impossible because of the diffuse hepatic involvement by this generalized disorder. Aspiration and incision have the disadvantage of high recurrence, while external drainage is of limited usefulness because of the prolonged drainage and morbidity. More permanent relief can be obtained by internal drainage if the deeply located cysts can be fenestrated so that communication to the liver surface is accomplished. Since the polycystic contents are sterile,

noninflammatory, and have similar electrolyte and enzyme content as serum, free flow into the peritoneal cavity and absorption from the peritoneal surface are acceptable. Instances of polycystic disease that are asymptomatic need no treatment.

III Other Therapy: —

Prognosis: Normal life span for isolated defect; otherwise related to the associated renal involvement

Detection of Carrier: ?

Special Considerations: —

References:
Henson, S.W., Jr. et al: Benign tumors of the liver. IV. Polycystic disease of surgical significance. Surg. Gynecol. Obstet. 104:63, 1957.
Lin, T.Y. et al: Treatment of non-parasitic cystic disease of the liver: A new approach to therapy with polycystic liver. Ann. Surg. 168:921, 1968.
Sedacca, C.M. et al: Polycystic liver: An unusual cause of bleeding esophageal varices. Gastroenterology 40:128, 1961.

Contributors: **Jay L. Grosfeld**
H. William Clatworthy, Jr.

Editor's Computerized Descriptors: GI., Liver, GU.

LIVER TRANSPOSITION

Includes: Transposition du foie
Situs inversus der Leber
Transposición del hígado
Hepatic situs inversus
Transposition of liver

Excludes: —

Minimal Diagnostic Criteria: Presence of liver in left side of the abdomen†

Clinical Findings: Mirror-image transposition places the liver on the left side rather than its usual right-upper quadrant position. Abdominal situs inversus may be complete or partial and is usually associated with dextrocardia. This anomaly should be suspected if the gastric air bubble is noted on the right on abdominal xray.

Complications
I Derived: —
II Associated: Related to associated congenital malformations. Congenital heart disease (tetralogy of Fallot, transposition of great vessels, pulmonic stenosis) and intraabdominal anomalies (duodenal atresia or stenosis, incomplete bowel fixation prone to midgut volvulus), preduodenal portal vein, biliary atresia, asplenia, and Kartagener triad of bronchitis, sinusitis, and situs inversus.

Etiology: ?

Pathogenesis: Related to presence of associated malformations.

Related Facts
I Sex Ratio: M1.5:F1
II Risk of Occurrence: ?
III Risk of Recurrence for
    Patient's Sib: Exact risk unknown but is more common in sibs of patients with situs inversus.
    Patient's Child: ?
IV Age of Detectability: 46% in the 1st month of life
V Prevalence: True prevalence unknown; 1 in 11,000 as per radiographic survey

Treatment
I Primary Prevention: —
II Secondary Prevention: —
III Other Therapy: Operations often required for associated correctable intraabdominal anomalies such as duodenal atresia, biliary atresia, etc. Important to place abdominal incision in the proper location because of situs inversus.

Prognosis: Depends on the presence and severity of associated anomalies of the cardiovascular and GI systems where mortality may be greater than 50%.

Detection of Carrier: —

†Special Considerations: The frequent association of cardiovascular and GI anomalies must be emphasized in these infants. Cases in which dextrocardia is observed should be carefully evaluated for a heart lesion, and in addition, have x-ray studies of the abdomen for possible abdominal manifestations of situs inversus. Similarly, in the newborn with intestinal obstruction, the presence of dextrocardia on chest xray should alert the surgeon to place his incision on the appropriate side of the abdomen. In regard to the liver itself, biliary atresia has been reported in approximately 8% of cases of situs inversus. The prognosis of the biliary atresia is not altered by the left-sided hepatic position.

References:
Fonkalsrud, E.W. et al: Abdominal manifestations of situs inversus in infants and children. Arch. Surg. 92:791, 1966.

Merklin, R.J. et al: Situs inversus and cardiac defects: A study of 111 cases of reversed asymmetry. J. Thorac. Cardiovasc. Surg. 43:334, 1963.

Contributors: **Jay L. Grosfeld**
H. William Clatworthy, Jr.

Editor's Computerized Descriptors: Resp., CV., Spleen, GI., Liver

LOBODONTIA

Includes: Lobodontie
Lobodoncia
Teeth, carnivore-like

Excludes: Dens in dente (276)
Hypodontia
Microdontia (660)
Enamel, hypoplasia (342)

Minimal Diagnostic Criteria: Multiple dental anomalies of the teeth resulting in a dentition resembling that of a carnivore.

Clinical Findings: Multiple anomalies of the teeth resulting in a dentition resembling that of a carnivore. Only one kindred has been reported to date. All observed cases have had multitubercular molar crowns, generalized reduction of crown size, accentuation of mesiobuccal cusps of molars and buccal cusps of premolars, accentuation of cingulum of premolars and incisors, suppression in height of other molar and premolar cusps and large diastemata in upper and lower canine regions. Some, but not all cases, have in addition multiple dens in dente or deep palatal invaginations, single conical molar roots, agenesis of teeth, ectopic eruption of teeth and shovel-shaped incisors.

Complications
I **Derived:** Pulpal inflammation, degeneration and periapical involvement in teeth with dens in dente
II **Associated:** —

Etiology: Autosomal dominant; McK *18700

Pathogenesis: ? The morphologic alterations peculiar to this entry are genetically determined and clinical complications such as pulpal degeneration in teeth with dens in dente probably occur after eruption into the oral cavity.

Related Facts
I **Sex Ratio:** M1:F1 (observed 7:5)
II **Risk of Occurrence:** Very rare
III **Risk of Recurrence for**
    Patient's Sib: If one parent is affected, 1 in 2; otherwise not increased
    Patient's Child: 1 in 2
IV **Age of Detectability:** At 2 years by clinical and x-ray examination of deciduous teeth
V **Prevalence:** Estimated to be less than 1 in 1,000,000 (very rare; only one kindred known, 1971).

Treatment
I **Primary Prevention:** Genetic counseling
II **Secondary Prevention:** Root canal therapy for teeth with dens in dente; use of occlusal sealants following eruption. Occlusal table should be restored, cusps preserved.
III **Other Therapy:** —

Prognosis: Apparently normal life span

Detection of Carrier: —

Special Considerations: —

References:
Dahlberg, A. A.: Evolutionary background of dental and facial growth. J. Dent. Res. (Suppl.) 44:151, 1965.
Mayhall, J. T.: Analysis of dental form regression syndrome. IADR Program and Abstract #373, 1967.
Robbins, I. M. and Keene, H. J.: Multiple morphologic dental anomalies: Report of a case. Oral Surg. 17:683, 1964.
Witkop, C.J., Jr.: Hereditary defects of dentin. In Poole, A.E. (ed.): Symposium on Genetics. Dent. Clin. North Am. 19: no. 1, 1975.

Contributors: **Harris J. Keene**
Albert A. Dahlberg

Editor's Computerized Descriptor: Teeth

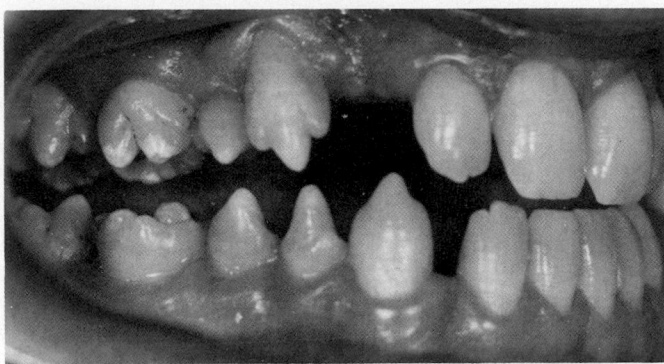

330. Note cone-shaped mandibular premolars and fang-like maxillary canine

608
LOCALIZED ABSENCE OF SKIN
603-500

Includes: Aplasie cutanée
Aplasia cutis congenita circumscripta
Aplasia cutánea
Aplasia cutis congenita
Skin, localized absence

Excludes: Ectodermal dysplasia
Localized absence of skin, blistering and nail abnormalities (609)
Dermal hypoplasia, focal (281)

Minimal Diagnostic Criteria: Localized absence of skin of scalp or lower legs.

Clinical Findings: Localized absence of skin at birth. Most commonly seen on scalp, usually at the apex on or near the midline. Presents as ulcer with absence of both skin and hair. Serous membrane may cover subcutaneous tissue. Crusting is followed by healing in a few weeks leaving a fine depressed hairless scar. In a rare form this condition may involve the trunk and limbs, particularly the lower legs.†

Complications
 I **Derived:** Underlying skull, meninges and brain may be included in defect.
 II **Associated:** Rarely associated with cleft lip-palate, polydactyly, ocular anomalies, hemangiomas, spina bifida with mental retardation, congenital heart defect.

Etiology: Suggestive autosomal dominant transmission of "scalp form."

Pathogenesis: Localized developmental abnormality of skin. Amniotic adhesions no longer accepted as cause.

Related Facts
 I   **Sex Ratio:** M1:F1
 II **Risk of Occurrence:** ?
 III **Risk of Recurrence for**
   Patient's Sib: If autosomal dominant and if parent is affected, 1 in 2 (50%) for each offspring to be affected; otherwise not increased.
   Patient's Child: If autosomal dominant, 1 in 2
 IV **Age of Detectability:** At birth by examination of skin
 V   **Prevalence:** Approximately 250 cases reported.

Treatment
 I   **Primary Prevention:** Genetic counseling
 II **Secondary Prevention:** If defect is large, skin grafting may be required.
 III **Other Therapy:** —

Prognosis: Excellent except in rare patients with associated complications.

Detection of Carrier: —

†**Special Considerations:** Localized absence of skin occasionally seen in trisomy D syndrome, focal dermal hypoplasia, and recessive dystrophic epidermolysis bullosa.

References:
Bart, B.J. et al: Congenital localized absence of skin and associated abnormalities resembling epidermolysis bullosa. Arch. Dermatol. 93:296, 1966.

Contributor: **Bruce J. Bart**

Editor's Computerized Descriptors: Skin, Hair

LOCALIZED ABSENCE OF SKIN, BLISTERING AND NAIL ABNORMALITIES

Includes: Anomalie cutanée et unguéale-épidermolyse
Aplasia cutis circumscripta, Blasenbildung und Nagelanomalien
Ausencia localizada de piel, vesiculización y anomalías ungüeales
Skin, localized absence, blistering and nail abnormalities
Nail abnormalities, localized absence and blistering of skin
Blistering, localized absence of skin and nail abnormalities

Excludes: Localized absence of skin (608)
Epidermolysis bullosa with skin and nail defects
Dermal hypoplasia, focal (281)
Ectodermal dysplasia

Minimal Diagnostic Criteria: Localized absence of skin of lower limbs plus nail abnormalities, or blistering.

Clinical Findings: Congenital localized absence of skin involving the lower limbs with blistering of skin and mucous membranes, and absence or deformities of thumb nails and great toenails. Of 26 affected members in 1 family, 14 had localized skin absence, 21 had blistering and 24 had nail absence or deformity. All but 4 members had a combination of the above.

Complications
I   **Derived:** Chronic ulceration in scarred areas of defect on legs. Death in 1 member of kindred from severe extensive blistering.
II   **Associated:** —

Etiology: Autosomal dominant transmission of single abnormal gene. Penetrance is complete but expressivity is variable.

Pathogenesis: ?

Related Facts
I   **Sex Ratio:** M1:F1
II   **Risk of Occurrence:** Very rare
III   **Risk of Recurrence for**
     Patient's Sib: If parent is affected 1 in 2 (50%) for each offspring to be affected; otherwise not increased.
     Patient's Child: 1 in 2
IV   **Age of Detectability:** At birth by examination of skin
V   **Prevalence:** Only 1 kindred reported to date.

Treatment
I   **Primary Prevention:** Genetic counseling
II   **Secondary Prevention:** —
III   **Other Therapy:** —

Prognosis: Good except for 1 member who died from extensive blistering.

Detection of Carrier: —

Special Considerations: —

References:
Bart, B.J. et al: Congenital localized absence of skin and associated abnormalities resembling epidermolysis bullosa. Arch. Dermatol. 93:296, 1966.
Pers, M.: Congenital absence of skin: Pathogenesis and relation to ring-constriction. Acta Chir. Scand. 126:388, 1963.

Contributor: **Bruce J. Bart**

————————————

Editor's Computerized Descriptors: Skin, Nails

LONG QT SYNDROME WITHOUT DEAFNESS

Includes: Syndrome QT long sans surdité
Syndrom des langen QT ohne Taubheit
Síndrome de QT largo sin sordera
Romano-Ward syndrome
Roman-Ward syndrome
Syncope and QT prolongation without deafness

Excludes: Cardioauditory syndrome† (123)

Minimal Diagnostic Criteria: Characteristic ECG findings. Normal hearing.

Clinical Findings: Syncopal episodes commonly begin in early childhood. These may be mild and transient, or severe leading to several minutes of unconsciousness or even to sudden death. Early mortality among reported cases is high. Most commonly the syncopal episodes are provoked by violent emotions or physical exercise. The frequency of the syncopal attacks varies from several per month in some individuals to only 1 or 2 episodes in a lifetime in others. In those who survive to early adulthood there appears to be a lessening of the episodes.

The ECG shows a long QT interval. Although this superficially appears to be a QT interval, in some cases there clearly is a Q-U interval with a low amplitude T wave and a large U wave. Episodes of spontaneous T wave alternation (from positive to negative in a given ECG lead) have been observed; and in 1 reported case this was followed in a few seconds by ventricular fibrillation. The QT interval may vary in the same individual. The basic sinus rhythm commonly shows a slow rate at rest. In the face of exercise, the sinus rate may show less acceleration than is appropriate for the amount of work performed, ie a relative sinus bradycardia.

Complications
I   **Derived:** Syncope and sudden death
II   **Associated:** —

Etiology: Autosomal dominant; McK *19250

Pathogenesis: Syncope and sudden death in this syndrome are consistent with either asystole or fibrillation. Postmortem examinations have shown damage to the SA node's arterial blood supply as well as to the Purkinje system. In addition, the clinical prolongation of the QT interval may be produced experimentally by causing imbalances of the sympathetic innervation to the heart (right stellate ganglion vs left stellate ganglion). The long QT interval increases the duration of the vulnerable period and would lower the fibrillation threshold. Patients with this syndrome exhibit abnormally low heart rates and an inability to increase their rate with exercise or atropine. It is possible that in the younger patients with smaller hearts, which would be resistant to fibrillation, the cause of death is asystole due to default of the SA node and failure of any secondary pacemaker to take over. In older patients with larger hearts, the cause of death is probably fibrillation initiated by an R on T phenomenon. This dual mechanism would explain the incomplete success of various rational therapeutic measures. Propranolol and sympathectomy prevent the fibrillation by raising fibrillation thresholds but suppress pacemaker function, whereas artificial electronic pacemakers prevent asystole but leave the patient vulnerable to fibrillation.

Related Facts
I   **Sex Ratio:** M1:F1

II Risk of Occurrence: Rare. Approximately 155 cases reported in the literature, most within the last 6 years with increased recognition of the syndrome.

III Risk of Recurrence for
Patient's Sib: If parent is affected 1 in 2 (50%) for each offspring to be affected; otherwise not increased.
Patient's Child: 1 in 2

IV Age of Detectability: At birth by ECG and theoretically in utero by fetal ECG with improved resolution for T wave analysis.

V Prevalence: Low, and falls with age due to nonsurvival of some.

Treatment

I Primary Prevention: Genetic counseling in those of familial occurrence

II Secondary Prevention: Propranolol increases the threshold for ventricular fibrillation and is the best therapeutic modality available at present. Left lower cervical and left upper thoracic ganglionectomy have been of benefit in some instances. The combination of the 2 therapies may be advantageous. Artificial pacemaker therapy employing the standby or demand mode, although theoretically useful, is difficult to maintain long-term. It has seemed more appropriate for interim therapy.

III Other Therapy: —

Prognosis: Poor: 50% of the cases reportedly died before adolescence. However, this figure is influenced by the fact that the more severe forms of the syndrome have been reported; also, most of these were in the period of time preceding the therapy listed above. The prognosis should be improved by earlier recognition and application of current concepts.

Detection of Carrier: QT interval on ECG is normal or long, but may be increased by exercising the subject.

†Special Considerations: There is considerable agreement in the findings in this syndrome, and the cardiac aspects of the cardioauditory syndrome. The syndrome of familial paroxysmal ventricular fibrillation, although excluded by the absence of a long QT interval, does have several features in common including prominent U waves and prolongation of the QT interval with exercise.

References:

Garza, L.A. et al: Heritable Q-T prolongation without deafness. Circulation 41:39, 1970.
Karhunen, P. et al: Syncope and QT prolongation without deafness: The Romano-Ward syndrome. Am. Heart J. 80:820, 1970.
Romano, C. et al: Artimie cardiache rare dell 'eta pediatrica. Clin. Pediatr. (Bologna). 45:656, 1963.
Schwartz, P.J. et al: The long-QT syndrome. Am. Heart J. 89:378, 1975.
Ward, O.C.: New familial cardiac syndrome in children. Ir. Med. J. 54:103, 1964.

Contributors: **B. Lynn Miller**
Philip Posner

Editor's Computerized Descriptor: CV.

LUNG, ABERRANT LOBE

Includes: Lobe aberrant du poumon
Akzessorischer Lungenlappen
Lóbulo pulmonar aberrante
Tracheal lobe
Esophageal lobe
Accessory lung arising from bronchial tree, esophagus, or stomach
Aberrant lobe of lung
Aberrant bronchus
Extrapulmonic lobe

Excludes: Azygous lobe
Lung lobe sequestration (612)
Congenital communication between bronchial tree and biliary system

Minimal Diagnostic Criteria: Evidence of aberrant bronchial origin from the trachea or from the esophagus using either direct vision or x-ray technic.

Clinical Findings: An aberrant bronchus arising from the trachea usually supplies normal lung tissue and thus gives rise to no symptoms or signs unless it becomes diseased. This is equally true of the aberrant bronchus that is rarely found to arise from the medial aspect of the intermediate bronchus. There are no roentgenologic findings, except with a special technic such as laminography or bronchography, which may reveal the aberrant origin of the bronchus. Bronchoscopy will also reveal the presence of the aberrant bronchial orifice.

An anomalous lobe arising from the esophagus usually contains no functioning pulmonic tissue. It remains asymptomatic until it becomes infected. On occasion the "bronchus" may arise from the stomach and pass through the diaphragm to supply pulmonic tissue.

Complications
I Derived: Infection, hemorrhage.
II Associated: —

Etiology: ?

Pathogenesis: ? There are many theories and these are described well by Spencer.

Related Facts
I Sex Ratio: M1:F1
II Risk of Occurrence: ?
III Risk of Recurrence for
Patient's Sib: ?
Patient's Child: ?
IV Age of Detectability: Not until infection or hemorrhage occurs or special testing is performed.
V Prevalence: ?

Treatment
I Primary Prevention: —
II Secondary Prevention: Aberrant lobes of nonfunctioning tissue as are typically associated with bronchi of esophageal or gastric origin are more apt to be the seat of complications and should be prophylactically excised. When they become symptomatic due to infection they may be treated with antibiotics and again may require excision.
III Other Therapy: Standard care for infection or hemorrhage, if and when it occurs.

Prognosis: Normal for life span and intelligence. Normal for function with tracheal aberrant bronchi; esophageal aberrant lobe is extremely rare but seems to have a great tendency to develop infection.

Detection of Carrier: —

Special Considerations: —

References:

Atwell, S. W.: An aberrant bronchus. Ann. Thorac. Surg. 2:438, 1966.

Chofnas, I.: Tracheal lobe of the right lung. Am. Rev. Respir. Dis. 87:280, 1963.

Levine, M. I. and Mascia, A. V.: Pulmonary Disease and Anomalies of Infancy and Childhood. New York: Harper and Row, 1966.

Spencer, H.: Pathology of the Lung. New York:Pergamon Press, 1968.

Thomson, N. B. and Aquino, T.: Anomalous origin of the right main-stem bronchus. Surgery 51:668, 1962.

Contributor: **William E. Bloomer**

Editor's Computerized Descriptor: Resp.

LUNG LOBE SEQUESTRATION

Includes: Séquestration d'un lobe pulmonaire
Extralobäre Lungensequestration
Secuestración del lóbulo pulmonar
Extra lobar sequestration
Aortic pulmonary lobe

Excludes: —

Minimal Diagnostic Criteria: Intrathoracic density displacing or replacing normal parenchyma associated with bronchial and vascular anomalies and consisting of lung components in various stages of development.

Clinical Findings: Usually asymptomatic in infancy. During childhood and early adulthood, infection or bleeding may occur in the involved region. Abnormalities on physical examination are usually absent. Increased density with or without cystic highlights is present on the chest radiogram, usually involving the base, more often on the left than on the right. Bronchography demonstrates rearrangement of the bronchial pattern, with loss or displacement of normal segment(s). Occasionally, filling of the sequestered region may occur. Aortography frequently demonstrates anomalous arterial blood supply originating from the descending thoracic or abdominal aorta. Laboratory findings are normal unless hemorrhage or infection have supervened.†

Complications
I **Derived:** Infection, infrequent; hemorrhage, rare.
II **Associated:** —

Etiology: ?

Pathogenesis: The intralobar and extralobar forms of sequestration are thought to be results of the same or a similar developmental abnormality, occurring at different times. Both occur because of the development of an extra foregut bud, which arises caudal to the normal bud as indicated by the frequent presence of a thoracic or abdominal aortic blood supply, by the association with esophageal cysts and fistulas and by the occasional presence of ectopic pancreas and liver in these. If the extra bud arises early enough (from the short foregut) it will be carried into the celomic cavity and incorporated into parts of normal lobes. Development at another time most likely leads to the extralobar type of sequestration which histologically matches the intralobar form.

Related Facts
I   **Sex Ratio:** M?:F?
II **Risk of Occurrence:** ?
III **Risk of Recurrence for**
     Patient's Sib: ?
     Patient's Child: ?
IV **Age of Detectability:** Variable; see Clinical Findings.
V   **Prevalence:** ?

Treatment
I   **Primary Prevention:** —
II **Secondary Prevention:** Surgical resection of involved tissue
III **Other Therapy:** For infection or hemorrhage as needful

Prognosis: Normal for life span, intelligence and function

Detection of Carrier: ?

†**Special Considerations:** These anomalies probably fit into a broader spectrum of developmental anomalies originating in the foregut. Esophageal duplication cysts, bron-

chogenic cysts and tracheoesophageal fistula with or without atresia probably all are different forms of the same or similar abnormalities of development. Sequestration, once diagnosed, does not represent a major surgical challenge. However, in the undiagnosed case the presence of anomalous arterial supply, particularly when infradiaphragmatic in origin, can present a grave danger because of unexpected damage to these vessels with ensuing retraction into the abdomen.

References:
Blesovsky, A.: Pulmonary sequestration: A report of an unusual case and a review of the literature. Thorax 22:351, 1967.
Gerle, R.D. et al: Congenital broncho-pulmonary-foregut malformation: Pulmonary sequestration communicating with the gastrointestinal tract. N. Engl. J. Med. 278:1413, 1968.
Halasz, N.A. et al: Esophago-bronchial fistula and bronchopulmonary sequestration: Report of a case and review of the literature. Ann. Surg. 155:215, 1962.

Contributor: **N. A. Halasz**

Editor's Computerized Descriptor: Resp.

LYMPHANGIOMA OF ALVEOLAR RIDGES

Includes: Lymphangiome gingival
Lymphangiom der Zahnleisten
Linfangioma de los bordes alveolares dentarios

Excludes: Epulis congenital (360)
Bohn nodules
Epstein pearls
Mucous retention cysts
Eruption cysts

Minimal Diagnostic Criteria: Lymphangioma on the alveolar ridges of newborns. This must be confirmed histologically.

Clinical Findings: These lymphangiomas are seen on the maxillary or mandibular alveolar ridges of newborn infants. When on the maxillary ridge they are on the crest at the site where the 1st molars are expected to erupt. When on the mandibular ridge, they are on the lingual surface at a site homologous to those on the maxillary ridge. The tongue may have to be displaced to see those on the mandibular ridge. The lymphangiomas are frequently bilateral and may exist in all 4 quadrants simultaneously.

They are fluid-filled, and their surfaces vary from slightly raised above adjacent mucosa to being raised 3-4 mm above adjacent mucosa. Their diameters vary from < 1 mm to several millimeters.

Complications
I **Derived:**   The lesions appear to bother infants during nursing.
II **Associated:**   —

Etiology: ? All affected infants have been black.

Pathogenesis: ? The histologic appearance of some biopsied lesions is similar to that of hemangioma, but the majority resemble lymphangioma. The lesions are composed of soft tissue with numerous endothelial-lined vascular channels. They collapse when biopsied and discharge a thin clear fluid. No teeth are evident in the tissue under the lesions.

Related Facts
I **Sex Ratio:**   M3:F2
II **Risk of Occurrence:**   Approximately 1:25 among blacks (4%); not reported among whites.†
III **Risk of Recurrence for**
    Patient's Sib: ?
    Patient's Child: ?
IV **Age of Detectability:**   At birth
V **Prevalence:**   ? Not reported in older children

Treatment
I **Primary Prevention:**   —
II **Secondary Prevention:**   Surgical excision
III **Other Therapy:**   —

Prognosis: Good. Since these lesions have not been reported in grown children, one should assume that they regress prior to intraoral examination by a physician or dentist. Such an assumption should be made cautiously, however. They may, in fact, regress, they may go unnoticed or they may evolve into some other intraoral lesion. Several cases that were followed showed variable changes in the lesions. In some, the lesions became smaller with time. In others, the lesions remained the same size, but changed color and surface character. In still others, the lesions became fibrotic masses. The longest follow-up was 6 1/2 months.

Detection of Carrier: —

†Special Considerations: The racial predilection and symmetric distribution of alveolar ridge lymphangiomas suggest the possibility of a developmental, perhaps genetic, etiology. Family studies have not been done.

References:
Levin, L.S. et al: Lymphangiomas of the alveolar ridges in neonates. Pediatrics 58:881, 1976.

Contributors: **Ronald J. Jorgenson**
                     L. Stefan Levin

Editor's Computerized Descriptor: Teeth

LYMPHEDEMA I

Includes: Lymphoédème congénitale
Frühmanifestes Lymphödem
Linfedema de instalación precoz
Early-onset lymphedema
Congenital hereditary lymphedema
Milroy disease
Nonne-Milroy type hereditary lymphedema

Excludes: Lymphedema II (615)

Minimal Diagnostic Criteria: Presence of edema at birth and a familial history of similarly affected individuals

Clinical Findings: Chronic, pitting edema of the lower limbs. Expressivity varies from minimal swelling of an ankle to greatly enlarged feet, legs and thighs. The overlying skin is attenuated, but otherwise normal.

Complications
I   **Derived:** —
II **Associated:** —

Etiology: Autosomal dominant with variable expressivity†; McK *15310

Pathogenesis: There is usually a slow, asymptomatic progression in the severity of the edema with age. Attempts to visualize lymphatics in involved areas have been unsuccessful. For this reason, the edema appears to be due to a defect in the development of lymphatic drainage rather than increased filtration, which may be secondary to edema of any type.

Related Facts
I   **Sex Ratio:** M1:F1
II   **Risk of Occurrence:** ? Very uncommon
III **Risk of Recurrence for**
     Patient's Sib: If parent is affected 1 in 2 (50%) for each sib; otherwise not increased.
     Patient's Child: 1 in 2
IV   **Age of Detectability:** Neonatal period
V   **Prevalence:** ? Rare. Twenty-three sibships have been described in a wide geographic distribution, including Caucasian, Negro and Oriental families but it probably is more frequent than has been appreciated.

Treatment
I   **Primary Prevention:** Genetic counseling
II   **Secondary Prevention:** —
III **Other Therapy:** Resection of subcutaneous tissues with subsequent skin autografts have been performed with variable results. Diuretics and bed rest are partially and temporarily effective.

Prognosis: Normal life span and intelligence. Some degree of disability may result from edema of lower limbs.

Detection of Carrier: †

†Special Considerations: Careful examination of some supposedly normal individuals with affected progeny may show minor involvement; all reported pedigrees are compatible with inheritance as a dominant trait. No linkage has been found between this defect and several common markers. Several families contain individuals with involvement of the hands. Historic evidence of individuals with late onset lymphedema II has been described in about 10% of pedigrees of the congenital, early onset lymphedema I.
Chronic lymphedema is primarily a cosmetic handicap. The potential complications of a proposed therapy should be evaluated accordingly.

References:
Esterly, J. R.: Congenital hereditary lymphoedema. J. Med. Genet. 2:93, 1965.
Schroeder, E. and Helweg-Larson, H. F.: Congenital hereditary lymphedema (Nonne-Milroy-Meige's disease). Acta Med. Scand. 137:198, 1950.

Contributor: **John R. Esterly**

Editor's Computerized Descriptor: Skin

LYMPHEDEMA II

Includes: Lymphoédème à début tardif
Spätmanifestes Lymphödem
Linfedema tardío
Familial lymphedema with onset after childhood
Idiopathic lymphedema
Primary noninflammatory lymphedema
Meige type lymphedema
Lymphedema forme tarde
Yellow nail syndrome with familial late-onset lymphedema
Lymphedema praecox
Late-onset lymphedema

Excludes: Lymphedema I (614)
Lymphedema of the Turner or Bonnevie-Ullrich syndrome
Secondary lymphedema from multiple causes
Tumorigenic lymphedema
Lymphangiosarcoma in chronic lymphedema of the lower limb

Minimal Diagnostic Criteria: Since the diagnosis is a clinical one an accurate family history must be obtained and all forms of secondary lymphedema ruled out. If the edema presents after the age of 40 years, one should suspect an underlying malignant lesion. For example, if lymphedema develops in one or both lower limbs of an elderly man, the most common cause is carcinoma of the prostate. Similarly a pelvic carcinoma should be suspected when lymphedema is first present in the leg of a middle-aged or elderly woman.

Lymphangiographic studies can be helpful in considering the differential diagnosis and, in cases of idiopathic lymphedema, may show aplasia, hypoplasia or dilated lymph trunks.

Clinical Findings: Late onset lymphedema II may make its appearance as early as the teens but the most common time of onset is between the ages of 20 and 40 years. Upper and lower limbs may be involved, but in the vast majority of cases it is the lower limbs that are affected. In one series of 131 cases only 5 patients had upper limb involvement. Bilateral lower limb lymphedema occurred in approximately half of those cases with lower limb involvement. The degree of involvement can be quite variable and may be so minimal as to go undetected, or, in contrast, may be so extensive that ambulation is a problem. Since there is no specific laboratory test to diagnose this form of lymphedema, it becomes imperative that all causes of secondary lymphedema be excluded. Namely, such processes as infection, postphlebitic lymphedema, postlymphangitic lymphedema and neoplasia should be ruled out. In general, other genetic abnormalities have not been associated with the hereditary form of late onset lymphedema II. However, in 1966 Wells described a family with affected members showing dystrophic yellow nails and lymphedema involving both lower limbs and occasionally the hands and face. Whether these 2 findings are related or represent a coincidental occurrence is not known.

Complications
I **Derived:** The most common complication is single or recurrent episodes of lymphangitis or cellulitis, and these may lead to ulceration. Trichophytosis has been found in approximately 10% of the cases. Lymphangiosarcoma may develop but this occurs in less than 1% of the cases.
II **Associated:** Possibly yellow, dystrophic nails

Etiology: Lymphedema II, autosomal recessive transmission; Lymphedema II with yellow nail syndrome has autosomal dominant transmission. The modes of transmission for lymphedema praecox and lymphedema forme tarde are unknown. McK *15320

Pathogenesis: ? Anatomically there seems to be a hypoplasia of the lymphatic system in all genetic forms of lymphedema.

Related Facts

I Sex Ratio: M1:F1. However, it is M1:F10 in lymphedema praecox and lymphedema forme tarde.

II Risk of Occurrence: ? Primary types more common than the genetic

III Risk of Recurrence for

    Patient's Sib: Lymphedema II, 1 in 4 (25%) for each sib; Lymphedema II with yellow nail syndrome, if parent is affected, 1 in 2 (50%) for each offspring to be affected; otherwise not increased.

    Patient's Child: Lymphedema II, not increased unless mate is heterozygote or homozygote. Lymphedema II with yellow nail syndrome, 1 in 2. Primary form is not genetically determined, therefore, other family members should not be affected unless by chance.

IV Age of Detectability: Late onset lymphedema II around puberty. Yellow nail syndrome with lymphedema - middle age. Primary form - detectable between the ages of 10 and 40 years, most common between 20 and 30 years.

V Prevalence: ?

Treatment

I Primary Prevention: Genetic counseling

II Secondary Prevention: —

III Other Therapy: Either type of edema may partially respond to a pararubber bandage or an elastic stocking. Some patients have been reported to have a reduction of the edema with the use of a diuretic. When the lymphedema is severe and uncontrollable, surgical intervention with removal of the diseased tissue may be indicated.

Prognosis: The lymphedema per se does not alter the normal life span or intelligence. However, such complications as lymphangitis or the development of lymphangiosarcoma may result in an early death. If the edema is extreme with an unsightly appearance, problems in ambulation coupled with various emotional difficulties usually are present.

Detection of Carrier: Heterozygote is affected in lymphedema II with yellow nail syndrome.

Special Considerations: —

References:

Goodman, R.M.: Familial lymphedema of the Meige type. Am. J. Med. 32:651, 1962.

Schirger, A. et al: Idiopathic lymphedema: Review of 131 cases. JAMA 182:14, 1962.

Wells, G.C.: Yellow nail syndrome: With familial primary hypoplasia of lymphatics, manifest late in life. Proc. R. Soc. Med. 59:447, 1966.

Contributor: **Richard M. Goodman**

Editor's Computerized Descriptors: Skin, Nails, Lymphatic

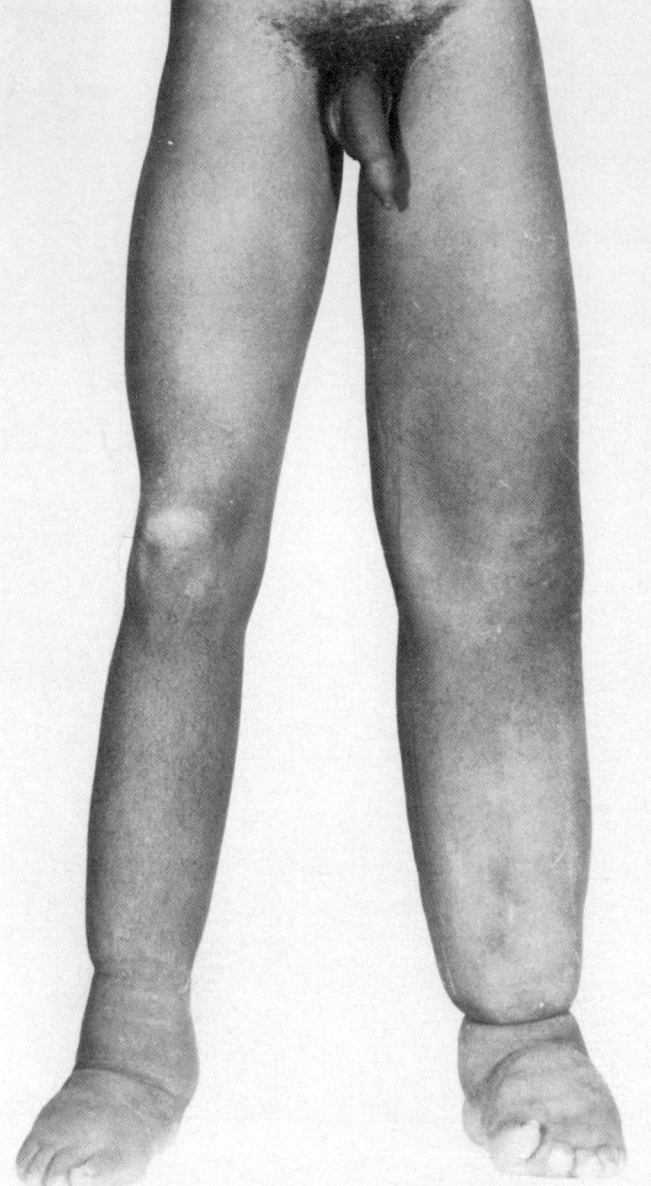

331. Lymphedema II

LYSINEMIA

Includes: Lysinémie
Lysinämie
Lisinemia
Hyperlysinemia

Excludes: Lysine intolerance

Minimal Diagnostic Criteria: Persistent lysinemia and lysinuria

Clinical Findings: In 7 reported cases, 5 were found to be mentally retarded, 3 were physically retarded and 3 exhibited synophrys. Impaired sexual development, prognathous jaw, high maxilla, and slight webbing of the fingers were each found in 2 patients; 1 patient had strabismus.

Laboratory findings include increased concentration of lysine in the blood, about or above 6 mg/100 ml and lysinuria due to lysinemia.†

Complications
I   **Derived:** Mental retardation
II **Associated:** —

Etiology: Probably autosomal recessive; McK *23870

Pathogenesis: Deficiency of lysine-α-ketoglutarate reductase.

Related Facts
I   **Sex Ratio:** M1:F1
II **Risk of Occurrence:** Very rare
III **Risk of Recurrence for**
    Patient's Sib: Probably 1 in 4 (25%) for each offspring to be affected
    Patient's Child: Not increased, unless mate is carrier or homozygote
IV **Age of Detectability:** Neonatal period by analysis of blood and urine
V   **Prevalence:** Very rare

Treatment
I   **Primary Prevention:** Genetic counseling
II **Secondary Prevention:** ?
III **Other Therapy:** —

Prognosis: ?

Detection of Carrier: ?

†Special Considerations: Lysinemia seems to be very rare. In congenital lysine intolerance, a clinical picture simulating ammonia intoxication while the patient is on a normal or high-protein intake has been reported. These episodes consist of vomiting, coma, spasticity and convulsions which are relieved by the withdrawal of protein intake. This phenomenon is presumably due to the inhibitory effect of lysine on arginase in Krebs urea cycle. In lysinemia such episodes have never been observed.

References:
Colombo, J.P. et al: Congenital lysine intolerance with periodic ammonia intoxication: A defect in L-lysine degradation. Metabolism 16:910, 1967.
Dancis, J. et al: Familial hyperlysinemia with lysine-ketoglutarate reductase insufficiency. J. Clin. Invest. 48:1447, 1969.
Ghadimi, H. and Zischka, R.: Hyperlysinemia and lysine metabolism. In Nyhan, W.L. (ed.): Amino Acid Metabolism and Genetic Variation. New York:McGraw-Hill, 1967, p.227.
Woody, N. C. and Ong, E. B.: Paths of lysine degradation in patients with hyperlysinemia. Pediatrics 40:986, 1967.

Contributor: **H. Ghadimi**

Editor's Computerized Descriptors: Eye, Face, Hair, Skel., GU., Nerve

MACRODONTIA

Includes: Macrodontie
Makrodontie
Macrodoncia
Teeth, enlarged

Excludes: Hemihypertrophy (458)
Teeth, fused (930)

Minimal Diagnostic Criteria: Absolute measurements of teeth exceed range of normal variation.

Clinical Findings: True macrodontia, where teeth are larger than normal, must be differentiated from relative macrodontia, wherein the teeth are of normal size but occur in small jaws. Individual teeth or groups of teeth may exceed normal dimensions. True macrodontia affecting all teeth is relatively rare.

Complications
I   **Derived:** Crowding of teeth in dental arches. Malocclusion. Impacted teeth with dentigerous cyst formation.
II **Associated:** Pituitary gigantism, hemihypertrophy, angiomas which affect the jaws.

Etiology: Essentially unknown. True macrodontia probably is ascribable to a genetic component. Large teeth are seen in some cases with poly-X states (XXXXY). Some cases are associated with pituitary hyperfunction. Macrodontia of individual teeth is most frequently the result of fusion with supernumerary teeth or partial twinning of tooth germ. Macrodontia of groups of teeth is found in association with angiomas of the jaws and hemihypertrophy. Occurs in various species of animals.

Pathogenesis: Essentially unknown. Local or general factors which influence growth result in enlarged teeth. Structure of enamel and dentin usually normal.

Related Facts
I   **Sex Ratio:** ?
II **Risk of Occurrence:** ? Rare
III **Risk of Recurrence for**
    Patient's Sib: ? Probably low
    Patient's Child: ? Probably low
IV **Age of Detectability:** Upon eruption of primary or permanent teeth
V   **Prevalence:** ? Rare

Treatment
I   **Primary Prevention:** Not necessary
II **Secondary Prevention:** Usually no treatment indicated. Extraction and orthodontic treatment if malocclusion or impacted teeth are present.
III **Other Therapy:** —

Prognosis: Usually good with no decrease in life span unless associated with pituitary gigantism, angiomas or hemihypertrophy

Detection of Carrier: —

Special Considerations: —

References:
None

Contributor: **Lawrence Meskin**

Editor's Computerized Descriptor: Teeth

MACROGLOSSIA

Includes: Macroglossie
Makroglossie
Macroglosia
Isolated congenitally enlarged tongue
Muscular macroglossia
Hemangiomatous macroglossia
Tongue gigantism
Primary macroglossia
Nodular macroglossia
Lymphangiomatous macroglossia

Excludes: Chromosome twenty-one trisomy syndrome (171)
Hypothyroidism
Glycogen storage diseases
Mucopolysaccharidoses
Mucolipidoses
Neurofibromatosis (712)
Hemihypertrophy (458)
Multiple mucosal neuroma syndrome
Beckwith-Wiedemann syndrome (104)

Minimal Diagnostic Criteria: Isolated enlargement of tongue

Clinical Findings: Enlarged tongue in the absence of anomalies associated with the conditions listed under Excludes.

Complications
I   **Derived:** Superficial ulceration and infection may occur in hemangiomatous and lymphangiomatous macroglossia. Later complications may include speech defects and malocclusion. In lymphangiomatous macroglossia, cystic hygroma and involvement of the oral floor may occur.
II **Associated:** —

Etiology: ?

Pathogenesis: Depends upon type of macroglossia. Hemangiomatous and lymphangiomatous macroglossia result from hamartomatous overgrowth of vascular and lymphatic tissue, respectively. In muscular macroglossia, hypertrophy of individual muscle fibers has been observed.

Related Facts
I   **Sex Ratio:** ?
II   **Risk of Occurrence:** ? Very low
III **Risk of Recurrence for**
     Patient's Sib: ?
     Patient's Child: ?
IV   **Age of Detectability:** At birth, by clinical evaluation
V   **Prevalence:** ? Very rare

Treatment
I   **Primary Prevention:** —
II   **Secondary Prevention:** Surgical treatment, reduction of tongue size with sclerosing agents
III **Other Therapy:** Speech therapy and orthodontic treatment may be indicated in some instances.

Prognosis: Excellent in most cases, probably does not reduce longevity.

Detection of Carrier: —

Special Considerations: —

References:
Bronstein, I.P. et al: Macroglossia in children; review of literature, report of case of true muscular hypertrophy and suggested classification. Am. J. Dis. Child. 54:1328, 1937.
Gorlin, R.J.: Developmental anomalies of the face and oral structures. In Gorlin, R.J. and Goldman, H.M. (eds.): Thoma's Oral Pathology, 6th Ed. St. Louis:C.V. Mosby Co., 1970, vol. 1, p. 37.

Contributor: **M. Michael Cohen, Jr.**

MACROTIA

Includes: Macrotie
Ear, enlarged scapha and lobule

Excludes: Microtia-atresia (664)
Atresia alone
Deafness and ear pits (247)
Darwin tubercle (Marker) (241)
Ear lobe pit (Marker) (322)
Ear flare

Minimal Diagnostic Criteria: Very much enlarged pinna, particularly in area of the scapha†

Clinical Findings: The patient has a very large, but generally well-shaped auricle without other malformations of the ear. The ear is, however, somewhat disproportionate in that the most exaggerated portion of the ear is the scapha. The other parts of the ear are also somewhat larger than normal, especially the lobule. Occasionally the ear may protrude somewhat. A variant of this may be seen in Marfan syndrome in which the cartilage is somewhat floppy as well as the ear being large. The condition is usually bilateral and symmetric.

Complications
I **Derived:** Embarrassment or psychologic disturbance due to the excessive size of the ears
II **Associated:** Marfan syndrome, ectopia lentis, defects of the media of arteries

Etiology: Autosomal dominant in some

Pathogenesis: ?

Related Facts
I **Sex Ratio:** M?:F?
II **Risk of Occurrence:** ?
III **Risk of Recurrence for**
   Patient's Sib: When autosomal dominant and if parent is affected < 1 in 2 (< 50%) for each offspring to be affected; otherwise not increased.
   Patient's Child: < 1 in 2
IV **Age of Detectability:** At birth
V **Prevalence:** ?

Treatment
I **Primary Prevention:** Genetic counseling
II **Secondary Prevention:** Plastic surgical repair may be indicated
III **Other Therapy:** —

Prognosis: Good for life span, intelligence and function if isolated defect of outer ear, otherwise dependent upon concomitant defects.

Detection of Carrier: —

†**Special Considerations:** Anomalies of the external ear should suggest the possibility of an anomaly of the middle ear as well. Hearing should be assessed as soon as possible and appropriate therapy instituted. The anatomy of the middle and inner ear should be determined by petrous pyramid polytomography.

References:
Ver Meulen, V.R.: Macrotia—the over-sized ear: A method for reduction. Laryngoscope 80:1053, 1970.

Contributor: **LaVonne Bergstrom**

Editor's Computerized Descriptor: Ear

MACULA, HETEROTOPIC

Includes: Hétérotopie de la macule
Heterotopie der Macula
Heterotopia de la mácula
Ectopia of macula
Heterotopia of macula

Excludes: —

Minimal Diagnostic Criteria: Abnormal position of the macula relative to the disk on ophthalmoscopic examination. The foveal reflex can often be best located with red-free light. Pseudostrabismus occurs in most cases.

Clinical Findings: The foveal reflex and the macula do not lie in their optically correct positions. Usually it is 2 disk diameters temporal to the optic disk. Ophthalmoscopically, it appears as if the macula were pulled temporally by some developmental or inflammatory condition. Minimal retinal traction associated with retrolental fibroplasia is probably the most common cause, but related defects include other retinal folds, vascular anomalies, colobomas of the optic disk and remnants of the hyaloid arterial system.

Despite accurate fixation on the light of the ophthalmoscope, a pseudostrabismus is seen with eccentric fixation. The visual acuity varies considerably but is frequently better than would be expected from the apparent eccentric fixation. On visual field plotting, the blind spot is in an abnormal location.

Complications
I **Derived:** —
II **Associated:** Retrolental fibroplasia and other developmental and inflammatory conditions

Etiology: ?

Pathogenesis: Details are unknown, but could be explained by irregular growth rates of the posterior segment of the eye either pre- or postnatally. Most cases are due to secondary displacement of the macula by traction bands which may result from chorioretinitis, retrolental fibroplasia or other pre- or postnatal defects.

Related Facts
I **Sex Ratio:** ?
II **Risk of Occurrence:** ?
III **Risk of Recurrence for**
   Patient's Sib: ?
   Patient's Child: ?
IV **Age of Detectability:** At birth in the primary cases, and later in life when secondary to other conditions.
V **Prevalence:** ?

Treatment
I **Primary Prevention:** —
II **Secondary Prevention:** —
III **Other Therapy:** —

Prognosis: Good for retention of existing vision

Detection of Carrier: —

Special Considerations: —

References:
Amalric, P. and Bessou, P.: Heterotopie maculaire. Bull. Soc. Ophthalmol. 10:646, 1960.
Cohen, I.J. and Weisberg, H.K.: Vertical heterotopia of macula. Arch. Ophthalmol. 44:419, 1950.
Duke-Elder, S.: System of Ophthalmology, vol. 3, part 2. Congenital Deformities. St. Louis: C.V. Mosby Co., 1963, p. 654.
Gröndahl, J.: Heterotopia maculae-probably caused by ablatio falciformis congenita. Acta Ophthalmol. (Kbh) 41:259, 1963.
Mann, I.: Developmental Abnormalities of the Eye. Philadelphia:

J.B. Lippincott, 1957, p. 143.

Nauheim, J.S.: Heterotopia of the macula. Arch. Ophthalmol. 63:144, 1960.

Rados, W.T. and Scholz, R.O.: Pseudostrabismus with heterotopia of the macula. Am. J. Ophthalmol. 45:683, 1958.

Willets, G.S.: Heterotopia of the macula. Br. J. Ophthalmol. 50:596, 1966.

Contributor: **Robert M. Ellsworth**

Editor's Computerized Descriptor: Eye

MACULAR COLOBOMA AND BRACHYDACTYLY

Includes: Colobome maculaire et brachydactylie
Makula-Kolobom und Brachydaktylie
Coloboma de la mácula y braquidactilia
Sorsby syndrome
Brachydactyly and macular coloboma

Excludes: Fetal toxoplasmosis syndrome (387)
Apical dystrophy of hands and feet, type MacArthur and McCullough

Minimal Diagnostic Criteria: Congenital macular colobomata and limb malformation on xrays

Clinical Findings: Characterized by 1) bilateral pigmented macular colobomata of 5 to 6 DD by 3 to 4 DD, with the larger diameter horizontally placed, and 2) an apical dystrophy of hands and feet. The latter consists of rudimentary nails on the index finger of each hand and hallux of each foot, plus an abnormal appearance of the terminal part of the thumb and big toe, which vary from extreme broadness to complete bifurcation. Xrays reveal diminution or actual suppression of the 2nd phalanx of the little finger, a variable bifurcation of the terminal phalanx of thumb and hallux with a considerable atrophy of all terminal phalanges of both hands and feet. There is variable absence of the small toe.

Complications
I **Derived:** Horizontal pendular nystagmus and visual acuity of maximally 10/200 corrected
II **Associated:** —

Etiology: Autosomal dominant with complete penetrance

Pathogenesis: ?

Related Facts
I **Sex Ratio:** M1:F1
II **Risk of Occurrence:** ? Rare
III **Risk of Recurrence for**
　Patient's Sib: If one parent is affected, 1 in 2 (50%) for each offspring to be affected; otherwise not increased
　Patient's Child: 1 in 2
IV **Age of Detectability:** Neonatal period
V **Prevalence:** ? Rare, only 1 family has been described.

Treatment
I **Primary Prevention:** Genetic counseling
II **Secondary Prevention:** ?
III **Other Therapy:** —

Prognosis: Normal for life span and intelligence. Lifelong visual acuity in the legally blind range

Detection of Carrier: —

Special Considerations: —

References:
Sorsby, A.: Congenital coloboma of the macula: Together with an account of the familial occurrence of bilateral macular coloboma in association with apical dystrophy of hands and feet. Br. J. Ophthalmol. 19:65, 1935.

Contributor: **Irene Hussels-Maumenee**

Editor's Computerized Descriptors: Vision, Eye, Nails, Skel.

MACULAR DEGENERATION, VITELLIRUPTIVE

Includes: Maladie de Best
Vitelliruptive Makuladegeneration
Degeneración macular congénita
Hereditary vitelliruptive macular degeneration
Vitelline macular degeneration
Vitelliform, macular degeneration
Best disease
Congenital macular degeneration
Central exudative detachment of retina
Macular cysts
Macular pseudocysts
Congenital vitelliform cysts of macula
Exudative central detachment
Central cystoid dystrophy

Excludes: Pseudovitelliform macular degeneration†
Progressive foveal dystrophy
Central serous retinopathy

Minimal Diagnostic Criteria: Typical appearing lesion in younger members of a family with macular degeneration of autosomal dominant inheritance

Clinical Findings: The age of onset of the macular lesion is usually between 5-15 years, but it has been seen as early as 1 week of age.

The typical features of the lesion are seen in early cases. It has been described as looking like "an egg with sunny-side up," at a somewhat later stage like a "scrambled egg," or like a "cystic lesion filled with exudates and precipitates, sometimes with a definite level, resembling a hypopyon." This early lesion is usually yellow or orange in color, elevated, has sharp borders and is frequently almost circular in outline. However, eventually it loses its cystic appearance and the exudate-like material disappears. A macular degeneration may then follow which is indistinguishable from other types of macular degenerations. Visual acuity, particularly in the early stages of the disease, is usually better than anticipated from the appearance of the macula. However, deep retinal hemorrhage may occur, probably from the choriocapillaris, with eventual hypertrophic scar formation so that vision can be reduced early in life.

However, visual acuity typically remains good until the 4th decade when a secondary macular degeneration frequently occurs. On the other hand, secondary intraretinal macular changes may be minimal and fairly good visual acuity may be maintained throughout life. Visual fields are normal except for central scotoma when acuity is abnormal. Dark adaptation and ERG are usually normal but minimal abnormality has been noted. The electrooculogram is always abnormal.

Complications
I   **Derived:**   Intraretinal macular degeneration, macular hemorrhage
II **Associated:**   —

Etiology: Autosomal dominant transmission with many examples of reduced penetrance and expressivity; McK *15370

Pathogenesis: The 1 published histologic study is from a patient in the late stages. This report noted extensive choroidal and retinal changes so that no conclusions could be drawn regarding the basic or initial pathology. The electrooculogram is markedly abnormal in all cases tested, even in younger members in early stages of the disease. This finding suggests that a diffuse abnormality of the pigment epithelium exists in this disease even though only the macular area shows ophthalmoscopic changes. With red light, which penetrates the retinal pigment epithelium, the typical lesion of younger subjects is observed. On the other hand, blue light, which does not penetrate beyond the retinal receptors, does not show the typical lesion. Therefore the typical lesion is probably external to the pigment epithelium. On the other hand, blue light shows the typical features of the secondary macular degeneration in older subjects indicating its intraretinal location. Fluorescence is not observed with the very early lesion. However, after an uncertain period of time, fluorescence characteristic of defective pigment epithelium is seen in the macula and is dependent on the size and position of the original lesion. In fact a precise correspondent between the early lesion and the total fluorescent defect implies close proximity of the original lesion to the pigment epithelium, either within or directly adjacent to the structure.

Related Facts
I   **Sex Ratio:** M1:F1
II   **Risk of Occurrence:**   ?
III **Risk of Recurrence for**
     Patient's Sib: If parent is affected, < 1 in 2 (< 50%) for each offspring to be affected; otherwise not increased
     Patient's Child: < 1 in 2
IV   **Age of Detectability:**   Usually detected between 5-15 years of age, but occasionally may not be noted until the 3rd or even beginning of the 4th decade of life
V   **Prevalence:**   ?

Treatment
I   **Primary Prevention:**   Genetic counseling
II   **Secondary Prevention:**   —
III **Other Therapy:**   —

Prognosis: Life span normal, guarded for vision

Detection of Carrier: A carrier of the gene with no macular abnormality can be identified by an abnormal EOG .

†Special Considerations: Patients with typical vitelliform fusions have been recently reported who have normal EOGs. These patients are not part of a familial disease, have visual loss associated with the lesions, and represent a different entity which has been called "pseudovitelliform degeneration."

References:
Braley, A.E. and Spivey, B.E.: Hereditary vitelline macular degeneration: A clinical and functional evaluation of a new pedigree with variable expressivity and dominant inheritance Arch. Ophthalmol. 72:743, 1964.
Deutman, A.F.: Electro-oculography in families with vitelliform dystrophy of the fovea. Arch. Ophthalmol. 81:305, 1969.
Fishman, G.A. et al: Pseudovitelliform macular degeneration. Arch ophthalmol. 95:73, 1977.
François, J.: Vitelliform degeneration of the macula. Bull. N.Y. Acad. Med. 44:18, 1968.
Krill, A.E. et al: Hereditary vitelliruptive macular degeneration. Am. J. Ophthalmol. 61:1405, 1966.
Krill, A.E.: Vitelliruptive macular dystrophy. In Krill, A.E. and Archer, D.B. (eds.): Krill's Hereditary Retinal and Choroidal Diseases. Hagerstown:Harper & Row, 1977, vol II.

Contributors: **Alex E. Krill‡**
                     Mitchel L. Wolf

___

Editor's Computerized Descriptor: Eye
Also see Section I, Fig. 33

MADAROSIS

Includes: Madarose
Isolated congenital hypotrichosis
Congenital underdevelopment of the lashes
Alopecia adnata
Eyelashes, underdeveloped

Excludes: Ectodermal dysplasia
Oculo-mandibulo-facial syndrome (738)
Hypotrichosis secondary to generalized disease

Minimal Diagnostic Criteria: Hypoplasia (severe diminution or absence) of lashes. Lack of primary cause such as trauma, inflammation, mycotic infection, neurotic epilation, or generalized disease such as congenital atrophy of the skin, general alopecia, idiopathic hypoparathyroidism, xeroderma pigmentosa, or mandibulofacial dysostosis.

Clinical Findings: In congenital underdevelopment of the lashes, the cilia are replaced by fine hairs and there is general atrophy of the skin. Complete absence of the lashes is usually accompanied by the absence of eyebrows and scalp hair. The nails and sweat glands are usually normal.

Complications
I **Derived:** —
II **Associated:** Atrophy of skin, alopecia, cataract, ectodermal dysplasia, faulty dentition

Etiology: ? A few families have displayed autosomal dominant inheritance.

Pathogenesis: ? The hair follicles are incomplete microscopically.

Related Facts
I **Sex Ratio:** ?
II **Risk of Occurrence:** Unknown, but rare
III **Risk of Recurrence for**
    Patient's Sib: When autosomal dominant, if parent is affected, 1 in 2 (50%) for each offspring to be affected; otherwise not increased.
    Patient's Child: When autosomal dominant, 1 in 2
IV **Age of Detectability:** At birth
V **Prevalence:** ? Very rare

Treatment
I **Primary Prevention:** —
II **Secondary Prevention:** —
III **Other Therapy:** —

Prognosis: Normal life span

Detection of Carrier: —

Special Considerations: —

References:
Duke-Elder, S.: System of Ophthalmology. vol. 3, pt. 2. Congenital Deformities. St. Louis: C.V. Mosby Co., 1963, p. 872.
Waardenburg, P.J. et al: Genetics and Ophthalmology. Oxford: Blackwell Scientific Publications, Ltd., 1961, vol. 1., p. 202.

Contributor: **Donald R. Bergsma**

Editor's Computerized Descriptors: Hair, Skin

MALATE DEHYDROGENASE, MITOCHONDRIAL (MARKER)

Includes: Malico-déhydrogénase mitochondriale
Lösliche Malatdehydrogenase
Malato deshidrogenasa mitocondrial (Marcador)
Mitochondrial malate dehydrogenase, genetic variant of

Excludes: Malate dehydrogenase, soluble (Marker) (625)

Minimal Diagnostic Criteria: Identification after starch-gel electrophoresis and specific enzymatic staining

Clinical Findings: No known physical, mental or other biochemical anomalies are known to be associated with individuals who are heterozygous for this enzyme variant. No homozygous individuals have been found.
    Starch-gel electrophoresis patterns of malate dehydrogenase from human tissue indicate a new genetic polymorphism for the mitochondrial form of the enzyme. Studies of families showed simple Mendelian segregation rather than maternal inheritance, suggesting that not all mitochondrial proteins are coded by mitochondrial DNA.

Complications
I **Derived:** —
II **Associated:** —

Etiology: Autosomal dominant transmission of biochemical variant; McK *15410

Pathogenesis: Inherited variant of a subunit of mitochondrial malate dehydrogenase leading to an alteration of electrophoretic mobility but no decrease in enzyme activity.

Related Facts
I **Sex Ratio:** M1:F1
II **Risk of Occurrence:** Approximately 1 in 100 live births, white
III **Risk of Recurrence for**
    Patient's Sib: If parent has the variant, 1 in 2 (50%) for each offspring to be affected
    Patient's Child: 1 in 2
IV **Age of Detectability:** At birth, using placental or leukocyte extract (mitochondrial enzymes cannot be detected in human erythrocytes).
V **Prevalence:** A genetic polymorphism: 1 in 100 of white individuals are heterozygotes.

Treatment
I **Primary Prevention:** Not needed
II **Secondary Prevention:** None needed
III **Other Therapy:** —

Prognosis: Normal life span

Detection of Carrier: Starch-gel electrophoresis

Special Considerations: —

References:
Davidson, R.G. and Cortner, J.A.: Mitochondrial malate dehydrogenase: A new genetic polymorphism in man. Science 157:1569, 1967

Contributors: **Jean A. Cortner**
R. G. Davidson

Editor's Computerized Descriptor: —

MALATE DEHYDROGENASE, SOLUBLE (MARKER)

Includes: Malico-déshydrogénase soluble
Lösliche Malatdehydrogenase
Malato deshidrogenasa soluble (Marcador)
Genetic variant of soluble malate dehydrogenase
Erythrocyte malate dehydrogenase supernatant

Excludes: Malate dehydrogenase, mitochondrial (Marker) (624)

Minimal Diagnostic Criteria: Identification after starch-gel electrophoresis and specific enzymatic staining

Clinical Findings: No known physical, mental or other biochemical anomalies are known to be associated with individuals who are heterozygous for this enzyme variant. No homozygous individuals have been found.†

Complications
I   **Derived:** —
II   **Associated:** —

Etiology: Autosomal dominant transmission of biochemical variant. Soluble-MDH also polymorphic in mice. McK *15420

Pathogenesis: Inherited variant of a subunit of soluble malate dehydrogenase leading to an alteration of electrophoretic mobility but no decrease in enzyme activity.

Related Facts
I   **Sex Ratio:** ? Only one family, M2:F1 among 3 affected persons
II   **Risk of Occurrence:** Extremely rare
III   **Risk of Recurrence for**
    Patient's Sib: If parent has variant, 1 in 2 (50%) for each offspring to have the variant.
    Patient's Child: 1 in 2
IV   **Age of Detectability:** At birth using placenta or cord blood
V   **Prevalence:** ? Found only in one Negro female and her 2 sons.

Treatment
I   **Primary Prevention:** None indicated
II   **Secondary Prevention:** None indicated
III   **Other Therapy:** —

Prognosis: Normal life span

Detection of Carrier: Starch-gel electrophoresis

†Special Considerations: An example of an extremely rare genetic variant with no apparent clinical significance

References:
Davidson, R. G. and Cortner, J. A.: Genetic variant of human erythrocyte malate dehydrogenase. Nature 215:761, 1967.

Contributors: **Jean A. Cortner**
R. G. Davidson

Editor's Computerized Descriptor: —

MANDIBULAR PROGNATHISM

Includes: Prognathisme
Progenie
Prognatismo mandibular
Class III skeletal malocclusion
Progenia
Hapsburg jaw

Excludes: Pseudoprognathism (functional prognathism resulting from dental interferences in centric relation or from habit)
Prognathism as a component of various syndromes

Minimal Diagnostic Criteria: Excessive anterior mandibular growth, insufficient anterior maxillary growth, or a combination of both

Clinical Findings: Excessive anterior mandibular growth, insufficient anterior maxillary growth, or a combination of both; protruding chin and lower lip; increased gonial angle; anterior and posterior crossbite; premature eruption of mandibular molar teeth in some cases.

Complications
I   **Derived:** —
II   **Associated:** —

Etiology: Polygenic inheritance; probably etiologically heterogeneous; an autosomal dominant type seems likely.† McK *17670

Pathogenesis: Defect produces imbalance in mandibular and maxillary growth.

Related Facts
I   **Sex Ratio:** M1:F1
II   **Risk of Occurrence:** 1% in Caucasian population
III   **Risk of Recurrence for**
    Patient's Sib: Approximately 10% risk assuming that prognathism occurs with a frequency of 1% in the general population
    Patient's Child: Approximately 10% risk assuming that prognathism occurs with a frequency of 1% in the general population
IV   **Age of Detectability:** The condition is rarely evident at birth, but becomes apparent with growth and development. In some cases, the condition is progressive.
V   **Prevalence:** A composite frequency of approximately 1% has been estimated for white populations. Reported frequencies have ranged from 0.48 to 4%. Frequencies of 3-5% have been reported in black populations. A frequency of 6% has been reported in a Japanese population. Variability of reported frequencies depends, in part, upon a) the use of different criteria by various investigators and b) the use of different age groups by different investigators.

Treatment
I   **Primary Prevention:** —
II   **Secondary Prevention:** Surgical correction and orthodontic treatment in patients who are dissatisfied with their physical appearance.
III   **Other Therapy:** —

Prognosis: Excellent, life span is not reduced.

Detection of Carrier: Carrier may be unaffected or mildly to severely affected.

†Special Considerations: Although the data of Litton et al are compatible with polygenic inheritance, the possibility of other modes of transmission in different families or in different populations has not been ruled out. Thus mandibular prognathism may be etiologically and genetically heterogeneous. It follows an autosomal dominant mode of inheritance in some families. Sometimes a distinction is made between absolute mandibular prognathism and relative mandibular prognathism (maxillary hypoplasia). Schulze noted that maxillary hypoplasia may occur even with so-called absolute prognathism in some cases. Horowitz and Converse found that mandibular length was not significantly increased in cases of mandibular prognathism, suggesting that a distinction between absolute and relative mandibular prognathism may be somewhat artificial. However, absolute mandibular prognathism occurs in some cases.

References:
Horowitz, S.L. et al: Craniofacial relationships in mandibular prognathism. Arch. Oral Biol. 14:121, 1969.
Litton, S.F. et al: A genetic study of class III malocclusion. Am. J. Orthod. 58:565, 1970.
Schulze, C.: Developmental abnormalities of the teeth and jaws. In Gorlin, R.J. and Goldman, H.M. (eds.): Thoma's Oral Pathology, 6th Ed. St. Louis: C.V. Mosby, 1970, vol. 1.

Contributor: **M. Michael Cohen, Jr.**

Editor's Computerized Descriptors: Face, Teeth, Skel.

MANDIBULOFACIAL DYSOSTOSIS

Includes: Dysostose mandibulofaciale
Dysostosis mandibulofacialis
Disostosis mandibulofacial
Treacher Collins syndrome†

Excludes: Hemifacial microsomia (457)
Oculo-auriculo-vertebral dysplasia (735)
Nager acrofacial dysostosis
Wildervanck-Smith syndrome
Achard syndrome

Minimal Diagnostic Criteria: Anomalies are not obligatory but facultative. See *Very frequent findings* below.

Clinical Findings: *Very frequent findings:* Downward obliquity of palpebral fissures, lower eyelid coloboma, hypoplastic or aplastic zygomatic arches, defect of orbital rim, hypoplastic supraorbital ridges, dysplastic ears, micrognathia and concave lower mandibular border and malocclusion.
Common findings: Defect of auditory canal, defects of auditory ossicles, conductive hearing loss, madarosis medial to coloboma, flattening of nasofrontal angle, high-arched or cleft palate, sclerotic, nonpneumatized mastoids and small paranasal sinuses.
Occasional findings: Auricular tags and fistulas, tongue-shaped extension of hair onto cheek, macrostomia or microstomia, choanal atresia, minor skeletal anomalies, cardiac anomalies, microphthalmia, iris and choroid coloboma, mental deficiency and absent parotid gland.

Complications
I **Derived:** Mental deficiency may be secondarily induced by conductive hearing loss in some cases.
II **Associated:** See *Occasional findings* under Clinical Findings.

Etiology: Autosomal dominant with high penetrance and variable expressivity. More than half the cases arise as fresh mutations.

Pathogenesis: Genetic defect leads to multiple congenital anomalies

Related Facts
I **Sex Ratio:** M1:F1
II **Risk of Occurrence:** ? Low
III **Risk of Recurrence for**
Patient's Sib: If parent is affected 1 in 2 (50%) for each offspring to be affected; otherwise not increased. If isolated case, risk is negligible.
Patient's Child: 1 in 2
IV **Age of Detectability:** At birth, by physical examination
V **Prevalence:** ? Uncommon

Treatment
I **Primary Prevention:** Genetic counseling
II **Secondary Prevention:** Early recognition of conductive hearing loss is important to prevent possible secondarily induced mental deficiency by the use of hearing aids or surgical intervention. Surgical repair of ear anomalies and cleft. Orthognathic surgical procedures can be employed to reconstruct zygomatic arches and supraorbital rims, as well as to correct mandibular deformity with micrognathia, open bite, and concave lower mandibular border.
III **Other Therapy:** Orthodontic treatment and speech therapy may be necessary in some cases.

Prognosis: Life span is not affected, except when severe cardiac defect is present.

Detection of Carrier: —

†**Special Considerations:** Mandibulofacial dysostosis per se is etiologically heterogeneous being observed in the autosomal

recessive Nager acrofacial dysostosis syndrome and also in the Wildervanck-Smith syndrome. A recent report suggests etiologic heterogeneity for the Nager syndrome with both dominant and recessive forms. Thus, the term Treacher Collins syndrome is more specific for the condition under discussion.

References:
Franceschetti, A. and Klein, D.: Mandibulo-facial dysostosis, new hereditary syndrome. Acta Ophthalmol. 27:143, 1949.
Gorlin, R.J. et al: Syndromes of the Head and Neck, 2nd Ed. New York: McGraw-Hill, 1976.

Contributor: **M. Michael Cohen, Jr.**

Editor's Computerized Descriptors: Eye, Hearing, Ear, Face, Oral, Teeth, Nasoph., Nose, Hair, Skel.

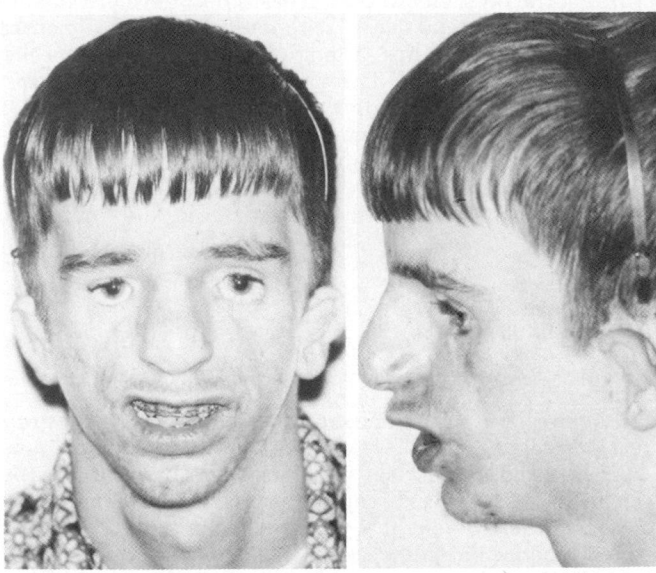

332. Note microtia, downward slant of palpebral fissures, and maxillary hypoplasia

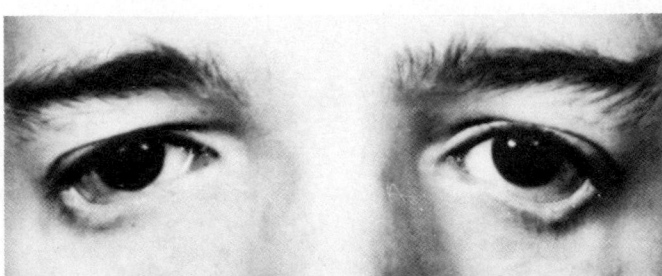

333. Note downward slant of plapebral fissures and coloboma of lower lid

MAPLE SYRUP URINE DISEASE

Includes: Maladie des urines à odeur de sirop d'érable
Ahornsirupkrankheit
Enfermedad urinaria a jarabe de arce
Branched-chain ketoaciduria
Branched-chain ketonuria
Intermittent branched-chain ketonuria

Excludes: Hypervalinemia (509)

Minimal Diagnostic Criteria: Elevation of the branched-chain amino acids or keto acids in the blood and increased excretion in the urine. The specific diagnosis is made by demonstrating the enzyme defect in the leukocytes or skin fibroblasts grown in tissue culture.

Clinical Findings: Early onset of symptoms occurs in most instances before the end of the 1st week of life with feeding difficulty, vomiting, shrill cry, and a characteristic odor of urine and other secretions. Neurologic signs - loss of tendon reflexes and Moro, alternating hypotonicity may be followed by convulsions, coma, respiratory difficulties and death. In the untreated child that survives, severe mental and neurologic damage are found.

Biochemical features include elevation of plasma concentrations of the branched-chain amino acids, leucine, isoleucine and valine to 5-40 times normal, and increased urinary excretion of these amino acids; elevation of plasma concentrations and increased urinary excretion of the keto acid derivatives of the branched chain amino acids. In white blood cells the activity of branched-chain keto acid decarboxylase is absent. Alloisoleucine is present in plasma.†

Complications
I   **Derived:** Severe neurologic manifestations, mental deficiency, and early death
II **Associated:** —

Etiology: Autosomal recessive; McK *24860

Pathogenesis: Inactivity of decarboxylase of the branched-chain keto acids. It is not yet known whether one or three enzymes are involved. Sequence which produces clinical findings is unknown.

Related Facts
I   **Sex Ratio:** M1:F1
II **Risk of Occurrence:** Reported variously as 1:125,000 to 1:300,000 live births
III **Risk of Recurrence for**
    Patient's Sib: Probably 1 in 4 (25%) for each offspring to be affected
    Patient's Child: Not increased, unless mate is carrier or homozygote
IV **Age of Detectability:** Before birth by enzymatic analysis following amniocentesis, or immediately after birth by enzyme assay of leukocytes. The branched-chain amino acids may be elevated in the blood within 48 hours of birth.
V   **Prevalence:** Described in many ethnic groups and in many geographic locations and racial backgrounds.

Treatment
I   **Primary Prevention:** Genetic counseling; antepartum diagnosis
II **Secondary Prevention:** Dietary therapy with control of intake of branched-chain amino acids to provide accurately the requirements of patient. Dietary therapy can be lifesaving; it must be instituted early in life and must be carefully monitored. Prevention of neurologic and mental damage seems possible, but experience is still limited.
III **Other Therapy:** Exchange transfusion or dialysis to treat acute toxic state.

Prognosis: Very poor if untreated. Death occurs almost invariably before the end of the 2nd year. With careful dietary control, normal growth and development are possible.

Detection of Carrier: By enzyme assay of the peripheral leukocyte, it is possible to distinguish a group of carriers from a group of controls with statistical accuracy. This has not been sufficiently accurate for genetic counseling of a specific individual.

†Special Considerations: Many variants have been described presenting a spectrum of severity of manifestations which generally correlates with the level of enzyme activity. The most severe is the classic disease as described above, with early onset of symptoms requiring prompt dietary treatment, including purified amino acids. Some infants have a later onset of less severe symptoms, which may be controlled by simply limiting protein intake. In a milder variety, patients may tolerate a normal diet but suffer from intermittent attacks of branched-chain aminoacidemia and ketoaciduria, associated with neurologic symptoms. It is suspected that several mutant forms of the enzyme are responsible for the varied clinical pictures. One patient has been reported who responded to pharmacologic doses of thiamine.

References:

Dancis, J. and Levitz, M.: Abnormalities of branched-chain amino acid metabolism (hypervalinemia, branched-chain ketonuria maple syrup urine disease, isovaleric acidemia). In Stanbury, J.B. et al (eds.): The Metabolic Basis of Inherited Disease, 3rd Ed. New York:McGraw-Hill, 1966, p. 426.

Dancis, J. et al: Enzyme activity in classical and variant forms of maple syrup urine disease. J. Pediatr. 81:312, 1972.

Scriver, C.R. et al: Thiamine-responsive maple syrup urine disease. Lancet 1:310, 1971.

Snyderman, S.E. et al: Maple syrup urine disease with particular reference to dietotherapy. Pediatrics 34:454, 1964.

Contributors: **Selma Snyderman**
Joseph Dancis

Editor's Computerized Descriptors: Speech, Muscle, Resp., GI., Nerve

MARDEN-WALKER SYNDROME

Includes: Syndrome de Marden-Walker
Síndrome de Marden-Walker

Excludes: Chondrodystrophic myotonia (155)

Minimal Diagnostic Criteria: Too few cases known.

Clinical Findings: Three additional children have been described who probably have the same syndrome as the newborn described by Marden and Walker. One was 6 months old; 2 were 2 years old. All 4 children had psychomotor retardation, blepharophimosis, hypertelorism, micrognathia, fixed facial expression, low-set ears, decreased muscle mass of the limbs and congenital contractures of the hips, elbows and knees. The 2 newborn infants had almost identical facies. Both had small pursed mouths with everted lower lips, a long philtrum, sagging cheeks, and upturned nose tips. Three of the children had kyphosis, 3 had no deep tendon reflexes, 2 had pectus excavatum, 1 had pectus carinatum. One had cleft palate, 3 had a high-arched palate. Features found only once include arachnodactyly, deeply set eyes, preauricular tag, dolichocephaly, hirsutism, low hairline, dextrocardia and epicanthic folds.

Complications
I   **Derived:** —
II **Associated:** —

Etiology: Probably autosomal recessive;† McK *24870

Pathogenesis: A pneumoencephalogram of 1 patient was performed at 9 months. It revealed a normal subarachnoid space around the cervical spinal cord, an enlarged cisterna magna, medullary cistern, 4th ventricle and suprapineal recess of the 3rd ventricle. This indicated a reduced size of the cerebellum and brainstem. Electromyography showed myopathic changes. A quadriceps muscle biopsy revealed that many muscle fibers of both Types I and II were reduced in diameter. The abnormal neuromuscular system probably accounts for the immobile face, everted lips, sagging cheeks, strabismus, blepharophimosis, joint contractures and kyphoscoliosis.

Related Facts
I   **Sex Ratio:** M3:F1
II **Risk of Occurrence:** Rare
III **Risk of Recurrence for**
    Patient's Sib: 1 in 4 (25%) for each offspring to be affected, if autosomal recessive.
    Patient's Child: Not increased unless mate is carrier or homozygote.
IV **Age of Detectability:** At birth by clinical examination
V   **Prevalence:** Rare

Treatment
I   **Primary Prevention:** Genetic counseling
II **Secondary Prevention:** —
III **Other Therapy:** Supportive

Prognosis: One child died of pneumonia at 3 weeks. Three others have severe psychomotor retardation.

Detection of Carrier: ?

†Special Considerations: The evidence for autosomal recessive inheritance is the report that 2 of the patients were cousins and each was the offspring of a consanguineous marriage. (Temtamy).

Roentgenograms of the infant described by Marden and Walker revealed a truncated chest configuration with an increased anteroposterior diameter but a normal cardiac silhouette. The heart progressively increased in size in the 2nd and 3rd months. Skull films revealed a small frontal region, a prominent parietal area and normal ossification. The metacarpals, phalanges and metatarsals were long and bilateral talipes equinovarus was present. The vertebrae in the lower thoracic and lumbar areas were tall and narrow. An IVP showed mild dilation of the collection system. An EEG was mildly abnormal with depression of voltage in the left posterior cerebrum.

At autopsy no entrance was found for the inferior vena cava which presumably had a common entrance with the superior vena cava. The musculature just inferior to the pulmonary valve was slightly hypertrophic. Gross examination of the brain revealed no abnormality. Microscopic examination of the kidneys revealed a diffuse dilation of the large collecting tubules and hydropic degeneration of the proximal and distal tubules (microcystic disease of the kidneys). Skeletal muscle appeared atrophic without infiltrate or degeneration.

Two older children have been described with what may be this syndrome, but at the present time, it is difficult to know whether or not this represents the same entity (Passarge, 1975, Younessian, 1964).

This syndrome should be distinguished from Chondrodystrophic Myotonia, the principal manifestations of which are shortness of stature, myotonia, congenital hip dysplasia and blepharophimosis or blepharospasm.

References:
Fitch, N. et al: Congenital blepharophimosis, joint contractures, and muscular hypotonia. Neurology 21:1214, 1971.
Marden, P.M. and Walker, W.A.: A new generalized connective tissue syndrome. Am. J. Dis. Child. 112:225, 1966.
Passarge, E.: Marden-Walker syndrome. Case report. In Bergsma, D. (ed.): Malformation Syndromes. Birth Defects: Orig. Art. Ser., vol. XI, no. 2. Amsterdam: Excerpta Medica for The National Foundation-March of Dimes, 1975, p. 470.
Temtamy, S.A. et al: Probable Marden-Walker syndrome: Evidence for autosomal recessive inheritance. In Malformation Syndromes, op. cit. p. 104.
Younessian, S. and Ammann, F.: Deux cas de malformations cranio-faciales: 1. Mecrophthalmie ("nani me oculo-palpebral") avec dysostose craniofaciale et status dysraphique; 2. Dysmorphie mandibulo-oculo-faciale (syndrome d'Hallermann-Streiff). Opthalmoloqica 147:108, 1964.

Contributors: **Philip M. Marden**
Naomi Fitch

Editor's Computerized Descriptors: Eye, Ear, Face, Oral, Nose, Hair, Skel., Muscle, CV., GU., Nerve

MARFAN SYNDROME

Includes: Syndrome de Marfan
Síndrome de Marfan
Arachnodactyly

Excludes: Homocystinuria (474)
Arachnodactyly, contractural (85)

Minimal Diagnostic Criteria: Arachnodactyly with ectopia lentis and no urinary homocystine. Other findings alone may be highly suggestive, if there is an established family history. No specific laboratory test is available.

Clinical Findings: Skeletal features include dolichostenomelia, kyphoscoliosis, loose joints including genu recurvatum and flat feet, pectus excavatum or carinatum, dolichocephaly, high-arched palate, and long narrow face. Eye features include bilateral ectopia lentis (in about 75% of cases) usually with upward displacement of the lens and associated iridodonesis. The lens is small and spherical. High myopia and spontaneous retinal detachment are frequent. Cardiovascular findings include dilatation of the ascending aorta with aortic regurgitation, dissecting aneurysm of the aorta, mitral regurgitation and calcification of the mitral annulus. Other findings are reduced subcutaneous tissue, muscle hypoplasia, inguinal hernia and lung cysts.

Complications
I   **Derived:** Loss of vision, heart failure, aortic rupture, and compromised respiration
II **Associated:** —

Etiology: Autosomal dominant transmission, rarely with incomplete penetrance but with considerable variation in expression; McK *15470

Pathogenesis: The early changes of the aorta are those of cystic medial necrosis with degeneration of elastic fibers and cystic areas filled with metachromatically staining material. Heart valves may show myxomatous degeneration. Metachromasia of cultured fibroblasts has been found.

Related Facts
I   **Sex Ratio:** M1:F1
II **Risk of Occurrence:** Uncommon
III **Risk of Recurrence for**
    Patient's Sib: If parent is affected, 1 in 2 (50%) for each offspring to be affected; otherwise not increased
    Patient's Child: 1 in 2
IV **Age of Detectability:** May be apparent clinically in infancy but often not until the 2nd decade.
V   **Prevalence:** 1 in 66,000 in most populations

Treatment
I   **Primary Prevention:** Genetic counseling
II **Secondary Prevention:** Prevention of aortic rupture with propranolol therapy in cases with aortic dilatation is under study. In females, early induction of puberty with estrogens can avert embarrassingly excessive height and perhaps severe scoliosis.
III **Other Therapy:** Surgery for severe pectus excavatum or kyphoscoliosis may be indicated after puberty. Experience with surgery for aortic and valvar abnormalities is accumulating.

Prognosis: Death from dissection of the aorta has occurred as early as age 4 3/4 years; another patient was killed in an accident at age 82. In one series the average age at death was 43 in males and 46 in females.

Detection of Carrier: Not applicable

Special Considerations: —

References:
Halpern, B. L. et al: A prospectus on the prevention of aortic rupture in the Marfan syndrome with data on survivorship without treatment. Johns Hopk. Med. J. 129:123, 1971.
McKusick, V. A.: Heritable Disorders of Connective Tissue. 4th Ed. St. Louis:C.V. Mosby Co., 1972.
Matalon, R. and Dorfman, A.: The accumulation of hyaluronic acid in cultured fibroblasts of the Marfan syndrome. Biochem. Biophys. Res. Commun. 32:150, 1968.
Robins, P.R. et al: Scoliosis in Marfan's syndrome, its characteristics and results of treatment in thirty-five patients. J. Bone Joint. Surg. 57:358, 1975.
Symbas, P.N. et al: Marfan's syndrome with aneurysm of ascending aorta and aortic regurgitation, surgical treatment and new histochemical observations. Am. J. Cardiol. 25:483, 1970.

Contributor: **Robert A. Norum**

Editor's Computerized Descriptors: Vision, Eye, Face, Oral, Skin, Skel., Muscle, Hernia not CNS, Resp., CV.
Also see Section I, Fig. 62

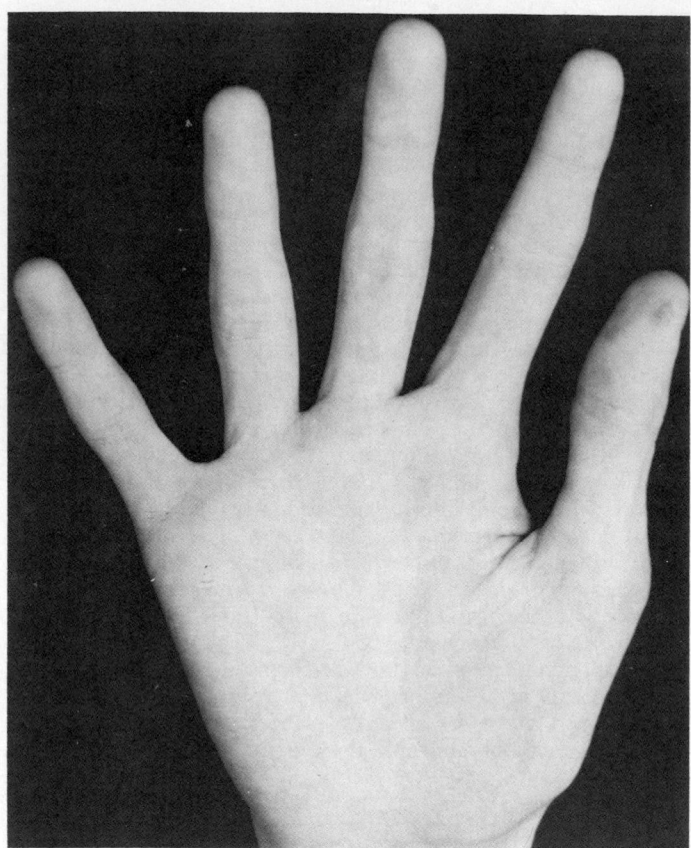

335. Note arachnodactyly

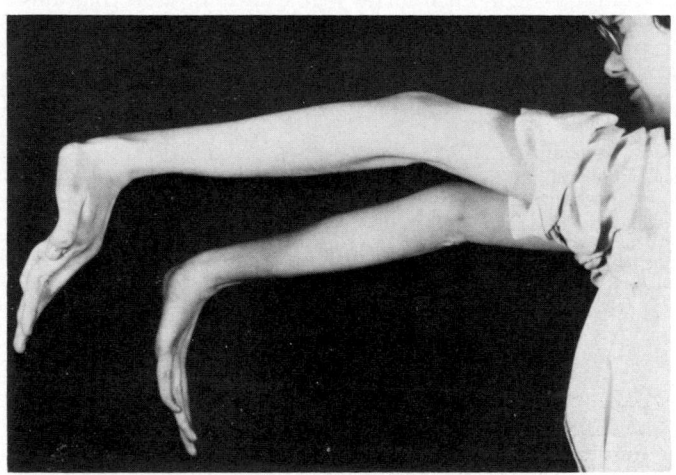

334. Note joint hyperextensibility

MAXILLA, MEDIAN ALVEOLAR CLEFT

Includes: Fente alvéolaire médiane du maxillaire supérieur
Mediane Overkieferspalte
Fisura alveolar mediana del maxilar
Cleft, maxillary median alveolar

Excludes: Lip, median cleft of upper (595)
Failure of formation of premaxillary portion of maxillary bone

Minimal Diagnostic Criteria: Radiographic evidence of a cleft of a minimum of 2 mm. This must be differentiated from the un-closed suture between the centers of the calcification of the pre-maxilla. The maxillary incisors must be or must have been present.†

Clinical Findings: Radiographic evidence of a cleft in the midline of premaxillary portion of the maxilla. There may or may not be a diastema between the central incisors present. There may or may not be a divergence of the roots of the central incisors.

Complications
I Derived: —
II Associated: —

Etiology: ? Postulated by Stout and Collett to be entrapment of epithelial rests that prevents fusion of the center of calcification of the premaxilla. Gier and Fast suggested the possibility of the influence of teratogenic agents, genetic factors or mechanical factors.

Pathogenesis: Failure of fusion of the primary ossification centers of the premaxilla during early embryonic development

Related Facts
I   Sex Ratio: ? Original report: 5 females
II Risk of Occurrence: ?
III Risk of Recurrence for
    Patient's Sib: ?
    Patient's Child: ?
IV Age of Detectability: ? Earliest reported case detected at 7 years. This case found in routine radiographic examination.
V   Prevalence: ? Rare

Treatment
I   Primary Prevention: —
II Secondary Prevention: None indicated. Orthodontic movement not recommended.†
III Other Therapy: —

Prognosis: Normal life span and function

Detection of Carrier: —

†Special Considerations: This condition can now be diagnosed only when all 4 maxillary incisors are present, indicating that there has been at least primary formation of premaxillary portion for the maxilla. Any attempts of orthodontic movement of these teeth would result in loss of the teeth because of lack of bone support.

References:
Gier, R.E. and Fast, T.B.: Median maxillary anterior alveolar cleft: Case reports and discussion. Oral Surg. 24:496, 1967.
Miller, A.S. et al: Median maxillary anterior cleft: Report of three cases. J. Am. Dent. Assoc. 79:896-7, 1969.
Stout, F.W. and Collett, W.K.: Etiology and incidence of median maxillary anterior alveolar cleft. Oral Surg. 28:66, 1969.

Contributor: Ronald E. Gier

Editor's Computerized Descriptors: Teeth Skel.

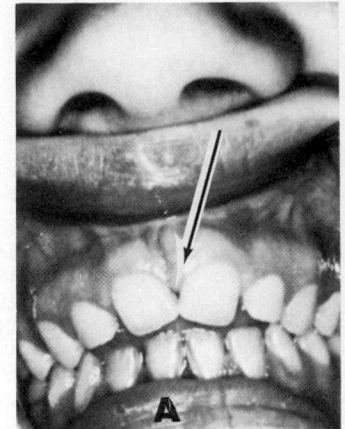
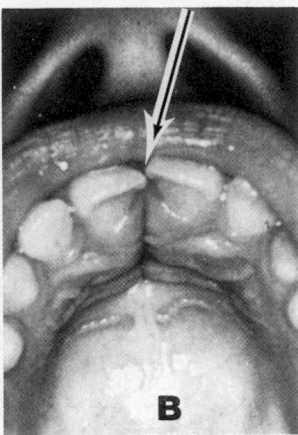

336. A) Median alveolar cleft; B) intraoral view

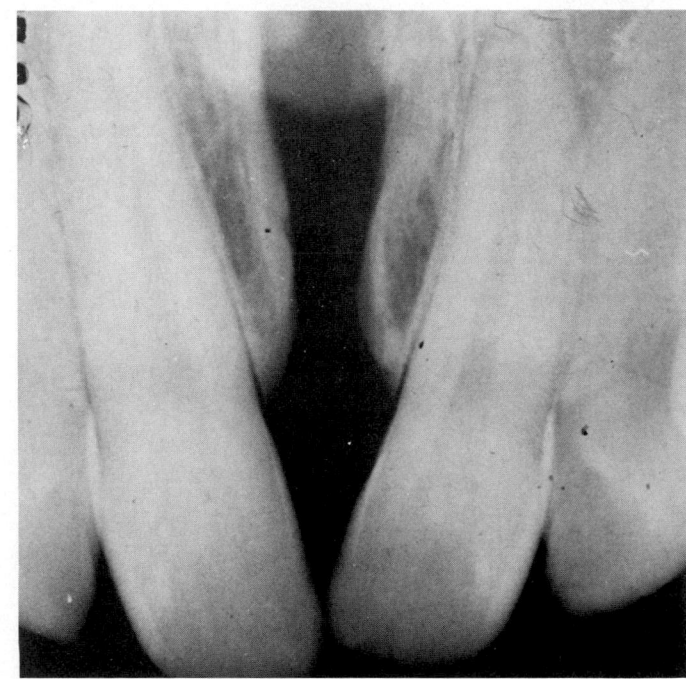

337. Periapical radiograph of maxillary median alveolar cleft

MCDONOUGH SYNDROME

Editor's Computerized Descriptors: Eye, Ear, Face, Teeth, Nerve, Hair, Skel., Muscle, CV., GU.

Includes: Syndrome de McDonough
Síndrome de McDonough

Excludes: Noonan syndrome (720)
Turner syndrome (977)

Minimal Diagnostic Criteria: Mental retardation, short stature, sternovertebral deformities, congenital heart defect, and characteristic facial features.

Clinical Findings: The McDonough syndrome was observed in 3 sibs, 2 boys and 1 girl, of nonconsanguineous parents. The affected children were mentally retarded with IQ scores of 50-70, verbal scores being lower than performance scores. They had a strikingly unusual facies, congenital heart defects (septal defects, stenosis of aorta and pulmonary artery), sternal deformity, diastasis recti, kyphosis, and short stature. Craniofacial anomalies included anteverted auricles, small upward slanted palpebral fissures, synophrys and strabismus. Cryptorchidism was present in both boys. †

Complications
I **Derived:** Heart failure, scoliosis
II **Associated:** —

Etiology: Autosomal recessive

Pathogenesis: ?

Related Facts
I **Sex Ratio:** M1:F1
II **Risk of Occurrence:** ?
III **Risk of Recurrence for**
  Patient's Sib: 1 in 4 (25%) for each offspring to be affected
  Patient's Child: Not increased unless mate is carrier or homozygote
IV **Age of Detectability:** Infancy or early childhood
V **Prevalence:** ? Obviously rare

Treatment
I **Primary Prevention:** Genetic counseling
II **Secondary Prevention:** Cardiac surgery, orthopedic measures
III **Other Therapy:** Special education

Prognosis: Influenced by heart defect.

Detection of Carrier: ? Minor manifestations of the syndrome may be present in heterozygotes.

†**Special Considerations:** The delineation of the phenotypic spectrum requires further observations. In the family described, a possible variant familial developmental pattern may be postulated as the explanation for similar features in 3 affected and 2 unaffected sibs and in the parents: Abnormal occipital hairline, maxillary prognathism and malocclusion of teeth, simian crease and distally located axial triradius. It seems possible, however, that some of these features are minor manifestations of the syndrome in heterozygotes. A coincidental finding was the ascertainment of Klinefelter syndrome (XXY constitution) in 1 of the brothers with the McDonough syndrome; the father was shown to be a mosaic for an XY and an XXY cell line.

References:
Neuhäuser, G. and Opitz, J.M.: Studies of malformation syndromes in man XXXX: Multiple congenital anomalies/mental retardation syndrome or variant familial developmental pattern: Differential diagnosis and description of the McDonough syndrome (with XXY son from XY/XXY father). Z. Kinderheilkd. 120:231, 1975.

Contributor: **Gerhard Neuhäuser**

MECKEL DIVERTICULUM

Includes: Diverticule de Meckel
Meckelsches Divertikel
Divertículo de Meckel
Vitelline duct, remnant
Omphalomesenteric duct

Excludes: Intestinal duplication (532)

Minimal Diagnostic Criteria: Positive diagnosis can only be made by the gross anatomic findings found at operation or autopsy. The diverticulum can vary in size, but arises from the antimesenteric border of the ileum, usually within 100 cm of the ileocecal valve. Ectopic gastric or pancreatic tissue is present in approximately two-thirds of the diverticula.

Clinical Findings: Asymptomatic, except if a complication occurs. The presenting symptoms are related to the complications and include, in order of frequency, hemorrhage, intestinal obstruction, inflammation (simulating appendicitis), perforation and peritonitis, and umbilical discharge. Very rarely can the diverticulum be demonstrated by roentgenologic examination. A new test has been proposed for the detection of the diverticulum, namely a 99 m technetium-pertechnetate scan of the abdomen, and has been found useful in demonstrating ectopic gastric mucosa, which is present in 64% of complicated Meckel diverticula.

Complications
I   **Derived:** Hemorrhage (40%), obstruction (25%), inflammation (23%), perforation (5%) or umbilical discharge (7%)
II **Associated:** —

Etiology: ?

Pathogenesis: Meckel diverticulum, or its variants, develops as a gross structural defect of the yolk stalk which is a normal structure in the 5-9 mm embryo. At this state, the yolk stalk constricts and separates from the intestine. A persistence of the yolk stalk appears in several forms. The stalk may remain patent and continuous, producing an umbilical-intestinal fistula. It may be patent at the outer end, producing a sinus. A cyst will form if the central portion is patent. Most commonly, a blind pouch occurs on the ileum, hanging free in the abdominal cavity or sometimes attached to the umbilicus by a fibrous cord.

Related Facts
I   **Sex Ratio:** M1:F1
II   **Risk of Occurrence:** 1 in 60
III **Risk of Recurrence for**
     Patient's Sib: ?
     Patient's Child: ?
IV   **Age of Detectability:** Detected only by complications, which occur more commonly before the age of 2 years (60%), but can occur at any age.
V   **Prevalence:** 1 in < 60

Treatment
I   **Primary Prevention:** —
II   **Secondary Prevention:** Excision of diverticulum. If obstruction exists, it may be necessary to resect a segment of necrotic ileum with the diverticulum and do an ileo-ileostomy. A patent or obliterated remnant of the omphalomesenteric duct should also be excised. An incidental removal of a Meckel diverticulum at time of laparotomy may be done to prevent the subsequent complications of the diverticulum if good surgical judgment permits it.
III **Other Therapy:** —

Prognosis: Excellent with recovery from surgical treatment. Most deaths occur from a delayed recognition of a perforation and obstruction in infants.

Detection of Carrier: —

Special Considerations: —

References:
Bremer, J.L.: Congenital Anomalies of the Viscera. Boston:Harvard University Press, 1957, p. 51.
Kiesewetter, W.B.: Meckel's diverticulum in children. Arch. Surg. 75:914, 1957.
Mustard, W.T. et al (eds.): Pediatric Surgery. Chicago:Year Book Medical Publ., 1969, p. 864.
Wine, C. et al: Role of the technetium scan in the diagnosis of Meckel's diverticulum. J. Pediatr. Surg. 60:885, 1974.

Contributor: **Paul W. Johnston**

Editor's Computerized Descriptor: GI.

MECKEL SYNDROME

Includes: Syndrome de Meckel
Síndrome de Meckel
Gruber syndrome
Dysencephalia splanchnocystica

Excludes: Chromosome thirteen trisomy syndrome (168)

Minimal Diagnostic Criteria: Microcephaly (with posterior exencephalocele), cleft palate, polydactyly, polycystic kidneys, external genital ambiguity in males.

Clinical Findings: Microcephaly with or without posterior exencephalocele and sloping forehead; capillary hemangiomata of forehead, occasional hypertelorism, rarely hypotelorism. Anencephaly has been seen at least twice. Eyes frequently malformed: microphthalmia, (rarely anophthalmia), colobomata, cataracts; upper eyelid may protrude over lower like eave of a roof. Rarely cleft lip or formation of a single nostril. Cleft palate is common; natal teeth have been observed. Tongue at times shows clefts and papillomatous processes (as in the orofaciodigital syndrome I), and at times heavy buccal frenula are present (as in the Ellis-van Creveld syndrome). The epiglottis may be cleft or hypoplastic. Micrognathia, minor ear anomalies are very common. Brain: frequent absence of olfactory lobes, dorsal or posterior exencephaloceles usually with some dilatation of ventricles, microencephaly, various types of associated cerebral and cerebellar dysgeneses. Premature craniosynostosis (secondary) and occipital cribriform plates (incipient cranial rachischisis) have been observed.

Heart may be normal or show one or more congenital malformations; at times complex cardiac defects are present. The liver usually is fibrotic and contains some cysts, rarely a great number of large cysts.

If renal dysgenesis is severe, the pulmonary manifestations (hypoplasia, atelectasis) of the "Potter syndrome" may be present.

Renal dysplasia, usually smaller than normal kidneys, reduced amount of renal parenchyma with numerous small cysts (Type III of Potter). Rarely renal aplasia, more commonly severe polycystic involvement which may at times produce huge polycystic kidneys that can be a birth impediment. Ureter is usually patent, proximal portions may be hypoplastic. Bladder may be hypoplastic, portions of ureter may be atretic. Adrenals may be small, rarely absent. Gonads are usually small and dysplastic, in males usually undescended. External genital ambiguity occurs commonly in males with the Meckel syndrome; female internal genitalia may be seen in such male pseudohermaphrodites. Imperforate anus and single umbilical artery have been described. The urachus may be patent. Females may have a septate vagina.

Polydactyly is very common, usually postaxial hexadactyly of all 4 limbs. However, higher degrees of polydactyly occur. At times syndactyly of the 2nd and 3rd, less commonly the other toes. Simian creases, camptodactyly, clinodactyly of fingers or toes, various clubfoot deformities are very common.

Death is usually due to renal insufficiency, with or without added pulmonary and cardiac complications.

Complications

I Derived: Huge polycystic kidneys may be a birth impediment; any woman who has had a child with congenital polycystic kidneys and who presents again with an infant in a breech position (with or without polyhydramnios) should be considered for possible cesarean section.

II Associated: —

Etiology: Presumed to be due to homozygous state of a rare recessive mutant gene, parental consanguinity is seen at times.†
McK *24900

Pathogenesis: ?

Related Facts

I Sex Ratio: M1:F1
II Risk of Occurrence: ?
III Risk of Recurrence for
  Patient's Sib: 1 in 4 (25%) for each sib
  Patient's Child: Reproductive fitness zero
IV Age of Detectability: In certain cases prenatally - absence of amniotic fluid and of neutral α-glucosidase indicates absence of proper renal function. Sonography, possibly supplemented with hyopaque x-ray contrast studies, may detect encephalocele. Sonography with greatly increased α-fetoprotein levels may indicate anencephaly. In any case, the syndrome is diagnosable at birth, in atypical cases if a previous sib was typically affected.
V Prevalence: Holmes et al found that 5 out of 106 cases of anencephaly, meningomyelocele, meningocele and encephalocele ascertained prospectively and retrospectively in Boston had the Meckel syndrome (4.7%). Fried et al found that three-fourths of Jewish-Israeli sibships with the syndrome were of Yemenite origin.

Treatment

I Primary Prevention: Genetic counseling, prenatal diagnosis
II Secondary Prevention: —
III Other Therapy: Supportive measures till death

Prognosis: Invariably fatal in infancy

Detection of Carrier: —

†**Special Considerations:** Some of the cases described as examples of "the Ullrich-Feichtiger syndrome" (UFS) may actually be mildly affected Meckel syndrome patients. Some patients with UFS probably had the chromosome 13 trisomy syndrome, others the Smith-Lemli-Opitz (SLO) syndrome. Certain cases simulating chromosome 13 trisomy syndrome but without the trisomy - ie with 46, XX or 46, XY constitution - probably represent cases of the Meckel syndrome. Extremely severely affected cases of the SLO syndrome may present differential diagnostic difficulties. The differential diagnosis should also consider 2 of the short rib-polydactyly (SRB) syndromes, ie the SRP syndrome type Majewski and the SRP syndrome type Saldino-Noonan which have many manifestations in common with the Meckel syndrome. A careful review of the Spranger et al reference is strongly recommended before a definitive diagnosis is made.

References:
Fried, K. et al: Polycystic kidneys associated with malformations of the brain, polydactyly, and other birth defects in newborn sibs. J. Med. Genet. 8:285, 1971.
Holmes, L.B. et al: Etiologic heterogeneity of neural tube defects. N. Engl. J. Med. 294:365, 1976.
Hsia, Y.E. et al: Genetics of the Meckel syndrome (dysencephalia splanchnocystica). Pediatrics 48:237, 1971.
Meckel, S. and Passarge, E.: Encephalocele, polycystic kidneys and polydactyly as an autosomal recessive trait simulating certain other disorders: The Meckel syndrome. Ann. Genet. 14:97, 1971.
Opitz, J.M. and Howe, J.J.: The Meckel syndrome (dysencephalia splanchnocystica, the Gruber syndrome). In Bergsma, D. (ed.): Part II. Malformation Syndromes. Birth Defects: Orig. Art. Ser., vol. V. no. 2. White Plains: The National Foundation-March of Dimes, 1969, p. 167.
Spranger J. et al: Short rib-polydactyly (SRP) syndromes Types Majewski and Saldino-Noonan. Z. Kinderheilkd. 116:73-94, 1974.

MEDIAN CLEFT FACE SYNDROME

Includes: Frontonasale Dysplasie
Síndrome de fisura media del rostro
Frontonasal dysplasia

Excludes: Hypertelorism-hypospadias syndrome (505)
Nose, glioma (726)
Ablepharon (3)

Minimal Diagnostic Criteria: True ocular hypertelorism, with a broad nasal root, median nasal groove, or true ocular hypertelorism with a broad nasal root and notching of the ala nasi, absent nasal tip.

Clinical Findings: Patients consistently manifest true ocular hypertelorism. Anterior cranium bifidum occultum may be present and the anterior hairline may assume a widow's peak configuration which is a V-shaped extension of the hair onto the center of the forehead.

The severity of median clefting varies from absence of the nasal tip to separation of the nose into 2 parts. Sedano et al divided patients into 4 groups depending on the severity of median clefting: A) ocular hypertelorism, broad nasal root, median nasal groove with absence of the nasal tip. True midline clefting is not present. B) ocular hypertelorism, broad nasal root, deep median facial groove or true clefting involving the nose or the nose and upper lip. Palatal clefting may be also be present. C) ocular hypertelorism, broad nasal root, notching of one or both ala nasi. D) a combination of B & C.

Less common physical features include brachycephaly, microphthalmia, epibulbar dermoids, colobomas of the upper eyelid, congenital cataracts, preauricular skin tags, hypoplastic frontal sinuses, clinodactyly, camptodactyly, and cryptorchidism. Approximately 20% of these patients may be mentally retarded, usually to a mild degree.

Complications
I **Derived:** Psychologic problems due to the facial appearance.
II **Associated:** Encephalocele associated with cranium bifidum frontalis, agenesis of the corpus callosum, meningocele or meningoencephalocele.

Etiology: Majority of cases are sporadic.

Pathogenesis: Abnormal embryologic development of the nose or face due to unknown cause(s). Possibly related to failure of normal anterior extension of ectomesenchyme from neural crest over frontonasal process.

Related Facts
I **Sex Ratio:** M1:F1 probably
II **Risk of Occurrence:** ?
III **Risk of Recurrence for**
   Patient's Sib: Probably nil
   Patient's Child: Probably nil
IV **Age of Detectability:** At birth
V **Prevalence:** ?

Treatment
I **Primary Prevention:** ?
II **Secondary Prevention:** Major maxillofacial, plastic and ophthalmologic surgery when indicated
III **Other Therapy:** Psychiatric help may be indicated. Special education may be required.

Prognosis: Longevity should not be compromised.

Detection of Carrier: —

Special Considerations: —

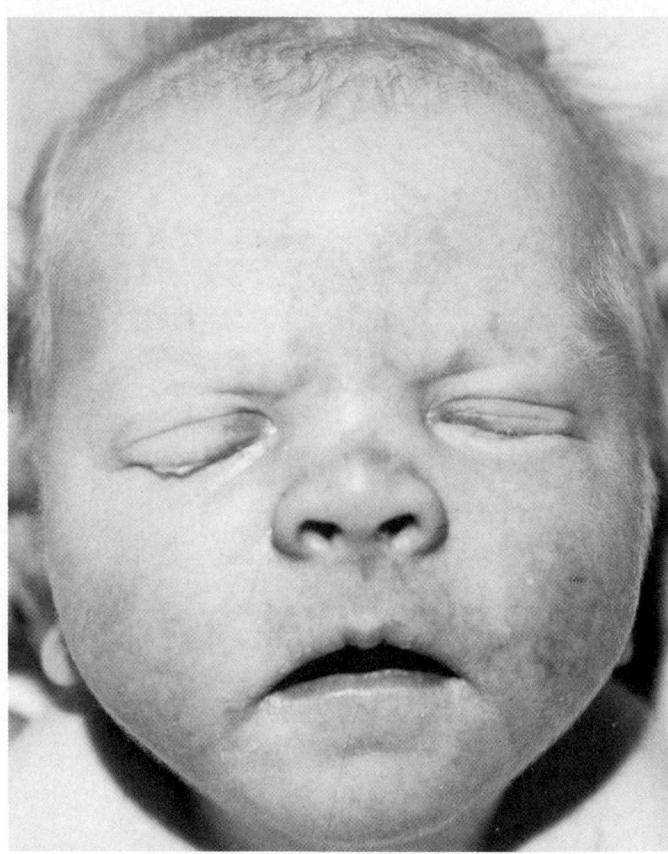

338. Note overlap of upper eyelids; capillary hemangiomas on forehead, bridge, and top of nose; down-turned angles of mouth

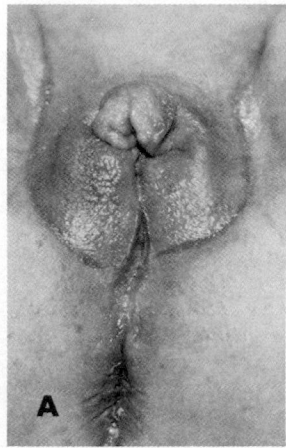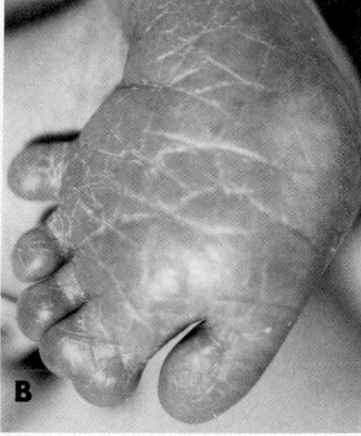

339. A) Hypoplastic phallus with dorsal prepuce, urethral opening at base of phallus, and fusion of labioscrotal swellings; B) short 1st toe, postaxial hexadactyly, complete cutaneous syndactyly of 2nd and 3rd toes, and severe valgus deformity

References:

DeMyer, W.: Median facial malformations and their implications for brain malformations. In Bergsma, D. (ed.): Morphogenesis and Malformation of Face and Brain. Birth Defects: Orig. Art. Ser., vol. XI, no. 7. New York: Alan R. Liss Inc. for The National Foundation-March of Dimes, 1975, p. 155.

Sedano, H. et al: Frontonasal dysplasia. J. Pediatr. 76:906, 1970.

Contributor: **R.S. Wilroy, Jr.**

Editor's Computerized Descriptors: Eye, Face, Oral, Nasoph., Nose, Hair, Skel., GU., Nerve

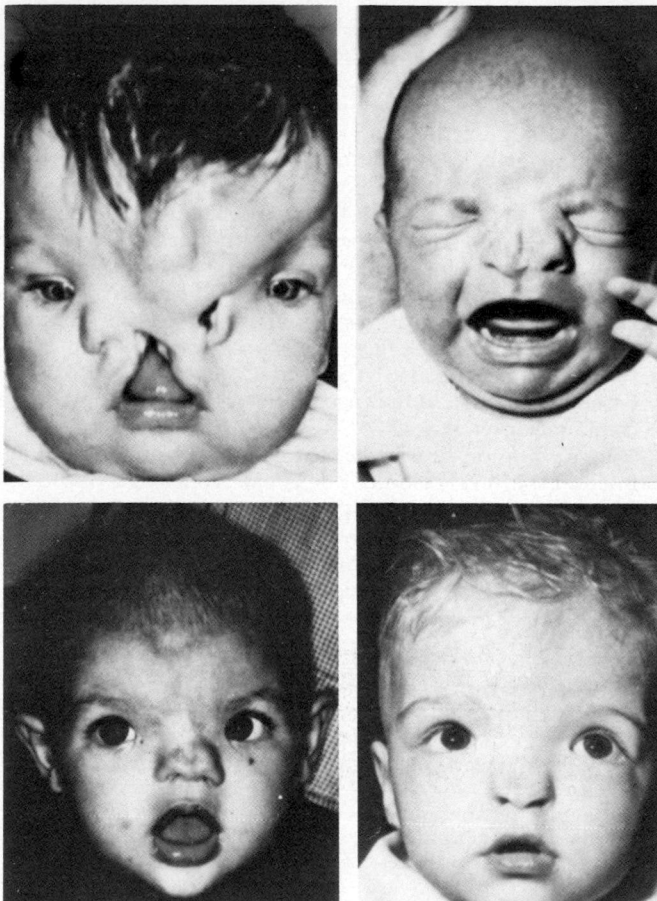

340. Variability in median facial cleft syndrome

MEDIAN CLEFTS OF LOWER LIP, MANDIBLE AND TONGUE

Includes: Fissure médiane labio-mandibule-linguale
Mittlere Unterlippen-Unterkiefer-Zungenspalte
Fisura mediana del labio inferior, de la mandíbula y de la lengua
Mandibular cleft, median
Tongue, median cleft

Excludes: Tongue, cleft (952)
Oro-facio-digital syndrome I (770)

Minimal Diagnostic Criteria: Median clefting of the lower lip and, in many cases, midline involvement of the mandible, tongue, and neck

Clinical Findings: Clefting is variable in degree, minimally involving the lower lip. In many cases, there is complete cleavage of the mandible, tongue, and structures of the midneck down to the hyoid bone. Clefting of the lower lip and mandible sometimes occurs without tongue involvement.

Complications
I   **Derived:** —
II **Associated:** Ankyloglossia, cleft upper lip, dysplastic ears, iris coloboma, cervical tags

Etiology: ?

Pathogenesis: Failure of development of the copula which arises between the paired mandibular processes or persistence of the central groove which, together with 2 lateral grooves, appears in the mandibular process of 5 - 6 mm embryos.

Related Facts
I   **Sex Ratio:** M1:F1, probably
II   **Risk of Occurrence:** ?
III **Risk of Recurrence for**
       Patient's Sib: ?
       Patient's Child: ?
IV   **Age of Detectability:** At birth, by physical examination
V   **Prevalence:** 1 in 600 cases of orofacial clefting

Treatment
I   **Primary Prevention:** —
II   **Secondary Prevention:** Surgical correction of defect
III **Other Therapy:** —

Prognosis: Fair - depends on extent of clefting

Detection of Carrier: —

Special Considerations: —

References:

Gorlin, R.J. and Goldman, H.M. (eds.): Thoma's Oral Pathology, 6th Ed. St. Louis:C.V. Mosby, 1970, vol. 1, p. 50.

Monroe, C.W.: Midline cleft of the lower lip, mandible and tongue with flexion contracture of the neck. Plast. Reconstr. Surg. 38:312, 1966.

Contributor: **M. Michael Cohen, Jr.**

Editor's Computerized Descriptors: Eye, Ear, Face, Oral, Neck Skel.,

MEGALOCORNEA

Includes: Mégalocornée
Megalokornea
Anterior megalophthalmos
Keratomegalia
Cornea, enlarged

Excludes: Buphthalmos
Glaucoma, congenital (414)
Keratoglobus

Minimal Diagnostic Criteria: Corneal diameter over 13 mm and normal intraocular pressure; no evidence of primary glaucoma

Clinical Findings: Symmetric, bilateral, nonprogressive increase in the corneal diameter (> 13 mm). The cornea is transparent, and occasionally has increased curvature resulting in astigmatism. The anterior chamber is deep, and there may be mesodermal abnormalities in the chamber angle and atrophy of the iris stroma. Attenuation of the dilator muscle of the pupil, which is relatively common, results in miosis. Cataract frequently occurs, and may cause reduction in visual acuity.

Complications
I **Derived:** Glaucoma, cataract
II **Associated:** †

Etiology: Usually X-linked recessive, but may be autosomal recessive or autosomal dominant.† McK *30930

Pathogenesis: ?

Related Facts
I **Sex Ratio:** M1:F< 1
II **Risk of Occurrence:** ?
III **Risk of Recurrence for**
    Patient's Sib: When X-linked recessive, autosomal recessive or autosomal dominant, see Table I X-linked R, AR or AD, respectively.
    Patient's Child: When X-linked recessive, autosomal recessive or autosomal dominant, see Table I X-linked R, AR or AD, respectively.
IV **Age of Detectability:** —
V **Prevalence:** ?

Treatment
I **Primary Prevention:** Genetic counseling
II **Secondary Prevention:** Correction of refractive error; therapy for the secondary glaucoma and cataract when indicated
III **Other Therapy:** —

Prognosis: Good

Detection of Carrier: —

†**Special Considerations:** An associated mosaic dystrophy of the cornea (possibly of different types) has been reported in three separate pedigrees. Megalocornea also occurs in Marfan syndrome. Two pedigrees have been described with mental retardation associated with megalocornea.

References:
Duke-Elder, S.: System of Ophthalmology. vol. 3, part 2. Congenital Deformities. London: Henry Kimpton, 1964.
Neuhäuser, G. et al: Syndrome of mental retardation, hypotonic cerebral palsy and megalocorneae, recessively inherited. Z. Kinderheilkd. 120:1, 1975.
Young, A. I.: Megalocornea and mosaic dystrophy in identical twins. Am. J. Ophthalmol. 66:734, 1968.

Contributors: **Morton F. Goldberg**
                      Joel Sugar

Editor's Computerized Descriptors: Vision, Eye

MEGALOCORNEA-MENTAL RETARDATION SYNDROME

Includes: Syndrome de mégalocornée et retard mental
Syndrom von Megalocornea und geistiger Retardierung
Síndrome de retardo mental y megalocórnea
Syndrome of mental retardation, seizures, hypotonic cerebral palsy and megalocornea

Excludes: Megalocornea and mental retardation in other syndromes and mesenchymal dysplasias (eg Marfan syndrome)

Minimal Diagnostic Criteria: Megalocornea, short stature and mental retardation.

Clinical Findings: The syndrome was observed in 2 boys and 1 girl of nonconsanguineous parents, and in at least 5 sporadic cases. All affected had short stature and mental retardation of moderate-to-severe range. Hypotonic cerebral palsy consisting of delayed motor development, muscular hypotonia and ataxia was present in most affected persons. Choreoathetotic movements were seen occasionally. Epileptic seizures occurred in most patients and EEG anomalies with generalized or focal discharges were noted. Megalocornea was present in all children, the corneal diameter being more than 12-15 mm, accompanied by deep anterior chamber (anterior megalophthalmus), iris hypoplasia and iridodonesis. Most patients were microcephalic from birth. Minor anomalies of the face included prominent forehead, telecanthus, epicanthus, and micrognathia.

Complications
I **Derived:** Glaucoma, cataracts
II **Associated:** ?

Etiology: ? Autosomal recessive

Pathogenesis: ?

Related Facts
I **Sex Ratio:** M1:F1
II **Risk of Occurrence:** ?
III **Risk of Recurrence for**
    Patient's Sib: ? If autosomal recessive 1 in 4 (25%) for each offspring to be affected.
    Patient's Child: If autosomal recessive not increased unless mate is carrier or homozygote.
IV **Age of Detectability:** Infancy or early childhood
V **Prevalence:** ? Rare

Treatment
I **Primary Prevention:** Genetic counseling
II **Secondary Prevention:** Early treatment of increased intraocular pressure and cataracts
III **Other Therapy:** Physiotherapy, anticonvulsant medication

Prognosis: Many of the patients were severely retarded and lived in an institution.

Detection of Carrier: ?

Special Considerations: —

References:
Frank, Y. et al: Megalocornea associated with multiple skeletal anomalies-new genetic syndrome. J. Genet. Hum. 21:67, 1973.
Neuhäuser, G. et al: Syndrome of mental retardation, seizures, hypotonic cerebral palsy and megalocornea, recessively inherited. Z. Kinderheilkd. 120:1, 1975.

Contributor: **Gerhard Neuhäuser**

Editor's Computerized Descriptors: Eye, Face, Skel., Muscle, Nerve

MELANOCYTOMA

Includes: Pigmentation congénitale du disque (optique)
Angeborene Pigmentation der Papille
Pigmentación congénita del disco óptico
Optic disk, melanocytoma
Fleck form pigmentation
Magnocellular nevus
Congenital pigmentation of optic disk

Excludes: Nevus of Ota (716)
Melanosis oculi, congenital (640)
Acquired melanosis oculi†

Minimal Diagnostic Criteria: See Clinical Findings

Clinical Findings: Congenital pigmentation of the optic disk is always benign and may take a variety of forms, the most important of which is the melanocytoma. The melanocytoma is a benign tumor, which tends to occur in a very deeply pigmented individual, eg Negroes and other non-Caucasians. The lesion is a small deeply pigmented tumor occurring eccentrically on the disk. It seldom, if ever, produces any effect on vision and may cause only an enlargement of the blind spot. It almost always remains stationary although there are some reports of possible growth; the latter perhaps related to a coincidental thromboembolic phenomenon.

Complications
I   **Derived:** Local invasiveness of the lesion has been reported, but there have been no reports of orbital extension or metastasis.
II **Associated:** —

Etiology: ?

Pathogenesis: This lesion is considered to be hamartomatous or progonomatous rather than neoplastic and can probably be regarded as atavistic, comparable with the tumor-like pigment formation in the optic nerve of certain reptiles.

Related Facts
I   **Sex Ratio:** ?
II   **Risk of Occurrence:** ?
III **Risk of Recurrence for**
      Patient's Sib: ?
      Patient's Child: ?
IV   **Age of Detectability:** ?
V   **Prevalence:** ?

Treatment
I   **Primary Prevention:** —
II   **Secondary Prevention:** —
III **Other Therapy:** —

Prognosis: Excellent; no visual impairment and no threat to life

Detection of Carrier: —

†**Special Considerations:** The practical significance of this tumor is that it must be differentiated from a malignant melanoma. Melanocytomas have also been reported in the uveal tract, and in these locations differentiation from malignant melanoma is even more difficult.

References:
Howard, G.M.: Melanocytoma of the disc complicated by hematoma under retinal pigment epithelium. Trans. Am. Acad. Ophthalmol. Otolaryngol. 70:281, 1966.
Howard, G.M. and Forest, A.W.: Incidence and location of melanocytomas. Arch. Ophthalmol. 77:61, 1967.
Tost, M.: Pigmentation of the optic disc in microphthalmic mice. J. Pediatr. Ophthalmol. 4:17, 1967.
Zimmerman, L.E. and Garron, L.K.: Melanocytoma of the optic disc. In Zimmerman, L.E. (ed.): International Ophthalmology Clinics, vol 2. Tumors of the Eye and Adnexa. Boston: Little, Brown, 1962. p. 431.

Contributor: **Morton E. Smith**

Editor's Computerized Descriptor: Eye
Also see Section I, Fig. 36

MELANOSIS OCULI, CONGENITAL

Contributor: **Morton E. Smith**

Editor's Computerized Descriptor: Eye

Includes: Mélanose oculaire congénitale
Melanosis bulbi congenitalis
Melanosis ocular congénita
Ocular melanocytosis

Excludes: Acquired melanosis oculi
Nevus of Ota (716)
Malignant melanoma
Nevus
Precancerous melanosis
Melanocytoma (639)

Minimal Diagnostic Criteria: Unilateral focal pigmentation of iris, fundus or sclera (rarely bilateral)†

Clinical Findings: This benign congenital pigmented lesion is usually unilateral and affects only the eye, not accompanied by skin pigmentation as in nevus of Ota. The iris often appears as brown velvet and the fundus is a uniform slate grey. The sclera may appear brown or slate grey. The cornea and conjunctiva are rarely affected. The optic nerve may be involved.

Complications
I   **Derived:** —
II **Associated:** There are reports suggesting a higher incidence of malignant melanoma occurring in the uveal tract (or orbit) in eyes with congenital melanosis oculi than in the normal population. One report (Blodi), however, questions this.

Etiology: ?

Pathogenesis: ?

Related Facts
I   **Sex Ratio:** M1:F>1
II   **Risk of Occurrence:** ?
III **Risk of Recurrence for**
     Patient's Sib: ?
     Patient's Child: ?
IV   **Age of Detectability:** —
V   **Prevalence:** Occurs more commonly in dark-complexioned individuals, eg Orientals. It occurs more frequently in females.

Treatment
I   **Primary Prevention:** —
II   **Secondary Prevention:** —
III **Other Therapy:** —

Prognosis: Good, no visual impairment

Detection of Carrier: —

†Special Considerations: There is excessive pigmentation of the mesodermal layers of the eye but the pigment-bearing epithelium is not involved.

References:
Blodi, F.C.: Ocular melanocytosis and melanoma. Am. J. Ophthalmol. 80:389, 1975.
Makley, T.A., Jr. and King, C.M.: Malignant melanoma in melanosis oculi. Trans. Am. Acad. Ophthalmol. Otolaryngol. 71:638, 1967.
Manschot, W.A.: Congenital ocular melanosis, conjunctival naevus, conjunctival melanosis, conjunctival melanoma. Ophthalmologica 152:495, 1966.
Reese, A.B.: Tumors of the Eye, 3rd Ed. New York: Harper and Row, 1976.
Reese, A.B.: Congenital melanomas. Trans. Am. Ophthalmol. Soc. 71:186, 1973.
Sabates, F.N. and Yamashita, T.: Congenital melanosis oculi complicated by two independent malignant melanomas of the choroid. Arch. Ophthalmol. 77:801, 1967.
Stafford, W.R.: Congenital melanosis oculi: Report of a case. Arch. Ophthalmol. 68:738, 1962.

MELORHEOSTOSIS

Includes: Mélorhéostose
Meloreostosis
Melorheostosis Leri
Flowing hyperostosis
Osteosis eburnisans monomelica

Excludes: Diaphyseal dysplasia (290)
Hyperostosis corticalis generalisata (497)

Minimal Diagnostic Criteria: Diagnosis of this disorder can be made only from the typical radiographic changes.

Clinical Findings: This disorder is a rare form of hyperostosis which has a linear distribution along the major axis of the long bones. Radiographically, the hyperostosis resembles melting wax dripping down the side of a candle, hence the term, melorheostosis, from the Greek words *melos* (member) and *rhein* (flow). The disease is almost always unilateral in its distribution, and usually affects a single limb. It is usually first detected in childhood or young adulthood, but has been diagnosed at birth because of deformities of the fingers. Patients usually present because of progressive pain, stiffness, and limitation of motion, or deformity such as contractures of the fingers. The pain ranges from a dull ache to sharp; it is not constant, and is often aggravated by activity. The overlying skin is often normal in appearance, but may be tense, shiny, or erythematous. Linear scleroderma has been described. The subcutaneous tissues are often indurated and edematous, and the overlying muscles may be atrophic and weak. The adjacent joints may be intermittently warm and swollen with eventual limitation of joint motion due to soft tissue fibrosis. The affected limb may be shorter or, less commonly, longer. It usually appears larger in circumference, and may be angulated or curved.

Radiographs reveal the typical molten wax appearance with streaked sclerotic thickening of 1 side of the long bone. This irregular linear opacity runs along the major axis of the long bone, and may extend from 1 bone to the adjacent bone. The limb girdle is usually involved as well. The sclerosis may extend into the epiphyseal regions as streaks, but the articular areas are usually unaffected. The hyperostosis may not be prominent in infancy or childhood, but becomes more apparent with age.

Biopsies of affected sclerotic bones have revealed irregularly arranged Haversian systems with dense thickened trabeculae and occasional islands of cartilage. Cellular fibrotic tissue is seen in the marrow spaces. Fibrosis of the subcutaneous tissues and skeletal muscle atrophy have been described. Degenerative, inflammatory, and obliterative changes have been noted in the surrounding blood vessels.

Complications
I **Derived:** This disorder can lead to painful limitation of motion and weakness of the affected limb, as well as fibrous contractures of the adjacent joints.
II **Associated:** —

Etiology: ?

Pathogenesis: ?

Related Facts
I **Sex Ratio:** M1:F1
II **Risk of Occurrence:** ?
III **Risk of Recurrence for**
    Patient's Sib: ? (All cases to date have been sporadic)
    Patient's Child: ?

IV **Age of Detectability:** Can be detected from birth if radiographs are performed. It is usually not diagnosed until late childhood or early adulthood when a limb is xrayed because of vague symptoms of pain or joint immobility.
V **Prevalence:** ?

Treatment
I **Primary Prevention:** —
II **Secondary Prevention:** Orthopedic procedures to prevent or correct limb deformities.
III **Other Therapy:** —

Prognosis: Apparently normal for life span. The pain and disability are usually progressive.

Detection of Carrier: —

Special Considerations: —

References:
Campbell, C.J. et al: Melorheostosis. J. Bone Joint Surg., 50A:1281, 1968.
Morris, J.M. et al: Melorheostosis. J. Bone Joint Surg. 45A:1191, 1963.
Patrick, J.H.: Melorheostosis associated with arteriovenous aneurysm of the left arm and trunk. J. Bone Joint Surg. 51B:126, 1969.

Contributors: **David L. Rimoin**
David W. Hollister

Editor's Computerized Descriptors: Skin, Skel., Muscle

MENINGOCELE

Includes: Meningozele
Spina bifida cystica without neurologic deficit
Cranial meningoceles

Excludes: Spina bifida occulta
Myelomeningocele (693)
Lipomeningocele (602)
Myelorachischisis
Encephalocele (343)

Minimal Diagnostic Criteria: Translucent skin mass with spina bifida and widening of interpedicular distance on xray.

Clinical Findings: Skin covered soft tissue mass over midline of back or slightly off to one side. Most commonly in the lumbar area. Herniation of meninges can occur over midline of cervical spine and cranium. In latter location they are called encephaloceles or cranial meningoceles. Overlying skin may have angiomatous or hairy patch. There is no paralysis or sensory loss. The head circumference is normal and hydrocephaly is rarely associated. On xray, spina bifida underlies the mass.

Complications
I **Derived:** Breakdown of skin covering. Rarely, nerve roots are trapped in sac causing leg weakness.
II **Associated:** May be a component of other syndromes.

Etiology: Polygenic

Pathogenesis: Failure of complete midline fusion of the vertebral arches with cystic distention of meninges, but without neural tissue in sac. Gardner's theory is based upon the existence of hydrocephalus and hydromyelia as a normal condition in early embryonic life as a result of fluid secreted by the neural epithelium in the first instance and then by the choroid plexus. By preventing the normal circulation of cerebrospinal fluid, the delay or failure of permeation of the roof of the 4th ventricle will produce all grades of anomalies seen in the dysraphic states. A meningocele results when the internal hydromyelia becomes external and the expanding subarachnoid space bulges beneath cutaneous ectoderm impeding at the same time proper mesodermal closure.

Related Facts
I **Sex Ratio:** M1:F1
II **Risk of Occurrence:** ? Possibly 1 in 20,000 live births
III **Risk of Recurrence for**
 Patient's Sib: ? Empiric risk
 Patient's Child: ? Empiric risk
IV **Age of Detectability:** At birth
V **Prevalence:** ? Possibly 1 in 20,000

Treatment
I **Primary Prevention:** Genetic counseling
II **Secondary Prevention:** Repair of cystic mass during 1st year of life
III **Other Therapy:** ?

Prognosis: Good

Detection of Carrier: ?

Special Considerations: —

References:
Gardner, W.J.: Myelocele: Rupture of the neural tube? Clin. Neurosurg. 15:57, 1968.
Shulman, K.: Defects of closure of the neural plate. In Barnett, H.L. (ed.): Pediatrics. 14th Ed. New York: Appleton-Century-Crofts, 1968, p. 853.

Contributor: **Kenneth Shulman**

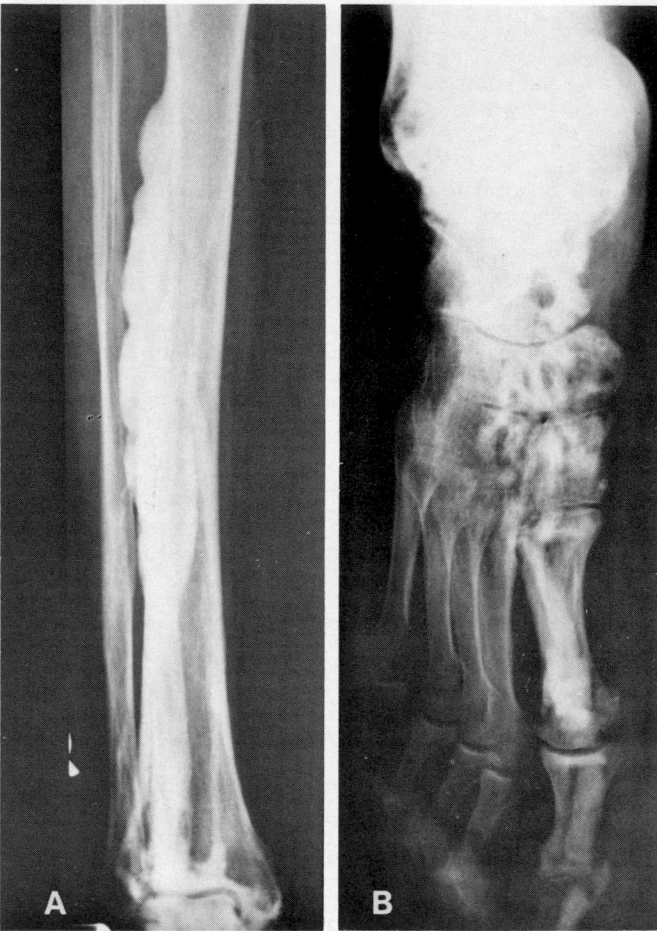

341. A) Striking streaks of increased density in right tibia; B) bands of increased density in right tarsal area but limited to the great toe

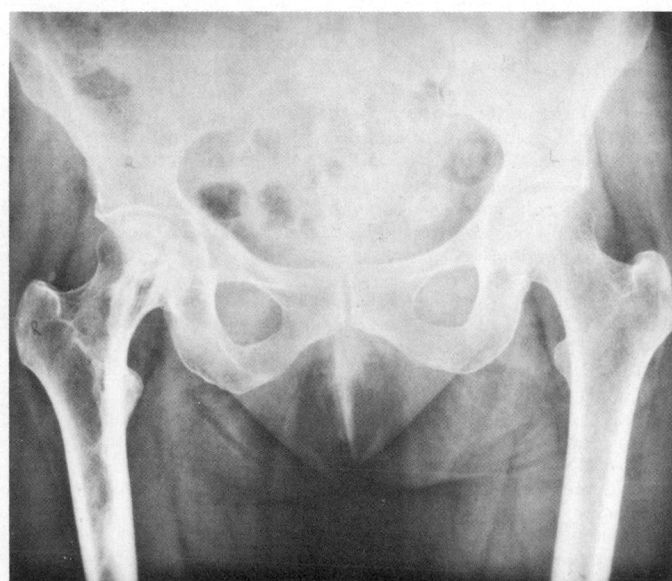

342. Longitudinal bands of increased density beginning in the femoral head

MENKES SYNDROME

Includes: Syndrome de Menkes
Síndrome de Menkes
Neurodegenerative disease
X-linked and kinky hair
Kinky hair disease

Excludes: —

Minimal Diagnostic Criteria: Severe mental retardation, seizures, abnormal hair and X-linked inheritance

Clinical Findings: Characterized in males by abnormal hair (trichorrhexis nodosa, pili torti, and monilethrix) which is fragile, sparse, and may be white; profound failure to thrive and growth retardation; severe retardation with failure of mental development, progressive spasticity and decerebration; as well as seizures. Radiologic features include metaphyseal spurring and diaphyseal periosteal reaction, flaring of rib ends and parietal wormian bones.†

Complications
I **Derived:** Seizures, retardation, death
II **Associated:** —

Etiology: X-linked recessive; McK *30940

Pathogenesis: ? An elevation of glutamic acid in plasma was reported in 2 families, but not in another. Abnormality of fatty acid oxidation was reported.

Related Facts
I **Sex Ratio:** M1:F0
II **Risk of Occurrence:** Rare
III **Risk of Recurrence for**
   Patient's Sib: If mother is a carrier 1 in 2 (50%) for each brother to be affected and 1 in 2 for each sister to be a carrier
   Patient's Child: 1 in 1 (100%) for carrier daughters; not increased for sons unless wife is a carrier
IV **Age of Detectability:** Has been noted within early months of life.
V **Prevalence:** Rare, 21 males from 5 families reported.

Treatment
I **Primary Prevention:** Genetic counseling
II **Secondary Prevention:** —
III **Other Therapy:** Anticonvulsant medication for seizures

Prognosis: Death usually occurs in 1st or 2nd years.

Detection of Carrier: —

†Special Considerations: Pathologic findings in these children consist of small head, often micrognathia, patchy degeneration of cortex and cerebellum as well as basal ganglia, with degeneration of white matter presumably secondary to gray matter disease. Purkinje cells showed irregular swelling and fluorescence under UV light. Abnormalities of the cerebral blood vessels have been seen on angiogram.

References:
Aguilar, M.J. et al: Kinky hair disease. I. Clinical and pathological features. J. Neuropathol. Exp. Neurol. 25:507, 1966.
Bray, P. F.: Sex-linked neurodegenerative disease associated with monilethrix. Pediatrics 36:417, 1965.
Menkes, J.H. et al: A sex-linked recessive disorder with retardation of growth, peculiar hair, and focal cerebral and cerebellar degeneration. Pediatrics 29:764, 1962.
Wesenberg, R.L. et al: Radiological findings in the kinky-hair syndrome. Radiology 92:500, 1969.
Yoshida, T. et al: A sex-linked disorder with mental and physical retardation characterized by cerebrocortical atrophy and increased glutamic acid in the cerebrospinal fluid. Tohoku J. Exp. Med. 83:261, 1961.

Contributor: **John Mark Freeman**

Editor's Computerized Descriptors: Hair, Nerve

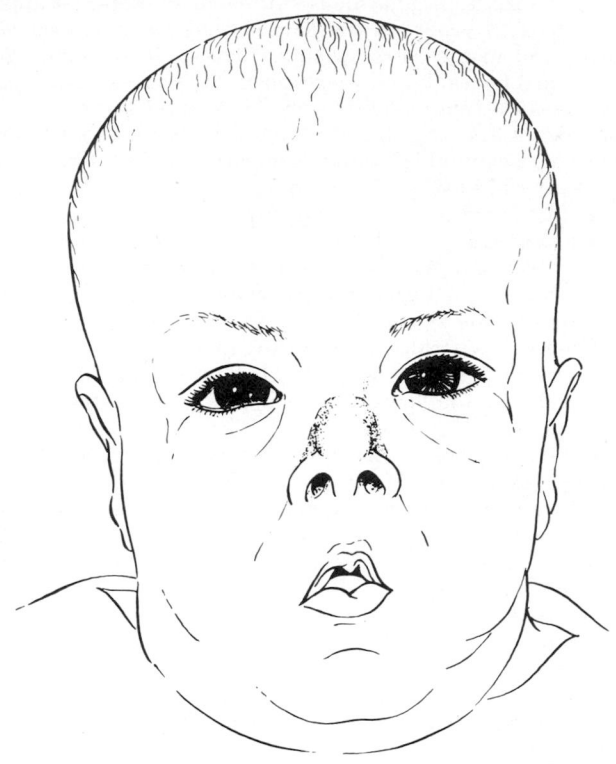

343. Note short sparse hair, short broad nose, micrognathia, and broad cheeks

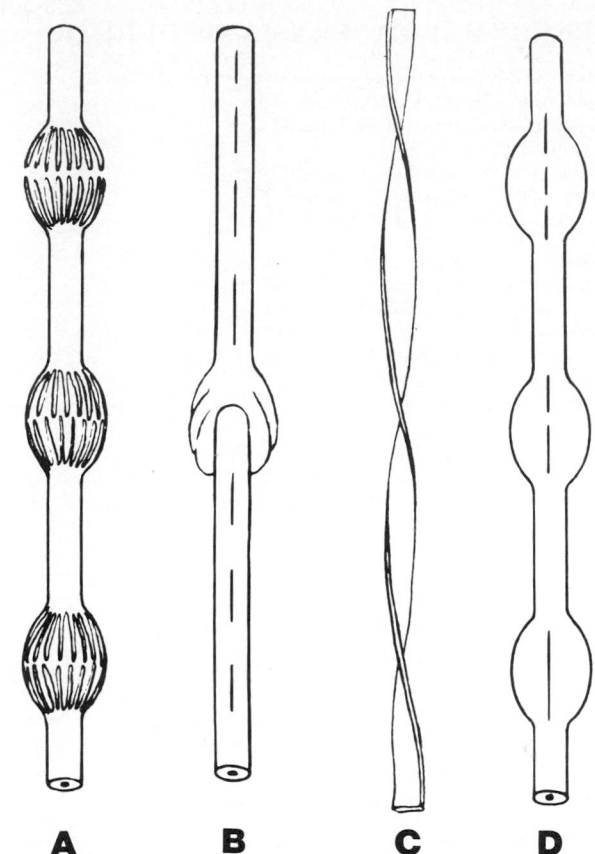

345. Diagram of hair defects: A) trichorrhexis nodosa; B) bamboo hair; C) congenital pili torti; D) congenital monilethrix

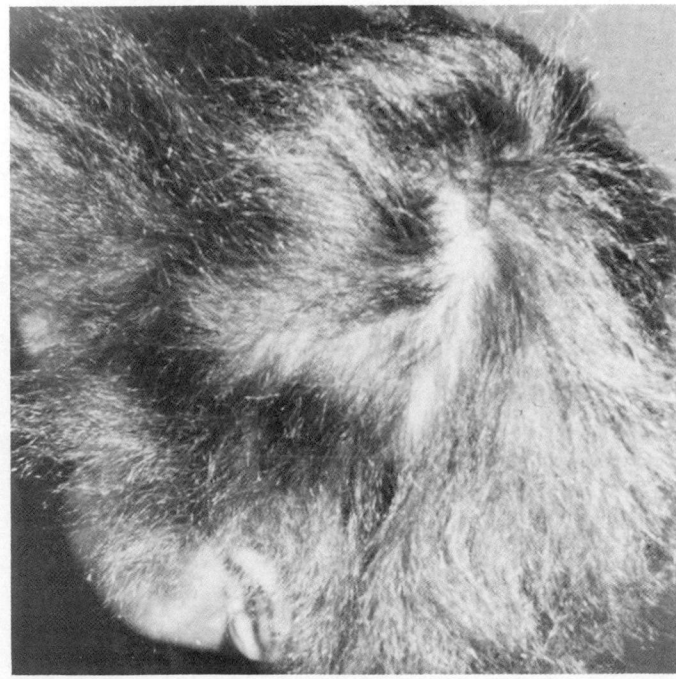

344. Pili torti. Note unruly spiral hair shafts

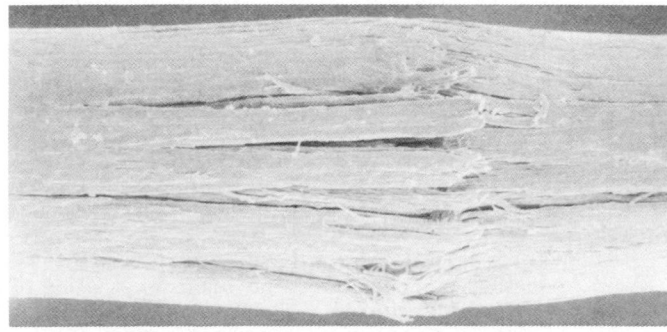

346. Trichorrhexis nodosa swelling with multiple longitudinal splits and a traverse or "paint brush" fracture in pili annulati

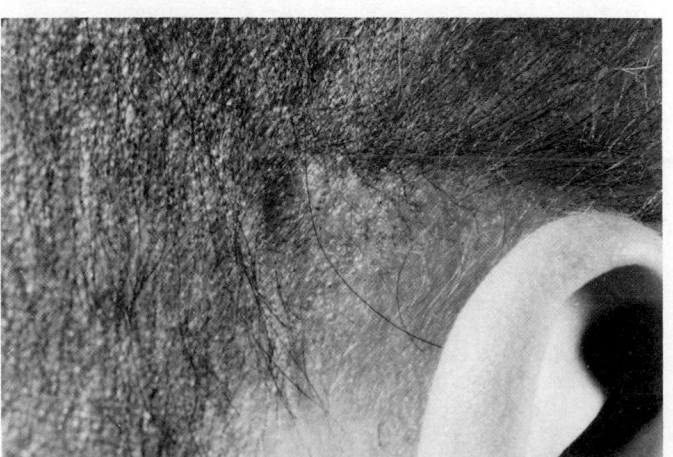

347. Monilethrix

695

MESENCHYMAL DYSPLASIA OF PURETIĆ

Includes: Dysplasie mésenchymale-syndrome de Puretić
Mesenchymale Dysplasie (Puretić)
Displasia mesénquimatica de Puretić
Puretić syndrome
Systemic familial mesenchymosis of Puretić et al
Systematized mesodermal dysplasia
"Systemic hyalinosis" Ishikawa-Hori

Excludes: Lipoid proteinosis (599)
Generalized lipid proteinosis of Crawford
Systemic amyloidosis of Gottron
Enchondromatosis (345)
Osteochondromatosis with hemangiomata
Mucopolysaccharidoses
Collagenoses (rheumatoid arthritis, scleroderma, dermatomyositis)
Familial dactylolysis of Harnasch
Disseminated calcinoses (calcinosis universalis, lipocalcinogranulomatosis of Teutschländer, Nievergelt syndrome, chondroangiopathia calcarea)
Skin dysembryomas of Achten
Histiocytosis X
Arthromyodysplasia congenita
Polyfibromatosis of Touraine

Minimal Diagnostic Criteria: Impossible to ascertain from 1 case report. Diagnosis can be made upon clinical grounds and confirmed by histologic examination of nodes. The epidermis overlying nodes is thin with flat epidermoid-ermal junction. At the periphery the epidermis is partly acanthotic. The corneal layer is well developed with scattered osteofollicular hyperkeratosis. The basal membrane is unequally PAS positive, with irregular interruptions over some nodes. The nodes extend from the deeper layers of dermis down into the subcutis. Hard, nonulcerated nodes are built of altered, swollen, homogeneous, highly PAS-positive collagen fibers, which are 2-4 times broader than normal. Between these fibers are some hydropically degenerated fibroblasts and numerous blood and lymph capillaries, mostly closed. Endothelium of capillaries is swollen; their nuclei stain well by hematoxylin.

Clinical Findings: Based upon the case of a boy born in 1948, published by Puretić et al in 1962, and followed up to the age of 22 years, the fully developed syndrome comprises:

Contractures of joints from early infancy, progressing to severe reduction of movements; and fusiform swelling of some joints. The patient appeared normal at birth. His 1st symptoms appeared when he was 3 months old. From age 14 years he could hardly stand, walk or feed himself. By age 18 years body stiffness was almost complete.

Muscle hypotrophy and reduced subcutaneous tissue.

Skin lesions include:

1) Multiple large cutaneous and subcutaneous nodes over the entire body, symmetric in distribution, some ulcerated and calcified. These lesions 1st appeared between the 6th and 9th years of the patient's life. They appeared mostly on those parts of the body where the skin was tense or repeatedly traumatized, such as the scalp, tip of the nose ("clown-like nose"), chin, and various parts of the trunk and limbs. The nodes were painless, mostly hard or of rubbery consistency, and reached a size of 2-2.5 cm after 1 to 2 years; those in the parietooccipital and temporal regions calcified and ulcerated. However, after 2-4 years the exudation of purulent and calcareous material ceased, leaving barely noticeable scars. Nodes in other regions continue to exude after more than 10 years. Over a period of 8 years, since the patient was 11 1/2 years old, 1 parietooccipital lesion has eroded the calvarium, leaving only a tiny lamella of internal table.

2) Diffuse and nodular infiltrations in the perioral region, in the alae nasi and in the nasolabial fold regions, beginning in the 6th year of life.

3) Transparent gelatinous cutaneous blisters, 1st apparent at age 9 years, on the palms, soles, fingers, toes, ear-lobes and in the retroauricular folds; transforming early into hard nodes. In 3-5 years most of these regressed spontaneously without leaving scars. However, those on the tips of fingers and toes have enlarged to twice the size of a normal terminal phalanx ("fingers looking like drumsticks") and have persisted to age 22.

4) Lichenoid infiltrations in the nuchal and perianal regions appearing at about 6 years of age and regressing slowly over 2-3 years with residual skin atrophy.

5) Dysseborrheic, poikilodermiform and sclerodermiform changes in the skin first noted at age 6 years.

Gingival hyperplasia, appearing at age 9 years, dark red, covering 2/3 of the upper teeth, and producing nodular swellings of the lower gingiva, protruding between the teeth.

Osteolysis of terminal phalanges, 1st noted at 6 1/2 years of age, appearing before visible fingertip nodules. This progressed to nearly complete lysis over 2-3 years. Osteoporosis of the long bones appeared at 10 years in periarticular regions, and had become generalized by age 18. Dorsolumbar scoliosis was also notable.

Stunted growth with height below the 3rd% by age 14 years and accompanied by delayed skeletal maturation.

Recurrent suppurative infections of the skin, eyes, nose and middle ears. This was associated with only slight regional lymphadenopathy. Antibody response to influenza A_2 was normal.

Degenerative changes including enlarged skull, coarse facies, dense eyebrows, protrusion of the lower portion of the sternum and camptodactyly of both 5th fingers. Despite the grotesque facies, Reilly-Alder granules were never seen in leukocytes and osseous signs of mucopolysaccharidosis were absent.

Normal mental development.

Delayed sexual development.

Complications
I **Derived:** Impossible to separate integral parts of condition from complications. The condition apparently renders the patient susceptible to secondary bacterial infections.
II **Associated:** None known

Etiology: The condition is probably due to the presence of an autosomal recessive mutant gene in the homozygous state. A previously born sister and brother of the proband developed painful contractures of elbows, knees, shoulders and hips prior to 3 months of age, along with perianal nodes (sister) and repeated febrile infections (brother). Both died at 8 months of age. One full sib and 1 half sib are healthy.

Pathogenesis: Two factors are hypothesized: 1) an inborn defect of mesenchymal tissue and, 2) a humoral factor originating from dilated blood or lymph capillaries. Immunoelectrophoresis has revealed increased IgG, normal-to-increased IgA and normal IgM. The karyotype is 46, XY.†

Related Facts
I **Sex Ratio:** M2:F1 in single reported family. Theoretically M1:F1 if autosomal recessive
II **Risk of Occurrence:** Very rare
III **Risk of Recurrence for**
  Patient's Sib: 1 in 4 if autosomal recessive
  Patient's Child: Not increased theoretically

IV **Age of Detectability:** First signs in early infancy, fully developed syndrome in early childhood.

V **Prevalence:** Very rare. Besides the case described by the authors, 1 additional case, probably of the same or a closely related condition, was reported by Ishikawa and Hori in a Japanese boy. Each patient had sibs, all of whom died in infancy, and each may have had the same or similar condition.

Treatment

I **Primary Prevention:** Genetic counseling

II **Secondary Prevention:** Avoidance or early treatment of bacterial infections.

III **Other Therapy:** Corticosteroids, ACTH and resochin have shown a satisfactory effect on joint lesions and motility. Testosterone and other anabolic steroids had no effect. In remission gentle physiotherapy, spa and sea baths. Irradiation of nodes or local injections of hyaluronidase without success. Total excision of nodes, if feasible, is most effective; there are no recurrences thereafter; however, partial excision results in prolonged suppuration and slow healing. General supportive measures include high vitamin and high protein diet, repeated blood transfusions, gamma globulins, liver extracts and iron.

Prognosis: For life: One patient now living at age 22 years; 2 sibs died in 1st year of life, 1 of diarrhea, the other of unknown cause. For function: Severe limitation because of contractures, deforming lesions and susceptibility to infections. For intelligence: Apparently no effect.

Detection of Carrier: —

†**Special Considerations:** At an early stage, 1-day-old cutaneous blisters or transparent nodes (with serous sticky content) show pronounced dilatation of lymphatic and blood capillaries beneath epidermis, but in the deeper layers of corium the formation of cleft-like blisters with remnants of tissue septa appear. Cutis is filled with a liquid which stains pink by eosin; collagenous fibers surrounded by exudate lose sharp contours, stain more deeply by eosin and become homogenized. At a later stage, blisters (a few days old, transformed into hard nodes) show analogous changes, but here the homogenization of collagenous fibers is more pronounced. Within the exuded liquid, red undulating fibrils are visible only here and there. They blend with the sedimentary liquid forming homogeneous masses. Histochemically those masses have analogous characteristics to those in earlier described nodes. There is a slight perivascular infiltration of lymphocytes, neutrophils, plasma cells and altered fibroblasts.

References:

Ishikawa, H. and Hori, Y.: Systematisierte Hyalinose im Zusammenhang mit Epidermolysis bullosa polydystrophica und Hyalinosis cutis et mucosae. Arch. Klin. Exp. Dermatol. 281:30, 1963.

McKusick, V.A.: Mendelian Inheritance in Man. 4th ed. Baltimore:- Johns Hopkins Press, 1975.

Puretic S. et al: A unique form of mesenchymal dysplasia. Br. J. Dermatol. 74:8, 1962.

Contributors: Štefanija Puretić
Božidar Puretić‡

Editor's Computerized Descriptors: Face, Oral, Nasoph., Skin, Hair, Skel., Muscle

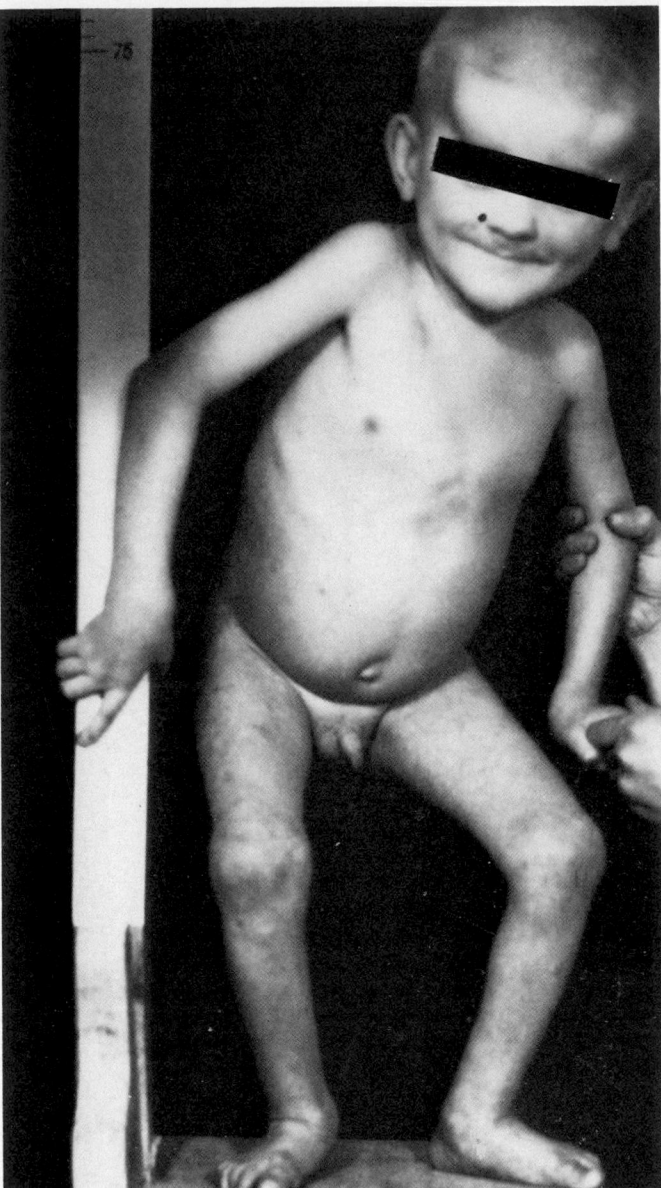

348. Puretić syndrome in young male

MESENTERIC CYSTS

Includes: Kystes mésentériques
Mesenterial Zysten
Quistes mesentéricos
Lymphangioma of mesentery
Cystic hygroma of mesentery
Lymphatic cyst of mesentery

Excludes: Intestinal duplication (532)

Minimal Diagnostic Criteria: Mass found at operation not sharing wall with intestine, no muscular lining of wall, alkaline media.

Clinical Findings: Abdominal mass, pain, partial or complete intestinal obstruction, fever of unknown etiology, singly or in combination may be presenting complaints.

Complications
I   Derived: —
II Associated: Chylous ascites may be associated with or caused by rupture of cyst. Intraabdominal abscess may result from infection in cyst. Volvulus of cyst with adjacent gut may result in obstruction or loss of viability of intestinal wall.

Etiology: ?

Pathogenesis: Anomaly of lymphatic tissue in mesentery with obstructed lymphatics and cyst formation

Related Facts
I   Sex Ratio: M1:F1
II   Risk of Occurrence: ?
III Risk of Recurrence for
    Patient's Sib: ?
    Patient's Child: ?
IV Age of Detectability: Any age; 25% under 10 years of age
V   Prevalence: ? (8 in 820,000 admissions at Mayo; 3 in 12,425 admissions at Children's Hospital, Los Angeles)

Treatment
I   Primary Prevention: —
II   Secondary Prevention: Resection of cyst from mesentery with or without adjacent bowel depending on blood supply. Marsupialization of cyst generally results in recurrence or ascites.
III Other Therapy: —

Prognosis: Excellent for complete recovery with resection.

Detection of Carrier: —

Special Considerations: —

References:
Benson, C.D.: Messenteric cysts. In Mustard, W.T. et al (eds.): Pediatric Surgery, 2nd Ed. Chicago:Year Book Medical Publishers, 1969, vol. 2, p. 872.

Contributor: Lawrence K. Pickett

Editor's Computerized Descriptor: GI.

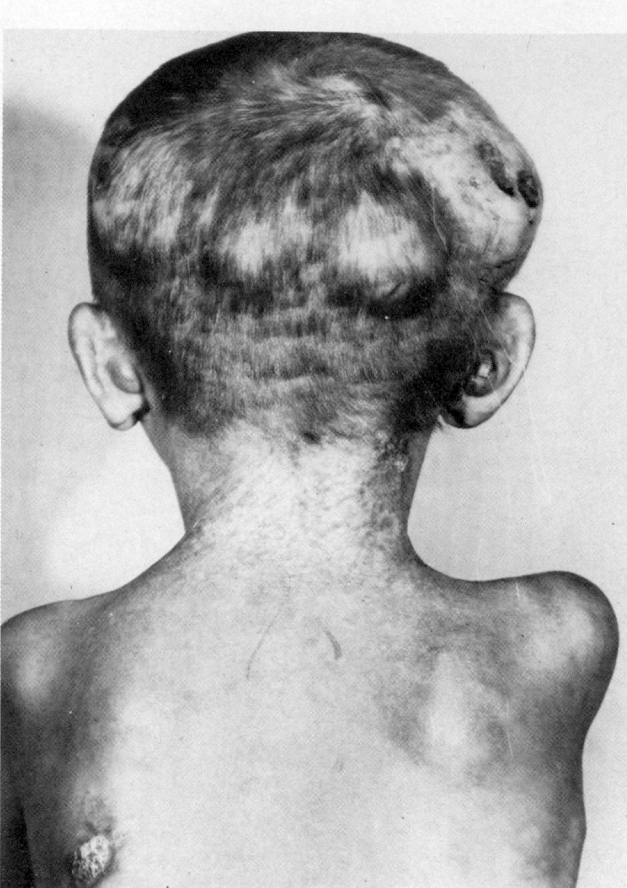

349. Mesenchymal displasia of Puretić

MESOMELIC DYSPLASIA, LANGER TYPE

Includes: Dysplasie mésomélique, type Langer
Mesomele Dysplasie, Typ Langer
Displasia mesomiélica, tipo Langer
Mesomelic dwarfism of the hypoplastic ulna, fibula, mandible type

Excludes: All other forms of mesomelic dysplasia
Dyschondrosteosis† (308)
Acromesomelic dysplasias
Acrodysostosis (16)
Chondroectodermal dysplasia (156)
Robinow syndrome (876)

Minimal Diagnostic Criteria: Disproportionate dwarfism with severe shortness of the middle segment of the limbs, and characteristic radiographic appearance of ulna, radius, tibia and fibula.

Clinical Findings: Disproportionate dwarfing with shortening of forearms and lower legs. There is moderate limitation of extension at the elbows and marked ulnar deviation of the hands at the wrists. The lumbar spine has an increased lordosis. The mandible is hypoplastic on occasion. Adult height is about 130 cm. Intelligence is normal. Radiologically, the hands are normal but there is severe hypoplasia of the distal ulna. The radius is short, thick and laterally curved. The carpal bones lie against a medially faced articular surface of the radius. The proximal fibula is aplastic with the remainder of the fibula hypoplastic to a variable degree. The tibia is short and wide. The feet, skull and spine are normal.

Complications
I **Derived:** —
II **Associated:** —

Etiology: Probably autosomal recessive. However, familial cases have been reported suggesting that the condition may be produced by homozygosity for the autosomal dominant dyschondrosteosis gene.† McK *24970

Pathogenesis: ?

Related Facts
I **Sex Ratio:** M1:F1
II **Risk of Occurrence:** ?
III **Risk of Recurrence for**
   Patient's Sib: 1 in 4 (25%) in both possible modes of inheritance. † If, indeed, homozygosity for the dyschondrosteosis gene is the case there is an additional risk of 1 in 2 (50%) for dyschondrosteosis to recur.
   Patient's Child: Possibly 50% chance for dyschondrosteosis.
IV **Age of Detectability:** At birth
V **Prevalence:** ?

Treatment
I **Primary Prevention:** Genetic counseling
II **Secondary Prevention:** Orthopedic procedures and physiotherapy to relieve the ulnar deviation of the hands if needed.
III **Other Therapy:** —

Prognosis: Normal intelligence and life span.

Detection of Carrier: The spouse of an individual with dyschondrosteosis should be clinically and radiologically examined to exclude the same condition.

†**Special Considerations:** The parents of the 2 patients described by Langer were considered normal. Two earlier reports by Böök (Hereditas 36:161, 1950) and by Brailsford (Br. J. Radiol. 8:533, 1953) and 2 recent reports by Silverman (Prog. Pediatr. Radiol. 4:546, 1973) and by Esperitu et al (Am. J. Dis. Child. 129:375, 1975) all describe probands with identical clinical and radiographic findings as Langer, and suggest that the parents had short stature of dyschondrosteosis type.

References:
Esperitu, C. et al: Mesomelic dwarfism as the homozygous expression of dyschondrosteosis. Am. J. Dis. Child. 129:375, 1975.
Kaitila, I.I. et al: Mesomelic skeletal dysplasias. Clin. Orthop. 114:94, 1976.
Langer, L.O.: Mesomelic dwarfism of the hypoplastic ulna, fibula, mandible type. Radiology 89:654, 1967.

Contributor: **Ilkka I. Kaitila**

Editor's Computerized Descriptors: Face, Skel.

MESOMELIC DYSPLASIA, NIEVERGELT TYPE

Includes: Dysplasie mésomélique, type Nievergelt
Mesomele Dysplasie, Typ Nievergelt
Displasia mesomiélica, tipo Nievergelt
Mesomelic dwarfism, Nievergelt type

Excludes: All other forms of mesomelic dysplasia
Dyschondrosteosis (308)
Robinow syndrome (876)
Acromesomelic dysplasias
Acrodysostosis (16)
Chondroectodermal dysplasia (156)

Minimal Diagnostic Criteria: Mesomelic shortness of the lower legs with a rhomboid radiographic appearance of the tibia and fibula.

Clinical Findings: Patients present with moderate to severe disproportionate dwarfism in which the forearms and the lower legs are deformed and shortened. Bony protuberances with cutaneous dimples are present at both medial and lateral aspects of the lower legs. At the knees there is a moderate valgus deformity, whereas the ankles and feet are often in an abducted equinovarus position. A bony protuberance and cutaneous dimple may be found at the lateral aspect of the forearms. Extension at the elbows and supination of the forearms are moderately limited and the hands deviate medially at the wrists. Finger extension is often limited by contractures. The adult height has been reported to be 135-147 cm. Intelligence is normal.

Radiographically, the middle segment bones of the limbs are rhomboid in appearance. The proximal head of the radius and often the ulna, as well, are dislocated and they may be synostotic. Metatarsal synostosis is common. The growth plates of the tibia and fibula are severely slanted. There is considerable clinical variability in the expression of this rare condition.

Complications
I **Derived:** —
II **Associated:** —

Etiology: Autosomal dominant with variable expressivity; McK *16340

Pathogenesis: The severely disturbed development of the tubular bones with anomalous slanting of the growth plates in the middle segment of the limbs results in marked growth retardation and deformity of the bones.

Related Facts
I   **Sex Ratio:** M1:F1
II **Risk of Occurrence:** ?
III **Risk of Recurrence for**
   Patient's Sib: If parent is affected, 1 in 2 (50%) for each offspring to be affected; otherwise not increased.
   Patient's Child: 1 in 2
IV **Age of Detectability:** At birth
V   **Prevalence:** ?

Treatment
I   **Primary Prevention:** Genetic counseling
II **Secondary Prevention:** Orthopedic surgery and physiotherapy for correction of the atypical clubfeet and possibly of the malaligned growth plates of the tibia and fibula.
III **Other Therapy:** —

Prognosis: Normal life span with orthopedic problems.

Detection of Carrier: —

Special Considerations: —

References:

Nievergelt, K.: Positiver Vaterschaftsnachweis auf Grund erblicher Missbildungen der Extremitäten. Arch. Julius Klaus-Stiftung 19:157. 1944.
Solonen, K.A. and Sulamaa, M.: Nievergelt syndrome and its treatment. Ann. Chir. Gynaecol. Fenn. 47:142, 1958.
Young, L.W. and Wood, B.P.: Nievergelt syndrome (mesomelic dwarfism-type Nievergelt). In Bergsma, D. (ed.): Limb Malformations. Birth Defects: Orig. Art. Ser., vol X, no. 5. Miami: Symposia Specialists for The National Foundation-March of Dimes, 1974, p. 81.

Contributor: **Ilkka I. Kaitila**

Editor's Computerized Descriptor: Skel.

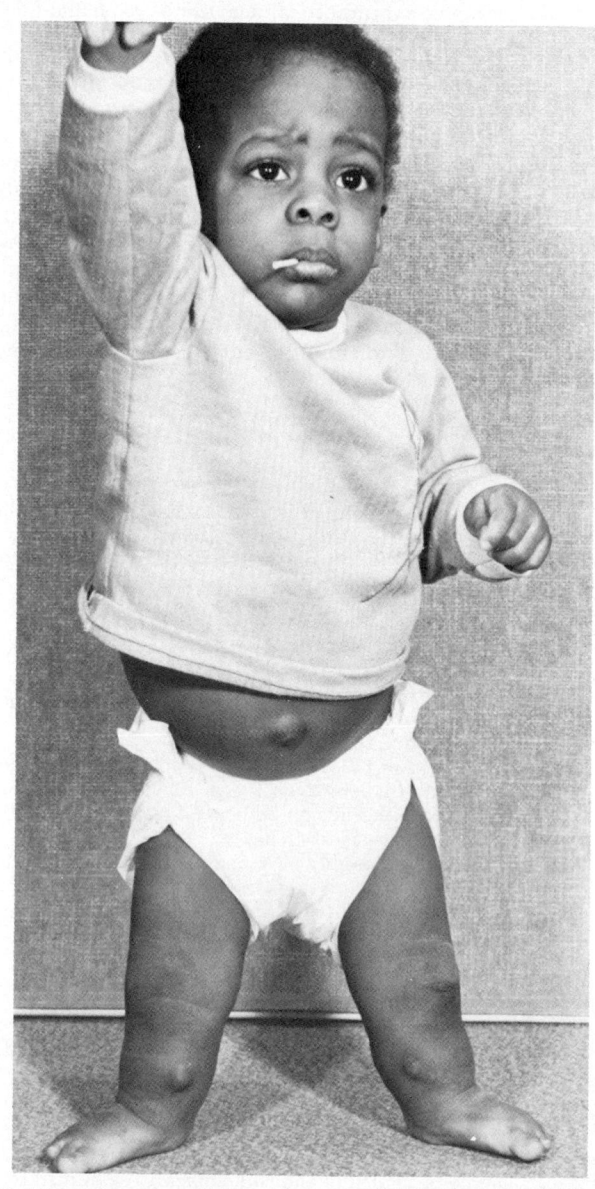

350. Note bilateral medial protuberance of the underlying tibial apices

MESOMELIC DYSPLASIA, REINHARDT-PFEIFFER TYPE

Includes: Dysplasie mésomélique, type Reinhardt-Pfeiffer
Mesomele Dysplasie, Typ Reinhardt-Pfeiffer
Displasia mesomiélica, tipo Reinhardt-Pfeiffer
Ulnofibular dysplasia, Reinhardt-Pfeiffer type
Hypoplasia of ulna and fibula

Excludes: All other forms of mesomelic dysplasia
Dyschondrosteosis (308)
Robinow syndrome (876)
Acromesomelic dysplasias
Acrodysostosis (16)
Chondroectodermal dysplasia (156)

Minimal Diagnostic Criteria: Moderate short stature with mesomelic shortening of the limbs. The lower legs are laterally bowed and at the apex of the angulation there is a cutaneous dimple. Short, triangular and thickened fibula radiographically. Dysplastic distal ulna and bowed radius with subluxation or dislocation at the elbows.

Clinical Findings: The stature is disproportionately and moderately short. Lateral bowing of the shortened forearms occurs with limited pronation and supination. Hands and fingers are normal but there is moderate ulnar deviation of the hands at the wrists. The lower legs are disproportionately short and the distal third is often thickened in diameter. They are laterally bowed with a brown pigmented cutaneous dimple at the bend. The feet are flat and often slightly adducted. Adult height is 150-169 cm. Intelligence is normal. Radiologically, marked shortening of the distal ulna occurs with a prominent interosseal ridge in the proximal portion. The radius is bowed and the distal end extends over the ulna and forms an anomalous articular surface for the carpal bones which are deformed and fused on occasion. The proximal head of the radius is subluxated or dislocated. The articulating distal humerus is often dysplastic. The proximal fibula is markedly shortened and only extends up to midshaft of the tibia. There is marked bowing and angulation of the shaft of the fibula which in the anteroposterior view has a triangular configuration. The tibia is thick and short, and in midshaft there may be a mild valgus deformity. The hypoplastic distal epiphysis of the tibia and the shortened distal fibula cause a marked lateral angulation of the distal articular surface towards the talus. Both the talus and the calcaneus are mildly deformed.

Complications
I   **Derived:** Some patients have a tendency for swelling of the lower legs. The skeletal deformities may progress with age.
II **Associated:** Mild myopia and strabismus

Etiology: Autosomal dominant with marked variation in the phenotypic expression.† McK *19140

Pathogenesis: —

Related Facts
I   **Sex Ratio:** M1:F1†
II **Risk of Occurrence:**   ?
III **Risk of Recurrence for**
    Patient's Sib: If parent is affected 1 in 2 (50%) for each offspring to be affected; otherwise not increased
    Patient's Child: 1 in 2
IV **Age of Detectability:** —
V   **Prevalence:** —

Treatment
I   **Primary Prevention:** Genetic counseling
II **Secondary Prevention:** Surgery may be indicated for correction of the cutaneous dimples
III **Other Therapy:** —

Prognosis: Normal life span

Detection of Carrier: Careful clinical and radiologic examination is required for detection of a mildly affected individual.

†**Special Considerations:** This condition has been described in only 1 family. Four males and 10 females, of 15 members studied in 4 generations, were affected. There was marked clinical and radiographic variation of the phenotypic expression between sibs in the same family and between the parents and sibs. In 2 of the affected members only the upper limbs were involved.

References:
Kaitila, I.I. et al: Mesomelic skeletal dysplasias. Clin. Orthop: 114:94, 1976.
Reinhardt, K. and Pfeiffer, R.A.: Ulno-fibulare Dysplasie. Eine autosomal dominant vererbte Mikromesomelie ähnlich dem Nievergelt-Syndrom. Fortschr. Geb. Roentgenstr. Nuklearmed. 107:379, 1967.

Contributor: Ilkka I. Kaitila

Editor's Computerized Descriptors: Skin, Skel.

MESOMELIC DYSPLASIA, WERNER TYPE

Includes: Dysplasie tibiale avec anomalies digitales
Mesomele Dysplasie, Typ Werner
Displasia mesomiélica, tipo Werner
Aplasia of tibia with polydactyly and absent thumbs

Excludes: Other forms of mesomelic dysplasia
Dyschondrosteosis (308)
Robinow syndrome (876)
Acromesomelic dysplasias
Acrodysostosis (16)
Chondroectodermal dysplasia (156)
Cleft hand and absent tibia syndrome
Unilateral absence of tibia with polydactyly†

Minimal Diagnostic Criteria: Absent or hypoplastic tibia with polydactyly and absence of the thumbs.

Clinical Findings: Dwarfism due to marked shortening of the lower legs with polydactyly and absence of the thumbs. In most cases there is aplasia or severe hypoplasia of the tibia, whereas the fibula is normal; the proximal head of the fibula is posteriorly and laterally dislocated and lies lateral to the middle shaft of the femur. The distal end of the fibula extends down to the lateral side of the foot. The patellae are hypoplastic. The forearms are normal, but the carpal bones may be fused; range of movement is limited at the wrists. The thumbs may be absent and replaced by 1 or 2 extra fingers. Similarly, there are 2-4 extra toes which are rudimentary and preaxially located. Intelligence is normal.

Radiologically, the tibia is rudimentary or totally absent and has no growth plates. The bones in the ankle are deformed and the number of metatarsals and phalanges increased. In the hand, even the extra fingers appear normal with 3 phalanges and normal metacarpal bones. There are no thumbs.

Complications
I **Derived:** The foot deformity with polysyndactyly has a functional resemblance to severe clubfoot deformity.
II **Associated:** —

Etiology: Autosomal dominant with marked variability in phenotypic expression.

Pathogenesis: The short stature presumably results from the absence of growth plates of the tibia.

Related Facts
I   **Sex Ratio:** M1:F1
II **Risk of Occurrence:** ?
III **Risk of Recurrence for**
    Patient's Sib: If parent is affected 1 in 2 (50%) for each offspring to be affected; otherwise not increased.
    Patient's Child: 1 in 2
IV **Age of Detectability:** At birth
V   **Prevalence:** ?

Treatment
I   **Primary Prevention:** Genetic counseling
II **Secondary Prevention:** —
III **Other Therapy:** Orthopedic surgery to remove the supernumerary digits.

Prognosis: Normal life span

Detection of Carrier: Careful clinical and radiographic examination of the parents and sibs in order to detect a mildly affected relative.

†Special Considerations: In order to elucidate the variability in phenotypic expression of this dysplasia, a report is cited: The father of 2 identically affected daughters with severely hypoplastic tibiae and with polydactyly and absent thumbs, had identical manifestations in his hands whereas the tibiae were completely normal.

Several reports describe association of unilateral absence of the tibia with other malformations such as poly(syn)dactyly. Instead of polydactyly, 1 report describes a dysplastic radius. A lethal congenital heart defect (truncus arteriosus and ventricular septal defect) was present in a newborn with unilateral aplasia of the tibia and polysyndactyly. The mode of inheritance of these dysplasias usually has been autosomal dominant; some may represent a form of the mesomelic dysplasia, Werner type.

References:
Eaton, G.O. and McKusick, V.A.: A seemingly unique polydactyly-syndactyly syndrome in four persons in three generations. In Bergsma, D. (ed.): Part III. Limb Malformations. Birth Defects: Orig. Art. Ser., vol. V, no 3. New York: The National Foundation-March of Dimes, 1969, p. 221.
Pashayan, H. et al: Bilateral aplasia of the tibia, polydactyly and absent thumbs in father and daughter. J. Bone Joint Surg. 53-B: 495, 1971.
Werner, P.: Ueber einen seltenen Fall von Zwergwuchs. Arch. Gynaekol. 104:278, 1915.

Contributor: **Ilkka I. Kaitila**

Editor's Computerized Descriptor: Skel.

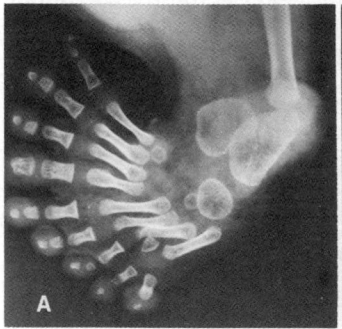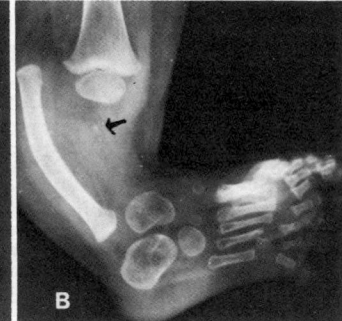

351. A) Preaxial polydactyly with 4th toe from medial aspect appearing as the hallux; postaxial polydactyly with a trapezoidal 8th metatarsal; B) absent tibia with rudimentary calcified proximal remnant; bowed and dislocated fibula

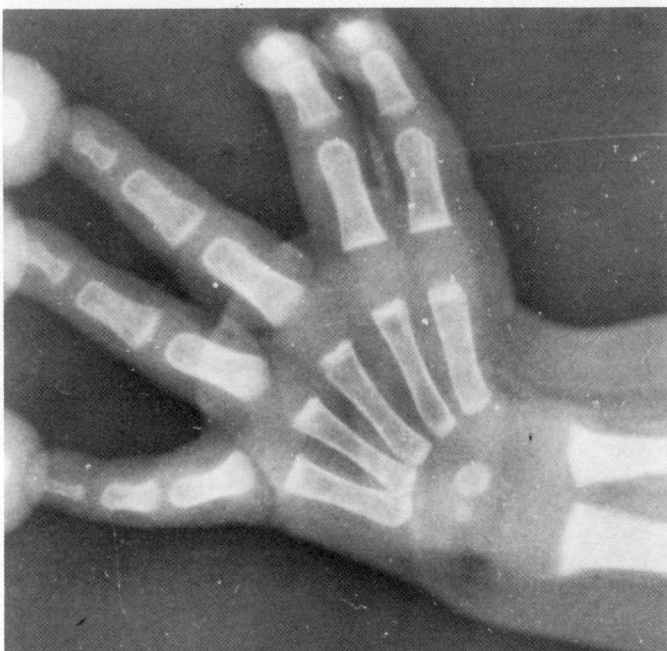

352. Digitalized thumb with syndactyly of 1st and 2nd digits

METACHONDROMATOSIS

Includes: Métachondromatose
Metacondromatosis

Excludes: Multiple cartilaginous exostoses† (685)
Enchondromatosis† (345)

Minimal Diagnostic Criteria: Both exostoses and enchondromata in the same patient.

Clinical Findings: Exostotic lesions in the hands and long bones in a patient who is unusually short. In contrast to multiple exostoses, the osteochondromata point toward the growth plate. Furthermore, they frequently regress and may actually disappear. Radiologic examination reveals evidence of both exostoses and enchondromata. The exostoses frequently involve the hands as well as the long bones and the enchondromata may be seen in various growth plates. The spine may be involved with irregularity of the end plates.

Complications
I   **Derived:**   Short stature secondary to enchondromata in the growth plates of the long bones. Deformity and limitation of function of fingers due to exostoses.
II **Associated:** —

Etiology: Autosomal dominant trait

Pathogenesis: Iliac crest biopsy has demonstrated typical lobulated enchondromata. The exostoses are histopathologically indistinguishable from both solitary and multiple exostoses.

Related Facts
I   **Sex Ratio:**   ?
II   **Risk of Occurrence:**   Rare
III **Risk of Recurrence for**
     Patient's Sib: 1 in 2 if parent is affected; otherwise negligible
     Patient's Child: 1 in 2
IV   **Age of Detectability:**   Infancy to early childhood
V   **Prevalence:** —

Treatment
I   **Primary Prevention:**   Genetic counseling
II   **Secondary Prevention:**   Orthopedic surgery to remove exostoses if they produce pain, deformity, or limitation of function.
III **Other Therapy:** —

Prognosis: ? No malignancies have been reported.

Detection of Carrier: —

†**Special Considerations:**   This disorder must be distinguished from both multiple cartilaginous exostoses and enchondromatosis. The presence of both lesions in the same patient, the fact that the exostoses point toward the epiphyses, and frequently occur in the hands are differentiating features of this disorder.

References:
Lachman, R.S. et al: Metachondromatosis. In Bergsma, D. (ed.): Skeletal Dysplasias. Birth Defect: Orig. Art. Ser., vol. X, no. 9. Miami: Symposia Specialists for The National Foundation-March of Dimes, 1974, p. 171.
Maroteaux, P.: La metachondromatose. Z. Kinderheilkd. 109:246, 1971.

Contributors: **Ralph S. Lachman**
David L. Rimoin

Editor's Computerized Descriptor: Skel.

METACHROMATIC LEUKODYSTROPHIES

Includes: Leucodystrophie métachromatique
Metachromatische Leukodystrophien
Leucodistrofias metacromáticas
Cerebral sclerosis, degenerative diffuse-Scholz type
Metachromatic form of diffuse cerebral sclerosis
Lipidosis, sulfatide
Cerebroside sulfatidosis

Excludes: Globoid cell leukodystrophy (415)
Sudanophilic leukodystrophy
Pelizaeus-Merzbacher syndrome (803)
Other leukodystrophies of nervous system
Other degenerative conditions of nervous system

Minimal Diagnostic Criteria: The late infantile form can be suspected on the basis of clinical progression and is aided by a positive family history. The laboratory findings which can be of help are an increase in CSF protein and a prolonged nerve conduction time.

In the juvenile and adult form the diagnosis is less evident clinically, and may be suspected on the basis of the clinical picture plus increased CSF protein, prolonged nerve conduction times or the demonstration of metachromatic material on peripheral nerve biopsy. In all forms of the disease the diagnosis can be established by demonstration of the enzymatic defect in white cells or skin fibroblasts.†

Clinical Findings: There are 3 clinical forms of this leukodystrophy: a late infantile form, a juvenile form and an adult form.

Late infantile metachromatic leukodystrophy: The child is usually normal until approximately 12-16 months of life. Early symptoms are a failure of further motor development particularly in terms of function of the lower limbs followed by progressive loss of the ability to walk. The child then regresses to hanging on to objects to stand with a genu recurvatum. Following these symptoms there is a progression of involvement of the upper limbs. Some patients may show nystagmus. By the age of 2 or 2 1/2 the patient is unable to pull himself to a sitting position, has dysarthria, is hypotonic and may have difficulty with swallowing. Since both the central and peripheral nervous systems are involved the child may have spasticity and hyperreflexia or hypotonicity and hyporeflexia. At times there are combinations of both the decreased reflexes in the lower limbs and increased reflexes in the upper limbs. Eventually the child loses speech and it is difficult to tell if the child is in contact with his surroundings. However, prior to loss of speech mentation seems to be relatively preserved and seizures are an uncommon phenomenon. There may be involvement of the retina with optic atrophy or retinal changes.

Juvenile metachromatic leukodystrophy: Is more likely to present as ataxia as an initial symptom. There is then progressive involvement of gait and a slower progression than one sees with the late infantile form.

Adult metachromatic leukodystrophy: May present as a dementia or may present with involvement of basal ganglia and long tract findings. The progression is one of increasing dementia often with behavioral disturbance.

Complications
I **Derived:** Progressive loss of motor function, aspiration pneumonia, urinary tract infections and a bedridden patient
II **Associated:** —

Etiology: The basic defect in the disease is a failure of the degradation of sulfatide (the sulfate ester of galactocerebroside). The enzymatic defect is the lack of the lysosomal enzyme, cerebroside sulfatase. This defect is inherited as an autosomal recessive. McK *25000, *25020

Pathogenesis: Metachromatic leukodystrophy is a turn-over disorder of sulfatide metabolism which is abnormally slow. The defective cerebroside sulfatase activity causes a widespread increase in sulfatides including brain, peripheral nerve, gallbladder, testes, liver and pancreas. Associated with the sulfatide accumulation is the progressive breakdown of membranes of the myelin sheath which itself contains abnormal amounts of sulfatide. The disease can be diagnosed in utero by demonstration of the enzymatic defect in amniotic cells as well as at birth from leukocytes or from skin fibroblasts.

Related Facts
I **Sex Ratio:** M1:F1
II **Risk of Occurrence:** 1 in 40,000 births in Northern Sweden
III **Risk of Recurrence for**
    Patient's Sib: 1 in 4 (25%) for each offspring to be affected
    Patient's Child: Not increased unless mate is carrier or homozygote. (Late infantile and juvenile forms are lethal prior to reproductive age.)
IV **Age of Detectability:** The condition can be diagnosed at birth using leukocytes or skin fibroblasts. In utero detection is feasible.
V **Prevalence:** ?

Treatment
I **Primary Prevention:** Genetic counseling
II **Secondary Prevention:** —
III **Other Therapy:** Supportive as indicated

Prognosis: Late infantile form: Death 2-4 years after time of diagnosis. Juvenile form: Death 4-6 years after diagnosis. Adult form: ?

Detection of Carrier: The heterozygote can be detected by enzymatic assay of leukocytes or skin fibroblasts using the arylsulfate assay. Carriers have 40-60% of the activity of control patients.

†**Special Considerations:** A special form of this disease exists in which there is the accumulation of not only sulfatide but also sulfated mucopolysaccharides. In addition there is also storage of gangliosides in cerebral cortex. The accumulated sulfated mucopolysaccharide resembles heparan sulfate. These patients have a distinctive granulation abnormality in their leukocytes and have a deficiency not only of sulfatase A but also of sulfatase B and sulfatase C (a trisulfatase deficiency).

References:
Austin, J. et al: Metachromatic leukodystrophy (MLD) VIII. MLD in adults; diagnosis and pathogenesis. Arch. Neurol. 18:225, 1968.
Kaback, M.M. and Howell, R.R.: Infantile metachromatic leukodystrophy. Heterozygote detection in skin fibroblasts and possible application to intrauterine diagnosis. N. Engl. J. Med. 282:1336, 1970.
Percy, A.K. and Brady, R.O.: Metachromatic leukodystrophy: Diagnosis with samples of venous blood. Science 161:594, 1968.

Contributor: **James H. Austin**

Editor's Computerized Descriptors: Eye, Speech, Skel., Muscle, Nerve

METAPHYSEAL CHONDRODYSPLASIA, TYPE JANSEN

Includes: Chondrodysplasie métaphysaire type Jansen
Metaphysäre Chondrodysplasie, Typ Jansen
Condrodisplasia metafisaria, tipo Jansen
Metaphyseal dysostosis, type Jansen

Excludes: Other rare types of severe metaphyseal chondrodysplasia
Enchondromatosis (345)
Marfucci syndrome
Hypophosphatasia (516)

Minimal Diagnostic Criteria: Dwarfism, peculiar facies, severe metaphyseal chondrodysplasia.

Clinical Findings: Progressive, short-limb dwarfism with contractural deformities of the joints and expansion of the ends of the long bones. Adult height about 120 cm. Peculiar facies. Often elevated serum calcium levels.† Diagnostic radiographic findings: expanded, cupped metaphyses with severely disorganized enchondral ossification, progressive sclerosis of the skull. Minor epiphyseal, diaphyseal and spinal changes.

Complications
I   **Derived:** Severe, early progressive osteoarthritic changes, kyphoscoliosis.
II **Associated:** —

Etiology: Autosomal dominant; McK *15640

Pathogenesis: Disorganized metaphyseal ossification with presence of irregular masses of abnormal cartilage in the metaphyseal regions.

Related Facts
I   **Sex Ratio:** M1:F1
II   **Risk of Occurrence:** Minimal
III **Risk of Recurrence for**
    Patient's Sib: If parent is affected 1 in 2 (50%) for each offspring to be affected; otherwise not increased.
    Patient's Child: 1 in 2
IV **Age of Detectability:** Infancy by radiographic features.
V   **Prevalence:** Very rare. About 10 verified cases have been reported.

Treatment
I   **Primary Prevention:** Genetic counseling
II   **Secondary Prevention:** Physiotherapy
III **Other Therapy:** Orthopedic treatment

Prognosis: Normal life span

Detection of Carrier: —

†**Special Considerations:** It is important to distinguish this disorder from metabolic disorders, especially rickets, as in presence of hypercalcemia, vitamin D therapy may be harmful.

References:
Holthusen, W. et al: The skull in metaphyseal chondrodysplasia, type Jansen. Pediatr. Radiol. 3:137, 1975.
Jansen, M.: Über atypische Chondrodystrophie (Achondroplasie) und über eine noch nicht beschriebene angeborene Wachstumsstörung des Knochensystems: Metaphysäre Dysostose. Z. Orthop. Chir. 61:253, 1934.
Sutcliffe, J. and Stanley, P.: Metaphyseal chondrodysplasias. Prog. Pediatr. Radiol. 4:250, 1973.

Contributor: **K.S. Kozlowski**

Editor's Computerized Descriptors: Face, Skel.

METAPHYSEAL CHONDRODYSPLASIA, TYPE MCKUSICK

Includes: Chondrodysplasie métaphysaire récessive autosomique, type McKusick
Metaphysäre Chondrodysplasie, Typ McKusick
Condrodisplasia metafisaria, tipo McKusick
Cartilage-hair hypoplasia

Excludes: Other rare types of moderately severe metaphyseal chondrodysplasia
Hypophosphatemic rickets and other types of "renal rickets"
Hypophosphatasia (516)
Hypochondroplasia (510)
Dyschondrosteosis (308)

Minimal Diagnostic Criteria: Short-limb dwarfism. Fine sparse hair. Metaphyseal chondrodysplasia with predominant peripheral involvement.

Clinical Findings: Progressive short-limb dwarfism with predominant peripheral involvement. Fine sparse hair, eyebrows, and lashes, otherwise normal head, and skull. Adult height about 120 cm. Often characteristic radiographic findings: metaphyseal chondrodysplasia with predominant hands, foot, and knee involvement; hypermobility of fingers; minimal-to-moderate spinal changes. There is considerable variability of expressivity of pleiotropic effects.

Complications
I   **Derived:** Early osteoarthritic changes. Equinovarus deformity of the feet subsequent to overgrowth of the fibula.
II **Associated:** Malabsorption, Hirschsprung disease and impaired cellular immunity with chronic neutro- and lymphopenia sometimes reported.†

Etiology: Autosomal recessive; McK *25025

Pathogenesis: Relation between ectodermal and bone defects and associated diseases unclear.

Related Facts
I   **Sex Ratio:** M1:F1
II   **Risk of Occurrence:** With exception of some inbred groups, minimal.
III **Risk of Recurrence for**
    Patient's Sib: 1 in 4 (25%) for each offspring to be affected.
    Patient's Child: Not increased unless mate is carrier or homozygote.
IV **Age of Detectability:** Early preschool age.
V   **Prevalence:** 170 in 100,000 among Amish population in the U.S.A. Increased gene frequency in some areas in Finland.

Treatment
I   **Primary Prevention:** Genetic counseling
II   **Secondary Prevention:** Physiotherapy
III **Other Therapy:** Orthopedic treatment.

Prognosis: Normal life span if treated.

Detection of Carrier: ?

†**Special Considerations:** Affected individuals should avoid smallpox vaccinations and be guarded against all viral infections.

References:
Lux, S.E. et al: Chronic neutropenia and abnormal cellular immunity in cartilage-hair hypoplasia. N. Engl. J. Med. 282:231, 1970.
Maroteaux, P. et al: Les formes partielles de la dysostose metaphysaire. Presse Med. 71:1523, 1963.
McKusick, V.A. et al: Dwarfism in the Amish. II. Cartilage-hair hypoplasia. Bull. Johns Hopk. Hosp. 116:285, 1965.
Ray, H.C. and Dorst, J.P.: Cartilage-hair hypoplasia. Prog. Pediatr. Radiol. 4:270, 1973.

Contributor: **K.S. Kozlowski**

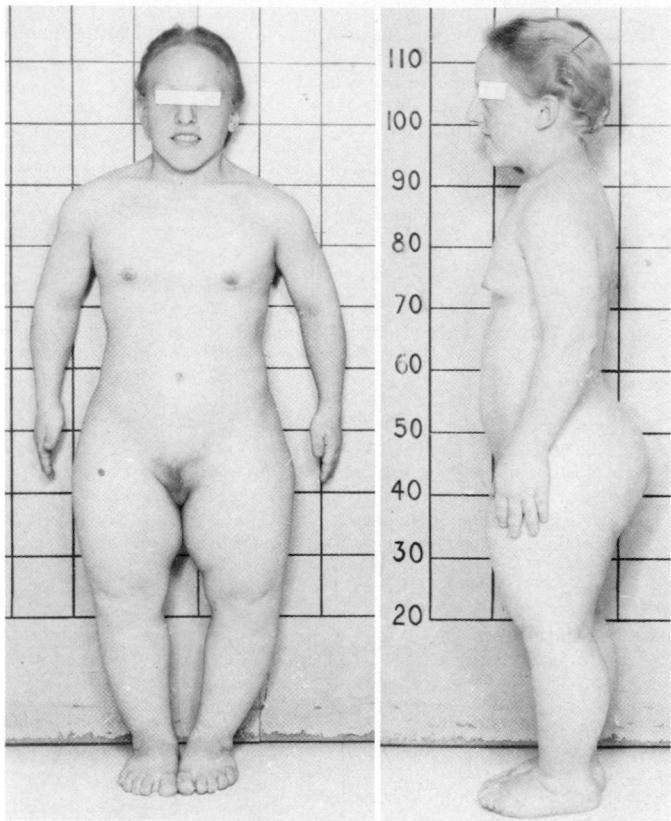

353. Note mild bowing of femurs and tibiae, excessively long fibulae, and sparse, short blond hair which has never been cut

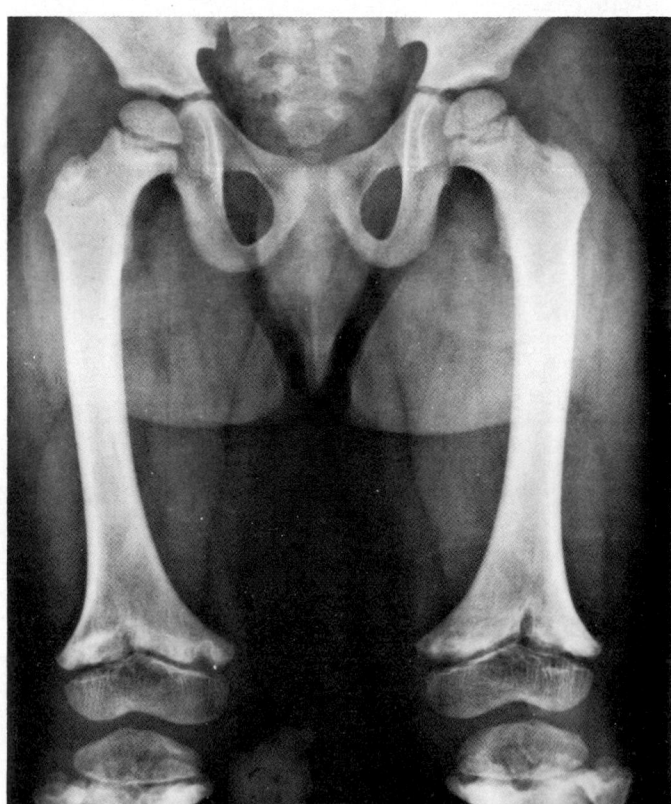

354. Long bones are short with flared ends; metaphyseal zones of provisional calcification are scalloped and irregular, but of normal density

METAPHYSEAL CHONDRODYSPLASIA, TYPE SCHMID

Includes: Chondrodysplasie métaphysaire dominante, type Schmid
Metaphysäre Chondrodysplasie, Typ Schmid
Condrodisplasia metafisaria, tipo Schmid
Metaphyseal dysostosis, type Schmid

Excludes: Other rare types of moderately severe metaphyseal chondrodysplasia
Hypophosphatemic rickets and other types of "renal rickets"†
Hypophosphatasia (516)
Hypochondroplasia (510)
Dyschondrosteosis (308)

Minimal Diagnostic Criteria: Shortening of stature. Normal head. Moderately severe metaphyseal chondrodysplasia.

Clinical Findings: Moderate, progressive shortening of stature with bowed legs and waddling gait. Adult height about 140 cm. Characteristic radiographic findings: expanded, cupped metaphyses with disorganized metaphyseal ossification. Minimal epiphyseal, diaphyseal and spinal changes. Coxa vara and genu varum. Normal skull.

Complications
I   **Derived:** Coxa and genua vara. Early progressive osteoarthritis.
II   **Associated:** —

Etiology: Autosomal dominant; McK *15650

Pathogenesis: Disorganized metaphyseal ossification, biochemical defect not defined.†

Related Facts
I   **Sex Ratio:** M1:F1
II   **Risk of Occurrence:** Minimal
III   **Risk of Recurrence for**
    Patient's Sib: If parent is affected 1 in 2 (50%) for each offspring to be affected.
    Patient's Child: 1 in 2
IV   **Age of Detectability:** Early preschool age
V   **Prevalence:** Rare

Treatment
I   **Primary Prevention:** Genetic counseling
II   **Secondary Prevention:** Physiotherapy
III   **Other Therapy:** Orthopedic treatment

Prognosis: Normal life span

Detection of Carrier: —

†**Special Considerations:** It is important to distinguish this disorder from metabolic diseases, especially rickets, as vitamin D therapy is unnecessary and may be harmful.

References:
Schmid, F.: Beitrag zur Dysostosis enchondralis metaphysaria. Monatschr. Kinderheilkd. 97:393, 1949.
Sutcliffe, J. and Stanley, P.: Metaphyseal chondrodysplasias. Prog. Pediatr. Radiol. 4:250, 1973.

Contributor: **K.S. Kozlowski**

Editor's Computerized Descriptor: Skel.

METAPHYSEAL CHONDRODYSPLASIA WITH THYMOLYMPHOPENIA

Includes: Chondrodysplasie métaphysaire avec thymolymphopé-
nie
Metaphysäre Chondrodysplasie mit Thymolymphopenie
Condrodisplasia metafisaria con timolinfopenia
Metaphyseal dysostosis with Swiss type agammaglobulinemia
Variant form of Swiss type agammaglobulinemia

Excludes: Swiss type agammaglobulinemia without bone disease
Other immunologic defects
Metaphyseal osteochondrodystrophies
Hypoparathyroidism

Minimal Diagnostic Criteria: Recurrent, severe infections in a
child with ectodermal dysplasia, absence of thymic-dependent and
thymic-independent lymphoid tissue, and metaphyseal chondrodysplasia.

Clinical Findings: At birth, short-limbed short stature, and ectodermal dysplasia. Cutis laxa, scalp alopecia and ichthyosiform dermatosis may be present. Within weeks, failure to thrive and recurrent bacterial, fungal and viral infections. Severe combined immune deficiency (lymphopenia, total or selective immunoglobulin
deficiency). Radiologically: metaphyseal chondrodysplasia, pelvic
dysplasia (flat acetabulae). Absent tonsils, adenoids and thymus.

Complications
I **Derived:** Recurrent, severe infections
II **Associated:** —

Etiology: Autosomal recessive; McK *20090

Pathogenesis: Relation between the thymo-lymphoid and bone
defects unclear.

Related Facts
I   **Sex Ratio:** M1:F1
II **Risk of Occurrence:** Low
III **Risk of Recurrence for**
    Patient's Sib: 1 in 4 (25%) for each offspring to be affected.
    Patient's Child: No long-term survival
IV **Age of Detectability:** In neonatal period with appropriate
    methods
V   **Prevalence:** —

Treatment
I   **Primary Prevention:** Genetic counseling
II **Secondary Prevention:** Reconstitution of the lymphoid
    stem cells may be attempted.
III **Other Therapy:** Protective isolation; antibiotics

Prognosis: Death in infancy

Detection of Carrier: —

Special Considerations: —

References:
Alexander W.J. and Dunbar J.S.: Unusual bone changes in thymic
  alymphoplasia. Ann. Radiol. 11:389, 1968.
Gatti R.A. et al: Hereditary lymphopenic agammaglobulinemia
  associated with a distinctive form of short-limbed dwarfism and
  ectodermal dysplasia. J. Pediatr. 75:675, 1969.
Sutcliffe J. and Stanley P.: Metaphyseal chondrodysplasias. Progr.
  Pediatr. Radiol. 4:250, 1973.

Contributor:　　**K.S. Kozlowski**

Editor's Computerized Descriptors: Nasoph., Skel., Lymphatic,
Thymus, Skin

METATROPIC DYSPLASIA

Includes: Nanisme métatropique
Metatropischer Zwergwuchs
Enanismo metatrófico
Hyperplastic form of chondrodystrophy
Metatropic dwarfism

Excludes: Achondroplasia (10)
Mucopolysaccharidosis IV (678)
Asphyxiating thoracic dysplasia (91)
Kniest dysplasia (557)

Minimal Diagnostic Criteria: Skeletal dysplasia with tongue-
like flattening of the vertebral bodies, short ribs, progressing kyphoscoliosis, crescent-like iliac wings, osseous hyperplasia of the
trochanteric region and the metaphyses of the tubular bones,
irregular metaphyses and epiphyses, normal cranial vault and
viscerocranium, dysplastic skull base.†

Clinical Findings: In infancy, long narrow thorax and relatively
short limbs; rapidly progressing kyphoscoliosis. In later infancy
and childhood, reversion of body proportions with development of
short-spine dwarfism. Radiologically, severe spondyloepimetaphyseal dysplasia of the skeleton.

Complications
I **Derived:** Severe progressive kyphoscoliosis, early arthroses
II **Associated:** —

Etiology: Heterogeneous. Both autosomal dominant and autosomal recessive transmission have been observed. McK *25060

Pathogenesis: ? Shortening of the tubular bones with irregular
metaphyseal and epiphyseal ossification. Irregular arrangement
of bone trabeculae which contain islands of cartilage. Endochondral ossification processes are grossly reduced in quantity.

Related Facts
I   **Sex Ratio:** M1:F1
II **Risk of Occurrence:** ?
III **Risk of Recurrence for**
    Patient's Sib: When autosomal recessive or autosomal
      dominant, see Table I AR or AD, respectively.
    Patient's Child: When autosomal recessive or autosomal
      dominant, see Table I AR or AD, respectively.
IV **Age of Detectability:** At birth by radiology of skeleton,
    especially lateral view of the spine
V   **Prevalence:** ?

Treatment
I   **Primary Prevention:** Genetic counseling
II **Secondary Prevention:** Intensive orthopedic care aiming at
    prevention of kyphoscoliosis and secondary position defects
III **Other Therapy:** —

Prognosis: Guarded because of incapacitating physical deformities. Death frequently occurs in early infancy. Surviving patients
may reach at least their 3rd decade of life. Ultimate body height
between 110 and 120 cm.

Detection of Carrier: —

†**Special Considerations:** Metatropic dwarfism has been confused with achondroplasia and Morquio mucopolysaccharidosis.
Cases of "hyperplastic chondrodystrophy" of the older literature
probably had metatropic dwarfism. There exist one or more
closely related, though ill-defined conditions (pseudometatropic
dwarfism) necessitating the observance of rigid diagnostic criteria. No criteria are available to distinguish the autosomal recessive from the autosomal dominant form.

References:
Maroteaux, P. et al: Der metatropische Zwergwuchs. Arch. Kinder-
  heilkd. 173:211, 1966.
Spranger, J. et al: Bone Dysplasias. Philadelphia: J.B. Saunders,
  Co., 1974.

Contributor: **Jürgen W. Spranger**

Editor's Computerized Descriptor: Skel.

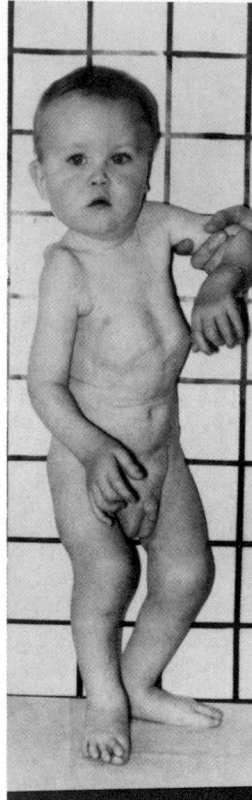 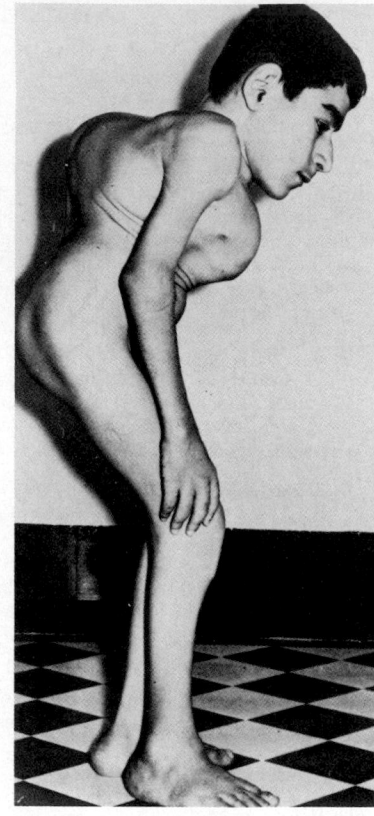

355. Note progressive skeletal changes

METHIONINE MALABSORPTION SYNDROME

Includes: Malabsorption de la méthionine
Methionin-Malabsorption
Síndrome de malabsorción de la metionina
Oast-house urine disease

Excludes: Hartnup disorder (453)

Minimal Diagnostic Criteria: Alpha-hydroxybutyric acid in urine and feces in amounts related to the methionine intake. This compound believed to account for odor. Its formation occurs in the intestine from bacterial degradation of methionine. Methionine excretion increased in feces but not in the urine under usual endogenous conditions. Loading by mouth with methionine increases fecal excretion of many amino acids; loading with branched-chain compounds does not affect methionine excretion.

Clinical Findings: Two probands (English and Belgian) with this trait have been described. At diagnosis, they were mentally retarded. Physical development was normal. Clinical findings included white hair, blue eyes, convulsions, intermittent diarrhea, and an intermittent sweet odor to the urine and the patient. The level of dietary intake of protein determined the presence or absence of intestinal symptoms, seizures and odor; a high intake provoked symptoms.

Complications
I   **Derived:**   Diarrhea; seizures and mental retardation seem related to metabolic disorder; whether they are incidental findings cannot be ruled out, but seems unlikely.
II   **Associated:**   —

Etiology: Presumed to be autosomal recessive.† McK *25090

Pathogenesis: Proposed deficiency of specific intestinal membrane transport system for L-methionine

Related Facts
I   **Sex Ratio:**   ?
II   **Risk of Occurrence:**   ?
III   **Risk of Recurrence for**
   Patient's Sib: Presumably 1 in 4 (25%) for each offspring to be affected
   Patient's Child: Not increased unless mate is carrier or homozygote.
IV   **Age of Detectability:**   Presumably at birth
V   **Prevalence:**   ?

Treatment
I   **Primary Prevention:**   Genetic counseling
II   **Secondary Prevention:**   Low methionine intake, eg low animal protein or soy protein diet, improves symptoms and EEG.
III   **Other Therapy:**   —

Prognosis: ?

Detection of Carrier: Evidence for partial intestinal transport defect.

†Special Considerations: Belgian male proband was youngest of 12. Both parents show partial trait. Smith and Strang's female infant with "oast-house" odor had similar appearance and clinical symptoms.Her urine contained α-hydroxybutyric acid, but phenylpyruvic acid was also present, plus many hydroxy-, keto- and amino acids.
   Only case of "oast-house urine syndrome" reported to date but probably similar to case reported by Hooft et al.

References:
Hooft, C. et al: Further investigation in the methionine malabsorption syndrome. Helv. Paediatr. Acta 23:334, 1968.
Jepson, J. B. et al: An inborn error of metabolism with the urinary excretion of hydroxyacids, ketoacids, and aminoacids. Lancet 2:1334, 1958.
Smith, A. J. and Strang, L. B.: An inborn error of metabolism with the urinary excretion of alpha-hydroxy-butyric acid and phenylpyruvic acid. Arch. Dis. Child. 33:109, 1958.

Contributor: **Charles R. Scriver**

Editor's Computerized Descriptors: Eye, Hair, GI., Nerve

METHYLMALONIC ACIDEMIA

Includes: Acidémie méthylmalonurique
Methylmalonacidämie
Acidemia metilmalónica
Methylmalonic aciduria

Excludes: Propionic acidemia† (826)
Pernicious anemia

Minimal Diagnostic Criteria: Elevation of the concentration of methylmalonic acid in blood or urine in the absence of pernicious anemia†

Clinical Findings: Onset early in life of symptoms which may be indistinguishable from ketotic hyperglycinemia. Repeated episodes of ketoacidosis may lead to coma and may be fatal. Neutropenia is prominent, and osteoporosis and thrombocytopenia may occur. Infections are common and may precipitate life-threatening ketoacidosis. Mental retardation has been observed regularly in those surviving early infancy. Growth retardation is striking. Convulsions and EEG abnormalities may be seen. Some patients have had chronic monilial infections. Red cells are normal and megaloblastosis is absent.

Concentrations of methylmalonic acid in the plasma are elevated; they tend to approximate 10 mg/100 ml. Urinary excretions of methylmalonic acid may be over 500 mg per day. This compound is not normally detectable in blood or urine. It has also been found in the cerebrospinal fluid and in tissues of patients dying of the disease. Increased quantities of glycine are found in the blood and urine. The amounts are usually less than those of ketotic hyperglycinemia and in the range of nonketotic hyperglycinemia. Normal concentrations of glycine are also found frequently in patients who manifest elevations at other times. Concentrations of B_{12} in the blood are not low.

Complications
I   **Derived:**   Death, mental retardation
II **Associated:**   —

Etiology: Probably autosomal recessive; McK *25100

Pathogenesis: Enzymatic site of the defect is in methylmalonyl CoA mutase. This may be primary, or secondary to a defect in B$_{12}$ metabolism.

Related Facts
I   **Sex Ratio:**   M1:F1
II   **Risk of Occurrence:**   ?
III **Risk of Recurrence for**
     Patient's Sib: Probably 1 in 4 (25%) for each offspring to be affected
     Patient's Child: Probably not increased unless mate is carrier or homozygote
IV   **Age of Detectability:**   Detectable in the first days of life. This disorder is detectable in the fetus by assay of methylmalonic acid in amniotic fluid or in maternal urine.
V   **Prevalence:**   Rare

Treatment
I   **Primary Prevention:**   Genetic counseling
II   **Secondary Prevention:** B_{12} should be used in those patients who are sensitive to the vitamin. The efficacy of diets low in isoleucine, valine, threonine and methionine is under study. Avoidance of exposure to and prompt treatment of infection.
III **Other Therapy:**   Deletion of protein-containing foods and substitution of electrolyte and glucose-containing fluids in the presence of ketosis.

Prognosis: Most patients have died very early in infancy.

Detection of Carrier: ?

†**Special Considerations:** This condition is closely related to propionic acidemia. Elucidation of the fundamental defect and the mechanisms of ketosis in either condition should lead to better understanding of both, and of normal metabolism.

Genetic heterogeneity has been established in that there are now at least three distinct forms of methylmalonic acidemia, two of which are responsive to vitamin B_{12}, the second of the B_{12} sensitive forms has associated homocystinuria and cystathionuria.

References:

Nyhan, W. L. et al: Response to dietary therapy in B_{12} unresponsive methylmalonic acidemia. Pediatrics 51:539, 1973.

Oberholzer, V. G. et al: Methylmalonic aciduria: An inborn error of metabolism leading to chronic metabolic acidosis. Arch. Dis. Child. 42:492, 1967.

Rosenberg, L. E.: Methylmalonic aciduria: An inborn error leading to metabolic acidosis, long-chain ketonuria and intermittent hyperglycinemia. N. Engl. J. Med. 278:1319, 1968.

Stokke, O. et al: Methylmalonic acidemia: A new inborn error of metabolism which may cause fatal acidosis in the neonatal period. Scand. J. Clin. Lab. Invest. 20:313, 1967.

Contributor: **William L. Nyhan**

Editor's Computerized Descriptors: Skel., Nerve

MICROCEPHALY

Includes: Microcéphalie
Mikrozephalie
Microcefalia
Microencephaly

Excludes: Premature closure of cranial sutures
Congenital diplegia with small head
Relative microcephaly associated with cerebral lesions of infancy
Fetal toxoplasmosis syndrome (387)
Fetal cytomegalovirus syndrome (381)
Fetal rubella syndrome (384)

Minimal Diagnostic Criteria: Head circumference very small. In infancy normal open sutures on xray. Mental retardation.

Clinical Findings: A head circumference smaller than 2 SD below the head circumference for age (always below 17 inches maximum). The forehead is often narrow with flattened occiput. Varying degrees of mental retardation, although there is usually severe amentia. In infancy, on x-ray examination, the cranial sutures will all appear to be open. Skull thickness may be normal or increased. EEG frequently normal. Seizures present in small percentage of cases. Sloping forehead.

Complications
I   **Derived:** Mental retardation
II   **Associated:** Chorioretinitis

Etiology: Heterogeneous; autosomal recessive for true microcephaly; may follow degenerative brain disorder, birth trauma, intrauterine infection or xrays in utero. McK *25120

Pathogenesis: Microcephaly may be secondary to growth of brain and may resemble that of a 3-4 month fetus. Occipital cortex is poorly developed. Growth arrest 3-4 month fetus.

Related Facts
I   **Sex Ratio:** M1:F1 probable
II   **Risk of Occurrence:** ?
III **Risk of Recurrence for**
     Patient's Sib: When autosomal recessive 1 in 4 (25%) for each offspring to be affected
     Patient's Child: Not increased unless mate is carrier or homozygote.
IV   **Age of Detectability:** Infancy
V   **Prevalence:** ?

Treatment
I   **Primary Prevention:** Genetic counseling
II   **Secondary Prevention:** ?
III **Other Therapy:** ?

Prognosis: Poor

Detection of Carrier: ?

Special Considerations: —

References:

Ford, F. R.: Diseases of the Nervous System in Infancy, Childhood and Adolescence. Springfield: Charles C Thomas, 1966.

McKusick, V.A. et al: Chorioretinopathy with hereditary microcephaly, Arch. Ophthalmol. 75:597, 1966.

Norman, R.M. and Tingey, A.H.: Syndrome of micrencephaly, strio-cerebellar calcifications and leucodystrophy. J. Neurol. Neurosurg. Psychiatry 29:157, 1966.

Contributor: **Kenneth Shulman**

Editor's Computerized Descriptors: Skel., Nerve

MICRODONTIA (MARKER)

Includes: Microdontie
Mikrodontie
Microdoncia (Marcador)

Excludes: Fetal radiation syndrome (383)
Ectodermal dysplasia, anhidrotic (333)
Incontinentia pigmenti (526)
Chondroectodermal dysplasia (156)
Chromosome twenty-one trisomy syndrome (171)
Goniodysgenesis (439)
Teeth, pegged or absent maxillary lateral incisor (934)

Minimal Diagnostic Criteria: The involved tooth or teeth must be small enough to be outside the usual limits of variation.

Clinical Findings: The involved tooth or teeth are small in size, well beyond usual limits of variation. Microdontia is manifested in 2 forms: true generalized microdontia which is extremely rare, occurring in some cases of pituitary dwarfism and, secondly, microdontia involving a single tooth or groups of teeth. The latter commonly affects the lateral incisors and maxillary molars and, along with the reduction in size, these teeth often exhibit a change in shape.

Complications
I   **Derived:** May precipitate psychologic problems due to altered esthetic harmony.
II **Associated:** Microdontia may occur as a partial manifestation in the conditions listed under Exclusions and small teeth have been reported associated with a number of conditions including: cleft lip, Turner syndrome, focal dermal hypoplasia, lipoid proteinosis, the mucopolysaccharidoses (especially Hurler, Hunter and San Fillipo types), oculoauriculovertebral dysplasia, progeria, craniofacial dysostosis, Ehlers-Danlos syndrome, encephalofacial angiomatosis, odontodysplasia, osteogenesis imperfecta, dentinogenesis imperfecta, oculomandibulodyscephaly and monilethrix.

The most common form of microdontia (1.2 to 3.2% of general population) are peg maxillary lateral incisors. This is a discrete genetic trait which is manifest as either peg or missing maxillary lateral incisors. This tooth is also found in microform in the craniooculodental syndrome. Loss of the central mamillon of developing incisors in patients with congenital syphilis results in small screwdriver-shaped teeth. Absent or small mandibular incisors are nearly a constant feature of the ankyloglossia superior syndrome. Microdontia of a specific tooth, the maxillary 2nd primary molar, occurs in the supravalvular aortic stenosis-elfin facies syndrome.

Etiology: Essentially unknown. As one manifestation of the pleiotropic effects of gene mutations when associated with syndromes. In some cases of individual teeth, it is probably due to a gene mutation resulting in a dominantly inherited trait with variable expressivity. In the supravalvular aortic stenosis-elfin facies syndrome, possibly due to sensitivity to or excessive doses of maternal vitamin D. See Teeth, Pegged or Absent Maxillary Lateral Incisor.

Pathogenesis: Essentially unknown. Some disturbance impeding the full development of the tooth germ or germs involved either by affecting the full development of the enamel organ or secondarily by faulty development of tooth structure such as dentin or enamel.

Related Facts
I   **Sex Ratio:** M1:F1 (for microdontia in general)
II   **Risk of Occurrence:** True generalized microdontia-very rare. Individual microdontia-fairly common especially among maxillary laterals and maxillary 3rd molars.
III **Risk of Recurrence for**
     Patient's Sib: ?
     Patient's Child: ?
IV   **Age of Detectability:** At eruption of teeth by dental examination
V   **Prevalence:** For general population: 4% for 3rd molars; other teeth combined-1%, excluding maxillary lateral incisors

Treatment
I   **Primary Prevention:** —
II   **Secondary Prevention:** —
III **Other Therapy:** Restorative dentistry

Prognosis: Excellent for isolated microdontia

Detection of Carrier: —

Special Considerations: —

References:
Shafer, W.G. et al: A Textbook of Oral Pathology, 2nd Ed. Philadelphia: W.B. Saunders, 1963, p. 34.
Steinberg, A.G. et al: Hereditary generalized microdontia. J. Dent. Res. 40;58, 1961.
Woolf, C.M.: Missing maxillary lateral incisors; a genetic study. Am. J. Hum. Genet. 23:289, 1971.

Contributors: **Satish R. Rao
Carl J. Witkop, Jr.**

Editor's Computerized Descriptor: Teeth

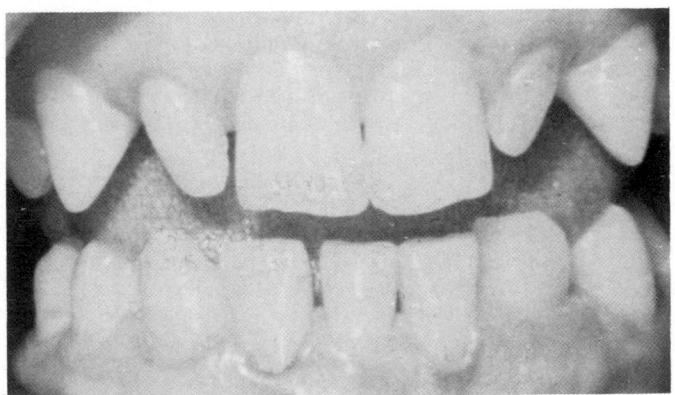

356. Peg-shaped maxillary lateral incisors

MICROPHTHALMIA

Includes: Microphtalmie
Mikrophthalmie
Microftalmia
Microphthalmos
Nanophthalmia
Eye, undersized

Excludes: Microphthalmia and digital anomalies (662)

Minimal Diagnostic Criteria: Smaller than normal eye

Clinical Findings: Microphthalmia in its pure, isolated and uncomplicated form is also known as nanophthalmia. In this case, the entire eye is smaller than normal, usually without defect except for ametropia and occasionally reduction in vision.

Fundus abnormalities have been reported such as absent or deficient retinal pigment epithelium in the posterior fundus, fluorescein perfusion delay, irregularity or patchy absence in the choriocapillaris, and mottled coloration of the fundus.

More commonly, microphthalmia is found as a small, malformed remnant of an eye within the orbit. The intraocular structures are often not grossly identifiable. The cornea may be opacified, the lens cataractous with posterior synechiae along with uveal disorganization and retinal detachment. The optic nerve may be small and abnormally shaped with poorly formed neural columns. Microphthalmia is often associated with cystic outpouchings occupying the inferior or entire orbital cavity. The small eye may be partially or totally overshadowed by an orbital cyst.

Complications
I Derived: —
II Associated: Colobomas of any portion of the eye, uveal effusion with secondary retinal and choroidal detachment, corectopia, foveal aplasia or hypoplasia, chorioretinitis, cataract, persistent hyperplastic primary vitreous, dyscranium, urogenital defects, astrocytoma of the optic nerve and chiasm, first-arch syndrome variant, glaucoma, nystagmus, hypospadias, cleft palate and trilocular heart with persistent left superior vena cava

Etiology: Autosomal recessive or autosomal dominant. Other causes include intrauterine infection, radiation, chemical agents, and chromosomal aberrations.

Pathogenesis: Usually from an involution of the primary optic vesicle and failure of closure of the fetal fissure. Failure of development of the surface ectoderm also is responsible for some cases.

Related Facts
I Sex Ratio: M1:F1
II Risk of Occurrence: Rare in its pure form
III Risk of Recurrence for
 Patient's Sib: When autosomal recessive or autosomal dominant, see Table I AR or AD, respectively.
 Patient's Child: When autosomal recessive or autosomal dominant, see Table I AR or AD, respectively.
IV Age of Detectability: At birth
V Prevalence: Relatively rare in the presence of other ocular anomalies

Treatment
I Primary Prevention: Genetic counseling
II Secondary Prevention: Correct refractive error with appropriate lenses, if possible.
III Other Therapy: Dependent upon associated abnormality. If glaucoma, medical therapy indicated; if uveal effusion, steroid therapy.

Prognosis: Visually good in the pure form. Visually poor in association with other ocular defects, depending upon the severity of the abnormalities.

Detection of Carrier: —

Special Considerations: —

References:
Bonner, J. and Ide, C.H: Astrocytoma of the optic nerve and chiasm associated with microphthalmos and orbital cyst. Br. J. Ophthalmol. 58:828, 1974.
Brockhurst, R.J.: Nanophthalmos with uveal effusion. Arch. Ophthalmol. 93:1289, 1975.
Cross, H.E. and Yoder, F.: Familial nanophthalmos. Am. J. Ophthalmol. 81:300, 1977
Warburg, M.: The heterogeneity of microphthalmia in the mentally retarded. In Bergsma, D. (ed.): Part VIII. Eye. Birth Defects: Orig. Art. Ser., vol. VII, no. 3. Baltimore:Williams & Wilkins for The National Foundation-March of Dimes, 1971, p. 136.

Contributor: **Elsa K. Rahn**

Editor's Computerized Descriptor: Eye

MICROPHTHALMIA AND DIGITAL ANOMALIES

Includes: Microphtalmie avec anomalies digitales
Mikrophthalmie und Fingerdeformitäten
Microftalmia con anomalías digitales
Dyscrania pygophalangea
Anophthalmia and digital anomalies
Digital anomalies and microphthalmia
Lenz microphthalmia

Excludes: Oculo-dento-osseous dyplasia (737)
Chromosome thirteen trisomy syndrome (168)
Meckel syndrome (634)
Microphthalmia without digital anomalies
Microphthalmia as part of other syndromes

Minimal Diagnostic Criteria: Smaller than normal or absent eye(s) with digital and possibly other defects

Clinical Findings: Characterized by microcephaly, microphthalmos with or without cyst in one or both orbits, anomalies of the pinna, cleft lip, cleft palate, sunken nose, hamartomas of the tongue, cleft epiglottis, rudimentary 6th fingers and toes, syndactyly, talipes equinovarus, cystic abnormalities of the internal organs, cardiac defects and malformations of the GU system.†

Complications
I   **Derived:** —
II   **Associated:** Widespread abnormalities throughout the body

Etiology: X-linked transmission unless part of another specific syndrome; McK *30980

Pathogenesis: Failure of development of the surface ocular ectoderm, more often an involution of the primary optic vesicle and failure of closure of the fetal fissure. Otherwise unknown or associated with other syndromes present.

Related Facts
I   **Sex Ratio:** M1:F0
II   **Risk of Occurrence:** Rare
III   **Risk of Recurrence for**
    Patient's Sib: If mother is a carrier 1 in 2 (50%) for each brother to be affected and 1 in 2 for each sister to be a carrier.
    Patient's Child: 1 in 1 (100%) for carrier daughters; not increased for sons unless wife is a carrier.
IV   **Age of Detectability:** At birth
V   **Prevalence:** Rare

Treatment
I   **Primary Prevention:** Genetic counseling
II   **Secondary Prevention:** Symptomatic and surgical treatment of presenting congenital anomalies when possible. Corrective therapy of refractive error, if indicated, and other treatment measures when feasible, such as multiple aspirations of cyst, excision of cyst alone, or excision of both the microphthalmic eye and cyst.
III   **Other Therapy:** Cosmetic improvement through progressive dilatation of the orbit by successive implants of increasingly larger size during the period of rapid growth for proper development and for maintenance of a prosthesis.

Prognosis: Varies greatly with degree of eye defects and associated defects.

Detection of Carrier: May manifest slight abnormalities.

†Special Considerations: This may represent a mild expression of more complex syndromes. Lenz reported an interesting pedigree in which the proband was born blind; the mother had only a deformity of the joints of the 5th finger, while other affected persons had narrow shoulders, double thumbs, defects of the teeth, skeleton, heart and GU system, and some had unilateral eye anomaly.

References:
Falls, H.F.: Congenital anomalies of the eye. In Symposium on Surgical and Medical Management of Anomalies of the Eye. St. Louis:C. V. Mosby Co., 1968, p. 49.
Gorlin, R.J. and Červenka, J.: Syndromes of facial clefting. Scand. J. Plast. Reconstr. Surg. 8:13, 1974.
Lenz, W.: Recessiv-geschlechtsgebundene Mikrophthalmie mit multiplen Missbildungen. Z. Kinderheilkd. 77:384, 1955.
Sugar, H.S. et al: The oculo-dento-digital dysplasia syndrome. Am. J. Ophthalmol. 61:1448, 1966.
Warburg, M.: The heterogeneity of microphthalmia in the mentally retarded. In Bergsma, D. (ed.): Part VIII. Eye. Birth Defects: Orig. Art. Ser., vol. VII, no. 3. Baltimore:Williams and Wilkins for The National Foundation-March of Dimes, 1971, p. 136.
Waring, G.O. et al: Clinicopathologic correlation of microphthalmos with cyst. Am. J. Ophthalmol. 82:714, 1976.
Yunis, J.J (ed.): Human Chromosome Methodology. New York Academic Press, 1965. p. 222.

Contributor: **Elsa K. Rahn**

Editor's Computerized Descriptors: Eye, Ear, Face, Oral, Skel., CV., GU.

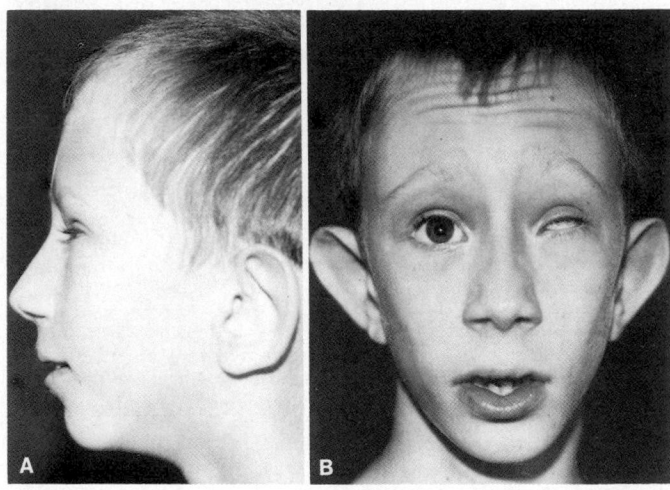

357. A) Microcephaly, micrognathia, posteriorly rotated and poorly differentiated auricles; B) microphthalmia on left; upward slanting of incompletely developed palpebral fissures; anteflexion of auricles

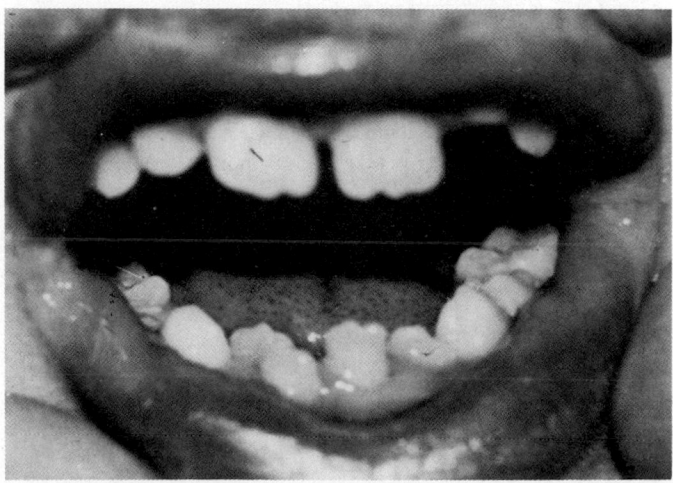

358. Agenesis of upper lateral incisors; maleruption of notched lower incisors

MICROSPHEROPHAKIA

Includes: Microsphérophakie
Mikrosphärophakie
Microesferofaquia
Congenital microphakia and spherophakia

Excludes: Acquired microphakia and spherophakia
Spherophakia-brachymorphia syndrome (893)

Minimal Diagnostic Criteria: Small spherical lens within the dilated pupil

Clinical Findings: Microphakia and spherophakia are usually concurrent. The lens has a smaller than normal diameter and is spherical in shape. The anterior-posterior measurement is increased and may cause the lens to protrude forward into the anterior chamber. This forward protrusion and close apposition of the lens to the iris may, in later life, result in glaucoma. Glaucoma in infancy is generally concomitant with abnormalities within the anterior chamber. The periphery of the lens is readily outlined with the pupil dilated. The zonules can also be visualized as radial strands between the pupillary and lens margins. Subluxation or luxation of the lens may occur from rupture of poorly developed, elongated and weakened zonules. Microspherophakia usually occurs bilaterally as an isolated phenomenon.

Complications
I   **Derived:** Myopia, cataract, glaucoma, subluxation or luxation of the lens
II **Associated:** Marchesani syndrome

Etiology: Autosomal recessive as isolated defect. May be sporadic. In association with other syndromes it follows the inheritance pattern of that symptom complex.

Pathogenesis: Arrest in development of the lens between the 5th or 6th fetal month. It has been postulated that an inadequate blood supply from the vascular tunic of the lens, or improper support secondary to faulty zonular development are possible mechanisms of pathogenesis.

Related Facts
I   **Sex Ratio:** M1:F1
II **Risk of Occurrence:** Rare
III **Risk of Recurrence for**
    Patient's Sib: When isolated defect, 1 in 4 (25%) for each offspring to be affected
    Patient's Child: Not increased unless mate is carrier or homozygote
IV **Age of Detectability:** At birth
V   **Prevalence:** Rare

Treatment
I   **Primary Prevention:** Genetic counseling
II **Secondary Prevention:** Correct existing refractive errors, usually myopia, due to the increased anterior-posterior diameter. Surgery is indicated if glaucoma occurs as a complication.
III **Other Therapy:** —

Prognosis: Generally good

Detection of Carrier: —

Special Considerations: —

References:
Duke-Elder, S.: System of Ophthalmology, vol. 3, part 2. Congenital Deformities. London:Henry Kimpton, 1963, p. 694.
Waardenburg, P. J. et al: Genetics and Ophthalmology. Springfield:C. C Thomas, 1961, vol. 1.

MICROTIA-ATRESIA

Includes: Atrésie et hypoplasie auriculaire
Mikrotie und Atresie
Microtía y atresia
Thalidomide external ear malformation
All forms of hypogenesis of pinna with or without associated atresia of the external auditory canal
Anotia
Ear, dysgenesis of

Excludes: Isolated atresia of the external auditory canal
Isolated pinna malformations
Posttraumatic or postsurgical auricular deformity with stenosis of the external auditory canal
Cryptotia (232)
Other auricular malformations
Stenosis of the external auditory canal

Minimal Diagnostic Criteria: Presence of a normal, deformed or absent pinna with or without an atretic ear canal and a maximum conductive hearing loss.†

Clinical Findings: The right ear is more frequently involved than the left. One-sixth of the patients have bilateral deformity. In a few instances microtia with or without atresia may be seen on 1 side and atresia alone on the contralateral side. The pinna may be only slightly smaller than normal and have the general configuration of a normal ear. In most instances the auricle appears crumpled and grossly deformed with only a few fleshy and cartilaginous remnants, resembling the embryologic hillocks which eventually form the pinna. In occasional patients the external ear is entirely absent. The external auditory canal may be absent, narrowed throughout its length, or show a funnel-like narrowing to complete atresia a few millimeters medial to the concha. Occasionally a tiny opening can be found anterior, inferior or in some instances posterior-superior to the normal canal position. Often these end blindly, but in rare instances may communicate with a tympanic membrane. Evidently some of these deformed misplaced canals contain ceruminous glands, since cerumen can be found in the lumen. However, others are more correctly termed preauricular pits.

Various parts of the ear may be deformed. In some instances the helix is deficient; in others the lobule is deformed. The tragus may show varying degrees of maldevelopment. Preauricular appendages may be associated. In the rare instances in which anotia occurs, there may be no palpable space between the mastoid tip and the condyloid process of the mandible due to growth of the temporomandibular joint posteriorly. In these instances, severe middle ear anomalies, hypoplasia or aplasia of the middle ear may be associated, making reconstruction of the hearing mechanism difficult or impossible. The mastoid process may be poorly developed. Occasionally thick soft tissue is found at surgery where the drumhead should be; but more commonly, a bony atresia plate of varying thickness is present. In extremely rare cases, a true tympanic membrane lies just medial to the atretic area, which may be associated with a cholesteatoma and widespread bone destruction.

A conductive hearing loss with an air-bone gap of 40-60 db is nearly always present even when the auditory canal is patent. This is due to associated ossicular or middle ear malformation. In some instances a sensorineural hearing loss is also present, caused by a concomitant inner ear anomaly. Vestibular evaluation by rotational testing has been reported to be normal. Roentgenographic study using petrous pyramid polytomography is essential in planning surgical therapy and in giving a prognosis. If xrays reveal a severely deformed or aplastic middle ear or significant inner ear malformations, surgery may not be beneficial. The xrays may also outline an abnormal course of the facial nerve in the temporal bone, an often associated anomaly.

At operation a narrow or nonexistent space for an external auditory canal may be found. The middle ear cleft and mastoid may be normal in size or hypoplastic. The malleus and incus are often deformed, fused or fixed to the bony atresia plate. The incus may be absent. Abnormal bony prominences are often present in the middle ear. The stapes may be deformed or the footplate fixed. There may be discontinuity at the incudostapedial junction. The round window may be absent.

Complications
I   **Derived:** Conductive hearing loss due to atresia or to associated middle ear anomalies. Frequency approaches 100%. Malposition, anomaly or hypoplasia of the facial nerve with or without partial or complete facial palsy.
II **Associated:** Hypoplasia of the ipsilateral mandible and face due to maldevelopment of the entire branchial arch complex; narrowing of the osseous portion of the eustachian tube, absence of the torus tubarius (very rare), abnormal widening of the eustachian tube.
    Inner ear anomalies. Found in 12-50%.
    Absence or hypoplasia of parotid gland. Absence of homolateral tonsil. Preauricular pits and appendages, branchial cysts, hypoplasia and displacement of the tensor tympani muscle and tendon, absence of the lesser petrosal nerve, cleft palate, teratoid tumors of the tonsil; various craniofacial, skeletal, spinal and visceral anomalies.

Etiology: Autosomal recessive or autosomal dominant inheritance. Chromosome 18q- and also 18 trisomy have been found in some patients. Thalidomide has caused microtia and anotia with cranial nerve palsies and aplasia of the inner ear. Rubella and other intrauterine infections have been implicated.
    Absence or malfunction of an inductive "organizer" has been postulated. Condition has been seen in pigs, cattle, goats, sheep, horses, rabbits and mice.

Pathogenesis: ? Disturbances of development of the 1st branchial groove and of the hillocks of the pinna, nearly all of which are also formed from 1st branchial arch structures. The core of mesoderm which forms in the primitive canal area may fail to recanalize and form an atresia plate. Since the 1st branchial arch develops abnormally, other structures derived from it (the malleus, incus, tensor tympani and mandible) may also be deformed. The 2nd branchial arch may also be involved, resulting in stapes and facial nerve anomalies.
    The pathogenesis of associated visceral or skeletal anomalies is probably related to exogenous factors which affect the growth of other organ systems that are developing at the same embryonic period.

Related Facts
I   **Sex Ratio:** M > 1:F1 Some investigators believe that the apparent increased incidence in males is due only to the fact that female patients cover the deformity with their hair.
II **Risk of Occurrence:** 1 in 20,000 to 1 in 30,000 births (Sullivan).
III **Risk of Recurrence for**
    Patient's Sib: In sporadic cases? When autosomal recessive or autosomal dominant see Table I AR or AD, respectively.
    Patient's Child: When autosomal recessive or autosomal dominant, see Table I AR or AD, respectively.
IV **Age of Detectability:** At birth. In cases in which the canal is patent, a middle ear anomaly is almost invariably present with maximum conductive hearing loss. In these cases the hearing loss may be overlooked for a long time, but it should

be suspected and can be diagnosed at birth.

V **Prevalence:** ? Said to be relatively frequent in Navajo Indians, 1 in 1200 live births (Jaffe).

Treatment

I **Primary Prevention:** Genetic counseling

II **Secondary Prevention:** Pinna, canal and middle ear reconstruction. Hearing aids should be fitted until the hearing mechanism is reconstructed, if the defect is bilateral.

III **Other Therapy:** If surgical restoration of hearing is not possible or fails, fitting of hearing aids, preferential seating in school and speech therapy are advisable.

Prognosis: Good for life unless serious associated defects exist. Restoration of serviceable hearing occurs in 50-67% of cases. Facial nerve injury or external ear canal stenosis occurs as a complication of surgery in some cases. In a few cases, inner ear damage resulting in total hearing loss occurs.

Detection of Carrier: —

†**Special Considerations:** The child with microtia-atresia deserves careful evaluation by polytomography of the anatomy of his external canal, middle and inner ear. His hearing should be thoroughly tested, even if there is no atresia. He should also have a careful general evaluation to rule out significant occult defects.

References:

Converse, J.M. (ed.): Reconstructive Plastic Surgery. Philadelphia: W.B. Saunders Co., 1964, vol. 3.

Crabtree, J.A.: Tympanoplastic techniques in congenital atresia. Arch. Otolaryngol. 88:63, 1968.

d'Avignon, M. and Barr, B.: Ear abnormalities and cranial nerve palsies in thalidomide children. Arch. Otolaryngol. 80:136, 1964.

Grimaud, R. et al: Anomalies morphologiques des chromosomes de la 16e paire et appareil auditif. Acta Otolaryngol. 63:144, 1967.

Jaffe, B.F.: The incidence of ear diseases in the Navajo Indians. Laryngoscope 79:2126, 1969.

Nauton, R.F. and Valvassori, G.E.: Inner ear anomalies: Their association with atresia. Laryngoscope 78:1041, 1968.

Contributor: **LaVonne Bergstrom**

Editor's Computerized Descriptors: Hearing, Ear, Face, Oral, Skel., Nerve

MITRAL VALVE ATRESIA

Includes: Atrésie mitrale
Mitralklappen-Atresie
Atresia mitral

Excludes: Mitral atresia associated with other major cardiac anomalies such as various forms of single ventricle, also aortic-mitral atresia

Minimal Diagnostic Criteria: Echocardiography is suggestive with selective left atrial angiocardiography being diagnostic. Ventriculography will delineate the associated anatomic abnormalities.

Clinical Findings: Mitral atresia is represented by a complete fusion of the mitral valve leaflets with no entry into the left ventricle. The left ventricle is almost always hypoplastic with a small cavity. The left atrium is similarly reduced in size. The communication between the atria is usually a patent foramen ovale rather than a defect of the secundum or primum variety. The atrial septum is rarely ($< 10\%$) intact and, under these circumstances, entry into the right side of the heart is via a levocardinal vein. The hemodynamic alterations are dependent on the presence or absence of pulmonary stenosis and the size of the atrial communication. Oxygenated blood in this malformation returns from the lungs into the left atrium and then passes into the right atrium via the foramen ovale or atrial defect to mix with the caval return. Following right ventricular filling, both great arteries receive blood: the pulmonary artery from the right ventricle, and the aorta through a VSD and the LV, or through a patent ductus arteriosus. The size of the aorta and pulmonary artery reflects the proportion of right ventricular output directed into each major vessel as determined by pulmonary and systemic vascular resistances.

The age of presentation and clinical picture depend largely on the size of the atrial patency and the status of pulmonary blood flow. In those patients with diminished pulmonary blood flow, ie associated pulmonary stenosis, cyanosis is the main finding. Auscultation in this group reveals a harsh systolic ejection murmur along the left sternal border secondary to pulmonary outflow tract obstruction. There is a single second heart sound. Signs of congestive heart failure are not present. In the group with augmented pulmonary blood flow or pulmonary venous obstruction, congestive heart failure is the dominant feature. Tachypnea and hepatomegaly are then the chief presenting findings along with nonspecific murmurs. On occasion, a continuous murmur has been described along the left upper sternal margin secondary to flow from the high pressure left atrium to the lower pressure right atrium.

No specific radiologic picture has been described and the findings vary according to the hemodynamic alterations present. In patients with increased pulmonary blood flow, cardiac enlargement with prominent pulmonary vascular markings is seen. If the size of the atrial communication is small, a predominantly pulmonary venous obstructive pattern will be noted. When pulmonary stenosis is present, the heart is usually of normal size and the vascularity of the lungs diminished. In cases with associated transposition of the great arteries, a narrow cardiac base has been observed.

The ECG commonly shows right axis deviation; right atrial enlargement and severe right ventricular hypertrophy. The latter is associated with a qR pattern in the right precordial leads.

The echocardiogram shows absence of the mitral leaflet motion pattern, a variable-sized left atrium and a dilated right ventricle, exaggerated tricuspid motion, a slit-like or absent left ventricular cavity and, generally, a hypoplastic aortic root in the anterior-posterior and superior-inferior echocardiographic axes. The echocardiogram, when all of the above are noted, is definitive in this diagnosis. (See also Aortic Valve Atresia.)

Cardiac catheterization with selective left atrial angiocardiography is crucial for the confirmation of the diagnosis. A left-to-right shunt is usually present at the atrial level. The right ventricular and pulmonary artery pressures are elevated to systemic levels in the absence of pulmonary stenosis. The left atrial pressure is variably increased, depending on the size of the left atrial communication and the magnitude of the pulmonary blood flow. Large prominent a waves are generally found. When a large opening exists, the pressures in both atria tend to be equal. Injection of contrast material into the left atrium will show a direct passage of the contrast media into the right atrium, right ventricle, and then simultaneous opacification of both great arteries. Right ventricular injection may also be helpful in the delineation of the origin of the great arteries and the presence or absence of pulmonary stenosis.

Complications
I **Derived:** Death is usually secondary to congestive heart failure or hypoxemia.
II **Associated:** Coarctation of the aorta or interruption of the aortic arch, complete transposition of the great vessels, and ventricular septal defect or single ventricle; a high incidence (40%) of noncardiac malformations has been reported. They are of wide variety, including horseshoe kidney, ectopic pancreas and cleft lip.

Etiology: ?

Pathogenesis: Congenital mitral atresia is due to fusion of left AV primordia at an early age. It has also been suggested by some authors that premature closure of the foramen ovale in utero is the primary event and the consequent hemodynamic changes result in the left ventricular underdevelopment.

Related Facts
I **Sex Ratio:** ? A slight predominance of females has been noted.
II **Risk of Occurrence:** 5 in 1000 cases of autopsied congenital heart disease.
III **Risk of Recurrence for**
   Patient's Sib: ?
   Patient's Child: ?
IV **Age of Detectability:** From birth, by cardiac catheterization and selective angiocardiography.
V **Prevalence:** ?

Treatment
I **Primary Prevention:** —
II **Secondary Prevention:** If the patient is in congestive heart failure, digitalis, diuretics, etc should be promptly instituted. Pulmonary artery banding is frequently required. In children with decreased pulmonary blood flow, an appropriate aorticopulmonary shunt is necessary. Attempt should be made during cardiac catheterization to enlarge the atrial septum using the balloon atrial septostomy technique as this is often a site of obstruction.
III **Other Therapy:** —

Prognosis: The overall prognosis is poor. In selective cases, palliation with pulmonary artery banding and atrial septostomies as well as systemic pulmonary artery shunts can lead to long-term survival.

Detection of Carrier: ?

Special Considerations: —

References:

Goldberg, S.J. et al: Pediatric and Adolescent Echocardiography. Chicago: Year Book Medical Publishers, 1975.
Meyer, R.A. and Kaplan, S.: Echocardiography in the diagnosis of hypoplasia of the left or right ventricles in the neonate. Circulation 46:55, 1972.
Noonan, J.A.: Hypoplastic left ventricle. In Moss, A.J. and Adams, F.H. (eds.): Heart Disease in Infants, Children, and Adolescents. Baltimore: Williams & Wilkins, 1968, p. 602.
Rudolph, A.M. et al: Hemodynamic considerations in the development of narrowing of the aorta. Am. J. Cardiol. 30:514, 1972.
Watson, D.G. et al: Mitral atresia with normal aortic valve: Report of 11 cases and review of the literature. Pediatrics 25:450, 1960.

Contributors: **William E. Hellenbrand**
Michael A. Berman
Robert M. Fineman
Norman S. Talner

Editor's Computerized Descriptors: Resp., CV.

MITRAL VALVE INSUFFICIENCY

Includes: Insuffisance mitrale
Mitral Insuffizienz
Insuficiencia mitral
Mitral regurgitation due to isolated cleft posterior leaflet of mitral valve
Anomalous shortened chordae tendineae
Shortened or defective valve tissue
Thickening and deformities of chordae tendineae

Excludes: Rheumatic and other acquired types of mitral insufficiency
Mitral insufficiency associated with endocardial cushion defects
Mitral valve prolapse (668)

Minimal Diagnostic Criteria: A maximal apical murmur indicates the diagnosis. Left heart catheterization with selective left ventricular angiocardiography is the procedure of choice to confirm the diagnosis and to establish the severity of the problem.

Clinical Findings: There are a number of anatomic abnormalities of the mitral (left atrioventricular) valve which may lead to incompetence of this valve. Several of these form part of more or less well-defined pathologic anatomic entities such as endocardial cushion defects, inversion of the ventricles, and some cases of endocardial fibroelastosis. At other times, the mitral incompetence is apparently due to dilatation of the valve ring or malfunction of the papillary muscles, eg in cases of myocardiopathy or anomalous origin of the left coronary artery from the pulmonary trunk.

There are, however, cases in which the anatomic abnormality only involves the mitral valve, but even here the pathologic anatomy varies greatly. There may be an isolated cleft in the posterior cusp of the mitral valve, or the chordae tendineae may be abnormally shortened or thickened. In other cases, the mitral valve is dysplastic and has a nodular and crimpled appearance, or the valve tissue appears to be deficient.

The clinical findings vary with the magnitude of valvar regurgitation. With significant regurgitation a history of easy fatigability, growth retardation and frequent respiratory infections is common. There is no history of rheumatic fever, and the sedimentation rate and ASO titers will be within normal limits. Left- and right-sided cardiac failure is a common feature of congenital mitral insufficiency during the 1st years of life.

Upon physical examination there is usually an enlarged heart, an apical pansystolic murmur and an accentuated third heart sound accompanied by an apical diastolic murmur. The systolic murmur is frequently accompanied by a thrill at the apex. The pulmonary component of the second heart sound is usually accentuated when severe regurgitation is present.

The radiologic findings in this group consist of signs of pulmonary venous hypertension and left atrial and left ventricular enlargement which, at times, may be considerable. The large left atrium may elevate the left main stem bronchi, and occasionally there may be bronchial obstruction with resulting atelectasis.

The ECG in isolated congenital mitral insufficiency shows an axis which is in the quadrant from 0° to +90°. The ECG cardiogram usually shows left ventricular hypertrophy. The P wave may be broad and bifid, suggesting left atrial enlargement.

The echocardiogram in mitral insufficiency shows left atrial and left ventricular enlargement. Mitral valve motion may be exaggerated; but the diagnosis cannot be made primarily by echocardiography. Only secondary effects can be assessed accurately by echocardiography.

Cardiac catheterization will demonstrate the presence of an elevated wedge and left ventricular end-diastolic pressures. In some instances, due to increased compliance of the left atrium, mean left atrial pressure may be within normal limits. The left atrial or wedge pressure is characterized by a tall, peaked v wave followed by a rapid y descent. A large a wave may also be present in some instances. The left ventricular pressure pulse shows a rapid fall after the ejection peak. The right ventricular and pulmonary artery pressures are usually elevated to some degree but are not abnormal in pulse contour.

Selective left ventricular angiocardiography will demonstrate systolic regurgitant flow of contrast material into the left atrium. It will also show the marked dilatation of the left atrium with each ventricular contraction. The left atrium may be of aneurysmal proportions and regurgitation of contrast material may extend back into the pulmonary veins as well.†

Complications
I **Derived:** Severe mitral regurgitation will result in signs of left ventricular failure as well as the development of pulmonary hypertension and right-sided congestive heart failure.
II **Associated:** Mitral insufficiency is commonly seen with left-sided obstructive lesions such as coarctation of the aorta, aortic stenosis, idiopathic hypertrophic subaortic stenosis, or with such left heart volume overload lesions as patent ductus arteriosus. Mitral regurgitation may also be seen in patients with anomalous origin of the left coronary artery from the pulmonary trunk as a consequence of papillary muscle infarction. Problems of mitral insufficiency have been described accompanying the Marfan syndrome and mucopolysaccharidoses I and II.

Etiology: Multiple causes including autosomal dominant and recessive connective tissue disorders, familial non-mendelian and sporadic cases.

Pathogenesis: The pathogenesis of the mitral valve defect varies with the particular anomaly present. Other lesions of the mitral valve are most probably due to some abnormality in the elaboration of the valve, its chordae and papillary muscles from the ventricular wall, or due to overgrowth of endocardial cushion type tissue or fibrous tissue in early development.

Related Facts
I **Sex Ratio:** M1:F1
II **Risk of Occurrence:** < 1 in 1000
III **Risk of Recurrence for**
    Patient's Sib: ?
    Patient's Child: ?
IV **Age of Detectability:** From birth with selective angiocardiography
V **Prevalence:** ?

Treatment
I **Primary Prevention:** —
II **Secondary Prevention:** Mitral valvuloplasty or replacement of the mitral valve with insertion of a prosthetic valve in symptomatic patients.
III **Other Therapy:** Symptomatic treatment for congestive heart failure and respiratory tract infections.

Prognosis: Several patients have been helped by mitral valvuloplasty or valve replacement, although prognosis in symptomatic infants is poor.

Detection of Carrier: ?

†**Special Considerations:** More recently the entity of mid-systolic click, "floppy" mitral valve or mitral valve prolapse syndrome, has been recognized (See Mitral Valve Pro-

lapse).

The secondary pathologic findings with mitral regurgitation reflect elevations in left atrial and pulmonary venous pressure, and consist of pulmonary vascular congestion with medial and intimal changes in the pulmonary vascular bed. With left-sided ventricular failure pulmonary edema may be present.

The hemodynamic alterations with mitral regurgitation result from the volume overload of the left ventricle and left atrium. Pulmonary congestion arises from elevation of left atrial and pulmonary venous pressures. With severe regurgitation systemic perfusion may be compromised.

References:

Edwards, J.E. and Burchell, H.B.: Pathologic anatomy of mitral insufficiency. Mayo Clin. Proc. 33:497, 1958.

Goldberg, S.J. et al: Pediatric and Adolescent Echocardiography. Chicago:Year Book Medical Publishers, 1975.

Talner, N.S. et al: Congenital mitral insufficiency. Circulation 23:339, 1961.

Weiss, A.N. et al: Echocardiographic detection of mitral valve prolapse. Circulation 52:1091, 1975.

Contributors: **William E. Hellenbrand
Michael A. Berman
Norman S. Talner**

Editor's Computerized Descriptors: Resp., CV.

MITRAL VALVE INSUFFICIENCY, DEAFNESS AND SKELETAL MALFORMATIONS

Includes: Cardiopathie congénitale, surdité et malformations squelettiques
Vitium cordis congenitum, Taubheit und Skelett Fehlbildungen
Cardiopatía congénita, sordera y malformaciones esqueléticas
Deafness, mitral insufficiency and skeletal malformations
Skeletal malformations, heart disease and conductive hearing loss

Excludes: Lentigines syndrome, multiple (586)
Pulmonic stenosis and deafness

Minimal Diagnostic Criteria: Conductive hearing loss, mitral insufficiency and osseous abnormalities. As more cases are described, variation in the syndrome may become apparent.

Clinical Findings: Three patients have been described with conductive hearing loss, congenital mitral insufficiency, and osseous abnormalities. All 3 were of short stature, had similar facies, and prominent freckling over the face and shoulders. External auditory canals were narrow and oblique; middle ear exploration in 2 cases revealed a fixed footplate. Audiograms prior to surgery demonstrated a conductive hearing loss with a normal bone line. Roentgenograms showed varying degrees of fusion of the cervical vertebrae, carpal and tarsal bones; phalanges appeared shortened. Mitral insufficiency was relatively mild. The ECG showed an incomplete right-bundle branch block and cardiac catheterization gave findings compatible with mitral insufficiency. On dermatoglyphic analysis all patients had 3rd interdigital whorls. All other laboratory studies including PBI, 24 hr urinary gonadotropins and karyotype were normal. All were of normal intelligence.

Complications
I **Derived:** Language delay may result from the hearing loss. In some cases, symptoms secondary to the mitral insufficiency may be expected.
II **Associated:** One child had a left exotropia. A high-arched palate and crowded dentition may be present. The thyroid was palpable in each case but thyroid function studies were normal.

Etiology: ? Possibly autosomal dominant with incomplete penetrance.

Pathogenesis: ?

Related Facts
I **Sex Ratio:** ? All 3 cases reported were female. This is probably biased by the small sample.
II **Risk of Occurrence:** ?
III **Risk of Recurrence for**
   Patient's Sib: ?
   Patient's Child: ? (Reproductive fitness probably normal)
IV **Age of Detectability:** Theoretically diagnosable at birth by physical examination and audiogram. The murmur and conductive hearing loss may easily be missed on initial examination and newborn audiometric screening.
V **Prevalence:** ?

Treatment
I **Primary Prevention:** ?
II **Secondary Prevention:** Middle ear surgery may improve hearing although amplification may be necessary prior to surgery. Cardiac surgery may also be necessary in symptomatic cases.
III **Other Therapy:** —

Prognosis: Good with normal or near-normal life span

Detection of Carrier: —

Special Considerations: —

References:
Forney, W.R. et al: Congenital heart disease, deafness and skeletal malformations: A new syndrome? J. Pediatr. 68:14, 1966.

Contributor: **Janet M. Stewart**

Editor's Computerized Descriptors: Eye, Hearing, Ear, Oral, Teeth, Dermatoglyphic, Skel., CV.

MITRAL VALVE PROLAPSE

Includes: Prolapsus mitral
Syndrom der ballonierenden Mitralklappe
Prolapso de la válvula mitral
Midsystolic click-late systolic murmur syndrome
Barlow syndrome
Balloon or billowing mitral valve
Congenital mitral valve insufficiency

Excludes: Endocardial cushion defects (347)
Rheumatic and other acquired types of mitral valve insufficiency

Minimal Diagnostic Criteria: An apical midsystolic click, particularly if it is followed by a late systolic murmur of mitral insufficiency suggests the diagnosis. Echocardiography can be diagnostic in the mitral valve prolapse syndrome, particularly when there is a classic late systolic posterior dipping with multiple systolic lines on the mitral valve complex. Selective left ventricular angiocardiography may be used to confirm the diagnosis and to establish the degree of valvar insufficiency.

Clinical Findings: This anomaly is characterized by an aneurysmal protrusion of the posterior or anterior mitral valve leaflet, or both, into the left atrium, usually late in ventricular contraction. Patients with isolated mitral valve prolapse are asymptomatic, or complain of mild exercise intolerance or vague chest pain. Upon physical examination there is an apical midsystolic click or a late systolic murmur of mitral valve insufficiency. Both auscultatory findings are highly influenced by postural changes and often can only be detected in the left decubitus or upright position. The roentgenographic findings usually are normal but thoracic skeletal anomalies ("straight back," scoliosis or pectus excavatum) are common. The ECG may show an indeterminate or left QRS axis and particularly biphasic or negative T waves in leads aVF or III.

Mitral valve prolapse often is associated with atrial septal defects of the ostium secundum or sinus venosus type. These patients have all the clinical and radiologic findings of an atrial septal defect. In addition, an apical click or a late systolic murmur of mitral insufficiency may be present. When an ASD coexists, the ECG shows right ventricular hypertrophy and sometimes an indeterminate QRS axis or mild left axis deviation. Abnormal T waves in leads aVF or III may be found.

The echocardiogram can support the clinical diagnosis of a prolapsing mitral valve by demonstrating an abrupt posterior dip in late systole or a pansystolic "hammock" type displacement of the mitral leaflets.

Selective left ventriculography will confirm the prolapsing of the valve leaflets into the left atrium during ventricular contraction. In some instances there is a mild-to-moderate degree of mitral valve insufficiency. Frequently, the left ventricle will show an asymmetric contraction with a convex bulging in the midaspect of the anterolateral wall, or a localized protrusion of the posteroinferior wall into the left ventricular cavity.

Complications
I **Derived:** Little is known about the natural history of a congenital prolapsing mitral valve identified in childhood. Adults, however, have been found to have significant complications as a result of similarly malformed atrioventricular valves. Dysfunction of the mitral apparatus may produce insufficiency that, once established, may become progressively worse. Infective endocarditis has been reported even when the valve is competent. Significant cardiac arrhythmias, mostly of ventricular origin, have been presumed to be the cause of sudden death in rare instances.
II **Associated:** Other congenital heart defects, particularly

atrial septal defects of the ostium secundum or sinus venosus type. Thoracic skeletal anomalies ("straight back" syndrome, scoliosis and pectus excavatum). Similarly malformed mitral valves have been described accompanying Marfan and Ehlers-Danlos syndromes.

Etiology: ? Several families have been described with an autosomal dominant mode of inheritance with increased expression among females. McK *15770

Pathogenesis: ? The end result is a myxomatous type degeneration of the valve leaflets.

Related Facts
I   **Sex Ratio:**   M1:F2
II **Risk of Occurrence:**   ?
III **Risk of Recurrence for**
    Patient's Sib: If parent is affected 1 in 2 (50%) for each offspring to be affected; otherwise not increased.
    Patient's Child: 1 in 2
IV **Age of Detectability:**   From infancy, with selective angiocardiography
V   **Prevalence:**   ?

Treatment
I   **Primary Prevention:**   —
II **Secondary Prevention:**   The susceptibility of these patients to bacterial endocarditis warrants prophylactic antibiotics for dental or surgical procedures.
III **Other Therapy:**   Antiarrhythmic therapy for symptomatic patients with signs of ventricular irritability. Mitral valve replacement may be necessary in case of severe insufficiency.

Prognosis: Good, particularly during childhood and adolescence.

Detection of Carrier: —

Special Considerations: —

References:
Barlow, J.B. and Bosman, C.K.: Aneurysmal protrusion of the posterior leaflet of the mitral valve. An auscultatory-electrocardiographic syndrome. Am. Heart J. 71:166, 1966.
Salomon, J. et al: Thoracic skeletal abnormalities in idiopathic mitral valve prolapse. Am. J. Cardiol. 36:32, 1975.
Shah, P.M. and Gramiak, R.: Echocardiographic recognition of mitral valve prolapse. Circulation 42(Suppl. III):111, 1970.
Victorica, B.E. et al: Ostium secundum atrial septal defect associated with balloon mitral valve in children. Am. J. Cardiol. 33:668, 1974.

Contributor: **Benjamin E. Victorica**

Editor's Computerized Descriptor: CV.

MITRAL VALVE STENOSIS

Includes: Rétrécissement mitral
Mitralstenose
Estenosis mitral

Excludes: Rheumatic and other forms of acquired mitral stenosis
Lutembacher syndrome
Hypoplastic left heart syndrome
Endocardial fibroelastosis (348, 349)

Minimal Diagnostic Criteria: The presence on auscultation of an accentuated first sound, a loud second sound and a low-pitched diastolic rumble at the apex with x-ray findings of pulmonary venous obstruction and left atrial enlargement with right ventricular hypertrophy on the ECG, should raise the possibility of 1) cor triatriatum, 2) supravalvar mitral stenosing ring, 3) congenital mitral stenosis, or 4) obstruction to left ventricular outflow. The echocardiogram and cardiac catheterization used in conjunction with angiocardiography should allow the definitive diagnosis to be made.

Clinical Findings: The pathologic anatomy is characterized by an abnormal left-sided atrioventricular valve with thickened leaflets which are often rubbery in texture. The commissures are frequently fused, leaving a small orifice. The chordae tendineae from the papillary muscles may be shortened and thickened. The valve leaflets are occasionally thin, with fused commissures and shortened chordae tendineae. Variation on the length of the chordae may produce either a funnel-shaped or flat discoid valve. This may allow only small openings in between the chordae for blood flow. Occasionally, a double orifice of the mitral valve may be associated with stenosis. A thickened left atrial wall and evidence of fibroelastosis will often accompany the deformity of the mitral valve. There will be varying degrees of right ventricular hypertrophy depending on the severity of mitral obstruction and resultant pulmonary hypertension.

The hemodynamic alterations and clinical manifestations will depend on the magnitude of the obstruction between the left atrium and left ventricle. Mitral valve stenosis causes an elevation of left atrial pressure which is reflected backwards into the pulmonary vascular bed as pulmonary hypertension. Mean left atrial pressure may average from 10 mm Hg in mild situations to 40 mm Hg in severe cases. The elevation of pulmonary artery pressure results in right ventricular hypertension. In longstanding cases of mitral stenosis, the right ventricle can fail and signs of systemic venous congestion will appear. The cardiac output may be normal or diminished; and it may not increase in response to exercise.

The symptoms of congenital mitral stenosis are usually present in the first few months of life. The common signs are tachypnea, exertional dyspnea and repeated severe pulmonary infections. Syncopal attacks related to low cardiac output have been reported. Growth is generally poor. The left chest is prominent due to right ventricular hypertrophy and decreased lung compliance. A xiphoid impulse may be felt. The signs of pulmonary and systemic venous congestion may be present. The first heart sound is increased in intensity. The second heart sound is often narrowly split with an accentuated pulmonic closure sound as a result of the elevated pulmonary artery pressure. An opening snap is occasionally heard in older patients as is a sharp, high-pitched sound which occurs during the maximal diastolic gradient across the mitral valve. The most common murmur is a low-pitched middiastolic rumble. This may be associated with an atrial presystolic murmur.

If pulmonary hypertension develops, the murmur of pulmonary insufficiency may be present. Fifteen percent of patients with mitral stenosis have no murmur.

The roentgenographic findings of mitral stenosis are often masked by the associated lesion, whether intracardiac or extracardiac. In mitral stenosis in its pure form and in the absence of a shunt lesion, there are almost invariably signs of pulmonary venous obstruction. The degree of pulmonary venous obstruction or hypertension depends upon the severity of the stenosis. This may range from mild redistribution of flow to interstitial Kerley B lines in the bases, hemosiderosis and ossification. Mitral stenosis in an uncomplicated form may show a normal size cardiac silhouette with a mitral configuration. This is in contrast to mitral insufficiency which usually presents with an enlarged cardiac silhouette. The left atrial enlargement is usually discrete, whereas that in mitral insufficiency is more diffuse. The pulmonary trunk is enlarged. The left main bronchus may be elevated as a result of left atrial enlargement. Secondary atelectasis may occur.

The ECG will demonstrate right axis deviation with a mean frontal axis between $+90°$ to $+150°$. Right ventricular hypertrophy usually is present with evidence of left atrial or combined atrial enlargement as manifested by bifid or peaked P waves. Atrial fibrillation is rare.

The vectorcardiogram will show a mean right axis in the frontal projection and right ventricular hypertrophy in the horizontal and sagittal leads. The frontal mean P axis is at $0°$ to $+60°$ and the T axis is at $0°$ to $+120°$

Phonocardiography has documented the accentuation of the first heart sound occasionally associated with a presystolic murmur at the apex. There is a rumbling, middiastolic murmur. The severity of mitral valve obstruction may be assessed by measuring the $Q\text{-}S_1$ interval, which is the time between the onset of electrical systole and the first heart sound (mechanical systole) and comparing this to the time between the aortic valve closure and the opening snap (OS). In a mild disease, the former is short and the latter is long. In a severe disease, the former is lengthened, while the $A_2\text{-OS}$ interval is short.

The characteristic echocardiographic features of mitral stenosis include a decreased E-F diastolic slope of mitral valve motion, anterior (instead of posterior) diastolic motion of the posterior mitral leaflet, and a dilated left atrium. If pulmonary artery pressure is increased, the characteristic pulmonary valve motion pattern (no "A" dip, flattening of diastolic slope and "W" pattern) may be observed.

Cardiac catheterization documents the level of pulmonary artery and pulmonary capillary wedge pressures. Simultaneous recording of pulmonary artery wedge or left atrial pressure and left ventricular enddiastolic pressure, along with the determination of cardiac output, allows assessment of the mitral valve orifice size. Left atrial pressure curves will show an elevation in the mean pressure as well as an increase in the a wave. If the lesion is well-established, there is a prominent x descent and the y descent will be slowed. Angiocardiography will reveal delayed emptying of the left atrium with a dilatation of the pulmonary veins. The thickened valve leaflets will often be seen and the left ventricular cavity appears smaller than normal.

Complications
I Derived: Pulmonary hypertension with development of pulmonary valvular insufficiency. Death from congestive heart failure and severe respiratory infections.
II Associated: This lesion is commonly associated with other left-sided heart lesions such as patent ductus arteriosus

(50%) and coarctation of the aorta (20-30%). Aortic stenosis and endocardial fibroelastosis are also present in 15-30% of cases.

Etiology: ?

Pathogenesis: Failure of the mitral valve commissures to develop and allow adequate area for blood flow.

Related Facts
I   Sex Ratio: Ml:Fl
II Risk of Occurrence: 5 in 1000 cases of autopsied congenital heart disease
III Risk of Recurrence for
    Patient's Sib: ?
    Patient's Child: ?
IV Age of Detectability: From birth with echocardiography and cardiac catheterization.
V   Prevalence: ?

Treatment
I   Primary Prevention: —
II Secondary Prevention: Mitral valvoplasty. Replacement of mitral valve with prosthetic valve.
III Other Therapy: Symptomatic therapy for congestive heart failure and respiratory tract infections.

Prognosis: The prognosis of symptomatic infants is poor, with or without surgery. Approximately 50% will die within the 1st year of life with 20% surviving to 3 years of age. If there are associated cardiac lesions, the survival rate is less.

Detection of Carrier: ?

Special Considerations: —

References:
Castaneda, A.R. et al: Congenital mitral stenosis resulting from anomalous arcade and obstructing papillary muscles: Report of correction by use of ball valve prosthesis. Am. J. Cardiol. 24:237, 1969.
Goldberg, S.J. et al: Pediatric and Adolescent Echocardiography. Chicago: Year Book Medical Publishers, 1975.
Lundstrom, N.R.: Echocardiography in the diagnosis of congenital mitral stenosis and in evaluation of the results of mitral valvotomy. Circulation 46:44, 1972.
Noonan, J.A.: Hypoplastic left ventricle. In Moss, A.J. and Adams, F.H. (eds.): Heart Disease in Infants, Children, and Adolescents. Baltimore:Williams & Wilkins, 1968, p. 660.
VanDerHorst, R. and Hastreiter, A.: Congenital mitral stenosis. Am. J. Cardiol. 20:773, 1967.

Contributors: **William E. Hellenbrand**
Michael A. Berman
Norman S. Talner

Editor's Computerized Descriptors: Resp., CV.

MOYNAHAN SYNDROME

Includes: Syndrome de Moynahan
Síndrome de Moynahan

Excludes: Oculo-mandibulo-facial syndrome (738)
Progeria (825)

Minimal Diagnostic Criteria: Diagnosis must be made mainly on clinical grounds, but the usual EEG findings are almost pathognomonic.

Clinical Findings: Two reported patients were hairless at birth. Very scanty, lanugo type hair and eyelashes may appear later. Grand mal convulsions form a prominent part of the symptomology usually at intervals of 2 to 3 weeks. Status epilepticus may supervene. There is a marked delay in the milestones; patient takes little interest in his surroundings or food until well on in 3rd year. Talking is delayed and speech limited to a few words. Features include large stature, gross features, short lanugo scalp hair, no eyebrows and few eyelashes. Skeletal changes include delay in bone development. EEG shows gross abnormality of unusual kind, with absence of alpha rhythm and generalized slow activity between 1 and 4 cycles per second, mixed with a small amount of low amplitude fast activity. No differences between anterior and posterior halves of the head and no spikes or complex wave forms have appeared at any time. Lumbar puncture reveals normal CSF pressure and protein, no cells; urine contains no abnormal amino acids. Blood chemistry is normal.

Biopsy of scalp shows scanty hair follicles, some of which contain a rim of keratin.

Complications
I Derived: —
II Associated: —

Etiology: Probably autosomal recessive. The single available family study reveals that the disorder is probably due to a mutant autosomal gene which produces an intermediate effect in the heterozygous state and the full-blown syndrome when homozygous.

Pathogenesis: ? Ultraphysiology studies have revealed a developmental anomaly involving both cerebral hemispheres, but there are other metabolic changes, such as delay in bone development as well as the absence or deficiency of hair follicles, which indicate that the gene in double dose has widespread effects.

Related Facts
I **Sex Ratio:** Both cases of complete syndrome are males; both parents had alopecia in first few years of life.
II **Risk of Occurrence:** Only one family reported.
III **Risk of Recurrence for**
   Patient's Sib: If autosomal recessive, 1 in 4 for full-blown syndrome; 1 in 2 for isolated childhood alopecia and 1 in 4 for unaffected sib.
   Patient's Child: 1 in 2 for isolated childhood alopecia, but not increased for full-blown syndrome unless mate is heterozygote or homozygote.
IV **Age of Detectability:** Early infancy
V **Prevalence:** Only one family known

Treatment
I **Primary Prevention:** Genetic counseling
II **Secondary Prevention:** Treatment for epilepsy
III **Other Therapy:** The severe mental retardation may necessitate permanent custodial care in an institution

Prognosis: For life: ? For intelligence: severe retardation.† For function: requires custodial care and management for life.

Detection of Carrier: Both parents suffer from congenital alopecia which regrew spontaneously during early childhood, and this holds true for the heterozygous sibs.

†**Special Considerations:** The mental deficit is severe enough to demand life-long custodial care. At times the child is difficult to restrain.

References:
None

Contributor: **Edmund J. Moynahan**

Editor's Computerized Descriptors: Hair, Skel., Nerve, Speech

MUCOLIPIDOSIS I

Includes: Mucolipidose de type I
Mucolipidose I
Lipomucopolysaccharidosis
Sialidosis
Cherry red spot - myoclonus syndrome

Excludes: Mucopolysaccharidoses
Mucolipidosis II (672)
Mucolipidosis III (673)
Other inborn errors of complex carbohydrate metabolism

Minimal Diagnostic Criteria: General physical resemblance to Hurler syndrome, with normal urinary mucopolysaccharides, elevated sialic acid containing oligosaccharides, mild mental retardation, cherry-red macular change, signs of white matter involvement in older children, decreased activity of N-acetyl-neuraminidase in cultured fibroblasts and in leukocytes.

Clinical Findings: This syndrome comprises a small group of children who develop some physical and radiologic resemblance to Hurler syndrome, exhibit signs of white matter disease, excrete abnormal amounts of sialic acid-containing oligosaccharides and have a deficient activity of α-N-acetyl-neuraminidase in cultured fibroblasts, in leukocytes and probably other organs. Moderate developmental retardation is noted in late infancy. As the disease progresses, the children have short stature (with disproportionately short trunk), hepatosplenomegaly, herniae, moderately severe mental retardation, impaired hearing and cherry-red macular spots. After about 5 years, there are progressive signs of white matter handicap, with myoclonic seizures, decreased muscle strength, hypotonia, ataxia, tremor, nystagmus, irregular reflexes, and reduced nerve conduction velocity. Peripheral lymphocytes contain abnormal granules and vacuoles, and large storage cells are found in the bone marrow. In older patients, the EEG shows peculiar complexes of high-frequency polyspikes and sharp waves. The activity of multiple lysosomal enzymes is elevated in cultured fibroblasts but the activity of α-N-acetyl-neuraminidase is absent or greatly diminished. There is a generalized bone dysplasia similar to that seen in moderately severe Hunter disease.

Complications
I **Derived:** Corneal opacities (inconsistent); seizures may occur in late childhood
II **Associated:** —

Etiology: Autosomal recessive inheritance.

Pathogenesis: The absent activity of α-N-acetyl-neuraminidase activity leads to the intralysosomal accumulation of sialic acid containing partially degraded glycopeptides. A considerable number of different sialic acid-containing oligosaccharides are excreted in the urine.†

Related Facts
I **Sex Ratio:** M1:F1
II **Risk of Occurrence:** Low
III **Risk of Recurrence for**
  Patient's Sib: 1 in 4 (25%) for each offspring to be affected.
  Patient's Child: Not pertinent
IV **Age of Detectability:** Symptoms begin in 1st year of life or early childhood. Prenatal diagnosis is possible.
V **Prevalence:** Rare

Treatment
I **Primary Prevention:** Genetic counseling
II **Secondary Prevention:** No basic treatment is known, but leads should be followed from the experience with other inborn errors of complex carbohydrate metabolism and sphingolipidoses.
III **Other Therapy:** Would be similar to that for any child with progressive CNS disease, including control of seizures where needed.

Prognosis: Longest survival known is for patient who died at 20 years of age.

Detection of Carrier: By enzyme assay in cultured fibroblasts.

†Special Considerations: There appear to exist more than one type of neuraminidase deficiency with slightly different clinical features and possibly longer survival. It has been suggested that in Mucolipidosis I there is a deficiency of α(2-6)neuraminidase and that a partial deficiency of that enzyme may lead to a milder clinical phenotype.

References:
Cantz, M. et al.: Mucolipidosis I: Increased sialic acid content and deficiency of an α-N-acetylneuraminidase in cultured fibroblasts. Biochem. Biophys. Res. Commun. 74:732,1977.
Kelly, T.E.: Isolated acid neuraminidase deficiency: A distinct lysosomal storage disease. Am. J. Med. Genet. 1:31, 1977.
Spranger, J. et al.: Mucolipidosis I - a sialidosis. Am. J. Med. Genet. 1:21, 1977.
Strecker, G. et al.: Structure of nine sialyl-oligosaccharides accumulated in urine of eleven patients with three different types of sialidosis. Eur. J. Biochem. 75:391, 1977.

Contributor: **Jürgen W. Spranger**

Editor's Computerized Descriptors: Hearing, Face, Skel., Spleen, Liver, Nerve

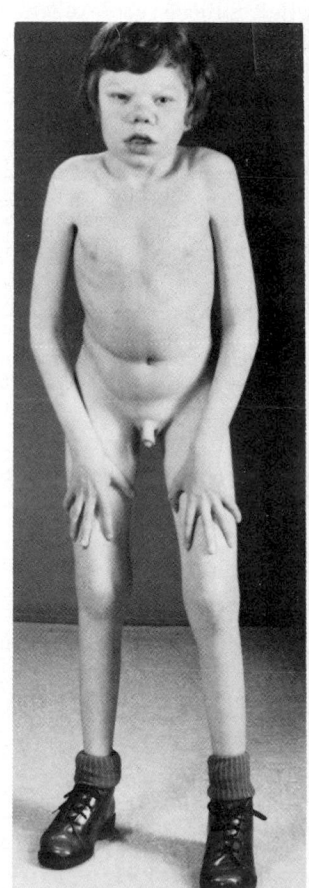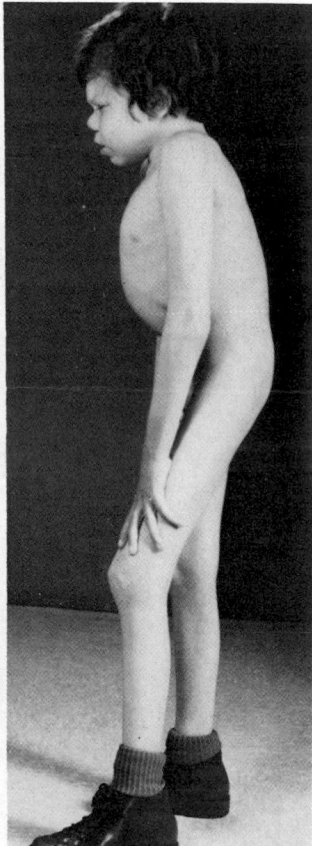

359. Note skeletal features

MUCOLIPIDOSIS II

Includes: Mucolipidose de type II
Mucolipidose II
I-cell disease

Excludes: Mucopolysaccharidoses I-VII (674, 675, 676, 677, 678, 679, 680)
Mucolipidoses I, III,† and IV (671, 673)
Mannosidosis
G_{M1}-gangliosidosis (431, 432)

Minimal Diagnostic Criteria: An appropriate clinical presentation and absence of mucoplysacchariduria are required. Markedly elevated levels of a variety of lysosomal enzymes including beta-N-acetylhexosaminidase and arylsulfatase A are found in serum, urine, and spinal fluid. Reduced levels of a whole battery of lysosomal enzymes are detected within cultured fibroblasts. S^{35} mucopolysaccharide degradation is markedly impaired in cultured fibroblasts, and numerous membrane-bound vacuolar inclusions can be observed by phase contrast microscopy of these cells.

Clinical Findings: Most patients have had coarse facial features similar to those seen in the Hurler syndrome, and severe skeletal changes including kyphoscoliosis, lumbar gibbus, anterior "beaking" and wedging of vertebral bodies, widening of the ribs, and proximal pointing of the metacarpals. Growth and psychomotor retardation are common. Frequent respiratory infections and severe joint contractures are major clinical problems. Corneal opacities are frequently observed but not often to the extent seen in the Hurler syndrome, and striking gingival hyperplasia is usually present. Clinical onset is quite early and most patients have had obvious problems by 6-10 months of age. In contrast to the mucopolysaccharidoses, increased urinary excretion of glycosaminoglycans has not been observed.

Complications
I **Derived:** Severe orthopedic deformities and psychomotor retardation
II **Associated:** Frequent respiratory infections

Etiology: Autosomal recessive; McK *25250

Pathogenesis: Lysosomal enzymes from affected patients appear to be deficient in a shared "recognition marker" necessary for the proper intracellular packaging of these hydrolases. This results in diminished levels of the relevant enzymes intracellularly in some tissues and the elevation of enzyme activity extracellularly. It is presumed that the pathology in this condition is due to intralysosomal storage of a variety of macromolecules or to the unrestrained activity of extracellular proteases and other enzymes.

Related Facts
I **Sex Ratio:** M1:F1
II **Risk of Occurrence:** Rare, less than 30 reported cases
III **Risk of Recurrence for**
   Patient's Sib: 1 in 4 (25%) for each offspring to be affected
   Patient's Child: Patients do not usually live to reproductive age.
IV **Age of Detectability:** Prenatal diagnosis possible
V **Prevalence:** ?

Treatment
I **Primary Prevention:** Genetic counseling and prenatal diagnosis
II **Secondary Prevention:** —
III **Other Therapy:** Supportive

Prognosis: Usually death by age 5.

Detection of Carrier: No reproducible abnormalities have been identified in heterozygotes.

†Special Considerations: Due to the biochemical similarities between these patients and those with the milder disorder, Mucolipidosis III, it is possible that these conditions are genetically related, and it is likely that phenotypes intermediate in severity will be identified.

References:
Leroy, J.G. and Martin, J.J.: Mucolipidosis II (I-cell disease): Present status of knowledge. In Bergsma, D. (ed.): Disorders of Connective Tissue. Birth Defects: Orig Art. Ser., vol. XI, no. 6. Miami: Symposia Specialists for The National Foundation-March of Dimes, 1975, p. 283.
Shapiro, L.J. et al: Biochemical studies in mucolipidoses II and III. Ibid, p. 301.
Spranger, J.W. and Wiedemann, H.R.: The genetic mucolipidoses. Humangenetik 9:113, 1970.

Contributors: **Larry J. Shapiro**
Kyrieckos Aleck

Editor's Computerized Descriptors: Eye, Face, Skin, Skel., Nerve, Oral, Resp., Hernia not CNS

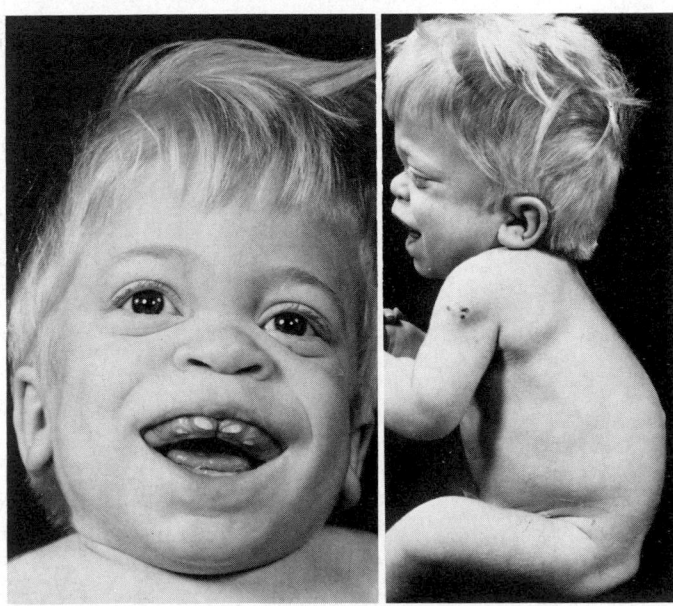

360. Note coarse facies with proptotic eyes, open wide mouth showing hyperplastic gums, abundant hair, scaphocephaly and gibbus

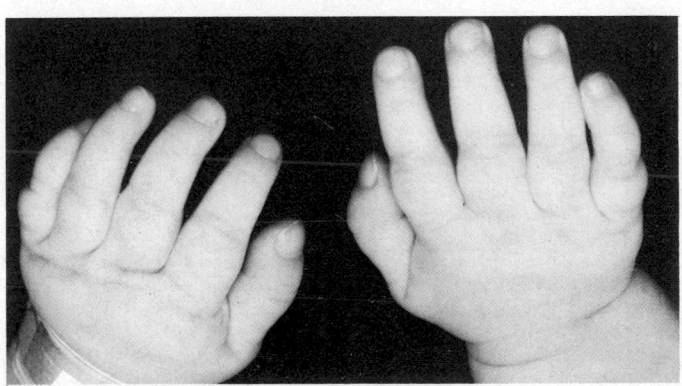

361. Short digits and the beginning of deformity.

MUCOLIPIDOSIS III

Includes: Mucolipidose de type III
Mucolipidose III
Pseudopolydystrophy
Pseudo-Hurler polydystrophy

Excludes: Mucopolysaccharidoses

Minimal Diagnostic Criteria: This condition should be suspected when the following features are present: early onset, painless joint stiffness and decreased mobility, short stature, some coarseness of the facial features suggesting a mild mucopolysaccharidosis, mild mental retardation, no excess urinary acid mucopolysaccharides and xray evidence of dysostosis multiplex.†

Clinical Findings: The clinical features include early childhood onset of joint stiffness without pain, swelling or tenderness; limitation of mobility is slowly progressive but seems to become stationary after puberty. Other characteristics are minimal-to-moderate coarseness of the facial features suggesting a mild mucopolysaccharidosis, corneal opacities by slit-lamp examination; short stature; mild mental retardation may be noted, and aortic regurgitation has been observed in several cases. The urinary excretion of acid mucopolysaccharides is normal. Skin fibroblast cultures are metachromatic and contain increased amounts of uronic acid; peripheral leukocytes are normal. Vacuolated plasma cells are found in the bone marrow. Xrays of the skeleton show abnormalities which resemble milder forms of the mucopolysaccharidoses.

Complications
I **Derived:** Easy fatigability. Congestive heart failure may occur.
II **Associated:** —

Etiology: Autosomal recessive; McK *25260

Pathogenesis: ?

Related Facts
I   **Sex Ratio:** M1:F1
II **Risk of Occurrence:** ? Very rare
III **Risk of Recurrence for**
    Patient's Sib: 1 in 4 (25%) for each offspring to be affected
    Patient's Child: Not increased unless mate is carrier or homozygote
IV **Age of Detectability:** Joint stiffness has been noted as early as 13 months
V   **Prevalence:** Very rare

Treatment
I   **Primary Prevention:** Genetic counseling
II **Secondary Prevention:** —
III **Other Therapy:** Orthopedic care as indicated

Prognosis: Joint stiffness typically is evident by 2-4 years of age. It can cause a significant handicap for the adult. Carpal tunnel compression may be present by late childhood. Aortic valvular disease is common. Progressive destruction of the hip joints results in the most disabling problems for these individuals by late teens. Survival to age 50 years is known but there is little information available on the course of the disease in adulthood.

Detection of Carrier: ?

†**Special Considerations:** Electron microscopy shows cellular changes consistent with a disturbance in both mucopolysaccharide and glycolipid metabolism, thus justifying classification as a mucolipidosis.
Lysosomal enzyme values may be elevated in serum. Activities of multiple lysosomal enzymes in fibroblasts are decreased and elevated in the cell culture medium. Serum and fibroblast studies in this disorder may be indistinguishable from those of patients with I-cell disease.

References:
Kelly, T.E.: The mucopolysaccharidoses and mucolipidoses. Clin. Orthop. 114:116, 1976.
Melhem, R. et al: Roentgen findings in mucolipidosis III (Pseudo-Hurler polydystrophy). Radiology 106:153, 1973.
Scott, C.I., Jr. and Grossman, M.S.: Pseudo-Hurler polydystrophy. In Bergsma, D. (ed.): Part IV. Skeletal Dysplasias. Birth Defects: Orig. Art. Ser., vol. V, no. 4. New York: The National Foundation-March of Dimes, 1969, p. 349.
Spranger, J.W. and Wiedemann, H.R.: The genetic mucolipidoses. Diagnosis and differential diagnosis. Humangenetik 9:113, 1970.
Spranger, J.W. et al: Bone Dysplasias. Philadelphia: W.B. Saunders, 1974.
Steinbach, H.L. et al: The Hurler syndrome without abnormal mucopolysacchariduria. Radiology 90:472, 1968.

Contributor: **Charles I. Scott, Jr.**

Editor's Computerized Descriptors: Eye, Face, Skel., CV., Nerve

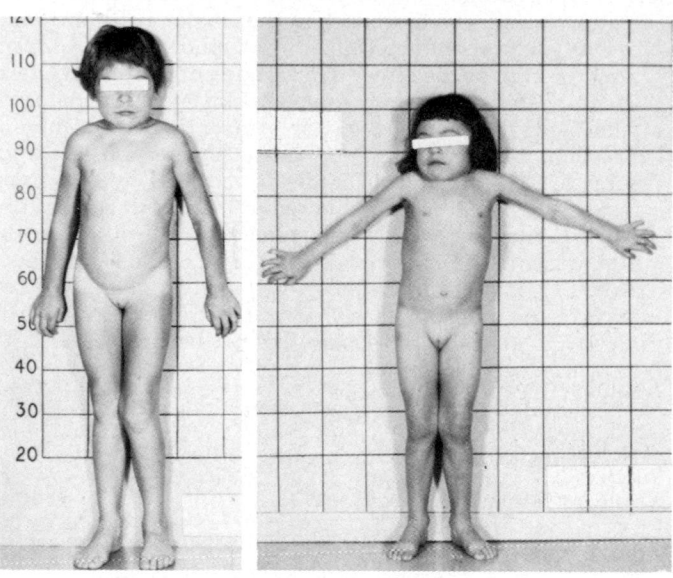

362. Pseudo-Hurler polydystrophy phenotype

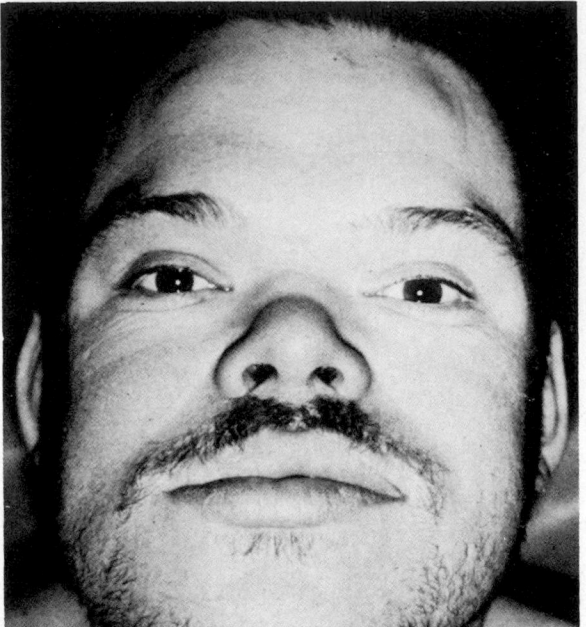

363. Note coarse facial features

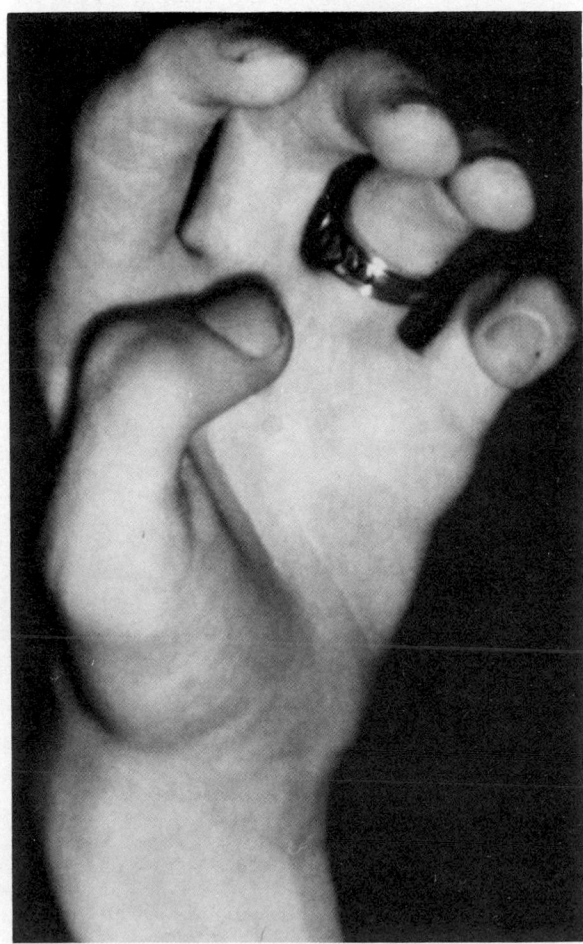

364. Note joint contractures

MUCOPOLYSACCHARIDOSIS I-H

Includes: Mucopolysaccharidose de type I
Mucopolysaccharidose I
Mucopolisacaridosis Tipo I
Hurler syndrome
Hurler-Pfaundler syndrome
MPS I
Gargoylism (undesirable term)

Excludes: Other mucopolysaccharidoses
Mucolipidosis III (673)
G_{M1}-Gangliosidosis, type 1 (431)
MPS I-H/I-S compound

Minimal Diagnostic Criteria: Presence of constant clinical signs, excess mucopolysacchariduria and either 1) deficient α-L-iduronidase in leukocytes or fibroblasts, or 2) abnormal sulfate incorporation and degradation by cultured fibroblasts which can be "corrected" by addition of "Hurler factor". Metachromatic staining of fibroblasts and leukocyte inclusions are nonspecific findings.

Clinical Findings: Normal appearance at birth but may have excessive birthweight. In early months of life onset of progressive coarsening of facial features, depressed nasal bridge, corneal clouding, hepatosplenomegaly, joint stiffness and thoracolumbar kyphosis. Other constant features seen by age 2 years: inguinal or umbilical herniae, abundance of fine body hair particularly over extensor areas and back, enlarged and scaphoid head, large tongue and lips, small spaced teeth, mucoid rhinorrhea, noisy respiration, limitation of joint mobility especially at phalanges, elbows, shoulders and hips. Later signs: cardiac murmurs, deafness, blindness, short stature. Growth normal or excessive during 1st year with decline thereafter. Short stature apparent by 3 years. Motor and mental development reach peak prior to 2 years and deteriorate thereafter.†

Roentgenologic findings include scaphocephaly, "shoe-shaped" and enlarged sella, diaphyseal widening of tubular bones most pronounced in upper limbs, expansion of shaft of the ribs, anterior beaking of the vertebrae.

Laboratory findings include mucopolysacchariduria with excessive excretion of dermatan sulfate and heparan sulfate; deficiency of the lysosomal enzyme, α-L-iduronidase, demonstrable in fibroblasts or leukocytes. Fibroblasts have abnormal sulfate kinetics in culture, incorporating excessive sulfate from the media and failing to normally degrade sulfated mucopolysaccharide when grown in sulfate-deficient media. 10% to 60% of leukocytes show metachromatic staining granules; metachromatic staining of fibroblasts.

Complications
I **Derived:** Loss of vision due to corneal clouding and retinal degeneration, mental deterioration due to deposits in CNS, and hydrocephaly, cardiac decompensation from MPS deposits in intima of coronary vessels and valves, deafness, skeletal incapacitation due to joint limitation, death usually from cardiorespiratory decompensation.
II **Associated:** —

Etiology: Autosomal recessive† McK *25280

Pathogenesis: The Hurler features develop because of progressive deposition of acid mucopolysaccharide in various tissues. Deficient function of α-L-iduronidase, an enzyme responsible for degradation of AMPS underlies this condition.

Related Facts
I **Sex Ratio:** M1:F1
II **Risk of Occurrence:** Not known with certainty; probably > 1 in 100,000 live births; described in Caucasians, Orientals

and Negroes.

III Risk of Recurrence for
    Patient's Sib: 1 in 4 (25%) for each offspring to be affected
    Patient's Child: (No patients have reproduced.)
IV Age of Detectability: At 14 weeks gestation by iduronidase assay or sulfate incorporation and "correction" studies using cultured amniotic cells.
V Prevalence: Less than frequency at birth due to early death

Treatment
I Primary Prevention: Genetic counseling, prenatal diagnosis and abortion
II Secondary Prevention: Curative therapy is not available. Evaluation of the benefits of plasma and leukocyte infusions must await more experience. Surgical correction of joint contractures and herniae offers cosmetic and functional improvement. Corneal transplantation and cardiac valvular replacement do not give lasting benefit. None of these surgical measures impede mucopolysaccharide deposition or progressive deterioration.
III Other Therapy: Physical therapy; special education with attention to deafness and physical handicaps.

Prognosis: Relentless physical and mental deterioration leads to death before age 10 in most patients. Death results from pneumonia or cardiac decompensation.

Detection of Carrier: The heterozygote can be identified by assay of α-L-iduronidase in cultured fibroblasts.

†Special Considerations: In the truest sense, the mucopolysaccharidoses are storage diseases. The signs are progressive, developing parallel to the accumulation of tissue mucopolysaccharide. In addition to the 6 generally acknowledged types of mucopolysaccharidosis, occasional patients are seen in whom the combination of clinical, roentgenologic and laboratory findings prevent easy classification.

MPS 1 (I-H) and MPS V (I-S) have deficiency of the same enzyme, α-L-iduronidase; hence the suggestion that they are allelic conditions. In keeping with this hypothesis, a group of patients with iduronidase deficiency who have intermediate clinical features has been identified. These patients, felt to have one Hurler mutant gene and one Scheie mutant gene, have the onset of signs between ages 1-2 years, normal or near normal intelligence, and intermediate progression of signs. The oldest recognized patient is in her 20s. This condition has been termed Hurler-Scheie compound or MPS 1-H/I-S compound.

References:
Leroy, J.G. and Crocker, A.C.: Clinical definition of the Hurler-Hunter phenotypes. Am. J. Dis. Child. 112:518, 1966.
Maroteaux, P. and Lamy, M.: Hurler's disease, Morquio's disease and related mucopolysaccharidoses. J. Pediatr. 67:312, 1965.
McKusick, V.A.: Heritable Disorders of Connective Tissue. 4th Ed. St. Louis: C.V. Mosby Co., 1972.
Stevenson, R.E. et al: The iduronidase deficient mucopolysaccharidoses. Clinical and roentgenographic features. Pediatrics, 57:111, 1976.

Contributor: **Roger E. Stevenson**

Editor's Computerized Descriptors: Eye, Hearing, Face, Oral, Nose, Hair, Skel., Hernia not CNS, Resp., CV., Nerve, Spleen, Liver

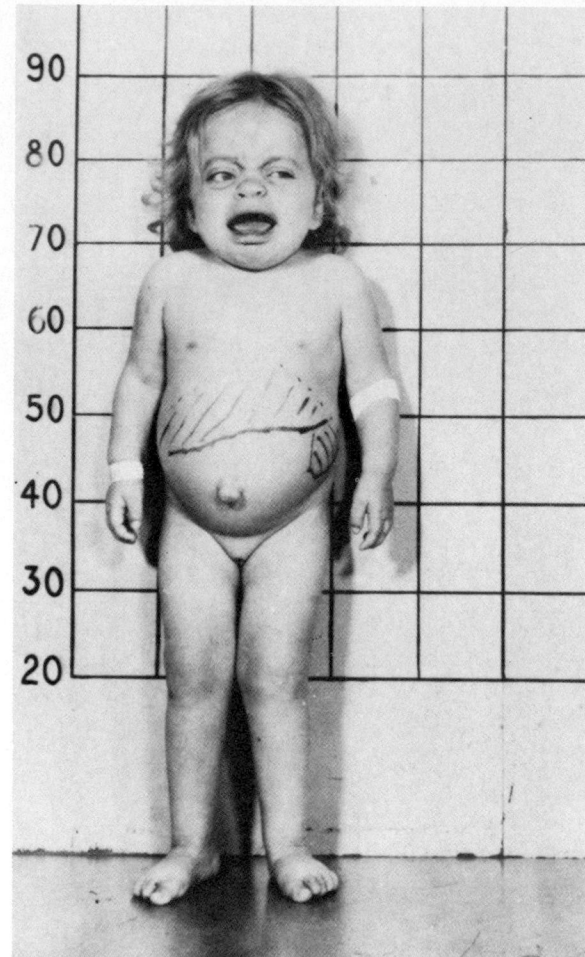

365. Note coarse facial features and hepatosplenomegaly

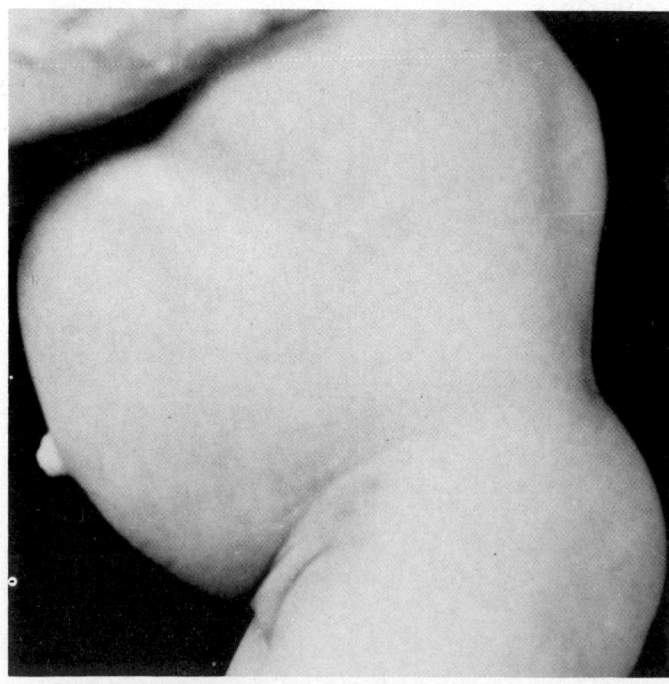

366. Note umbilical hernia, protruding abdomen, and gibbus

MUCOPOLYSACCHARIDOSIS I-S

Includes: Mucopolysaccharidose de type V
Mucopolysaccharidose V
Mucopolisacaridosis Tipo V
Scheie syndrome
MPS V

Excludes: Other mucopolysaccharidoses
MPS I-H/I-S compound
Mucolipidosis III (673)
G_{M1}-Gangliosidosis, type 1 (431)

Minimal Diagnostic Criteria: Corneal clouding, mild or absent intellectual impairment, variable but generally mild somatic features plus mucopolysacchariduria plus specific abnormal sulfate kinetics in fibroblast culture or deficiency of α-L-iduronidase activity in fibroblasts or leukocytes.

Clinical Findings: Corneal clouding and herniae may be present at birth or soon thereafter; otherwise signs of mucopolysaccharide disease are absent during infancy. By early school age, joint stiffness with limitation at phalanges, elbows and shoulders. Genu valgum is the rule. Cardiac murmurs often aortic in origin appear, corneal clouding, retinal degeneration and skeletal involvement increase, auditory and visual acuity decrease and carpal tunnel signs and psychotic episodes may develop; hepatosplenomegaly, mental retardation and stunting of growth are not features. Hurloid features, if present at all, are mild.

Roentgenologic findings include mild changes of dysostosis multiplex. Laboratory findings include excessive heparan sulfate and dermatan sulfate excretion in the urine; fibroblasts and leukocyte inclusions may stain metachromatically; leukocytes and fibroblasts have deficient α-L-iduronidase activity.

Complications
I **Derived:** Aortic regurgitation, carpal tunnel syndrome, blindness from corneal clouding and retinal degeneration, hearing loss, psychotic episodes.
II **Associated:** —

Etiology: Autosomal recessive†

Pathogenesis: Deficiency of α-L-iduronidase, one of the lysosomal enzymes responsible for mucopolysaccharide degradation, leading to deposition of AMPS in soft tissues and interruption of normal bone development.

Related Facts
I **Sex Ratio:** M1:F1
II **Risk of Occurrence:** ? Must be exceedingly rare
III **Risk of Recurrence for**
   Patient's Sib: 1 in 4 (25%) for each offspring to be affected
   Patient's Child: (No patients have reproduced; all offspring should be carriers.)
IV **Age of Detectability:** Theoretically at about 14 weeks gestation by assay of α-L-iduronidase using cultured amniotic fluid cells.
V **Prevalence:** ?

Treatment
I **Primary Prevention:** Genetic counseling
II **Secondary Prevention:** No specific therapy available. Surgical release of joint contractures and carpal tunnel syndrome, herniorrhaphy.
III **Other Therapy:** Hearing aids, medical management of cardiac decompensation, physical therapy for skeletal contractures.

Prognosis: The few cases reported have survived into adulthood.

Detection of Carrier: Carriers have intermediate levels of α-L-iduronidase.

†**Special Considerations:** Scheie syndrome is considered allelic to Hurler syndrome because both lack α-L-iduronidase.

References:
Scheie, H.G. et al: A newly recognized forme fruste of Hurler's disease (Gargoylism): The Sanford R. Gifford Lecture. Am. J. Ophthalmol. 53:753, 1962.

Contributor: **Roger E. Stevenson**

Editor's Computerized Descriptors: Vision, Eye, Hearing, Skel., Hernia not CNS, CV., Nerve, Liver, Spleen

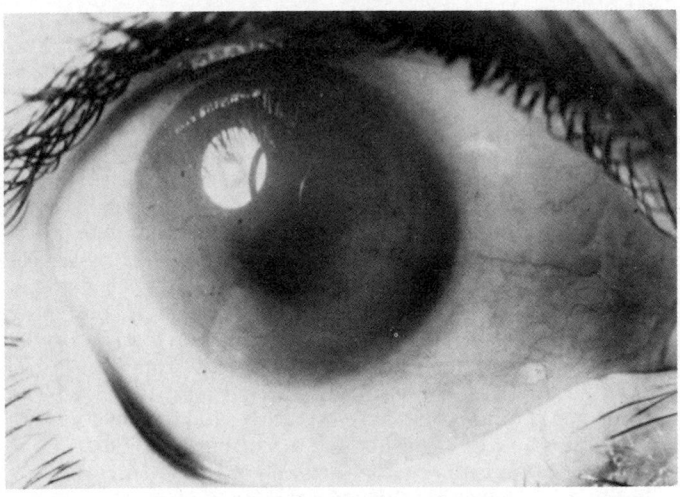

367. Diffuse corneal clouding involving the entire stroma

MUCOPOLYSACCHARIDOSIS II

Includes: Mucopolysaccharidose de type II
Mucopolysaccharidose II
Mucopolisacaridosis Tipo II
Hunter syndrome
MPS II

Excludes: Other mucopolysaccharidoses
Mucolipidosis III (673)
G_{M1}-Gangliosidosis, type 1 (431)

Minimal Diagnostic Criteria: Male with the below-described clinical findings, mucopolysacchariduria and 1) abnormal sulfate kinetics in cultured fibroblasts corrected by Hunter factor, or 2) sulfoiduronate sulfatase deficiency in fibroblasts, serum, or lymphocytes.

Clinical Findings: Normal appearance at birth with normal or excessive growth during first 1-2 years. Paucity of clinical signs except respiratory symptoms (noisy breathing from upper airway obstruction, recurrent rhinorrhea), large scaphoid head and herniae (inguinal and umbilical) during infancy. Coarsening of facial features with thickening of the nostrils, lips and tongue, joint stiffness, growth failure, excessive growth of fine body hair and hepatosplenomegaly become obvious at about 2 years and progress in severity. Thick skin, short neck, widely spaced teeth, hearing loss of some degree, and papilledema commonly present; nodular skin lesions on the arms or posterior chest wall, retinal pigmentation, mild pectus excavatum, pes cavus, mucoid diarrhea and seizures less common. The spine is straight, corneas clear grossly, and intellect may be normal but with a tendency to disruptive, destructive behavior. Mentation, valvular and coronary heart disease, hearing and joint mobility slowly deteriorate.

Two other less distinctive types are recognized clinically: in the "mild form" (MPS II-B) mentation may be normal and deterioration of mental function only slowly progressive; in the "severe form" (MPS II-A) profound mental retardation becomes obvious by late childhood. Other clinical features may be the same, but with slower progression in the "mild form."†

Roentgenologic findings include scaphoid skull, enlarged sella with anterior excavation, skeletal findings of dysostosis multiplex, minimal vertebral changes, precocious osteoarthritis of femoral head.

Laboratory findings include acid mucopolysacchariduria with excessive excretion of dermatan sulfate and heparan sulfate; leukocytes and fibroblasts are deficient in the enzyme sulfoiduronate sulfatase; metachromatic staining of leukocyte granules and fibroblasts; cultured fibroblasts accumulate sulfated mucopolysaccharides at an enhanced rate and can be "corrected" with purified Hunter factor or with fibroblast secretion from non-Hunter individuals.

Complications
I **Derived:** Coronary and valvular cardiac disease from AMPS deposition, hydrocephaly, progressive hearing loss, immobilization by joint contractures, degenerative hip disease.
II **Associated:** —

Etiology: X-linked recessive; McK *30990

Pathogenesis: Accumulation of acid mucopolysaccharide in tissues underlies most of the observed clinical features.
The block in mucopolysaccharide metabolism has been shown to be a deficiency of the enzyme sulfoiduronate sulfatase.

Related Facts
I **Sex Ratio:** M1:F0

II **Risk of Occurrence:** ? 1 in 100,000 live births known in Caucasians, Negroes, Orientals, and American Indians.
III **Risk of Recurrence for**
   Patient's Sib: If mother is a carrier, 1 in 2 (50%) for each brother to be affected and 1 in 2 for each sister to be a carrier.
   Patient's Child: 1 in 1 (100%) for carrier daughters; not increased for sons unless wife is a carrier.
IV **Age of Detectability:** At 14 weeks gestation by sulfate metabolism or sulfoiduronate sulfatase assay of cultured amniotic cells.
V **Prevalence:** ? Less than birth frequency because of early death.

Treatment
I **Primary Prevention:** Genetic counseling, prenatal diagnosis
II **Secondary Prevention:** Surgical correction of herniae and joint contractures for functional and cosmetic improvement; ventricular shunting for hydrocephaly.
III **Other Therapy:** Hearing devices, physical therapy, special education.

Prognosis: Compatible with survival to adult life. However, the majority of patients die prior to age 20 years of cardiac decompensation, pulmonary infection or neurologic complications. The longest survivor died at age 60. One known affected has reproduced.

Detection of Carrier: May be identified by enzyme assay or sulfate incorporation studies of fibroblasts. Utilizing cloning techniques, two cell lines, one with the mucopolysaccharide abnormality and the other normal, can be discerned. Consistent selection of Hunter cells in culture after thawing carrier cells frozen in liquid nitrogen offers another means of carrier detection.

†**Special Considerations:** Individuals with MPS I and MPS II excrete the same acid mucopolysaccharides qualitatively and quantitatively; yet they are quite distinct genetically and clinically. MPS II has all the features of MPS I but to a remarkably milder degree - the corneal changes can be seen only with the slit lamp, intellect may be normal at least initially, the skeletal changes are less severe, and outlook for longevity is greater. The mild and severe subtypes both lack the same enzyme; hence are probably allelic conditions.

References:
Hunter, C.: A rare disease in two brothers. Proc. R. Soc. Med. 10:104, 1917.
Leroy, J.G. and Crocker, A.C.: Clinical definition of the Hurler-Hunter phenotypes. Am. J. Dis. Child. 112:518, 1966.
McKusick, V.A.: Heritable Disorders of Connective tissue. 4th ed. St. Louis: C.V. Mosby Co., 1972.

Contributor: **Roger E. Stevenson**

Editor's Computerized Descriptors: Eye, Hearing, Face, Oral, Teeth, Nasoph., Nose, Neck, Skin, Hair, Skel., Hernia not CNS, Resp., Spleen, Liver, Nerve, CV.

MUCOPOLYSACCHARIDOSIS III

Includes: Mucopolysaccharidose de type III
Mucopolysaccharidose III
Mucopolisacaridosis Tipo III
Sanfilippo syndrome
MPS III
Polydystrophia oligophrenia

Excludes: Other mucopolysaccharidoses†
Mucolipidosis I, II and III (671, 672, 673)
G_{M1}-Gangliosidosis, type 1 (431)

Minimal Diagnostic Criteria: Severe mental deterioration, mild somatic defects, and the urinary excretion of heparan sulfate alone are findings sufficient for the diagnosis of MPS III. Metachromatic staining is nonspecific. Confirmatory enzyme assay or sulfate kinetic studies on cultured fibroblasts are necessary to distinguish the 2 types.

Clinical Findings: Normal appearance at birth, initial developmental milestones normal. Slowing of development usually obvious within 1-2 years but may not become apparent until early school age. Mental and motor development reach a peak by early school age followed by behavioral disturbances and dramatic intellectual decline thereafter. Mental and motor skills are lost and the often agitated, demented patient becomes bedridden. Growth is minimally affected, the head enlarged, hirsutism present. The mild coarsening of facial features, limitation of joint mobility, and hepatosplenomegaly never become prominent features. Deafness, although hard to evaluate, is thought to occur. Corneal clouding and cardiac abnormalities have not been described. The A and B subtypes have identical features, but can be distinguished by enzymatic assay.

    Roentgenologic findings: all bone changes, except for the skull, are similar but milder than in MPS I. The calvarium is remarkably thickened and sellar enlargement is not pronounced.

    Laboratory findings: urinary excretion of heparan sulfate: Sanfilippo A lacks heparan sulfate sulfatase; Sanfilippo B lacks N-acetyl-α-glucosaminidase, both lysosomal enzymes that degrade mucopolysaccharide; fibroblasts and lymphocyte granules stain metachromatically.

Complications
I   **Derived:** Severe mental deterioration
II   **Associated:** —

Etiology: Both subtypes autosomal recessive; McK *25290

Pathogenesis: An enzymatic error in degradation of acid mucopolysaccharide underlies both subtypes.

Related Facts
I   **Sex Ratio:** M1:F1
II   **Risk of Occurrence:** ? Perhaps 1 in 150,000
III   **Risk of Recurrence for**
     Patient's Sib: 1 in 4 (25%) for each offspring to be affected
     Patient's Child: (No patients have reproduced.)
IV   **Age of Detectability:** 14 weeks gestation by enzyme assay or by sulfate incorporation of cultured amniotic cells.
V   **Prevalence:** ?

Treatment
I   **Primary Prevention:** Genetic counseling, prenatal diagnosis and abortion
II   **Secondary Prevention:** ? Plasma and lymphocyte infusions currently under investigation.
III   **Other Therapy:** —

Prognosis: Death in bedridden, severely demented state by age 20. Few survivors to age 30.

Detection of Carrier: Intermediate enzyme levels in asymptomatic carriers.

†**Special Considerations:** MPS III carries the grave prognosis of severe CNS involvement but is largely spared the pronounced skeletal, corneal, and visceral involvement of the other mucopolysaccharidoses. The 2 subtypes although identical clinically, are separable biochemically.

References:
Maroteaux, P. and Lamy, M: Hurler's disease, and related mucopolysaccharidoses. J. Pediatr. 67:312, 1965.
Sanfilippo, S.J. et al: Mental retardation associated with acid mucopolysacchariduria (heparitin sulfate type). J. Pediatr. 63:837, 1963.
Terry, K. and Linker, A.: Distinction among four forms of Hurler's syndrome. Proc. Soc. Exp. Biol. 115:394, 1964.

Contributor: **Roger E. Stevenson**

Editor's Computerized Descriptors: Face, Hair, Skel., Nerve

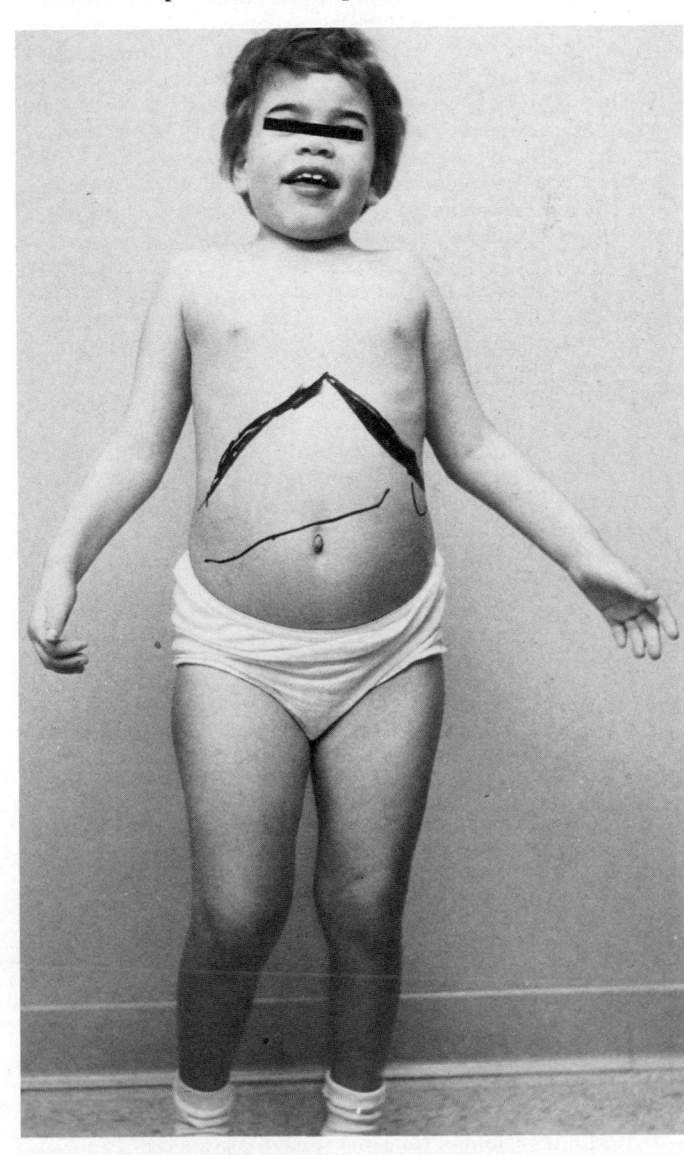

368. MPS III. Note mild coarsening of facial features, hepatosplenomegaly

MUCOPOLYSACCHARIDOSIS IV

Includes: Mucopolysaccharidose de type IV
Mucopolysaccharidose IV
Mucopolisacaridosis Tipo IV
Morquio syndrome†
Brailsford syndrome
Morquio-Ullrich syndrome
MPS IV
Chondroosteodystrophy
Keratosulfaturia

Excludes: Other mucopolysaccharidoses
Mucolipidosis I, II and III (671, 672, 673)
G_{M1}-Gangliosidosis, type 1 (431)
Other forms of short-trunk dwarfism
β-Galactosidase deficiency

Minimal Diagnostic Criteria: Pathognomonic roentgenologic findings plus clinical features and keratosulfaturia. Confirmatory enzyme assay (6-sulfate sulfatase) is desirable.†

Clinical Findings: The normal intrauterine growth and development continues during the early postnatal months. By 18 months growth retardation and skeletal changes (genu valgum, flaring of lower ribs, kyphoscoliosis) become obvious. Intellectual development proceeds at a normal pace and may remain relatively normal despite progressive somatic changes; marked growth retardation, diffuse steamy corneal clouding, prominent lower face, enamel hypoplasia in deciduous and secondary teeth, short neck, pectus carinatum, exaggerated lumbar lordosis, laxity and subluxation of joints, eg wrists, and flat feet. Aortic regurgitation is present in most patients by age 20. Hearing loss present in many patients and cardiac signs in a minority.

Roentgenologic findings: X-ray changes predate clinical abnormalities and progressively worsen. Vertebral flattening with central anterior projections in the thoracic area and hook-shaped projections in lumbar area, aplasia or hypoplasia of odontoid, increased intervertebral spaces, ossification centers delayed, epiphyses irregular, proximal pointing of metacarpals, wide ribs, generalized osteoporosis, normal skull.

Laboratory findings: keratosulfaturia in the presence of normal or increased total urinary AMPS excretion; deficiency of n-acetyl-hexosamine 6-sulfate sulfatase in cultured fibroblasts; granular inclusions in small percentage of granulocytes.

Complications
I   **Derived:** Neurologic signs from spinal cord and nerve root compression, hearing loss, aortic regurgitation, compensatory hyperpnea. Atlantoaxial subluxation due to aplasia of the odontoid and ligamentous laxity may lead to acute or chronic neurologic signs. Weakness in the legs is usually due to this and paraplegia is frequent.
II   **Associated:** —

Etiology: Autosomal recessive; McK *25300

Pathogenesis: A deficiency of galactose 6 sulfatase leads to lysosomal accumulation of keratin sulfate in susceptible tissues.

Related Facts
I   **Sex Ratio:** M1:F1
II   **Risk of Occurrence:** Probably < 1 in 100,000
III   **Risk of Recurrence for**
    Patient's Sib: 1 in 4 (25%) for each offspring to be affected
    Patient's Child: No patients have reproduced.
IV   **Age of Detectability:** Prior to 1 year of age by roentgenologic changes and keratosulfate excretion.
V   **Prevalence:** ?

Treatment
I   **Primary Prevention:** Genetic counseling
II   **Secondary Prevention:** No curative therapy available. Surgical correction of herniae, upper cervical spinal fusion to avert or remedy spinal cord compression. Corneal transplantation not helpful, cardiac valve replacement not appropriate.
III   **Other Therapy:** Physical therapy, hearing aids

Prognosis: May survive to early adulthood; most die prior to age 20 usually with cardiac or neurologic complications.

Detection of Carrier: ?

†Special Considerations: Designation of Morquio disease as a mucopolysaccharidosis is based on urinary excretion of keratosulfate. Excessive keratosulfaturia may occur in the absence of elevated total urinary mucopolysaccharides. Keratosulfaturia may decrease or disappear entirely in older patients. Study of the kinetics of sulfate metabolism has not been useful in the diagnosis of MPS IV. There exists at least 2 subtypes; the classic form described above and a type with less severe skeletal and extraskeletal features and no excessive mucopolysacchariduria. Additionally a third group of patients having very mild features with keratosulfaturia and β-galactosidase deficiency of fibroblasts has been identified.

References:
Langer, L.O., Jr. and Carey, L.S.: The roentgenographic features of the KS mucopolysaccharidosis of Morquio (Morquio-Brailsford disease). Am. J. Roentgenol. Radium Ther. Nucl. Med. 97:1, 1966.
Robins, M.M. et al: Morquio's disease: An abnormality of mucopolysaccharide metabolism. J. Pediatr. 62:881, 1963.

Contributor: **Roger E. Stevenson**

Editor's Computerized Descriptors: Eye, Hearing, Face, Teeth, Neck, Skel., Resp., CV., Nerve

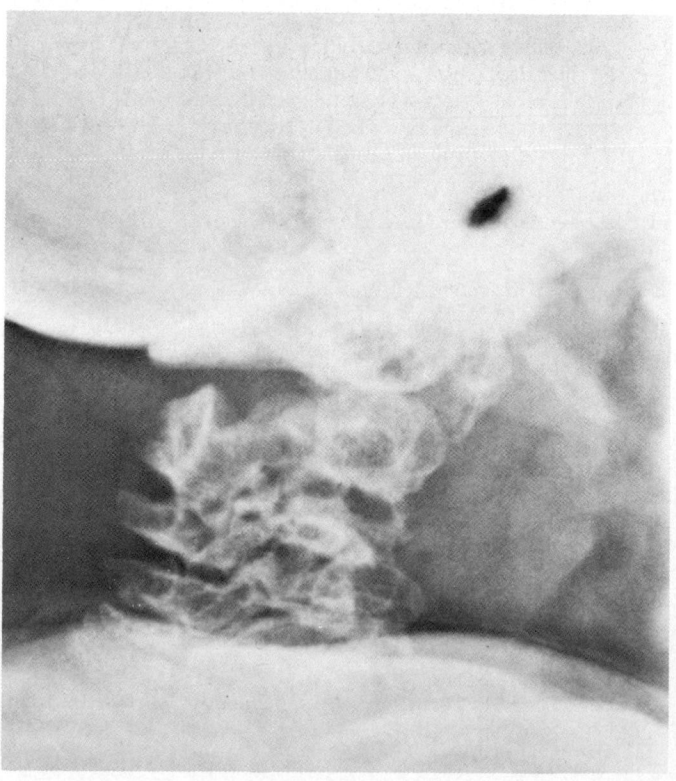

369. Lateral roentgenogram of cervical spine shows rudimentary dens; atlas closely applied to the occiput

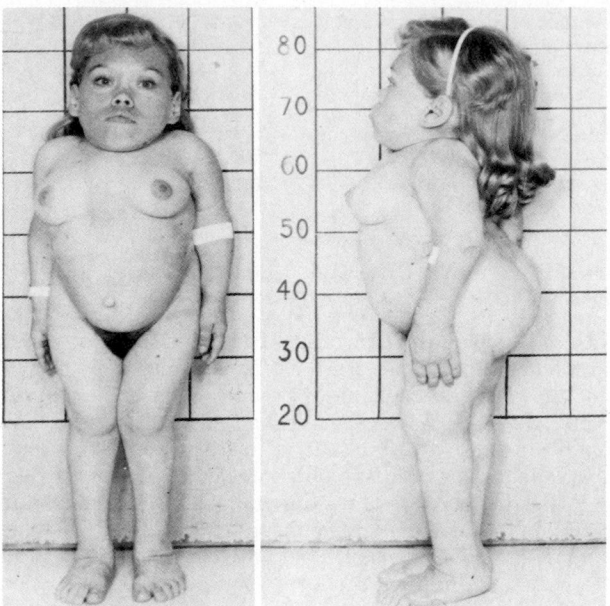

370. Note prominent lower face, short neck, short-trunk dwarfism and skeletal deformities secondary to MPS IV

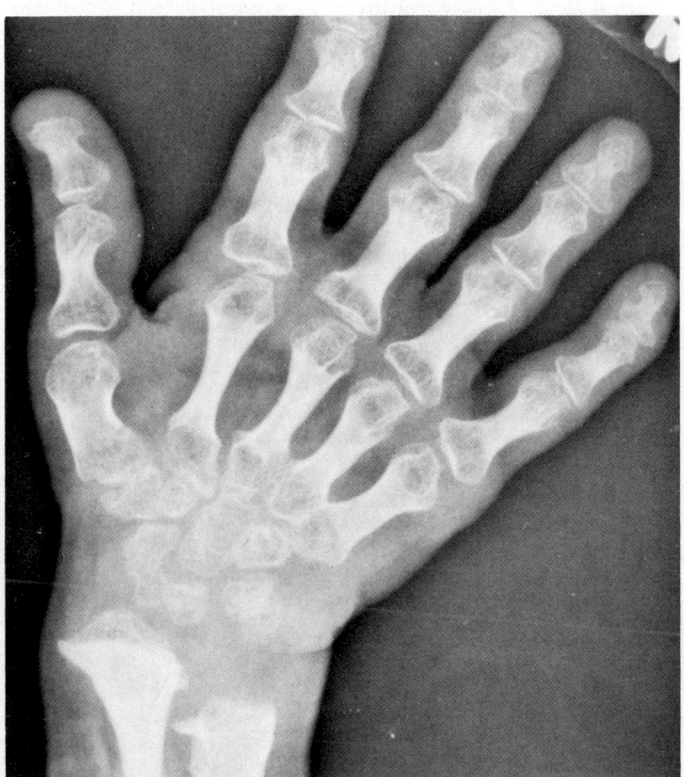

371. Note small, extremely irregular carpals; short ulna and ulnar deviation; short metacarpals and phalanges with wide ends, but well-constricted shafts

MUCOPOLYSACCHARIDOSIS VI

Includes: Mucopolysaccharidose de type VI
Mucopolysaccharidose VI
Mucopolisacaridosis Tipo VI
Maroteaux-Lamy syndrome
MPS VI

Excludes: Other mucopolysaccharidoses
Mucolipidosis I, II and III (671, 672, 673)
G_{M1}-Gangliosidosis, type 1 (431)

Minimal Diagnostic Criteria: Severe Hurler-like somatic features with normal intelligence, urinary dermatan sulfate excess, arylsulfatase B deficiency or abnormal sulfate kinetics in cultured fibroblasts.†

Clinical Findings: Normal appearance at birth. Mental development normal or nearly so, growth retardation noted by 2-3 years. Slowly progressive clouding of corneas, hearing loss, joint stiffness, coarsening of facial features with thick nostrils and lips obvious by early school age; hepatosplenomegaly, lumbar kyphosis, genu valgum; herniae.

Roentgenologic findings: calvarium with greatly enlarged sella, fragmented epiphyses, mild flattening of vertebrae with wedging of lumbar vertebrae, expanded ribs.

Laboratory findings include urinary excretion of dermatan sulfate; metachromatic staining of fibroblasts and leukocyte inclusions; fibroblasts and leukocytes have deficient arylsulfatase B activity.

Complications
I   **Derived:** Blindness, progressive hearing loss, cardiac and respiratory decompensation, hydrocephaly
II **Associated:** —

Etiology: Autosomal recessive; McK *25320

Pathogenesis: Deficiency of arylsulfatase B preventing normal lysosomal degradation of mucopolysaccharide, allowing accumulation of AMPS in soft tissues and disruption of bone development.

Related Facts
I   **Sex Ratio:** M1:F1
II **Risk of Occurrence:** ? < 1 in 100,000 live births
III **Risk of Recurrence for**
   Patient's Sib: 1 in 4 (25%) for each offspring to be affected
   Patient's Child: Not increased unless mate is carrier or homozygote. (Fertility not known, patients die early.)
IV **Age of Detectability:** Theoretically at 14 weeks gestation by assay of arylsulfatase B or by sulfate incorporation and "correction" studies in cultured amniotic cells.
V   **Prevalence:** ?

Treatment
I   **Primary Prevention:** Genetic counseling, prenatal diagnosis
II **Secondary Prevention:** Plasma and leukocyte infusions presently under investigation. Surgical correction of herniae and contractures benefit patients.
III **Other Therapy:** Physical therapy, hearing aids.

Prognosis: Death prior to 20 years, generally of cardiorespiratory complications.

Detection of Carrier: Not possible with certainty using currently available laboratory techniques.

†**Special Considerations:** There appears to be a milder form which is less common than the classic form described above. Sulfate incorporation, "correction" studies and enzyme analysis indicate the 2 subtypes to be allelic.

References:

Maroteaux, P. and Lamy, M.: Hurler's disease, Morquio's disease, and related mucopolysaccharidoses. J. Pediatr. 67:312, 1965.

McKusick, V.A.: Heritable Disorders of Connective Tissue, 4th Ed. St. Louis: C.V. Mosby Co., 1972.

Contributor: Roger E. Stevenson

Editor's Computerized Descriptors: Eye, Hearing, Face, Nose, Skel., Hernia not CNS, Liver, Spleen, Resp.

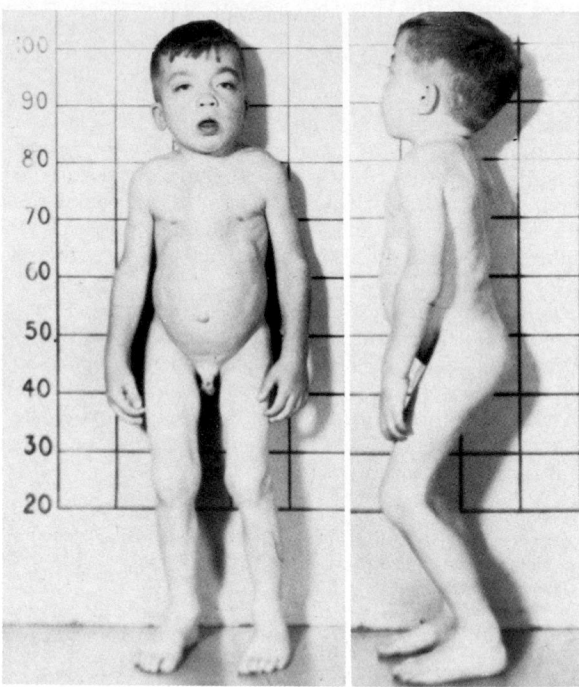

372. Note short stature, coarse facies, protruding tongue, disproportionately short neck, deformed chest, and semicrouching stance

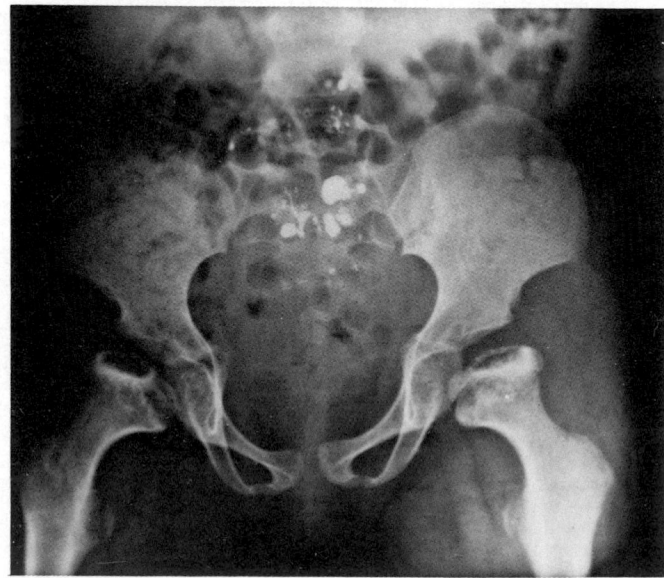

373. Note flat femoral capital epiphyses with large, cyst-like radiolucencies; surrounding sclerosis; narrow necks; gracile pelvic bones; oblique acetabular roofs

MUCOPOLYSACCHARIDOSIS VII

Includes: Mucopolysaccharidose de type VII
Mucopolysaccharidose VII
Mucopolisacaridosis Tipo VII
β-glucuronidase deficiency

Excludes: Mucopolysaccharidoses I-VI†
Mucolipidoses I-IV
Aspartylglycosylaminuria
Fucosidosis (398)
Mannosidosis

Minimal Diagnostic Criteria: β-glucuronidase deficiency in tissues, fibroblasts, leukocytes, and serum.

Clinical Findings: This clinical description is based on the first 6 described cases of MPS VII. Although this disease is not yet well defined, 2 major groups appear to be emerging. Some patients (4 cases) have had clinical signs either at birth or within the 1st year of life. These patients exhibit coarsened facies, hepatosplenomegaly, corneal clouding (3/4), frequent respiratory infections, umbilical or inguinal herniae, leukocyte inclusions, short stature (3/4), and developmental retardation. The radiologic features of the early-onset form include moderate-to-severe bony abnormalities, J-shaped sella, vertebral beaking, and broadening of tubular bones, (dysostosis multiplex). A 2nd form, presenting in the 2nd decade of life, has been recognized in 2 patients. A 13-year-old male presented with normal mentation and growth, and without hepatosplenomegaly. He manifested a coarsened face, mild bony changes, granulocyte inclusions and minimal corneal opacification. His major medical problem, however, was fibromuscular dysplasia of the aorta with mucopolysaccharide infiltration, resulting in severe aortic regurgitation and left heart failure. A 17-year-old girl has been reported with β-glucuronidase deficiency but no other stigmata.

Complications
I **Derived:** Moderate retardation in those cases presenting early. Orthopedic problems including joint contractures and spinal malformations. Severe aortic infiltration resulting in fibromuscular dysplasia and aortic regurgitation.
II **Associated:** Frequent respiratory illnesses and dislocated hips.

Etiology: Autosomal recessive; McK *25322

Pathogenesis: Absence of lysosomal enzyme β-glucuronidase in all tissues examined and storage of mucopolysaccharides in various organs. The clinical variability is not yet explained.

Related Facts
I **Sex Ratio:** M3:F3
II **Risk of Occurrence:** Rare. Only 6 cases reported to date.
III **Risk of Recurrence for**
   Patient's Sib: 1 in 4 (25%) for each offspring to be affected.
   Patient's Child: Approximately 0, but depends upon the carrier frequency which is unknown.
IV **Age of Detectability:** Midtrimester of pregnancy by analysis of amniotic fluid cells.
V **Prevalence:** Rare

Treatment
I **Primary Prevention:** Genetic counseling
II **Secondary Prevention:** Prenatal diagnosis; enzyme replacement therapy is being investigated but is not yet feasible.
III **Other Therapy:** Surgical procedures for correction of herniae, orthopedic, ophthalmologic and cardiac problems.

Prognosis: The disease course exhibits marked variability and, as such, accurate prediction of the prognosis is not yet possible.

Detection of Carrier: Possible by fibroblasts or leukocyte assays for β-glucuronidase activity.

†**Special Considerations:** Mucopolysaccharidosis VII differs from the other mucopolysaccharidoses in that it was defined as a biochemical entity as quickly as it was clinically recognized. Subsequent cases therefore were identified on biochemical grounds and not on the basis of clinical findings. It has been suggested that the clinical forms represent allelic disorders; however, the genetic and molecular basis for phenotypic heterogeneity is unknown.

References:

Beaudet, A.L. et al: Variation in the phenotypic expression of β-glucuronidase deficiency. J. Pediatr. 86:388, 1975.

Gehler, J. et al: Mucopolysaccharidosis VII: β-glucuronidase deficiency. Humangenetik 23:149, 1974.

Glaser, J.H. and Sly, W.S.: β-glucuronidase deficiency mucopolysaccharidosis: Methods for enzymatic diagnosis. J. Lab Clin. Med. 83:969, 1973.

Contributors: **Kyrieckos Aleck**
Larry J. Shapiro

Editor's Computerized Descriptors: Eye, Face, Skel., Hernia not CNS, Resp., CV., Spleen, Liver

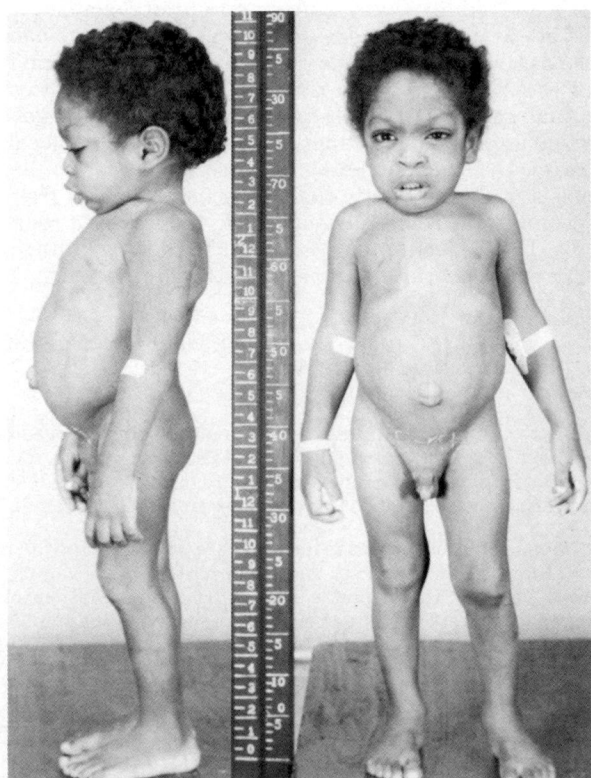

374. Note short stature, coarse facial features, chest configuration, and abdominal protuberance

MUCOSA, WHITE FOLDED DYSPLASIA

Includes: Leucokératose esfobrante des muqueuses
Leukoplakische epitheliale Naevi
Mucosa plegada, blanca displásica
White sponge nevus
White folded dysplasia of mucosa

Excludes: Leukoplakia†
Intraepithelial dyskeratosis (538)
Pachyonychia congenita (789)
Leukoedema
Focal epithelial hyperplasia of oral mucosa
Dyskeratosis congenita
Dermal hypoplasia, focal (281)
Oral epithelial nevus of Cooke

Minimal Diagnostic Criteria: Congenital white folded soft hyperplastic oral mucosal lesions without eye involvement and a history of similar mucosal lesions in other family members.

Clinical Findings: Congenital, asymptomatic, white, folded, soft, hyperplastic mucosal lesions reported to involve the following mucosal sites in the percentages given. It is not known if all sites listed were examined in all cases.

Oral mucosa	100%
Vaginal mucosa	60%
Anal mucosa	40%
Penile mucosa	30%
Nasal mucosa	10%

No roentgenologic changes. Cytologic smears (Papanicolaou stain) show that majority of mucosal cells contain a perinuclear or cytoplasmic condensation in the cytoplasm (by electron microscopy, tonofibrils) which stain intensely (H & E and Papanicolaou). Tissue sections demonstrate hyperplasia of prickle cell layer, moderate acanthosis, intracellular edema giving a "chicken wire" appearance to section, perinuclear or cytoplasmic condensations best seen on Papanicolaou or PAS stains with little or no changes in lamina propria or submucosa.

Complications
I **Derived:** None except iatrogenic effects resulting from surgical or x-ray therapy for supposed precancerous lesion when treatment is initiated while lesion is mistaken for leukoplakia especially with vaginal involvement.
II **Associated:** —

Etiology: A gene mutation resulting in an autosomal dominantly inherited trait. No linkage with ABO, MNS, P, Rh, Fy, Jk, Se, Hp, Gc, PGM. McK *19390

Pathogenesis: ? Essentially an intracellular lesion with alterations in the cytoplasmic distribution of tonofibrils in epithelial cells.

Related Facts
I **Sex Ratio:** M1:F1
II **Risk of Occurrence:** ? Rare
III **Risk of Recurrence for**
    Patient's Sib: If parent is affected 1 in 2 (50%) for each offspring to be affected; otherwise not increased
    Patient's Child: 1 in 2
IV **Age of Detectability:** Diagnosed in neonatal period by visual examination confirmed by cytologic or histologic examination. Most cases not diagnosed until late childhood.
V **Prevalence:** ? Rare (100 reported cases)

Treatment
I **Primary Prevention:** Genetic counseling
II **Secondary Prevention:** ?
III **Other Therapy:** Stripping and other surgical procedures,

especially for vaginal and penile lesions should be avoided as there is no indication that this is a precancerous lesion.

Prognosis: Excellent. Does not predispose to malignant disease. No demonstrable reduction in reproductive fitness or longevity. Main complications result when lesions treated by surgery or radiation on the basis of a mistaken diagnosis.

Detection of Carrier: —

†Special Considerations: Must be differentiated from leukoedema which is acquired, usually found in debilitated conditions and is usually not folded; from leukoplakia which is acquired, not congenital and usually a firm hard lesion of the mucosa. (Any patient with atypical vaginal "leukoplakia" should be examined for lesion at other mucosal sites as a possible example of this condition and radical therapy avoided.) Must also be differentiated from focal hypoplasia of oral mucosa which is the same color as the adjacent normal mucosa and histologically shows only increased thickness of epithelial cell layer; from intraepithelial dyskeratosis which has perilimbal gelatinous plaques of the bulbar conjunctivae and from oral epithelial nevus of Cooke which is not familial and histologically has a basket weave pattern of the superficial cornified layer and a granular layer absent in normal oral mucosa. Diagnosis of this condition can be made on smears which show the perinuclear or cytoplasmic condensations giving this disease the designation of the "spotted cell disease." Distribution of cytoplasmic condensation is the opposite of that seen in pemphigus which has a perinuclear halo and peripheral cytoplasmic condensation.

References:
Browne, W.G. et al: White sponge naevus of the mucosa: Clinical and linkage data. Ann. Hum. Genet. 32:271, 1969.
Whitten, J. B.: The electron microscopic examination of congenital keratoses of the oral mucous membranes. I. White sponge nevus. Oral Surg. 29:69, 1970.
Witkop, C. J., Jr. and Gorlin, R. J.: Four hereditary mucosal syndromes: Comparative histology and exfoliative cytology of Darier-White's disease, hereditary benign intraepithelial dyskeratosis, white sponge nevus, and pachyonychia congenita. Arch. Dermatol. 84:762, 1961.
Zegarelli, E.V. et al: Familial white folded dysplasia of the mucous membranes. Arch. Dermatol. 80:59, 1959.

Contributor: **Carl J. Witkop, Jr.**

Editor's Computerized Descriptors: Oral, Nasoph., GI., GU.

MÜLLERIAN APLASIA

Includes: Syndrome de Rokitansky-Küster-Hauser
Aplasie von Uterus und Vagina
Aplasia de los conductos de Müller
Rokitansky-Küster-Hauser syndrome†
Congenital absence of uterus and vagina

Excludes: Androgen insensitivity syndrome, complete (49)
Incomplete transverse vaginal septum
Müllerian fusion, incomplete (684)

Minimal Diagnostic Criteria: Congenital absence of the uterus in a 46,XX individual with normal ovarian development and normal female external genitalia. Müllerian remnants or fallopian tubes may persist.

Clinical Findings: Individuals with müllerian aplasia show normal sexual development except for absence of müllerian derivatives; thus, fallopian tubes, uterine corpus, uterine cervix and the upper portion of the vagina are absent. Occasionally fibromuscular remnants or rudimentary fallopian tubes persist. The external genitalia are those of a normal female. The hymen is intact, but the vagina ends blindly. At puberty, normal female secondary sexual development occurs, including breast enlargement, pubic and axillary hair, and an appropriate increase in the size of external genitalia. Pelvic examination at puberty reveals a blindly ending vaginal pouch, usually 4-5 cm long, but occasionally no more than 1-2 cm long. Ovaries are normal; sex steroid levels are normal and plasma gonadotropin levels respond appropriately to normal feedback control. Urologic anomalies are associated with müllerian aplasia more frequently than expected; the most frequent are unilateral renal aplasia, pelvic kidney, and renal ectopia. The frequency of certain skeletal abnormalities, particularly vertebral abnormalities, is increased.

Complications
I   **Derived:** Lack of adequate vaginal length may cause difficulties with coitus; infertility.
II **Associated:** Renal and vertebral anomalies

Etiology: Cytogenetic studies are normal and no teratogenic factors have been demonstrated. There are several reports of multiple affected sibs. Recurrence risk figures are not available, but polygenic/multifactorial etiology seems most likely. McK *27700

Pathogenesis: The müllerian ducts differentiate into the fallopian tubes, uterus, uterine cervix, and upper portion of the vagina. The lower portion of the vagina is derived from invaginations of the urogenital sinus. Thus, the phenotype observed in these individuals can be explained completely by absence or aplasia of müllerian ducts.

Related Facts
I   **Sex Ratio:** M0:F1
II   **Risk of Occurrence:**   ?
III **Risk of Recurrence for**
     Patient's Sib: Slightly increased riks for 46,XX sibs, compared to the general population, but probably no more than 5%; no risk for XY sibs.
     Patient's Child: All patients are infertile.
IV   **Age of Detectability:** At puberty because of primary amenorrhea.
V   **Prevalence:** ? Approximately 20% of women with primary amenorrhea have müllerian aplasia.

Treatment
I   **Primary Prevention:** Genetic counseling
II   **Secondary Prevention:** —
III **Other Therapy:** Construction of artificial vagina may be necessary. Hormonal therapy is not necessary, nor is laparotomy or laparoscopy necessary to confirm the diagno-

Prognosis: Presumably normal life span, unless renal abnormalities are severe.

Detection of Carrier: —

†Special Considerations: A few individuals who otherwise conform to the diagnosis of müllerian aplasia show rudimentary müllerian structures—relatively undifferentiated fibromuscular elements, rudimentary fallopian tubes, or occasionally a small uterine-like structure. If such müllerian remnants persist, many investigators apply the term Rokitansky-Küster-Hauser syndrome. It seems likely that müllerian aplasia and the Rokitansky-Küster-Hauser syndrome represent the same entity.

A second group of individuals show absence of the lower portion of the vagina. The caudal portion is replaced by 2-3 cm of fibrous tissue, superior to which are a well-differentiated upper vagina, uterine cervix, uterine corpus and fallopian tubes. These individuals have vaginal atresia.

A phenotypic female with normal secondary sexual development but without a uterus has either müllerian aplasia or complete testicular feminization. These 2 disorders are readily distinguished by cytogenetic studies.

References:
Jones, H.W., Jr. and Mermut, S.: Familial occurrence of congenital absence of the vagina. Am. J. Obstet. Gynecol. 114:1100, 1972.
Jones, H.W., Jr. and Scott, W.M.: Hermaphroditism, Genital Anomalies, and Related Endocrine Disorders, 2nd ed. Baltimore: Williams & Wilkins, 1971.
Sarto, G.E. and Simpson, J.L.: Abnormalities of the müllerian and wolffian duct systems. In Summitt, R.E. and Bergsma, D. (eds.): Annual Review of Birth Defects 1977. New York:Alan R. Liss for The National Foundation-March of Dimes, l978, vol. XIV (6C).
Simpson, J.L.: Disorders of Sexual Differentiation: Etiology and Clinical Delineation. New York: Academic Press, 1976.

Contributor: **Joe Leigh Simpson**

Editor's Computerized Descriptor: GU.

MÜLLERIAN DERIVATIVES IN MALES, PERSISTENT

Includes: Syndrome de hernie utérine
Uterus-Hernie
Síndrome de hernia uterina
Uterine inguinal hernia syndrome
Persistence of oviducts in males
Tubular male pseudohermaphroditism
Hernia uteri inguinale syndrome
Uterine hernia syndrome

Excludes: Chromosome 45,X/46,XY mosaicism (173)
True hermaphroditism (971)
All other forms of male pseudohermaphroditism

Minimal Diagnostic Criteria: 46,XY individual with normal male external genitalia and testes who has a uterus and fallopian tubes.

Clinical Findings: A uterus and fallopian tubes are present in otherwise normal males. Affected individuals have normal male external genitalia, normal wolffian derivatives (vasa deferentia, epididymides, seminal vesicles) and usually normal testes. No somatic anomalies are present. At puberty virilization occurs. Endocrine studies produce results expected of a normal male. The disorder is often detected because the uterus and fallopian tubes prolapse into an inguinal hernia; thus, these patients are often said to have the uterine inguinal hernia syndrome. However, many affected patients do not have inguinal herniae and for that reason this contributor prefers the designation cited in the title.

Complications
I   **Derived:** Herniation of the uterus and fallopian tubes into the inguinal canal; neoplastic transformation of cryptorchid testes.
II **Associated:** None

Etiology: Probably an autosomal recessive or X-linked recessive gene. McK *26155. In 1 family, maternal half-sibs were affected.

Pathogenesis: ? but müllerian derivatives presumably fail to regress because of either 1) failure of the fetal testes to elaborate the müllerian suppressive factor, or 2) inability of the müllerian ducts to respond to the müllerian suppressive factor.

Related Facts
I   **Sex Ratio:** M1:F0
II   **Risk of Occurrence:** ?
III **Risk of Recurrence for**
     Patient's Sib: If trait is autosomal recessive, 1 in 4 for 46,XY sibs, and 1 in 8 for all sibs. If trait is X-linked recessive, 1 in 2 for 46,XY sibs and 1 in 4 for all sibs.
     Patient's Child: Zero unless the patient's mate is heterozygous, in which case risk of 1 in 2 for 46,XY sibs and 1 in 4 for all sibs.
IV   **Age of Detectability:** Usually after puberty or later in life, when herniation occurs.
V   **Prevalence:** ? but rare. Many cases may never be ascertained. About 100 cases have been reported.

Treatment
I   **Primary Prevention:** Genetic counseling
II   **Secondary Prevention:** Inguinal herniorrhaphy. Uterus and fallopian tubes should be removed if discovered. Orchiopexy may be necessary.
III **Other Therapy:** —

Prognosis: Presumably normal life span, provided neoplastic transformation does not occur.

Detection of Carrier: —

Special Considerations: —

References:
Brook, C.G.D. et al: Familal occurrence of persistent Müllerian structures in otherwise normal males. Br. Med. J. 1:771, 1973.
Simpson, J.L.: Disorders of Sexual Differentiation: Etiology and Clinical Delineation. New York; Academic Press, 1976.
Sloan, W.R. and Walsh, P.C.: Familial persistent Müllerian duct syndrome. J. Urol. 115:459, 1976.

Contributor: **Joe Leigh Simpson**

Editor's Computerized Descriptors: Hernia not CNS, GU.

MÜLLERIAN FUSION, INCOMPLETE

Includes: Utérus bifide
Fussionsstörung der Müllerschen Gänge
Fusión incompleta de los conductos de Müller
Rudimentary uterine horn
Uterus unicornus
Uterus arcuatus
Arcuate uterus
Uterus subseptus
Uterus bicornus
Bicornuate uterus
Uterus bipartitus
Uterus bilocularis
Uterus didelphys
"Double uterus" (misnomer)
Uterus pseudodidelphys
Uterus bicornus unicollis

Excludes: Vaginal septum, transverse (985)
Hymen, imperforate (483)
Müllerian aplasia (682)
True duplication of müllerian ducts†

Minimal Diagnostic Criteria: Broadening and medial depression of the superior portion of the uterine septum (arcuate uterus) or more severe fusion defects in a 46,XX individual with normal ovarian and external genital development. Diagnosis should be confirmed by radiographic studies or laparoscopic visualization.

Clinical Findings: Failure of fusion of the paired müllerian ducts results in 2 hemiuteri; each hemiuterus has a single fallopian tube. Sometimes 1 müllerian duct fails to contribute to the definitive uterus or produces only a rudimentary horn. The extent of müllerian fusion may vary from slight broadening and medial depression of the superior portion of the uterine septum (arcuate uterus) to completely separated hemiuteri with separate cervices, vaginas, and perineal orifices. The most frequent types of incomplete müllerian fusion include uterine arcuatus, uterus unicornus (absence of 1 uterine horn), uterus septus (persistence of the entire uterine septum), uterus bicornis unicollis (2 hemiuteri, each leading to the same cervix), and uterus bicornus bicollis (2 hemiuteri, each leading to separate cervices). Paired vaginal septa and paired perineal orifices are relatively uncommon.

The external genitalia usually are normal, but a vaginal septum may be present. Ovarian development and puberty are normal.

Complications
I **Derived:** A rudimentary uterine horn may retain blood, produce pain and possibly rupture. Pregnancy in a rudimentary uterine horn may lead to uterine rupture or missed abortion.†
Pregnancies may be complicated by an increase in the incidences of 2nd trimester abortion and premature labor. Malpresentations are not uncommon. Following delivery the placenta may fail to separate readily from the uterus.
II **Associated:** Urologic anomalies may occur ipsilateral to a rudimentry or absent uterine horn. Incomplete müllerian fusion may be present in the Meckel syndrome, the Rüdiger syndrome, and the hand-foot-genital syndrome.

Etiology: Reported familial aggregates have included several kindreds with multiple affected sibs, and several kindreds in which both a mother and her daughters were affected. Available data are probably most consistent with polygenic or multifactorial etiology.

Pathogenesis: The müllerian ducts are originally paired organs that fuse and subsequently canalize to form the upper vagina, uterus, and fallopian tubes. Failure of fusion or canalization results in uterine septa or hemiuteri, each associated with no more than 1 fallopian tube. More incomplete fusion results in persistence of vaginal septa.

Related Facts
I Sex Ratio: F1:M0

II Risk of Occurrence: ?

III Risk of Recurrence for
  Patient's Sib: ? Probably slightly increased for 46,XX sibs (?2-5%, based upon polygenic/multifactorial etiology).
  Patient's Child: Probably slightly increased for 46,XX offspring (?2-5%).

IV Age of Detectability: Variable. Retention of menstrual blood in rudimentary horns may produce symptoms shortly after puberty, but affected indivudals are usually detected at a later age because of recurrent 2nd trimester abortions, abnormal uterine contour during labor, or other intrapartum or postpartum abnormalities. Many affected individuals are probably never detected, particularly those with uterus arcuatus or uterus subseptus.

V Prevalence: An estimated 0.1% of females, although very minor uterine anomalies have been claimed in as many as 2-3% of women whose uteri are examined immediately following delivery. A relatively high proportion of the latter have uterus arcuatus or uterus subseptus.

Treatment
I Primary Prevention: Genetic counseling.

II Secondary Prevention: Many patients with hemiuteri or septal defects have normal pregnancies and require no treatment. Extirpation of a rudimentary uterine horn may be necessary. Reunification of paired hemiuteri or removal of a septum may permit full-term pregnancy; however, surgery should not be undertaken unless the patient has had a least one 2nd trimester abortion.

III Other Therapy: —

Prognosis: Normal life span, provided rupture of a uterine horn does not lead to life-threatening complications.

Detection of Carrier: ?

†Special Considerations: Incomplete müllerian fusion should be distinguished from true müllerian duplication, an anomaly that probably results from division of 1 or both müllerian ducts early in embryogenesis. Such individuals have 2 separate uteri, each of which may have 2 fallopian tubes.

Several unusual clinical situations may result from the presence of a rudimentary horn. Menstrual blood may be retained, producing a pelvic mass and pelvic pain. Pregnancy occurring in a rudimentary tube that communicates with the uterus may terminate in uterine rupture or missed abortion; the latter may lead to lithopedian formation. A canal between hemiuteri may exist, even if a septum extends to the cervix or if 2 cervices are present. Finally, a vaginal septum bulging with blood from a rudimentary horn may obscure identification of the cervix.

References:
Jones, H.W., Jr. and Wheeless, C.R.: Salvage of the reproductive potential of women with anomalous development of the Müllerian ducts: 1868-1968 - 2068. Am. J. Obstet. Gynecol. 104:348, 1960.

Jones, H.W., Jr. and Scott, W.M.: Hermaphroditism, Genital Anomalies, and Related Endocrine Disorders, 2nd Ed. Baltimore: Williams & Wilkins, 1971.

Polishuk, W.Z. and Ron, M.A.: Familial bicornuate and double uterus. Am. J. Obstet. Gynecol. 119:982, 1974.

Sarto, G.E. and Simpson, J.L.: Abnormalities of the müllerian and wolffian duct systems. In Summitt, R.E. and Bergsma, D. (eds.-):Annual Review of Birth Defects 1977. New York:Alan R. Liss for The National Foundation-March of Dimes, l978, vol. XIV (6C).

Simpson, J.L.: Disorders of Sexual Differentiation: Etiology and Clinical Delineation. New York: Academic Press, 1976.

Contributor: **Joe Leigh Simpson**

Editor's Computerized Descriptor: GU.

MULTIPLE CARTILAGINOUS EXOSTOSES

Includes: Multiple Kartilaginäre Exostosen
Diaphyseal aclasis
Multiple exostoses

Excludes: Enchondromatosis (345)

Minimal Diagnostic Criteria: Cartilage-capped exostoses at site of actively growing bone

Clinical Findings: Characterized by numerous cartilage-capped exostoses clustered around areas of actively growing bone. The most common sites of involvement are the juxtaepiphyseal areas of the tubular bones, ribs, pelvis and scapula, while the vertebral bodies, the patella, and the carpal and tarsal bones are usually unaffected. Seventy-five percent of patients have recognizable bony deformities. Most commonly these are forearm deformities (50%), bowed radius with shortened ulna (43%), valgus ankles (45%), short stature (41%), conical ulna (25%), genu valgum (21%), radiohumeral dislocation (8%), scoliosis (4%), pelvic deformities (4%) and thoracic deformities (3%). The short stature is mild and due to shortness of the lower limbs. The arm span is also decreased. Bony deformities occur in bones affected with exostoses and are thought to be due to a "squandering" of linear growth for lateral growth. The exostoses may be recognized at birth and 80% of lesions will be recognized in the 1st decade of life. Growth of the exostoses keeps pace with active skeletal growth by enchondral growth and ceases with calcification of the cartilage cap. Radiographically, an isolated exostosis jutting from the diaphyseal shaft or a characteristic club-shaped appearance may be observed. The acid mucopolysaccharide levels are normal in adults, but mildly elevated in affected children; this increase is thought to be due to the increased bulk of cartilaginous tissue.

Complications
I   **Derived:** Vertebral exostoses may cause spinal cord compression; pelvic exostoses may cause urinary obstruction or fetal malposition; exostoses may be fractured and require removal; peripheral nerves and tendons may be compressed. Malignant degeneration occurs in about 10% of cases. Subcutaneous bursa may develop over the exostosis in about 10% of cases.
II **Associated:** Osteoma cutis

Etiology: Autosomal dominant and completely penetrant†; McK *13370

Pathogenesis: Radiographically the lesions are initially recognized as an asymmetric or beaked overgrowth of the cortex immediately adjacent to the epiphyseal plate. Thereafter, this projection may be followed by normal bone growth, leaving an isolated exostosis jutting from the diaphyseal shaft or an asymmetric increase in width may occur producing the characteristic club-shaped appearance. The exostosis, grossly and microscopically is identical to the adjacent bone, with an outer cortex, inner marrow and covering cartilage cap. Growth proceeds by enchondral ossification. The exostosis migrates with the diaphysis.†

Related Facts
I   **Sex Ratio:** Probably M1:F1, but earlier literature reported a male preponderance.
II   **Risk of Occurrence:** Krooth et al reported an incidence of 1 in 1000 on Guam. The incidence in the United States is unknown.
III **Risk of Recurrence for**
     Patient's Sib: If parent is affected, 1 in 2 (50%) for each offspring to be affected; otherwise not increased
     Patient's Child: 1 in 2
IV   **Age of Detectability:** May be detected at birth, 80% detected by the 1st decade.
V   **Prevalence:** ? Reported as 1 in 90,000 patient visits per year in a general hospital; 1 in 7000 patient visits per year in an orthopedic hospital. No ethnic predisposition known.

Treatment
I   **Primary Prevention:** Genetic counseling
II   **Secondary Prevention:** Resection of exostoses which interfere with movement, are painful, fractured, and compress nerves or tendons, or for cosmesis. Chondrosarcomas are resistant to radiotherapy and should be treated by surgical excision
III **Other Therapy:** —

Prognosis: Normal life expectancy unless chondrosarcomas develop. Malignant degeneration has been reported to occur after trauma. Chondrosarcomas increase in size slowly and metastasize late.

Detection of Carrier: —

†Special Considerations: About 40% of cases are the result of new mutations. Males and females are probably equally severely affected. The pattern of involvement with exostoses is usually not transmitted, ie an offspring may not show the same distribution of the exostoses as his affected parent.

References:
Jaffe, H.L.: Hereditary multiple exostoses. Arch. Pathol. 36:335, 1943.
Krooth, R.S. et al: Diaphyseal aclasis (multiple exostoses) on Guam. Am. J. Hum. Genet. 13:340, 1961.
McKusick, V.A.: Heritable Disorders of Connective Tissue, 4th Ed. St. Louis: C.V. Mosby Co., 1972.
Solomon, L.: Hereditary multiple exostoses. Am. J. Hum. Genet. 16:351, 1964.
Solomon, L.: Hereditary multiple exostoses. J. Bone Joint Surg. 45B:292, 1963.
Stocks, P. and Barrington, A.: Hereditary disorders of bone development. Treasure of Human Inheritance 3: Part I, 1925.

Contributor: Jack R. Lichtenstein

Editor's Computerized Descriptor: Skel.

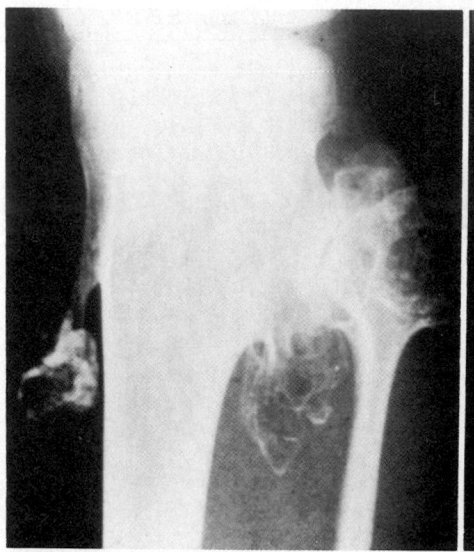
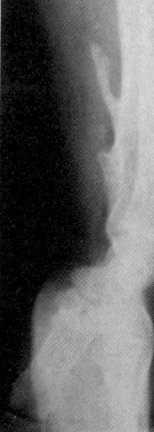
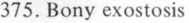

375. Bony exostosis

MUSCLE HYPOPLASIA, CONGENITAL UNIVERSAL

Includes: Hypoplasie musculaire généralisée congénitale
Angeborene generalisierte Muskelhypoplasie
Hipoplasia muscular universal congénita

Excludes: All other forms of congenital hypotonia and weakness

Minimal Diagnostic Criteria: Diffuse or universal muscular weakness, nonprogression, and normal muscle biopsy

Clinical Findings: Very few of this type of case have been described and it is not at all clear if this condition represents a single entity. It may be a syndrome with multiple causes. In 1958 Krabbe described the case of a man who had shown delayed postural control in infancy and muscular weakness and cramps, a myopathic gait and a limited capacity for exercise in childhood. There was no progression or deterioration in muscular capability. All of the skeletal muscles were very small, and tone and reflexes were reduced. Biopsy showed small bundles of muscle fibers, but no degenerative or inflammatory changes. There was no proliferation of connective tissue. The serum enzymes such as creatine phosphokinase (CPK) tend to be normal and there are no other laboratory abnormalities disclosed. It has been postulated that this condition represents either a failure in full maturation of muscle, or the presence of a lesser number of otherwise normal fibers. Certain other cases of this possible syndrome have also been described.

Complications
I   Derived: —
II Associated: —

Etiology: ?

Pathogenesis: ?

Related Facts
I   Sex Ratio: ?
II   Risk of Occurrence: ?
III Risk of Recurrence for
     Patient's Sib: ?
     Patient's Child: ?
IV   Age of Detectability: In early infancy due to delayed postural control and other evidence of universal muscular weakness
V   Prevalence: ?

Treatment
I   Primary Prevention: —
II   Secondary Prevention: —
III Other Therapy: —

Prognosis: ?

Detection of Carrier: —

Special Considerations: —

References:
Fukuma S. et al: A case of generalized muscular atrophy. Brain Nerve 13:261, 1961.
Krabbe, K. H.: Congenital generalized muscular atrophies. Acta Psychiatr. Scand. 33:94, 1958.
Schrier, K. and Huperz, R.: Über die Hypoplasia musculorum generalistata congenita. Ann. Paediatr. (Basel) 186:241, 1956.

Contributor: Carl M. Pearson

Editor's Computerized Descriptor: Muscle

MUSCULAR DYSTROPHY, ADULT PSEUDOHYPERTROPHIC

Includes: Myopathie pseudo-hypertrophique de l'adulte
Pseudohypertrophische Muskeldystrophie Typ Becker
Distrofia muscular pseudohipertrófica del adulto
Benign X-linked recessive muscular dystrophy
Muscular dystrophy, Becker
Pseudohypertrophic muscular dystrophy, adult type
Adult pseudohypertrophic muscular dystrophy

Excludes: Muscular dystrophy, childhood pseudohypertrophic (689)
Muscular dystrophy, autosomal recessive pseudohypertrophic (688)

Minimal Diagnostic Criteria: Positive family history in at least one additional male subject; elevated serum enzymes, weakness especially in proximal muscle groups.†

Clinical Findings: Clinical diagnosis in males almost invariably characterized by gradual progression of weakness and wasting of pelvic and later of the pectoral muscles. Inability to walk by 25 or more years after time of clinical onset. Absence of cardiac deformities in most families. Absence of contractures or deformities in most families. Often a normal life span. Invariably enlargement of the calf muscles with characteristic hypertrophy or "pseudohypertrophy." The weakness is predominantly proximal in distribution involving the pelvic girdle, the thigh muscles and to a lesser extent the proximal muscles of the upper limbs. There is, in addition, progressive development of lumbar lordosis, development of a waddling gait and progressive difficulty in arising from the floor, or from the chair and a progressive decrease in the ability first to run and then to walk.

Diagnostic laboratory features include elevated serum enzymes especially CPK (creatine phosphokinase), aldolase and transaminase. Muscle biopsy will show "myopathic changes" and the EMG will also disclose evidence of a myopathy.

Complications
I   Derived: Slowly progressive weakness of the skeletal musculature
II Associated: —

Etiology: X-linked recessive; McK *31010

Pathogenesis: Unknown except that the clinical and pathologic features are associated with progressive deterioration of the striated musculature of the body due to some unknown cause. The increase in elevation of the serum enzyme levels is a secondary event due to muscle fiber necrosis, or to a defect in the sarcolemmal membrane of striated muscle fibers.

Related Facts
I   Sex Ratio: M100:F0.1 (or less are symptomatic)
II   Risk of Occurrence: ?
III Risk of Recurrence for
     Patient's Sib: If mother is a carrier, 1 in 2 (50%) for each brother to be affected and 1 in 2 for each sister to be a carrier. Probably less than 1 in 1000 sisters or mothers are symptomatic.
     Patient's Child: 1 in 1 (100%) for carrier daughters; not increased for sons unless wife is a carrier. Less than 1 in 1000 are symptomatic.
IV   Age of Detectability: Approximately age 25 years by clinical manifestations, possibly earlier by serum enzyme measurements
V   Prevalence: ?

Treatment

I Primary Prevention: Genetic counseling

II Secondary Prevention: Supportive orthopedic aids and physical therapy

III Other Therapy: —

Prognosis: May live normal life span but with progressive decrease in muscular strength and difficulty in ambulation.

Detection of Carrier: Uncertain, but possibly mild elevation of serum enzymes in female carrier or possibly small increased frequency of EMG abnormalities.

†Special Considerations: There may be several variations of the Becker type of dystrophy occurring in different family groups, in which the age of onset may be as early as the 4th or 5th year (Emery and Dreifuss) or another type may have severe cardiac involvement (Mabry et al).

References:

Becker, P.E.: Two new families of benign sex-linked recessive muscular dystrophy. Rev. Can. Biol. 21:551, 1962.

Dreifuss, F.E. and Hogan, G.R.: Survivial in X-chromosomal muscular dystrophy. Neurology (Minneap.) 11:734, 1961.

Mabry, C.C. et al: X-linked pseudohypertrophic muscular dystrophy with a late onset and slow progression. N. Engl. J. Med. 273:1062, 1965.

Contributor: Carl M. Pearson

Editor's Computerized Descriptors: Skel., Muscle

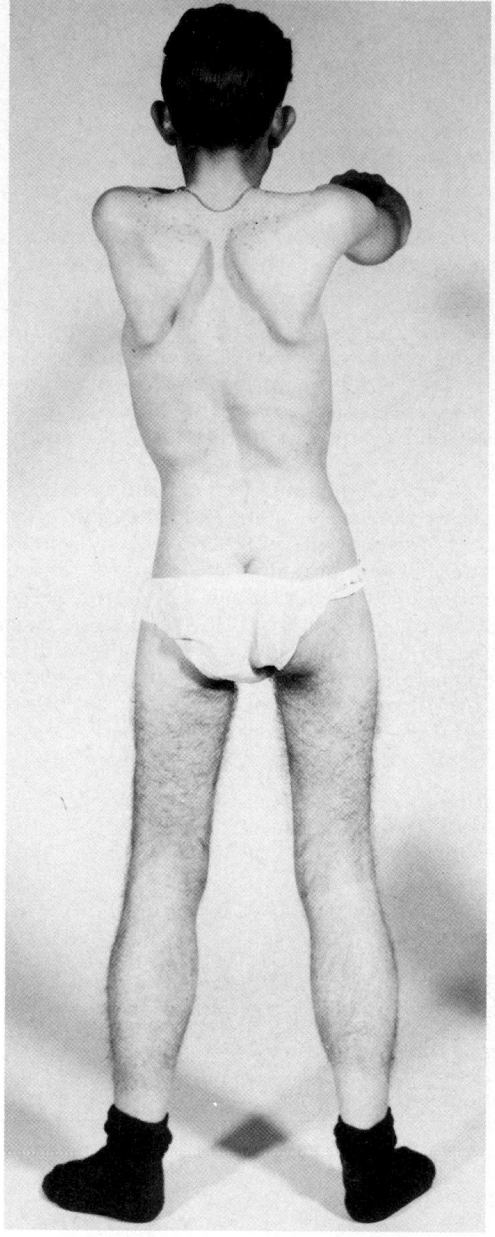

376. Note enlargement of calf muscles compared to other muscles

683-500

MUSCULAR DYSTROPHY, AUTOSOMAL RECESSIVE PSEUDOHYPERTROPHIC

Includes: Dystrophie musculaire pseudohypertrophique (de transmission autosomique)

Pseudohypertrophische Muskel-dystrophie, autosomal-rezessive Form

Distrofia muscular pseudohipertrófica recesiva autosómica

Pseudohypertrophic muscular dystrophy

Excludes: Muscular dystrophy, childhood pseudohypertrophic (689)

Muscular dystrophy, adult pseudohypertrophic (687)

Other forms of childhood muscular dystrophy

Minimal Diagnostic Criteria: Proximal weakness; hypertrophy, especially of the calf muscles; occurrence in both male and female children; moderate elevation of serum CPK and muscle biopsy consistent with myopathy or dystrophy.†

Clinical Findings: The onset may be in the 2nd year or as late as the 14th year but often is in the 2nd half of the 1st decade. Progression is comparatively slow and patients usually become unable to walk in their early 20s sometimes as early as 15 years or as late as 43 years. Weakness is chiefly proximal and does not appear to differ clearly from that of classic Duchenne dystrophy. Pseudohypertrophy is frequent. The muscle biopsies are classic for muscular dystrophy. The serum enzymes including CPK (creatine phosphokinase) are usually only moderately raised (up to 3 times the normal limit) but this may perhaps not be so in the early stages of the disease. Since so few pedigrees have been described in this form, little more is known of it.†

Complications
I   Derived: —
II   Associated: —

Etiology: Autosomal recessive

Pathogenesis: ? Progressive deterioration of striated muscle fibers, predominantly in the early years in the proximal muscle groups. The condition is slowly progressive.

Related Facts
I   **Sex Ratio:** M1:F1
II   **Risk of Occurrence:** ?
III **Risk of Recurrence for**
     Patient's Sib: 1 in 4 (25%) for each offspring to be affected
     Patient's Child: Not increased unless mate is carrier or homozygote
IV   **Age of Detectability:** Varies from 3 to 15 years
V   **Prevalence:** ? Too few cases have been described.

Treatment
I   **Primary Prevention:** Genetic counseling
II   **Secondary Prevention:** Orthopedic measures and physical therapy
III **Other Therapy:** —

Prognosis: ? Usually slowly progressive condition but mortality figures are not available.

Detection of Carrier: ?

†Special Considerations: Of the various forms of childhood muscular dystrophy this is the most difficult one to clearly define because proof of autosomal recessive inheritance in the family must be obtained and this is difficult at best. There have, however, been a number of families which seem to fulfill this criteria and it has been stated that this type of case makes up between 3-5% of all cases of pseudohypertrophic muscular dystrophy.

References:
Blyth, H. and Pugh, R. J.: Muscular dystrophy in childhood: The genetic aspect; a field study in the Leeds region of clinical types and their inheritance. Ann. Hum. Genet. 23:127, 1959.

Jackson, C. E. and Carey, J. H.: Progressive muscular dystrophy: Autosomal recessive types. Pediatrics 28:77, 1961.

Johnston, H. A.: Severe muscular dystrophy in girls. J. Med. Genet. 1:79, 1964.

Contributor: **Carl M. Pearson**

Editor's Computerized Descriptor: Muscle

MUSCULAR DYSTROPHY, CHILDHOOD PSEUDOHYPERTROPHIC

Includes: Dystrophie musculaire pseudohypertrophique de l'enfant
Muskeldystrophie, Typ Duchenne
Distrofia muscular pseudohipertrófica infantil
Classic X-linked recessive muscular dystrophy
Progressive muscular dystrophy of childhood
Duchenne muscular dystrophy
Childhood pseudohypertrophic muscular dystrophy

Excludes: All other forms of muscular dystrophy
Muscular dystrophy, autosomal recessive pseudohypertrophic (688)
Muscular dystrophy, adult pseudohypertrophic (687)

Minimal Diagnostic Criteria: Demonstration of muscular weakness, predominantly proximal; maleness; onset within the first decade of life; elevated serum enzymes, especially CPK.

Clinical Findings: Onset is usually in the first 3 years of life. The earliest symptom is clumsiness in walking with a tendency to fall. In many cases, the first attempts to walk are delayed and are awkward from the beginning. In others, progress may be apparently normal until the 3rd year and, rarely, parents report nothing abnormal until the 6th or 7th year. Frequently the parents will note that the child's walking begins to lack freedom of movement; the child may have difficulty in running or runs awkwardly. He may also begin to experience difficulty in arising from the floor and frequent falling. The inability to run is often a useful guide in the early stages. Invariably this disease occurs in boys and extremely rarely in girls. When there is difficulty in arising, the method of "climbing up the legs" to reach a standing position is characteristic (Gowers sign). In more advanced stages the boy walks with a waddling gait, with a protruding abdomen and with his toes and feet wide apart and his shoulders and chin drawn back. There is frequently significant lumbar lordosis. Physical examination discloses "pseudohypertrophy" or rubbery enlargement of the calf muscles out of proportion to the other body musculature. Occasionally other muscles also show unusual enlargement including the gluteii and deltoids.

The disease is relentlessly progressive so that the child usually becomes confined to a bed or a wheelchair by the 10th or 11th year. There is progressive wasting initially of the proximal and later the distal muscles and development also of weakness of the shoulder girdle muscles so that elevating the arm to the horizontal becomes difficult, usually by the 6th or 7th year. The hypertrophy of the calves may remain, despite significant wasting of the more proximal muscles. However, strength in the calf muscles progressively decreases (after being maintained early) and fatty replacement of muscle occurs later, therefore the term pseudohypertrophy was originally utilized for this clinical and anatomic feature. Progressive contractures of the hip flexors develop in many cases, and to a lesser extent of the knee flexors and of the muscles of the upper limbs. In addition, shortening of the heel cords develops so the child has a tendency to walk up on the toes, even early. The deep tendon reflexes are usually diminished in the upper limbs early and the knee jerks also disappear or diminish soon. The ankle jerks, however, remain brisk until a comparatively late stage. There is a tendency for some mental backwardness in cases of muscular dystrophy, although many children are of normal intelligence and some are well above average. The general consensus is that the average intelligence of these children, as revealed by formal meas-

urements of the IQ, is approximately 10% lower than a sample population of boys of similar age and social standing. Deep tendon reflexes are frequently depressed or are absent altogether with the exception of the ankle jerks, which are usually preserved or are even unusually brisk (Dubowitz). The disease is progressive and the vital musculature, including the respiratory musculature and the bulbar musculature, becomes involved soon. Survival beyond the age of 20 is unusual, and beyond age 35 is unheard of. Death usually results from pulmonary infection or cardiac failure.

Laboratory studies with which to diagnose this condition consist of: 1) characteristic changes in the muscle biopsy; 2) electromyographic features of a myopathy in most muscles; 3) elevation of serum enzymes which apparently leak from muscle into the serum. The most helpful of these enzymes is the CPK (creatine phosphokinase) but others, such as aldolase, and either transaminase or lactic dehydrogenase, are also elevated. Tests for serum and urine creatine and creatinine measurements have been suggested in the past but are of little value, when compared with the 3 features mentioned before.

Complications
I   **Derived:** Cardiac muscle involvement occurs in many children, but because of marked reduction in physical activity it is usually not a problem. ECG abnormalities indicative of myocardial involvement are frequent. Congestive heart failure is uncommon. Skeletal deformity occurs primarily as a consequence of muscular wasting and weakness and includes narrowing of shaft and rarefaction of the ends of the long bones, in some cases. In a later stage there is frequently a severe spinal scoliosis relating to lack of symmetry of muscle pull on the spine. Widespread decalcification also occurs associated with inactivity.
II **Associated:** Possible mild mental retardation in some

Etiology: X-linked recessive; McK *31020

Pathogenesis: Uncertain, the disease appears to be one of a primary structural or possibly membrane, or specific organelle defect within striated muscle fibers leading to progressive structural breakdown of muscle fibers, attempts at regeneration, and eventual gradual replacement of striated muscle by fat and fibrous connective tissue. During this process enzymes leak out, and may be used as diagnostic tools. No specific biochemical defect has so far been uncovered in this disease. There are recent suggestions that the disease may be due, at least in part, to a neural or neuronal defect (McComas et al).

Related Facts
I   **Sex Ratio:** M999:F1 or less, (the latter refers to minimally symptomatic females).
II **Risk of Occurrence:** Approximately 1 in 100,000 live births. 30% of cases appeared to arise by "spontaneous mutation."
III **Risk of Recurrence for**
    Patient's Sib: If mother is a carrier, 1 in 2 (50%) for each brother to be affected and 1 in 2 for each sister to be a carrier, less than 1% symptomatic.
    Patient's Child: Theoretically 1 in 1 (100%) for carrier daughters; not increased for sons unless wife is a carrier. (Males do not live sufficiently long to reproduce.)
IV **Age of Detectability:** At birth (by serum enzyme measurements); usually by age 3 by other features.
V   **Prevalence:** Approximately 1 in 200,000 in population under age 20 years and practically 0 thereafter.

Treatment
I   **Primary Prevention:** Genetic counseling
II **Secondary Prevention:** Rehabilitation, surgical corrective measures and physical therapy to avoid contractures
III **Other Therapy:** No specific diet or drug therapy is available for treatment of this form of dystrophy, even though a multitude of methods have been tested.

Prognosis: For life: invariably fatal, usually by age 20. For function: progressive decline in muscular capability, usually wheelchair and bed-confined by ages 10-12 with progressive decrease in function of all body musculature.

Detection of Carrier: Asymptomatic female carriers, possessing minor striated muscle defects which do not compromise everyday activities and function of muscular work may occur. Detection is by careful history, elevation of serum enzymes (especially CPK). Mild focal EMG alterations and mild muscle biopsy alterations are found in some carrier females.†

†Special Considerations: Carriers defined as *definite* are mothers of an affected son who have an affected brother, maternal uncle, sister's son or other male relative in the female line of inheritance; also mothers of affected sons by different, nonconsanguineous fathers. As *probable* are mothers of two or more affected sons, and who have no other affected relatives. *Possible* are the mothers of isolated carriers and the sisters and other female relatives of affected males.

References:

Dubowitz, V.: The reflexes in progressive muscular dystrophy. Dev. Med. Child Neurol. 6:621, 1964.

McComas, A. J. et al: Evidence for a neural factor in muscular dystrophy. Nature 226:1263, 1970.

Pearson, C. M. et al: X-chromosome mosaicism in females with muscular dystrophy. Proc. Natl. Acad. Sci. USA 50:24, 1963.

Steinberg, A. G. and Bearn, A. G. (eds.): Progress in Medical Genetics. New York: Grune and Stratton, 1967, vol. 5.

Walton, J. N. and Nattrass, F. F.: On classification, natural history and treatment of myopathies. Brain 77:169, 1954.

Contributor: **Carl M. Pearson**

Editor's Computerized Descriptors: Skel., Muscle, CV., Nerve

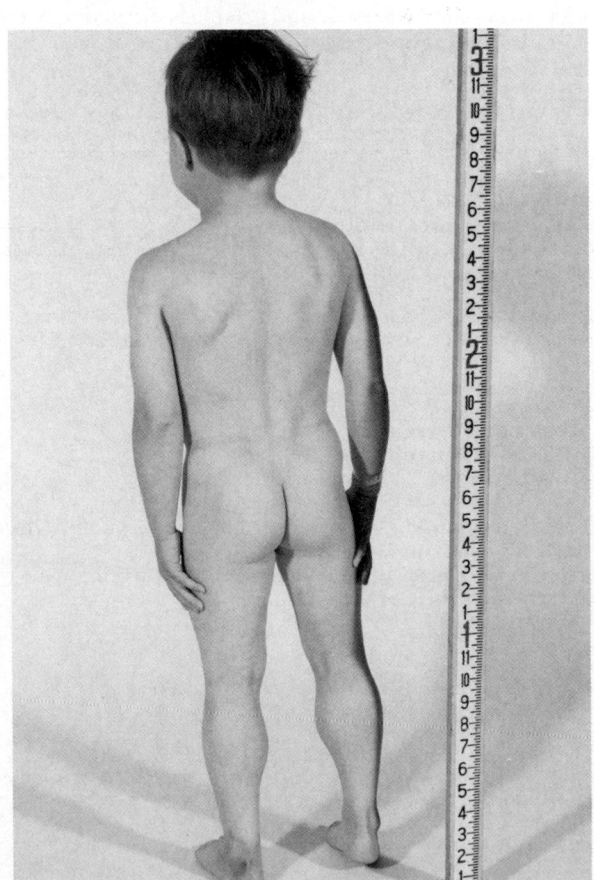

377. Note relatively large calf muscles

MUSCULAR DYSTROPHY, DISTAL

Includes: Dystrophie musculaire distal
Muskeldystrophie, Typ Welander
Distrofia muscular distal
Gowers form of dystrophy
Welander type of muscular atrophy
Distal muscular dystrophy

Excludes: Muscular dystrophy, limb-girdle (691)
Peroneal muscular atrophy of Charcot-Marie-Tooth
All other forms of muscular dystrophy

Minimal Diagnostic Criteria: Weakness in the distal limb muscles. Electromyogram consistent with a myopathy. Muscle biopsy consistent with a myopathy or muscular dystrophy.

Clinical Findings: Initial involvement is of the peripheral limb muscles. It usually appears with weakness in the small muscles of the hands and it slowly spreads proximally. In the legs, the anterior tibial muscles and the calves are affected first. The condition is comparatively benign, but proximal weakness occurs in a few of the more severe cases. These may be homozygous for the dominant gene.

In the early stages the appearance in the limbs is similar to that of peroneal muscular atrophy. However, in the latter condition, there is usually impairment of vibratory sense in the limbs and a prolongation of nerve conduction. Neither of these features appear in distal muscular dystrophy.

Complications
I   **Derived:** Progressive weakness with increasing disability upon ambulation
II   **Associated:** —

Etiology: Autosomal dominant or autosomal recessive; McK *15860, *25340

Pathogenesis: ? There is a specific and slowly progressive deterioration of muscle fibers, primarily in the peripheral muscles.

Related Facts
I   **Sex Ratio:** M1:F1
II   **Risk of Occurrence:** ?
III   **Risk of Recurrence for**
    Patient's Sib: When autosomal dominant or autosomal recessive, see Table I AD or AR, respectively.
    Patient's Child: When autosomal dominant or autosomal recessive, see Table I AD or AR, respectively.
IV   **Age of Detectability:** Detectable only when first signs of peripheral weakness appear, usually between the ages of 40 and 60 years.
V   **Prevalence:** ? Frequent in Scandinavia, especially in Sweden, but rare in other parts of the world.

Treatment
I   **Primary Prevention:** Genetic counseling
II   **Secondary Prevention:** Various physical measures such as supportive bracing, exercises and physical therapy might slightly retard the progression of the disease.
III   **Other Therapy:** —

Prognosis: Generally good for life but guarded for ambulation because of progressive distal, and, to a lesser extent, proximal weakness.

Detection of Carrier: —

Special Considerations: —

References:
Welander, L.: Homozygous appearance of distal myopathy. Acta Genet. Med. Gemellol. (Roma) 7:321, 1957.
Welander, L.: Myopathia distalis tarda hereditaria: 249 examined cases in 72 pedigrees. Acta Med. Scand. 141:Suppl. 265:1, 1951.

Contributor: **Carl M. Pearson**

Editor's Computerized Descriptor: Muscle

MUSCULAR DYSTROPHY, LIMB-GIRDLE

Includes: Myopathie (forme des ceintures)
Schulter-Beckengürtelform der Muskeldystrophie
Distrofia muscular escápulo-pélvica
Limb-girdle muscular dystrophy

Excludes: Muscular dystrophy, childhood pseudohypertrophic (689)
All other forms of muscular dystrophy

Minimal Diagnostic Criteria: Muscular weakness of one or both groups of girdle muscles in a symmetric fashion. Electromyographic evidence of myopathic response. Possibly elevation of serum enzymes, especially CPK (creatine phosphokinase). The enzyme elevations in this disease may be significant, but oftentimes are minimal by contrast with the rises in serum enzymes in childhood pseudohypertrophic muscular dystrophy (X-linked Duchenne type). A positive muscle biopsy indicating evidence of a myopathy.

Clinical Findings: Characterized by primary involvement of either the shoulder girdle muscles or of the pelvic girdle, with usual progression to the other areas after a variable period of time. Muscular pseudohypertrophy occurs in the calves and other muscles in a small proportion of cases. Abortive cases are uncommon but do occur. There are variable degrees of severity and rates of progression. Severe disability is usually present about 20 years after clinical onset. Muscular contractures and skeletal deformities occur only late in the course of the disease, or sometimes not at all. When the shoulder muscles are involved the patient develops a typical slope of the shoulders, which often become somewhat hunched forward. The patient then has difficulty in lifting the arms above the head. Pelvic girdle weakness is characteristic and produces difficulty in climbing stairs and arising from low chairs.†

Complications
I **Derived:** Skeletal malformations occasionally develop associated with asymmetric involvement of the skeletal musculature.
II **Associated:** —

Etiology: ? Usually inherited as an autosomal recessive character, but in rare instances as an autosomal dominant trait. A few cases may be sporadic.† McK *25360

Pathogenesis: ? The mechanisms of weakness involve structural breakdown of the striated musculature in the affected muscles.

Related Facts
I **Sex Ratio:** Probably M1:F1
II **Risk of Occurrence:** ?
III **Risk of Recurrence for**
    Patient's Sib: When autosomal recessive or autosomal dominant, see Table I AR or AD, respectively.
    Patient's Child: When autosomal recessive or autosomal dominant, see Table I AR or AD, respectively.
IV **Age of Detectability:** Usually in the 3rd to 5th decade when weakness develops.
V **Prevalence:** ?

Treatment
I **Primary Prevention:** Genetic counseling
II **Secondary Prevention:** —
III **Other Therapy:** —

Prognosis: Most patients become severely disabled in middle life and have a shortened life span.

Detection of Carrier: —

†Special Considerations: This disorder is probably a composite of several different conditions.

References:
Walton, J. N.: Clinical aspects of human muscular dystrophy. In Bourne, G.H. and Golarz, M.N. (eds.): Muscular Dystrophy in Man and Animals. New York:Hafner Publishing Co., 1963, p. 263.

Contributor: **Carl M. Pearson**

Editor's Computerized Descriptor: Muscle

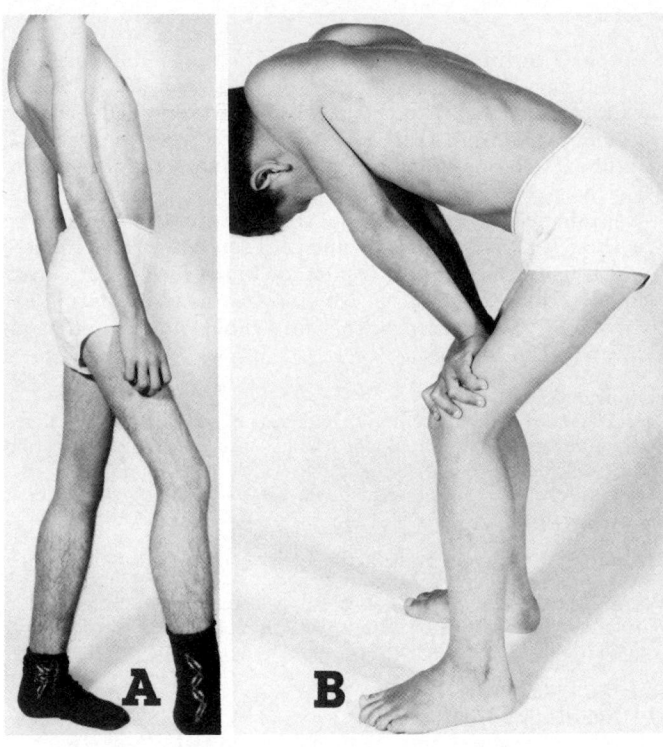

378. Limb-girdle dystrophy: A) hypererect stance; B) arising pattern

MUSCULAR DYSTROPHY, OCULOPHARYNGEAL

Includes: Dystrophie musculaire oculopharyngée
Okulopharyngeale Form der Muskeldystrophie
Distrofia muscular óculofaringea
Oculopharyngeal myopathy
Ocular muscular dystrophy
Pharyngeal muscular dystrophy
Oculopharyngeal muscular dystrophy

Excludes: Myotonic dystrophy (702)
Myasthenia gravis
Other causes for bulbar weakness and ptosis
Other forms of dystrophy

Minimal Diagnostic Criteria: Evidence of ptosis and pharyngeal muscle weakness along with a positive family history of this condition, or a muscle biopsy disclosing myopathic or dystrophic features

Clinical Findings: This syndrome is characterized by late-onset bilateral ptosis of the eyelids and progressive dysphagia. The onset of weakness of those involved muscle groups may occur anywhere from the 4th to the 8th decades. There may be progressive ptosis with the necessity to correct the ptotic defect. Dysphagia often proves to be progressive with increasing difficulty in handling solid foods and eventually in handling fluids. After being present for 1 - 2 decades in the above mentioned muscle groups, mild evidence of proximal muscle weakness develops in the shoulder and pelvic girdles.

There are no definitive laboratory tests aside from muscle biopsies which are helpful in this condition. Serum enzymes such as creatine phosphokinase (CPK) are invariably normal or only mildly elevated. Electromyography of the involved muscles may disclose a "myopathic pattern" but this type of study is rarely done.

Complications
I **Derived:** Aspiration pneumonitis or other problems associated with serious swallowing difficulty may supervene at any time, especially late in the course of the disease.
II **Associated:** —

Etiology: Autosomal dominant; McK *16430

Pathogenesis: ? There is progressive deterioration of the muscle fibers.

Related Facts
I **Sex Ratio:** M1:F1
II **Risk of Occurrence:** ?
III **Risk of Recurrence for**
Patient's Sib: If parent is affected, 1 in 2 (50%) for each offspring to be affected; otherwise not increased.
Patient's Child: 1 in 2
IV **Age of Detectability:** Clinical signs usually between the 3rd and 5th decades
V **Prevalence:** ?

Treatment
I **Primary Prevention:** Genetic counseling
II **Secondary Prevention:** Supportive measures such as eyelid crutches to overcome ptotic defect, operative partial correction of ptosis. Careful nursing and other management to avoid spillover aspiration pneumonitis from dysphagia.
III **Other Therapy:** —

Prognosis: Generally good for life unless the patient develops aspiration pneumonia associated with the dysphagia problem.

Detection of Carrier: —

Special Considerations: —

References:
Barbeau, A.: The syndrome of hereditary late onset ptosis and dysphagia in French Canadians. In Kuhn, E. (ed.): Progressive Muskeldystrophie Myotonie, Myasthenie. New York: Springer Verlag, 1966.
Hayes, R. et al: Oculopharyngeal muscular dystrophy. N. Engl. J. Med. 268:163, 1963.
Victor, M. et al: Oculopharyngeal muscular dystrophy: A familial disease of late life characterized by dysphagia and progressive ptosis of the eyelids. N. Engl. J. Med. 267:1267, 1962.

Contributor: Carl M. Pearson

Editor's Computerized Descriptors: Eye, Nasoph., Muscle, Resp.

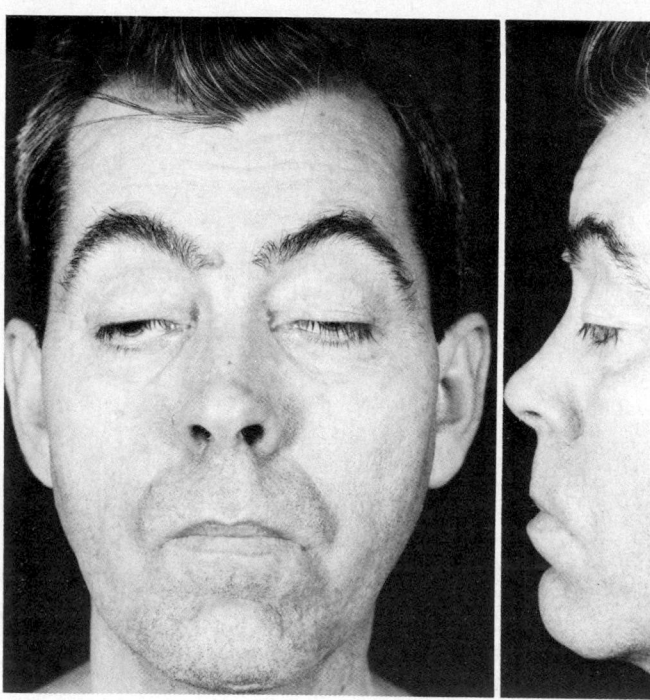

379. Note bilateral ptosis and expressionless face

MYELOMENINGOCELE

Includes: Meningomyelocele
Myeloschisis
Spina bifida cystica with paralysis

Excludes: Meningocele (642)
Lipomeningocele (602)
Hydrocephaly (481)

Minimal Diagnostic Criteria: Midline defect with neurologic deficit

Clinical Findings: A visible sac or epithelial defect in which nerve tissue can be seen and associated with neurologic deficit caudal to the level of the lesion. The surface lesion varies from that nearly completely skin covered to fully exposed lower spinal cord and cauda equina. In myeloschisis the paravertebral muscle mass is also exposed. Neurologic loss is generally of the lower motor neuron type with absent reflexes and segmental sensory loss. Sphincter loss is usual. Of greatest frequency in the lumbosacral area followed by cervical area. An enlarged head indicating hydrocephaly associated with the Arnold-Chiari malformation is often found.

Complications
I   **Derived:** Hydrocephaly, hydronephrosis secondary to urinary retention, hip dislocations related to unopposed action of hip flexors
II **Associated:** Congenital heart disease, GU anomalies, cleft palate

Etiology: Polygenic, multifactorial

Pathogenesis: Failure of neural tube closure at 4 weeks gestation or later cleft formation and cord splitting due to central cord distention with overgrowth of neural elements.

Related Facts
I   **Sex Ratio:** M1:F1
II   **Risk of Occurrence:**   1 in 500 to 1 in 200 live births
III **Risk of Recurrence for**
       Patient's Sib: Up to 7% chance in subsequent pregnancies
       Patient's Child: Up to 7% chance
IV   **Age of Detectability:** At birth
V   **Prevalence:** Most common of CNS malformations

Treatment
I   **Primary Prevention:** Genetic counseling
II   **Secondary Prevention:** Repair of open defects to prevent meningitis and loss of neural function. Treatment of hydrocephaly. Prevention of urologic and orthopedic acquired deformities.
III **Other Therapy:** —

Prognosis: Good in patients with minimal neurologic defects without hydrocephaly. Poor in those with complete lower limb paralysis, severe hydrocephaly, or other congenital defects.

Detection of Carrier: ?

Special Considerations: —

References:
Bark, D.J.H. and Sutcliff, R.G.: Alpha fetal protein in the antenatal diagnosis of anencephaly and spina bifida. Lancet 2:197, 1972.
Bark, D.J.H. et al: Prenatal diagnosis of anencephaly through maternal serum alpha fetal protein measurement. Lancet 2:923, 1973.
Lorber, J.: Editorial. Pediatrics 53:307, 1974.
Lorber, J.: The family history of spina bifida cystica. Pediatrics 35:589, 1965.
Shulman, K. and Ames, M.: Intensive treatment of fifty children born with myelomeningocele. N.Y. J. Med. 68:2656, 1968.

Contributor: **Kenneth Shulman**

Editor's Computerized Descriptors: Skin, GI., GU., Nerve

MYOPATHY, MITOCHONDRIAL

Includes: Myopathie mitochondriale
Mitochondrale Myopathie
Miopatía mitocondrial
Pleoconial myopathy
Myopathy, megaconial
Mitochondrial myopathy

Excludes: All other forms of nonprogressive congenital or infantile myopathy

Minimal Diagnostic Criteria: Infantile weakness. Abnormal mitochondria by electron microscopy.

Clinical Findings: These extremely rare conditions have only been described recently. The clinical feature consists of a nonprogressive diffuse muscular weakness which is associated with alterations of mitochondria as demonstrated electron microscopically in biopsied muscle.

Probably these disorders comprise a series of clinical syndromes rather than a single entity, but because they are so rare, insufficient information is available to more fully delineate them.

The only way that the diagnosis can be made is by electron microscopic examination of biopsied striated muscle which shows abnormalities of mitochondria, the details of which are yet to be fully delineated. In one of the conditions the mitochondria were large, they contained many cristae and appeared to be abnormal in form and structure. In another patient there appeared to be large numbers of relatively normal sized mitochondria, primarily located around sarcolemmal nuclei. Light microscopy has shown collections of subsarcolemmal granules. Some mitochondria were extremely large and contained abnormal rectangular inclusion structures. In many of the cases so far described the abnormality could have been suspected in histochemical preparations since stains for oxidative enzymes showed aggregates of prominent mitochondria, especially in the subsarcolemmal regions.

Complications
I   Derived: —
II Associated: —

Etiology: ?

Pathogenesis: ? Presumably there is a structural defect in mitochondria or mitochondrial metabolism leading to a decrease in energy contribution to muscle fibers, and possibly structural defects in the maintenance of normal muscle fiber integrity.

Related Facts
I   Sex Ratio: ?
II   Risk of Occurrence: ?
III Risk of Recurrence for
     Patient's Sib: ?
     Patient's Child: ?
IV   Age of Detectability: Infancy
V   Prevalence: ?

Treatment
I   Primary Prevention: —
II   Secondary Prevention: —
III Other Therapy: —

Prognosis: ? Probably normal life span

Detection of Carrier: ?

Special Considerations: —

References:
Price, H.M. et al: Myopathy with atypical mitochondria in type I

skeletal muscle fibers: A histochemical and ultrastructural study. J. Neuropathol. Exp. Neurol. 26:475, 1967.

Shy, G.M. et al: Two childhood myopathies with abnormal mitochondria: I. megaconial myopathy; II. pleoconial myopathy. Brain 89:133, 1966.

van Wijngaarden, G.K. et al: Skeletal muscle disease with abnormal mitochondria. Brain 90:577, 1967.

Contributor: **Carl M. Pearson**

Editor's Computerized Descriptor: Muscle

MYOPATHY, MYOTUBULAR

Includes: Myopathie myotubulaire
Myotubuläre Dystrophie
Miopatía miotubular
Myotubular myopathy
Centronuclear myopathy

Excludes: All other forms of nonprogressive myopathy of infancy and early childhood

Minimal Diagnostic Criteria: Infantile weakness. Centronuclear histopathology.

Clinical Findings: This rather rare disorder has been described only in several infants who manifest either a nonprogressive or a mildly progressive weakness and diffuse hypotonia of musculature which often occurs in conjunction with cardiac abnormalities (including arrhythmia) and CNS manifestations (including seizures). Several patients appear to have had a slowly progressive disease. Two patients have died of severe respiratory disease or myocardial failure at ages 9 and 11, respectively.

There are no clinical laboratory alterations and the creatine phosphokinase (CPK) and other muscle enzymes which appear in serum are always relatively at normal. Electromyography demonstrates "myopathic" potentials. The diagnosis can be established only by muscle biopsy. The biopsy reveals striking histologic characteristics since, even in an H and E section there is demonstrated a striking centrally placed prominence of the muscle nuclei, much like those which are seen in fetal muscle, thus the name "myotubular myopathy." In most of the very few cases that have been described so far the majority of the muscle fibers (up to 85% of them) resembles fetal fibers, being smaller in diameter and containing central nuclei. Histochemical studies have shown that oxidative enzyme activity may be either increased or decreased in the central region of the fibers and that myofibrillar ATPase activity is usually absent. Electron microscopic studies have demonstrated that, in addition to the presence of central nuclei, the central region of the fibers is usually devoid of myofibrils.

Complications
I **Derived:** Aspiration pneumonitis; congestive heart failure.
II **Associated:** Epilepsy, ptosis, respiratory or cardiac failure.

Etiology: ? There is probably a genetic basis for this disease, but this has not as yet been determined.

Pathogenesis: ?

Related Facts
I **Sex Ratio:** ?
II **Risk of Occurrence:** ?
III **Risk of Recurrence for**
   Patient's Sib: ?
   Patient's Child: ?
IV **Age of Detectability:** At birth or early infancy
V **Prevalence:** ?

Treatment
I **Primary Prevention:** —
II **Secondary Prevention:** —
III **Other Therapy:** —

Prognosis: Fair to poor. Most children die of pulmonary or cardiac complications in the 1st decade.

Detection of Carrier: —

Special Considerations: —

References:

Kinoshita, M. and Cadman, T. E.: Myotubular myopathy. Arch. Neurol. 18:265, 1968.

Sher, J.H. et al: Familial centronuclear myopathy: A clinical and pathological study. Neurology (Minneap.) 17:727, 1967.

Spire, A.J. et al: Myotubular myopathy: Persistence of fetal muscle in an adolescent boy. Arch. Neurol. 14:1, 1966.

Contributor: **Carl M. Pearson**

Editor's Computerized Descriptors: Muscle, CV., Resp.

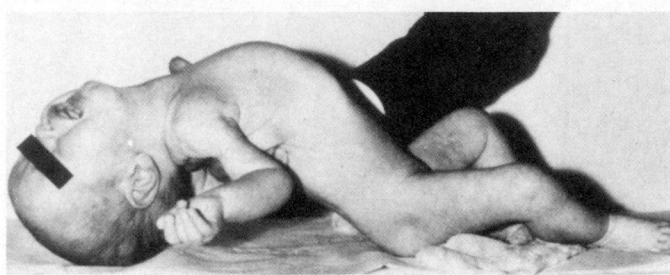

380. Note generalized weakness and hypotonia

MYOPATHY, NEMALINE

Includes: Myopathie némaline
Nemalin-Myopathie
Miopatía por alteracíon enzimológica parcial vermiforme de la fibra muscular esquelética
Nemaline myopathy
Rod body myopathy

Excludes: All other forms of diffuse nonprogressive congenital or infantile forms of muscular weakness

Minimal Diagnostic Criteria: Infantile weakness, hypotonia and muscle underdevelopment. Nemaline rods in muscle fibers with appropriate stains.

Clinical Findings: Persons who manifest this nonprogressive myopathy are usually recognized in infancy because of diffuse smallness or underdevelopment of their skeletal musculature, as well as weakness and hypotonia of all of the limb and trunk muscles. Such weakness is present from birth or early in infancy. The proximal limb muscles are mainly affected, although the neck and face may also be involved. The tendon reflexes are depressed, and are sometimes absent. In general the condition is nonprogressive, although there are 1 or 2 examples of possible progression during the 1st year of life causing complications from severe diaphragmatic and intercostal muscle weakness. Many affected individuals show skeletal changes reminiscent of arachnodactyly. Especially notable is a high-arched palate in most affected patients.

Routine clinical laboratory tests are normal. Serum enzymes such as creatine phosphokinase (CPK) are invariably normal or only slightly elevated and there are no other abnormal serum, chemical or other abnormalities. Electromyogram may demonstrate a "myopathic" picture.

Histologic examination of affected muscle tissue is the only way in which the diagnosis can be clearly established.†

Complications
I   **Derived:** Occasionally respiratory failure from severe diaphragmatic and intercostal muscle weakness
II   **Associated:** —

Etiology: ? Probably inherited as an autosomal dominant trait, although this has not as yet been clarified fully. This reviewer knows of at least 1 family of 7 children in which 3 were affected with the disease, and the mother demonstrated some histologic characteristics of its presence also. There was no consanguinity in this family. McK *16180

Pathogenesis: ? There are abnormal structural characteristics in muscle fibers, but it should be noted that nemaline-like rods are also found in other types of myopathic or neuropathic diseases of muscle on rare occasions.

Related Facts
I   **Sex Ratio:** Probably M1:F1, but too few cases in the literature to be certain
II   **Risk of Occurrence:** ?
III   **Risk of Recurrence for**
    Patient's Sib: ? Probably 1 in 2 (50%) for each offspring to be affected.
    Patient's Child: ? Probably 1 in 2
IV   **Age of Detectability:** Infancy by muscle biopsy
V   **Prevalence:** ?

Treatment
I   **Primary Prevention:** ?
II   **Secondary Prevention:** ?
III   **Other Therapy:** —

Prognosis: Normal life span, probably

Detection of Carrier: Probably by muscle biopsy and special stains

†Special Considerations: The muscle fibers show no degenerative changes, and on routine H and E sections, little or no change is usually seen. However, when special stains are utilized, such as a modified trichrome stain (Gomori) on frozen sections of muscle, or on an overdifferentiated PTAH stain, they show the presence of small rods or threads which are displaced longitudinally or obliquely in some fibers, often in clusters, and frequently bridging 2 to 4 sarcomeres. These nemaline rods are devoid of enzyme activity and in the modified trichrome stain they appear as dark green masses against the lighter green background of the major portion of the muscle fiber. The electron microscope has further differentiated and delineated the character of the nemaline rods. These studies reveal that the rods appear to be "cross hatched" due to the presence of transverse and axial striae. The transverse striae have a periodicity of approximately 145Å, and the axial striae have a periodicity ranging from 120 to 180Å. It appears from the various studies that have been done that the rod body in most of the material so far studied corresponds reasonably well with the crystal lattice that is also found in the Z-band of the sarcomere.

References:

Lindsey, J.R. et al: Pathology of nemaline myopathy: Studies of two adult cases including an autopsy. Bull. Johns Hopk. Hosp. 119:387, 1966.

Price, H.M. et al: New evidence for excessive accumulation of Z-band material in nemaline myopathy. Proc. Natl. Acad. Sci. USA 54:1398, 1965.

Shy, G.M. et al: Nemaline myopathy: A new congenital myopathy. Brain 86:793, 1963.

Contributor: **Carl M. Pearson**

Editor's Computerized Descriptors: Oral, Skel., Muscle, Nerve

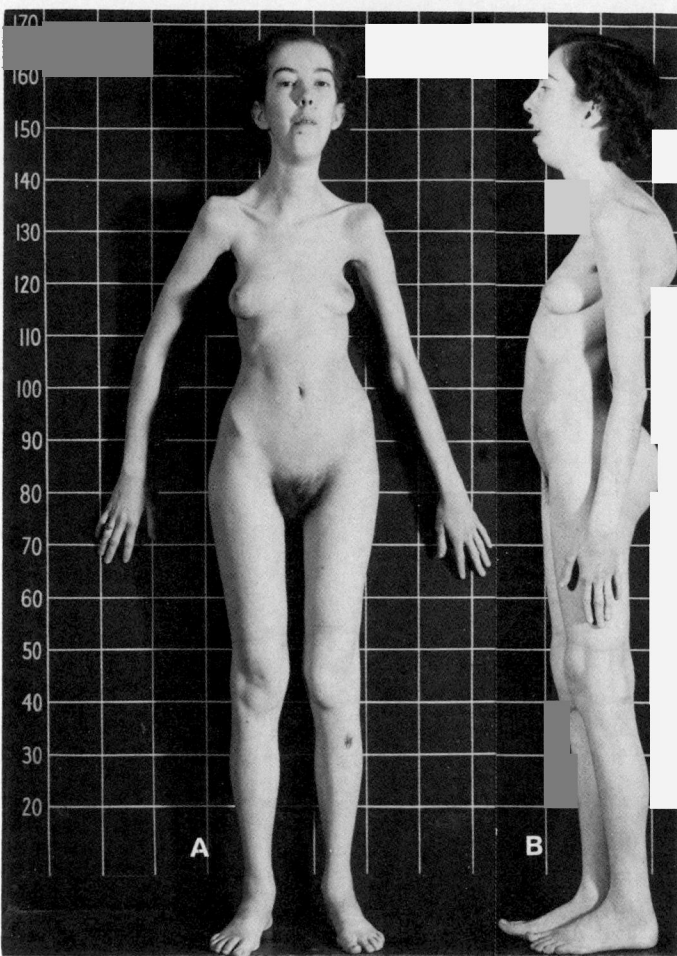

381. A) Expressionless facies, muscle loss and extremely narrow thorax; B) marked kyphosis and lordosis

MYOPATHY WITH LACTIC ACIDEMIA

Includes: Myopathie avec acidémie lactique
Myopathie mit Laktatacidämie
Miopatía con acidemia láctica

Excludes: Pyruvate dehydrogenase deficiency (851)
Fructose-1-phosphate aldolase deficiency (395)
Fructose-1,6-diphosphatase deficiency (396)
Lactate elevation secondary to other causes
Pyruvate carboxylase deficiency with lactic acidemia (850)

Minimal Diagnostic Criteria: Myopathy with a disproportionate lactate increase during exercise.

Clinical Findings: Clinical findings in the mitochondrial myopathies with lactate elevation have included: onset in the 1st decade; exercise intolerance; weakness; vomiting, headaches, and cramps with exercise; growth failure; myoglobinuria; rapid pulse rate; neurologic degeneration; seizures; ptosis and facial muscle weakness; and cardiomyopathy. The condition has frequently been fatal after progressing over a period of years. Two instances of sibs with sideroblastic anemia have been reported, as well as a group with cataracts of early onset.

Muscle disease associated with abnormalities of muscle mitochondria seen on histochemical or electron microscopic study has been recognized with increasing frequency in recent years. The great heterogeneity in this group of disorders has been emphasized by the widely disparate clinical pictures reflected in age of onset, severity, progression, simultaneous nervous system involvement, episodicity, apparent mode of inheritance, and in some few cases, by the results of biochemical studies of the muscle mitochondria. In several instances, distinct elevations of lactate and pyruvate have been seen without association with a single clinical picture. In all instances, however, where lactate and pyruvate elevation has been present in 1 family member, it has been found in all other affected members of that family. The presence of elevated lactate levels appears to have no bearing on the prognosis of the disease.

Lactate has varied from normal at rest to well over 100 mg/dl with minimal exercise. During exercise especially, the lactate/pyruvate ratio has tended to be elevated. Elevated CPK and myoglobinuria are seen. The histology is described in the references noted below.

Complications
I **Derived:** Neurologic and intellectual deterioration and death after several years in some cases. Severe, life-threatening episodes of weakness occur in others whose symptoms may remit completely with supportive care.

II **Associated:** —

Etiology: Instances of both autosomal recessive and autosomal dominant inheritance have been documented. In other families with multiple affected members, the mode of inheritance has been difficult to specify with certainty.

Pathogenesis: Patients have been described with reduced oxygen consumption while others have had increased oxygen consumption compatible with uncoupling of oxidative phosphorylation. The stimulus to lactate and pyruvate accumulation is a matter of speculation.

Related Facts
I **Sex Ratio:** M1:F1
II **Risk of Occurrence:** ?
III **Risk of Recurrence for**
  Patient's Sib: When autosomal dominant or autosomal recessive see Table I AD or AR, respectively.

Patient's Child: When autosomal dominant or autosomal recessive, see Table I AD or AR, respectively.
IV **Age of Detectability:** ?
V **Prevalence:** ?

Treatment
I **Primary Prevention:** Genetic counseling
II **Secondary Prevention:** Corticosteriods in pharmacologic doses have proved beneficial in some cases. Exercise restriction may prevent many of the most severe acute symptoms.
III **Other Therapy:** —

Prognosis: Very poor in some patients; good in others.

Detection of Carrier: Some heterozygotes have much milder symptoms. Families with autosomal dominant inheritance show a broad range of symptoms in different family members.

Special Considerations: —

References:
Hackett, T.N. et al: A metabolic myopathy associated with chronic lactic acidemia, growth failure and nerve deafness. J. Pediatr. 83:426, 1973.
Shapira, Y. et al: Familial poliodystrophy, mitochondrial myopathy, and lactate acidemia. Neurology 25:614, 1975.
van Wijngaarden, G.K. et al: Skeletal muscle disease with abnormal mitochondria. Brain 90;577, 1967.

Contributors: **Stephen D. Cederbaum**
John P. Blass

Editor's Computerized Descriptors: Eye, Muscle, CV., GI., Nerve

MYOPHOSPHORYLASE DEFICIENCY

Includes: Déficit en myophosphorylase
Myophosphorylase Mangel
Deficiencia en miofosforilasa
Muscle phosphorylase deficiency
McArdle disease
Glycogen storage disease, type V
Glycogenosis V

Excludes: Glycogenosis, types VII and VIII (428, 429)
All other types of glycogen storage disease

Minimal Diagnostic Criteria: Muscle cramping and rapid fatigue upon minimal or moderate exercise. Failure of rise of serum lactate and pyruvate in venous blood from exercised arm following ischemic exercise. Histochemical absence of muscle phosphorylase.

Clinical Findings: Characterized by muscle pain, weakness and stiffness, plus muscle cramping which occurs during slight or moderate exertion usually in the 2nd decade, or before. The muscles involved are those that are exercised, and nonexercised muscles do not participate in these symptoms. The symptoms usually date from early childhood. Pain on exercise is the most prominent feature, and it can occur in any muscles, even those of the jaw. Rest rapidly relieves the symptoms following moderate exercise, but after more severe exercise, or the longer the painful exercise is continued, the longer the symptoms tend to persist in those muscles. The pain may sometimes disappear on continued moderate exercise provided the exertion is not strenuous, and that stiffness has not occurred. The latter has been called the "second wind" phenomenon and may be related in some way to this physiologic state. A frequent and characteristic sign and symptom is the inability to extend the fingers after powerful, long-sustained, or frequently repeated gripping movements. After such exercise full recovery may take many minutes. Rarely, pain, weakness and swelling of the muscle may persist for a number of days after vigorous exercise. More than half of the cases so far described have given a history of occasional myoglobinuria following exercise. An occasional case has been described of "late onset variety" in which symptoms did not develop until the 5th decade or later.

Physical examination does not usually reveal any abnormality but about 1/3 of the 30 or more cases so far described in the literature have demonstrated some degree of myopathic weakness, usually mild. This weakness preferentially affects the upper limbs. Moderate exercise, such as climbing stairs, may cause not only pain and obvious stiffness but also marked tachycardia, dyspnea and exhaustion. Ischemic exercise of the forearm muscles results in rapid fatigue and shortening of the forearm flexors which may persist for some minutes after release of the circulation. This shortening of muscle develops when muscular stiffness becomes severe and it is not a true "cramp" but rather a physiologic "contracture", since electromyographically it is silent.

The characteristic laboratory features of this condition are an inability to produce lactic acid in the venous circulation during exercise, and this is best shown by an absence of rise in lactate in venous blood from the forearm muscles after release of the circulation following adequate ischemic exercise. Pathologically a muscle biopsy will demonstrate an increase in muscle glycogen to a level of usually between 2 and 5% (normal 1% or less). Histochemical staining will demonstrate a complete absence of the enzyme phosphorylase in muscle. Other pathologic changes may be found in muscle and these will include localized swelling of mitochondria, blebs or vacuoles within muscle and intermittent or spotty necrosis of muscle fibers.

Complications
I **Derived:** Slowly progressive myopathic weakness in upper and lower limbs after many years of persistent disease. Acute myoglobinuria following intensive exercise, sometimes with acute renal failure due to acute tubular necrosis. Congestive heart failure and other signs of cardiac decompensation with increased age, due to the inability of the myocardium to cope with an abnormally large muscle blood flow caused by exercise. It is also possible that in rare instances there may be a partial defect in myocardial phosphorylase content.
II **Associated:** —

Etiology: Probably autosomal recessive. Hereditary absence of muscle phosphorylase.

Pathogenesis: Defect in ability to utilize glycogen stored in muscle during more than minimal exercise, due to myophosphorylase defect in the glycolytic pathway. Secondary "myopathic" alterations may occur from progressive accumulation of glycogen in muscle.

Related Facts
I **Sex Ratio:** Probably M1:F1
II **Risk of Occurrence:** ?
III **Risk of Recurrence for**
  Patient's Sib: ?
  Patient's Child: ?
IV **Age of Detectability:** Usually within the 1st or 2nd decades of life. Occasional families have been described in which clinically described detectability has been delayed until the 5th or 6th decades.
V **Prevalence:** Extremely rare, about 30 patients to date

Treatment
I **Primary Prevention:** Genetic counseling
II **Secondary Prevention:** Logically it should be possible partially to replace carbohydrate in the glycolytic circuit by adequate ingestion of glucose or fructose prior to undertaking exercise. Even with such attempts, however, adequate amounts of these carbohydrates cannot get into the circuit with sufficient rapidity to prevent all of the muscular side effects. The long-term ingestion of either glucose or fructose has generally proved to be disappointing. They are difficult to take, they predispose to obesity, and in the case of fructose may cause colicky GI pain. Isoprenaline, 10 to 20 mg, taken about 15 minutes before exercise has helped in one or 2 cases over a two-year period, but in another case it was discontinued because of side effects. Its action is transient, but it is theoretically possible to prolong this action by giving a slow release form. The patients should keep within limits exertion which causes significant pain. As far as possible, any vigorous exertion should be preceded by a moderately lengthy period of more gentle activity which will slowly increase the rate of circulation to muscle and allow for better and more efficient muscle metabolism.
III **Other Therapy:** —

Prognosis: Must be guarded in most cases, especially those having an associated myopathy or myoglobinuria. Where these features are not present, the condition does not appear to be progressive in the usual case. Nevertheless, with increasing age the myocardium may be less able to cope with the abnormally large muscle blood flow caused by exercise.

Detection of Carrier: ?

Special Considerations: —

References:
McArdle, B.: Myopathy due to a defect in muscle glycogen breakdown. Clin. Sci. 10:13, 1951.
Pearson, C.M. et al: A metabolic myopathy due to absence of mus-

cle phosphorylase. Am. J. Med. 30:502, 1961.
Rowland, L.P. et al: The clinical diagnosis of McArdle's disease: Identification of another family with deficiency of muscle phosphorylase. Neurology (Minneap.) 16:93, 1966.

Contributor: **Carl M. Pearson**

Editor's Computerized Descriptors: Muscle, CV., GU.

MYOPIA

Includes: Myopie
Miopía
Severe infantile myopia
Nearsightedness
Congenital myopia

Excludes: —

Minimal Diagnostic Criteria: Myopia at or shortly after birth which does not shift to hyperopia during the first few months of life.

Clinical Findings: Myopia at or shortly after birth which persists. A positive family history often alerts the parents to watch for mannerisms of nearsightedness which may be confirmed by retinoscopy under cycloplegia and ophthalmoscopy. The average age of diagnosis is 3 years. Congenital myopia has a tendency to remain relatively stationary and shows no sex predilection. The average amount of myopia is approximately - 8.00 diopters. The visual acuity may be correctable to 20/30 or better, however, on the average, the visual acuity ranges between 20/50 and 20/60. Not infrequently, strabismus is also present in congenital myopia. Fundus changes occur in about 50% of cases and include posterior sclerectasia, choroidal crescents, tilted optic nerve head, choroidal mottling, pigment thinning or deficiency, and vitreous floaters.

Complications
I   **Derived:** —
II   **Associated:**   Retinal detachment, mesodermal dysplasia, retrolental fibroplasia, subluxation of lens, osteogenesis imperfecta, anterior chamber anomalies, keratoconus, lateral spinal curvatures, umbilical and inguinal hernias, flat feet, various syndromes, mongolism, strabismus and nystagmus

Etiology: Multifactorial. Usually autosomal recessive but may be autosomal dominant. There also appears to be an association between high irreversible myopia and prematurity; need for oxygen administration after birth even in full-term infants. An association has also been implicated with maternal disease in pregnancy including toxemia, renal disease, hypertension and hyperemesis gravidarum. McK *16070

Pathogenesis: It has been postulated by Ida Mann that the mechanism of development of congenital myopia of increased axial length might be related to delayed scleral condensation during embryonic life with resultant stretching of the posterior pole under normal intraocular tension. Contributing factors include corneal curvature and lens structure and position.

Related Facts
I   **Sex Ratio:**   M1:F1
II   **Risk of Occurrence:**   ?
III   **Risk of Recurrence for**
    Patient's Sib: When autosomal recessive or autosomal dominant, see Table I AR or AD, respectively.
    Patient's Child: When autosomal recessive or autosomal dominant, see Table I AR or AD, respectively.
IV   **Age of Detectability:**   Infancy
V   **Prevalence:**   Relatively rare

Treatment
I   **Primary Prevention:**   Genetic counseling
II   **Secondary Prevention:**   Correct refractive error with appropriate lenses as young as feasible. Avoid physically injurious occupational and vocational activities.
III   **Other Therapy:**   —

Prognosis: Favorable, since most cases of myopia are stationary. Visually guarded if myopia is progressive.

Detection of Carrier: —

References:
Curtin, B.J.: The pathogenesis of congenital myopia: A study of 66 cases. Arch. Ophthalmol. 69:166, 1963.
Hiatt, R.L. et al: Clinical evaluation of congenital myopia. Arch. Ophthalmol. 74:31, 1965.
Zauberman, H. and Merin, S.: Unilateral high myopia with bilateral degenerative fundus changes. Am. J. Ophthalmol. 67:756, 1969.

Special Considerations: —

Contributor: **Elsa K. Rahn**

Editor's Computerized Descriptors: Vision, Eye

MYOSITIS OSSIFICANS

Includes: Myosite ossifiante
Miositis osificante
Myositis ossificans, progressive
Fibrodysplasia ossificans progressiva
Localized myositis ossificans

Excludes: Traumatic myositis ossificans
Myositis ossificans circumscripta

Minimal Diagnostic Criteria: Pain and swelling in muscles, primarily those of the trunk, shoulders and pelvic girdle. Biopsy evidence of fibrosing myositis. X-ray evidence of calcification or bone deposition in muscle. Foreshortening of the great toes or other digits including the thumbs.

Clinical Findings: This condition is usually limited to children or young adults who demonstrate involvement of aponeuroses, tendons and fascia in addition to the connective tissue of the muscle itself. Commonly, the child presents with the swelling or swellings in the neck, mimicking congenital torticollis. The swellings may be fluctuant or hard and tend to vary in size and consistency. Ultimately, with progression of the condition, the swellings become hardened as bone is deposited within the edematous connective tissue. Although frequently painless, in some cases swellings are very sensitive and this, together with the swellings of joints and fever, may closely resemble the pattern of acute rheumatic fever or juvenile rheumatoid arthritis. It is frequent to see children afflicted with this problem demonstrating significant bilateral swellings of the trapezius and paraspinal muscles in the upper back with redness, edema, tenderness and representing a rather hunched shoulder posture. The neck cannot be turned because of pain and the child or young adult therefore turns his entire body when looking to one side or another. Although almost any voluntary muscle may be involved in the process, in the majority of cases the most severely affected muscles are those of the back, shoulder and pelvic girdles. Ultimately large groups of muscles may become ossified and the bone tends to conform in the shape of the replaced muscle. Ulceration of the tense, overlying skin may expose ossified muscle and may result in secondary infection. This is a rare occurrence. Although the diaphragm itself is rarely involved, the general fixation of the ribs results frequently in a terminal aspiration pneumonia and death from infection or asphyxia.

In conjunction with the ossifying myositis there are also congenital skeletal anomalies in most cases. The anomalies are those of the great toes or other digits which demonstrate foreshortening and absence of one or more phalanges. Pathologically, in the acute stages, muscle biopsy may demonstrate massive edema and fibroblastic proliferation with some cellular infiltration. These changes completely encroach upon and replace the striated muscle fibers which appear to be only secondarily involved in the fibroplastic process. Somewhat later, a metaplastic process occurs in which the connective tissue is converted into mature appearing bone, sometimes even with marrow elements and cartilage. Bone and cartilage are frequently surrounded by dense fibrous connective tissue and the muscle fibers are therefore replaced or pushed aside in the process. X-ray examination of the affected areas may show calcification or bone formation, generally conforming to the shape of the muscle or muscles involved. Other laboratory studies have not been particularly helpful and there is no evidence of articular disease or other systemic disease.

Complications

I **Derived:** Aspiration pneumonia or asphyxia from general fixation of the rib cage

II **Associated:** Hypoplasia of the phalanges of the thumbs, the 1st metacarpals, and the phalanges of the great toes. Some cases have also shown hypoplasia of the middle phalanges of the little fingers.

Etiology: Autosomal dominant with strong selection pressure. Almost all cases are new mutants. McK *13510

Pathogenesis: ?

Related Facts

I **Sex Ratio:** M1:F1

II **Risk of Occurrence:** ?

III **Risk of Recurrence for**

Patient's Sib: ? If parent is affected, possibly < 1 in 2 (< 50%) for each offspring to be affected; otherwise not increased.

Patient's Child: ? Possibly < 1 in 2

IV **Age of Detectability:** Usually in childhood by signs and symptoms of the disease as well as x-ray evidence of calcification in muscle.

V **Prevalence:** Rare. About 350 cases have been described in the literature.

Treatment

I **Primary Prevention:** Theoretically genetic counseling

II **Secondary Prevention:** None, possibly respiratory assistance and careful feeding of a liquid diet to avoid aspiration pneumonitis.

III **Other Therapy:** —

Prognosis: Fair to poor. If severe ankylosis and bridging of bones and muscles occur then severe respiratory restriction occurs and secondary complications arise. If, however, this does not occur the ossifying process may slow down or stop, and then prognosis for life improves with continuous limitation of movement of some muscles and disability. Death occurs in about 25% of patients within 5 years of the diagnosis.

Detection of Carrier: —

Special Considerations: —

References:

Eaton, W.L. et al: Early myositis ossificans progressiva occurring in homozygotic twins; a clinical and pathological study. J. Pediatr. 50:591, 1957.

McKusick, V. A.: Heritable Disorders of Connective Tissue. St. Louis:C.V. Mosby, 1956, p.184.

Tünte, W. et al: Zur Genetik der Myositis ossificans progressiva. Humangenetik 4:340, 1967.

Contributor: **Carl M. Pearson**

Editor's Computerized Descriptors: Skin, Skel., Muscle

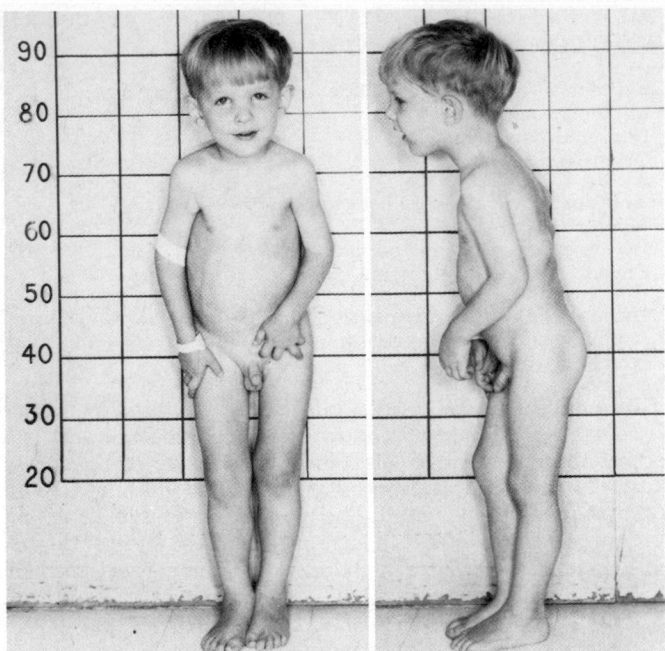

382. Characteristic posture with stiff spine and arms held close to sides

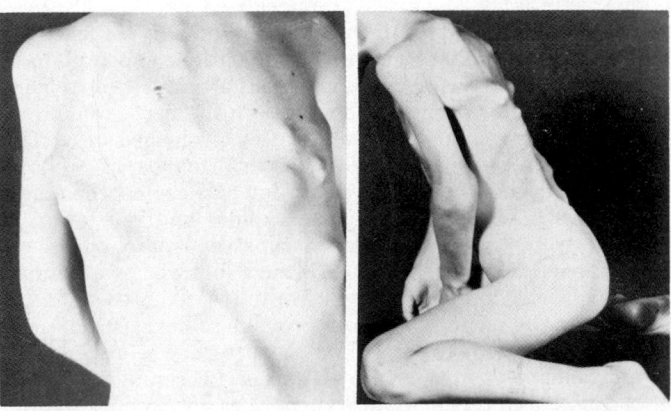

383. Bony ridges and nodules are evident the entire length of back

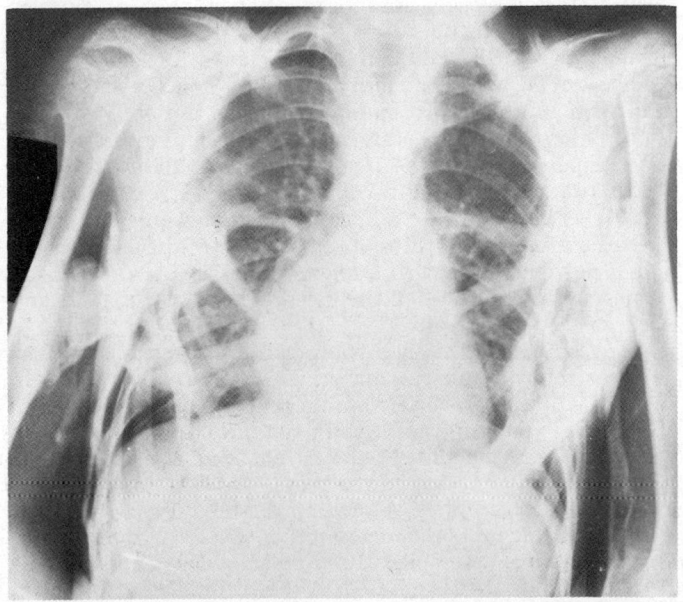

384. Bone bridges between humerus and rib cage, bilaterally

MYOTONIA CONGENITA

Includes: Myotonie congénitale
Miotonía congénita
Congenital myotonia
Thomsen disease

Excludes: Paramyotonia congenita (796)
Myotonic dystrophy (702)
Paralysis, hyperkalemic periodic (794)
Chondrodystrophic myotonia (155)

Minimal Diagnostic Criteria: Clinically and electromyographically demonstrable myotonia with a family history of a similar condition

Clinical Findings: Myotonia (decreased power of rapid relaxation of muscle following a firm contraction) is a prominent feature of this condition and is more widespread than in myotonic dystrophy or in other conditions in which myotonia may be found. The myotonia is demonstrated by percussion of skeletal muscle as a brief dimpling or depression of the muscle which may last for several seconds, before relaxation occurs. The myotonia is particularly evident upon percussion of the thenar eminence or of the tongue. It is especially prominent in the lower limbs and in some cases has been limited to the legs. It frequently may also affect the grip and the ocular movements and most characteristically causes a generalized painless stiffness which is accentuated by rest and gradually relieved by exercise. It is characteristic for the patient to complain of difficulty in initiating any movement after rest, and a painless stiffening of the limb occurs with the first attempts to make alternating movements after prolonged rest. The movement is initially slow in performance as well as delayed in cessation. With repetition of the effort the movement is gradually made more rapidly and relaxation is more prompt until, after many repetitions, the movement can be quickly and freely performed, followed by a natural relaxation. After a rest of some minutes, renewed attempts to make the movement again provoke some degree of muscular spasm, but prolonged rest is necessary before another movement initiates severe myotonia. Loosening of one set of muscles by repeated movement does not necessarily prevent the appearance of myotonia in another movement, even though closely similar muscles or parts of muscles may be used in the latter. The first grasp of the hand is made awkwardly and cannot be relaxed for 30 to 60 seconds, during which the muscles of the whole limb stand out in firm contraction. Small movements initiate myotonia only after prolonged rest, but any powerful effort sets up correspondingly severe myotonia with inability to relax. Blinking may occur naturally, whereas a strong closure of the eyes may initiate a spasm which continues for more than a minute after attempted opening of the eyes. A sudden movement such as a sneeze may set up a prolonged spasm of the muscles of the face, tongue, larynx, neck and chest.

In conjunction with myotonia there is usually diffuse hypertrophy of muscles, and this usually persists throughout life, although the myotonia tends to gradually diminish. The hypertrophy affects particularly the muscles of the thighs, forearms and shoulders, but may also involve the muscles of the neck and the masseters. The tongue is not enlarged. In complete relaxation the muscles have a natural consistency, but if myotonia is severe and persistent, they feel firm and tense. Muscular power may appear to be reduced, but this is related to the difficulty in initiating movements, possibly owing to inability to relax antago-

nists. Power to resist passive movement is strong, and is in proportion to the size of the muscles.

There are no abnormal laboratory findings except the presence of striking myotonia upon electromyography. Serum enzymes such as creatine phosphokinase (CPK) are invariably normal or only slightly elevated. Muscle biopsy is not abnormal, and in fact may show some measurable enlargement of individual muscle fibers.

Complications
I   **Derived:** —
II **Associated:** —

Etiology: Autosomal dominant; McK *16080

Pathogenesis: ? Probably a defect in the sarcolemmal membrane, or in the sarcoplasmic reticulum membranous structures. There is a possibility that there may be a defect in the "relaxing factor" in muscle, but this is yet to be proved.

Related Facts
I   **Sex Ratio:**   M1:F1
II **Risk of Occurrence:**   ?
III **Risk of Recurrence for**
    Patient's Sib: If parent is affected, 1 in 2 (50%) for each offspring to be affected; otherwise not increased.
    Patient's Child: 1 in 2
IV **Age of Detectability:**   Usually at birth, or soon thereafter, by myotonic features especially noticeable around the face, eyes and throat. Should be detectable in all patients by electromyography in infancy.
V   **Prevalence:**   ?

Treatment
I   **Primary Prevention:**   Genetic counseling
II **Secondary Prevention:**   Symptomatic management of the myotonic phenomenon can be achieved moderately satisfactorily with the use of certain drugs. The two most successful ones are quinine sulfate, generally used in a dosage of 0.3 gm 3-5 times a day or diphenylhydantoin (Dilantin), usually recommended in dosage of 0.1 gm 3-6 times daily. Other medications have been recommended but are not in general use now.
III **Other Therapy:**   —

Prognosis: Generally excellent for life with no increase in mortality rate. In fact, the myotonia gradually diminishes in later years, and usually weakness is not a feature at all.

Detection of Carrier: There is an occasional individual who is clinically asymptomatic and who may manifest myotonia only electromyographically.

Special Considerations: —

References:
Caughey, J. E. and Myrianthopoulos, N. C.: Dystrophia Myotonica and Related Disorders. Springfield: Charles C Thomas, 1963.
Thomsen, E.: Myotonia: Thomsen's Disease (Myotonia Congenita), Paramyotonia, and Dystrophia Myotonica; a Clinical and Heredobiologic Investigation. Copenhagen:Munksgaard, 1948.

Contributor: **Carl M. Pearson**

_____

Editor's Computerized Descriptor: Muscle

MYOTONIC DYSTROPHY

Includes: Dystrophie myotonique
Myotone Dystrophie
Miotonía distrófica
Dystrophia myotonica
Myotonia atrophica
Steinert disease

Excludes: Myotonia congenita (701)
Paramyotonia congenita (796)
Other causes of myotonia
Paralysis, hyperkalemic periodic (794)
Other forms of muscular dystrophy

Minimal Diagnostic Criteria: Wasting and weakness of facial and neck muscles and those of the limbs distally. Myotonia to percussion as demonstrated in the thenar eminence and on the tongue. Myotonia and myopathic changes by EMG. Family history of a similar disorder in most cases.

Clinical Findings: The presenting symptoms are usually a weakness of the hands, difficulty in walking, or a tendency to fall. However, upon questioning the patient, it will often be revealed that myotonia, (inability to relax a firm grip) or muscular stiffness has been present for many years. Myotonia is the presenting symptom in about 1/3 of all cases. The weakness in myotonia primarily involves the facial and neck muscles and the distal muscles of all 4 limbs. The facial appearance is characteristic. Ptosis is almost invariable and there also may be symmetric impairment of ocular movement. Frequently difficulty occurs in closing the eyes due to weakness of the orbicularis oculi. There is also difficulty in retracting the corners of the mouth and pursing the lips. Often the lower lip droops. Wasting of the masseters, temporal muscles and sternocleidomastoids gives a characteristic haggard appearance. Dysarthria is common due to weakness of the facial muscles or because of myotonia of the tongue. Weakness and wasting of the limbs affect mainly the muscles of the forearms, the anterior tibial group (leading to foot drop) and to a lesser extent of the calves and peronei. The distal weakness is quite different from the proximal weakness that usually occurs in the other common forms of muscular dystrophy. Abdominal wall muscular weakness is invariable. Later, during the progression of the disease, more proximal limb muscles are also involved. Myotonia is often clinically limited to the tongue, forearm and hand muscles, but on rare occasions it may be generalized. It tends to become less apparent as the disease progresses. The tendon reflexes are reduced in the affected muscles and contractures occur in the later stages.

The condition has many nonmuscular symptoms. It is really a diffuse systemic disorder in which myotonia and muscular atrophy are accompanied by cataracts (typically composed of white and greenish colored posterior subcapsular particles), frontal baldness in the male, gonadal atrophy, and sometimes heart disease, and impaired pulmonary ventilation, mild endocrine abnormalities, bone changes, mental defects or dementia and abnormalities of the serum immunoglobulins. Cardiac involvement is common so that about 65% of patients have electrocardiographic abnormalities, usually conduction defects. Pulmonary vital capacity and especially maximum breathing capacity are often impaired. The consequent alveolar hypoventilation may partially account for the apathy and somnolence which is often found. Weak esophageal contraction may be demonstrated by contrast radiography. The testes are small and their histology resembles that found in Klinefelter syndrome, although the nuclear sex is male and chromosomal abnormalities have not been demonstrated. Females may have irregular menstruation and infertility, and parturition may be prolonged in fully developed cases. There is often a mild hypofunction of the pituitary, thyroid, adrenal cortex or of the pancreatic islets, the latter leading to a mild diabetic state.

Laboratory abnormalities are minimal but fairly characteristic. The electromyogram reveals characteristic myotonia as well as some "myopathic" electrical discharges. The myotonia may be present in many muscles, not only those which demonstrate the myotonic phenomenon clinically. Serum enzymes such as creatine phosphokinase (CPK) may be mildly elevated, or are normal. A muscle biopsy shows myopathic changes including irregularity of size of muscle fibers and central positioning of muscle nuclei. In the later stages muscle fibers may be replaced by fibrous tissue and fat. The ECG may demonstrate abnormalities, especially conduction defects. An excessive catabolism of immunoglobulins have been demonstrated in this disorder.

Complications
I   **Derived:** Cardiac irregularities. Dyspnea because of cardiac or respiratory mechanism involvement, sudden death from cardiac arrhythmia or aspiration pneumonitis.
II **Associated:** Mild or severe mental deficiency, diminished endocrine glandular function, hypofertility, diminished vision due to progressive cataracts.

Etiology: Autosomal dominant; McK *16090

Pathogenesis: Uncertain. There is progressive deterioration of muscle fibers due to an unknown defect or defects in them. There is also slowly progressive fibrosis of myocardium and partial atrophy or selective replacement of some endocrine glands by connective tissue. This is most notable in the testes, which are small and demonstrate progressive replacement of the seminiferous tubules.

Related Facts
I   **Sex Ratio:** M1:F1
II **Risk of Occurrence:** ?
III **Risk of Recurrence for**
    Patient's Sib: If parent is affected, 1 in 2 (50%) for each offspring to be affected; otherwise not increased.
    Patient's Child: 1 in 2
IV **Age of Detectability:** Potentially at birth, occasionally in the 2nd decade, but most usually between ages 20 and 50 years. Myotonia, electromyographically, may be detected long before clinical signs and features are apparent.
V   **Prevalence:** ?

Treatment
I   **Primary Prevention:** Genetic counseling
II **Secondary Prevention:** Physical therapeutic and orthopedic measures directed against muscle weakness. Mechanical devices or surgical procedures to correct ptosis. Surgical resection of cataracts in some patients. Supporting therapy for mild endocrine glandular deficiency, correction of mild diabetes, hypothyroidism or hypoadrenocorticalism. External cardiac pacemaker in selective cases where arrhythmia presents a serious problem. Supportive respiratory assistance in some patients because of alveolar hypoventilation.
III **Other Therapy:** —

Prognosis: Generally fair for many years after clinical onset. Then, however, death usually occurs before the normal age, usually from pulmonary infection or cardiac failure. Sudden death due to cardiac arrhythmia or pulmonary failure has been reported. These patients are particularly at risk during anesthesia.†

Detection of Carrier: —

†Special Considerations: Affected families frequently show progressive social decline in successive generations.

References:
Caughey, J. E. and Myrianthopoulos, N. C.: Dystrophia Myotonica and Related Disorders. Springfield: Charles C Thomas, 1963.
Pearson, C.M. et al: Myotonic dystrophy: Its variable clinical, histological and biochemical expressions. In Barbeau, A. and Brunetpe, J.R. (eds.): Progress in Neurogenetics. Amsterdam: Excerpta Medica, 1969, p.199.
Pruzanski, W.: Variants of myotonic dystrophy in preadolescent life (the syndrome of myotonic dysembryoplasia). Brain 89:563, 1966.
Thomsen, E.: Myotonia: Thomsen's Disease (Myotonia Congenita) Paramyotonia, and Dystrophia Myotonica; a Clinical and Heredobiologic Investigation. Copenhagen:Munksgaard, 1948.

Contributor: **Carl M. Pearson**

Editor's Computerized Descriptors: Eye, Face, Neck, Hair, Muscle, Resp., CV., GI., GU., Nerve

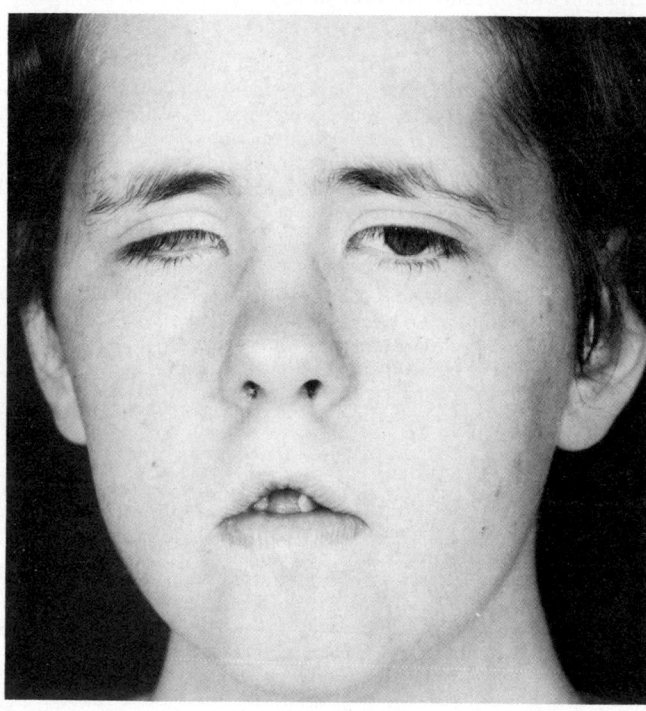

385. Note ptosis and corneal opacification OD

NAEGELI SYNDROME

Includes: Syndrome de Naegeli
Síndrome de Naegeli
Chromatophore nevus of Naegeli
Franceschetti-Jadassohn syndrome
Reticular pigmented dermatosis
"Transitional" cases presenting some clinical manifestations of both classic incontinentia pigmenti and Naegeli syndrome

Excludes: Incontinentia pigmenti (526)

Minimal Diagnostic Criteria: Reticular cutaneous pigmentation, discomfort provoked by heat. Plantar and palmar hypohidrosis and hyperkeratosis.

Clinical Findings: Characterized by cutaneous reticular pigmentation without preliminary inflammatory stages, dental signs consisting of yellow spotting of the enamel, disturbances of sweating, and palmar and plantar keratoses.
"Transitional" cases present spattered pigmentation with keratoses or reticular pigmentation with ocular signs, nail changes, dwarfism, inflammatory beginnings, disturbances of sweating.

Complications
I **Derived:** Abnormal EEG, osteoporosis, cataract, nail disturbances, alopecia, and stunted growth.
II **Associated:** —

Etiology: Autosomal dominant; McK *16100

Pathogenesis: ? Reticular pigmentation appears around the 2nd year.

Related Facts
I **Sex Ratio:** M1:F1
II **Risk of Occurrence:** Rare
III **Risk of Recurrence for**
Patient's Sib: If parent is affected, 1 in 2 (50%) for each offspring to be affected; otherwise not increased.
Patient's Child: 1 in 2
IV **Age of Detectability:** The 2nd year
V **Prevalence:** Rare

Treatment
I **Primary Prevention:** Genetic counseling
II **Secondary Prevention:** —
III **Other Therapy:** —

Prognosis: Average life span, reproductive fitness seems unimpaired.

Detection of Carrier: ?

Special Considerations: —

References:
Curth, H.O.: Incontinentia pigmenti. In Jadassohn, J. (ed.): Handbuch der Haut -und Geschlectskrankheiten. New York: Springer-Verlag, 1966, vol. 7, p. 820.
Curth, H.O. and Warburton, D.: The genetics of incontinentia pigmenti. Arch. Dermatol. 92:229, 1965.
Franceschetti, A. and Jadassohn, W.: A propos de "l'incontinentia pigmenti", délimination de deux syndromes différents figurant sous le même terme. Dermatologica 108:1, 1954.
Naegeli, O.: Familiärer chromatophorennävus. Schweiz. Med. Wochenschr. 57:48, 1927.

Contributor: **Helen Ollendorff Curth**

Editor's Computerized Descriptors: Eye, Teeth, Skin, Sweating, Hair, Nails, Skel., Nerve

NAIL-PATELLA SYNDROME

Includes: Onychoostéodysplasie
Nagel-Patella-Syndrom
Síndrome ónico-patelar
Arthroosteoonychodysplasia
Onychoosteodysplasia
Iliac horns

Excludes: Turner syndrome (977)

Minimal Diagnostic Criteria: Hypoplastic nails and hypoplastic patella

Clinical Findings: Characterized by dysplasia of the nails, absent or hypoplastic patellae, abnormality of the elbows interfering with supination, pronation or extension, and iliac horns. The nails of both hands and feet may be affected; those of the index and middle fingers and thumb being the most frequent. Hypoplasia, narrowness and splitting of the nails are the usual findings. The patella may be small, tripartite, polygonal or absent; lateral dislocation of the patella occurs. Iliac horns are seen, arising from the posterior ilium. There may be webbing of the elbow preventing full extension. Nephropathy occurs in some 30% of patients and may be either glomerulonephritic or nephrotic in type. Scoliosis occasionally occurs.

Complications
I Derived: Subluxation of the knee, genu varus, early onset osteoarthritis of the knee. Lateral dislocation of the patella may complicate walking, especially down the stairs. The elbow may subluxate. The nephropathy, though usually benign, may cause death at an early age.
II Associated: Deformity of sternum, spina bifida occulta, shoulder anomalies, anomalies of pectoralis minor, triceps and biceps, hyperostosis frontalis interna, clinodactyly of 5th finger, partial symphalangism of distal interphalangeal joints, hypothyroidism and goiter, mental retardation, cataracts, microcornea, microphthalmia, calcaneal and valgus foot deformities.

Etiology: Autosomal dominant, probably full penetrance but variable expressivity.† McK *16120

Pathogenesis: Electron microscopic studies have shown many collagen fibrils in thickened basement membranes and in mesangial matrix of otherwise normal glomeruli.

Related Facts
I Sex Ratio: M1:F1
II Risk of Occurrence: ?
III Risk of Recurrence for
Patient's Sib: If parent is affected, 1 in 2 (50%) for each child to be affected; otherwise not increased.
Patient's Child: 1 in 2
IV Age of Detectability: At birth because of nail defects
V Prevalence: ?

Treatment
I Primary Prevention: Genetic counseling
II Secondary Prevention: Orthopedic treatment for problems arising in the knee or elbow.
III Other Therapy: Patients should be repeatedly assessed for renal abnormalities.

Prognosis: The renal complications have caused death as early as 8 years of age. A total of 8% of patients reported in the literature reviewed in 1970 had died of renal disease.

Detection of Carrier: —

†Special Considerations: The locus for the nail-patella syndrome is linked with the locus for ABO blood group. The recombination fraction is about 10% but it is higher in females than in males. The locus for adenylate kinase is in the same linkage group.

References:
Hawkins, C.F. and Smith, O.E.: Renal dysplasia in a family with multiple hereditary abnormalities including iliac horns. Lancet 1:803, 1950.
Morita, T. et al: Nail-patella syndrome. Light and electron microscopic studies of the kidney. Arch. Intern. Med. 131:271, 1973.
Renwick, J.H. and Lawler, S.O.: Genetical linkage between the ABO and nail-patella loci. Ann. Hum. Genet. 19:312, 1955.
Similä, S.; et al: Hereditary onycho-osteodysplasia (the nail-patella syndrome) with nephrosis-like renal disease in a newborn boy. Pediatrics 46:61, 1970.
Williams, H.J.: Radiographic diagnosis of osteoonychodystrophy in infancy. Radiology 109:151, 1973.

Contributor: **David C. Siggers**

Editor's Computerized Descriptors: Nails, Skel., GU.

Includes: Absence des conduits lacrymaux
Tränengangsstenose
Conducto nasolacrimal impermeable
Atresia of nasolacrimal ducts
Lacrimal duct impatency

Excludes: Lacrimal canaliculus atresia (563)

Minimal Diagnostic Criteria: Clinical findings below may be confirmed by irrigation and xray with contrast media, if diagnosis is in doubt.

Clinical Findings: Infants present with tearing, mucocele of the lacrimal sac, or dacryocystitis. Impatency usually occurs at the junction of the duct with the nasal mucosa. This condition is differentiated from atresia of the lacrimal canaliculus by easier passage of a probe into the lacrimal sac in the former condition.

Complications
I   **Derived:** Epiphora, mucocele, dacryocystitis
II **Associated:** —

Etiology: Unknown, although 1 family shows autosomal dominant inheritance.

Pathogenesis: Delay in normal canalization of the embryonic epithelial core

Related Facts
I   **Sex Ratio:** M1:F1
II **Risk of Occurrence:** 1 in 17 of unselected term babies; much more frequent if premature; the overwhelming majority open spontaneously in the 1st week of life. Incidence of significant delay unknown but not uncommon.
III **Risk of Recurrence for**
    Patient's Sib: When autosomal dominant, if parent is affected 1 in 2 (50%) for each offspring to be affected; otherwise not increased.
    Patient's Child: When autosomal dominant 1 in 2
IV **Age of Detectability:** 1st weeks of life
V   **Prevalence:** Unknown but not uncommon

Treatment
I   **Primary Prevention:** Genetic counseling
II **Secondary Prevention:** Massage to break membrane, antibiotic drops to prevent infection, irrigation and probing to break membrane,† resection of nasal bone if imperforate
III **Other Therapy:** Systemic antibiotics if dacryocystitis supervenes

Prognosis: Most are cured by increasing therapy as outlined above. However, dacryocystitis will be recurrent until patency and flow are established.

Detection of Carrier: —

†Special Considerations: Irrigation and probing should be attempted through the superior canaliculus, which is of less functional importance than the lower. These maneuvers are simple procedures before the age of 6 months but require general anesthesia thereafter (until adulthood). Because of the ever present risk of dacryocystitis, early referral to an ophthalmologist is advisable.

References:
Duke-Elder, S.: System of Ophthalmology, vol. 3, pt. 2. Congenital Deformities. St. Louis: C.V. Mosby, 1963, p. 934.
Hurwitz, J.J. and Welham, R.A.N.: Role of dacryocystography in management of congenital nasolacrimal duct obstruction. Can. J. Ophthalmol. 10:346, 1975.

Contributor: **Donald R. Bergsma**

Editor's Computerized Descriptor: Eye

Includes: Kystes nasopharyngiens
Nasopharyngeale Zysten
Quistes nasofaríngeos
Intraadenoidal cysts
Congenital cysts of the nasopharynx
Extraadenoidal cysts
Branchial cleft cysts, Bailey type IV

Excludes: Intraadenoidal pseudocyst secondary to incomplete adenoidectomy or sealed over crypt secondary to repeated inflammatory episodes
Retention cysts of seromucinous glands, excretory ducts of which are occluded by a collar of lymphatic tissue
Interstitial pseudocysts, devoid of epithelium, due to tissue edema
Pseudocyst secondary to inflammation of fascial envelope of longus capitis muscle

Minimal Diagnostic Criteria: The differential diagnostic problem of the intraadenoidal cyst is difficult and trivial. With the extraadenoidal cyst, the excised velum of tissue theoretically should show appropriate epithelial coverings on both surfaces but careful pathologic examinations are rarely carried out in such cases. The true branchial cyst is lateral and often bilateral. Lack of an inner epithelial lining entitles one to call these lesions merely pseudocysts. Inasmuch as the pharyngeal tubercle may hide the essential lesion, direct nasopharyngeal examination is desirable.

Clinical Findings: Symptoms include purulent postnasal discharge not coming through the choanae. Aching pain high in the throat or at the base of the skull with a feeling of pressure or fullness, periodically relieved by evacuation of secretion.

Intraadenoidal cysts derive from the medial pharyngeal recess, present an elliptical opening on the nether surface of the adenoid, axis anteroposterior, lying in the midline, differing from the usual crypt opening in that it is more regular. Usually there is no special swelling, but pus and debris may be extruded on suction or pressure in the untreated state.

Extraadenoidal cysts located deep to the pharyngobasilar fascia are derived from bursa pharyngea embryonalis (midline). They will not be diagnosed in children until the adenoid is removed, but, in the adult may be seen caudal to the lowermost extent of any adenoid present. Again, usually no swelling is seen in the nasopharynx, but a small hole in the midline, slightly rostral to the pharyngeal tubercle. In the untreated state, this hole may be surrounded by a cuff of granular, inflamed mucosa. It may exude pus intermittently. The hole usually leads to a small cavity, separated from the general nasopharyngeal space by a thin velum of tissue. In rare instances, the space in question can enlarge caudally to the level of the epiglottis. Indentation of the basiocciput has been described but must be quite rare.

Branchial cleft cysts, Bailey type IV are derived from first and dorsal portion of 2nd pharyngeal pouch. They are often paired, present on the lateral aspects of the nasopharyngeal wall. The branchial nature is not easy to establish. Cystic nature may be established by injection of radiopaque material but this may deceive. Lateral location and bilaterality strongly suggest branchial origin. Pathologic findings are more cogent.

It is of the utmost importance to evaluate sinonasal disease as a cause of symptoms. This can only be done with reasonable certainty by careful clinical examination supplemented by x-ray study of the sinuses.

Complications

I **Derived:** Chronic or subacute bronchitis; chronic blepharoconjunctivitis; subacute or chronic tubotympanitis, sometimes with conductive hypacusis; rarely, paranasal sinusitis; fever intermittently; recurring pharyngitis. In one case metastatic cervical lymphosarcoma observed in the neck complicating lymphosarcoma in a paratubal branchial sinus present bilaterally.

II **Associated:** —

Etiology: ?

Pathogenesis: The true bursa pharyngea is due to the inductive effect of chorda mesoderm upon the pharyngeal epithelium in the fornix region where bundles of pharyngobasilar fascia do not commingle to form a barrier, as more anteriorly, to extrusion of pharyngeal entoderm.

Intraadenoidal midline cysts may be due to such an embryonic disturbance of the median pharyngeal recess which precedes development of the pharyngeal tonsil itself, but products of which may nevertheless be incorporated within the adenoid.

Branchial cleft cysts arise here, as elsewhere, but much more rarely. They are prone to remain intramural (Bailey type IV) and not to migrate into the neck.

Related Facts
I **Sex Ratio:** ?
II **Risk of Occurrence:** ?
III **Risk of Recurrence for**
Patient's Sib: ?
Patient's Child: ?
IV **Age of Detectability:** Nasopharyngeal cysts are discovered either at the time of adenoid or adenotonsil surgery in childhood; or, less commonly, on careful investigation of postnasal pus in adults which cannot be demonstrated to come from the nose or paranasal sinuses.
V **Prevalence:** ?

Treatment
I **Primary Prevention:** ?
II **Secondary Prevention:** *Intraadenoidal cyst* is cured through thorough adenoidectomy under direct visual control, whether it is of true bursal origin or not.
Extraadenoidal cyst is usually cured by marsupialization or saucerization.
Branchial cleft cysts are best treated by excision under direct vision.
III **Other Therapy:** Aspiration and injection of sclerosing agents or marsupialization are temporizing only and recurrence may be expected.

Prognosis: Normal for life span and intelligence; functionally good in all types with proper treatment

Detection of Carrier: —

Special Considerations: —

References:
Guggenheim, P.: Cysts of the nasopharynx. Laryngoscope 77:2147, 1967.
Taylor, J. N. S. and Burwell, R. G.: Branchiogenic nasopharyngeal cysts. J. Laryngol. Otol. 68:677, 1954.
Wilson, C. P.: A case of bilateral congenital sinuses of the nasopharynx. Acta Otolaryngol. (Stockh.) 48:76, 1957.
Wilson, C. P.: Observations on the surgery of the nasopharynx. Ann. Otol. Rhinol. Laryngol. 66:5, 1957.

Contributor: Paul Guggenheim

—

Editor's Computerized Descriptors: Eye, Hearing, Ear, Nasoph., Resp.

NASOPHARYNGEAL STENOSIS

Includes: Sténose nasopharyngée
Estenosis nasofaríngea
Nasopharyngeal atresia

Excludes: Nose, anterior atresia (723)
Nose, posterior atresia (727)

Minimal Diagnostic Criteria: Complete or incomplete attachment of the soft palate to the posterior nasopharynx.†

Clinical Findings: The posterior soft palate and posterior nasopharynx are connected by a thin membrane. Although respiratory distress in the newborn with a complete membrane would be expected, it has not been reported. The patients do have excessive nasal discharge.

Complications
I **Derived:** Reduced nasal airway proportional to the amount of obstruction produced by the membrane. Nasal discharge due to impaired flow of the nasal mucous into the pharynx.
II **Associated:** Shallow nasopharynx reported in about one-half of cases.

Etiology: ? One case of congenital syphilitic nasopharyngeal stenosis has been reported.

Pathogenesis: ? Incomplete rupture of buccopharyngeal membrane has been proposed; however, this is questionable since the buccopharyngeal membrane is thought to rupture prior to fusion of the lateral palatal processes to form the soft palate, and the buccopharyngeal membrane should not be attached to the posterior nasopharynx.

Related Facts
I **Sex Ratio:** ? (Sex reported in only 2 cases, both of which were female.)
II **Risk of Occurrence:** ? Rare
III **Risk of Recurrence for**
Patient's Sib: No increased risk
Patient's Child: No increased risk
IV **Age of Detectability:** At birth by palpation between the soft palate and posterior pharyngeal wall
V **Prevalence:** ? Rare

Treatment
I **Primary Prevention:** —
II **Secondary Prevention:** The cases of membranous connection between the palate and pharynx have responded to blunt penetration of the membrane followed by a digital dilation without recurrence of the stenosis. If a cicatricial stenosis or thick membrane is encountered it can be treated with a seton suture as described by Nichols or by mucosal flaps as described by MacKenty and others.†
III **Other Therapy:** Although respiratory difficulties have not been reported, they would be expected in cases of complete or severe obstruction of the nasopharynx. This should be treated with an oral airway pending definitive treatment of the stenosis.

Prognosis: *Treated:* Membranous stenosis-excellent prognosis for permanent establishment of a nasal airway. Cicatricial stenosis-tends to recur; however, permanent establishment of a nasal airway has been accomplished with the seton procedure and with mucosal flaps.
Untreated: Danger of death from complete or severe nasopharyngeal stenosis because the newborn does not breathe through his mouth except when crying or gasping for air.

Detection of Carrier: —

†**Special Considerations:** There are 2 primary considerations: Nasopharyngeal stenosis should be considered in the newborn with obstruction of the nasal airway without choanal atresia. Although membranous occlusion of the nasopharynx will re-

spond to simple penetration and dilation of the stenotic segment, cicatricial stenosis will almost surely recur with this form of therapy.

References:

MacKenty, J.E.: Nasopharyngeal atresia. Arch. Otolaryngol. 6:1, 1927.

Stevenson, E.W.: Cicatricial stenosis of the nasopharynx. Laryngoscope. 79:2035, 1969.

Contributor: **Raymond O. Smith, Jr.**

Editor's Computerized Descriptor: Nasoph.

NEPHRITIS AND NERVE DEAFNESS, HEREDITARY

Includes: Néphropathie héréditaire avec surdité
Hereditäre Nephritis und Schalleitungsschwerhörigkeit
Nefritis hereditaria y sordera neural
Nephropathy with deafness, hereditary
Alport syndrome
Nephritis with hearing loss
Hereditary chronic nephritis
Hereditary interstitial pyelonephritis
Hearing loss and nephritis

Excludes: Hereditary nephropathy without deafness
Benign familial hematuria
Nephrosis, familial (710)
Nephronophthisis
Medullary cystic disease

Minimal Diagnostic Criteria: Persistent urinary findings of hematuria (100%) and proteinuria (70-80%), at times variable, with hearing loss of sensorineural type or nephritis in patient, parent or sibs and family history of other members with deafness or nephritis. Renal function may be normal or depressed, renal biopsy may show no definite pathology or chronic membranoglomerulonephritis and foam cells.

Clinical Findings: When first recognized it may present with variable hematuria, proteinuria, and occasional pyuria. Renal function is then usually normal but progressive loss of renal function occurs usually causing renal failure in males by the 2nd to 3rd decade with a more benign course in females. Tubular defects and the nephrotic syndrome are rarely seen. May present as acute or chronic glomerulonephritis. Evidence of urinary tract infection is usually absent. Urinary findings are microscopic hematuria, proteinuria and hyaline, granular and cellular casts. Bilateral sensorineural hearing loss is present in about 50% of the cases. It may begin in the first few years of life, is more common in males, and is slowly progressive. Audiometric studies show high-tone sensorineural hearing loss with recruitment, high SISI scores, absent tone decay, type II Bekesy tracings typical of cochlear pathology. Hearing loss and renal involvement can occur separately in affected members. Ocular defects occur in about 15% of patients and include anterior or posterior lenticonus; spherophobia and congenital cataracts.

Complications
I **Derived:** Those of chronic renal disease
II **Associated:** Hearing loss 40-60%, ocular defects in 15%

Etiology: Autosomal dominant with unusual segregation; McK *10420

Pathogenesis: Unknown; renal pathology is variable even in members of same family. Earliest alteration is glomerular basement membrane thickening. In some, pattern is similar to glomerulonephritis, in others there is periglomerular fibrosis with tubular atrophy and interstitial infiltrate resembling pyelonephritis. Foam cells, though not pathognomonic are frequently seen in later stages of disease. Initial lesion is mild and progresses slowly. Immunofluorescence is negative. Temporal bone histologic findings inconsistent; atrophy of organ of Corti and hyalinization and thinning of the tectorial membrane have been described.

Related Facts
I Sex Ratio: M1:F1
II Risk of Occurrence: ?
III Risk of Recurrence for

  Patient's Sib: Heterozygous mothers transmit the gene to more than 50% of daughters and probably to more than 50% of their sons.

  Patient's Child: Heterozygous mothers transmit the gene to more than 50% of daughters and probably to more than 50% of their sons. (Males usually die early.)

IV Age of Detectability: As early as 1st few weeks of life by intermittent albuminuria and microscopic hematuria
V Prevalence: ?

Treatment
I Primary Prevention: Genetic counseling
II Secondary Prevention: —
III Other Therapy: Supportive as may be indicated

Prognosis: Males have poorest outlook with death from uremia likely before age 30 and often in their teens; females variable but usually benign though renal abnormalities persist. Death from uremia does however occur in females.

Detection of Carrier: Presence of either nephritis or deafness with other affected family members.

Special Considerations: —

References:
Johnson W.J. and Hagan, P.J.: Hereditary nephropathy and loss of hearing. Arch. Otolaryngol. 82:166, 1965.

McCrory, W.W. et al: Hereditary renal glomerular disease in infancy and childhood. Adv. Pediatr. 14:253, 1966.

Perkoff, G.T.: The hereditary renal diseases. N. Engl. J. Med. 277:79, 1967.

Contributors: **David A. Dolowitz**
William J. Johnson
P. John Hagan
Wallace W. McCrory

Editor's Computerized Descriptors: Eye, Hearing, GU.

NEPHROSIS, CONGENITAL

Includes: Néphrose congénitale
Angeborene Nephrose
Nefrosis congénita
Congenital nephrotic syndrome
Microcystic renal disease
Neonatal nephrosis

Excludes: Nephrosis, familial (710)
Fetal syphilis syndrome (385)
Nephrotic syndrome associated with mercury poisoning, malaria or toxoplasmosis
Fetal cytomegalovirus syndrome (381)
Renal vein thrombosis
Congenital nephrosis with histopathology of diffuse mesangial sclerosis

Minimal Diagnostic Criteria: Edema; hypoproteinemia; hypoalbuminemia; onset before 2 months of age; usually hypercholesterolemia and proteinuria. Negative tests for syphilis, malaria, mercury, toxoplasma and cytomegalovirus.

Clinical Findings: Newborns present as small for date infants with edema, hypoproteinemia and proteinuria. Occasionally the edema is absent at birth, but shortly thereafter becomes generalized, severe and persistent. Congenital nephrosis may be suspected in the absence of persistent edema when the placenta is large and heavy and the infant has low birthweight. Laboratory findings consist of proteinuria; hypoproteinemia with serum protein of 2.5-3.7 gm%; low serum albumin of 0.4-0.9 gm%; serum cholesterol may be lower than 200 mg% initially; in most cases, this value varies between 200-400 mg% with tendency to rise as high as 800 mg%. The disease is invariably fatal with death occurring by age of 1 year as result of infection or renal failure.

Complications
I Derived: Electrolyte imbalance, infections, renal failure, retardation of growth and development.
II Associated: —

Etiology: Evidence for autosomal recessive transmission was shown in a study of 57 Finnish families by Norio. In nearly one-third of the marriages, consanguinity was noted. McK *25630

Pathogenesis: ?

Related Facts
I Sex Ratio: M1:F1
II Risk of Occurrence: ?
III Risk of Recurrence for
  Patient's Sib: 1 in 4 (25%) for each offspring to be affected
  Patient's Child: (Early death precludes reproduction.)
IV Age of Detectability: At birth or shortly thereafter by clinical picture. Mothers at risk of bearing a child with congenital nephrosis have been noted to have markedly elevated alpha-fetoprotein in their own sera and amniotic fluid starting from 15th week of gestation.
V Prevalence: ? Greatest number of cases from Finland and areas outside Finland where there is large aggregation of people of Finnish extraction.

Treatment
I Primary Prevention: Genetic counseling
II Secondary Prevention: Steroid and other immunosuppressive drugs not of demonstrated value. Successful renal transplantations have been reported.
III Other Therapy: Adequate therapy for infections

Prognosis: Very poor. Most succumb within 1st year of life. Longest known life span is 3 years, 10 months.

Detection of Carrier: —

Special Considerations: —

References:
Hallman, N. et al: Main features of the congenital nephrotic syndrome. Acta Paediatr. Scand. (Suppl.) 172:75, 1967.

Hoyer, J.R. et al: The nephrotic syndrome of infancy; clinical, morphological, and immunological studies of four infants. Pediatrics 40:233, 1967.

Hoyer, J.R. et al: Successful renal transplantation in 3 children with congenital nephrotic syndrome. Lancet 1:1410, 1973.

Huttunen, N.P.: Congenital nephrotic syndrome of Finnish type. Arch. Dis. Child. 51:344, 1976.

Norio, R.: Heredity in the congenital nephrotic syndrome. Ann. Paediatr. Fenn. (Suppl.) 12:27:1, 1966.

Seppala, M. et al: Congenital nephrotic syndrome: Prenatal diagnosis and genetic counseling by estimation of amniotic fluid and maternal serum alpha-fetoprotein. Lancet 2:123, 1976.

Contributor: **Madoka Shibuya**

Editor's Computerized Descriptors: Skin, GU.

NEPHROSIS, FAMILIAL

Includes: Néphrose familiale
Familiäre Nephrose
Nefrosis familiar
Familial nephrotic syndrome occurring postnatally

Excludes: Nephrosis, congenital (709)
Nephritis and nerve deafness, hereditary (708)
Other types of hereditary nephritis

Minimal Diagnostic Criteria: Sib with nephrosis, edema, hypoproteinemia, hypercholesterolemia, and proteinuria. Renal biopsy may reveal minimal findings or evidence of membranoproliferative focal sclerosing glomerulonephritis.

Clinical Findings: The manner of onset of familial nephrosis is similar to all other types of nephrosis with the insidious onset of edema. It is not present at birth but may appear as early as 2 months of age. There may be a history of an upper respiratory infection prior to the onset of edema. With increasing edema, there is often history of a decrease in urinary output. The physical examination reveals generalized edema, at times including ascites. Hypertension and hematuria are generally absent at onset. Laboratory studies reveal severe-to-moderate proteinuria, hypoproteinemia, hypercholesterolemia, normal BUN and no marked reduction in creatinine clearance at onset. Serum complement levels are normal. It is not until the same type of nephrosis develops in a sib that one becomes aware of the fact that one is dealing with a familial form of nephrosis. Familial nerve deafness is not associated with this form of renal disease and if present suggests hereditary nephritis and nerve deafness (Alport syndrome).

The course may follow 2 patterns as to response to steroid therapy and to outcome. In 1 group, steroid therapy produces little or no improvement and death from infection or renal failure ultimately results. Alternatively, the patient responds to steroid with evidence of complete remission and thereafter may have 1 or more relapses which respond to steroid therapy but eventually there is complete recovery. The pattern of response in the 2nd involved member of the family usually follows a course similar to that of the 1st affected sib.

Complications
I **Derived:** For those who do not respond to steroid, infection or renal failure may be the cause of death. For those who are steroid-responsive, the clinical course may be relatively uncomplicated.
II **Associated:** —

Etiology: ? Autosomal recessive mode of inheritance seems likely

Pathogenesis: ? †

Related Facts
I **Sex Ratio:** ? More reported cases among males
II **Risk of Occurrence:** ?
III **Risk of Recurrence for**
   Patient's Sib: ? If autosomal recessive 1 in 4 (25%) for each offspring to be affected
   Patient's Child: ? If autosomal recessive not increased unless mate is carrier or homozygote.
IV **Age of Detectability:** Anytime after the age of 2 months
V **Prevalence:** ?

Treatment
I **Primary Prevention:** —
II **Secondary Prevention:** Steroid therapy
III **Other Therapy:** Antibiotics

Prognosis: The prognosis is favorable among those who are steroid-responsive. If there is no response to steroid therapy, the prognosis is unfavorable.

Detection of Carrier: ?

†**Special Considerations:** The pathologic findings are variable and do not provide a means to distinguish this form of the nephrotic syndrome from nonfamilial forms. Some may show no abnormalities on routine light microscopy of the kidney; however, on electron microscopy there is fusion of the foot processes (so-called minimal change). In others, the microscopic features are those of membranous glomerulonephritis with or without lobular nephritis or focal sclerosing glomerulonephritis. The form with minimal change renal pathology is the steroid-responsive form with a good outlook for ultimate recovery.

References:

Braun, F.C., Jr. and Bayer, J.F.: Familial nephrosis associated with deafness and congenital urinary tract anomalies in siblings. J. Pediatr. 60:33, 1962.
Friderich, J. et al: Häufigkeit, Prognose und Behandlung des Nephrosesyndroms. Helv. Paediatr. Acta. 9:109, 1954.
McCrory, W.W. et al: Hereditary renal glomerular disease in infancy and childhood. Adv. Pediatr. 14:253, 1966.

Contributor: **Wallace W. McCrory**

Editor's Computerized Descriptors: Skin, GU.

NEUROECTODERMAL PIGMENTED TUMOR

Includes: Tumeur neuro-ectodermique pigmentée
Pigmentierter neuroektodermaler Tumor
Tumor neuroectodérmico pigmentado
Progonoma†

Excludes: Ameloblastoma
Oral melanoma
Oral nevi
Epulis, congenital (360)

Minimal Diagnostic Criteria: Must be differentiated by microscopic examination. Nonencapsulated infiltrating tumor characterized by moderately vascularized fibrous connective tissue stroma with tumor cells aggregated into alveolar spaces. Cells are cuboidal about alveolar periphery and decrease in size centrally. Nuclei are round, deeply basophilic and surrounded by scanty cytoplasm. Pigment may be prominent or inconspicuous. Special stains dramatize presence of melanin pigment.

Clinical Findings: Nonulcerated, rapidly growing tumor in jaws of infants almost invariably less than 1 year of age. It locally destroys bone and displaces teeth. Most cases occur in the maxilla - 80%, occasionally in the mandible - 10%, both exhibiting midline predilection. Other sites - 10%. These include anterior fontanel, shoulder and epididymis. Two cases reported high urinary vanilmandelic acid excretion which returned to normal upon removal of the tumor.

Complications
I **Derived:** Natural history of untreated lesion not known, however, disfigurement, displacement of associated teeth and possible problem of impaired sucking can occur.
II **Associated:** —

Etiology: Hypotheses include:
Neuroectodermal: arises from cells of the neural crest which migrate to the site of tumor origin during embryogenesis. Identification of high urinary excretion of vanilmandelic acid which falls to normal upon tumor removal supports this hypothesis. Odontogenic: histogenic hypothesis. Melanocarcinoma: original concept, now disbelieved.

Pathogenesis: Tumor often present at birth, grows rapidly destroying bone locally and displacing associated teeth.

Related Facts
I **Sex Ratio:** M1:F1
II **Risk of Occurrence:** ?
III **Risk of Recurrence for**
Patient's Sib: ? None reported
Patient's Child: ?
IV **Age of Detectability:** Often present at birth, almost invariably recognized during the 1st year of life.
V **Prevalence:** ?

Treatment
I **Primary Prevention:** —
II **Secondary Prevention:** Surgical extirpation indicated
III **Other Therapy:** —

Prognosis: Following surgical extirpation (slightly in excess of 10% have been irradiated as well) recurrence has occurred in 20% of the treated cases. Recurrences have only been associated with maxillary or mandibular examples of the tumor. Except for local surgical disfigurement, prognosis is excellent.

Detection of Carrier: —

†**Special Considerations:** This tumor has been reported under a wide variety of titles which include: melanotic ameloblastoma, melanotic progonoma, retinal anlage tumor, melanotic neuroectodermal tumor of infancy, pigmented ameloblastoma, pigmented adamantinoma, heterotropic pigmented retinoblastoma, retinal choristoma, con-

genital pigmented epulis, melanotic odontoma.

In view of the x-ray appearance of irregular, ragged lytic lesion of bone and the clinical feature of rapid growth, care must be exercised to prevent an erroneous diagnosis of malignant neoplasm. Histopathologic examination should precede therapeutic assault whenever pigmented neuroectodermal tumor of infancy is included in the differential diagnosis.

References:

Borello, E. D. and Gorlin, R. J.: Melanotic neuroectodermal tumor of infancy - a neoplasm of neural crest origin: Report of a case associated with high urinary excretion of vanilmandelic acid. Cancer 19:196, 1966.

Brekke, J.H. and Gorlin, R.J.: Melanotic neuroectodermal tumor of infancy. J. Oral Surg. 33:858, 1975.

Kerr, D. A. and Pullon, P. A.: A study of the pigmented tumors of jaws of infants (melanotic ameloblastoma, retinal anlage tumor, progonoma). Oral Surg. 18:759, 1964.

Contributors: **Nathaniel H. Rowe**
John J. Sauk, Jr.

Editor's Computerized Descriptors: Face, Skel., Teeth

NEUROFIBROMATOSIS

Includes: Neurofibromatose
von Recklinghausen disease

Excludes: Tuberous sclerosis (975)
Other phakomatoses

Minimal Diagnostic Criteria: The presence of more than 5 café-au-lait spots 1.5 cm in diameter associated with the typical cutaneous tumors is sufficient evidence to clarify the diagnosis in approximately 90%.

Clinical Findings: Café-au-lait spots may be present at birth. They may increase in size and number with age, and tend to occur on the unexposed areas of the body. A diagnosis of neurofibromatosis must be considered if more than 5 café-au-lait spots measuring greater than 1.5 cm in diameter are found. Cutaneous tumors are common. They tend to be widespread usually escaping the palmar surfaces. They may occur in nodules along a peripheral nerve, oftentimes causing a violaceous hue of the overlying skin. The tumors, because of their relation to the nerve trunks, occasionally produce motor or sensory disturbances. Some tumors become pedunculated and massive. Plexiform neurofibromata may be associated with hypertrophy of a body part. The patient's skin color may be darker than that of other family members and heavy freckling may be present.

Virtually every part of the CNS has been affected by this disease process. Cranial nerve signs may be the result of a glioma or neuroma. Optic nerve and chiasm gliomas or acoustic neuromas, particularly in children, are the most frequent cranial nerve tumors. The eye or orbit does not escape. Tumors of the lids, optic nerve, neurofibromata of the iris, conjunctiva, cornea and ciliary nerves have been reported. Intraorbital neurofibromatosis may produce proptosis and muscle palsies. Neurofibromatosis is occasionally associated with glaucoma. Tumors may develop on spinal nerves producing variable neurologic signs depending on the level of involvement. The frequency of seizures is increased, probably secondary to central pathology. The incidence of mental retardation is increased, but good data is lacking as to numbers and degree.

Congenital defects of the skeleton such as elevation of the scapula, asymmetries and absence of long bones are found in this disease. The sella turcica is box shaped. Pseudoarthroses are frequently encountered. The roentgenologic findings are numerous. There may be kyphoscoliosis due to scalloping of the posterior vertebral bodies or secondary to a spinal nerve tumor. Erosive changes of bones are common, probably secondary to pressure exerted by a tumor. Disorders of bony growth producing marked asymmetry occasionally occurs. There may be bowing or pseudoarthrosis of long bones, particularly the tibia. Intraosseous cystic bone lesions may present as spontaneous fractures. Bony defects of the sphenoid bone, orbital roof, sutures, and temporal fossa may be seen in conjunction with a plexiform neuroma of the eyelid. Enlargement of the optic canal occurs with an optic glioma. Biopsy of a cutaneous or neural tumor is usually diagnostic.

Complications
I   **Derived:** The cutaneous tumors rarely undergo sarcomatous degeneration. The incidence of brain tumors, including meningiomas and gliomas, is increased in this patient population. Spinal cord compression may result due to bony involvement or tumors of the spinal nerves. Increased intracranial pressure may be secondary to an intracranial tumor. Optic atrophy may be the end result.

Masses of the mediastinum and GI tract may occur due to

neurofibroma of the automatic nervous system.
II **Associated:** The incidence of pheochromocytoma is increased so that a patient may present with hypertensive crisis.

Etiology: Autosomal dominant; McK *16220

Pathogenesis: ?

Related Facts
I **Sex Ratio:** M1:F1
II **Risk of Occurrence:** 1 in 3300 live births
III **Risk of Recurrence for**
    Patient's Sib: If parent is affected, 1 in 2 (50%) for each offspring to be affected; otherwise not increased.
    Patient's Child: 1 in 2
IV **Age of Detectability:** Usually in 1st decade, occasionally at birth, by physical examination.
V **Prevalence:** About 1 in 3000. No ethnic differences noted.

Treatment
I **Primary Prevention:** Genetic counseling
II **Secondary Prevention:** Surgical excision of cutaneous tumors is suggested when sudden rapid growth occurs. If malignancy is demonstrated, extensive local resection is mandatory. Tumors involving the CNS should be fully investigated and removed if feasible.
III **Other Therapy:** Anticonvulsants are used if seizures occur. Special education may be helpful with mild retardation.

Prognosis: Usually a slowly progressive disease compatible with a full and useful life. Malignant degeneration of cutaneous tumors or central nervous involvement may cause death.

Detection of Carrier: —

Special Considerations: —

References:
Crowe, F.W. et al: A Clinical, Pathological, and Genetic Study of Multiple Neurofibromatosis. Springfield: C. C Thomas, 1956.

Contributors: **Robert H. A. Haslam**
                        Kenneth Shulman

Editor's Computerized Descriptors: Eye, Ear, Skin, Skel., CV., Nerve
Also see Section I, Fig. 56

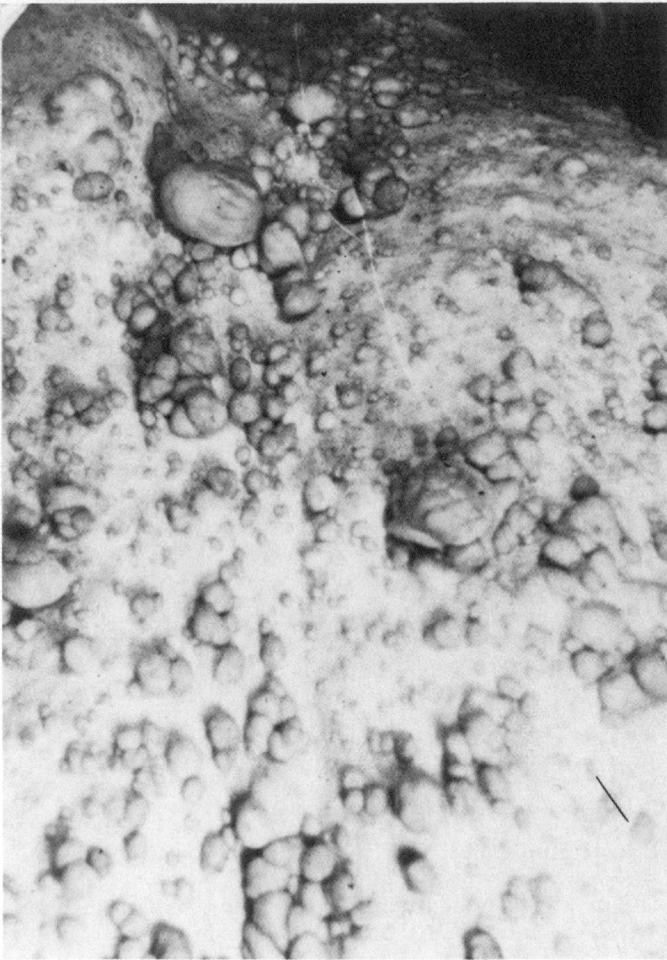
386. Pedunculated neurofibromatosis

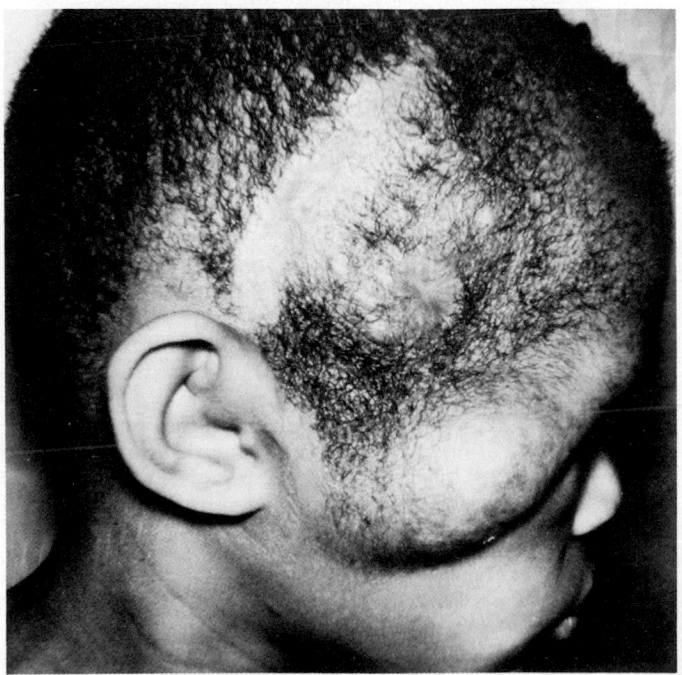
387. Large neurofibromas of scalp and face

NEURONAL CEROID-LIPOFUSCINOSES

Includes: Lipofuschinose du système nerveux
Neuronale ceroid-lipofuscinose
Lipofuscinosis neuronal ceroidea
Amaurotic familial idiocy, all three types
Cerebromacular degeneration
Batten-Vogt syndrome
Neuronal storage disease with curvilinear bodies
Jansky-Bielschowsky syndrome
Myoclonic variant of cerebral lipoidosis
Maculocerebral degeneration
Pigmentary retinal lipoid neuronal heredodegeneration
Spielmeyer-Vogt disease
Kufs disease

Excludes: Niemann-Pick disease (717)
Gaucher disease (406)
Hand-Schüller-Christian syndrome
G_{M1}-Gangliosidosis, types 1 and 2 (431 & 432)
G_{M2}-Gangliosidosis with hexosaminidase A deficiency (434)
G_{M2}-Gangliosidosis with hexosaminidase A and B deficiency (433)
Other neuronal storage and degenerative diseases

Minimal Diagnostic Criteria: The diagnosis is aided by a positive family history of a child with a similar progressive disease. A child with a progressive dementia, seizures and myoclonic jerks can be suspected of having this particular syndrome. The diagnosis in each instance may be proven by analysis of neurons obtained either by rectal biopsy or brain biopsy. Electron microscopic evaluation of the neurons may show inclusions which have the appearance of curvilinear bodies, or bodies with fingerprint profile inclusions. Until further biochemical information is available age of onset is also used as a guide for classification.†

Clinical Findings: There are 3 clinical forms of this syndrome.

Late infantile neuronal ceroid-lipofuscinosis begins between the ages of 2 and 5 years with seizures usually being the first indication of disease. The progression is fairly rapid with loss of mental function and motor coordination. The seizures are an ever increasing problem and may be quite refractory to anticonvulsant medications. Some patients develop myoclonic jerks which may be quite sensitive to a variety of stimuli such as turning the light on, a loud noise or eliciting a tendon reflex.

The retina may be involved and may show abnormalities in the macular area or a retinitis pigmentosa around the macular area. Progressive loss of vision may be a problem but is not quite as prominent as in the juvenile form. The course of the disease is usually 3-5 years and the terminal stages are marked by loss of contact with surroundings, myoclonic jerks, difficulty with feeding, and death usually from aspiration pneumonia.

Juvenile neuronal ceroid-lipofuscinosis has an onset around ages 8-12 years. There are 2 patterns of onset. Some children start with visual disturbance with retinitis pigmentosa which may be progressive, followed after 2-3 years by seizures and progressive mental deterioration. As the disease progresses the children may develop myoclonic jerks and seizures which can be quite refractory to anticonvulsant medications. The course of the disease is slower than the late infantile form and many of these children survive for 6-8 years. Ataxia may be a prominent symptom and one is sometimes hard pressed to tell whether the ataxia is from anticonvulsant medications or progression of the disease.

In an alternate juvenile form of this disease the dementia is a leading symptom starting as behavioral difficulties and progressing to a more global dementia. Seizures are a later manifestation and retinal involvement may not occur at all.

Adult neuronal ceroid-lipofuscinosis is rare and the diagnosis is seldom made during life. There is one form in which the patient appears to have ataxia and dementia as prominent clinical symptoms and in another form there may be evidence of basal ganglia involvement as well as dementia. These cases may be extremely difficult to differentiate from other progressive degenerative diseases of the nervous system.

There are no distinctive x-ray or routine laboratory findings that aid in the diagnosis of any of these conditions. Diagnosis can be established by rectal biopsy in some children or may require brain biopsy.

Complications
I Derived: Seizures occur in practically all patients at some stage of the disease. Retinal involvement occurs in almost all forms of the juvenile condition and is usually retinitis pigmentosa with decreasing vision a prominent symptom. Children usually die from complications of aspiration pneumonia.
II Associated: —

Etiology: The condition is marked by the storage of a fluorescent lipopigment. It has been suggested that this pigment, which is somewhat similar to lipofuscin which also occurs in a number of organs during aging, is related to defects in the oxidation of polyunsaturated and saturated fatty acids. The mode of transmission in the late infantile and juvenile forms is autosomal recessive. It is not known for the adult form. McK *25673

Pathogenesis: ?

Related Facts
I Sex Ratio: M1:F1
II Risk of Occurrence: Late infantile form? Juvenile form? Adult form?
III Risk of Recurrence for
   Patient's Sib: Late infantile and juvenile forms: 1 in 4 (25%) for each offspring to be affected
   Patient's Child: (Late infantile and juvenile forms are lethal.)
IV Age of Detectability: Late infantile form, 2-3 years of age on clinical criteria. Juvenile form, 8-10 years of age on clinical criteria.
V Prevalence: Juvenile form: 1 in 25,000 in Sweden

Treatment
I Primary Prevention: Genetic counseling
II Secondary Prevention: —
III Other Therapy: Supportive measures

Prognosis: Late infantile form: The life expectancy is 2-5 years after diagnosis. Juvenile form: The life expectancy is 4-8 years after time of diagnosis.

Detection of Carrier: —

†**Special Considerations:** Final classification of this syndrome will require biochemical information about the nature of the stored material and the underlying biochemical defect or defects.

References:
Hagberg, B. et al: Late infantile progressive encephalopathy with disturbed polyunsaturated fat metabolism. Acta Paediatr. (Uppsala) 57:495, 1968.
Herman, M.M. et al: Additional electron microscopic observations on two cases of Batten-Spielmeyer-Vogt disease (neuronal ceroid- lipofuscinosis). Acta Neuropathol. (Berl.) 17:85, 1971.
Zeman, W. et al: The neuronal ceroid-lipofuscinoses (Batten-Vogt syndrome). In Vinken, P.J. et al (eds.): Handbook of Clinical Neurology. Amsterdam:North Holland Publishing Co., 1970, vol. 10, p. 588.

Contributor: **Guy M. McKhann**

NEUTROPENIA, CYCLIC

Includes: Neutropénie cyclique
Zyklische Neutropenie
Neutropenia cíclica
Periodic neutropenia
Cyclic neutropenia

Excludes: Periodic fever
Mediterranean fever

Minimal Diagnostic Criteria: Repeated white cell and differential counts over a 4-6 week period to establish neutropenia and oscillation of the neutrophil count at regular intervals.†

Clinical Findings: Episodes of fever, malaise and oral ulcerations lasting for 3-10 days and recurring at approximately 21 day intervals. Mild splenomegaly is occasionally observed. Onset is usually during infancy or childhood.
The peripheral blood neutrophil count is severely depressed during the symptomatic period. Symptoms are rare when neutrophils are greater than 500/mm^3.

Complications
I   **Derived:** During neutropenic periods, infection of superficial skin lacerations may develop. Chronic gingivitis and periodontal disease are common. Recurrent boils, otitis media, cervical adenitis, bronchitis and pneumonia have been reported.
II   **Associated:** Anemia, thrombocytopenia have occurred in some patients. Other periodic complaints - arthralgia, abdominal pain, diarrhea - may coexist.

Etiology: Probably transmitted as an autosomal dominant with high penetrance and variable expressivity but familial nature not always demonstrable.

Pathogenesis: Prior to peripheral blood neutropenia, the bone marrow shows a decrease in neutrophil precursors. At the nadir, there are early myeloid precursors in the absence of mature neutrophils. The periodic failure to differentiate suggests either an intrinsic defect in the stem cells themselves or in feedback control mechanisms.†

Related Facts
I   **Sex Ratio:** M1:F1
II   **Risk of Occurrence:** ?
III **Risk of Recurrence for**
     Patient's Sib: If parent is affected, 1 in 2 (50%) for each offspring to be affected; otherwise not increased.
     Patient's Child: 1 in 2
IV   **Age of Detectability:** From birth
V   **Prevalence:** Less than 1 in 100,000

Treatment
I   **Primary Prevention:** Genetic counseling
II   **Secondary Prevention:** Prompt recognition and treatment of serious infection. No therapy has yet resulted in a cure but clinical or hematologic improvement has been reported following ACTH, corticosteroids, testosterone, staphylococcal vaccine and infusion of normal plasma or plasma from a volunteer given typhoid vaccine. Following splenectomy, objective and subjective improvement has been noted in some patients.
III **Other Therapy:** May be curable by marrow transplantation.†

Prognosis: The disease is often relatively benign and consistent with a normal life span. However it varies widely and severe infections with a fatal outcome have been reported. There is a tendency for moderation of illness with time.

Detection of Carrier: —

†Special Considerations: Total leukocyte counts may fluctuate or may be fairly constant due to the monocytosis which occurs in about 50% of cases at the nadir of the neutrophil cycle. Periodic variation in lymphocytes, eosinophils, platelets and reticulocytes, described in some patients, suggests that the defect in cyclic neutropenia is not confined to the neutrophil series.

Cyclic neutropenia occurs as an autosomal recessive disorder in the grey collie dog and can be viewed as a model of cyclic neutropenia in man. Cyclic changes of other hematologic elements also occur in these dogs. Transplants of normal bone marrow into a neutropenic dog and neutropenic marrow into a normal dog have shown that the disease may be abolished or established by appropriate allografting and suggest that the disease is secondary to defective hematopoietic stem cells.

References:
Dale, D.C. and Graw, R.E.: Transplantation of allogeneic bone marrow in canine cyclic neutropenia. Science 183:83, 1974.

Guerry, D. et al: Periodic hematopoiesis in human cyclic neutropenia. J. Clin. Invest. 52:3220, 1973.

Morley, A.A. et al: Familial cyclical neutropenia. Br. J. Haematol. 13:719, 1967.

Page, A.R. and Good, R.A.: Studies on cyclic neutropenia: A clinical and experimental investigation. Am. J. Dis. Child. 94:623, 1957.

Reimann, H.A.: Periodic Diseases. Philadelphia:F.A. Davis Co., 1963, p. 94.

Weiden, P.L. et al: Canine cyclic neutropenia: A stem cell defect. J. Clin. Invest. 53:950, 1974.

Contributor: **Elizabeth M. Smithwick**

Editor's Computerized Descriptor: Oral

NEVUS FLAMMEUS

Includes: Naevus flammeus
Nape nevus
Nevus telangiectatica
Salmon patch
Erythema nuchae
Capillary nevus
Port-wine stain
Capillary hemangioma
"Birthmark" †
Nevi flammei

Excludes: Larger strawberry or cavernous hemangiomas, though nevus flammeus may occur in conjunction with these.

Minimal Diagnostic Criteria: Vascular skin lesions

Clinical Findings: Salmon patches, so common in infants, consist of pinkish-red, macular, telangiectatic linear skin lesions. On the forehead, the overall shape is that of a wedge or tornado funnel tapered onto the glabellum. Eyelids are often involved in the neonate. Involvement of the posterior surface of the neck and of the occiput is often partially retained in later life. Port-wine marks tend to have a more intense hue (purplish-red) and may become papulonodular.

Complications
I **Derived:** Rarely, nevi flammei portend an underlying disorder of the nervous system, eg Sturge-Weber syndrome, epidural hemangiomatosus of the spinal cord in conjunction with nevus flammeus of corresponding dermatomes. Telangiectatic nevi are an inconstant feature of cerebroretinal arteriovenous aneuryism, neuroretinoangiomatosis, and other neuroophthalmic defects. Tissue hypertrophy may accompany nevi flammei of the limbs (see Angioosteohypertrophy syndrome), genitalia, lips and other sites.
II **Associated:** Glaucoma, phocomelia, chromosome 13 trisomy syndrome, chromosome 4 p- syndrome, underlying arteriovenous communication, ? congenital heart disease.

Etiology: In their development, appearance and distribution, nevi flammei may be under neural influences. Salmon patches have followed pedigree patterns of autosomal dominant type but high prevalence precludes a definite conclusion regarding all cases. Phocomelic "thalidomide babies" and infants with various chromosome anomalies have exhibited facial nevi flammei, and rarely nevi flammei first appear following exposure to intense cold or other physical injury (multifactorial). Nevi flammei of trunk and limbs have been reported infrequently following irregularly dominant patterns. McK *16310

Pathogenesis: Facial salmon patches disappear early in life. Nape nevi also fade early, but remnants commonly persist. Port-wine stains tend to increase in size and intensify in hue.

Related Facts
I **Sex Ratio:** M1:F1 for most types
II **Risk of Occurrence:** Salmon patch in over 50% of neonates (ie "normal anatomic variants"). Port-wine stains fairly uncommon.
III **Risk of Recurrence for**
  Patient's Sib: When autosomal dominant and if parent is affected 1 in 2 (50%) for each offspring to be affected; otherwise not increased.
  Patient's Child: 1 in 2
IV **Age of Detectability:** Usually neonatal period
V **Prevalence:** Nape nevi in about 30% of adults. Lower figures reported in Negroes but lesions are less visible.

Treatment
I **Primary Prevention:** Genetic counseling
II **Secondary Prevention:** —
III **Other Therapy:** Port-wine stain: cosmetic coverage, excision and graft, CO_2 ice, electrodesiccation, dermabrasion, tattooing, thorium X, grenz ray, radiophosphorus.

Prognosis: Normal for life span, intelligence and function when uncomplicated.

Detection of Carrier: —

†Special Considerations: The theory that salmon patches are caused by trauma directly to the lesional area has been dispelled; the expression "pressure marks" should no longer be in use.

References:
Bettley, F.R.: Erythema nucae. Br. J. Dermatol. 52:363, 1940.
Selmanowitz, V.J.: Nevus flameus of the forehead. J. Pediatr. 73:755, 1968.

Contributor: **Victor J. Selmanowitz**

Editor's Computerized Descriptor: Skin

NEVUS OF OTA

Includes: Mélanose oculaire
Otas Nävus
Melanosis ocular
Congenital oculodermal melanocytosis
Nevus fuscocaeruleus maxillofacialis
Oculocutaneous pigmentation syndrome

Excludes: Congenital melanosis oculi without dermal involvement
Acquired melanosis oculi
Malignant melanoma
Nevus
Precancerous melanosis
Melanocytoma (639)

Minimal Diagnostic Criteria: See Clinical Findings.

Clinical Findings: This benign pigmented lesion usually appears unilaterally and affects the skin, eye, and adnexa supplied by the 1st and 2nd divisions of the trigeminal nerve. Occasionally the eardrum, buccal mucosa, palate, and nasopharynx may be involved. It is usually noted at birth, frequently increasing with puberty or pregnancy.

The conjunctival pigmentation consists of bluish-grey spots in the palpebral region. The sclera is usually most heavily involved, the pigment appearing as discrete, dark blue spots. Heterochromia irides may be present and the trabecular meshwork may be involved. The fundus has a uniform dark slate-grey appearance.

Complications
I **Derived:** —
II **Associated:** There are reports suggesting a higher incidence of malignant melanoma in the uveal tract of eyes with nevus of Ota than in the normal population. Rarely, the disease is accompanied by cutaneous, ocular, vascular, osseous, neurologic, or general problems.

Etiology: ? †

Pathogenesis: ? †

Related Facts
I **Sex Ratio:** M>F
II **Risk of Occurrence:** ?
III **Risk of Recurrence for**
Patient's Sib: ?
Patient's Child: ?
IV **Age of Detectability:** Usually at birth
V **Prevalence:** ?

Treatment
I **Primary Prevention:** —
II **Secondary Prevention:** —
III **Other Therapy:** —

Prognosis: Good

Detection of Carrier: —

†Special Considerations: Nevus of Ota is much more common in the deeper pigmented races such as Orientals and Negroes. Histologically there is an abundance of melanocytes with many melanin granules. The nevus of Ota is structurally comparable to the aberrant and persistent Mongolian spot.

References:
Duke-Elder, S.: System of Ophthalmology, vol. 3, pt. 2. Congenital Deformities, London: Henry Kimpton, 1964.
Fishman, G.R.A. and Anderson, R.: Nevus of Ota: Report of two cases, one with open-angle glaucoma. Am. J. Ophthalmol. 54:453, 1962.
Font, R.L. et al: Diffuse malignant melanoma of the iris in the nevus of Ota. Arch. Ophthalmol. 77:513, 1967.

Guerin, T.C. and Daudon-Couteaux, R.: Nevus of Ota. Arch. Ophthalmol. (Paris) 34:359, 1974.

Hagler, W.S. and Brown, C.C.: Malignant melanoma of the orbit arising in a nevus of Ota. Trans. Am. Acad. Ophthalmol. Otolaryngol. 70:817, 1966.

Reese, A.B.: Tumors of the Eye, 3rd Ed. New York: Harper & Row, 1976.

Contributor: **Morton E. Smith**

Editor's Computerized Descriptors: Eye, Skin

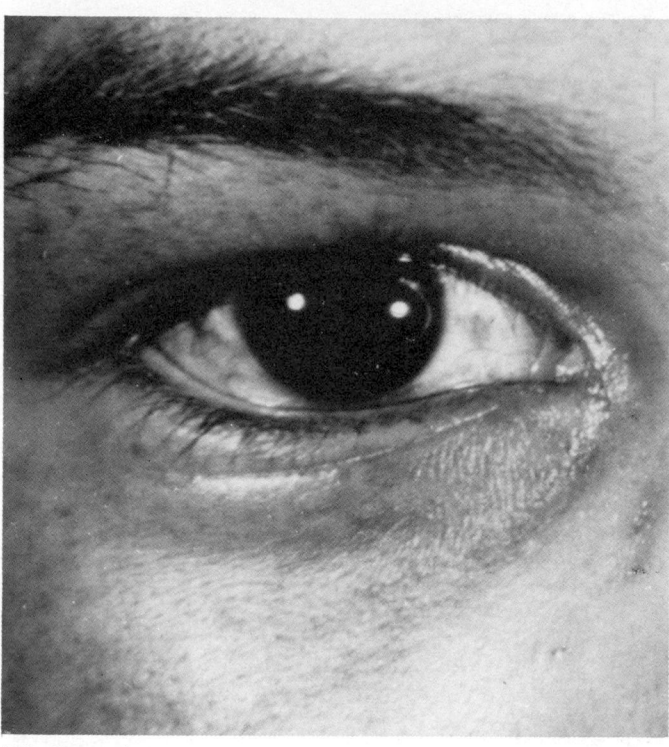

388. Nevus of ota

NIEMANN-PICK DISEASE

Includes: Maladie de Niemann-Pick
Niemann-Picksche Krankheit
Enfermedad de Niemann-Pick
Sphingomyelin lipidosis

Excludes: G_{M2}-Gangliosidosis with hexosaminidase A deficiency (434)
Wolman disease (1003)
Gaucher disease (406)
G_{M1}-Gangliosidosis, type 1 (431)

Minimal Diagnostic Criteria: Enlargement of liver or spleen; presence of foam cells in marrow, liver or spleen; demonstration of abnormal intracellular accumulation of sphingomyelin and a negative search for other situations which may produce secondary formation of similar foam cells.

Clinical Findings: The term "Niemann-Pick disease" is applied to at least 4 phenotypes which have areas of clinical difference but a presumed biochemical relationship.† Enlargement of the spleen and liver is common to all types and usually quite notable, while lymphadenopathy is not prominent. The hematologic effects of the splenomegaly ("hypersplenism") are common, but less intense than in Gaucher disease. Pulmonary infiltration (xray) is characteristic in the circumstances where organomegaly is of high order, and growth impairment is of varying degree. All forms except the remarkable "adult" type (Group B) have increasingly serious neurologic involvement—including developmental slowing, arrest of development, and then deterioration of general function. Occasional patients have seizures and the older children may show ataxia or other cerebellar signs. Cherry-red macular changes are noted in some of the patients, especially the younger ones. It is usual to find vacuolization of some of the lymphocytes in the peripheral blood. Occasional children develop small papular or nodular skin xanthomas, which are apparently not secondary to hyperlipidemia, the latter being seen only in Group A and Group B patients.

Complications
I **Derived:**   Chronic nutritional failure eventually ensues, as well as progressive debility and mental retardation except, as mentioned, in the Group B patients. Bronchopneumonia is usual in the terminal patients, as are anemia and ascites.
II **Associated:**   Prolonged jaundice of moderate degree in the first 6 months of life is reported in about one-quarter of the patients and is of unknown pertinence.

Etiology: Autosomal recessive inheritance for all forms of Niemann-Pick disease. Specific sphingomyelinase deficiency has been identified in the tissues, cultured fibroblasts, and WBC of patients from Group A and Group B; studies currently underway suggest that other assay systems will be available soon to document similar enzymopathies for the other Groups. McK *25720

Pathogenesis: It appears reasonable to assume that local tissue sphingomyelin accumulation can be adequately explained on the basis of the lysosomal enzyme insufficiency. An explanation is also needed, however, for the simultaneous cholesterol increase in tissues, unless, as Fredrickson has suggested, a specific intermolecular complex is formed. The specific origin of the CNS defect is incompletely understood. Only in Group A patients is there a cortical increase in sphingomyelin, per se, and in Group B patients (with the same enzymopathy) the brain is normal.

Related Facts
I **Sex Ratio:**   M1:F1
II **Risk of Occurrence:**   Uncommon, but not rare. About half of the Group A patients are of Ashkenazi Jewish ancestry. It is estimated that the carrier rate among Jews is about 1:100.

The majority of the Group D patients are of French-Canadian (Yarmouth County, Nova Scotia) background.

III Risk of Recurrence for
  Patient's Sib: 1 in 4 (25%) for each offspring to be affected
  Patient's Child: Not increased unless mate is carrier or homozygote.
      A number of persons with Group B involvement are now known to have had normal children.
IV Age of Detectability: Prenatal diagnosis is possible for Group A patients. Hepatosplenomegaly is detectable after 2-3 months of age, and developmental delays shortly thereafter. Groups C and D patients have often shown prolonged jaundice in the early months of life.
V Prevalence: About 200 patients have been described to date.

Treatment
I Primary Prevention: Genetic counseling
II Secondary Prevention: —
III Other Therapy: Supportive treatment is important for the child and family. This includes assistance in feeding, control of infection, anticonvulsants where needed, transfusion or splenectomy.

Prognosis: Variable†

Detection of Carrier: Parents and uninvolved sibs have no known clinical handicaps. The level of sphingomyelinase activity in the WBC and cultured fibroblasts from Group A heterozygotes is reduced, but the range overlaps with normal figures and a firm diagnosis may not be possible.

†Special Considerations: As mentioned, the eponymic designation currently encompasses 4 clinical situations not genetically interrelated. With the exception of the sphingomyelinase levels, there are no objective studies on the tissues (chemical, histologic) of these various phenotypes which would allow their further separate classification. Group A patients present the so-called classic picture, with onset of symptoms in early infancy, marked organomegaly, rapidly advancing CNS handicaps, and death by 3 years of age. More than half of the cases reported in the literature belong to this group and a half of them are of Ashkenazi Jewish ancestry.

Group B patients show the same massive sphingomyelin accumulation in the liver and spleen, and the pulmonary changes, as seen in the classically-involved infants (Group A), but the nervous system seems to be spared. A number of such patients, followed since early childhood, are now young adults and doing well clinically, so that statements on ultimate prognosis cannot be made.

Group C patients show a pattern now being identified with reasonable frequency, characterized by developmental slowing beginning in late infancy, moderate chemical changes, enlargement of the liver and spleen and gradual debilitation leading to death by 3 to 9 years of age.

Group D involvement has been found most notably in French ancestry patients from Nova Scotia, with neurologic difficulties in middle childhood (including cerebellar and athetoid symptoms), with survival until 12-20 years of age.

References:
Brady, R.O. et al: The metabolism of sphingomyelin. II. Evidence of an enzymatic deficiency in Niemann-Pick disease. Proc. Natl. Acad. Sci. USA 55:336, 1966.
Callahan, J.W. and Khalil, M.: Sphingomyelinases and the genetic defects in Niemann-Pick disease. In Wolk, B.W. and Schneck, L. (eds.). Current Trends in Sphingolipidoses and Allied Disorders. New York:Plenum Press, 1976, p. 367.
Crocker, A. C. and Farber, S.: Niemann-Pick disease: A review of 18 patients. Medicine (Baltimore) 37:1, 1958.
Fredrickson, D.S. and Sloan, H.R.: Sphingomyelin lipidosis: Niemann-Pick disease. In Stanbury, J.B. et al: (eds.): The Metabolic Basis of Inherited Disease, 3rd Ed. New York:McGraw-Hill, 1972, p. 783.
Lachman, R. et al: Radiological findings in Niemann-Pick disease. Radiology 108:659, 1973.

Contributor: **Allen C. Crocker**

Editor's Computerized Descriptors: Eye, Skin, Resp., Lymphatic, Spleen, Liver, Nerve

NIGHTBLINDNESS

713-500

Includes: Héméralopie
Nachtblindheit
Ceguera nocturna
Nyctalopia

Excludes: Oguchi disease (740)
Dayblindness
Nightblindness with myopia
Vitamin A deficiency
Retinitis pigmentosa (869)

Minimal Diagnostic Criteria: Visual difficulty in dim light.

Clinical Findings: Nyctalopia is the opposite of hemeralopia.† Nightblindness is a visual impairment that expresses itself only in dim light. There is no obvious anatomic eye abnormality. The eye has reduced adaptation and hence is relatively insensitive in the dark. The visual field may be normal or concentrically diminished. In the presence of retinal macular abnormality, dense central scotomas can be demonstrated. The ERG is helpful in the differential diagnosis. The scotopic responses of the ERG are either extinguished or show diminished amplitude of the b-wave. Photopic activity is retained. Fundus reflectometer studies have shown the presence of normal rod visual purple or rhodopsin. Supportive evidence indicates that the rod defect is proximal to the rod photoreceptor inner segment and that parts of the cone system are preserved throughout life.

Complications
I **Derived:** —
II **Associated:** ? Chorioretinal degeneration

Etiology: Autosomal dominant with variable penetrance

Pathogenesis: The scotopic mechanism may be somewhat impaired with resulting loss of adaptation and relative insensitivity to darkness. This may be due to a defect of the rods or inefficient associated pigment.

Related Facts
I **Sex Ratio:** M1:F1
II **Risk of Occurrence:** ?
III **Risk of Recurrence for**
  Patient's Sib: If parent is affected, 1 in 2 (50%) for each offspring to be affected; otherwise not increased.
  Patient's Child: 1 in 2
IV **Age of Detectability:** Preschool by repeated accidents in dim light
V **Prevalence:** ?

Treatment
I **Primary Prevention:** Genetic counseling
II **Secondary Prevention:** Avoidance of motion, hence accidents, in dim light
III **Other Therapy:** —

Prognosis: Life expectancy normal unless death by accident in dim light

Detection of Carrier: Affected parent and patient

†Special Considerations: Unfortunately, the words nyctalopia (nightblindness) and hemeralopia (dayblindness) are incorrectly used synonymously. Hemeralopia exists when vision is better in dim than in bright illumination. Contrariwise, nyctalopia exists when vision is good in moderate illumination but deficient in feeble illumination.

References:
François, J. et al: A new pedigree of idiopathic congenital nightblindness transmitted as a dominant hereditary trait. Am. J. Ophthalmol. 59:621, 1965.
Hill, D.A. et al: Cone electroretinograms in congenital nyctalopia with myopia. Am. J. Ophthalmol. 78:127, 1974.
Nettleship, E.: A history of congenital stationary night-blindness in nine consecutive generations. Trans. Ophthalmol. Soc. U. K. 27:269, 1907.
Weale, R.A.: Fundus reflectometry. Ophthalmologica 169:30, 1974.

Contributor: **Elsa K. Rahn**

Editor's Computerized Descriptor: Vision

NIGHTBLINDNESS, STATIONARY

Includes: Héméralopie stationnaire
Stationäre Nachtblindheit
Ceguera nocturna estacionaria
X-linked congenital nightblindness with myopia
Autosomal dominant nightblindness
Nougaret nightblindness
Autosomal recessive nightblindness
Essential nightblindness
Riggs type nyctalopia
Schubert-Bornschein type nyctalopia

Excludes: Oguchi disease (740)
Fundus albipunctatus (399)
Retinitis pigmentosa (869)
Vitamin A deficiency

Minimal Diagnostic Criteria: Normal eyegrounds and normal daylight visual fields with absent or reduced secondary adaptation demonstrated on subjective testing.†

Clinical Findings: There is marked inability to see at night because of poor or absent rod (secondary) adaptation. The affected patients have no fundus changes, and all genetic subtypes have been described. The autosomal dominant form, also known as Nougaret Nyctalopia, has been traced from the 17th century proband in France through 11 generations and over 2000 relatives. Central vision and fields are normal. The X-linked and recessive forms are often associated with myopia of 4 or more diopters. Acuity is often reduced and, in severe cases, nystagmus is present.

Subjective dark adaptometry most often shows a monophasic curve with no rod limb. A milder form with some rod function was described by Riggs. Abnormalities of the cone system are frequent implying a widespread, though stationary retinal disease. The ERG has been used to subclassify the patients with stationary nightblindness. The differentiation between stationary and progressive disease, such as retinitis pigmentosa, is relatively simple, but there have been conflicting reports on the type of ERG seen with each of the stationary subtypes. In general the light-adapted responses are normal in dominant disease while those types associated with poor vision and myopia have reduced amplitudes and altered wave forms. The dark-adapted responses in the forms with some rod adaptation show a slow increase in amplitude with progressive adaptation and a reduced final amplitude. The more common forms with absent rod adaptation have an electronegative response with normal or subnormal a-wave amplitudes but only minimal b-waves. The EOG is normal. Fundus reflectometry and both rhodopsin and cone kinetics are normal implying a defect which is distal to the outer segments.

Complications
I   **Derived:** An occasional case will have macular degeneration.
II   **Associated:** —

Etiology: Autosomal recessive, autosomal dominant, and X-linked recessive transmission occur. McK *16350, *31050

Pathogenesis: Only 1 eye has been studied histologically in stationary nightblindness. The patient was from a dominant pedigree and although there was weak staining of the outer segments with McManus stain for mucopolysaccharide, the remainder of the structures were normal.

On the basis of the electrophysiology and receptor kinetics, it is most probable that the diseases do not originate in the outer segments of the receptors. The possibilities are then disease of inner segments when ERG a- and b-waves are affected, bipolar disease if the a-wave is normal, or even problems in neural transmission.

Related Facts
I   **Sex Ratio:** In autosomal recessive and dominant types M1:F1; in the X-linked recessive type M1:F0
II   **Risk of Occurrence:** ?
III **Risk of Recurrence for**
     Patient's Sib: When autosomal recessive, dominant or X-linked recessive, see Table I AR, AD or X-linked R, respectively.
     Patient's Child: When autosomal recessive, dominant or X-linked recessive, see Table I AR, AD or X-linked R, respectively
IV   **Age of Detectability:** Can be detected as soon as behavior in reduced illumination is observed.
V   **Prevalence:** ?

Treatment
I   **Primary Prevention:** Genetic counseling
II   **Secondary Prevention:** —
III **Other Therapy:** Night vision pocketscope

Prognosis: Normal life span

Detection of Carrier: Pedigree analysis may reveal obligate carriers

†**Special Considerations:** Some patients with Oguchi disease or fundus albipunctatus have no secondary or rod dark adaptation similar to patients in the essential nightblindness group. These patients are excluded on the basis of typical fundus changes. Also patients with early retinitis pigmentosa may have no ophthalmologic findings (retinitis pigmentosa, sine pigmentosa) and may have a similar dark adaptation profile to patients in the essential nightblindness group. However, these patients are usually distinguished on the basis of abnormal visual fields, and a usual extinguished or minimal ERG.

References:
Auerbach, E. et al: An electrophysiological and psychophysical study of two forms of congenital night blindness. Invest. Ophthalmol. 8:332, 1969.
Carr, R.E. et al: Visual functions in congenital night blindness. Invest. Ophthalmol. 5:508, 1966.
Carr, R.E.: Congenital stationary night blindness. Trans. Am. Ophthalmol. Soc. 72:448, 1974.
Franceschetti, A. et al: Chorioretinal Heredodegenerations. Springfield: Charles C Thomas, 1974.
Hill, D.A. et al: Cone electroretinograms in congenital nyctalopia with myopia. Am. J. Ophthalmol. 78:127, 1974.

Contributors: **Alex E. Krill‡**
                      Mitchel L. Wolf

Editor's Computerized Descriptor: Vision

NOONAN SYNDROME

Includes: Syndrome de Noonan
Síndrome de Noonan
Male Turner syndrome
Female Turner syndrome with normal XX sex karyotype
Female pseudo-Turner syndrome
Turner phenotype with normal karyotype
Ullrich syndrome
Ullrich-Noonan syndrome

Excludes: Klippel-Feil syndrome
Turner syndrome (977)
Lentigines syndrome, multiple (586)
Pterygium syndrome
Aarskog syndrome (1)

Minimal Diagnostic Criteria: The syndrome must be delineated principally at the clinical level. A combination of most of the below-mentioned features should strongly suggest the Noonan syndrome. Historically and for practical purposes, most females thought to have the Turner syndrome, but who are of normal stature, or who are mentally retarded, or who have a right-sided cardiac lesion, or who manifest gonadal function should be strongly suspected of having the Noonan syndrome. The finding of an XX sex karyotype in such a patient will confirm the diagnosis.†

Clinical Findings: Based on a review of 260 published and personally observed cases, the clinical findings of the Noonan syndrome include the following: *short stature* has been observed in 72% of cases; *gonadal function* may vary from complete agonadism, in 2 reported cases, to normal gonadal function and fertility in the majority of cases. A number of affected females have reproduced. Every adolescent female under our observation has developed normally and has regular menses, although pubescence and menarche have been delayed in some. On the other hand, a number of reported females have had *primary or early secondary amenorrhea. Cryptorchidism,* unilateral or more commonly bilateral, occurs in 70% of affected males. However, fertility has been documented in several affected males, and masculinization at puberty is the rule. *Mental retardation* has been encountered in 61% of 210 cases in which mentality was noted. This may vary from mild to profound. *Lesions of the heart or great vessels* occur in approximately 55% of cases, the most commonly encountered lesion being pulmonic valvular or infundibular stenosis. Others include peripheral pulmonary artery stenosis, patent ductus arteriosus, atrial septal defect and tetralogy of Fallot. Approximately 80% of cardiac lesions involve the right side of the heart; most other patients have had either aortic stenosis or coarctation of the aorta. Recently described lesions of interest have been eccentric hypertrophy of the left ventricle and asymmetric septal hypertrophy. An unusual ECG abnormality has been described in such patients, involving a superiorly oriented QRS axis in the frontal plane. Echocardiography has been established as a useful procedure in the investigation of left ventricular or septal hypertrophy, even in patients without clinical signs of cardiac disease. Craniofacial features include *excessively folded auricular helices* 84%, *low-set ears* 62%, *hypertelorism* 84%, *epicanthal folds* 51%, *ptosis* of the eyelids 66%, *downward slanting palpebral fissures* 83%, *narrow* or *high palatal arch* 65% with occasional clefts of the uvula, *open bite* or other *dental malocclusion* 52% and *micrognathia* 69%. *Scalp defects* at the vertex have been described in several cases. The *hair* is often light in color in white patients, is curly to kinky, and *extends low* on the posterior neck in 81% of cases. The *neck is webbed* in 78% of cases and has

been described as "broad", "short", or "thick" in others. The thorax has the appearance of widely spaced nipples, although studies have shown this to be more apparent than real. More striking is a peculiar combination of *proximal pectus carinatum-distal pectus excavatum* 77%. *Cubitus valgus* is encountered in 86% of cases, with minor anomalies of the hands and feet being uncommon. Kyphosis or scoliosis, and vertebral anomalies occur in a small but significant percentage of cases. *Urinary tract anomalies* are found in about 27% of cases. These include obstructive uropathy with hydronephrosis, duplication of the collecting system and renal hypoplasia. *Downy hirsutism* is common, especially over the cheeks, shoulders, arms, and forearms. *Peripheral lymphedema* occurs at some time in life in 37% of cases. While some reports have suggested that total fingertip ridge counts of affected patients are lower than in unaffected relatives, this is not consistent, and even in those reports, ridge counts did not differ from the population means for either sex. Thus, characteristic dermatoglyphic changes have not been found, although distal placement (t') of the axial triradius is not uncommon.

As is apparent, the severity of the Noonan syndrome is quite variable. Furthermore, less severely affected cases can often be found in presumably unaffected 1st-degree relatives of obviously affected probands. While patients, both male and female, share some phenotypic features with females having the Turner syndrome, careful clinical evaluation with attention to the TOTAL phenotype allows differentiation of the 2 conditions.

Complications
I **Derived:** Complications due to the commonly encountered mental retardation, cardiac failure or pulmonary changes resulting from the cardiac defect, sterility in the presence of gonadal dysgenesis or agonadism. Myopia is not uncommon. Neoplasms of various types may be more common than in the normal population.
II **Associated:** Not yet discernible

Etiology: The Noonan syndrome is known to occur in familial aggregations-in several members of the same sibship, and in multiple generations of the same family. A number of reports document the transmission of the Noonan syndrome from mother to son and daughter, and a few indicate its transmission from father to son. It has been described in multiple offspring of apparently unaffected but consanguineous parents. While nosologic-etiologic heterogeneity must be considered, the available evidence seems to favor an autosomal dominant mode of inheritance. As has been suggested, the low frequency of male-to-male transmission may be attributable to the frequent occurrence of cryptorchidism with its potentially adverse effect on fertility. It should be emphasized that no evidence exists to indicate that the Noonan syndrome is the result of a chromosome abnormality.† McK *16395

Pathogenesis: The mutant gene(s) affect(s) multiple systems. A basic defect has not been discovered. In those patients exhibiting hypogonadism, histologically apparent gonadal dysgenesis is a primary pathogenetic factor.

Related Facts
I **Sex Ratio:** Probably M1:F1. The predominance of male cases in the material reviewed (165 of 260 cases) is probably due to bias of ascertainment.
II **Risk of Occurrence:** ? But may be as high as 1 in 1000 live births
III **Risk of Recurrence for**
Patient's Sib: Approximately 1 in 2 for sib to be affected in autosomal dominant cases if parent is affected; negligible if patient represents a fresh mutation.

Patient's Child: Approxiamtely 1 in 2 for child, male or female, to be affected in autosomal dominant cases.

IV Age of Detectability: In early infancy, if lymphedema or webbing of the neck is present. Diagnosis may not be apparent until later when shortness of stature, facial features, and other anomalies draw attention to the patient.

V Prevalence: ? But possible as high as 1 in 1000. No race influence apparent.

Treatment

I Primary Prevention: Genetic counseling

II Secondary Prevention: If indicated, repair of cardiac defect, surgical correction of cryptorchidism, hormonal substitution therapy.

III Other Therapy: If indicated, surgery for webbing of the neck, scoliosis or urinary tract anomaly, or orthodontic therapy

Prognosis: Life span should probably be normal unless shortened by cardiac defect and its complications. Some degree of mental defect in about 60% of the cases. Retardation may be mild, but some have IQs < 50. Patients may or may not reproduce, depending upon many factors. Associated skeletal anomalies may also hamper function.

Detection of Carrier: In retrospect some "apparently normal" relatives of affected persons reveal "microstigmata" of the condition and can thus be said to be affected.

†Special Considerations: The term "Noonan syndrome" is employed primarily to avoid the confusing use of the Turner and Ullrich eponyms, which immediately suggest a chromosome abnormality. The absence of evidence to support a chromosome abnormality, as well as the frequent familial distribution of the disorder (its presence in multiple sibs and in multiple generations of the same family) and the presence of "microstigmata" in apparently unaffected relatives point to a single gene mutation.

The Noonan syndrome bears some resemblance to the multiple lentigines syndrome, especially when patients with the latter do not have lentigines. However, Gorlin reported twin sisters who lacked lentigines and both of whom had offspring with lentigines. The autosomal dominant pattern of the multiple lentigines syndrome, its associated profound deafness, its commonly associated hypospadias, and its lentigines should serve in most cases to differentiate it from the Noonan syndrome. However, isolated patients with the multiple lentigines syndrome who lack lentigines may be confused with the Noonan syndrome.

Some reports call attention to the similarities between the Noonan syndrome and the Aarskog syndrome.

No characteristic biochemical or metabolic abnormality has been detected. Immunoreactive growth hormone response to insulin and arginine challenge is normal in those tested who are short of stature. Testicular biopsies have revealed varying degrees of seminiferous tubule dysgenesis and poor differentiation of Leydig cells or of Sertoli cells. Some are, of course, normal with normal spermatogenesis.

References:

Char, F. et al: The Noonan syndrome-A clinical study of forty-five cases. In Bergsma, D. (ed.): Part XV. The Cardiovascular System, Birth Defects: Orig. Art. Ser., vol. VIII, no 5. Baltimore: Williams & Wilkins for The National Foundation-March of Dimes, 1972, p.110.

Collins, E. and Turner, G.: The Noonan syndrome-A review of the clinical and genetic features of 27 cases. J. Pediatr. 83:941, 1973.

Engle , M.A. and Ehlers, K.H.: Cardiovascular malformations in the syndrome of Turner phenotype with normal karyotype. In The Cardiovascular System, op. cit. p. 104.

Kaplan, M.S. et al: Noonan's syndrome. A case with elevated serum alkaline phosphatase levels and malignant schwannoma of the left forearm. Am. J. Dis. Child. 116:359, 1968.

Noonan, J.A.: Hypertelorism with Turner phenotype: A new syndrome with associated congenital heart disease. Am. J. Dis. Child. 116:373, 1968.

Nora, J.J. et al: The Ullrich-Noonan syndrome (Turner phenotype). Am. J. Dis. Child. 127:48, 1974.

Nora, J.J. et al: Echocardiographic studies of left ventricular disease in Ullrich-Noonan syndrome. Am. J. Dis. Child. 129:1417, 1975.

Polani, P.: Turner's, Ullrich's and Noonan's syndromes. Br. Med. J. 1:177, 1974.

Summitt, R.L.: Turner syndrome and Noonan's syndrome. J. Pediatr. 74:155, 1969.

Wright, N.L. et al: Noonan's syndrome and Ebstein's malformation of the tricuspid valve. Am. J. Dis. Child. 116:367, 1968.

Contributor: **Robert L. Summitt**

Editor's Computerized Descriptors: Vision, Eye, Ear, Face, Oral, Teeth, Neck, Skin, Nerve, Hair, Skel., CV., Lymphatic, GU.

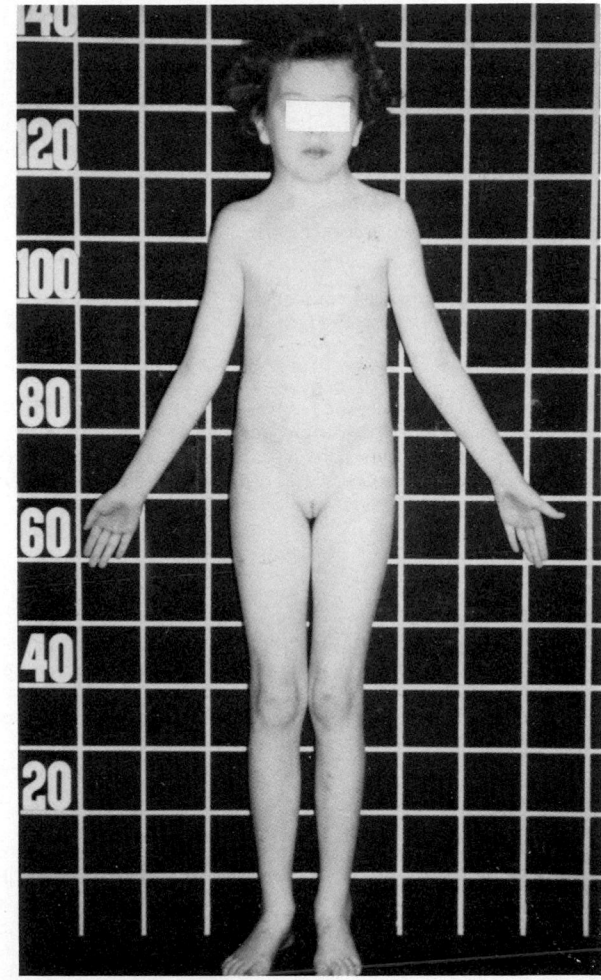

389. Note webbed neck and cubitus valgus

NORRIE DISEASE

Includes: Maladie de Norrie
Mb. Norrie
Enfermedad de Norrie
Congenital bilateral pseudoglioma of retina with recessive X-linked inheritance†
Vitreoretinal dysplasia with recessive X-linked inheritance

Excludes: Retinal dysplasia (866)
Chromosome thirteen trisomy syndrome† (168)
Encephaloretinal dysplasia
Vitreous, persistent hyperplastic primary (994)

Minimal Diagnostic Criteria: Recessive X-linked dysplasia of the retina existing bilaterally in boys blind from birth

Clinical Findings: Both globes are affected and typically show some degree of microphthalmos. The anterior chamber is shallow and the pupil is commonly dilated with no light reflex. Posterior synechia, ectropion of the iris pigment fringe, and a hypoplastic iris usually are present. A grey membrane or a grey-yellow opaque mass with vessels is apparent behind the lens. Elongated ciliary processes are often visible and in cases where the fundus can be seen, retinal folds, detachment of the retina, and pseudotumor formations may be observed. The affected patients are totally blind from birth. The lens is initially clear but may become cataractous. Phthisis bulbi is the usual end result and has usually supervened by age of 10 years. Most of the observed patients are mentally retarded and severe deafness frequently develops later in life.

Complications
I **Derived:** Complicated cataract
II **Associated:** Mental retardation and sensorineural deafness

Etiology: X-linked recessive; McK *31060

Pathogenesis: Hypoplasia and necrosis of the inner retinal layers occur. Hyperplasia of the retinal pigment epithelium may be present along with optic atrophy, complicated cataract and phthisis bulbi. Associated persistence and hyperplasia of the primary vitreous has been reported.

Related Facts
I **Sex Ratio:** M1:F0
II **Risk of Occurrence:** ?
III **Risk of Recurrence for**
   Patient's Sib: If mother is a carrier 1 in 2 (50%) for each brother to be affected and 1 in 2 for each sister to be a carrier.
   Patient's Child: 1 in 1 (100%) for carrier daughters; not increased for sons unless wife is a carrier
IV **Age of Detectability:** At birth
V **Prevalence:** ?

Treatment
I **Primary Prevention:** Genetic counseling
II **Secondary Prevention:** Sound amplification and habilitation for hearing loss
III **Other Therapy:** —

Prognosis: Blind from birth

Detection of Carrier: —

†**Special Considerations:** The ocular picture in Norrie disease is somewhat similar to the retinal dysplasia which occurs in chromosome thirteen trisomy syndrome and in other conditions. It is distinguished by the absence of other systemic abnormalities, by the concomitant mental retardation and deafness and by the X-linked recessive mode of inheritance. Pseudoglioma is a clinical term describing a number of conditions which produce a white reflex or amaurotic "cat's eye reflex" in the pupil. Reese has grouped these conditions as "leukokoria" which may be produced by developmental abnormalities such as persistent hyperplastic primary vitreous, retinal dysplasia, congenital retinal folds, or by inflammatory conditions such as metastatic endophthalmitis, larval granulomatosis, and toxoplasmosis, by retrolental fibroplasia or by retinoblastoma.

References:
Andersen, S.R. and Warburg, M.: Norrie's disease: Congenital bilateral pseudotumor of the retina with recessive X-chromosomal inheritance; preliminary report. Arch. Ophthalmol. 66:614, 1961.
Dahlberg-Parrow, R.: Congenital sex-linked pseudoglioma and grave mental deficiency. Acta Ophthalmol. (Kbh). 34:250, 1956.
Franceschetti, A. et al: Les Hérédo-dégénérescences Chorio-rétiniennes (Dégénerescences Tapéto-retiniennes). Paris:Masson et Cie, 1963, p. 878.
Warburg, M.: Norrie's disease: A congenital progressive oculo-acoustico- cerebral degeneration. Acta Ophthalmol. (Kbh.) 89:1, 1966.
Warburg, M.: Norrie's disease. In Bergsma, D. (ed.): Part VIII. Eye, Birth Defects: Orig. Art. Ser., vol. VII, no. 3. Baltimore: Williams & Wilkins for The National Foundation-March of Dimes, 1971, p. 117.

Contributor: **Robert M. Ellsworth**

Editor's Computerized Descriptors: Vision, Eye, Hearing, Nerve

NOSE AND NASAL SEPTUM DEFECTS

Includes: Anomalie du nez et de la cloison nasale
Aussere Fehlbildungen von Nase und Nasenseptum
Defectos de la nariz y del tabique nasal
Absence of nose
Absence of nasal septum
Persistent frontonasal process
Absence of half of nose
Half nose plus proboscis
Triple nares
Dermoid cysts of nose of both skin and dural origin

Excludes: Nose, bifid (724)
Nose, duplication (725)
Nasal deformities secondary to cleft lip or cleft palate
Abnormalities of growth of the maxillary processes, nasal glioma,
encephaloceles, neurofibroma or hemangiomas
Nose, anterior atresia (723)

Minimal Diagnostic Criteria: Specific evidence of a nasal defect
other than bifid nose or nasal duplication

Clinical Findings: The degree of nasal deformity can vary from
a small notch in one ala to total absence of the nose. The more
minor abnormalities are much more frequent.

Complications
I **Derived:** Total nasal obstruction may be associated with
asphyxia at birth. Intermediate degrees of nasal obstruction
may also lead to a higher incidence of acquired ear disease.
Speech defects are occasionally present. Psychologic complications may occur due to the cosmetic deformity.
II **Associated:** Hypertelorism and abnormal location of the anterior fontanel are frequently seen with major deformities
and are probably directly related to an abnormality of development of the frontonasal process.

Etiology: ? Some cases appear to be genetic.

Pathogenesis: The external nose and nasal septum are derived
from a prolongation of the frontonasal process together with an
infolding which produces the nasal septum. Unequal growth of
the 2 sides of the nasal septum or excessive infolding of the septal
portion without fusion of the 2 parts can account for the majority
of the abnormalities of the nose and septum. The unusual inclusion dermoids of dural origin can be accounted for by dural extensions which have become included in the frontonasal process as
it grows out from the anterior cranium.

Related Facts
I **Sex Ratio:** M1:F1
II **Risk of Occurrence:** ?
III **Risk of Recurrence for**
   Patient's Sib: ?
   Patient's Child: ?
IV **Age of Detectability:** Usually at birth
V **Prevalence:** ?

Treatment
I **Primary Prevention:** —
II **Secondary Prevention:** Operative repair of defect or recon-
struction is indicated if either functional or cosmetic prob-
lems are present.
III **Other Therapy:** —

Prognosis: Generally good except for cases with total nasal obstruction occurring at birth when asphyxia may lead to death, if
not properly managed. Newborn infants are obligate nose breath-
ers and temporary measures to keep the mouth open should be
used until definitive surgery can be performed.

Detection of Carrier: —

Special Considerations: —

References:

Badrawy, R.: Mid-line congenital anomalies of the nose. J. Laryngol. Otol. 81:419, 1967.

Contributors: **R. Storey Fenton**
W.S. Goodman

Editor's Computerized Descriptors: Eye, Nose, Speech, Skel.,
Resp.

NOSE, ANTERIOR ATRESIA

Includes: Atrésie nasale antérieure
Vordere Nasengangsatresie
Atresia nasal anterior
Stenosis of anterior nares
Atresia of anterior nares
Choanal atresia, anterior
Bony choanal atresia, anterior
Membranous choanal atresia, anterior
Anterior nasal atresia

Excludes: Nose and nasal septum defects (722)
Nasopharyngeal stenosis (707)
Nose, posterior atresia (727)

Minimal Diagnostic Criteria: Bony or membranous atresia of the anterior nares with underdeveloped nostril†

Clinical Findings: There is a narrowing or stenosis of the anterior nares, usually unilateral, either membranous or bony. The newborn may have respiratory distress when not crying if lesion is bilateral. The nasolacrimal duct is present and normal but x-ray examination may show lack of anterior ethmoid and maxillary sinuses.

Complications
I   **Derived:** Respiratory distress of the newborn when bilateral
II   **Associated:** —

Etiology: ?

Pathogenesis: The anterior nares are closed by epithelial plugs from the 2nd-6th month of intrauterine life. Failure of absorption of these plugs results in anterior atresia or stenosis of varying degrees.

Related Facts
I   **Sex Ratio:** Apparently M1:F1
II   **Risk of Occurrence:** Very rare
III   **Risk of Recurrence for**
    Patient's Sib: ?
    Patient's Child: ?
IV   **Age of Detectability:** At birth
V   **Prevalence:** ? Very rare

Treatment
I   **Primary Prevention:** —
II   **Secondary Prevention:** Reconstructive surgery to provide an epithelial lined nasal cavity with cosmetically acceptable nostrils can be performed.
III   **Other Therapy:** —

Prognosis: Good for life span, intelligence and function unless bilateral and associated with respiratory distress, not recognized and not corrected.

Detection of Carrier: —

†**Special Considerations:** Anterior nasal atresia can be differentiated from half-nose by the presence of posterior choanae on examination of the nasopharynx, absence of purulent dacrocystitis and presence of a partial nasal chamber and paranasal sinuses on x-ray examination.

References:
Ballenger, J.J.: Diseases of the Nose, Throat and Ear. Philadelphia:Lea & Febiger, 1969.
Maloney, W.H. (ed): Otolaryngology. Hagerstown: Harper & Row, 1969. Vol 3.

Contributor: **Daniel R. Miller**

Editor's Computerized Descriptors: Nasoph., Nose

NOSE, BIFID

Includes: Nez de dogue
Doggennase
Nariz de dogo
Bifid nose
Congenital median fissure of nose
Median cleft of nose "doggennose"

Excludes: Nose, duplication (725)
Nose and nasal septum defects (722)
Median cleft face syndrome (635)
Cranium bifidum occultum
Hypertelorism (504)

Minimal Diagnostic Criteria: Vertical midline cleft of the nose

Clinical Findings: The tip and dorsum of the nose are divided by a vertical central sulcus of variable width, resulting in a broad and flat nose. The columella is broad and short, separating abnormally shaped nostrils. The septum may be duplicated and the nasal bones may be normal or excessively broad. Radiologic examination is helpful in determining presence of choanal atresia or associated abnormalities of skull and sinuses.

Complications
I   **Derived:** Bifid nose is almost always found in association with hypertelorism, a real or illusory increase in interpupillary distance, and can be associated with other congenital midline defects of the face, such as cranium bifidum occultum (32%), median cleft lip (16%), and triad of bifid nose, cranium bifidum occultum and cleft lip (12%). Incidence of severe mental retardation is 8%, and of borderline retardation 12%.
II   **Associated:** —

Etiology: Pedigrees of 2 reported families indicate autosomal recessive transmission of trait. Three of 25 patients with bifid nose had ancestors with hypertelorism without bifid nose. One reported patient with bifid nose had a normal twin.

Pathogenesis: In the 5-week embryo the medial nasal processes are widely separated by the frontal process. Normally the frontal process grows upward and away from the lower face, and the paired medial nasal processes grow toward the midline, over the frontal process to form the mesodermal structures of the midface. Failure of these processes to merge or failure of obliteration of ectodermal remnants may result in midline clefts of the nose.

Related Facts
I   **Sex Ratio:** M1:F1
II   **Risk of Occurrence:** 1 in 1000 congenital defects of the face
III   **Risk of Recurrence for**
    Patient's Sib: 1 in 4 (25%) for each offspring to be affected
    Patient's Child: Not increased unless mate is carrier or homozygote
IV   **Age of Detectability:** At birth
V   **Prevalence:** ?

Treatment
I   **Primary Prevention:** Genetic counseling
II   **Secondary Prevention:** Plastic surgical procedure to remove excess midline tissue and approximate nostrils. Use of flaps or skin grafts may be necessary to fill cleft defect.
III   **Other Therapy:** —

Prognosis: Normal for life span, intelligence and function if an isolated defect

Detection of Carrier: ?

Special Considerations: —

References:
Baibak, G. and Bromberg, B.E.: Congenital midline defects of the midface. Cleft Palate J. 3:392, 1966.
Boo-Chai, K.: The bifid nose; with a report of 3 cases in siblings.

Plast. Reconstr. Surg. 36:626, 1965.

DeMeyer, W.: The median cleft face syndrome: Differential diagnosis of cranium bifidum occultum, hypertelorism, and median cleft nose, lip and palate. Neurology 17:961, 1967.

Glanz, S.: Hypertelorism and the bifid nose. Sthn. Med. J. 59:631, 1966.

Contributors: **Daniel R. Miller**
LaVonne Bergstrom

Editor's Computerized Descriptors: Eye, Face, Nasoph., Nose, Skel.

NOSE, DUPLICATION

Includes: Nez bifide
Doppelnase
Duplicación nasal
Duplication of nose
Nasal duplication

Excludes: Nose and nasal septum defects (722)
Supernumerary nostrils

Minimal Diagnostic Criteria: Two distinct and complete noses, each with 2 nostrils and 2 nasal cavities.†

Clinical Findings: In the newborn with nasal duplication, preliminary inspection reveals what appears to be a bifid nose with 2 well-developed nostrils; however, in addition, there exist between the nares 2 small sinus openings that, on careful examination, prove to be definite nostrils leading into separate nasal cavities. As the child grows, these openings develop into unmistakable nostrils with obvious alar cartilages. Finally, with further development, 2 separate and complete noses become distinctly evident. Although the small mesial nostrils usually open into definite nasal cavities separate from the lateral larger nasal cavities, the former spaces may be nothing more than blind pouches without a posterior opening. However, the lateral nasal cavities extend through choanae into the nasopharynx. Roentgenograms of this curious deformity are difficult to interpret but do reveal an indeterminate nasal defect.

Complications
I   Derived: —
II Associated: —

Etiology: ?

Pathogenesis: From nasal embryology, one can assume that various forms of bifid nose, median clefts of the upper lip, notches in the nostrils, dermoid cysts, sinuses, and other ectodermal inclusions on the bridge of the nose are the result of arrested development of the frontonasal process (especially the globular processes) and the olfactory sacs.

Although it seems apparent that failure of the nasal laminae to consolidate into a single nasal septum is the cause of a bifid nose, it is most difficult to understand the faulty embryologic processes that initiate the formation of 2 noses with 4 nostrils and 4 nasal cavities. One can theorize that some irregularity in the evolution of the 2 olfactory placodes causes them to bring forth 4 olfactory pits, all in a horizontal plane, rather than 2; such an anomaly would alter the developmental pattern of the medial nasal process. If such were the case, it would tend to explain why the lateral nostrils are larger and more normal in size than are the mesial nostrils, since the lateral nasal processes have not been involved in the developmental defect. Furthermore, I would like to suggest that the 2 medial olfactory pits probably form olfactory sacs which are interposed between the 2 nasal laminae. These sacs, which become medial nasal cavities, thus prevent the laminae from fusing into 1 nasal septum; instead, they stay divided and form 2 septa. With the presence of 2 septa, 4 nostrils, and 4 nasal cavities, the developmental anomaly goes on to form 2 separate noses.

Related Facts
I **Sex Ratio:** Only 2 cases have been recorded, both of females.
II **Risk of Occurrence:** ? Rare
III **Risk of Recurrence for**
  Patient's Sib: ?
  Patient's Child: ?
IV **Age of Detectability:** At birth
V **Prevalence:** Only 2 cases have been recorded.

Treatment
I **Primary Prevention:** —
II **Secondary Prevention:** Surgical rectification of the deformity. The correction of nasal duplication requires 3 or 4 surgical procedures several years apart.
III **Other Therapy:** —

Prognosis: Normal for life span and intelligence

Detection of Carrier: —

†Special Considerations: Several cases of supernumerary nostrils have been reported in the literature, but in all instances, the accessory nostrils were situated above rather than between the normal nares. Then too, in almost all of these cases, the secondary nostril opened into the same nasal cavity as did the normal nostril. Moreover, in none were there 2 septa or 2 columellae.

References:
Erich, J.B.: Nasal duplication: Report of case of patient with two noses. Plast. Reconstr. Surg. 29:159, 1962.
Muecke, F.F. and Souttar, H.S.: Double nose. Proc. R. Soc. Med. 17:8, 1924.

Contributor: **John B. Erich**

Editor's Computerized Descriptors: Nasoph., Nose

NOSE, GLIOMA

Includes: Gliome nasal
Nasengliom
Glioma nasal
Encephalochoristoma nasofrontalis
Nasal glioma

Excludes: Nasal polyps
Nasal neurofibroma
Dermoid cyst or teratoma of head and neck (283)
Hemangioma of nose
Meningocele (642)
Encephalocele (343)

Minimal Diagnostic Criteria: A unilateral intra- or extranasal mass present at birth producing a broad nasal bridge and wide-set eyes is the characteristic clinical picture. Nasal gliomas have no fluid connection with the subarachnoid space. If the mass pulsates or increases in size with straining or crying, a spinal fluid communication may exist and then meningocele or encephalocele must be ruled out. Biopsy of the mass with histopathologic study will help establish the diagnosis.†

Clinical Findings: These congenital neurogenic tumors are often located externally at the nasal bridge; however, they can present as an intranasal or nasopharyngeal tumor. Rarely a combination of locations will be evident. A nasal bridge that is broader in width, and eyes that are more widely separated than normal suggest an intranasal tumor. The external tumor is raised and usually covered with intact skin. These tumors vary from 1 to 5 cm in diameter, are firm, mobile, round and smooth. Color varies from pink to red.

Intranasal tumors are located high in the nasal cavity, but may extend down to the anterior nares. These tumors appear to arise from above the middle turbinate or olfactory fissure, and they should not be confused with nasal polyps. They are nearly always unilateral and cause airway obstruction.

Nasal gliomas are benign in clinical behavior. They rarely enlarge, and recurrence after complete excision is rare. Communication between the tumor and the anterior cranial fossa is not present in true nasal glioma.†

Complications
I **Derived:** Nasal cosmetic deformities, rhinitis, meningitis, encephalitis, sinusitis, nasal obstruction, cerebrospinal fluid rhinorrhea and epistaxis.
II **Associated:** Meningocele, encephalocele

Etiology: ? These tumors probably arise from congenital malformations of the nose, base of the skull, and CNS in the region of the foramen cecum. Glial tissue is separated from the CNS and remains outside the calvarium.

Pathogenesis: These abnormalities result from developmental defects in the frontal, nasal, ethmoid or sphenoid bones of the skull. Tumors composed of CNS tissues arise from such defects. Nasal gliomas contain glial tissues, are separated from the brain, and are occasionally connected to the base of the skull with a fibrous stalk. Nasal gliomas per se have no fluid connection with the CNS and hence contain no spinal fluid that circulates between it and the subarachnoid space.†

Related Facts
I **Sex Ratio:** M3:F2
II **Risk of Occurrence:** ?
III **Risk of Recurrence for**
  Patient's Sib: ?
  Patient's Child: ?
IV **Age of Detectability:** At or shortly after birth
V **Prevalence:** ?

Treatment
I   **Primary Prevention:** —

II **Secondary Prevention:** Complete surgical excision usually results in a cure. Intracranial communication must be ruled out before excising the tumor.

III **Other Therapy:** Antibiotics for infections and rhinoplasty for nasal deformities may be necessary.

Prognosis: The prognosis is good when total excision is performed.

Detection of Carrier: —

†**Special Considerations:** X-ray examination, including tomography, will often reveal a defect in the calvarium when a fluid communication does exist. The mass can be " tapped" with a needle to determine the presence of spinal fluid, but careful aseptic techniques must be used to avoid subsequent infections. When spinal fluid is present in the tumor, air or dye contrast studies of the CNS should be performed. The presence or absence of fluid communication must be determined before considering surgical therapy.

Encephaloceles may be difficult to differentiate from nasal gliomas, though they are quite different in structure. The encephalocele contains an ependyma-lined space that is filled with cerebrospinal fluid that communicates with the ventricles of the brain. Glial and fibrous tissues are present beneath the ependymal lining. A biopsy from the wall of such a tumor may not reveal the true nature of this tumor. A defect in the base of the skull on x-ray examination helps make this diagnosis. These tumors pulsate and increase in size when the infant strains or cries.

Meningoceles are rare and consist of meninges that herniate through a developmental defect in the cranium. They have clinical characteristics that are similar to those of the encephalocele. There are 2 types of meningocele that occur about the nose. The sphenopharyngeal dehiscence involves the sphenoid or ethmoid bones with a tumor presenting in the orbit, nasal cavity, nasopharynx, or medial to the ramus of the mandible. An intranasal (sincipital) dehiscence involves the cribriform plate with a tumor either in the nasal cavity, or externally at the medial canthus of the eye, or in the orbit.

References:
Black, B. K. and Smith, D. E.: Nasal glioma: Two cases with recurrence. Arch. Neurol. Psychiatry 64:614, 1950.
Converse, J. M. (ed.): Reconstructive Plastic Surgery. Philadelphia: W. B. Saunders Co., 1964, p. 777.
Proctor, B. and Proctor, C.: Congenital lesions of the head and neck. Otolaryngol. Clin. North Am. 3(2):221, 1970.

Contributor: **Gerald M. English**

Editor's Computerized Descriptors: Eye, Nasoph., Nose

NOSE, POSTERIOR ATRESIA

Includes: Atrésie choanal postérieure
Choanalatresie
Atresia coanal posterior
Bony choanal atresia, posterior
Membranous choanal atresia, posterior
Choanal atresia, posterior
Atresia of posterior nares
Posterior nasal atresia

Excludes: Nasopharyngeal stenosis (707)
Nose, anterior atresia (723)

Minimal Diagnostic Criteria: A lateral xray of the head demonstrating radiopaque dye in the nasal cavities and air in the unoccluded nasopharynx behind the obstructing membrane.

Clinical Findings: The newborn infant gets into acute respiratory distress every time he attempts to breathe quietly with the mouth closed. Cyanosis, struggling, exhaustion and death can occur unless an oral airway is obtained. When crying, the infant does well because the mouth is open. The newborn normally tends to breathe with the mouth closed. Nursing becomes a problem as the infant frequently has to stop feeding to gasp for breath.

There is mucus in the anterior nasal cavities. A catheter cannot be passed into the oral pharynx. If the airways are cleaned and decongested, an obstructing membrane will be seen in the depths of the nostril posteriorly with a dimple in the center. Lateral xrays of the head with radiopaque dye in the anterior portion of the nose will demonstrate the soft tissue between the dye and the air in the nasopharynx.

Complications
I   **Derived:** Death occurs occasionally unless an oral airway is maintained. Collection of mucus in the nose with discharge onto the face associated with complete mouth breathing.

II **Associated:** Cardiac defects (25%), branchial arch abnormalities (21%), abnormalities of pinna (15%), microcephaly (15%), micrognathia (15%), miscellaneous palatal abnormalities (15%), nasopharyngeal abnormalities (15%), mandibulofacial dysostosis (11%), cleft palate (10%), conductive or mixed hearing loss (3.5-7%), digital abnormalities (7%), miscellaneous tongue abnormalities (7%), cleft lip and palate (4%), tracheoesophageal fistula (3%), cervical meningocele, cleidocranial dysostosis, hiatus hernia, diaphragmatic hernia, oxycephaly, hypertelorism, facial cleft, absent nasal septum, imperforate anus, hydronephrosis, facial nerve paralysis, mental retardation, absent spleen, ileal atresia, cerebral agenesis, and micropenis.

Twenty-five percent of cases have a single minor associated abnormality; 25% have a single major associated abnormality and 50% have multiple associated abnormalities. Unilateral choanal atresia: 45% have associated anomalies. Bilateral choanal atresia: 60% have associated anomalies. Sex incidence of associated anomalies: M2:F1.

Etiology: ?

Pathogenesis: Failure of the nasal cavities as they form to complete excavation.

Related Facts
I   **Sex Ratio:** M1:F2
II **Risk of Occurrence:** 1 in 5000 live births
III **Risk of Recurrence for**
    Patient's Sib: Not increased
    Patient's Child: Not increased
IV **Age of Detectability:** At birth by lack of a nasal airway causing acute respiratory distress with the mouth closed.
V   **Prevalence:** 1 in 14,000 in general population

Treatment
I Primary Prevention: —
II Secondary Prevention: If the condition is bilateral, then an oral airway must be maintained until the bilateral choanal atresia is surgically corrected. By the intranasal route the correction may be made immediately after birth; by the transpalatal route the correction should be put off until the infant is 6 months of age.†
III Other Therapy: —

Prognosis: Normal for life span, intelligence and function if the infant survives the 1st few days or weeks of life when he tends to breathe entirely through his nose. Death occurring in the 1st days of life usually is from acute respiratory obstruction.

Detection of Carrier: —

†Special Considerations: The application of modern otologic techniques including micro instrumentation and the operating microscope allow safe surgical correction in the 1st few days of life with a relatively minor operative procedure. Nonreactive silastic tubes maintain the patency of the corrected defect until reepithelialization occurs and simultaneously allows for a patent airway.

References:
Baker, M.C.: Congenital atresia of posterior nares. Arch. Otolaryngol. 58:431, 1953.
Durward, A. et al: Congenital choanal atresia. J. Laryngol. 40:461, 1945.
Evans, J.N.G. and MacLachlan, R.F.: Choanal atresia. J. Laryngol. 85:903, 1971.
Singleton, G.T. and Hardcastle, B.: Congenital choanal atresia. Arch. Otolaryngol. 87:620, 1968.

Contributors: **G. T. Singleton**
B. Hardcastle

Editor's Computerized Descriptors: Face, Oral, Nasoph., Neck, Skel., Resp., CV.

NOSE, TRANSVERSE GROOVE (MARKER)

Includes: Sillon nasal transversal
Quere Nasenfurche
Surco nasal transverso
Nasal groove, familial transverse
Transverse nasal stripe
Nasal crease
Transverse nasal groove (Marker)

Excludes: —

Minimal Diagnostic Criteria: See Clinical Findings

Clinical Findings: A horizontal depression or groove 1-3 mm wide and about 1 mm deep, located just caudad to ala nasi.

Complications
I Derived: —
II Associated: Otosclerosis, hyperelasticity of the joints, severe dental caries

Etiology: Autosomal dominant with variable penetrance; McK *16150

Pathogenesis: ?

Related Facts
I Sex Ratio: M1:F1
II Risk of Occurrence: ?
III Risk of Recurrence for
 Patient's Sib: If parent is affected 1 in 2 (50%) for each offspring to be affected; otherwise not increased.
 Patient's Child: 1 in 2
IV Age of Detectability: Becomes prominent in childhood
V Prevalence: ?

Treatment
I Primary Prevention: Genetic counseling possible but not necessary
II Secondary Prevention: Not necessary
III Other Therapy: Not necessary

Prognosis: Normal for life span, intelligence and function; the groove disappears after puberty.

Detection of Carrier: —

Special Considerations: —

References:
Anderson, P.C.: Familial transverse nasal groove. Arch. Dermatol. 84:316, 1961.

Contributor: **Raymond P. Wood, II**

Editor's Computerized Descriptors: Ear, Teeth, Nose, Skel.

NUCLEOSIDE-PHOSPHORYLASE DEFICIENCY

Includes: Déficit en nucléoside-phosphorylase
Nukleosidphosphorylase-Mangel
Deficiencia de nucleósido fosforilasa
Defective T-cell and normal B-cell immunity in nucleoside-phosphorylase deficiency

Excludes: Adenosine deaminase deficiency

Minimal Diagnostic Criteria: Absent to severely reduced red blood cell, lymphocyte, and fibroblast nucleoside-phosphorylase activity, defective cell-mediated immunity with normal antibody-mediated immunity and a history of recurrent infections consistent with immunodeficiency disease.

Clinical Findings: Seven patients with nucleoside-phosphorylase deficiency have been identified. Patients may be asymptomatic for periods of several years. Initial manifestations usually include recurrent infection. Patients have succumbed to overwhelming infection with varicella or variola (following immunization). A fatal graft-versus-host reaction has been observed. Severe anemia was described in a single patient. The oldest identified patient is age 10 and continues to have recurrent infection. Immunologic studies have demonstrated normal B-cell immunity with absent to severely depressed T-cell immunity. Although enzyme activity is absent at birth, immunologic function may be normal and subsequently declines with age. Measurement of purine nucleosides in the urine and blood reveals increased amounts of inosine, deoxyinosine, guanosine, deoxyguanosine and decreased amounts of uric acid. Orotic aciduria has been found in some patients. Treatment has included transfer factor, thymus transplantation, thymosin and uridine given orally. Only partial reconstitution has been achieved. Infusions of red blood cells as a possible source of enzyme have not resulted in enhanced immune function. Patients should not be immunized with attenuated live viral vaccines or receive unirradiated blood products.

Complications
I **Derived:** —
II **Associated:** Associated with underlying immunodeficiency disease.

Etiology: Autosomal recessive

Pathogenesis: ? Because a similar disorder, adenosine deaminase deficiency, also is associated with immunodeficiency disease, it is postulated that the purine salvage pathway is involved in some way in immunodeficiency disease. However, the mechanism whereby a deficiency of enzymes in this pathway results in immunodeficiency is unknown. Pyrimidine "starvation" secondary to the accumulation of adenine nucleotides or elevated levels of cyclic nucleotides or deoxynucleotides might impair lymphocyte function. Alternatively, increased nucleosides or deoxynucleosides may impair lymphocyte function.

Related Facts
I **Sex Ratio:** ? Theoretically M1:F1
II **Risk of Occurrence:** ?
III **Risk of Recurrence for**
  Patient's Sib: 1 in 4 (25%) for each offspring to be affected
  Patient's Child: All offspring are obligate carriers, but their children are unlikely to manifest the disease as the frequency of the mutant gene must be low in the population.
IV **Age of Detectability:** At birth. Nucleoside-phosphorylase activity may be quantitated in fibroblasts; therefore, the diagnosis could be made in utero.
V **Prevalence:** ?

Treatment
I **Primary Prevention:** Genetic counseling
II **Secondary Prevention:** At present, nucleoside-phosphorylase cannot be replaced in the patient, either directly or by transfusion.
III **Other Therapy:** Appropriate immunologic reconstitution for the defined immunodeficiency disease may modify or prevent recurrent infections.

Prognosis: ? Guarded

Detection of Carrier: By analysis of red blood cells for nucleoside-phosphorylase concentration. Carrier has approximately 50% normal concentration.

Special Considerations: —

References:
Cohen, A. et al: Abnormal purine metabolism and purine overproduction in a patient deficient in purine nucleoside phosphorylase. N. Engl. J. Med. 295:1449, 1976.
Giblett, E.R. et al; Nucleoside-phosphorylase deficiency in a child with severely defective T-cell immunity and normal B-cell immunity. Lancet 1:1010, 1975.
Hirschhorn, R.: Defects of purine metabolism in immunodeficiency diseases. Prog. Clin. Immunol. 3:67, 1977.
Osborne, W.R.A. et al: Purine nucleoside phosphorylase deficiency: Evidence for molecular heterogeneity in two families with enzyme-deficient members. J. Clin. Invest. 60:741, 1977.
Stoop, J.W. et al: Purine nucleoside phosphorylase deficiency associated with selective cellular immunodeficiency. N. Engl. J. Med. 296:651, 1976.

Contributors: **Diane W. Wara**
Arthur J. Ammann

Editor's Computerized Descriptor: —

OBESITY, HYPERTHERMIA, OLIGOMENORRHEA AND PAROTID SWELLING

Includes: Obésité, hyperthermie oligomenorrhée et tuméfaction de la parotide
Fettsucht-Hyperthermie-Oligomenorrhoe-Parotis-Schwellung
Adiposidad-hipertermia-oligomenorrea y tumefacción de la parótida
Diencephalic parotitis
AOP syndrome
AHOP syndrome

Excludes: Froehlich syndrome

Minimal Diagnostic Criteria: Presumably the items listed below

Clinical Findings: The only known cases are those of Rauch. Recurrent bilateral swelling of the parotid gland begins at puberty. This is followed, within 2-5 years, by obesity of the Froehlich type, oligomenorrhea, hyperthermia and psychic disturbances such as melancholia and oligophrenia. All reported cases are female.

Complications
I   Derived: ?
II Associated: ?

Etiology: Rauch has suggested an autosomal dominant, sex-limited mutant gene.

Pathogenesis: Rauch has suggested an hereditary alteration of some portion of the diencephalon.

Related Facts
I   Sex Ratio: M0:F1
II Risk of Occurrence: ?
III Risk of Recurrence for
    Patient's Sib: Presumably 1 in 2 for a sister if the mother is affected, but not increased in about 1/3 of cases which are the result of fresh mutation; and 0 for a brother.
    Patient's Child: Presumably 1 in 2 for a daughter and 0 for a son.
IV Age of Detectability: Puberty to 21st year
V   Prevalence: ?

Treatment
I   Primary Prevention: Genetic counseling
II Secondary Prevention: ?
III Other Therapy: —

Prognosis: For life: presumably normal. For intelligence: mental deterioration is an integral part of the condition and this interferes with function.

Detection of Carrier: Presumably females who have the mutant gene will manifest its effects. No means known in males who carry the gene.

Special Considerations: —

References:
Rauch, S.: Die Speicheldrüsen des Menschen: Anatomie, Physiologie und klinische Pathologie. Stuttgart:G. Thieme Verlag, 1959, p.309.
Rauch, S.: Die rezidiviernde abakterielle Parotitis bilateralis dienzephaler Genese - AOP Syndrom. Pract. Oto-rhino-laryng. (Basel) 17:359, 1955.

Contributor: Robert J. Gorlin

Editor's Computerized Descriptors: Face, GU., Nerve

OBSTRUCTION WITHIN RIGHT VENTRICLE OR ITS OUTFLOW TRACT

Includes: Sténose ventriculaire droite
Einengung des rechten Ventrikels oder seiner Ausflussbahn
Estenosis infundibular del ventrículo derecho
Two-chambered right ventricle
Anomalous muscle bundle of right ventricle
Aberrant right ventricular muscle bands
Isolated infundibular pulmonary stenosis
Stenosis of ostium infundibulum

Excludes: Tetralogy of Fallot (938)
Pulmonary valve stenosis (839)

Minimal Diagnostic Criteria: A pulmonary ejection murmur with ECG evidence of right ventricular hypertrophy should suggest the diagnosis. Angiocardiography confirms the diagnosis.

Clinical Findings: Four anatomic types of infundibular pulmonary stenosis have been identified: 1) a fibrous band at the site of the juncture of the infundibulum and right ventricle; 2) diffuse narrowing of the infundibulum by thickened myocardium; 3) anomalous muscle bundles which are proximal to the infundibulum. These bundles are hyperplastic muscle bands passing from the area near the septal leaflet of the tricuspid valve to the anterior ventricular wall. Also, the moderator band may be hyperplastic; and 4) as part of a diffuse idiopathic myocardial hypertrophy in which the hypertrophied ventricular septum obstructs the lumen of the right ventricular outflow tract. Since the location of the right ventricular outflow obstruction varies, differences in the size of the distal or infundibular chamber and the proximal right ventricular cavity result. The right ventricle proximal to the obstruction is hypertrophied, as is the right atrium. Unlike cases with stenosis of pulmonary valve, the pulmonary artery is not dilated.

Infundibular stenosis may also occur secondary to severe stenosis of the pulmonary valve. Here, also, the clinical features vary with the degree of right ventricular outflow obstruction. With mild stenosis, the patients are asymptomatic; in those with severe stenosis, easy fatigability and at times right-sided congestive cardiac failure occur. Cyanosis may be present in the latter group, if a right-to-left shunt occurs through an anatomically patent foramen ovale. A pulmonic systolic ejection murmur is present. It may be located lower along the left sternal border than in valvar stenosis, particularly when the obstruction is located low in the right ventricle. Both the length of the murmur and the point in systole of maximum intensity of the murmur are increased in severe stenosis. Likewise, the degree of splitting of the second heart sound increases with increasing severity, and the intensity of the pulmonary component is diminished. In contrast to valvar pulmonic stenosis, an ejection click is uncommon.

Roentgenographic findings of infundibular stenosis are similar to those of valvar pulmonary stenosis, except that poststenotic dilatation of the pulmonary trunk or left pulmonary artery is not usually present.

The ECG demonstrates right ventricular hypertrophy, the severity of which is directly related to the degree of stenosis. Progression of ECG evidence of right ventricular hypertrophy is more frequently observed in this condition than in stenosis of the pulmonary valve.

The outflow tract of the right ventricle can be visualized by echocardiography, but its precise character is difficult to assess. In this condition, right ventricular and septal hypertrophy are present. In some instances, an abnormal muscle band may be imaged. The pulmonary valve frequently has an early subtotal closure followed by reopening.

Cardiac catheterization typically reveals a systolic pressure gradient within the right ventricle, although this may be missed if the obstruction is located close to the pulmonary valve. In patients with anomalous muscle bundle, the pressure gradient may be found close to the tricuspid valve. Since the obstruction is generally caused by myocardial tissue, it is dynamic in nature. With exercise or isoproterenol infusion, the degree of obstruction may increase, thereby reducing the effective right ventricular outflow area. The end diastolic right ventricular and right atrial pressures may be elevated, and in severe cases, a right-to-left shunt exists at the atrial level.

Biplane right ventriculography confirms the diagnosis. This demonstrates the muscular narrowing in the infundibular area. Although the obstruction is visualized throughout the cardiac cycle, it is more marked during systole than diastole, again indicating its dynamic nature. Whereas most pulmonary outflow obstructions are best visualized in the lateral projection, an anomalous muscle bundle is best seen in the anteroposterior projection. Since the muscle bundles' course is primarily an anteroposterior direction, they are seen end on as circular nonopacified areas low in the right ventricle. The pulmonary valve is normal and poststenotic dilatation of the pulmonary artery is usually not present.

Complications
I **Derived:** Right-sided cardiac failure, myocardial fibrosis, bacterial endocarditis, tricuspid valve insufficiency.
II **Associated:** —

Etiology: ?

Pathogenesis: Anomalous or hyperplastic muscle bundles may be due to incomplete involution of the embryonic right ventricular trabeculae.

Related Facts
I **Sex Ratio:** M1:F1
II **Risk of Occurrence:** ? Less than 1% of congenital cardiac defects
III **Risk of Recurrence for**
  Patient's Sib: ?
  Patient's Child: ?
IV **Age of Detectability:** From birth
V **Prevalence:** ?

Treatment
I **Primary Prevention:** —
II **Secondary Prevention:** If stenosis is severe, surgical excision of obstructive mechanism under cardiopulmonary bypass.
III **Other Therapy:** —

Prognosis: Data regarding the natural history of these conditions are scanty. There is, however, one report with serial cardiac catheterizations which shows that anomalous muscle bundles become more obstructive with time. The other forms are also believed to be progressive, but there is little evidence to support this.

Detection of Carrier: —

Special Considerations: —

References:
Emmanouilides, G.C.: Primary infundibular stenosis. In Moss, A.J. and Adams, F.H. (eds.): Heart Disease in Infants, Children, and Adolescents. Baltimore: Williams & Wilkins Co., 1968, p. 468.
Goldberg, S.J. et al: Echocardiographic observations regarding pulmonary valve motion in children with pulmonary vascular obstructive disease. Reflections 1:28, 1975.
Hartmann, A.F., Jr. et al: Development of right ventricular obstruction by aberrant muscular bands. Circulation 30:679, 1964.
Lucas, R.V., Jr. et al: Anomalous muscle bundle of the right ventricle: Hemodynamic consequences and surgical considerations. Circulation 25:443, 1962.

Contributor:　　**James H. Moller**

Editor's Computerized Descriptors: Resp., CV.

OCULAR AND FACIAL ANOMALIES WITH PROTEINURIA AND DEAFNESS

727-500

Contributors: **Agnes M. Ickenroth
Cor W.R.J. Cremers**

Includes: Myopie, hypertélorisme et surdité de perception sévère
Myopie, Telecanthus (Hypertelorismus) und Innenohr-Schwerhörigkeit
Miopía, telecanto secundario (hipertelorismo) y pérdida severa de la audición neurosensorial

Editor's Computerized Descriptors: Vision, Eye, Hearing, Oral, Teeth, Nose, Speech, GU.

Excludes: Waardenburg syndrome (997)
Oro-facio-digital syndrome II (771)
Deafness, myopia, cataract and saddle nose (261)

Minimal Diagnostic Criteria: Ocular and facial anomalies, proteinuria and deafness.

Clinical Findings: Two patients, a sister and brother, have been described. The most prominent eye symptoms were myopia(11-27D), cataract, and total retinal detachment causing blindness. Furthermore posterior staphyloma, small corneas, hypoplasia of iris stroma, choroidal atrophy, coloboma of iris and lens, rubeosis iridis, heterochromia, congenital pupillary membrane, underdeveloped filtration angle and laterally displaced inferior canaliculi were reported. Telecanthus, hypertelorism, a flat bridge of the nose, an arched palate and brownish teeth were noted in both patients. Proteinuria was revealed in both, bilateral ureteral reflux and dilatation in one. Severe sensorineural hearing loss was diagnosed in both.

Complications
I **Derived:** Low psychomotor development was seen in 1/2. No speech was present in either.
II **Associated:** —

Etiology: Possibly autosomal recessive

Pathogenesis: —

Related Facts
I   **Sex Ratio:**   M1:F1
II   **Risk of Occurrence:** —
III **Risk of Recurrence for**
     Patient's Sib: If autosomal recessive, 1 in 4 (25%) for each offspring to be affected.
     Patient's Child: Not increased unless mate is carrier or homozygote
IV   **Age of Detectability:**   In early infancy
V   **Prevalence:** —

Treatment
I   **Primary Prevention:**   Genetic counseling
II   **Secondary Prevention:** —
III **Other Therapy:** —

Prognosis: The severe eye anomalies will eventually lead to blindness.

Detection of Carrier: —

Special Considerations: —

References:
Holmes, L.B. and Schepens, C.L.: Syndrome of ocular and facial anomalies, telecanthus and deafness. J. Pediatr. 81:552, 1972.
Murdoch, J.L. and Mengel, M.C.: An unusual eye-ear syndrome with renal abnormality. In Bergsma, D. (ed.): Part IX. Ear. Birth Defects: Orig. Art. Ser., vol. VII, no. 4. Baltimore: Williams & Wilkins for The National Foundation-March of Dimes, 1971, p. 136.
Özer, F.L.: A possible "new" syndrome with eye and renal abnormalities. In Bergsma, D. (ed.): Part XVI. Urinary System and Others. Birth Defects: Orig. Art. Ser., vol. X, no. 4. Baltimore: Williams & Wilkins for The National Foundation-March of Dimes, 1974, p. 168.

OCULAR COLOBOMAS

Includes: Colobomes de l'iris, de la rétine
Okuläre Kolobome
Colobomas oculares
Typical iris colobomas, ciliary body, choroid, retina, optic nerve
Anomalous closure of embryonic cleft

Excludes: Aniridia (57)
Atypical ocular colobomas

Minimal Diagnostic Criteria: Depends on total ophthalmologic evaluation.

Clinical Findings: Defects in any or all of the ocular tissues associated with the embryonic cleft occur downward and inward. These may be complete or partial and are usually present at birth. In the fundus, segmental absence of the choroid and retina result in exposure of bare sclera anywhere along the aforementioned axis with resultant field scotomas and often decreased visual acuity, strabismus and nystagmus. The defect may touch or involve the disk which can appear deeply cupped, excavated or pitted. If the optic nerve is involved, a posterior ectatic cyst forms. Colobomas of the ciliary body, iris, lens and zonules also occur in this area and can be best visualized by slit-lamp biomicroscopy. More frequently, isolated colobomas of the iris are atypical in other locations, and due to other causes. If proliferating retina protrudes through the colobomatous embryonic cleft, an orbital cyst with microphthalmos results in the most extreme cases.

Complications
I **Derived:** —
II **Associated:** Microphthalmos, persistent pupillary membrane, macular dysplasia, high myopia, lens opacities, optic atrophy, myelination of nerve fibers, posterior lenticonus

Etiology: Multifactorial. Iris coloboma may be autosomal dominant. Embryonic fissure derived ocular colobomas uncertain. Expressivity is quite variable and penetrance said to be 20 to 30%. Environmental factors cannot be ruled out as in colobomatous cysts where transmission has been documented.†

Pathogenesis: Accentuation of inversion of the inner layer of the optic cup anywhere along the fetal fissure results in nonclosure of varied degree and position yielding the diverse colobomas described.

Related Facts
I **Sex Ratio:** M1:F1
II **Risk of Occurrence:** ?
III **Risk of Recurrence for**
    Patient's Sib: When autosomal dominant and if a parent is affected, 1 in 2 (50%) for each offspring to be affected; otherwise not increased.
    Patient's Child: 1 in 2 when autosomal dominant
IV **Age of Detectability:** Usually at birth
V **Prevalence:** ?

Treatment
I **Primary Prevention:** Genetic counseling
II **Secondary Prevention:** ?
III **Other Therapy:** —

Prognosis: Normal life span, visual prognosis variable with extent of defect

Detection of Carrier: Affected parent and patient when autosomal dominant

†**Special Considerations:** Typical colobomata have been documented and studied in a variety of animals with similar pathology and hereditary transmission as in man. In rabbits and pigs, genetic dominance characterizes the defective embryonic fissure closure resulting from hyperplasia of the ectodermal edge. However, similar defects in animals have been produced by xrays, naphthalene, actinomycin, oxygen deficiency and a host of other exogenous factors.

References:
Cogan, D. G.: Congenital anomalies of the retina. In Bergsma, D. (ed.): Part VIII, Eye. Birth Defects: Orig. Art. Ser. vol. VII, no. 3. Baltimore:Williams & Wilkins for The National Foundation-March of Dimes, 1971, p.41.
Duke-Elder, S.: System of Ophthalmology. Vol. 3, Pt. 2. Congenital Deformities. London:Henry Kimpton, 1964. p. 456.

Contributor: **Harold E. Cross**

Editor's Computerized Descriptors: Vision, Eye

OCULAR DRUSEN

Includes: Drusen oculaires
Okuläre Drusen
Drusen ocular
Familial drusen
Familial colloid bodies
Doyne honeycombed retinal degeneration
Malattia levantinese
Hutchinson-Tay choroiditis

Excludes: Fundus flavimaculatus (400)
Fundus albipunctatus (399)
Drusen secondary to disease of choroid
Giant drusen of optic disk

Minimal Diagnostic Criteria: Drusen beginning in the 3rd or 4th decade with no evidence of other choroidal disease and seen in more than 1 member of family.†

Clinical Findings: The eyegrounds are characterized by deep yellowish lesions usually round or oval in configuration and varying in size from small, dot-like to larger foci about 4 times the caliber of the 1st order retinal arterioles. They may have pigment flecks in the center or around their borders, and frequently show secondary changes such as calcification. The lesions are usually of greatest concentration in the posterior polar region. They are frequently present in the periphery and are sometimes widespread over most of the retina. These lesions may become confluent, particularly in or near the macular area into well-defined cloverleaf shapes or multilevel plaques. With fluorescein angiography, the lesions are well defined and overwhelmingly of distinct round shape with little tendency for confluence. These deposits are usually first seen in the 3rd or 1st half of the 4th decade.

White or yellowish plaques may be seen in the macula and numerous clusters of drusen elsewhere. Secondary macular degeneration occurs frequently in the last stage. Not all cases follow the typical sequence. There is considerable variation in the ophthalmoscopic appearance even within the same family.

Visual acuity is affected when drusen appear in the fovea. The loss is often moderate with vision maintained at 20/30 to 20/60. However, widespread macular degeneration can occur either with extensive drusen or serous retinal detachment.

Peripheral vision remains good but central scotomas are present when macular degeneration supervenes. Dark adaptation may be mildly abnormal but the ERG is normal. The EOG was initially reported as severely affected but recent data do not support those claims and most patients have a normal EOG.

Complications
I **Derived:** Macular degeneration
II **Associated:** —

Etiology: Autosomal dominant with occasional report of autosomal recessive

Pathogenesis: These deposits are hyaline excrescences in the cuticular portion of Bruch membrane—numerous discrete, round, fluorescent spots of varying size which far outnumber the drusen seen with the ophthalmoscope and are compatible with a diffuse pigment epithelium alternation. Pigment epithelium changes may be seen even in areas where there are no drusen, suggesting a widespread disturbance of the pigment epithelium in this condition. The drusen probably represent a secretion of the abnormal pigment epithelium.

Related Facts

I **Sex Ratio:** M1:F1
II **Risk of Occurrence:** ?
III **Risk of Recurrence for**
  Patient's Sib: When autosomal dominant or autosomal recessive see Table I AD or AR, respectively.
  Patient's Child: 1 in 2 if autosomal dominant, not increased markedly if autosomal recessive unless mate is carrier or homozygote.
IV **Age of Detectability:** Usually between 25-35 years of age
V **Prevalence:** ?

Treatment
I **Primary Prevention:** Genetic counseling
II **Secondary Prevention:** —
III **Other Therapy:** —

Prognosis: Normal life span with frequent minimal reduction of vision in later life. Occasional moderate to severe reduction of vision.

Detection of Carrier: Affected parent and patient when autosomal dominant

†**Special Considerations:** Drusen may be secondary to numerous diseases of the choroid and are frequently noted in patients over 60 years of age on this basis. Melanoma of the choroid is a frequent cause of secondary drusen in younger patients.

Fundus flavimaculatus and fundus albipunctatus are both of autosomal recessive inheritance. Fluorescein characteristics particularly distinguish fundus flavimaculatus from drusen. The lesions of fundus albipunctatus are white or yellow-white, uniform, dot-like, discrete and are usually present over most of the fundus with greatest density in the midperiphery. Their size usually corresponds to a 2nd or-der arteriole. The early lesions of drusen may be confused with the typical lesions of fundus albipunctatus. Drusen, however, are eventually characterized by variability in size, shape, color and a tendency to confluence. The ERG and dark adaptation are always affected in fundus albipunctatus but these tests are normal in drusen.

References:
Bird, A.C.: Bruch's membrane degenerations. In Krill, A.E. and Archer, D.B. (eds.): Krill's Hereditary and Choroidal Diseases, vol. II. Clinical Characteristics. Hagerstown: Harper & Row, 1977.
Ernest, J.T. and Krill, A.E.: Fluorescein studies in flavimaculatus and drusen. Am. J. Ophthalmol. 62:1, 1966.
Fishman, G.A. et al: The electrooculogram in diffuse (familial) drusen. Arch. Ophthalmol. 92:231, 1971.
Krill, A.E. and Klein, B.A.: Flecked retina syndrome. Arch. Ophthalmol. 74:496, 1965.
Pearce, W.G.: Doyne's honeycomb retinal degeneration: Clinical and genetic features. Br. J. Ophthalmol. 52:73, 1968.

Contributors: **Alex E. Krill‡**
Mitchel L. Wolf

Editor's Computerized Descriptors: Vision, Eye

OCULO-AURICULO-VERTEBRAL DYSPLASIA

Includes: Dysplasie oculo-auriculo vertébrale
Okuloaurikulovertebrale Dysplasie
Displasia óculo-aurículo-vertebral
Goldenhar syndrome

Excludes: Hemifacial dysostosis
Hemifacial microsomia (457)
Mandibulofacial dysostosis (627)
Oro-facio-digital syndrome I (770)

Minimal Diagnostic Criteria: There is no accepted definition of what constitutes the oculoauriculovertebral dysplasia syndrome. It is a variation of the 1st and 2nd arch syndromes. The distinguishing features of this syndrome include unilateral facial hypoplasia, dermoids, lipodermoids, or lipomas of the eyes, colobomas of the upper eyelid, ear abnormalities, and vertebral abnormalities.

Clinical Findings: Eye abnormalities: epibulbar dermoids (may be unilateral or bilateral) - 70%, subconjunctival lipodermoids or lipomas - 40%, colobomas of the upper lid - 25%, extraocular muscle defects - 25%, antimongoloid obliquity 30%, microcornea - 4%, iris colobomas - 5%, ptosis - 5%, colobomas of the eyebrow - 2%.

Auricular abnormalities: preauricular tags - 95%, abnormal size or shape of the ear - 80%, hearing loss - 55%, unilateral posteriorly placed ears - 50%, atresia or stenosis of external auditory meatus - 40%, blind-ended fistulas - 10%.

Oral abnormalities: unilateral facial hypoplasia of the ramus and condyle - 85%, high-arched palate - 50%, micrognathia - 45%, open bite - 30%, cleft palate - 25%, macrostomia - 20%.

Musculoskeletal abnormalities: vertebral abnormalities - 40%, scoliosis - 40%, spina bifida - 30%, rib abnormalities - 30%, clubfoot - 20%.

Congenital heart disease - 35%.

Mental retardation - 25%.

Less commonly found eye manifestations include anophthalmia, iris atrophy, and polar cataracts. Infrequent oral manifestations include bifid tongue, bifid uvula, and double lingual frenum. Less common vertebral abnormalities are cuneiform vertebrae, fused vertebrae, supernumerary vertebrae, lumbarization of the 1st sacral vertebra, and sacral fovea. Roentgenographic findings include minimal-to-marked asymmetry of the mandibular ramus and articular condyles, a small temporomandibular fossa on the involved side, hypoplasia of the zygomatic arch, aplasia or hypoplasia of the maxillary sinus, low positioning of the orbit, and hypoplasia of the temporal bone on the involved side with diminished development of the mastoid cells. Also present are the vertebral anomalies already mentioned, and elongation of the odontoid.

Complications

I **Derived:** Irregular astigmatism has been found in approximately 20% of the patients. Profound deafness does not occur. Various dental abnormalities are present due to aplasia of the ramus and condyle on the involved side. The vertebral abnormalities usually do not cause any difficulties.

II **Associated:** See Minimal Diagnostic Criteria and Clinical Findings.

Etiology: It is possibly secondary to a vascular abnormality during embryogenesis. Although there are 2 possible cases of the syndrome occurring in sibs, it does not appear to be an inherited disorder. Chromosomal analyses have been normal.

Pathogenesis: It is postulated that a vascular insufficiency or abnormality disrupts the normal embryologic development of 1st and 2nd arches.

Related Facts
I **Sex Ratio:** M1:F1
II **Risk of Occurrence:** ?
III **Risk of Recurrence for**
Patient's Sib: ? Extremely unlikely with only 2 possible reported cases occurring in sibs.
Patient's Child: ?
IV **Age of Detectability:** At birth, by noting the various clinical manifestations.
V **Prevalence:** ?

Treatment
I **Primary Prevention:** —
II **Secondary Prevention:** The dental abnormalities, especially repair of the cleft palate and malocclusion, should be done early. Plastic surgery can improve the patient's cosmetic appearance.
III **Other Therapy:** The various manifestations should be treated appropriately.

Prognosis: Normal life span.

Detection of Carrier: —

Special Considerations: —

References:
Berkman, M. D. and Feingold, M.: Oculoauriculovertebral dysplasia (Goldenhar's syndrome). Oral Surg. 25:408, 1968.
Darling, D. B. et al: The roentgenological aspects of Goldenhar's syndrome (oculoauriculovertebral dysplasia). Radiology 91:254, 1968.
Greenwood, R.D. et al: Cardiovascular malformations in oculoauriculovertebral dysplasia (Goldenhar syndrome). J. Pediatr. 85:816, 1974.
Lamba, P.A. and Ramamurthy, S.: Oculoauriculovertebral dysplasia (Goldenhar syndrome). Clin. Pediatr. (Phila.) 12:631, 1973.
Smithells, R. W.: Oculo-auriculo-vertebral syndrome (Goldenhar's syndrome). Dev. Med. Child. Neurol. 6:406, 1964.

Contributor: **Murray Feingold**

Editor's Computerized Descriptors: Eye, Hearing, Ear, Face, Oral, Teeth, Nasoph., Skel.
Also see Section I, Figs. 66, 67

OCULO-CEREBRO-RENAL SYNDROME

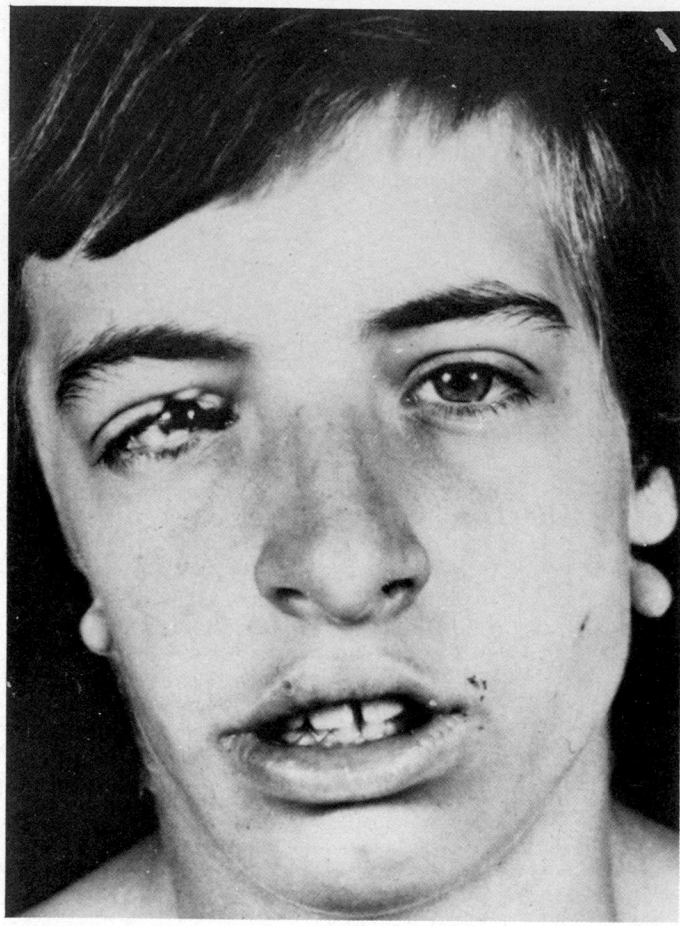

390. Note coloboma of upper eyelid, abnormal auricles, and unilateral facial hypoplasia

Includes: Syndrome oculo-cérébro rénal
Okulozerebrorenales Syndrom
Síndrome óculocerebrorenal
Lowe syndrome

Excludes: Renal tubular syndrome, Fanconi (864)

Minimal Diagnostic Criteria: Bilateral cataracts at birth, mental retardation and hypotonia in a male child are the clinical hallmarks. Laboratory findings, which may vary in intensity, stem from the evidence of renal tubular dysfunction, including: generalized renal hyperaminoaciduria; "tubular" proteinuria (soluble with heat after initial precipitation with 20% sulfosalicylic acid) comprising β-globulins; low-T_m glucosuria; high renal clearance of inorganic phosphate with hypophosphatemia; renal tubular acidosis with impaired bicarbonate conservation and with evidence for a particular defect in H^+ secretion and ammonia production; titratable organic aciduria not totally accounted for by the α-aminoaciduria, but as yet unidentified as to composition. The tubular dysfunction increases in severity with age, beginning in early infancy; its manifestations are believed to be absent at birth, although only a few patients have yet been studied from birth onwards. Rickets is considered to be secondary to the hypophosphatemia. Progressive glomerular and interstitial fibrosis have been reported in the syndrome.

Clinical Findings: Limited to males, characterized by dense to mature cataracts (100%), glaucoma† with or without buphthalmos, corneal scarring or superficial granulations (> 50%), enophthalmos, growth failure (100%), severe mental retardation (100%), hypotonia and reduced or absent deep tendon reflexes after early infancy, metabolic acidosis, generalized hyperaminoaciduria and tubular proteinuria. Cryptorchidism may be present. Hypophosphatemic rickets appears as a later manifestation.

All patients are said to have a characteristic appearance, derived from their blindness and caused by cataracts, mental retardation and hypotonia. A high-pitched scream is the common utterance. When rickets develops, typical signs of this complication emerge.

Most patients die in childhood; a few have survived beyond adolescence.

Complications
I **Derived:** The major clinical triad is apparent from birth. Renal tubular dysfunction then appears. Inability to offset the latter is followed by predictable complications. Death is usually the result of intercurrent infection or dehydration and electrolyte imbalance.
II **Associated:** —

Etiology: X-linked recessive; McK *30900

Pathogenesis: It is presumed that all features of trait are related to an undefined derangement of energy metabolism. Trait is expressed prenatally since the patient is born with some manifestation eg cataracts. Deficient γ-glutamyl transpeptidase activity predicted but not yet substantiated.

Related Facts
I   **Sex Ratio:** M1:F0
II **Risk of Occurrence:** ? Rare
III **Risk of Recurrence for**
    Patient's Sib: If mother is a carrier, 1 in 2 (50%) for each brother to be affected and 1 in 2 for each sister to be a carrier.
    Patient's Child: Theoretically, 1 in 1 (100%) for carrier daughters; not increased for sons unless wife is a carrier

(patients either die or are incapacitated).

IV Age of Detectability: At birth for cataracts; 3 to 6 months for tubular manifestations

V Prevalence: Rare

Treatment

I Primary Prevention: Genetic counseling

II Secondary Prevention: Correction of acidosis, hypophosphatemia and other manifestations of tubulopathy

III Other Therapy: Care of ocular manifestations as may be indicated

Prognosis: Poor; all patients have loss of vision and are severely retarded mentally. Majority die in 1st decade.

Detection of Carrier: None

†Special Considerations: Histopathologic examination of eyes reveals warty excrescences and defects of the capsule of microphakic lenses. It has been postulated that the glaucoma is secondary to the small lens pulling on the ciliary body centrally and thus preventing normal anterior chamber angle cleavage. Heterozygotes show no evidence of the trait. (Holmes, L.B. et al: Pediatrics 44:358, 1969.)

References:

Abbassi, V. et al: Oculo-cerebro-renal syndrome: A review. Am. J. Dis. Child. 115:145, 1968.

Chutorian, A. and Rowland, L. P.: Lowe's syndrome. Neurology (Minneap.) 16:115, 1966.

François, J.: Congenital Cataracts. Assen, Netherlands:Charles C. Thomas, 1963, p. 265.

Witzleben, C.L. et al: Progressive morphologic renal changes in the oculo-cerebro-renal syndrome of Lowe. Am. J. Med. 44:319, 1968.

Contributors: **Charles R. Scriver**
Steven M. Podos

Editor's Computerized Descriptors: Vision, Eye, Speech, Muscle, GU., Nerve

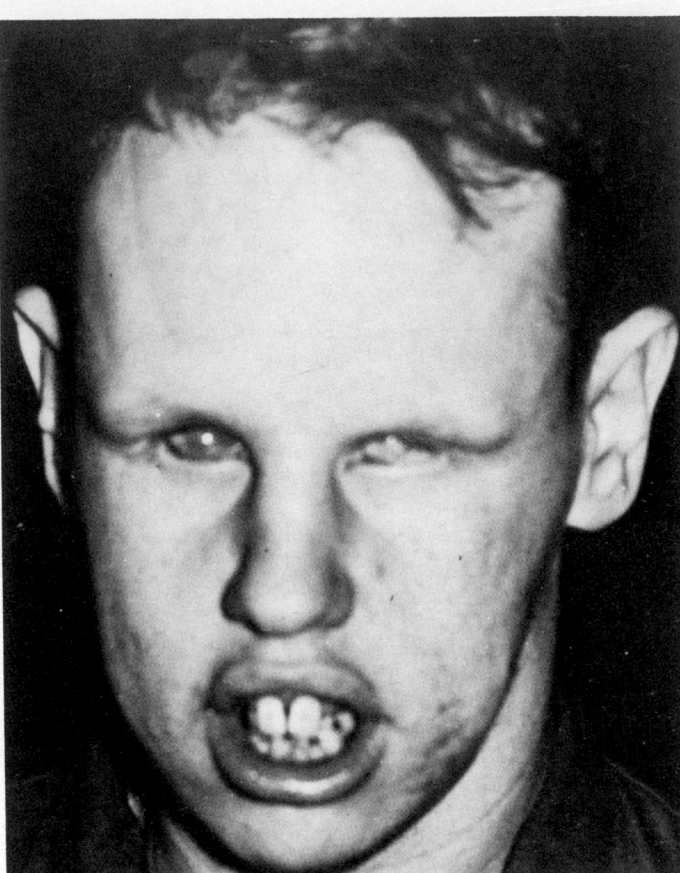

391. Oculocerebrorenal syndrome

OCULO-DENTO-OSSEOUS DYSPLASIA

Includes: Dysplasie oculo-dento-osseuse
Okulo-dento-ossäres Dysplasie
Síndrome óculo-óseo-dentario
Oculodentodigital dysplasia

Excludes: Microcornea
Amelogenesis imperfecta (46)
Oro-cranio-digital syndrome (769)
Cranio-oculo-dental syndrome (229)

Minimal Diagnostic Criteria: Characteristic facies, microcornea, syndactyly of the 4th and 5th fingers

Clinical Findings: Characteristic facies exhibiting thin nose with hypoplastic alae and narrow nostrils, microcornea, soft tissue syndactyly and camptodactyly of 4th and 5th fingers and hypoplasia of enamel. There may be associated ocular hypertelorism, microphthalmos and various other eye findings such as secondary glaucoma, persistence of pupillary membranes and optic atrophy. Head circumference has been noted to be small and the lip and palate to be cleft in a few cases. The hair may be dry and lusterless. Constant skeletal alterations include thickened mandible, metaphyseal widening of long bones, lack of formation of middle phalanges of toes.

Complications
I   **Derived:** Secondary glaucoma
II **Associated:** —

Etiology: Autosomal dominant; McK *16420

Pathogenesis: ?

Related Facts
I   **Sex Ratio:** M1:F1
II **Risk of Occurrence:** ?
III **Risk of Recurrence for**
     Patient's Sib: If parent is affected 1 in 2 (50%) for each offspring to be affected; otherwise not increased.
     Patient's Child: 1 in 2
IV **Age of Detectability:** At birth by physical examination
V   **Prevalence:** ?

Treatment
I   **Primary Prevention:** Genetic counseling
II **Secondary Prevention:** Surgical correction of syndactyly, crowning of teeth
III **Other Therapy:** —

Prognosis: Excellent. No indication of reduced longevity. Blindness may result.

Detection of Carrier: —

Special Considerations: —

References:
Reisner, S. H. et al: Oculodentodigital dysplasia. Am. J. Dis. Child. 118:600, 1969.

Contributor: **Robert J. Gorlin**

Editor's Computerized Descriptors: Eye, Face, Oral, Teeth, Nose, Hair, Skel.

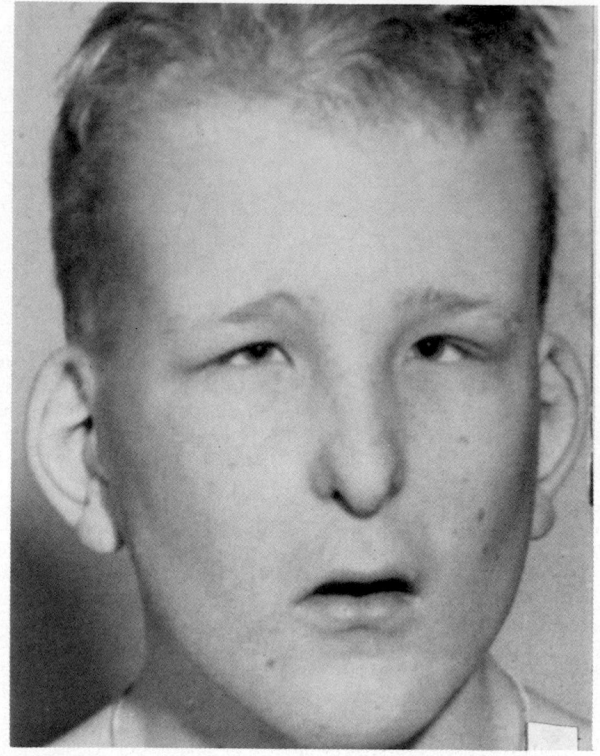

392. Typical facies characterized by pinched nose and small mouth with overlapping upper lip

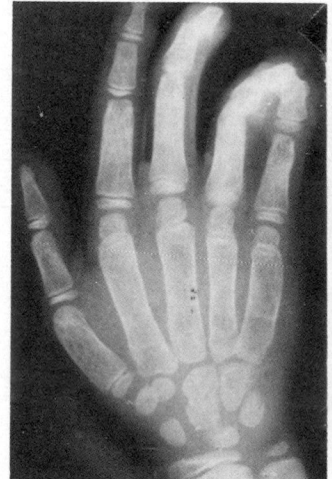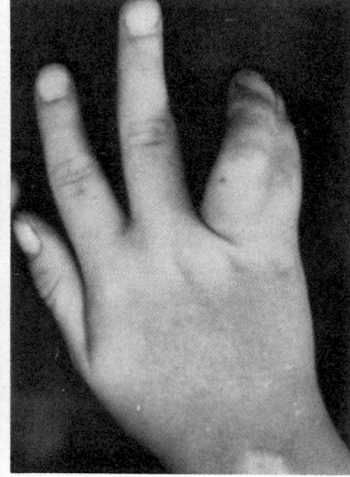

393. Typical 4–5 syndactyly with ulnar deviation of involved fingers. Note lack of modeling; tiny cube-shaped middle phalanges in involved fingers; bony terminal syndactyly

OCULO-MANDIBULO-FACIAL SYNDROME

Includes: Syndrome oculo-mandibulo faciale
Okulomandibulofazialen Syndrom
Síndrome óculomandíbulofacial
Hallermann-Streiff syndrome
François dyscephaly
Dyscephalia oculomandibulofacialis
Dyscephaly with congenital cataract and hypotrichosis
Oculomandibulodyscephaly

Excludes: Progeria (825)
Mandibulofacial dysostosis (627)
Pyknodysostosis (846)
Cleidocranial dysplasia (185)
Oculo-dento-osseous dysplasia (737)
Chondroectodermal dysplasia (156)
Seckel syndrome (881)

Minimal Diagnostic Criteria: Proportionate nanism, normal mentation, congenital cataracts, microphthalmia, dyscephaly with mandibular and nasal cartilage hypoplasia, hypotrichosis, cutaneous atrophy limited to scalp and nose, and dental anomalies.

Clinical Findings: Proportionate dwarfism is a constant feature. Brachycephaly with frontal and parietal bossing is common. The face appears small in relation to the skull. A hypoplastic mandible and narrow, beaked nose give the face a somewhat bird-like appearance. The rami of the mandible are hypoplastic with the condylar head displaced anteriorly. Bilateral congenital cataract and variable degrees of microphthalmia are present. The palate has been reported as being highly arched. Dental anomalies include natal teeth, supernumerary teeth, hypodontia and enamel hypoplasia. Hypotrichosis is generalized, but more pronounced over the scalp. Alopecia may be present. The skin is markedly atrophic over the scalp and nasal area.

Occasionally found are microcephaly, shallow sella turcica, blue sclerae, nystagmus, strabismus, downward obliquity of the palpebral fissures, malar hypoplasia, glossoptosis, syndactyly, lordosis, scoliosis, hypogenitalism and cryptorchidism.

Mentation is usually within normal limits.

Complications
I **Derived:** Vitiligo, respiratory and feeding difficulties in infancy, blindness, psychologic disturbances, deafness.
II **Associated:** Death in childhood has been recorded in a few instances from pulmonary infection.

Etiology: The mode of transmission is unclear. The majority of over 50 cases reported in the literature are sporadic. An affected father and daughter and also 2 of 3 sibs from a consanguineous marriage have been reported. Affected monozygotic twins are also known. There appears to be variable expression, and incomplete penetrance has not been ruled out. The chromosomes have been normal.

Pathogenesis: ? The syndrome results from a developmental defect early in embryonic life (perhaps as early as the 5th week). During early infancy, feeding difficulties and respiratory embarrassment present the greatest problems and may be fatal. Respiratory tract infections are common. Vision is diminished and may relate to the reported association of nystagmus and strabismus. The congenital cataracts which contribute to decreased vision may resorb spontaneously or visual acuity may decrease to the point of total blindness.

Related Facts
I **Sex Ratio:** Apparently M1:F1
II **Risk of Occurrence:** Rare
III **Risk of Recurrence for**

Patient's Sib: ? Usually sporadic. When autosomal dominant or autosomal recessive see Table I AD or AR, respectively.
Patient's Child: If autosomal dominant 1 in 2; if autosomal recessive, not increased unless mate is carrier or homozygote (reproductive fitness is greatly reduced).
IV **Age of Detectability:** Within 1st year of life
V **Prevalence:** Rare

Treatment
I **Primary Prevention:** —
II **Secondary Prevention:** Tracheostomy in cases of severe respiratory embarrassment
III **Other Therapy:** —

Prognosis: Average life span treated, unknown; untreated, unknown (adult cases reported); usual cause of death, unknown; normal for intelligence

Detection of Carrier: —

Special Considerations: —

References:
Carones, A. V.: François dyscephalic syndrome. Ophthalmologica 142:510, 1961.
François, J.: A new syndrome: Dyscephalia with bird face and dental anomalies, nanism, hypotrichosis, cutaneous atrophy, microphthalmia, and congenital cataract. Arch. Ophthalmol. 60:842, 1958.
Gorlin, R. J. and Pindborg, J. J.: Syndromes of the Head and Neck. New York:McGraw-Hill, 1964.
Hoefnagal, D. and Bernirschke, K.: Dyscephalia mandibulo-oculofacialis (Hallermann-Streiff syndrome). Arch. Dis. Child. 40:57, 1965.
Steele, R. W. and Bass, J. W.: Hallermann-Streiff syndrome. Am. J. Dis. Child. 120:462, 1970.

Contributor: **Ronald J. Jorgenson**

Editor's Computerized Descriptors: Eye, Face, Teeth, Nose, Skin, Hair, Skel.

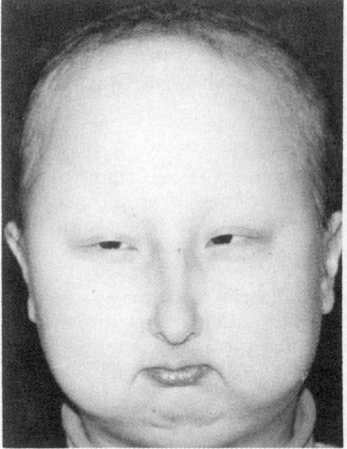 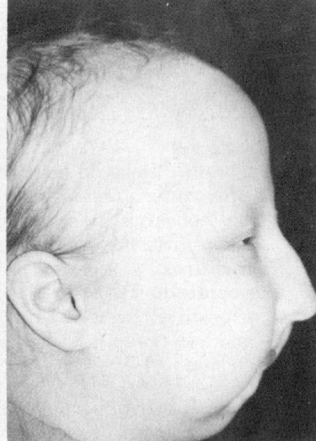

394. Note hypotrichosis; narrow, beaked nose; small mandible; microphthalmia

ODONTODYSPLASIA

Includes: Amelogenesis imperfecta nonhereditaria segmentalis
Zahndysplasie
Odontodisplasia
Localized arrested tooth development
Odontogenesis imperfecta
Odontogenic dysplasia
Regional odontodysplasia
Teeth, ghost
Unilateral dental malformation

Excludes: Amelogenesis imperfecta (46)
Dentin dysplasia, coronal (277)
Dentin dysplasia, radicular (278)
Dentinogenesis imperfecta (279)
Pulpal dysplasia (843)
Teeth, shell

Minimal Diagnostic Criteria: Segments of primary or permanent dentitions exhibit hypoplasia and hypocalcification of enamel and dentin. Affected teeth show reduced radiodensity (" ghostly") and abnormally large pulp chambers with calcific inclusions.

Clinical Findings: Dysgenesis of enamel, dentin and pulp with hypoplasia and hypocalcification of enamel and dentin. Primary or secondary teeth may be affected independently, with only a portion of the teeth being involved. It is unlikely that the succedaneous tooth will be formed normally if the primary tooth is involved. Condition appears to occur more frequently in the maxillary arch; it affects the primary teeth equally, but of the permanent teeth the incisors and cuspids are more commonly involved. Affected teeth may remain unerupted with associated enlarged follicles. Affected teeth are characterized by defective formation of both enamel and dentin; and are 1) smaller than normal, 2) of abnormal morphology, and 3) delayed or partially erupted. Histologically there may be califications within the pulp or follicle. Corpuscular structures comprising concentric layers of collagenous connective tissue may occur in the follicle.

Radiographs exhibit reduced radiodensity, abnormally large pulpal chambers with calcific inclusions and short or hypoplastic roots. Root formation may be near-normal or much delayed.

Complications
I   **Derived:**   Delayed eruption of primary or secondary teeth. Unesthetic anterior teeth may predispose toward psychosocial concerns. Dental caries may occur in hypoplastic defects. Brittleness of teeth may predispose towards coronal fractures.
II   **Associated:**   Subsequent to dental caries there may be pulpal exposure, periapical infection, granuloma, cyst formation, and loss of teeth with possible drifting and resultant malocclusion.

Etiology: ? However because of distribution of affected teeth, both prenatal and early postnatal influences appear to be important. Intrinsic causative factors suggested are localized viral infection, abnormal vascular supply, and localized tissue ischemia. Trauma or ionizing radiation do not appear to be tenable causes.

Pathogenesis: Initial event unknown; affected teeth show thin, hypoplastic and hypocalcified enamel exhibiting irregular, aprismatic, matrix formation with embedded cellular debris. Dentin shows tubular irregularity with amorphous clefts of debris. The pulp may exhibit inflammation and calcific inclusions. The dental follicle may show corpuscular structures comprising concentric layers of collagenous connective tissue and calcifications. There may be delayed root formation with large pulp chambers and root canals.

Related Facts
I   **Sex Ratio:**   Probably M1:F2
II   **Risk of Occurrence:**   Extremely rare
III   **Risk of Recurrence for**
    Patient's Sib: Not increased
    Patient's Child: Not increased
IV   **Age of Detectability:**   Detected preeruptively by radiographs or posteruptively by clinical examination
V   **Prevalence:**   Very rare (less than 60 reported cases, 1975)

Treatment
I   **Primary Prevention:**   —
II   **Secondary Prevention:**   Removal of affected primary teeth. Removal of affected, pulpally-involved secondary teeth and fabrication of artificial replacements for function and esthetics.†
III   **Other Therapy:**   —

Prognosis: Treated: excellent for primary dentition but succedaneous teeth may be involved. Untreated: associated complications may occur. Oral condition does not appear to interfere with patient's longevity.

Detection of Carrier: —

†Special Considerations: An affected secondary tooth bud may be removed, attached to soft tissue of affected primary tooth, during extraction. Teeth may fracture readily. Affected teeth may be associated with a firm, painless, soft tissue swelling of the labial and lingual gingiva.

References:
Gardner, D.G. and Sapp, J.P.: Regional odontodysplasia. Oral Surg. 35:351, 1973.
Gibbard, P.D. et al: Odontodysplasia. Br. Dent. J. 135:525, 1973.
Lustmann, J. et al: Odontodysplasia. Report of two cases and reveiw of the literature. Oral Surg. 39:781, 1975.

Contributors: **Jay T. Cline**
                     Louise Brearley Messer

Editor's Computerized Descriptor: Teeth
Also see Section 1, Fig. 85

OGUCHI DISEASE

Includes: Maladie d'Oguchi
Mb. Oguchi
Enfermedad de Oguchi
Oguchi disease types 1, 2A and 2B

Excludes: Nightblindness, stationary (719)

Minimal Diagnostic Criteria: Abnormal fundus discoloration in patient with nightblindness with usual disappearance of discoloration and occurrence of secondary dark-adaptation after prolonged period in the dark.

Clinical Findings: This is a form of stationary nightblindness associated with a peculiar discoloration of the fundus, which, with prolonged dark-adaptation, will usually lead to a disappearance of the abnormal fundus coloration and marked improvement or normalization of subjective dark-adaptation. The coloration is described as grey or yellow and may be homogenous or streaky in appearance. The abnormal coloration may be found throughout the entire eyegrounds, only in the midperipheral area or mainly in the posterior eyegrounds. The abnormal zones of coloration are brilliant with more pronounced reflexes than normal. The underlying choroid is usually invisible under areas of abnormal coloration and it may be difficult to distinguish retinal veins from retinal arterioles in such areas.

The various patients with Oguchi disease have been divided into 2 major types. Most patients fall into type 1 and are characterized by the occurrence of secondary or rod dark-adaptation after a sufficient period of time in the dark. The final threshold may be normal or elevated. With time in the dark, the abnormal fundus discoloration disappears. This latter event is known as Mizuo phenomenon. Patients with type 2 show no secondary or rod dark-adaptation. These patients have less striking abnormal fundus coloration than those classified as type 1. Some of these patients, type 2A, show Mizuo phenomenon, whereas others, type 2B, do not.

The disorder is stationary. Although some patients have been reported to have mild color defects and some visual field constriction, there is usually no other impairment of vision associated with the disease. The ERG shows a normal cone response. The rod response after several minutes of dark adaptation is grossly abnormal with mainly an A wave seen. Even after the patient is allowed to achieve a secondary dark adaptation and the Mizuo phenomenon, the ERG has been reported as abnormal by some investigators but a normal scotopic response to a single flash of light has been reported. The EOG is normal, reflection densitometry and rhodopsin kinetics are normal as is fluorescein angiography. The disorder is most likely one of neural transmission rather than a structural rod abnormality.

Complications
I **Derived:** —
II **Associated:** —

Etiology: Autosomal recessive; McK *25810

Pathogenesis: In 2 reports, light microscopy showed an abnormal number of cones, many of them larger than normal, in the posterior eyegrounds. Many of these cones were arranged in double rows and contained vesicular spaces between them. In addition there was an abnormal positioning of the cone nuclei, many lying outside of the external limiting membrane. Also, an extra layer with a syncytial structure and strongly pigmented was described between the photoreceptors and the true pigment epithelium. The pigment epithelium cells had dense and shrunken nuclei. However, in a recent histologic examination the extra layer was not detected. Although displaced cone nuclei were seen, the authors noted that in controls without Oguchi disease cone nuclei could sometimes be detected beyond the external limiting membrane. A nodular bulging of the inner side of the pigment epithelium was noted in some areas. This bulging was due to aggregates of fuchsin granules. These same granules were also seen to an abnormal degree among the rods and cones. In areas the pigment epithelium showed thinning and irregularities in cellular structure in many sites.

Related Facts
I   **Sex Ratio:** M1:F1
II **Risk of Occurrence:** ?
III **Risk of Recurrence for**
    Patient's Sib: 1 in 4 (25%) for each offspring to be affected
    Patient's Child: Not increased markedly unless mate is carrier or homozygote
IV **Age of Detectability:** ?
V   **Prevalence:** ? (Has been reported in all races, but most patients were Japanese.)

Treatment
I   **Primary Prevention:** Genetic counseling
II **Secondary Prevention:** —
III **Other Therapy:** —

Prognosis: Normal life span

Detection of Carrier: —

Special Considerations: —

References:
Carr, R.E. and Gouras, P.: Oguchi's disease. Arch. Ophthalmol. 73:646, 1965.
Carr, R.E. and Ripps, H.: Rhodopsin kinetics and rod adaptation in Oguchi's disease. Invest. Ophthalmol. 6:426, 1967.
François, J. and Verriest, G.: La maladie d'Oguchi. Bull. Soc. Belge. Ophtalmol. 108:465, 1955.
Gouras, P.: Electroretinography: Some basic principles. Invest. Ophthalmol. 9:557, 1970.

Contributors: **Alex E. Krill‡**
Mitchel L. Wolf
Donald R. Bergsma

Editor's Computerized Descriptors: Vision, Eye

OLIGOPHRENIA, EPILEPSY AND ICHTHYOSIS SYNDROME

Includes: Syndrome oligophrénie-épilepsie ichtyose
Oligophrenie-Epilepsie-Ichtyose Syndrom
Síndrome de oligofrenia, epilepsia, ictiosis
Rud syndrome†
Ichthyosis, epilepsy and oligophrenia

Excludes: Xeroderma and mental retardation (1004)
Sjögren-Larsson syndrome

Minimal Diagnostic Criteria: Diagnosis must be based upon clinical findings and it would appear that the presence of all 3 named signs is essential. However, the syndrome may be suspected when there is onset of ichthyosis (usually within the first months of life) coupled with somatic and mental development retardation. The onset of epilepsy may be delayed beyond the first 10 years of life, but in some instances, has appeared as early as the 1st year of life. To date, only 1 case has been reported in the Negro race. At present, there is controversy regarding the criteria required for diagnosis of Rud syndrome.†

Clinical Findings: There may be none at birth. Ichthyosis is usually the first sign to be noticed. Mental retardation is rarely suspected until milestones of development are delayed. Epilepsy may not occur until patient is in teens. Associated findings (based upon about 20 reported cases) occur in various combinations and include: retarded somatic development and hypogonadism (probably in most cases); sexual infantilism (about half of reported cases).

Complications

I **Derived:** Severe cases of ichthyosis may show heat prostration in hot weather due to reduced sweating. The only other likely complications are those secondary to epilepsy and mental retardation.

II **Associated:** The following conditions have each been reported once: macrocytic anemia, polyneuritis, partial gigantism of long bones, arachnodactyly, retinitis pigmentosa, hyperglycemia, hypothyroidism, macular atrophy, and alopecia totalis. In 2 patients the existence of talipes equinovarus has been reported.

Etiology: Possibly autosomal recessive

Pathogenesis: The only gross structural defect is the ichthyotic skin. The only reported case which came to autopsy showed CNS changes of a nonspecific nature typical of those associated with profound mental defect. Functional disorders are mental retardation and epilepsy (or EEG evidence of an epileptic diathesis in most cases where EEGs were made).

A 5 1/2-year-old boy diagnosed as having the Rud syndrome by Nissley and Thomas (ichthyosis, hypogonadism, mental retardation but no epilepsy as yet) had a consistent abnormality on karyotyping. A C group chromosome was found to have an abnormal morphology, resulting in a chromosome indistinguishable from the number 3 chromosomes of the A group. This finding was interpreted as being an isochromosome for the long arm of a C group chromosome or a C group chromosome with extra genetic material translocated onto the short arm. The relationship, if any, between this chromosomal abnormality and the clinical findings was unclear.

Related Facts

I **Sex Ratio:** M1:F1
II **Risk of Occurrence:** ? Rare
III **Risk of Recurrence for**
   Patient's Sib: In 2 recorded instances, a sib apparently had a similar syndrome. (Other genetic abnormalities are said to be more common in such families.)

Patient's Child: Kissel, André and André have described Rud syndrome in a mother and Sjögren-Larsson syndrome in her daughter.
IV **Age of Detectability:** Usually in childhood when all 3 clinical features are present.
V **Prevalence:** Apparently rare

Treatment

I **Primary Prevention:** —
II **Secondary Prevention:** —
III **Other Therapy:** Infrequent bathing and cleansing. Use of ointments for the ichthyosis, general treatment measures for epilepsy and mental retardation.

Prognosis: Life expectancy is probably shortened. No progressive mental impairment has been noted but mental retardation appears to vary from severe to mild.

Detection of Carrier: —

†**Special Considerations:** The concept of the Rud syndrome involves the perpetuation of what probably began as a translator's error. All complications over the misconceptions about Rud's original case descriptions can be resolved if we call the present syndrome the "Oligophrenia, Epilepsy and Ichthyosis Syndrome" and do not claim that it is necessarily the same as that described by Rud. See Maldonaldo et al for a recent discussion of the neuroichthyoses.

References:
Butterworth, T. and Strean, L. P.: The ichthyosiform genodermatoses. Postgrad. Med. 37:175, 1965.
Hilliard, L. T. and Kirman, B. H.: Mental deficiency. Boston:Little, Brown and Co., 1965.
Kissel, P. et al: Coexistance dans la même famille d'un syndrome de Sjögren-Larsson et d'un syndrome de Rud. J. Genet. Hum. 21:15, 1973.
Maldonaldo, R.R. et al: Neuroichthyosis with hypogonadism (Rud's syndrome). Int. J. Dermatol. 14:347, 1975.
Nissley, P.S. and Thomas, G.H.: The Rud syndrome. In Bergsma, D. (ed.): Part XII. Skin, Hair and Nails. Birth Defects: Orig. Art. Ser., vol. VII, no. 8. Baltimore:Williams & Wilkins for The National Foundation-March of Dimes, 1971, p. 246.
Wells, R. S. and Kerr, C. B.: Genetic classification of ichthyosis. Arch. Dermatol. 92:1, 1965.

Contributor: **John A. Ewing**

Editor's Computerized Descriptors: Skin, GU., Nerve

OLIVOPONTOCEREBELLAR ATROPHY, DOMINANT MENZEL TYPE

Includes: Atrophie olivopontocérébelleuse dominante (type Menzel)

Dominante olivopontozerebellare Atrophie, Typ Menzel

Atrofia olivopontocerebelosa dominante (tipo Menzel)

Olivopontocerebellar atrophy I†

Excludes: Olivopontocerebellar atrophy of other types

Minimal Diagnostic Criteria: Adult life onset of progressive ataxia, pneumoencephalographic or autopsy findings of olivopontocerebellar atrophy (OPCA), and evidence of autosomal dominant transmission.

Clinical Findings: Onset in the 2nd-5th decades of life, usually about 30 years of age, of a slowly progressive unsteadiness of gait, and later of all limbs. There is progressive dysarthria with scanning speech, tremors, involuntary movements often of choreiform type, and sensory impairment. Later there may develop upper motor neuron signs with extensor plantar responses.†

Complications
I   **Derived:** Patients become bedridden and are unable to care for themselves.
II   **Associated:** —

Etiology: Autosomal dominant. Penetrance is complete, as far as we know, but the age of onset is variable. McK *16440

Pathogenesis: The brain shows the changes of olivopontocerebellar atrophy with sparing of the cerebellar vermis and marked loss of cerebellar Purkinje cells and less striking granule cell loss in the remainder of the cerebellum. The dentate nucleus is usually involved and there is decreased size of the superior cerebellar peduncles and cerebellar white matter. The basis pontis is small with loss of transverse fibers and fiber loss in the middle cerebellar peduncles. There is marked neuronal loss in the inferior olivary nuclei. The substantia nigra also frequently shows neuronal loss. In most cases the spinal cord shows loss of fibers in the posterior funiculus, spinocerebellar tracts and, on occasion, in the pyramidal tracts. Sometimes neuronal loss is found in the posterior horns, Clarke column, or anterior horns. No biochemical abnormalities have been identified.

Related Facts
I   **Sex Ratio:** M1:F1
II   **Risk of Occurrence:** Only 9 kindreds with this disease have been described in the literature. The risk is small, unless one is a member of 1 of these families.
III   **Risk of Recurrence for**
    Patient's Sib: If parent is affected, 1 in 2 (50%) for each offspring to be affected; otherwise not increased.
    Patient's Child: 1 in 2
IV   **Age of Detectability:** At the time of onset of symptoms at about 30 years of age.
V   **Prevalence:** Unknown, but very small. Only 61 cases have been described in the United States.

Treatment
I   **Primary Prevention:** Genetic counseling
II   **Secondary Prevention:** None
III   **Other Therapy:** Only supportive therapy for the patient's ataxia and finally his inability to care for himself in bed.

Prognosis: Patients may die in their 4th-7th decades of life, usually of debilitation and pneumonia.

Detection of Carrier: At present the carrier can be identified only when signs of this disease develop. This may be after he or she has had children.

†Special Considerations: OPCA Type I includes some cases previously called hereditary cerebellar ataxia, type A of Greenfield, and of cerebellar ataxia I of McKusick. There is moderate variability in some of the signs of this disease. Some cases may have no sensory loss. Some patients may show weakness due to lower motor neuron loss, while others have normal strength.

References:
Gray, R.C. and Oliver, C.P.: Marie's hereditary cerebellar ataxia (olivopontocerebellar atrophy). Minn. Med. 24:327, 1941.
Hassin, G.B. and Harris, T.H.: Olivopontocerebellar atrophy. Arch. Neurol. Psychiatr. 35:43, 1936.
Konigsmark, B.W. and Weiner, L.P.: The olivopontocerebellar atrophies: A review. Medicine 49:227, 1970.
Menzel, P.: Beitrag zur Kenntniss der hereditären Ataxie und Kleinhirnatrophie. Arch. Psychiatr. Nervenkr. 22:160, 1890.
Waggoner, R.W. et al: Hereditary cerebellar ataxia. Report of a case and genetic study. Arch. Neurol. Psychiatr. 39:570, 1938.

Contributor: **Bruce W. Konigsmark‡**

Editor's Computerized Descriptors: Speech, Nerve

OLIVOPONTOCEREBELLAR ATROPHY, DOMINANT SCHUT-HAYMAKER TYPE

Includes: Atrophie olivopontocérébelleuse dominante (type Schut-Haymaker)
Dominante olivopontozerebellare Atrophie, Typ Schut-Haymaker
Atrofia olivopontocerebelosa dominante (tipo Schut-Haymaker)
Olivopontocerebellar atrophy IV†

Excludes: Olivopontocerebellar atrophy of other types

Minimal Diagnostic Criteria: Adult life onset of cerebellar ataxia and variable upper motor neuron signs; pneumoencephalographic or autopsy findings of olivopontocerebellar atrophy with variable anterior motor horn cell and spinocerebellar tract loss, loss of neurons in 9th, 10th and 12th cranial nerves; and evidence of autosomal dominant transmission.

Clinical Findings: Onset between about 17 and 35 years of age of a slowly progressive cerebellar ataxia. Tendon reflexes vary from completely absent to hyperactive. Plantar responses are flexor in most cases, but extensor in a few. Muscle tone varies from minimal to marked rigidity. Sensation varies from normal to moderate loss of position and pain sensation. Some cases may show clinical signs of Friedreich ataxia with absent deep reflexes and mild coordination defect; others may show more prominent cerebellar ataxia with variable deep tendon reflexes and moderate coordination disturbances, and some will show prominent pyramidal signs suggesting spastic quadriplegia.†

Complications
I **Derived:** Patients become incapacitated and bedridden.
II **Associated:** —

Etiology: Autosomal dominant, penetrance is complete. McK
*16460

Pathogenesis: The brain shows the changes of olivopontocerebellar atrophy with moderate to severe cerebellar atrophy and cerebellar cortical cell loss. There is marked neuronal and fiber loss in the inferior olivary nuclei. The basis pontis shows some variation from case to case with moderate atrophy in some cases and no changes in others. In the brainstem, neuronal loss varies from none to severe in the 9th, 10th and 12th cranial nerves and substantia nigra. The white matter of the spinal cord varies from normal to severe fiber loss in the posterior funiculus and spinocerebellar tracts. The anterior motor horn cells may be normal or show moderate loss. Most severely affected in all cases are the inferior olivary nuclei, restiform bodies, brachium conjunctivum, cerebellum and 12th nerves. No biochemical abnormalities are known.

Related Facts
I **Sex Ratio:** M1:F1
II **Risk of Occurrence:** Only 42 affected persons, all in 1 kindred, are identified.
III **Risk of Recurrence for**
   Patient's Sib: If parent is affected, 1 in 2 (50%) for each offspring to be affected; otherwise not increased.
   Patient's Child: 1 in 2
IV **Age of Detectability:** At about 25 years
V **Prevalence:** Unknown, but very small

Treatment
I **Primary Prevention:** Genetic counseling
II **Secondary Prevention:** —
III **Other Therapy:** Only supportive therapy for the patient's inability to care for himself in bed.

Prognosis: Patients die about 15 years after onset, usually of debilitation and infection.

Detection of Carrier: The carrier can be identified only when signs of this disease become evident, often after 1 or more of his children are born.

†Special Considerations: OPCA type IV includes some cases previously called hereditary cerebellar ataxia and of type A of Greenfield. Of all the olivopontocerebellar degenerations, this disease shows the greatest variation in clinical signs and pathologic changes. Schut and Haymaker divided the clinical types in this family into 3 groups: Friedreich ataxia type, cerebellar ataxia type and spastic paraplegia type. The pathologic findings showed a similar variation with a variable degree of severity of involvement of different structures.

References:
Konigsmark, B.W. and Weiner, L.P.: The olivopontocerebellar atrophies: A review. Medicine 49:227, 1970.
Schut, J.W.: Hereditary ataxia; clinical study through six generations. Arch. Neurol. Psychiatr. 63:535, 1950.
Schut, J.W. and Haymaker, W.: Hereditary ataxia; pathologic study of five cases of common ancestry. J. Neuropathol. Clin. Neurol. 1:183, 1951.

Contributor: **Bruce W. Konigsmark‡**

Editor's Computerized Descriptor: Nerve

OLIVOPONTOCEREBELLAR ATROPHY, DOMINANT WITH OPHTHALMOPLEGIA

Includes: Atrophie olivopontocérébelleuse avec ophtalmoplégie et démence
Dominante olivopontozerebellare Atrophie mit ophthalmoplegie und Demenz
Atrofia olivopontocerebelosa dominante con oftalmoplegia y demencia
Olivopontocerebellar atrophy V
Familial cerebelloolivary degeneration with late development of rigidity and dementia

Excludes: Olivopontocerebellar atrophy of other types

Minimal Diagnostic Criteria: Adult life onset of progressive ataxia, tremor, rigidity, ophthalmoplegia and severe mental deterioration; pneumoencephalographic or autopsy findings of olivopontocerebellar atrophy and cerebral cortical atrophy; and evidence of autosomal dominant transmission

Clinical Findings: Adult onset of progressive ataxia, dysarthria, rigidity, tremor and mental deterioration. Patients may be diagnosed as having Parkinson disease when the rigidity and tremor are prominent. Generally walking, writing and speech become difficult. Patients in their 3rd decade of life show mental deterioration with disorientation to time and place and are only able to follow simple commands. Dysarthria is characterized by a high-pitched scanning voice. Eye movements become involved first with paresis of upward and lateral gaze and then complete external ophthalmoplegia. Marked rigidity and coarse resting and intention tremor become evident.†

Complications
I **Derived:** Patients become bedridden and are unable to care for themselves.
II **Associated:** —

Etiology: Autosomal dominant, penetrance is complete. McK *16470

Pathogenesis: The gross brain is small, ranging from 700-1200 gm. There is olivopontocerebellar atrophy as well as cerebral cortical atrophy. There is a severe loss of neurons in the inferior olivary nuclei, the basis pontis, and the cerebellar cortex. In the spinal cord there is loss of posterior funiculus fibers. The substantia nigra shows marked neuronal loss and there is a mild neuronal loss in the globus pallidus, caudate nuclei and cerebral cortex. No biochemical abnormalities are known.

Related Facts
I **Sex Ratio:** M1:F1
II **Risk of Occurrence:** There are only 3 kindreds known with this disease.
III **Risk of Recurrence for**
　Patient's Sib: If parent is affected, 1 in 2 (50%) for each offspring to be affected; otherwise not increased.
　Patient's Child: 1 in 2
IV **Age of Detectability:** At about 20 years
V **Prevalence:** Unknown, but very small.

Treatment
I **Primary Prevention:** Genetic counseling
II **Secondary Prevention:** —
III **Other Therapy:** Supportive therapy for ataxia and for the mental deterioration and disorientation.

Prognosis: Affected persons die about 10 years after onset of symptoms, usually because of debility and infection.

Detection of Carrier: The carrier can be identified only when symptoms of ataxia develop, sometimes after 1 or more of his children are born.

†Special Considerations: This disease differs from the other olivopontocerebellar atrophies clinically because of the marked mental deterioration, and pathologically because of the marked brain atrophy with olivopontocerebellar degeneration and cerebral cortical neuronal loss. Some patients have been diagnosed as having Parkinson disease because of prominent rigidity and tremor.

References:
Carter, H.R. and Sukavajana, C.: Familial cerebelloolivary degeneration with late development of rigidity and dementia. Neurology (Minneap.) 6:876, 1956.
Chandler, J.H. and Bebin, J.: Hereditary cerebellar ataxia - olivopontocerebellar type. Neurology (Minneap.) 6:187, 1956.
Konigsmark, B.W. and Lipton, H.L.: Dominant olivopontocerebellar atrophy with dementia and extrapyramidal signs: Report of a family through three generations. In Bergsma, D. (ed.): Part VI. Nervous System. Birth Defects: Orig. Art. Ser., vol. VII, no. 1. Baltimore: Williams & Wilkins for The National Foundation March of Dimes, 1971, p. 178.

Contributor: **Bruce W. Konigsmark‡**

Editor's Computerized Descriptors: Eye, Speech, Nerve

OLIVOPONTOCEREBELLAR ATROPHY, DOMINANT WITH RETINAL DEGENERATION

Includes: Atrophie olivopontocérébelleuse avec dégénérescence rétinienne
Dominante olivopontozerebellare Atrophie und Retina degeneration
Atrofia olivopontocerebelosa con degeneración retineana
Olivopontocerebellar atrophy III
Cerebellar-macular abiotrophy
Retinal degeneration associated with spinocerebellar ataxia
Infantile cerebellar atrophy with retinal degeneration

Excludes: Olivopontocerebellar atrophy of other types

Minimal Diagnostic Criteria: Infancy or adult life onset of ataxia, dysarthria and tremor; progressive visual loss, beginning about the same time as the ataxia and involving the macula and then remainder of retina; evidence of autosomal dominant transmission, and pneumoencephalogram or neuropathologic findings of OPCA.

Clinical Findings: This disease is characterized by a remarkably variable age of onset of cerebellar ataxia and retinal degeneration. The disease may first show signs from the age of 1 year to over 50 years of age; however, the usual age of onset is about 20 years. The syndrome is characterized by a progressive visual loss, ataxia and tremor. Clinically, eye signs are prominent with an unusual retinal pigmentary degeneration and sometimes with ophthalmoplegia and nystagmus. The retinal changes begin with pallor and degeneration in the macula which gradually enlarges and in which numerous granules of pigment are found. Peppery granules of pigment then are found throughout the remainder of the retina. Cerebellar ataxia involving the limbs and speech begin about the same time as the retinal changes. The ataxia and rigidity progress leading to confinement in bed about 10 years after onset. The syndrome in infancy is characterized by tremor, ataxia, retinal degeneration and weakness.†

Complications
I   **Derived:** Affected persons become bedridden, dying usually of an infection.
II **Associated:** —

Etiology: Autosomal dominant. Penetrance is complete with a remarkably variable age of onset. McK *16450

Pathogenesis: The changes of olivopontocerebellar atrophy are seen grossly and histologically. Cerebellar Purkinje cells are markedly decreased in numbers, particularly in the vermis, while granule cells are relatively preserved. There is also moderate loss of substantia nigra neurons. The retina shows marked loss of ganglion cells and of rods and cones, with some preservation of bipolar cells. There are numerous adhesions of retina to choroid with loss of pigment epithelium in the areas of adhesion. Some pigment cells contain increased amounts of pigment. No biochemical abnormalities have been identified.

Related Facts
I   **Sex Ratio:** M1:F1
II **Risk of Occurrence:** Only 5 kindreds affected with this disease have been described in the United States.
III **Risk of Recurrence for**
    Patient's Sib: If parent is affected, 1 in 2 (50%) for each offspring to be affected; otherwise not increased.
    Patient's Child: 1 in 2
IV **Age of Detectability:** Very variable, usually about 20 years
V   **Prevalence:** Unknown, but very small

Treatment
I   **Primary Prevention:** Genetic counseling
II **Secondary Prevention:** —
III **Other Therapy:** Only supportive therapy, particularly when the patient is bedridden.

Prognosis: Affected persons generally die of debilitation and infection about 15 years after onset.

Detection of Carrier: The carrier can be identified only when symptoms begin, or if an affected child is born.†

†Special Considerations: This disease shows a greater variation in the age of onset than practically any other of the hereditary nervous system diseases. In 1 family we studied, 2 sibs died of this disease before the diagnosis was made in the affected father, who had only minimal retinal changes. Clinically this disease generally shows more rigidity than the other types of OPCA and ophthalmoplegia is a prominent feature.

References:
Carpenter, S. and Schumacher, G.A.: Familial infantile cerebellar atrophy associated with retinal degeneration. Arch. Neurol. 14:82, 1966.
Havener, W.H.: Cerebellar-macular abiotrophy. Arch. Ophthalmol. 45:40, 1951.
Konigsmark, B.W. and Weiner, L.P.: The olivopontocerebellar atrophies: A review. Medicine 49:227, 1970.
Weiner, L.P. et al: Herediatary olivopontocerebellar atrophy with retinal degeneration. Report of a family through six generations. Arch. Neurol. 16:364, 1967.
Woodworth, J.A. et al: A composite of hereditary ataxias: A familial disorder with features of olivopontocerebellar atrophy, Leber's optic atrophy, and Friedreich's ataxia. Arch. Intern. Med. 104:594, 1959.

Contributor: **Bruce W. Konigsmark‡**

Editor's Computerized Descriptors: Vision, Eye, Speech, Nerve

OLIVOPONTOCEREBELLAR ATROPHY, LATE-ONSET

Contributor: Bruce W. Konigsmark‡

Editor's Computerized Descriptors: Eye, Face, Speech, Nerve

Includes: Atrophie olivopontocérébelleuse
Sporadische olivopontocerebellare Atrophie
Atrofia olivopontocerebelosa esporádica

Excludes: Hereditary olivopontocerebellar atrophies
Holmes cerebelloolivary atrophy
Marie ataxia

Minimal Diagnostic Criteria: Adult life onset of progressive ataxia, tremor, dysarthria, pneumoencephalographic or autopsy findings of olivopontocerebellar atrophy (OPCA), absence of family history of consanguinity or of similar disorder.

Clinical Findings: Onset is in the 5th or 6th decades of life with a progressive cerebellar ataxia of the limbs and trunk, slowness of voluntary movements, scanning speech, nystagmus, and tremor of the head and trunk. In some cases, signs of Parkinson disease are prominent, with rigidity, tremor, bradykinesia and immobile facies. Reflexes are usually normal though there may be loss of knee and ankle jerks or an extensor plantar response.

Complications
I   **Derived:**   Patients become incapacitated in 5-10 years.
II   **Associated:**   —

Etiology: ? May be recessive olivopontocerebellar atrophy (OPCA II) with very late expressivity. Other etiologic possibilities include toxic factors or a specific deficiency.

Pathogenesis: There is atrophy and neuronal loss in the inferior olives, basis pontis, and cerebellar cortex. Secondary to the basis pontis neuronal loss, there is atrophy of the middle cerebellar peduncles and loss of cerebellar white matter. There may be neuronal loss in the cerebellar dentate nuclei or substantia nigra. The spinal cord is generally normal.

Related Facts
I   **Sex Ratio:**   M1:F1
II   **Risk of Occurrence:**   ?
III   **Risk of Recurrence for**
    Patient's Sib: ? If autosomal recessive, 1 in 4 (25%) for each offspring to be affected.
    Patient's Child: ? Not increased unless mate is carrier or homozygote.
IV   **Age of Detectability:**   Onset of symptoms at about 45 years
V   **Prevalence:**   Unknown, but about 1 case will be diagnosed every several years in a large medical center.

Treatment
I   **Primary Prevention:**   —
II   **Secondary Prevention:**   —
III   **Other Therapy:**   Supportive therapy for ataxia and incapacitation

Prognosis: Signs slowly progress with incapacitation in 5-10 years and death due to debility and infection about 5 years later.

Detection of Carrier: —

Special Considerations: —

References:
Critchley, M. and Greenfield, J.G.: Olivo-ponto-cerebéllar atrophy. Brain 71:343, 1948.
Déjerine, J. and Thomas, A.: L'atrophie olivo-ponto-cérébelleuse. Nouv. Inconogr. Salpêtr. 13:330, 1900.
Geary, J.R. et al: Olivopontocerebellar atrophy. Neurology 6:218, 1956.
Greenfield, J.G.: Spino-cerebellar Degenerations. Springfield: Charles C Thomas, 1954, p. 45.
Hassin, G.B.: Marie's ataxie (olivopontocerebellar atrophy); clinical and pathologic considerations. Arch. Neurol. Psychiatr. 37:1371, 1937.

OLIVOPONTOCEREBELLAR ATROPHY, RECESSIVE FICKLER-WINKLER TYPE

Contributor: **Bruce W. Konigsmark‡**

Editor's Computerized Descriptors: Speech, Nerve

Includes: Atrophie olivopontocérébelleuse récessive, de type Fickler-Winkler
Olivopontocerebellare Atrophie Typ Fickler-Winkler
Atrofia olivopontocerebelosa recesiva (tipo Fickler-Winkler)
Olivopontocerebellar atrophy II†

Excludes: Olivopontocerebellar atrophy of other types

Minimal Diagnostic Criteria: Progressive cerebellar ataxia and dysarthria, pneumoencephalographic or autopsy findings of olivopontocerebellar atrophy, and evidence of autosomal recessive transmission

Clinical Findings: Variable age of onset, between about 7 and 50 years of age, of a slowly progressive cerebellar ataxia, head tremor and dysarthria with scanning speech. There are no choreiform movements; strength and sensation are normal.†

Complications
I Derived: Patients gradually become bedridden and debilitated.
II Associated: —

Etiology: Autosomal recessive. Penetrance appears to be complete, but more cases need to be described to define this disease more clearly. McK *25830

Pathogenesis: There is olivopontocerebellar atrophy with neuronal loss in the inferior olivary nuclei, basis pontis, and cerebellar cortex. Purkinje cells in the cerebellar hemispheres are most strikingly affected. The spinal cord and other brain structures are normal. There are no known biochemical abnormalities.

Related Facts
I Sex Ratio: M1:F1
II Risk of Occurrence: Only 2 sibs are documented with this disease.
III Risk of Recurrence for
   Patient's Sib: 1 in 4 (25%) for each offspring to be affected
   Patient's Child: Not increased unless mate is carrier or homozygote.
IV Age of Detectability: At onset of symptoms, from about 7-50 years
V Prevalence: Unknown, but very small

Treatment
I Primary Prevention: Genetic counseling
II Secondary Prevention: —
III Other Therapy: Only supportive therapy is available.

Prognosis: Affected persons die from 5-15 years after onset, usually of debilitation and infection.

Detection of Carrier: —

†Special Considerations: OPCA type II includes cases previously called hereditary cerebellar ataxia, type A of Greenfield and of cerebellar ataxia I of McKusick, and some cases of sporadic olivopontocerebellar atrophy. Since only 4 cases of this disease have been described, the clinical and pathologic variations are not clearly defined. However, the age of onset generally is younger than that of OPCA I. Also there is no sensory loss or involuntary movements, as found in OPCA I.

References:
Fickler, A.: Klinische und pathologischanatomische Beiträge zu den Erkrankungen des Kleinhirns. Dtsch. Z. Nervenheilk. 41:306, 1911.
Konigsmark, B.W. and Weiner, L.P.: The olivopontocerebellar atrophies: A review. Medicine 49:227. 1970.
Winkler, C.: A case of olivo-pontine cerebellar atrophy and our conceptions of neo- and palaio-cerebellum. Schweiz. Arch. Neurol. Neurochir. Psychiatr. 13:684, 1923.

OMPHALOCELE

Includes: Omfalocele
Exomphalos
Ruptured omphalocele
Umbilical hernia

Excludes: Ventral hernia
Gastroschisis (405)
Ectopia cordis (335)

Minimal Diagnostic Criteria: Wide umbilical ring with visual evidence of intestine in the substance of the cord, evisceration of the intestine through the umbilical ring with remnant of sac present or umbilical defect with skin covered mass (umbilical hernia).

Clinical Findings: Sacular malformation of the umbilical cord containing various portions of the intestinal tract, with the umbilical ring widely open. This is generally covered by a membrane made up of Wharton jelly as an extension of the peritoneum. Elements of the umbilical cord may be present in the wall of the sac. The umbilical defect varies in size, small, 1-2 cm, to massive and obliterating most of the abdominal wall. Contents of the omphalocele may be just 1 loop of bowel or the entire intestinal tract with the liver, spleen, etc included. The membrane may be thin and translucent or substantial and opaque. The skin of the abdominal wall may extend up on the eviscerated intestine to make up one-third to one-half of the sac wall, or in the case of congenital umbilical hernia, the mass will be covered with skin. The sac may have ruptured during or before birth, the remnants of sac present or nonexistent. The difference between a ruptured omphalocele and gastroschisis remains in dispute. They will be considered as different entities in this discussion.†

Complications

I   **Derived:** Atresia of the intestine secondary to vascular impairment of the mesentery, 3-4%; incomplete rotation of the intestine with abnormal fixation of the gut 100%; duodenal band causing obstruction frequent; malformation or abnormal fixation of the liver.

When the defect is eccentric in the epigastrium an associated diaphragmatic defect in the subxyphoid area should be suspected. There is an inferior pericardial defect demonstrable with intestines in the pericardium or ectopia cordis, ie a portion of the heart in the abdomen, generally a ventricular aneurysm; exstrophy of the bladder or exstrophy of the cloaca associated low-lying defect in the hypogastrium with separation of the symphyses pubis.

II **Associated:** Remote anomalies of the cardiovascular system 16-20%; GU system 40%; CNS 4%.

Etiology: ?

Pathogenesis: The body of the embryo is joined by infolding of the borders of the original flat disk. Failure of this infolding process causes a number of anomalies of the anterior abdominal wall depending on which folds have been effected. Failure of lateral folds causes umbilical defect covered by amnion-omphalocele. Failure of cephalic fold causes high defect, sternal and diaphragmatic defects, ectopia cordis, etc. Failure of caudal fold causes ectopia vesical or vesicointestinal fissure (exstrophy of cloaca).

Related Facts

I   **Sex Ratio:** M3:F2
II   **Risk of Occurrence:** 1 in 6000 live births
III **Risk of Recurrence for**
     Patient's Sib: ?
     Patient's Child: ?
IV   **Age of Detectability:** At birth, or for umbilical hernia, neonatal period
V   **Prevalence:** ?

Treatment

I   **Primary Prevention:** —
II **Secondary Prevention:** Operative correction by replacement of the viscera within the abdomen for the small defects and small masses. Primary repair of the umbilical hernia with closure of the umbilical defect is possible at any age. In larger defects when the return of the viscera to hypoplastic or underdeveloped abdominal cavity will result in respiratory deficiency, ie elevation of the diaphragm and diminished respiratory exchange, the fascia should remain open, the defect enlarged and a staged repair employed using temporary synthetic material, ie silastic rubber sheeting. Ultimate closure can be accomplished in stages by 2-4 weeks of age. Skin coverage only with later abdominal wall repair now is infrequently employed. Continuity with intestinal tract must be insured with appropriate repair of atresias or division of bands due to incomplete rotation. Central venous feedings for support may be used where GI function is delayed.
III **Other Therapy:** —

Prognosis: Excellent once the repair is accomplished and intestinal function established. Late obstruction due to adhesions are not a frequent problem in the larger lesions. Mortality rate: 20-30%. Causes of death are infections, inanition or unrelated congenital abnormalities.

Detection of Carrier: —

†**Special Considerations:** Syndrome of macroglossia, macrosomia, umbilical defect, and hypoglycemia should be investigated in the infant with omphalocele. The life-threatening hypoglycemia is generally of short duration and responds to replacement and supportive therapy with glucose. Macroglossia can require hemiglossectomy at an early date and growth does not compensate for the disproportionate size of the tongue.

References:
Rickham, P.P.: Exomphalos and gastroschisis. In Rickham, P.P. et al (eds.): Neonatal Surgery. New York: Appleton-Century-Crofts, 1969, p. 254.

Contributor: **Lawrence K. Pickett**

Editor's Computerized Descriptors: Hernia not CNS, CV., GI., Liver, GU., Nerve

OPHTHALMO-MANDIBULO-MELIC DYSPLASIA

Includes: Dysplasie oculo-mandibulaire
Ophthalmomandibulomele Dysplasie
Displasia oftalmo-mandibulomélica

Excludes: —

Minimal Diagnostic Criteria: The salient clinical features are blindness from corneal opacity, temporomandibular fusion leading to inability to move the lower or upper jaw with the mouth kept half open (an anterior open bite) and deformities of the limbs.

Clinical Findings: Three cases in a single family have been described. Clinical findings have included blindness due to corneal opacity, temporomandibular fusion with anterior open bite leading to difficulty in mastication, shortening and bowing of the forearm which is held fixed in midpronation, ulnar-deviated clubhands, flexion deformity in the fingers, dislocated radial head with limitation of elbow flexion and a mild degree of genu valgum.

Radiologic abnormalities are seen in the mandible and limb bones. In the mandible the condyloid process is conical and the temporomandibular joint ankylosed. The coronoid process is absent and the angle of the jaw obtuse. In the upper limb the glenoid fossa is shallow, the lateral condyle of the humerus is aplastic and the trochlea is abnormal. The olecranon and coronoid processes of the ulna are absent; the radial head is absent and the proximal end of the radius is pointed and positioned posterolateral to the distal end of the humerus. The radial shaft is bowed and short. The distal third of the ulna is absent and the distal end notched. At the wrists the radius articulates irregularly and solely with the carpal lunate. The carpal navicular is hypoplastic. The interphalangeal joints of the long, ring, and little fingers show narrowing of the joint spaces and fusion. The hip shows coxa valga and absence of the lesser trochanter. At the knee the distal end of the femur is concave with a hypoplastic lateral condyle. The tibial spine is absent and the upper surface of the tibia is convex and congruent with the concave femoral surface. The fibula is short with the lateral malleolus situated higher than the medial.

Complications
I   **Derived:** Affected patients cannot take solid food since laryngeal obstruction may result.
II **Associated:** —

Etiology: Autosomal dominant; McK *16490

Pathogenesis: ?

Related Facts
I   **Sex Ratio:** (Only 3 reported cases) M2:F1
II **Risk of Occurrence:** ?
III **Risk of Recurrence for**
   Patient's Sib: If parent is affected, 1 in 2 (50%) for each sib; otherwise not increased.
   Patient's Child: 1 in 2
IV **Age of Detectability:** At birth from clinical features
V   **Prevalence:** Only 3 reported cases

Treatment
I   **Primary Prevention:** Genetic counseling
II **Secondary Prevention:** —
III **Other Therapy:** The value of early corneal grafting to restore vision is questionable.

Prognosis: For life: The condition does not seem to influence life span or intelligence. For function: Blindness, defective mastication and limb abnormalities impair function.

Detection of Carrier: Parents of affected child and patients

Special Considerations: —

References:
Pillay, V. K.: Ophthalmo-mandibulo-melic dysplasia: An hereditary syndrome. J. Bone Joint Surg. 46A:858, 1964.

Contributor: **V. K. Pillay**

Editor's Computerized Descriptors: Vision, Eye, Face, Oral, Teeth, Skel.

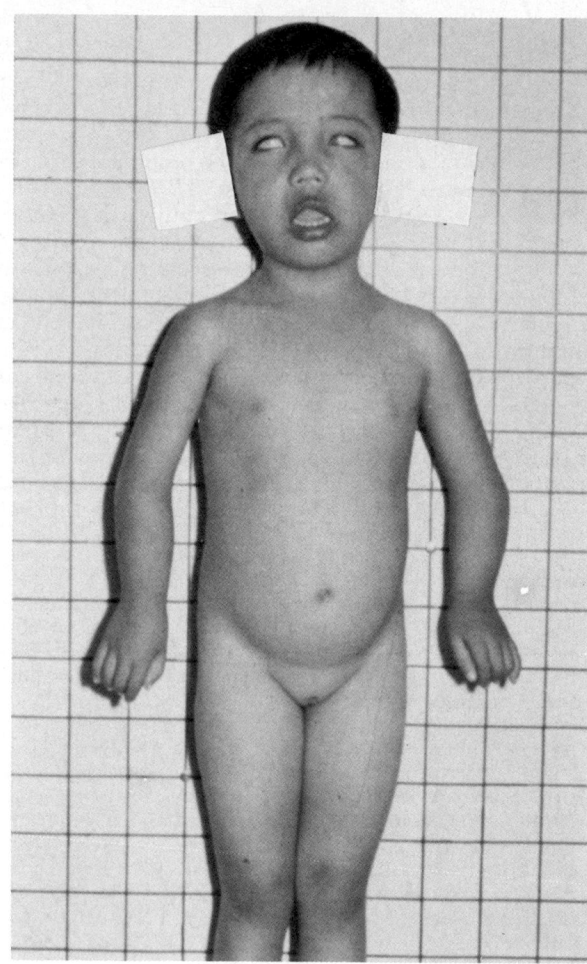

395. Note corneal opacities; open mouth; short, bowed forearm with ulnar-deviated clubhand

OPHTHALMOPLEGIA EXTERNA AND MYOPIA

Includes: Ophtalmoplégie externe avec myopie
Äussere Ophthalmoplegie und Myopie
Oftalmoplejía externa y miopía
Myopia and external ophthalmoplegia
External ophthalmoplegia and myopia

Excludes: Ophthalmoplegia progressive, external (752)
Ophthalmoplegia, familial static (751)
Ophthalmoplegia secondary to generalized myopathy or neuropathy
Ocular myasthenia gravis
Ptosis, congenital (834)

Minimal Diagnostic Criteria: Ophthalmoplegia, high myopia and absent tendon-jerk reflexes

Clinical Findings: This syndrome is expressed in males who display bilateral ptosis, weakness of the extraocular muscles, high myopia, ectopic pupils, absent tendon-jerks, anomalous occlusion of the teeth, and scoliosis. Electromyography of the upper limbs is normal.

Complications
I **Derived:** Strabismus; myopic degeneration of the choroid and retina
II **Associated:** Cardiopathy, hernia, enuresis, flatfoot, spina bifida

Etiology: X-linked recessive transmission of mutant gene. (Technically an X-linked intermediate gene, because the female carriers are identifiable.) McK *31100

Pathogenesis: ?

Related Facts
I **Sex Ratio:** M1:F0
II **Risk of Occurrence:** Extremely low. Only 1 extended family described in literature.
III **Risk of Recurrence for**
  Patient's Sib: If mother is a carrier, 1 in 2 (50%) for each brother to be affected and 1 in 2 for each sister to be a carrier.
  Patient's Child: 1 in 1 (100%) for carrier daughters; not increased for sons unless wife is a carrier.
IV **Age of Detectability:** First months of life
V **Prevalence:** Unknown but extremely low

Treatment
I **Primary Prevention:** Genetic counseling
II **Secondary Prevention:** Strabismus surgery is usually contraindicated, orthodontia, eyeglasses.
III **Other Therapy:** Supportive

Prognosis: ? Apparently no threat to life

Detection of Carrier: Female carriers display areflexia and signs of hyperthyroidism.

Special Considerations: —

References:
François, J.: Heredity in Ophthalmology. St. Louis: C.V. Mosby Co., 1961, p. 104.
Ortiz de Zárate, J.C.: Recessive sex-linked inheritance of congenital external ophthalmoplegia and myopia coincident with other dysplasias: A reappraisal after 15 years. Br. J. Ophthalmol. 50:606, 1966.
Salleras, A. and Ortiz de Zárate, J.C.: Recessive sex-linked inheritance of external ophthalmoplegia and myopia coincident with other dysplasias. Br. J. Ophthalmol. 34:662, 1950.

Contributor: **Donald R. Bergsma**

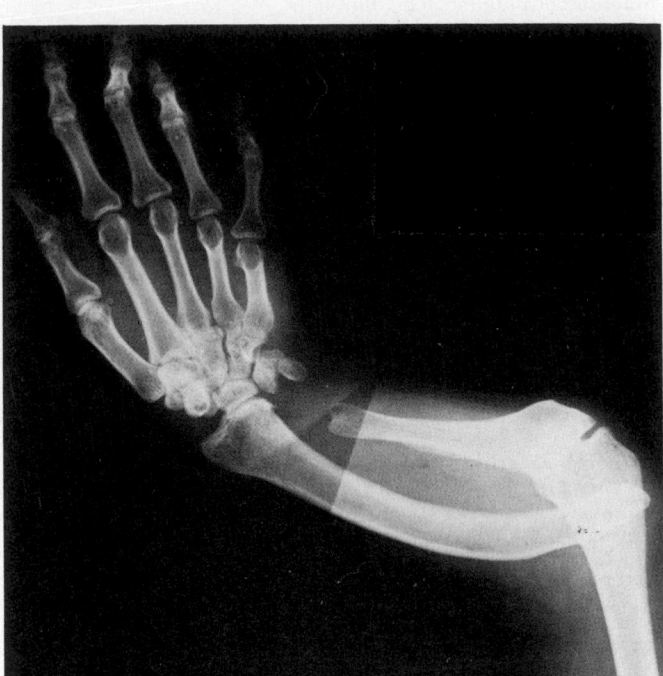

396. Aplasia of lateral humeral condyle, radial head, and distal ulna. Radio humeral and proximal radio ulnar dislocation

OPHTHALMOPLEGIA, FAMILIAL STATIC

Includes: Ophtalmoplégie familiale
Familiäre statische Ophthalmoplegie
Oftalmoplejía estática familiar
External ophthalmoplegia congenita
Hereditary congenital ophthalmoplegia
Ophthalmoplegia totalis
Ophthalmoplegia externa, complete or incomplete

Excludes: Ophthalmoplegia, progressive external (752)
Ophthalmoplegia externa and myopia (750)
Ophthalmoplegia secondary to generalized myopathy or neuropathy
Ocular myasthenia gravis

Minimal Diagnostic Criteria: Weakness of the extraocular muscles may be minimal as manifest by nystagmus in certain fields of gaze. Electromyography may help in borderline cases.†

Clinical Findings: Unilateral or, more frequently, bilateral congenital ophthalmoplegia of variable degree but usually of fairly uniform severity within family groups. Ptosis may or may not accompany the extraocular muscle weakness. Ophthalmoplegia totalis implies paralysis of the pupillary sphincter and of accommodation. This latter form is rare.

Complications
I   **Derived:** Postural anomalies due to hyperextension of the head. Amblyopia secondary to ptosis or strabismus.
II **Associated:** Hereditary ataxia of the Friedreich or Marie types, facial nerve weakness, syndactyly and clubfoot.

Etiology: Usually a mutant autosomal dominant gene. Some families display irregular autosomal dominant inheritance. Rare families display X-linked and autosomal recessive inheritance. Occasional sporadic cases may be phenocopies secondary to exogenous causes. McK *16500

Pathogenesis: The early literature favors nuclear aplasia of the nerves involved. More recent studies favor extraocular myopathy as the primary defect in a majority of cases with variable degrees of aplasia, atrophy and fibrosis. Some cases have been demonstrated to be secondary to anomalous insertion of extraocular muscles.

Related Facts
I   **Sex Ratio:** Probably close to M1:F1, although there are several reports of families where males predominate.
II   **Risk of Occurrence:** ? The syndrome is considered uncommon, not rare. Congenital ophthalmoplegia accounts for approximately 15% of extraocular muscle paralysis.
III **Risk of Recurrence for**
     Patient's Sib: When autosomal dominant or X-linked, see Table I AD or X-linked R, respectively.
     Patient's Child: When autosomal dominant or X-linked, see Table I AD or X-linked R, respectively.
IV   **Age of Detectability:** At birth or soon thereafter
V   **Prevalence:** ?

Treatment
I   **Primary Prevention:** Genetic counseling after diagnosis and pedigree study
II   **Secondary Prevention:** Many procedures for surgical repair of ptosis are described. Early treatment is necessary to prevent postural deformity from backwards head tilt. Surgery on the extraocular muscles is usually contraindicated.
III **Other Therapy:** Crutch spectacles

Prognosis: Usually nonprogressive. Normal life span.

Detection of Carrier: —

†**Special Considerations:** A similar condition with onset in childhood may be classified either with this condition or with progressive ophthalmoplegia.

References:
Duke-Elder, S.: System of Ophthalmology, vol. 3, pt. 2. Congenital Deformities, St. Louis: C.V. Mosby, Co., 1963.
François, J.: Heredity in Ophthalmology. St. Louis: C.V. Mosby, 1961.
Waardenburg, P.J. et al: Genetics and Ophthalmology. Oxford: Blackwell Scientific Publications, Ltd., 1961, vol. 2. p. 1090.

Contributor: **Donald R. Bergsma**

Editor's Computerized Descriptor: Eye

OPHTHALMOPLEGIA, PROGRESSIVE EXTERNAL

Includes: Ophthalmoplégie progressive
Progressive Ophthalmoplegie
Oftalmoplejía progresiva
Progressive ophthalmoplegia
Myopathic ophthalmoplegia externa
Ophthalmoplegia plus
Progressive extraocular muscular dystrophy
Abiotrophic ophthalmoplegia externa
Chronic progressive external ophthalmoplegia
Ocular myopathy
Oculo-cranio-somatic neuromuscular disease with ragged-red fibers
Kearns-Sayre-Shy-Daroff syndrome

Excludes: Ptosis, congenital (834)
Ophthalmoplegia externa and myopia (750)
Ocular myasthenia gravis
Ophthalmoplegia, familial static (751)
Ophthalmoplegia secondary to thyroid disease
Ophthalmoplegia secondary to generalized myopathy or neuropathy
Facial diplegia, congenital (376)
Ophthalmoplegia totalis with ptosis and miosis (753)
Congenital fibrotic syndromes
Oculopharyngeal dystrophy
Phytanic acid storage disease (810)

Minimal Diagnostic Criteria: Although frequently a 1st sign, ptosis is not necessary for the diagnosis. Compatible family history is helpful but need not be positive. Differentiation from other causes of acquired ophthalmoplegia is necessary. Myasthenia gravis can usually be distinguished by its characteristic response to anticholinesterases. Laboratory evidence of thyroid dysfunction should be sought. Rarely other neuromuscular diseases may have an associated ophthalmoplegia (type I hypotrophy with central nuclei, myotonic atrophy, and even isolated case reports of polymyositis and spinal muscular atrophy).

Clinical Findings: The 1st sign is usually bilateral but often asymmetric ptosis which presents at almost any age. This is followed by the insidious onset of ophthalmoplegia which may become complete over months to years. Diplopia is uncommon because of the gradual onset and ptosis, although strabismus and nystagmus can occur in certain fields of gaze. The pupillary reactions remain normal. Orbicularis weakness is usually associated. Backward head tilt often develops to compensate for the ptosis.

Complications
I **Derived:** Exposure keratitis may occur because of the absence of the normal Bell phenomenon and orbicularis weakness with lagophthalmos. Visual difficulties may occur either due to the ptosis covering the pupil or the associated retinal pigmentary degeneration present in some cases.
II **Associated:** There are a number of associations, some of which define separate nosologic entities: abetalipoproteinemia (Bassen-Kornzweig), ataxia, spastic quadriparesis, pharyngeal weakness, hearing loss. A syndrome of retinal pigmentary degeneration, cardiac conduction abnormalities, and variably small stature, ataxia, hearing loss, EEG abnormalities, high cerebrospinal fluid protein, is called Kearns-Sayre.

Etiology: The large number of associated findings forces consideration of progressive external ophthalmoplegia as a clinical complex with multiple etiologies. Some cases are clearly inherited as autosomal dominants; these familial cases often have no associated findings. Most cases are sporadic, and in the Kearns-Sayre variant there is an association with a previous meningitis which suggests the possibility of a slow virus infection, but this has not been demonstrated by animal inoculations.

Pathogenesis: A considerable debate has occurred over

whether this entity is neurogenic or myogenic in origin. Autopsied cases have demonstrated both normal brain stem nuclei and a spongiform degeneration. Skeletal muscle biopsies subjected to histochemical examination have shown an abnormality of type I fibers with increased lipids and an accumulation of material which on electron microscopy can be seen to be abnormal mitochondria. When viewed by light microscopy after histochemical staining with a modified trichrome, these fibers have been described as "ragged-red." This and other systemic manifestations suggest a generalized metabolic abnormality.

Related Facts
I   **Sex Ratio:**   M1:F1
II   **Risk of Occurrence:**   ?
III **Risk of Recurrence for**
     Patient's Sib: If parent is affected, 1 in 2 (50%) for each offspring to be affected; otherwise not increased significantly.
     Patient's Child: 1 in 2
IV   **Age of Detectability:**   Infancy to old age
V   **Prevalence:**   ?

Treatment
I   **Primary Prevention:**   Genetic counseling
II   **Secondary Prevention:**   Surgical treatment of strabismus is rarely indicated. Ptosis surgery should be approached with great caution because of the risk of exposure keratitis postoperatively.
III **Other Therapy:**   Crutch spectacles, pacemaker for heart block if indicated.

Prognosis: When unassociated with other problems, the prognosis is good, and the disease is compatible with a normal life span. In patients with retinal pigmentary degeneration the visual prognosis is better than in the usual retinitis pigmentosa. Children with the Kearns-Sayre variant have a poor prognosis with progression of weakness, intellectual deterioration, and visual loss with death from cardiac complications or intercurrent infection.

Detection of Carrier: —

Special Considerations: —

References:
Daroff, R.B.: Chronic progressive external ophthalmoplegia: A critical review. Arch. Ophthalmol. 82:845, 1969.
Drachman, D.A.: Ophthalmoplegia plus: The neurodegenerative disorders associated with progressive external ophthalmoplegia. Arch. Neurol. 18:654, 1968.
Duke-Elder, S.: System of Ophthalmology, vol. 3, part 2. Congenital Deformities. St. Louis: C.V. Mosby Co., 1963, p. 986.
Malbrán, E.S.: Myopathic ophthalmoplegia externa. Int. Ophthalmol. Clin. 6:711, 1966.
Rowland, L.P.: Progressive external ophthalmoplegia. In Vinken, P.J. and Bruyn, G.W. (eds.): Handbook of Clinical Neurology. System Disorders and Atrophies. Amsterdam: North-Holland Publishing Co., 1975, vol. 22, part II, p. 177.
Walsh, F.B. and Hoyt, W.F.: Progressive muscular dystrophy principally affecting extraocular muscles: Chronic progressive external ophthalmoplegia. In Walsh, F.B. and Hoyt, W.F. (eds.): Clinical Neuro-ophthalmology, 3rd Ed. Baltimore: Williams & Wilkins, 1969, vol. I, p. 1254.

Contributors: **Donald R. Bergsma**
                        John W. Gittinger

Editor's Computerized Descriptors: Eye, Nerve

OPHTHALMOPLEGIA TOTALIS WITH PTOSIS AND MIOSIS

Includes: Ophtalmoplégie avec ptosis et miosis
Ophthalmoplegia totalis mit Ptose und Miosis
Oftalmoplejía total con ptosis y miosis
Ptosis and miosis with ophthalmoplegia totalis

Excludes: Ophthalmoplegia, progressive external (752)
Ophthalmoplegia externa and myopia (750)
Ophthalmoplegia, familial static (751)
Ophthalmoplegia secondary to generalized myopathy or neuropathy
Ptosis, congenital (834)
Ocular myasthenia gravis

Minimal Diagnostic Criteria: See Clinical Findings.

Clinical Findings: Severe weakness of the extraocular muscles associated with ptosis and miosis

Complications
I   **Derived:**   Postural anomalies due to hyperextension of the head. Amblyopia secondary to ptosis or strabismus.
II   **Associated:**   —

Etiology: Autosomal recessive; McK *25840

Pathogenesis: ?

Related Facts
I   **Sex Ratio:**   M1:F1
II   **Risk of Occurrence:**   Extremely low. Only 3 families, 2 of which are interrelated, are described in the literature.
III **Risk of Recurrence for**
     Patient's Sib: 1 in 4 (25%) for each offspring to be affected
     Patient's Child: Not increased unless mate is carrier or homozygote
IV   **Age of Detectability:**   1st month of life
V   **Prevalence:**   Unknown, but extremely low

Treatment
I   **Primary Prevention:**   Genetic counseling
II   **Secondary Prevention:**   Many procedures for surgical repair of ptosis are described. Early treatment is necessary to prevent postural deformity from backwards head tilt. Surgery on the extraocular muscles is usually contraindicated.
III **Other Therapy:**   Crutch spectacles

Prognosis: Normal life span

Detection of Carrier: —

Special Considerations: —

References:
François, J.: Heredity in Ophthalmology. St. Louis: C.V. Mosby, Co, 1961, p. 242.
Waardenburg, P.J.: Over een recessieven vorm van aangeboren ophthalmoplegie. Genetica 6:487, 1924.

Contributor: **Donald R. Bergsma**

Editor's Computerized Descriptors: Vision, Eye, Nerve

OPITZ-KAVEGGIA FG SYNDROME

Includes: FG syndrome
Síndrome FG

Excludes: Acropectorovertebral dysplasia (22)

Minimal Diagnostic Criteria: Male sex, characteristic facies, hypotonia, with or without imperforate anus.

Clinical Findings: Summary based on 15 known cases. The patients, all males, usually have normal intrauterine growth, an OFC which ranges from normal to >98th percentile at birth and postnatally, and may lead to the false impression of hydrocephaly; postnatal growth failure, with adult heights of 145-160 cm; congenital hypotonia of variable degree with squints and ptosis; hypotonic mouth-breathing facies with highly arched palate, micrognathia, inverted V shape of upper lip, protruding tongue with drooling, and malocclusion; sloping shoulders with winged scapulae, mild-to-moderate pectus excavatum and repeated attacks of pneumonia; lumbar hyperlordosis, distended abdomen with marked constipation; at times cryptorchidism; hyperextensible joints, clubfeet, simian creases, crowding of toes and deep creases of soles; at times with a history of hypoactive fetal movements; a characteristic facial appearance with a high broad forehead, hypertelorism with prominent nose, upsweep of frontal hair, relatively large mouth with thick lips; mild posterior rotation of small auricles with minor anomalies of auricular differentiation; minor anomalies of limbs with broad thumbs and big toes, minimal cutaneous syndactyly of 3rd and 4th fingers, at times mild joint contractures; imperforate anus (usually membranous) in 7/12 cases; and severe constipation in all surviving patients.

Patients have mild-to-severe MR with IQ around 50; agenesis of corpus callosum was seen in 1 patient and suspected in another; 1 patient had seizures. All survivors have a somewhat hyperactive, mischievous, easy-going and affable personality. Pyloric stenosis has been seen in 2 patients; hypoplastic left heart, VSD, generalized dilatation of the urinary tract, and severe craniosynostosis were each seen in 1 patient.†

Complications
I **Derived:** Pneumonia and constipation due to hypotonia.
II **Associated:** ? Breech presentation

Etiology: X-linked recessive mutant gene.

Pathogenesis: ? True multiple congenital anomaly/mental retardation (MCA/MR) syndrome.†

Related Facts
I **Sex Ratio:** M1:F0; to date 15 males
II **Risk of Occurrence:** Rare
III **Risk of Recurrence for**
    Patient's Sib: If mother is a carrier 1 in 2 (50%) for each brother to be affected and 1 in 2 (50%) for each sister to be a carrier.
    Patient's Child: Theoretically, 1 in 1 (100%) for carrier daughters; not increased for sons unless wife is a carrier. However, patient's ability to reproduce is doubtful.
IV **Age of Detectability:** At birth
V **Prevalence:** ?

Treatment
I **Primary Prevention:** —
II **Secondary Prevention:** Imperforate anus surgery as indicated neonatally (colostomy usually not required); treatment of CHD, seizures, constipation and pneumonia.
III **Other Therapy:** —

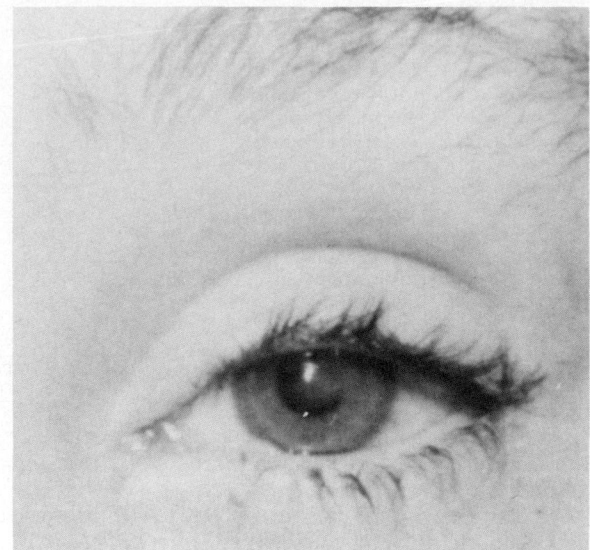

397. Ptosis and miosis

Prognosis: Four of 15 died neonatally (1 of CHD and 1 of amniotic aspiration and hyaline membrane disease), 1 at 4 1/2 months of unstated cause, and 2 others around 2 years of pneumonia. The remainder had mental retardation.

Detection of Carrier: Not accomplished to date, but carriers should be studied in greater detail.

†**Special Considerations:** Another patient had unusual histologic brain abnormalities: dense, subependymal infiltrates of glial cells, granulocytes, lymphocytes and histiocytes especially in a perivascular distribution.

References:
Keller, M.A. et al: A new syndrome of mental deficiency with craniofacial, limb and anal abnormalities. J. Pediatr. 88:589, 1976.

Opitz, J.M. and Kaveggia, E. G.: Studies of malformation syndromes of man XXXIII: The FG syndrome. An X-linked recessive syndrome of multiple congenital anomalies and mental retardation. Z. Kinderheilkd. 117:1, 1974.

Riccardi, V.M. et al: Studies of malformation syndromes of man XXXIII B: The FG syndrome: Further characterization, report of a third family, and of a sporadic case. Am. J. Med. Genet. 1:47, 1977.

Contributor: **John M. Opitz**

Editor's Computerized Descriptors: Eye, Ear, Face, Oral, Teeth, Nose, Skin, Dermatoglyphic, Hair, Skel., Muscle, Resp., CV., GI., GU., Nerve

OPTIC ATROPHY, INFANTILE HEREDOFAMILIAL

Includes: Atrophie optique hérédo-familiale infantile
Heredofamiliäre Opticusatrophie, infantile Form
Atrofia óptica infantil heredo familiar
Autosomal recessive optic atrophy
Autosomal dominant optic atrophy
Simple recessive optic atrophy
Congenital optic atrophy
Behr syndrome (complicated optic atrophy)
Infantile recessive optic atrophy

Excludes: Leber optic atrophy (579)
Optic neuritis
Tumor of optic nerve

Minimal Diagnostic Criteria: Optic atrophy occurring at birth or in the 1st decade of life.

Clinical Findings: Simple or complicated optic atrophy occurs with various patterns of transmission and graded symptomatology.

The term congenital optic atrophy is usually reserved for the rare optic atrophy of recessive inheritance. It is occasionally noted in the neonate but more frequently discovered at some point before the patient is 3-4 years of age. Vision is quite poor and there is often a pendular nystagmus as well as achromatopsia. The condition is stable and has no pyramidal tract involvement. A normal ERG distinguishes congenital optic atrophy from a tapetoretinal degeneration. Consanguineous parentage is often discovered.

Complicated optic atrophy is also referred to as infantile recessive optic atrophy or Behr syndrome. This disorder has its onset in childhood (between 1 and 9 years of age) and is associated with mild mental deficiency, spasticity, hypertonia, and ataxia. Pallor of the disks tends to be temporal; nystagmus and strabismus are common associated findings. This disorder tends to stabilize after a variable period of progression.

Dominant optic atrophy is characterized by dominant autosomal inheritance, an insidious onset between the ages of 4-8 years, moderately reduced visual acuity, temporal pallor of disks, field defects, and acquired blue-yellow dyschromatopsia. Nystagmus is unusual. This type of optic atrophy is more common and milder than recessive type.

Complications
I Derived: —
II Associated: Pyramidal tract signs in certain cases.

Etiology: — McK *16540, *21000

Pathogenesis: ?

Related Facts
I Sex Ratio: M1:F1 probable
II Risk of Occurrence: ?
III Risk of Recurrence for
  Patient's Sib: When autosomal recessive or autosomal dominant, see Table I AR or AD, respectively.
  Patient's Child: When autosomal recessive or autosomal dominant, see Table I AR or AD, respectively.
IV Age of Detectability: In the 1st decade of life
V Prevalence: ?

Treatment
I Primary Prevention: Genetic counseling
II Secondary Prevention: —
III Other Therapy: —

Prognosis: Poor in the autosomal recessive types, fair to poor in the autosomal dominant types; visual rehabilitation needed.

Detection of Carrier: —

Special Considerations: —

References:
Glazer, J.: Heredofamilial disorders of the optic nerve. In Goldberg, M. (ed.): Genetic and Metabolic Eye Disease. Boston:Little, Brown, 1974.
Hereditary optic atrophies, symposium 6. In 2nd Int. Congr. Neurogenetics and Neuro-ophthalmology, Montreal, Canada, 1967. New York:Excerpta Medica, 1967, p. 69.
Jaeger, W.: Hereditary optic atrophies in childhood. J. Genet. Hum. 15:312, 1966.
Kjer, P.: Infantile optic atrophy with dominant mode of inheritance. Acta Ophthalmol. (Suppl.) 54, 1959.
Smith, D.P.: Diagnostic criteria in dominantly inherited juvenile optic atrophy. Am. J. Optom. Physiol. Opt. 49:183, 1972.

Contributor:　**Morton E. Smith**

Editor's Computerized Descriptors: Vision, Eye, Muscle, GU., Nerve

OPTIC DISK PITS

Includes: Fossettes de la macule
Grubenpapillen
Fóveas del disco óptico
Holes in optic disk
Crater-like cavities in optic disk
Optic disk fossae

Excludes: Ocular colobomas (733)

Minimal Diagnostic Criteria: Sharp-edged pits in optic disk

Clinical Findings: These pits occur ophthalmoscopically as oval holes, 1/8 to 1 disk diameters in size, with sharp edges and of varying depth, some 1.5 to 20 diopters. They usually occur in the lower temporal quadrant of the disk, and the floor may be covered by soft grey tissue; occasionally, there is some pigmentation in the bottom of the pit. In the majority of cases, the pits are single and unilateral. The arrangement of the retinal vessels is usually not disturbed, but in some cases, branches of the central retinal vessels may run down through the hole and occasionally cilioretinal arteries emerge from it, or opticociliary veins descend into it.

Symptoms may be absent, but frequently there is enlargement of the blind spot or sector defects in the visual field. If the maculopapillary bundle is involved, acuity may be diminished and a partial or complete paracentral or central scotoma may be present. In about 25% of these cases, associated macular degeneration is observed. Fluorescein studies reveal a leak of fluid of unknown source and composition from the pit in the nerve to the macula.

Complications
I Derived: Macular degeneration
II Associated: Retinal cysts, abnormalities of the cilioretinal vasculature, and true colobomas of the optic disk or retina and choroid.

Etiology: ?

Pathogenesis: A developmental defect of the optic nervehead. During abnormal differentiation of the primitive epithelial papilla, the pluripotential neuroepithelial cells of the wall of the optic vesicle may form atypical transparent retinal tissue instead of neuroglial supporting tissue at about the 15 mm stage. The cause of the macular lesion associated with 25% of cases is not clear but is probably due to involvement of the maculopapillary bundle, which nonspecifically lowers the resistance of this area to noxious agents or vascular disturbance.

Optic disk pits may represent atypical colobomas and the macular disturbance is caused by a mechanical phenomenon with leak of fluid from the pit into the subretinal space.

Related Facts
I Sex Ratio: ?
II Risk of Occurrence: 1 in 11,000 patients with ocular complaints
III Risk of Recurrence for
Patient's Sib: ?
Patient's Child: ?
IV Age of Detectability: The pit in the optic nerve is present at birth, but the related macular lesion occurs later, usually in the 2nd or 3rd decade.
V Prevalence: ?

Treatment
I Primary Prevention: —
II Secondary Prevention: The use of photocoagulation to the macula remains controversial to date.

III Other Therapy: —

Prognosis: Good except in cases with secondary degenerative macular lesions in which central acuity is lost. In a relatively large series of cases, the vision was good in 40% of cases, diminished but useful in 35% and seriously diminished in 25%.

Detection of Carrier: —

Special Considerations: —

References:
Duke-Elder, S.: System of Ophthalmology, vol. 3, part 2. Congenital Deformities. St. Louis: C.V. Mosby Co., 1963, p. 678.
Gordon, R. and Chatfield, R.: Pits in the optic disc associated with macular degeneration. Br. J. Ophthalmol. 53:481, 1969.
Kranenburg, E.W.: Crater-like holes in the optic disc and central serous retinopathy. Arch. Ophthalmol. 64:912, 1960.
Mann, I.: Developmental Abnormalities of the Eye. Philadelphia: J.B. Lippincott, 1957, p. 113.
Mustonen, E. and Varonen, T.: Congenital pit of the optic nerve-head associated with serous detachment of the macula. Acta Ophthalmol. 50:689, 1972.
Savin, H. and Rosen, E.: Congenital pit of the optic disc with acquired retinal cyst. Ann. Opthalmol. 4:756, 1972.
Sugar, H.S.: Congenital pits in the optic disc with acquired macular pathology. Am. J. Ophthalmol. 53:307, 1962.
Sugar, H.S.: Congenital pits in the optic disc. Am. J. Ophthalmol. 63:298, 1967.

Contributor: **Robert M. Ellsworth**

Editor's Computerized Descriptor: Eye

OPTIC DISK, SITUS INVERSUS

Includes: Inversion du disque optique
Situs inversus der Papille
Situs inversus del disco óptico
Dysversion of optic disk

Excludes: Congenital pit of optic nerve
Coloboma of optic nerve

Minimal Diagnostic Criteria: Typical ophthalmoscopic findings in the nervehead. Various field defects including hemianopia, arcuate scotomas, concentric contraction and enlargement of the blind spot may be noted.

Clinical Findings: Normally, the excavation in the optic disk is directed toward the lens or is tilted temporally in the direction of the macula. In situs inversus, the disk is tilted in another direction, usually nasally or below, and the central retinal vessels stream out in that direction. The condition is frequently bilateral and typical crescents may appear above, nasally or below the nervehead. The condition is often associated with a major refractive error, particularly myopic astigmatism. In some cases, bizarre defects have been noted in the visual field. These patients frequently have headaches of variable severity.†

Complications
I   **Derived:** Skull xrays may occasionally reveal oxycephaly.
II **Associated:** Myopia; rare associated conditions include atypical chorioretinal atrophy, corneal opacities, ectopia of the macula and cilioretinal arteries. Strabismus, Duane syndrome and mild glaucoma have been noted in association with situs inversus of the optic disk.

Etiology: Cause of the visual field defect may be mechanical compression of the optic nerve fibers or abnormalities in the vascularization of the nervehead.

Pathogenesis: Not known in detail but involves an anomalous insertion of the optic stalk into the optic vesicle.
The field defects may be related to ectasia of the posterior portion of the globe and in other cases to hypoplasia of the retina and choroid with fewer receptors per unit area.

Related Facts
I   **Sex Ratio:** M1:F1
II   **Risk of Occurrence:** ?
III **Risk of Recurrence for**
      Patient's Sib: —
      Patient's Child: —
IV   **Age of Detectability:** At birth
V   **Prevalence:** ?

Treatment
I   **Primary Prevention:** —
II   **Secondary Prevention:** —
III **Other Therapy:** —

Prognosis: The field defects usually show no progression.

Detection of Carrier: —

†Special Considerations: The nature of the field defects with situs inversus of the disks differs from that of chiasmal lesions relative to the vertical meridian; chiasmal lesions tend to respect the midline and end in a sharp edge which, in the early stages, does not cross the nasal side. Ocular lesion defects, on the other hand, tend to slope obliquely across the midline and frequently involve part of the upper nasal quadrant.

References:
Duke-Elder, S.: System of Ophthalmology, vol. 3, part 2. Congenital Deformities. St. Louis: C.V. Mosby, 1963, p. 677.
Graham, M. and Wakefield, G.: Bitemporal visual field defects associated with anomalies of the optic discs. Br. J. Ophthalmol. 57:307, 1973.
Mann, I.: Developmental Abnormalities of the Eye. Philadelphia:

J.B. Lippincott, 1957, p. 113.

Manor, R.S.: Temporal field defects due to nasal tilting of the discs. Ophthalmologica 168:269, 1974.

Rucker, C.W.: Bitemporal defects in visual fields resulting from developmental anomalies of optic disks. Arch. Ophthalmol. 35:546, 1946.

Veirs, E.R.: Inversio papillae with altitudinal fields; report of a case. Am. J. Ophthalmol. 34, 1596, 1951.

Contributor: **Robert M. Ellsworth**

Editor's Computerized Descriptors: Vision, Eye

OPTIC NERVE HYPOPLASIA

Includes: Hypoplasie du nerf optique
Hypoplasie des n. opticus
Hipoplasia del nervio óptico
Partial absence of optic nerve
Hypoplasia of optic nerve

Excludes: Optic nerve aplasia

Minimal Diagnostic Criteria: Ophthalmoscopic appearance in conjunction with reduced vision

Clinical Findings: Hypoplasia of the optic nerve is not uncommon and may be unilateral or bilateral in equal frequency. It is more often found with other anomalies than as an isolated entity. The optic nerve appears small, pale, and misshapen. It may have a greyish or brownish-black pigment crescent on the temporal side, a deep physiologic cup, a peripapillary cuff or may appear mottled throughout. The foveolar reflex may be absent. The retinal vasculature is normal or attenuated. The visual acuity, if diminished in the affected eye, is proportionate to the severity of the hypoplastic disk with or without strabismus on the same side. Visual field defects and radiologically, a small optic foramen has been noted on the involved side.

Complications
I   **Derived:** —
II **Associated:** Microphthalmia, nystagmus, partial 4th or 6th nerve palsies, dacryostenosis, cyclopia, anencephaly, hydrocephaly, orbital encephalomeningocele, ptosis, blepharophimosis, hypopituitarism, and agenesis of the septum pellucidum, deafness, and anomalies of the urinary and skeletal systems.

Etiology: A familial tendency has been observed in bilateral cases. It may be inherited as an autosomal dominant. Maternal diabetes causing an adverse intrauterine environment may also be a cause.

Pathogenesis: Embryologic defect of differentiation in the ganglion cell layer. Some of the optic nerve fibers fail to develop and reach the disk but mesoderm has invaginated the optic stalk, and retinal vessels exist. Teratogenic substances, for example drugs such as quinine and possibly sulfonaamides, have been implicated if taken during the early weeks of gestation.

Related Facts
I   **Sex Ratio:** Probably Ml:Fl
II   **Risk of Occurrence:** Relatively common when found in association with hypopituitarism.
III **Risk of Recurrence for**
    Patient's Sib: If autosomal dominant and if parent is affected, 1 in 2 (50%) for each offspring to be affected; otherwise not increased.
    Patient's Child: 1 in 2 if autosomal dominant
IV   **Age of Detectability:** Infancy by ophthalmoscopic examination
V   **Prevalence:** Rare

Treatment
I   **Primary Prevention:** Genetic counseling
II   **Secondary Prevention:** —
III **Other Therapy:** —

Prognosis: Visual prognosis dependent upon degree of severity of the hypoplasia and associated anomalies

Detection of Carrier: Affected parent and patient when autosomal dominant

Special Considerations: —

References:
Ewald, R. A.: Unilateral hypoplasia of the optic nerve. Am. J. Oph-

thalmol. 63:763, 1967.

Hackenbrauch, Y. et al: Familial bilateral optic nerve hypoplasia. Am. J. Ophthalmol. 79:314, 1975.

Helveston, E. M.: Unilateral hypoplasia of the optic nerve. Arch. Ophthalmol. 76:195, 1966.

Patel, H. et al: Optic nerve hypoplasia with hypopituitarism. Am. J. Dis. Child. 129:175, 1975.

Petersen, R.A. and Walton, D.S.: Optic nerve hypoplasia with good visual acuity and visual field defects. Arch. Ophthalmol. 95:254, 1977.

Whinery, R. D. and Blodi, F. C.: Hypoplasia of the optic nerve: A clinical and histopathologic correlation. Trans. Am. Acad. Ophthalmol. Otolaryngol. 67:733, 1963.

Contributor: **Elsa K. Rahn**

Editor's Computerized Descriptors: Vision, Eye, Nerve

OPTICO-COCHLEO-DENTATE DEGENERATION

Includes: Dégénérescence systématisée optico-cochléo-dentelée
Degeneration der Opticus-, cochlearis-, Dentatun- und Schleifensysteme
Degeneración óptico-cócleo-dentata
Nyssen and van Bogaert syndrome

Excludes: Huntington chorea (478)
Progressive optic atrophy and congenital sensorineural deafness
GM₂-gangliosidosis (433, 434)
Pelizaeus-Merzbacher disease (803)
Optic atrophy, ataxia, and progressive sensorineural hearing loss
Optic atrophy, polyneuropathy and sensorineural deafness

Minimal Diagnostic Criteria: Optic atrophy, deafness and spastic quadriplegia.

Clinical Findings: Twelve cases have been recorded; 2 or more sibs have been involved in each family. Cases presented before age 1 in 9/12 and during early childhood in 3/12. The disorder presents with motor disturbances in early-onset cases; poor head control, decreased lower limb use, inability to sit or stand, flexion contractures of the legs and kyphoscoliosis are seen. Spastic quadriplegia developed progressively with marked involvement of lower limbs in late-onset cases; ataxic gait, intention tremor with spasticity and cerebellar myoclonus were present. Tendon stretch reflexes were hyperactive or absent. All patients have a thin wasted appearance with disuse atrophy. Blindness occurred in 11, 9 before age 3. In 2 cases nystagmus was seen before age 1. All developed deafness, 10 before age 9. Eight patients never developed speech. Neuropathologic lesions included atrophy and demyelination of the primary optic and cochlear pathways, atrophy of the nerve cells of dorsal and ventral cochlear nuclei, disseminated nerve cell loss of the dentate nucleus, degeneration of the medial lemnisci and, in some cases, of the pyramidal tracts. Nonspecific parenchymal losses (diffuse cortical nerve cell loss producing brain atrophy) and alteration of blood vessels may be seen. It appears that the severity of the disorder, head circumference, level of mental functioning and degree of neuronal loss correlate with the age of onset.

Complications
I **Derived:** Microcephaly, speech disturbances, mental retardation.
II **Associated:** In late-onset cases, deafness and blindness may cause psychologic isolation, which may give rise to affective disturbances. Intercurrent infections.

Etiology: Autosomal recessive; variability of expressivity is demonstrated.† McK *25870

Pathogenesis: ?

Related Facts
I **Sex Ratio:** M7:F5 of the 12 patients described
II **Risk of Occurrence:** —
III **Risk of Recurrence for**
  Patient's Sib: 1 in 4 (25%) for each offspring to be affected
  Patient's Child: Not increased unless mate is carrier or homozygote.
IV **Age of Detectability:** Most often in early infancy
V **Prevalence:** ?

Treatment
I **Primary Prevention:** Genetic counseling
II **Secondary Prevention:** Physical therapy, positioning to prevent decubitus ulcers.
III **Other Therapy:** —

Prognosis: Progression varies and may be very rapid or slow, 4/5 deaths have occurred before puberty.

Detection of Carrier: —

†Special Considerations: This syndrome represents a nosologic entity, but genetic heterogeneity is possible.

References:
Konigsmark, B.W. and Gorlin, R.J.: Genetic and Metabolic Deafness. Philadelphia: W.B. Saunders, 1976.
Müller, J. and Zeman, W.: Dégénérescence systématisée optico-cochléo-dentelée. Acta Neuropathol. (Berl.) 5:26, 1965.
Zeman, W.: Dégénérescence systématisée optico-cochléo-dentelée. Handbook. Clin. Neurol. 21:535, 1975.

Contributors: **Agnes M. Ickenroth**
Cor W.R.J. Cremers

Editor's Computerized Descriptors: Vision, Eye, Hearing, Skel., Muscle, Nerve

ORAL DERMOIDS

Includes: Kystes dermoïdes de la bouche
Dermoide der Mundhöhle
Quistes dermoides orales
Epidermoid cyst
Dermoids, oral
Dysontogenetic cyst
Teratoma
Developmental cyst
Cystic teratoma
Teratoid cyst

Excludes: Ranula
Thyroglossal duct remnant (945)
Cystic hygroma
Branchial cleft cysts or sinuses (117)
Cellulitis of the floor of the mouth

Minimal Diagnostic Criteria: An elevation of the floor of the mouth, or a slight fullness in the submental area usually eliciting the complaint of a "fullness" of the floor of the mouth which interferes with speaking or eating.

Clinical Findings: Dermoids present as sublingual masses and are located either above or below the mylohyoid muscle, usually in the midline. They may occasionally be on one side only. They may displace the tongue upward and cause difficulty in eating, speaking, and, rarely, in breathing. When below the mylohyoid muscle, they will present as pendulous submental masses beneath the mandible.

Oral dermoids generally feel "doughlike", but may feel cystic, depending on the consistency of the contents, which may vary from a cheesy, sebaceous-like substance to a more liquified material. They may contain hair, nails, keratin and may contain pus when secondarily infected.

These lesions vary in weight from one gram to several hundred grams, and may vary from a small pea-sized growth to the size of a grapefruit. Fistulous tracts may develop which open either intraorally into the floor of the mouth, or extraorally into the skin beneath the chin.

Dermoids may undergo malignant degeneration and metastasize to lymph nodes.†

Complications
I **Derived:** Interference with speaking, eating or breathing. Disfigurement. Secondary infection with or without cellulitis. Fistulae.
II **Associated:** —

Etiology: ?

Pathogenesis: Oral dermoids occur when oral epithelium is trapped during midline closure of the oral cavity, or through closure of channels or clefts which during fetal life were covered with epithelium, or through abnormal deposits of epidermis in deeper tissues.

The majority of the oral dermoids are developmental cysts derived from epithelial rests enclaved during the midline closure of the bilateral mandibular (first) and hyoid (second) branchial arches. Some of these dermoid cysts may possibly be formed by remnants of the tuberculum impar of His, which together with the lateral processes from the inner surface of each mandibular arch, form the body of the tongue and the floor of the mouth. These developments take place during the 3rd and 4th weeks of embryonic life.

The growth of these cysts may be either gradual or sudden. It is suggested that the development of oral dermoids occurs during the period of increased activity of epithelial tissues, such as sweat glands or hair which fill the lumen of the cyst. This increased growth activity coincides with the ages of 15-35 years, when most of these lesions become clinically evident.†

Related Facts
I **Sex Ratio:** M1:F1
II **Risk of Occurrence:** < 175 cases reported to date in the world literature. Of 1495 dermoid cysts at Mayo Clinic (1910-1935), 103 (6.94%) were in the head and neck and of these only 24, or 0.6%, were in the floor of the mouth.
III **Risk of Recurrence for**
   Patient's Sib: ?
   Patient's Child: ?
IV **Age of Detectability:** Clinically from birth on. Most come to clinical attention from 15-35 years.
V **Prevalence:** ? Extremely rare. There is no known predilection for race or ethnic group.

Treatment
I **Primary Prevention:** —
II **Secondary Prevention:** Either intraoral or extraoral surgical removal depending on the position of the dermoid in relation to the mylohyoid muscle. Those lying between the mylohyoid muscle and oral mucous membrane (sublingual) are best removed by an intraoral approach while those lying between the mylohyoid muscle and platysma muscle are approached through an extraoral or skin incision.
III **Other Therapy:** —

Prognosis: Excellent, if the tumor is surgically removed in its entirety. If the lesion is incompletely removed, the remaining epithelial cells may proliferate to form a new lesion.
   Dermoids may undergo malignant degeneration and may even metastasize to lymph nodes, and, therefore, should be completely removed when first diagnosed.

Detection of Carrier: —

†**Special Considerations:** A classification of oral dermoids based upon embryology and histopathology has been presented by Meyer as follows: *Dysontogenetic cysts of the floor of the mouth*
   a. *Epidermoid* - An epithelial-lined cavity surrounded by a capsule with no skin appendages; this is a simple-type lesion with embryologic ectodermal elements.
   b. *Dermoid* - An epithelial-lined cavity with 1) skin appendages of hair, hair follicles, sebaceous glands, sweat glands and 2) connective tissue and fat tissue, etc. This is a compound-type of cyst with ectodermal and mesodermal derivatives.
   c. *Teratoid* - An epithelial-lined cavity with the following elements present in the capsule: 1) skin appendages including hair follicles, sebaceous glands, keratin, etc, 2) connective tissue derivatives such as fibers, bone, muscle, blood vessels, etc and 3) respiratory and GI tissues. This is a complex cyst with derivatives of all 3 embryologic tissues of ectoderm, mesoderm and endoderm.
   Because of its long usage and presence in the literature, the term "dermoid" should be retained as a clinical term for all types of dysontogenetic or developmental cystic lesions of the floor of the mouth.

References:
Meyer, I.: Dermoid cysts (dermoids) of the floor of the mouth. Oral Surg. 8:1149, 1955.
New, G. B. and Erich, J. B.: Dermoid cysts of the head and neck. Surg. Gynecol. Obstet. 65:48, 1937.
Yoshimura, Y. et al: Congenital dermoid cyst of the sublingual region: Report of a case. J. Oral Surg. 28:366, 1970.

Contributor: **Irving Meyer**

Editor's Computerized Descriptor: Oral

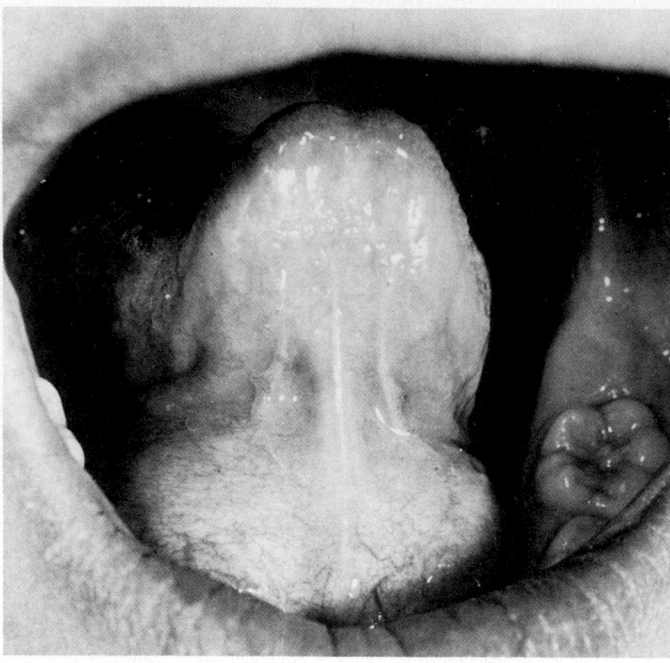

398. Sublingual oral dermoid

ORBITAL AND PERIORBITAL DERMOID CYSTS

Includes: Kystes dermoïdes orbitaires et périorbitaires
Orbitale und periorbitale Dermoidzysten
Quistes dermoides orbitarios y periorbitarios
Dermoid cysts, orbital and periorbital

Excludes: Congenital orbital cyst with microphthalmia
Dermolipoma (284)
Limbal dermoid (591)

Minimal Diagnostic Criteria: Clinical findings plus biopsy confirmation

Clinical Findings: Dermoid cysts are relatively common in the orbit and periorbit. Of those cysts occurring in the head and neck region, 50% are in the orbital region, and of these 60% are in the outer one-third of the upper lid and brow. Periorbital dermoids are also noted with relative frequency in the inner and upper angle of the orbit.

Although congenital, only 7% are noticed within the 1st year of life. Growth is often accelerated about the time of puberty.

They are smooth, tense, rounded or hourglass-shaped tumors which may vary in size from pea-size to a large orange. The overlying skin is freely movable over them, but they are often adherent to the underlying bone. Occasionally there is a depression or absence of the bone underlying them and these features are noted with xray.

Complications
I **Derived:** Inflammation and pressure changes may involve secondary adhesions to the muscles, optic nerve or other orbital contents. A large retrobulbar dermoid may cause proptosis or displacement of the eye.
II **Associated:** Rarely, malignant change may occur in the wall.

Etiology: ?

Pathogenesis: The cyst probably arises from the inclusion of a pouch of skin which becomes sequestrated in the deeper tissues during fetal life. The surface epithelium and the dura mater are originally in contact and become separated by the formation of the cranial bones; but if an adhesion occurs between the two in the region of the sutures, the surface epithelium becomes cut off and buried and may become the origin of a cystic growth.

Related Facts
I **Sex Ratio:** ?
II **Risk of Occurrence:** ?
III **Risk of Recurrence for**
    Patient's Sib: ?
    Patient's Child: ?
IV **Age of Detectability:** Infancy for only 7%; others at or after puberty
V **Prevalence:** ?

Treatment
I **Primary Prevention:** —
II **Secondary Prevention:** Complete operative extirpation
III **Other Therapy:** —

Prognosis: Good; but incomplete excision may result in formation of a granuloma within the orbit.

Detection of Carrier: —

Special Considerations: —

References:
Dayal, Y. and Hameed, S.: Periorbital dermoid. Am. J. Ophthalmol. 53:1013, 1962.
Duke-Elder, S.: System of Ophthalmology, vol. 3, pt. 2. Congenital Deformities. London: Henry Kimpton, 1964. p. 956.
Reese, A.B.: Tumors of the Eye, 3rd Ed. New York: Harper & Row, 1976, p. 416.

Contributor: **Morton E. Smith**

Editor's Computerized Descriptor: Eye

ORBITAL CEPHALOCELES

Includes: Méningocèle de l'orbite
Orbitale Zephalozele
Cefalocele orbitario
Meningocele, orbital
Encephalocele, orbital
Orbital hydrencephalocele†

Excludes: —

Minimal Diagnostic Criteria: Clinical findings plus proptosis or palpable mass.

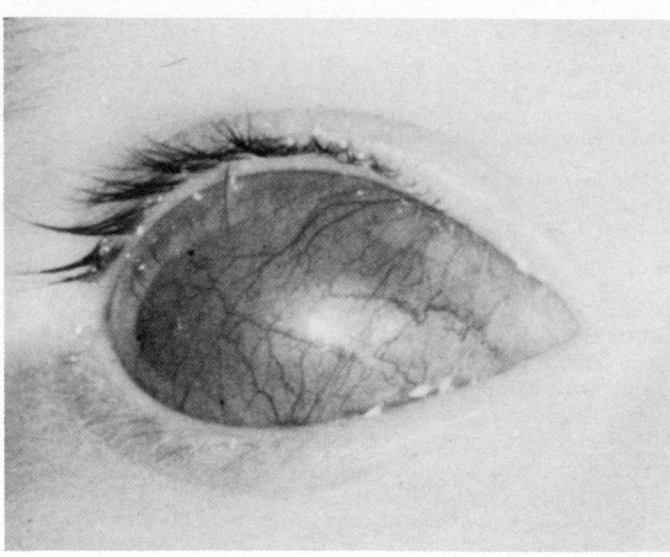

399. Encephalocele in orbit

Clinical Findings: This entity represents protrusion of cranial contents through a defect in the orbital wall. The herniations most commonly occur through the upper and medial wall of the orbit near the root of the nose and are usually unilateral. The protruding mass is fluctuant and covered with normal or purplish-red thinned skin. The eye is often displaced down and out. Communication with the cranial chamber is present when it is demonstrated that reduction of the mass produces bulging at the fontanels. Pressure may produce an oculocardiac reflex. The progressive proptosis may be pulsating, and increases upon straining, sneezing or coughing. X-rays often show the bony defect.

Complications
I **Derived:** Papilledema, optic atrophy, oculomotor palsies
II **Associated:** Associated anomalies include acrocephaly, microphthalmus, anophthalmos, colobomas, nystagmus, and atresia of the lacrimal passages.

Etiology: ?

Pathogenesis: ?

Related Facts
I **Sex Ratio:** ?
II **Risk of Occurrence:** ?
III **Risk of Recurrence for**
   Patient's Sib: ?
   Patient's Child: ?
IV **Age of Detectability:** —
V **Prevalence:** —

Treatment
I **Primary Prevention:** —
II **Secondary Prevention:** Neurosurgical repair
III **Other Therapy:** —

Prognosis: Guarded

Detection of Carrier: —

†**Special Considerations:** The protrusion is named according to the contents of the material. If the herniation contains only the meningeal membranes it is referred to as an orbital meningocele; if cerebral tissue is also herniated it is called orbital encephalocele; if cerebral fluid is included, it is an orbital hydrencephalocele.

References:
Esilä, R. et al: Unilateral orbital anterior hydroencephalocele and bilateral atresia of the lacrimal passages. Acta Ophthalmol. (Kbh.) 45:390, 1967.
Walsh, F. and Hoyt, W.: Clinical Neuroophthalmology, 3rd Ed. Baltimore: Williams and Wilkins, 1969.

Contributor: **Morton E. Smith**

————————

Editor's Computerized Descriptor: Eye

Includes: Gliome de l'orbite
Glioma opticum
Glioma orbitario
Optic nerve glioma

Excludes: —

Minimal Diagnostic Criteria: Optic atrophy or papilledema, unilateral proptosis in patient less than 15 years of age, supported by typical x-ray findings.

Clinical Findings: These tumors usually occur in the 1st decade of life and arise from astrocytes or spongioblasts of the optic nerve, chiasm or optic tract. Intraorbital gliomas occur early and precede the onset of proptosis. The proptosis is straight ahead, nonpulsating and progressive. There is resistance to retrodisplacement of the globe. Ocular motility is usually not restricted, but diplopia may be a complaint in older children. About two-thirds of cases show optic atrophy while a third show papilledema. There may also be retinal hemorrhages or exudates. Intracranial tumors are characterized by visual loss and visual field defects. Radiographic enlargement of the optic foramen is present in approximately 85% of orbitocranial lesions. A pear-shaped anterior extension of the sella may be present with involvement of the chiasm. About 20% of gliomas occur with neurofibromatosis or are associated at least with significant numbers of café-au-lait spots.

Complications
I   **Derived:** Blindness (partial or total), cosmetic defect, death
II **Associated:** Neurofibromatosis

Etiology: ?

Pathogenesis: ?

Related Facts
I   **Sex Ratio:** ?
II **Risk of Occurrence:** ?
III **Risk of Recurrence for**
    Patient's Sib: ?
    Patient's Child: ?
IV **Age of Detectability:** First 2 decades of life
V   **Prevalence:** ?

Treatment
I   **Primary Prevention:** —
II **Secondary Prevention:** Treatment consists of surgical excision when possible. Radiotherapy should be used following incomplete surgical removal or in cases of surgical inaccessibility, eg chiasmal or tract invasion. Recent reports support the approach that no therapy at all may be warranted in some cases.
III **Other Therapy:** —

Prognosis: Prognosis is good if the tumor is confined to 1 nerve and if excision is complete. Some untreated cases may extend into cranium and become fatal.

Detection of Carrier: —

Special Considerations: —

References:
Condon, J.R. and Rose, F.C.: Optic nerve glioma. Br. J. Ophthalmol. 51:703, 1967.
Glazer, J. et al: Visual morbidity with chiasmal glioma. Arch. Ophthalmol. 85:3, 1971.
Hovland, K.R. and Ellis, P.P.: Hemorrhagic glaucoma with optic nerve glioma. Arch. Ophthalmol. 75:806, 1966.
Hoyt, W. and Baghdassarian, S.: Optic glioma of childhood. Br. J. Ophthalmol. 53:793, 1969.
Lloyd, L.: Gliomas of optic nerve and chiasm in childhood. Trans. Am. Ophthalmol. Soc. 71:488, 1973.
Reese, A.B.: Tumors of the Eye, 3rd. Ed. New York: Harper & Row, 1976.
Saran, N. and Winter, F.C.: Bilateral gliomas of the optic discs associated with neurofibromatosis. Am. J. Ophthalmol. (Suppl.) 64:607, 1967.
Udvarhelyi, G.B. et al: Gliomas of the optic nerve and chiasm in children: An unusual series of cases. Clin. Neurosurg. 13:204, 1965.
Walsh, F. and Hoyt, W.: Clinical Neuroophthalmology, 3rd Ed. Baltimore: Williams & Wilkins, 1969.

Contributor: **Morton E. Smith**

Editor's Computerized Descriptors: Vision, Eye, Skin, Skel., Nerve

ORBITAL HEMANGIOMA

Includes: Hémangiome de l'orbite
Hämangiom der orbita
Hemangioma de la órbita
Hemangioma of lids and orbit

Excludes: Orbital lymphangioma (765)

Minimal Diagnostic Criteria: Hemangioma of eye or adnexa

Clinical Findings: These are the most common orbital tumors in children. Any portion of the eye or adnexa may be involved. They present as a soft compressible purplish mass often palpable through the lids or conjuctiva. The child may have unilateral exophthalmos. Visual acuity may be unaltered or the tumor may be so extensive as to cause papilledema, retinal hemorrhage and reduced vision.

Complications
I   **Derived:** Visual defects secondary to papilledema; retinal hemorrhages. The lid may be so involved that it will cover the eye and amblyopia may result.
II **Associated:** Occasionally there are hemangiomas elsewhere in the body, or the hemangioma of the orbit may actually be part of a Sturge-Weber syndrome or Hippel-Lindau syndrome.

Etiology: ?

Pathogenesis: The lesion is considered to be a congenital hamartoma.

Related Facts
I   **Sex Ratio:** M?:F?
II   **Risk of Occurrence:** ? Not rare
III **Risk of Recurrence for**
     Patient's Sib: ?
     Patient's Child: ?
IV **Age of Detectability:** At birth
V   **Prevalence:** ? Not rare

Treatment
I   **Primary Prevention:** —
II   **Secondary Prevention:** The overwhelming majority of these lesions will spontaneously subside within the 1st few years of life. If a lesion is so extensive to produce jeopardy to the eye (papilledema, optic nerve compression, covering of the eye, etc), then intervention is necessary. Recent reports show that treatment with high doses of steroids may be of great benefit in early cases. Surgery is at times necessary.
III **Other Therapy:** —

Prognosis: Normal for life and intelligence; good for vision

Detection of Carrier: —

Special Considerations: —

References:
de Venecia, G. and Lobeck, C.C.: Successful treatment of eyelid hemangioma with prednisone. Arch. Ophthalmol. 84:98, 1970.
Henderson, J.W.: Orbital Tumors. Philadelphia: W.B. Saunders, 1973.
Reese, A.B.: Tumors of the Eye, 3rd Ed. New York: Harper & Row, 1976.

Contributor: **Morton E. Smith**

Editor's Computerized Descriptors: Vision, Eye

ORBITAL LYMPHANGIOMA

Includes: Lymphangiome de l'orbite
Orbitales Lymphangiom
Linfangioma orbitario
Capillary lymphangiomas of orbit
Cavernous lymphangiomas of orbit
Cystic lymphangiomas of orbit
Ocular lymphangioma

Excludes: Orbital hemangioma (764)
Elephantiasis

Minimal Diagnostic Criteria: Biopsy confirmation of the lesion reveals a tumor composed of variable-sized thin-walled channels lined with endothelium and filled with proteinaceous material consistent with lymph.

Clinical Findings: These lesions are benign and usually congenital although they may first present at any age. They are soft, cystic, fluctuant, compressible tumors which are present in the orbit, within the lids or beneath the conjunctiva. A bluish-purple color is common. The eye may be proptosed and ocular motility may be impaired. It is not uncommon to find other lymphangiomas in nearby locations, eg nasal cavity, oropharynx, etc. It is slowly progressive. Xrays may show asymmetry if the lymphangioma involves much of 1 side of the face. Orbital lymphangioma may show enlargement of the orbit by xray.

Complications
I   **Derived:** Repeated hemorrhage within the tumor is not uncommon. Cellulitis, either with or without a concurrent URI is another characteristic complication.
II **Associated:** Lymphangiomas in other areas, eg oropharynx, may produce symptoms relevant to that area.

Etiology: ?

Pathogenesis: ?

Related Facts
I   **Sex Ratio:** ?
II   **Risk of Occurrence:** ?
III **Risk of Recurrence for**
     Patient's Sib: ?
     Patient's Child: ?
IV **Age of Detectability:** ?
V   **Prevalence:** 1 in 33,000; represents a small percentage of causes of unilateral exophthalmos; rarer than hemangiomas.

Treatment
I   **Primary Prevention:** —
II   **Secondary Prevention:** Surgical extirpation. Recurrences are common with incomplete removal, and repeated surgical excisions with appropriate plastic repair are often necessary.
III **Other Therapy:** Sclerosing solutions and x-ray therapy are seldom indicated.

Prognosis: Prognosis for cure is poor unless the lesion is small enough to be completely excised. The absence of any middle-aged or elderly patients still undergoing treatment suggests that the progression of these lesions ceases early in childhood.

Detection of Carrier: —

Special Considerations: —

References:
Jones, I.S. Lymphangiomas of the ocular adnexa: An analysis of 62 cases. Trans. Am. Ophthalmol. Soc. 57:602, 1959.
Reese, A.B.: Tumors of the Eye, 3rd Ed. New York: Harper & Row, 1976.

Contributor: **Morton E. Smith**

ORIGIN OF LEFT PULMONARY ARTERY FROM RIGHT PULMONARY ARTERY

Includes: Origine de l'artère pulmonaire gauche dans l'artère pulmonaire droite
Atypischer Ursprung der linken Pulmonalarterie von der rechten a. pulmonalis
Origen de la arteria pulmonar izquierda en la arteria pulmonar derecha
Pulmonary vascular sling
Aberrant left pulmonary artery

Excludes: Other vascular rings

Minimal Diagnostic Criteria: An ovid-shaped density on the lateral chest film between the lower trachea and esophagus, causing an anterior indentation on the barium-filled esophagus, is diagnostic. A pulmonary arteriogram is confirmatory.

Clinical Findings: The pathologic anatomy of this defect shows the main pulmonary artery arising in normal fashion and coursing undivided toward the right. At a point just anterior and to the right of the carina of the trachea, the left pulmonary artery arises from the posterior aspect of the right pulmonary artery. The left pulmonary artery courses toward the left lung passing over the right main stem bronchus posterior to the trachea (but anterior to the esophagus) to the left lung. It is the only vascular anomaly that passes between the trachea and the esophagus. This left pulmonary artery may compress the tracheobronchial tree as it crosses the right bronchus (most often and most severely involved), as it passes behind the trachea, or rarely, as it crosses the left bronchus. It may also obstruct the esophagus and sometimes cause choking or regurgitation in these infants.

More than 90% of the patients present with severe symptoms, the most common being wheezing or stridor, or both. These infants may be misdiagnosed as having asthma, tracheobronchial foreign body, primary tracheal or laryngeal abnormalities or aortic arch vascular rings. The stridor is usually more inspiratory than expiratory, which helps to differentiate it from the other vascular rings. Some patients have only dyspnea, and mild cyanosis which may be intermittent. These patients' clinical symptoms resemble those with congenital lobar emphysema or asthma. Half of the reported patients had acute episodes of dyspnea and cyanosis, or severe exacerbations of respiratory obstruction of short duration. Many of these episodes are associated with unconsciousness or convulsions, and death may occur. The symptoms may be accelerated during feeding. Respiratory infections are not a prominent part of the clinical picture.

The diagnosis can be supported in chest roentgenograms with a barium-filled esophagus. The characteristic finding is an indentation on the left lateral and the anterior wall of the esophagus near the level of the tracheal bifurcation. This may be seen only in lateral view. The esophageal course may appear entirely normal. The definitive diagnosis is made by selective angiocardiography from the right ventricle, or, preferably, the main pulmonary artery. Bronchography will not establish this diagnosis.

Complications
I   **Derived:** Obstructive emphysema or atelectasis of that part of the lung supplied by a compressed bronchus. Death from hypoxia due to severe obstruction of the trachea. Narrowing or stenosis of the trachea or bronchus may occur other than at the site of vessel compression.
II **Associated:** Occasionally (about 10%), complete tracheal rings may occur. The right upper lobe bronchus may arise

from the trachea rather than from the right main bronchus (bronchus suis). Rarely a single-lobed lung may occur on one side. Eighteen of the 41 cases reported in the literature had no associated intracardiac defect. Aside from cardiovascular and respiratory tract anomalies, this anomaly has been associated with imperforate anus, diaphragmatic hernia, absent gallbladder, partial malrotation of the intestines, asplenia, Hirschsprung disease, cleft lip and palate, absent left lobe of the thyroid, thymic rest, hemivertebrae, biliary atresia, forearm anomalies and chromosome 21 trisomy.

Etiology: ?

Pathogenesis: The left 6th arch has developed as evidenced by the presence of a ductus arteriosus or its remnant in the normal position. The left pulmonary artery has apparently failed to meet the left lung normally. Explanations for this vary. One theory is that the anomalous artery was late in developing or left lung development was accelerated, upsetting the timing and not allowing them to meet in the usual manner. Another theory is that the left pulmonary artery is not formed from the 6th arch but rather from collateral vessels in the fetal mediastinal plexus.

Related Facts
I   **Sex Ratio:** Ml:Fl
II   **Risk of Occurrence:** ?
III **Risk of Recurrence for**
      Patient's Sib: ?
      Patient's Child: ?
IV   **Age of Detectability:** From birth
V   **Prevalence:** ?

Treatment
I   **Primary Prevention:** —
II   **Secondary Prevention:** Division of the aberrant vessel with reanastomosis to the main pulmonary artery so the left pulmonary artery is anterior to the trachea.
III **Other Therapy:** Good respiratory toilet in symptomatic cases prior to definitive surgery

Prognosis: Poor in severe cases if surgery is not done. Most of those patients die in the 1st year of life. Some children are only mildly symptomatic and may not require surgery. Successful therapy should establish a normal prognosis in the absence of other anomalies.

Detection of Carrier: —

Special Considerations: —

References:
Clarkson, P.M. et al: Aberrant left pulmonary artery. Am. J. Dis. Child. 113:373, 1967.
Nora, J.J. and McNamara, D.G.: Vascular rings and related anomalies. In Watson, H. (ed.): Paediatric Cardiology. St. Louis: C.V. Mosby Co., 1968, p. 233.
Tan, P.M. et al: Aberrant left pulmonary artery. Br. Heart J. 30:110, 1968.

Contributors: **Barbara J. Bourland**
                    Dan G. McNamara

Editor's Computerized Descriptors: Resp., GI., CV.

ORIGIN OF PULMONARY ARTERY FROM ASCENDING AORTA

Includes: Artère pulmonaire anormale partie de l'aorte ascendante
Ursprung des Pulmonalarterie von der Aorta ascendens
Origen de la arteria pulmonar en la aorta ascendente
Origin of one pulmonary artery from ascending aorta, anterior or posterior, right or left
Hemitruncus arteriosus
Cases of congenital origin of either the right or left pulmonary artery in which the affected lung in actual fact is supplied by a vessel arising from the ascending aorta proximal to the take-off of the first (brachio) cephalic vessel with or without other cardiac defects.

Excludes: Those cases of congenital absence of right or left pulmonary artery in which the affected lung is supplied either by multiple bronchial-arterial collateral vessels or by a patent ductus arteriosus

Minimal Diagnostic Criteria: Diagnosis must be established by cardiac catheterization with angiography in the aortic root, showing a pulmonary artery arising from the ascending aorta.

Clinical Findings: Origin of a pulmonary artery from the ascending aorta may occur either on the right or left side. Those on the right tend to be posterior in origin and those on the left anterior. Abnormal origin of 1 of the pulmonary arteries is usually, not always, contralateral to the aortic arch. The branching pattern of the other aortic arch vessels is usually normal for the situs of the arch.

Symptomatology follows that of a large left-to-right shunt, usually occurring in early infancy. Heart failure is common while pulmonary resistances allow a large flow. Most cases have elevated pressures in both pulmonary arteries. If pulmonary resistances increase, as is usual in untreated cases, pulmonary flow will decrease and eventually cyanosis and hemoptysis will occur with pulmonary vascular obstructive disease.

The ECG will usually reveal biventricular hypertrophy in early cases, evolving to right ventricular hypertrophy if pulmonary vascular obstructive disease develops.

Roentgenograms of the chest may show increased vascularity and cardiomegaly in cases with large left-to-right shunts. Progressive pulmonary vascular obstruction results in decreased heart size and vascularity.†

Radioactive isotopes injected intravenously will result in no uptake in the affected side.

Complications
I   **Derived:** Congestive heart failure in cases with large pulmonary blood flow. Hypoxia and hemoptysis resulting from pulmonary vascular obstructive disease.
II   **Associated:** If the defect is associated with tetralogy of Fallot, ventricular septal defect or patent ductus arteriosus, additional complications of those defects may be present.

Etiology: ? Presumably multifactorial inheritance

Pathogenesis: Anterior type: In these cases the anomalous pulmonary artery is made up of the left 4th arch (in cases with a right aortic arch), a segment of the dorsal aorta, the distal portion of the left 6th arch, and the left embryonic pulmonary artery. Presumably, in such cases, the segment of the left dorsal aorta between the 6th arch and the 7th intersegmental artery is interrupted, resulting in a left subclavian artery arising anomalously from the descending aorta.

Posterior type: The artery is made up of the proximal portion of the 6th arch and the embryonic pulmonary artery. Apparently, at the time of partitioning of the truncus and truncoaortic sac, it was left "stranded." It may therefore be expected to be located always on the right side in situs solitus individuals with either a right or left aortic arch.

Related Facts
I   **Sex Ratio:**   M1:F1
II **Risk of Occurrence:** ?
III **Risk of Recurrence for**
    Patient's Sib: Predicted Risk - < 1 in 100; Empiric Risk ?
    Patient's Child: Predicted Risk - < 1 in 100; Empiric Risk ?
IV **Age of Detectability:** Infancy
V   **Prevalence:** ? Most commonly the right pulmonary artery is anomalous. With tetralogy of Fallot the left pulmonary artery is more commonly anomalous, regardless of situs of aortic arch.

Treatment
I   **Primary Prevention:** —
II **Secondary Prevention:** Surgical anastomosis of the anomalous artery to the main pulmonary trunk either primarily or with a prosthetic graft has been successful and must be undertaken early to avoid pulmonary vascular obstructive disease. Ligation and division of an associated patent ductus arteriosus on the unaffected side is recommended. If associated with tetralogy of Fallot repair of this defect must also be undertaken.
III **Other Therapy:** —

Prognosis: If diagnosis and surgical correction are undertaken early, prognosis, according to recent reports, is good.

Detection of Carrier: —

†**Special Considerations:** Pulmonary function studies may show that the involved lung contributes very little, if any, to gas exchange, although ventilation is normal.

References:
Cumming, G.R. et al: Aortic origin of the right pulmonary artery. Am. J. Cardiol. 30:674, 1972.
Keane, J.F. et al: Anomalous origin of one pulmonary artery from the ascending aorta. Circulation 50:588, 1974.
Netter, F.H.: The Ciba Collection of Medical Illustrations. Vol. 5. The Heart. Ciba Publications Dept., New Jersey, 1969, p. 162.

Contributor: **Donald A. Riopel**

Editor's Computerized Descriptors: Resp., CV.

ORIGIN OF PULMONARY ARTERY FROM DUCTUS ARTERIOSUS

Includes: Artère pulmonaire anormale partie du canal artériel
Abgang des Pulmonalarterie von Ductus Botalli
Origen de la arteria pulmonar en el conducto arterioso
Origin of a pulmonary artery from the ipsilateral (to aortic arch) ductus arteriosus
Origin of a pulmonary artery from the contralateral (to aortic arch) ductus arteriosus
Congenital absence of one pulmonary artery with blood supplied to the affected lung by means of a ductus arteriosus

Excludes: Origin of pulmonary artery from ascending aorta (767)
Congenital absence of right or left pulmonary artery with blood supplied to the affected lung by multiple collateral channels other than the ductus arteriosus

Minimal Diagnostic Criteria: Discrepancy in the vascular pattern between the 2 lungs may suggest the diagnosis, particularly in patients in whom the symptoms and signs suggest presence of tetralogy of Fallot. Aortic angiography is the procedure of choice in establishing the diagnosis.

Clinical Findings: The distal pulmonary artery receives its blood supply not from the pulmonary trunk but from a ductus arteriosus. Such a ductus arteriosus originates from the aortic arch if the arch is on the same side, or from the innominate artery if the aortic arch is on the opposite side. There is a tendency for the ductus arteriosus to close at least partially, and thus, as a rule, a large left-to-right shunt is not present. The anomaly is uncommon as an isolated lesion. The clinical findings are largely determined by other cardiovascular anomalies, usually some form of tetralogy of Fallot. Although it most commonly occurs on the left, there have been cases reported on the right side. Recently a case was reported of both pulmonary arteries arising from a normally septated truncus, the right originating from the aorta and the left pulmonary artery from a ductus arteriosus. If no associated lesions are present, symptoms and signs depend on the magnitude of the left-to-right shunt. If the shunt is small, or if the blood supply to the affected lung is actually decreased, patients are asymptomatic. Xrays of the chest may show discrepancy in the vascularity of the lung fields. If so, the affected lung generally shows a reduced vascular pattern. The unaffected side may show hypervascularity if no significant intracardiac right-to-left shunt is present, such as is seen in cases associated with various forms of tetralogy of Fallot. The lung on the affected side may be smaller than normal. ECG findings are usually determined by associated cardiovascular defects and may be normal if the anomaly occurs as an isolated lesion.

    Pulmonary function tests may show that the involved lung participates very little, if any, in oxygen exchange, although ventilation is normal.

Complications
I   **Derived:** In the unusual case where the lesion is isolated and the ductus arteriosus remains widely patent causing a large left-to-right shunt, congestive heart failure and respiratory infections may occur.
II **Associated:** Symptoms of additional lesions such as tetralogy of Fallot may be present.

Etiology: Presumably multifactorial inheritance

Pathogenesis: In both forms, the anomaly appears to be due to early obliteration and disappearance of the proximal portion of one or the other 6th arch. The corresponding embryonic pulmonary artery, therefore, will be supplied instead by the distal 6th arch segment, ie the ductus arteriosus. In some cases it may be difficult to distinguish the precise origin of the anomalous vessel, ie cases of origin of the pulmonary artery from the ascending aorta may occur so close to the innominate artery that a ductal origin is implicated, especially if the origin of the vessel has a narrow caliber.

Related Facts
I **Sex Ratio:** M1:F1
II **Risk of Occurrence:** ?
III **Risk of Recurrence for**
  Patient's Sib: ?
  Patient's Child: ?
IV **Age of Detectability:** Depends largely on associated lesions. Can be detected at birth.
V **Prevalence:** ?

Treatment
I **Primary Prevention:** —
II **Secondary Prevention:** Surgery might be considered in those cases where the lesion is isolated and a large left-to-right shunt is present. Anastomosis of the anomalous vessel to the pulmonary trunk may be attempted. In patients who in addition, however, have tetralogy of Fallot, the anomalous vessel may represent the main pulmonary blood supply. Then no such surgical procedure is indicated until complete correction of the tetralogy is accomplished.
III **Other Therapy:** —

Prognosis: Depends largely on associated cardiovascular anomalies. If the anomaly is the sole cardiovascular defect, prognosis depends on the magnitude of any left-to-right shunt and on the pulmonary arteriolar resistance in the affected lung.

Detection of Carrier: —

Special Considerations: —

References:
Bricker, D.L. et al: Anomalous aortic origin of the right and left pulmonary arteries in a normally septated truncus arteriosus. Chest 68:591, 1975.
Netter, F.H.: The Ciba Collection of Medical Illustrations. Vol. 5. The Heart. Ciba Publications Department, New Jersey, 1969, p. 162.
Pool, P.E. et al: Congenital unilateral absence of a pulmonary artery. Am. J. Cardiol. 10:706, 1962.
Wagenvoort, C.A. et al: Origin of right pulmonary artery from ascending aorta. Circulation 23:84, 1961.

Contributor: **Donald A. Riopel**

Editor's Computerized Descriptors: Resp., CV.

ORO-CRANIO-DIGITAL SYNDROME

Includes: Dysostose cranio-oculo-digitale
Orokraniodigitales Syndrom
Síndrome oro-cráneo-digital

Excludes: Oto-palato-digital syndrome (786)
Cranio-oculo-dental syndrome (229)
Oculo-dento-osseus dysplasia (737)
Oro-facio-digital syndrome I (770)

Minimal Diagnostic Criteria: For an isolated case: bilateral or unilateral cleft lip, cleft palate, or occult cleft of the lip; microcephaly; anomaly of the thumbs such as hypoplasia, distal placement or inflexibility; anomaly of the toes such as mediodorsal curvature or syndactyly. Fewer criteria apparently are needed once the syndrome is recognized in a sibship.

Clinical Findings:
Mediodorsal curvature of the 4th toes	4/5
Minimal syndactyly of the 2nd and 3rd toes	4/5
Growth retardation	3/5
Microcephaly	3/5
Hypoplasia and inflexibility of thumbs	3/5
Low birthweight	3/5
Dislocation and shortening of radii	2/5
Cleft lip or palate	2/5
Mental retardation	1/5
Occult cleft lip	1/5

Complications
I **Derived:** Difficulty in running
II **Associated:** —

Etiology: Autosomal recessive

Pathogenesis: ?

Related Facts
I **Sex Ratio:** M2:F3 in one sibship
II **Risk of Occurrence:** One sibship reported
III **Risk of Recurrence for**
  Patient's Sib: 1 in 4 (25%) for each offspring to be affected
  Patient's Child: Not increased unless mate is carrier or homozygote
IV **Age of Detectability:** Neonatal by clinical findings
V **Prevalence:** One sibship reported

Treatment
I **Primary Prevention:** Genetic counseling
II **Secondary Prevention:** Plastic and orthopedic operative procedures
III **Other Therapy:** Speech correction, physical therapy

Prognosis: Probably normal life expectancy

Detection of Carrier: ? Parents of the one reported sibship were phenotypically normal.

Special Considerations: —

References:
Juberg, R. C. and Hayward, J. R.: A new familial syndrome of oral, cranial, and digital anomalies. J. Pediatr. 74:755, 1969.

Contributor: **Richard C. Juberg**

Editor's Computerized Descriptors: Face, Oral, Skel., Nerve

ORO-FACIO-DIGITAL SYNDROME I

Includes: Syndrome oro-facio-digital I
Oro-fazio-digitales Syndrom I
Síndrome oro-facio-digital I
OFD I syndrome
Papillon-Léage and Psaume syndrome
Gorlin-Psaume syndrome
Orodigitofacial dysostosis

Excludes: Oro-facio-digital syndrome II (771)

Minimal Diagnostic Criteria: Patient should be female (except in the case of Klinefelter syndrome). To make diagnosis, patient should have multiple hyperplastic frenula.

Clinical Findings: Hyperplastic frenula (ca 100%), tongue cleft into two or more lobes (ca 100%), hamartoma of tongue (50%), ankyloglossia (30%), grooved anterior alveolar process of mandible (60%), agenesis of lower lateral incisor teeth (50%), lateral grooving of maxillary alveolar process (90%), cleft palate (80%), median cleft of upper lip (40%), broad nasal root (95%), hypoplasia of malar bone (75%), clinodactyly, brachydactyly or syndactyly (90%), mental retardation (? %), evanescent facial milia (100%), dryness or alopecia of scalp (65%).

Complications
I   **Derived:** —
II **Associated:** —

Etiology: X-linked dominant gene, lethal in male; McK *31120

Pathogenesis: ?

Related Facts
I   **Sex Ratio:** M0:F1
II   **Risk of Occurrence:** ?
III **Risk of Recurrence for**
    Patient's Sib: 50% if a sister; 0 if a brother. (If male receives mutant gene from mother, pregnancy is not completed.)
    Patient's Child: 50% if a daughter; 0 if a son. Hence there is a M1:F2 ratio in all offspring of affected females. The overall ratio of affected to unaffected offspring of affected mothers is 1:2
IV **Age of Detectability:** At birth from phenotype
V   **Prevalence:** Possibly 1 in 50,000 population

Treatment
I   **Primary Prevention:** Genetic counseling
II **Secondary Prevention:** —
III **Other Therapy:** —

Prognosis: Normal life span with average IQ about 70 and functional limitations primarily due to mental retardation

Detection of Carrier: Carrier of mutant gene should manifest phenotype.

Special Considerations: —

References:
Fuhrmann, W. et al: Das oro-facio-digitale Syndrom: Zugleich eine Diskussion der Erbgänge mit geschlechtsbegrenztem Letaleffekt. Humangenetik 2:133, 1966.
Gorlin, R. J.: The oral-facial-digital (OFD) syndrome. Cutis 4:1345, 1968.
Gorlin, R. J. and Psaume, J.: Orodigitofacial dysostosis- a new syndrome, a study of 22 cases. J. Pediatr. 61:520, 1962.

Contributor: **Robert J. Gorlin**

Editor's Computerized Descriptors: Face, Oral, Teeth, Nose, Skin, Hair, Skel.

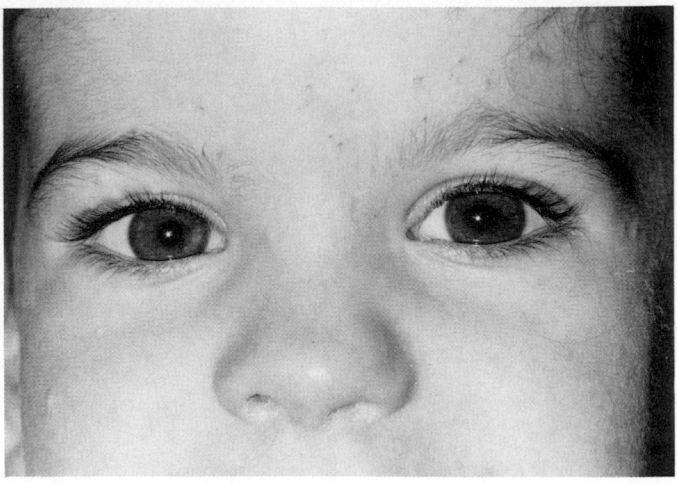

400. Note milia, dystopia canthorum, and asymmetric alar cartilages

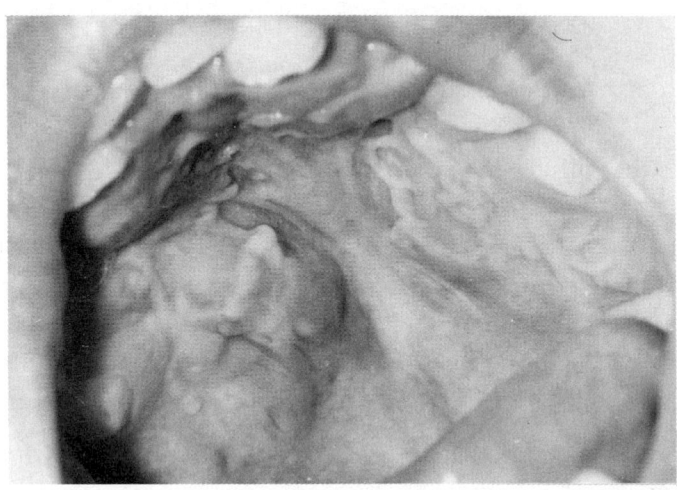

401. Note bizarre cleft palate

ORO-FACIO-DIGITAL SYNDROME II

Includes: Syndrome de Mohr
Mohr-Syndrom
Síndrome de Mohr
OFD II syndrome
Mohr syndrome

Excludes: Oro-facio-digital syndrome I (770)

Minimal Diagnostic Criteria: Diagnosis of this syndrome can be made only upon clinical grounds by the association of the below mentioned oral, facial and digital anomalies. This syndrome can be distinguished from OFD I by the occurrence of the former in males, its autosomal recessive inheritance, the bilateral polysyndactyly of the halluces, a wide rather than hypoplastic nasal tip, absence of the central rather than the lateral incisors and the absence of several features which are typical of OFD I such as thick fibrous bands clefting the alveolar ridge, and skin and hair abnormalities.

Clinical Findings: This syndrome consists of oral, facial and digital malformations. These include a lobate tongue with nodules at the bases of the clefts, midline clefts of the lip, high-arched or cleft palate, hypertrophied frenula, absent central incisors, broad nasal root, broad bifid nasal tip, dystopia canthorum, hypoplasia of the body of the mandible, bilateral polysyndactyly of the halluces, brachydactyly, syndactyly, clinodactyly or polydactyly. Conductive hearing loss associated with a malformed incus may be a feature.

Radiographs may reveal hypoplasia of the zygomatic arch and maxilla, absence of central incisors and a midline maxillary cleft, hypoplasia of the body of the mandible, brachydactyly, clinodactyly and bilateral polysyndactyly of the halluces associated with short, broad naviculars and first metatarsals. The medial cuneiform bones may be broad or duplicated. Audiograms may reveal a bilateral conductive hearing deficit. Laboratory studies are normal.

Complications
I **Derived:** Recurrent otitis media may occur secondary to the cleft palate.
II **Associated:** —

Etiology: The occurrence of this syndrome in sibs of both sexes with unaffected parents and the presence of consanguinity in one family suggest an autosomal recessive mutant gene.† McK *25210

Pathogenesis: ?

Related Facts
I **Sex Ratio:** M1:F1
II **Risk of Occurrence:** ?
III **Risk of Recurrence for**
    Patient's Sib: If autosomal recessive, 1 in 4 (25%) for each sib
    Patient's Child: Not increased unless mate is heterozygote or homozygote.
IV **Age of Detectability:** At birth by clinical features
V **Prevalence:** ?

Treatment
I **Primary Prevention:** Genetic counseling
II **Secondary Prevention:** Repair of cleft lip and palate, release of hypertrophied frenulae, amputation of extra halluces. A hearing aid if conductive hearing loss is present. Surgery to correct the middle ear anomaly might be feasible in some instances.
III **Other Therapy:** —

Prognosis: For life: No effect on life span. The Mohr syndrome is a nonprogressive birth defect. For intelligence: No effect upon intelligence. For function: Hearing loss may interfere with func-

tion. Oral anomalies may interfere with speech.

Detection of Carrier: Parents of affected persons

†Special Considerations: The clinical distinction between OFD I, which is inherited as an X-linked or sex-limited autosomal dominant trait and the Mohr syndrome (OFD II) which is inherited as an autosomal recessive trait, has important implications in genetic counseling.

References:
Gorlin, R. J.: The oral-facial-digital (OFD) syndrome. Cutis 4:1345, 1968.
Rimoin, D. L. and Edgerton, M. T.: Genetic and clinical heterogeneity in the oral-facial-digital syndromes. J. Pediatr. 71:94, 1967.

Contributor: **David L. Rimoin**

Editor's Computerized Descriptors: Hearing, Ear, Face, Oral, Teeth, Nose, Skel.

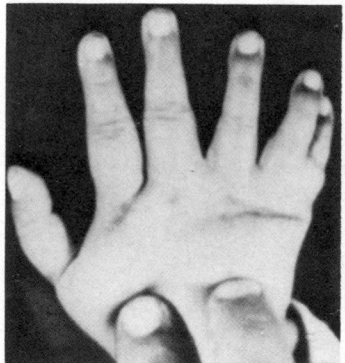 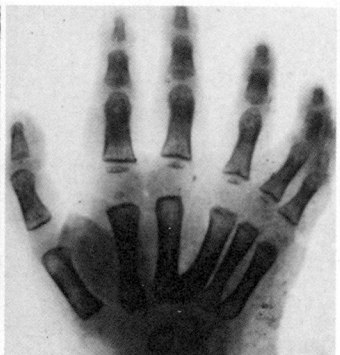

402. Note postaxial polydactyly

OROTICACIDURIA

Includes: Oroticacidurie

Excludes: Acquired oroticaciduria produced by 6- azauridine

Minimal Diagnostic Criteria: The diagnosis is suggested by megaloblastic anemia unresponsive to B_{12} or folic acid and confirmed by the documentation of orotic acid in large amounts in the urine. Erythrocytes and fibroblasts in cell culture are deficient in both orotidylic pyrophosphorylase and orotidylic decarboxylase.

Clinical Findings: Patients with oroticaciduria have a megaloblastic anemia which is unresponsive to treatment with B_{12} or folic acid. They also have retardation in growth. They excrete large amounts of orotic acid in the urine and may present with crystalluria. One patient has been reported with only a deficiency of orotidylic decarboxylase (OMP-DC) with an increased activity of orotidylic pyrophosphorylase (OMP-PP). Two surviving patients are mentally retarded.

Complications
I   **Derived:** The first patient described died of generalized varicella, suggesting that resistance to infectious disease may be abnormal.
II **Associated:** —

Etiology: Autosomal recessive biochemical defect; McK *25890, *25892

Pathogenesis: Deficiency of OMP-PP and OMP-DC suggests gene linkage or that one defect is secondary. 5-Azaorotic acid or dihydroorotic acid induces higher levels of both enzymes, thus providing evidence for posttranslational change. The pathogenesis of the clinical findings is unknown.

Related Facts
I   **Sex Ratio:** All of the patients described have been male.
II **Risk of Occurrence:** ?
III **Risk of Recurrence for**
    Patient's Sib: 1 in 4 (25%) for each offspring to be affected
    Patient's Child: Not increased unless mated to heterozygote.
IV **Age of Detectability:** Presumably at birth by enzyme assay of erythrocytes or fibroblasts.
V   **Prevalence:** ?

Treatment
I   **Primary Prevention:** Genetic counseling
II **Secondary Prevention:** Partial remissions have been observed with glucocorticoid administration. Replacement therapy with a mixture of yeast nucleotides led to a complete remission and a decrease in urinary orotic acid. This preparation was poorly tolerated. Surviving patients are being successfully maintained on oral uridine therapy.
III **Other Therapy:** —

Prognosis: ?

Detection of Carrier: Assay of OMP-DC in the erythrocyte or fibroblast.

Special Considerations: —

References:
Smith, L.H., Jr. et al: Hereditary orotic aciduria. In Stanbury, J.B. et al (eds.): The Metabolic Basis of Inherited Disease. 3rd Ed. McGraw-Hill:New York, 1972, p. 1003.

Contributor: **William L. Nyhan**

Editor's Computerized Descriptor: —

OSSICLE AND MIDDLE EAR MALFORMATIONS

Includes: Malformations des osselets et de l'oreille moyenne
Fehlbildungen von Gehörknöchelchen und Mittelohr
Malformaciones de los huesesillos auriculares y del oído medio
Vascular malformations of middle ear
Middle ear malformations with hearing loss
Middle ear and ossicle malformations
Nerve malformations of middle ear

Excludes: Middle ear malformations associated with or found in conjunction with other anomalies of the external and internal ear or other branchial derivatives, ie severe atresia or agenesis of the external auricle and canal

Minimal Diagnostic Criteria: If malformation involves the ossicular conductive mechanism, there will be a hearing loss of a conductive nature observed since birth or early childhood. If malformation does not involve the conductive mechanism, there may be no signs or symptoms, but one may observe the defects during surgery for unrelated subsequent pathology.

Clinical Findings: Malformations of the middle ear may be functionally significant in that a conductive hearing impairment may cause a serious social handicap. Secondly, many of these malformations may not impair hearing, but are of significance from the standpoint of surgical anatomy. These asymptomatic malformations may first be observed only incidentally after a normal tympanic membrane has been elevated for the purpose of correcting a hearing loss produced by a progressive pathologic process such as otosclerosis.

Middle ear malformations with hearing loss: Nonfluctuating hearing impairment since birth. The tympanic membrane and external ear may be normal, but one may occasionally see ossicular malarrangement behind a transparent normal tympanic membrane. The hearing loss is conductive in nature unless associated with a congenital or acquired cochlear deficit. Usually, both air and bone conduction curves are typically flat through the speech frequencies but this is not an infallible diagnostic sign. The conductive hearing impairment is usually greater than is seen associated with common inflammatory complications.

Middle ear malformations with no hearing loss attributable to the malformation: These defects are silent until concomitant disease causes sufficient hearing impairment to justify surgery. The defect is then unexpectedly discovered during operative exploration. X-ray evidence of ossicular malformation may be obtained through polytomographic technique. Interpretation of films must be done by one skilled in the study of these anatomic shadows. Even then, definitive description is gross and can be misleading. Exploratory tympanotomy with direct visualization of the middle ear is necessary for appraisal of the defect.

Complications
I   **Derived:** Due to hearing impairment, delayed or slow mental development may occur. Severity is proportional to hearing impairment.
II **Associated:** Defects of other derivatives of the same branchial arches (I and II).

Etiology: ?

Pathogenesis: The middle ear structures are derived from mesenchymal tissue of the 1st and 2nd branchial arches. The middle ear begins to form in the 3rd embryonic week and the tympanic cavity is almost completely formed by the 13th week. The ossicular chain continues to develop, but has completely matured to its adult size by the time of birth.

Soft tissue malformations: Probably the most common anomaly observed is the absence of the stapedius muscle, tendon and pyramidal eminence. This occurs in approximately 1 in each 100 ears explored. It is unilateral in almost 50%. A dehiscence of the fallopian canal causing exposure of the sheath of the facial nerve in the middle ear is so common that it should be considered a variation of normal, but is still widely classified as a malformation. (In over 50% of ears, there is a dehiscence of the fallopian canal immediately superior to the oval window.) Marked variation of the position of the facial nerve is extremely rare, but on rare instances, the nerve trunk may be found inferior to the oval window on the promontory or between the stapedial crura passing through the obturator foramen. It may thus be found completely covering the oval window. An extremely large chorda tympani branch may signal a marked malformation of the main trunk of the facial nerve. Vascular malformations may be of great surgical significance. Persistent stapedial arteries are common, but are usually small. A very large artery may hinder, or entirely prevent, proper stapedial surgical techniques. This occurs in approximately 1 ear per 1000. A dangerous herniation of the jugular bulb through a dehiscence in the floor of the middle ear may occur in approximately 1 in 400 ears. Usually, the vascular projection is not too high, but may extend superiorly to cover the round window. Accidental entry into the bulb may occur when the tympanic membrane is being elevated from its annulus inferiorly or during a myringotomy.

Ossicular malformations: Defects in development of the 1st branchial arch may produce abnormalities of the upper ossicular chain which is composed of the body and short process of the incus and the head of the malleus. Fusion of the incudomalleolar joint or bony union with the epitympanic wall or complete distortion of the size and shape of the 2 ossicles may occur. Malformations principally associated with the 2nd arch involve the lower ossicular chain (the handle of the malleus, the long process of the incus and the stapes). Malformations of the stapes are more often seen than of any other ossicle. Lack of oval window and stapedial footplate development is the most frequent cause of congenital conductive deafness (estimated to be over 75% of all cases). This is a combined maldevelopment of the otic capsule and the stapedial footplate. All stages of nondevelopment in the region of the oval window may be seen. Fusion of the long process of the incus, the head of the stapes and the handle of the malleus is rare.

Related Facts

I   Sex Ratio: M1:F1

II Risk of Occurrence: Not precisely calculated. Defect sufficient to interfere with hearing function probably occurs 1 in 40,000 live births. A surgically significant malformation sufficient to distort surgical landmarks may occur 1 in 100 births.

III Risk of Recurrence for
   Patient's Sib: Not increased
   Patient's Child: Not increased

IV Age of Detectability: If there is significant hearing impairment, detectability is possible from birth to 5 years.

V   Prevalence: 1 in 50,000 to 1 in 33,000

Treatment

I   Primary Prevention: —

II Secondary Prevention: Otologic surgery or amplification

III Other Therapy: Speech and language training

Prognosis: Normal for life span. After birth, there is no progression of the congenital structural malformation. Hearing should remain stable.

Detection of Carrier: —

Special Considerations: —

References:
   Hough, J.V.: Congenital malformations of the middle ear. Arch. Otolaryngol. 78:335, 1963.
   Hough, J.V.: Malformations and anatomical variations seen in the middle ear during the operation for mobilization of the stapes. Laryngoscope 68:1337, 1958.
   Hough, J.V.: Malformations and anatomical variations seen in the middle ear during operations on the stapes. Am. Acad. Ophthalmol. Otolaryngol. Rochester, Minn., 1961. (Monograph)

Contributor: **Jack Van Doren Hough**

Editor's Computerized Descriptors: Hearing, Ear

OSTEOCHONDRITIS DISSECANS

Includes: Ostéochondrite disséquante
Osteocondritis disecante

Excludes: Anomalies of ossification and tangential osteochondral fractures

Minimal Diagnostic Criteria: Characteristic radiographic appearance of excavation of bone and a loose body†

Clinical Findings: This process may occur at any of a number of sites such as the head of the femur, the tibial tubercle, the phalangeal epiphysis, the semilunar bone of the wrist, the capitellum of the humerus, the spine, the tarsal scaphoid, the 2nd metatarsal and the patella. Pain, swelling and limitation of motion may develop in the affected joints, but the lesion may be asymptomatic. The patient may feel a loose body in the joint. The knee is most commonly affected. Radiographs of joints show characteristic excavation of bone and a loose body. In the knee the classic site of detachment is in the infralateral aspect of the medial femoral condyle.

Complications
I **Derived:** Pain, limitation of motion and instability of affected joints
II **Associated:** —

Etiology: ? Some familial cases suggest autosomal dominant inheritance.

Pathogenesis: Trauma frequently precedes presentation but the primary or secondary role of trauma is debated. Detached pieces of bone and articular cartilage separate from dead bone suggesting a change in bone preceding the separation. Ischemia has been proposed as a mechanism, but arterial injection studies of the knee have shown no defect.

Related Facts
I **Sex Ratio:** In the second metatarsal M1:F4; in the elbow M8:F1
II **Risk of Occurrence:** Common
III **Risk of Recurrence for**
    Patient's Sib: If autosomal dominant and parent is affected 1 in 2 (50%) for each offspring to be affected; otherwise not increased.
    Patient's Child: 1 in 2
IV **Age of Detectability:** Most cases affecting the knee present clinically in the 2nd decade or later; cases affecting the femoral head present at age 2-13 years with peak at 6.5 years.
V **Prevalence:** Common. Patients with affected epiphysis of femoral head in U.S.A. number 15,000 to 20,000; rare in Negroes.

Treatment
I **Primary Prevention:** Genetic counseling when autosomal dominant
II **Secondary Prevention:** In most cases affecting the knee, loose bodies in the joint should be removed. Attempts to return the detached piece to its origin have been unsatisfactory.
III **Other Therapy:** Surgery is indicated in some cases.

Prognosis: Normal life span. There is some disability occasionally.

Detection of Carrier: —

†**Special Considerations:** Some families show osteochondritis dissecans of multiple sites. In one family, knees or elbows were affected in 9 persons in 3 generations. In another family with normal parents, knees and elbows were affected in 2 brothers who also had hypertelorism, finger contractures, peculiarly shaped ears, sternal deformity and cryptorchidism.

References:
Goff, C. W.: Legg-Calvé-Perthes Syndrome and Related Osteochondroses of Youth. Springfield:Charles C Thomas, 1954.
Hanley, W.B. et al: Osteochondritis dissecans and associated malformations in 2 brothers. A review of familial aspects. J. Bone Joint Surg. 49A:925, 1967.
Siegel, I. M.: The osteochondroses. Am. J. Orthop. Surg. 10:246, 1968.
Smillie, I. S.: Osteochondritis dissecans. Edinburgh: E. & S. Livingstone Ltd., 1960.
Stougaard, J.: The hereditary factor in osteochondritis dissecans. J. Bone Joint Surg. 43B:256, 1961.

Contributor: **Robert A. Norum**

Editor's Computerized Descriptor: Skel.

OSTEODYSPLASTY

Includes: Ostéodysplastie
Osteodisplastia
Melnick-Needles syndrome

Excludes: Weissman-Netter syndrome

Minimal Diagnostic Criteria: Generalized bone dysplasia characterized chiefly by cortical irregularities. In the adult, the bony changes may be quite mild.

Clinical Findings: This rare disorder of the skeleton primarily affects membranous bone. Early there is failure to gain well in height and weight, although adult height is only mildly affected. The facies are unusual and are characterized by exophthalmos, full cheeks, micrognathia, marked malocclusion and the ears tend to be large. The gait may be abnormal. The anterior fontanel closes late. Serum chemistries are generally normal although the serum phosphorus may be slightly elevated. In children xrays show a severe bone dysplasia with cortical irregularity of the long bones, flaring of the metaphyses, coxa valga, bowing of the radius and tibia, ribbon-like appearance of the ribs and deformities of the iliac bones. The calvarium is thickened in the adult. Intelligence is normal.

Complications
I   **Derived:** Gait disturbances and arthrosis of the hips in the adult
II   **Associated:** —

Etiology: Autosomal dominant; McK *16610

Pathogenesis: ?

Related Facts
I   **Sex Ratio:** Probably M1:F1 (The majority of reported cases have been female)
II   **Risk of Occurrence:** ?
III   **Risk of Recurrence for**
   Patient's Sib: If parent is affected, 1 in 2 (50%) for each offspring to be affected; otherwise not increased.
   Patient's Child: 1 in 2
IV   **Age of Detectability:** At birth by physical and radiologic examination. It has also been recognized in utero by xrays.
V   **Prevalence:** ?

Treatment
I   **Primary Prevention:** Genetic counseling
II   **Secondary Prevention:** Appropriate dental and orthopedic management including bracing and surgery for coxa vara.
III   **Other Therapy:** —

Prognosis: Normal for life span and intelligence. Function variable.

Detection of Carrier: —

Special Considerations: —

References:
Maroteaux, P. et al: L'Ostéodysplastie (syndrome de Melnick et de Needles). Presse Med. 76:715, 1968.
Melnick, J.C. and Needles, C.F.: An undiagnosed bone dysplasia. A two family study of 4 generations and 3 generations. Am. J. Roentgenol. Radium Ther. Nucl. Med. 97:39, 1966.

Contributor: **Charles I. Scott, Jr.**

Editor's Computerized Descriptors: Eye, Ear, Face, Teeth, Skel.

OSTEOECTASIA

Includes: Ostéoectasie
Osteoectasis
Osteoectasia with macrocranium (with hyperphosphatasia)
Hyperostosis corticalis deformans
Osteochalasia desmalis familiaris
Juvenile Paget disease
Chronic osteopathy with hyperphosphatasia

Excludes: Cortical hyperostosis, infantile (221)
Endosteal hyperostosis

Minimal Diagnostic Criteria: Calvarial thickening; demineralization and expansion of the tubular bones; hyperphosphatasia.

Clinical Findings: Small stature, large skull, progressive bowing of the legs and arms with pain, tenderness and muscular weakness; tendency to bone fractures.
   Radiographs show a thickened calvaria with loss of normal bone structure and changes reminiscent of Paget disease; generalized demineralization; expansion and bowing of the long bones, widening of the short tubular bones. In some patients and some sites there is dissolution of the normal cortical architecture of the tubular bones.
   Laboratory findings include an elevated activity of serum alkaline and acid phosphatase, and of serum aminopeptidase; uric acid levels are increased in serum and urine. There is an elevation of the urinary peptide-bound hydroxyproline.

Complications
I   **Derived:** Angioid streaks of the retina, macular atrophy, vascular hypertension. Hearing deficit and optic atrophy due to continued new bone formation at the skull base.
II   **Associated:** —

Etiology: Autosomal recessive with considerable variability of expression. McK *23900

Pathogenesis: There is excessive bone turnover which leads to decreased amounts of mature lamellar bone. The defect is possibly related to a defective production or action of calcitonin.

Related Facts
I   **Sex Ratio:** M1:F1
II   **Risk of Occurrence:** Rare
III   **Risk of Recurrence for**
   Patient's Sib: 1 in 4 (25%) for each offspring to be affected.
   Patient's Child: Negligible
IV   **Age of Detectability:** 3rd-18th month of life.
V   **Prevalence:** ?

Treatment
I   **Primary Prevention:** Genetic counseling
II   **Secondary Prevention:** Long-term treatment with calcitonin seems to be highly effective
III   **Other Therapy:** Surgical correction of bone deformities; removal of excessive bone compressing the optic nerves, if necessary.

Prognosis: Untreated, most patients are severely deformed and incapacitated by the age of 14 years. Vascular hypertension may lead to cerebrovascular accidents and death.

Detection of Carrier: ? Perhaps by checking activities of serum phosphatases

Special Considerations: —

References:

Caffey, J.: Familial hyperphosphatasemia with ateliosis and hypermetabolism of growing membranous bone. Progr. Pediat. Radiol. 4:438, 1973.

Woodhouse, N.J.Y. et al: Paget's disease in 5-year-old. Acute response to human calcitonin. Br. Med. J. II:267, 1972.

Contributor: Jürgen W. Spranger

Editor's Computerized Descriptors: Eye, Hearing, Skel., Muscle, CV.

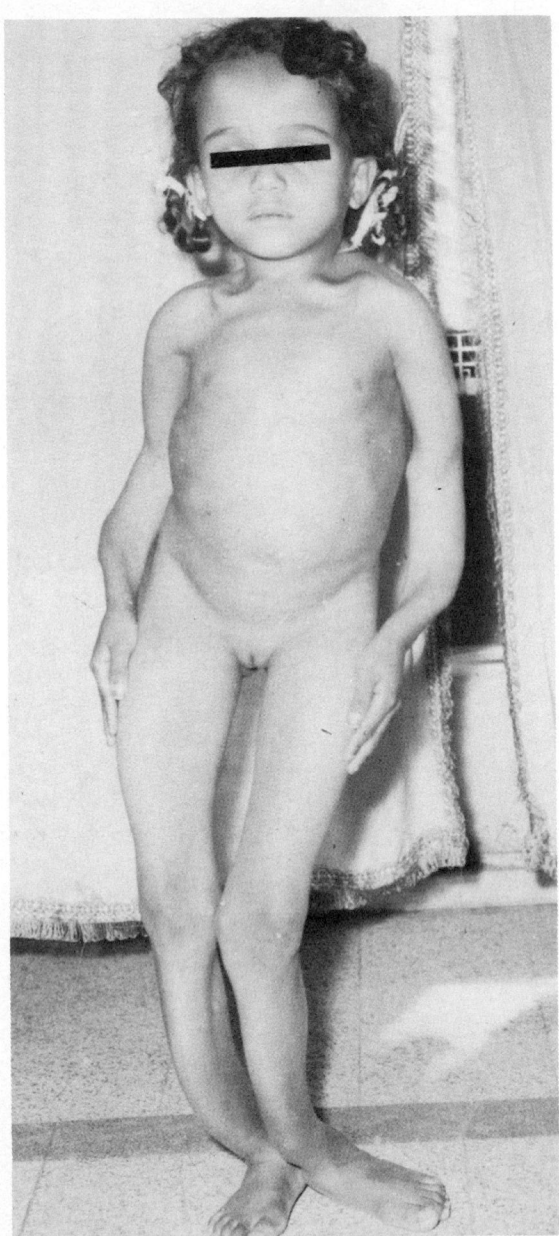

403. Typical bowing of long bones and clavicles, pigeon breast deformity, and enlarged cranium

OSTEOGENESIS IMPERFECTA

Includes: Osteogenesis imperfecta congenita
Osteogenesis imperfecta tarda
Mollities ossium
Fragilitas ossium
Osteopsathyrosis idiopathica
Trias fragilitis ossium hereditaria
Lobstein syndrome
Vrolik disease

Excludes: Hypophosphatasia (516)
Osteoporosis, juvenile idiopathic (782)

Minimal Diagnostic Criteria: Evidence of blue sclerae, skeletal fractures with minimal trauma, typical radiographic changes or otosclerosis.

Clinical Findings: Osteogenesis imperfecta (OI) is a descriptive term applied to a multisystem disease complex involving the skeletal, ocular, cutaneous, otologic, dental and vascular tissues with the greatest morbidity arising from the skeletal manifestations. The spectrum of severity varies considerably, ranging from a severe neonatal form characterized by multiple intrauterine fractures of the limbs and ribs, soft membranaceous cranium, and usually neonatal death from intracranial hemorrhage or respiratory embarrassment to a very mild form manifesting only a slight tendency toward bone fractures, blue sclerae or mild deafness. The traditional scheme of dividing the syndrome into osteogenesis imperfecta congenita (the severe neonatal form) and osteogenesis imperfecta tarda (later onset of symptoms) does not appear to be wholly adequate because there is a great deal of intrafamilial variability; and families manifesting both mild and severe forms are known. Several other classifications have been proposed; however, none has been completely satisfactory. Furthermore, it is not clear how many distinct disorders are included under the term of OI.

The majority of patients have some or all of the following features. The single most characteristic feature of OI is an increased susceptibility to bone fracture, and the resultant deformities may include pseudoarthrosis, saber shins and marked bowing of the legs. Short stature may result from these deformities, as well as growth retardation from repeated epiphyseal fractures. Other skeletal anomalies include kyphoscoliosis and pectus excavatum and carinatum. The face is usually triangular in shape due to the broad-domed forehead, temporal bulge and overhanging occiput. The teeth are often yellow-brown or opalescent and break easily (dentogenesis imperfecta). The skin is thin and translucent. Joint laxity is increased and hernie are frequently observed. Blue sclerae occur frequently but not in all patients. Beyond the 2nd decade, otosclerosis often leads to varying degrees of deafness. Aortic regurgitation has been reported. Some patients, however, may have nothing more than blue sclerae and yet have severely affected 1st-degree relatives.

Radiographically, generalized osteopenia with thin cortices and multiple fractures and excessive callous formation are observed. Long bones often show thin diaphyses with an abrupt expansion at the metaphyseal ends. In some cases, however, the diaphyses may be thickened and demonstrate a cystic appearance. The vertebrae usually have the typical codfish appearance. Skull xrays reveal multiple wormian bones.

Complications

I   **Derived:** In addition to those mentioned above, other complications include tendon evulsion, wide scars, increased capillary fragility, subcutaneous hemorrhage, hemorrhagic diathesis, hypermetropia, keratoconus, and neurologic dysfunction due to platybasia.

II **Associated:** Elastosis perforans.

Etiology: The majority of cases appear to follow an autosomal dominant inheritance pattern with a wide range of expressivity and incomplete penetrance. However, autosomal recessive inheritance has been documented in severe neonatal cases, and in some progressive cases.† McK *16620

Pathogenesis: The manifestations result from abnormal connective tissue. A defect in collagen synthesis has been postulated, but no consistent abnormality has yet been described. It is quite likely that OI represents a heterogeneous group of collagen defects.

Related Facts

I **Sex Ratio:** M1:F1
II **Risk of Occurrence:** ?
III **Risk of Recurrence for**

Patient's Sib: If parent affected, 1 in 2 (50%) for each offspring to be affected: otherwise not increased. If no consanguinity and neither parent has evidence of the disorder, ie blue sclerae, excessive fractures, then risk is probably negligible unless patient has severe neonatal lethal crumpled bone variety.

Patient's Child: 1 in 2

IV **Age of Detectability:** Because of clinical variability, detection may range from birth through adulthood
V **Prevalence:** ?

Treatment

I **Primary Prevention:** Genetic counseling
II **Secondary Prevention:** Oral magnesium oxide therapy, calcitonin, sodium fluoride, phosphate and vitamin C have been suggested to be potentially useful; however, definite improvement of clinical symptoms with any of these treatments is yet to be documented. Immobilization should be avoided. Orthopedic surgery may improve bone deformities.
III **Other Therapy:** Because of hormonal effects, pregnancy may be deleterious to severely affected females and cesarean section is usually required.

Prognosis: Dependent upon severity of involvement. Ranges from death in perinatal period to normal life span with little if any morbidity.

Detection of Carrier: It is possible that serum and urine pyrophosphate levels may serve to distinguish the carrier with mild expressivity from the normal sib. There is a wide range of expressivity of this disorder within families. An affected member may demonstrate only blue sclera while sibs or offspring may demonstrate the full manifestations of the disorder.

†**Special Considerations:** The vast majority of cases appear to be inherited in an autosomal dominant manner from the previous generation or represent new dominant mutations. When parents are consanguineous and clinically normal, autosomal recessive inheritance should be suspected, in which case the risk of the patient's sibs would be 25%. It is likely that 4 or more distinct disorders have been included under the term "osteogenesis imperfecta".

References:

Bauze, B.J. et al: A new look at osteogenesis imperfecta. A clinical, radiological and biochemical study of forty-two patients. J. Bone Joint Surg. 57B:2, 1975.
McKusick, V.A.: Heritable Disorders of Connective Tissue, 4th Ed. St. Louis: C.V. Mosby 1972, p. 390.
Sillence, D. and Danks, D.: The differentiation of genetically distinct varieties of osteogenesis imperfecta in the newborn period. Clin. Res. 26:178A, 1978.

Contributors: **William A. Horton**
Jouni Uitto
Jack R. Lichtenstein

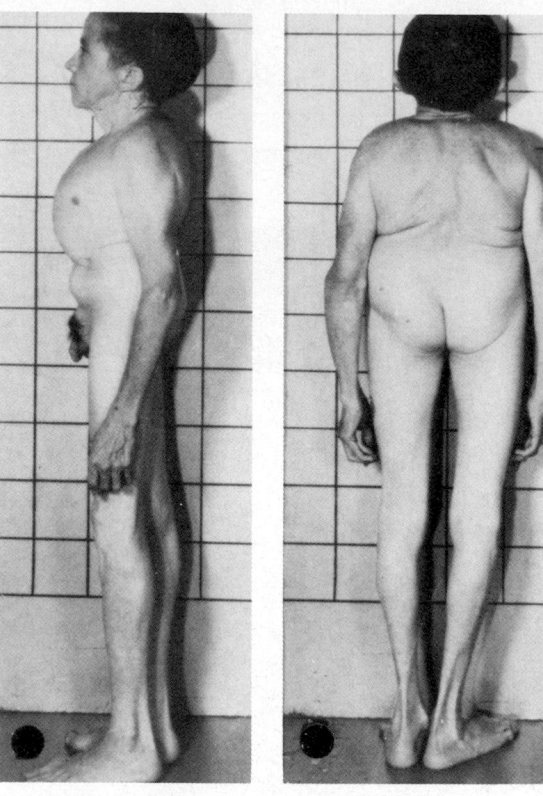

404. Note short barrel-shaped chest and short neck

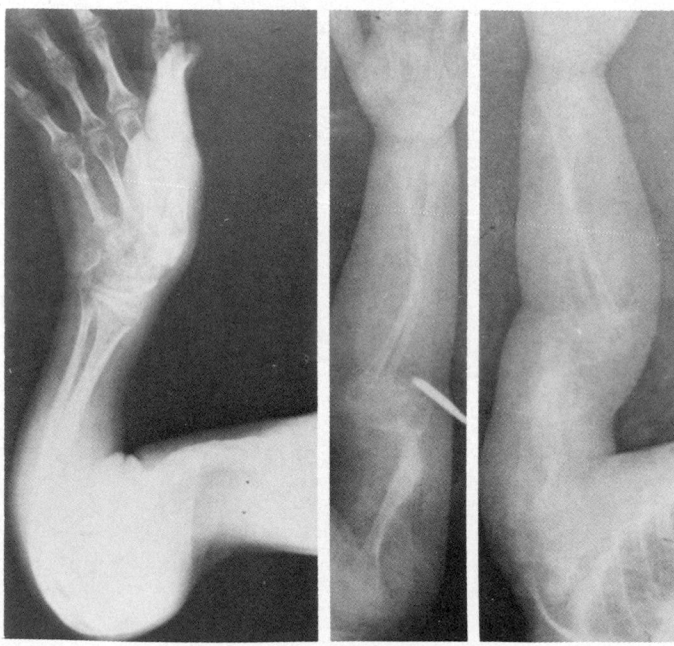

405. Note thin, severely bowed long bones

OSTEOPATHIA STRIATA

Includes: Ostéopathie striée
Osteopatía estrida
Voorhoeve disease
Hyperostosis generalisata with striation

Excludes: Osteopetrosis, dominant (779)
Enchondromatosis (345)
Hyperostosis corticalis generalisata (497)

Minimal Diagnostic Criteria: The typical roentgenologic appearance of longitudinal striations

Clinical Findings: There are no definite clinical findings due to this disease. Indeed, there is some question as to whether this is a distinct entity or merely a variant of osteopoikilosis. Patients with striated bony lesions have been reported with dermatofibrosis lenticularis, and in families with osteopoikilosis.

Radiographs show longitudinal striations in the long bones, beginning at the epiphyseal line and most prominent in the metaphyses. Irregular fan-like striations are seen in the ilium. Increased bone density has been reported in the skull and ribs. Thickening of the cranial vault, with projection of dense bone from the inner table and obliteration of the sinuses has been observed. No abnormal laboratory results have been reported.

Complications
I **Derived:** Conductive deafness has been reported in 2 cases, probably resulting from the narrow auditory canals, fixation of the ossicular chain and loss of mastoid air cells.
II **Associated:** Reduced intelligence has been reported in 2 patients and premature cortical cataracts have been reported in 1 patient. Dermatofibrosis lenticularis has also been reported. Other radiologic findings which have been reported are: small areas of translucency in the metaphysis, localized thinning of the cortex and small exostoses.

Etiology: ? Although this disorder is thought to be inherited as an autosomal dominant, there is no supportive information. All definite cases have been sporadic, except for the cases occurring in families with osteopoikilosis (where the bony abnormalities are inherited as an autosomal dominant).

Pathogenesis: ? The pathology has been reported to be similar to osteopetrosis in involved areas, with loss of lamellar structure due to the obliteration of canaliculi. The pathogenesis is unknown, although similar lesions have been produced in mice by inhibition of resorption of metaphyseal spongiosa with estrogens.

Related Facts
I **Sex Ratio:** ?
II **Risk of Occurrence:** ? Certainly rare
III **Risk of Recurrence for**
  Patient's Sib: ?
  Patient's Child: ?
IV **Age of Detectability:** Usually detected in adults as an incidental radiographic finding, although it most likely is detectable in childhood.
V **Prevalence:** ? Certainly rare

Treatment
I **Primary Prevention:** —
II **Secondary Prevention:** Hearing aid and surgical mobilization of the ossicles may be necessary for accompanying deafness.
III **Other Therapy:** —

Prognosis: Normal for life span, probably normal for intelligence and function except for possible loss of hearing or sight.

Detection of Carrier: —

Special Considerations: —

References:
Hurt, R. L.: Osteopathia striata-Voorhoeve's disease; report of a case presenting the features of osteopathia striata and osteopetrosis. J. Bone Joint Surg. 35B:89, 1953.
Walker, B. A.: Osteopathia striata with cataracts and deafness. In Bergsma, D. (ed.): Part IV. Skeletal Dysplasias. Birth Defects: Orig. Art. Ser., vol. V, no. 4, White Plains: The National Foundation-March of Dimes, 1969, p. 295.

Contributor: **Jack R. Lichtenstein**

Editor's Computerized Descriptor: Skel.

OSTEOPETROSIS, DOMINANT

Includes: Ostéopétrose à manifestation précoce
Frühmanifeste Osteopetrose
Osteopetrosis precoz
Albers-Schönberg disease
Benign adult form of osteopetrosis
Marble bone disease
Dominant osteopetrosis
Osteopetrosis with late manifestation

Excludes: Osteopetrosis, recessive (780)
Pyknodysostosis (846)
Hyperostosis generalisata
Osteopoikilosis (781)
Craniometaphyseal dysplasia (228)
Diaphyseal dysplasia (290)
Dysosteosclerosis (310)

Minimal Diagnostic Criteria: This disorder can only be diagnosed on the basis of the distinct radiographic features in an individual who does not show the severe clinical symptomatology of the recessive form of the disorder.†

Clinical Findings: This disorder is characterized by a generalized sclerotic process of bone with marked variability in its clinical features. Close to 50% of the patients are asymptomatic and are diagnosed on incidental xrays or because of genetic analysis of their family due to a more severely affected relative. The most common problem in this disorder is pathologic fractures; 40% of the reported cases had a history of fractures. Osteomyelitis, primarily of the mandible occurs in 10% of cases. This may be a severe problem in management and commonly follows dental extractions or infections. Bone pain, primarily of the lumbar spine, occurs in 20% of the patients. The cranial hyperostosis may result in cranial nerve palsies which have been described in 16% of the cases. The nerves most commonly affected are the 2nd, 3rd, and 7th cranial nerves, resulting in optic atrophy, extraocular muscle palsies, and facial palsy. Frontal bossing, exophthalmos or facial palsies may result in a peculiar facial appearance. There is marked intrafamilial variability in the clinical features of this disorder and nonpenetrance has been described. Hepatosplenomegaly and severe anemia are usually not features of the dominant form of osteopetrosis. Elevated serum acid phosphatase levels have been found in almost all reported cases, but other serum chemistries and calcium balance studies have been normal.

Skeletal xrays reveal a generalized sclerotic process. The earliest radiographic features are an increase in the density of the diaphyseal regions of the growing bone with parallel radiolucent striations in the metaphyseal regions. The vertebral bodies may develop a "sandwich" appearance with sclerosis of the upper and lower plates with an intervening less dense appearance. The tubular bones, especially the metacarpals, may show a "bone within a bone" appearance. The skull is thickened and dense, especially at the base.

Histologic examination of the affected bones shows absence of a true medullary cavity with noncalcified hyaline cartilage remnants scattered diffusely within the bone. The bone itself is made up primarily of Haversian systems with scanty fibrillar composition. Foci of osteoblastic and osteoclastic activity can be seen.

Complications
I   **Derived:** —
II **Associated:** Pathologic fractures, cranial nerve palsies with blindness, strabismus or facial palsy, osteomyelitis of the mandible.

Etiology: Autosomal dominant

Pathogenesis: ? Several theories have been advanced including defective resorption of primary spongiosa or overproduction of bone of abnormal composition.

Related Facts
I   **Sex Ratio:** M1:F1
II **Risk of Occurrence:** ?
III **Risk of Recurrence for**
    Patient's Sib: If parent is affected 1 in 2 (50%) for each offspring to be affected; otherwise not increased.
    Patient's Child: 1 in 2
IV **Age of Detectability:** In early childhood by skeletal radiographs. This disease is often not diagnosed until adolescence or adulthood.
V **Prevalence:** The prevalence of this disorder has been estimated to be about 1 in 100,000 in a Brazilian population.

Treatment
I   **Primary Prevention:** Genetic counseling
II **Secondary Prevention:** Avoidance of contact sports, etc to prevent pathologic fractures. Surgical reaming has been tried for cranial nerve involvement.
III **Other Therapy:** —

Prognosis: Life expectancy is apparently normal except if severe osteomyelitis and sepsis are uncontrolled.

Detection of Carrier: —

†Special Considerations: This disorder is distinct from the congenital malignant form of the disease, both clinically and genetically. Severe anemia and hepatosplenomegaly are not features of this dominant disorder. The dominant and recessive forms of osteopetrosis, however, cannot be differentiated radiographically. Any individual with the radiographic features of osteopetrosis in the adolescent or adult ages will almost certainly have the dominant form of the disease. This disease must be differentiated from the other forms of skeletal sclerosis such as fluorosis, heavy metal intoxication, craniometaphyseal dysplasia, osteopoikilosis, Engelmann disease, etc.

References:
Johnston, C.C., Jr. et al: Osteopetrosis. Medicine 47:149, 1968.
Salzano, F.M.: Osteopetrosis: Review of dominant cases and frequency in a Brazilian state. Acta Genet. Med. Gemellol (Roma) 10:353, 1961.
Welford, N.P.: Facial paralysis associated with osteopetrosis (marble bones). J. Pediatr. 55:67, 1959.

Contributors: **David L. Rimoin**
David W. Hollister

Editor's Computerized Descriptors: Eye, Face, Skel., Nerve

OSTEOPETROSIS, RECESSIVE

Includes: Ostéopétrose à manifestation tardive
Spätmanifeste Osteopetrose
Osteopetrosis tardía
Albers-Schönberg disease
Marble bone disease
Malignant congenital osteopetrosis
Osteosclerosis fragilis generalisata
Osteopetrosa generalisata
Recessive osteopetrosis

Excludes: Osteopoikilosis (781)
Diaphyseal dysplasia (290)
Craniometaphyseal dysplasia (228)
Dysosteosclerosis (310)
Osteopetrosis, dominant (779)

Minimal Diagnostic Criteria: The malignant clinical features may suggest the diagnosis, but it can only be confirmed by skeletal radiographs.

Clinical Findings: Osteopetrosis as a rare autosomal recessive disorder is associated with dense brittle bones, macrocephaly, progressive deafness and blindness, hepatosplenomegaly, and severe anemia beginning in early infancy or in utero. The diagnosis can be made in utero by xrays revealing the generalized sclerotic skeletal system. These children may be stillborn or exhibit failure to thrive and die in infancy or early childhood. The osteosclerotic process impinges on the marrow cavity resulting in severe anemia and pancytopenia with extramedullary hematopoiesis producing hepatosplenomegaly and lymphadenopathy, often with nucleated red blood cells in the peripheral blood (myeloid metaplasia). Cranial sclerosis may result in macrocephaly and hydrocephaly, as well as impingement on the cranial nerve foramina, leading to blindness with optic atrophy, deafness, facial palsies, and strabismus. Dentition may be delayed and severe dental caries are common. Growth and developmental retardation are common, but intelligence is normal in over 75% of the cases. The sclerotic skeletal system predisposes to pathologic factors and osteomyelitis. Serum chemistries are usually normal, but hypocalcemia, hyperphosphatemia and tetany have been described.

Skeletal xrays reveal uniformly dense sclerotic bones with associated metaphyseal splaying and clubbing. The medullary canals and trabecular patterns are obliterated. Radiolucent streaks appear in the long bone metaphyses, while the epiphyses are sclerotic but of normal contour. The skull is thickened, particularly at the base, with narrowing of the cranial foramina. The mastoids and paranasal sinuses are poorly aerated. The metacarpals and metatarsals may appear block-shaped with a "bone in bone" appearance, and there may be partial aplasia of the distal phalanges. The vertebrae are of normal shape, but the ribs appear flared.

Histologic examination of bone reveals obliteration of the medullary cavity with a lattice-like network of hyaline cartilage surrounded by thick bone which exhibits a paucity of fibrils. Foci of osteoblastic and osteoclastic activity can be seen.

Complications
I **Derived:** Pancytopenia, cranial nerve palsies and failure to thrive
II **Associated:** —

Etiology: Autosomal recessive†; McK *25970

Pathogenesis: A variety of theories have arisen to explain the pathogenesis of this disorder, including faulty resorption of primary spongiosa, poorly formed hypofibrillar bone, or thyrocalcitonin hypersecretion; none of which have been substantiated to date.

Related Facts
I **Sex Ratio:** M1:F1
II **Risk of Occurrence:** ?
III **Risk of Recurrence for**
 Patient's Sib: 1 in 4 (25%) for each offspring to be affected
 Patient's Child: They do not live to reproduce.
IV **Age of Detectability:** In utero or infancy by skeletal xrays
V **Prevalence:** ?

Treatment
I **Primary Prevention:** Genetic counseling
II **Secondary Prevention:** Steroid therapy has been reported to be of some value by 1 group of investigators, but this has not been tested by others.
III **Other Therapy:** —

Prognosis: Death in infancy or childhood, usually due to anemia or secondary infection.

Detection of Carrier: ?

†Special Considerations: The congenital autosomal recessive form of osteopetrosis is a distinct disorder which differs from the benign dominant form both clinically and genetically. It must be distinguished from other disorders with bony sclerosis such as fluorosis, heavy metal intoxication, craniometaphyseal dysplasia, Engelmann disease, and osteopoikilosis.

References:
Johnston, C.C., Jr. et al: Osteopetrosis. Medicine 47:149, 1968.
Moe, P.J. and Skjaeveland, A.: Therapeutic studies in osteopetrosis. Acta Paediatr. Scand. 58:593, 1969.
Tips, R.L. and Lynch, H.T.: Malignant congenital osteopetrosis resulting from a consanguineous marriage. Acta Paediatr. 51:585, 1962.

Contributors: **David L. Rimoin**
David W. Hollister

Editor's Computerized Descriptors: Vision, Eye, Hearing, Teeth, Skel., Spleen, Liver, Nerve

OSTEOPOIKILOSIS

Includes: Ostéopoecilie
Osteopoikilose
Osteopoiquilosis
Osteopathia condensans disseminata
Osteopoecilia
Osteitis condensans, generalisata
"Spotted bones"
Osteodermatopoikilosis
Osteodysplasia enostotica

Excludes: Osteopetrosis, dominant (779)
Osteosclerosis of other etiologies
Osteoblastic metastases
Chondrodysplasia punctata, Conradi-Hünermann type (153)

Minimal Diagnostic Criteria: Typical grain-to-pea size densities on radiographs.

Clinical Findings: This disorder is usually discovered accidently, by radiographs. The typical appearance is oval or round densities, oriented in longitudinal directions, most abundant in the pelvis and shoulder girdles and the epiphyses and metaphyses of the long bones. The skull is rarely involved. Although the round densities are rarely seen in the diaphyses, the distinct parallel lines of density extending from the epiphyseal line down into the diaphyses, as seen in osteopathia striata, may be found in patients with osteopoikilosis or in their relatives. This has led some observers to consider them as the same process. Dermatofibrosis lenticularis is the skin manifestation of the disorder, occurring in over 50% of cases with radiographic changes. These are raised, yellowish lesions, which may coalesce and form stripes. The common locations are the buttocks, thighs, back and abdominal skin but not the face. The skin lesions have been reported without the radiographic changes in families with osteopoikilosis.

Complications
I **Derived:** Keloids
II **Associated:** Fibrous nodules of the peritoneal lining. Associations which have been reported and may not be real are short stature, diabetes, cleft lip, scleroderma, palmar and plantar keratosis, subcutaneous fibrous nodules and hyperostosis frontalis interna.

Etiology: Autosomal dominant inheritance with incomplete penetrance. Skipped generations are common. The skin lesions and bony lesions may occur separately in the same family. McK *16670

Pathogenesis: The basic defect appears to be a spotty hyperplasia of collagen in the corium and bone matrix. The bony lesions are due to a thickening of the trabecular spongiosa.

Related Facts
I **Sex Ratio:** Probably M1:F1, although males are more frequently detected because they more frequently have radiographs for trauma, etc.
II **Risk of Occurrence:** 1 in 20,000 in Germany
III **Risk of Recurrence for**
    Patient's Sib: If parent is affected 1 in 2 (50%) for each offspring to be affected; otherwise not increased.
    Patient's Child: 1 in 2
IV **Age of Detectability:** At birth (has been detected prenatally)
V **Prevalence:** 12 cases per 211,000 radiographs, in a survey in Germany (Jonaseh), ie about 1 in 20,000.

Treatment
I **Primary Prevention:** Theoretically, genetic counseling
II **Secondary Prevention:** —
III **Other Therapy:** —

Prognosis: Normal for life span, intelligence and function

Detection of Carrier: —

Special Considerations: —

References:
Busch, K. F. B.: Familial disseminated osteosclerosis. Acta Radiol. (Stockh.) 18:693, 1937.
Danielsen, L. et al: Osteopoikilosis associated with dermatofibrosis lenticularis disseminata. Arch. Dermatol. 100:465, 1969.
Jonaseh, E.: 12 Falle von Osteopoikilie. Fortschr. Roentgenstr. 82 :344, 1955.
McKusick, V. A.: Heritable Disorders of Connective Tissue, 3rd Ed. St. Louis:C.V. Mosby, 1966, p. 415.

Contributor: **Jack R. Lichtenstein**

Editor's Computerized Descriptors: Skin, Skel.

OSTEOPOROSIS, JUVENILE IDIOPATHIC

776-500

Includes: Ostéoporose juvénile
Juvenile Osteoporose
Juvenile osteoporosis
Idiopathic juvenile osteoporosis

Excludes: Osteopetrosis
Osteoporosis secondary to any identifiable cause, particularly lymphoma and leukemia
Osteogenesis imperfecta (777)

Minimal Diagnostic Criteria: 1) Radiologic evidence of diminished bone density in the absence of any defined underlying disease. 2) Onset in childhood or adolescence in a previously normal individual. 3) Spontaneous remission after a variable course. 4) Absence of evidence suggestive of osteogenesis imperfecta in other family members.

Clinical Findings: Juvenile osteoporosis is a disease of childhood and adolescence exhibiting marked clinical variability. The disease usually begins in the peripubertal period (age 8-13), but several younger cases (age 3-8) have been reported. The affected patients are clinically (and presumably radiologically) normal until the onset of fractures following minor trauma. The fractures are usually of the vertebrae, but long bone fractures are also common. Metabolic studies indicate negative calcium balance but serum calcium, phosphorus and alkaline-phosphatases are often normal. Radiographs typically show marked diminution in bone density. The disease can persist for many years, but usually remits, or markedly improves, within 5 years. Even after remission, one can be left with severe sequellae due to spinal cord compression, malaligned long bones, and pseudoarthroses. It is unknown if these patients have an increased propensity for senile osteoporosis.

Complications
I **Derived:** Bony deformities secondary to fractures leading to decreased height, kyphosis, protuberant sternum and malalignment of long bones and pseudoarthroses.
II **Associated:** None

Etiology: Autosomal recessive inheritance has been suggested by some but a clear inheritance pattern has not been ascertained.†

Pathogenesis: Unknown, but negative calcium balance studies have been documented.

Related Facts
I **Sex Ratio:** M1:F1
II **Risk of Occurrence:** Rare. Only 24 cases reported, but may be more common because of mild unrecognized or unreported cases.
III **Risk of Recurrence for**
   Patient's Sib: ?
   Patient's Child: ?
IV **Age of Detectability:** Variable; childhood to adolescence.
V **Prevalence:** 24 cases reported by 1976.

Treatment
I **Primary Prevention:** None
II **Secondary Prevention:** Avoidance of any activity which might cause fractures or exacerbate old fractures. No pharmaceutic agents have been helpful to date, but a complete evaluation of the effects of establishment of positive calcium balance has not been completed.
III **Other Therapy:** —

Prognosis: Normal life span and intelligence. Spontaneous remission is usual, but long standing cases have had severe residual damage.

Detection of Carrier: Not applicable

†**Special Considerations:** This condition might not represent a single entity but rather a heterogeneous group of disorders with a common clinical appearance.

References:
Dent, C.E. and Friedman, M.: Idiopathic juvenile osteoporosis. Q. J. Med. 34:177, 1965.
Dent, C.E.: Idiopathic juvenile osteoporosis. In Bergsma, D. (ed.): Part IV. Skeletal Dysplasias. Birth Defects: Orig. Art. Ser., vol. V, no. 4. New York: The National Foundation-March of Dimes, 1969, p. 134.

Contributors: **Kyrieckos Aleck**
Larry J. Shapiro

Editor's Computerized Descriptor: Skel.

OSTEOPOROSIS-PSEUDOGLIOMA SYNDROME

Includes: Syndrome d'ostéoporose et pseudogliome
Syndrom von Osteoporose und Pseudogliom
Síndrome de pseudogliomas y osteoporosis
Syndrome of pseudogliomatous blindness, osteoporosis and mild mental retardation
Osteoporosis with ocular pseudoglioma

Excludes: Osteogenesis imperfecta (777)
Other forms of osteoporosis

Minimal Diagnostic Criteria: Blindness from "pseudogliomatous" retinal detachment causing phthisis bulbi; osteoporosis; fractures from minor accidents and deformities; mild mental retardation.†

Clinical Findings: At least 5 families are known in which 2 or more sibs were affected. Blindness in infancy is probably due to "pseudogliomatous" retinal detachment or from fetal uveitis, resulting in microphthalmia, phthisis bulbi, corneal opacity and cataracts. Osteoporosis of variable severity is manifested at age 2-3 years, sometimes resulting in incapacitating deformities secondary to multiple fractures from minor trauma. Vertebral deformities result in a short trunk. Ligaments are lax. Microcephaly is present in some. Mental retardation when present usually is of mild-to-borderline degree; special verbal abilities were occasionally seen (idiot savant); hearing is usually normal. Radiographic findings include osteoporosis, thin cortex and coarse trabecular structure of long bones, spontaneous fractures, bowing of limbs, metaphyseal cysts, codfish vertebrae, and wormian bones.

Complications
I Derived: Blindness, deformities, physical handicap, mental deficiency
II Associated: ?

Etiology: Autosomal recessive; McK *25977

Pathogenesis: ?

Related Facts
I Sex Ratio: M1:F1
II Risk of Occurrence: ?
III Risk of Recurrence for
Patient's Sib: 1 in 4 (25%) for each offspring to be affected
Patient's Child: Not increased unless mate is carrier or homozygote
IV Age of Detectability: Infancy (blindness) and early childhood (fractures and osteoporosis)
V Prevalence: ? Obviously rare

Treatment
I Primary Prevention: Genetic counseling
II Secondary Prevention: Treatment of osteoporosis, care for fractures and deformities. Prevention of retinal detachment in patients at risk.
III Other Therapy: —

Prognosis: Osteoporosis may be progressive during childhood; later stabilization occurs.

Detection of Carrier: ? Incomplete manifestation of the syndrome may be seen in heterozygotes.

†Special Considerations: "Pseudoglioma" is a nonspecific term; usually retinal detachment is the cause of blindness. The syndrome is probably a connective tissue dysplasia primarily involving eyes, bones, and ligaments. Biochemical findings reported from some cases include hypercalcinuria and hydroxyprolinuria as nonspecific secondary manifestations of osteoporosis. A decreased rate of bone formation and an increased rate of bone resorption have been shown by microautoradiographic studies.

References:
McKusick, V.A.: Heritable Disorders of Connective Tissue, 4th Ed. St. Louis: C.V. Mosby, 1972.
Neuhäuser, G. et al: Autosomal recessive syndrome of pseudogliomatous blindness, osteoporosis and mild mental retardation. Clin. Genet. 9:324, 1976.

Contributor: Gerhard Neuhäuser

Editor's Computerized Descriptors: Vision, Eye, Skel.

OTODENTAL DYSPLASIA

778-500

Includes: Dento-auriculaire
Oto-dentales Syndrom
Síndrome otodentario
Globodontia with high frequency hearing loss
Otodental syndrome

Excludes: Macrodontia (617)
Molarization of premolar teeth

Minimal Diagnostic Criteria: Large globe-shaped molar teeth and sensorineural hearing loss.

Clinical Findings: Large globe-shaped tooth crowns occur in both dentitions affecting the canine teeth and teeth posterior to the canines. Some affected persons have only molar teeth involved. The incisor teeth are spared and are of normal size and shape. Over half have 1 or more congenitally missing premolars or the premolars may be small. Age of onset of hearing loss varies from birth to 3rd and 4th decade. It is sensorineural, high frequency and moderate to profound (50 db or greater hearing loss). Patients with only isolated hearing loss have transmitted the full syndrome. Data from 1 kindred show 30/37 had full syndrome, 3/37 had globodontia only and 4/37 had only hearing loss. The latter had offspring affected with both defects.† Local spots of yellow hypomature enamel have been noted in those with large teeth. Radiographs show duplication of pulp chambers in molar teeth.

Complications
I **Derived:** Malocclusion, full-face appearance, long philtrum, delayed eruption of teeth and impacted teeth.
II **Associated:** Some families have shown thin enamel with large interrod spaces.

Etiology: Autosomal dominant; McK *16675

Pathogenesis: ? Abnormal tooth form appears to be result of massive development of each tooth mamelon, or twinning-fusion of tooth germ.

Related Facts
I **Sex Ratio:** M1:F1
II **Risk of Occurrence:** Rare
III **Risk of Recurrence for**
  Patient's Sib: If parent is affected, 1 in 2 (50%) for each offspring to be affected; otherwise not increased.†
  Patient's Child: 1 in 2†
IV **Age of Detectability:** At time of eruption of posterior primary teeth, 18 months-2 years.
V **Prevalence:** ? Rare - 6 kindreds known.

Treatment
I **Primary Prevention:** Genetic counseling
II **Secondary Prevention:** Orthodontic treatment with selected tooth extraction. Hearing aids.
III **Other Therapy:** —

Prognosis: Does not appear to affect longevity. Hearing loss may be progressive and eventually involve conversational frequencies.

Detection of Carrier: —

†**Special Considerations:** Patients within affected kindreds with isolated hearing loss have had offspring with the complete syndrome. High requency hearing loss is common and can be due to a number of other genetic and environmental causes. Thus within kindreds, isolated hearing loss may indicate incomplete expression of the ODS gene but also may not indicate those bearing the ODS gene.

References:
Levin, L.S. et al: Otodental dysplasia. A new ectodermal dysplasia. Clin. Genet. 8:136, 1975.
Witkop, C.J., Jr. et al: Globodontia in the otodental syndrome. Oral Surg. 41:472, 1976.

Contributors: **Carl J. Witkop, Jr.**
L. Stefan Levin

Editor's Computerized Descriptors: Hearing, Face, Teeth

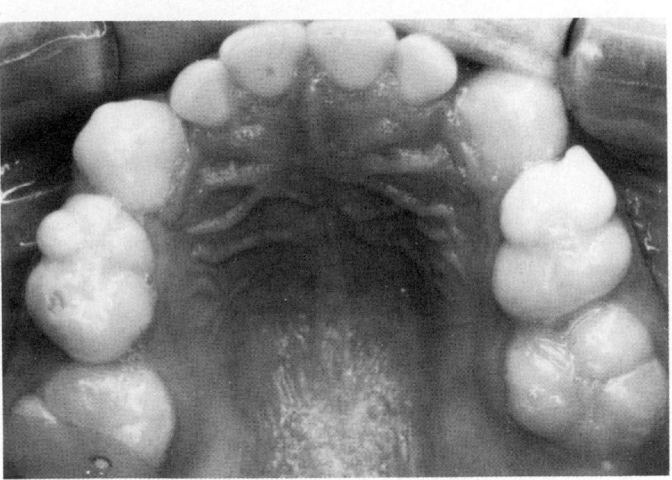

406. Teeth in otodental dysplasia

OTO-OCULO-MUSCULO-SKELETAL SYNDROME

Includes: Syndrome de Nathalie
Nathalie Syndrom
Síndrome de Nathalie
Deafness and cataract with muscular atrophy and skeletal defects

Excludes: Other syndromes with deafness and cataract

Minimal Diagnostic Criteria: Early childhood deafness, cataract, muscular atrophy, ECG abnormalities

Clinical Findings: This syndrome is reported in 4 of 7 sibs. Early childhood deafness was present in 4/4, cataract in 4/4, muscular atrophy in 3/4, skeletal defects in 3/4, retardation of growth in 3/4, ECG abnormalities in 4/4 and underdeveloped sexual characteristics in 2/4. The proposita suffered intermittently from regular and very frequent palpitations of the heart. The ECG showed ventricular extrasystoles, possibly multifocal in origin or supraventricular extrasystoles with an aberrant intraventricular conduction. The proposita died during an attack of these palpitations.

Deafness was diagnosed at the age of 5 in 3/4 and by the age of 4 in 1/4. Audiograms since that age showed no progression in the hearing loss. Radiographs of the temporal bones in the proposita were normal. Vestibular function examined in 2/4 was normal.

Complications
I **Derived:** Death secondary to extrasystoles
II **Associated:** Enuresis, nocturia in some cases and some family members.

Etiology: Autosomal recessive.

Pathogenesis: ?

Related Facts
I **Sex Ratio:** M1:F1 theoretic; actual: M1:F3
II **Risk of Occurrence:** Rare
III **Risk of Recurrence for**
 Patient's Sib: 1 in 4 (25%) for each offspring to be affected
 Patient's Child: Not increased unless mate is carrier or homozygote
IV **Age of Detectability:** First years of life
V **Prevalence:** Rare

Treatment
I **Primary Prevention:** Genetic counseling
II **Secondary Prevention:** Special education for deafness. Lens discission for cataract and orthopedic treatment of skeletal defects.
III **Other Therapy:** Medication because of extrasystoles

Prognosis: Possibly diminished life span

Detection of Carrier: ?

Special Considerations: —

References:
Cremers, C.W.R.J. et al: The Nathalie syndrome, a new hereditary syndrome. Clin. Genet. 8:330, 1975.

Contributor: **Cor W.R.J. Cremers**

Editor's Computerized Descriptors: Eye, Hearing, Skel., Muscle, CV., GU.

OTO-PALATO-DIGITAL SYNDROME

Includes: Syndrome oto-palato-digital
Otopalatodigitales Syndrom
Síndrome oto-pálato-digital

Excludes: Cleft palate, flattened facies and multiple congenital dislocations
Oro-cranio-digital syndrome (769)

Minimal Diagnostic Criteria: Unknown, but clinical change in face, hands and feet together with radiographic alteration of hands and feet seem to be minimal criteria.

Clinical Findings: Cleft palate, antimongoloid obliquity of palpebral fissures, conduction deafness, toes like those of a tree frog, flattened shortened terminal phalanges, subluxation of head of radius, wide-spaced nasal bridge giving pugilistic facies.

Roentgenographic alterations include vertical clivus, lack of normal flare of ilia, mild coxa valga, secondary ossification centers of proximal 2nd metacarpal and 2nd and 3rd metatarsals which fuse with cuneiform bones producing paddle-shaped structures.

Otologic surgical findings include abnormalities of the ossicles and chronic serous otitis media.

Complications
I **Derived:** —
II **Associated:** —

Etiology: X-linked recessive; McK *31130

Pathogenesis: ?

Related Facts
I **Sex Ratio:** M1:F0
II **Risk of Occurrence:** ?
III **Risk of Recurrence for**
 Patient's Sib: If mother is a carrier 1 in 2 (50%) for each brother to be affected and 1 in 2 for each sister to be a carrier
 Patient's Child: 1 in 1 (100%) for carrier daughters; not increased for sons unless wife is a carrier
IV **Age of Detectability:** Unknown, but probably by 2 or 3 years of age
V **Prevalence:** ?

Treatment
I **Primary Prevention:** Genetic counseling
II **Secondary Prevention:** Treatment of deafness has been (to date) limited to 2 cases- variable improvement. No therapy needed for feet or hands. Repair cleft palate.
III **Other Therapy:** —

Prognosis: Good, except for deafness

Detection of Carrier: Facial features in the female heterozygote are variable. Most constant is overhanging brow with prominent supraorbital ridges, depressed nasal bridge, and flat midface. Other skeletal alterations are variable. Females have higher frequency of greater multangular navicular fusion.

Special Considerations: —

References:
Dudding, B. et al: The otopalato-digital syndrome: A new symptom-complex consisting of deafness, dwarfism, cleft palate, characteristic facies, and a generalized bone dysplasia. Am. J. Dis. Child. 113:214, 1967.
Gall, J.C., Jr.: et al: Oto-palato-digital syndrome. Comparison of clinical and radiographic manifestations in males and females. Am. J. Hum. Genet. 24:24, 1972.
Gorlin, R. J. et al: The oto-palato-digital syndrome in females. Heterozygous expression of an X-linked trait. Oral Surg. 35:218, 1973.

Contributor: **Robert J. Gorlin**

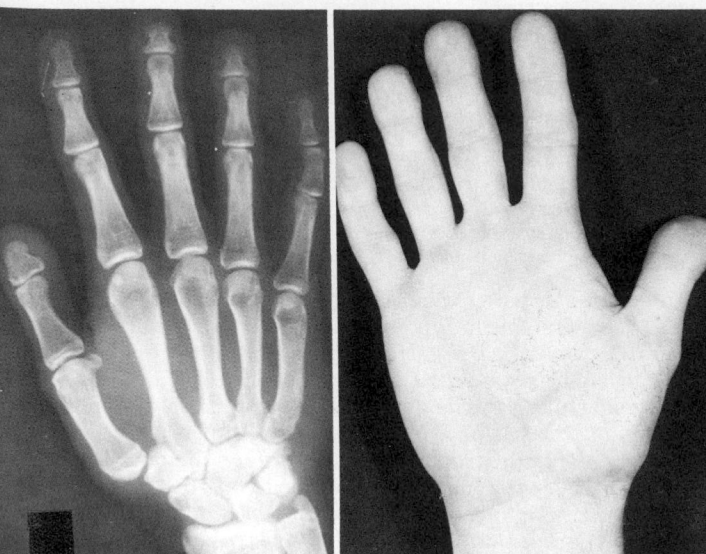

407. Xray and photo showing short distal phalanges of thumb and digits 3 and 4. Note fusion of hamate and capitate bones

OTOSCLEROSIS

Includes: Otosclérose
Otosklerose
Otoesclerosis
Labyrinthine otosclerosis
Labyrinthine otosclerosis with fixed stapes footplate

Excludes: Congenital ossicular fixation
Tympanosclerosis
Postinflammatory conductive hearing loss
Stapes fixation due to Paget osteitis deformans
Osteogenesis imperfecta (777)

Minimal Diagnostic Criteria: Progressive conductive hearing loss in a young or middle-aged adult without evidence of other middle ear disease.

Clinical Findings: There is a slowly progressive conductive hearing loss of insidious onset unrelated to inflammatory middle ear findings. Approximately 75% of cases are bilateral. The patient may volunteer a history of hearing better in noisy situations-'paracusis Willisiani." Tinnitus is a frequent complaint and is usually a low frequency type sometimes accompanied by an audible pulse. Vertigo is found in about 5-8% of patients with otosclerosis.

The tympanic membranes are normal to inspection and mobility is unaltered. There may be a pink flush seen through the eardrum caused by increased vascularity of the mucosa over the otosclerotic focus on the promontory of the middle ear-'Schwartze sign." This sign is believed to be correlated with increased vascularity in the mucosa of the promontory overlying the focus, and is believed to signify an "active" focus. An "inactive" focus is thought to be a healed area of otosclerosis and grossly appears whiter than the surrounding normal area. Audiometry reveals a conductive hearing loss of varying severity, initially more marked in the lower frequencies, but as the lesion progresses with increased stapes fixation all frequencies are affected. Middle ear impedance is increased as measured by an acoustic bridge. Labyrinthine or cochlear otosclerosis results in a sensorineural hearing loss. This may or may not be accompanied by a conductive component. The pathology is not clear but seems to be related to destruction of the endosteal membrane of the cochlea adjacent to spiral ligament. Radiologic examination by polytomography is generally not necessary clinically, but may be helpful in distinguishing otosclerotic stapes fixation from other acquired ossicular fixation or identifying an otosclerotic focus in a patient with a pure sensorineural loss.

At surgery the stapes footplate is found to be partially or completely fixed to the otic capsule by an otosclerotic focus. This most commonly occurs at the anterior footplate but can be at any other location, may be circumscribed, or the lesion may obliterate the oval window niche.

Complications
I   **Derived:** Labyrinthine or cochlear otosclerosis has been suspected to be a cause of severe sensorineural hearing loss. There has been evidence that sensorineural hearing losses are not increased in otosclerosis compared to the normal population, but there is a small percentage of these patients who show a severe progressive sensorineural hearing loss long before presbycusis could be assumed to be an explanation.
II **Associated:** Vestibular disturbances are more common in patients with otosclerosis than in the general population. There is a statistically significant correlation with the ability to taste phenylthiocarbamide, but the significance of this is unknown.

Etiology: Autosomal dominant with incomplete penetrance, estimated at between 25-40%, depending on the series studied.

Pathogenesis: Otosclerosis is a focal, progressive replacement of the endochondral bone of the otic capsule with abnormal bone which has the microscopic appearance of healing fibrous bone, but is normally calcified. The site of predilection is the otic capsule anterior to the stapes footplate, and the process progresses to involve and fix the stapes footplate to the surrounding bone. The pathogenesis of the sensorineural hearing loss is not yet completely understood.

Related Facts
I   **Sex Ratio:** M1:F1
II **Risk of Occurrence:** ?
III **Risk of Recurrence for**
      Patient's Sib: If only 1 parent is affected, 1 in 5 to 1 in 8 depending on penetrance.
      Patient's Child: If spouse is not affected, 1 in 5 to 1 in 8. Reproductive fitness of proband is not affected
IV **Age of Detectability:** A conductive hearing loss is first seen at age 11-15 in 10% of cases, progressing to 50% at age 21-25, and reaching 100% at age 40. Earlier detectability could possibly be achieved with temporal bone tomograms in the absence of clinical findings, but the significance of this in terms of morbidity is unclear.
V   **Prevalence:** Clinical otosclerosis is 1 in 330 in the Caucasian population, about 1 in 3300 in the Negro population, and estimated to be 1 in 33,000 in the Oriental. Series of temporal bone specimens which show histologic otosclerosis, not necessarily with hearing loss, have shown histologic otosclerosis to be present in 1 in 14 to 1 in 10 of Caucasian subjects studied in the United States and approximately 1 in 100 in Negroes.

Treatment
I   **Primary Prevention:** Genetic counseling
II **Secondary Prevention:** Stapedectomy to restore hearing in those with a conductive loss secondary to otosclerosis has been highly developed and is generally very successful. The most common procedure is removal of the fixed stapes from the oval window and replacement with a wire or teflon prosthesis. The oval window is cleaned of otosclerotic bone and covered with Gelfoam, fat or vein and the prosthesis placed between the incus and this new membrane. Improvement in hearing occurs in approximately 90+% with an incidence of surgical complications about 3%.
III **Other Therapy:** —

Prognosis: Normal for life span and intelligence

Detection of Carrier: —

Special Considerations: —

References:
Kelemen, G. and Linthicum, F.H., Jr.: Labyrinthine otosclerosis. Acta Otolaryngol. (Suppl.) 253:1, 1969.
Morrison, A.W. and Bundey, S.E.: The inheritance of otosclerosis. J. Laryngol. Otol. 84:921, 1970.
Schuknecht, H.F. (ed.): Otosclerosis. Henry Ford Hospital International Symposium. Boston:Little, Brown and Co., 1962.

Contributors: Daniel R. Miller
LaVonne Bergstrom

———————————

Editor's Computerized Descriptors: Hearing, Ear

PACHYDERMOPERIOSTOSIS

Includes: Pachydermopériostose
Paquidermoperiostosis
Idiopathic hypertrophic osteoarthropathy
Touraine-Solente-Golé syndrome
Osteoarthropathy, idiopathic hypertrophic

Excludes: Secondary (pulmonary) hypertrophic osteoarthropathy
Thyroid acropachy

Minimal Diagnostic Criteria: The presence of at least 2 of the 3 major abnormalities (clubbing, periostosis, cutis gyrata) in an individual with a negative family history and no sign of a predisposing lesion (eg bronchogenic carcinoma), or the presence of 1 of these major lesions in a close relative of a typical case.†

Clinical Findings: Clubbing of the fingers and toes; periosteal new bone formation, especially over the distal ends of the long bones; coarse facial features with thickening, furrowing and excessive oiliness of the skin of the face and forehead (cutis verticis gyrata); hyperhidrosis of the hands and feet and occasional intermittent swelling or pain in the large joints. Radiographs reveal irregular subperiosteal ossification over the long bones, primarily at the distal ends and most pronounced at the insertion of tendons and ligaments. There is marked variability in expressivity, the disorder being more severe in males than in females.

Complications
I   **Derived:** Ptosis due to hypertrophy of the eyelids, skeletal pain secondary to periostosis, seborrheic dermatitis and secondary folliculitis associated with large open skin pores
II **Associated:** —

Etiology: Autosomal dominant with marked variability in phenotypic expression, usually more severe in males

Pathogenesis: This syndrome usually appears around puberty and slowly progresses for about 10 years being self-limited thereafter. Periostosis and clubbing may well be related to an autonomic nervous system defect, since there is a decrease in peripheral blood flow and vagal resection has been reported to improve the symptoms of joint swelling. Skin histopathology is characterized by a proliferation of fibrocytes, and increased collagen and acid mucopolysaccharide production in the dermis.

Related Facts
I   **Sex Ratio:** M7:F1 among reported cases but probably related to increased severity of the disease in males
II **Risk of Occurrence:** ?
III **Risk of Recurrence for**
      Patient's Sib: If parent is affected, 1 in 2 (50%) for each offspring to be affected; otherwise not increased.
      Patient's Child: 1 in 2
IV **Age of Detectability:** Childhood or adolescence by clinical features
V   **Prevalence:** ?

Treatment
I   **Primary Prevention:** Genetic counseling
II **Secondary Prevention:** Plastic surgery to improve facial appearance; vagotomy is said to relieve skeletal pain and swelling.
III **Other Therapy:** —

Prognosis: Normal life span

Detection of Carrier: Skeletal radiographs may detect periosteal new bone formation in otherwise unaffected female relatives.

†Special Considerations: It is important to distinguish this disorder from secondary hypertrophic osteoarthropathy as the latter condition may be associated with a treatable primary lesion (eg bronchogenic carcinoma, bronchiectasis, ulcerative colitis). A full clinical work-up for a primary lesion must be performed on all sporadic cases of pachydermoperiostosis as the diagnosis of this genetic disorder in isolated cases can only be made by exclusion.

The unequal sex ratio is probably due to the variable expression of this dominant trait, which is much more severe in males. The phenotypic expression of this trait in females may be limited to asymptomatic periosteal new bone formation, and these individuals would go undetected unless skeletal radiographs were obtained.

References:
Hambrick, G.W. Jr. and Carter, B.M.: Pachydermoperiostosis. Touraine-Solente-Golé syndrome. Arch. Dermtol. 94:594, 1966.

Rimoin, D.L.: Pachydermoperiostosis (idiopathic clubbing and periostosis): Genetic and physiologic considerations. N. Engl. J. Med. 272:923, 1965.

Vogl, A. and Goldfischer, S.: Pachydermoperiostosis: Primary or idiopathic hypertrophic osteoarthropathy. Am. J. Med. 33:166, 1962.

Contributor: **David L. Rimoin**

Editor's Computerized Descriptors: Eye, Face, Skin, Sweating, Nails, Skel.

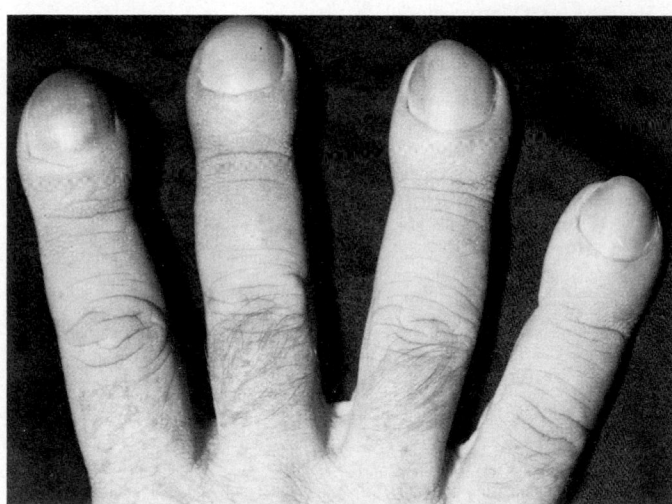

408. Note clubbing of fingers

PACHYONYCHIA CONGENITA

Includes: Pachyonychie congénitale
Kongenitale Pachyonychie
Paquioniquia congénita
Pachyonychia congenita types I, II and III

Excludes: Dyskeratosis
Keratoderma of palms and soles
Pityriasis rubra pilaris (811)

Minimal Diagnostic Criteria: Thick nails on all digits beginning soon after birth.

Clinical Findings: Greatly thickened nails, angling upward, on all digits. Nail plates appear pinched up so that the free edges are distally raised, narrowed and pointed, giving appearance of claw or knob. Scalloped edges on tongue. Tender bullae and callosities especially on plantar pressure areas. Three clinical types may be observed as follows:

Type I- symmetric palmar and plantar callosities with follicular keratoses of the trunk.

Type II- type I plus oral or lingual mucosal lesions resembling leukokeratosis or leukoplakia and scalloped tongue. This is the Riehl type and is most frequent.

Type III- type I with corneal changes.

Complications
I **Derived:**   Traumatic injury to nail roots; infection, either monilial or bacterial; paronychial infection. Difficult walking due to painful calluses. Blindness (type III)
II **Associated:**   —

Etiology: Autosomal dominant; McK *16720

Pathogenesis: Probably congenital misalignment of nail root so that nails grow up instead of out. Hyperkeratosis of ventral nail and hyper- and parakeratosis of matrix.

Related Facts
I **Sex Ratio:**   M1:F1
II **Risk of Occurrence:**   Rare
III **Risk of Recurrence for**
Patient's Sib: If parent is affected, 1 in 2 (50%) for each offspring to be affected; otherwise not increased.
Patient's Child: 1 in 2
IV **Age of Detectability:**   As neonate or infant
V **Prevalence:**   ?

Treatment
I **Primary Prevention:**   Genetic counseling
II **Secondary Prevention:**   Filing or grinding nails. Surgical avulsion may result in regrowth with further nail distortion. Amputation of distal phalanges reported in one case.
III **Other Therapy:**   Specially fitted shoes, treatment of infections

Prognosis: Defects remain for life.

Detection of Carrier: —

Special Considerations: —

References:
Cosman, B. et al: Plastic surgery in pachyonychia congenita and other dyskeratoses: Case report and review of the literature. Plast. Reconstr. Surg. 33:226, 1964.

Joseph, H.L.: Pachyonychia congenita. Arch. Dermatol. 90:594, 1964.

Kumer, L. and Loos, H.O.: Über Pachyonychia congenita (Typus Riehl). Wien. Klin. Wochenschr. 48:174, 1935.

Wright, C.S. and Guequierre, J.P.: Pachyonychia congenita: Report of two cases, with studies on therapy. Arch. Dermatol. Syph. 55:819, 1947.

Contributor: **Herbert L. Joseph**

PALATE FISTULA (MARKER)

Includes: Fistule palatine
Gaumenfistel
Fistula palatina (Marcador)
Fistula of palate

Excludes: Nasoalveolar fistula and cyst
Median palatal fistula and cyst

Minimal Diagnostic Criteria: Small openings in anterior pillars at junction of soft palate and pharynx

Clinical Findings: Bilateral or unilateral fistulas at junction of soft palate and pharynx in the anterior pillars without cicatrization

Complications
I   **Derived:** —
II **Associated:** Absence of palatine tonsils

Etiology: ?

Pathogenesis: Maldevelopment of 2nd branchial pouch with failure of complete obliteration of pouch. Resultant fistula lined by stratified squamous epithelium with lymphoid tissue adjacent.

Related Facts
I   **Sex Ratio:** Insufficient data
II   **Risk of Occurrence:** ?
III **Risk of Recurrence for**
     Patient's Sib: ?
     Patient's Child: ?
IV   **Age of Detectability:** At birth by visual examination
V   **Prevalence:** ?

Treatment
I   **Primary Prevention:** —
II   **Secondary Prevention:** —
III **Other Therapy:** —

Prognosis: Excellent

Detection of Carrier: —

Special Considerations: —

References:
Claiborne, J. H., Jr.: Hiatus in the anterior pillar of the fauces of the right side with congenital absence of tonsil on either side. Am. J. Med. Sci. 89:490, 1885.
Gorlin, R. J. and Pindborg, J. J.: Syndromes of the Head and Neck. New York:McGraw-Hill, 1964.
Neuss, O.: Anatomische Varianten und Fehlbildungen der Mundhöhle mit Darstellung eines Falles symmetrischer Fistelbildung in den vorderen Gaumenbögen. Z. Laryngol. Rhinol. 35:411, 1956.

Contributor: **Jan E. Jirásek**

Editor's Computerized Descriptors: Oral, Nasoph.

PALLISTER-W SYNDROME

Includes: Syndrome W
W Syndrom
Síndrome de Pallister tipo W

Excludes: OPD syndrome

Minimal Diagnostic Criteria: Mental retardation, some manifestations of a median oral cleft, the characteristic facial appearance, and mild skeletal abnormalities of the upper limbs.

Clinical Findings: Presently the syndrome is defined on the basis of 2 male sibs having a malformation-mental retardation syndrome with the following features: moderate mental retardation, grand mal seizures, tremor, mild spasticity, an incomplete median cleft in the palate and upper lip, broad tip of nose, broad and flat maxilla, telecanthus, alternating esotropia and high forehead. Skeletal abnormalities in the upper limbs included cubitus valgus, shortness of the ulnae, bowing of the radii and clinocamptodactyly. One patient had pes cavus, the other metatarsus varus and pes planus.

Complications
I **Derived:** Broad uvula, absent incisors, and nasal speech secondary to oral cleft; antimongoloid slant of palpebral fissures secondary to hypoplastic maxillae anterior cowlick secondary to high forehead. Injury secondary to seizures and mental retardation.
II **Associated:** Prematurity

Etiology: Autosomal dominant (with manifestations expressed more severely in males than in females),, or X-linked recessive (with some expression in female heterozygotes).

Pathogenesis: A number of the facial manifestations can be related to incomplete median clefting.

Related Facts
I **Sex Ratio:** 2 brothers had severe, their mother and sister had mild manifestations.
II **Risk of Occurrence:** Small
III **Risk of Recurrence for**
 Patient's Sib: If autosomal dominant or X-linked recessive, see Table I AD or X-linked R, respectively.
 Patient's Child: If autosomal dominant or X-linked recessive, see Table I AD or X-linked R, respectively.
IV **Age of Detectability:** At birth
V **Prevalence:** Apparently rare

Treatment
I **Primary Prevention:** Genetic counseling
II **Secondary Prevention:** Cleft palate care and repair, correction of strabismus, orthopedic surgery
III **Other Therapy:** Special education, speech therapy, seizure control

Prognosis: Survival into adulthood

Detection of Carrier: Females at-risk for producing affected males may show mild craniofacial manifestations.

Special Considerations: —

References:
Pallister, P.D. et al: The W syndrome. In Bergsma, D. (ed.): Malformation Syndromes, Birth Defects: Orig. Art. Ser., vol. X, no. 7. Miami:Symposia Specialists for The National Foundation-March of Dimes, 1974, p. 51.

Contributor: **Jürgen Herrmann**

Editor's Computerized Descriptors: Eye, Face, Oral, Teeth, Nose, Hair, Skel., Nerve

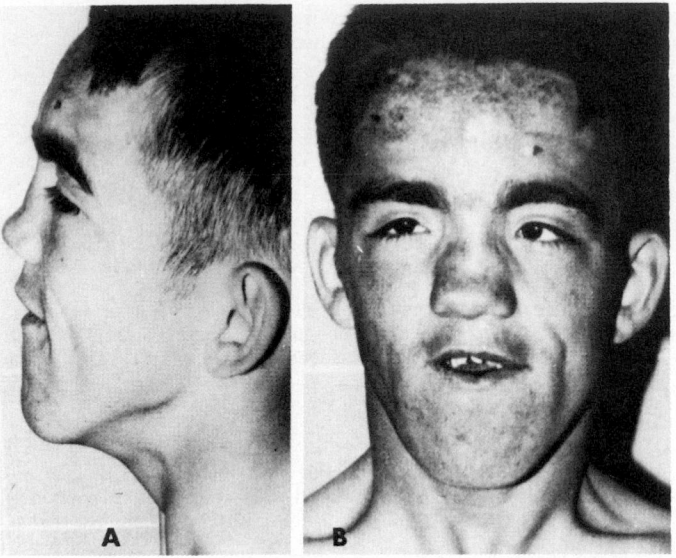

409. A) Lateral view of face in Pallister syndrome; B) frontal view

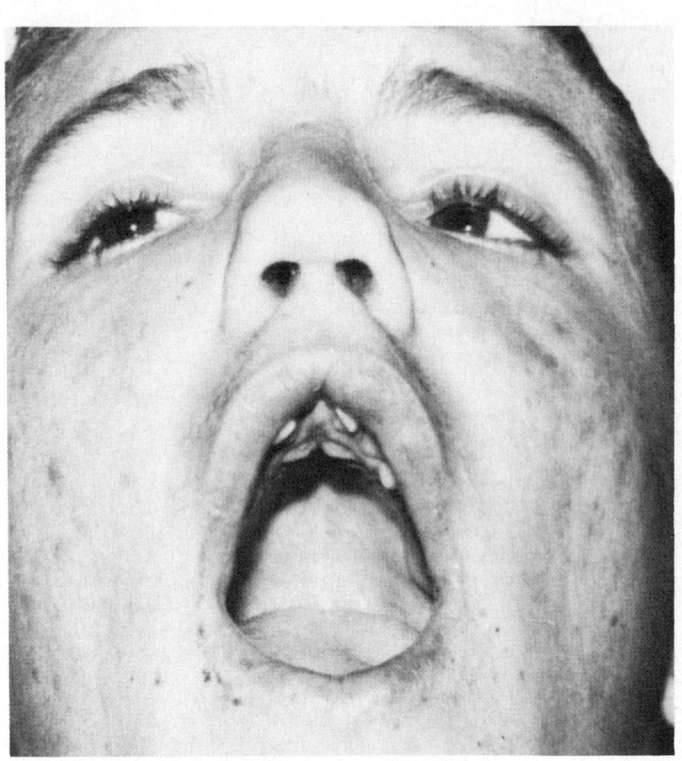

410. Incomplete median cleft of palate and upper lip

PALMO-PLANTAR ERYTHEMA

Includes: Erythéme palmo-plantaire
Hereditäres palmo-plantares erythem
Eritema palmo-plantar
Hereditary palmo-plantar erythema
Erytheme palmare hereditarium
Lane disease
Red palms

Excludes: —

Minimal Diagnostic Criteria: Constant erythema of palmar surfaces of fingers†

Clinical Findings: Constant bright mottled erythema over the thenar and hypothenar eminence, palmar surface at the base of the fingers, and the palmar surfaces of the fingers. May involve the soles.

Complications
I   **Derived:** —
II **Associated:** Keratosis palmaris et plantaris in certain affected families. May be related with liver disease, rheumatoid arthritis, chronic immunologic diseases, aging, pregnancy.†

Etiology: ? Possibly autosomal dominant†; McK *13300

Pathogenesis: ?

Related Facts
I   **Sex Ratio:** M?:F?
II   **Risk of Occurrence:** Rare
III **Risk of Recurrence for**
    Patient's Sib: ? If autosomal dominant and if parent is affected, 1 in 2 (50%) for each offspring to be affected; otherwise not increased.
    Patient's Child: ? If autosomal dominant, 1 in 2
IV **Age of Detectability:** ?
V   **Prevalence:** ?

Treatment
I   **Primary Prevention:** —
II   **Secondary Prevention:** —
III **Other Therapy:** —

Prognosis: ?

Detection of Carrier: —

†**Special Considerations:** The condition was first described in 2 patients in 1929. The lesion is indistinguishable from, if not precisely the same phenomenon as, palmar erythema of liver disease, normal pregnancy, rheumatoid arthritis and perhaps many other diseases. Even such nonspecific states as aging may show red palms. The evidence that it is hereditary is very thin indeed; the heritable etiology of palmar erythema seems to be unfortunately perpetuated from book to book and in published papers since its first casual appearance in 1929.

References:
Bland, J.H. et al: Palmar erythema and spider angiomata in rheumatoid arthritis. Ann. Intern. Med. 48:1026, 1958.
Lane, J.E.: Erytheme palmare hereditarium. Arch. Dermatol. Syph. (Chic.) 20:445, 1929.

Contributor: **John H. Bland**

Editor's Computerized Descriptor: Skin

PANCREATITIS, HEREDITARY

Includes: Pancréatite héréditaire
Hereditäre Pankreatitis
Pancreatitis hereditaria
Familial pancreatitis

Excludes: Chronic relapsing pancreatitis associated with hyperlipidemia or hyperparathyroidism
Idiopathic acute pancreatitis
Cystic fibrosis (237)

Minimal Diagnostic Criteria: Increased serum amylase and lipase during the acute phase of illness will serve to diagnose pancreatitis. Increased urinary amylase to creatinine clearance ratio helps confirm serum values and should be performed when possible.

Calcifications in the distribution of the pancreas, especially if apparent in childhood, strongly suggests hereditary pancreatitis.

The diagnosis can be made if there is documentation of repeated episodes of acute pancreatitis and a family history of similar illness. Analysis of serum lipoproteins and evaluation of parathyroid function are necessary to exclude familial hyperlipidemia and hyperparathyroidism.

Clinical Findings: Hereditary pancreatitis presents with episodes of recurrent epigastric or abdominal pain that may radiate through to the back and subscapular area. The pain is often initiated by a large fatty or spicy meal. The attack progresses to maximal intensity in 24-48 hours and abates in 4 days to several weeks. Nausea and vomiting frequently accompany the pain and may result in serum electrolyte disturbances. Serum and urinary amylase and lipase will be elevated during the active phase. The attacks of acute pancreatitis are separated by symptom-free periods of days to years in duration. During the symptom-free periods there will be no disturbance in serum amylase and lipase.

In time, the repeated episodes of pancreatitis result in pancreatic fibrosis with exocrine insufficiency (30-50%) or glucose intolerance (30%). Pancreatic exocrine insufficiency produces steatorrhea in most instances, but subclinical disease may be diagnosed by measurement of pancreatic peptidases or lipase obtained at duodenal intubation. Secretin stimulation may provide another degree of discrimination of exocrine funciton.

Pancreatic calcifications observed on abdominal xray are of diagnostic importance. Some patients (50%) will exhibit coarse, rounded calcifications in the head of the pancreas. Linear distribution is consistent with the anatomic finding of calcifications in the major pancreatic ducts.

Involvement of multiple family members has been documented in all series.

Complications
I   **Derived:** Acute dehydration and serum electrolyte disturbances (common in acute attacks); pancreatic exocrine insufficiency (often with steatorrhea); pancreatic endocrine insufficiency (glucose intolerance); pancreatic carcinoma (25%); portal or splenic vein thrombosis (rare); acute hemorrhagic pancreatitis (with or without hemorrhagic pleural and peritoneal effusions) (rare); and pancreatic pseudocyst.
II **Associated:** Aminoaciduria (cystine and lysine) has been documented in 2 families. Abnormal sweat electrolytes have been found in 1 family.

Etiology: Hereditary pancreatitis is inherited as an autosomal dominant trait with incomplete penetrance and variable expressivity. McK *16780

Pathogenesis: The biochemical or anatomic abnormality responsible for recurrent bouts of pancreatitis has not been established.

Related Facts
I Sex Ratio: M1:F1

II Risk of Occurrence: ? Rare

III Risk of Recurrence for
Patient's Sib: If parent is affected 1 in 2 (50%) for each offspring to be affected.
Patient's Child: 1 in 2

IV Age of Detectability: The majority of cases have their onset in childhood, often in infancy.

V Prevalence: ? 231 known or suspected cases have been reported.

Treatment
I Primary Prevention: Genetic counseling

II Secondary Prevention: —

III Other Therapy: Supportive measures during acute attacks include restorative and maintenance IV fluids and electrolytes, NPO, nasogastric suction and narcotic pain medication. Enzyme replacement and low fat diet for pancreatic exocrine insufficiency. Appropriate measures for control of glucose intolerance.

Prognosis: Life expectancy is generally normal, if acute attacks are managed appropriately and pancreatic carcinoma is not a complicating factor.

Detection of Carrier: Asymptomatic parents of affected individuals have been shown to have abnormalities in pancreatic exocrine function.

Special Considerations: —

References:
Gross, J.B. et al: Hereditary pancreatitis. Am. J. Med. 33:358, 1962.
Kattwinkel, J. et al: Hereditary pancreatitis. Pediatrics 51:55, 1973.

Contributor: **Peter F. Whitington**

Editor's Computerized Descriptor: GI.

PARALYSIS, HYPERKALEMIC PERIODIC

Includes: Paralysie périodique hyperkaliémique
Hyperkaliämische Paresen
Parálisis periódica hipercaliémica
Periodic paralysis, hyperpotassemic
Adynamia episodica hereditaria
Hyperkalemic periodic paralysis

Excludes: Paralysis, hypokalemic periodic (795)
Normokalemic periodic paralysis
Paramyotonia congenita (796)

Minimal Diagnostic Criteria: Episodes of flaccid paralysis associated with an elevated serum potassium on at least one occasion during an attack. Positive family history.

Clinical Findings: In this condition typical appearance of paralytic attacks occur proximally. The condition is usually first detected by the parents in infancy or in childhood. The attacks occur most commonly and with greatest frequency and severity when the child is at school, becoming less frequent later in life with the avoidance of unnecessary exercise. A typical attack characteristically develops when the individual is sitting in a chair or is in bed after exercise. If the exercise has been severe, resting for 30 minutes is often sufficient to induce an attack. Weakness is usually noticed first in the lower back, in the thighs and calves, and in the arms and legs. In severe attacks the neck muscles are affected and, very occasionally, there may be difficulty in swallowing and coughing. The muscles innervated by the cranial nerves are rarely affected. Clinical myotonia, and especially electromyographically demonstrated myotonia occur especially during attacks.

Although severe attacks may occasionally last 2 or more days, most attacks are short; even in the more severe episodes the weakness is usually at its worst within 30 to 40 minutes and it has largely vanished within 3 hours. Mild, variable weakness may persist for many hours at a time. Recovery may be enhanced by exercise and developing attacks can be terminated or aborted in the same way, although they are then likely to recur (sometimes with increased severity) after resting. The number and severity of attacks can vary markedly, even in a single family. Some patients may have very rare attacks, while others may have one or more severe attacks every day. Other factors aside from exercise which can precipitate clinical attacks include emotion, cold, hunger, infections and general anesthesia.

Physical examination between attacks usually shows no abnormality. In some families, a proximal myopathy develops later in life when the attacks or paralysis lessen. Weakness during the attacks may be variable in incidence and distribution, but generally it tends to affect the trunk and proximal muscles and it may develop into a severe flaccid quadriplegia. Swallowing may be difficult but respiratory muscles are only rarely involved. Reflexes are diminished or absent in severe attacks, but excitability to direct percussion may be increased, although usually diminished or absent.

Laboratory features demonstrate, generally, a rise in serum potassium during attacks and a normal serum potassium between attacks. There are no other significant abnormalities aside from electromyographically demonstrated myotonia, usually during attacks or during the administration of a thiazide diuretic.

Complications
I Derived: Dysphagia with aspiration pneumonitis and occa-

sionally marked hypoventilation during attacks.

II Associated: —

Etiology: Autosomal dominant

Pathogenesis: ? Possibly some alteration in sarcolemmal membrane permeability to electrolytes, or a defect in the sarcoplasmic reticulum membrane. Evidence of marked depolarization of the muscle cell membrane has been demonstrated during attacks, and partial depolarization has also been demonstrated between attacks by intrafiber electrode studies.

Related Facts
I   Sex Ratio: M1:F1
II Risk of Occurrence: ?
III Risk of Recurrence for
   Patient's Sib: If parent is affected, 1 in 2 (50%) for each offspring to be affected; otherwise not increased.
   Patient's Child: 1 in 2
IV Age of Detectability: Usually at birth or early infancy with episodes of weakness, or even by minimally demonstrable facial or ocular myotonia.
V   Prevalence: ?

Treatment
I   Primary Prevention: Genetic counseling
II Secondary Prevention: Treatment of the acute attack has been said to be benefitted by calcium gluconate, 1 - 2 gm orally. Intravenous chlorothiazide, or glucose and insulin may be helpful. Prophylactic treatment consists of regular gentle exercise after exertion, liberal carbohydrate feedings and the use of carbonic anhydrase inhibitors regularly, including acetozalamide or the longer acting carbonic anhydrase inhibitor dichlorphenamide, the latter in a dosage of 50 to 100 mg daily. Chlorothiazide, about 500 to 750 mg daily or hydrochlorothiazide, in a dosage of 100 to 150 mg daily may prove to be beneficial. In some patients on diuretic therapy, mild supplementation with oral potassium may be required to avoid bothersome myotonia.
III Other Therapy: —

Prognosis: Generally good for life, although a very small percentage (less than 1%) of individuals may die during an acute attack of weakness. Significant myopathic weakness of primarily the proximal variety may develop late in life in a small percentage of patients afflicted with this disorder. In those individuals, the muscle biopsy may demonstrate a significant vacuolar myopathy.

Detection of Carrier: By inducing attacks, or occasionally by demonstration of myotonia during weakness, or after the administration of an oral diuretic.

Special Considerations: —

References:
  Layzer, R. R. et al: Hyperkalemic periodic paralysis. Arch. Neurol. 16:455, 1967.
  Pearson, C. M.: The periodic paralyses: Differential features and pathological observations in permanent myopathic weakness. Brain 87:341, 1964.
  Pearson, C. M. and Kalyanaramen, K.: The periodic paralyses. In Stanbury, J. B. et al (eds.): The Metabolic Basis of Inherited Disease, 3rd Ed. New York:McGraw-HIll, 1972, p. 1181.

Contributor: **Carl M. Pearson**

Editor's Computerized Descriptors: Muscle, Resp.

PARALYSIS, HYPOKALEMIC PERIODIC

Includes: Paralysie périodique hypokaliémique
  Hypokaliämische Paresen
  Parálisis periódica hipocaliémica
  Periodic paralysis, hypopotassemic
  Familial periodic paralysis
  Hypokalemic periodic paralysis

Excludes: Paralysis, hyperkalemic periodic (794)
  Normokalemic periodic paralysis
  Paramyotonia congenita (796)

Minimal Diagnostic Criteria: Attacks of minimal or severe paralysis in conjunction with lowered serum potassium levels. Positive family history.

Clinical Findings: Characterized by attacks of flaccid quadriplegia, commonly lasting for several hours. In most families the attacks begin during the 2nd decade and are at their greatest frequency between the ages of 20 and 35 years. They then tend to decrease in number and severity, and especially in females they may completely disappear. The attacks can vary in severity from slight transient weakness of a single muscle group to almost complete paralysis. In a typical severe attack an otherwise healthy young adult awakens in the early morning hours unable to move his limbs or trunk. He is able to breathe, talk, and swallow and show facial movements almost normally. Most moderate or severe attacks last 6-24 hours, but especially severe paralysis may last for 2-3 days or longer. Rapid complete recovery then almost invariably occurs within 1 or 2 hours. If the patient is awakened at an early stage, or if the onset is during the daytime, it is often possible by exercising the weak muscles to abort the attack. It is characteristic for the lower limbs to be affected first, then the arms, the trunk, the neck and sometimes the face. Death occurs very rarely in an attack. The proximal muscles of the limbs are the first to be affected and, even in severe attacks, slight movement of the fingers is often possible.

The most important predisposing factors are prolonged rest after vigorous exercise, a heavy meal a few hours before, anxiety, emotion or cold. A heavy carbohydrate meal seems to be particularly apt to be followed by paralysis. Giving frequent doses of glucose, or preferably glucose and insulin is one of the most certain methods of inducing an attack.

Examination during an attack shows flaccid paralysis to occur predominantly in the proximal distribution. The paralyzed muscles fail to respond to direct mechanical or electrical stimulation. Bradycardia is not uncommon and the ECGs show prominent U waves, and flattening of the T waves in conjunction with the lowered serum potassium to the level of 2.0 to 2.5 MEq/L. Between attacks, patient's strength and serum potassium level are invariably within the normal range, although sometimes at the lower normal level.

Complications
I   Derived: During attacks severe dysphagia with aspiration pneumonitis occurs very rarely, and respiratory failure (because of respiratory muscle weakness) occurs extremely rarely.
II Associated: Occasionally electromyographic myotonia may be demonstrated during attacks.

Etiology: Autosomal dominant with complete penetrance.
  Males are somewhat more symptomatically affected than females.

Pathogenesis: ? There probably is a defect in muscle cell membrane polarization or impermeability to electrolytes, especially potassium, sodium and chloride. A defect in the membrane of the sarcoplasmic reticulum has been postulated.

Related Facts

I **Sex Ratio:** M1:F1 actual, but manifesting M1:F0.7
II **Risk of Occurrence:** ? Relatively rare
III **Risk of Recurrence for**
    Patient's Sib: If parent is affected, male 1 in 2; female 1 in 2.5 to be affected.
    Patient's Child: Male 1 in 2; female 1 in 3
IV **Age of Detectability:** Second decade. Theoretically an attack of weakness could be precipitated anytime after birth by an infusion of glucose and insulin.
V **Prevalence:** ?

Treatment

I **Primary Prevention:** Genetic counseling
II **Secondary Prevention:** Treatment of attacks with infusion or administration of potassium salts. 10 gm of KC1 may be given orally, in an adult, and an additional 5 gm may be required. If this cannot be tolerated its equivalent in another quickly absorbed K-containing solution can be given or intravenous infusion of potassium may be given. It must be absolutely certainly established that the paralysis is of the hypokalemic variety before such therapy is undertaken.

    Prophylactic treatment consists of continuous high level potassium administration, although this treatment alone is often not beneficial. Others have managed prophylactic treatment with spironolactone (Aldactone-A) 100 to 200 mg daily, a thiazide diuretic such as chlorothiazide (250 to 750 mg daily), or a carbonic anhydrase inhibitor such as acetozalamide or dichlorphenamide, the latter in a dosage of 50 to 100 mg daily.

III **Other Therapy:** —

Prognosis: Generally good for life, but about 2-5% of persons may die in a severe attack. Rarely, a slowly progressive myopathy with myopathic weakness, predominantly proximal in distribution, may develop late in life after paroxysmal attacks have almost completely disappeared.

Detection of Carrier: Difficult to do, but it is theoretically possible to precipitate an attack of weakness in an otherwise asymptomatic carrier by intravenous administration of glucose and insulin or even with large quantities of carbohydrate, given orally in conjunction with prolonged inactivity.

Special Considerations: —

References:
McArdle, B.: Metabolic myopathies: The glycogenoses affecting muscle and hypo- and hyperkalemic periodic paralysis. Am. J. Med. 35:661, 1963.
Pearson, C. M. and Kalyanaramen, K.: The periodic paralyses. In Stanbury, J.B. et al (eds.): The Metabolic Basis of Inherited Disease, 3rd Ed. New York:McGraw-Hill, 1972, p. 1180.
Shy, G. M. et al: Studies in familial periodic paralysis. Exp. Neurol. 3:53, 1961.

Contributor: **Carl M. Pearson**

Editor's Computerized Descriptors: Muscle, CV.

PARAMYOTONIA CONGENITA

Includes: Paramyotonie congénitale
Paramiotonía congénita
Myotonia congenita intermittens
Eulenburg disease

Excludes: Myotonic dystrophy (702)
Myotonia congenita (701)
Paralysis, hyperkalemic periodic (794)
All other conditions in which myotonia exists

Minimal Diagnostic Criteria: Myotonia initiated by cold. Often fluctuation in serum potassium level in conjunction with periodic attacks of weakness. Positive family history of a similar disturbance.

Clinical Findings: The affected individual suffers from myotonia (an inability to rapidly release a firm grasp) which is apparent only upon exposure to cold. In addition, some of the patients experienced attacks of unexplained generalized muscular weakness. The problem is somewhat difficult to resolve completely since *all forms of myotonia* are always made somewhat worse by exposure to general body chilling or cold. Thus the criteria may not be completely sufficient to distinguish paramyotonia from myotonia congenita. The attacks of muscular weakness which occur in affected individuals serve, to some extent, to distinguish this condition from myotonia congenita (in which paroxysmal weakness rarely occurs) and it is now recognized that the attacks of weakness are *quite similar* to those which occur in hyperkalemic periodic paralysis. The weakness that occurs in paramyotonia is accompanied by a rise in serum potassium. However, there are other families and patients that have been described in whom the myotonia is accompanied by a *drop* in the serum potassium. Thus, although the nosologic status of paramyotonia congenita is somewhat confused, it still remains a useful diagnostic category for all patients in whom myotonic weakness is induced by cold.

Complications
I **Derived:** —
II **Associated:** —

Etiology: Autosomal dominant; McK *16830

Pathogenesis: ? There is usually no evidence of pathologic change in muscle fibers, although occasionally vacuolization of mild degree has been described. There may be some type of membrane defect either of the sarcolemmal membrane or of the sarcoplasmic reticulum membranes, although this is yet to be classified.

Related Facts
I **Sex Ratio:** M1:F1
II **Risk of Occurrence:** ?
III **Risk of Recurrence for**
    Patient's Sib: If parent is affected, 1 in 2 (50%) for each offspring to be affected; otherwise not increased.
    Patient's Child: 1 in 2
IV **Age of Detectability:** Potentially at birth, commonly within the first several years of life, especially by electromyographic studies, and particularly when the patient is chilled.
V **Prevalence:** ?

Treatment
I **Primary Prevention:** Genetic counseling
II **Secondary Prevention:** Regulation of serum potassium levels by acetozalamide or the thiazide diuretics has proved, in some families, to be helpful in decreasing the number of attacks but not in preventing myotonia. Myotonia may respond to treatment with either quinine or diphenylhydantoin.

III Other Therapy: —

Prognosis: Generally good for life

Detection of Carrier: Demonstration of myotonia, electromyographically or clinically, often at room temperature and always upon exposure to cold.

Special Considerations: —

References:

Drager, G.A. et al: Paramyotonia congenita. Arch. Neurol. 80:1, 1958.

Erb, W.: Ueber die "Juvenil Form" der progressiven Muskelatrophie und ihre Beziehungen zur sogenannten Pseudohypertrophie der Muskeln. Dtsch. Arch. Klin. Med. 34:467, 1884.

Magee, K. R.: A study of paramyotonia congenita. Arch. Neurol. 8:461, 1963.

Contributor: **Carl M. Pearson**

Editor's Computerized Descriptor: Muscle

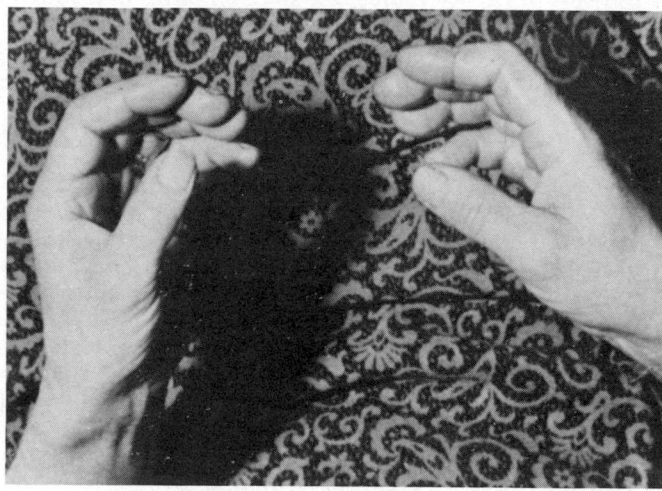

411. Paramyotonia congenita. After a short exposure to cold, fingers become stiff, then weak and paralyzed

PARANASAL SINUSES, ABSENT

Includes: Agénésie des sinus de la face
Aplasie der Nasennebenhöhlen
Ausencia de los senos paranasales
Paranasal sinuses, panagenesis
Agenesis of paranasal sinuses, unilateral
Sinuses, absence of frontal

Excludes: Hypoplastic paranasal sinuses
Absence of frontal sinuses, microcornea and glaucoma

Minimal Diagnostic Criteria: Absence of paranasal sinuses radiographically, if the patient is past the age at which the sinuses are present on xrays. (The average age at which the paranasal sinuses become identifiable on xrays is maxillary—2 years; frontal—6-8 years; ethmoid—2 years; sphenoid—4 years.)

In adults with absence radiographically of only 1 sinus, the possibility of neoplastic and inflammatory disease must be eliminated before a diagnosis of agenesis can be assumed. This may necessitate surgical exploration.

Clinical Findings: Transillumination of involved frontal or maxillary sinuses is not possible. However, this is of little help in small children because the sinuses are not large enough normally to transilluminate well. Palpation of the face over the paranasal sinuses will be normal. Examination of the nose may reveal abnormalities of the turbinates on the ipsilateral side of the unilateral agenesis. Waters view, lateral view, Caldwell view and basal view xrays will show absence of some or all paranasal sinuses.†

Complications

I **Derived:** —

II **Associated:** A single family study with hereditary microcornea, glaucoma, and absent frontal sinuses.

Etiology: ?

Pathogenesis: ?

Related Facts

I **Sex Ratio:** M?:F?

II **Risk of Occurrence:** Extremely rare

III **Risk of Recurrence for**
Patient's Sib: ?
Patient's Child: ?

IV **Age of Detectability:** 2-8 years when paranasal sinuses appear radiographically.

V **Prevalence:** Very rare

Treatment

I **Primary Prevention:** —

II **Secondary Prevention:** None for absent paranasal sinuses, but in patients with absent frontal sinuses, microcornea and open angle glaucoma, insidious blindness may develop unless the glaucoma is treated.

III **Other Therapy:** —

Prognosis: Normal for life span and intelligence

Detection of Carrier: —

†Special Considerations: There is 1 reported case of panagenesis of paranasal sinuses and 1 known case of unilateral absent paranasal sinuses. The case of unilateral agenesis was associated with an ipsilateral hypertrophied middle turbinate resulting in obstruction of the nasal airway on that side. There was also an absence of the inferior turbinate on the same side. A single family presented microcornea, glaucoma and absent frontal sinuses. In this particular family, no male-to-male transmission was present in the 3 generations affected; therefore, the type of dominant transmission is unknown.

References:
Goh, A.S. and Acquarelli, M.J.: Unilateral absent paranasal sinuses with hypertrophied middle turbinate. West. J. Med. 7:239, 1966.
Holmes, L.B. and Walton, D.S.: Hereditary microcornea, glaucoma and absent frontal sinuses: A family study. J. Pediatr. 74:968, 1969.
Mocellin, L.: Panagenesia of the paranasal sinuses: Report of a case. Arch. Otolaryngol. 88:311, 1968.

Contributors: **Robert N. Gebhart**
M. J. Acquarelli

Editor's Computerized Descriptor: Nasoph.

PARASTREMMATIC DYSPLASIA

Includes: Nanisme parastrémmatique
Parastremmatischer Zwergwuchs
Enanismo parastremático
Distorted limb dwarfism

Excludes: Metatropic dysplasia (656)
Other short-trunk types of skeletal dysplasias

Minimal Diagnostic Criteria: Platyspondyly, kyphoscoliosis, irregular ossification of the iliac crest; severe epiphyseal and metaphyseal deformities.

Clinical Findings: Short-trunk type of dwarfism with adult height below 110 cm; kyphoscoliosis; severe genu varum or valgum; bowing of the legs; multiple joint contractures.
Radiographs show flat vertebral bodies with irregularly ossified end-plates; small iliac wings bordered by a wide lace of irregular calcifications; small or unossified femoral heads and necks; severe shortening and distortion of the tubular bones with striking ossification defects of the epiphyses and metaphyses.

Complications
I   **Derived:** Delayed motor development, secondary arthrosis
II **Associated:** —

Etiology: Autosomal dominant

Pathogenesis: ?

Related Facts
I   **Sex Ratio:** M1:F1
II **Risk of Occurrence:** Very rare
III **Risk of Recurrence for**
    Patient's Sib: If parent is affected 1 in 2 (50%) for each offspring to be affected; otherwise not increased.
    Patient's Child: 1 in 2
IV **Age of Detectability:** Infancy
V   **Prevalence:** Very rare

Treatment
I   **Primary Prevention:** Genetic counseling
II **Secondary Prevention:** Symptomatic orthopedic procedures
III **Other Therapy:** —

Prognosis: Though severely incapacitated, the patients survive to adulthood and may reproduce.

Detection of Carrier: Skeletal surveys reveal characteristic deformities.

Special Considerations: —

References:
Langer, L.O. et al: An unusual bone dysplasia: Parastremmatic dwarfism. Am. J. Roentgenol. Radium Ther. Nucl. Med. 110:550, 1970.

Contributor: **Jürgen W. Spranger**

Editor's Computerized Descriptor: Skel.

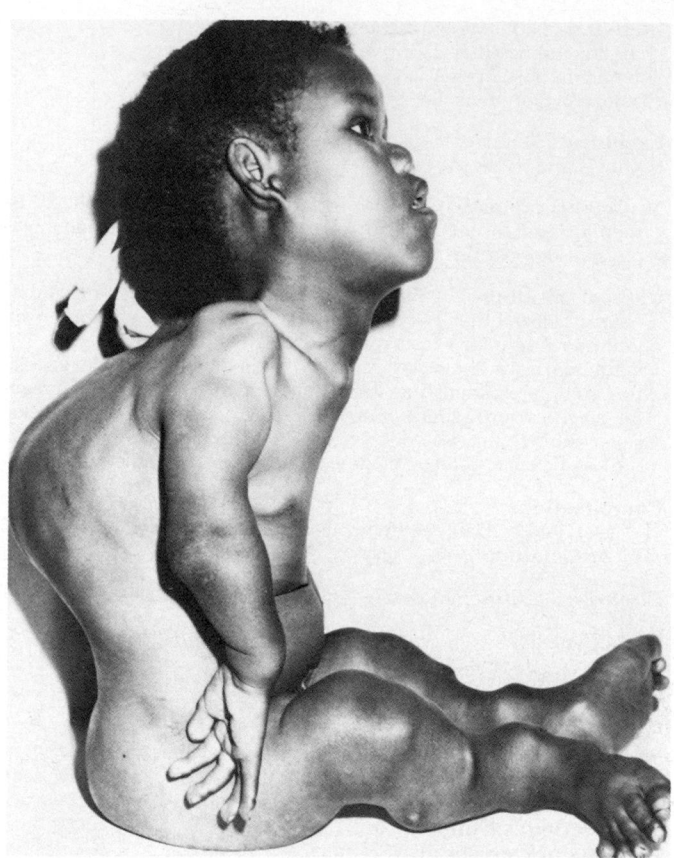

412. Note short trunk, marked kyphosis, bowed legs, and joint contractures

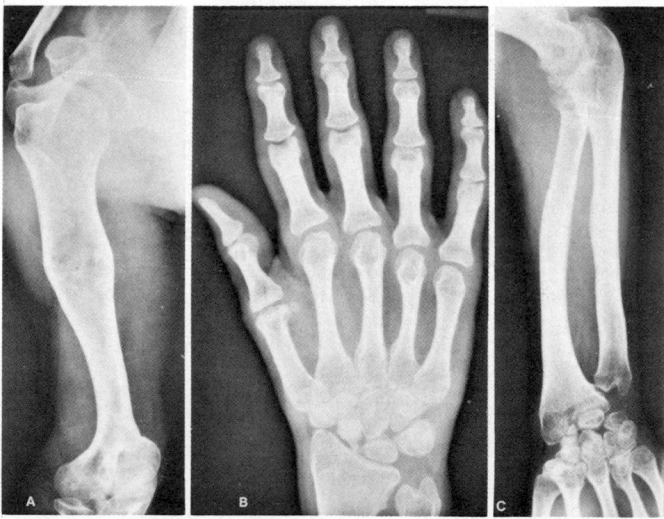

413. A& C) Shortening of tubular bones with flared, irregular ends; B) small, deformed carpal bones with cupped distal ends of proximal and middle phalanges

PAROTITIS, PUNCTATE

Includes: Parotidite ponctuée
Parotitis punctata
Parotiditis punctata
Parotitis of childhood, chronic recurrent
Sialangiectasis
Sialectasis
Mikulicz disease
Parotitis associated with Sjögren syndrome

Excludes: Other forms of chronic or recurrent forms of parotid infection; eg viral, sarcoid, bacterial, etc

Minimal Diagnostic Criteria: Evidence of punctate sialectasis on sialography. If possible, a tissue examination of the gland should be done to confirm the pathology.

Clinical Findings: This is an interesting and possibly unique pathologic process which appears to occur in 3 different clinical forms:

Chronic recurrent parotitis of childhood which is usually misdiagnosed as "recurrent mumps." It is not infectious or contagious. Attacks subside about the time of puberty in about 90% of cases.

Mikulicz disease occurs in adults who have no evidence of systemic disease. Nearly always only the parotid gland is involved. There may be recurrent attacks of parotid swelling or there may be a chronic diffuse enlargement or a discrete mass. Involvement may be unilateral or bilateral.

Punctate parotitis is a very frequent, if not a constant, component of a systemic disease—Sjögren syndrome. The parotitis may be recurrent or present as a chronic, diffuse enlargement. Clinically only 1 gland may be involved, but radiologically and pathologically, both are affected.

Pathologic and radiologic findings in the parotid gland are similar in all 3 clinical types. The authors feel that there are 3 primary histopathologic lesions, namely: hyperplasia of the epithelial and myoepithelial cells of the intralobular ducts, disappearance of acinar structures, replacement of the glandular parenchyma by a diffuse infiltration of lymphoid cells.

Involvement of larger ducts and gross glandular destruction with increased fibrosis is thought to be associated with secondary infection. Occasionally cystic lesions develop from the hyperplastic ducts. In longstanding cases the pathology may undergo involution and fatty replacement.

The classic radiologic findings are demonstrated by sialography in which terminal or punctate sialectasis is seen. Some workers have reported that the lesion then progresses through globular, cavitary and destructive stages. These may be caused by bacterial infection secondary to reduced salivary flow. Although there is no unanimity of opinion, many feel that the punctate areas are an artifact due to extravasation of contrast material, but nevertheless they are a valuable diagnostic sign.

Complications
I **Derived:** Secondary bacterial infection due to diminution of salivary flow from acinar destruction.
II **Associated:** —

Etiology: This is an inflammatory lesion but not a bacteriologic disease. A chronic viral infection is possible but this has not been adequately evaluated. Evidence for a genetic etiology in at least some cases is as follows: definite familial incidence, occurrence in very young children, preliminary studies indicating hereditary factors in Sjögren syndrome with which punctate parotitis is usually associated.

Pathogenesis: —

Related Facts

I **Sex Ratio:** Varies by clinical type, namely: chronic recurrent parotitis of childhood M>1:F1, Mikulicz disease M1:F>1, Sjögren syndrome M1:F19.

II **Risk of Occurrence:** ? Fairly rare, but probably more common than generally thought.

III **Risk of Recurrence for**
   Patient's Sib: ?
   Patient's Child: ?

IV **Age of Detectability:** Whenever clinical involvement of the parotid occurs.

V **Prevalence:** ?

Treatment

I **Primary Prevention:** —

II **Secondary Prevention:** The type of treatment depends on the gross pathology and severity of clinical symptoms. Mild cases may require only observation and management of secondary infection. Among available treatments are: massage of the gland, stimulation of salivary flow by chewing gum or wax, treating infections of the teeth or tonsils, antibiotics for the acute attack, sialography (because the iodides it contains may be beneficial); injection of antibiotics into the duct system, and small doses (800-1800r) of x-ray therapy, with or without duct ligation. Surgical treatment includes tympanic neurectomy to eliminate the parasympathetic nerve supply to the gland and either subtotal or total parotidectomy, sparing the facial nerve.

III **Other Therapy:** —

Prognosis: Chronic recurrent parotitis of childhood subsides around the age of puberty in about 90% of cases. The parotitis of Mikulicz disease and Sjögren syndrome seems to subside spontaneously after a variable length of time.

Detection of Carrier: —

Special Considerations: —

References:
Blatt, I.M.: On sialectasis and benign lymphosialadenopathy (the pyogenic parotitis, Goujerot-Sjögren's syndrome, Mikulicz's disease complex), a 10-year study. Laryngoscope 74:1684, 1964.

Bunim, J.J.: A broader spectrum of Sjögren's syndrome and its pathogenic implications. Ann. Rheum. Dis. 20:1, 1961.

Hemenway, W.G.: Chronic punctate parotitis. Laryngoscope 81:485, 1971.

Contributor: **LaVonne Bergstrom**

Editor's Computerized Descriptor: Oral

800
794-500
PATENT DUCTUS ARTERIOSUS

Includes: Persistance du canal artériel
Offener Ductus arteriosus
Persistencia del canal arterial
Persistent ductus arteriosus

Excludes: Aortico-pulmonary septal defect (83)
Truncus arteriosus (972)

Minimal Diagnostic Criteria: The presence of classic clinical and laboratory findings with the characteristic continuous murmur. Selective aortogram, if necessary, is the procedure of choice to confirm the diagnosis.

Clinical Findings: Patent ductus arteriosus (PDA), in its pathologic manifestation, represents the postnatal patency of a normal fetal vessel between the left pulmonary artery and the aorta. In fetal life, most of the blood from the right ventricle bypasses the nonaerated lungs through this channel. Functional closure of the ductus usually occurs within hours or days after birth. The hemodynamic changes and clinical manifestations of its persistence depend on the magnitude of the pulmonary blood flow. The amount of left-to-right shunt is related to the size of the ductal lumen and the resistance in the pulmonary vascular bed. Infants and small children with a large ductus and low pulmonary vascular resistance have the highest pulmonary blood flow and pressures. The large pulmonary venous return results in relative mitral valve stenosis and increases in left ventricular end diastolic pressure and volume. The degree of right ventricular overloading depends on the magnitude of pulmonary artery pressure. The aortic diastolic runoff lesion characteristically results in widening of the systemic arterial pulse pressure. These patients are usually symptomatic early in life with the clinical findings of a large extracardiac left-to-right shunt. Tachypnea, frequent respiratory infections, growth retardation and congestive heart failure (sometimes resulting in pulmonary edema) are common findings. Bounding peripheral pulses or pulses of normal amplitude in the presence of congestive heart failure are highly suggestive of this lesion. Infants with PDA have variable murmurs, depending on the systolic and diastolic pressure differences between the aorta and pulmonary artery. The majority lack the diastolic component of the continuous murmur typically heard in older children or the diastolic component is short. A diastolic mitral flow murmur of the apex is usually present.

After 1 year of age, the great majority of cases are asymptomatic with normal growth and development. The left-to-right shunt is of small-to-moderate size and the pulmonary artery pressure is usually normal. The typical and diagnostic continuous machinery-like murmur is present in more than 90% of the cases. This murmur is maximal in the 2nd and 3rd left intercostal space and left subclavian area. It is often associated with a systolic thrill also present over the suprasternal notch area. The characteristic ductus murmur has a crescendo-decrescendo configuration peaking around the second sound and often obscures it. The second sound is normally split and the pulmonic component may be slightly accentuated.

The roentgenologic findings are dependent on the hemodynamic situation. Infants with left-to-right shunts usually reveal cardiomegaly, increased vascular markings and left atrial enlargement. The ascending aorta may appear enlarged and the pulmonary trunk prominent. Sometimes the ductus itself is visible as a short, convex density just below the aortic knob. In older children, the xrays are often normal or show mild cardiomegaly with only slight increase of the pulmonary arterial markings. The ductus (or ductus infundibulum) is often apparent as a discrete density distal to the aortic knob or as an extra density between the aortic knob and pulmonary trunk. This may be apparent in patients with otherwise normal roentgenographic findings. The ECG in infancy commonly shows biventricular hypertrophy and left atrial enlargement. In contrast, older children's ECGs are normal or show left ventricular hypertrophy of the volume overload type.

Echocardiac findings of a PDA result from the increased pulmonary blood flow. PDA itself is not recognizable by M-mode echocardiography. The left atrium enlarges as a function of increased pulmonary venous return. The left ventricle, as measured by echocardiography, may increase. Valvular motion is usually normal. Thickening of the right ventricle is unusual in children without pulmonary vascular obstructive disease.

Cardiac catheterization is sometimes necessary to demonstrate the presence of the extracardiac left-to-right shunt and rule out associated cardiac lesions. Direct passage of the catheter through the ductus is often possible.

Complications
I **Derived:** Death from congestive heart failure and pneumonia; development of high pulmonary vascular resistance resulting in the reversal of the shunt (Eisenmenger physiology); aneurysm of the ductus arteriosus; subacute bacterial endocarditis later in life.
II **Associated:** Approximately 15% have an additional cardiac lesion. The most common are ventricular septal defect, coarctation of the aorta, aortic stenosis, pulmonic stenosis or multiple pulmonary artery coarctations. A high incidence of extracardiac congenital anomalies are present as part of the postrubella syndrome.

Etiology: Presumably multifactorial inheritance. Since the ductus arteriosus represents the distal left 6th aortic arch, a normal vessel during fetal life, the question of etiology is concerned not with its existence but with the possible causes of its patency. Rubella, prematurity and hypoxia are the main known factors. Rubella infection in the 1st trimester of pregnancy leads to congenital defects in 70-80%. About half of these include heart malformations of which patent ductus or pulmonary artery coarctations are by far the most common. The importance of arterial oxygen tension after birth for the closure of the ductus seems to be established from the clinical and experimental experience. Perinatal respiratory distress or a reduced oxygen tension at high altitude leads to a higher frequency of the malformation. There is also some evidence for genetic factors in its presence (families with several cases of PDA have been reported).

Pathogenesis: ?

Related Facts
I **Sex Ratio:** M1:F2 (M1:F1 in rubella-related PDA)
II **Risk of Occurrence:** Approximately 1 in 830 live births
III **Risk of Recurrence for**
   Patient's Sib: Predicted risk - 3.5 in 100; Empiric risk - 3.4 in 100
   Patient's Child: Predicted risk - 3.5 in 100; Empiric risk - 4.3 in 100
IV **Age of Detectability:** From birth by heart murmur or aortogram
V **Prevalence:** Approximately 1 in 830 in pediatric population

Treatment
I **Primary Prevention:** Vaccine for rubella; prevention of prematurity and neonatal hypoxemia.
II **Secondary Prevention:** Operation - division or ligation of the ductus.†

III **Other Therapy:** —

Prognosis: Generally good. After successful surgical repair, normal life expectancy. Surgical mortality less than 1%, higher in infancy (in particular when associated with other cardiac lesions). In undetected cases, increasing mortality in the 4th decade of life and onwards due to the development of pulmonary vascular changes or subacute bacterial endocarditis.†

Detection of Carrier: —

†**Special Considerations:** PDA in a premature infant is likely to close spontaneously even if heart failure has occurred. In symptomatic full-term infants, spontaneous closure seldom occurs.

References:
Krovetz, L.J. and Warden, H.E.: Patent ductus arteriosus: An analysis of 515 surgically proved cases. Dis. Chest. 42:46, 1962.
Krovetz, L.J. et al: Handbook of Pediatric Cardiology. New York: Harper and Row, 1969.
Marquis, R.M.: Persistence of the ductus arteriosus. In Watson, H. (ed.): Paediatric Cardiology. St. Louis: C.V. Mosby, 1968, p. 242.
Silverman, N.A. et al: Echocardiographic assessment of ductus arteriosus shunt in premature infants. Circulation 50:821, 1975.

Contributor: **Benjamin E. Victorica**

Editor's Computerized Descriptors: Resp., CV.

PECTUS CARINATUM

Includes: Thorax en carène
Tórax en quilla
Pigeon breast
Congenital chondrosternal prominence
Chicken breast

Excludes: Pectus excavatum (802)

Minimal Diagnostic Criteria: Prominence of sternum with lateral depression of ribs

Clinical Findings: There are two types of pigeon breast, the "pouter" breast and the "keel" breast. The rare "pouter" type has a prominent forward tilting of the manubrium with abnormal fusion of all sternal segments and a depression of the sternum below the manubrium. The more common "keel" breast has considerable prominence of the entire body of the sternum with lateral depression of the ribs and costal cartilages. There is considerable variation in this type of defect. The condition manifests itself at birth and becomes more obvious as the child grows. There is usually no limitation of function or diminution of pulmonary reserve.

Complications
I **Derived:** It is possible to have a diminution of the intrathoracic space due to the depression of costal cartilages. The "pouter" type deformity has been associated in one patient with paroxysmal tachycardia and a heart displaced to the left.
II **Associated:** Marfan syndrome, homocystinuria, mucopolysaccharidoses, rickets

Etiology: ?

Pathogenesis: Several theories have been proposed but none proven. Brodkin believes that the various sternal deformities are the result of failure of the development of muscle in the ventral segment of the diaphragm and that these portions of the muscle exert a pull on the attached chest wall as a result of the unopposed action of muscles on the other side. Others believe this deformity is due to an overgrowth of the costal cartilages.

Related Facts
I **Sex Ratio:** ?
II **Risk of Occurrence:** ?
III **Risk of Recurrence for**
  Patient's Sib: ?
  Patient's Child: ?
IV **Age of Detectability:** At birth by physical examination
V **Prevalence:** ? Reported as 1 in 1660 in school population of Newark, N. J. (Brodkin).

Treatment
I **Primary Prevention:** —
II **Secondary Prevention:** —
III **Other Therapy:** Surgery is usually for cosmetic effect and because of the variety of defects, ingenuity and individuality of approach are required.†

Prognosis: Normal for life and intelligence. Function may depend on severity of "pouter" type.

Detection of Carrier: —

†**Special Considerations:** Although it appears that pectus carinatum does not interfere with normal activity, there have been no good reported studies of intrathoracic gas volumes or mechanics of breathing. The deformity is not caused by or related to airway obstruction. It is generally agreed by surgeons that surgical correction should be deferred until the chest wall is stable.

References:

Brodkin, H. A.: Congenital chondrosternal prominence (pigeon breast); new interpretation. Pediatrics 3:286, 1949.
Ravitch, M. M.: Congenital deformities of the chest wall. In Benson, C.D. et al (eds.): Pediatric Surgery. Chicago:Year Book Medical Publishers, 1962, vol. 1, p. 227.

Contributor: **Patricia S. Zelkowitz**

Editor's Computerized Descriptor: Skel.

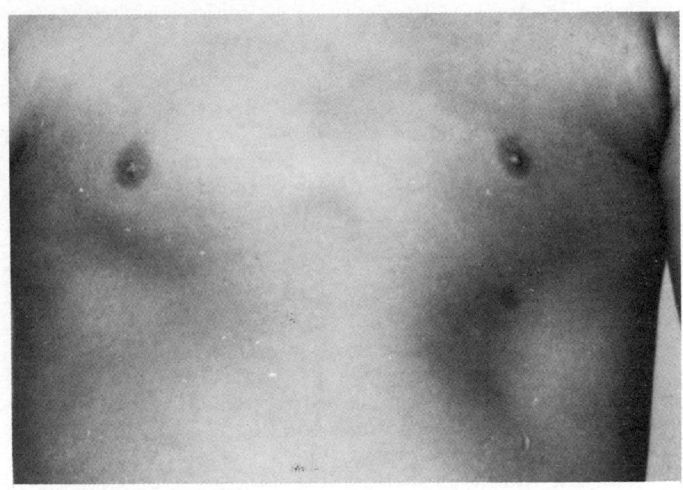

414. Asymmetric pectus carinatum

PECTUS EXCAVATUM

Includes: Thorax en entonnoir
Pecho excavado
Funnel chest
Trichterbrust
Schusterbrust
Pectum recurvatum
Chonechondrosternon

Excludes: Pectus carinatum (801)

Minimal Diagnostic Criteria: Central depression of the chest at the level of the sternum.

Clinical Findings: The AP diameter of the lower thorax is decreased by the posterior dislocation of the lower sternum, which carries the costal cartilages and the anterior part of the ribs with it. The affected portion of the sternum is concavely deformed as well as displaced. The manubrium is generally normally situated, whereas the xiphoid may extend so far posteriorly as to impinge on either the vertebral bodies or the paravertebral gutters. The frontal left side of the chest is usually slightly bulging because of an underlying heart.

Children with this anomaly are usually asymptomatic, unless they have primary lung or heart disease. Only occasionally are vague complaints heard about decreased exercise tolerance and discomfort in the chest, yet many patients claim improved physical performance after operation. The validity of such symptoms is doubtful particularly in adolescents, because of the frequently associated psychologic disturbance related to the cosmetic defect.

Objective evidence for cardiopulmonary involvement is usually lacking. However, in the presence of independent heart or lung disease, the deformity may have an unmeasurable aggravating effect.

Complications
I   **Derived:** Psychologic effects are noted. In the presence of chronic lung disease, congenital or acquired heart conditions, old age when calcification of cartilages has progressed, a severe chest deformity can further impair the function of the intrathoracic organs, by dislocation, distortion, compression or restriction of mobility of certain parts.
II **Associated:** Occasional abnormalities found by heart catheterization or by pulmonary function studies never proved to be convincing in causal relationship with pectus excavatum. Occurs in association with Marfan syndrome, Noonan syndrome and chronic obstruction of airways in infants.

Etiology: Possibly autosomal dominant transmission; there are many sporadic cases.

Pathogenesis: Disputed, but the most probable mechanism is an intrinsic failure of osteogenesis. Other theories include a partial weakness of the diaphragm, with the stronger portions causing an asymmetric pull on the chest wall; an abnormally short tendon or fibrous central portion of the diaphragm; and persistent obstructive respiratory disease causing an increased transpulmonary pressure gradient during respiration.

Related Facts
I   **Sex Ratio:** Probably M1:F1
II **Risk of Occurrence:** ?
III **Risk of Recurrence for**
    Patient's Sib: ? If autosomal dominant and if parent is affected, 1 in 2 (50%) for each offspring to be affected; otherwise not increased.
    Patient's Child: ? If autosomal dominant, 1 in 2.
IV **Age of Detectability:** Usually present at birth, often undetected until some months later.
V   **Prevalence:** ?

Treatment
I   **Primary Prevention:** Genetic counseling
II **Secondary Prevention:** —
III **Other Therapy:** Surgical repair of deformity by mobilization and repositioning of the body of the sternum after a perichondrial resection or morcellation of costal cartilages; by replacing deformed portions or correcting contours with bone grafts or with prosthetic materials. Temporary internal support with steel brace is often necessary.†

Prognosis: Probably normal life span. May be progressive or stationary; recurrence after operation not uncommon unless internal strut is used.

Detection of Carrier: —

†Special Considerations: This anomaly, in the vast majority of cases, presents only cosmetic problems. Therefore, it often will not be reported to the physician. The lack of statistical data about the anomaly can thus be explained. The approach toward surgical repair depends on individual assessment of the relative significance of physiologic and psychologic indications, and of the balance between operative risks and expectable results. In case of independent heart or lung diseases the same factors must be weighed with particular care and in some cases a more radical approach may be indicated.

References:
Brown, J. J. M.: Surgery of Childhood. London: E. Arnold, Ltd., 1962.
Koop, C. E.: The management of pectus excavatum. Surg. Clin. North Am. 36:1627, 1956.
Polgar, G. and Koop, C. E.: Pulmonary function in pectus excavatum. Pediatrics 32:209, 1963.

Contributor: **George Polgar**

Editor's Computerized Descriptor: Skel.

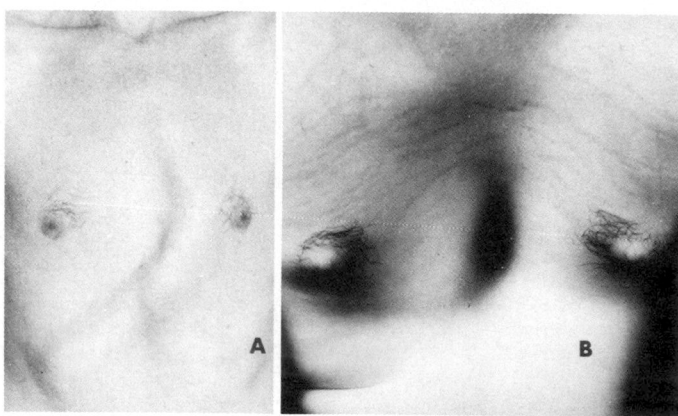

415. Pectus excavatum: A) asymmetric, B) with striae cutis distensae

PELIZAEUS-MERZBACHER SYNDROME

Includes: Sclérose cérébrale-type I
Mb. Pelizaeus-Merzbacher
Esclerosis cerebral I
Cerebral sclerosis I

Excludes: Cockayne syndrome (189)
Schilder disease
Orthochromatic leukodystrophy
Metachromatic leukodystrophies (651)
Globoid cell leukodystrophy (415)
Brain, spongy degeneration (115)
Other leukodystrophies of nervous system
Other degenerative diseases of nervous system

Minimal Diagnostic Criteria: The pattern of involvement of males, the onset around age 4-6 months with peculiar rolling nystagmus followed by delay in motor development should strongly suggest the diagnosis. A family history compatible with a pattern of inheritance as an X-linked recessive is also suggestive.†

Clinical Findings: The disease is a slowly progressive one with onset around age of 4-6 months. The distinctive clinical feature is often a peculiar rolling nystagmus of the eyes. The patients are delayed in motor milestones in terms of sitting and standing and, in the later stage of disease, may develop contractures and spasticity of the lower limbs. Movements of the arms are jerky and clumsy, particularly fine motor movements. Speech development may be slightly delayed but is often within the normal range. The children's mentation seems to be relatively normal early in the course of the disease. The progression is a gradual one with increasing involvement of lower limbs and then upper limbs. The nystagmus persists and ataxia may become a prominent symptom. There is a slow progression and death often occurs around the 16th-25th year of life. In this form of the disease the pattern of inheritance is that of an X-linked recessive.

Complications
I   **Derived:** Progressive neurologic disease; terminally pneumonia is frequent.
II   **Associated:** —

Etiology: This appears to be inherited as an X-linked recessive. McK *31160

Pathogenesis: ? No precise biochemical information yet available. The pathology is distinctive with a marked loss of myelin except for relatively well-preserved areas or islands of normal myelin.

Related Facts
I   **Sex Ratio:** M1:F0
II   **Risk of Occurrence:** ?
III   **Risk of Recurrence for**
    Patient's Sib: If X-linked recessive and if mother is carrier, 1 in 2 (50%) for each brother to be affected and 1 in 2 for each sister to be a carrier.
    Patient's Child: (Condition is lethal for patient.)
IV   **Age of Detectability:** 12-18 months
V   **Prevalence:** ?

Treatment
I   **Primary Prevention:** Genetic counseling
II   **Secondary Prevention:** —
III   **Other Therapy:** —

Prognosis: This is a slowly progressive leukodystrophy; patients live to 15-25 years of age.

Detection of Carrier: —

†**Special Considerations:** There is considerable confusion about this entity in the literature. We have restricted ourselves to the X-linked form with early onset with nystagmus, a prominent part of the picture. There are, however, closely related processes with sporadic appearance, without nystagmus as a prominent early sign, but which do have a slowly progressive course compatible with a leukodystrophy. In addition pathologically these other cases do have these islands of normal myelin and the presence of rather marked demyelination. The final characterization of this group of diseases will require biochemical clues as to the mechanisms of the failure of formation or maintenance of myelin.

References:
Seitelberger, F.: Pelizaeus-Merzbacher disease. In Vinken, P.J. et al (eds.): Handbook of Clinical Neurology. Amsterdam:North Holland Publishing Co., 1970, vol. 10, p. 150.
Zeman, W. et al: Pelizaeus-Merzbacher disease. J. Neuropathol. Exp. Neurol. 23:334, 1964.

Contributor: **Guy M. McKhann**

Editor's Computerized Descriptors: Eye, Speech, Skel., Nerve

PENTOSURIA (MARKER)

Includes: Pentosurie
L-xylulosuria

Excludes: Alimentary pentosuria

Minimal Diagnostic Criteria: Pentosuric individuals excrete 1 to 4 gm of L-xylulose per day. Unlike glucose or galactose, xylulose (as well as ketoses such as fructose) reduces Benedict's solution at low temperatures. Consequently the Lasker and Enklewitz Benedict's test (55°, 10 minutes) should be used as the first and most convenient diagnostic test. Paper chromatography will provide direct evidence that the urinary sugar is xylulose. It is unnecessary to demonstrate that the xylulose is of the L form since D-xylulosuria has never been reported. However, when desired, the osazone of L-xylulose can be prepared and characterized by its melting point behavior upon a mixture with D-xylosazone. The derivative mixture melts approximately 40° higher than the separate isomers.

Clinical Findings: Pentosuria is not accompanied by any functional disturbances or symptoms other than the daily excretion of gram quantities of the pentose, L-xylulose. The pentose is present in only trace quantities in normal urine. However, presumably as a result of a defect in the liver enzyme system which acts on this ketopentose, the sugar is poorly metabolized and is largely excreted in the urine. The condition is usually discovered when patients with high levels of urinary sugar are found to be without diabetic symptoms. Analysis of the urine discloses that the reducing sugar is not glucose.

Complications
I Derived: None. Early reports of unusual psychologic manifestations were very probably a consequence of the uncertainty of diagnosis and of unnecessary or ineffective attempts at treatment. Diabetes mellitus is occasionally found in pentosuric individuals, but as yet there is no valid data on whether the coincidence of the 2 conditions is other than rare and random.

II Associated: —

Etiology: Autosomal recessive deficiency of the enzyme NADP-xylitol (L-xylulose) dehydrogenase. McK *26080
The exception is one study suggesting that in a particular Lebanese family the mechanism of inheritance appeared to be that of a dominant gene with reduced penetrance. The condition has been encountered almost exclusively in Ashkenazi Jews of Polish-Russian extraction and, occasionally, in individuals of Lebanese descent.

Pathogenesis: No specific pathology has been demonstrated. Although it has been stated that the pentosuric condition persists relatively unchanged throughout life, members of one Lebanese family were reported to show pentosuria after earlier urine tests for pentose had been negative. The urinary level of xylulose is not markedly influenced by ordinary variations in diet. A direct test of pentosuric liver has not as yet been possible. Although there is no well-established relationship between pentosuria and diabetes mellitus, there is suggestive evidence that the latter disease may be accompanied by a disturbance in the glucuronate-xylulose pathway. Further work on this possible interrelationship is required. Wang and van Eys (N. Eng. J. Med. 282:892, 1970) have shown a decrease of NADP-linked xylitol dehydrogenase in red cells of patients with pentosuria.

Related Facts
I Sex Ratio: M1:F1
II Risk of Occurrence: 1 in 2500 births among Ashkenazim;
otherwise rare
III Risk of Recurrence for
Patient's Sib: 1 in 4 (25%) for each offspring to excrete pentose
Patient's Child: Not increased unless mate is carrier or homozygote.
IV Age of Detectability: Infants, as early as 2 weeks of age
V Prevalence: 1 in 2500 among Ashkenazim

Treatment
I Primary Prevention: —
II Secondary Prevention: —
III Other Therapy: —

Prognosis: Normal life span

Detection of Carrier: Carriers appear to be capable of handling the normal load of L-xylulose produced in normal metabolism. However, by stressing the glucuronic acid-xylulose metabolic pathway by the administration of a large test dose of D-glucuronolactone, it has been found that the heterozygous carrier of the pentosuric gene is less able than homozygous normal individuals to metabolize the L-xylulose produced from the glucuronolactone.

Special Considerations: —

References:
Hiatt, H.H.: Pentosuria. In Stanbury, J.B. et al (eds.): The Metabolic Basis of Inherited Disease. New York:McGraw-Hill, 1972, p.119.
Hollman, S. and Touster, O.: Non-glycolytic Pathways of Metabolism of Glucose. New York:Academic Press, 1964, p. 95.
Touster, O.: Essential pentosuria and the glucuronate-xylulose pathway. Fed. Proc. 19:977, 1960.
Touster, O.: Pentose metabolism and pentosuria. Am. J. Med. 26:724, 1959.

Contributor: **Oscar Touster**

Editor's Computerized Descriptor: —

PERICARDIUM AGENESIS

Includes: Agénésie péricardique
Perikard-Agenesie
Agenesia del pericardio
Congenital pericardial defects
Congenital partial or complete absence of the pericardium
Left atrial herniation
Agenesis of pericardium

Excludes: Ectopia cordis (335)

Minimal Diagnostic Criteria: Characteristic radiologic findings after diagnostic pneumothorax. See below.

Clinical Findings: Although this entity was first described in 1559, almost half of the cases have appeared in the literature during the past decade, suggesting that pericardial agenesis is not as rare as once believed. Saint Pierre and Froment reviewed 153 cases from the literature up to 1970, and subdivided them as follows:

Total absence of pericardium	9%
Left-sided defect	70%
Partial	35%
Total	35%
Right-sided defect	4%
Partial	4%
Total	0%
Diaphragmatic pericardial aplasia	17%

Clinically, most patients are asymptomatic, but when symptoms occur, they are thought to be related to the specific defect. For example, in partial left-sided defects (foramen type) herniation of the left ventricle through the foramen can result in chest pain or even sudden death. Pressure on the coronary arteries from the rim of the foramen may produce angina. Some authors suggest that chest pain is related to mediastinal adhesions, torsion of the great vessels due to lack of stability of the heart, or the previously mentioned pressure on the coronary arteries.

In a review of the isolated partial left-sided type of defect, 16 of 27 cases were asymptomatic. Chest pain, occasionally associated with radiation to the left arm and dyspnea, were present in 8 cases. Other symptoms included occasional syncopal attacks, dyspnea without pain, and small hemoptyses.

Physical findings have also been vague and variable. Sometimes cardiac enlargement or hypermobility of the heart is present. Soft systolic murmurs are sometimes reported. ECG findings are present only in cases with associated heart malformations or malrotation of the heart.

The most useful diagnostic features are radiographic findings. Absence of the left side of the pericardium produces a very prominent aortic arch, pulmonary artery, and left atrial shadows. If herniation of the left atrium through a foramen has occurred, the radiograph may be interpreted as a dilatation of the pulmonary artery, atrial tumor or various hilar tumors, or lymph node enlargement. The xray frequently suggests cardiac enlargement. Complete defects produce morbid shifting of the heart without shifting of the trachea. A case of partial right-sided defect revealed radiolucent herniation of the lung into the pericardial cavity.

Fluoroscopy may reveal asynchronous pulsation of the left atrium with either partial or complete defects. A diagnostic pneumothorax may be useful in showing air entering the pericardial cavity. If positive, this procedure is diagnostic, but a negative result does not rule out a pericardial defect as it is sometimes difficult to introduce air through small pericardial defects or if pleuropericardial adhesions are present.

Cardiac catheterization and angiography may reveal a displaced left atrium if herniation has occurred and will rule out other cardiac abnormalities. In one case angiocardiography suggested an encysted pericardial effusion which on echocardiogram was disproved.

Complications

I **Derived:** Sudden death has been associated with herniation and strangulation of the left ventricle. In the preantibiotic era, pleuropericarditis resulted from exposure of the unprotected heart to pulmonary infections.

II **Associated:** 30-40% have associated anomalies. Bronchogenic cyst is probably the most common followed by associated cardiac defects including patent ductus arteriosus, bifid heart, tetralogy of Fallot, ventricular septal defect, tricuspid incompetence, and bicuspid aortic valve. Cerebral anomalies have occurred in 2 patients. Congestive heart failure, when it occurs, is usually related to associated intracardiac defects.

Etiology: ?

Pathogenesis: Unknown, but generally thought to result from incomplete development of either the transverse septum or of the pleuropericardial folds which in turn may be due to premature atrophy of the duct of Cuvier of the left side. This theory supports the left-sided defects but fails to explain the infrequent right-sided defect.†

Related Facts

I **Sex Ratio:** M3:F1

II **Risk of Occurrence:** ?

III **Risk of Recurrence for**
  Patient's Sib: No reported cases have occurred in more than one member of a family or in twins.
  Patient's Child: No reported cases have occurred in more than one member of a family or in twins.

IV **Age of Detectability:** Infancy, by roentgenogram

V **Prevalence:** Approximately 160 cases reported

Treatment

I **Primary Prevention:** —

II **Secondary Prevention:** There has been no treatment in many cases. Partial defects, if small, may be closed primarily. In other cases adjacent tissues such as pleura have been used to close partial defects. In cases of left atrial herniation, some surgeons have done left atrial appendectomy. Some have favored the creation of a complete defect, if a partial defect exists, in hopes of preventing entrapment or incarceration of portions of the heart. The best treatment is probably restoration of normal anatomy if possible, thus preventing other complications of complete defects such as pleuropericarditis or adhesions of the heart, lung tissue and other adjacent tissues. Various surgical techniques have been discussed by Fosburg et al who favor anatomic closure.

III **Other Therapy:** —

Prognosis: For life: the defects may be well tolerated and compatible with a normal life span. There is no effect on intellect and usually none on function. However, fatal complications such as herniation and strangulation of the left ventricle or left atrium and pleuropericarditis have been reported.†

Detection of Carrier: ?

†**Special Considerations:** Reported cases continue to show the high incidence of complete left-sided defects (70%). The frequent lack of clinical symptoms and laboratory findings make the diagnosis difficult, but when suspected, a diagnostic pneumothorax may be performed and the size ascertained by cardiac catheterization. If symptoms are persistent or threatening, surgical exploration may be indicated.

References:

Fosburg, R.C. et al: Congenital partial absence of the pericardium. Ann. Thorac. Surg. 5:171, 1968.

Haider, D. et al: Congenital pericardio-peritoneal communication with herniation of omentum into the pericardium. A rare cause of cardiomegaly. Br. Heart J. 35:981, 1973.

Hipona, F.A. and Crummy, A.B.: Congenital pericardial defect associated with tetralogy of Fallot. Herniation of normal lung into the pericardial cavity. Circulation 29:132, 1964.

Moene, R.J. et al: Congenital right-sided pericardial defect with herniation of part of a lung into the pericardial cavity. Am. J. Cardiol. 31:519, 1973.

Saint Pierre, A. and Froment, R.: Absence totales et partielles du pericarde. Arch. Mal. Couer. 63:638, 1970.

Contributors: **Audrey H. Nora**
James J. Nora

Editor's Computerized Descriptors: Resp., CV.

PERIODONTOSIS, JUVENILE

Includes: Periodontose juvénile
Juvenile paradentose
Juvenile periodontosis

Excludes: Hyperkeratosis palmoplantaris and periodontoclasia (494)
Scleroderma
Chromosome twenty-one trisomy syndrome (171)
Neutropenia, cyclic (714)
Juvenile diabetes
Traumatogenic occlusion
Hypophosphatasia (516)
Histiocytosis
Hypophosphatemia (517)
Acatalasemia (6)
Ectodermal dysplasia
Acrosclerosis
Leukemia

Minimal Diagnostic Criteria: Loosening and migration of the teeth usually first involving the maxillary 1st molars and incisors. Roentgenographically, widening of the periodontal ligament space and loss of lamina dura are apparent. Vertical patterns of bone loss are characteristic and horizontal resorption may also be observed. Marrow spaces of supporting bone are enlarged reducing osseous trabeculation, presenting an appearance of radiologic osteoporosis.

Clinical Findings: Juvenile periodontosis is a condition seen infrequently in children in the prepubertal, pubertal and early postpubertal periods. The age of onset may occur early and involve the primary dentition as has been reported recently by Jorgenson et al. It is a chronic destructive disease which at first is characterized by degenerative noninflammatory destruction of the periodontium. The periodontal tissues of all of the teeth may be affected but in most instances the mandibular or maxillary 1st permanent molars and the incisors are the 1st teeth to be involved. Clinically, the development and the progress of periodontosis is at first a painless condition, followed by tooth migration and mobility in the absence of gingival inflammation. As the condition progresses gingival inflammation, pocket formation and exudation are complicating factors.

Complications
I **Derived:**   Premature loss of teeth. May be of concern to patient particularly when there is pathologic wandering of maxillary or mandibular incisor teeth.
II **Associated:**   —†

Etiology: ? Viral and genetic factors suggested, also response to occlusal stress in young individuals. Recent reports suggest a functional defect in leukocytes.

Pathogenesis: ? A rapid loss of bone and the widening of the periodontal space in young individuals most often involving the molar and incisor teeth. As the condition progresses, the teeth become very mobile, and migration of the involved teeth occurs.

Related Facts
I **Sex Ratio:**   M1:F1
II **Risk of Occurrence:**   Uncommon
III **Risk of Recurrence for**
  Patient's Sib: When autosomal dominant or autosomal recessive, see Table I AD or AR, respectively.
  Patient's Child: When autosomal dominant or autosomal recessive, see Table I AD or AR, respectively.
IV **Age of Detectability:**   Prepubertal and pubertal periods
V **Prevalence:**   ? Rare

Treatment
I **Primary Prevention:** ?
II **Secondary Prevention:** Early, thorough and continuous periodontal therapy
III **Other Therapy:** Prosthetic replacement of teeth

Prognosis: Poor. Usually the disease progresses with early loss of teeth.

Detection of Carrier: ?

†**Special Considerations:** A clinically similar condition may occur as a sign in the following conditions: Papillon-Lefèvre syndrome, scleroderma, chromosome 21 trisomy, cyclic neutropenia, juvenile diabetes mellitus, traumatogenic occlusion, hypophosphatasia, histiocytosis, acatalasemia, hypophosphatemia, ectodermal dysplasia, acrosclerosis and leukemia.

References:
Butler, J.H.: A familial pattern of juvenile periodontitis (periodontosis). J. Periodont. 40:115, 1969.
Cianciola, L.J. et al: Defective polymorphonuclear leukocyte function in a human periodontal disease. Nature 265:445, 1977.
Fourel, J.: Periodontosis: A periodontal syndrome. J. Periodont. 42:240, 1972.
Hawes, R.R.: Report of three cases of juvenile periodontosis with early loss of teeth. J. Dent. Child. 27:169, 1960.
Jorgenson, R.J. et al: Periodontosis in sibs. Oral Surg. 39:396, 1975.
Ruben, M.P. et al: Diseases of the periodontium. In Gorlin, R.J. and Goldman, H.M. (eds.): Thoma's Oral Pathology, 6th Ed. St. Louis: C.V. Mosby, 1970, p. 433.

Contributor: **M. Michael Cohen, Sr.**

Editor's Computerized Descriptor: Teeth

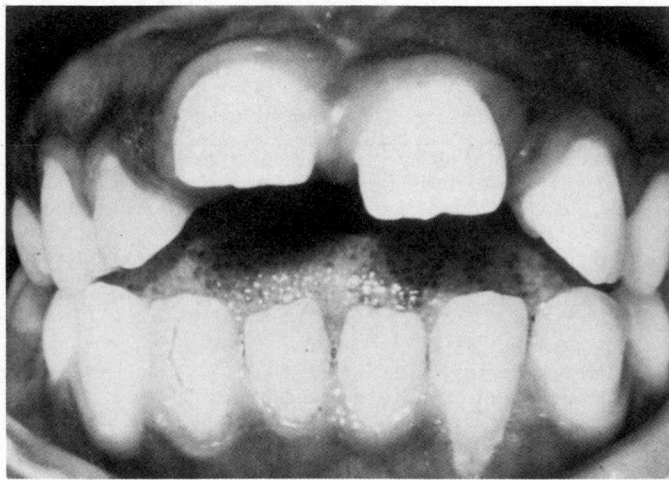

416. Note malpositioned teeth in periodontosis

PERSISTENT LEFT SUPERIOR VENA CAVA CONNECTED TO CORONARY SINUS

Includes: Persistance de la veine cave supérieure gauche unie à l'atrium droit par l'intermédiaire du sinus coronarien
Persistenz der linken Vena cava superior mit Verbindung zum rechten Vorhof über den Sinus coronarius
Persistencia de la vena cava superior izquierda comunicada con la aurícula derecha por medio del seno coronario
Persistent left superior vena cava connecting to right atrium via coronary sinus

Excludes: Persistent left superior vena cava (LSVC) connecting to left atrium
Total anomalous pulmonary venous connection to the left superior vena cava

Minimal Diagnostic Criteria: A persistent LSVC is virtually always an incidental finding. Angiography or catheter passage confirms the diagnosis.

Clinical Findings: In this anomaly, a persistent LSVC connects to the coronary sinus. The physiology is normal. Its importance lies in the frequent coexistence of other congenital cardiac defects and in the technical complications it may engender during cardiac catheterization or cardiac surgery. From the junction of the left subclavian and left internal jugular veins the LSVC descends vertically in front of the aortic arch. A short distance from its origin, it receives the superior left intercostal vein, then passes in front of the left pulmonary hilum. It receives the hemiazygos vein, penetrates the pericardium and crosses the posterior wall of the left atrium obliquely, receives the greater cardiac vein and enters the coronary sinus.

The coronary sinus and its right atrial ostium are larger than normal. As a rule, the persistent LSVC is part of a bilateral superior caval system. Rarely the RSVC may be absent.

Radiologic features: The shadow of the LSVC may be seen along the left upper border of the mediastinum. Diagnosis may be confirmed by passage of a cardiac catheter into the LSVC via the left subclavian vein or by way of the coronary sinus from the heart.

Echocardiographic features: The enlarged coronary sinus may produce an abnormal echo in the left atrium. This echo is similar to the left atrial echoes produced by TAPVC to coronary sinus and cor triatriatum.

Complications
I **Derived:** Utilization of the LSVC for catheter passage in a right heart study may interfere with the satisfactory completion of the procedure. At operation, ligation of the LSVC may be fatal when the RSVC is absent. Cannulation of the LSVC via the coronary sinus is necessary during cardiopulmonary bypass.
II **Associated:** Tetralogy of Fallot, ventricular septal defect, sinus venosus atrial septal defect, cyanotic congenital cardiac defects, particularly those with malposition of the heart or abdominal viscera. A high incidence of leftward P axis is found in patients with persistent LSVC.

Etiology: ?

Pathogenesis: Embryologically, persistence of the LSVC is a consequence of simple failure of obliteration of the left common cardinal vein.

Related Facts
I **Sex Ratio:** ?
II **Risk of Occurrence:** ?
III **Risk of Recurrence for Patient's Sib:** ?

IV Age of Detectability: From birth by catheterization or angiography

V Prevalence: 1 in 330 in the normal population. 1 in 30 in patients with congenital heart disease.

Treatment
I Primary Prevention: —
II Secondary Prevention: —
III Other Therapy: —

Prognosis: Excellent when occurring as an isolated anomaly

Detection of Carrier: —

Special Considerations: —

References:
Lucas, R.V., Jr. and Schmidt, R.E.: Anomalous venous connection, pulmonary and systemic. In Moss, A.J. and Adams, F.H. (eds.): Heart Disease in Infants, Children, and Adolescents. Baltimore: Williams & Wilkins, 1968, p. 672.

Contributor: **Russell V. Lucas, Jr.**

Editor's Computerized Descriptor: CV.

PHENYLKETONURIA

Includes: Phenylcetonurie
Phenylketonurie
Fenilcetonuria
Phenylalanine hydroxylase deficiency
Hyperphenylalanemia†

Excludes: Transient hyperphenylalanemia†

Minimal Diagnostic Criteria: Persistent elevation of blood phenylalanine concentrations above 6 mg/100 ml with normal blood tyrosine.†

Clinical Findings: The major problem in untreated phenylketonuria, and sometimes the only problem, is mental retardation. During the first few weeks of life, there may be severe vomiting and epileptic seizures. Irritability may be seen in infancy. Some children have an eczematoid eruption; others have dry skin. Children may have a "mousy" smell due to phenylacetic acid in the urine and sweat. Although there are exceptions, phenylketonuric individuals tend to have blue eyes, blond hair and fair skin.

Approximately two-thirds of those with concentrations of phenylalanine in serum above 6 mg/100 ml will develop moderate-to-severe mental retardation.† Neurologic examination in these children may reveal a mild microcephaly, hand posturing with purposeless movements, and increased reflexes. Many have abnormal EEG patterns.

Biochemical characteristics are elevated blood phenylalanine (mean 2.0 mg% with range 115-2.5 mg), urinary excretion of o-hydroxyphenylacetic acid (mean 1.6 μ M/g creatinine), and excretion of urinary phenylpyruvic acid.

Complications
I Derived: Mental retardation, seizures
II Associated: —

Etiology: Autosomal recessive transmission; McK *26160

Pathogenesis: Deficiency of liver phenylalanine hydroxylase reduces ability to form tyrosine. The accumulation of phenylalanine, phenylpyruvic acid and other metabolites must in some way lead to mental retardation, for prevention of accumulation through dietary restriction of phenylalanine prevents mental retardation.

Related Facts
I Sex Ratio: M1:F1
II Risk of Occurrence: 1 in 15,000 live births in the U.S. in general (lower in Negroes and Ashkenazi Jews).
III Risk of Recurrence for
  Patient's Sib: 1 in 4 (25%) for each offspring to be affected
  Patient's Child: Not increased unless mate is carrier or homozygote. Heterozygous offspring of an unrelated homozygous patient are usually mentally retarded.
IV Age of Detectability: At 48 hours, by measurement of blood phenylalanine if protein intake is normal. By the 6th day, the diagnosis should virtually always be clear.
V Prevalence: ?

Treatment
I Primary Prevention: Genetic counseling
II Secondary Prevention: The low-phenylalanine diet is effective in preventing mental retardation, but treatment must be started during the early weeks of life.
III Other Therapy: —

Prognosis: In the untreated patient with mental retardation and seizures, reduced life span may be expected. With treatment, the prognosis should be excellent.

Detection of Carrier: Phenylalanine tolerance test (0.1 gm/kg

Patient's Child: ?

body weight) is helpful in distinguishing a group of carriers from a group of controls. However, there is about a 20% overlap. Hence, this test cannot reliably be used to identify the carrier.

†**Special Considerations:** In a collaborative study of newborn screening programs of patients with high concentrations of phenylalanine and normal tyrosine, it was found that about one quarter have had persistent phenylalaninemia between 6 and 19.9 mg/100, and the remainder have had phenylalaninemia greater than 20 mg%. Among untreated patients, normal mental development has been found in almost all of those with phenylalanine concentrations less than 19.9 mg/100. In treated patients, a diet low in phenylalanine was effective in preventing mental deficiency, particularly if started at less than 30 days of age. A number of terms have been employed in hyperphenylalaninemic patients including phenylketonuria, hyperphenylalanemia, persistent hyperphenylalanemia, phenylalanemia and atypical phenylketonuria. These patients may represent heterogeneity in the phenylalanine hydroxylase enzyme.

References:

Berman, J.L. et al: Causes for high phenylalanine with normal tyrosine in newborn screening programs. Am. J. Dis. Child. 117:54, 1969.

Koch, R. et al: Phenylalaninemia and phenylketonuria. In Nyhan, W.L. (ed.): Heritable Disorders of Amino Acid Metabolism. New York:J. Wiley & Sons, 1974, pp. 109-140.

Lyman, F.L. (ed.): Phenylketonuria. Springfield:C.C Thomas, 1963.

Shear, C.S. et al: Phenylketonuria: Experience with diagnosis and management. In Heritable Disorders of Amino Acid Metabolism. op. cit., pp. 141-159.

Contributor: **William L. Nyhan**

Editor's Computerized Descriptors: Eye, Skin, Hair, Skel., GI, Nerve

PHENYLTHIOCARBAMIDE TASTING (MARKER)

Includes: Sensibilité gustative à la thio-urée
Phenylthiokarbamid
Catación de la feniltiocarbamida (Marcador)
Hereditary differences of taste threshold to bitter compounds containing the N-C=S group
Phenylthiourea sensitivity
Taste blindness

Excludes: Hereditary differences of taste threshold to other substances
Unconfirmed associations with TB, diabetes mellitus and other medical or dental conditions
Spurious linkage data

Minimal Diagnostic Criteria: Much work on PTC-taste-testing has been invalidated by faulty techniques, in particular by attempts at short cuts. It is urgently recommended that the measurement of taste sensitivity to phenylthiourea by Harris and Kalmus (see reference) be adhered to.

Clinical Findings: The taste thresholds for most substances of individuals in population samples are approximately normally distributed around a mean value, indicating the involvement of many environmental as well as genetic factors. The only exception to this which has so far been firmly established concerns numerous substances containing one or several N-C=S groups, which in many human populations show bimodal taste threshold distributions; the best known of these substances are phenylthiourea (phenylthiocarbamide, PTC) and the therapeutically used antithyroid thiouracil derivatives. Only one other substance, anetholtrithione, has a similar threshold distribution, while no other sapid substance, bitter or otherwise, has shown a similar behavior. N-C= S substances occur in many plants, among them some vegetables, such as cabbage, kale and rutabaga. Rabbits fed entirely on cabbage develop goiter, and milk of cows fed on kale has caused slight goiter in infants.

Testing for PTC thresholds in sample populations of West Europeans which are also characteristic for many North American Indian and Chinese populations, show that 2 groups of people can be recognized; those having a high threshold, the "nontasters" (about 30%) and those with a low threshold, the "tasters" (about 70%). Family and sib studies have shown that tasting is almost entirely determined by an autosomal dominant gene T, so that the genotypes *TT* and *Tt* are tasters and the homozygous recessives, *tt*, nontasters. There may be a slight superiority in the general tasting ability of women, but the proportion of tasters and nontasters is the same in both sexes. Taster mode and nontaster mode, as well as the divisive antimode in a threshold distribution, shift with the increasing age of a population sample towards a lower sensitivity. Smoking may have only a slight effect on tasting, but xrays in therapeutic doses temporarily destroy the perception of any taste, including that for PTC. In samples of isolated tribal populations of Africans, Amerindians, and presumably of other remote people, nontasters may be completely absent.

PTC sensitivity has been widely tested in attempts to find and, if possible, to measure linkage with other marker genes, such as those responsible for the blood antigens and the enzyme polymorphism, as well as linkage with morbid genes, which are responsible for autosomally transmitted diseases. Regrettably none of the numerous claims for PTC linkage has withstood critical scrutiny.

The finding that rabbits fed predominantly on cabbage

from a hospital kitchen developed goiter and the subsequent isolation of the responsible goitrogens (antithyroid substances) from vegetables which were N-C=S containing substances suggested that the "taster" status of a person may in some way be connected with his propensity to develop thyroid disease. Such connections do indeed exist but their interpretation is rather complex. Whether a person is a taster or a nontaster does not seem to affect his overall propensity to develop goiter, but it seems that in areas where goiter is not endemic, nontasters are more prone to develop adenomatous nodular goiters, while tasters are more likely to develop diffuse toxic goiter. Furthermore, compensated athyrotic cretins, but not metabolic ones, have so far all been nontasters and there was an excess of nontasters among the relatives of these cretinoid patients. Association (pleiotropism) with taster status has been claimed for a great number of common diseases, eg TB and diabetes mellitus and for some other rarer medical conditions, but again most of these claims unfortunately cannot be accepted. Nevertheless, the search for genes linked or associated with the taster locus must be continued; sooner or later "tasting" will play some part in mapping man's autosomes.

Complications
I Derived: —
II Associated: Thyroid disease

Etiology: Ability to taste PTC requires 1 autosomal dominant gene T. McK *17120

Pathogenesis: —

Related Facts
I Sex Ratio: M1:F1
II Risk of Occurrence: About 1 in 3 to 1 in 4 nontasters in Western Europeans; < 1% in some isolated tribal populations
III Risk of Recurrence for
  Patient's Sib: If one parent TT and other TT, Tt, or tt all offspring will be tasters; if one parent Tt and other tt, 1 in 2 (50%) chance of being taster; if both parents Tt, 3 in 4 (75%) chance of being taster. See above
  Patient's Child: —
IV Age of Detectability: When patient can fully cooperate
V Prevalence: About 30% nontasters in Western Europeans and < 1% in some isolated tribal populations

Treatment
I Primary Prevention: Not necessary
II Secondary Prevention: —
III Other Therapy: —

Prognosis: Excellent if associated disease is absent

Detection of Carrier: Parents of nontaster

Special Considerations: —

References:
Dawson, W. and West, G.B.: Taste polymorphism to anetholtrithione and phenylthiocarbamate. Ann. Hum. Genet. 30:273, 1967.

Fraser, G.R.: Cretinism and taste sensitivity to phenylthiocarbamide. Lancet 1:964, 1961.

Harris, H.: Measurement of taste sensitivity to phenylthiourea (PTC). Ann. Eugen. (London) 15:24, 1949.

Harris, H. and Kalmus, H.: Chemical specificity in genetical differences of taste sensitivity. Ann. Eugen. (London) 15:32, 1949.

Harris, H. and Trotter, W.R.: Taste sensitivity to phenylthiourea in goitre and diabetes; preliminary communication. Lancet 2:1038, 1949.

Kalmus, H.: Genetical taste polymorphism and thyroid disease. In Proc. 2nd Int. Congr. Human Genetics. Rome:Instituto G. Mendel, 1963, vol. 3, p. 1856.

Contributor: **Hans Kalmus**

Editor's Computerized Descriptor: —

PHYTANIC ACID STORAGE DISEASE

Includes: Syndrome de l'acide phytanique
Phytansäure-Speicherkrankheit
Tesaurismosis de ácido fitánico
Refsum disease
Heredopathia atactica polyneuritiformia

Excludes: Similar clinical syndromes with retinal pigmentation but without demonstrated accumulation of phytanic acid or deficiency in phytanic acid oxidation

Minimal Diagnostic Criteria: Demonstration should be made of abnormal concentrations of phytanic acid in plasma or tissues. The major "clinical triad" consists of retinitis pigmentosa, peripheral neuropathy, and cerebellar ataxia. CSF protein level is increased without cells present.

Clinical Findings: The clinical features found at the time of reporting are listed here for patients in whom the actual biochemical defect was confirmed. Retinal degeneration, with nightblindness, concentric narrowing of visual fields and an atypical retinal pigmentation, are virtually always found. There is peripheral neuropathy in 90% of the patients, with motor weakness, muscular atrophy, loss of deep tendon reflexes, electromyographic evidence of denervation, and loss of superficial sensation to pain, touch or temperature. Muscle pain, or paresthesias, are infrequent. Other neurologic features include cerebellar signs (75%), nerve deafness (50%), pupillary abnormalities (40%), anosmia (35%), and nystagmus (25%). Cardiac involvement can sometimes be shown, with nonspecific ST-T changes in the precordial ECG or left ventricular enlargement. Cataracts were seen in 40% of the patients, and 60% have some skeletal malformations (shortening of the metatarsals, osteochondritis dissecans, pes cavus, etc). Some patients have ichthyotic skin changes, occasionally florid (trunk, palms, soles). Spinal fluid protein levels are increased in 85% of the patients (55-730 mgm%, mean: 275), without increased cells present.

Complications
I **Derived:** Four patients have had sudden death, possibly from cardiac arrhythmias, and 2 have died with respiratory paralysis. Renal function has been impaired in 4 patients, and increased urine lipid noted in 1 (with severe fatty infiltration of the kidneys).
II **Associated:** Aminoaciduria has been reported in two patients, of uncertain relationship to the primary defect.

Etiology: Autosomal recessive inheritance is established, by the usual genetic criteria (occurrence in sibships, high consanguinity incidence, etc.) and further indicated by demonstration of a partial defect in heterozygotes. McK *26650
Phytanic acid accumulation has been shown to be secondary to deletion of a phytanic acid oxidizing system, with the specific metabolic block involving the initial α-oxidation. This probably involves specifically an α-hydroxylating system that converts phytanic acid to α-hydroxyphytanic acid.

Pathogenesis: It is likely, but not proved, that the accumulation of phytanic acid in itself leads to the clinical manifestations of the disease. Animal feeding experiments have been negative, however, and rare instances of moderately elevated plasma phytanic acid levels have been found in parents of patients without clinical signs. It is pertinent that in some patients the course of the illness has been favorably influenced by dietary restriction of phytanic acid.
The possibility of other primary gene effects than that on phytanic acid oxidation has not been ruled out. It is of interest that the nervous system is a natural site of high concentrations of α-hydroxy fatty acids, but skin and nerve tissue from patients analyzed to date have not shown alteration in concentration or composition of these acids.

Related Facts
I **Sex Ratio:** M1:F1
II **Risk of Occurrence:** ?
III **Risk of Recurrence for**
Patient's Sib: 1 in 4 (25%) for each offspring to be affected
Patient's Child: Not increased unless mate is carrier or homozygote.
IV **Age of Detectability:** The earliest clinical manifestations (eg nightblindness) usually occur within the first 2 decades.
V **Prevalence:** ?

Treatment
I **Primary Prevention:** Genetic counseling
II **Secondary Prevention:** It is possible to limit the accumulation of phytanic acid and to decrease body stores by a diet from which phytanic acid and its precursors have been removed. Dairy products (butter, milk, cheese) and ruminant fats (beef and sheep) are the major sources, but phytanic acid is rather widely distributed in foodstuffs, including lipids of marine animals. Phytol in its unesterified form is a precursor for phytanic acid, but when esterified in the chlorophyll molecule it is apparently minimally absorbed. Plasma phytanate levels have dropped in all patients who have adhered to the special diet, and in none of those adhering has there been a clinical relapse. In 4 patients follow-up data are now available up to 10 years; some improvement in symptomatology occurs over the first 6-12 months (excluding cranial nerve manifestations), after which the clinical picture seems to stabilize. Obviously one would anticipate that institution of the diet in childhood would be most advantageous.
III **Other Therapy:** Supportive measures for consequences of neuropathy (physiotherapy, orthopedic devices); cataract extraction when indicated.

Prognosis: The course of the untreated disease is slowly progressive with frequent exacerbations and remissions of symptoms (occasionally correlated with intercurrent viral infection).
Life expectancy is shortened, but the age at death varies greatly. Expiration in childhood is rare, but death before age 40 occurred in 6 of the 33 chemically-established cases. Cardiac and respiratory problems appear to be the major threat to survival.

Detection of Carrier: Parents, sibs and children of known patients are clinically unaffected, and their plasma phytanic acid levels have been normal except in 2 instances (mothers of patients). Cell cultures from skin biopsies of patients show oxidation of phytanic acid at 1-2% of the normal rate. Cultures from heterozygote individuals have a partial defect, and hence this technique could be utilized in the detection of heterozygosity.

Special Considerations: —

References:
Refsum, S.: Heredopathia atactica polyneuritiformis; familial syndrome not hitherto described; contribution to clinical study of hereditary diseases of nervous system. Acta Psychiatr. Scand. (Suppl.) 38:1, 1946.
Steinberg, D. et al: Refsum's disease: Nature of the enzyme defect. Science 156:1740, 1967.
Steinberg, D. et al: Refsum's disease - a recently characterized lipidosis involving the nervous system. Ann. Intern. Med. 66:365, 1967.
Steinberg, D.: Phytanic acid storage disease (Refsum's syndrome). In Stanbury, J.B. et al (eds.): The Metabolic Basis of Inherited Disease, 4th Ed. New York:McGraw-Hill, Inc., 1978, p. 688.

Contributor: **Daniel Steinberg**

Editor's Computerized Descriptors: Vision, Eye, Skin, Skel., Muscle, Resp., CV., GU., Nerve

PITYRIASIS RUBRA PILARIS

Includes: Pityriasis rubra pilaire
Pitiriasis rubra pilaris
Lichen acuminatus
Lichen ruber acuminatus
Pityriasis pilaris

Excludes: Phrynoderma
Ichthyosis
Keratosis pilaris
Exfoliative dermatitis with pityriasis rubra pilaris
Psoriasis vulgaris (833)

Minimal Diagnostic Criteria: Pathognomonic black horny follicular plugs on the backs of the fingers; hyperkeratosis of palms and soles: the yellowish or greyish red to orange or salmon-yellow color of the plaques, with islands of normal skin and the dry scaliness of the face and scalp.

Clinical Findings: Persistent dry horny acuminate follicular papules on the dorsal surfaces of the 1st and 2nd phalanges. Symmetrically distributed, pinhead in size, brownish red to rosy yellow in color and enclose a dry lusterless atrophic hair in their keratotic centers. The horny central plugs are often capped by a black point. Multiplication and coalescence of papules form plaques which are symmetrically distributed. The plaques are sharply marginated with small islands of normal skin within the affected areas. The skin looks like goose flesh and feels like a nutmeg grater.

Nails are dull, rough, brittle, and frequently transversely striated. They are lusterless, and grey or yellow in color. Palms and soles exhibit firm thick reddish-yellow hyperkeratosis which scales freely and often become fissured. Face is red, thickened, inelastic, and often there is ectropion of lower lids.

Complications
I **Derived:** —
II **Associated:** May be associated with liver disease, neuromuscular dysfunction, rheumatism, psoriasis, and hormonal dysfunction.

Etiology: Autosomal dominant with incomplete penetrance; McK *17320

Pathogenesis: —

Related Facts
I **Sex Ratio:** M1:F1
II **Risk of Occurrence:** ?
III **Risk of Recurrence for**
    Patient's Sib: If parent is affected < 1 in 2 (< 50%) for each offspring to be affected; otherwise not increased.
    Patient's Child: < 1 in 2
IV **Age of Detectability:** Birth to 70 years without any significant age predilection.
V **Prevalence:** Rare

Treatment
I **Primary Prevention:** Genetic counseling
II **Secondary Prevention:** Difficult to evaluate because of natural exacerbations and remissions. Vitamin A by mouth ranging from 50 M to 200 M units per day. Metrotrexate has been used. Vitamin A alcohol in lubriderm topically has been used successfully.
III **Other Therapy:** —

Prognosis: In 75 patients, 8% resolved completely; improved in 60%; remitted and exacerbated in 24%; did not change in 7%; became worse in 1%. True prognosis unknown. Information unavailable concerning the possible predisposition of patients to develop other diseases and ultimate cause of death.

Detection of Carrier: —

Special Considerations: —

References:
Butterworth, T. and Strean, L. P.: Clinical Genodermatology. Baltimore:Williams & WIlkins Co., 1962, p. 38.
Davidson, C.L., Jr. et al: Pityriasis rubra pilaris; a follow-up study of 57 patients. Arch. Dermatol. 100:175, 1969.
Gross, D.A. et al: Pityriasis rubra pilaris: Report of a case and analysis of the literature. Arch. Dermatol. 99:710, 1969.
Lamar, L. M. and Gaethe, G.: Pityriasis rubra pilaris. Arch. Dermatol. 89:515, 1964.

Contributor: **George Gaethe**

Editor's Computerized Descriptors: Skin, Nails

PLASMA-ASSOCIATED DEFECT OF PHAGOCYTOSIS

Includes: Absence de phagocytose
Leinersche Krankheit
Defecto de la fagocitosis relacionado con el plasma
Complement C5 deficiency
Leiner disease
Neonatal seborrheic diathesis

Excludes: Other complement deficiency diseases

Minimal Diagnostic Criteria: Demonstration in vitro of defective phagocytosis of yeast particles or staphylococci by normal polymorphonuclear leukocytes in the presence of serum or plasma from the patient.

Clinical Findings: Repeated severe infections occur shortly after birth including generalized seborrheic dermatitis with a marked inflammatory component, persistent diarrhea usually associated with bacterial infection and resistant to antibiotic and dietary management, and marked wasting or dystrophic appearance of the patient.

Of particular significance is the finding of almost exclusively gram-negative bacteria on culture material. Staphylococcus aureus is the only gram-positive organism seen with any frequency. Patients with the syndrome are likely to be markedly cachectic and show a generalized failure to thrive.

Common laboratory findings include neutrophilia, diffuse hyperglobulinemia and elevated sedimentation rate. Despite treatment with systemic antibiotics, the patients show little change in their clinical state.

Complications
I **Derived:** Disability, marked weakness and death resulting from uncontrolled infection most usually by gram-negative bacteria.
II **Associated:** —

Etiology: Probably autosomal recessive

Pathogenesis: The basic abnormality involves a dysfunction of the fifth component of complement (C5). The ability of patient's serum to enhance phagocytosis of yeast particles can be restored to normal by the addition of highly purified C5.†

Related Facts
I **Sex Ratio:** M1:F1
II **Risk of Occurrence:** ?
III **Risk of Recurrence for**
   Patient's Sib: 1 in 4 (25%) for each offspring to be affected
   Patient's Child: Not increased unless mate is carrier or homozygote
IV **Age of Detectability:** At birth by phagocytosis test
V **Prevalence:** Rare

Treatment
I **Primary Prevention:** Genetic counseling
II **Secondary Prevention:** The only effective way of treating this disorder to date is by the infusion of fresh plasma or blood. This contains C5 in adequate amounts that have proved life saving to 2 severely afflicted infants. The usual bank blood is not a satisfactory source of active C5, hence the requirement for fresh blood or plasma. Antibiotics as specific as possible for the infecting organism should be administered.
III **Other Therapy:** —

Prognosis: Based upon the experience of Leiner and with the present families, the mortality rate of this disorder is somewhere in the range of 40%. The use of plasma as a source of active C5 is life saving and may enable such patients to eventually enjoy normal life expectancy.

Detection of Carrier: The carrier state has been identified by use of the phagocytic assay of yeast particles. However, the values obtained with this assay have shown the carrier to be as low as the patient. Hence, with the presently available measurements the patient and clinically normal members of the family sharing the defect cannot be differentiated.

†**Special Considerations:** Although only a few children have been shown to date to have this defect, the implications of a humoral deficiency state causing impaired cellular function such as phagocytosis are of crucial importance in the understanding of normal inflammation.

References:
Jacobs, J.C. and Miller, M.E.: Total familial Leiner's disease. A deficiency of the opsonic activity of serum complement. Pediatrics 49:225, 1972.
Leiner, C.: Über erythrodermia desquamativa, eine eigenartige universelle Dermatose der Brustkinder. Arch. Dermatol. Syph. 89:163, 1908.
Miller, M.E. et al: A familial, plasma-associated defect of phagocytosis. Lancet 2:60, 1968.
Miller, M.E. and Nilsson, U.R.: A familial deficiency of the phagocytosis enhancing activity of serum related to a dysfunction of the fifth component of complement (C5). N. Engl. J. Med. 282:354, 1970.

Contributor: **Michael E. Miller**

Editor's Computerized Descriptor: Skin

POLAND SYNDROME

Includes: Syndactylie de type Poland
Sindactilia de Poland
Symbrachydactyly with ipsilateral aplasia of sternal head of pectoralis major muscle
Poland syndactyly

Excludes: Syndactyly (923)
Miscellaneous syndactyly
Symbrachydactyly without associated muscle defect
Syndactyly as a part of the acrocephalosyndactylies

Minimal Diagnostic Criteria: The association of symbrachydactyly with ipsilateral aplasia of the sternal head of pectoralis major is diagnostic. The muscle defect is observed clinically as absence of the normal well-developed curved anterior axillary fold.

Clinical Findings: The two main components of the syndrome are symbrachydactyly and pectoral muscle defect. Symbrachydactyly is a specific hand malformation, always unilateral, characterized by the association of short digits and syndactyly. The phalanges are short or absent. The middle phalanges are affected more frequently and in severe cases they are absent or fused with the distal phalanges (terminal symphalangism and assimilation hypoplasia). The distal phalanges are minimally affected and rarely absent. The thumb is usually least affected. Syndactyly is either partial or complete, usually involving the soft tissues and not associated with bone synostosis. Syndactyly frequently involves the index and middle fingers.

The associated muscle defect is ipsilateral aplasia of the sternal head of the pectoralis major while its clavicular head is always present and sometimes hypertrophied.

Asymmetry of breast development, ipsilateral absence of the breast and subcutaneous tissue, as well as ipsilateral webbing of the axilla are sometimes noted.

Complications
I **Derived:** Associated defects in other muscles are occasional features. Muscles affected are the pectoralis minor, rectus abdominis, latissimus dorsi, serratus anterior and intercostal. Associated bone defects have also been noted; examples are hypoplasia of upper ribs, Sprengel deformity of the scapula and shortening of arm and forearm bones. Ipsilateral hypoplasia of the kidney was noted in one patient.
II **Associated:** —

Etiology: ? Practically all reported cases are sporadic.

Pathogenesis: ? No progressive development.

Related Facts
I **Sex Ratio:** M1:F1
II **Risk of Occurrence:** ?
III **Risk of Recurrence for**
    Patient's Sib: Not increased
    Patient's Child: Not increased
IV **Age of Detectability:** At birth by clinical examination
V **Prevalence:** Among 33 cases with symbrachydactyly, Pol in 1921 found 21 cases with ipsilateral aplasia of sternal head of pectoralis major. Among 102 cases with absent sternal head of pectoralis major, Bing in 1902 found 14 cases with associated symbrachydactyly. Sigiura et al (1962) found one boy with Poland syndactyly among 6297 Japanese primary school children.

Treatment
I **Primary Prevention:** —
II **Secondary Prevention:** Surgical correction
III **Other Therapy:** —

Prognosis: Normal life span

Detection of Carrier: —

Special Considerations: —

References:
Clarkson, P.: Poland's syndactyly. Guys Hosp. Rep. 111:335, 1962.
Temtamy, S. A.: Genetic factors in hand malformations. Unpublished doctoral dissertation. Johns Hopkins University, 1966.
Temtamy, S.A. and McKusick, V.A.: The Genetics of Hand Malformations. Birth Defects: Orig. Art. Ser., Bergsma, D. (ed.). New York: Alan R. Liss, Inc. for The National Foundation-March of Dimes, 1978, vol. XIV, no. 3.

Contributor: **Samia A. Temtamy**

Editor's Computerized Descriptors: Skin, Skel., Muscle

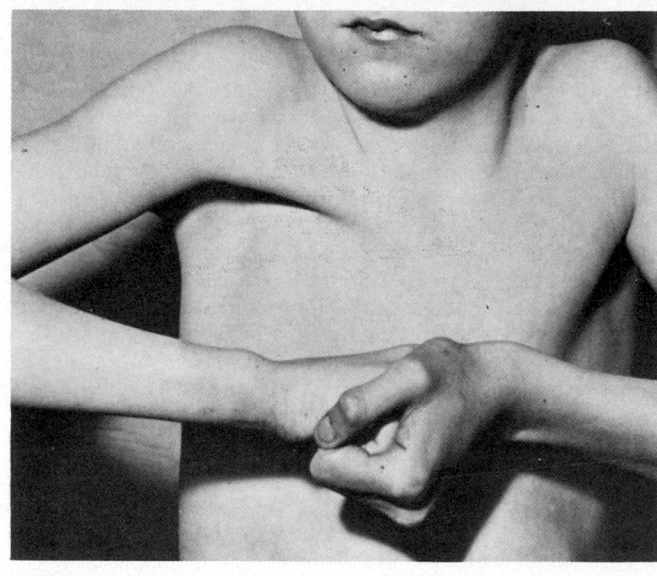

417. Absence of sternal head of right pectoral major muscle

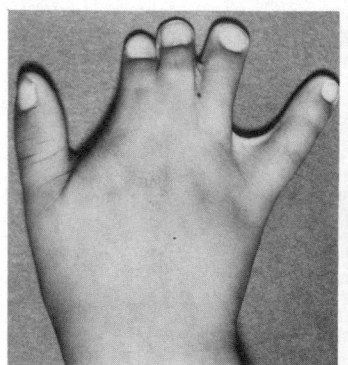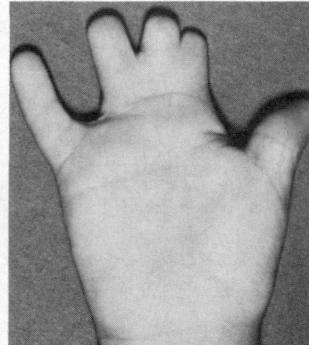

418. Digital hypoplasia and syndactyly

POLYDACTYLY

Includes: Polydactylie
Polydaktylie
Polidactilia
Preaxial polydactyly
Thumb polydactyly
Polydactyly of index finger and polysyndactyly
Postaxial polydactyly, types A and B

Excludes: Laurence-Moon-Biedl syndrome (578)
Chondroectodermal dysplasia (156)
Syndactyly (923)
Chromosome thirteen trisomy syndrome (168)
Numerous syndromes with pre- or postaxial polydactyly

Minimal Diagnostic Criteria: An extra digital triradius is found at the base of the extra digit. When it is a pedunculated postminimus that was surgically removed or fell out spontaneously, the extra triradius in the dermatoglyphics may be the only evidence of postaxial polydactyly.

Clinical Findings: In *preaxial polydactyly* the extra digit is on the radial side of the hand. The deformity in polydactyly of the thumb is duplication of all or part of the components of a thumb. In polydactyly of a triphalangeal thumb, the thumb has 3 phalanges with duplication of all or part of its components. In polydactyly of the index finger, the thumb is present and the index finger is duplicated. Dermatoglyphic findings in this case are diagnostic, since an extra A triradius and an A line are present, corresponding to the extra index finger.

In *postaxial polydactyly*, the extra digit is on the postaxial side or ulnar side in the upper limb and the fibular side in the lower limb. Two phenotypic and possibly genetically different varieties exist. In one of them, postaxial polydactyly type A, the extra digit is rather well formed and articulates with the 5th or extra metacarpal. In postaxial polydactyly type B, or pedunculated postminimus, the extra digit is not well formed and is frequently in the form of a skin tag.

Complications
I **Derived:** —
II **Associated:** —

Etiology: Polydactyly of a triphalangeal thumb, polydactyly of index finger and postaxial polydactyly are autosomal dominant traits with variable penetrance and expressivity. Thumb polydactyly is frequently unilateral and the cases are sporadic with no evidence of inheritance. McK *17420

Pathogenesis: —

Related Facts
I **Sex Ratio:** M1:F1
II **Risk of Occurrence:** Postaxial polydactyly is about 10 times more frequent in Negroes than in Caucasians. In American whites, incidence figures vary from 1 in 3300 to 1 in 630 live births, and in American Negroes figures vary from 1 in 300 to 1 in 100 live births.
III **Risk of Recurrence for**
Patient's Sib: If parent is affected, 1 in 2 (50%) for each offspring to be affected; otherwise not increased.
Patient's Child: 1 in 2
IV **Age of Detectability:** At birth
V **Prevalence:** ?

Treatment
I **Primary Prevention:** Genetic counseling
II **Secondary Prevention:** Surgical removal of the extra digit
III **Other Therapy:** —

Prognosis: Polydactyly as an isolated malformation does not affect life span.

Detection of Carrier: —

Special Considerations: —

References:
Mohan, J.: Postaxial polydactyly in three Indian families. J. Med. Genet. 6:196, 1969.
Temtamy, S. A.: Genetic factors in hand malformations. Unpublished doctoral dissertation. Johns Hopkins University, 1966.
Temtamy, S.A. and McKusick, V.A.: The Genetics of Hand Malformations. Birth Defects: Orig. Art. Ser., Bergsma, D. (ed.). New York: Alan R. Liss, Inc. for The National Foundation-March of Dimes, 1978, vol. XIV, no. 3.

Contributor: **Samia A. Temtamy**

Editor's Computerized Descriptors: Dermatoglyphic, Skel.

POLYMASTIA

Includes: Polymastie
Polimastia
Presence of complete supernumerary mammary glands
Presence of aberrant gland tissue without nipple or areola
Supernumerary nipples without obvious glandular tissue
Polythelia

Excludes: Intraareolar polythelia
Supernumerary nipples on the normal breast

Minimal Diagnostic Criteria: A supernumerary nipple with histologic appearance of breast tissue. They must be distinguished from congenital moles or stains, plane warts, or papillomata.

Clinical Findings: Complete supernumerary mammary glands are very rare. They usually appear as polythelia. A vast majority occur along a line extending from the axilla to the groin, along the so-called "milkline." Most such glands are observed in the thoracic region. They may be unilateral or bilateral, and may occur above or below the normal mammae. They occur more frequently on the left side than on the right. When they are situated above the normal mammae they are usually lateral to them, whereas when placed below the normal mammae they are medial. The laterally situated glands are well-formed, of considerable size, and can lactate; while medial ones are usually small, imperfectly developed and incapable of lactation.

Single supernumeraries are more common than multiple ones; the incidence decreases inversely to the number of mammae. Patients with 8 or 9 supernumerary breasts have been described. In some rare cases the accessory breasts appear outside the mammary ridge, in such locations as the face, neck, arm, thigh, buttock and back.

The supernumerary breasts undergo cyclic changes in size and density of the normal breast, and are subject to the same diseases including carcinoma. They generally attract attention at the time of puberty or in association with pregnancy and lactation. However, they may remain unnoticed and quiescent through puberty and repeated pregnancies.

Complications
I   **Derived:** Pain or dribbling of milk during the period of lactation, esthetic and psychologic embarrassment to the patient. Although carcinomatous changes occur, it is not established whether tumors arise with greater frequency in ectopic mammary glands than in normally situated ones.
II **Associated:** Association of supernumerary breasts with multiple births, tuberculosis, and left-handedness has been reported in the earlier literature but more careful evaluation of statistical data failed to bear any such relationship. Boenheim found high incidence of congenital abnormalities of skin, eye, teeth, palate, chin, etc coincident with supernumerary nipples. Evans found polythelia to be commonly associated with systemic hypertension, pulmonary hypertension and cardiomyopathy.

Etiology: Familial occurrence of supernumerary breasts has been generally recognized. Iwai found hereditary transmission in 6% of the cases. Klinkerfuss recorded a hereditary incidence through 4 generations of a family. The condition has also been observed in identical twins, and is known to affect both sexes. In certain families it shows autosomal dominant mode of inheritance.

Pathogenesis: The supernumerary breasts occurring along the milkline result when the embryonic mammary ridge fails to undergo normal regression. There is no satisfactory explanation for the supernumeraries occurring outside of the milkline.

Related Facts
I   **Sex Ratio:** M > F in Caucasians, F > M in Japanese
II **Risk of Occurrence:** Approximately 1 in 100†

III **Risk of Recurrence for**
Patient's Sib: When autosomal dominant, if parent is affected 1 in 2 (50%) for each offspring; otherwise not increased.
Patient's Child: When autosomal dominant, 1 in 2
IV **Age of Detectability:** Neonatal period; in certain instances the supernumeraries will remain unnoticed till after puberty or after pregnancies.
V   **Prevalence:** 1 in 250 in British children
1 in 20 in British population
1 in 36 in Finnish population
1 in 27 in Japanese population
1 in 17 in New York females
1 in 100 generally accepted figure

Treatment
I   **Primary Prevention:** —
II **Secondary Prevention:** —
III **Other Therapy:** Excision for cosmetic purposes

Prognosis: Normal for life span, intelligence and function with normal reproductive fitness.

Detection of Carrier: —

†**Special Considerations:** Racial differences have been observed for sex distribution and site of occurrence of the supernumerary breasts. In Caucasians more than 90% of the accessory breasts are found below the normally situated mammae, while in Japan 88% of the supernumeraries are above the normal one. Among Japanese the incidence of supernumeraries among females was 3 times as great as among males, in contrast to Caucasians in whom there is preponderance of supernumeraries among males.

References:
Iwai, T.: A statistical study on the polymastia of the Japanese. Lancet 2:753, 1907.
Klinkerfuss, G. H.: Four generations of polymastia. JAMA 82:1247,1924.
Speert, H.: Supernumerary mammae, with special reference to the Rhesus monkey. Q. Rev. Biol. 17:59, 1942.

Contributors: **Eduardo Orti**
Qutub H. Qazi

Editor's Computerized Descriptor: Skin

POLYSPLENIA SYNDROME

Includes: Polysplenie
Polisplenia
Syndrome of bilateral left-sidedness

Excludes: Asplenia syndrome† (92)

Minimal Diagnostic Criteria: Evidence for partial visceral heterotaxy in individuals with or without congenital heart disease in whom the erythrocytes are normal and in whom azygos return of the inferior vena caval bed is present. Occasionally, abdominal aortography will demonstrate the presence of multiple splenules.

Clinical Findings: The term "polysplenia syndrome" is used to indicate a characteristic constellation of visceral anomalies of which the outstanding feature, in addition to the presence of a number of more or less individual splenules, is a strong tendency for normally asymmetric organs (or pairs of organs) to develop more or less symmetrically. The right-sided organs or parts of organs assume the morphologic characteristics of their left-sided counterparts, but in mirror image (isomerism). In at least 70% of cases, no eparterial bronchus is present on either side and the lobation of both lungs resembles that of a normal bilobed left lung. The right and left lobes of the liver are commonly about equal in size and the stomach may be located on either side. Partial or complete failure of rotation of the intestinal tract is common and the mesentery may be free and located in the midline. Splenic tissue is present on *both* sides of the dorsal mesogastrium, rather than only on the left side. Two relatively large spleens, 1 on either side of the dorsal mesogastrium, are usually present. Generally 1 or more small accessory spleens are also found.

Cardiovascular anomalies are commonly, but not always present. While in some cases these anomalies may be extremely complex and similar to those seen in asplenia syndrome, by and large the cardiovascular malformations tend to be much simpler in polysplenia syndrome. Transposition of the great arteries and obstruction to pulmonary arterial blood flow are unusual. A very characteristic systemic venous anomaly present in the great majority of cases is azygos return of the inferior vena caval bed. The hepatic segment of the inferior cava is either absent or markedly hypoplastic. The azygos vein may be located either on the right or left side of the spine. The pulmonary venous connection in cases with severe anomalies is interesting in that commonly the right and left pulmonary veins enter their corresponding atria. As in asplenia syndrome, there may be isomerism of the atria; in this case, however, the morphology of the atria resembles that of a normal left atrium. Atrial septal defects are common as are endocardial cushion defects of some type. A *coronary* sinus may be present in contradistinction to the asplenia syndrome.

The clinical picture depends largely on the complexity and severity of the cardiovascular lesions. Severe forms of the syndrome may present themselves within days or weeks after birth with cyanosis, respiratory distress, feeding difficulties and congestive heart failure. Early death is common in such infants. In individuals in which the heart is normal or nearly normal, symptoms may be slight or absent. The ECG in patients with the more severe forms of polysplenia syndrome usually shows inverted P waves in leads II, III, and aVF. Left axis deviation is present in cases with some form of endocardial cushion defect. Radiographs commonly demonstrate partial visceral heterotaxy. The air-filled tracheobronchial tree, particularly in older children and young adults, may be seen to be symmetric, both right and left main bronchi resembling a normal left bronchus. This sign is not, however, pathognomonic since bilateral absence of an eparterial bronchus may occasionally be seen in individuals without the syndrome. The enlarged azygos vein may be visible as a convexity of the upper mediastinal border. Cardiac catheterization and angiocardiography demonstrate the azygos return of the inferior vena caval bed and the nature of the cardiovascular lesions, if any.

The multiple spleens are not observed during cardiac examination, but might be found by abdominal ultrasonography. With respect to the heart, polysplenia syndrome has many of the cardiac features of the asplenia syndrome. See Asplenia Syndrome.

Complications
I **Derived:** These depend largely on the severity of the cardiovascular anomalies present.
II **Associated:** —

Etiology: —

Pathogenesis: ?

Related Facts
I **Sex Ratio:** Uncertain at present; male predominance seen in asplenia syndrome is apparently not found in polysplenia syndrome.
II **Risk of Occurrence:** Exact figures not available, but syndrome is being recognized with increasing frequency and is not as rare as was originally thought.
III **Risk of Recurrence for**
  Patient's Sib: Probably negligible
  Patient's Child: ?
IV **Age of Detectability:** Shortly after birth
V **Prevalence:** ?

Treatment
I **Primary Prevention:** —
II **Secondary Prevention:** Pulmonary banding may be considered in patients with large shunts in order to forestall the development of other pulmonary vascular changes.
III **Other Therapy:** In young infants with severe forms of syndrome, probably none. In others, surgical therapy is indicated where feasible.

Prognosis: Varies greatly depending upon the severity of syndrome in any individual case.

Detection of Carrier: —

†**Special Considerations:** While polysplenia syndrome is very probably in some ways related etiologically and pathogenetically to asplenia syndrome, the 2 syndromes should be considered distinct entities.

References:
Anderson, R.C. et al: Anomalous inferior vena cava with azygos continuation (infrahepatic interruption of the inferior vena cava): Report of 15 new cases. J. Pediatr. 59:370, 1961.
Campbell, M. and Deuchar, D.C.: Absent inferior vena cava, symmetrical liver, splenic agenesis, and situs inversus, and their embryology. Br. Heart J. 29:268, 1967.
Moller, J.H. et al: Congenital cardiac disease associated with polysplenia: A developmental complex of bilateral "left-sidedness." Circulation 36:789, 1967.
Ongley, P.A. et al: Anomalous connection of pulmonary veins to right atrium associated with anomalous inferior vena cava, situs inversus and multiple spleens: A developmental complex. Mayo Clin. Proc. 40:609, 1965.
Van Mierop, L.H.S. et al: Asplenia and polysplenia syndrome. In Bergsma, D. (ed.): Congenital Cardiac Defects - Recent Advances. Birth Defects: Orig. Art. Ser., vol. VIII, no. 1. Baltimore: Williams & Wilkins, Co. for The National Foundation-March of Dimes, 1972, pp. 74-82.

Contributor: **L. H. S. Van Mierop**

Editor's Computerized Descriptors: Resp., CV., Spleen, GI.

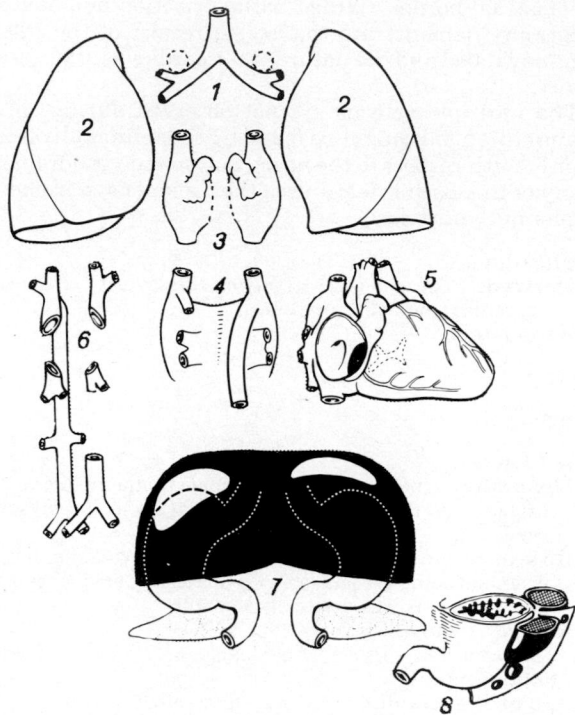

419. Note partial or complete failure of bowel rotation. 1) Bilateral hyparterial bronchi; 2) bilateral bilobed lungs; 3) bilateral morphologic left atria; 4) pulmonary venous anomalies; 5) cardiac malformations; 6) systemic venous anomalies; 7) symmetric liver and right- or left-sided stomach; 8) stomach and double spleen

POLYSYNDACTYLY

Includes: Polydactylie avec syndactylie
Polysyndaktylie
Polisindactilia
Preaxial polydactyly of toes associated with syndactyly

Excludes: Syndactyly (923)
Acrocephalopolysyndactyly (13)
Polysyndactyly with peculiar skull shape

Minimal Diagnostic Criteria: See Clinical Findings.

Clinical Findings: In the feet, preaxial polydactyly or duplication of the 1st or 2nd toes is associated with syndactyly of various degrees. In the hands, the most common malformation is syndactyly of the 3rd and 4th fingers; the terminal phalanx of the thumb is usually malformed, broad and short or bifid and sometimes radially deviated. Pedunculated post minimi is a feature in some families. While hand malformation is mild and variable, malformation of the feet is constant and nearly uniform.

Complications
I Derived: —
II Associated: —

Etiology: Autosomal dominant; McK *17470

Pathogenesis: ?

Related Facts
I Sex Ratio: M1:F1
II Risk of Occurrence: ?
III Risk of Recurrence for
  Patient's Sib: If parent is affected, 1 in 2 (50%) for each offspring to be affected; otherwise not increased.
  Patient's Child: 1 in 2
IV Age of Detectability: At birth
V Prevalence: ?

Treatment
I Primary Prevention: Genetic counseling
II Secondary Prevention: Surgical correction of malformations
III Other Therapy: —

Prognosis: Normal life span

Detection of Carrier: —

Special Considerations: —

References:
Goodman, R. M.: A family with polysyndactyly and other anomalies. J. Hered. 56:37, 1965.
Temtamy, S. A.: Genetic factors in hand malformations. Unpublished doctoral dissertation. Johns Hopkins University, 1966.
Temtamy, S.A. and Loutfy, A.H.: Polysyndactyly in an Egyptian family. In Bergsma, D. (ed.): Limb Malformations. Birth Defects: Orig. Art. Ser., vol X, no. 5, Miami: Symposia Specialists for The National Foundation-March of Dimes, 1974, p. 207.

Contributor: **Samia A. Temtamy**

Editor's Computerized Descriptor: Skel.

POPLITEAL PTERYGIUM SYNDROME

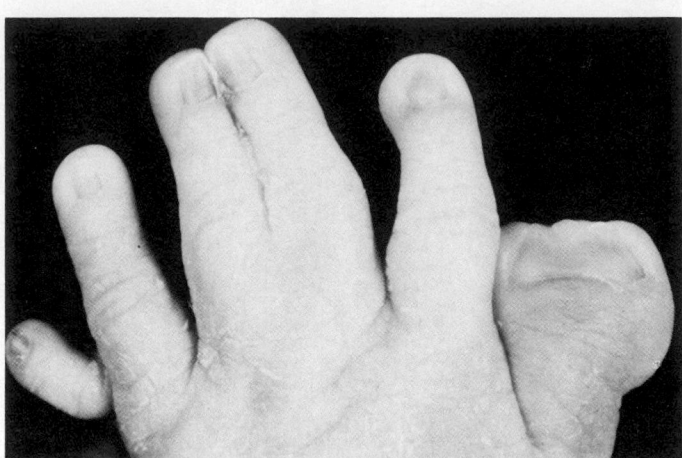

420. Pre- and postaxial polydactyly with syndactyly

Includes: Ptérygium poplité
Kniepterygium-Syndrom
Síndrome de pterigión poplíteo
Webbing, popliteal
Cleft lip-palate, popliteal pterygium, digital and genital anomalies

Excludes: Arthrogryposis (88)
Caudal regression
Cleft lip or palate and median lip pits
Multiple pterygium syndrome

Minimal Diagnostic Criteria: Popliteal pterygium, pits of lower lip, cleft lip-palate or cleft palate and genital anomalies

Clinical Findings: Bilateral, rarely unilateral, popliteal pterygium extending from the heel to the ischial tuberosity. Intercrural pterygia. Cleft lip-palate. Pits or fistulas of the lower lip. Genital anomalies in the male include: cryptorchidism and absent or cleft scrotum, and in the female: absence of labia majora and enlarged clitoris. Syndactyly of hands or feet, filiform adhesions between the upper and lower lids and hypoplasia or agenesis of digits may also be present.

Complications
I   **Derived:** Walking difficulties, limited extension, rotation and abduction of the legs; speech impairment
II **Associated:** —

Etiology: Autosomal dominant with incomplete penetrance and variable expressivity. McK *11950

Pathogenesis: Essentially unknown. Failure of fusion of primary and secondary palate.

Related Facts
I   **Sex Ratio:** M1:F1
II   **Risk of Occurrence:** ? Rare
III **Risk of Recurrence for**
    Patient's Sib: If parent is affected 1 in 2 (50%) for each offspring to be affected; otherwise not increased
    Patient's Child: < 1 in 2
IV **Age of Detectability:** Neonatal
V   **Prevalence:** ? Rare

Treatment
I   **Primary Prevention:** Genetic counseling
II   **Secondary Prevention:** Plastic reparative surgery for cleft lip-palate, lip pits, popliteal pterygium,† ankyloblepharon and syndactyly
III **Other Therapy:** Speech therapy

Prognosis: After surgery, walking will improve as well as speech. General health is not impaired.

Detection of Carrier: —

†Special Considerations: The sciatic nerve lies free within the pterygium. If plastic surgery of the webbing is attempted and this fact unrecognized, sectioning of the nerve may occur.

References:
Bixler, D. et al: Phenotypic variation in the popliteal pterygium syndrome. Clin. Genet. 4:220, 1973.
Gorlin, R.J. et al: Popliteal pterygium syndrome: Syndrome comprising cleft lip-palate, popliteal and intercrural pterygia, digital and genital anomalies. Pediatrics 41:503, 1968.
Hecht, F. and Jarvinen, J. M.: Heritable dysmorphic syndrome with normal intelligence. J. Pediatr. 70:927, 1967.
Kind, H.P.: Popliteales pterygium syndrom. Helv. Paediatr. Acta 25:508, 1970.

Contributor: **Heddie O. Sedano**

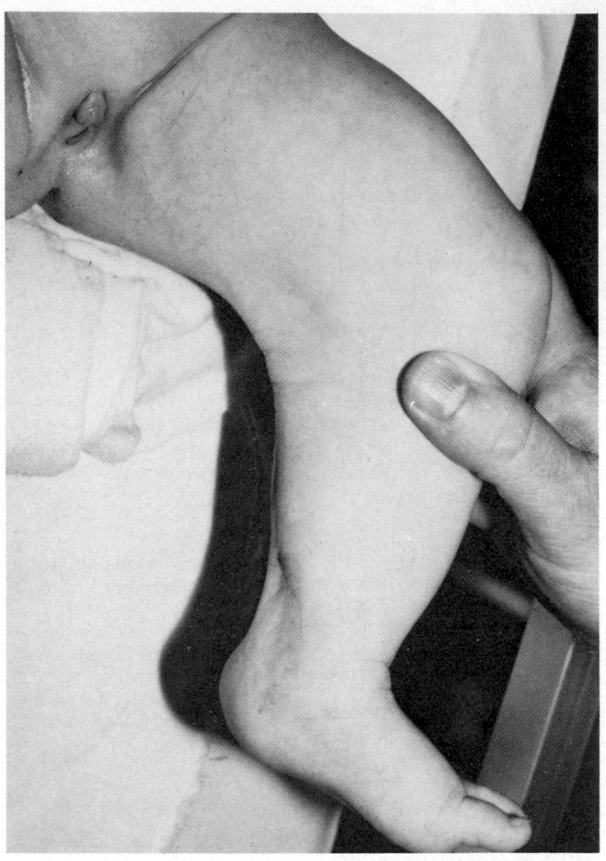

421. Popliteal pterygium extending over the popliteal space to the intercrural area, with hypoplasia of the labia majora

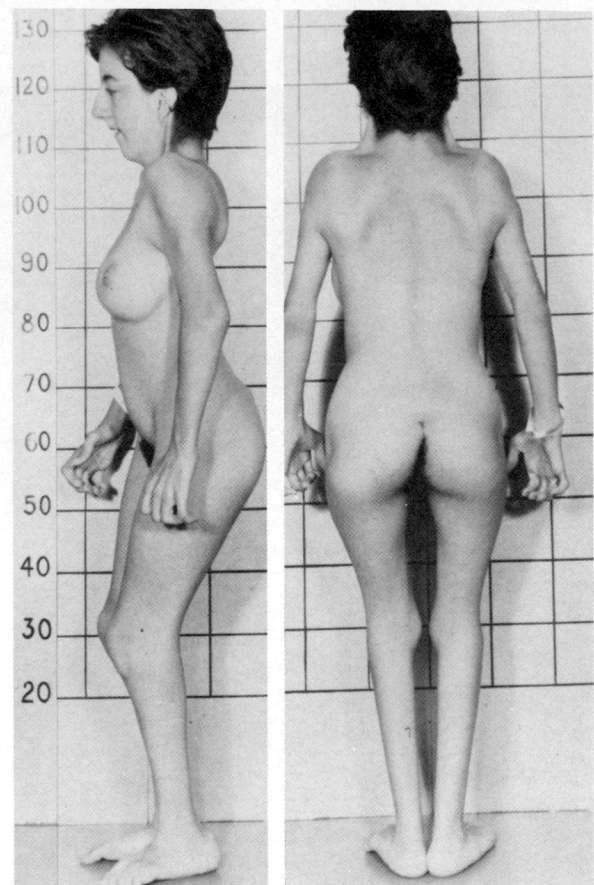

423. Note short stature; marked webbing of neck, low posterior hairline; flexion contractures of fingers and knees; foot deformities

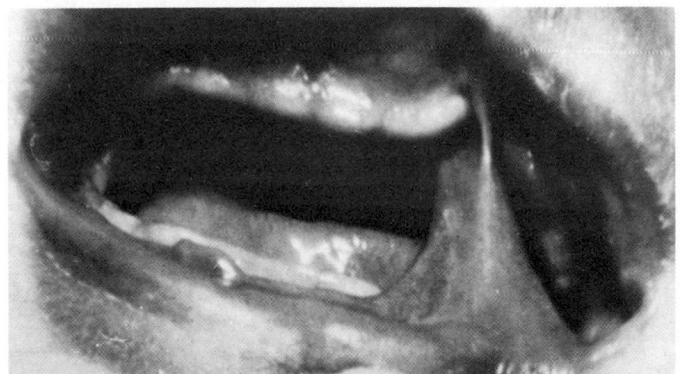

422. Note soft tissue band extending from lower lip to maxillary alveolus at site of incomplete cleft lip

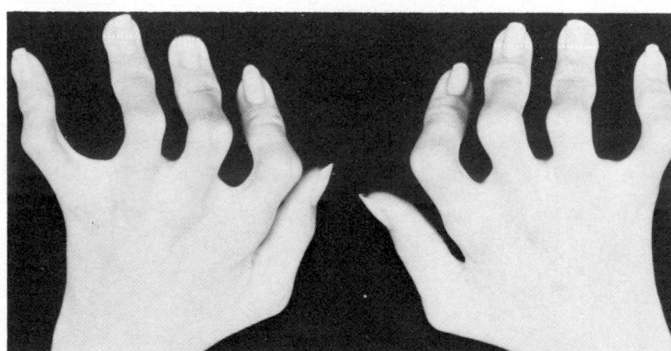

424. Maximal extension of fingers with flexion contractures

Includes: Porokeratose
Poroqueratosis
Porokeratosis of Mibelli
Chronic progressive keratoatrophoderma
Hyperkeratosis eccentrica

Excludes: Keratoderma of palms and soles
Ichthyosis hystrix

Minimal Diagnostic Criteria: Demonstration of the cornoid lamella in histologic sections in all types.

Clinical Findings: The primary lesion is a small hyperkeratotic papule which gradually enlarges to form a plaque with a raised wall-like border and a depressed center. Some lesions remain small while others may attain a large size. Any part of the integument, even the mucosa, may be involved. The areas most affected are the hands and feet, especially the dorsal surfaces, and the face and neck.

Since the early classic description of porokeratosis by Mibelli, several clinical variants of the disease have been reported: 1) Superficial disseminated eruptive form (Respighi). The lesions are faint and may be easily overlooked. 2) Disseminated superficial actinic porokeratosis. This form is essentially the same as that described by Respighi and may be considered a variant of it. 3) Hyperkeratotic verrucous type. May undergo ulceration and may simulate carcinoma. 4) Forma minima (Freund) is nonfamilial and is considered by certain authors as a form of lichen striatus. Recently, another clinical variant, linear porokeratosis, has been reported in which the lesions occur in a linear distribution. Horn-like giant cornoid lamellae have also been described.

Complications
I **Derived:** Malignant degeneration (epidermoid carcinoma) has been reported.
II **Associated:** —

Etiology: Autosomal dominant; McK *17580

Pathogenesis: ? No relationship to sweat duct, contrary to what is implied by the present name of the disease.

Related Facts
I **Sex Ratio:** M2:F1 ?
II **Risk of Occurrence:** Rare
III **Risk of Recurrence for**
   Patient's Sib: If parent is affected 1 in 2 (50%) for each offspring to be affected; otherwise not increased.
   Patient's Child: 1 in 2
IV **Age of Detectability:** Any age
V **Prevalence:** Rare. Many cases are mild and may escape notice.

Treatment
I **Primary Prevention:** Genetic counseling
II **Secondary Prevention:** Excision if feasible
III **Other Therapy:** —

Prognosis: Normal for life span and intelligence. Involvement of face cosmetically disagreeable. Although characteristically progressive, lesions may spontaneously involute.

Detection of Carrier: —

Special Considerations: —

References:
Chernosky, M. E. and Freeman, R. G.: Disseminated superficial actinic porokeratosis (DSAP). Arch. Dermatol. 96:611, 1967.
McMillan, G.L. et al: Linear porokeratosis with giant cornoid lamella. Arch. Dermatol. 112:515, 1976.
Mikhail, G. R. and Wertheimer, F. W.: Clinical variants of porokeratosis (Mibelli). Arch. Dermatol. 98:124, 1968.
Rahbari, H. et al: Linear porokeratosis - a distinctive clinical variant of porokeratosis of Mibelli. Arch. Dermatol. 109:526, 1974.

Contributor: **George R. Mikhail**

Editor's Computerized Descriptor: Skin

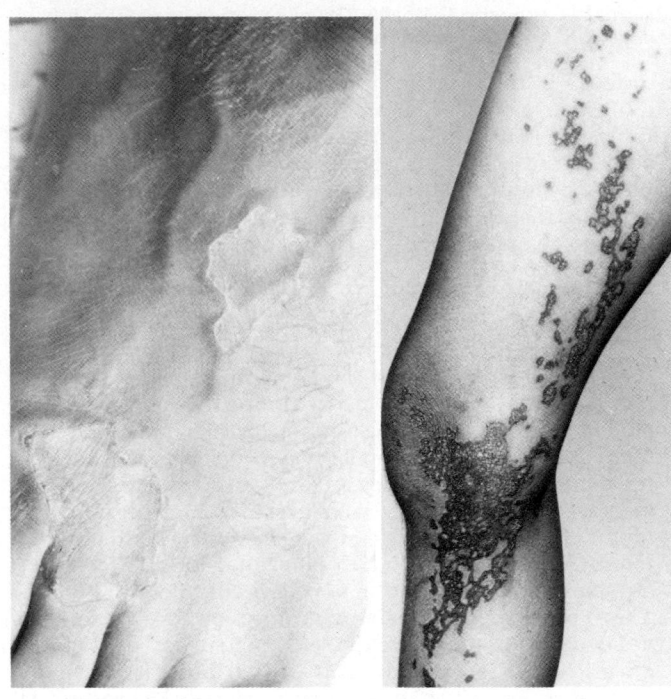

425. Porokeratosis. Note dike-like border of lesion

PORPHYRIA, ACUTE INTERMITTENT

Includes: Porphyrie aiguë intermittente
Akute intermittierende Porphyrie
Porfiria aguda intermitente
Swedish genetic porphyria
Pyrroloporphyria

Excludes: Porphyria, variegate (822)
Coproporphyria (203)

Minimal Diagnostic Criteria: Demonstration of significantly increased porphobilinogen excretion

Clinical Findings: The disease may exist in latent form for a lifetime or may be manifest by attacks of neurologic dysfunction. Four known groups of precipitating causes include: drugs (barbiturates, sulfonamides, griseofulvin, diphenylhydantoin, etc); estrogen and possibly progesterone, oral contraceptives in certain cases; infections; and starvation. Some attacks occur without obvious precipitating factors. In about 10-20% of women with this disease attacks occur in a cyclic pattern, usually beginning about 3 days before the menstrual periods.

The acute attack results from damage in any portion of the nervous system. Signs and symptoms of the acute attack which are attributable to autonomic neuropathy include abdominal pain, constipation (occasionally diarrhea), tachycardia, sweating, labile hypertension, postural hypotension, retinal artery spasm, and vascular spasm in the skin of the limbs. Peripheral neuropathy may be sensory or motor. There may be pain in the back or limbs (more commonly in the legs) which may persist for long periods without motor involvement or may precede motor paralysis. There may be paresthesias, but objective sensory findings are usually absent unless the sensory neuropathy is of long duration. Motor involvement is variable in terms of symmetry, severity and rate of progress of the process. All peripheral nerves, including cranial, are subject to the neuropathy. CNS manifestations include bulbar paralysis, cerebellar and basal ganglion manifestations, hypothalamic dysfunction, seizures, acute and chronic psychoses, hallucinations and coma.

Medullary and phrenic nerve involvement may cause respiratory paralysis, which is the most common cause of death. Hyponatremia, sometimes of severe degree, may result from excessive sodium loss from the GI tract or may be associated with the classic findings of the syndrome of inappropriate release of antidiuretic hormone. Hypomagnesemia, occasionally sufficient to produce tetany, may accompany the hyponatremia.

The 2 most significant psychiatric syndromes associated with this disease are organic brain syndrome (irritability, restlessness, confusion, disorientation, hallucinations) and depression. BSP excretion may be normal or decreased during asymptomatic periods, but it is usually impaired during activity of the disease. Other frequent laboratory findings include hypercholesterolemia (40-50% of patients), increased serum PBI and thyroxin-binding globulin (TBG) and hyper-β-lipoproteinemia. During acute attacks a diabetic glucose tolerance test is often demonstrable.

Complications
I   **Derived:** Chronic pain syndrome (peripheral or abdominal), motor paralysis (including respiratory paralysis), seizures, organic brain syndrome, depression.
II **Associated:** —

Etiology: Autosomal dominant biochemical defect; McK *17600

Pathogenesis: An increase of δ-amino-levulinic acid synthetase,

the first and rate-controlling enzyme of the heme biosynthetic pathway has been demonstrated in the livers of patients with this disease. Recent evidence also indicates a decreased level of porphobilinogen deaminase (uroporphyrinogen I synthetase). However, it is not clear how these findings relate to the acute attacks of neurologic dysfunction.

Related Facts
I   **Sex Ratio:** For the manifest disease it is thought to be M1:F1.5
II   **Risk of Occurrence:** ?
III **Risk of Recurrence for**
     Patient's Sib: When parent is affected, 1 in 2 (50%) for each offspring to be affected; otherwise not increased.
     Patient's Child: 1 in 2
IV   **Age of Detectability:** The disease is usually not manifest clinically and sometimes not evident biochemically before puberty.
V   **Prevalence:** In past series it has been given as about 1 in 66,000 in the British Isles, etc, but in certain areas such as Lapland it is much higher than this. Probably exceeds 1 in 66,000 worldwide.

Treatment
I   **Primary Prevention:** Genetic counseling
II   **Secondary Prevention:** Abdominal pain may be relieved by chlorpromazine. Demerol may be useful if chlorpromazine does not completely alleviate pain. The cause of hyponatremia must be determined before it is treated. If caused by primary salt loss from the GI tract, salt replacement is essential. If associated with the findings of the syndrome of inappropriate release of ADH, water restriction has been successful in raising serum sodium levels. The problem has been complicated by the frequent finding of hypovolemia, which, if sufficiently pronounced in the presence of hyponatremia, is an indication for hypertonic saline administration. Some patients have responded well to a high carbohydrate intake —as high as possible (up to 400 gm/day or more). Since the response is not uniform or predictable, a high carbohydrate intake should be attempted in all patients experiencing an attack of acute intermittent porphyria.

Supportive care during acute attacks is of great importance. When there is peripheral neuropathy, respiratory paralysis, dysphagia or coma, careful attention to nursing care, avoidance of aspiration, assisted respiration, early recognition of pneumonia, and physiotherapy are of great importance. Splints and sandbags should be used for wrist and foot drop.

In those women who experience regularly recurrent attacks in relation to menstrual cycles, administration of oral contraceptive preparations have been useful in preventing attacks. The schedule used is similar to that used for contraception, but the dosage required may or may not be higher. This approach should be used with caution, since experience with it in this type of patient is limited and oral contraceptives sometimes precipitate attacks in women who do not experience the regularly recurring cyclic attacks.

Prophylaxis is of great importance and involves warning patients and members of their families about avoiding the known precipitating factors.
III **Other Therapy:** —

Prognosis: A mortality rate of 24% over a 5-year observation period was previously reported. In the patient with known disease who has been warned about the precipitating factors, the prognosis is now much better than this.

Detection of Carrier: Detected by quantitative urinary porphobilinogen determination.

Special Considerations: —

References:

Tschudy, D. P.: Porphyrin metabolism and the porphyrias. In Duncan, G.G. (ed.): Diseases of Metabolism. Philadelphia:W. B. Saunders Co., 1969, p. 600.

Wetterberg, L.: A Neuropsychiatric and Genetical Investigation of Acute Intermittent Porphyria. Stockholm:Bokforlaget, 1968.

Contributor: **Donald P. Tschudy**

Editor's Computerized Descriptors: Eye, Skin, Sweating, Resp., CV., GI., Nerve

PORPHYRIA, ERYTHROPOIETIC

Includes: Porphyrie érythropoïètique congénitale
Porphyria erythropoetica (Günther)
Porfiria eritropoyética congénita
Erythropoietic uroporphyria
Porphyria, congenital erythropoietic
Günther disease
Hematoporphyria congenita
Erythrodontia
Enamel and dentin staining from erythropoietic porphyria

Excludes: Porphyria, acute intermittent (820)
Enamel and dentin defects from erythroblastosis fetalis (340)
Erythropoietic protoporphyria and the other photosensitizing porphyrias discussed below
Nonporphyric photodermatoses such as xeroderma pigmentosum

Minimal Diagnostic Criteria: Demonstration by quantitative methods of greatly increased uroporphyrin I in the urine and fluorescence of red cells and marrow normoblasts. In addition it is desirable to demonstrate increased erythrocyte uroporphyrin levels by direct analysis. Fluorescence of the teeth should be sought when erythrodontia is not obvious. Clinical pigmentation of teeth may be minimal in some cases but an extract of ground tooth structure with 0.5 N HC1 will normally exhibit brilliant red fluorescence.

Clinical Findings: The two organ systems mainly affected are the skin and bone marrow. The onset of symptoms is usually between birth and age 5 years. Pink or red urine may be the first obvious sign. Photosensitivity may be manifest in infancy and may cause the child to cry when exposed to sunlight. The vesicles or bullae which appear on the exposed portions of the body often ulcerate and heal with scarring. Secondary infections in the skin lesions and repeated episodes of ulceration and scarring lead to severe deformities of the nose, ears, eyes and fingers. Conjunctivitis, keratitis, ectropion, loss of fingernails and phalanges may occur. Hypertrichosis often is seen on the face and limbs, but areas of alopecia may occur on the scalp. Areas of pigmentation and depigmentation develop in exposed areas.

Hemolysis occurs in the majority of patients with this disease, some of whom can increase red cell production sufficiently to prevent the normochromic anemia seen in others. The more active periods of hemolysis are accompanied by increased fecal urobilinogen, normoblastic hyperplasia of the marrow, and circulating normoblasts. Splenomegaly is present in about 3/4 of the patients with this disease. Thrombocytopenia, presumably secondary to hypersplenism, and clinically evident jaundice occur rarely.

Bones are red-brown in color and fluoresce red in UV light.

Teeth vary in color from yellow-brown to red-brown to violet. Teeth fluoresce distinctly red in Wood's (UV) light. Both enamel and dentin contain porphyrins. However, higher concentrations are found in dentin.

Complications

I **Derived:** Varying degrees of deformity of nose, ears, eyes and fingers. Areas of pigmentation and depigmentation occur on exposed areas. Ectropion, loss of nails and terminal phalanges may occur. Areas of alopecia in the scalp and hypertrichosis of face and limbs. Hemolytic anemia and occasionally hypersplenism.

II **Associated:** —

Etiology: Autosomal recessive biochemical defect; McK *26370

Pathogenesis: Deficiency of uroporphyrinogen III cosynthetase which ranges from 1/10 to 1/3 normal levels of activity.

Insufficient production or utilization of uroporphyrinogen isomerase resulting in the production of unusable isomer uroporphyrinogen I. This isomer and its oxidized or decarboxylased products (uroporphyrin I, coproporphyrin I) have a high degree of physical affinity for calcium phosphate and are, therefore, incorporated into the bones and teeth during osteo- and odontogenesis. The pigmentation of the teeth is thus dependent primarily upon the level of circulating abnormal porphyrins at the time of initial calcification. In one reported case, a female with proven erythropoietic porphyria gave birth to a basically unaffected infant whose primary teeth which formed and calcified in utero were pigmented reddish-brown.

Related Facts

I   **Sex Ratio:** M1:F1
II **Risk of Occurrence:** Unknown, rare
III **Risk of Recurrence for**
    Patient's Sib: 1 in 4 (25%) for each offspring to be affected
    Patient's Child: Not increased unless mate is carrier or homozygote
IV **Age of Detectability:** Clinical signs are always evident from as early as birth up to age 5 years at the latest. Probably urinary porphyrin analysis will detect the disease within the first year in most cases.
V   **Prevalence:** Less than 100 authenticated cases were published in the world literature up to 1975.

Treatment

I   **Primary Prevention:** Genetic counseling
II **Secondary Prevention:** Avoidance of light with a wavelength around 4000 A as much as possible. Use of protective clothing, etc. A sunscreen filter chemically induced in skin may be useful (see Fusaro et al for details). Splenectomy for severe hemolytic anemia has sometimes been useful. Porcelain or acrylic crowns may be useful.
III **Other Therapy:** —

Prognosis: Death usually occurs before middle age.

Detection of Carrier: In 2 of 3 families studied, the level of uroporphyrinogen III cosynthetase in hemolysates of parents or children of patients was intermediate between normal and homozygotic levels, whereas in a 3rd family these levels were normal. It remains to be determined how useful this procedure will be in detecting heterozygotes, but the majority probably will be detectable by this complicated method.

Special Considerations: —

References:

Fusaro, R.M. et al: Sunlight protection in normal skin: By absorptive filter chemically induced in stratum corneum. Arch. Dermatol. 93:106, 1966.

Goldberg, A. and Rimington, C.: Diseases of Porphyrin Metabolism. Springfield: Charles C Thomas, 1962.

Schmid, R.: The porphyrias. In Stanbury, J.B. et al (eds.): The Metabolic Basis of Inherited Disease. New York: McGraw-Hill, 1966, p. 813.

Townes, P. L.: Transplacentally acquired erythrodontia. J. Pediatr. 67:600, 1965.

Tschudy, D. P.: Porphyrin metabolism and the porphyrias. In Duncan, G.G. (ed.): Diseases of Metabolism. Philadelphia: W. B. Saunders Co., 1969, p. 600.

Contributors: **Donald P. Tschudy**
John N. Trodahl

Editor's Computerized Descriptors: Eye, Ear, Teeth, Nose, Skin, Hair, Nails, Skel., Spleen, GU.

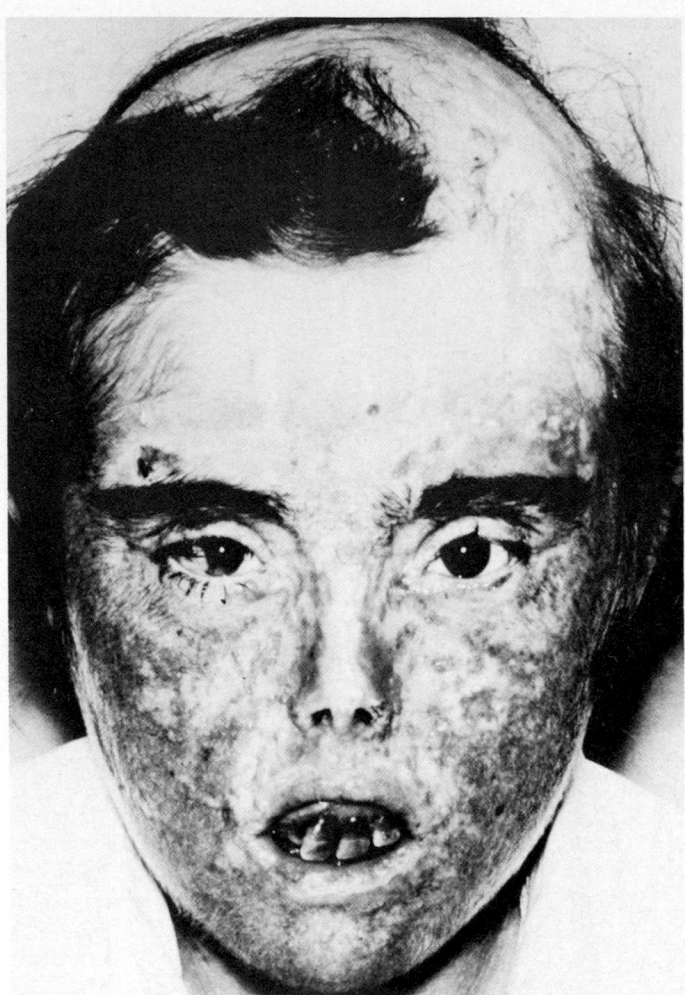

426. Note severe scarring from photosensitivity and tooth pigmentation

PORPHYRIA, VARIEGATE

Includes: Porfiria variegada
Porphyria variegata
Mixed porphyria
Protocoproporphyria
South African genetic porphyria

Excludes: Porphyria, acute intermittent (820)
Coproporphyria (203)

Minimal Diagnostic Criteria: Increased urinary excretion of porphobilinogen during an acute attack. Increased fecal protoporphyrin with normal red cell protoporphyrin.

Clinical Findings: This disease may present either cutaneous manifestations of photosensitivity or neurologic aspects identical to those described for acute intermittent porphyria or both.†

The skin lesions may be vesicles, bullae or erosions, with variable degrees of scarring and pigmentation of the skin exposed to sunlight. There may be increased skin fragility. Hypertrichosis on the face or chronic thickening of skin may occur with diffuse yellowish papules. Azotemia and electrolyte abnormalities are frequent and often result from the GI manifestations of the acute attack.

Complications
I   **Derived:** Chronic skin lesions, chronic pain syndrome (peripheral or abdominal), motor paralysis (including respiratory paralysis), seizures, organic brain syndrome, depression.
II **Associated:** —

Etiology: Autosomal dominant biochemical defect; McK *17620

Pathogenesis: Increased levels of hepatic δ-aminolevulinic acid synthetase have been demonstrated, but the relationship of this finding to the attacks of neurologic dysfunction is unknown.

Related Facts
I   **Sex Ratio:** M1:F1.3 in one series of 66 cases
II   **Risk of Occurrence:** ?
III **Risk of Recurrence for**
     Patient's Sib: If parent is affected, 1 in 2 (50%) for each offspring to be affected; otherwise not increased.
     Patient's Child: 1 in 2
IV   **Age of Detectability:** Usually after puberty
V   **Prevalence:** In the total white population of South Africa it has been estimated as 1 in 330. Its incidence is probably somewhat less than 1 in 66,000 in most parts of the world.

Treatment
I   **Primary Prevention:** Genetic counseling
II   **Secondary Prevention:** Avoidance of sunlight. (For neurologic manifestations see †)
III **Other Therapy:** —

Prognosis: ?

Detection of Carrier: Demonstration of increased fecal protoporphyrin in members of family with the known disease.

†Special Considerations: See Acute Intermittent Porphyria for more detailed Clinical Findings and for Treatment II Secondary Prevention re: neurologic manifestations.

References:
Eales, L.: Porphyria as seen in Cape Town: A survey of 250 patients and some recent studies. S. Afr. J. Lab. Clin. Med. 9:151, 1963.
Waldenstrom, J. and Haeger-Aronsen, B.: The porphyrias: A genetic problem. Prog. Med. Genet. 5:58, 1967.

Contributor: Donald P. Tschudy

Editor's Computerized Descriptors: Eye, Skin, Sweating, Hair, Muscle, CV., GI., Nerve

PRADER-WILLI SYNDROME

Includes: Syndrome de Prader-Willi
Síndrome de Prader-Willi
Hypotonia, hypomentia, hypogonadism and obesity
HHHO
Hypogenital dystrophy with diabetic tendency
Prader-Labhart-Willi syndrome

Excludes: Other forms of infantile hypotonia
Laurence-Moon-Biedl syndrome (578)
Adiposogenital dystrophy
Congenital myopathies
Congenital spinal muscular atrophies
Early-onset myotonic dystrophy
Atonic diplegia and other severe supranuclear hypotonias
Syndrome of hypotonia, obesity, mental deficiency, facial, oral, ocular, and limb anomalies (Cohen)
Alström syndrome (41)

Minimal Diagnostic Criteria: 1st phase: Severe muscular atonia, hypo- to areflexia, feeding difficulties, and in males micropenis, hypoplastic scrotum and cryptorchidism. Diagnosis of 1st phase of PW is more difficult in girls, although small labia majora and absent labia minora in combination with the above symptoms may suggest PW.

2nd phase: Polyphagia, delayed psychomotor development, mental subnormality, friendly childish behavior with spells of stubbornness and occasional temper tantrums, muscular hypotonia, obesity, short stature, hypogonadism.

Clinical Findings: A decrease of fetal movements in the last months of pregnancy is noticed at times. Breech deliveries occur in 10-40% of the cases. The mean birthweight is several hundred grams less than the average birthweight of term babies. Mean duration of gestation is within the normal range. Some Prader-Willi Syndrome (PW) babies are born with dislocated hips or talipes valgoplanus.

The clinical course can be divided into 2 phases. The 1st phase is characterized by severe hypotonia or even atonia. There is evidence of facial diplegia with a flat face and a triangular mouth (tented upper lip). Young infants with PW are almost motionless; Moro response, withdrawal reflex and tendon reflexes are decreased or absent. Sucking and swallowing reflexes are very poorly developed and usually necessitate feeding by gavage, dropper, spoon or premature nipple for weeks or even months. There is a tendency to hypothermia in early infancy. Penis and scrotum are hypoplastic, the latter often consists of no more than an area of corrugated skin in the anterior perineum. Testes are not descended. The external genitalia of the female PW show small labia majora and practically nonexistent labia minora.

After some weeks or more often months, the PW infants enter the 2nd phase. They become more lively and responsive, and feeding difficulties subside, in fact they become hungry and cry for food. Some PW children have a constant painful hunger feeling which forces them to seek incessantly for food. They pilfer the refrigerator and are capable of eating the food of the house pets or even eat out of the garbage can. Other PW patients may not seek food, but are unable to recognize satiety and eat as long as food is in sight. PW children, as a consequence of their eating habits, become extremely obese. The obesity involves particularly the trunk and proximal limbs. In some children forearms and lower legs become obese as well, but hands and feet are always spared and remain disproportionately small (acromicria). Longitudinal growth is impaired. Height is always below the 50th percentile. The prepubertal growth spurt does not occur, thus growth retardation becomes even more conspicuous at that age.

Psychomotor development is delayed. Prader-Willi children sit and walk late. Their intellectual development is far below that of their normal sibs; psychometric tests yield IQs between 20 and 90. Their speech development is particularly retarded, their vocabulary is limited, and articulation is poor, slurred, and barely understandable. They are happy and content children and lack drive and initiative. They show a peculiar deficiency in the control of their emotions. Phases of exuberant joy and friendliness alternate with reactions of uncontrollable negativism and even destructiveness. Adult PW patients with lesser degrees of mental subnormality are able to perform menial tasks under sheltered conditions. The muscular hypotonia has a tendency to become less pronounced with increasing age.

Other manifestations are microdontia, dental caries, enamel defects (notably in the 1st dentition), strabismus, high-arched palate, dry oral mucosa, mesobrachyphalangy, simian creases. Poorly modeled ears and narrow external ear canals are occasionally encountered. Scoliosis is not infrequent.

Complications
I **Derived:** Diabetes mellitus, adult type, without tendency to ketosis appears often during 2nd decade.

Gastric perforations as a consequence of overeating. Early development of arteriosclerosis has been described in a few cases.†

II **Associated:** —

Etiology: ? The overwhelming majority of the cases are sporadic. Two instances of PW in sibs and 1 instance of PW in 1st cousins have been reported. Moreover PW in a pair of monozygotic twins has been described and parental consanguinity was observed twice. Thus, a genetic component seems to be present: autosomal recessive as well as multifactorial inheritance has been considered, yet an autosomal dominant mutation has not been excluded.

Pathogenesis: A hypothalamic dysfunction has been assumed, yet postmortem examinations of the diencephalon have so far not revealed any pathologic alterations. A defect in the fat metabolism in association with an altered action of insulin has been conjectured as well.

Related Facts
I **Sex Ratio:** Reports on PW include twice as many males as females. However, this sex difference is probably spurious because PW (sexual hypoplasia) is more easily recognized in the male than in the female, notably during the early phase of the condition.

II **Risk of Occurrence:** ?

III **Risk of Recurrence for**
Patient's Sib: Negligible
Patient's Child: ? No PW is known to have reproduced yet

IV **Age of Detectability:** Diagnosis can be suspected in male infants at birth or shortly thereafter. Accurate diagnosis of PW in females is possible in the 2nd phase only.

V **Prevalence:** ? But quite frequent

Treatment
I **Primary Prevention:** —

II **Secondary Prevention:** Since excessive obesity is indeed a life-threatening manifestation of PW, prevention of obesity or treatment of obesity is mandatory by:

1. Drugs which have an appetite decreasing effect such as Dexedrine sulfate (PW children show at times a strong reaction to Dexedrine sulfate; even small doses make them extremely sleepy. Thus Dexedrine sulfate should be given in very small doses.) It has been shown to be effective only in some cases. Prolonged Dexedrine sulfate medication may cause further growth retardation.

2. Restriction of caloric intake has been advocated by some investigators, yet many PW patients may vehemently resist such restrictions.

3. Surgical bypass of small intestine leads to considerable weight loss, yet the procedure is not without complications such as dehydration, electrolyte imbalance, protein malnutrition and liver damage.

4. Gastric bypass is preferable, since it does not involve the above complications and yields excellent results in some PW patients.

5. Jaw wiring may be considered in older children and adults, if overeating cannot be otherwise controlled. It allows only intake of a liquid diet supplemented by vitamins.

III **Other Therapy:** ?

Prognosis: Life expectancy is shortened. Sudden death due to respiratory insufficiency may occur. Early development of diabetic glomerulosclerosis has been reported as well.

Detection of Carrier: ?

†**Special Considerations:** Obesity may in rare cases reach such proportions that manifestations of the Pickwickian syndrome, with life-threatening cardiorespiratory difficulties and hypercapnia may develop.

Normal laboratory examinations include serum electrolytes, urinalysis and blood morphology. Endocrinologic studies of the pituitary-adrenal and pituitary-thyroid axis show no consistent abnormalities.

Studies of the hypothalamic-pituitary-gonadal axis yield variable results. Most male and female PW patients show evidence of congenital hypogonadotropic hypogonadism with increased or normal, rarely decreased, urinary gonadotropins and no or subnormal reponses to Clomiphene. Male PW patients are infertile. The penis is small-to-minute; cryptorchidism is frequent. In some instances the gubernaculum is too short to permit orchidopexy. Anorchia has been reported in rare instances and in some cases the testicles are descended but are very small. The development of secondary sex characteristics is delayed and incomplete. The voice remains high-pitched. Histology of the testes shows immature seminiferous tubules with decreased or even absent spermatogenesis. Leydig cells are present in normal or increased amounts. Plasma testosterone levels are below the normal range and remain subnormal after Clomiphene administration. There are, however, exceptional cases where prolonged Clomiphene treatment led to normal plasma testosterone levels and normal spermatogenesis.

Female PW patients show either primary amenorrhea, or delayed menarche with subsequent irregular anovulatory cycles. Estrogenization of the vaginal mucosa varies between moderately decreased and normal. Secondary sex characteristics are few or-in some instances-normal.

ECG studies are normal in some cases, while in other cases nonspecific abnormalities are found.

Pneumoencephalography is normal in most instances. Light microscopic examination of muscle shows normal findings as well, while aberrations comparable to those seen in disuse atrophy are found by electron microscopy. Various chromosomal aberrations have been described in less than 10% of the cases, for example, XYY, mosaicism, elongation of the Y chromosome and D-D interchange heterozygosity. They have no causal significance for the condition.

References:
Bistrian, B.R. et al: Metabolic aspects of a protein sparing modified fast in the dietary management of Prader-Willi obesity. N. Engl. J. Med. 296:774, 1977.
Cohen, M.M. et al: A new syndrome with hypotonia, obesity, mental deficiency, and facial, oral, ocular, and limb anomalies. J. Pediatr. 83:280, 1973.
Hall, B.D. and Smith, D.W.: Prader-Willi syndrome. J. Pediatr.

81:286, 1972.

Hamilton, C.R. et al: Hypogonadotropinism in Prader-Willi syndrome. Am. J. Med. 52:322, 1972.

Katcher, M.L. et al: Absence of spermatogonia in the Prader-Willi syndrome. Eur. J. Pediatr. 24:257, 1977.

Wannarachue, N. et al: Hypogonadism in Prader-Willi syndrome. Am. J. Ment. Defic. 79:592, 1975.

Zellweger, H. and Schneider, H.J.: Syndrome of hypotonia-hypomentia-hypogonadism-obesity (HHHO) or Prader-Willi syndrome. Am. J. Dis. Child. 115:588, 1968.

Contributor: **Hans Zellweger**

Editor's Computerized Descriptors: Eye, Ear, Face, Oral, Teeth, Speech, Dermatoglyphic, Skel., Muscle, GI., GU., Nerve

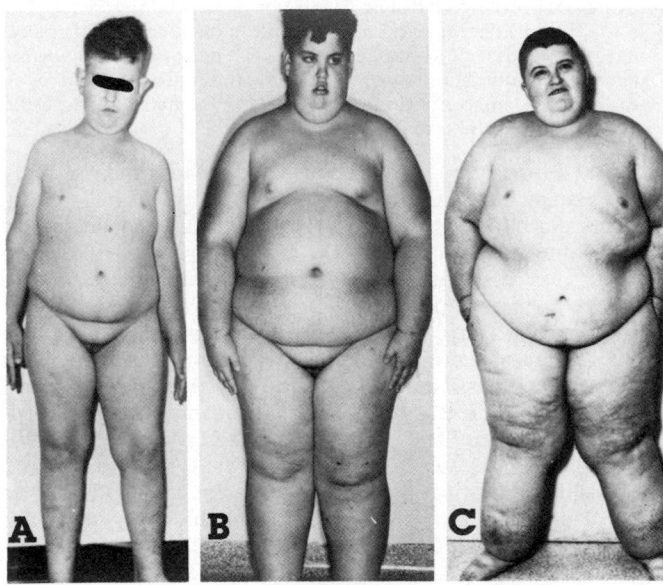

427. Obesity in Prader-Willi: A) mild; B) moderate; C) marked

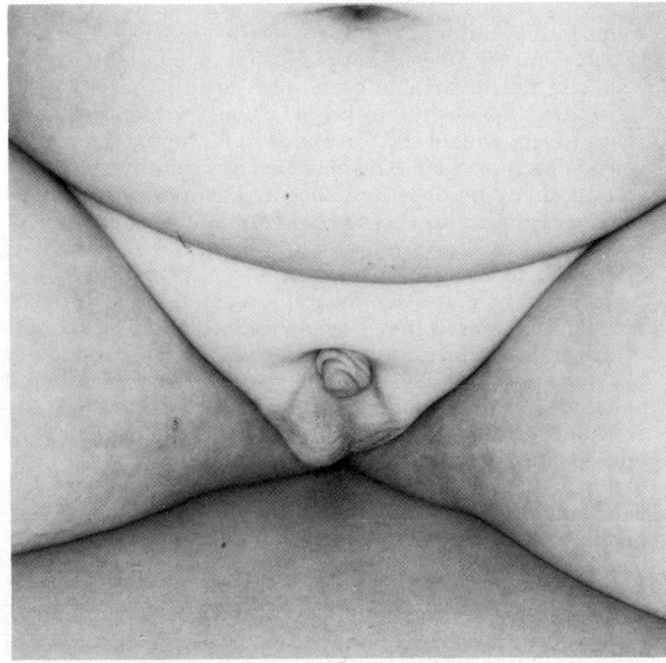

428. Genital hypoplasia in male

PROBOSCIS LATERALIS

Includes: Nez latérale
Proboscis lateral
Arrhinencephalia unilateralis
Lateral nasal proboscis

Excludes: Nose and nasal septum defects (722)
Nose, bifid (724)

Minimal Diagnostic Criteria: Presence of the soft tissue proboscis suspended from the medial orbital roof

Clinical Findings: The patient is born with a soft, trunk-like process which is suspended from the medial portion of the orbital roof. Distally, the process is club-shaped and contains the opening of a canal which traverses the entire proboscis and ends proximally in a cul-de-sac. There is usually an associated deficiency of the ipsilateral nasal wall that varies from total absence to a small tissue defect; however, the proboscis may occur without other anomalies. Histologically the proboscis is similar to the lateral nasal wall except that the reported cases have not contained bone. Proximally, the central canal is lined by columnar epithelium; the distal portion of the canal may be lined by stratified squamous epithelium. The connective tissue stroma contains muscle fibers and cartilaginous elements. Bilateral nasal probosci have been reported on one occasion.

Complications
I **Derived:** There is usually some deficiency of the ipsilateral lateral nasal wall.
II **Associated:** Ophthalmic - 44% of cases - including: unilateral anophthalmia, iris coloboma, upper or lower lid cleft, and choroidal cleft. Facial bone anomalies other than nasal bones - 38% of cases. Brain and cranial vault anomalies - 19% of cases.

Etiology: ?

Pathogenesis: Structurally the proboscis is apparently derived from the lateral nasal process, which is derived from the frontonasal process. The abnormal development of the lateral nasal process may be further reflected by total or partial absence of the lateral nasal wall.

Related Facts
I **Sex Ratio:** M1:F1
II **Risk of Occurrence:** Rare, less than 1 in 100,000 live births
III **Risk of Recurrence for**
  Patient's Sib: No reported increased risk
  Patient's Child: No reported increased risk
IV **Age of Detectability:** At birth by gross appearance
V **Prevalence:** Less than 1 in 100,000 - no known geographic or ethnic prevalence

Treatment
I **Primary Prevention:** —
II **Secondary Prevention:** If there is no associated deficiency of the nasal wall, the proboscis may be excised. The proboscis should be utilized in the plastic reconstruction of the nose if there is a tissue deficiency. Closure of the defect is usually best performed as a 2-stage procedure, utilizing the proboscis as a pedicle flap.†
III **Other Therapy:** —

Prognosis: Normal life span unless there are associated severe cerebral or cranial vault anomalies.

Detection of Carrier: —

†**Special Considerations:** It is important that the proboscis be retained if there is a nasal defect, since the proboscis contains the ideal tissue for the nasal reconstruction. Biber has suggested

delaying the repairs until the child reaches adolescence in order to achieve a better definitive reconstruction; however, this presents the problems of a prolonged cosmetic defect and probably psychologic problems for the patient.

References:
Biber, J.J.: Proboscis lateralis: Rare malformation of nose; its genesis and treatment. J. Laryngol. Otol. 63:734, 1949.
Rosen, Z. and Gitlin, G.: Bilateral nasal proboscis associated with unilateral anophthalmia, unilateral diffuse pigmentation of the conjunctiva, and anomalies of the skull and brain. Arch. Otolaryngol. 70:545, 1959.

Contributor: **Raymond O. Smith, Jr.**

_____

Editor's Computerized Descriptors: Eye, Nasoph., Skel., Nerve

PROGERIA

Includes: Progerie
Hutchinson-Gilford syndrome
Progeronanism
Senile nanism

Excludes: Werner syndrome (998)
Cockayne syndrome (189)
Oculo-mandibulo-facial syndrome (738)
Seckel syndrome (881)
Acrogeria
Various "gerodermata"
Cutis laxa (233)
Leprechaunism (587)

Minimal Diagnostic Criteria: Onset of growth failure in 1st year of life, weight decreased for height, permanent failure of sexual maturation, loss of "all" subcutaneous fat, delayed and abnormal dentition, craniofacial disproportion with small head but even smaller face, micrognathia, alopecia, prominent eyes and scalp veins, normal intelligence.

Clinical Findings: At birth affected infants may already have suspicious findings ("sclerodermatous skin," midfacial cyanosis, sculptured nose) but are usually considered to be normal infants. During the 2nd half-year of life a profound and progressive retardation in weight gain and growth becomes apparent. Since the facial bones share in this growth failure, the cranium remains relatively large and the eyes prominent. The nose stays small, perhaps beaked, with nasal cartilage contours visible under the thin skin. The mandible grows slowly, resulting in true micrognathia. At about the same time the scalp hair becomes sparse and the scalp veins prominent. Eyebrows and eyelashes may disappear during the 1st and 2nd year of life. The result is total alopecia from the early years on, apart from a few downy small white or blonde hairs which persist throughout life. The net effect is to produce what has been called a "plucked-bird appearance." Concurrent with the failure to gain and grow is the gradual disappearance of all subcutaneous fat except in the suprapubic area. This absence of subcutaneous fat, along with failure of long bones to grow in girth as well as in length, results in spindly limbs with prominent joints, especially the knees. Stiffness of the joints and resultant limitation of motion develop. This and the invariable coxa valga are the basis for the wide-based "horse-riding stance" usually evident by 2 or 3 years of age which adds to the striking appearance. The voice is high-pitched. The clavicles are usually short and thin and may become radiolucent. The anterior fontanel remains patent and there are occasional Wormian bones. The short clavicles are associated with narrow shoulders and pyriform thorax. Abnormal nails are apparent by 2 or 3 years of age. These are dystrophic, small and short. The terminal phalanges may become radiolucent. The skin develops an aged appearance, being thin, shiny, taut and dry in some areas and dry, dull and wrinkled in others. Small blotchy brownish pigmentations tend to develop with increasing age. There is a marked delay in dentition, with crowded maloccluded teeth which may be rotated, displaced or overlapping. Intelligence is normal or above average. There are no ocular abnormalities as in oculomandibulofacial syndrome. Atherosclerosis may result in early death by myocardial infarction or cerebral vascular accident.

There are no consistent abnormalities of serum lipids. No endocrine or metabolic abnormality has been documented other than an increase in metabolic rate without hyperthyroidism. Growth hormone responses are normal but insulin tolerance may be increased. Collagen fiber bundles are disorganized, thickened and "hyalinized." The extracted collagen has decreased solubility, abnormal thermal shrinkage and decreased uptake of oxygen, proline, and glucose. Chromosomal studies have been normal. Deficient DNA repair after cobalt 60 gamma radiation, altered HL-A antigens and increased levels of heat-labile enzymes have been demonstrated in cultured skin fibroblasts. Decreased growth capacity of these fibroblasts has been universally noted.

Complications
I **Derived:** Myocardial infarcts, congestive heart failure; less commonly cerebrovascular occlusions secondary to atherosclerosis; limitation of motion of large and small joints; cephalohematoma.
II **Associated:** —

Etiology: ? 2 out of 8 sibs whose parents were 1st cousins were affected: There are insufficient cases in all other sibships to document autosomal recessive inheritance. Significant increase in paternal age in many families with cases of progeria suggests possibility of autosomal dominant mutation. Multifactorial inheritance cannot be excluded.

Pathogenesis: ?

Related Facts
I **Sex Ratio:** M2:F1
II **Risk of Occurrence:** In U.S. about 1 in 250,000 live births; cases reported from all continents except Australia; no documented cases reported in Orientals except for 1 case born to a Chinese mother and a Caucasian father; several cases have been reported in Blacks.
III **Risk of Recurrence for**
 Patient's Sib: ?
 Patient's Child: ? Since reproduction has not been reported
IV **Age of Detectability:** Latter part of 1st year of life, possibly at birth if "sclerodermatous" skin, glyphic nose, midfacial cyanosis present.
V **Prevalence:** 73 patients since 1886 either reported or known to the contributor. Incidence in various population or ethnic groups not calculable, but in the U.S. there should be about 10-15 cases at any given time.

Treatment
I **Primary Prevention:** —
II **Secondary Prevention:** —
III **Other Therapy:** Protection against physical trauma, wig or hat, possible psycho- and physiotherapy, therapy for congestive heart failure.

Prognosis: General health usually good with few infections. Physical handicaps due to size are usual, due to joint problems less likely. Psychologic problems related to appearance and self-image are common. Of 18 patients whose age of nontraumatic death is known, death ranged from 7-27 1/2 years with a median age of 12 years and a mean of 13.4 years.

Detection of Carrier: —

Special Considerations: —

References:
DeBusk, F.L.: The Hutchinson-Gilford progeria syndrome. J. Pediatr. 80:697, 1972.
Goldstein, S. and Moerman, E.: Heat-labile enzymes in skin fibroblasts from subjects with progeria. N. Engl. J. Med. 292:1305, 1975.

Contributor: **Franklin DeBusk**

Editor's Computerized Descriptors: Eye, Face, Teeth, Nose, Speech, Skin, Hair, Nails, Skel., Resp., CV., GU., Nerve

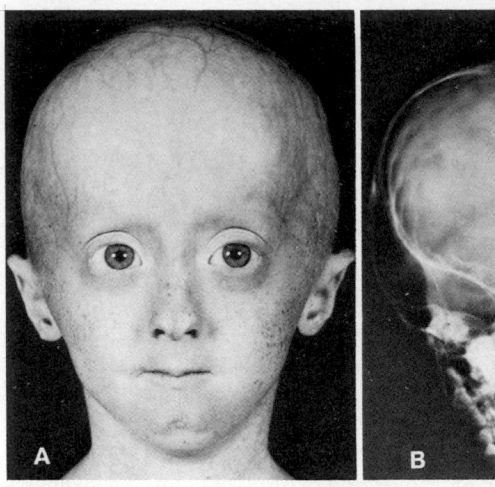

429. A) Note hairlessness and prominent venous pattern; B) open fontanels and small facial bones relative to calvarium

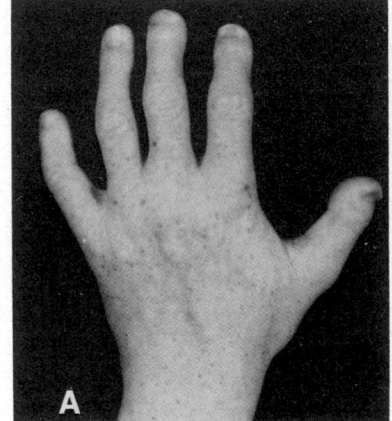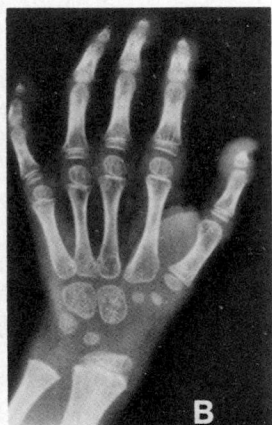

430. A) inability to extend fingers fully, somewhat knobby interphalangeal joints; stubby terminal phalanges of several digits; B) retarded bone age and hypoplastic terminal phalanges

PROPIONIC ACIDEMIA

Includes: Hyperglycinémie
Ketotische Form der Hyperglyzinämie
Hiperglicinemia cetónica
Hyperglycinemia, ketotic
Glycinosis

Excludes: Glycinuria without hyperglycinemia
Glucoglycinuria (418)
Hyperglycinemia, nonketotic (492)
Methylmalonic acidemia (658)

Minimal Diagnostic Criteria: Increased concentrations of glycine in the blood and recurrent episodes of ketoacidosis, elevated concentration of propionate in serum. Definitive diagnosis requires the determination that propionyl CoA carboxylase activity is deficient.

Clinical Findings: Onset early in life of vomiting, acidosis and ketonuria. Episodes of ketoacidosis are recurrent; they lead to coma and often to death in infancy. Mental retardation and variable neurologic findings are observed in those surviving early infancy. Neutropenia and thrombocytopenia occur as do frequent infections and transient purpura. Osteoporosis may be followed by pathologic fractures.

Plasma concentrations of glycine are usually greater than 5 mg/100 ml, tend to approximate 10 mg/100 ml, and may be as high as 70 mg/100 ml. Normal mean concentrations approximate 1 mg/100 ml. Mean urinary excretion of glycine, even in a patient less than 3 years of age, was over 400 mg/100 ml or 5.5 mg of glycine/mg creatinine. Glycine excretion in controls was 0.2 mg/100 ml of creatinine. Glycine concentration in the cerebrospinal fluid is also elevated. Concentrations of propionic acid in the blood are high. Even remission levels approximate 10-20 mM. In relapse they may be 100 times that. These patients have sizeable amounts of methylcitrate and hydroxypropionate in the urine, methylcitrate in concentration of 2-6 μM/mg creatinine.

Complications
I   **Derived:** Mental retardation and early death
II **Associated:** —

Etiology: Autosomal recessive deficiency of propionyl CoA carboxylase. McK *23200

Pathogenesis: Accumulation of methylcitrate, hydroxypropionate or tiglate may relate to the development of clinical disease.

Related Facts
I   **Sex Ratio:** M1:F1
II **Risk of Occurrence:** ?
III **Risk of Recurrence for**
    Patient's Sib: Probably 1 in 4 (25%) for each offspring to be affected
    Patient's Child: Patients die before reproductive age.
IV **Age of Detectability:** Birth to 7 days. Method: quantitative assay of the plasma concentration of glycine or propionate, urinary methylcitrate.
V   **Prevalence:** ?

Treatment
I   **Primary Prevention:** Genetic counseling
II **Secondary Prevention:** These patients are abnormally sensitive to leucine, isoleucine, threonine, valine and methionine. Two patients have been successfully treated with a low-protein diet (0.5 g/kg). Whether or not supplementation with nontoxic amino acids is helpful has not been determined. Avoidance of exposure to, and prompt treatment of, infection.
III **Other Therapy:** Deletion of protein-containing foods and the use of electrolyte-containing solutions in the presence of ketosis.

Prognosis: All but 4 patients have died very early in life. The exceptions are still quite young.

Detection of Carrier: ? Reliable methods are not available.

Special Considerations: —

References:

Ando, T. et al: Propionic acidemia in patients with ketotic hyperglycinemia. J. Pediatr. 78:827, 1971.

Ando, T. et al: The oxidation of glycine and propionic acid in propionic acidemia with ketotic hyperglycinemia. Pediatr. Res. 6:576, 1972.

Ando, T. et al: Isolation and identification of methylcitrate, a major metabolic product of propionate in patients with propionic acidemia. J. Biol. Chem. 247:2200, 1972.

Ando, T. et al: 3-Hydroxypropionate: Significance of β-oxidation of propionate in patients with propionic acidemia and methylmalonic acidemia. Proc. Natl. Acad. Sci. USA 69:2807, 1972.

Ando, T. and Nyhan, W.L.: Propionic acidemia and the ketotic hyperglycinemia syndrome. In Nyhan, W.L. (ed.): Heritable Disorders of Amino Acid Metabolism. New York:J. Wiley & Sons, 1974.

Childs, B. et al: Idiopathic hyperglycinemia and hyperglycinuria: A new disorder of amino acid metabolism. Pediatrics 27:522, 1961.

Hsia, Y.E. et al: Defective propionate carboxylation in ketotic hyperglycinaemia. Lancet 1:757, 1969.

Nyhan, W.L. et al: Tiglicaciduria in propionic acidemia. Biochem. J. 126:1035, 1972.

Rasmussen, K. et al: Excretion of tiglylglycine in propionic acidemia. J. Pediatr. 81:970, 1972.

Rasmussen, K. et al: Excretion of propionylglycine in propionic acidaemia. Clin. Sci. 42:665, 1972.

Wadlington, W.B. et al: Hyperglycinemia and propionyl CoA carboxylase deficiency and episodic severe illness without consistent ketosis. J. Pediatr. 86:707, 1975.

Contributor: **William L. Nyhan**

Editor's Computerized Descriptors: Skel., GI., Nerve

PRURITUS, HEREDITARY LOCALIZED

Includes: Prurit héréditaire localisé
Hereditärer lokalisierter Pruritus
Prurito localizado hereditario

Excludes: —

Minimal Diagnostic Criteria: A localized, familial pruritus unassociated with other causes and without significant skin changes.

Clinical Findings: Hereditary localized area of pruritus unassociated with any significant skin changes. In the 2 families reported to date, it occurred on the back. The age of onset is usually in the 3rd decade but ranges from 4 to 41 years.

Complications
I   **Derived:** —
II **Associated:** —

Etiology: Autosomal dominant or possibly X-linked dominant; McK *17710

Pathogenesis: ?

Related Facts
I   **Sex Ratio:** In the 1st family reported, there were 7 females and 1 male affected, and 1 male carrier without symptoms. This male had 5 affected daughters and 2 unaffected sons
II **Risk of Occurrence:** ?
III **Risk of Recurrence for**
    Patient's Sib: If autosomal dominant or X-linked dominant, see Table I AD or X-linked D, respectively.
    Patient's Child: If autosomal dominant or X-linked dominant, see Table I AD or X-linked D, respectively.
IV **Age of Detectability:** Generally in the 2nd-3rd decade
V   **Prevalence:** ?

Treatment
I   **Primary Prevention:** Genetic counseling
II **Secondary Prevention:** —
III **Other Therapy:** —

Prognosis: Normal life span

Detection of Carrier: —

Special Considerations: —

References:
Comings, D.E. and Comings, S.N.: Hereditary localized pruritus. Arch. Dermatol. 92:236, 1965.

Contributor: **David E. Comings**

Editor's Computerized Descriptor: Skin

PSEUDOACHONDROPLASTIC DYSPLASIA

Includes: Dysplasie pseudo-achondroplastique
Pseudoachondroplasie
Displasia pseudoacondroplástica
Pseudoachondroplastic spondyloepiphyseal dysplasia

Excludes: Achondroplasia (10)
Spondyloepiphyseal dysplasia congenita (897)
Spondyloepiphyseal dysplasia tarda (898)
Epiphyseal dysplasia, multiple (358)
Hypochondroplasia (510)

Minimal Diagnostic Criteria: Normal skull, disproportionate short stature with long trunk and short limbs, typical vertebral and epiphyseal dysplasia during growth.

Clinical Findings: Disproportionate dwarfism with relatively long trunk, short arms and legs, and normal skull and facies; normal appearing at birth (xrays taken at birth have been normal); growth retardation and disproportion usually present by 2 years of age; limbs generally shortened particularly hands and feet; joint laxity except at elbows; knees may be bowed or knocked; trunk relatively long, but absolutely normal or mildly shortened with marked lumbar lordosis and mild-to-moderate scoliosis in some individuals; moderate-to-severe short stature (91.5-137.2 cm adult height). Radiographs in childhood show moderate flattening of the vertebral bodies, irregularity and tongue-like projections of central portion of vertebral body; during adolescence markedly irregular calcification of vertebrae occurs with partial restoration of normal vertebral form by adulthood. Generalized epiphyseal dysplasia particularly in weight bearing joints; capital femoral epiphyses, knees, wrists, and short tubular bones with small, irregular, flat epiphyses, as well as mildly irregular metaphyses during childhood leading to flattening and irregularity of joint when epiphyses fuse.

Complications
I   **Derived:** Arthritis, particularly hip and knee; scoliosis; ulnar deviation of hand, and joint laxity making functional fixation of joints difficult; slow developmental landmarks or waddling gait; social and psychologic adjustments to short stature.
II **Associated:** Cord compression has been described.

Etiology: Almost all cases have autosomal dominant inheritance or represent new dominant mutations. 100% penetrance occurs. Cases previously reported as autosomal recessive inheritance represented parental gonadal mosaicism.

Pathogenesis: ? Cartilage histology shows characteristic pattern of chondrocyte inclusion bodies.

Related Facts
I   **Sex Ratio:** M1:F1
II **Risk of Occurrence:** Rare
III **Risk of Recurrence for**
    Patient's Sib: If parent is affected, 1 in 2 (50%) for each offspring to be affected; otherwise not increased.
    Patient's Child: 1 in 2
IV **Age of Detectability:** Usually 2-4 years of age. If previously affected child, parents may suspect diagnosis at about one year because of short fingers, short arms or inability to straighten elbow completely.
V   **Prevalence:** Rare

Treatment
I   **Primary Prevention:** Genetic counseling
II **Secondary Prevention:** Avoid vigorous athletics since trauma to joints seems to hasten arthritis.

III Other Therapy: Symptomatic orthopedics for arthritis and bowing

Prognosis: Normal for life span and intelligence; fairly severe degenerative arthritis; many social, emotional and vocational problems.

Detection of Carrier: —

Special Considerations: —

References:

Hall, J.G.: Pseudoachondroplasia. In Bergsma, D. (ed.): Disorders of Connective Tissue. Birth Defects: Orig. Art. Ser., vol. XI, no. 6. Miami: Symposia Specialists for The National Foundation-March of Dimes, 1975, p. 187.

Maroteaux, P. and Lamy, M.: Les formes pseudo-achondroplastiques des dysplasias spondylo-epiphysaires. Presse Med. 67:383, 1959.

Spranger, J.W. et al: Bone Dysplasias. Philadelphia:W.B. Saunders, 1974, p. 124.

Contributor: **Judith G. Hall**

Editor's Computerized Descriptor: Skel.

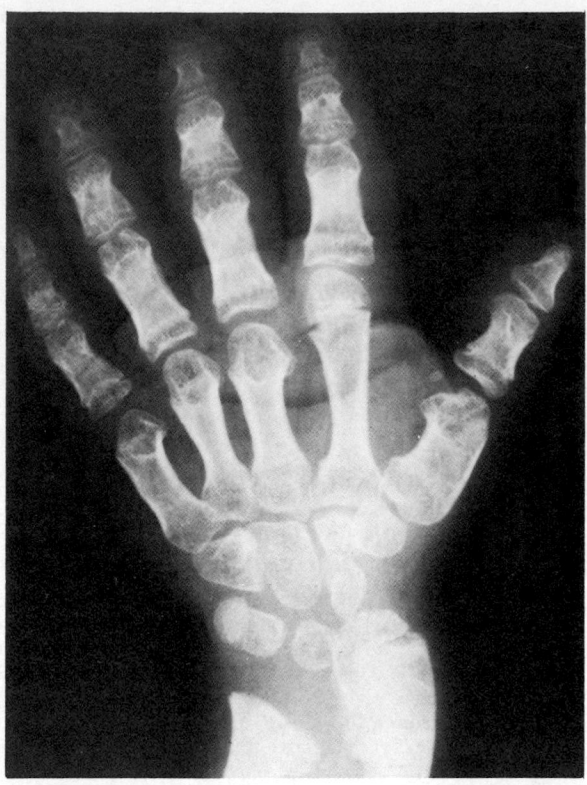

432. Abnormality in epiphyseal formation of the distal ulna results in relative overgrowth of the radius and ulnar deviation of the hand

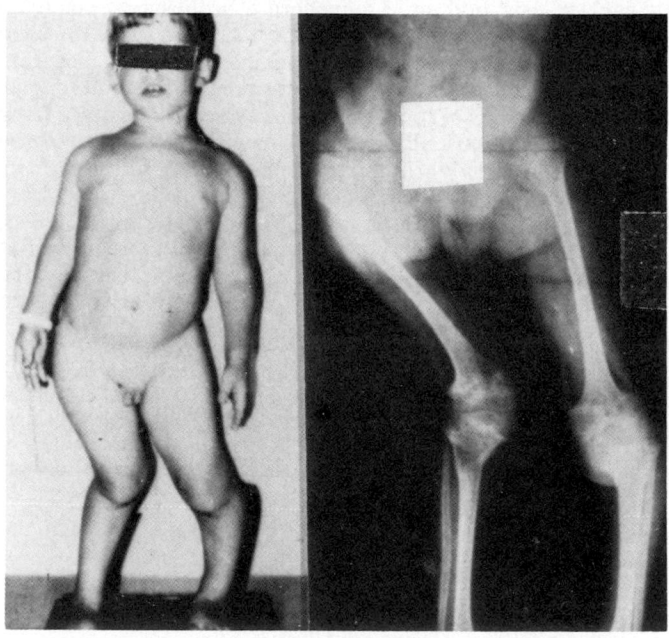

431. Note "windswept" appearance of legs with knock-knee on the right and bowleg on the left

PSEUDOHYPOALDOSTERONISM

Includes: Pseudohypoaldostéronisme
Pseudohypoaldosteronismus
Pseudohipoaldosteronismo
Aldosterone unresponsiveness

Excludes: Adrenal hypoplasia, congenital (24)
Adrenal hypoaldosteronism of infancy, transient (23)
Isolated hypoaldosteronism due to adrenal 18-hydroxysteroid dehydrogenase deficiency
Isolated hypoaldosteronism due to adrenal 18-hydroxylase deficiency
Steroid 21-hydroxylase deficiency (908)
Steroid 3β-hydroxysteroid dehydrogenase deficiency (909)
Steroid 20-22 desmolase deficiency (907)
Renal diseases with salt wasting

Minimal Diagnostic Criteria: Hyponatremia, hyperkalemia, urinary salt wasting, in the absence of renal or adrenal disease, and with normal or high aldosterone levels are essential to make the diagnosis.

Clinical Findings: Pseudohypoaldosteronism is the name given to a salt-wasting syndrome of infancy and early childhood in which there appears to be renal tubular unresponsiveness to the metabolic effects of aldosterone. Failure to thrive, anorexia, lethargy, vomiting, dehydration and circulatory collapse are almost universal findings in early infancy. The external genitalia are normal. Hyponatremia, often severe, hyperkalemia, and urinary sodium wasting are also characteristic. Renal function is otherwise normal, as is adrenal function determined by cortisol levels which are normal or high, and respond appropriately to administration of ACTH. Plasma aldosterone concentrations and secretion rate are markedly elevated to 10-fold normal levels, and plasma renin concentrations are also extraordinarily high. There is no correction of urinary salt loss following mineralocorticoids such as deoxycorticosterone or 9α-fluorohydrocortisone. A variant of this syndrome, in which plasma aldosterone levels are normal or modestly elevated, and in which there is a clinical response to salt-retaining steroids has also been described. In this latter form parental consanguinity has been prominent in the families of affected individuals. There is a tendency for spontaneous amelioration of salt loss with increasing age, so that treatment sometimes may be discontinued in the 2nd or 3rd year of life.

Complications
I   **Derived:** —
II   **Associated:** —

Etiology: Most cases previously described have been sporadic in nature, without familial aggregation. However, in the variant described by Rössler et al the familial aggregation and parental consanguinity suggest an autosomal recessive form of an inherited disorder.

Pathogenesis: The syndrome is explicable on the basis of renal tubular unresponsiveness to the action of aldosterone, and secondary homeostatic adjustments due to salt loss and dehydration in stimulating the renin-angiotensin-aldosterone system. As such, the syndrome would represent a further example of end-organ unresponsiveness to a hormone, akin to pseudohypoparathyroidism and nephrogenic diabetes insipidus. However complete unresponsiveness is unlikely since in some of the reported cases an aldosterone inhibitor, spironolactone, aggravated salt loss, and a partial response to high doses of mineralocorticoids has been observed. Alternatively, the clinical findings are explicable on the basis of a defect in salt reabsorption in the proximal renal tubule or ascending limb of the Henle loop, thus flooding the distal renal tubule with sodium beyond its reabsorptive capacity and resulting in secondary hyperaldosteronism with some response to mineralocorticoids.

Related Facts
I   **Sex Ratio:** M1:F1
II   **Risk of Occurrence:** ?
III   **Risk of Recurrence for**
    Patient's Sib: 1 in 4 (25%) for each offspring to be affected if autosomal recessive.
    Patient's Child: Not increased unless mate is carrier or homozygote, if autosomal recessive.
IV   **Age of Detectability:** Usually the disease is detected in the neonatal period or first 3 years of life.
V   **Prevalence:** ?

Treatment
I   **Primary Prevention:** Genetic counseling is probably indicated, and screening of other sibs should be performed.
II   **Secondary Prevention:** In most cases, supplemental salt intake of up to 5 gm daily corrects the electrolyte disturbance and restores growth to normal. Some patients may respond to mineralocorticoids with appropriate reduction in salt intake. A potassium exchange resin has been necessary in 1 case to correct severe hyperkalemia.
III   **Other Therapy:** —

Prognosis: With correction of electrolyte disturbance the prognosis appears to be very good for growth and development.

Detection of Carrier: —

Special Considerations: —

References:
Cheek, D.B. and Perry, J.W.: A salt wasting syndrome in infancy. Arch. Dis. Child. 33:252, 1958.
Proesmans, W. et al: Pseudohypoaldosteronism. Am. J. Dis. Child. 126:510, 1973.
Rössler, A. et al: Salt wastage, raised plasma-renin activity, and normal or high plasma-aldosterone: A form of pseudohypoaldosteronism. Lancet 1:959, 1973.
Savitt, H. et al: Pseudohypoaldosteronism. Clin. Res. 23:165A, 1975.

Contributor: **Mark A. Sperling**

Editor's Computerized Descriptors: CV., GI., GU.

PSEUDOHYPOPARATHYROIDISM

Includes: Ostéodystrophie
Albrightsche Osteodystrophie
Pseudohipoparatiroidismo
Pseudohypoparathyroidism, Type 1 (PHP-1)
Pseudohypoparathyroidism, Type 2 (PHP-2)
Albright hereditary osteodystrophy
Pseudo-pseudohypoparathyroidism

Excludes: Brachydactyly (114)
Hypoparathyroidism

Minimal Diagnostic Criteria: *PHP-1:* Low serum calcium, high levels of serum parathyroid hormone (PTH) and impaired urinary excretion of phosphate and cAMP in response to PTH challenge.
PHP-2: Same as PHP-1 but urinary excretion of cAMP in response to PTH challenge is normal.
Pseudo-PHP-1: During pseudo-PHP (normocalcemic) state, there is high basal urinary cAMP and normal phosphate and cAMP excretion responses to PTH. Pseudo-PHP patients retain the somatotype at all times.

Clinical Findings: Pseudohypoparathyroidism (Albright hereditary osteodystrophy) is characterized by skeletal and developmental abnormalities, signs and symptoms of "hypoparathyroidism" and evidence for endorgan unresponsiveness to high endogenous parathyroid hormone activity. The clinical condition comprises 2 different phenotypes: Pseudohypoparathyroidism, type-1 (PHP-1) and type-2 (PHP-2). PHP-1 also has a temporal, normocalcemic-normophosphatemic form known as pseudo-pseudohypoparathyroidism (pseudo-PHP-1, which includes latent PHP-1). The phenotypes can be subdivided into an unexplained and variable somatotype, and events related to abnormal mineral metabolism.

Short stature, short neck, round facies, brachydactyly (in particular, shortened 4th and 5th metacarpals or metatarsals) and mental retardation are the major somatotypic findings. Hypocalcemia, hyperphosphatemia, tetany, muscle cramps, convulsions, skeletal abnormalities, delayed dental eruption and enamel hypoplasia, ectopic calcification are findings related to the abnormal mineral metabolism. The major biochemical findings in PHP-1 and PHP-2 are summarized as follows:

Feature	PHP-1	PHP-2
Serum calcium	low	low
Serum phosphorus	high	normal or high
Serum immunoreactive parathyroid hormone (iPTH)	high	high
Renal response to PTH challenge		
a) phosphate excretion	decreased	decreased
b) 3'-5' AMP (cAMP) excretion	decreased	normal

Complications
I **Derived:** Tetany convulsions, cataracts and poor dentition
II **Associated:** A low thyroxine level with elevated TSH response to TRF has been reported.

Etiology: *PHP-1* (and pseudo-PHP-1): Absence of any proved example of male-to-male transmission and M1:F2 sex distribution is compatible with X-linked dominant inheritance. Sex-limited autosomal dominant inheritance has also been considered. Genetic heterogeneity for PHP-1 is probable. McK *30080
PHP-2: Inheritance is undefined but autosomal recessive is a possibility.

Pathogenesis: Unresponsiveness of the target organ to a bovine PTH challenge (or to the normal cellular effects of PTH-initiated responses) characterizes PHP-1 and PHP-2. Adenylcyclase activity is intact in renal cortex of PHP-1 patients. Failure of the intracellular interpretation of the PTH and cAMP mediated "message" may explain the findings in PHP-1 and PHP-2. Restoration of serum (and tissue?) calcium levels permits the renal response to bovine PTH to occur in PHP-1 (in some patients) and in PHP-2. The pseudo-PHP stage still eludes interpretation. Bone responsiveness to PTH in PHP has not been as quantitatively defined as the renal response. Hypocalcemia is not exclusively related to the unresponsiveness to PTH: treatment with $1,25(OH)_2D_3$ at "physiologic" doses restores serum calcium to normal suggesting that the intrarenal abnormality in PHP impairs synthesis of $1,25(OH)_2D_3$.

Related Facts
I **Sex Ratio:** M1:F2 for mixed populations
II **Risk of Occurrence:** ?
III **Risk of Recurrence for**
   Patient's Sib: PHP-1: When autosomal dominant or X-linked dominant see Table 1 AD or X-linked D, respectively.
   PHP-2: If autosomal recessive, 1 in 4 (25%) for each offspring to be affected.
   Patient's Child: PHP-1: When autosomal dominant or X-linked dominant, see Table 1 AD or X-linked D, respectively.
   PHP-2: If autosomal recessive, not increased unless mate is carrier or homozygote.
IV **Age of Detectability:** Possible in infancy
V **Prevalence:** ?

Treatment
I **Primary Prevention:** Genetic counseling
II **Secondary Prevention:** Treatment of hypocalcemia can be achieved with $1\alpha,25(OH)_2D_3$ (0.04-0.08 µg per kg body weight per day): requirements for $25\text{-}OHD_3$ are approximately 100 times higher (vs 3 times in the normal state). Renal responsiveness to bovine PTH may be restored with normocalcemia in PHP-1 and PHP-2.
III **Other Therapy:** Excision of foci of ectopic calcification is necessary occasionally

Prognosis: Normal life span. Occurrence of mental retardation cannot be predicted because of variable experience and uncertain pathogenesis.

Detection of Carrier: —

Special Considerations: —

References:
Chase, L.R. et al: Pseudohypoparathyroidism: Defective excretion of 3'-5'-AMP in response to parathyroid hormone. J. Clin. Invest. 48:1832, 1969.
Kooh, S.W. et al: Treatment of hypoparathyroidism and pseudohypoparathyroidism with metabolites of vitamin D: Evidence for impaired conversion of 25-hydroxyvitamin D to 1α25 dihydroxyvitamin D. N. Engl. J. Med. 293:840, 1975.
Potts, J.T., Jr.: Pseudohypoparathyroidism. In Stanbury, J.B. et al (eds.): The Metabolic Basis of Inherited Disease, 3rd Ed. New York: McGraw-Hill, 1972, p. 1305.
Rodriguez, M.J. et al: Pseudohypoparathyroidism type II: Restoration of normal renal responsiveness to parathyroid hormone by calcium administration. J. Clin. Endocrinol. Metab. 39:693, 1974.

Contributor: **Charles R. Scriver**

Editor's Computerized Descriptors: Face, Teeth, Neck, Skel., Nerve

PSEUDOVAGINAL PERINEOSCROTAL HYPOSPADIAS

Includes: Hypospadias périnéo-scrotal
Pseudovaginale perineoskrotale Hypospadie
Hipospadia pseudovaginal perineoescrotal
PPSH†
Incomplete male pseudohermaphroditism, type 2 (Wilson and Goldstein)†
17-ketosteroid reductase deficiency (some cases)†
Familial perineal hypospadias (Van Wyck and Grumbach)†
5α-reductase deficiency†
Masculinizing male pseudohermaphroditism (Jones)†
Masculinizing male hermaphroditism (Jones)†

Excludes: Androgen insensitivity syndrome, incomplete (50)
Androgen insensitivity syndrome, complete (49)
Reifenstein syndrome (855)
Chromosome 45,X/46,XY mosaicism (173)
Adrenal lipoid hyperplasia
3β-ol dehydrogenase deficiency
Steroid 17α-hydroxylase deficiency (903)
Steroid 17,20-desmolase deficiency (904)
Müllerian derivatives in males, persistent (683)

Minimal Diagnostic Criteria: Androgen sensitive 46,XY individuals with genital ambiguity, normal size testes, no müllerian derivatives, puberal virilization and normal plasma testosterone. The diagnosis is historically one of exclusion, applied only to 46,XY individuals with phenotype described below.

Clinical Findings: The term pseudovaginal perineoscrotal hypospadias (PPSH) has been employed to describe an intersex state in which 46,XY individuals have ambiguous external genitalia but otherwise develop like normal males. Somatic anomalies are absent. The external genitalia consist of a phallus that resembles a clitoris more than a penis, perineal urethral orifice, and usually a separate blindly ending perineal orifice that resembles a vagina (pseudovagina). At puberty, these androgen-sensitive individuals virilize. Phallic enlargement, increased facial hair, muscular hypertrophy, and lowering of the voice occur but breast development does not. The testes are relatively normal in size, and may be located in the inguinal canals or in the labioscrotal folds. Plasma testosterone is normal in cases adequately studied. Testes may show pachytene spermatogonia and even a few spermatozoa, but more often the testes resemble immature cryptorchid testes. Wolffian derivatives, but not müllerian derivatives, are present.

Complications
I   **Derived:** Misassignment of sex. Neoplastic transformation of testes could occur but apparently is rare.
II **Associated:** Usually none

Etiology: Autosomal recessive mutant allele; McK *26460

Pathogenesis: Previous reports have suggested that PPSH is the result of resistance of the undifferentiated fetal external genitalia to androgens. Such reports predated the availability of techniques for the detailed investigation of testosterone biosynthesis and metabolism. Recent reports reflect the nosologic-pathogenetic heterogeneity in the phenotype termed PPSH. A defect in 17-ketosteroid reductase has been documented in affected sibs, and, more recently, diminished 5α-reductase activity has been demonstrated in other affected patients. Moreover, in a large inbred isolate multiple affected patients with 5α-reductase deficiency conformed to the diagnostic criteria for PPSH. As other cases of PPSH are investigated thoroughly, other

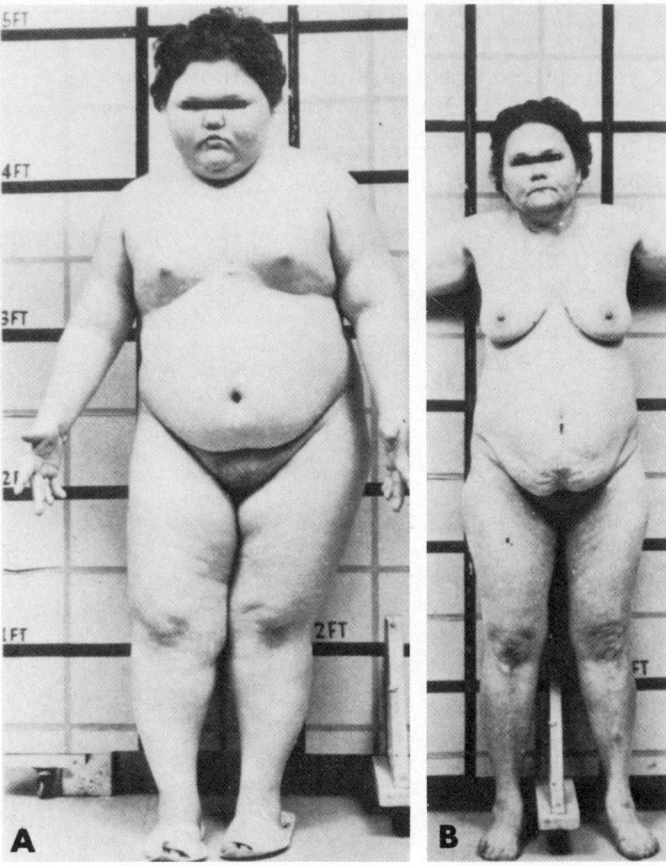

433. A) Thirteen-year-old girl with pseudohypoparathyroidism who was the daughter of B) with pseudo-pseudohypoparathyroidism

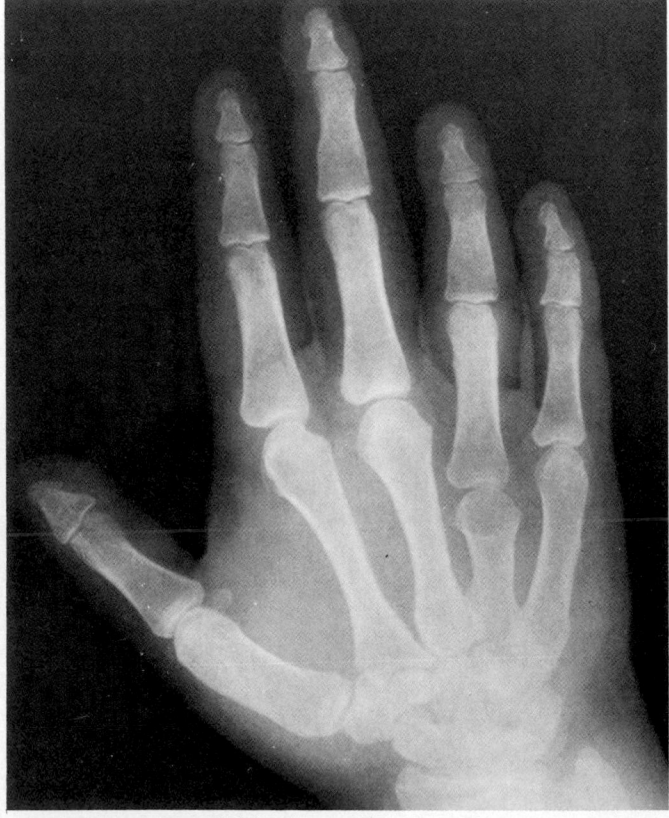

434. Note shortened 4th metacarpal

metabolic defects will doubtless be documented. No familial cases have been found which do not conform to an autosomal recessive mode of inheritance.

Related Facts

I   **Sex Ratio:**   M1:F0
II **Risk of Occurrence:**   ? But relatively rare
III **Risk of Recurrence for**
   Patient's Sib: 1 in 4 (25%) for 46,XY sib to be affected; 1 in 8 for all sibs.
   Patient's Child: All patients are presumed sterile. If not sterile, risk would be very low unless mate were heterozygous for same allele, in which case the risk would be 1 in 2 for 46,XY offspring.
IV **Age of Detectability:**   At birth because of genital ambiguity, if appropriate diagnostic studies are carried out.
V   **Prevalence:**   ? But relatively rare

Treatment

I   **Primary Prevention:**   Genetic counseling
II **Secondary Prevention:**   Depends upon sex of rearing. If diagnosis is made in early infancy, a female sex assignment is appropriate according to some authorities. In that instance, surgical reconstruction of the external genitalia and gonadectomy are in order, and vaginoplasty may be necessary. Estrogen substitution therapy will be necessary beginning in the 2nd decade of life.
   A male sex assigment, on the other hand, must be followed by surgical reconstruction of the external genitalia to produce a functional penis. Orchidopexy may be necessary, but androgen supplementation is not ordinarily necessary.
III **Other Therapy:**   —

Prognosis: Presumably normal life span

Detection of Carrier: ?

†Special Considerations: As is the case for terms such as Reifenstein syndrome and Lubs syndrome, the term pseudovaginal perineoscrotal hypospadias is based on a clinical phenotype. Evidence is accumulating that this clinical phenotype can be produced by any one of several enzymatic defects in the biosynthesis of testosterone or its conversion to dihydrotestosterone. Although several enzymatic defects in testosterone biosynthesis and its conversion to dihydrotestosterone may produce the PPSH phenotype, on the other hand, those same enzymatic defects may not always produce the PPSH phenotype. For example, some patients with the 17-ketosteroid reductase deficiency have the PPSH phenotype while others may not, but instead may exhibit breast development at puberty. (See also Pathogenesis.) The placement of the daggered terms (†) in the Includes and Excludes categories is thus tentative. Although the term, PPSH, may serve a useful nosologic purpose for the present, it should ultimately be replaced by terms that explicitly describe the etiology for those cases of male pseudohermaphroditism heretofore termed PPSH.

References:
Imperato-McGinley, J. and Peterson, R.E.: Male pseudohermaphroditism. The complexities of male phenotypic development. Am. J. Med. 61:251, 1976.
Moore, R.J. et al: Diminished 5α-reductase activity in extracts of fibroblasts cultured from patients with familial incomplete male pseudohermaphroditism, type 2. J. Biol. Chem. 250:7168, 1975.
Opitz, J.M. et al: Pseudovaginal perineoscrotal hypospadias. Clin. Genet. 3:1, 1972.
Peterson, R.E. et al: Male pseudohermaphroditism due to steroid 5α-reductase deficiency. Am. J. Med. 62:170, 1977.
Simpson, J.L.: Disorders of Sexual Differentiation: Etiology and Clinical Delineation. New York: Academic Press, 1976.
Summitt, R.L.: Disorders of sex differentiation. In Givens, J.R. (ed.): Gynecologic Endocrinology. Chicago: Year Book Publishers, 1977, p. 69.
Walsh, P.C. et al: Familial incomplete male pseudohermaphroditism, type 2. N. Engl. J. Med. 291:944, 1974.

Contributors: **Joe Leigh Simpson**
Robert L. Summitt

Editor's Computerized Descriptor: GU.

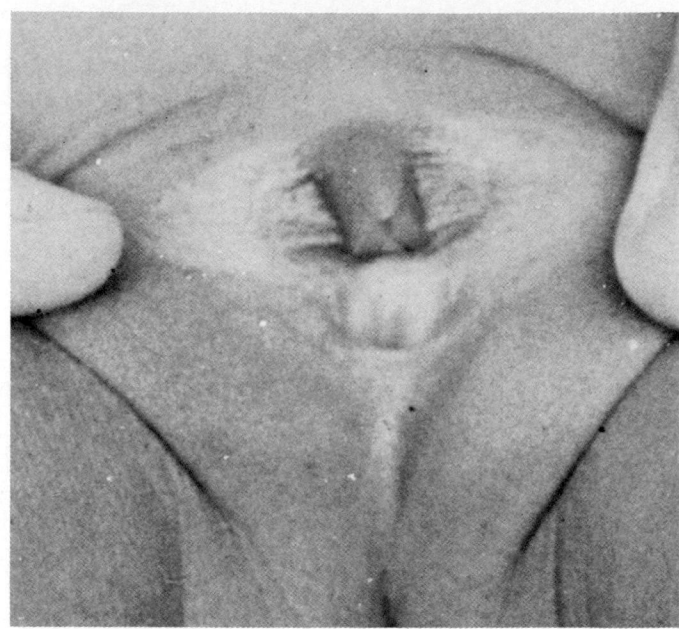

435. Young male with 5α-reductase deficiency illustrating urogenital sinus, clitoral-like phallus, and labial-like scrotum

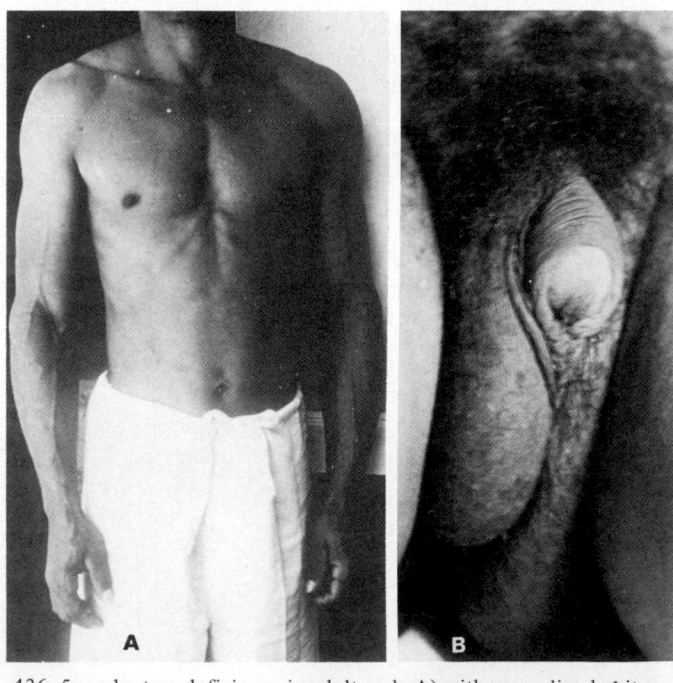

436. 5α-reductase deficiency in adult male A) with masculine habitus, B) illustrating growth of phallus and scrotum with testes of normal size

PSEUDOXANTHOMA ELASTICUM

Includes: Pseudoxanthome élastique
Pseudoxantoma elástico
Angioid streaks with skin changes
Systemic elastorrhexis
Groenblad-Strandberg syndrome
PXE
Elastosis dystrophica

Excludes: Senile elastosis

Minimal Diagnostic Criteria: Angioid streaks and PXE skin changes in the absence of Paget disease of bone.†

Clinical Findings: Changes occur in the skin, eyes and arteries. The name used for this condition refers to the skin changes which superficially resemble xanthoma and histologically show degeneration of elastic fibers. The skin lesions are usually discernible by the 2nd decade at the latest and are most striking around the neck and in the axilla. The skin of the antecubital area, groin, penis and periumbilical area may be affected also. The changes consist of yellowish nodular or reticular thickening. The skin about the mouth and chin and in the areas of the nasolabial folds is loose and thickened. The mucosa on the inside of the lower lip may be thickened and yellow with a superficial vascular network.

In the eyes, the hallmark is angioid streaks-irregular streaking radiating from the disk and lying behind the retinal vessels. These superficially resemble vessels-hence the name. They are likely to disappear when pressure is applied to the globe. Histologically they can be shown to result from breaks in the Bruch membrane. Hemorrhages also occur in the fundus and threaten vision especially when they are located in the region of the macula.

Degeneration in the elastic fibers of arteries is accompanied by rupture (especially in the submucosa of the alimentary tract so that GI bleeding is a major complication in terms of frequency and clinical significance) or occlusion (eg in coronary arteries, cerebral arteries or arteries of limbs).

Complications
I **Derived:** Blindness, rarely complete. Occlusion of cerebral, coronary or peripheral arteries with expected clinical results.
II **Associated:** —

Etiology: Autosomal recessive and autosomal dominant forms occur. McK *26480, *17785

Pathogenesis: Earliest discernible change in elastic fibers of corium is accretion of calcium salts. The fibers, as well as Bruch membrane, seem to become brittle and fracture. An inborn error of metabolism with secondary damage to the connective tissue elements (as in alkaptonuria and homocystinuria) is theoretically plausible but none has been demonstrated.

Related Facts
I **Sex Ratio:** Probably M1:F1 (More females come to medical attention.)
II **Risk of Occurrence:** ?
III **Risk of Recurrence for**
 Patient's Sib: 1 in 4 (25%) for each offspring to be affected
 Patient's Child: Not increased unless mate is carrier or homozygote
IV **Age of Detectability:** Varies from birth to 3rd or 4th decade
V **Prevalence:** ?

Treatment
I **Primary Prevention:** Genetic counseling
II **Secondary Prevention:** Both vitamin E and vitamin C have been recommended but there is no evidence of benefit and little rationale for their use.
III **Other Therapy:** ?

Prognosis: Normal for intelligence and early function but survivorship is significantly reduced by GI bleeding and arterial occlusion.

Detection of Carrier: —

†**Special Considerations:** Angioid streaks also occur with Paget disease of bone and with sickle cell anemia. Encrustation of a normal Bruch membrane by calcium and iron, respectively, may be responsible.

The autosomal recessive form may be less prone to vascular complications than the autosomal dominant form. Indeed 2 distinct autosomal dominant forms may exist. One has severe vascular and ocular changes. The 2nd is accompanied by mild ocular changes, blue sclerae, high palate, and loose jointedness.

References:
McKusick, V.A.: Heritable Disorders of Connective Tissue. 4th Ed. St. Louis:C.V. Mosby Co., 1972.
Pope, F.M.: Autosomal dominant pseudoxanthoma elasticum. J. Med. Genet. 11:152, 1974.

Contributor: **Victor A. McKusick**

Editor's Computerized Descriptors: Eye, Skin, CV., GI.

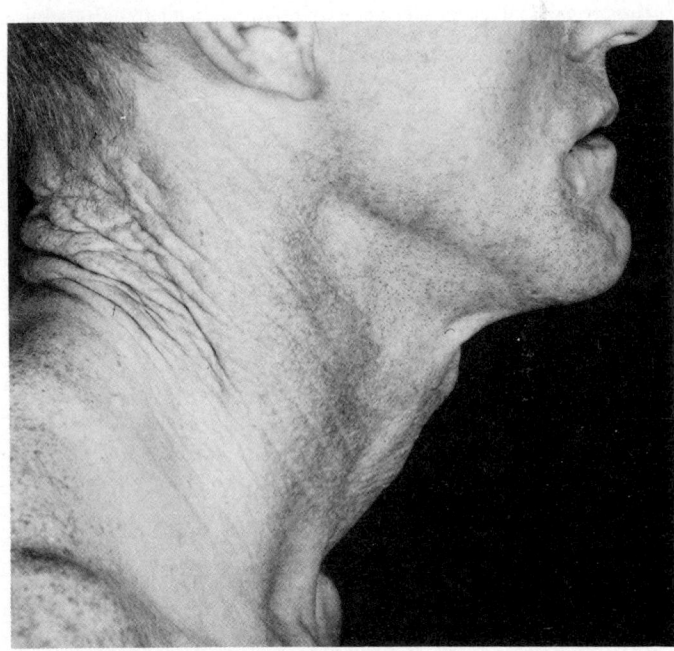

437. Note excess loose skin of neck

PSORIASIS VULGARIS

Includes: Psoriasis vulgaire
Pustular psoriasis

Excludes: Seborrheic dermatitis

Minimal Diagnostic Criteria: Typical erythematous, scaling plaques in symmetric distribution. In atypical cases, biopsy affirmation.

Clinical Findings: Symmetric erythematous plaques on skin with silvery micaceous scale. Most common on scalp, elbows, knees. May be generalized. Pitting of nails with dystrophy, onycholysis. Pinpoint bleeding upon removal of scale. Isomorphic response (Koebner phenomenon); appearance of psoriatic lesion at point of trauma to skin. Lesions may be pustular. Unpredictable and capricious in its course, usually chronic, with remissions and exacerbations. Microscopically parakeratosis and epidermal hyperplasia with relatively little inflammation. No consistent laboratory abnormalities. Serum uric acid often elevated.

Complications
I **Derived:** Generalized exfoliative erythroderma possibly associated with high output cardiac failure, hypoalbuminemia, hypothermia. Generalized pustular psoriasis.
II **Associated:** Debatable associated rheumatoid-like arthritis.

Etiology: Multifactorial†

Pathogenesis: Lesions characterized by increased epidermal mitotic rate and decreased cell turnover time, parakeratosis, epidermal hyperplasia, minimal inflammation, and prominent subepidermal capillaries.

Related Facts
I **Sex Ratio:** M1:F1
II **Risk of Occurrence:** 1 in 100 to 1 in 33 in Caucasians in Europe and the United States. Less common in Negro and American Indian.
III **Risk of Recurrence for**
   Patient's Sib: 7.5% if neither parent is affected; 16% if 1 parent is affected; 50% if both parents are affected.
   Patient's Child: 16% if 1 parent affected; 50% if both parents affected.
IV **Age of Detectability:** Mean age of onset: 27 years; range: infancy to old age.
V **Prevalence:** 1 in 100 to 1 in 33 in Caucasians in Europe and United States. Less frequent in Negro and American Indian.

Treatment
I **Primary Prevention:** —
II **Secondary Prevention:** Avoid trauma to skin and emotional stress.
III **Other Therapy:** Substances which reduce mitotic rate in epidermis include: topically applied coal tar and derivatives or corticosteroids, systemic agents such as antimetabolites eg methotrexate, corticosteroids, physical agents including ultraviolet light.†

Prognosis: Normal for life span and intelligence. Some degree of functional disability may result from extensive involvement.

Detection of Carrier: —

†Special Considerations: Careful examination of relatives may reveal minor undetected involvement. Even when these individuals are included, pedigrees do not fit any simple mode of inheritance and are highly variable.

Psoriasis is primarily a cosmetic handicap, but it can be disabling if severe on hands and feet or generalized. Diligent topical therapy is advised rather than treatment with systemic antimetabolites or corticosteroids due to possible severe complications from these agents.

References:
Farber, E. M. and McClintock, R. P., Jr.: A current review of psoriasis. Calif. Med. 108:440, 1968.
Rook, A.J. et al: Textbook of Dermatology. Oxford:Blackwell Scientific, 1968.
Watson, W. et al: Genetics of psoriasis. Arch. Dermatol. 105:197, 1972.

Contributor: **William Watson**

Editor's Computerized Descriptors: Skin, Nails

PTOSIS, CONGENITAL

Includes: Angeborene Ptose
Ptosis congénita
Congenital blepharoptosis
Myogenic stiff ptosis
Neurogenic flaccid ptosis
Ptosis with superior rectus weakness

Excludes: Blepharophimosis
Sixth nerve paralysis (889)
Jaw-winking syndrome (548)
Periodic ptosis with cyclic oculomotor spasm
Pseudoptosis
Ptosis secondary to myasthenia gravis or myotonic dystrophy
Ptosis with epicanthus
Ophthalmoplegia, progressive external (752)
Secondary ptosis
Horner syndrome (475)
Ophthalmoplegia totalis and ptosis

Minimal Diagnostic Criteria: No sharp cutoff exists for diagnosing mild bilateral cases. Unilateral cases can be detected by comparison with the fellow lid. Diagnosis is most obvious on upward gaze.†

Clinical Findings: Simple ptosis is characterized by drooping of and inability to raise the upper eyelid associated in one-third of cases with weakness of upward movement of the eye. Approximately 80% are unilateral. This type of simple ptosis accounts for approximately 80% of all congenital ptosis. It is stationary throughout life and unaccompanied by visual defects unless the lid covers the pupil causing amblyopia, or weakness of the recti muscles causes strabismus. The degree of ptosis varies among cases and may be noticeable only on upward gaze. Elevation of the eyebrow and backward head tilt are frequent compensatory maneuvers. The skin of the lid is smooth without the normal tarsal fold.

Complications
I **Derived:** Postural anomalies due to hyperextension of the head (particularly in bilateral cases). Amblyopia (particularly in unilateral cases or with associated strabismus).
II **Associated:** See Exclusions cited above. There is probable linkage to the genes for the MN blood group system. Occasional association with endognathia, hereditary edema of the limbs, general mental and physical degeneration, arachnodactyly, Turner syndrome, chromosome 18q- and a wide variety of congenital neurologic and cranial malformations has been described.

Etiology: Autosomal dominant with approximately 60% penetrance; McK *17830

Pathogenesis: Most cases are due to abnormal peripheral differentiation of the levator muscle (which embryologically develops from the superior rectus). Other cases, particularly those with ophthalmoplegia (other than paresis of the superior rectus), are due to agenesis or aplasia of the appropriate midbrain nuclei. Fibrosis of the atrophic muscle usually occurs.

Related Facts
I **Sex Ratio:** M1:F1
II **Risk of Occurrence:** Relatively common, exact incidence unknown
III **Risk of Recurrence for**
 Patient's Sib: If parent is affected 1 in 3 (30%) for each offspring to be affected, 1 in 2 for inheriting mutant gene; otherwise not increased.
 Patient's Child: 1 in 3 (30%) for each offspring to be affected, 1 in 2 for inheriting mutant gene.
IV **Age of Detectability:** Most cases are diagnosable at birth.
V **Prevalence:** Relatively common, exact prevalence unknown

Treatment
I **Primary Prevention:** Genetic counseling
II **Secondary Prevention:** Many surgical procedures are described. Results are good on simple ptosis but often poor when accompanied by defective eye motility. Early treatment is necessary to prevent amblyopia or postural changes where these are a threat.
III **Other Therapy:** Crutch spectacles

Prognosis: Normal life span. Condition stationary throughout life.

Detection of Carrier: Affected parent and patient

†**Special Considerations:** Differentiation between myogenic and neurogenic ptosis is best made by electromyographic examination.

References:
Beard, C.: Ptosis. St. Louis: C.V. Mosby, 1969, pp. 40-50, 81-107.
Berke, R. N.: Congenital ptosis: A classification of 200 cases. Arch. Ophthalmol. 41:188, 1949.
Duke-Elder, S.: System of Ophthalmology. Vol. 3, pt. 2. Congenital Deformities. St. Louis: C.V. Mosby, Co., 1963, p. 887.
Smith, B. et al: Surgical treatment of blepharoptosis. Am. J. Ophthalmol. 68:92, 1969.

Contributor: **Donald R. Bergsma**

Editor's Computerized Descriptors: Vision, Eye

PULMONARY ARTERY COARCTATION

Includes: Sténose de l'artère pulmonaire
Supravalvuläre Pulmonalstenose
Coarctación de la arteria pulmonar
Pulmonary branch stenosis (839)
Pulmonary artery stenosis
Supravalvular pulmonary stenosis

Excludes: Primary or secondary pulmonary hypertension
Occlusive pulmonary vascular disease
Pulmonary artery atresia
Infundibular pulmonary stenosis
Pulmonary valve stenosis (839)

Minimal Diagnostic Criteria: The characteristic systolic murmurs, heard equally well in both axillae and back as over the base, should suggest the diagnosis, particularly when the patient has the fetal rubella, Williams, or Ullrich-Noonan syndrome. Pulmonary artery angiocardiography may be used to demonstrate anatomic constrictions.

Clinical Findings: The murmurs of pulmonary artery coarctations are the most common murmurs encountered in the newborn nursery (5% of newborns in the experience of the authors). In the great majority of cases, these murmurs represent a transient benign condition which disappears with the normal growth and maturation of the pulmonary vascular bed. In a small percentage of cases, the murmurs are produced by the high pulmonary flow of a left-to-right shunt or true anatomic constriction of the pulmonary arteries. In the case of true coarctation the pathologic anatomy varies from a discrete, abrupt narrowing (often at a bifurcation) to a diffuse elongation. Generalized hypoplasia is rarely present in 1 or both main branches. Stenoses often are multiple, but in most cases are only mildly obstructive. Histologically there is intimal thickening and fibrosis with fragmentation of the internal elastic laminae at the site of the obstruction with vein-like dilatation of the distal artery. There may be calcification of the intima in later stages. Four anatomic groups have been described: Type I: in which the stenosis is in the main pulmonary trunk or near its point of bifurcation into the main pulmonary arteries; Type II: stenosis at the bifurcation extending into the left or right branch, or both; Type III: multiple peripheral stenoses; and Type IV: main pulmonary trunk plus peripheral stenoses. Associated cardiac anomalies are common, particularly pulmonary valvar stenosis, patent ductus arteriosus, ventricular septal defect, atrial septal defect and tetralogy of Fallot. The likelihood that the coarctations are anatomically significant is greatly increased if the patient has any 1 of the following syndromes: fetal rubella, Williams, or Ullrich-Noonan. In fact, most patients who have severe pulmonary artery coarctations have 1 of these 3 syndromes.

The hemodynamic alterations, and consequently the clinical picture, will vary with the degree of obstruction of the pulmonary artery coarctation(s). The presence of an associated lesion will influence the clinical picture. The presence of branch stenosis may be masked by pulmonary valvar or infundibular stenosis, or accentuated by increased pulmonary flow.

The pathophysiology resembles that of pulmonary valve stenosis. With increasing degrees of obstruction there is increased right ventricular hypertension and, consequently, hypertrophy. Certain cases may be progressive and eventually lead to severe and extensive stenosis. Cardiac failure may then occur, resulting in cardiomegaly and right atrial hypertension. A right-to-left shunt across a pat-

ent foramen ovale then causes cyanosis.

Continuous murmurs are rarely heard. The usual murmur in pulmonary artery coarctation consists of high-pitched ejection murmur(s) heard in the right axilla, left axilla and back, as well as over the base. There is usually no ejection click and the second heart sound is normal in most cases. The murmurs resemble the peripheral lung murmurs caused by very large atrial level left-to-right shunts. It should be emphasized that, although the great majority of newborns who have murmurs of peripheral pulmonary artery coarctation have a benign, transient condition, these newborns should be followed through sequential visits until the murmurs disappear. If the murmurs are present for more than 3 months, anatomic coarctation or increased pulmonary flow from a shunt should be suspected. Atrial septal defect is not infrequently misdiagnosed as benign pulmonary artery coarctation (until congestive heart failure becomes manifest).

The ECG may be normal in the presence of very mild obstruction. Usually right ventricular hypertrophy of the pressure overload type is present (the degree depending on the severity of the obstruction).

The roentgenographic findings in isolated pulmonary artery stenosis are not characteristic. With severe bilateral stenosis, the pulmonary arterial vascular workings are diminished. The cardiac silhouette may assume a right ventricular contour, but the pulmonary artery segment is not enlarged.

At cardiac catheterization, a consistent peak systolic pressure gradient within the pulmonary arterial bed of 10 mm Hg is consistent with anatomic pulmonary artery coarctation (but may also be found in high pulmonary flow from left-to-right shunts). With severe bilateral stenoses, the morphology of the proximal main pulmonary artery pressure pulse often exhibits a wide pulse pressure characterized by a fast upstroke, a depressed dicrotic notch and a slow diastolic runoff. Indeed, it may show "ventricularization," ie resemble the right ventricular pressure tracing, very similar to when massive pulmonic valve regurgitation is present. The degree of right ventricular and right atrial hypertension depends on the severity of the obstruction. In the presence of an associated lesion, the above findings will be changed. For example, an increase in the pressure difference across the coarctation is seen with a large left-to-right shunt.

Complications

I **Derived:** Right heart failure, right-to-left shunt at atrial level with desaturation and elevated hematocrit, progressive stenosis of coarctations with increasing right ventricular hypertension, pulmonary artery thrombosis, rupture of distal dilated arteries with hemoptysis, and persistent right ventricular hypertension after total correction of the associated cardiac defect (such as tetralogy of Fallot).

II **Associated:** Pulmonary artery coarctations are particularly common in certain syndromes. These include fetal rubella, Williams, and Ullrich-Noonan syndromes.

Etiology: Multifactorial inheritance postulated in Williams syndrome and sporadic cases. Found in the autosomal dominant Ullrich-Noonan syndrome. Found following profound teratogenic maternal exposure to rubella virus. McK *18550

Pathogenesis: A teratogenic insult (eg rubella) may cause a defect in the internal elastic laminae of the artery, producing a localized weakness in the wall in response to pulsatile pressure at systemic levels in utero. Resultant medial damage will then cause intimal hyperplasia and fibrosis.

Other theories advocated include: an inflammatory lesion in an area of turbulent flow (arterial branch) may cause intimal fibrosis, or a teratogenic insult may cause slowing of the maturation and development of certain segments of the pulmonary vascular bed.

Related Facts
I **Sex Ratio:** M1:F1
II **Risk of Occurrence:** The occurrence of hemodynamically significant branch stenosis is small—of the order of 1:20,000. The frequency of transient benign disease in the newborn is about 5%.
III **Risk of Recurrence for**
Patient's Sib: Depends on etiology
Patient's Child: Depends on etiology
IV **Age of Detectability:** Infancy
V **Prevalence:** Varies from higher rates during the rubella pandemic of 1964-65 to lower rates at present.

Treatment
I **Primary Prevention:** Rubella vaccination
II **Secondary Prevention:** Arterial reconstruction if stenosis is severe enough and repair is anatomically feasible; lobectomy if multiple peripheral stenoses are localized to 1 area of lung.
III **Other Therapy:** Symptomatic therapy for relief of congestive heart failure.

Prognosis: The severity, location and extent of the stenoses, and the presence or absence of associated syndromes and cardiac defects, determine the prognosis.†

Detection of Carrier: Depends on etiologic category.

†**Special Considerations:** Differentiation between transient, anatomic, hemodynamic and syndrome categories.

References:
Dunkle, L.M. and Rowe, R.D.: Transient murmur simulating pulmonary artery stenosis in premature infants. Am. J. Dis Child. 124:666, 1972.
Nora, J.J. et al: The Ullrich-Noonan syndrome (Turner phenotype). Am. J. Dis. Child. 127:48, 1974.
Toews, W.H. et al: Presentation of atrial septal defect in infancy. JAMA 234:1250, 1975.
Watson, H.: Stenosis of the pulmonary arteries. In Watson, H. (ed.): Paediatric Cardiology. St. Louis:C.V. Mosby Co., 1968, p. 534.

Contributors: **James J. Nora**
Audrey H. Nora

_____

Editor's Computerized Descriptors: Resp., CV.

PULMONARY VALVE ABSENT

Includes: Absence congénitale de valvules pulmonaires
Fehlen der Pulmonalklappe
Ausencia de la válvula pulmonar
Tetralogy of Fallot with absent pulmonary valve
Ventricular septal defect with absent pulmonary valve
Absent pulmonary valve

Excludes: Pulmonary valve atresia (837)

Minimal Diagnostic Criteria: A diastolic murmur in the 2nd and 3rd left intercostal space at the sternal border, with enlarged pulmonary artery on xray with normal pulmonary vascularity and a normal ECG, or one showing right ventricular hypertrophy suggests the diagnosis.

Selective pulmonary artery angiocardiography is confirmatory as it will show absence of pulmonary valve tissue or a thickened ridge of tissue with massive reflux of contrast media from the large pulmonary artery into the right ventricle.

Clinical Findings: At the site of the pulmonary valve, a ring of nodular tissue is present which has no structural characteristics of a pulmonary valve. Histologically, this tissue is composed of large pale-staining, myxomatous appearing cells. The pulmonary valvar annulus is frequently hypoplastic and therefore stenotic. Because of the pulmonic regurgitation, the right ventricle is enlarged. In addition, the pulmonary trunk and major pulmonary arterial branches are dilated, often appearing aneurysmal. The pulmonary trunk has been studied histologically and found in some cases to present a mosaic of fibers, rather than normal lamellar configuration. In the majority of patients with absent pulmonary valve a ventricular septal defect coexists, usually as part of a tetralogy of Fallot malformation.

The clinical findings vary depending upon the type of associated cardiac malformation. In patients with absent pulmonary valve coexisting with ventricular septal defect, the signs and symptoms of congestive cardiac failure occur in infancy. Most patients with absent pulmonary valve present with the pathologic anatomy of tetralogy of Fallot. The predominant shunt in infancy is left to right with minimal cyanosis. Addition of pulmonary insufficiency due to absent valve usually results in severe congenital heart failure early in infancy or even in utero. Patients with isolated absence of the pulmonary valve are generally asymptomatic until adulthood. The major bronchi may be partially compressed by the aneurysmally dilated pulmonary arteries which may lead to obstructive emphysema.

Cardiac findings are those of pulmonary stenosis and pulmonary insufficiency. A to-and-fro murmur is present along the left upper sternal border. The systolic portion of the murmur is of the ejection type and may be harsh and loud, especially in those with coexistent cardiac anomalies, whereas it is softer in patients with the isolated anomaly. A diastolic murmur of pulmonary insufficiency is present and its intensity is related to the degree of reflux. The second heart sound is single. A pulmonic systolic ejection click may be present. ECG may be normal if pressures are normal, regurgitation is not gross, and there are no complicating conditions. The ECG of patients with isolated absence of the pulmonary valve reveals right ventricular hypertrophy. Among those with coexistent ventricular septal defect, biventricular hypertrophy is observed, and in those with tetralogy of Fallot, right ventricular hypertrophy of pressure overload type. In patients with ventricular septal defect and absent pulmonary valve, generalized cardiomegaly is present on the roentgenogram. The pulmonary trunk and pulmonary vessels, especially the right pulmonary artery, are greatly enlarged and may be misinterpreted as a tumor mass. Tetralogy of Fallot with absent pulmonary valve reveals enlarged pulmonary trunk, but near normal sized cardiac silhouette. With the isolated pulmonary valve anomaly the cardiac size is usually normal, but the pulmonary trunk is dilated.

A major echocardiographic finding is inability to image pulmonary valve. However, a failure to find this structure is relatively weak evidence for diagnosis. Additionally, the right pulmonary artery and right ventricle are usually dilated. Paradoxical septal motion may be present. The tricuspid valve may flutter. The remainder of the echocardiographic examination is normal.

For patients with a ventricular septal defect, additional findings specific for that condition may be present. See Ventricular Septal Defect.

In patients with absent pulmonary valve associated with tetralogy of Fallot, the catheterization data are similar to those of patients with tetralogy of Fallot. Whether the shunt is right to left or left to right depends entirely upon the degree of right ventricular obstruction. In isolated absent pulmonary valve, the right ventricular systolic pressure may be normal or slightly elevated with a small systolic pressure difference across the valve related to increased pulmonary flow. In all cases, the pulmonary arterial pulse pressure contour is characteristic, showing a wide pulse pressure, low diastolic pressure (similar to the right ventricular end diastolic pressure) and a low dicrotic notch. Angiography assists in identifying the presence of associated cardiac malformations. The pulmonary trunk and major pulmonary vessels are greatly dilated and pulsatile. The right ventricular chamber is enlarged and may remain opacified for a prolonged period. The pulmonary valve is not distinct and the pulmonary annulus is narrowed. Pulmonary arteriography reveals reflux of opaque material into the right ventricle.

Complications
I   Derived: Congestive cardiac failure, obstructive emphysema
II Associated: —

Etiology: ?

Pathogenesis: ?

Related Facts
I   Sex Ratio: M1:F1
II   Risk of Occurrence: Rare
III Risk of Recurrence for
     Patient's Sib: ?
     Patient's Child: ?
IV   Age of Detectability: At birth
V   Prevalence: ?

Treatment
I   Primary Prevention: —
II   Secondary Prevention: Pulmonary arterial banding is the palliative treatment for the infant in cardiac failure. This procedure reduces the magnitude of the left-to-right shunt and the degree of pulmonary insufficiency. Corrective surgery includes closing the ventricular septal defect and replacing the pulmonary trunk by an aortic homograft or valved conduit.
III Other Therapy: Treatment of congestive cardiac failure and the pulmonary complications. Patients with isolated absence of pulmonary valve or with coexistent malformations who are asymptomatic do not require operation.

Prognosis: The prognosis is poor in patients with coexistent defects, with many dying in infancy from congestive cardiac failure complicated by pulmonary disorders. Patients with tetralogy of Fallot may survive relatively symptom free into teens and 20s. Patients with isolated absent pulmonary valve survive until their 70s, although there is increasing evidence that this is not always as benign a condition as once believed. Particularly, in adults who develop unrelated pulmonary diseases resulting in pulmonary hypertension, symptoms may develop because of the increased right ventricular pressure and volume work.

Detection of Carrier: —

Special Considerations: —

References:
Goldberg, S.J. et al: Pediatric and Adolescent Echocardiography: A Handbook. Chicago: Year Book Medical Publishers, 1975.
Miller, R.A. et al: Congenital absence of the pulmonary valve: The clinical syndrome of tetralogy of Fallot with pulmonary regurgitation. Circulation 26:266, 1962.
Venables, A.W.: Absence of the pulmonary valve with ventricular septal defect. Br. Heart J. 24:293, 1962.

Contributor: **James H. Moller**

Editor's Computerized Descriptors: Resp., CV.

PULMONARY VALVE ATRESIA

Includes: Atrésie des valvules pulmonaires
Pulmonalklappen-Atresie
Atresia de la válvula pulmonar
Pulmonary valve atresia with intact ventricular septum
Pulmonary atresia with normal aortic root
Pulmonary atresia with hypoplastic right ventricle
Atresia of pulmonary valve

Excludes: Pulmonary valve stenosis (839)
Tetralogy of Fallot with pulmonary valve atresia

Minimal Diagnostic Criteria: Selective right ventricular angiocardiography is needed to establish the pathologic anatomy of pulmonary atresia.

Clinical Findings: The pulmonary valve presents as an imperforate membrane, with 2 or 3 small raphae or the pulmonary root is hypoplastic or atretic. The pulmonary trunk is usually hypoplastic and patent to the level of the pulmonary valve. The right ventricle is generally thick walled and hypoplastic. The lumen is small, the wall hypertrophied and the endocardium may be fibroelastotic. The tricuspid valve is also hypoplastic and at times incompetent, in which case occasionally the right ventricle may be dilated. Secondary anatomic features include enlarged myocardial sinusoids which connect with the coronary arterial branches. During systole, blood leaves the right ventricle via the sinusoids and flows into the coronary arterial system. The right atrium is enlarged and hypertrophied. An atrial communication is present, usually a patent foramen ovale, or less frequently, an ostium secundum type atrial septal defect. A patent ductus arteriosus may be present, offering a means of pulmonary perfusion. Generally, it closes early in infancy and flow depends on an enlarged bronchial collateral circulation.

Regardless of the size of the right ventricular cavity, the clinical manifestations are similar. Cyanosis is present at birth or shortly thereafter. If the ductus remains patent, however, only mild cyanosis is present. Cyanosis increases quickly as the ductus closes. The other prominent finding is dyspnea. The signs of cardiac failure are prominent only in patients with tricuspid regurgitation. Physical examination reveals a cyanotic, dyspneic infant with cardiomegaly. The second heart sound is single. In more than half the patients, there is a systolic murmur which is usually soft, and may be related to either the ductus arteriosus or tricuspid regurgitation. Ventricular size has been broadly classified as either hypoplastic or normal. The pulmonary vascularity is decreased with markedly ischemic lung fields. There is a tendency for the cardiac silhouette to be larger in patients with an enlarged right ventricle, especially in those with tricuspid insufficiency. The pulmonary arterial segment is concave and the right atrium is grossly enlarged. The upper mediastinum often is narrow and the aortic knob inapparent.

The ECG reveals normal or right axis deviation. This serves to distinguish this condition from tricuspid atresia in which left axis deviation is the rule. Furthermore, a qR pattern in lead AVF suggests pulmonary atresia, whereas such a qR pattern is seen in lead aVL in tricuspid atresia. Right atrial enlargement is present although not always in the 1st week of life. A few older cases show left atrial enlargement. The precordial leads are useful in distinguishing the 2 types of pulmonary valvar atresia. With a hypoplastic right ventricle, a pattern of "absence of right ventricular forces" is present with an rS in lead V_1 and an R in V_6. Normal or enlarged right ventricles are associated with classic patterns of right ventricular hypertrophy.

The pulmonary valve will not be imaged. However, this finding is not conclusive, for the pulmonary valve may have merely been missed. The right ventricular outflow tract usually appears narrowed, and this is appreciated as a more anterior than normal position of the anterior aortic wall. In most instances, the aorta will be larger than normal. Right ventricular cavity size will depend upon the exact anatomy of a particular patient. Right ventricular hypertrophy almost always is present. If pulmonary blood flow is low, left atrial size would be expected to be small. If the right pulmonary artery is present, it can be imaged and measured via the suprasternal notch approach.

Cardiac catheterization is useful in establishing the diagnosis. It is not always possible to advance the catheter tip into a hypoplastic right ventricle. The right ventricular pressure is elevated with the peak systolic pressure exceeding the systemic arterial pressure. Right atrial pressure is elevated and shows large "a" waves. Oxygen saturations on the right side of the heart are low and blood from the left atrium is desaturated. Indicator dilution curves performed from either atrium are practically identical, showing a common pathway of circulation.

Angiocardiography confirms the diagnosis and yields information regarding right ventricular size. The angiocardiogram reveals no passage of contrast material from the right ventricle into the pulmonary artery. Contrast may be seen escaping from the right ventricle either through an insufficient tricuspid valve or through myocardial sinusoids with retrograde filling of coronary arteries. In some cases, opacification of the aortic root occurs as well with such retrograde flow. Right atrial injections show passage of contrast from right-to-left atrium but frequently fail to distinguish this condition from tricuspid atresia. The pulmonary arteries fill by way of a patent ductus arteriosus or enlarged bronchials.

Complications
I **Derived:** Acidosis secondary to hypoxia, cardiac failure.
II **Associated:** —

Etiology: Unknown but presumably multifactorial inheritance

Pathogenesis: Pulmonary atresia is probably due to early fusion of the pulmonary valvar primordia.

Related Facts
I **Sex Ratio:** M1:F1
II **Risk of Occurrence:** Approximately 1 in 10,000 live births
III **Risk of Recurrence for**
    Patient's Sib: Predicted risk - 1:100; Empiric risk - undetermined.
    Patient's Child: The anomaly does not permit survival to the reproductive age.
IV **Age of Detectability:** From birth
V **Prevalence:** 1 in 1000 at birth diminishes to only the rare survivors of palliative surgery.

Treatment
I **Primary Prevention:** —
II **Secondary Prevention:** Supportive therapy with oxygen and treatment of acidosis. Digitalis is indicated in patients with congestive heart failure. This condition represents a surgical emergency. Following cardiac catheterization, operation is mandatory. If the ventricle is normal or enlarged, pulmonary valvotomy can be performed under conditions of inflow occlusion. When the right ventricle is hypoplastic, an ascending aorta - right pulmonary artery anastomosis is indicated.
III **Other Therapy:** —

Prognosis: The prognosis is poor, as most infants die within the first 3 months, except if the ductus remains patent. The operative mortality is high.

Detection of Carrier: —

Special Considerations: —

References:
Benton, J.W., Jr. et al: Pulmonary atresia and stenosis with intact ventricular septum. Am. J. Dis. Child. 104:161, 1962.
Chung, K. et al: Echocardiography in truncus arteriosus: The value of pulmonic valve detection. Circulation 48:281, 1973.
Davignon, A.L. et al: Congenital pulmonary atresia with intact ventricular septum: Clinicopathologic correlation of two anatomic types. Am. Heart J. 62:591, 1961.
Goldberg, S.J. et al: Pediatric and Adolescent Echocardiography: A Handbook. Chicago: Year Book Medical Publishers, 1975.

Contributor: **James H. Moller**

Editor's Computerized Descriptors: Resp., CV.

PULMONARY VALVE INCOMPETENCE

Includes: Insuffisance de la valvule pulmonaire
Pulmonalinsuffizienz
Insuficiencia de la válvula pulmonar
Pulmonary regurgitation due to intrinsic abnormality of pulmonary valve
Incompetence of pulmonary valve

Excludes: Absent pulmonary valve with associated defects
Secondary incompetence of pulmonary valve with lesions which primarily cause dilatation of pulmonary artery

Minimal Diagnostic Criteria: An early diastolic murmur along the left sternal border with ECG evidence of right ventricular hypertrophy suggests the diagnosis. Pulmonary artery angiocardiography confirms the diagnosis.

Clinical Findings: Incompetence of the pulmonary valve results from a structural abnormality of the valve which may be bicuspid, tricuspid or quadricuspid. Functional pulmonary incompetence may also be present in patients with idiopathic dilatation of the pulmonary artery or other lesions which cause dilatation of the pulmonary artery.

Because of incompetence of the pulmonary valve, the right ventricular stroke volume is increased. As a result, the main pulmonary artery, its major branches and the right ventricular chamber are dilated. The degree of dilatation of the right side of the heart is dependent not only upon the degree of pulmonary incompetence but also on the level of pulmonary arterial pressure. If sufficient regurgitation occurs and marked right ventricular dilatation develops, congestive cardiac failure may occur.

The clinical findings are related primarily to the degree of incompetence and the level of pulmonary arterial pressure. Patients with minor degrees of incompetence are asymptomatic. The elevated pulmonary vascular resistance that is normally present in the neonatal period, or that may develop secondarily later in life, tends to augment the degree of regurgitation, thereby imposing an excessive pressure load upon the right ventricle and leading to congestive cardiac failure. Newborn infants with pulmonary insufficiency can thus present with signs of severe cardiac failure. A systolic ejection type murmur is present, which is related to increased right ventricular stroke volume. This murmur is followed by a medium to low-pitched diastolic regurgitant murmur along the left sternal border. The pulmonary component of the second heart sound may be absent if the valve is rudimentary. If both components of the second sound are present, the degree of splitting may be increased because of the increased right ventricular stroke volume. When pulmonary arterial hypertension is present, the pulmonic component is accentuated. A pulmonary ejection click may be present.

Thoracic roentgenograms in most children show a normal-sized cardiac silhouette with prominent pulmonary trunk and major arterial branches. With severe incompetence or pulmonary hypertension, the right-sided cardiac chambers are enlarged. Cardiac fluoroscopy shows increased pulsations of the pulmonary trunk and main arteries.

The ECG findings may reflect the volume overload on the right ventricle. It may either be normal or reveal mild right ventricular hypertrophy. The latter is manifested as an rSR' pattern in lead V_1, a larger than normal S wave in lead V_6, and terminal slowing of the QRS electrical forces.

The pulmonary valvular abnormality cannot be visualized directly. If the insufficiency is of moderate or greater degree, the right ventricular cavity will be dilated. In more advanced instances, paradoxical septal motion may be present. Tricuspid flutter has been reported but it is relatively rare. Thickness of the right ventricular wall is related to the etiology of the pulmonary insufficiency. The right pulmonary artery is usually dilated.

In the presence of significant pulmonary valve incompetence, cardiac catheterization characteristically reveals a wide pulmonary arterial pulse pressure with the diastolic pressure similar to that of right ventricular end diastolic pressure. The dicrotic notch is low. Small systolic pressure gradients may be present between the right ventricle and the pulmonary artery secondary to the increased forward flow.

Angiocardiography shows an enlarged right ventricle especially the infundibulum. The pulmonary trunk is dilated. In severe cases, the main pulmonary arteries may show considerable dilatation as well. Pulmonary arteriography shows retrograde opacification of the right ventricle.

Complications
I **Derived:** Congestive cardiac failure
II **Associated:** —

Etiology: ?

Pathogenesis: ?

Related Facts
I **Sex Ratio:** M1:F1
II **Risk of Occurrence:** ? Less than 1% of all cases of congenital heart defects
III **Risk of Recurrence for**
  Patient's Sib: ?
  Patient's Child: ?
IV **Age of Detectability:** From birth
V **Prevalence:** ?

Treatment
I **Primary Prevention:** —
II **Secondary Prevention:** Medical treatment if cardiac failure is present. Surgical therapy is rarely indicated. It could, however, be accomplished by homograft replacement of the pulmonary valve or other type of valvar prosthesis.
III **Other Therapy:** —

Prognosis: Pulmonary valve incompetence has been generally considered a benign condition, but reports of death in the neonatal period and in later life have been reported. Short-term animal studies of surgically induced insufficiency have indicated its benign nature. Longer periods of observation are needed to determine the future course of the child or younger adult with symptom-free isolated pulmonary valvar incompetence.

Detection of Carrier: —

Special Considerations: —

References:
Collins, N.P. et al: Isolated congenital pulmonic valvular regurgitation; diagnosis by cardiac catheterization and angiocardiography. Am. J. Med. 28:159, 1960.
Gasul, B.M. et al: Congenital isolated pulmonary valvular insufficiency. In Heart Disease in Children: Diagnosis and Treatment. Philadelphia:J.B. Lippincott Co., 1966, p. 807.
Goldberg, S.J. et al: Pediatric and Adolescent Echocardiography: A Handbook. Chicago:Year Book Medical Publishers, 1975.
Vlad, P. et al: Congenital pulmonary regurgitation: A report of six autopsied cases. Am. J. Dis. Child. 100:640, 1960.

Contributor: **James H. Moller**

Editor's Computerized Descriptors: Resp., CV.

PULMONARY VALVE STENOSIS

Includes: Sténose des valvules pulmonaires
Pulmonalstenose
Estenosis de la válvula pulmonar
Pulmonary valvar stenosis with intact ventricular septum
Pulmonary valvar stenosis with normal aortic root
Trilogy of Fallot

Excludes: Infundibular pulmonic stenosis
Pulmonary artery coarctation (835)

Minimal Diagnostic Criteria: A harsh systolic murmur, maximal in the 2nd left intercostal space, with an enlarged main pulmonary artery on xray with normal pulmonary vascularity, plus right ventricular hypertrophy on the ECG, indicate the diagnosis. Selective right ventricular angiocardiography is confirmatory.

Clinical Findings: In the majority of patients with pulmonary valvar stenosis, the pulmonary valve is dome-shaped, with partial commissural fusion, resulting in a central circular orifice of variable size. Less frequently, the valve shows no commissural fusion. In this particular form, called pulmonary valvar dysplasia, 3 distinct cusps and commissures are present, the valvar tissue being greatly thickened and redundant. The sinuses of Valsalva are partly obliterated by tissue composed of large, pale-staining myxomatous-like cells. In this form, pulmonary stenosis results from the mass of valvar tissue encroaching on the pulmonary orifice. Secondary anatomic features of pulmonary valve stenosis include poststenotic dilatation of both the pulmonary trunk and usually also the left pulmonary artery. The right ventricle is hypertrophied in proportion to the severity of the stenosis. With time, 2 alterations occur in the right ventricle which significantly alter right ventricular function. One of these is the development of myocardial fibrosis and the 2nd is the development of infundibular stenosis. Right atrial enlargement and hypertrophy are present in the more severe cases, and this may be of sufficient degree to open a previously competent patent foramen ovale.

The clinical and laboratory findings are dependent in part upon the severity of the stenosis. The majority of patients with pulmonary valve stenosis are asymptomatic and show normal growth and development. With moderate stenosis, easy fatigability may be present. Congestive cardiac failure and cyanosis (related to a right-to-left atrial shunt) may develop but usually only in patients with severe pulmonary valvar stenosis. These findings may be present in the infant with severe stenosis or may develop gradually in the adult with significant pulmonary valve stenosis. The prominent physical finding is a loud pulmonary systolic ejection murmur, which is usually associated with a thrill along the upper left sternal border and in the suprasternal notch. The murmur is usually introduced by a pulmonic systolic ejection click, but this may be absent in severe cases. Other auscultatory features may be indicative of the severity of the stenosis. With significant pulmonary stenosis the murmur becomes longer and the peak intensity of the murmur is delayed further into systole. The development or presence of a murmur of tricuspid insufficiency is indicative of severe pulmonary stenosis. The components of the second heart sound are normal in mild stenosis, but with increasing degrees of severity, the pulmonic component becomes delayed and softer, or even inaudible.

Attention must be directed to the general appearance and physical characteristics of the child. They may indicate the etiology of the pulmonary valve stenosis, as in post-rubella syndrome. Children with a dysplastic pulmonary valve are generally small in stature, retarded in sexual development, and have a rather typical triangular shaped face with ptosis, hypertelorism and low-set ears. Pulmonic systolic ejection clicks are rarely heard among these patients. Usually the heart size is normal as is the pulmonary vasculature. There is prominence of the pulmonary trunk and left pulmonary artery. In patients with severe stenosis, the pulmonary artery segment is usually inapparent. With severe or long-standing moderate pulmonary stenosis, the overall cardiac size may be slightly enlarged, representing primarily right ventricular and right atrial enlargement. In patients with cyanosis related to right-to-left atrial shunt, the pulmonary vasculature is diminished, but left atrial enlargement is then present. Combination of decreased pulmonary vascularity and left atrial enlargement should suggest a large right-to-left shunt at atrial level.

In mild pulmonary valvar stenosis, the ECG is normal, or shows only minimal evidence of right ventricular hypertrophy (T wave positive in V_1). With more severe stenosis, there is progressively more right axis deviation and right ventricular hypertrophy. Right atrial enlargement may be observed. There is a rough correlation between the height of the R wave in right precordial leads and the severity of the stenosis. In children with dysplastic pulmonary valves, Noonan syndrome with pulmonary stenosis, and rubella patients with stenotic pulmonary valves, the ECG findings of severe right axis deviation and r^S deflections in all precordial leads suggest a degree of right ventricular hypertrophy which is not actually present.

In most instances, the echocardiographic "a" wave amplitude of the pulmonary valve is excessive in some beats; in other beats, the "a" wave appears normal. In some children with pulmonary valvular stenosis, the "a" wave appears normal. Right ventricular anterior wall thickness is related to the severity of the disease. Right ventricular cavity size may vary from small to dilated. If the right ventricular cavity is dilated, paradoxical septal motion may be present even in the absence of a right ventricular volume overload. The right pulmonary artery is usually dilated.

Cardiac catheterization reveals a systolic pressure difference across the pulmonary valve and there may be right-to-left shunt at the atrial level. Simultaneous measurement of the cardiac output and the gradient across the pulmonary valve permit calculation of the size of the stenotic pulmonary valvar orifice. Measurement of hemodynamic parameters during exercise permits assessment of right ventricular function. Right ventricular angiography demonstrates a dome-shaped pulmonary valve with a jet of contrast passing through the small central orifice. The angiocardiogram reveals hypertrophy of the right ventricle, especially the crista supraventricularis, which forms the posterior wall of the right ventricular infundibulum. Generally, the infundibulum narrows during systole, but widens sufficiently during diastole. In patients with a dysplastic pulmonary valve, the valve cusps do not dome and there is no jet. The thickened cusps maintain a fixed position in both diastole and systole; the sinuses of Valsalva are nearly occluded.

Complications
I **Derived:** Congestive cardiac failure, tricuspid valvar insufficiency, development of myocardial fibrosis, increased hematocrit.
II **Associated:** May be seen as part of the congenital rubella, Noonan, and the multiple lentigines syndromes.

Etiology: Presumably multifactorial. May be seen as part of the congenital rubella, Noonan, and the multiple lentigines syndromes.

Pathogenesis: Dome-shaped pulmonary valve probably results from fusion of the embryonic valvar cusps. Dysplastic pulmonary valve probably results from failure of reabsorption of the embryonic cusp tissue that normally occurs in the formation of the sinuses of Valsalva.

Related Facts
I **Sex Ratio:** M1:F1
II **Risk of Occurrence:** ?
III **Risk of Recurrence for**
    Patient's Sib: 2.9% (predicted); 2.9% (empiric)
    Patient's Child: 2.9% (predicted); 3.6% (empiric)
IV **Age of Detectability:** From birth by clinical means and cardiac catheterization.
V **Prevalence:** Approximately 1 in 1250 of the general population.

Treatment
I **Primary Prevention:** Genetic counseling.
II **Secondary Prevention:** Medical, symptomatic treatment of congestive cardiac failure, when this is present. Pulmonary valvotomy should be performed in any patient with a calculated pulmonary valve area less than 0.5 cm^2/meter^2 of body surface area. With a normal cardiac output this valve area usually generates a right ventricular pressure in the range of 75 mm Hg. In patients with significant infundibular stenosis, it may be necessary to resect a portion of the obstructing muscle as well as open the pulmonary valve. In patients with a dysplastic pulmonary valve, the operation involves excision of the valvar tissue or the placement of an outflow patch across the pulmonary annulus.
III **Other Therapy:** Infants with severe pulmonary stenosis and cardiomegaly represent surgical emergencies. Prompt performance of diagnostic procedures and pulmonary valvotomy may be lifesaving.

Prognosis: Serial cardiac catheterization studies have indicated that beyond infancy patients with mild-to-moderate pulmonary valvar stenosis show no increase in the level of right ventricular pressure. There are suggestions, however, that the incidence of coexistent infundibular pulmonary stenosis increases in each decade of life. As a result, the infundibular stenosis may result in increased levels of right ventricular pressure and complicate operation. With time, right ventricular myocardial fibrosis develops which may significantly alter the compliance and function of the right ventricle. The results of operation in children are excellent and pulmonary valvotomy can be performed successfully at low risk. In adults, particularly those with poor right ventricular function, the operative risk is higher, and the postoperative catheterization data frequently reveal continued poor right ventricular myocardial performance.

Detection of Carrier: —

Special Considerations: —

References:
Emmanouilides, G. C.: Obstructive lesions of the right ventricle and pulmonary arterial tree. In Moss, A.J. and Adams, F.H. (eds.): Heart Disease in Infants, Children, and Adolescents. Baltimore:Williams and Wilkins, 1968.
Goldberg, S.J. et al: Pediatric and Adolescent Echocardiography. Chicago:Year Book Medical Publishers, 1975.
Koretzky, E.D. et al: Congenital pulmonary stenosis resulting from dysplasia of valve. Circulation 40:43, 1969.
Levine, O.R. and Blumenthal, S.: Pulmonic stenosis. Circulation 32(Suppl. 3):33, 1965.
Weymann, A.E. et al: Echocardiographic patterns of pulmonic valve motion in pulmonic stenosis. Am. J. Cardiol. 33:178, 1974.

Contributor: **James H. Moller**

PULMONARY VALVE, TETRACUSPID

Includes: Valve pulmonaire tétracuspide
Vierklappiges Pulmonalostium
Válvula pulmonar tetracuspídea
Quadricuspid pulmonary valve
Tetracuspid pulmonary valve

Excludes: —

Minimal Diagnostic Criteria: Selective pulmonary artery angiocardiography is necessary to establish the diagnosis. Even then, exact delineation of a tetracuspid pulmonary valve is difficult. Thus, necropsy is required definitively to document the diagnosis.

Clinical Findings: The pulmonary valve has 4 valve cusps. The cusps may each be of equal size or one may be smaller. Often it is the supernumerary cusp that is deformed, imperfect or smaller. When present as an isolated anomaly, the right-sided cardiac chambers are normal. If the valve is insufficient, the pulmonary artery and right ventricle may be dilated. Symptoms and signs are only present if the pulmonary valve is incompetent or stenotic.

Complications
I **Derived:** Pulmonary valve insufficiency, bacterial endocarditis
II **Associated:** —

Etiology: ?

Pathogenesis: This anomaly probably results from the formation of an additional intercalated pulmonary valve swelling.

Related Facts
I **Sex Ratio:** Ml:Fl
II **Risk of Occurrence:** Extremely rare
III **Risk of Recurrence for**
   Patient's Sib: ?
   Patient's Child: ?
IV **Age of Detectability:** From birth
V **Prevalence:** ?

Treatment
I **Primary Prevention:** —
II **Secondary Prevention:** —
III **Other Therapy:** —

Prognosis: Good, the anomaly usually being an incidental finding at necropsy.

Detection of Carrier: —

Special Considerations: —

References:
Kissin, M.: Pulmonary insufficiency with a supernumerary cusp in the pulmonary valve: Report of a case with review of the literature. Am. Heart J. 12:206, 1936.

Contributor: **James H. Moller**

PULMONARY VENOUS CONNECTION, PARTIAL ANOMALOUS

Includes: Anomalie partielle des veines pulmonaires
Partielle Lungenvenenfehlmündung
Conexión anómala de las venas pulmonares parcial
Partial anomalous venous return
Partial transposition of great veins
Partial anomalous pulmonary venous connection

Excludes: Pulmonary venous connection, total anomalous (842)

Minimal Diagnostic Criteria: Typical physical, electrocardiographic and roentgen features of ASD. Cardiac catheterization, including selective pulmonary arteriography, confirms the diagnosis when the clinical features are atypical.

Clinical Findings: Anatomy: Partial anomalous pulmonary venous connection (PAPVC) exhibits a wide anatomic spectrum. Almost every conceivable connection between the pulmonary veins and the proximal systemic veins has been reported. Left-sided pulmonary veins usually connect anomalously to derivatives of the left cardinal system (coronary sinus and innominate vein). Anomalous connections of the right pulmonary veins are usually to derivatives of the right cardinal system, (superior vena cava, right atrium, and occasionally inferior vena cava). However, the embryologic splanchnic plexus is a midline structure and this explains the developmental possibility for the crossed drainage. An atrial septal defect usually accompanies PAPVC. Major additional cardiac anomalies (exclusive of atrial septal defect) are present in approximately 20% of the cases.

Physiology: The fundamental physiologic disturbance of PAPVC is similar to that of atrial septal defect; ie increased pulmonary blood flow with consequent recirculation of oxygenated blood through the lungs. Factors determining the precise hemodynamic state include: 1) the number of anomalously connected veins, 2) the site of anomalous connection, 3) the presence or absence of atrial septal defect, 4) the size and location of atrial septal defect, and 5) associated anomalies.

When the atrial septum is intact, the number of anomalously connected veins and the state of the pulmonary parenchyma determine the amount of blood which drains anomalously. When a single pulmonary vein is anomalously connected, the anomalously draining blood approximates 20% of total pulmonary blood flow. This amount is clinically inapparent. When veins from one lung drain anomalously and the pulmonary resistance is normal, the PBF:SBF = 3:1. This higher than expected pulmonary flow is due to the fact that pressure in the right atrium, into which the anomalously connected lung drains, is less than left atrial pressure, thus resulting in preferential flow through the anomalously connected lung. When PAPVC and atrial septal defect coexist, the hemodynamic picture is identical to that of uncomplicated atrial septal defect. The left-to-right shunt is usually large (PBF:SBF = 3:1).

Clinical features: These depend on the size of the shunt, the state of the atrial septum, the state of the pulmonary vascular bed and the presence of associated anomalies. The age of recognition of PAPVC is usually 5-6 years. Symptoms are uncommon in childhood, but there may be some dyspnea on exertion. Right heart failure occurs rarely in the child but is not uncommon in adults. Cyanosis is unusual during childhood. In the presence of an associated atrial septal defect, the findings are identical to those noted in the uncomplicated atrial septal defect. These are right ventricular lift, pulmonary systolic ejection murmur, diastolic tricuspid flow murmur at the lower left sternal border and wide splitting of the second sound which is unaltered by respiration. The presence of an intact atrial septum results in normal variation of splitting of the second heart sound on respiration.

Thoracic roentgenograms reveal pulmonary vascularity of the shunt type, dilatation of the main pulmonary artery and both major branches and evidence of right heart (atrial and ventricular) enlargement. In addition, there may be distinctive features dependent on the site of anomalous connection. The patient with anomalous connection of the right pulmonary veins to the inferior vena cava has a vertically oriented, crescent-like shadow in the right lower lung field (scimitar syndrome). In addition, the right lung is almost invariably hypoplastic, there are signs of chronic infection secondary to bronchial anomalies, and the heart is shifted to the right. Connection to the azygos vein results in a rounded bulge in the right upper mediastinum. A prominent supracardiac shadow may be recognized when partial connection is to the left superior vena cava (snowman silhouette).

ECG findings include a rR' pattern or rSR' pattern in the right precordial leads. Peaked P waves and right ventricular hypertrophy of the systolic overload pattern occur in older patients exhibiting pulmonary hypertension. A frontal P wave axis of +15° or less is commonly seen in patients with PAPVC to the SVC or with sinus venosus type atrial septal defect.

Echocardiographic features: The echocardiogram is normal if one vein connects anomalously and the atrial septum is intact. When the veins of one lung connect anomalously or there is an associated ASD, the echo features are similar to those found in ASD.

Heart catheterization findings are similar, and at times, identical to those in uncomplicated atrial septal defect. There is increased oxygenation at the right atrial level. Depending on the site of anomalous connection, the catheter tip may detect increased saturation in a systemic vein. Indicator dilution techniques may also demonstrate drainage into a systemic vein. Separate injections of an indicator substance into the right and left pulmonary arteries, respectively, allow an assessment of the drainage of the right and left pulmonary veins. However, since in uncomplicated atrial septal defect a greater portion of blood from the right lung drains anomalously, the demonstration of anomalous drainage does not indicate PAPVC. When the atrial septum is intact and all the blood from 1 lung drains anomalously into the right atrium directly and the blood from the other lung drains normally, a diagnosis of PAPVC can be definitely confirmed by indicator dilution studies. Selective pulmonary arteriography or pulmonary vein angiography allows identification of the vast majority of forms of PAPVC. This includes those to peripheral veins, coronary sinus and the majority of PAPVC to the right atrium. When the pulmonary veins insert just to the right atrial side of the atrial septum, definition is difficult when the PAPVC is associated with an atrial septal defect. However, insertion of the catheter into the anomalous pulmonary veins with selective angiography in the left anterior oblique position will usually determine the relationship of the veins to the atrial septum.

Complications

I **Derived:** As a consequence of increased pulmonary blood flow, pulmonary vascular disease is not uncommon in middle age and may be followed by right-to-left shunting and right ventricular failure. In the presence of an intact atrial septum, disease or surgical resection of normally draining pulmonary tissue may result in severe disability or death.

II Associated: No significant association except in the scimitar syndrome where pulmonary sequestration, anomalous systemic arterial supply to the right lung and pulmonary hypoplasia are common.

Etiology: ?

Pathogenesis: The embryologic basis for PAPVC is failure of some of the pulmonary veins to gain connection with the embryonic common pulmonary vein with persistence of one or more of the still present systemic venous channels as a route for pulmonary venous drainage.

Related Facts
I **Sex Ratio:** Ml:Fl
II **Risk of Occurrence:** ?
III **Risk of Recurrence for**
   Patient's Sib: ?
   Patient's Child: ?
IV **Age of Detectability:** From birth
V **Prevalence:** Authorities have quoted figures from 1 in 166 to 1 in 16,000 in the general population.

Treatment
I **Primary Prevention:** —
II **Secondary Prevention:** Surgical repair utilizing cardiopulmonary bypass. Anomalous connections to SVC, right atrium and coronary sinus are corrected by utilizing a pericardial patch to close the atrial septal defect in such a way so as to include the anomalously connecting veins. In connections to the IVC or to the innominate vein, the anomalously connecting vein must be transected and reanastomosed. Pulmonary parenchyma is excised only if the parenchyma is distinctly abnormal, and should not be done as a method of treating PAPVC with normal parenchyma.
III **Other Therapy:** —

Prognosis: Many patients have minimal symptoms and survive into late adult life. On the other hand, pulmonary vascular disease as a consequence of high flow is not uncommon in middle age. The long-term postoperative prognosis is undefined.

Detection of Carrier: —

Special Considerations: —

References:
Brody, H.: Drainage of pulmonary veins into right side of heart. Arch. Pathol. 33:221, 1942.
Lucas, R.V., Jr. and Schmidt, R.E.: Anomalous venous connection, pulmonary and systemic. In Moss, A.J. and Adams, F.H. (Eds.): Heart Disease in Infants, Children and Adolescents. Baltimore:-Williams and Wilkins, 1977.
McCormack, R.J. et al: Partial anomalous pulmonary venous drainage and its surgical correction. Scott. Med. J. 5:357, 1960.

Contributor: **Russell V. Lucas, Jr.**

Editor's Computerized Descriptor: CV.

PULMONARY VENOUS CONNECTION, TOTAL ANOMALOUS

Includes: Retour veineux pulmonaire anormal total
Komplette Lungenvenen-Transposition
Anomalía total del drenaje venoso pulmonar
Total anomalous pulmonary venous return
Complete transposition of great veins

Excludes: Subtotal pulmonary venous connection
Pulmonary venous connection, partial anomalous (841)
Scimitar syndrome (879)

Minimal Diagnostic Criteria: *TAPVC without pulmonary venous obstruction:* Cyanotic infant with venous hum at the left base, cyanotic infant with ECG signs of right atrial and pure right ventricular hypertrophy together with roentgenologic findings of shunt vascularity and pure right heart enlargement, roentgen signs showing shunt vascularity and "snowman" configuration. Selective pulmonary arteriography will indicate the type of anomalous connection.

TAPVC with pulmonary venous obstruction: Cyanotic infant who exhibits an increase in cyanosis during feeding, roentgen signs of pulmonary venous obstruction, normal sized heart, and the above roentgen signs with discrete indentation in the barium-filled esophagus just above the diaphragm.

Selective pulmonary arteriography demonstrates the site of anomalous connection. Areas of obstruction may be seen, but, as a consequence of the obstruction to the venous drainage, there may be significant delay in the passage of opaque material through the pulmonary vasculature and the angiogram must be programmed so as to allow films to be taken up to 15-20 seconds after injection.

Clinical Findings: Anatomy: All pulmonary veins from both lungs connect anomalously directly or indirectly to the right atrium. In the majority of patients, total anomalous pulmonary venous connection (TAPVC) is an isolated anomaly. The presence of an atrial communication is necessary to sustain life and therefore an atrial septal defect or patent foramen ovale is considered part of the complex. The specific site of anomalous connection may be to right atrium directly, to a derivative of the cardinal venous system (right superior vena cava, azygos vein, innominate vein, left superior vena cava, or coronary sinus), or to a derivative of the umbilico-vitelline system (portal vein, ductus venosus, hepatic vein or inferior vena cava).

The hemodynamic state and clinical features in TAPVC vary according to the presence or absence of obstruction to pulmonary venous blood flow. The anatomic sites of obstruction include obstruction at the atrial septum (inadequate size foramen ovale), obstruction in the anomalous venous channel (secondary to intrinsic narrowing of the channel or to extrinsic pressure) and the interposition of the hepatic sinusoids in TAPVC below the diaphragm.

TAPVC without pulmonary venous obstruction: At birth the distribution of blood between the pulmonary and systemic circuits is approximately equal since resistance in these vascular beds is equal. In the 1st few weeks of life maturation of the pulmonary vascular bed results in a dramatic decrease in pulmonary vascular resistance and an increase in pulmonary blood flow to 3-5 times the systemic blood flow. Due to the high proportion of fully saturated blood entering the right atrium, oxygen saturation of the right atrium may be 80% or higher. Adequate mixing in the right atrium is the rule. Thus, oxygen saturations in the right atrium, right ventricle, pulmonary artery and aorta are equal. Dilatation and hypertrophy of the right atrium and right ventricle and dilatation of the pulmonary artery are consequences of increased pulmonary blood flow. Right heart failure is commonly seen. Pulmonary artery pressure may be slightly elevated or systemic.

Clinically, the babies may be asymptomatic at birth, but in the first month of life develop tachypnea and fail to thrive. They are subject to repeated respiratory infections and usually have cardiac failure in the 1st few months of life. Cyanosis is mild or clinically inapparent.

Physical examination reveals a scrawny, irritable baby who may be slightly dusky. Dyspnea, tachypnea and tachycardia are usual as is a right ventricular heave. A characteristic feature is the presence of multiple cardiac sounds. The 1st sound is loud and distinct and is followed by a systolic ejection click. The second sound may be widely split, particularly in older children or adults, and does not vary with respiration. The pulmonary component of the second sound is accentuated. A third heart sound is almost always present and a fourth heart sound is frequent. In the infant with rapid heart rates, the third and fourth sounds usually blend into a loud consummation sound. Characteristically, a grade II/VI soft blowing systolic murmur is heard in the pulmonary area; occasionally, no murmur is heard. A diastolic tricuspid flow murmur at the lower left sternal border is present in about half the patients. Occasionally, when the anomalous connection is to the left innominate vein, a venous hum at the left or right base is present.

Radiologic Features: Certain features are common to all cases: increased pulmonary vascular markings of the shunt type, right atrial and right ventricular enlargement and enlargement of the pulmonary artery segment. In addition, the specific site of anomalous connection may result in characteristic roentgenographic signs. The "snowman" or "figure-of-eight" cardiac silhouette appears in TAPVC to the left innominate vein. When the anomalous connection is to the azygos vein, a characteristic rounded shadow is seen in the upper right mediastinum. Connection to the right superior vena cava results in the dilatation of the lower portion of the superior vena cava and blurring of the right superior vena cava-atrial junction. Connection to the coronary sinus may result in a discrete indentation in the barium-filled esophagus just below the left atrium.

The ECG is characterized by tall P waves in lead II and right precordial leads. Right axis deviation is usual. Right ventricular hypertrophy is invariably present, usually manifested by high voltage R waves in the right precordial leads, occasionally by incomplete right bundle branch block pattern. A QR pattern in V_1 is seen in about one-third of the cases.

Echocardiographic features: TAPVC is one of the entities that produce signs of right ventricular diastolic volume overload. These are increased right ventricular dimension index and paradoxical ventricular septal motion. The presence of an echo-free space posterior to the left atrium appears to be a reliable sign of the venous confluence (common pulmonary vein) almost always present in TAPVC. Rarely there is no venous confluence posterior to the left atrium in TAPVC and the sign is absent. An echo-free space may be detected in atresia of the common pulmonary vein and some of the variants of cor triatriatum. In TAPVC to the coronary sinus an additional linear echo is present within the left atrium. This echo cannot be distinguished from the left atrial echoes produced by persistent left superior vena cava to coronary sinus and cor triatriatum.

Cardiac catheterization may allow identification of the site of anomalous connection if highly saturated blood is obtained from a systemic vein. The characteristic feature is high and equal oxygen saturations in the right atrium, the right ventricle and pulmonary artery and aorta. Pressures in the right atrium, right ventricle and pulmonary artery are elevated. Pulmonary arteriography defines the anatomy of the anomalous connection.

TAPVC with pulmonary venous obstruction: Typically, pulmonary venous obstruction occurs when the connection is to a structure below the diaphragm. However, intrinsic or extrinsic obstruction can develop in any anomalous channel. The presence of pulmonary venous obstruction does not identify the site of the anomalous connection. Cyanosis and tachypnea are present at birth or occur within the 1st few days of life. There is rather rapid progression of dyspnea, feeding difficulties, hypoxia and cardiac failure. In spite of these alarming symptoms, the cardiovascular findings may be minimal. The heart is not enlarged. There is no right ventricular heave. The second sounds are normally split and the pulmonary component accentuated. A cardiac murmur is often absent; when present, it is usually a soft, blowing systolic murmur in the pulmonic area. Rales are usual at the lung bases. Hepatomegaly is almost always present, and occasionally peripheral edema is noted.

Radiologic features include a heart that is normal or nearly normal in size and contour. The lung fields have diffuse stippled densities that form a reticular pattern which fans out from the hilar region. The ECG invariably reveals right ventricular hypertrophy. Unlike TAPVC without venous obstruction, however, right heart enlargement is not a usual feature. The confluence of pulmonary veins situated just above the diaphragm may result in a discrete indentation of the esophagus.

Echocardiographic features: The signs of right ventricular diastolic volume overload are not present. The echo-free space posterior to left atrium and the echo within the left atrium may be present as noted above.

Cardiac catheterization: Oximetry may be helpful if fully saturated blood is obtained from a systemic vein. Interpretation of the oximetry must be cautious, however, since pulmonary blood flow is decreased and its volume may not be sufficient to allow high saturation when mixed with systemic venous blood. Moreover, streaming of renal vein blood may result in the appearance of highly oxygenated blood in the inferior vena cava. Right ventricular pressures are usually systemic or higher. Right atrial pressures are usually normal. Pulmonary arteriography allows anatomic definition of the anomalous connection.

Complications
I **Derived:** Death from congestive heart failure, death secondary to inadequate systemic blood flow, hypoxia and shock; progression of pulmonary vascular disease in older children.
II **Associated:** A particularly high incidence of TAPVC occurs in patients with the asplenia syndrome.

Etiology: ?

Pathogenesis: The embryologic basis of the anomaly is aplasia or early obliteration of the common pulmonary vein, while primitive pulmonary systemic venous connections still exist. The persistence of 1 or more of these channels allows an alternate route for pulmonary venous drainage.

Related Facts
I **Sex Ratio:** M1.4:F1
II **Risk of Occurrence:** 1 in 5000 live births
III **Risk of Recurrence for**
    Patient's Sib: ?
    Patient's Child: ?

IV Age of Detectability: From birth
V Prevalence: ?

Treatment
I   Primary Prevention: —
II Secondary Prevention: Surgical correction utilizing cardiopulmonary bypass is usually necessary in infancy. Occasionally a patient does well enough to allow later surgical intervention.
III Other Therapy: Symptomatic therapy for congestive heart failure and infection. Palliation by creation of an atrial septal defect by balloon septostomy appears warranted in the child under 6 months of age without pulmonary venous obstruction.

Prognosis: Influenced by the size of the atrial communication and by obstructive lesions in the anomalous venous pathways. Overall, approximately 50% of the patients are dead by 3 months; 80% do not survive the 1st year of life. When the atrial communication is not adequate or obstruction exists in the anomalous venous channel, prognosis is more grim. Death usually occurs within the 1st weeks of life and it is unusual for a patient with obstruction to survive past 3 months. Rarely, when a large atrial communication is present, the patient may reach adulthood with few symptoms. Infants under 12 months of age have a surgical mortality of at least 50%. This figure seems to be improving. In the older patient, the surgical risk is significantly less.

Detection of Carrier: —

Special Considerations: —

References:
Burroughs, J.T. and Edwards, J.E.: Total anomalous pulmonary venous connection. Am. Heart J. 59:913, 1960.
Lucas, R.V., Jr. and Schmidt, R.E.: Anomalous venous connection, pulmonary and systemic. In Moss, A.J. and Adams, F.H. (eds.): Heart Disease in Infants, Children, and Adolescents. Baltimore: Williams & Wilkins, 1977.
Paquet, M. and Gutgesell, H.: Echocardiographic features of total anomalous pulmonary venous connection. Circulation 51:599, 1975.
Wukasch, D.C. et al: Total anomalous pulmonary venous return. Ann. Thorac. Surg. 19:622, 1975.

Contributor: **Russell V. Lucas, Jr.**

——————————————

Editor's Computerized Descriptors: Resp., CV., Liver

PULPAL DYSPLASIA

Includes: Displasie pulpaire
Dysplasia pulpae
Displasia pulpar

Excludes: Dentinogenesis imperfecta (279)
Osteogenesis imperfecta (777)
Dentin dysplasia, radicular (278)
Dentin dysplasia, coronal (277)
Dentino-osseous dysplasia (280)
Teeth, thistle-shaped pulp chambers (937)
Calcinosis
Ehlers-Danlos syndrome (338)
Fibrous dysplasia of dentin
Odontodysplasia (739)
Shell teeth
Pulp stones

Minimal Diagnostic Criteria: Teeth with large ovoid pulp chambers with multiple pulp stones.†

Clinical Findings: On roentgenographs the teeth of both dentitions have ovoid crowns, relatively small roots with large root canals, large ovoid or flame-shaped pulp chambers extending into the tooth root and multiple pulp stones. The pulp calcifications are present in developing and unerupted teeth as well as those in occlusion. The pulp calcifications may fill the pulp chambers in older persons.

Complications
I   Derived: —
II Associated: Three patients have had growth retardation with stature 3 SD below normal. One had idiopathic oligophrenia.

Etiology: ? All cases nonfamilial.

Pathogenesis: ? Pulp calcifications begin around blood vessels in the developing dental papilla and by a process of apposition, tubular dentin is deposited around these calcifications.

Related Facts
I   Sex Ratio: ? All have been female.
II   Risk of Occurrence: ?
III Risk of Recurrence for
     Patient's Sib: ? All have been isolated cases.
     Patient's Child: ? All have been isolated cases.
IV   Age of Detectability: By dental radiographic examination at time of eruption of teeth.
V   Prevalence: ? Very rare

Treatment
I   Primary Prevention: None required
II Secondary Prevention: —
III Other Therapy: —

Prognosis: ? Growth retardation

Detection of Carrier: —

†Special Considerations: The original report included what is now known to be two different disorders, pulpal dysplasia which has been nonfamilial and dentin dysplasia type II (coronal dentin dysplasia).

References:
Rao, S. R. et al: Pulpal dysplasia. Oral Surg. 30:682, 1970.
Shields, E.P. et al: A proposed classification for heritable human dentine defects with a description of a new entity. Arch. Oral Biol. 18:543, 1973.
Witkop, C.J., Jr.: Hereditary defects of dentin. Dent. Clin. North Am. 19:25, 1975.

Contributors: **Satish R. Rao**
Carl J. Witkop, Jr.

844
838-500

PUNCTA AND CANALICULI, SUPERNUMERARY

Includes: Canalicules lacrymaux surnuméraires
Überzählige Tränenpunktchen und-gänge
Canalículos y orificios lacrimales supernumerarios
Diverticula of canaliculus
Canaliculi and puncta, supernumerary
Supernumerary puncta and canaliculi

Excludes: Lacrimal sac fistula (565)
Lacrimal sac fistula secondary to trauma

Minimal Diagnostic Criteria: Supernumerary puncta or canaliculi.†

Clinical Findings: The extra puncta and canaliculi usually are situated on the lower lid nasal to the normal structures but all combinations of placement have been recorded. More than 1 extra punctum and canaliculus may be present. They may end blindly, run independently to the lacrimal sac, or (more frequently) join with the normal canaliculus. Most are benign, a few become inflamed. Diverticula of the canaliculi without external opening are detected by xray with contrast media. Some cases of double puncta may represent side openings from a single canaliculus.

Complications
I **Derived:** Inflammation of the lacrimal passage is more frequent when malformations exist than in the normal patient.†
II **Associated:** Abnormalities of the orbital bones, colobomata of the lid and auricular deformation

Etiology: ? In 1 kindred it has displayed autosomal dominant transmission over 3 generations.

Pathogenesis: Irregular outbudding of the superior end of the ectodermal core which sinks into the mesoderm at the facial fissure.

Related Facts
I **Sex Ratio:** ?
II **Risk of Occurrence:** ?
III **Risk of Recurrence for**
    Patient's Sib: When autosomal dominant and if parent is affected, 1 in 2 (50%) for each offspring to be affected; otherwise not increased.
    Patient's Child: 1 in 2 when autosomal dominant
IV **Age of Detectability:** At birth
V **Prevalence:** Estimates vary from 1 in 60,000 eye cases to 1 in 800 eye cases. Since it is seldom looked for, the latter higher estimate is probably the better.

Treatment
I **Primary Prevention:** —
II **Secondary Prevention:** Surgical excision of the anomalous tract if symptoms arise
III **Other Therapy:** Topical and, if necessary, systemic antibiotics and hot compresses if inflammation occurs.

Prognosis: Normal life span. Repeated inflammation can be expected if it once occurs.

Detection of Carrier: ?

†**Special Considerations:** Blockage of the lacrimal passages into the nose should be searched for, if inflammation or epiphora occurs.

References:
Chignell, A.H.: Double punctum and canaliculus. Am. J. Ophthalmol. 65:736, 1968.
Duke-Elder, S.: System of Ophthalmology, vol. 3, pt. 2. Congenital Deformities. St. Louis: C.V. Mosby Co., 1963, p. 930.

Contributor: **Donald R. Bergsma**

PUPILLARY MEMBRANE PERSISTENCE

Includes: Persistance de la membrane pupillaire
Persistierende Pupillarmembran
Persistencia de la membrana pupilar
Anterior tunica vasculosa lentis persistence

Excludes: Mesodermal dysgenesis of anterior segment
Anterior capsular cataract

Minimal Diagnostic Criteria: Strands of iris with one or both ends attached to the iris collarette and usually crossing a portion of the pupil, most clearly seen with the slit lamp following dilatation.

Clinical Findings: A variety of tissue remnants in the pupillary space are found in 95% of newborns and lesser percentages in older age groups. These are usually asymptomatic. Most often the fine strands are attached to the iris collarette (lesser circle). Occasionally, hyperplasia of the iris stroma or imperforate pupil membrane results, but mostly iris-attached residues have no functional significance.

Less often strands attach to the anterior lens capsule at which point there may be a white plaque dense enough to require surgery. Isolated pigment splotches on the lens capsule also occur. Rarely, central anterior synechiae to the posterior cornea are the end result. When white opacities of the cornea are associated, the picture is not unlike mesodermal dysgenesis of the anterior segment.

Complications
I **Derived:** —
II **Associated:** Corneal and lenticular opacities

Etiology: A defect in embryogenesis of unknown cause for which a few pedigrees have been reported. Autosomal dominance was noted in one kindred which had persons in 4 generations with irregular tissue in the pupillary space. McK *17890

Pathogenesis: Failure of the normal process of atrophy of the pupillary arcades and associated mesodermal tissue

Related Facts
I **Sex Ratio:** M1:F1
II **Risk of Occurrence:** ?
III **Risk of Recurrence for**
   Patient's Sib: When autosomal dominant, and if parent is affected, 1 in 2 (50%) for each offspring to be affected; otherwise not increased.
   Patient's Child: When autosomal dominant, 1 in 2
IV **Age of Detectability:** At birth
V **Prevalence:** ?

Treatment
I **Primary Prevention:** —
II **Secondary Prevention:** —
III **Other Therapy:** —

Prognosis: Life span normal; excellent ocular prognosis

Detection of Carrier: —

Special Considerations: —

References:
Cassady, J.R. and Light, A.: Familial persistent pupillary membranes. Arch. Ophthalmol. 58:438-448, 1957.
Duke-Elder, S.: System of Ophthalmology, vol. 3, part 2. Congenital Deformities. London:Henry Kimpton, 1964, p. 775.

Contributor: **Harold E. Cross**

PYKNODYSOSTOSIS

Includes: Pycnodysostose
Pyknodysostose
Picnodisostosis
Pycnodysostosis

Excludes: Osteogenesis imperfecta (777)
Cleidocranial dysplasia† (185)
Osteopetrosis†

Minimal Diagnostic Criteria: Short stature, dysplasia of the skull, obtuse mandibular angle, dysplastic clavicles, partial or total aplasia of the terminal phalanges and generalized increased roentgenographic density of the skeleton.†

Clinical Findings: Short stature, usually less than 5 feet; craniofacial disproportion as a result of underdeveloped facial bones and prominence of the frontal and parietal bones; obtuse angle of the mandible; widening of the cranial sutures, persistence of the fontanels; delayed exfoliation of deciduous teeth; permanent teeth appear on schedule but may be malformed or malpositioned; narrow grooved palate; the clavicles are dysplastic with partial aplasia of the acromial ends; short terminal phalanges of the digits with wrinkling of the skin over the dorsal surfaces distally; flattened nails. Radiographic examination shows an increased density of bone of the entire skeleton, eg osteosclerosis; delayed closure of sutures, wormian bones, open fontanels, hypoplastic facial bones and sinuses, an obtuse mandibular angle and dental irregularities are present on skull film; there is tapering of the distal phalanges with absence of the ungual tufts; segmentation anomalies of the vertebrae; long bone deformities due to fractures may be present.

Complications
I   **Derived:** Due to increased bone density, fractures are common, occurring in approximately two-thirds of the patients. Persistent open fontanels and progressive loss in the distal phalanges and outer clavicles may occur.
II **Associated:** Mental retardation was observed in 6 of 33 cases. Kyphosis, scoliosis, increased lumbar lordosis and a narrow or deeply grooved chest have also been reported.

Etiology: Autosomal recessive inheritance is supported by consanguinity in 7 of 32 families and sibship occurrence from unaffected parents. X-linked recessive inheritance has been suggested in 1 family in which the maternal uncle of an affected male also had pyknodysostosis. McK *26580

Pathogenesis: ?

Related Facts
I   **Sex Ratio:** Of 33 cases reported M23:F10
II **Risk of Occurrence:** Very rare
III **Risk of Recurrence for**
    Patient's Sib: 1 in 4 (25%) for each offspring to be affected.
    Patient's Child: Not increased unless mate is carrier or homozygote.
IV **Age of Detectability:** Theoretically could be detected at birth; the diagnosis has been reported in a child 9 months old.
V   **Prevalence:** ?

Treatment
I   **Primary Prevention:** Genetic counseling
II **Secondary Prevention:** Special dental care and orthopedic management of any fractures
III **Other Therapy:** —

Prognosis: Normal life span

Detection of Carrier: —

†**Special Considerations:** In cleidocranial dysplasia there is normal bone density, normal distal phalanges, a normal mandibular angle and inheritance is autosomal dominant. Osteopetrosis is usually associated with some degree of anemia, hepatosplenomegaly, diminished or absent marrow space in the long bones and, often, deafness.

References:
Elmore, S.M.: Pycnodysostosis: A review. J. Bone Joint Surg. 49A:153, 1967.
Maroteaux, P. and Lamy, M.: La pycnodysostose. Presse Méd. 70:999, 1962.
Shuler, S.E.: Pycnodysostosis. Arch. Dis. Child. 38:620, 1963.
Spranger, J.W. et al: Bone Dysplasias. Philadelphia: W.B. Saunders, 1974.

Contributor: **Charles I. Scott, Jr.**

Editor's Computerized Descriptors: Face, Oral, Teeth, Skin, Nails, Skel.

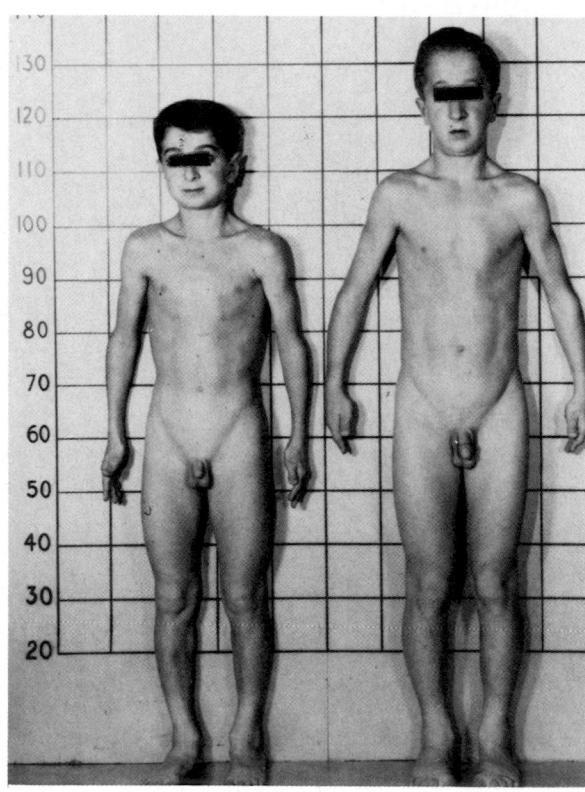

438. Pyknodysostosis in cousins

PYLE DISEASE

Includes: Dysplasie métaphysaire de Pyle
Mb. Pyle
Enfermedad de Pyle
Metaphyseal dysplasia, familial

Excludes: Craniometaphyseal dysplasia (228)
Craniodiaphyseal dysplasia (224)
Dysosteosclerosis (310)
Diaphyseal dysplasia (290)

Minimal Diagnostic Criteria: This disease can only be diagnosed on the basis of typical x-ray changes involving severe "Erlenmeyer flask" deformities of the tubular bone metaphyses with minimal changes in the skull.†

Clinical Findings: This disorder is characterized by marked flaring of the tubular bone metaphyses with few clinical signs. The major clinical characteristic of this disorder is genu valgum which develops early in life, and may hinder running. Muscular weakness and joint pain have also been observed and in a few patients there has been associated scoliosis, and mild limitation of extension at the elbows. The legs may be somewhat longer than average, but trunk length is normal. There is somewhat increased tendency to fracture long bones. Dental malocclusion may be present. Skeletal xrays reveal a marked, abrupt "Erlenmeyer flask" flare to the metaphyses of the tubular bones with diaphyseal endostosis. This lack of modeling of tubular bones is most marked in the long bones, but is also observed in the metacarpals and phalanges as a mild flaring of the ends of the bones. The ribs, clavicles, pubic and ischial bones are widened. The vertebrae are usually normal, but mild platyspondyly may be seen. The skull is only mildly involved with a supraorbital bulge and perhaps mild hyperostosis of the calvarium. The mandible has a rounded obtuse angle and there may be mild prognathism.

Complications
I **Derived:** Genu valgum may produce difficulty in running; dental malocclusion; occasional muscular weakness and joint pain.
II **Associated:** —

Etiology: Autosomal recessive; McK *26590

Pathogenesis: The most likely pathogenetic mechanism in this disorder is a lack of resorption of secondary spongiosa.

Related Facts
I **Sex Ratio:** M1:F1
II **Risk of Occurrence:** ?
III **Risk of Recurrence for**
 Patient's Sib: 1 in 4 (25%) for each offspring to be affected
 Patient's Child: Not increased unless mate is carrier or homozygote
IV **Age of Detectability:** This disorder is usually detected by chance radiographic observation. The metaphyseal flaring may be seen in early childhood.
V **Prevalence:** ?

Treatment
I **Primary Prevention:** Genetic counseling
II **Secondary Prevention:** Orthopedic surgical procedures may be performed for genu valgum, but this is usually unnecessary.
III **Other Therapy:** —

Prognosis: Normal for life span

Detection of Carrier: ?

†**Special Considerations:** This disease is associated with marked changes in the metaphyses of the long bones with little or no changes in the cranium. Although the term "Pyle disease" has been used for the various forms of craniometaphyseal dyplasia, it should be restricted to this autosomal recessive disorder with minimal cranial changes.

References:
Bakwin, H. and Krida, A.: Familial metaphyseal dysplasia. Am. J. Dis Child. 53:1521, 1937.
Feld, H. et al: Familial metaphyseal dysplasia. Radiology 65:206, 1955.
Gorlin, R.J., et al: Genetic craniotubular bone dysplasias and hyperostoses-a critical analysis. In Bergsma, D. (ed.): Part IV. Skeletal Dysplasias. Birth Defects: Orig. Art. Ser., vol. V, no. 4. New York: The National Foundation-March of Dimes, 1969, p. 79.

Contributors: **David L. Rimoin**
David W. Hollister

Editor's Computerized Descriptors: Eye, Face, Teeth, Skel., Muscle

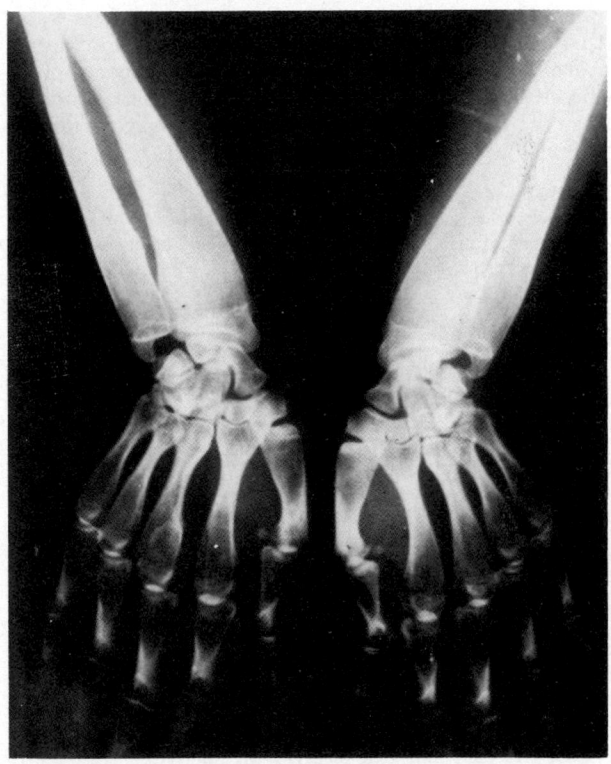

439. Distal portions of radius, ulna and metacarpals 2–4 are splayed; 1st metacarpals and phalanges show splaying of proximal portions

PYLORIC STENOSIS

Includes: Sténose du pylore
Pylorusstenose
Estenosis pilórica
Hypertrophic pyloric stenosis
Congenital hypertrophic pyloric stenosis

Excludes: Pylorospasm

Minimal Diagnostic Criteria: Nonbilious vomiting and pyloric hypertrophy identified by palpation or roentgen examination.

Clinical Findings: Nonbilious projectile vomiting characteristically beginning at 2-3 weeks of age progresses to almost complete gastric outlet obstruction associated with constipation, weight loss, dehydration, and electrolyte imbalance (hypokalemic alkalasia). Eagerness to nurse after vomiting is common. Visible gastric peristaltic waves proceed from left to right following feeding. The thickened hypertrophied muscular pylorus can be palpated in the epigastrium as an olive-sized and shaped movable mass or "tumor." Contrast roentgen studies (using barium-water mixture) identify an elongated, curved, pyloric channel with proximal and distal protrusion of the hypertrophied pyloric musculature into the duodenal and gastric lumena to cause the so-called "shoulder" sign. Delayed gastric emptying is not a valid specific diagnostic sign.

Complications
I **Derived:** Starvation, dehydration, and severe electrolyte imbalance, jaundice, (unusual, less than 3%) indirect bilirubin predominates, hematemesis
II **Associated:** —

Etiology: Probably polygenic and sex modified†

Pathogenesis: The edematous, hypertrophy of the circular (and some longitudinal) musculature of the pylorus is progressive to some extent. Variations in mucosal edema account for changes in the degree of obstruction.

Related Facts
I **Sex Ratio:** M4:F1
II **Risk of Occurrence:** 1 in 250 births (1 in 200 males; 1 in 1000 females) highest in Caucasians, uncommon in non-Caucasians, rare in Asiatics, especially Chinese.
III **Risk of Recurrence for**
    Patient's Sib: If mother was affected, 1 in 5 (20%) for brothers and 1 in 14 (7%) for sisters. If father was affected, 1 in 20 (5%) for brothers and 1 in 40 (21/2 %) for sisters.
    Patient's Child: If patient is female, 1 in 5 (20%) for sons and 1 in 14 (7%) for daughters. If patient is male, 1 in 20 (5%) for sons and 1 in 40 (21/2 %) for daughters.
IV **Age of Detectability:** Usually 2-4 weeks of age
V **Prevalence:** 1 in 250 infants; the most common problem requiring abdominal surgery in infancy.

Treatment
I **Primary Prevention:** —
II **Secondary Prevention:** Laparotomy and Ramstedt pyloromyotomy are curative.
III **Other Therapy:** Nonsurgical treatment with antispasmodics is generally unsatisfactory.

Prognosis: Excellent. Following pyloromyotomy symptoms vanish and the pyloric hypertrophy disappears. Some evidence suggests that these patients have a higher incidence of peptic ulcer in later life.

Detection of Carrier: —

†**Special Considerations:** In this defect it is improbable that a single mutant gene makes a major contribution to the genetic liability.

References:
Benson, C.D.: Infantile hypertrophic pyloric stenosis. In Mustard, W.T. et al (eds.): Pediatric Surgery. 2nd Ed. Year Book Medical Publishers, 1969. vol. 2, p. 818.
Carter, C.O. and Evans, K.A.: Inheritance of congenital pyloric stenosis. J. Med. Genet. 6:233, 1969.
Rickham, P.P.: Congenital hypertrophic pyloric stenosis. In Rickham, P.P. et al (eds.): Neonatal Surgery. New York:Appleton-Century Crofts, 1969, p. 271.
Scharli, A. et al: Hypertrophic pyloric stenosis at the Children's Hospital of Pittsburgh from 1912 to 1967: A critical review of current problems and complications. J. Pediatr. Surg. 4:108, 1969.

Contributor: **William K. Sieber**

Editor's Computerized Descriptor: GI.

PYROGLUTAMIC ACIDEMIA

Includes: Acidémie pyroglutamique
Pyroglutar-Azidämie
Acidemia piroglutámica
5-oxoprolinuria
Glutathione synthetase deficiency

Excludes: Prolinemia, types I and II
Erythrocyte γ-glutamylcysteine synthetase deficiency?
Glutathionuria (422)

Minimal Diagnostic Criteria: The finding of large amounts of pyroglutamic acid (5-oxoproline) in the urine.

Clinical Findings: Onset early in life. The 3 patients described have shown variable signs and symptoms. Severe metabolic acidosis and episodes of hemolytic anemia with no mental retardation were seen in 2 children. The 3rd (adult) patient had an episode of jaundice in the newborn period, but has since had no signs of hemolytic anemia. However, he has severe metabolic acidosis, is mentally retarded, has cerebellar ataxia, and epileptogenic seizures. He has frequent episodes of vomiting in spite of surgical correction of his esophageal hiatus hernia. His clinical condition has gradually deteriorated over the last 5 years, and he is now institutionalized.

Plasma concentrations of pyroglutamic acid are usually about 50 mg/100 ml (4 mmole/l), and the urinary excretion of the metabolite is about 0.5 gm (4 mmole)/kg body weight/24 hours. The urinary excretion of urea is only one-third of the normal. The concentration of potassium in serum is reduced. The erythrocyte glutathione level is less than 0.001 μmole/gm of wet cells, and the glutathione content of muscle tissue is about 0.04 μmole/gm wet weight (3% of the normal). The amino acid content of the erythrocytes is reported to be increased by a factor of 20-100. The enzyme glutathione synthetase is deficient, with erythrocyte and tissue activities less than 3% of the normal. The pattern of amino acids in serum and CSF are normal, except for elevation of proline (3 times normal) in the adult patient.

Complications
I   Derived: Metabolic acidosis
II Associated: Hemolytic anemia, mental retardation, cerebellar ataxia.

Etiology: Probably autosomal recessive; McK *26613

Pathogenesis: All patients described to date have a defect in the ability to synthesize glutathione synthetase. The last enzyme needed in the glutathione pathway, catalyzing the conversion of γ-glutamylcysteine to glutathione, is deficient. Production of pyroglutamic acid is most likely secondary to the glutathione synthetase deficiency.

Related Facts
I   Sex Ratio: M1:F1
II Risk of Occurrence: ?
III Risk of Recurrence for
   Patient's Sib: 1 in 4 (25%) for each offspring to be affected, if autosomal recessive.
   Patient's Child: Not increased unless mate is carrier or homozygote.
IV Age of Detectability: Neonatal period to adult years by detection of elevated amounts of pyroglutamic acid in the urine; or metabolic acidosis (acid-base status) and reduced excretion of urea in the urine.
V   Prevalence: ?

Treatment
I   Primary Prevention: Genetic counseling

II Secondary Prevention: Treatment with bicarbonate to compensate for the metabolic acidosis. The patients should not be exposed to amino acids intravenously, and should not be given large amounts of ascorbic acid or drugs known to precipitate hemolysis.
III Other Therapy: —

Prognosis: The 3 patients detected to date are still alive. The children are behaving well on bicarbonate treatment, the adult patient is now 24 years old. Due to the gradually increasing neurologic symptoms he is now institutionalized.

Detection of Carrier: Fibroblast culture experiments by assay of glutathione synthetase activity in parents.

Special Considerations: —

References:
Eldjarn, L. et al: Pyroglutamic aciduria: Rate of formation and degradation of pyroglutamate. Clin. Chim. Acta 49:311, 1973.
Eldjarn, L. et al: Pyroglutamic acidemia. In Nyhan, W.L. (ed.): Heritable Disorders of Amino Acid Metabolism. New York: John Wiley & Sons, 1974, p. 479.
Hagenfeldt, L. et al: Pyroglutamic aciduria. Acta Paediatr. Scand. 63:1, 1974.
Jellum E. et al: Pyroglutamic aciduria-A new inborn error of metabolism. Scand. J. Clin. Lab. Invest. 26:327, 1970.
Larsson, A. et al: Pyroglutamic aciduria (5-oxoprolinuria) an inborn error in glutathione metabolism. Pediatr. Res. 8:852, 1974.
Marstein, S. et al: Biochemical studies of erythrocytes in a patient with pyroglutamic acidemia. N. Engl. J. Med. 295:406, 1976.
Wellen, W.P. et al: Glutathione synthetase deficiency, an inborn error of metabolism involving the γ-glutamyl cycle in patients with 5-oxoprolinuria (pyroglutamic aciduria). Proc. Natl. Acad. Sci. USA 71:2505, 1974.

Contributors: **Egil Jellum**
                   Oddvar Stokke
                   Lorentz Eldjarn

Editor's Computerized Descriptor: —

PYRUVATE CARBOXYLASE DEFICIENCY WITH LACTIC ACIDEMIA

Includes: Déficit en pyruvate carboxylase avec acidémie lactique
Pyruvatkarboxylase-Mangel mit Laktatacidämie
Deficiencia de piruvato carboxilasa con acidemia láctica
Lactic acidemia without hypoxemia

Excludes: Pyruvate dehydrogenase deficiency (851)
Fructose-1-phosphate aldolase deficiency (395)
Fructose-1,6-diphosphatase deficiency (396)
Myopathy with lactic acidemia (697)
Lactate elevation secondary to other causes

Minimal Diagnostic Criteria: Neurologic deterioration with lactic and pyruvic acidemia.

Clinical Findings: Most patients have appeared normal at birth and during infancy, but development has tended to be slow. More serious difficulties have become apparent by 1 year of age. Abnormalities have included "failure to thrive," vomiting, irritability, apathy, inactivity, hypotonia, areflexia, spasticity, cerebellar ataxia, abnormal eye movements, and seizures. The course has usually been progressive with neurologic and intellectual deterioration and death within several years. Some of the children have been considered to have subacute necrotizing encephalomyelopathy (Leigh syndrome).

Lactate, pyruvate, and alanine are elevated on most occasions and the lactate/pyruvate ratio is usually in the normal range. Lactates as high as 100 mg/dl have caused chronic metabolic acidosis, while other patients have had levels in the range of 20-40 mg/dl. EEG abnormalities have occurred in some of the patients. Pyruvate carboxylase activity has been decreased or absent on liver biopsy specimens.†

Complications
I   **Derived:** Neurologic and intellectual deterioration and death in most instances.
II **Associated:** —

Etiology: Probably autosomal recessive; McK *26615

Pathogenesis: Pyruvate carboxylase is important both in gluconeogenesis and in maintaining adequate levels of oxaloacetate to support full activity of the tricarboxylic acid cycle. Hypoglycemia has not been a prominent part of the clinical picture in most patients.

Related Facts
I   **Sex Ratio:** M1:F1
II   **Risk of Occurrence:** ?
III **Risk of Recurrence for**
     Patient's Sib: 1 in 4 (25%)
     Patient's Child: None have survived to procreate
IV   **Age of Detectability:** Earliest diagnoses were made within the first several months. Lactate and pyruvate theoretically should be elevated within the 1st week of life. Diagnosis is confirmed by liver biopsy.
V   **Prevalence:** ?

Treatment
I   **Primary Prevention:** Genetic counseling
II   **Secondary Prevention:** Thiamine, lipoic acid, glutamine, and aspartic acid in pharmacologic doses have all been reported to be helpful in reducing lactate and pyruvate levels and mitigating the symptoms and their rate of progression.
III **Other Therapy:** —

Prognosis: Poor. Death usually occurs within several years.

Detection of Carrier: Reliable methods have not been reported.

†Special Considerations: The signs and symptoms of this disorder are nonspecific and inconsistent. Primary suspicion is caused by elevated lactate, pyruvate, or alanine, and the diagnosis must be confirmed by liver biopsy. It cannot be readily distinguished from pyruvate dehydrogenase deficiency (QV) on clinical or biochemical grounds alone. The assay for pyruvate carboxylase is reported to be difficult and is best performed in a laboratory with experience in the methodology.

Lactic acidemia is defined by the presence of a blood lactate in excess of 15 mg/dl and becomes lactic acidosis when compensatory mechanisms no longer are able to maintain the arterial pH in the normal range. Lactate exists in equilibrium with pyruvate and with alanine. The NADH/NAD ratio reflects the ratio of lactate to pyruvate. In some instances, the L/P ratio provides a clue to the nature of the primary metabolic error. Blood drawn from the external jugular vein of a child may have artifactually elevated levels of lactate and pyruvate.

Elevation of blood lactate is a laboratory abnormality which may be due to a variety of inherited and acquired conditions. Within each entity, the severity may vary with the nature and degree of the enzyme deficiency.

Because lactate and pyruvate are readily measured in most clinical laboratories, elevations in these compounds may be detected in cases of acidosis, even though the primary cause of the acidosis may be an entirely different disorder. Conversely, significant elevations in both lactate and pyruvate may cause no obvious alteration in plasma bicarbonate and thus be overlooked entirely.

The assessment of patients with elevations of lactate must include measurement of the lactate/pyruvate ratio, urinary lactate excretion, urinary ketone excretion, association between lactate and pyruvate levels and meals, blood sugar measurement in the fasting and postprandial state, a history for the sensitivity to dietary factors or minor environmental stress and efforts to determine the possible involvement of other organic acids in cases of acidosis. High levels of pyruvate may cause an apparent false-positive test for ketones when using a commercial nitroprusside reagent (acetest, Ames).

In a decreasing but still significant number of patients with an apparently primary elevation of lactate and pyruvate, no definite enzymatic diagnosis is made. In these instances, some people use empiric dietary therapy or pharmacologic doses of thiamine, biotin or lipoic acid. False-positive and nonspecific chemical responses to thiamine have been reported.

In most cases in which no enzymatic diagnosis is made, it is most prudent to assume that the inheritance is autosomal recessive. Exceptions include those instances of a similar disease in a parent or those cases of primary myopathy in which autosomal dominant or other inheritance mechanisms may be operating.

References:
DeGroot, C.J. and Hommes, F.A.: Further speculation on the pathogeneis of Liegh's encephalomyelopathy. J. Pediatr. 82:541, 1973.
Tada, K. et al: Hyperalaninemia with pyruvicemia in a patient suggestive of Leigh's encephalomyelopathy. Tohoku J. exp. Med. 109:13, 1973.
Tang, T.T. et al: Pathogenesis of Leigh's encephalomyelopathy. J. Pediatr. 81:189, 1972.

Contributors: **Stephen D. Cederbaum**
John P. Blass

Editor's Computerized Descriptors: Eye, Muscle, GI., Nerve

PYRUVATE DEHYDROGENASE DEFICIENCY

Includes: Déficience en pyruvate déshydrogénase
Pyruvat-Dehydrogenase-Mangel
Deficiencia de piruvato deshidrogenasa
Lactic and pyruvic acidemia with carbohydrate sensitivity
Lactic and pyruvic acidemia with episodic ataxia and weakness
Alaninuria

Excludes: Lactic and pyruvic acidemia due to other causes
Lactic acidosis due to fructose-1, 6-diphosphatase deficiency
Lactic acidosis with persistently increased lactate: pyruvate ratio

Minimal Diagnostic Criteria: Persistent or recurrent pyruvic acidemia; enzyme deficiency must be confirmed using skin fibroblasts or other tissue.

Clinical Findings: May vary from severe acidosis appearing in the 1st few days of life to recurrent episodes of ataxia and weakness following upper respiratory infection or other minor stress. Growth retardation has been frequent. Varying permanent neurologic deficits and mental retardation have been seen in most patients. Near normal resting levels of lactate and pyruvate have been associated with severe neurologic damage in several patients.

Biochemical findings vary from severe lactic acidosis appearing shortly after birth to minimal pyruvic acidemia (1.5-1.8mg/dl; n1 < 1.2) 2 hours following a meal high in carbohydrate. In some instances elevation of blood pyruvate levels is seen only during the acute episodes of ataxia and weakness. The blood lactate:pyruvate ratio has almost always been normal (< 20). Alanine excretion of greater than 100mg/gm creatine is a variable finding and often is present only during acute episodes. Blood alanine has been elevated above 6mg/dl only with pyruvate values persistently greater then 2.0 mg/dl. CSF pyruvate and lactate also have been elevated. Increased lactate in the urine (> 0.7 mg/mg creatine) is seen when blood lactate is 2-4 times normal.

Complications
I **Derived:** Mental retardation, neurologic damage; in some instances early death from lactic acidosis.
II **Associated:** —

Etiology: Autosomal recessive; McK *20880

Pathogenesis: Defective oxidation of pyruvate and deficiency of pyruvate dehydrogenase have been demonstrated in cultured skin fibroblasts. Increased dietary carbohydrates typically precipitate lactic acidosis in the more severely affected patients.

Related Facts
I **Sex Ratio:** Males predominate thus far. 1:1 expected.
II **Risk of Occurrence:** ?
III **Risk of Recurrence for**
    Patient's Sib: 1 in 4 (25%) for each offspring to be affected.
    Patient's Child: Not increased unless mate is carrier or homozygote.
IV **Age of Detectability:** Shortly after birth by skin fibroblast assay. Age at which pyruvate and lactate elevation is detected will probably depend on the nature and severity of the biochemical defect.
V **Prevalence:** ?

Treatment
I **Primary Prevention:** Genetic counseling.
II **Secondary Prevention:** The disorder is exacerbated by increased carbohydrate intake and improved by increased dietary fat. Avoidance of infection and undue stress is desirable. High doses of thiamine have not been proved to be of benefit.†
III **Other Therapy:** Corticosteriod therapy has been reported to

abort the acute episodes of ataxia and weakness in several instances.

Prognosis: In most instances irreversible neurologic damage and mental retardation have occurred by the time of diagnosis. The impact of a high fat diet instituted at an early age has not been assessed. The ultimate risk of permanent neurologic handicap to those patients with only episodic symptoms is unknown.

Detection of Carrier: Skin fibroblasts. Discrimination incomplete.

†Special Considerations: Blood pyruvate levels have always been abnormal following a meal high in carbohydrate. The long-term-impact of a high fat diet has not been determined. Dietary trial for pyruvic and lactic acidemia should be undertaken with care, since other causes of pyruvic acidemia may lead to carbohydrate dependence.

References:
Blass, J.P. et al: A defect in pyruvate decarboxylase in a child with an intermittent movement disorder. J. Clin. Invest. 49:423, 1970.
Blass, J.P. et al: Clinical and metabolic abnormalities accompanying deficiencies in pyruvate oxidation. In Hommes, F.A. and VandenBerg, C.J. (eds.): Normal and Pathological Development of Energy Metabolism. New York: Academic Press, 1975, p. 193.
Cederbaum, S.D. et al: Sensitivity to carbohydrate in a patient with familial intermittent lactic acidosis and pyruvate dehydrogenase deficiency. Pediatr. Res. 10:713, 1976.
Falk, R.E. et al: Ketonic diet in the treatment of pyruvate dehydrogenase deficiency. Pediatrics, 58:713, 1976.

Contributors: **Stephen D. Cederbaum**
John P. Blass

Editor's Computerized Descriptors: Muscle, Nerve

PYRUVATE KINASE DEFICIENCY

Includes: Déficit en pyruvate-kinase
Pyruvatkinasemangel
Deficiencia en piruvato quinasa
Congenital nonspherocytic hemolytic anemias associated with diminished activity or kinetic abnormalities of erythrocyte pyruvate kinase

Excludes: Congenital nonspherocytic hemolytic anemias associated with deficiencies of other enzymes, or with unstable hemoglobin, or of unknown cause

Minimal Diagnostic Criteria: Hemolytic anemia with reticulocytosis. No specific abnormality of erythrocyte morphology. Increased autohemolysis of affected erythrocytes in vitro usually demonstrable, usually uncorrected by glucose but corrected by ATP. Erythrocyte 23DPG levels are unusually high, in severely anemic patients reaching levels greater than 3 times normal. Erythrocyte pyruvate kinase activity reduced, usually to 5-20% of normal. Occasionally, maximal pyruvate kinase activity normal but enzyme catalytically inefficient at low substrate (phospho-enol-pyruvate) concentrations.

Clinical Findings: Signs of excessive hemolysis of varying grades of severity in different patients and changing from time to time: chronic hemolytic anemia, hyperbilirubinemia, splenomegaly, reticulocytosis.

Complications
I **Derived:** Gallstones secondary to chronic hyperbilirubinemia. Exacerbations of anemia resulting from transient marrow erythroid hypoplasia, usually associated with infections. Leg ulcers, rarely.
II **Associated:** Leukocyte pyruvate kinase normal but liver pyruvate kinase activity may be reduced.

Etiology: Autosomal recessive; McK *26620

Pathogenesis: The sequence of events preceding hemolysis of pyruvate kinase deficient erythrocytes is poorly understood. Deficient erythrocytes usually have low glycolytic rates in vitro (particularly when compared to control erythrocytes of similar age) and are unable to maintain intracellular ATP levels. However, in vivo erythrocyte ATP levels may be normal. Nevertheless, ATP depletion as a result of inadequate glycolysis is thought to be the central event resulting in premature hemolysis. The almost immediate destruction of a portion of newly formed reticulocytes in the spleen or elsewhere in the reticuloendothelial system contributes importantly to the observed hemolysis. Molecular variants of erythrocyte pyruvate kinase have been characterized by their abnormal substrate kinetics, but no detailed studies of molecular structure are as yet available. The low activity variant has normal substrate kinetics indicating that diminished synthesis of the enzyme, a structural alteration, or a combination of both may be the basic defect.†

Related Facts
I **Sex Ratio:** M1:F1
II **Risk of Occurrence:** Unknown but low
III **Risk of Recurrence for**
 Patient's Sib: 1 in 4 (25%) for each offspring to be affected
 Patient's Child: None unless mate is carrier or homozygote
IV **Age of Detectability:** At birth (assay of erythrocyte pyruvate kinase).
V **Prevalence:** Rare. Most affected individuals thus far described have been of European origin.

Treatment
I **Primary Prevention:** Genetic counseling
II **Secondary Prevention:** Splenectomy reduces or eliminates the need for blood transfusions in severely anemic patients but is not curative. Anemia persists, but usually a higher hemoglobin level can be maintained.† Postsplenectomy reticulocyte counts usually rise rather than fall and may occasionally exceed 90%.
III **Other Therapy:** Supportive blood transfusions. Cholecystectomy if gallstones form.

Prognosis: Varies with severity of anemia (eg high mortality in early childhood described in unsplenectomized Amish kindred). Most patients survive to adulthood and mildly anemic patients may expect to have a near-normal life span unless complications (eg gallstones) supervene.

Detection of Carrier: Carriers are clinically and hematologically normal, but their erythrocyte pyruvate kinase activity is usually half that found in normals. Alternatively, carriers may have normal enzyme activity but abnormal substrate kinetics (altered Km PEP).

†**Special Considerations:** Pyruvate kinase deficient reticulocytes are protected from the consequences of their glycolytic defect by the availability of alternate metabolic pathways (oxidative phosphorylation).
Oxidative phosphorylation in such reticulocytes may be inhibited during sequestration in hypoxic, acidic regions of the spleen whereupon glycolysis alone is inadequate to support their increased ATP requirements. The result is ATP depletion which induces a membrane lesion characterized by massive prelytic loss of intracellular potassium and water, cell shrinkage, and increased cell rigidity. The shrunken rigid cell produced is presumed to be susceptible to further sequestration because of difficulty in traversing the 3 micron pores separating splenic cords from sinuses. Eventually, cell lysis occurs. Splenectomy, by removal of a stagnant, hypoxic trap, allows reticulocytes to survive and partially alleviates the anemia.

References:
Keitt, A. S.: Pyruvate kinase deficiency and related disorders of red cell glycolysis. Am. J. Med. 41:762, 1966.
Mentzer, W.C., Jr.: Pyruvate kinase deficiency and disorders of glycolysis. In Nathan, D.G. and Oski, F.A. (eds.): Hematology of Infancy and Childhood. Philadelphia: W.B. Saunders Co., 1974, p. 315.
Tanaka, K.R. and Paglia, D.E.: Pyruvate kinase deficiency. Semin. Hematol. 8:367, 1971.

Contributors: **William C. Mentzer, Jr.**
Louis K. Diamond

Editor's Computerized Descriptor: GI.

RADIAL DEFECTS

Includes: Aplasie radiale
Radius defekte
Defectos del radio
Radial hemimelia
Deficient radial rays and phocomelia
Radial aplasia
Radial dysplasia

Excludes: Heart-hand syndrome (455)
Fanconi anemia
Thrombocytopenia with absent radius (941)
Fetal thalidomide syndrome (386)
Radial dysplasia - craniosynostosis syndrome
Aplasia of the radius and cleft lip syndrome
Ventriculoradial dysplasia
Vater association (987)

Minimal Diagnostic Criteria: Hypoplasia of the thumb or 1st metacarpal in the absence of other malformations.

Clinical Findings: Several degrees of severity occur. In the mildest form, there is hypoplasia of the 1st metacarpal often combined with hypoplasia of the thumb. With increasing severity, there is complete loss of the 1st metacarpal producing a small flail thumb attached to the index finger by soft tissue. The next level of severity is characterized by hypoplasia or aplasia of the radius associated with varying degrees of thumb and 1st metacarpal hypoplasia. Both the radius and ulna are absent in the most severe form which is associated with variable radial ray abnormalities and often hypoplasia of the humerus. Approximately 20% of all affected individuals have radial defects alone, of which about two-thirds are unilateral.

Complications
I **Derived:** Dysfunction of upper limbs related to severity of malformation.
II **Associated:** —

Etiology: If all cases of radial defects with associated anomalies are excluded, most cases are sporadic.†

Pathogenesis: Suppression of developing limb structures.

Related Facts
I **Sex Ratio:** M1:F1
II **Risk of Occurrence:** ? Very low
III **Risk of Recurrence for**
  Patient's Sib: ? Probably very low
  Patient's Child: ? Probably very low
IV **Age of Detectability:** At birth
V **Prevalence:** ?

Treatment
I **Primary Prevention:** —
II **Secondary Prevention:** Surgery may improve function in certain cases.
III **Other Therapy:** —

Prognosis: Normal for intelligence and life span. Dysfunction is related to severity of deformity.

Detection of Carrier: —

†Special Considerations: For accurate genetic counseling as well as proper treatment, it is important to exclude the many complex syndromes in which radial defects occur. (See Exclusions above.) In particular, the cardiovascular, GU, and hematologic systems should be carefully examined. Although families have been reported showing autosomal dominant inheritance of isolated radial defects, it is very difficult to completely rule out the more complex syndromes, ie heart and hand syndrome with only minor heart manifestations.

References:
Carroll, R.E. and Louis, D.S.: Anomalies associated with radial dysplasia. J. Pediatr. 84:409, 1974.
Temtamy, S.A.: On anomalies associated with radial dysplasia. J. Pediatr. 85:585, 1974.
Temtamy, S. A. and McKusick, V. A.: Synopsis of hand malformations with particular emphasis on genetic factors. In Bergsma, D. (ed.): Part III. Limb Malformations. Birth Defects: Orig. Art. Ser., vol. 5, no. 3. New York:The National Foundation-March of Dimes, 1969, p. 125.

Contributor: **William A. Horton**

Editor's Computerized Descriptor: Skel.

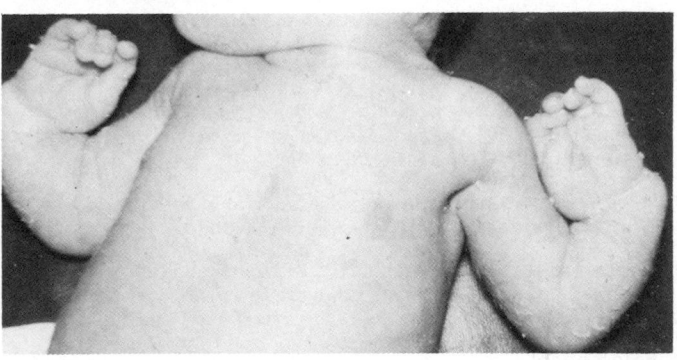

440. Bilateral radial aplasia

RADIOULNAR SYNOSTOSIS

Includes: Synostose radiale cubitale
Radio-ulno-Synostose
Sinostosis radial cubital
Congenital pronation

Excludes: Humeroradial synostosis (477)
Synostosis secondary to injury

Minimal Diagnostic Criteria: Restriction of motion of the elbow and characteristic radiographic appearance.

Clinical Findings: Restriction of pronation-supination movement to less than half of normal range, often fixed in pronation. Some cases show mild limitation of extension and flexion at the elbow. Radiographs show synostosis at the proximal ends of the radius and ulna. Bilateral in more than 80%.

Complications
I   **Derived:**   Restriction of pronation-supination
II **Associated:** Clubfoot, congenital dislocated hip, hand malformation and exostoses

Etiology: Autosomal dominant; also associated with the 48,XXXY syndrome, and other syndromes. McK *17930

Pathogenesis: Unknown; there is atrophy and fibrosis of the supinator muscles as well as pronator teres and pronator quadratus. The interosseous membrane is thickened and tight.

Related Facts
I   **Sex Ratio:**   M1:F1
II   **Risk of Occurrence:**   Rare
III **Risk of Recurrence for**
    Patient's Sib: If parent is affected with hereditary form 1 in 2 (50%) for each offspring to be affected; otherwise not increased.
    Patient's Child: 1 in 2, if simply inherited form
IV **Age of Detectability:** At birth, by examination and xray
V   **Prevalence:** Rare

Treatment
I   **Primary Prevention:** Genetic counseling
II   **Secondary Prevention:** Surgery does not restore active pronation-supination but can be used to put the forearm in a fixed position more favorable for hand function.†
III **Other Therapy:** Not needed

Prognosis: Normal life span

Detection of Carrier: —

†**Special Considerations:** Surgical release of the fusion between ulna and radius may increase passive range of motion, but active pronation-supination is rarely improved, probably due to the effect of the synostosis on the forearm muscle development.

References:
Davenport, C. B. et al: Radio-ulnar synostosis. Arch. Surg. 8:705, 1924.
Hansen, O. H. and Anderson, N. O.: Congenital radio-ulnar synostosis. Report of 37 cases. Acta Orthop. Scand. 41:225, 1970.

Contributor: **Robert A. Norum**

Editor's Computerized Descriptor: Skel.

REIFENSTEIN SYNDROME

Includes: Syndrome de Reifenstein
Síndrome de Reifenstein
Some cases of incomplete androgen insensitivity syndrome

Excludes: Hypospadias (518)
Chromosome 45,X/46,XY mosaicism (173)
Adrenal lipoid hyperplasia
Pseudovaginal perineoscrotal hypospadias (831)
3β-ol dehydrogenase deficiency
Steroid 17α-hydroxylase deficiency (903)
Steroid 17,20-desmolase deficiency (904)
17-ketosteroid reductase deficiency
Androgen insensitivity syndrome, complete (49)

Minimal Diagnostic Criteria: Historically, a diagnosis of the Reifenstein syndrome has been limited to 46,XY individuals with small testes, elevated plasma FSH and LH as adults, perineoscrotal hypospadias involving a phallus of nearly normal size, and the lack of virilization at puberty, usually with gynecomastia.†

Clinical Findings: The term Reifenstein syndrome has been employed since its first description to delineate an intersex state in which 46,XY individuals have small testes and a phallus of relatively normal size but with perineoscrotal hypospadias. No other vaginal or vagina-like orifice exists, although the scrotum may be bifid. Affected adults do not have a facial beard, and in such patients lowering of the voice and temporal hair recession do not occur. Gynecomastia may occur, but the amount of parenchymal tissue is much less than that in the complete or in most other cases of the incomplete androgen insensitivity syndrome. Somatic anomalies are absent. The testes may be located in the scrotum or in the inguinal canals, and have been characterized by 1) Leydig cell hyperplasia, 2) small atrophic, hyalinized seminiferous tubules and 3) interstitial fibrosis. Spermatogenesis may be demonstrable. Epididymides, vasa deferentia and seminal vesicles may or may not be present. Lack of virilization at puberty has in the past been attributed to inadequate testosterone synthesis. However, recent evidence indicates that in some, and possibly in all, cases the failure of virilization is due not to decreased testosterone synthesis but instead to decreased sensitivity to androgens.

Complications
I   **Derived:** Misassignment of sex; complications of hypoandrogenism; sterility; psychologic problems.
II **Associated:** Possibility of gonadal neoplasia, but this appears to be rare.

Etiology: Probably an X-linked recessive mutant gene, or, less likely, a male sex-limited autosomal dominant mutant gene.

Pathogenesis: Although previous reports have indicated that the incomplete virilization in 46,XY patients with the Reifenstein syndrome was the result of a defect in testosterone biosynthesis, or that the cause was unknown, recent evidence indicates otherwise. Wilson et al recently investigated 1 of the families previously reported as the Reifenstein syndrome by Bowen et al. Two important points were noted: 1) within that 1 family, the degree of deficient masculinization varied among those affected, and 2) the responsible pathogenetic mechanism was not a defect in testosterone biosynthesis but rather hyposensitivity to androgen. Furthermore, Griffin et al have demonstrated deficient dihydrotestosterone binding to cultured genital skin fibroblasts from 3 patients of the family reported by Wilson. Other patients (and families) previously described as having the Reifenstein syndrome have not been so extensively investigated; however, in those families in which multiple members are affected and in which an X-linked recessive mode of inheritance is operative, the pathogenesis will also probably be found to involve androgen hyposensitivity. The pathogenesis in sporadic cases will probably be heterogeneous, since the description of the Reifenstein syndrome is based on clinical phenotype.

For further information on pathogenesis, the reader is referred to the discussion of the Androgen Insensitivity Syndrome, Incomplete.

Related Facts
I **Sex Ratio:** M1:F0
II **Risk of Occurrence:** ? but relatively rare
III **Risk of Recurrence for**
  Patient's Sib: 1 in 2 (50%) for 46,XY sib to be affected; 1 in 4 (25%) for all sibs, assuming mother is heterozygous for X-linked recessive mutant allele.
  Patient's Child: No patient has ever reproduced.
IV **Age of Detectability:** Genital anomalies are apparent at birth, and diagnosis of androgen insensitivity can be proven by proper diagnostic studies. If diagnosis is delayed, hypoandrogenism will again become apparent at puberty.
V **Prevalence:** ? But rare

Treatment
I **Primary Prevention:** Genetic counseling, possibly intrauterine diagnosis (see discussion of Androgen Insensitivity Syndrome, Incomplete).
II **Secondary Prevention:** Depends on sex of rearing. If diagnosis is made in early infancy, a female sex assignment may in some cases be appropriate. In that instance, surgical reconstruction of the external genitalia, gonadectomy and creation of a vaginal opening are in order. Estrogen substitution therapy will be necessary beginning in the 2nd decade of life.
  A male sex assignment, on the other hand, must be followed by surgical reconstruction of the external genitalia to produce a functional penis and may involve orchidopexy. Androgen administration may be necessary beginning in adolescence.
III **Other Therapy:** —

Prognosis: Presumably normal life span provided neoplastic transformation of gonads does not supervene. All patients reported to date have been infertile.

Detection of Carrier: So far not accomplished. However, if the genetic mode is X-linked recessive, it may be feasible in familial cases to demonstrate androgen hyposensitivity (deficiency of androgen-binding protein) in cultured genital skin fibroblasts from heterozygous females.

†**Special Considerations:** The Reifenstein syndrome has historically been designated a clinical phenotype and, when it was 1st described as a syndrome, its etiology and pathogenesis were unknown. It was apparent that it was genetically determined and was transmitted apparently in an X-linked recessive manner. Sporadic cases were also described, again strictly on the basis of phenotype. As improved methodology became available for the study of testosterone biosynthesis and metabolism, nosologic heterogeneity became apparent in what had previously been called the Reifenstein syndrome. At least 1 sporadic case has been attributed to 17-ketosteroid reductase deficiency. Reinvestigation of 1 of the families originally described by Reifenstein has demonstrated a defect in androgen response by target tissues. As more cases of the Reifenstein syndrome are completely investigated, further heterogeneity will doubtless be discovered. Androgen hyposensitivity is likely to be the pathogenetic mechanism in most if not all of those familial cases inherited in an X-linked recessive manner. Terms such as Reifenstein syn-

drome are rapidly losing their usefulness in the nosology of male pseudohermaphroditism, and will probably soon become obsolete. If diagnostic measures necessary to define the metabolic defect be undertaken in *all* cases of male pseudohermaphroditism, descriptive metabolic terminology could be used to classify the disease in question, thus allowing terms such as Reifenstein syndrome to be deleted from the "intersex" vocabulary.

References:
Amrhein, J.A. et al: Partial androgen insensitivity. The Reifenstein syndrome revisited. N. Engl. J. Med. 297:350, 1977.
Bowen, P. et al: Hereditary male pseudohermaphroditism with hypogonadism, hypospadias, and gynecomastia (Reifenstein's syndrome). Ann. Intern. Med. 62:252, 1965.
Griffin, J.E. et al: Dihydrotestosterone binding by cultured human fibroblasts. Comparison of cells from control subjects and from patients with hereditary male pseudohermaphroditism due to androgen resistance. J. Clin. Invest. 57:1342, 1976.
Knorr, D. et al: Reifenstein's syndrome. A 17β-hydroxysteroid-oxidoreductase deficiency? Acta Endocrinol. (Suppl.) (Kbh) 137:37, 1973.
Opitz, J.M., et al: Pseudovaginal perineoscrotal hypospadias. Clin. Genet. 3:1, 1972.
Simpson, J.L.: Disorders of Sexual Differentiation: Etiology and Clinical Delineation. New York: Academic Press, 1976.
Summitt, R.L.: Disorders of sex differentiation. In Givens, J.R. (ed.): Gynecologic Endocrinology. Chicago: Year Book Publishers, 1977, p. 69.
Wilson, J.D. et al: Familial incomplete male pseudohermaphroditism, type 1. Evidence for androgen resistance and variable clinical manifestations in a family with the Reifenstein syndrome. N. Engl. J. Med. 290:1098, 1974.

Contributors: **Joe Leigh Simpson**
Robert L. Summitt

Editor's Computerized Descriptor: GU.

RENAL AGENESIS, BILATERAL

Includes: Agénésie rénale bilatérale
Beiderseitige Nierenagenesie
Agenesia renal bilateral
Congenital bilateral absence of kidneys
Potter syndrome
Kidneys, absence of

Excludes: Potter syndrome associated with renal dysplasia or infantile polycystic kidney

Minimal Diagnostic Criteria: No kidneys

Clinical Findings: At birth, infants may show the following features: Potter facies: appears as if there is redundant and dehydrated skin, wide-set eyes, prominent fold arising at inner canthus of each eye, "parrot-beak" nose, receding chin, facial expression is that of an older infant; large, low-set ears with deficient auricular cartilages; no urine output; no kidneys palpable. About 40% of these infants are stillborn. Majority of those born alive die within 4 hours. A very rare infant survives more than 2 days. Incompatible with life.

Complications
I Derived: Death shortly after birth is attributed to asphyxia secondary to pulmonary hypoplasia. Renal failure is reason for death in the others.
II Associated: History of oligohydramnios or total absence of amniotic fluid or amnion nodosum. Often premature onset of labor, breech delivery and birthweight disproportionately low. The patient may have multiple malformations including: bilateral pulmonary hypoplasia; genital organ abnormalities such as absence of vas deferens and seminal vesicles or absence of uterus and upper vagina; GI malformations such as anal atresia, absent sigmoid and rectum, esophageal and duodenal atresia; single umbilical artery; major deformities of lower part of body or lower limbs.

Etiology: ? Schmidt et al reported its occurrence in 2 sisters. However, no hereditary factor has been defined.

Pathogenesis: ? Failure of embryogenesis of kidney and other systems

Related Facts
I Sex Ratio: M2:F1
II Risk of Occurrence: ? Davidson and Ross reviewed autopsies among children and reported the frequency of bilateral renal agenesis as follows: 28 of 25,354 children-0.1%; 10 of 4512 stillborns-0.2%; 15 of 4880 infants dying during first 6 weeks-0.3%.
III Risk of Recurrence for
Patient's Sib: ?
Patient's Child: ?
IV Age of Detectability: At birth
V Prevalence: ?

Treatment
I Primary Prevention: —
II Secondary Prevention: —
III Other Therapy: —

Prognosis: Inevitably fatal

Detection of Carrier: —

Special Considerations: —

References:
Cain, D.R. et al: Familial renal agenesis and total dysplasia. Am. J. Dis. Child. 128:377, 1974.
Davidson, W.M. and Ross G.I.M.: Bilateral absence of kidneys and related congenital anomalies. J. Pathol. Bact. 68:459, 1954.
Passarge, E. and Sutherland, J.M.: Potter's syndrome; chromosomal analysis of three cases with Potter's syndrome or related syndromes. Am. J. Dis. Child. 109:80, 1965.

Potter, E.L.: Bilateral absence of ureters and kidneys; a report of 50 cases. Obstet. Gynecol. 25:3, 1965.
Rizza, J.M. and Downing, S.E.: Bilateral renal agenesis in two female siblings. Am. J. Dis. Child. 121:60, 1971.
Schmidt, E.C.H. et al: Renal aplasia in sisters. Arch. Pathol. 54:403, 1952.

Contributor: **Madoka Shibuya**

Editor's Computerized Descriptors: Eye, Ear, Face, Nose, Skel., Resp., CV., GI., GU.

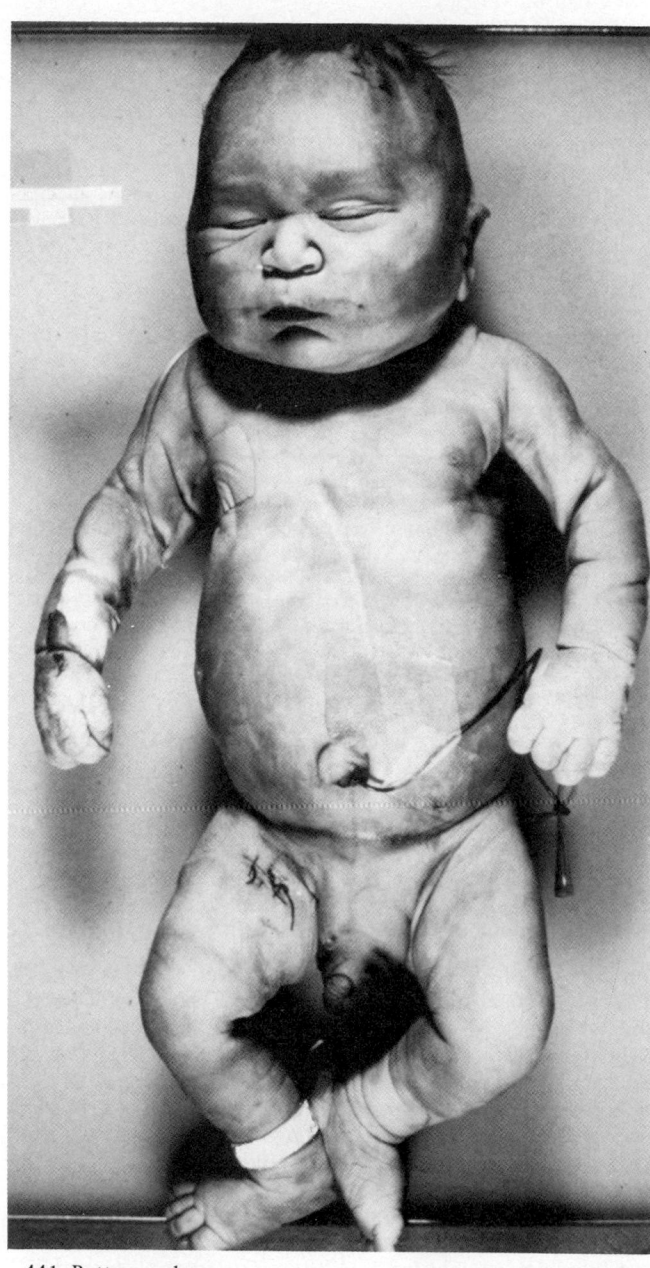

441. Potter syndrome

RENAL AGENESIS, UNILATERAL

Includes: Agénésie rénale unilatérale
Einseitige Nierenagenesie
Agenesia renal unilateral
Renal aplasia, unilateral
Kidney, congenital solitary

Excludes: Renal agenesis, bilateral (856)
Renal dysgenesis
Renal atrophy
Renal hypoplasia

Minimal Diagnostic Criteria: X-ray findings: absence of 1 renal outline most commonly on the left side; enlarged renal shadow on opposite side; asymmetry of the outlines of the psoas muscles; renal pelvis of moderate size, which does not parallel the degree of parenchymal hypertrophy; ectopy or malrotation of the single kidney in 5-10% of the cases. Cystoscopy reveals absence of a ureteral orifice on 1 side and often absence or deformity of the corresponding half of the interureteral ridge of the trigone. Ultrasonography shows the presence of only 1 kidney.

Clinical Findings: The affected infant usually appears normal at birth. In a few an anomaly of the genital tract, such as absence of vagina or unilateral cryptorchidism, may be present. Most frequently clinical recognition of unilateral renal agenesis results from an incidental examination during an illness.

Complications
I **Derived:** Unless the solitary kidney becomes infected, obstructed, or exposed to toxins, the condition is not clinically significant. Sterility has been noted.
II **Associated:** Usually the ipsilateral ureter is absent or poorly developed; adrenal gland on the side of anomaly may be absent. Multiple congenital anomalies of cardiac, skeletal or GI systems may be present. *Female:* various gynecologic anomalies including: true unicornuate uterus, double uterus, absent or double vagina, absence of fallopian tube or ovary of the homolateral side. *Male:* often ipsilateral absence of testis; on the affected side, vas deferens and seminal vesicle may be absent

Etiology: ?

Pathogenesis: ? Failure of normal embryologic development of unknown etiology. Had occurred following thalidomide ingestion early in pregnancy.

Related Facts
I **Sex Ratio:** ? Autopsy studies indicate solitary kidney to be more common among males; however, clinical studies indicate it to be more common among females. This apparent difference in sex incidence is attributable to fact that associated complications and other anomalies are more frequently recognized in females.
II **Risk of Occurrence:** Uncertain, recent estimate of 1 in 1500
III **Risk of Recurrence for**
 Patient's Sib: ? Gorvoy reported unilateral renal agenesis in 2 male sibs in a family.
 Patient's Child: ?
IV **Age of Detectability:** Whenever renal damage occurs or chance finding is made.
V **Prevalence:** ?

Treatment
I **Primary Prevention:** —
II **Secondary Prevention:** —
III **Other Therapy:** If indicated, relief of obstruction, or treatment of infection. If severely diseased, renal transplantation.

Prognosis: If uncomplicated, prognosis is good. Otherwise, the prognosis may be fair to poor.

Detection of Carrier: —

Special Considerations: —

References:
Bound, J.P.: Two cases of congenital absence of one kidney in same family. Br. Med. J. 2:747, 1943.
Emanuel B. et al: Congenital solitary kidney: A review of 74 cases. Am. J. Dis Child. 127:17, 1974.
Gorvoy, J.D. et al: Unilateral renal agenesis in two siblings: Case report. Pediatrics 29:270, 1962.
Ruderman, R.L. and Meyer, J.M.: Unilateral renal agenesis with unicornuate uterus. Can. Med. Assoc. J. 87:235, 1962.
Thompson, D.P. and Lynn, H.B.: Genital anomalies associated with solitary kidney. Mayo Clin. Proc. 41:538, 1966.

Contributor: **Madoka Shibuya**

Editor's Computerized Descriptor: GU.

RENAL BICARBONATE REABSORPTIVE DEFECT

Includes: Défaut de réabsorption rénale du bicarbonate
Renaler Bikarbonat-Resorptions-Defekt
Defecto de reabsorción renal del bicarbonato
Acidosis renal tubular (proximal)
Proximal renal tubular acidosis
Renal tubular bicarbonate-losing syndrome

Excludes: Renal tubular acidosis (862)
Renal tubular syndrome, Fanconi (864)
Oculo-cerebro-renal syndrome (736)
Fructose-1-phosphate aldolase deficiency (395)

Minimal Diagnostic Criteria: Hyperchloremic metabolic acidosis; reduced renal threshold and T_m for bicarbonate; absence of other proximal or distal tubule abnormalities

Clinical Findings: Several unrelated children have demonstrated hyperchloremic acidosis and failure to thrive; urine pH was acid but bicarbonate titration studies revealed distinctly reduced renal threshold and T_m for bicarbonate; no glycosuria, aminoaciduria, hyperphosphaturia or reduction in glomerular filtration rate were demonstrated; response to ammonium chloride administration was normal.

Complications
I **Derived:** Failure to thrive
II **Associated:** —

Etiology: Paucity of cases and absence of affected family members make specific genetic hypothesis difficult; preponderance of males raises possiblility of X linkage.†

Pathogenesis: Defective proximal tubular reabsorption of bicarbonate leads to cation loss and acidosis; mechanism of tubular defect unclear but more than one type is likely.

Related Facts
I **Sex Ratio:** ? More reported males than females.
II **Risk of Occurrence:** Very rare
III **Risk of Recurrence for**
    Patient's Sib: ?
    Patient's Child: ?
IV **Age of Detectability:** ?
V **Prevalence:** ?

Treatment
I **Primary Prevention:** —
II **Secondary Prevention:** Administration of large amounts of bicarbonate solution required to correct hyperchloremic acidosis.
III **Other Therapy:** —

Prognosis: ?

Detection of Carrier: Not studied

†Special Considerations: These patients demonstrate that renal tubular acidosis may be caused by proximal tubular abnormality of bicarbonate reabsorption, as well as by distal tubular defect in maintenance of hydrogen ion gradient; demonstration of familial nature of disease would be of great importance.

References:

McSherry, E. et al: Renal tubular acidosis in infants: The several kinds including bicarbonate-wasting and classic renal tubular acidosis. J. Clin. Invest. 51:499, 1972.

Morris, R.C., Jr.: Renal tubular acidosis: Mechanisms, classification and implications. N. Engl. J. Med. 281:1405, 1969.

Soriano, J.R. et al: Proximal renal tubular acidosis: A defect in bicarbonate reabsorption with normal urinary acidification. Pediatr. Res. 1:81, 1967.

Contributor: **Leon E. Rosenberg**

RENAL DISEASE, POLYCYSTIC ADULT TYPE

Includes: Polykystose rénale du type adulte
Zystennieren-Erwachsenenform
Enfermedad renal poliquística tipo adulto
Polycystic renal disease, adult type
Kidney, adult polycystic disease of

Excludes: Polycystic renal disease, infantile type
Congenital hepatic fibrosis
Multicystic renal dysplasia
Medullary cystic disease (nephronophthisis)
Medullary sponge kidney
Nephrosis, congenital (709)
Simple renal cysts
Multilocular renal cysts

Minimal Diagnostic Criteria: Familial occurrence; bilateral or unilateral masses in the flank with or without hypertension; hematuria and proteinuria; radiologic evidence on IVP of cystic disease.

Clinical Findings: Adult polycystic renal disease is a familial disease which occurs in both sexes. The disease is characterized by progressive renal insufficiency. The vast majority of cases become clinically apparent after the 4th decade and the average age at death is about 50 years. Fewer than 10% of individuals die in the 1st decade of life.

The presenting feature is often the feeling of abdominal fullness, discomfort or pain. Bilateral abdominal masses may be detected on examination. Hypertension is present in 50-60% of the cases. Urinalysis shows varying degrees of proteinuria and hematuria. Pyuria and bacteriuria may be present. Blood chemistries may still be normal or may be indicative of renal failure. Anemia is common but polycythemia may be occasionally observed. Some patients may present with ureteral colic resulting from passage of a blood clot from a ruptured cyst. Rarely subarachnoid hemorrhage from a ruptured aneurysm is the presenting symptom.

Diagnosis of polycystic disease may be confirmed by IVP which usually shows bilaterally enlarged kidneys with lobulated margins. Occasionally, 1 kidney may be larger than the other, and rarely, the kidneys may be of normal size. The renal pelvis may be normal or elongated, occasionally with cystic impressions on its margins. The calyceal configuration is very variable. The calyces may appear to be deformed with elongation, distention, flattening, or cystic impressions. The nephrogram will demonstrate numerous radiolucent cysts within the kidney and the angiogram will usually demonstrate stretching and narrowing of the vessels with loss of the terminal branching. Occasionally, the radiographic findings are dominant on 1 side with the other side appearing relatively normal, making the diagnosis difficult.

Complications
I **Derived:** Patients with polycystic kidney disease are prone to pyelonephritis and arteriolar nephrosclerosis. Rupture of cysts and hemorrhage into cysts may occur. Renal colic due to renal calculi or blood clots are not infrequent. Compression of the ureter by the large cystic kidney may lead to hydronephrosis.

Bone and joint disorders are fairly common. Attacks of gout often precede symptoms of significant uremia. Approximately 8% of patients show bone disease consisting of demineralization, trabeculation and spontaneous fractures.

Subarachnoid hemorrhage secondary to rupture of cerebral aneurysm is not infrequent.

Neoplasms (carcinoma, sarcoma) in polycystic kidneys are relatively rare.

II **Associated:** Approximately 1/3 of patients with adult polycystic renal disease have 1 or more cysts of the liver. These are lined with biliary epithelium. Hepatic cysts produce no functional impairment.

Less frequently, cysts are found in the pancreas (10%), spleen and lungs (5%); cysts of the ovary, endometrium, seminal vesicles, epidydimis, bladder and thyroid have been reported. Aneurysm of cerebral arteries are frequently associated with polycystic kidney disease (15%) as are other malformations of the CNS, especially hydrocephaly.

Etiology: Autosomal dominant with high degree of penetrance. McK *17390

Pathogenesis: ? There are many theories implicating developmental retention or malformation abnormalities or a combination of these. More recently, a toxic metabolic defect has been postulated. None of these theories are generally accepted.

In polycystic kidney disease, the kidney tissue is displaced by many cysts of varying size which are scattered throughout the parenchyma, gradually leading to gross enlargment of kidneys and to progressive renal failure.†

Related Facts
I **Sex Ratio:** M1:F1
II **Risk of Occurrence:** 1 in 250 live births (Campbell based this figure on 47,402 autopsies and included infantile type polycystic disease).
III **Risk of Recurrence for**
Patient's Sib: If parent is affected 1 in 2 (50%) for each offspring to be affected; otherwise not increased
Patient's Child: 1 in 2
IV **Age of Detectability:** Usually after 4th decade of life
V **Prevalence:** ? In a review of 7 hospital admission series, it varied from 1 in 342 to 1 in 4933; in 10 autopsy series it varied from 1 in 222 to 1 in 1019 (Daalgard, Strauss and Welt). No ethnic group variation has been reported.

Treatment
I **Primary Prevention:** Genetic counseling
II **Secondary Prevention:** —
III **Other Therapy:** Conservative management of renal insufficiency (protein restricted diet, correction of electrolyte and acid-base imbalance) and of cardiovascular complications and infection. In advanced cases, dialysis treatment and renal transplantation.

Prognosis: In the majority of cases the cystic conversion of renal parenchyma is progressive and the patients gradually develop uremia. However, there are wide variations in the course of the disease. Some patients may remain asymptomatic; in some, the disease progresses very slowly; however, once renal function has become impaired, most patients die within 3 years. Fifty to 60% of patients die from uremia. Myocardial infarcts, congestive heart failure, and cerebral hemorrhage each account for approximately 10% of deaths. The remaining patients die of unrelated causes.

Detection of Carrier: The condition has a high degree of penetrance in heterozygotes with late expressivity. The severity of polycystic kidney disease in homozygote states is unknown. In affected families urinalysis and IVP should be obtained on each family member to identify a mutant gene carrier.

†**Special Considerations:** Polycystic kidneys are found in several disease entities and multiple malformation syndromes. Cortical involvement usually predominates but medullary cysts are also occasionally present. The renal cysts in these conditions may thus resemble the cysts seen in adult cystic disease.

References:

Bernstein, J.: Heritable cystic disorders of the kidney: The mythology of polycystic disease. Pediatr. Clin. North Am. 18:435, 1971.

Crocker, J.F.S. et al: Developmental defects of the kidney: A review of renal development and experimental studies of maldevelopment. Pediatr. Clin. North Am. 18:355, 1971.

Daalgard, O.Z.: Polycystic disease of the kidney. In Strauss, M.B. and Welt, L.G. (eds.): Diseases of the Kidney. Boston: Little, Brown and Co., 1963.

Kissane, J.M.: Congenital malformations. In Heptinstall, R.H. (ed.): Pathology of the Kidney. Boston: Little, Brown and Co., 1966.

Contributors: **Edward Wasserman**
Inge Sagel
Nesrin Bingol

Editor's Computerized Descriptors: Skel., GU., CV.

860   854-500

RENAL, GENITAL AND MIDDLE EAR ANOMALIES

Includes: Anomalies rénale génitale et de l'oreille moyenne
Urogenital-und Mittelohrfehlbildungen
Anomalías renales, genitales y del oído medio
Genital, renal and middle ear anomalies
Middle ear, genitourinary anomalies

Excludes: Renal agenesis, unilateral (857)
Renal agenesis, bilateral (856)
Nephritis and nerve deafness, hereditary (708)
Deafness, renal and digital anomalies (264)

Minimal Diagnostic Criteria: Conductive hearing loss, variable renal anomalies and vaginal atresia. As new cases are reported, individuals may be found without the complete manifestations of the syndrome.†

Clinical Findings: Renal abnormalities vary from unilateral hypoplasia to unilateral or bilateral renal agenesis. Vaginal atresia may be associated with normal external genitalia, uterus, fallopian tubes and ovaries or with extensive internal genital anomalies. Hearing loss is conductive and associated with stenotic external auditory canals. Audiogram shows a conductive loss with a normal bone line. An absent or malformed incus has been described in 2 patients who had middle ear explorations. Variable features include a beaked nose, micrognathia, low-set small ears, clinodactyly and mild mental retardation.

Complications
I **Derived:** Delayed development of language secondary to the hearing loss. If renal anomalies are extensive enough, they may be incompatible with life. Undiagnosed vaginal atresia can lead to hydrometrocolpos at menarche.
II **Associated:** Mild mental retardation, beaked nose, micrognathia, low-set small ears, congenital heart disease, pulmonary hypoplasia.

Etiology: Possibly autosomal recessive with variable expressivity, and possibly sex-influenced. Very few patients have been described to date. It is not known if there is a form of this syndrome present in males.

Pathogenesis: ?

Related Facts
I **Sex Ratio:** M0:F1 (4 and possibly 5 cases reported, all female)
II **Risk of Occurrence:** ?
III **Risk of Recurrence for**
    Patient's Sib: (Expression of this defect in males is as yet unknown.) Possibly 1 in 4 (25%) for each offspring to be affected.
    Patient's Child: Possibly not increased unless mate is carrier or homozygote. (Reproductive fitness unknown although those with more severe abnormalities are probably infertile.)
IV **Age of Detectability:** At birth by careful examination although the vaginal atresia and conductive hearing loss may easily be missed.
V **Prevalence:** ?

Treatment
I **Primary Prevention:** Genetic counseling
II **Secondary Prevention:** Middle ear surgery may improve the hearing although amplification and special training may be necessary prior to middle ear surgery. Plastic surgery can create a vagina.
III **Other Therapy:** As required for secondary renal complications

Prognosis: Death may occur in infancy if renal abnormalities are severe or if associated abnormalities are present. Milder forms probably compatible with a normal life span.

Detection of Carrier: ?

†**Special Considerations:** Turner has reported a patient with a narrow external auditory meatus with mild deafness, vaginal atresia and an absent left kidney. In addition she had crowded dentition, lacrimal duct stenosis and an anteriorly placed rectum with mild rectal stenosis. This girl may represent an additional example of this syndrome.

References:

Turner, G.: A second family with renal, vaginal and middle ear anomalies. J. Pediatr. 76:641, 1970.

Winter, J.S. et al: A familial syndrome of renal, genital and middle ear anomalies. J. Pediatr. 72:88, 1968.

Contributor: **Janet M. Stewart**

Editor's Computerized Descriptors: Hearing, Ear, Nose, Resp., GU., Nerve

RENAL GLYCOSURIA (MARKER)

Includes: Glycosurie rénale
Renale Glucosurie
Glucosuria renal (Marcador)
Renal glycosuria A and B
Benign mellituria

Excludes: Diabetes mellitus
Renal tubular syndrome, Fanconi (864)
Glucose-galactose malabsorption (419)

Minimal Diagnostic Criteria: Demonstration that reducing substance in urine is glucose; glycosuria during an otherwise normal oral glucose tolerance test; excretion of > 300 mg glucose per 24 hr on standard carbohydrate diet; demonstration of reduced renal threshold for glucose by renal titration techniques; Type A renal glycosuria characterized by reduced threshold and reduced tubular maximum for glucose reabsorption (T_mG) while Type B renal glycosuria demonstrates reduced threshold, exaggerated "splay" and normal T_mG; absence of other proximal or distal tubular abnormalities.

Clinical Findings: Asymptomatic glucosuria; none other except for rare episodes of hypoglycemia reported during pregnancy; condition usually detected on routine urinalysis.

Complications
I **Derived:** None, except for iatrogenically induced hypoglycemic attacks in patients misdiagnosed as diabetics and treated with insulin.
II **Associated:** —

Etiology: Autosomal recessive transmission. Possibly several distinct autosomal mutations affecting specific glucose "carrier" system in proximal renal tubule.† McK *23310

Pathogenesis: Transport defect leads to reduced threshold or reduced T_m for glucose.

Related Facts
I **Sex Ratio:** M1:F1
II **Risk of Occurrence:** ?
III **Risk of Recurrence for**
   Patient's Sib: 1 in 4 (25%) for each offspring to be affected.
   Patient's Child: Not increased unless mate is carrier or homozygote.
IV **Age of Detectability:** Neonatal period
V **Prevalence:** ?

Treatment
I **Primary Prevention:** Genetic counseling
II **Secondary Prevention:** —
III **Other Therapy:** —

Prognosis: No apparent effect on longevity or health

Detection of Carrier: No reliable means; some demonstrate mild renal glycosuria†

†**Special Considerations:** Early studies using glucose tolerance tests suggested that renal glycosuria is inherited as a dominant trait; recent pedigree analyses using glucose titration techniques indicate that the disorder is inherited in an autosomal recessive fashion and that Type A and Type B renal glycosurics may be found in a single sibship; thus several different mutations affecting one or more glucose transport systems in the kidney may be responsible; gut transport system for glucose is not affected in pedigrees studied so far.

References:

Elsas, L. J. and Rosenberg, L. E.: Familial renal glycosuria: A genetic reappraisal of hexose transport by kidney and intestine. J. Clin. Invest. 48:1845, 1969.

Elsas, L.J. et al: Autosomal recessive inheritance of renal glycosuria. Metabolism 20:968, 1971.

Krane, S.M.: Renal glycosuria. In Stanbury, J.B. et al (eds.): The

Metabolic Basis of Inherited Disease, 4th Ed. New York: McGraw-Hill, 1978, p. 1607.

Contributor: **Leon E. Rosenberg**

Editor's Computerized Descriptor: GU.

RENAL TUBULAR ACIDOSIS

Includes: Acidose rénale
Renale tubuläre Azidose
Acidosis renal tubular (distal)
Lightwood syndrome
Albright-Butler syndrome

Excludes: Renal tubular syndrome, Fanconi (864)
Renal bicarbonate reabsorptive defect (858)
Oculo-cerebro-renal syndrome (736)

Minimal Diagnostic Criteria: Persistent hyperchloremic acidosis with failure to acidify urine to pH 5 or less after an ammonium chloride load; absence of glycosuria, pathologic aminoaciduria, hyperphosphaturia or excessive bicarbonate excretion.

Clinical Findings: Hyperchloremic metabolic acidosis with inability to acidify the urine below pH 5.5-6.0 (100%); hypokalemia, hyperkaluria, hypercalciuria occur frequently; bilateral neural deafness observed in families with carbonic anhydrase B defect.

Complications
I **Derived:** Nephrocalcinosis, destruction of renal parenchyma and renal insufficiency (frequency unknown)
II **Associated:** —

Etiology: Probably variable; 1 type is considered to show autosomal dominant transmission, a 2nd type is inherited as an autosomal recessive.† McK *17980

Pathogenesis: The recessive form is probably due to a defect in carbonic anhydrase B; in the dominant form increased permeability of distal renal tubule membrane to hydrogen ion may lead to increased back diffusion of hydrogen ion into systemic circulation with resultant acidosis. The latter being responsible secondarily for the hypercalciuria, hyperkaluria, nephrocalcinosis and renal insufficiency.†

Related Facts
I **Sex Ratio:** M1:F1 for both forms
II **Risk of Occurrence:** ?
III **Risk of Recurrence for**
   Patient's Sib: If autosomal dominant or autosomal recessive, see Table I AD or AR, respectively.
   Patient's Child: If autosomal dominant or autosomal recessive, see Table I AD or AR, respectively.
IV **Age of Detectability:** ?
V **Prevalence:** ?

Treatment
I **Primary Prevention:** Genetic counseling
II **Secondary Prevention:** Correction of acidosis with oral or parenteral citrate or bicarbonate therapy; supplementary potassium, calcium and vitamin D may be necessary to prevent potassium depletion or metabolic bone disease, respectively.
III **Other Therapy:** Management of renal insufficiency

Prognosis: Variable, depending on age of detection and secondary manifestations; usual cause of death is uncontrolled acidosis or renal insufficiency.

Detection of Carrier: In dominant form, heterozygotes appear to manifest the disease process leading to dominant pattern of inheritance; expression varies widely within a family; no current carrier detection for recessive form.

†**Special Considerations:** Theories about mechanism of classic, dominant form based on exclusion, ie lack of abnormalities in bicarbonate reabsorption, ammonia secretion, or glomerular filtration; several different disorders may still be included in this present delineation.

References:
Morris, R.C., Jr.: Renal tubular acidosis: Mechanisms, classification and implications. N. Engl. J. Med. 281:1405, 1969.

Seldin, D. W. and Wilson, J. D.: Renal tubular acidosis. In Stanbury, J.B. et al (eds.): The Metabolic Basis of Inherited Disease, 3rd Ed. New York:McGraw-Hill, 1972, p. 1548.

Shapira, E. et al: Enzymatically inactive red cell carbonic anhydrase B in a family with renal tubular acidosis. J. Clin. Invest. 53:59, 1974.

Wrong, O. and Davies, H. E. F.: The excretion of acid in renal disease. Q. J. Med. 28:259, 1959.

Contributor: **Leon E. Rosenberg**

Editor's Computerized Descriptors: Hearing, GU.

RENAL TUBULAR ACIDOSIS AND SENSORINEURAL DEAFNESS

Includes: Acidose rénale tubulaire et surdité neurosensorielle
Tubuläre Azidose und Innenohrschwerhörigkeit
Acidosis renal tubular y sordera neuro-sensorial
Infantile renal tubular acidosis and congenital sensorineural deafness
Adolescent or young adult renal tubular acidosis, and slowly progressive sensorineural deafness

Excludes: Autosomal dominant renal tubular acidosis, type I
Renal tubular acidosis with other associated defects
Oculo-cerebro-renal syndrome (736)

Minimal Diagnostic Criteria: Renal tubular acidosis with a defect in tubular HCO_3-reabsorption and sensorineural hearing loss or deafness.

Clinical Findings: Twelve patients in 7 families are described with this syndrome. Most presented at birth or soon thereafter with vomiting, dehydration, polydipsia, polyuria, hyposthenuria and failure to thrive. Nephrocalcinosis was observed in some cases.

Renal tubular acidosis is a clinical syndrome of disordered renal acidification which is out of proportion to the impairment of glomerular filtration and in which metabolic acidosis results from abnormalities of renal tubular function. This type of renal tubular acidosis is associated with a defect in tubular HCO_3-reabsorption. Deficient carbonic anhydrase B (CA-B) activity in the affected individuals of 1 family has been observed.

Deafness is variable. In most cases a sensorineural deafness is present in early childhood. In 2 sibs the onset of hearing loss was during late childhood and in 2 other sibs there was a striking difference in the degree of hearing loss.

Complications
I   **Derived:** Nephrocalcinosis
II **Associated:** Mild mental retardation

Etiology: Autosomal recessive; McK *26730

Pathogenesis: ?

Related Facts
I   **Sex Ratio:** M5:F4
II   **Risk of Occurrence:** ?
III **Risk of Recurrence for**
     Patient's Sib: 1 in 4 (25%) for each offspring to be affected.
     Patient's Child: Not increased unless mate is carrier or homozygote.
IV   **Age of Detectability:** Early childhood
V   **Prevalence:** The multiple independent reports of this syndrome suggest that it may not be excessively rare.

Treatment
I   **Primary Prevention:** Genetic counseling
II   **Secondary Prevention:** Treatment with alkalinizing solutions and high fluid intake. Hearing aid; special training if the hearing loss is severe.
III **Other Therapy:** —

Prognosis: Probably normal life span with good medical care.

Detection of Carrier: ?

Special Considerations: —

References:
Cohen, T. et al: Familial infantile renal tubular acidosis and congenital nerve deafness: An autosomal recessive syndrome. Clin. Genet. 4:275, 1973.

Donckerwolcke, R.A. et al: The syndrome of renal tubular acidosis with nerve deafness. Acta Paediatr. Scand. 65:100, 1976.

Konigsmark, B.W. and Gorlin, R.J.: Infantile renal tubular acidosis and congenital sensorineural deafness; adolescent or young adult renal tubular acidosis and slowly progressive sensorineural deafness. In Genetic and Metabolic Deafness. Philadelphia: W.B. Saunders Co., 1976, p. 290.

Nance, W.E. and Sweeney, A.: Evidence for autosomal recessive inheritance of the syndrome of renal tubular acidosis with deafness. In Bergsma, D. (ed.): Part IX. Ear. Birth Defects: Orig. Art. Ser., vol. VII, no. 4. Baltimore: Williams & Wilkins for The National Foundation-March of Dimes, 1971, p. 70.

Shapira, E. et al: Enzymatically inactive red cell carbonic anhydrase B in a family with renal tubular acidosis. J. Clin. Invest. 53:59, 1974.

Walker, W.G. et al: Syndrome of perceptive deafness and renal tubular acidosis. In Bergsma, D. (ed.): Part XVI. Urinary System and Others. Birth Defects: Orig. Art. Ser., vol. X, no. 4. Baltimore: Williams & Wilkins for The National Foundation-March of Dimes, 1974, p. 163.

Contributor: **Cor W.R.J. Cremers**

———————————————

Editor's Computerized Descriptors: Hearing, GI., GU.

RENAL TUBULAR SYNDROME, FANCONI

Includes: Maladie de Fanconi
Fanconi-Syndrom
Síndrome de Fanconi

Excludes: Fanconi aplastic anemia

Minimal Diagnostic Criteria: All aspects of the syndrome reflect impaired renal tubular transport. These comprise: generalized hyperaminoaciduria resembling plasma ultrafiltrate; hypophosphatemia and hyperphosphaturia; low T_m glucosuria; type II (proximal) renal tubular acidosis with bicarbonate loss; high free water clearance; high renal clearance of other filtered solutes (eg uric acid, potassium).

According to recent work, an analogous impairment of intestinal transport may also exist.

The morphologic lesion which affects the proximal tubule, often called a "swan neck lesion," is probably secondary to the functional deficit; it represents atrophy of epithelial cells and loss of volume of proximal tubular mass.

Progressive nephron failure and decreased glomerular filtration can ablate phenotypic expression of the Fanconi syndrome in its later stages in some traits (eg cystinosis).

Clinical Findings: A syndrome of many causes, some of which are inherited, yet often unidentified. The clinical manifestations are, in essence, peripheral, being dependent either on the condition causing the syndrome, or on the sequelae of the syndrome itself. The fully expressed syndrome comprises a generalized disturbance of proximal renal tubular transport. The most frequent clinical consequences include hypophosphatemic rickets (phosphate loss), acidosis (bicarbonate loss), weakness (potassium loss), and dehydration (water loss). Growth failure or weight loss may also occur in the uncompensated syndrome.

Time of onset of the trait depends on its cause. Exposure to toxic agents directly precedes most acquired causes, which must be eliminated before attributing the syndrome to an inherited cause. Inherited traits may produce the Fanconi syndrome either early in life, or not until much later in life; galactosemia and fructosemia produce the syndrome rapidly after the metabolite accumulates in the blood, while prolonged copper accumulation is required in Wilson disease before the syndrome is found. The recessively inherited Fanconi syndrome associated with cystinosis appears in the first 6 months of life; the noncystinotic adult idiopathic syndrome caused by a nonallelic mutation may not appear until the 4th decade.

Complications
I **Derived:** All clinical manifestions (eg rickets or osteomalacia, renal tubular acidosis and dehydration) can be considered as "complications" of the transport defect. Death secondary to uncorrected hypokalemia or dehydration can occur in infants.
II **Associated:** Complications of the primary trait (eg cystinosis, "tyrosinosis," Wilson disease) should be considered in their own terms. Death may be end stage of a number of the primary traits associated with the syndrome.

Etiology: May be acquired or inherited; rarely is autosomal dominant. Autosomal recessive transmission of many mutant alleles at numerous autosomal loci determine the various forms of the syndrome. Some mutant alleles are easily recognized as primary traits, such as "hereditary tyrosinemia," "infantile cystinosis," "galactosemia," "fructosemia," "Wilson disease." In these, the syndrome is clearly secondary to the expression of the primary trait. Other mutant alleles are identifiable only through the presence of the Fanconi syndrome itself, as in the adult idiopathic Fanconi syndrome. McK *22770

Pathogenesis: Impaired ability to *transfer* solute and water across the tubular cell membrane seems to be the fundamental lesion of the syndrome; *affinity* of the solutes for their binding site is apparently not altered.†

The inhibition of membrane transport is probably linked to specific forms of impaired availability or transduction of metabolic energy for transport.

Related Facts
I   **Sex Ratio:** Ml:Fl
II **Risk of Occurrence:**   ?
III **Risk of Recurrence for**
   Patient's Sib: If autosomal recessive or autosomal dominant, see Table I AR or AD, respectively.
   Patient's Child: If autosomal recessive or autosomal dominant, see Table I AR or AD, respectively.
IV **Age of Detectability:** Varies with primary cause.
V   **Prevalence:** Varies with primary cause.

Treatment
I   **Primary Prevention:** Genetic counseling; or elimination of acquired cause.
II **Secondary Prevention:** Offset phenotypic effects of trait; eg phosphate supplementation of diet to prevent hypophosphatemia; potassium and bicarbonate replacement to prevent hypokalemia and renal tubular acidosis; high fluid intake to prevent dehydration.
III **Other Therapy:** —

Prognosis: Depends on cause of trait.

Detection of Carrier: Depends on cause of trait. The syndrome is usually never expressed in carriers, except in unusual pedigrees, such as those described by Luder and Sheldon (Arch. Dis. Child. 30:160, 1955), and Ben-Ishay et al (Am. J. Med. 31:793, 1965), where a dominantly inherited trait was identified.

†**Special Considerations:** Little has been done to identify the functional mechanism of the syndrome. Rosenberg and Segal (Biochem. J. 92:345, 1964) showed that maleic acid, which causes the syndrome in vivo, acts as a noncompetitive inhibitor of transport by kidney slices in vitro. Scriver et al (Pediatrics 34:357, 1964) showed the transfer component of membrane transport, but not the component of solute binding by transport sites, was impaired in vivo in a patient with a partial expression of the syndrome. Low T_m values are anticipated in the syndrome if classic titration studies are done. Morris et al (J. Clin. Invest. 52, 57a, 1973 (Abstract)) have submitted evidence that cellular depletion of inorganic phosphate is critical to the development of the tubulopathy upon exposure to fructose in hereditary fructose intolerance.

It is not known whether cases of hypophosphatemic rickets with glucosuria and different forms of hyperaminoaciduria (Dent: J. Bone Jt. Surg. 34B:266, 1952; Dent & Harris: J. Bone Jt. Surg. 38B:204, 1965) represent partial expression of the Fanconi syndrome and the capacity for transport at the normal endogenous substrate loads could remain unimpaired, whereas the T_m might be depressed in such patients. Attempts to identify the actual biochemical lesion responsible for inhibition of the transfer component of membrane transport in the syndrome are essential for its further interpretation.

References:
Leaf, A.: The syndrome of osteomalacia, renal glucosuria, aminoaciduria, and increased phosphorus clearance (the Fanconi syndrome). In Stanbury, J.B. et al (eds.): The Metabolic Basis of Inherited Disease, 2nd Ed. New York:McGraw-Hill, 1966, p.1205.
Rosenberg, L. E.: Hereditary diseases with membrane defects. In Dowben, R.M. (ed.): Biological Membranes. Boston:Little-Brown, 1969, p. 255.
Scriver, C. R. and Hechtman, P.: Human genetics of membrane transport with emphasis on amino acids. In Harris, H. and Hirschhorn, K. (eds.): Advances in Human Genetics. New York: Plenum Press, 1970, vol. 2, p. 211.

Contributor: **Charles R. Scriver**

Editor's Computerized Descriptors: Skel., Muscle, GU.

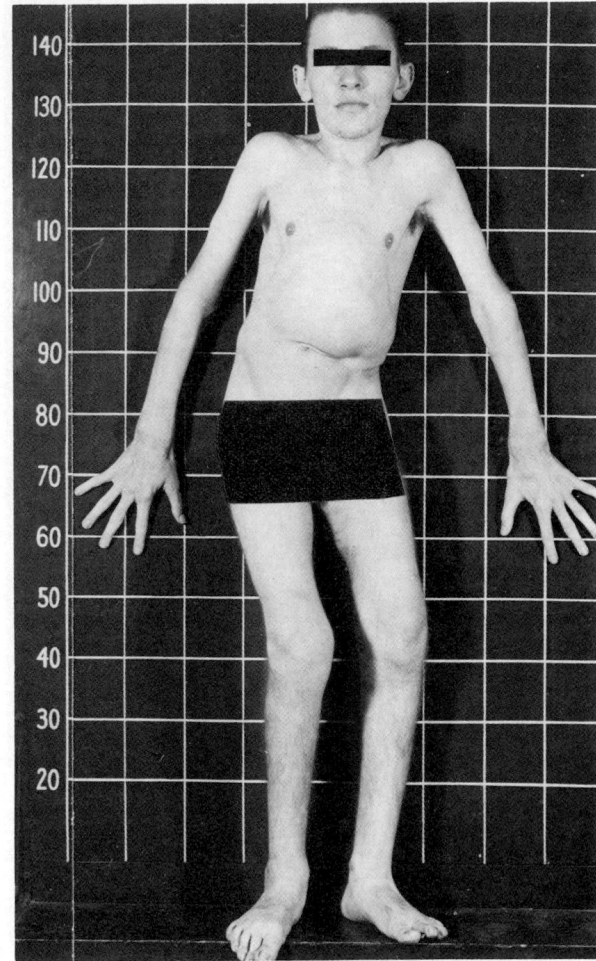

442. Skeletal changes of hypophosphatemia

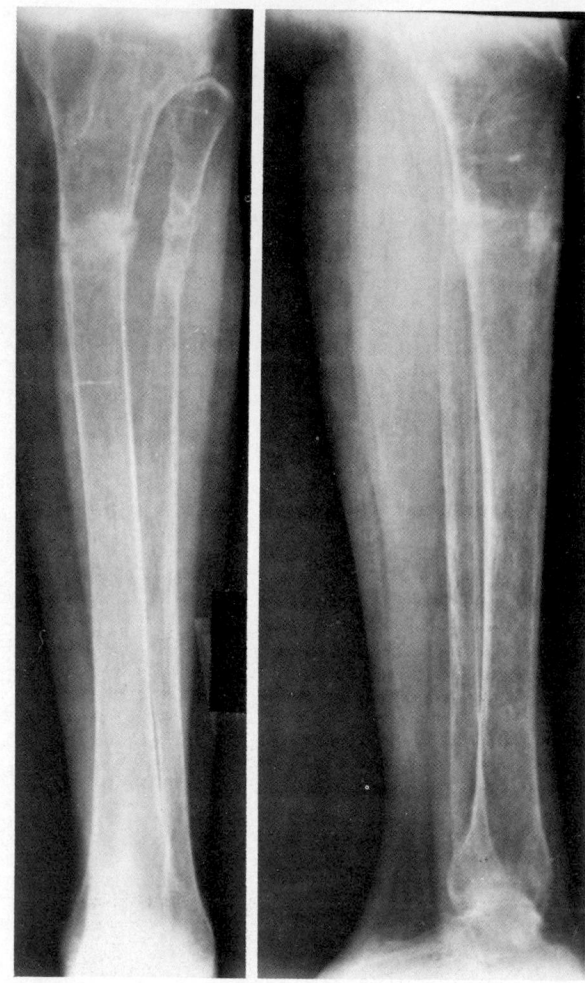

443. Hypophophatemic rickets. Note severe nonmineralization (osteomalacia) with "looser zones" of healing fractures in proximal tibia and fibula

RETINAL APLASIA

Includes: Aplasie rétinienne
Retina-Aplasie
Aplasia retineana

Excludes: Amaurosis congenita of Leber (43)
Retinitis pigmentosa (869)

Minimal Diagnostic Criteria: Evident absence of vision, absence or minimal pupillary reflexes, extinct ERG

Clinical Findings: Rarely seen unassociated with other ocular anomalies. Frequently confused with "cerebral blindness". At birth or shortly thereafter, affected individuals show evidence of lack of vision, absence of or minimal pupillary reflexes, occasionally nystagmus and photophobia.

The ophthalmoscopic findings present an interesting variability. The retina may appear essentially normal at birth, or exhibits pigmentary clumping either in or about the macular area, or limited to the periphery. Later, a generalized tapetoretinal degeneration may appear presenting salt and pepper-like changes, punctata albescens-like deposits or a retinitis pigmentosa picture. Optic nerve pallor and retinal vasculature alteration may subsequently evolve. Juvenile onset of cataracts and keratoconus or keratoglobus are frequently encountered. Massaging of the eyes with the knuckles (digitooculo reflex) is almost constant. The photopic and scotopic electroretinogram (ERG) responses are absent and fairly diagnostic. Early in the course of the disease there may be an absence of the b wave.

Complications
I **Derived:** Frequent development of keratoconus, acquired cataracts
II **Associated:** Ehlers-Danlos syndrome, mental retardation

Etiology: Genetic heterogeneity exists. Mode of transmission demonstrated to be both autosomal dominant and autosomal recessive. McK *17990

Pathogenesis: Initial dysfunction may be due to absence or dysfunction of rods and cones.†

Related Facts
I **Sex Ratio:** Ml:Fl
II **Risk of Occurrence:** ? Very rare
III **Risk of Recurrence for**
    Patient's Sib: When autosomal dominant or autosomal recessive, see Table I AD or AR, respectively.
    Patient's Child: When autosomal dominant or autosomal recessive, see Table I AD or AR, respectively.
IV **Age of Detectability:** Shortly after birth
V **Prevalence:** ? Isolated condition is very rare.

Treatment
I **Primary Prevention:** Genetic counseling
II **Secondary Prevention:** Special education for blind persons
III **Other Therapy:** There is no treatment other than management of the complications, if and when indicated (cataract, keratoconus, corneal ulceration and corneal rupture). Institutionalization may be indicated for those patients also having severe mental retardation.

Prognosis: Normal or slightly shortened life span-total blindness is the ultimate result.

Detection of Carrier: —

†**Special Considerations:** The finding of an "elastic diathesis" (Ehlers-Danlos syndrome) in many of the affected patients may help to explain the fairly high incidence of keratoconus or kerato-

globus- particularly in these children who are constantly traumatizing their eyes by rubbing.

References:
Alström, C.H. and Olson, O.: Heredo-retinopathia congenitalis: Monohybrida recessiva congenitalis autosomalis; a genetical-statistical study. Hereditas 43:1, 1957.
François, J.: Heredity in Ophthalmology. St. Louis: C.V. Mosby, 1961, p. 452.
Rahn, E.K. et al: Leber's congenital amaurosis with an Ehlers-Danlos-like syndrome: Study of an American family. Arch. Ophthalmol 79:135, 1968.

Contributor: **Harold F. Falls**

———————————————

Editor's Computerized Descriptors: Vision, Eye

RETINAL DYSPLASIA

Includes: Dysplasie rétinienne
Retinale Dysplasie
Displasia de la retina
Dysplastic retina

Excludes: Retinoblastoma (870)
Vitreous, persistent hyperplastic primary (994)

Minimal Diagnostic Criteria: —

Clinical Findings: This condition may occur as a unilateral ocular finding alone or may be part of a syndrome in which the ocular condition is bilateral and anomalies are present elsewhere in the body as expounded by Reese. The eye may be of normal size or may be microphthalmic. There is a characteristic leukocoria and for this reason the eyes are removed for a suspected retinoblastoma.

Complications
I **Derived:** Secondary glaucoma, cataract, retinal detachment
II **Associated:** *Ocular:* Goniodysgenesis, congenital glaucoma, persistent hyperplastic primary vitreous, coloboma
Systemic: Syndactyly, polydactyly, cleft palate, congenital anomalies of the heart. Retinal dysplasia has been described in 13-15 trisomy, chromosome 18 deletion defect, and with triploidy 69,XXY, Norrie disease, and Meckel syndrome.

Etiology: ? The underlying cause of retinal dysplasia is usually unknown: but it has been associated with blue tongue virus, herpesvirus, bovine virus, fetal irradiation, vitamin A deficiency, and photocoagulation of the chick embryo retina. Retinal dysplasia has been induced by experimental intrauterine trauma.

Pathogenesis: Abnormal development of the retina resulting in aimless retinal hyperplasia producing heaped areas with nonspecific rosette formation and immature cells.

Related Facts
I **Sex Ratio:** M?:F?
II **Risk of Occurrence:** ? Rare
III **Risk of Recurrence for**
 Patient's Sib: ?
 Patient's Child: ?
IV **Age of Detectability:** At birth
V **Prevalence:** ? Rare

Treatment
I **Primary Prevention:** —
II **Secondary Prevention:** Enucleation for suspected retinoblastoma and cosmetic purposes.
III **Other Therapy:** —

Prognosis: Good for life if the situation is limited to the eye. Visual prognosis, however, is poor. Prognosis for life is poor in those cases where there are other systemic anomalies.

Detection of Carrier: —

Special Considerations: —

References:
Hunter, W. and Zimmerman, L.E.: Unilateral retinal dysplasia. Arch. Ophthalmol. 74:23, 1965.
Lahov, M. et al: Clinical and histopathologic classification of retinal dysplasia. Am. J. Ophthalmol. 75:648, 1973.
Reese, A.B. and Blodi, F.C.: Retinal dysplasia. Am. J. Ophthalmol. 33:23, 1950.
Reese, A.B. and Straatsma, B.R.: Retinal dysplasia. Am. J. Ophthalmol. 45:119, 1958.
Silverstein, A.M. et al: The pathogenesis of retinal dysplasia. Am. J. Ophthalmol. 72:13, 1971.
Silverstein, A.: Retinal dysplasia and rosettes induced by experimental intrauterine trauma. Am. J. Ophthalmol. 77:51, 1974.

Contributor: **Morton E. Smith**

RETINAL FOLD

Includes: Plicature rétinienne
Retina-Falte
Pliegue retineano
Ablatio falciformis congenita
Congenital retinal septum

Excludes: True retinal detachment
Chromosome thirteen trisomy syndrome (168)
Grade III retrolental fibroplasia
Acquired folds secondary to intraocular foreign bodies or inflammatory disease

Minimal Diagnostic Criteria: A typical retinal fold running from the disk into the periphery.†

Clinical Findings: These folds occur in otherwise normal eyes and are occasionally bilateral. Ophthalmoscopically, they are seen as elevated, grey folds or ridges running from the nervehead into the retinal periphery where they commonly expand in a grey fan over the peripheral retina and the pars plana. These folds occur most commonly in the lower temporal quadrant of the retina, and occasionally send strands forward to the posterior capsule of the lens. Often, there is considerable disturbance in the retinal pigment epithelium along the edges of the fold and there may be traction detachment at various places along its course. Remnants of the hyaloid arterial system may be adherent to the surface of the fold. The normal retinal blood vessels appear to be pulled up into this fold and vessels may be absent from other areas of the retina. The visual acuity is minimal from birth and the first signs of the condition are strabismus or poor vision if the folds are bilateral.

Complications
I **Derived:** —
II **Associated:** None

Etiology: ?

Pathogenesis: These folds may be caused by a localized persistence of the primary vitreous with adherence to the retina. Other possibilities include an overgrowth of a localized area of the retina or a difference in the growth rate of the 2 layers of the optic cup.

Related Facts
I **Sex Ratio:** M1:F1
II **Risk of Occurrence:** ?
III **Risk of Recurrence for**
    Patient's Sib: ?
    Patient's Child: ?
IV **Age of Detectability:** At birth
V **Prevalence:** ?

Treatment
I **Primary Prevention:** —
II **Secondary Prevention:** —
III **Other Therapy:** —

Prognosis: The condition is static and generally shows no progression. Vision in the involved eye remains static and there is no threat to the normal fellow eye or to life.

Detection of Carrier: —

†**Special Considerations:** The condition may essentially represent a persistence of the posterior primary vitreous but the clinical presentation is distinctly different from anterior persistent hyperplastic primary vitreous. In 13-15 trisomy, there are many other associated congenital defects, along with the retinal fold. Coats disease is characterized by retinal telangiectasia and more widespread detach-

ment without a discrete, isolated fold.

Any inflammatory disease, and especially toxoplasmosis, can cause a retinal fold. In this case, however, the fold runs from the area of the granulomatous focus to the retinal periphery and usually does not run from the disk to the periphery unless the granuloma is in the peripapillary area.

References:

Badtke, G. and Domke, H.: Klinisch-histologischer Beitrag zur formalen Genese und Entwicklungsphysiologie der Ablatio falciformis congenita. Mit 16 Abbildungen. Klin. Monatsbl. Augenheilkd. 149:593, 1966.

Bardelli, A.: Presence of regression phenomena in ablatio falciformis retinae. Minerva Oftalmol. 10:33, 1968.

Bronner, A. et al: Falciform fold with retinal detachment. Bull. Soc. Ophthalmol. Fr. 72:391, 1972.

Duke-Elder, S.: System of Ophthalmology, vol. 3, pt. 2. Congenital Deformities. St. Louis: C.V. Mosby Co., 1963, p. 634.

Mann, I.: Developmental Abnormalities of the Eye. Philadelphia: J.B. Lippincott Co., 1957, p. 200.

Zakharchenko, V.: Congenital fold of the retina. Oftalmol. Zh. 27:445, 1972.

Contributor: **Robert M. Ellsworth**

Editor's Computerized Descriptors: Vision, Eye

RETINAL TELANGIECTASIA AND HYPOGAMMAGLOBULINEMIA

Includes: Télangiectasie rétinienne et hypogammaglobulinémie
Telangiektasie der Retina und Hypogammaglobulinämie
Telangiectasia retineana e hipogamaglobulinemia
Hypogammaglobulinemia and retinal telangiectasia

Excludes: Ataxia-telangiectasia (94)
Waldenström macroglobulinemia
Coats disease
Leber miliary retinal aneurysms

Minimal Diagnostic Criteria: Retinal telangiectasia plus hypogammaglobulinemia

Clinical Findings: Frenkel and Russe reported 2 sibs with retinal telangiectasia in 1967. The male had absence of IgA and IgM immunoglobulins and reduction of IgG immunoglobulin. The female had normal immunoglobulin levels but had a deficiency in delayed hypersensitivity. Both individuals had normal karyotypes. Six other unrelated individuals with hypogammaglobulinemia were found to have normal retinal vasculature.†

Complications
I Derived: Recurrent infections
II Associated: —

Etiology: ?

Pathogenesis: ?†

Related Facts
I Sex Ratio: ?
II Risk of Occurrence: ?
III Risk of Recurrence for
Patient's Sib: ?
Patient's Child: ?
IV Age of Detectability: —
V Prevalence: ?

Treatment
I Primary Prevention: —
II Secondary Prevention: Avoidance of pathogens
III Other Therapy: Treatment of infections as indicated

Prognosis: ?

Detection of Carrier: —

†Special Considerations: Possibly a type of cavernous hemangioma of the retina.

References:

Frenkel, M. and Russe, H. P.: Retinal telangiectasia associated with hypogammaglobulinemia. Am. J. Ophthalmol. 63:215, 1967.

Klein, M. et al: Cavernous hemangioma of the retina. Ann. Ophthalmol. 7:1213, 1975.

Contributors: **Morton F. Goldberg**
Joel Sugar

Editor's Computerized Descriptor: Eye

RETINITIS PIGMENTOSA

Includes: Rétinite pigmentaire
Tapetoretinal degeneration
Tapetoretinal dystrophy
Retinitis pigmentosa sine pigmenta
Rod-cone dystrophy
Pigmentary retinal degeneration

Excludes: Usher syndrome (983)
Gyrate atrophy (449)
Malignant myopia
Tapetochoroidal dystrophy (925)
Nightblindness, stationary (719)
Retinitis punctata albescens
Cone-rod degeneration (201)

Minimal Diagnostic Criteria: Characteristic impaired visual function and evidence of retinal disease by ERG in the presence or absence of morphologic retinal changes.

Clinical Findings: Decreased night vision and constricted visual fields are the earliest signs of retinitis pigmentosa (RP) and those often occur prior to the onset of morphologic retinal changes. The common ocular complications which add to the severity of the disease are posterior subcapsular cataracts and a macular degeneration often of the cystic type. There are several genetic variants of RP and the severity of the disease varies according to the subtype.

1) The most common form is autosomal recessive, and if sporadic cases are included, this comprises 80% of all cases. The onset is during the first 2 decades and progression is moderate with severe visual loss by the 5th decade. A slowly-progressive adult onset form of recessive disease has been noted with a recordable ERG, unlike the usual case where the ERG is often unrecordable even at a stage when visual impairment is only mild. This type is uncommon and is compatible with nearly normal visual function.

2) The autosomal dominant form also has an onset in the 1st or 2nd decade. The initial findings are mild, progression is slow, and although night vision and peripheral vision end up severely affected, central vision may be maintained into the 6th or 7th decade. Although complete penetrance is more common, families with incomplete penetrance have been described with characteristic changes in the temporal aspects of the ERG. A sectorial form of RP is seen in some dominant pedigrees. This progresses very slowly and is compatible with good function in the normal patches of retina. The sectorial form can masquerade as a nerve fiber bundle defect if corresponding pigmentary changes are not noted in the fundus.

3) The X-linked form is the least common type of RP but is also the most severe with profound visual loss by the 4th decade. The female carrier will often show signs of retinal involvement and may even be symptomatic. A less severe form of X-linked RP also occurs.

The typical retinal changes are clumps of pigment resembling bone corpuscles in the equatorial region, attenuated arterioles and a waxy somewhat pale disk. The pigment epithelium often develops white dots or diffuse depigmentation easily seen on fluorescein angiography. The pigment dispersion in the retina may take the form of round clumps and, rarely, no pigment is seen. The initial changes are often fine pigment stippling with accumulations over the retinal vessels. Fine salt and pepper changes characterized by tiny pigment clumps surrounded by rings of depigmentation help to distinguish the pathologic fundus of early RP from normal blonde fundi.

Dark adaptometry invariably shows elevated thresholds.

However, mild and atypical cases may demonstrate normal dark adaptation in some areas of the retina with elevated thresholds elsewhere. The visual field is often first affected in the equatorial region producing an encircling ring-type scotoma which widens toward the periphery and the center with resulting tubular vision. Arcuate or sector defects are also possible. Color vision may be affected with a tendency towards acquired tritanopia. Electrophysiologic studies are abnormal early in the course of the disease. A reduced or absent ERG is the rule, and the EOG and early receptor potential (ERP) are also reduced.

Complications
I **Derived:** —
II **Associated:** Ocular: Myopia, macular degeneration, cataracts, glaucoma, retinal detachment, keratoconus, drusen of the optic nerve, microphthalmia, achromatopsia, ophthalmoplegia.

Extraocular: Impaired hearing is common. There are a host of genetic disorders with associated RP including abetalipoproteinemia, Refsum syndrome, ceroid lipofuscinoses, micropolysaccharidoses types I-H, I-S, II and III, Bardet-Biedl syndrome, hereditary ataxias and myotonic dystrophy.

Etiology: Autosomal recessive, autosomal dominant, and X-linked recessive transmission. Unilateral cases are rare, sporadic, and probably of distinct etiology, possibly vascular; McK *26800, *18010, *31260

Pathogenesis: There is a progressive degeneration of the receptors with associated glial overgrowth and an eventual narrowing of the retinal vessels. Depigmentation of the retinal epithelium with a migration of its pigment into the retina is characteristic.

The main area of pathology is the neuroepithelium with progressive loss of rods and cones and abnormal pigment epithelium. Degenerated receptors may become partly replaced by neuroglia. The ganglion cells and the nerve fiber layer remain relatively unchanged. The retinal vessels, arterioles and veins alike, always show marked changes, generally atrophic.

Electron microscopic studies in RP emphasize the relationship between the pigment epithelium and the neural retina. A recent study on an autosomal dominant eye showed only a few abnormal cones left in the fovea. The pigment epithelium had increased lipofuscin near the macula while in the periphery, the cells contained only melanin. Recently, absence of 1 of 2 receptors for the alcohol form of vitamin A was demonstrated in the retina of an eye with severe X-linked RP.

Related Facts
I **Sex Ratio:** M1:F1 for autosomal dominant and autosomal recessive. M1:F0 for X-linked form.
II **Risk of Occurrence:** Varies with mode of transmission.
III **Risk of Recurrence for**
Patient's Sib: Whether autosomal recessive, autosomal dominant, or X-linked recessive, see Table I AR, AD, or X-linked R, respectively.
Patient's Child: Whether autosomal recessive, autosomal dominant, or X-linked recessive, see Table I AR, AD, or X-linked R, respectively.
IV **Age of Detectability:** Dependent on type of transmission with most frequent onset at the end of the 1st decade or beginning of 2nd decade
V **Prevalence:** Varies from 1:2000 to 1:7000 with an estimated carrier rate of 1:80

Treatment
I **Primary Prevention:** Genetic counseling
II **Secondary Prevention:** —
III **Other Therapy:** Night vision aids and optical field wideners

may help some symptoms. Protecting the retina from bright light by sunglasses or occlusion has been advocated. Appropriate therapy for hearing loss is also needed.

Prognosis: Normal life span unless influenced by an associated systemic problem. There is always impairment of visual fields and night vision but acuity may be normal.

Detection of Carrier: In the X-linked form the carrier may show a golden glistening "spotty" or "streaky" reflex in the macular area or throughout most of the eyegrounds. This change has been called a "tapetal" reflex. A few carriers will show some of the changes seen in males, but usually, in general, no functional disturbances are noted. Occasionally a mild abnormality, particularly of dark adaptation, or of the ERG is found. Rarely the female carrier will show marked symptoms. The ERP has also been used to identify carriers. Carriers generally cannot be detected in the autosomal recessive form. Pedigree analysis may reveal obligate carriers.

Special Considerations: —

References:
Deutman, A.F.: Rod-cone dystrophy: Primary hereditary, pigmentary retinopathy, retinitis pigmentosa. In Krill, A.E. and Archer, D.B. (eds.): Krill's Hereditary Retinal and Choroidal Diseases. Hagerstown:Harper & Row, 1977, vol. 2.
Duke-Elder, S. and Dobree, J.H.: System of Ophthalmology. vol. 10. Diseases of the Retina. St. Louis:C.V. Mosby Co., 1967.
Franceschetti, A. et al: Chorioretinal Heredodegeneration. Springfield: Charles C Thomas, 1974.
Klein, D.: Genetic approach to the nosology of retinal disorders. In Bergsma, D. (ed.): Part VIII. Eye. Birth Defects: Orig. Art. Ser., vol. VII, no. 3. Baltimore: William & Wilkins for The National Foundation-March of Dimes, 1971, p. 52.
Merin, S. and Auerbach, E.: Retinitis pigmentosa. Surv. of Ophthalmol. 20:303, 1976.

Contributors: **Mitchel L. Wolf**
Donald R. Bergsma
Alex E. Krill‡

Editor's Computerized Descriptors: Vision, Eye, Hearing

RETINOBLASTOMA

Includes: Rétinoblastome
Retinoblastom
Endophytum type retinoblastoma
Exophytum type retinoblastoma

Excludes: Retinal astrocytoma
Diktyoma

Minimal Diagnostic Criteria: Characteristic ophthalmoscopic appearance of a tumor arising in the retina of 1 or both eyes, usually occurring in a young infant. When the tumor is obscured by overlying detachment or inflammatory reaction in the vitreous, diagnostic xray and ultrasonography may be useful.†

P-32 uptake studies may be useful in special situations although the injection of P-32 into infants must be regarded with great circumspection. Computerized axial tomography has been of great value both in detecting a mass lesion within the eye and appreciating calcific densities that cannot be demonstrated by other techniques. CT scanning is also useful in detecting extension of tumor into the optic nerve, into the orbit, and into the middle cranial fossa.

Increased levels of lactic acid dehydrogenase have been found in almost all patients with retinoblastoma. The absolute level of this enzyme is increased in the aqueous. The aqueous:serum ratio is always greater than 1 and there is a fairly characteristic isoenzyme pattern. Simulating lesions rarely give an elevated aqueous LDH level.

Clinical Findings: The average age at the time of tumor diagnosis is 17 months. The most common presenting sign is a white "cat's eye reflex" in the pupil, and the 2nd most common sign is strabismus. Occasionally, spontaneous necrosis in the tumor will lead to a red, painful eye, with or without secondary glaucoma. In older children, poor vision or vitreous floaters are occasionally a presenting complaint. Because of a family history, sibs are examined early in life, and about 3% of these tumors are apprehended on routine examination.

The tumor arises multifocally in the retina and at least three-fourths of all cases have more than 1 tumor in an involved eye. The tumor arises bilaterally in one-third to one-fourth of all cases with a greater chance for bilaterality in the inherited cases. Retinoblastoma occurs in eyes of normal size and cataract is never seen except as a rare, late complication. The tumor may grow from the retina forward into the vitreous space, the endophytum type, when it can be clearly seen with an ophthalmoscope during the early stages. The tumors usually have a very characteristic creamy-pink color with numerous blood vessels on the surface. The exophytum type, however, grows beneath the retina, in the potential subretinal space, and a lesion may be obscured by an overlying detachment, and the borders and surface characteristics cannot be clearly seen. Two clinical findings are more or less pathognomonic of retinoblastoma. The first of these is calcification within the tumor which can be appreciated either with the ophthalmoscope or by xray. Pfeiffer has reported that approximately 75% of retinoblastomas will show intraocular calcification if the radiographs are properly exposed. When the tumor has achieved a relatively large size, the stroma breaks down and portions of the tumor float about in the vitreous as "seeds". The only other clinical condition that faintly resembles this is the "snowball floaters" seen in sarcoidosis, but the associated vascular findings in that disease in the absence of a tumor usually make the differentiation easy.

Complications
I Derived: Ocular: Retinal detachment. Inflammatory reaction due to spontaneous necrosis. Secondary glaucoma. Phthisis bulbi.

Systemic complications: This tumor may spread directly by way of the optic nerve into the subarachnoid space when the base of the brain can be seeded with tumor material, which then produces CNS symptoms and death. It also may metastasize hematogenously, usually following extension into the choroid, and may then appear in various organs within the body. The bone marrow is probably the tissue first invaded, but multiple viscera may be involved later. It is curious that the lung parenchyma is rarely involved. When the tumor extends out of the eye into the orbit it may then spread lymphogenously to the regional nodes.

II Associated: Many observers have been alerted to associated clinical defects, but none have been found. There is a suggestion that the excretion of HVA or VMA may be elevated in this disease.

Although about 5% of patients with retinoblastoma have mental retardation, the vast majority of cases seem to have a high IQ and excellent intellectual development.

Patients with the germinal mutation for retinoblastoma seem to have both increased susceptibility to radiation-induced tumors at relatively low dosage levels and a high incidence of second primary neoplasms later in life unrelated to retinoblastoma or the treatment thereof. Osteogenic sarcoma is the most common 2nd tumor although a great variety of other lesions have been reported.

Etiology: Probably autosomal dominant transmission with incomplete penetrance. Some reports of chromosome 13q-.

All patients with a family history and all patients with bilateral disease are assumed to be germinal mutations. Approximately 15% of unilateral sporadic cases eventually are revealed to be germinal mutations but the remainder are not transmitted as would be expected of an autosomal dominant disease. These latter may represent somatic mutation and the clinical picture seems to be 1 tumor in 1 eye. McK *18020

Pathogenesis: The tumors arise in 1 or both eyes from multiple foci in the retina, and then grow at variable rates, until the globe is entirely filled with tumor. At variable times during this course, extension into the optic nerve and subarachnoid space, or into the bloodstream with hematogenous metastasis may occur.

Related Facts
I Sex Ratio: Ml:Fl
II Risk of Occurrence: The tumor now appears to arise in 1 in 20,000 births (approximately 200 new cases are seen in the United States each year).

As more patients with germinal mutations live to reproductive age, an increase in incidence may be expected.
III Risk of Recurrence for
Patient's Sib: With no family history, 1%; with a positive family history: 50%
Patient's Child: 8-25% if parent had unilateral involvement; almost 50% if parent had bilateral retinoblastoma.
IV Age of Detectability: Birth to old age. At least 2 cases with metastatic retinoblastoma at birth are known and an occasional patient with spontaneous regression has been identified up to the age of 62 years.

The vast majority of patients are detected before the age of 2 years. It is extremely unlikely to see the appearance of a new tumor beyond the age of 3 years.
V Prevalence: ?

Treatment
I Primary Prevention: Genetic counseling
II Secondary Prevention: In families with a positive history, strenuous efforts must be made to examine all children within 1 week of birth. Supervoltage radiation is the most effective form of treatment, as this tumor is radiocurable.

The average tumor dose is 3500-4000 r delivered over 3-4 weeks. Radioactive cobalt applicators, light coagulation, diathermy and cryotherapy are valuable adjunctive measures.
III Other Therapy: The tumor is highly sensitive to various chemotherapeutic agents including nitrogen mustard, TEM, thio-TEPA, methotrexate, Cytoxan, actinomycin-D and vincristine. These agents are not curative however, and should be used only in conjunction with radiation or in the treatment of as yet incurable metastatic disease.

Prognosis: Overall mortality in the United States: 20%-much higher in less-developed countries. The stage of the disease at the time that diagnosis is made is the most significant factor in the eventual outcome.

For practical purposes, all fatal cases have 1 or both eyes in group 5 of the Reese-Ellsworth classification. If cases are detected at any earlier stage and adequate treatment is undertaken, there is virtually no mortality.

Prognosis appears to be better correlated with size and extent of tumor than with the histologic types.

Several articles have claimed that the mortality is greater in Negroes than in Caucasians, but on careful analysis it appears that this is due to the stage of the disease at the time treatment is undertaken.

Detection of Carrier: The chromosome pattern is normal in most families with hereditary retinoblastoma, and at this time, there is no way to identify the normal carriers of the abnormal genes.

†**Special Considerations:** This is a highly dangerous, hereditary tumor in which early diagnosis is vital. Leukokoria must be regarded as perhaps the most dangerous sign in all of ophthalmology and should lead to thorough investigation for retinoblastoma. Once the tumor has extended outside the eye into the orbit the chances of cure are minimal and no patients with metastatic retinoblastoma have ever survived. The differential diagnosis can be quite complex, and the most commonly confused conditions are larval granulomatosis, Coats disease, angiomatosis retinae and granulomatous uveitis. Persistent hyperplastic vitreous, retrolental fibroplasia, congenital retinal folds, medullated nerve fibers and colobomas can usually be readily identified when the children are examined under anesthesia.

The second most common presenting sign is strabismus and all children with this condition should have careful ophthalmoscopic examination of the retina even if this requires examination under anesthesia with an indirect ophthalmoscope.

References:
Bishop, J. and Madson, E.C.: Retinoblastoma. Review of the current status. Surv. Ophthalmol. 19:342, 1975.
Duke-Elder, S.: System of Ophthalmology, vol. 10. Diseases of the Ocular Media. St. Louis: C.V. Mosby, 1967, p. 672.
Ellsworth, R.M.: The practical management of retino-blastoma. Trans. Am. Ophthalmol. Soc. 67:462, 1969.
Reese, A.B.: Tumors of the Eye, 3rd Ed. New York: Harper and Row, 1976.

Contributor: **Robert M. Ellsworth**

Editor's Computerized Descriptors: Vision, Eye

RETINOSCHISIS

Includes: Retinosquisis
Congenital vascular veils in the vitreous
Vitreoretinal dystrophy
Congenital retinal cyst
Giant cyst of the retina
Juvenile retinoschisis, X-linked
Senile retinoschisis, autosomal recessive
Typical retinoschisis, autosomal dominant

Excludes: Retinal detachment

Minimal Diagnostic Criteria: The retinal findings noted below are usually easily seen and are entirely typical.

Clinical Findings: The clinical signs and symptoms usually fit into 1 of 3 common pictures:

Typical retinoschisis commonly occurs in hyperopic young males, is frequently bilateral and is often strikingly symmetric. The lesion begins most commonly in the inferior temporal quadrant, or somewhat less commonly in the superior temporal quadrant and appears ophthalmoscopically as a thin, translucent, veil-like membrane extending up as a dome into the vitreous. The translucent membrane contains the retinal vessels and often has small white dots which represent glial strands extending across the cystic area. The vitreous is usually fluid and posterior vitreous detachment is common. The process is often static for many years or very slowly progressive.

Senile retinoschisis, the 2nd clinical variant, is related to the 1st. It is commonly noted in older patients on routine examination and is rarely symptomatic. It is bilateral in approximately 90% of cases and may develop as a coalescence of peripheral cysts of Blessig. In the early stage, the cystic space is spanned by thin, grey fibers which gradually break, allowing the inner and outer leaves to separate forming an elevated cyst. In senile retinoschisis the split retina may extend 360° around the retinal periphery, but it does not commonly progress posteriorly and may remain static for many years.

Juvenile retinoschisis, the 3rd type of retinoschisis, is the one that causes serious problems. The area involved by the schisis is much more extensive and often extends back over the macular area and may involve the entire retina, resulting in a total retinal detachment with preretinal organization and a hopeless surgical prognosis. In the earlier stages, the areas of schisis often exhibit large holes in the anterior leaf between vessels, and, if breaks develop in both the anterior and the posterior leaf of the schisis, a true retinal detachment may occur. These eyes, with a combination of retinoschisis and retinal detachment, are particularly difficult to manage surgically. Patients with juvenile retinoschisis commonly have cystic macular degeneration which adds to the visual defect and makes a surgical prognosis for useful vision more questionable. Both macular degeneration and splitting of the retina through the macula may contribute to the visual defect in some patients. The visual field shows a complete scotoma with a sharp edge in the area of the schisis and the electroretinogram (ERG) is markedly depressed but not obliterated.

Complications
I **Derived:** Retinal detachment may complicate retinoschisis if holes are present in both the anterior and the posterior leaf. Hemorrhage into the vitreous may occur as a result of traction on the retinal vessels but may be mild and self-limited.
II **Associated:** Cystic macular degeneration, hyperopia.

Etiology: Typical retinoschisis is usually autosomal dominant.

Senile retinoschisis is usually autosomal recessive. Juvenile retinoschisis is X-linked. McK *31270

Pathogenesis: Hereditary lamellar splitting in the layers of the retina usually occurs in the plane of the outer plexiform layer. Juvenile retinoschisis may be related to congenital vascular veils in the vitreous and may be due to a condensation of the vitreous which was in contact with the inner layers of the optic cup. It is possible, too, that there is some persistence of the secondary branches of the vasa propria hyaloidae.

The more common type of retinoschisis resulting in "giant retinal cysts" is probably caused by the secretion of hyaluronic acid-sensitive mucopolysaccharide by some of the cells in the inner portion of the retinal cyst. Once retinoschisis has begun on the basis of this secretory mechanism it may easily spread to peripheral areas of cystoid degeneration and may progress posteriorly through normal retina.

Senile retinoschisis, especially the very mild nonprogressive type, may simply represent a coalescence of peripheral microcysts without the secretory mechanism that commonly causes progression.

Related Facts
I **Sex Ratio:** Both common and senile types M1:F1; juvenile retinoschisis M1:F0
II **Risk of Occurrence:** ?
III **Risk of Recurrence for**
    Patient's Sib: For typical retinoschisis, see Table I AD. For senile retinoschisis, see Table I AR. For juvenile retinoschisis, see Table I X-linked R.
    Patient's Child: For typical retinoschisis, see Table I AD. For senile retinoschisis, see Table I AR. For juvenile retinoschisis, see Table I X-linked R.
IV **Age of Detectability:** Juvenile retinoschisis may be seen at birth; the more common type of retinal cyst is usually seen in young men; and the senile type is seen in the 5th, 6th and 7th decades.
V **Prevalence:** ?

Treatment
I **Primary Prevention:** Genetic counseling
II **Secondary Prevention:** Light coagulation or cryotherapy for juvenile retinoschisis and for selected other patients.

The fluid in the area of schisis is extremely viscid and it is very difficult to drain this fluid off by conventional detachment procedures. Since, in many instances, especially in older adults there is no progression of the disease, treatment may not be necessary. In general, the indications for treatment are as follows: a) Any child with retinoschisis should be treated. This form of disease invariably progresses and can possibly be arrested before the macula is threatened. b) Documented progression of the schisis behind the equator in adult patients, especially when the temporal retina is involved. c) Any case that has demonstrable holes in both the inner and outer leaf of the schisis. It is in these patients that complicated detachments can occur. d) Retinal detachment in the fellow eye.

Two treatment modalities are effective. Light coagulation has been shown to cause collapse of these cysts. There are 2 rational approaches using light coagulation. The area of the "giant cyst" can be delimited with coagulations which may pose a temporary barrier, but cannot be relied upon to contain retinoschisis. If, in addition to a delimiting row of coagulations, the entire area of the schisis is treated, the fluid will often absorb over a period of weeks or months. Apparently the heat has some effect on the intraretinal fluid causing its resorption. The 2nd approach is cryotherapy, again treating the entire area of the schisis from the scleral side. At the present state of our knowledge, it would seem that either light coagulation or cryotherapy is equally effective.
III **Other Therapy:** —

Prognosis: Normal for life; guarded for vision in the juvenile type

Detection of Carrier: —

Special Considerations: —

References:
Broderick, J.D. and Wyatt, H.T.: Hereditary sex-linked retinoschisis. Br. J. Ophthalmol. 57:551, 1973.
Byer, N.: Clinical study of senile retinoschisis. Arch. Ophthalmol. 79:36, 1968.
Cibis, P.A.: Retinoschisis-retinal cysts. Trans. Am. Ophthalmol. Soc. 63:417, 1965.
Duke-Elder, S.: System of Ophthalmology, vol. 3, part 2. Congenital Deformities. St. Louis: C.V. Mosby, 1963, p. 643.
Ewing, C.C. and Jones, E.: Juvenile hereditary retinoschisis. Trans. Ophthalmol. Soc. UK 89:29, 1969.
Falls, H.: Retinoschisis. In Kimura, S.J. and Caygill, W.M. (eds.): Symposium on Differential Diagnostic Problems of Posterior Uveitis: Retinal Diseases. Philadelphia: Lea and Febiger, 1966.
Forsius, H. et al: A genetic study of three rare retinal disorders: Dystrophia retinae dysacusis syndrome, X-chromosomal retinoschisis and grouped pigments of the retina. In Bergsma, D. (ed.): Part VIII. Eye, Birth Defects:Orig. Art. Ser., vol. VII, no 3. Baltimore: Williams & Wilkins for The National Foundation-March of Dimes, 1971, p. 83.
Klein, D.: Genetic approach to the nosology of retinal disorders. Ibid, p. 52.
Mann, I: Developmental Abnormalities of the Eye. Philadelphia: J.B. Lippincott, 1957, p. 217.

Contributor: **Robert M. Ellsworth**

Editor's Computerized Descriptors: Vision, Eye

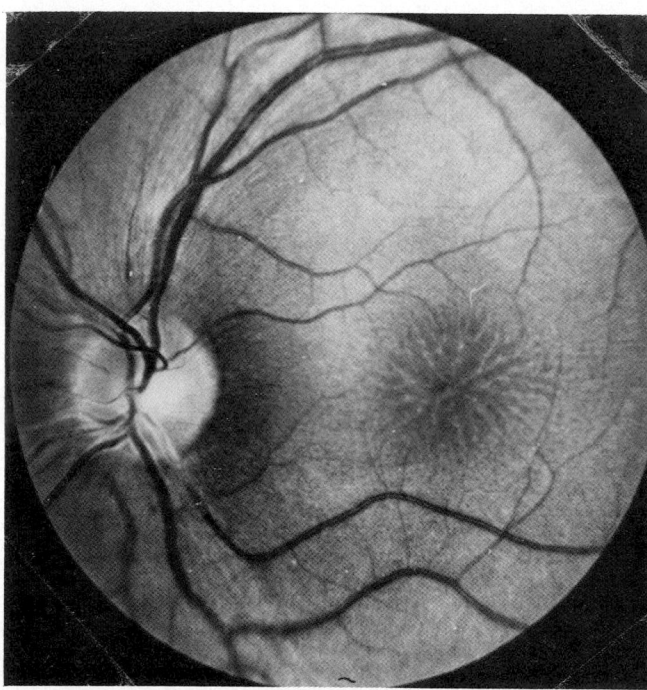

444. Cystic foveal degeneration with radial distribution in X-linked recessive retinoschisis

RETROLENTAL FIBROPLASIA

Includes: Fibroplasie rétro-cristallinienne
Retinolentale Fibroplasie
Fibroplasia retrolental
Retinopathy of prematurity

Excludes: Other causes of retrolental membranes

Minimal Diagnostic Criteria: Bilateral retinal pathology as noted below in premature children of low birthweight who have received oxygen. The earliest stages of the disease usually appear within the 1st month of life.

Classification of retrolental fibroplasia (see reference).

Active Stages: Stage 1. Dilatation and tortuosity of retinal vessels. Stage 2. Stage 1 plus neovascularization and some peripheral retinal clouding. Stage 3. Stage 2 plus retinal detachment of the periphery of the fundus and frequently a retinal fold extending from the disk to the retinal periphery. Of these folds, approximately 90% occur on the temporal side of the globe. Vitreous hemorrhage often occurs during this stage. Stage 4. Hemispheric or circumferential retinal detachment. Stage 5. Complete retinal detachment with contracture and organization into a retrolental membrane. Massive vitreous hemorrhage may occur during retinal organization.

Late cicatricial grades:

Grade I: Small mass of opaque, grey tissue in the periphery of the retina without visible retinal detachment. There may be some floating grey vitreous opacities and some pigment disturbance in the retinal periphery. Myopia is common but vision may be normal or near normal.

Grade II: A larger mass of opaque, grey tissue in the retinal periphery with some localized retinal detachment. The disk may show moderate distortion with "dragging" of the major retinal vessels toward the periphery so that they are straighter than usual. This usually occurs toward the temporal side and the macula may be displaced with obvious heterotopia and vision in the range of 20/40 to 20/200.

Grade III: Large mass of opaque tissue in the retina with a fold extending from this mass to the nervehead. When a retinal fold is present, the vision is usually in the 20/200 to hand motion range. As the fold forms, there is often some hemorrhage along the edges of the fold which later is represented by proliferation of the retinal pigment epithelium.

Grade IV: More extensive circumferential retinal pathology with a retrolental membrane covering part of the retrolental space: the vision in these eyes is usually at the hand motion to light perception level.

Grade V: A total retrolental membrane covering the entire posterior surface of the lens. The entire retina is incorporated into the retrolental membrane and these patients are totally blind.

Clinical Findings: This condition occurs in premature, but generally otherwise normal infants, usually born between 26 and 31 weeks gestation, of low birthweight from 800-1500 gm, who have received supplementary oxygen. The disease rarely occurs in full-term children of normal birthweight who have not received oxygen therapy. With some exceptions the disease is bilateral and is usually symmetric. There is an active phase early in life which becomes clinically evident at 3-5 weeks, postnatally. The earliest sign is constriction of the retinal arterioles which is then followed by venous dilatation, increased tortuosity, neovascularization and retinal and vitreous hemorrhage, occurring commonly in the periphery and most commonly in the temporal half of the retina. An exudative phase appears in the vitreous and white patches of edema occur in the peripheral retina followed by retinal detachment. The process may end spontaneously at any stage and if only peripheral cicatrization occurs, useful vision may be retained. In about 25% of the cases a progressive cicatricial phase develops from the 2nd to the 5th month of life, characterized by organization and contracture of the entire retina. The end result is formation of retinal folds or the formation of a dense, grey-white membrane lying behind the lens and obscuring all view of the fundus. As the retina undergoes progressive contraction, the ciliary processes are drawn into the mass and may be visible all around the circumference of the lens without indentation of the globe. The retrolental membrane is frequently vascularized and it is possible that progressive traction on this membrane accounts for the deep hemorrhage that occasionally occurs. The iris is also involved in the process of neovascularization and large radial iris vessels and posterior synechiae are common. The eyes may pass through a transient stage of glaucoma but the final end result of the contracture is phthisis bulbi. After the age of 6 years the condition of the eyes is usually stationary, although detachments can occur to about age 10 in patients having classifications Grade III or IV.

Complications
I **Derived:** Secondary glaucoma may occur during the phase of vasoproliferation and intraocular hemorrhage. Heterochromia may follow anterior segment hemorrhage. Eccentric fixation may occur following contracture of a temporal fold with ectopia of the macula.
II **Associated:** High myopia may occur along with retrolental fibroplasia as a feature of prematurity. Mental retardation, in some degree, is present in about 40% of cases.

Etiology: In premature infants the retinal vasculature is not fully developed at birth and is abnormally sensitive to the vasoconstrictive effect of ambient oxygen.†

Pathogenesis: The arterioles contract producing hypoxia of the peripheral retina and in response to this, vasoproliferation occurs on the retinal surface with hemorrhage into the retina and vitreous, followed by secondary organization with detachment, which may progress to total retinal detachment and contracture to phthisis bulbi. In addition to vasoproliferation, the hypoxia may produce areas of complete vasoobliteration and considerable capillary endothelial damage.

Related Facts
I **Sex Ratio:** M1:F1
II **Risk of Occurrence:** Now rare
III **Risk of Recurrence for**
 Patient's Sib: None
 Patient's Child: None
IV **Age of Detectability:** Birth to 6 weeks
V **Prevalence:** Rare

Treatment
I **Primary Prevention:** The ambient oxygen level in the incubator should be kept as low as possible concomitant with the well-being of the infant, in general, at a level of 40% or below. Catheterization of the umbilical artery is useful to monitor the blood pO₂ levels. Indirect ophthalmoscopy is not an effective way to monitor oxygen levels since persistent vitreous haze in premature infants may make visualization difficult and there is very poor correlation between the arterial caliber as viewed with the opthalmoscope and arterial oxygen tension values. Fluorescein angiography may detect early pathologic changes but has not been useful in the practical monitoring of premature infants.
II **Secondary Prevention:** Radiation and steroids have been used but without definite effect. Light coagulation employed early in the active stages may arrest progression. Cryotherapy may also be useful in obliterating peripheral neovas-cular tufts in eyes that are technically difficult to treat with light coagulation.
III **Other Therapy:** —

Prognosis: Normal life span. In Stage 1 and Stage 2 the active phase may regress spontaneously without serious retinal pathology. The healed Grades I and II eyes may have normal maculae and essentially normal vision. In Grade III and Grade IV eyes, there may be later retinal detachment occurring at age 5 through 10 years which causes progressive loss of vision. In Grade V eyes-total loss of vision.

Detection of Carrier: —

†**Special Considerations:** In premature infants with an essentially normal cardiovascular system there is fairly good data indicating that retinal changes will not occur if the ambient oxygen concentration is maintained at a level of 40% or less. The incidence of retrolental fibroplasia is definitely related to prematurity (and birthweight) and is more frequent and more severe in smaller infants.

The rate of withdrawal from oxygen does not seem to be related to the occurrence of retrolental fibroplasia. The retina shows a unique type of vascularization. At the 4th month of gestation, vessels from the embryonic hyaloid system extend into the retina and the retina does not receive its full normal vascularization until shortly after birth in the full-term infant. Perhaps < 1% of all cases of retrolental fibroplasia have occurred in infants receiving no significant oxygen therapy and this appears to be related to immaturity of the retinal vessels and peripheral anoxia in the absence of the vasoconstrictive effect of oxygen. In utero, the arterial oxygen saturation is only 50% or so and it is possible that the relative increase in oxygen saturation following birth may be enough to stimulate the sensitive premature retinal vessels to cause vasoproliferation and retrolental fibroplasia.

Current interest in retrolental fibroplasia centers around infants with the respiratory distress syndrome where there is pulmonary pathology and frequently right-to-left shunts. In these infants the level of ambient oxygen does not reflect arterial oxygen concentration, and it is only by monitoring arterial pO₂ that we may appreciate the oxygen levels in the retina. Safe limits of oxygen therapy have not been defined but at the moment it would seem that retinal pO₂ should be maintained at 100 mm Hg or less to avoid retinal pathology.

References:
Ashton, N. et al: Effect of oxygen on developing retinal vessels with particular reference to problem of retrolental fibroplasia. Br. J. Ophthalmol. 38:397, 1954.
Brockhurst, R.J. and Chishti, M.L.: Cicatrical retrolental fibroplasia: Its occurrence without oxygen administration and in full term infants. Albrecht von Graefes Arch. Klin. Ophthalmol. 195:113, 1975.
Cohen, J. et al: Clinical evaluation of school-age children with retrolental fibroplasia. Am. J. Ophthalmol. 57:41, 1964.
Duke-Elder, S.: System of Ophthalmology, vol. 3, part 2. Congenital Deformities. St. Louis.C.V. Mosby, 1963, p. 187.
Flynn, J.T.: Acute proliferative retrolental fibroplasia: Evolution of the lesion. Albrecht von Graefes Arch. Klin. Ophthalmol. 195:101, 1975.
Foos, R.Y.: Acute retrolental fibroplasia. Albrecht von Graefes Arch. Klin. Ophthalmol. 195:87, 1975.
Kinsey, E.: Retrolental fibroplasia; cooperative study of retrolental fibroplasia and use of oxygen. Arch. Ophthalmol. 56:481, 1956.
National Soc. Prev. of Blindness (Subcommittee, A.B. Reese, Chairman): Classification of retrolental fibroplasia. Am. J. Ophthalmol. 36:1333, 1953.
Patz, A.: New role of the ophthalmologist in prevention of retrolental fibroplasia. Arch. Ophthalmol. 78:565, 1967.

Patz, A.: The role of oxygen in retrolental fibroplasia. Albrecht von Graefes Arch. Klin. Ophthalmol. 195:77, 1975.

Stern, L.: Oxygen toxicity in premature infants. Albrecht von Graefes Arch. Klin. Ophthalmol. 195:71, 1975.

Tasman, W.: Retinal detachment in retrolental fibroplasia. Albrecht von Graefes Arch. Klin. Ophthalmol. 195:129, 1975.

Contributor: **Robert M. Ellsworth**

Editor's Computerized Descriptor: Eye

RICKETS, VITAMIN D-DEPENDENT

Includes: Rachitisme vitamino dépendant
Vitamin-D-abhängige Rachitis (Prader)
Raquitismo vitamino D-dependiente
Hereditary pseudovitamin D-deficiency rickets (PDR)
Hereditary vitamin D-dependent rickets
Autosomal recessive vitamin D-dependency (ARVDD)
Hypocalcemic, hypophosphatemic rickets with aminoaciduria
Type III, A, ii vitamin D refractory rickets with aminoaciduria (Classification of Fraser and Slater)

Excludes: Vitamin D-deficiency rickets
Hypophosphatemia (517)
Renal rickets
Hypophosphatemic rickets associated with glucosuria, renal tubular acidosis and cystinosis

Minimal Diagnostic Criteria: Radiologic rickets with hypocalcemia and elevated alkaline phosphatase in which the vitamin D requirement is 10- 100- fold greater than that needed to prevent vitamin D-deficiency rickets. Exclusion of other disorders including intestinal malabsorption, renal insufficiency and renal tubular abnormalities.

Clinical Findings: The clinical course is similar to that of vitamin D-deficiency rickets. Symptoms usually appear before the age of 2 years and commonly include growth failure, hypotonia, weakness and motor retardation. Pathologic fractures may occur. Often there is a history of convulsions or tetany and in some children this may be the presenting clinical feature. A history of adequate intake of vitamin D is often obtained.

Physical findings include thickening of the wrists and ankles, frontal bowing of lower limbs, and positive Trousseau and Chvostek signs. Skeletal xrays reveal signs of classic rickets that may vary in severity and are indistinguishable from those seen in vitamin D-deficiency rickets.

The serum calcium is low and serum phosphate low or normal, while the serum alkaline phosphatase and parathyroid hormone levels are elevated. Generalized aminoaciduria and elevated urinary cyclic AMP are probably secondary to increased circulating parathyroid hormone. Antirachitic activity, as measured by bioassay, is normal while serum 1,25 dihydroxy vitamin D_3 has been reported to be low. GI absorption of calcium and phosphorus are depressed. Mild hyperchloremic acidosis may be present.

Complications
I   **Derived:** Rachitic deformities and growth failure.
II **Associated:** Hypotonia, muscle weakness, tetany and convulsions. Enamel hypoplasia of teeth that form postnatally.

Etiology: Autosomal recessive; McK *26470

Pathogenesis: Probable genetic defect in renal 25-hydroxycholecalciferol 1-hydroxylase, the enzyme responsible for the conversion of 25 hydroxy vitamin D_3 to 1,25 dihydroxyvitamin D_3. This results in an attenuated response to normal amounts of vitamin D with subsequent development of classic rickets and hypocalcemia.

Related Facts
I   **Sex Ratio:** M1:F1
II **Risk of Occurrence:**   ?
III **Risk of Recurrence for**
   Patient's Sib: 1 in 4 (25%) for each offspring to be affected.
   Patient's Child: Not increased unless mate is carrier or homozygote.
IV **Age of Detectability:** Usually before the age of 2 years and as early as the 3rd or 4th month of life.
V   **Prevalence:**   ?

Treatment
I   Primary Prevention: Genetic counseling
II   Secondary Prevention: Early recognition of affected infants with early and continuous treatment with 10 to 100 times the normal requirement of vitamin D_2 or D_3. Limited experience has demonstrated that small amounts, possibly physiologic quantities, of 1,25 dihydroxyvitamin D_3 or 1-α-hydroxyvitamin D_3 are effective. These compounds do not require 1-α-hydroxylation and appear to be the most promising form of therapy. Discontinuation of treatment with either preparation results in the reappearance of vitamin D-depletion syndrome within a few days, this is of obvious advantage in minimizing or avoiding vitamin D intoxication.
III   Other Therapy: Calcium therapy for hypocalcemic tetany and convulsions. Orthopedic correction of deformities.

Prognosis: Treatment results in complete healing of rickets with normalization of plasma calcium and phosphate concentrations, remission of muscle hypotonia and weakness and normalization of growth. Continuous treatment required throughout childhood and possibly for life.

Detection of Carrier: ?

Special Considerations: —

References:
Fraser, D. et al: Pathogenesis of hereditary vitamin D-dependent rickets: An inborn error of vitamin D metabolism involving defective conversion of 25-hydroxycholecalciferol to 1α,25-dihydroxyvitamin D. N. Engl. J. Med. 289:817, 1973.
Fraser, D. and Salter, R.B.: The diagnosis and management of the various types of rickets. Pediatr. Clin. North Am. 5:417, 1958.
Hamilton, R. et al: The small intestine in vitamin D-dependent rickets. Pediatrics 45:364, 1970.
Prader, A. et al: Eine besondere Form der primären vitamin D-resistenten Rachitis mit Hypocalcamie und Autosomaldominantem Erbgang: Die hereditare Pseudo-mangelrachitis. Helv. Paediatr. Acta 16:452, 1961.
Scriver, C.R. Vitamin D dependency. Pediatrics 45:361, 1970.

Contributors: **David W. Gardner**
Constantine S. Anast

Editor's Computerized Descriptors: Teeth, Skel., Muscle, Nerve

RING CONSTRICTIONS

Includes: Brides, sillons (amniotiques)
Ringförmige Strikturen
Constricciones anulares congénitas
Congenital amputations
Annular grooves
Amniotic bands
Streeter dysplasia

Excludes: Agenesis of limbs or parts of limbs due to primary failure to form
Congenital amelia or partial amelia due to focal or intercalary defects
Ainhum
Congenital deafness with childhood appearance of keratopachydermia with constricting bands about fingers and toes

Minimal Diagnostic Criteria: Presence of scarred ring encircling limb or digit. Interruption of normal skin whorls at stumps of amputated digits and presence of cicatrix with absence of digital whorls in limb stumps proximal to digital level. Presence of whorls on tips of nondigital stumps suggests primary agenesis.†

Clinical Findings: Disorder present at birth and involves 1 or more limbs; not symmetric. May have multiple rings on the 1 limb. Limb may be involved both proximally and distally. Narrow ring of scar tissue encircles digit, or limb constriction may extend to contact with bone. Distal to constriction, part may be distended due to lymphedema or large quantity of fat and may be distorted in shape (ie clubfoot). Growth may be stunted. Fenestrated syndactyly is frequent. Complete amputation of digit or limb may occur in utero. Stump heals with cicatrix with interference with normal digital whorls. Amputated part is occasionally found in amniotic fluid. Lesions are usually epithelialized by the time of birth but active process has been observed with black eschars and hanging shreds of fibrous tissue. The face and calvarium may also be involved with facial clefts, asymmetric encephaloceles and grotesque features.

Complications
I   Derived: Skeletal deformities distal to constrictions due to interrupted neuromuscular and muscular functions and entrapment in scar, including clubfeet, synostosis of phalanges, nail bed defects, syndactyly. Lymphedema or lipoma distal to ring, and decreased vascular supply with cyanosis and poor response to cold.
II   Associated: Cleft lip and palate, other midline facial defects and congenital heart disease

Etiology: Increasing evidence supports the theory of Torpin of entanglement with mesodermic fibrous strings arising from the raw surfaces of the amnion and chorion after early rupture of the amnion. The fetus then develops in a fluid-filled chorionic sac, and its limbs and digits having been encircled and constricted by the stringy bands of chorionic connective tissue, develop deep grooves, and ultimately may be lost by spontaneous amputation distal to the point of encirclement. Entanglement with the umbilical cord or with true bands from an intact amnion have not been found. Streeter (1931) proposed either a primary cellular defect or an extrinsic insult to the fetus at the time of differentiation of the limb buds with resultant secondary degeneration of groups of cells with limited viability with local cell death and repair by scarring. Most recent work in this field, however, does not support the concept of Streeter. It should be noted, however, that rupture of the amnion has not been documented in every reported case of ring constrictions, and in some cases no information at all is available as to the status of the amnion.

Pathogenesis: Circumscribed areas of limb-bud tissue are maintained in viable form for only a brief period, whether due to intrinsic or extrinsic cause. Degeneration occurs primarily in the mesenchymal tissues, especially the subcutaneous connective tissue, but also involves ectodermal structures including skin and nails. The lesion may be deep enough to involve muscle and bone. Endarteritis and rarifying osteitis may occur distal to the primary lesion. The lesion heals by cicatrization leading to the characteristic ring constriction. If the defect is sufficiently profound, the part distal to the ring may be spontaneously amputated. Shreds of hyalinized connective tissue often hang from the open lesions, entrapping adjacent digits and producing fenestrated syndactyly after epithelialization. Interference with normal sequential development, both by interruption of neuromuscular and muscular supplies and by prevention of normal rotatory changes, produces clubfeet and other skeletal positional distortions.

Related Facts

I   **Sex Ratio:** M1:F1
II   **Risk of Occurrence:** ?
III **Risk of Recurrence for**
    Patient's Sib: Not increased
    Patient's Child: Not increased
IV   **Age of Detectability:** At birth
V   **Prevalence:** ?

Treatment

I   **Primary Prevention:** —
II   **Secondary Prevention:** —
III **Other Therapy:** Deep constrictions should be released early by Z-plasty. Function depends on rehabilitative orthopedic and plastic surgery and prosthetic replacement of missing limbs.

Prognosis: Life span is normal. Process stops at birth with subsequent healing and epithelialization of eschars. Occasionally, small portions of digits distal to the rings may be lost soon after birth if circulation is severely compromised by the process.

Detection of Carrier: —

†Special Considerations: Care should be taken clearly to differentiate this disorder from primary limb agenesis because of the etiologic character of the latter disease. The 3 most valuable methods of distinction are: active eschars present at birth, encircling ring constrictions, and interruption by scar of normal whorls on involved digits. Amputation stumps proximal to wrists and ankles also have cicatrized tips rather than the digital whorl pattern seen in true agenesis.

References:
Aker, C. and Rudolph, A.: Congenital ring constrictions and intra-uterine amputations. Am. J. Dis. Child. 121:393, 1971.
Field, J.H. and Krag, D.: Congenital constricting bands and congenital amputation of the fingers: Placental studies. J. Bone Joint Surg. 55A:1035, 1973.
Krag, D.: Amniotic rupture and birth defects of the extremities. Hum. Pathol. 5:69, 1974.
Streeter, G.L.: Focal deficiencies in fetal tissues and their relation to intrauterine amputation. Contrib. Embryol. Carneg. Instn. 22:(414):1, 1930.
Temtamy, S. and McKusick, V.A.: Synopsis of hand malformations with particular emphasis on genetic factors. In Bergsma, D. (ed.): Part III. Limb Malformations. Birth Defects: Orig. Art. Ser. vol. V, no. 3. White Plains: The National Foundation-March of Dimes, 1969, p. 125.
Torpin, R.: Amniochorionic mesablastic fibrous strings and amnionic bands: Associated constricting fetal malformations or fetal death. Am. J. Obstet. Gynecol. 91:65, 1965.

Contributor: **Liebe Sokol Diamond**

Editor's Computerized Descriptors: Skin, Dermatoglyphic, Skel.

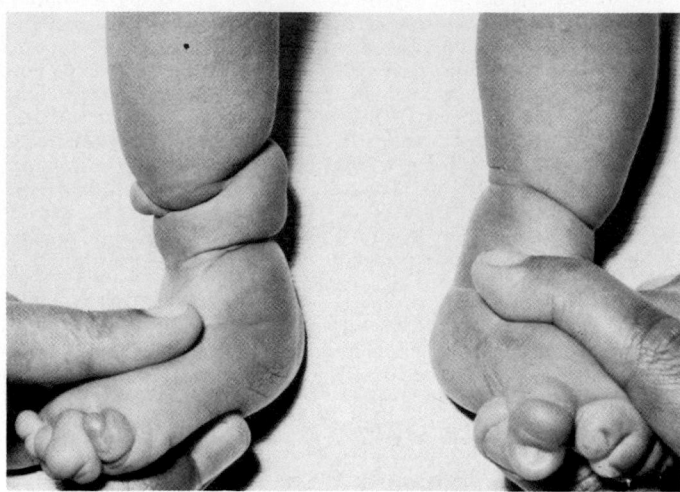

445. Ring constrictions and digital anomalies

ROBERTS SYNDROME

Includes: Syndrome de Roberts
Síndrome de Roberts
Tetraphocomelia with cleft lip and palate (and penis or clitoris hypertrophy)
Appelt-Gerken-Lenz syndrome
(SC) Pseudothalidomide syndrome†
Hypomelia-hypotrichosis-facial hemangioma syndrome

Excludes: Fetal thalidomide syndrome (386)
Heart-hand syndrome (455)
Femoral hypoplasia syndrome (type Daentl)
Caudal regression syndrome

Minimal Diagnostic Criteria: Midfacial clefting (usually severe) or hypoplastic nasal alae, facial hemangioma, silvery hair with absence/shortness-type limb malformations.

Clinical Findings: As indicated below, the Roberts syndrome and the pseudothalidomide syndrome may or may not be separate conditions. In any case, there exist a severe phenotype and a significantly less severe phenotype, corresponding to the Roberts syndrome and pseudothalidomide syndrome, respectively. The craniofacial manifestations in mildly affected patients include silvery-blond hair, facial hemangiomas and hypoplastic nasal alae. Severely affected patients show bilateral cleft lip and palate, hypertelorism, ocular proptosis and microcephaly. The limb malformations are regularly severe in the Roberts syndrome, they may be severe or significantly less severe in the pseudothalidomide syndrome. They are generally symmetric and more severe in the upper than in the lower limbs. The malformations consist of an absence/shortness-type defect involving, in order of decreasing severity and frequency, the ulna, radius, metacarpals, thumb, 5th finger and humerus. The corresponding order for the bones in the lower limbs is: fibula, tibia, metatarsals, hallux, 5th toe and femur. In severe cases humerus, radius and ulna are absent and a 3-digit hand is attached virtually to the shoulder. Variation between cases is due to the length of the long bones and the number of absent fingers and toes. Usually the upper limbs are apparently half the normal length, and the length of the lower limbs varies from half normal to near complete. Variation is increased by secondary manifestations, bowing of the legs, humeroradial or femoral-tibial synostosis, ankyloses, flexion contractures at elbows and knees, various types of clubfoot deformities, syndactyly, nail hypoplasia and dermatoglyphic abnormalities. Other abnormalities include enlargement of clitoris or penis, cryptorchidism, congenital heart disease, various renal anomalies and lumbar spina bifida.

Complications
I **Derived:** Prenatal or perinatal death; neonatal respiratory and feeding difficulties due to cleft lip and palate; physical limitations due to limb defects.
II **Associated:** High neonatal mortality; mental retardation; decreased vision due to corneal clouding.

Etiology: Autosomal recessive; McK *26830

Pathogenesis: ?

Related Facts
I **Sex Ratio:** M1:F1
II **Risk of Occurrence:** Small, but differs in various ethnic populations.
III **Risk of Recurrence for**
   Patient's Sib: 1 in 4 (25%) for each offspring to be affected
   Patient's Child: Not increased unless mate is carrier or homozygote

IV **Age of Detectability:** At birth; prenatal diagnosis has not been attempted but is perhaps possible.
V **Prevalence:** ? About 30 families have been described.

Treatment
I **Primary Prevention:** Genetic counseling
II **Secondary Prevention:** —
III **Other Therapy:** Surgical repair of facial and limb defects; special education

Prognosis: Increased pre- and perinatal mortality especially in more severely affected patients. Surviving patients may be mentally retarded.

Detection of Carrier: —

†Special Considerations: A severe phenotype (the Roberts syndrome) and a less severe phenotype (the pseudothalidomide syndrome) exist, although it is not possible to differentiate these on the basis of any single feature. More severely affected patients have a birth length of less than 37 cm. Less severely affected patients, who survive neonatal period, do not manifest cleft palate and have relatively long arms and hypoplastic nasal alae. In at least 2 instances the severe and the less severe phenotypes were observed in the same family, suggesting that they represent a different degree of severity of the same condition.

References:
Freeman, M.V.R. et al: The Roberts syndrome. Clin. Genet. 5:1, 1974.
Herrmann, J. et al: A familial dysmorphogenetic syndrome of limb deformities, characteristic facial appearance and associated anomalies: The "pseudothalidomide" or "SC-syndrome." In Bergsma, D. (ed.): Part III. Limb Malformations. Birth Defects: Orig. Art. Series., vol V, no. 3. New York: The National Foundation-March of Dimes, 1969, p. 81.
Herrmann, J. and Opitz, J.M.: The SC phocomelia and the Roberts syndrome: Nosologic aspects. Eur. J. Pediatr. 125:117, 1977.

Contributor: **Jürgen Herrmann**

Editor's Computerized Descriptors: Eye, Face, Oral, Nose, Skin, Hair, Skel., CV., GU., Nails, Dermatoglyphic

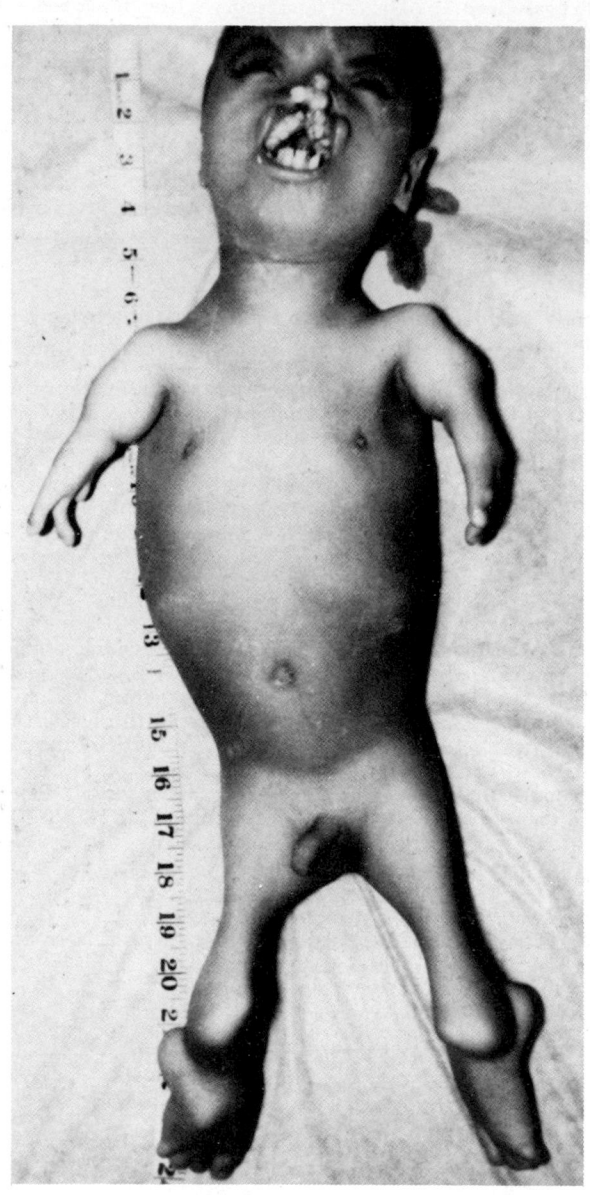

446. Note cleft of lip and palate with protrusion of premaxilla and limb defects

ROBINOW SYNDROME

Includes: Syndrome de figure foetale
Fetalgesicht-Minderwuchs Syndrom
Síndrome de rostro fetal
Robinow-Silverman-Smith syndrome
Mesomelic dwarfism, type Robinow
Mesomelic dwarfism with hemivertebrae and small genitalia
Fetal face syndrome

Excludes: Other mesomelic dwarfing syndromes
Other types of micropenis
Aarskog syndrome (1)

Minimal Diagnostic Criteria: Fetal face, forearm brachymelia, genital hypoplasia and moderate dwarfing.

Clinical Findings: The following description is based on the findings in 15 published cases. The syndrome can be recognized at birth. Constant findings are:

1) The "fetal face", so termed because it resembles the face of the fetus at 8 weeks. The neurocranium is disproportionately large, the forehead bulging. There is moderate hypertelorism, the mid-face is hypoplastic, the nose short and upturned, the mouth wide and triangular, with down-turned corners ("fish-mouth").

2) Forearm brachymelia. Mesomelic shortening of the lower limbs is less marked, or absent.

3) Genital hypoplasia. In males, the penis is invisible at birth unless the surrounding skin is retracted. Testicles and scrotum are usually normal. In females, the clitoris and labia minora are hypoplastic.

4) Moderate dwarfing. Length, usually within the lower part of the normal range at birth, falls below the 3rd percentile before the age of 2 years.

Intelligence is normal in most cases, mildly impaired in a few. Less constant findings are: vertebral or costovertebral anomalies, acrodysostosis, gingival hyperplasia, delayed eruption of the permanent teeth, dental malalignment. Infrequent findings are congenital heart disease, dislocated hips, inguinal hernia, undescended testicles, and penile agenesis.

The female pelvis is spacious enough to permit spontaneous delivery.

Though the penis becomes more visible as the infantile pubic fat disappears, the penile hypoplasia does not seem to improve with age, at least not during childhood. Knowledge of sexual development during puberty is insufficient for generalization.

Complications
I **Derived:** Scoliosis due to vertebral anomalies. Psychosocial problems related to the dysmorphic appearance and, in males, to the penile hypoplasia.
II **Associated:** —

Etiology: The etiology is probably always genetic. In the index family, the syndrome was inherited as an autosomal dominant. In several other families, some as yet unreported, autosomal recessive inheritance is strongly suggested. The dominant and recessive forms cannot yet be distinguished on the basis of clinical or radiographic features. Chromosomal studies have been performed in almost all cases. The results have invariably been normal.

Pathogenesis: ? The association of findings suggests a disturbance before the 8th week of embryonic development.

Related Facts
I **Sex Ratio:** M10:F5 in the 15 reported cases. Because of the striking penile hypoplasia males are more likely to be recognized and reported.

II Risk of Occurrence: Probably not less than 1 in 3,000,000 births, ie about 1 case/year in the U.S.

III Risk of Recurrence for

Patient's Sib: 1:2 - 1:4 according to mode of inheritance. Some of the sporadic cases may represent new mutations. The risk of recurrence in such cases cannot be assessed at this time.

Patient's Child: Depends on mode of inheritance in patient's family.

IV Age of Detectability: At birth.

V Prevalence: Probably about 10% lower than the risk of occurrence. Early death has occurred in one reported and in one unreported case.

Treatment

I Primary Prevention: Genetic counseling

II Secondary Prevention: Orthopedic treatment of vertebral anomalies, as indicated.

III Other Therapy: Penoplasty and androgen therapy have been tried with indifferent success.

Prognosis: In most cases general health has been good. Severe skeletal defects or congenital heart disease may cause morbidity or early death.

Detection of Carrier: —

Special Considerations: —

References:

Robinow, M. et al: A newly recognized dwarfing syndrome. Am. J. Dis. Child, 117:645, 1969.

Seel, R.E. et al: Das Fetalgesicht-Minderwuchs-Syndrom nach Robinow. Monatsschr. Kinderheilkd. 123:663, 1974.

Vera-Roman, J.M.: Robinow dwarfing syndrome accompanied by penile agenesis and hemivertebrae. Am. J. Dis. Child. 26:206, 1973.

Wadlington, W.B. et al: Mesomelic dwarfism with hemivertebrae and small genitalia (the Robinow syndrome). Am. J. Dis. Child. 126:202, 1973.

Contributor: **Meinhard Robinow**

Editor's Computerized Descriptors: Eye, Face, Oral, Nose, Skel., GU.

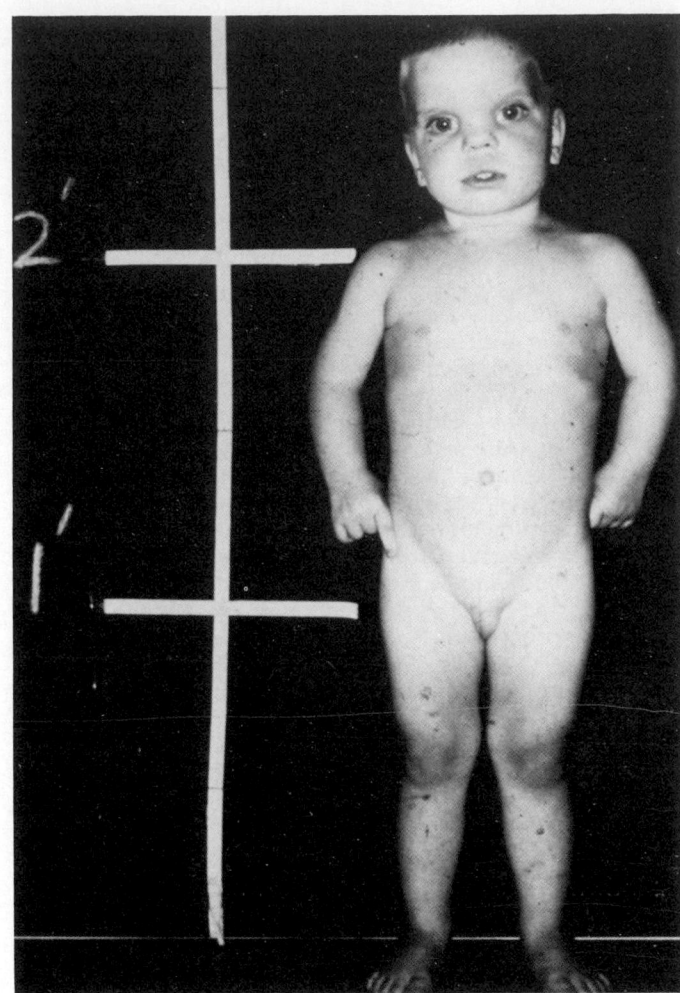

447. Note prominent forehead, ocular hypertelorism, short upturned nose, triangular mouth, and brachymelia

SACROCOCCYGEAL TERATOMA

Includes: Tératome sacrococcygienne
Sakrococcygeal teratome
Teratoma sacrocoxígeo
Teratoma sacrococcygeal (benign or malignant)

Excludes: Sacromeningocele

Minimal Diagnostic Criteria: Lobulated tumor mass in presacral space†

Clinical Findings: Sacrococcygeal teratomas are classified by their location. The most common type (47%) is predominantly external (sacrococcygeal) with only a minimal presacral component; type 2 (34%) tumors present externally but with a significant intrapelvic extension; type 3 (9%) are apparent externally but the predominant mass is pelvic and extends into the abdomen; the type 4 (10%) tumor is entirely presacral with no external presentation. The visible tumor presents as a lobulated mass, bulging into the perineum, distorting and displacing the anus and external genitalia to a more anterior position. The tumors are composed of both solid and cystic areas and enclosed within a fibrous capsule. The extent of presacral extension can be ascertained by rectal digital examination and plain roentgenography demonstrating anterior displacement of the rectal gas column. The majority (76%) of sacrococcygeal teratomas present within the first 2 months of life at which time the incidence of pelvic obstructive symptoms, including bowel and bladder dysfunction, is 7%, and the risk of malignancy 10.1%. Symptoms are present in 80% of infants when the teratoma is discovered after 2 months of age and the incidence of malignancy in this group is 91.7%.

Complications
I   **Derived:** a) Ulceration and infection; b) Ulceration and hemorrhage usually in association with hemangiomatous component; c) Malignancy (related to age of first detection: newborn and first 2 months of life 10.1%; after first 2 months 91.7%).
II   **Associated:** —

Etiology: ? A sacrococcygeal teratoma begins as a zone of totipotent cells derived from the distal primitive streak and remnants of Hensen node which undergo disorganized growth in contiguity with the developing coccygeal area.

Pathogenesis: Benign tumors, while arising from the sacrococcygeal region, have both an intrapelvic and external perineal component. Approximately 6% will grow outward and be pedunculated in appearance. The malignant tumors are primarily intrapelvic in location.

Related Facts
I   **Sex Ratio:** M1:F3 1 in 40,000 live births
II   **Risk of Occurrence:** —
III   **Risk of Recurrence for**
    Patient's Sib: ?
    Patient's Child: ?
IV   **Age of Detectability:** Two months and under, 76%; older than 2 months, 24%
V   **Prevalence:** ?

Treatment
I   **Primary Prevention:** —
II   **Secondary Prevention:** Treatment is operative removal of the tumor with reconstruction of the perineal region. Since these tumors are intimately associated with the perichondrium of the coccyx, coccygectomy is mandatory to avoid local recurrence of the tumors. The entire mass can be excised through a perineal incision in most patients; a combined abdominosacral procedure is necessary to remove all the intrapelvic component of large dumbbell-shaped tumors.
III   **Other Therapy:** Reexcision of recurrent tumors, plus radiotherapy and chemotherapy, if recurrence is malignant.

Prognosis: Overall operative mortality is 4%. 1) Benign teratoma: cure following complete excision of tumor with coccygectomy (100%). Recurrence rate without coccygectomy is 31.3%; 2) Malignant teratoma; 60% are dead within 10 months of operation; only 11% survive without apparent residual disease.

Detection of Carrier: —

†**Special Considerations:** All teratomas include cellular elements derived from embryonic ectoderm, endoderm and mesoderm. The most common tissues observed in the mature (benign) form of teratoma are those of the respiratory, GI and nervous systems and are clearly recognizable as to cell type and organ system. Fully developed limbs, segments of normal intestine and well-formed teeth have been found in benign tumors. The incidence of calcification with benign tumors is 35%. Incomplete maturation of various components is observed in immature teratomas while neoplastic tissue, usually adenocarcinomas (53%) is identified in patients with malignant teratomas.

References:
Altman, R.P. et al: Sacrococcygeal teratoma; American Academy of Pediatrics Surgical Section Survey - 1973. J. Pediatr. Surg. 9:389, 1974.
Dillard, B.M. et al: Sacrococcygeal teratoma in children. J. Pediatr. Surg. 5:53, 1970.
Donnellan, W. A. and Swenson, O.: Benign and malignant sacrococcygeal teratomas. Surgery 64:834, 1968.

Contributor: **Robert J. Touloukian**

Editor's Computerized Descriptors: GI., GU.

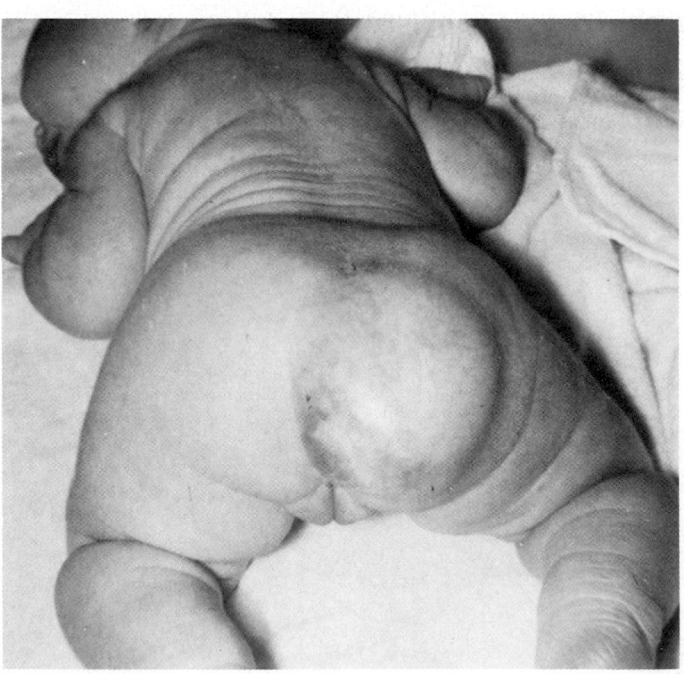

448. Sacrococcygeal teratoma

SALIVARY GLAND, MIXED TUMOR

Includes: Tumeur mixte des glandes salivaires
Hereditäre Mischtumoren der Speicheldrüsen
Tumor mixto hereditario de las glándulas salivares
Adenoma, hereditary pleomorphic salivary
Mixed tumor, salivary gland

Excludes: Branchogenic cyst
Other salivary gland tumors

Minimal Diagnostic Criteria: Presence of mixed tumor of salivary gland in more than 1 member of a family

Clinical Findings: A firm, well-circumscribed mass in the parotid gland without facial nerve involvement is found in the patient in the 3rd decade of life. Excisional biopsy reveals pathologic findings of a typical mixed benign tumor. In a series of 401 mixed tumors, Cameron found 3 families with tumors affecting more than 1 member. In 1 family, brother, sister and father were affected; in another, mother and daughter and in the 3rd, father and son. In this last family, the diagnosis of the father's tumor was made on clinical grounds, as he refused biopsy or excision. All the offspring were between 21 and 25 years of age.

Complications
I   **Derived:** Rarely malignant and rarely metastasize. Involvement of facial nerve with resultant paralysis is rare.
II **Associated:** —

Etiology: ? Possibly autosomal dominant

Pathogenesis: ?

Related Facts
I   **Sex Ratio:** Appears to be M1:F1
II   **Risk of Occurrence:** ?
III **Risk of Recurrence for**
    Patient's Sib: If autosomal dominant and if parent is affected, 1 in 2 (50%) for each offspring to be affected; otherwise not increased.
    Patient's Child: If autosomal dominant 1 in 2
IV **Age of Detectability:** All patients were over 20 years old.
V   **Prevalence:** ?

Treatment
I   **Primary Prevention:** Genetic counseling when autosomal dominant
II   **Secondary Prevention:** Surgical excision by superficial or total parotidectomy
III **Other Therapy:** —

Prognosis: Generally good for normal life span, intelligence and function if proper surgical treatment is employed. Metastases are rare and untreated mixed tumors usually enlarge slowly.

Detection of Carrier: —

Special Considerations: —

References:
Cameron, J.M.: Familial incidence of 'mixed salivary tumors.' Scott. Med. J. 4:455, 1959.

Contributor: Daniel R. Miller

Editor's Computerized Descriptor: Oral

SCIMITAR SYNDROME

Includes: Syndrome de scimitar
Síndrome de scimitar
Hypoplastic lung with systemic arterial supply and venous drainage
Partial anomalous pulmonary venous return

Excludes: Pulmonary venous connection, total anomalous (842)

Minimal Diagnostic Criteria: A scimitar shadow on chest xray in the right hemithorax. Cardiac catheterization must demonstrate the anomalous right pulmonary vein draining caudally into the inferior vena cava. The right lower lobe, in some cases, has received its arterial supply from an anomalous vessel arising from the aorta below the diaphragm.

Clinical Findings: A large variety of malformations of the pulmonary venous system have been reported. In the pediatric age group, the scimitar syndrome has been diagnosed most frequently in children being evaluated for recurrent respiratory infections or the presence of the heart in the right chest. In its most complete form, this syndrome consists of: anomalous pulmonary venous connection and drainage of part or the entire lung into the inferior vena cava, hypoplasia of the right lung, hypoplasia of the right pulmonary artery, dextrorotation or dextroposition of the heart and anomalous subdiaphragmatic systemic arterial supply to the lower lobe of the right lung from the aorta or its main branches. The symptoms of this syndrome are related to the degree of hypoplasia of the right lung or associated cardiac anomalies. The presence of the anomalous pulmonary vein of the right lung draining into the inferior vena cava by itself does not usually give rise to symptoms. The diagnosis can be made on plain frontal roentgenogram of the chest. On the xray, in the right hemithorax, a paracardiac shadow which is vertical, gently curved, and increased in width as it approaches the right cardiophrenic angle is seen. The shape of this shadow is similar to the shape of a scimitar. Also on xray, the heart is usually in a dextroposition and hypoplasia of the right lung in variable degrees may be seen. Bronchogram will demonstrate a variety of anomalies.†

Complications
I   **Derived:** Recurrent pneumonia
II **Associated:** Cardiac malformations are common. Ventricular septal defect, patent ductus arteriosus, tetralogy of Fallot, coarctation of the aorta, and absent right pulmonary artery have all been reported.

Etiology: ?

Pathogenesis: Unlike other pulmonary vein anomalies, the scimitar syndrome is accompanied by abnormalities of the right lung of varying degrees of severity. It should probably be considered as an abnormal development of the right lung bud and representing a more primitive type of malformation than the usual anomalies of the pulmonary venous system.

Related Facts
I   **Sex Ratio:** ? Preponderance of females in pediatric age group, but not in adults.
II   **Risk of Occurrence:** ?
III **Risk of Recurrence for**
    Patient's Sib: ?
    Patient's Child: ?
IV **Age of Detectability:** Infancy by xray
V   **Prevalence:** ?

Treatment
I   **Primary Prevention:** —
II   **Secondary Prevention:** —

III Other Therapy: Antibiotics for recurrent pneumonia. Surgical resection of involved tissue or correction of cardiac anomalies.

Prognosis: Dependent on associated cardiac anomalies

Detection of Carrier: —

†Special Considerations: The scimitar syndrome is only one of a large variety of pulmonary vein anomalies. These anomalies are diverse in nature and frequently associated with other cardiac malformations. The clinical manifestations are varied but are frequently due to pulmonary venous and arterial hypertension. These anomalies have been classified on an anatomic basis into groups: stenotic lesions, accessory veins, and anomalous connection, either partial or total, in a variety of combinations.

References:
Jue, K.L. et al: Anomalies of great vessels associated with lung hypoplasia- the scimitar syndrome. Am. J. Dis. Child. 111:35, 1966.
Nakib, A. et al: Anomalies of the pulmonary veins. Am. J. Cardiol. 20:77, 1967.

Contributor: **Patricia S. Zelkowitz**

Editor's Computerized Descriptors: Resp., CV.

SCLEROSTEOSIS

Includes: Sclérostéose
Sklerosteose
Esclerosteosis

Excludes: Osteopetrosis, dominant (779)
Osteopetrosis, recessive (780)
Dysosteosclerosis (310)
Other sclerosing bone dysplasias

Minimal Diagnostic Criteria: Skeletal sclerosis; lack of diaphyseal constriction of the tubular bones; cutaneous syndactyly of the fingers

Clinical Findings: Peculiar facies with broad, flat nasal bridge, ocular hypertelorism and broad mandible; cutaneous syndactyly of the fingers; radial deviation of the 2nd and 3rd fingers with absent or dysplastic nails. Radiographs reveal hyperostosis of the calvaria and base of the skull, lack of diaphyseal constriction and cortical sclerosis of the tubular bones.

Complications
I   Derived: Neurosensory deafness, facial nerve paralysis, rarely optic atrophy due to cranial nerve compression by excessive bone growth
II Associated: —

Etiology: Autosomal recessive; McK *26950

Pathogenesis: ?

Related Facts
I   Sex Ratio: M1:F1
II Risk of Occurrence: ? Apparently more frequent in South African Bantu population
III Risk of Recurrence for
     Patient's Sib: 1 in 4 (25%) for each offspring to be affected
     Patient's Child: Not increased unless mate is carrier or homozygote
IV Age of Detectability: Late infancy
V   Prevalence: ?

Treatment
I   Primary Prevention: Genetic counseling
II Secondary Prevention: —
III Other Therapy: Operative decompression of cranial nerve canals; symptomatic therapy for hearing loss.

Prognosis: Apparently normal life span

Detection of Carrier: —

Special Considerations: —

References:
Spranger, J. et al (eds.): Bone Dysplasias. Philadelphia: W.B. Saunders, 1974, p. 302.
Sugiura, Y. and Yashuhare, T.: Sclerosteosis. J. Bone Joint Surg. 57A:273, 1975.

Contributor: **Jürgen W. Spranger**

Editor's Computerized Descriptors: Eye, Hearing, Face, Nose, Nails, Skel., Nerve

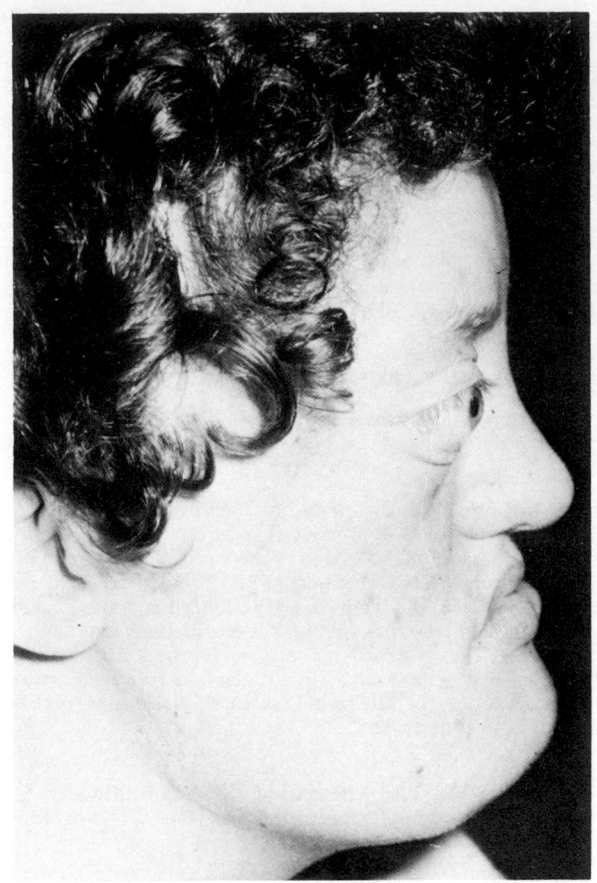

449. Note facial profile with broad mandible

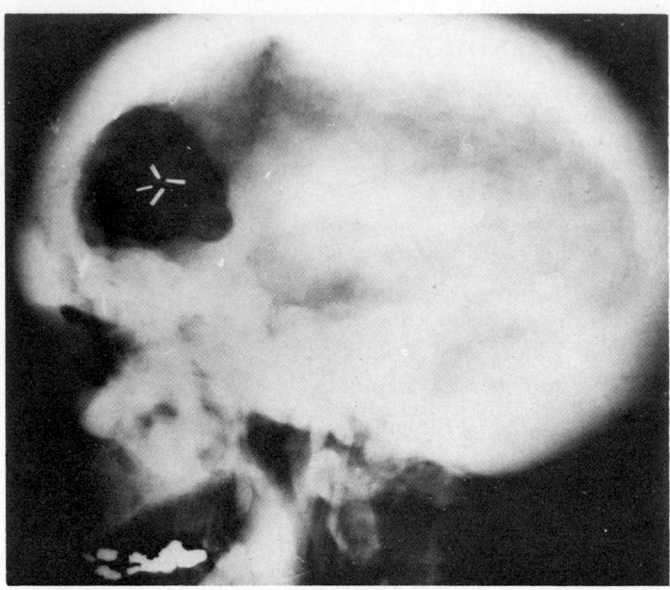

451. Hyperostosis of calvaria and skull base

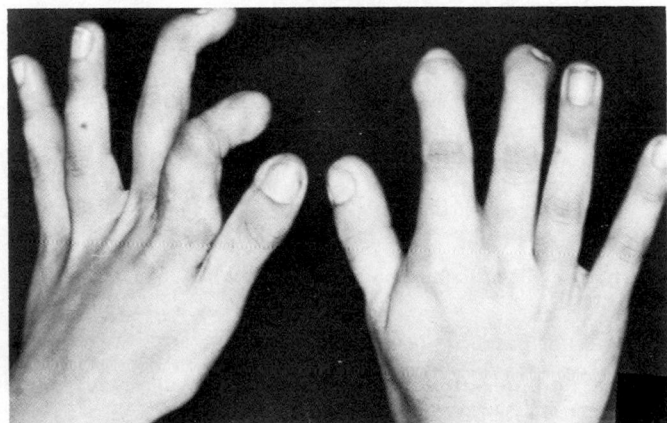

450. Hand deformities in sclerosteosis

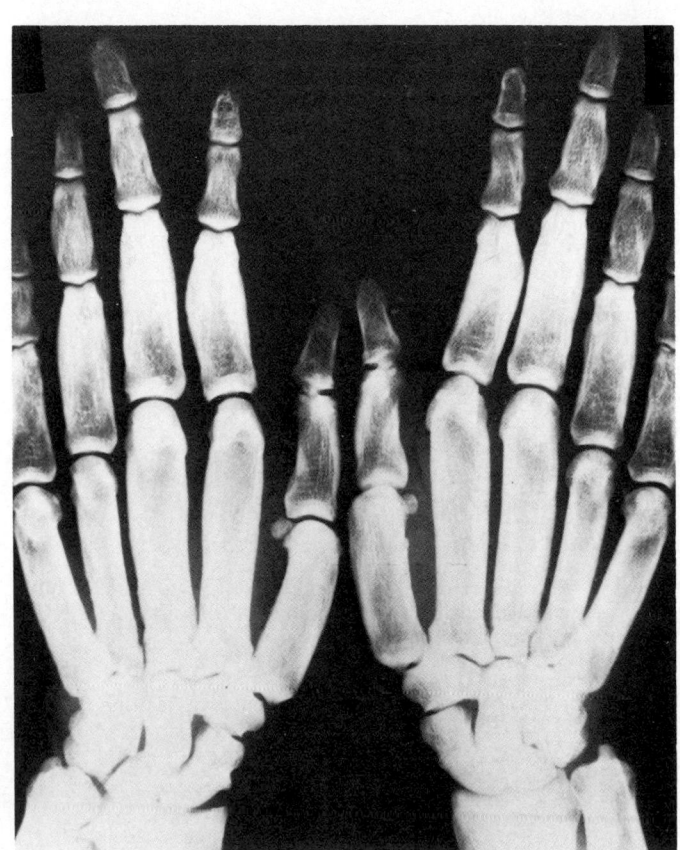

452. Note sclerosis and lack of diaphyseal constriction

SECKEL SYNDROME

Includes: Nanisme à tête d'oiseau
Vogelkopf-Zwergwuchs
Enanismo tipo "Cabeza de Pájaro"
Bird-headed dwarfism
Dwarfism, Seckel

Excludes: Microcephaly (659)
Virchow bird-headed dwarfism†

Minimal Diagnostic Criteria: The diagnosis depends upon characteristic craniofacial configuration with mental retardation, low birthweight dwarfism, plus other malformations.

Clinical Findings: Features of the syndrome include low birthweight for length of gestation, microcephaly, mental retardation, large eyes, large beaklike nose, narrow face, receding lower jaw, multiple malformations such as hypoplastic thumb, dislocation of femoral heads, clubfoot, scoliosis, strabismus and GU malformations. The brain shows a much simplified gross cerebral structure (pongidoid micrencephaly) with relatively intact cerebellum.

Complications
I **Derived:** —
II **Associated:** —

Etiology: Autosomal recessive; McK *21060

Pathogenesis: ?

Related Facts
I **Sex Ratio:** M1:F1
II **Risk of Occurrence:** Very low; probably 1 in 10,000 live births
III **Risk of Recurrence for**
   Patient's Sib: 1 in 4 (25%) for each offspring to be affected
   Patient's Child: Not increased unless mate is carrier or homozygote.
IV **Age of Detectability:** At birth
V **Prevalence:** Very rare

Treatment
I **Primary Prevention:** Genetic counseling
II **Secondary Prevention:** —
III **Other Therapy:** —

Prognosis: For life: Good. For intelligence: Mental retardation is a feature of the syndrome. For function: Function may be impaired by various anomalies such as dislocated femoral heads, clubfoot and scoliosis.

Detection of Carrier: —

†**Special Considerations:** Virchow described a form of bird-headed dwarfism with low birthweight, but without mental retardation and associated malformations.

References:
McKusick, V.A. et al: Seckel's bird-headed dwarfism. N. Engl. J. Med. 277:279, 1967.

Contributor: **Victor A. McKusick**

Editor's Computerized Descriptors: Eye, Face, Nose, Skel., GU., Nerve

SHORT FINGER-FLEXOR-TENDONS AND INABILITY TO OPEN MOUTH FULLY

Includes: Brièveté des tendons fléchisseurs des doigts avec incapacité d'ouverture complètement de la bouche
Verkürzte Beugesehnen der Finger und Unterkieferkontraktur
Tendones flexores cortos de los dedos e incapacidad para abrir la boca en forma completa
Camptodactyly and limited jaw excursion
Camptodactyly, facultative
Jaw excursion, limitation of
Finger flexor tendons, short

Excludes: Other types of camptodactyly
Cranio-carpo-tarsal dysplasia (223)

Minimal Diagnostic Criteria: Shortening of the flexor tendons of the wrist or deformity of the feet with inability to open the mouth fully.

Clinical Findings: Characterized by inability to open the mouth fully, curved fingers (camptodactyly) which occur at all the interphalangeal joints on dorsiflexion of the wrist. Volar flexion of the wrist allows complete extension of the fingers; forearm flexor tendons are short. Deformities of the feet also occur, including talipes equinovarus, pes planus, metatarsus varus and calcaneovalgus. The gastrocnemii and hamstrings are short. The latter causes a pelvic tilt. The affected individuals were all beneath the 3rd percentile in height. Intelligence is normal. Mild torticollis is also described.

Complications
I **Derived:** Difficulty with eating, locomotor difficulty
II **Associated:** One affected child died when 13 days old with intestinal obstruction.

Etiology: Autosomal dominant. Described in at least 2 kindreds and through 4 generations. McK *15830

Pathogenesis: ? †

Related Facts
I **Sex Ratio:** M1:F1
II **Risk of Occurrence:** ?
III **Risk of Recurrence for**
   Patient's Sib: If one parent affected, 1 in 2 (50%) for each offspring to be affected; otherwise not increased.
   Patient's Child: 1 in 2
IV **Age of Detectability:** Infancy
V **Prevalence:** ?

Treatment
I **Primary Prevention:** Genetic counseling
II **Secondary Prevention:** Orthopedic care for the foot deformities. Surgery has not been required for the flexor tendon shortening at the wrist.
III **Other Therapy:** —

Prognosis: Good for normal life span and intelligence. Variable for function.

Detection of Carrier: —

†**Special Considerations:** The cause of the inability to fully open the mouth has also not been established.

References:
De Jong, J.G.Y.: A family showing strongly reduced ability to open mouth and limitation of some movements of the extremities. Humangenetik 13:210, 1971.
Hecht, F. and Beals, R.K.: Inability to open the mouth fully: An autosomal dominant phenotype with facultative campylodactyly and short stature (Preliminary Note). In Bergsma, D. (ed.): Part III. Limb Malformations, Birth Defects: Orig. Art. Ser., vol. V, no. 3. White Plains: The National Foundation-March of Dimes, 1969, p. 96.

Wilson, R.V. et al: Autosomal dominant inheritance of shortening of the flexor profundus muscle-tendon unit with limitation of jaw excursion. Ibid. p. 99.

Contributor: **David C. Siggers**

Editor's Computerized Descriptors: Face, Skel.

SHORT RIB-POLYDACTYLY SYNDROME, MAJEWSKI TYPE

Includes: Chondrodysplasie léthale avec polydactylie, type Majewski
Thoraxdysplasie-Polydaktylie-Syndrom Typ Majewski
Síndrome de costillas cortas y polidactilia tipo Majewski

Excludes: Short rib-polydactyly syndrome, Saldino-Noonan type (884)
Chondroectodermal dysplasia (156)
Asphyxiating thoracic dysplasia (91)
Meckel syndrome (634)

Minimal Diagnostic Criteria: Short ribs, polydactyly, disproportionately short tibia, normal pelvis.

Clinical Findings: Hydropic appearance at birth; narrow thorax, short limbs, pre- or postaxial polydactyly; craniofacial abnormalities with cleft upper lip or palate, short flat nose, low-set deformed ears; multiple internal anomalies including hypoplastic epiglottis, cardiovascular defects, renal cysts, genital abnormalities.
Radiographs show short ribs, disproportionately short tibia, polydactyly and normal pelvis.

Complications
I   **Derived:** Respiratory insufficiency due to small thoracic cage and decreased pulmonary volume.
II **Associated:** —

Etiology: ?

Pathogenesis: ?

Related Facts
I   **Sex Ratio:** ?
II **Risk of Occurrence:** Very rare
III **Risk of Recurrence for**
    Patient's Sib: ?
    Patient's Child: ?
IV **Age of Detectability:** At birth
V   **Prevalence:** Very rare

Treatment
I   **Primary Prevention:** —
II **Secondary Prevention:** —
III **Other Therapy:** —

Prognosis: Death in early infancy from respiratory failure

Detection of Carrier: —

Special Considerations: —

References:
Spranger, J. et al: Short rib-polydactyly syndromes, types Majewski and Saldino-Noonan. Z. Kinderheilkd. 116:73, 1974.
Majewski, F. et al: Polysyndaktylie, verkürzte Gliedmassen und Genitalfehlbildungen. Z. Kinderheilkd. 111:118, 1971.

Contributor: **Jürgen W. Spranger**

Editor's Computerized Descriptors: Ear, Face, Oral, Nose, Larynx, Skin, Skel., Resp., CV., GU.

SHORT RIB-POLYDACTYLY SYNDROME, SALDINO-NOONAN TYPE

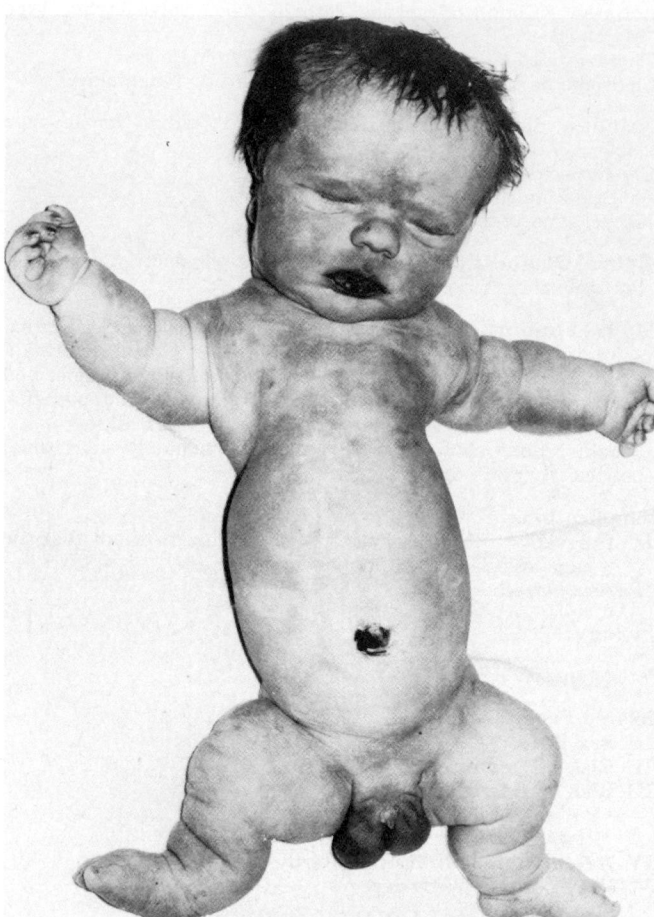

453. Shortening and postaxial polydactyly of all limbs; large head; narrow thorax; hypoplastic penis

Includes: Chondrodysplasie léthale avec polydactylie, type Saldino-Noonan
Thoraxdysplasie-Polydaktylie-Syndrom Typ Saldino-Noonan
Síndrome de costillas cortas y polidactilia tipo Saldino-Noonan

Excludes: Short rib-polydactyly syndrome, Majewski type (883)
Chondroectodermal dysplasia (156)
Asphyxiating thoracic dysplasia (91)
Meckel syndrome (634)
Chromosome thirteen trisomy syndrome (168)

Minimal Diagnostic Criteria: Narrow thorax, short ribs, scapular and pelvic dysplasia; ragged appearance of the ends of the tubular bones.

Clinical Findings: Hydropic appearance at birth; narrow thorax, protuberant abdomen; short, flipper-like limbs; postaxial polydactyly; anal atresia, renal and pancreatic cysts.†
Radiographs reveal short, horizontal ribs, small rounded scapulae, small iliac bones with flattened acetabular roofs, shortened tubular bones with periosteal spurs projecting longitudinally from the lateral aspects of the metaphyseal margins; incomplete and irregular ossifcation of the metacarpal and metatarsal bones and phalanges.

Complications
I **Derived:** Respiratory insufficiency due to small thoracic cage and decreased pulmonary volume.
II **Associated:** —

Etiology: Autosomal recessive; McK *26353

Pathogenesis: ?

Related Facts
I **Sex Ratio:** M1:F1
II **Risk of Occurrence:** Rare
III **Risk of Recurrence for**
  Patient's Sib: 1 in 4 (25%) for each offspring to be affected
  Patient's Child: Not increased unless mate is carrier or homozygote
IV **Age of Detectability:** At birth
V **Prevalence:** Rare

Treatment
I **Primary Prevention:** Genetic counseling
II **Secondary Prevention:** —
III **Other Therapy:** —

Prognosis: The patients are born dead or die within hours after birth from respiratory insufficiency.

Detection of Carrier: ?

†Special Considerations: A single case is known to me with characteristic features of the Saldino-Noonan syndrome but no polydactyly. Renal and pancreatic cysts have been observed. In 1 patient, the pancreatic changes were described as "inflammatory" lesions. Cases with the Saldino-Noonan syndrome were originally described as lethal forms of chondroectodermal dysplasia (Ellis-van Creveld syndrome). The skeletal changes are, however, different in the 2 conditions; renal cysts and anal atresia have not been reported in the Ellis-van Creveld syndrome.

References:
Saldino, R.M. and Noonan, C.D.: Severe thoracic dystrophy with striking micromelia, abnormal osseous development, including the spine, and multiple visceral anomalies. Am. J. Roentgenol. Radium Ther. Nucl. Med. 114:257, 1972.
Spranger, J. et al (eds.): Bone Dysplasias. Philadelphia:W. B. Saunders, 1974.

Contributor: **Jürgen W. Spranger**

SHWACHMAN SYNDROME

Includes: Chondrodysplasie métaphysaire avec insuffisance pancréatique exocrine et neutropénie cyclique
Pankreasdysplasie, Knochenmarksdysfunktion und metaphysäre Dysplasie
Hipoplasia pancreática, disfunción de la médula ósea y displasia metafisaria
Shwachman-Diamond-Oski-Khaw syndrome
Congenital pancreatic aplasia
Pancreatic hypoplasia, bone marrow dysfunction and metaphyseal dysplasia

Excludes: Cystic fibrosis (237)
Isolated deficiency of pancreatic exocrine enzymes
Secondary pancreatic exocrine insufficiency

Minimal Diagnostic Criteria: Subnormal basal and stimulated concentration of all pancreatic enzymes in the absence of cystic fibrosis, or recurrent episodes of pancreatitis. Hematologic disturbances or x-ray evidence of metaphyseal dysplasia is confirmatory.

Clinical Findings: Malabsorption as a result of pancreatic exocrine insufficiency begins in infancy (100%). Steatorrhea, diarrhea and failure to thrive are almost always present. Hypoproteinemia, low serum β-carotene levels and a low coefficient of fat absorption are usual clinical findings.

Bone marrow dysfunction most often presents as chronic or intermittent neutropenia (70%). A cyclic pattern of neutropenia is reported in some cases. Neutropenia is associated with recurrent bacterial infections. Sepsis (28%) is the most common cause of death and almost always occurs in the neutropenic infant. Anemia (50%) may be so severe as to be life threatening. Thrombocytopenia occurs in 16% and pancytopenia in 14%. Metaphyseal dysplasia (22%) may result in coxa vara deformity necessitating surgical correction. Generalized metaphyseal dysplasia involving ribs and limbs has been reported.

Dwarfism (50%) probably results from bony abnormalities and early malnutrition. There is usually no significant increase in growth velocity with pancreatic enzyme replacement, suggesting to some authors that growth failure is a primary part of the syndrome.

Complications
I   **Derived:** Malabsorption of fat and protein, diarrhea, failure to thrive, hypoproteinemia, recurrent bacterial infections, coxa vara deformity, short stature, xerophthalmia, diabetes mellitus and cirrhosis of liver.
II   **Associated:** Hirschprung disease, mental retardation, endocardial fibrosis, syndactyly, supernumerary metatarsals, imperforate anus with recto-urethral fistula, galactosuria, clitoral hypertrophy, microcephaly, increased circulating fetal hemoglobin.

Etiology: Autosomal recessive; McK *26040

Pathogenesis: The pancreatic disease appears to be a primary defect in histogenesis. The ductular structures are normal, as are the islets of Langerhans. There is an absence of acinar tissue. Since the islets and acinar elements arise from the same epithelial cords, it appears that there is selective interference with formation of acinar elements at about the 8th week of gestation.

The reason for the association between pancreatic insufficiency, bone marrow dysfunction and metaphyseal dysplasia is unclear. These associated disturbances do not resolve with improvement in nutrition and thus do not seem attributable to malabsorption.

Related Facts
I   **Sex Ratio:**   M1:F1

II Risk of Occurrence: ?
III Risk of Recurrence for
Patient's Sib: 1 in 4 (25%) for each offsrping to be affected
Patient's Child: Not increased unless mate is carrier or homozygote
IV Age of Detectability: Infancy
V Prevalence: ? It is the 2nd most common cause of pancreatic insufficiency in childhood. From 1964-1969, 56 cases were reported.

Treatment
I Primary Prevention: Genetic counseling
II Secondary Prevention: Orally administered pancreatic enzyme replacement improves digestion and absorption of peρtide and fats. Dietary fat restriction helps to improve symptomatic steatorrhea. Elemental formulas are useful in providing nutrition during infancy. Early attention to febrile illness including multiple bacterial cultures and appropriate use of antibiotics is necessary to prevent overwhelming infection. No therapy has been successful in reversing the hematologic disorder. Appropriate orthopedic attention to the metaphyseal dysplasia, especially that involving the hip, may prevent deformity.
III Other Therapy: —

Prognosis: Although these children have a better prognosis than those with cystic fibrosis, it is not good. The severity of the hematologic disturbance affects overall outcome.

Detection of Carrier: —

Special Considerations: —

References:
Reginster, L. et al: Hypoplasie de la fonction exocrine du pancreas. Acta Paediatr. Belg. 23:166, 1969.
Shmerling, D.H. et al: The syndrome of exocrine pancreatic insufficiency, neutropenia, metaphyseal dysostosis and dwarfism. Helv. Paediatr. Acta 24:547, 1969.
Shwachman, H. et al: The syndrome of pancreatic insufficiency and bone marrow dysfunction. J. Pediatr. 65:645, 1964.

Contributor: **Peter F. Whitington**

Editor's Computerized Descriptors: Eye, Skel., GI., Liver

SICKLE CELL ANEMIA

Includes: Anémie drépanocytaire
Sichelzellanämie
Anemia falciforme
Homozygous sickle hemoglobinopathy
Drepanocytic anemia
Chwechweechwe
Ahotutuo
Nuidudui
Lakuregebee
Orengua

Excludes: Sickle cell trait (sickle hemoglobin heterozygosity)
Sickle β-thalassemia†
Sickle hemoglobin in combination with other structurally abnormal hemoglobins†

Minimal Diagnostic Criteria: Hemoglobin electrophoresis demonstrating sickle hemoglobin with an absence of hemoglobin A or other structurally abnormal hemoglobins. Variable quantities of hemoglobin F (fetal hemoglobin) may be present. The presence of β-thalassemia, hereditary persistence of fetal hemoglobin, and other abnormal hemoglobins with electrophoretic mobility similar or identical to that of hemoglobin S may require additional studies for exclusion. The presence of hemoglobin S demonstrated in each parent, and confirmed by a sickling test, provides the most reliable means for establishing the diagnosis with certainty.†

Clinical Findings: The earliest manifestation of sickle cell anemia is often a dactylitis of the phalanges of the hands and feet presenting in infancy as a swelling of the affected areas, and associated with fever and irritability. In the older child and adult the *pain crisis* is the most characteristic clinical expression. In relatively younger children pain most commonly occurs in the limbs; painful episodes involving the back, thorax, abdomen, and head occur more often in older children and adults. Acidosis, dehydration, and fever, frequently associated with intercurrent infections, often precipitate these episodes of pain crisis. Clinical features associated with chronic hemolysis are present, including pallor, jaundice, and increase in the reticulocyte count, and erythroid hyperplasia of the bone marrow. Stained smears of peripheral blood demonstrate polychromatophilia, target cells, and frequently include sickled erythrocytes. Howell-Jolly bodies are frequently present in peripheral blood erythrocytes in the older child and adult. Hyposthenuria is a constant feature in the older child.

Complications
I Derived: *Infarction:* Occlusion of major blood vessels by masses of sickled cells may produce gross infarction leading to major degrees of organ dysfunction. Infarction of bone may lead to avascular necrosis. Massive liver necrosis and kidney failure may develop. Major insults to the CNS are frequent, and severe sequelae including hemiparesis have been described in up to 25% of reported cases.

Splenic enlargement is often present in younger children, and may produce the hematologic picture of hypersplenism. In the older child and adult the spleen undergoes a process of involution attributable to multiple episodes of infarction. The pattern of blood circulation through the spleen is altered in these patients so as to shunt the circulating blood away from the active follicles. The result of this alteration is a "functional asplenia" a change that helps to explain the increased susceptibility of these patients to pneumococcal and *H. influenzae* infections.

Osteomyelitis: For reasons that are poorly understood, children with sickle cell anemia have an unusual predisposition to develop osteomyelitis, most commonly due to Salmonella and other enteropathic organisms.

Gallstones are related to the chronic hemolytic process, are uncommon in younger children but occur with a substantial, increasing frequency in teenagers and adults.

Aplastic crisis is seen in all forms of chronic hemolytic anemia, results from a transient period of erythroid aplasia in the bone marrow. These episodes appear related to communicable infections. Rapidly increasing anemia, sometimes life-threatening, is present associated with an absence or major reduction in the reticulocyte count.

Sequestration crisis is seen almost exclusively in infants and young children, occurs as a sudden onset of severe anemia, and is accompanied by evidence of active erythropoiesis and an acutely enlarged spleen. Transfusions may be life-saving.

Priapism is rather uncommon, results from pooling of sickle cells in the corpora cavernosa resulting in obstruction of the venous outflow.

Leg ulcers are unusual in children, but occur with considerable frequency in adults. Blood stasis, perhaps accompanied by trauma, is held responsible.

II Associated: —

Etiology: An autosomal recessive trait resulting in a substitution of valine for glutamate at position number 6 of the hemoglobin beta chains.

Pathogenesis: As a consequence of the structural abnormality of the hemoglobin in this condition, under conditions of deoxygenation, a process of molecular aggregation of the hemoglobin occurs resulting in the formation of a rigid fiber-like structure. This change imparts a major distortion to the red blood cell causing it to assume an elongated shape and rigid, brittle properties. Under circumstances of deoxygenation, primarily involving the venous side of the circulation, masses of these sickled cells bring about varying degrees of vascular obstruction. Conditions of acidosis, dehydration, and hypoxia all potentiate this process.

Related Facts
I Sex Ratio: M1:F1
II Risk of Occurrence: 1:625 births in the American black population has been estimated. A considerably higher risk has been established particularly in certain areas of West Africa. Other populations of substantial risk include areas of Greece, Italy, several Mid-Eastern populations, Southern Turkey, and certain populations of Southern India.
III Risk of Recurrence for
Patient's Sib: 1 in 4 (25%) for each offspring to be affected
Patient's Child: Not increased unless mate is carrier or homozygote
IV Age of Detectability: Normally not clinically expressed until 3-6 months of age. Can be detected at birth, and by special studies can be detected in the 2nd trimester fetus.
V Prevalence: Estimated to be 1:1875 in the American black population.

Treatment
I Primary Prevention: Genetic counseling; antenatal detection.
II Secondary Prevention: Many complications seem not to be preventable. However, a generally less severe clinical course is observed in patients with good nutrition, and who receive prompt attention and treatment of intercurrent infection, dehydration, and other intercurrent problems.
III Other Therapy: Specific forms of therapy are not available. In addition to therapeutic measures indicated above, transfusions often provide a major temporary supportive role of various complications of this disease.

Prognosis: The clinical course is extremely variable and often unpredictable. Patients having access to adequate medical care most often survive into adulthood, and the majority lead productive lives.

Detection of Carrier: The heterozygous carrier can be readily identified by any of a variety of sickling tests. A positive test requires confirmation by hemoglobin electrophoresis.

†Special Considerations: Of major diagnostic importance is the need to distinguish this condition from a variety of phenotypically similar sickling syndromes. Many of these are indistinguishable from sickle cell anemia by application of usual hematologic studies, and in some cases can be distinguished only by family studies and other special forms of testing. Some of the known phenocopies of sickle cell anemia carry strikingly different implications for treatment and prognosis, and for this reason need to be distinguished from sickle cell anemia. In general, if both parents are available for study, the finding in each parent of a positive sickling test and an electrophoresis study consistent with sickle trait will allow the diagnosis to be established with certainty.

References:
Honig, G.R.: Sickling syndromes in children. Adv. Pediatr. 23:271, 1976.
Motulsky, A.G.: Frequency of sickling disorders in U.S. blacks. N. Engl. J. Med. 288:31, 1973.
Serjeant, G.R.: The Clinical Features of Sickle Cell Disease. New York: American Elsevier Publishing Co., 1974.

Contributors: **George R. Honig**
Wayne H. Borges

Editor's Computerized Descriptors: Skin, Skel., Spleen, GI., GU., Nerve

Also see Section I, Fig. 108.

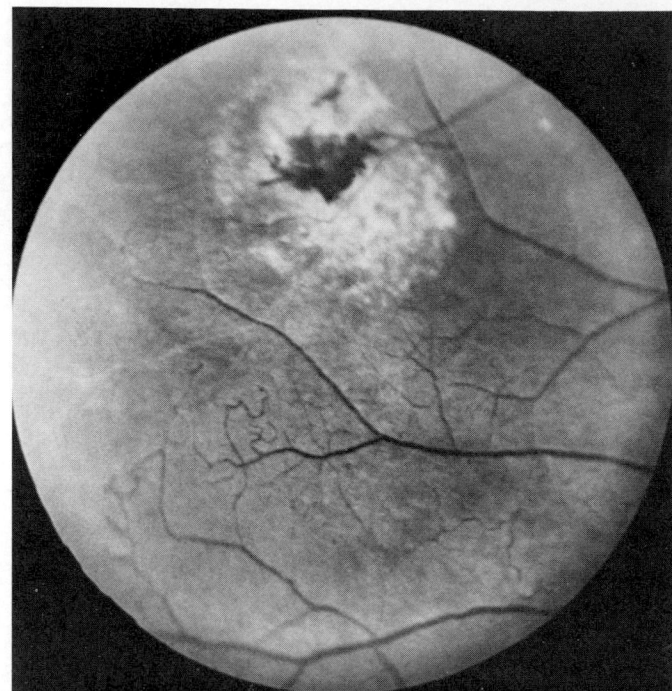

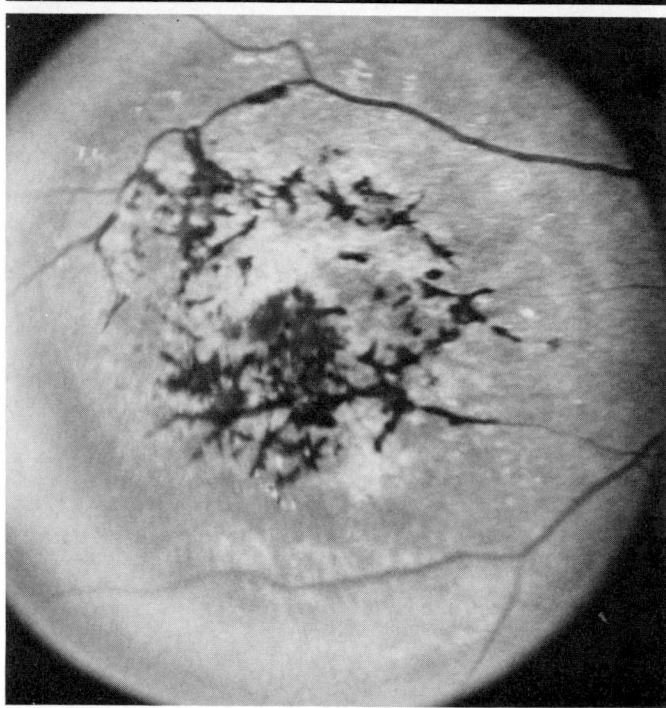

454. Examples of black sunburst in sickle cell anemia

SILVER SYNDROME

Includes: Syndrome de Silver
Síndrome de Silver
Syndrome of congenital asymmetry, short stature and variations
in sexual development
Russell-Silver syndrome

Excludes: Hemihypertrophy (458)
Diffuse static cerebral defects
Neurofibromatosis (712)
Turner syndrome (977)
Fibrous dysplasia, polyostotic (391)
Hemihypertrophy due to specific causes

Minimal Diagnostic Criteria: The major manifestations include significant asymmetry, shortness of stature, small size despite being born at term and variations in the clinical and laboratory pattern of sexual development. A combination of 3 or more of these findings probably should be present for a clinical diagnosis to be made. The presence of several of the minor manifestations (short incurved 5th fingers, triangular facies, turned-down corners of the mouth, café-au-lait spots and syndactyly) tend to make the diagnosis more certain.†

Clinical Findings: Based upon more than 100 reported cases of the Silver syndrome, the principal features are shortness of stature, significant asymmetry, variations in the pattern of sexual development, and small size despite being born at term. Other findings include: café-au-lait areas of the skin, unusually short and incurved 5th fingers, triangular shape of the face, turned-down corners of the mouth and syndactyly of the toes. Variable combinations of findings have been reported and no single finding was noted in all patients.

At birth affected infants are unusually small for gestational age. In those cases where the pattern of growth could be evaluated, it usually paralleled the normal growth curve but remained below the 3rd percentile level. Where children were observed into puberty, they continued to be short.

The asymmetry noted has been quite variable in extent and degree. In some, one entire side of the body was significantly larger than the other; in others, the extent of the asymmetry was limited and involved only the skull, spine, or all or part of a limb. The asymmetry is probably present at birth, but may not be appreciated for variable periods of time.

Variations in the pattern of sexual development include: elevated levels of serum or urinary gonadotropins in prepubertal children of both sexes. Sexual development may be precocious or may occur disproportionately early in relation to other physiologic evidences of maturity. Precocious sexual development is much more likely to occur in affected girls than in boys.

The café-au-lait spots are usually sharply circumscribed, smooth, light brown and vary in size from less than 1 cm to over 30 cm in diameter. The spots are usually not raised, but in one instance, the entire pigmented area was wrinkled and slightly elevated. The borders of some café-au-lait areas are smooth while others have jagged edges.

The heads of children with the Silver syndrome may be disproportionately large for the small facial mass ("pseudohydrocephaly") tapering to a narrow jaw and producing the characteristic triangular-shaped face. The lips are often thin with the corners of the mouth turned down ("shark mouth").

Abnormalities of the limbs include incurving of the 5th fingers and variable, usually slight, syndactyly between the 2nd and 3rd toes. Other variations in the size and configuration of the toes are not uncommon.

Most of the children have normal intelligence. Bone age is retarded but generally to a lesser degree than height age.

In children who do not exhibit significant asymmetry or variations in the pattern of sexual development, the combination of small size at birth, shortness of stature, café-au-lait areas of the skin and unusually short and incurved 5th fingers, is relatively common and may represent a partial form of the syndrome.

Complications
I Derived: Although a significant association between hemihypertrophy in children who are not short, and tumors of the kidneys (Wilms tumor) and adrenals (neuroblastoma), and adrenal hyperplasia has been noted, none of the reported cases of the Silver syndrome has been associated with malignancy. Asymmetry of the spine and lower limbs may produce disturbances of gait. Precocious puberty may be psychologically disturbing to the child and her parents.

II Associated: Urinary tract abnormalities and cardiac defects have been described in a few cases.

Etiology: ?

Pathogenesis:
The finding of elevated levels of growth hormone in a few cases suggests that the short stature may result in part from a relative unresponsiveness to this hormone. In general, however, there has been a normal response to the administration of human growth hormone.

The pathogenesis of both the asymmetry and the other clinical findings is unknown. Investigations of the presence of other endocrine or metabolic defects have failed to reveal any additional abnormalities.

Related Facts
I Sex Ratio: M1:F1
II Risk of Occurrence: Rare, but all races and ethnic groups appear susceptible.
III Risk of Recurrence for
   Patient's Sib: Extremely unlikely. A family history has been noted in 2 instances; in one the mother of a girl with the syndrome had extreme short stature at birth and extending into adult life along with precocious sexual development, café-au-lait areas, and mild syndactyly. In the other, 3 affected sibs were reported.
   Patient's Child: ?
IV Age of Detectability: Ordinarily at birth but may not be recognized for several months.
V Prevalence: ?

Treatment
I Primary Prevention: —
II Secondary Prevention: —
III Other Therapy: Treatment is symptomatic. Corrective shoes, braces and physical therapy may be necessary, but functional impairment may be minimal despite significant asymmetry. Patients, especially female patients and their parents, should be prepared for the precocious sexual development which may occur. Periodic examination should be carried out to determine the possible presence of a tumor of the kidney or adrenal.

Prognosis: Apparently normal life span. Approximately one-third of patients have been reported as showing some degree of mental retardation. Functional impairment will depend on the degree of asymmetry. In most instances no functional disturbance occurs.

Detection of Carrier: —

†Special Considerations: Serum gonadotropins and the excretion of urinary gonadotropins may be increased for age. In the 1st decade, the level of urinary gonadotropins may be increased to that found in normal women during the reproductive period of life.

Epiphyseal maturation has been retarded in approximately half of the cases. There may be a difference in osseous maturation on the 2 sides of the body.

In at least 2 instances of the Silver syndrome, elevated serum levels of growth hormone have been found.

Defects of the skeleton including poorly formed thoracic vertebrae (which differed from those seen in the ordinary type of hemivertebra), surface irregularities of the lumbar vertebrae which resemble those seen in juvenile kyphosis, irregularity and indentation of the metaphyses of the phalanges and hypoplasia of various phalanges, the sacrum and the coccyx have all been described.

No consistent chromosomal abnormality has been noted. In several instances, the analysis was reported to be normal, but in one instance there was a diploid-triploid mosaicism in the skin and fascia lata and a normal diploid complement in the lymphocytes.

References:
Fuleihan, D.S. et al: The Russell-Silver syndrome: Report of three siblings. J. Pediatr. 78:654, 1971.
Haslam, R.H.A. et al: Renal abnormalities in the Russell-Silver syndrome. Pediatrics 51:216, 1973.
Moseley, J.E. et al: The Silver syndrome: Congenital asymmetry, short stature and variations in sexual development; roentgen features. Am. J. Roentgenol. Radium Ther. Nucl. Med. 97:74, 1966.
Silver, H. K.: Asymmetry, short stature, and variations in sexual development: A syndrome of congenital malformations. Am. J. Dis. Child. 107:495, 1964.
Tanner, J. M. and Ham, T. J.: Low birth weight dwarfism with asymmetry (Silver's syndrome): Treatment with human growth hormone. Arch. Dis. Child. 44:231, 1969.
Tanner, J.M. et al: The natural history of the Silver-Russell syndrome: A longitudinal study of thirty-nine cases. Pediatr. Res. 9:611, 1975.

Contributor: **Henry K. Silver**

Editor's Computerized Descriptors: Face, Skin, Skel., GU.

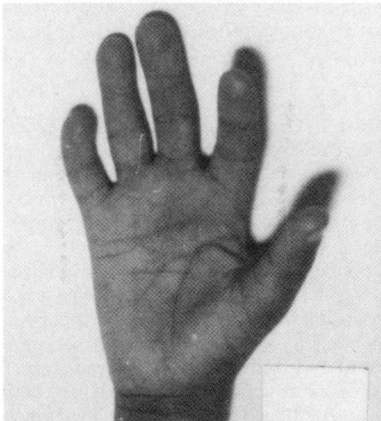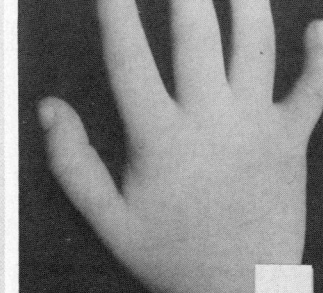

455. Clinodactyly of 5th finger

SITUS INVERSUS VISCERUM

Includes: Situs inversus (complet, partiel)
Viszeraler Situs inversus
Situs inversus visceral
Situs inversus intestinalis

Excludes: Dextrocardia

Minimal Diagnostic Criteria: Roentgenographic evidence in infants showing the gastric bubble in the right upper abdomen. Air insufflation of the stomach will assist in this diagnostic evaluation. Passage of the nasogastric tube into the stomach will show the tube passing into the right upper quadrant on abdominal roentgenograms. The presence of dextrocardia on the chest roentgenogram assists greatly in the diagnosis of situs inversus intestinalis with dextrocardia. Abdominal examination will reveal the liver to be present in the left upper abdomen. Barium enema roentgenograms show the sigmoid colon in the right lower quadrant.

Clinical Findings: The birthweight is only slightly lower than average. Based upon 37 reported cases, 2/3 of the patients with situs inversus viscerum had congenital obstructions of the GI tract. Atresia or stenosis of the duodenum or jejunum and incomplete fixation of the small bowel mesentery are common accompaniments. Biliary atresia is much more common than is seen in the general population. Cardiac anomalies are also common accompaniments of situs inversus viscerum. Fifteen of the 37 patients had major cardiac anomalies associated with situs inversus. The major malformations were tetralogy of Fallot in 5; transposition of the great vessels in 4; pulmonary stenosis in 4; ventricular septal defect in 4; patent ductus arteriosus in 4; single ventricle in 3; cor biloculare in 3; hypoplastic pulmonary artery in 3; anomalous pulmonary venous return in 3; atrioventricular canal in 2; atrial septal defect in 1. External malformations associated with situs inversus include clubfoot in 2; choanal atresia in 1; cleft palate in 1; absent humerus in 1; cutaneous hemangioma in 1; and meningomyelocele in 1.

Complications

I   **Derived:** None. Complications are based largely on the problems developing from the many associated malformations that accompany situs inversus. Serious complications have resulted from failure to recognize the presence of situs inversus viscerum while attempting surgical correction of other visceral malformations.

II   **Associated:** Based on experience with 37 patients with situs inversus, 78% of the patients had other malformations. Dextrocardia was approximately twice as common as levocardia or partial cardiac transposition. Fifteen of the 37 patients had major intraabdominal anomalies which required operative correction within the first few months of life. More than 85% of the lesions were surgically correctable. The most common malformations were: malrotation - 5, (with volvulus - 2), biliary atresia - 3, splenic agenesis - 3, duodenal atresia - 3, duodenal web - 2, annular pancreas - 2, imperforate anus - 2, anterior portal vein - 2, left vena cava - 2, jejunal atresia - 1, jejunal web - 1, gastric duplication - 1, and inguinal hernia - 1.

Etiology: ?

Pathogenesis: Mirror image transposition of the internal organs may affect thoracic and abdominal viscera together or independently. It is believed that the development of the embryonic organs occurs in definite dependent sequences. If for any reason the initial organ of such an interdependent system undergoes a reversal in position, all the succeeding stages are correspondingly affected: for example, rotation of the stomach to the right results automatically in transposition of the intestine. The left vitelline vein and the left umbilical vein are larger than their mates and have long been regarded as determining the early positions of the heart and liver which then act as such key organs. More recent studies, however, suggest that the problem of asymmetry in the viscera may depend upon controlling factors in the gut and that they may become operative even before the liver bud appears.

Related Facts

I   **Sex Ratio:** M22:F15

II   **Risk of Occurrence:** ?

III   **Risk of Recurrence for**
     Patient's Sib: ?
     Patient's Child: ?

IV   **Age of Detectability:** Usually within the first few weeks of life based upon the severity of the associated malformations

V   **Prevalence:** Reliable figures unavailable. Thirty-seven patients recorded in a 15-year-experience in a large children's hospital.

Treatment

I   **Primary Prevention:** —

II   **Secondary Prevention:** Early recognition and prompt, accurate management of the associated congenital malformations.†

III   **Other Therapy:** —

Prognosis: The prognosis depends upon the associated congenital malformations. Situs inversus viscerum alone is associated with normal life expectancy, productivity, intelligence and function.

Detection of Carrier: —

†Special Considerations: Abdominal malformations are almost as likely to occur as are cardiac malformations with situs inversus viscerum. The majority of the malformations are very serious and prompt diagnosis and surgical management are indicated. Recognition of situs inversus is imperative if surgical management is to be accurate.

References:
Fonkalsrud, E.W. et al: Abdominal manifestations of situs inversus in infants and children. Arch. Surg. 92:791, 1966.
Kilcoyne, R. F.: Situs inversus: A review. Marquette Med. Rev. 29:90, 1963.
Torgersen, J.: Genetic factors in visceral asymmetry in development and pathologic changes of lungs, heart, and abdominal organs. Arch. Pathol. 47:566, 1949.

Contributor: **Eric W. Fonkalsrud**

Editor's Computerized Descriptors: CV., GI., Liver

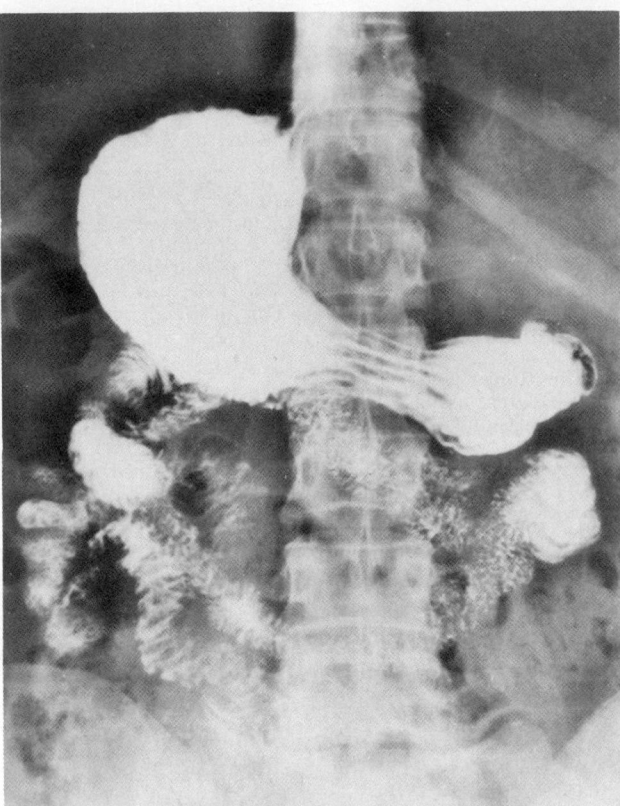

456. Upper GI series showing mirror image positioning of liver, stomach, and intestines in visceral situs inversus

SIXTH NERVE PARALYSIS

Includes: Paralysie de la sixième paire
Abduzensparese
Parálisis congénita del sexto par
Paralysis of sixth nerve, congenital
Stilling-Türk-Duane syndrome
Duane retraction syndrome
Ocular retraction syndrome

Excludes: Acquired sixth nerve paralysis
Other cranial nerve involvement
Jaw-winking syndrome (548)

Minimal Diagnostic Criteria: Limitation of abduction on lateral gaze of affected eye(s).

Clinical Findings: Congenital paralysis of the 6th nerve is manifested by a partial or complete failure of abduction on lateral gaze of the affected eye(s). Esotropia may or may not be present in the primary position of gaze. These findings as a pure form are extremely rare. Sixth nerve paralysis is usually part of the Duane retraction syndrome which also includes limited adduction, retraction of the globe in adduction, narrowing of the palpebral fissure in adduction creating a pseudoptosis, occasional vertical deviation of the eye in adduction, convergence insufficiency, and widening of the palpebral fissure in attempting abduction. The condition is usually unilateral (85%) and over 60% occur in the left eye.

Complications
I   **Derived:**   Strabismus, diplopia, amblyopia. Diplopia is often avoided by head turn and amblyopia is rare.
II **Associated:**   Spina bifida; familial dysgenesis of the elbows; oculofacial palsies; paradoxical movement of upper lids; deafness; defects of the muscles of the head, neck and tongue; keratoconus; cataract; colobomas of eye; microphthalmos; syringomyelia and Klippel-Feil synostosis. Nystagmus, epibulbar dermoid, myelinated nerve fibers, and Wildervanck syndrome.

Etiology: Heterogeneity almost certainly exists; autosomal dominant transmission occurs; pedigrees sometime also show minor manifestations of the syndrome. May possibly result from birth trauma. McK *12680

Pathogenesis: Related to central innervational disturbances, anomalies of the fascia or lateral rectus muscle, aberration of the 6th nerve or of innervation from other oculomotor nerves associated with or independent of developmental defects of the brainstem. May arise from arrest of embryonic development.

Related Facts
I   **Sex Ratio:**   M2:F3
II **Risk of Occurrence:**   Relatively rare, but the most common of all isolated congenital oculomotor nerve paralyses
III **Risk of Recurrence for**
    Patient's Sib: When autosomal dominant, if parent is affected, 1 in 2 (50%) for each offspring to be affected; otherwise not increased.
    Patient's Child: 1 in 2 when autosomal dominant
IV **Age of Detectability:**   In infancy
V   **Prevalence:**   Rare

Treatment
I   **Primary Prevention:**   Genetic counseling
II **Secondary Prevention:**   If any tropia in the primary position of gaze exists, surgery is indicated
III **Other Therapy:**   —

Prognosis: Good in the isolated condition since affected individuals learn to adapt to the inability to abduct the eye by compensatory turning of the head.

Detection of Carrier: —

Special Considerations: —

References:
Bielschowsky, A.: Lectures on motor anomalies; paralysis of individual eye muscles: Abducens-nerve paralysis. Am. J. Ophthalmol. 22:357, 1939.
Duke-Elder, S.: System of Ophthalmology, vol. 3, part 2 Congenital Deformities. London:Henry Kimpton, 1964, p. 991.
Hoyt, W. F. and Nachtigäller, H.: Anomalies of ocular motor nerves; neuroanatomic correlates of paradoxical innervation in Duane's syndrome and related congenital ocular motor disorders. Am. J. Ophthalmol. 60:443, 1965.
Isenberg, S. and Urist, M.J.: Clinical observations in 101 consecutive patients with Duane's retraction syndrome. Am. J. Ophthalmol. 84:419, 1977.
Pfaffenback, D.D. et al: Congenital anomalies in Duane's retraction syndrome. Arch. Ophthalmol. 88:635, 1972.
Sevel, D. and Kassar, B.S.: Bilateral Duane syndrome. Arch. Ophthalmol. 91:492, 1974.

Contributor: **Elsa K. Rahn**

Editor's Computerized Descriptor: Eye

SKIN LEIOMYOMAS, MULTIPLE

Includes: Léiomyome multiple de la peau
Leiomyomatosis cutis
Leiomioma cutáneo múltiple
Leiomyoma, multiple of skin
Multiple leiomyomas of skin
Hereditary multiple leiomyoma of skin

Excludes: Angiomyomas

Minimal Diagnostic Criteria: Skin lesions. See Clinical Findings.

Clinical Findings: Skin eruption of pink, red or dusky brown, firm, dermal nodules of varying size. These may be painful. May occur on any cutaneous surface but most commonly on thighs, hips and buttocks.

Complications
I   Derived: —
II Associated: —

Etiology: Autosomal dominant gene with reduced penetrance

Pathogenesis: May arise from arrectores pilorum muscles

Related Facts
I   **Sex Ratio:** M1:F1
II **Risk of Occurrence:** Rare
III **Risk of Recurrence for**
    Patient's Sib: If parent is affected, 1 in 2 (50%) for each offspring to be affected; otherwise not increased.
    Patient's Child: 1 in 2
IV **Age of Detectability:** 50% are detectable before the age of 20 years
V   **Prevalence:** About 100 reported cases

Treatment
I   **Primary Prevention:** Genetic counseling
II **Secondary Prevention:** —
III **Other Therapy:** Surgical excision if symptomatic

Prognosis: Normal for life span and health

Detection of Carrier: —

Special Considerations: —

References:
Fisher, W.C. and Helwig, E.B.: Leiomyomas of the skin. Arch. Dermatol. 88:510, 1963.
Kloepfer, H.W. et al: Hereditary multiple leiomyoma of the skin. Am. J. Hum. Genet. 10:48, 1958.
Rudner, E.J. et al: Multiple cutaneous leiomyoma in identical twins. Arch. Dermatol. 90:81, 1964.

Contributor: **R. W. Blaine**

Editor's Computerized Descriptor: Skin

SMITH-LEMLI-OPITZ SYNDROME

Includes: Syndrome de Smith-Lemli-Opitz
Síndrome de Smith-Lemli-Opitz

Excludes: —

Minimal Diagnostic Criteria: Anteverted nostrils +/- ptosis of the eyelids, syndactyly of the 2nd-3rd toes, and male genital anomaly in a mentally retarded patient with small stature would seem to be reasonable diagnostic criteria at the present time.†

Clinical Findings: Growth deficiency 100%, of prenatal onset with mean birthweight 2551 gm. Moderate-to-severe mental retardation 100% with variable alteration of muscle tone. Vomiting in early infancy, tendency toward a shrill cry. Microcephaly with moderate scaphocephaly. Ptosis of eyelids, inner epicanthic folds, strabismus, broad nasal tip with anteverted nostrils 100%, broad lateral palatine ridges and mild-to-moderate micrognathia 100%. Limbs frequently show simian crease, syndactyly 2nd-3rd toes, high frequency of whorls on finger tips. Genitalia reveal cryptorchidism, hypospadias, small penis. Other frequently reported abnormalities include: EEG abnormality, dysplasia epiphysialis punctata, acrocyanosis of hands and feet, and hypoplasia of thymus.

Occasional features include: broad nasal bridge, cleft palate, clenched hand with index finger overlying the 3rd, asymmetric short finger, distal palmar axial triradius, metatarsus adductus, dislocation of hip, deep sacral dimple, pit anterior to anus, wide-spread nipples, cardiac defect, inguinal hernia, pyloric stenosis and dilated renal calyces.

Complications
I **Derived:** Upper and lower respiratory infection, irritable behavior with shrill screaming, pyloric stenosis
II **Associated:** —

Etiology: Autosomal recessive; McK *27040

Pathogenesis: ?

Related Facts
I **Sex Ratio:** The majority of patients reported have been males, but this may simply represent an ascertainment bias because of the genital anomalies in the affected males.
II **Risk of Occurrence:** ?
III **Risk of Recurrence for**
Patient's Sib: Presumed 1 in 4 (25%) for each sib
Patient's Child: Probably not applicable because of reproductive unfitness
IV **Age of Detectability:** At birth
V **Prevalence:** Rare

Treatment
I **Primary Prevention:** Genetic counseling
II **Secondary Prevention:** ?
III **Other Therapy:** —

Prognosis: About half of the reported cases have died by 14 months of age, usually with pneumonia or other infectious complication. There is inadequate data on longevity for those patients who survive infancy. Moderate-to-severe mental retardation in all cases. The intellectual deficit and failure to thrive severely impair function. Two adults have IQs in the 20s.

Detection of Carrier: —

†Special Considerations: There is frequently a history of relatively late advent of fetal activity and the majority of patients have been born in a breech presentation - indications of a serious problem in fetal development and function.

References:

Garcia, C.A. et al: Neurological involvement in the Smith-Lemli-Opitz syndrome. Dev. Med. Child. Neurol. 15:48, 1973.
Park, S. C. et al: Congenital heart disease in an infant with Smith-Lemli-Opitz syndrome. J. Pediatr. 73:896, 1968.
Smith, D.W. et al: A newly recognized syndrome of multiple congenital anomalies. J. Pediatr. 64:210, 1964.

Contributor: **David W. Smith**

Editor's Computerized Descriptors: Eye, Face, Nerve, Nose, Dermatoglyphic, Skel., Muscle, GI., GU.

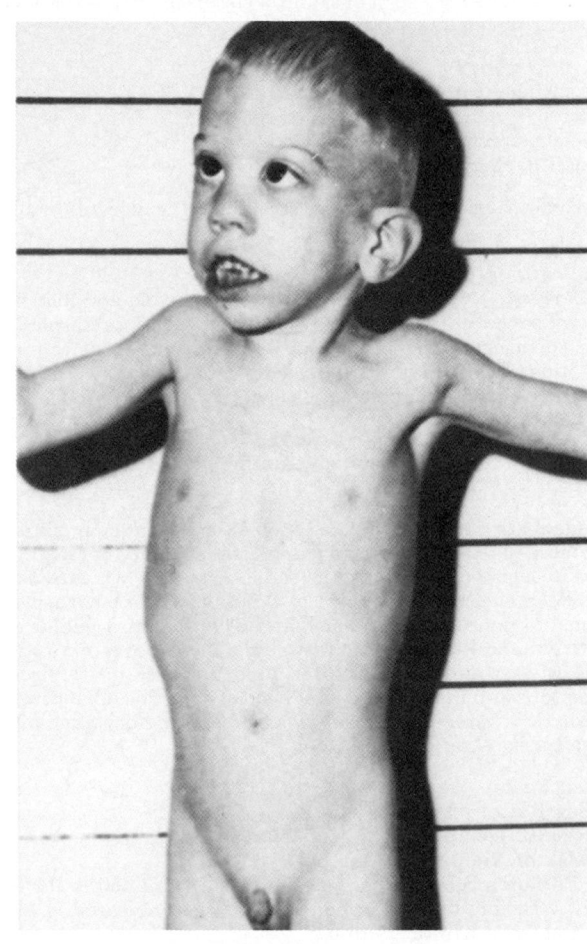

457. Smith-Lemli-Opitz syndrome

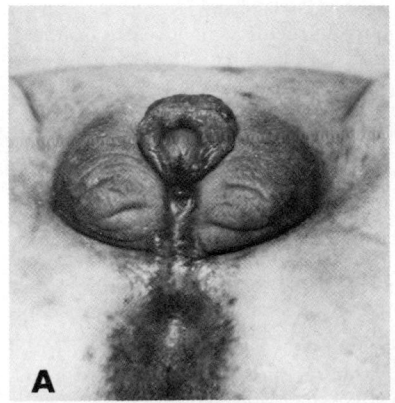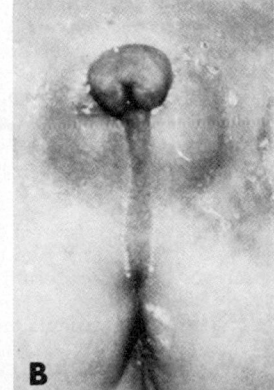

458. A) Hypospadias; B) hypospadias and hypoplastic scrotum

SPHEROCYTOSIS

Includes: Maladie de Minkowski-Chauffard
Sphärozytose
Esferocitosis
Hereditary spherocytosis
Spherocytic anemia congenital

Excludes: Nonspherocytic anemias congenital

Minimal Diagnostic Criteria: Hemolytic anemia with spherocytosis; increased osmotic fragility of erythrocytes; increased tendency of erythrocytes to undergo autohemolysis in vitro; shortened life span of erythrocytes from affected patient in normal recipient.

Clinical Findings:

Chronic hemolytic anemia	100%
Numerous microspherocytic erythrocytes demonstrable in peripheral blood	100%
Modest hyperbilirubinemia and splenomegaly	75-100%

No abnormalities of number or structure of leukocytes or platelets

Complications
I Derived: Aplastic crisis with severe anemia and hemolytic crises in childhood. Massive splenomegaly predisposes to splenic rupture; chronic hemolytic anemia leads to formation of bilirubin stones in gallbladder; aplastic crisis seen occasionally; chronic leg ulcers.

II Associated: —

Etiology: Autosomal dominant transmission with variable penetrance; McK *18290

Pathogenesis: Intrinsic defect of some component of erythrocyte membrane leads to increased passive permeability of cells to water and solutes; as a result, the sodium "pump," which requires metabolic energy in the form of ATP, must work harder than normal to remove sodium and water from the intracellular compartment and keep cells from swelling; increased pump activity appears to result in accelerated lipid turnover in erythrocyte membrane and in increased likelihood of depletion of glucose and glycolytic intermediates; formation of microspherocytes enhances splenic sequestration and hemolysis.†

Related Facts
I Sex Ratio: M1:F1
II Risk of Occurrence: 1 in 4500 (?)
III Risk of Recurrence for
    Patient's Sib: If parent is affected, 1 in 2 (50%) for each offspring to be affected; otherwise not increased.
    Patient's Child: 1 in 2
IV Age of Detectability: ?
V Prevalence: ? Estimated at 1 in 4500

Treatment
I Primary Prevention: Genetic counseling
II Secondary Prevention: Splenectomy ameliorates dramatically the hemolytic anemia; blood transfusions in severe hemolytic episodes
III Other Therapy: Cholecystectomy if choleliathiasis supervenes.

Prognosis: Splenectomy is invariably curative clinically leading to normal life span.

Detection of Carrier: Disease is transmitted as an autosomal dominant trait implying that heterozygous carriers for the mutant gene are the affected patients. Since trait is probably genetically heterogeneous, incomplete penetrance may be explained for populations of patients on this basis. Phenocopies also occur.

†Special Considerations: Although the exact nature of the membrane defect is obscure, its effects on water and cation permeability, cation pump activity and anaerobic glycolysis demonstrate sequence of pathophysiologic events; increased lipid turnover could reflect primary abnormality in erythrocyte lipid content but more likely reflects accelerated cation pump activity; a primary defect in the structure of the microfilamentous, membrane protein, spectrin has been proposed.

References:
Jacob, H. S.: Abnormalities in the physiology of the erythrocyte membrane in hereditary spherocytosis. Am. J. Med. 41:734, 1966.
Jacob, H.S. et al: Cyclic nucleotide-membrane protein interaction in the regulation of erythrocyte shape and survival: Defect in hereditary spherocytosis. In Brewer, G.J. (ed.): Erythrocyte Structure and Function. New York: Alan Liss, Inc., 1975, p. 235.
Jandl, J. H. and Cooper, R. A.: Hereditary spherocytosis. In Stanbury, J.B. et al (eds.): The Metabolic Basis of Inherited Disease. New York: McGraw-Hill, 1972, p. 1323.
Mackinney, A.A. et al: Ascertaining genetic carriers of hereditary spherocytosis by statistical analysis of multiple laboratory tests. J. Clin. Invest. 41:554, 1962.

Contributor: **Leon E. Rosenberg**

Editor's Computerized Descriptors: Spleen, GI.

SPHEROPHAKIA-BRACHYMORPHIA SYNDROME

Includes: Syndrome de sphérophakie-brachymorphie
Sphärophakie-Brachymorphie-Syndrom
Síndrome de esferofaquia y braquimorfia
Weill-Marchesani syndrome
Congenital mesodermal dysmorphodystrophy, brachymorphic type

Excludes: Constitutional short stature; dislocated lens and pupil

Minimal Diagnostic Criteria: Congenital spherophakia with or without dislocated lenses and short stature.

Clinical Findings: Characterized by congenital microspherophakia and dislocation of the lens in patients of pyknic habitus. The height may be below the 3rd percentile. The patients show brachycephaly, pug nose, depressed nasal bridge, short pudgy hands and feet, there may be articular stiffness and limitation of extension. The patients are high myopes.

Complications
I   **Derived:** Glaucoma
II   **Associated:** —

Etiology: Autosomal recessive with partial expression in the heterozygote; McK *27760

Pathogenesis: ?†

Related Facts
I   **Sex Ratio:** M1:F1
II   **Risk of Occurrence:** ? 1 in 100,000
III **Risk of Recurrence for**
     Patient's Sib: 1 in 4 (25%) for each offspring to be affected
     Patient's Child: Not increased unless mate is carrier or homozygote.
IV   **Age of Detectability:** At birth by slit-lamp examination, if suspected
V   **Prevalence:** ? 1 in 100,000 world-wide distribution

Treatment
I   **Primary Prevention:** Genetic counseling
II   **Secondary Prevention:** Control of intraocular pressure; iridotomy or lens extraction in case of glaucoma
III **Other Therapy:** —

Prognosis: Good for life span and intelligence, reduced visual function

Detection of Carrier: Distinctly short pyknic habitus without the ocular findings

†Special Considerations: The glaucoma may arise with or without dislocation of the lens. The anterior displacement of the lens may block the pupil and hinder the flow of aqueous from the posterior into the anterior chamber. Glaucoma may also arise as a complication of a dislocated lens through irritation of the ciliary body, blocking of the angle or by complete luxation into the anterior chamber.

References:
Kloepfer, H. W. and Rosenthal, J. W.: Possible genetic carriers in the spherophakia - brachymorphia syndrome. Am. J. Hum. Genet. 7:398, 1955.
Rennert, O. M.: The Marchesani syndrome. A brief review. Am. J. Dis. Child. 117:703, 1969.

Contributor: Irene Hussels-Maumenee

———————————

Editor's Computerized Descriptors: Vision, Eye, Nose, Skel.

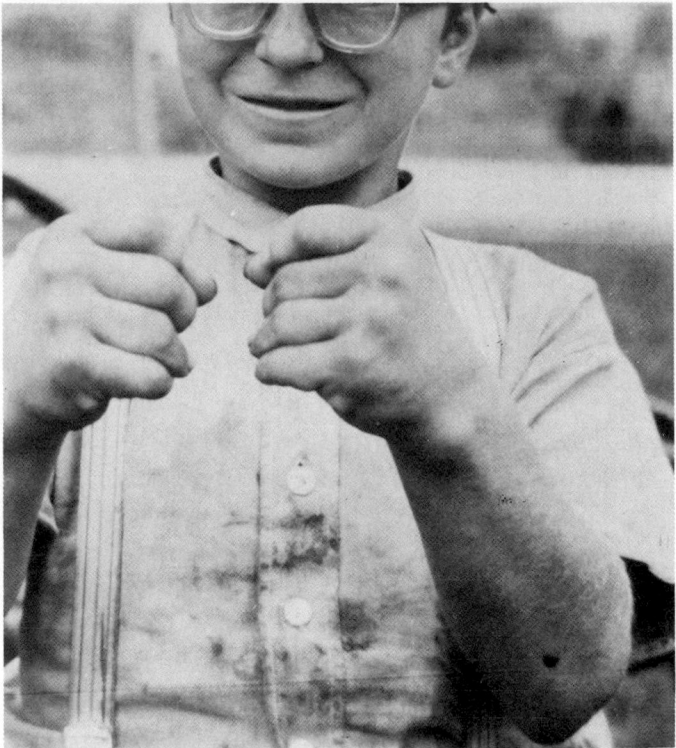

459. Note pug nose, short hands with knobby joints, and restriction in flexion

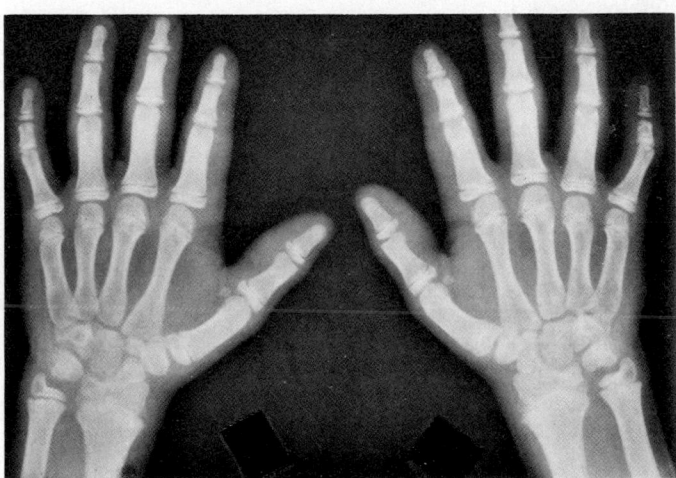

460. All bones are short, especially middle phalanges of 5th fingers

SPINAL CORD, NEURENTERIC CYST

888-500

References:
Bale, P.M.: A congenital intraspinal gastroenterogenous cyst and diastematomyelia. J. Neurol. Neurosurg. Psychiatry 36:1011, 1973.

Includes: Kyste neuro-entéritique
Neurenterische Rückenmarkszysten
Quiste neurentérico de la médula espinal
Cord cyst associated with posterior mediastinal cyst
Neurenteric cyst of spinal cord

Contributor: Kenneth Shulman

Editor's Computerized Descriptors: Sweating, Skel., GI., GU., Nerve

Excludes: Diastematomyelia (292)

Minimal Diagnostic Criteria: Depends upon suspicion of lesion on clinical grounds with definitive diagnosis made by myelography and surgical exploration

Clinical Findings: Progressive neurologic loss depending upon the level of the persisting embryologic defect, paralysis of legs, bladder and bowel with sensory loss in newborn or during first few years of life. If there is an associated posterior mediastinal cyst, cardiothoracic symptoms are present. There is generally no skin lesion over the area of affected spinal cord. Butterfly vertebrae.

Complications
I **Derived:** Paralysis of legs, bladder and bowel; with loss of ability to sweat below the level of the lesion, temperature control is difficult.
II **Associated:** Bowel duplications, mediastinal or cervical cysts. Diastematomyelia.

Etiology: ?

Pathogenesis: Persistent connection between alimentary tract and midline neural structures with mesodermal defect. One hypothesis is that primitive notocordal plate tissue carries entoderm into the vertebral canal and enterogenous cysts occur within the spinal canal in lower cervical or upper thoracic level. Association of enterogenous cyst with vertebral anomalies suggests errors in embryologic development. A midline ecto-endodermal adhesion is postulated obstructing the axial mesoderm and persisting as a neurenteric connection through the vertebral defect in the 2nd week of life. During the 3rd week the axial mesoderm would have to split or detour to pass the ectodermal-endodermal adhesion. This might result in defects in the vertebral bodies with the adhesion remaining as a postnatal cyst, diastematomyelia or band between the alimentary canal and spinal cord.

Related Facts
I **Sex Ratio:** ?
II **Risk of Occurrence:** ?
III **Risk of Recurrence for**
  Patient's Sib: ?
  Patient's Child: ?
IV **Age of Detectability:** ?
V **Prevalence:** ?

Treatment
I **Primary Prevention:** —
II **Secondary Prevention:** Surgical excision or drainage of spinal cyst. If a cyst is present in mediastinum or neck, it is removed at secondary operation.
III **Other Therapy:** Prevention of kidney disease secondary to bladder paralysis

Prognosis: Will depend upon the degree of paralysis and rapidity of onset. If paralysis is incomplete, prognosis is better.

Detection of Carrier: ?

Special Considerations: —

SPINAL MUSCULAR ATROPHY

Includes: Atrophie musculaire spinale
Spinale Muskelatrophie
Atrofia muscular espinal
Werdnig-Hoffman disease
Kugelberg-Welander disease

Excludes: Muscular dystrophy
Charcot-Marie-Tooth syndrome
Guillian-Barre syndrome
Benign congenital hypotonia

Minimal Diagnostic Criteria: Hypotonia, weakness, decreased or absent deep tendon reflexes with characteristic EMG and muscle biopsy findings.

Clinical Findings: At least 2 forms of spinal muscular atrophy can be distinguished: Infantile (Werdnig-Hoffman) and juvenile (Kugelberg-Welander).

In the early infantile form, symptoms may begin in utero, (decreased fetal movement), at birth or in the 1st months of life with hypotonia, weakness, decreased spontaneous activity and decreased or absent deep tendon reflexes. Intercostal muscles are nearly always involved while the diaphragm is spared resulting in "paradoxical" respirations. Muscle atrophy, fasciculations (particularly of the tongue) and a characteristic "frog" position with hips abducted and knees flexed are seen. There is failure to attain age-appropriate motor milestones. The course is rapidly progressive with death, usually due to pulmonary infection or respiratory insufficiency, occurring within 1-2 years of diagnosis.

A late-onset infantile form beginning after 6 months of age has a more prolonged course extending over several years. Intellectual development is normal.

In the juvenile form, the onset is usually after age 2 years and may occur as late as adolescence or adulthood. The course occasionally seems static and may improve slightly with age. The proximal muscles are affected first and may initially mimic Duchenne muscular dystrophy. Involvement is usually symmetric with slow progression. Life span may be normal.

Laboratory findings: Cerebrospinal fluid values are normal. Muscle enzymes are normal but may be mildly elevated in the juvenile form. Electromyogram (EMG) shows a denervation pattern with large amplitude, polyphasic potentials of long duration, reduced interference pattern on voluntary movement and fibrillation potentials at rest. Nerve conduction times are normal or minimally prolonged. Muscle biopsy shows groups of atrophied fibers interspersed with large bundles. "Type grouping" can be demonstrated with appropriate histochemical stains. Disorganized fibrils, sarcomeres, filaments and band structure; nuclear clumping; and areas of regeneration are seen by electron microscopy. Atrophy of anterior horn cells of spinal cord as well as peripheral nerve degeneration are seen.†

Complications
I **Derived:** Recurrent lower respiratory infection, scoliosis, osteoporosis and other orthopedic deformities.
II **Associated:** Urinary incontinence, cardiomyopathy, cardiac arrhythmia, arthrogryposis.

Etiology: Autosomal recessive. In rare instances there appears to be an autosomal dominant mode of inheritance. McK *15860, *25330, *25340

Pathogenesis: Degeneration of anterior horn cells of the spinal cord and brain stem with subsequent distinctive changes in the associated muscles.†

Related Facts
I **Sex Ratio:** M1:F1
II **Risk of Occurrence:** 1 per 25,000 live births in England (infantile form).
III **Risk of Recurrence for**
  Patient's Sib: 1 in 4 (25%) for each offspring to be affected, if autosomal recessive. If dominant, 1 in 2.
  Patient's Child: In most families not increased unless mate is a carrier or is also affected. If dominant, 1 in 2 (50%).
IV **Age of Detectability:** Before age 2 in the infantile form; 2 years to adulthood in juvenile form.
V **Prevalence:** ?

Treatment
I **Primary Prevention:** Genetic counseling
II **Secondary Prevention:** Physical therapy, respiratory care, agressive treatment of respiratory infections, supportive orthopedic care.
III **Other Therapy:** —

Prognosis: Werdnig-Hoffman: Death within 1-2 years of diagnosis in early infantile form, 3-5 years for late infantile form. Kugelberg-Welander: Prolonged survival and sometimes normal life span in juvenile form.

Detection of Carrier: —

†Special Considerations: Spinal muscular atrophy probably includes more than 1 genetic and clinical entity and may represent several distinct conditions. Until the basic defect is identified, distinctions remain imprecise. Families have been described in which members have been affected by apparently distinct forms of the disease. Age of onset and length of course are useful distinguishing characteristics for prognostic and counseling purposes but must be interpreted carefully, since overlapping certainly occurs among the various forms.

References:
Emery, A.E.H.: The nosology of the spinal muscular atrophies. J. Med. Genet. 8:481, 1971.
Fried, K. and Emery, A.E.: Spinal muscular atrophy type II. A separate genetic and clinical entity from type I (Werdnig-Hoffman disease) and type III (Kugelberg-Welander disease). Clin. Genet. 2:203, 1971.
Hausmanowa-Petrusewicz, I. et al: Genetic investigations on chronic forms of infantile and juvenile spinal muscular atrophy. J. Neurol. 213:335, 1976.
Meadows, J.C. et al: Chronic spinal muscular atrophy in adults. 1. The Kugelberg-Welander syndrome. J. Neurol. Sci. 9:527, 1969.
Munsat, T.L. et al: Neurogenic muscular atrophy of infancy with prolonged survival. The variable course of Werdnig-Hoffman disease. Brain. 92:9, 1969.
Pearn, J.H.: The gene frequency of acute Werdnig-Hoffman disease (SMA type I). A total population survey in Northeast England. J. Med. Genet. 10:260, 1973.

Contributors: **Louis E. Bartoshesky**
William Singer

Editor's Computerized Descriptors: Skel., Muscle, Resp., GU.

SPONDYLOCOSTAL DYSPLASIA

Includes: Dysplasie spondylo-costale
Spondylokostale Dysplasie
Displasia espóndilocostal
Autosomal dominant multiple hemivertebrae

Excludes: Spondylothoracic dysplasia (900)
Klippel-Feil syndrome

Minimal Diagnostic Criteria: A shortened trunk associated with segmentation anomalies of the vertebrae and ribs with a normal skull and limbs†

Clinical Findings: Short-trunked dwarfism associated with multiple anomalies of the vertebrae and ribs. The skull and limbs are normal. The U/L segment ratio is decreased for age and the arm span is greater than the height. The neck is thick and short and rotatory movements are limited. Patients are asymptomatic in childhood but increasing limitation of motion of the spine with back pain can occur in adults. Radiographs reveal gross disorganization of vertebral segmentation with a reduced number of vertebrae, fused or "block" vertebrae, hemivertebrae and sagitally cleft or "butterfly" vertebrae. The ribs and their vertebral pedicles are reduced in number and many of those present are hypoplastic or fused. The bones of the skull and limbs are normal.

Complications
I   **Derived:** Increasing limitation of spinal movement associated with back pain and referred pain secondary to nerve root compression
II **Associated:** —

Etiology: Autosomal dominant; McK *12260

Pathogenesis: ?

Related Facts
I   **Sex Ratio:** M1:F1
II   **Risk of Occurrence:** ?
III **Risk of Recurrence for**
    Patient's Sib: If parent is affected, 1 in 2 (50%) for each offspring to be affected; otherwise not increased.
    Patient's Child: 1 in 2
IV **Age of Detectability:** At birth by clinical and radiographic examination
V   **Prevalence:** ?

Treatment
I   **Primary Prevention:** Genetic counseling
II   **Secondary Prevention:** The effects of bracing or spinal fusion to prevent scoliosis and nerve root compression have not been evaluated.
III **Other Therapy:** —

Prognosis: Normal life span

Detection of Carrier: Diagnosed patients and their phenotypic parents

†Special Considerations: This syndrome must be distinguished from other disorders associated with hemivertebrae such as: nongenetic forms of hemivertebrae, which are usually more limited in their distribution; spondylothoracic dysplasia which is associated with more severe truncal shortening and deformity and early death from respiratory infection; and syndromes associated with limited segmentation anomalies of the spine, such as oculoauriculovertebral dysplasia, lateral facial cleft syndrome, Larsen syndrome, basal cell nevus syndrome, incontinentia pigmenti, Klippel-Feil syndrome, and the oculovertebral syndrome.

References:
Caffey, J.P.: Pediatric X-ray Diagnosis, 5th Ed. Chicago: Year Book Medical Publishers, 1967, p. 1109.
Rimoin, D.L. et al: Spondylocostal dysplasia: A dominantly inherited form of short-trunked dwarfism. Am. J. Med. 45:948, 1968.
van der Sar, A.: Hereditary multiple hemivertebrae. Docum. Med. Geogr. Trop. (Amst.) 4:23, 1952.

Contributor: **David L. Rimoin**

Editor's Computerized Descriptors: Neck, Skel.

SPONDYLOEPIPHYSEAL DYSPLASIA CONGENITA

Includes: Dysplasie spondylo-épiphysaire congénitale
Dysplasia spondyloepiphysaria congenita
Displasia espóndiloepifisaria congénita
SED congenita

Excludes: Spondyloepiphyseal dysplasia tarda (898)
Other spondyloepiphyseal dysplasias
Mucopolysaccharidosis IV (678)

Minimal Diagnostic Criteria: Short-trunk type of dwarfism; retarded ossification of the vertebral bodies and proximal femur; coxa vara; normally shaped hand bones.

Clinical Findings: Flat face, myopia or retinal detachment (approximately 50% of cases); muscular hypotonia in infancy; occasionally cleft palate or clubfoot; short-trunk type of dwarfism, barrel-chest, genu valga or vara; waddling gait, normal-sized hands and feet.

Radiographs show retarded ossification of the spine and proximal femora with flattened, anteriorly pointed vertebral bodies, lack of ossification of the pubic and ischial bones in young infants; grossly retarded or absent ossification of the femoral head and neck in older patients; severe varus deformity of the femoral neck, varying degrees of epiphyseal and metaphyseal irregularities of the long tubular bones; retarded ossification of the hand bones which are normally shaped.

Complications
I **Derived:** Retinal detachment may lead to blindness. Premature and severe arthritic changes occur in the hips. Hypoplasia of the odontoid process of C2 and lax ligaments predispose to atlantoaxial instability and spinal cord compression. Kyphoscoliosis, hyperextensible finger joints and joint dislocation.
II **Associated:** Recurrent otitis has been observed. Moderate sensorineural hearing loss (30-60 db) especially marked in high tones. Associated ocular findings include myopia, strabismus, cataracts, buphthalmos and secondary glaucoma.

Etiology: Autosomal dominant with considerable variability in phenotypic expression.† McK *18390

Pathogenesis: Histologic studies show a hypocellular matrix and lack of column formation with an irregular array of broad, short spicules of calcified cartilage and bone. Electron microscopic examination of cartilage reveals widely distended cisterns of rough endoplasmic reticulum in the chondrocytes.

Related Facts
I **Sex Ratio:** M1:F1
II **Risk of Occurrence:** ? Probably more frequent than mucopolysaccharidosis IV
III **Risk of Recurrence for**
  Patient's Sib: If parent is affected 1 in 2 (50%) for each offspring to be affected; otherwise not increased.
  Patient's Child: 1 in 2
IV **Age of Detectability:** At birth
V **Prevalence:** ?

Treatment
I **Primary Prevention:** Genetic counseling
II **Secondary Prevention:** Early correction of clubfoot deformity, closure of cleft palate; prevention of retinal detachment by regular ophthalmologic examinations and coagulation of early retinal tears.
III **Other Therapy:** Careful neurologic examinations to detect early signs of cervical cord compression. Symptomatic orthopedic care.

Prognosis: The patients reach adulthood and may reproduce. The adult height varies between 84 cm and 128 cm. Mental development is normal.

Detection of Carrier: The phenotype is usually well expressed and easily detectable by clinical and radiographic studies.†

†Special Considerations: A family with multiple affected sibs has been observed in which the father was clinically and radiographically normal and the mother had only a moderately severe scoliosis and short stature. If she was a carrier, scoliosis was the only phenotypic expression of the mutation. Other explanations include genetic heterogeneity of spondyloepiphyseal dysplasia congenita, germinal mosaicism and an unstable premutation.

References:
Spranger, J. and Langer, L.O.: Spondyloepiphyseal dysplasias. In Bergsma, D. (ed.): Skeletal Dysplasias. Birth Defects: Orig. Art. Ser., vol. X, no. 9. Miami: Symposia Specialists for The National Foundation-March of Dimes, 1974, p. 19.
Spranger, J. and Langer, L.O.: Spondyloepiphyseal dysplasia congenita. Radiology 94:313, 1970.

Contributor: **Jürgen W. Spranger**

Editor's Computerized Descriptors: Vision, Eye, Face, Oral, Skel., Muscle

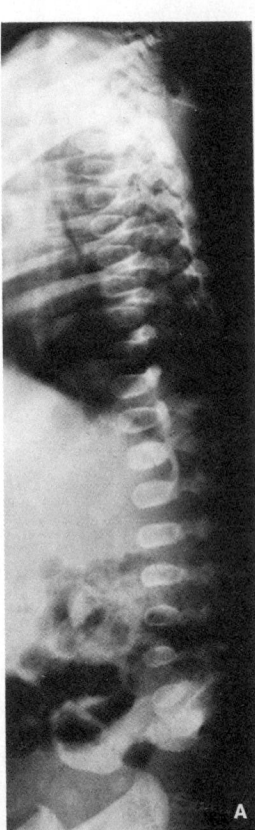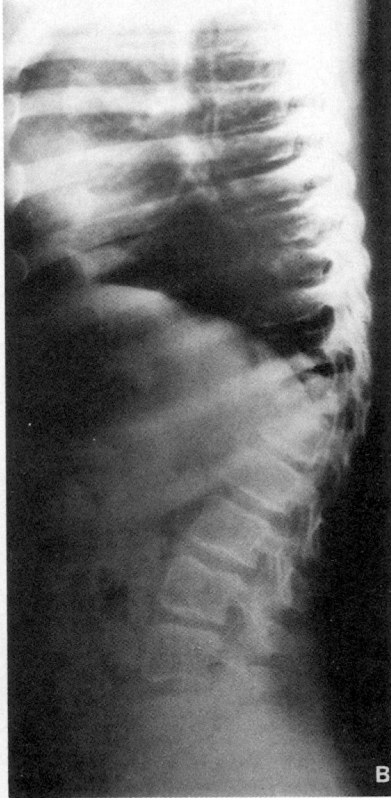

461. A) At 2 months: note flat vertebral bodies, dorsal wedging of thoracic and upper lumbar bodies; B) at 13 years: platyspondyly in dorsal spine and kyphosis

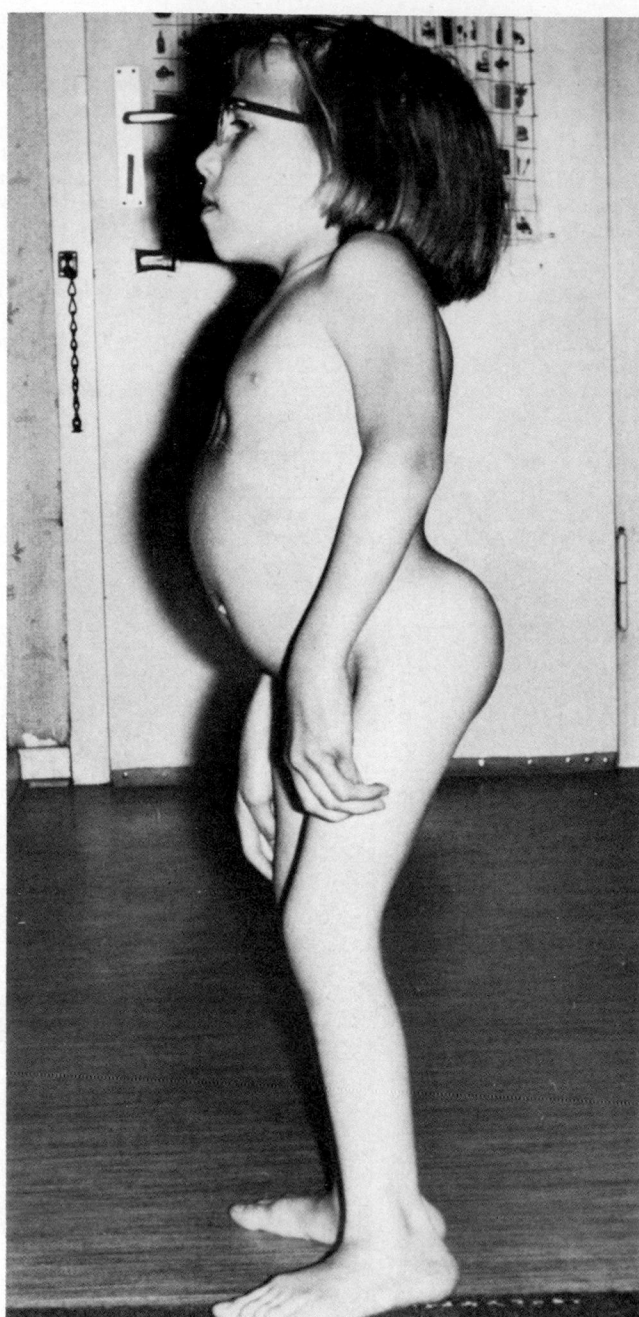

462. Short-trunk type dwarfism. Lumbar lordosis is accentuated, face is flat, and glasses are worn to correct myopia

SPONDYLOEPIPHYSEAL DYSPLASIA TARDA

Includes: Dysplasie spondylo-épiphysaire tardive
Dysplasia spondyloepiphysaria tarda
Displasia espóndiloepifisaria tardía
X-linked form of spondyloepiphyseal dysplasia
SED

Excludes: Mucopolysaccharidosis IV† (678)
Other forms of spondyloepiphyseal dysplasia
Epiphyseal dysplasia, multiple (358)

Minimal Diagnostic Criteria: This syndrome should be suspected in males who present with short-trunked dwarfism with onset in late childhood or early adolescence. The diagnosis is confirmed by skeletal xrays which reveal the typical humped-up appearance of the platyspondylotic vertebral bodies. Radiographic changes, however, are not diagnostic until at least adolescence.

Clinical Findings: This is a form of short-trunked dwarfism found only in males, associated with premature osteoarthrosis primarily of the spine and hips. Affected individuals are normal at birth, and failure of normal growth does not become apparent until 5-10 years of age. At this time, growth of the spine appears to stop. The shoulders assume a hunched-up appearance, the neck appears to shorten, and the chest broadens. As adults, they have a mild form of dwarfism with a short trunk, large chest cage, and relatively normal length to their limbs. The hands, feet, and head appear normal. Mild kyphoscoliosis may occur. Adult height ranges from 4'4"-5' 2". During late childhood or adolescence, vague back pain may occur; and in early adulthood, painful osteoarthrosis with limitation of motion of the back and hips is usually present. Symptoms may also affect the shoulders and less commonly, the knees and ankles. There are no extraskeletal manifestations of the disease. All laboratory studies have been normal.

Skeletal xrays reveal a distinct and diagnostic configuration to the lumbar vertebrae in adolescence and adulthood. This consists of generalized flattening of the vertebral bodies with a hump-shaped build-up of eburnated bone in the central and posterior portions of the superior and inferior plates. There is complete lack of visible bone in the areas of the ring apophyses. The disk spaces appear narrow, and at first glance may appear calcified, but the calcification is really part of the vertebral body itself. Premature disk degeneration does occur. The platyspondyly extends throughout the thoracic and cervical spine to the C-2 level with less marked involvement of the end plates. Superimposed osteospondylotic changes develop in early childhood. The thoracic cage appears increased in both transverse and AP diameters. The bony pelvis is small and on full trunk xrays, a marked discrepancy between the size of the rib cage and pelvis is obvious. The acetabulae are deep and the femoral necks short. Mild dysplastic changes are seen in all large joints, especially the hips. Premature osteoarthrosis of the hips with extensive cyst formation may develop in the 3rd-4th decade. Premature osteoarthrosis is also frequent in the shoulders and less common in the knees and ankles. The bones of the hands appear normal. Skeletal xrays, however, are completely normal in infancy and early childhood.

Complications
I   **Derived:** Premature osteoarthrosis of the hips almost always occurs in adulthood and may lead to disabling pain and limitation of motion. Pain in the back and shoulders may also present problems.
II **Associated:** —

Etiology: This syndrome has been described in multiple male members of several families, transmitted through unaffected females, indicating X-linked recessive inheritance.† McK *31340

Pathogenesis: ?

Related Facts
I **Sex Ratio:** M1:F0
II **Risk of Occurrence:** ?
III **Risk of Recurrence for**
   Patient's Sib: If mother is a carrier 1 in 2 (50%) for each brother to be affected and 1 in 2 for each sister to be a carrier.
   Patient's Child: 1 in 1 (100%) for carrier daughters; not increased for sons unless wife is a carrier.
IV **Age of Detectability:** Late childhood or early adolescence by short-trunked dwarfism and typical skeletal xrays.
V **Prevalence:** ?

Treatment
I **Primary Prevention:** Genetic counseling
II **Secondary Prevention:** Physical therapy to relieve joint stiffness and pain. Total hip replacement may be eventually the treatment of choice for severely disabling premature osteoarthrosis of the hips.
III **Other Therapy:** —

Prognosis: No effect on life span or intelligence, premature osteoarthrosis may lead to disabling pain and limitation of motion in mid to late adulthood.

Detection of Carrier: —

†**Special Considerations:** This disorder has been confused in the past with the mucopolysaccharidoses. The late age of onset, the typical radiographic features, the lack of extraskeletal manifestations, and the lack of elevated mucopolysaccharide excretion in urine allow for ready diagnosis of this disorder. Rare autosomal recessive and dominant varieties of late onset spondyloepiphyseal dysplasia have also been reported.

References:
Langer, L.O.: Spondyloepiphyseal dysplasia tarda. Radiology 82:833, 1964.
Maroteaux, P. et al: La dysplasie spondylo-epiphysaire tardive. Presse Med. 65:1205, 1957.
Poker, N. et al: Spondyloepiphysial dysplasia tarda. Radiology 85:474, 1965.
Spranger, J. and Langer, L.O. Spondyloepiphyseal dysplasias. In Bergsma, D. (ed.): Skeletal Dysplasias. Birth Defects: Orig. Art. Ser., vol. X, no. 9. Miami: Symposia Specialists for The National Foundation-March of Dimes, 1974, p. 19.

Contributors: **David L. Rimoin**
David W. Hollister

Editor's Computerized Descriptors: Neck, Skel.

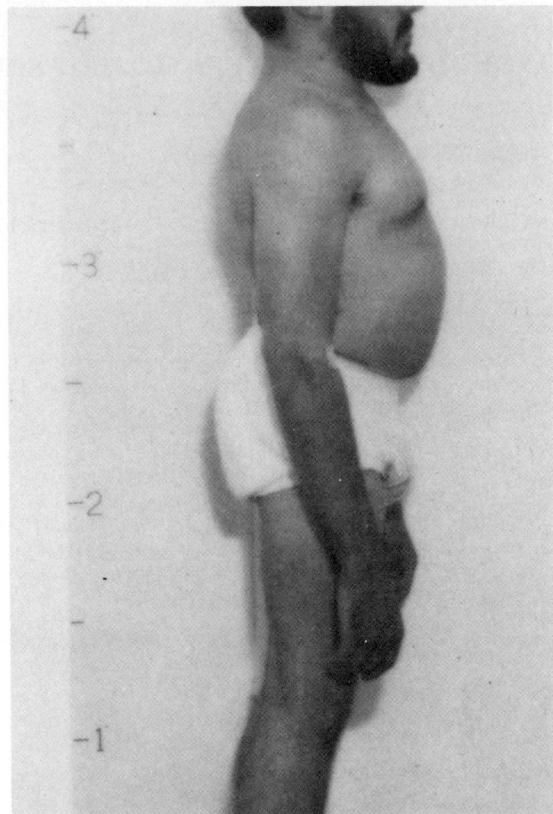

463. Note relatively large broad chest, short neck, exaggerated lumbar lordosis, and short trunk

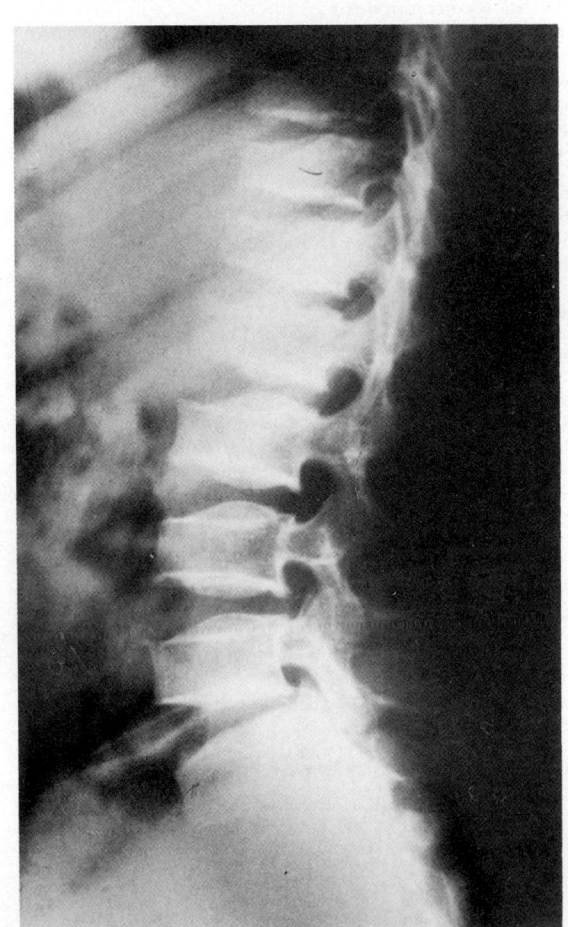

464. Note flat vertebral bodies; hump-shaped bone buildup in central and posterior portions of upper and lower plates; narrowing of disk spaces

SPONDYLOMETAPHYSEAL CHONDRODYSPLASIA, TYPE KOZLOWSKI

Includes: Chondrodysplasie spondylométaphysaire, type Kozlowski

Spondylometaphysäre Dysplasie, Typ Kozlowski

Condrodisplasia espóndilometafisaria, tipo Kozlowski

Excludes: Other types of spondylometaphyseal chondrodysplasias

Spondyloepimetaphyseal dysplasias

Spondylometaepiphyseal chondrodysplasias

Mucopolysaccharidosis IV (678)

Metatropic dysplasia (656)

Minimal Diagnostic Criteria: Shortening of stature and radiographic signs of platyspondyly and metaphyseal osteochondrodysplasia.

Clinical Findings: Progressive, moderate shortening of stature with predominant shortening of the trunk; waddling gait; kyphosis; normal head; adult height about 140 cm. Diagnostic radiographic findings characterized by generalized platyspondyly with unique shape of the vertebral bodies, metaphyseal osteochondrodysplasia and retarded carpal and tarsal bone age.†

Complications
I **Derived:** Kyphosis; scoliosis; early, severe osteoarthritic changes
II **Associated:** —

Etiology: Autosomal dominant

Pathogenesis: Fibrous appearance of cartilage matrix.

Related Facts
I **Sex Ratio:** M1:F1
II **Risk of Occurrence:** Minimal
III **Risk of Recurrence for**
  Patient's Sib: If parent is affected 1 in 2 (50%) for each offspring to be affected; otherwise not increased.
  Patient's Child: 1 in 2
IV **Age of Detectability:** Preschool age by radiographic features
V **Prevalence:** ?

Treatment
I **Primary Prevention:** Genetic counseling
II **Secondary Prevention:** Physiotherapy
III **Other Therapy:** Orthopedic treatment

Prognosis: Normal life span

Detection of Carrier: —

†**Special Considerations:** A number of patients with spine and metaphyseal dysplastic changes have been described who differ from the Kozlowski type of SMD in the appearance and distribution of the lesions radiographically. Although an attempt has been made to divide these cases into certain subtypes (eg Sutcliffe, Schmidt and Murdock types), their classification is still in question.

References:
Kozlowski, K.: Spondylo-metaphyseal dysplasia. Prog. Pediatr. Radiol. 4:299, 1973.
Kozlowski, K.: Metaphyseal and spondylo-metaphyseal dysplasias. Clin. Orthop. In press.
Kozlowski, K. et al: La dysostose spondylo-metaphysaire. Presse Méd. 75:2769, 1967.

Contributor: **K.S. Kozlowski**

Editor's Computerized Descriptor: Skel.

SPONDYLOTHORACIC DYSPLASIA

Includes: Dysplasie spondylo-thoracique

Spondylothorakale Dysplasie

Displasia espóndilotoraxica

Autosomal recessive multiple hemivertebrae

Occipito-facial-cervico-thoracic-abdomino-digital dysplasia

Jarcho-Levin syndrome

Excludes: Spondylocostal dysplasia (896)

Minimal Diagnostic Criteria: Severe vertebral dysplasia and fusion giving markedly short trunk and "crab-like" radiographic appearance.

Clinical Findings: Congenital short trunk with protuberant abdomen and relatively long limbs which may be of normal length. The trunk is short because of anomalous vertebral development (hemivertebrae, partially absent vertebral bodies, fused vertebrae) and incomplete segmentation of the ribs. The thorax has a bizarre "crab-like" radiographic appearance with ribs splaying out from fused vertebrae. The neck is short, also because of anomalous vertebrae, with a low posterior hairline and limited movement. The occiput is prominent. The facies is round, somewhat puffy with the chin resting on the chest. Long fingers and toes, even hammer toes have been reported. Many patients have herniae.

Complications
I **Derived:** Affected children die in infancy as a result of pulmonary insufficiency and pneumonia.
II **Associated:** —

Etiology: Autosomal recessive inheritance most likely because of consanguinity, affected sibs of both sexes, and most patients are Puerto Rican.† McK *27730

Pathogenesis: These spinal and rib anomalies probably have their origin in early embryonic development during vertebral segmentation about the 4th - 6th weeks. Secondary anomalies in trunk and thorax shape occur.

Related Facts
I **Sex Ratio:** M5:F12 - fewer males have been reported. This may reflect the small number of reported cases or that affected males may die in utero.
II **Risk of Occurrence:** ? Rare
III **Risk of Recurrence for**
  Patient's Sib: 1 in 4 (25%); may be slightly less for males
  Patient's Child: Theoretically would only be carrier, but affected individuals die in infancy
IV **Age of Detectability:** Prenatal, or at birth
V **Prevalence:** Very rare, most cases have been Puerto Rican

Treatment
I **Primary Prevention:** Genetic counseling; prenatal diagnosis with xray or ultrasound may be attempted.
II **Secondary Prevention:** Respiratory support
III **Other Therapy:** —

Prognosis: Poor, all reported cases have died in infancy

Detection of Carrier: ?

†**Special Considerations:** Less severe vertebral segmentation anomalies have been reported with autosomal dominant and recessive inheritance.

References:

Jarcho, S. et al: Hereditary malformation of the vertebral bodies. Bull. Johns Hopk. Hosp. 62:216, 1938.

Lavy, N. W. et al: A syndrome of bizarre vertebral anomalies. J. Pediatr. 69:1121, 1966.

Perez-Comas, A. et al: Occipito-facial-cervico-thoracic-abdomino-digital dysplasia; Jarcho-Levin syndrome of vertebral anomalies. J. Pediatr. 85:388, 1974.

Contributor: **Judith G. Hall**

Editor's Computerized Descriptors: Face, Hair, Skel., Neck, Resp.

SPRENGEL DEFORMITY

Includes: Surélévation de l'omoplate
Sprengelsche Difformität
Deformación de Sprengel
Scapula elevata
High scapula

Excludes: Klippel-Feil anomaly

Minimal Diagnostic Criteria: Clinical or radiologic evidence of elevated scapula.

Clinical Findings: The scapula is located higher than its usual T^2-T^7 position and is usually hypoplastic, having the "fetal shape" of an equilateral triangle. It lies closer to the midline producing a lump in the web of the neck and is rotated such that the glenoid fossa faces downward restricting abduction of the affected arm. Involvement may be bilateral. A communication of bone, cartilage or fibrous tissue between the scapula and adjacent vertebrae is found in 25-50% of patients. Over half the cases (67%) have associated anomalies which include scoliosis, hemivertebrae, fused vertebrae, spina bifida occulta, cervical ribs, missing ribs, fused ribs, clavicular anomalies and hypoplasia of the muscles of the shoulder girdle.†

Complications
I **Derived:** Limitation of motion (elevation) of ipsilateral arm, related to degree of scapular deformity.
II **Associated:** See under Clinical Findings.

Etiology: Most cases occur sporadically, but autosomal dominant transmission has been reported.† McK *18440

Pathogenesis: The defect presumably results from failure of the mesenchymal anlage of the scapula to descend from its cervical position to the normal thoracic position during the 2nd month of gestation.

Related Facts
I **Sex Ratio:** M1:F2 in sporadic cases.
II **Risk of Occurrence:** ? Very low Very low
III **Risk of Recurrence for**
   Patient's Sib: Very low in general; but when autosomal dominant and if parent is affected, 1 in 2 (50%) for each offspring to be affected; otherwise not increased.
   Patient's Child: If autosomal dominant, 1 in 2
IV **Age of Detectability:** At birth, or during childhood.
V **Prevalence:** ?

Treatment
I **Primary Prevention:** Genetic counseling in autosomal dominant cases.
II **Secondary Prevention:** Surgery may not be needed in mild cases, however, in those severely affected, both function and cosmetic appearance can be improved by reconstructive surgery. This usually involves removal of the omovertebral communication when present and excision of the superomedial part of the scapula.
III **Other Therapy:** Conservative treatment including exercise, passive stretching and voluntary elevation of the unaffected scapula have been used but appear to be of little value.

Prognosis: Life span and intelligence are normal. Functional disability is related to degree of scapula deformity and associated anomalies.

Detection of Carrier: —

†Special Considerations: Among those families showing autosomal dominant transmission, some demonstrate the scapula deformity alone in all affected members, while in other families the entire spectrum of associated anomalies (as listed under Clinical Findings) may be found with wide variation between affected members.

References:
Cavendish, M.E.: Congenital elevation of the scapula. J. Bone Joint Surg. 54B:395, 1972.
Chung, S.M. and Nissenbaum, M.M.: Congenital and developmental defects of the shoulder. Orthop. Clin. North Am. 6:381, 1975.
Wilson, M.G. et al: Dominant inheritance of Sprengel's deformity. J. Pediatr. 79:818, 1971.

Contributor: **William A. Horton**

Editor's Computerized Descriptors: Skel., Muscle

STEROID 11 β-HYDROXYLASE DEFICIENCY

Includes: Hyperplasie congénitale des surrénales par déficit en 11 β-hydroxylase
Angeborene Nebennieren-Hyperplasie 11β-Hydroxylase-Mangel
Hiperplasia suprarrenal congénita deficiencia de 11β-hidroxilasa
Adrenogenital syndrome with hypertension
Adrenal hyperplasia, congenital: 11β-hydroxylase deficiency

Excludes: Other enzyme deficiencies in adrenal steroid biosynthesis

Minimal Diagnostic Criteria: Progressive virilization, excessive 17-KS and 17-OHCS excretion, and markedly elevated concentration of Compound-S in plasma or urine which suppresses during glucocorticoid replacement.

Clinical Findings: This condition is characterized by progressive virilization, and all the sequelae of excessive androgen formation, including ambiguity of the external genitalia in genetic and gonadal females, as described for 21-hydroxylase deficiency. However, salt loss, hyponatremia and hyperkalemia do not occur; indeed, hypertension may occur but is not universally present, suggesting a spectrum in the severity of enzyme deficiency. The enzyme involved catalyzes the conversion of 11-deoxycortisol (Compound-S) to cortisol (Compound-F) in the glucocorticoid pathway, and deoxycorticosterone (DOC) to corticosterone (Compound-B) in the mineralocorticoid pathway. Consequently, the plasma concentrations of Compount-S and DOC are elevated, as are the respective urinary excretion products, whereas plasma and urinary cortisol and aldosterone may be diminished. Urinary excretion of 17-ketosteroids is elevated, reflecting excessive adrenal androgen production which is unaffected by the enzyme block and stimulated by excessive ACTH resulting from inadequate cortisol secretion. Urinary 17-hydroxycorticosteroids (17-OHCS) are also elevated since Compound-S and its urinary metabolite tetrahydro-S, both contain the 17, 21 dihydroxy, 20 keto grouping which reacts in the standard 17-OHCS measurements. Pregnanetriol excretion in urine may be modestly elevated.

Salt restriction is not associated with a rise in aldosterone, even after suppression of DOC by administered cortisol, suggesting that the same enzyme is involved in both glucocorticoid and mineralocorticoid pathways. Plasma renin levels are low. Mild cases may present in adult life and simulate the Stein-Leventhal syndrome.

Complications
I **Derived:** Ambiguity of the external genitalia may result in false gender allotment in genetic females; lack of electrolyte disturbances may delay the diagnosis in males. Progressive virilization, premature epiphyseal closure and final short stature, as well as preclusion of normal puberty and fertility may result from the untreated condition. Hypertension is a direct result of excessive production of DOC, a potent mineralocorticoid.
II **Associated:** Gynecomastia has been described in an affected male infant.

Etiology: Autosomal recessive; McK *20201

Pathogenesis: The enzyme block prevents the normal synthesis of cortisol, resulting in excessive ACTH stimulation and adrenal hyperplasia. The androgenic pathway is unaffected by the block; consequently production of dehydroepiandrosterone, androstenedione and testosterone is increased, producing virilization, rapid growth and accelerated bone maturation. DOC also is secreted in large quantities, resulting in salt and water retention, volume expansion and hypertension with low renin secretion. Both the enzymatic block and suppressed renin contribute to low aldosterone secretion.†

Related Facts

I **Sex Ratio:** M1:F1
II **Risk of Occurrence:** ?
III **Risk of Recurrence for**
   Patient's Sib: 1 in 4 (25%) for each offspring to be affected
   Patient's Child: Increased (1/2 times gene frequency in the population)
IV **Age of Detectability:** May be detected from birth to adult life.† Intrauterine diagnosis has not been demonstrated.
V **Prevalence:** ?

Treatment

I **Primary Prevention:** Genetic counseling
II **Secondary Prevention:** Replacement therapy with cortisol arrests virilization and restores blood pressure to normal. Intrauterine diagnosis has not been demonstrated but is theoretically feasible, as is intrauterine therapy with cortisol to minimize virilization.
III **Other Therapy:** Primary and definitive surgical repair may be required for ambiguous genitalia in genetic females.

Prognosis: The prognosis is normal for life span, reproduction and intelligence when diagnosed early and appropriate treatment is instituted.

Detection of Carrier: This has not been demonstrated, but theoretically might be attempted via levels of Compound-S achieved after ACTH stimulation.

†**Special Considerations:** A block in 11-hydroxylation may occur in some adrenocortical carcinomas, thus totally simulating the clinical features, and plasma and urinary steroid patterns observed with the congenital enzyme deficiency. However, under these circumstances glucocorticoid replacement will not suppress the oversecretion of the specific steroids. The possibility of carcinoma must always be considered in "late" presenting cases. Metapyrone (SU4885) is a drug which also blocks 11-hydroxylation; use is made of this agent in studying the intactness of the hypothalamic-pituitary-adrenal axis.

References:

Bongiovanni, A.M.: Disorders of adrenocortical steroid biogenesis. In Stanbury, J.B. et al (eds.): The Metabolic Basis of Inherited Disease, 3rd Ed. New York: McGraw-Hill, 1972, p. 857.

Frasier, S.D. et al: Androgen metabolism in congenital adrenal hyperplasia due to 11β-hydroxylase deficiency. Pediatrics 44:201, 1969.

Gabrilove, J.L. et al: Adrenocortical 11-β-hydroxylase deficiency with virilism first manifest in the adult woman. N. Engl. J. Med. 272:1189, 1965.

McLaren, N.K. et al: Gynecomastia with congenital virilizing adrenal hyperplasia (11-β-hydroxylase deficiency). J. Pediatr. 86:597, 1975.

New, M.I. and Seaman, M.P.: Secretion rates of cortisol and aldosterone precursors in various forms of congenital adrenal hyperplasia. J. Clin. Endocrinol. 30:361, 1970.

Contributor: **Mark A. Sperling**

Editor's Computerized Descriptors: Skel., CV., GU.

STEROID 17 α-HYDROXYLASE DEFICIENCY

Includes: Hyperplasie congénitale des surrénales par déficit en 17 α-hydroxylase
Angeborene Nebennieren-Hyperplasie 17α-Hydroxylase-Mangel
Hiperplasia suprarrenal congénita deficiencia de 17α-hidroxilasa
Hypertensive congenital adrenal hyperplasia
Adrenal hyperplasia, congenital: 17α-hydroxylase deficiency

Excludes: Glucocorticoid-responsive hyperaldosteronism
Other forms of congenital adrenal hyperplasia

Minimal Diagnostic Criteria: Diminished 17-hydroxylated steroids and sex steroids, hypertension, and lack of secondary sexual characteristics, in phenotypic females or males with ambiguous genitalia. Secretion of DOC is elevated but suppresses with administration of glucocorticoids. The cortisol response to ACTH and sex steroid hormone responses to chorionic gonadotropin are diminished or absent.

Clinical Findings: This disorder is characterized by hypertension and absence of secondary sexual characteristics. The enzyme defect prevents the formation of cortisol or any of its 17-hydroxylated precursors, as well as the formation of sex steroids, the latter defect apparently shared by the gonad. Mineralocorticoid formation is not affected.

In females, there is no ambiguity of the external genitalia at birth, but secondary sexual characteristics (breasts, pubic and axillary hair) fail to develop and primary amenorrhea may be the presenting complaint. Acute abdominal pain secondary to infarction of cystic enlarged ovaries has been reported in sibs. As could be expected from a defect interfering with adrenal and testicular androgen formation and thus male sexual differentiation, genotypic males have congenitally ambiguous genitalia. The penis is small or rudimentary, hypospadias is present, and the labia majora fail to fuse creating a shallow vagina. Cryptorchidism may be present.

Laboratory tests reveal hypokalemic alkalosis, low cortisol concentrations in plasma or 17-OHCS excretion in urine, and low-to-absent 17 ketosteroids, estrogens and testosterone. Plasma ACTH levels are elevated, and there is no response or a subnormal response in serum cortisol, or urinary 17-OHCS, or 17 KS following administration of ACTH. Similarly there is little or no gonadal response to administration of chorionic gonadotropin. Endogenous serum gonadotropin concentrations are high in older individuals. In contrast, circulating corticosterone (compound-B) and deoxycorticosterone (DOC) levels are elevated. Plasma renin is low, as is aldosterone, suggesting salt and water retention and volume expansion by DOC, with resultant suppression of the renin angiotensin/aldosterone pathway. This is confirmed by finding normal renin and aldosterone concentrations after suppressive doses of glucocorticoids. Partial defects with normokalemia have been described, but hypertension, diminished or absent sexual hair, and amenorrhea have been characteristic in all females, who consequently present in the mid-to-late teen years. In genetic males with the complete defect, the external genitalia will be entirely female and diagnosis can be delayed till puberty unless hypertension and hypokalemia are recognized. Males with the partial defect will be recognized earlier by virtue of ambiguity in the external genitalia.†

Complications

I **Derived:** Hypertension and hypokalemia result from excessive DOC secretion. Phenotypically normal female external genitalia in genetic males may result in false gender assignment. Impaired sexual development and fertility occur in both sexes.

II Associated: —

Etiology: Autosomal recessive; McK *20211

Pathogenesis: The clinical features and sequelae are a direct consequence of a defect in 17-hydroxylation affecting adrenal and gonadal steroidogenesis.

Related Facts

I **Sex Ratio:** M1:F1
II **Risk of Occurrence:** Not clearly delineated
III **Risk of Recurrence for**
    Patient's Sib: 1 in 4 (25%) for each offspring to be affected
    Patient's Child: ? Fertility impaired
IV **Age of Detectability:** May be detected from birth to adult life with the most frequent age of detection in the 2nd decade as a result of lack of pubertal development. Antenatal diagnosis has not yet been demonstrated.
V **Prevalence:** ?

Treatment

I **Primary Prevention:** Genetic counseling
II **Secondary Prevention:** Therapy with replacement doses of glucocorticoids returns blood pressure and serum potassium level to normal, and corrects inhibition of the renin/angiotensin/aldosterone pathway. Estrogen therapy in females and testosterone treatment in males brings about normal secondary sexual development.
III **Other Therapy:** Corrective surgery may be necessary in males with ambiguity of the external genitalia.

Prognosis: Normal for life span and intelligence, but fertility may be impaired.

Detection of Carrier: Hypertension and mild elevation of aldosterone partially supppressible by glucocorticoids were reported in the mother of an affected patient in whom the 17-hydroxylase defect seemed limited to the adrenal.

†Special Considerations: A defect in 17-hydroxylation has been found in an infant with a corticosterone secreting adrenal tumor nonsuppressible by glucocorticoids. Glucocorticoid-responsive hyperaldosteronism should and can be differentiated because 17-hydroxy corticosteroids and 17 ketosteroids are intermittently elevated.

References:
Bongiovanni, A.M.: Disorders of adrenocortical steroid biogenesis. In Stanbury, J.B. et al (eds.): The Metabolic Basis of Inherited Disease, 3rd Ed. New York: McGraw-Hill, 1972, p. 857.
DeLange, W.E. et al: Primary amenorrhea with hypertension due to 17-hydroxylase deficiency. Acta Med. Scand. 193:565, 1973.
New, M.I.: Male pseudohermaphroditism due to 17α-hydroxylase deficiency. J. Clin. Invest. 49:1930, 1970.
Weinstein, R.L. et al: Deficient 17-hydroxylation in a corticosterone producing adrenal tumor from an infant with hemihypertrophy and visceromegaly. J. Clin. Endocrinol. 30:457, 1970.

Contributor: **Mark A. Sperling**

Editor's Computerized Descriptors: Hair, CV., GU.

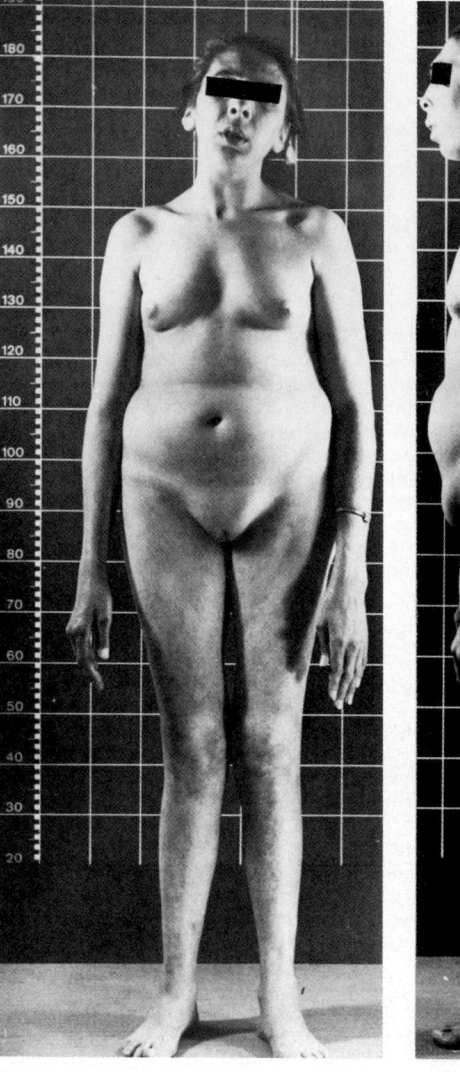
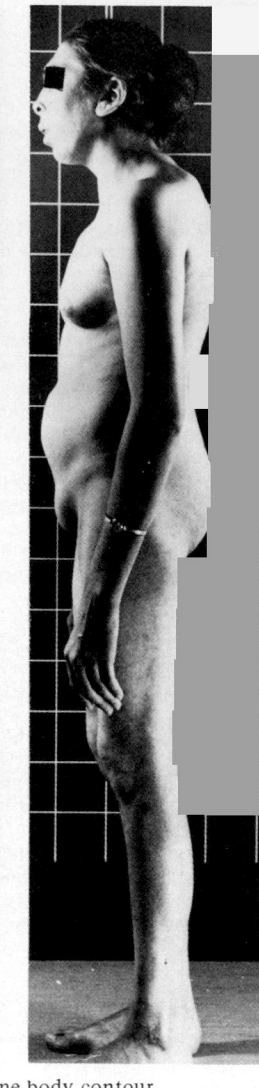

465. Note eunochoid appearance of feminine body contour

STEROID 17,20-DESMOLASE DEFICIENCY

Includes: Déficit en stéroïde 17-20-desmolase
17,20-Desmolase-Mangel
Deficiencia de 17 esteroide 20 desmolasa
Male pseudohermaphroditism due to steroid 17,20-desmolase deficiency

Excludes: Other enzymatic defects in testosterone biosynthesis
17-hydroxylase deficiency (903)
3β-hydroxysteroid dehydrogenase deficiency (909)
17-ketoreductase deficiency

Minimal Diagnostic Criteria: Low to absent 17-ketosteroids with no response to HCG or ACTH stimulation. Other steroids normal, adrenals and gonads present. Infant with ambiguous genitalia whose karyotype is 46,XY and demonstration of the inability of testicular tissue to convert precursors at the 17,20-desmolase step.

Clinical Findings: The hallmark of this syndrome is ambiguous genitalia in genetic males. Although long suspected, the condition has only recently been described in 1 family. The propositi were male cousins with ambiguous genitalia and XY karyotype. A maternal uncle had been reared as a female; karyotype was XY, testicles had been surgically removed, and a rudimentary uterus was present as well as 1 fallopian tube. Excretion of all androgens including dehydroepiandrosterone and testosterone was minimal or undetectable even after administration of human chorionic gonadotropin (HCG) at a dose of 5000 U/m^2 for 5 days. In contrast, secretion of glucocorticoids and mineralocorticoids was essentially normal. In vitro, testicular tissue from an affected patient readily converted 17-ketosteroids to testosterone, excluding 17-ketoreductase deficiency, but testosterone could not be formed from other precursors such as pregnenolone, progesterone, or their 17-hydroxylated equivalents. Thus, the defect appears to be at the 17,20-desmolase step. Infertility is to be expected in these individuals. Females with this condition have not been described, but would be expected to have normal internal and external genitalia and failure of pubertal development with infertility due to inability to form estrogen.

Complications
I **Derived:** —
II **Associated:** —

Etiology: A familial and probably autosomal recessive inherited disorder.

Pathogenesis: The clinical features are explicable on the basis of 17,20-desmolase deficiency affecting the adrenal and gonad. In 1 of the reported cases the testis also appeared to lack müllerian inhibiting substance, since a fallopian tube was present.†

Related Facts
I **Sex Ratio:** M1:F1 - probably, although only males have been reported.
II **Risk of Occurrence:** ?
III **Risk of Recurrence for**
  Patient's Sib: 1 in 4 (25%) for each offspring to be affected
  Patient's Child: Affected individuals are infertile.
IV **Age of Detectability:** Birth to adult life, males are likely to present in the perinatal period because of ambiguous genitalia; females will present because of lack of puberty.
V **Prevalence:** ?

Treatment
I **Primary Prevention:** Genetic counseling
II **Secondary Prevention:** In females, treatment with estrogen should permit sexual development but will not restore fertility. In males with severe ambiguity, plastic reconstruction of female external genitalia, removal of testes, and rearing in the female role would seem to be indicated, since construction of male genitalia and repair of hypospadias may be technically impossible. When ambiguity is less severe, plastic repair of external genitalia, and treatment with testosterone to bring about pubertal changes at the appropriate time are indicated.
III **Other Therapy:** —

Prognosis: Normal life span but fertility is severely impaired.

Detection of Carrier: Not possible

†**Special Considerations:** It is not clear why a fallopian tube should have been present, since müllerian-inhibiting substance produced by the fetal testis does not appear to be a steroid.

References:
Zachmann, M. et al: Testicular 17,20-desmolase deficiency causing male pseudohermaphroditism. Acta Endocrinol. (Suppl) (Kbh) 155:65, 1971.
Zachmann, M. et al: Steroid 17,20-desmolase deficiency: A new cause of male pseudohermaphroditism. Clin. Endocrinol. (Oxf) 1;369, 1972.

Contributor: **Mark A. Sperling**

Editor's Computerized Descriptor: GU.

Includes: Déficit de la 18-hydroxylase surrénalienne
18-Hydroxylase-Mangel
Deficiencia suprarrenal de 18-hidroxilasa
Hereditary hypoaldosteronism due to 18-oxidation defect
Familial aldosterone deficiency with enzyme defect
Adrenal 18-hydroxylase deficiency

Excludes: Steroid 18-hydroxysteroid dehydrogenase deficiency
(906)
Adrenal hypoaldosteronism of infancy, transient isolated (23)
Adrenal hypoplasia, congenital (24)
Angiotensin-unresponsive hypoaldosteronism

Minimal Diagnostic Criteria: Clinical features of hypoaldosteronism with no abnormalities in production of glucocorticoids and sex steroids, but overproduction of corticosterone and little or no 18-OH corticosterone.

Clinical Findings: These patients characteristically present in infancy with features of mineralocorticoid deficiency: dehydration, vomiting, failure to thrive, hyponatremia and hyperkalemia. The original report concerned 3 cousins from an inbred family-2 girls and 1 boy, all with normal external genitalia. There was no abnormal hyperpigmentation. Investigation revealed normal urinary excretion of 17-hydroxycorticosteroids and 17-ketosteroids with a normal response to stimulation by ACTH. Aldosterone excretion was undetectable and there was no response to ACTH or salt deprivation. However, urinary excretion of corticosterone and its metabolites was markedly increased, whereas only small amounts of 11-deoxycorticosterone (DOC) were detected even after ACTH stimulation, and 18-hydroxycorticosterone or its metabolites was absent. The defect therefore involves the 18-hydroxylation step from corticosterone to 18-OH corticosterone; the second to last step in aldosterone biosynthesis.† The adrenal gland of 1 affected patient showed a poorly developed zona glomerulosa and a hypertrophied juxtaglomerular apparatus. Despite the severe reduction in aldosterone synthesis, patients on a normal salt intake can maintain marginal sodium balance with serum sodiums of 120-130 mEq/1; salt deprivation is poorly tolerated. There is an excellent response to supplementation with salt and a mineralocorticoid. As with other defects involving aldosterone secretion there is an amelioration of the salt-losing tendency with increasing age so that electrolyte balance can be maintained by a high salt intake without addition of mineralocorticoid, although the basic biochemical defect persists. Milder forms of this entity also exist since hypoaldosteronism and increased excretion of corticosterone consistent with an 18-hydroxylase defect has been reported in young adults. The possibility that transient hypoaldosteronism of infancy represents a maturational delay in 18-hydroxylation has been separately discussed (see Adrenal Hypoaldosteronism of Infancy, Transient Isolated).

Complications
I   **Derived:** In newborns, death may result without replacement of fluid salt, and mineralocorticoid.
II **Associated:** —

Etiology: An autosomal recessively inherited enzyme defect is likely, in view of the fact that both males and females are affected and the reported parental consanguinity in affected families. McK *20340

Pathogenesis: The final 2 steps in aldosterone biosynthesis involve the hydroxylation of carbon 18 of corticosterone followed by oxidation (dehydrogenation) of the same carbon to produce aldosterone. Since cortisol and sex steroid synthesis is unaffected there is no elevation in ACTH or hyperpigmentation, and the external genitalia are normal. Although large quantities of corticosterone and some DOC are produced, they are weak mineralocorticoids relative to aldosterone. Hyponatremia, hyperkalemia, and volume depletion ensue, with an attempt to stimulate aldosterone via the renin-angiotensin system, thus accounting for renal juxtaglomerular hyperplasia. The reduced or absent 18-OH corticosterone with overproduction of corticosterone confirms the locus of the defect.

Related Facts
I   **Sex Ratio:** M1:F1
II   **Risk of Occurrence:** ?
III **Risk of Recurrence for**
     Patient's Sib: 1 in 4 (25%) for each offspring to be affected.
     Patient's Child: Not increased unless mate is carrier or homozygote.
IV   **Age of Detectability:** Usually in the newborn period or in the 1st year of life, but milder defects may be detected at any age.
V   **Prevalence:** ?

Treatment
I   **Primary Prevention:** Genetic counseling and screening of existing and future sibs.
II   **Secondary Prevention:** Treatment with salt supplementation and a mineralocorticoid such as DOC is necessary in the first few years of life. Later, patients appear able to maintain normal electrolyte balance by adjusting their sodium intake without mineralocorticoid supplements.
III **Other Therapy:** —

Prognosis: Excellent for life span, intelligence and reproduction if electrolyte disturbance is recognized and appropriately treated.

Detection of Carrier: Not reported

†Special Considerations: Hypoaldosteronism, with apparent selective inhibition of the 18-hydroxylation step has been reported after prolonged administration of heparin. In adults over 40 years of age with hypoaldosteronism and biochemical findings compatible with defective aldosterone synthesis, cardiovascular complications of hypokalemia have been a prominent presenting feature.

References:
Degenhart, H.J. et al: Further investigation of a new hereditary defect in the biosynthesis of aldosterone: Evidence for a defect in 18-hydroxylation of corticosterone. Acta Physiol. Pharmacol. Neerl. 14:1, 1966.
Jacobs, D.R. and Posner, J.B.: Isolated analdosteronism. Metabolism 13:522, 1964.
Visser, H.K.A.: Hypoadrenocorticism. In Gardner, L.I. (ed.): Endocrine and Genetic Diseases of Childhood. Philadelphia: W.B. Saunders, 1969, p. 442.
Wilson, I.D. and Goetz, F.C.: Selective hypoaldosteronism after prolonged heparin administration. Am. J. Med. 36:635, 1964.

Contributor: **Mark A. Sperling**

Editor's Computerized Descriptor: GI.

STEROID 18-HYDROXYSTEROID DEHYDROGENASE DEFICIENCY

Includes: Déficit de la 18-hydroxystéroïde-deshydrogénase surrénalienne
18-Hydroxysteroid-Dehydrogenase-Mangel
Deficiencia suprarrenal de 18-hidroxisteroide dehidrogenasa
Hereditary hypoaldosteronism due to 18-oxidation defect
Familial aldosterone deficiency with enzyme defect
Adrenal 18-hydroxysteroid dehydrogenase deficiency

Excludes: Steroid 18-hydroxylase deficiency (905)
Adrenal hypoaldosteronism of infancy, transient isolated (23)
Adrenal hypoplasia, congenital (24)
Angiotensin-unresponsive hypoaldosteronism

Minimal Diagnostic Criteria: Clinical features of hypoaldosteronism with elevated production of 18-hydroxycorticosterone and normal cortisol and sex steroids.

Clinical Findings: This defect is identical in its chemical findings to that caused by adrenal 18-hydroxylase deficiency. Growth failure with hyponatremia and hyperkalemia ameliorating with increasing age, and hypoaldosteronism are its hallmarks. The genitalia are normal, and the response to salt and mineralocorticoid supplementation is excellent.

Complications
I **Derived:** The degree of salt loss, and hyperkalemia will determine the extent of early complications.
II **Associated:** —

Etiology: Probably a recessively inherited disorder but X-linked inheritance cannot be excluded since only males have been reported.

Pathogenesis: Identical to that described for adrenal 18-hydroxylase deficiency except that the defect involves the final step in aldosterone biosynthesis. Biochemically, the defect involves the final oxidation (dehydrogenation) of 18-hydroxycorticosterone to aldosterone. Thus, the steroid patterns differ only in that production of 18-hydroxycorticosterone is increased but that of aldosterone remains low, despite stimuli such as ACTH.

Related Facts
I   **Sex Ratio:** Hitherto only affected males have been reported.
II **Risk of Occurrence:** ?
III **Risk of Recurrence for**
    Patient's Sib: When autosomal recessive or X-linked recessive, see Table I AR or X-linked R, respectively.
    Patient's Child: When autosomal recessive or X-linked recessive, see Table I AR or X-linked R, respectively.
IV **Age of Detectability:** Usually in the newborn period or in the 1st year of life but milder defects may be detected at any age.
V   **Prevalence:** ?

Treatment
I   **Primary Prevention:** Genetic counseling. Screening of existing and future sibs.
II **Secondary Prevention:** Treatment with salt supplementation and a mineralocorticoid such as DOC is necessary in the first few years of life. Later patients appear able to maintain normal electrolyte balance by adjusting their sodium intake without mineralocorticoid supplements.
III **Other Therapy:** —

Prognosis: Excellent if treatment with mineralocorticoid and salt is instituted.

Detection of Carrier: Not reported.

Special Considerations: —

References:
David, R. et al: Familial aldosterone deficiency: Enzyme defect, diagnosis and clinical course. Pediatrics 41:403, 1968.
Ulick, S. et al: Aldosterone biosynthetic defect in salt-losing disorder. J. Clin. Endocrinol. Metab. 24:669. 1964.
Visser. H.K.A.: Hypoadrenocorticism. In Gardner, L.I. (ed.): Endocrine and Genetic Diseases of Childhood. Philadelphia: W.B. Saunders, 1969, p. 442.

Contributor: **Mark A. Sperling**

Editor's Computerized Descriptor: GI.

STEROID 20-22 DESMOLASE DEFICIENCY

Includes: Hyperplasie congénitale des surrénales par déficit en 20-22 desmolase
Angeborene Nebennieren-Hyperplasie 20-22 Desmolase-Mangel
Hiperplasia suprarrenal congénita deficiencia de 20-22 desmolasa
Lipoid adrenal hyperplasia
Desmolase deficiency
Adrenal hyperplasia, congenital: 20-22 desmolase-deficiency

Excludes: Other forms of congenital adrenal hyperplasia

Minimal Diagnostic Criteria: Virtual absence of all steroids in urine or blood in patients with salt and water loss who may have ambiguity of the external genitalia. Definitive diagnosis is not feasible without performing stimulation tests with ACTH and HCG; both should be abnormal without a rise in pregnenolone. A presumptive diagnosis can be made if the adrenals show the characteristic histology.

Clinical Findings: This defect affects the critical initial reaction in the conversion of cholesterol to pregnenolone, a step involving cleavage of the cholesterol side chain from carbon 20 to carbon 22. The entire cleavage process, although termed a desmolase, may represent a series of enzyme reactions shared by the adrenal and gonad. Because of the early site in the assembly of all steroids, salt and water loss, and glucocorticoid insufficiency are universal findings. The external genitalia are normal in females but males may have ambiguity, supporting the contention that the gonad is affected and thus precluding masculinization during fetal life.

Laboratory investigation reveals virtual absence of urinary steroids, including pregnenolone and low secretion rates of cortisol and aldosterone. Extended survival is possible but death is frequent, despite seemingly adequate replacement with glucocorticoids, mineralocorticoids, and salt. At necropsy, the adrenals are markedly enlarged, and the cells are distended with cholesterol. Consanguinity is frequent in the parents of affected individuals.†

Complications
I **Derived:** Death is frequent even with adequate therapy.
II **Associated:** —

Etiology: Autosomal recessive; McK *20171

Pathogenesis: The clinical features are explicable from the site and severity of the enzyme block affecting the adrenal and gonad, and the deficiency of glucocorticoids, mineralocorticoids and sex steroids.

Related Facts
I **Sex Ratio:** M1:F1
II **Risk of Occurrence:** ? Rare
III **Risk of Recurrence for**
   Patient's Sib: 1 in 4 (25%) for each offspring to be affected
   Patient's Child: Surviving affected individuals will probably be infertile.
IV **Age of Detectability:** Most frequently detected in the newborn period because of salt loss or ambiguous genitalia. Antenatal diagnosis has not been demonstrated.
V **Prevalence:** ? Rare

Treatment
I **Primary Prevention:** Genetic counseling
II **Secondary Prevention:** Early recognition and replacement therapy with glucocorticoid, mineralocorticoid, and salt are essential for survival. Replacement therapy with estrogen or testosterone will be required to achieve secondary sexual characteristics in those reaching the age of puberty.†
III **Other Therapy:** In genetic males with severe ambiguity of the external genitalia closely resembling a female, plastic reconstruction to achieve male characteristics is, at best, difficult. Consideration should therefore be given to raising the individual as a female with appropriate surgical correction of the external genitalia.

Prognosis: Prognosis has been poor in severely affected individuals. Infertility is likely in those surviving to adult life.

Detection of Carrier: Has not been demonstrated

†Special Considerations: Aminoglutethimide, a toxic drug used rarely to inhibit steroidogenesis in adrenal carcinoma, acts by inhibiting the desmolase system and can experimentally simulate lipoid adrenal hyperplasia.

References:
Bongiovanni, A.M.: Disorders of adrenocortical steroid biogenesis. In Stanbury, J.B. et al (eds.): The Metabolic Basis of Inherited Disease, 3rd Ed. New York: McGraw-Hill, 1972, p. 857.
Camacho, A.M. et al: Congenital adrenal hyperplasia due to deficiency of one of the enzymes involved in biosynthesis of pregnenolone. J. Clin. Endocrinol. 28:153, 1968.
Moragas, A. and Ballabriga, A.: Congenital lipoid hyperplasia of the fetal adrenal gland. Helv. Paediatr. Acta 24:226, 1969.

Contributor: Mark A. Sperling

_____

Editor's Computerized Descriptor: —

STEROID 21-HYDROXYLASE DEFICIENCY

Includes: Hyperplasie congénitale des surrénales par déficit en 210hydroxylase
Angeborene Nebennieren-Hyperplasie 21-Hydroxylase-Mangel
Hiperplasia suprarrenal congénita deficiencia de 21-hidroxilasa
Adrenogenital syndrome: nonsalt-losing form, simple virilizing form, salt-losing form
Congenital virilizing adrenal hyperplasia
Female pseudohermaphroditism
Male pseudo-precocious puberty
Macrogenitosomia praecox
Adrenal hyperplasia, congenital: 21-hydroxylase deficiency

Excludes: Other enzyme deficiencies in adrenal steroidogenesis

Minimal Diagnostic Criteria: Elevated 17 KS and pregnanetriol excretion or markedly elevated plasma 17α-hydroxyprogesterone (50-450 times normal) and ACTH levels in patients with progressive virilization from birth. Abnormal steroid secretion must suppress following glucocorticoid administration.

Clinical Findings: This is the most common variant of congenital adrenal hyperplasia (CAH) resulting from a defect in the enzyme catalyzing the conversion of progesterone or 17α-hydroxy progesterone to deoxycorticosterone and 11-deoxycortisol, respectively; a step requiring hydroxylation of the carbon at the 21 position of the steroid nucleus. The androgen pathway is not blocked so that the fetus is exposed to excessive androgens from about the 3rd month of intrauterine life. Consequently, newborn females show variable degrees of masculinization of the external genitalia ranging from mild clitoral hypertrophy to complete labioscrotal fusion simulating a scrotum, male phallus with urethra opening at its tip, absence of palpable gonads within the "scrotal sac," and presence of a prostate. However, ovaries and a uterus are present and the chromosomal sex is female. Excessive skin pigmentation may be present around the genitalia or nipples reflecting increased ACTH (MSH). In newborn males no abnormality is apparent. However, progressive virilization occurs in both sexes resulting in rapid initial growth, accelerated bone age development with premature fusion of epiphyses and a final short stature, progressive clitoral or penile enlargement, early development of pubic and axillary hair, acne, hirsutism, voice changes, male habitus and male gender identification. Males have been referred to as an infant "Hercules." Untreated females fail to undergo pubertal changes due to suppression of gonadotropins by androgen excess. In males, this same mechanism prevents testicular enlargement, allowing differentiation from true precocious puberty secondary to ectopic or inappropriate pituitary gonadotropin secretion. However, rarely adrenal rests within the testes, subject to ACTH stimulation, may result in symmetric or nodular testicular enlargement and suggest precocious puberty or testicular neoplasia. In females with ambiguous genitalia the diagnosis is usually established in infancy or early childhood; occasional cases have been identified in the 2nd decade and as late as the 6th decade of life. Complete external virilization of newborn females may delay diagnosis and lead to false gender assignment with consequent psychologic sequelae.

Patients with partial or mild defects in 21-hydroxylase deficiency have normal serum electrolytes and may have normal levels of cortisol and aldosterone production, the latter rising with a low salt diet. The serum cortisol response to ACTH may be minimal indicating existing maximal stimulation by endogenous ACTH. Adrenal capacity is limited however, since many of these patients develop salt loss during stress or during diagnostic sodium restriction, with hyponatremia, hyperkalemia, vomiting, severe dehydration and vascular collapse.

Complete or severe 21-hydroxylase deficiency manifests early in the neonatal period with vomiting, renal salt loss, hyponatremia, hyperkalemia and dehydration. A misdiagnosis of pyloric stenosis may be made in newborn males; death of an older sib in infancy, particulary during stress, is often recorded. There is no direct correlation between the degree of virilization or external genital ambiguity and completeness of the 21-OH defect. However, plasma and urinary cortisol and its metabolites are decreased as is aldosterone; salt restriction is poorly tolerated and does not produce further increments in aldosterone secretion. The mild and severe forms may represent a spectrum of severity of a single enzyme deficiency; alternatively 2 separate enzyme deficiencies for the aldosterone and cortisol pathways have been proposed, as has the presence of factors promoting renal tubular salt loss.

Irrespective of clinical type, all affected patients have elevated urinary excretion of 17 ketosteroids and pregnanetriol, the excretory product of 17α-hydroxy progesterone. Plasma levels of these substances as well as testosterone, derived from peripheral conversion of androgen precursors, are elevated. Urinary 17 OHCS or plasma cortisol may be low or normal depending on the severity of the block.

Complications
I **Derived:** Lack of cortisol and aldosterone may result in hypoglycemia, severe electrolyte distrubances with dehydration and shock, particularly during stress. Ambiguity of genitalia may result in false gender assignment for genetic females. Progressive virilization, early epiphyseal closure with short stature, preclusion of normal pubertal changes, and infertility are direct sequelae of the untreated condition.
II **Associated:** Renal anomalies have been associated with this syndrome

Etiology: Autosomal recessive; McK *20191

Pathogenesis: The pathogenesis of all the features is explicable from the site and severity of the enzyme block, deficiency of cortisol or aldosterone, and oversecretion of androgens.

Related Facts
I **Sex Ratio:** M1:F1
II **Risk of Occurrence:** ?
III **Risk of Recurrence for**
    Patient's Sib: 1 in 4 (25%) for each offspring to be affected
    Patient's Child: Increased (1/2 times gene frequency in the population)
IV **Age of Detectability:** At birth. Successful antenatal detection has been reported.
V **Prevalence:** Varies on geographic locale from 1:500 in certain Eskimos, 1:5000 in Switzerland, 1:40,000 in the USA.

Treatment
I **Primary Prevention:** Genetic counseling
II **Secondary Prevention:** Replacement therapy with cortisol arrests the progressive virilization. A mineralocorticoid (DOC or 9α-fluorohydrocortisone), with additional salt intake may be necessary in the salt-losing form. Supplemental cortisol is necessary during acute stress. Antenatal diagnosis with cortisol injections into the amniotic fluid or fetus may minimize virilization.
III **Other Therapy:** Initial plastic surgical repair of ambiguous genitalia is achieved between the 1st-3rd years of life in order to permit appropriate gender identification and sex rearing. Definitive plastic repair can be achieved after puberty. Psychologic counseling may be required for parents and in late-diagnosed cases with ambiguous genitalia.†

Prognosis: Normal for life span, reproduction, and intelligence, when diagnosed early and appropriately treated.

Detection of Carrier: Urinary pregnanetriol excretion after ACTH infusion has been reported to be elevated in the parents of affected children when compared to controls. This test has not been commonly employed.

†Special Considerations: It is generally agreed that if diagnosis is missed for the first 3-4 years, a completely virilized female with penile urethra and apparent cryptorchidism be perpetuated in male rearing and identification.

References:

Bartter, F.C. et al: Aldosterone hypersecretion in "non-salt-losing" congenital adrenal hyperplasia. J. Clin. Invest. 47:1742, 1968.

Bongiovanni, A.M.: Disorders of adrenocortical steroid biogenesis. In Stanbury, J.B. et al (eds.): The Metabolic Basis of Inherited Disease, 3rd Ed. New York: McGraw-Hill, 1972, p. 857.

Childs, B. et al: Virilizing adrenal hyperplasia-a genetic and hormonal study. J. Clin. Invest. 35:213, 1956.

Lippe, B.M. et al: Serum 17-α-hydroxyprogesterone, progesterone, estradiol and testosterone in the diagnosis and management of congenital adrenal hyperplasia. J. Pediatr. 85:782, 1974.

Nichols, J. and Gibson, B.B.: Antenatal diagnosis of the adrenogenital syndrome. Lancet 2:1068, 1969.

Simpoulos, A.P. et al: Studies on the deficiency of 21-hydroxylation in patients with congenital adrenal hyperplasia. J. Clin. Endocrinol. Metab. 32:438, 1971.

Sperling, M.A. et al: Linear growth and growth hormonal responsiveness in treated congenital adrenal hyperplasia. Am. J. Dis. Child. 122:408, 1971.

Contributor: **Mark A. Sperling**

Editor's Computerized Descriptors: Speech, Skin, Hair, Skel., GU.

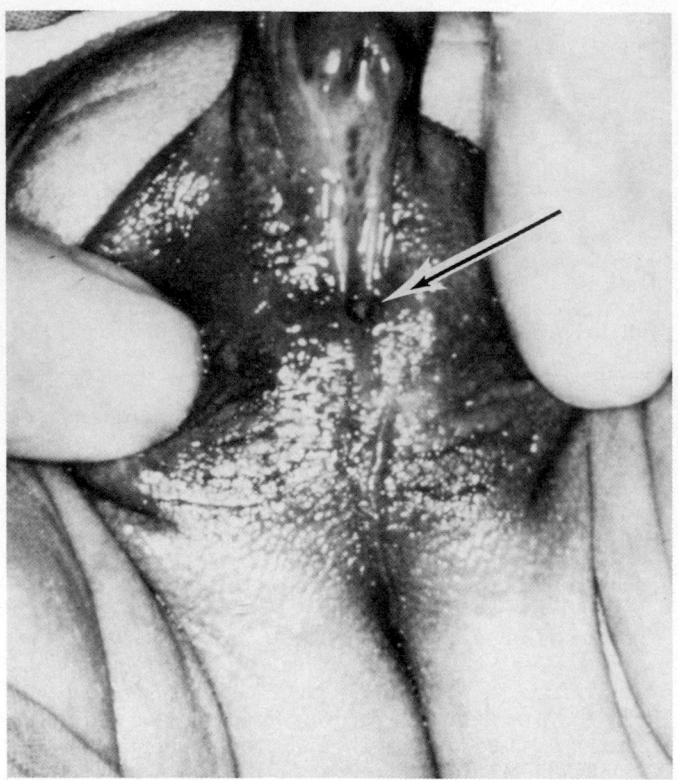

467. Genetic female with marked virilization of external genitalia

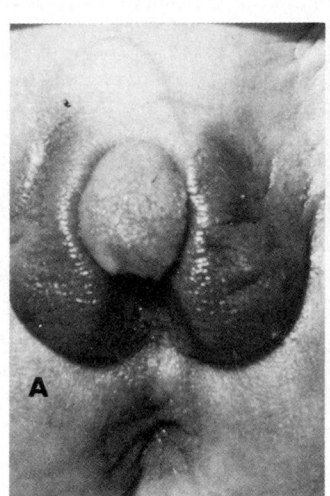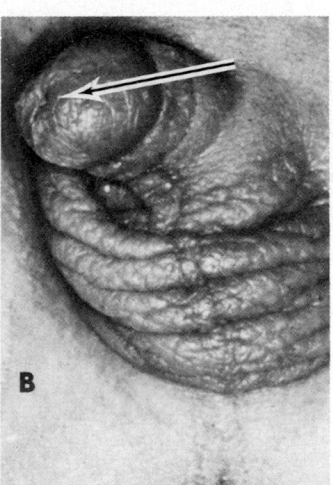

466. A) Moderate virilization of external genitalia; hyperpigmentation of labia. B) Complete virilization; urethral meatus (arrow) is located at tip of phallus

STEROID 3β-HYDROXYSTEROID DEHYDROGENASE DEFICIENCY

Includes: Hyperplasie congénitale des surrénales par déficit en 3 β-hydroxystéroïde-deshydrogénase

Angeborene Nebennieren-Hyperplasie: 3β-Hydroxysteroid-Dehydrogenase-Mangel

Hiperplasia suprarrenal congénita deficiencia de 3β-hidroxisteroide dehidrogenasa

3β-HSD deficiency

3β-Ol deficiency

3β-hydroxysteroid dehydrogenase and isomerase deficiency

Adrenal hyperplasia, congenital: 3β-hydroxysteroid dehydrogenase deficiency

Excludes: Other enzyme deficiencies in adrenal steroidogenesis

Minimal Diagnostic Criteria: Elevated 17 KS excretion, predominately DHEA or its derivatives, preponderance of δ5 urinary steroid compounds, mild virilization or under-masculinization, and suppression of abnormal steroids with exogenous glucocorticoids.

Clinical Findings: This is a rare form of congenital adrenal hyperplasia (CAH) in which the enzyme defect occurs early in adrenal steroidogenesis and affects the mineralocorticoid, glucocorticoid and sex steroid pathways. Thus, in severe enzyme deficiency, salt loss, hyponatremia, hyperkalemia, vomiting and dehydration are characteristic. In patients with partial defects, mineralocorticoid deficiency may not become apparent without stress, but hyponatremia becomes manifest during salt deprivation, particularly during withdrawal of supplemental glucocorticoids. Gradation in the severity of salt loss occurs even in affected sibs emphasizing the clinical heterogeneity in this syndrome, which has been diagnosed in a 40-year-old woman. The external genitalia show variable degrees of abnormality in both males and females; males have hypospadias, often perineal or 2nd degree in type, and a bifid scrotum with or without cryptorchidism; females have labial fusion, clitoral hypertrophy which is often mild, and mild but progressive hirsutism. This inadequate masculinization in males and mild virilization in females results from the accumulation and defective conversion of dehydroepiandrosterone (DHEA) a weak androgen, to androstenedione and subsequently testosterone. Laboratory tests reveal a high urinary excretion of 17 ketosteroids in which DHEA or its metabolites predominate. 17 OHCS and aldosterone excretion are typically low but may be normal in patients with partial defects, where plasma cortisol and cortisol production rates have been shown to be within the normal range. Pregnenolone and its derivatives (δ5-pregnenetriol; 16α-OH pregnenolone, 17α-OH pregnenolone) rather than pregnanolone derivatives (pregnanetriol) predominate in urine, reflecting the lack of enzyme isomerase activity required to shift the double bond from the C5-C6 position in the B-ring, to the C4-C5 position in the A ring of the steroid nucleus. The enzyme defect also occurs in the fetal testes (and ovary) and persists into later life, so that the response to exogenous (and presumably endogenous) gonadotropin is subnormal. However, in individuals with partial defects, there is evidence for increasing 3β-HSD activity with age, the enzyme activity being extra adrenal, and probably hepatic in origin. Consequently with increasing age, a large amount of pregnanetriol may appear in the urine, but does not represent the coexistence of a double enzyme defect in 3β-HSD and 21-OH activity. It is to be noted that in severe enzyme deficiency, 6 of the 7 initially reported cases died despite adequate glucocorticoid and salt replacement. The adrenal glands are hypertrophied and histologically appear to be laden with lipid.

Complications

I **Derived:** Salt loss, dehydration, hypoglycemia and death all may occur. Involvement of the gonads may preclude spontaneous puberty or fertility.

II **Associated:** —

Etiology: Autosomal recessive; McK *20181

Pathogenesis: The enzyme defect appears to affect the adrenals as well as the gonads. There is a difference in the timing of maximal enzyme activity in the testis and ovary. Thus 3β-HSD activity in the testes is maximal at about the 3rd intrauterine month, whereas in the ovaries and adrenal glands it becomes maximal at about the 4th month. Consequently, the abnormalities in male external genitalia are more severe.†

Related Facts

I **Sex Ratio:** M1:F1

II **Risk of Occurrence:** ?

III **Risk of Recurrence for**

Patient's Sib: 1 in 4 (25%) for each offspring to be affected

Patient's Child: Presumably increased (1/2 times gene frequency if fertility is normal)

IV **Age of Detectability:** May be detected from birth to adult life; most frequently in the first years of life, by virtue of salt loss with ambiguity of external genitalia. Antenatal diagnosis has not been demonstrated.

V **Prevalence:** ?

Treatment

I **Primary Prevention:** Genetic counseling

II **Secondary Prevention:** Treatment with glucocorticoid and mineralocorticoids should be instituted early, particularly in view of the reported high mortality in severly affected patients. Because the defect affects the gonads, replacement with sex steroids at puberty will be required.

III **Other Therapy:** Surgical correction of hypospadias or clitoromegaly may be required.

Prognosis: Normal for life in patients with partial defects; death has been reported in severely affected infants despite adequate replacement therapy. Reproductive function will be imparied.

Detection of Carrier: This has not been demonstrated.

†Special Considerations: An animal model of 3β-HSD deficiency has been produced in rats by the administration of a C-19 substrate analog to the mother. Partial prevention of hypospadias in affected male rats has been achieved by testosterone administration in utero, and prevention of the anatomic defect in affected female offspring by in utero administration of corticosterone. These studies confirm the pathogenesis of human disease.

References:

Axelrod, L.R. et al: Concurrent 3-beta-hydroxystéroid dehydrogenase deficiency in adrenal with sclerocystic ovary. Acta Endocrinol. 48:392, 1965.

Bongiovanni A.M.: The adrenogenital syndrome with deficiency of 3β-hydroxysteroid dehydrogenase. J. Clin. Invest. 41:2086, 1962.

Bongiovanni, A.M. et al: Urinary excretion of pregnanetriol and δ5-pregnenetriol in two forms of congenital adrenal hyperplasia. J. Clin. Invest. 50:2751, 1971.

Bongiovanni, A.M.: Disorders of adrenocortical steroid biogenesis. In Stanbury, J.B. et al (eds.): The Metabolic Basis of Inherited Disease, 3rd Ed. New York: McGraw-Hill, 1972, p. 857.

Goldman, A.S.: Experimental congenital adrenocortical hyperplasia: Persistent postnatal deficiency in activity of 3β-hydroxysteroid dehydrogenase produced in utero. J. Clin. Endocrinol. 27:1041, 1967.

Kenny, F.M. et al: Partial 3β-hydroxysteroid dehydrogenase (3β-HSD) deficiency in a family with congenital adrenal hyperplasia: Evidence for increasing 3β-HSD activity with age. Pediatrics 48:756, 1971.

Zachmann, M. et al: Unusual type of congenital adrenal hyperplasia probably due to deficiency of 3β-hydroxysteroid dehydrogenase. Case report of a surviving girl with steroid studies. J. Clin. Endocrinol. 30:719, 1970.

Contributor: **Mark A. Sperling**

Editor's Computerized Descriptors: Hair, GI., GU.

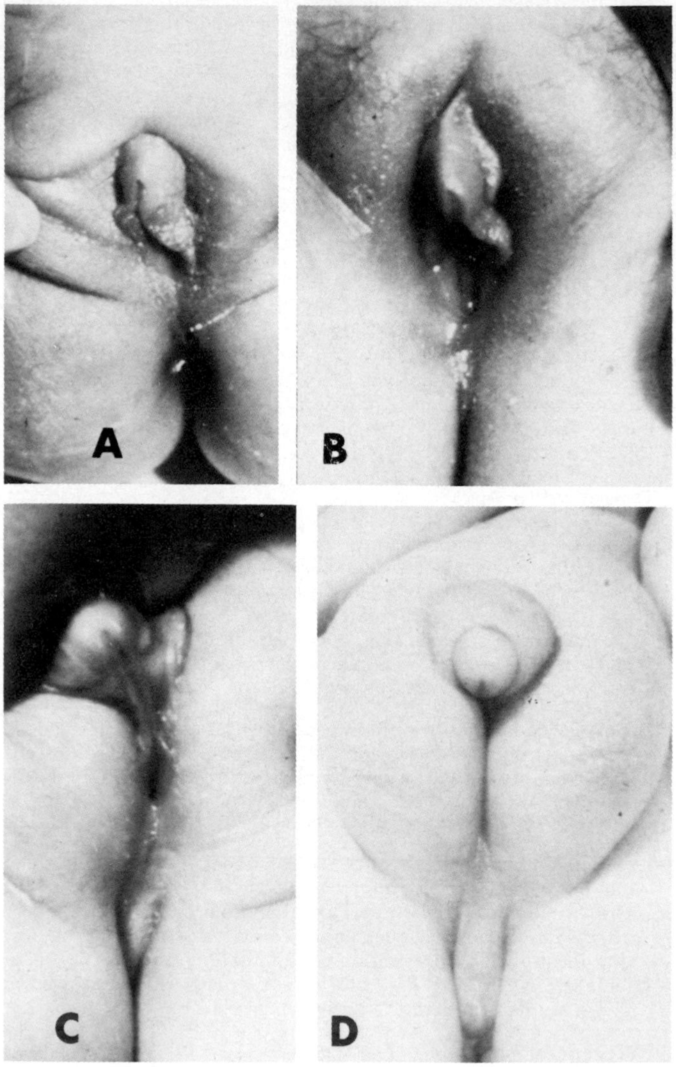

468. A & B) Note mild clitoral hypertrophy and pubic hair development in female. C& D) Bifid scrotum, severe hypospadias, and small phallus in male

910 **904-500**

STOMACH ATRESIA

Includes: Atrésie de l'estomac
Magenatresie
Atresia gástrica
Prepyloric atresia
Pyloric atresia
Antral atresia
Prepyloric membrane
Incomplete pyloric diaphragm
Congenital aplasia of pylorus
Fibromuscular atresia of antrum
Gastric atresia

Excludes: Duodenal atresia (supraampullary)
Pyloric stenosis (848)

Minimal Diagnostic Criteria: Nonbilious vomiting, roentgen identification of the pylorus as the site of obstruction or often identified only at time of surgery.

Clinical Findings: Nonbilious vomiting in a newly born infant with a scaphoid lower abdomen and a distended stomach. Maternal hydramnios common. Roentgen examination discloses only a large air-filled stomach with no second "bubble." Incomplete diaphragms can be identified only by upper GI series. In such infants partial obstruction produces clinical findings identical with pyloric stenosis but originating at birth.

Complications
I **Derived:** Hypokalemic alkalosis, dehydration, starvation
II **Associated:** Two of 29 reported cases had chromosome 21 trisomy.

Etiology: ?

Pathogenesis: ?

Related Facts
I **Sex Ratio:** M11:F15
II **Risk of Occurrence:** 1% of reported atresias
III **Risk of Recurrence for**
Patient's Sib: 2 instances of sibs among 29
Patient's Child: ?
IV **Age of Detectability:** At birth, clinically and radiologically.
V **Prevalence:** ?

Treatment
I **Primary Prevention:** —
II **Secondary Prevention:** Laparotomy, gastroduodenostomy, gastrojejunostomy, or excision of pyloric membrane have all been successful in relieving the obstruction.
III **Other Therapy:** —

Prognosis: 21 of 29 reported cases have survived surgical correction and presumably remain well.

Detection of Carrier: —

Special Considerations: —

References:
Bronsther, B. et al: Congenital pyloric atresia: A report of three cases and a review of the literature. Surgery 69:130, 1971.

Contributor: **William K. Sieber**

Editor's Computerized Descriptor: GI.

STOMACH DIVERTICULUM

Includes: Diverticule de l'estomac
Magendivertikulum
Divertículo gástrico congénito
Congenital gastric diverticulum

Excludes: Stomach duplication (912)
Gastric cysts

Minimal Diagnostic Criteria: Roentgen finding using contrast material

Clinical Findings: No characteristic clinical findings. Usually a radiologic diagnosis with outpouching from juxtacardiac posterior gastric wall involving all layers of gastric wall. This may occur near the pylorus in the presence of high small bowel obstruction probably as an acquired lesion.

Complications
I   **Derived:** Severe vomiting. In one instance, intussusception of the diverticulum resulted in gangrenous perforation and peritonitis.
II **Associated:** —

Etiology: ?

Pathogenesis: May originate as a duplication or secondary to pressure effects of pyloric or duodenal obstruction.

Related Facts
I   **Sex Ratio:** M?:F?
II   **Risk of Occurrence:** Very rare
III **Risk of Recurrence for**
     Patient's Sib: Small
     Patient's Child: Small
IV   **Age of Detectability:** At any age
V   **Prevalence:** Very rare

Treatment
I   **Primary Prevention:** —
II   **Secondary Prevention:** Surgical excision rarely indicated.
III **Other Therapy:** —

Prognosis: —

Detection of Carrier: —

Special Considerations: —

References:
Ogur, G.L. and Kolarsick, A.J.: Gastric diverticula in infancy. J. Pediatr. 39:723, 1951.

Contributor: **William K. Sieber**

Editor's Computerized Descriptor: GI.

STOMACH DUPLICATION

Includes: Duplication de l'estomac
Duplikation der Magen
Duplicación gástrica
Gastric enterocystoma
Reduplication of stomach
Cardioduodenal duct

Excludes: Mediastinal gastric cysts
Esophageal duplication (368)
Dorsal enteric remnants
Ectopic pancreas involving gastric wall
Vitelline remnants

Minimal Diagnostic Criteria: Palpable abdominal mass with roentgen evidence of origin from the gastric wall. Usually gastric origin can be established only at operation.

Clinical Findings: May present as an asymptomatic upper abdominal mass, a mass with vomiting or GI bleeding; may simulate pyloric stenosis (with symptoms beginning at birth and an easily palpable pyloric "tumor"), or may present as diffuse peritonitis due to rupture of the duplication. An abdominal mass is almost always palpable. Roentgen studies with contrast material sometimes clarify the diagnosis but usually demonstrate only pressure effects along the greater curvature and obstruction. These findings with depression of the splenic flexure are suggestive of gastric duplication.

Complications
I   **Derived:** Pyloric obstruction, rupture of duplication and resulting generalized peritonitis, sepsis and autodigestion with erosion into surrounding viscera may cause gastrocolic fistula and other bizarre fistulizations.
II **Associated:** Carcinomatous degeneration of the duplication

Etiology: ?

Pathogenesis: ?

Related Facts
I   **Sex Ratio:** M1:F8 in 1 series
II   **Risk of Occurrence:** Very rare
III **Risk of Recurrence for**
     Patient's Sib: ?
     Patient's Child: ?
IV   **Age of Detectability:** Neonate by physical examination but small cysts may be detected only if they become symptomatic in later life.
V   **Prevalence:** Only 55 cases in literature up to 1967

Treatment
I   **Primary Prevention:** —
II   **Secondary Prevention:** Laparotomy and surgical excision of the duplication and associated site of attachment to the normal gastric wall may require simple excision, subtotal, or even total gastrectomy. Internal drainage by anastomosis of cyst to the true gastric lumen has relieved symptoms.
III **Other Therapy:** —

Prognosis: When surgically removed, recovery results. Carcinoma has been reported in long-standing duplications.

Detection of Carrier: —

Special Considerations: —

References:
Brami, G.A. and Dennison, W.M.: Duplication of the stomach. Surgery 49:794, 1961.
Kammerer, G.T.: Duplication of the stomach resembling hypertrophic pyloric stenosis. JAMA 207:2101, 1969.
Kremer, R.M. et al: Duplication of the stomach. J. Pediatr. Surg. 5:360, 1970.

Contributor: **William K. Sieber**

STOMACH HYPOPLASIA

Includes: Hypoplasie gastrique
Hypoplasie der Magen
Hipoplasia gástrica
Microgastria

Excludes: —

Minimal Diagnostic Criteria: A roentgen diagnosis by upper GI examination with contrast material always associated with failure of rotation of the stomach without differentiation into fundus, body, and pyloric areas. The esophagus is usually dilated and takes over some storage function.

Clinical Findings: Vomiting, hematemesis, malnutrition, and secondary anemia are noted at birth and intensify.

Complications
I   **Derived:** Malnutrition
II **Associated:** —

Etiology: ?

Pathogenesis: ?

Related Facts
I   **Sex Ratio:** M?:F?
II   **Risk of Occurrence:** Very rare
III **Risk of Recurrence for**
       Patient's Sib: ?
       Patient's Child: ?
IV **Age of Detectability:** Usually as neonate, radiologically
V   **Prevalence:** Very rare

Treatment
I   **Primary Prevention:** —
II   **Secondary Prevention:** —
III **Other Therapy:** —

Prognosis: In a few followed cases, general poor health has been noted.

Detection of Carrier: —

Special Considerations: —

References:
Caffey, J.P.: Pediatric X-ray Diagnosis, 3rd Ed. Chicago:Year Book Medical Publishers, 1956, p. 496.

Contributor: **William K. Sieber**

Editor's Computerized Descriptor: GI.

STOMACH TERATOMA

Includes: Tératome gastrique
Teratom der Magen
Teratoma gástrico
Gastric teratoma
Tridermal gastric teratoma
Tridermic teratoma of stomach
Dermoid cyst of stomach

Excludes: —

Minimal Diagnostic Criteria: Large upper abdominal mass with calcification suggests diagnosis. Confirmed only by gross and microscopic pathology.

Clinical Findings: Abdominal mass. GI bleeding sometimes present (3 of 17 cases). Roentgen studies characteristically show areas of calcification in large bulky tumors that may cause gastric obstruction. Secondary to pressure of the large abdominal mass, respiratory difficulty and intestinal obstruction may be present.

Complications
I Derived: —
II Associated: —

Etiology: ?

Pathogenesis: ?

Related Facts
I Sex Ratio: M1:F0
II Risk of Occurrence: Rare
III Risk of Recurrence for
  Patient's Sib: Small
  Patient's Child: Small
IV Age of Detectability: Usually at birth or infancy
V Prevalence: Only 17 recorded cases

Treatment
I Primary Prevention: —
II Secondary Prevention: Surgical excision of the tumor by partial or total gastrectomy.
III Other Therapy: —

Prognosis: Fifteen of 16 patients are well following surgical resection of the tumor.

Detection of Carrier: —

Special Considerations: —

References:
DeAngelis, V.R.: Gastric teratoma in a newborn infant: Total gastrectomy with survival. Surgery 66:794, 1969.

Contributor: **William K. Sieber**

Editor's Computerized Descriptors: Resp., GI.

STURGE-WEBER SYNDROME

Includes: Maladie de Sturge-Weber
Mb. Sturge-Weber
Enfermedad de Sturge-Weber
Encephalofacial angiomatosis
Meningeal capillary angiomatosis
Encephalotrigeminal angiomatosis

Excludes: Neurofibromatosis (712)
Tuberous sclerosis (975)
von Hippel-Lindau syndrome (995)

Minimal Diagnostic Criteria: Facial angioma and intracranial anomaly as demonstrated by ECG and skull xray.

Clinical Findings: Cavernous angioma over the first or all of the 3 divisions of the 5th cranial nerve, always present at birth. There may be glaucoma on the side of the angioma due to the outflow occlusion of the angle. Generalized seizures beginning at age 1-2 years. Intracranial calcifications do not appear until after 2 years of age. Skull size smaller on site of abnormality.

Complications
I Derived: Seizures, mental retardation
II Associated: Progressive neurologic deficit

Etiology: ?

Pathogenesis: The intracranial calcifications are not in blood vessel walls but in the 2nd and 3rd layers of cortex due to tissue anoxia. The homolateral eye may be enlarged because of congenital glaucoma (buphthalmos). The iris of such an eye may remain blue, although the normal eye is brown, due to angiomatosis of choroid. Hemiplegia present in many cases opposite the side of the nevus. Hemianopia frequently present if child can be tested. Alternate explanation for calcification is transudation of protein through abnormal vessels and calcium binding. Degeneration of neurons and gliosis follows.

Related Facts
I Sex Ratio: ?
II Risk of Occurrence: ?
III Risk of Recurrence for
  Patient's Sib: ?
  Patient's Child: ?
IV Age of Detectability: At birth for facial lesion; in seizure work-up 50% detected before 1 year of age.
V Prevalence: ?

Treatment
I Primary Prevention: —
II Secondary Prevention: ?
III Other Therapy: In uncontrolled seizure states cortical resection or hemispherectomy is indicated. Results of this therapy are reasonably good.

Prognosis: If seizures become frequent, mental retardation occurs. Normal development may occur in slowly progressive patients or those without major CNS involvement.

Detection of Carrier: ?

Special Considerations: —

References:
Hendrick, E. B. et al: Hemispherectomy in children. Clin. Neurosurg. 16:315, 1969.
Weber, F.P.: Notes on association of extensive haemangiomatous naevus of skin with cerebral (meningeal) haemangioma, especially cases of facial vascular naevus with contralateral hemiplegia. Proc. R. Soc. Med. 22:25, 1929.

Contributor: **Kenneth Shulman**

Editor's Computerized Descriptors: Eye, Skin, Skel., Nerve

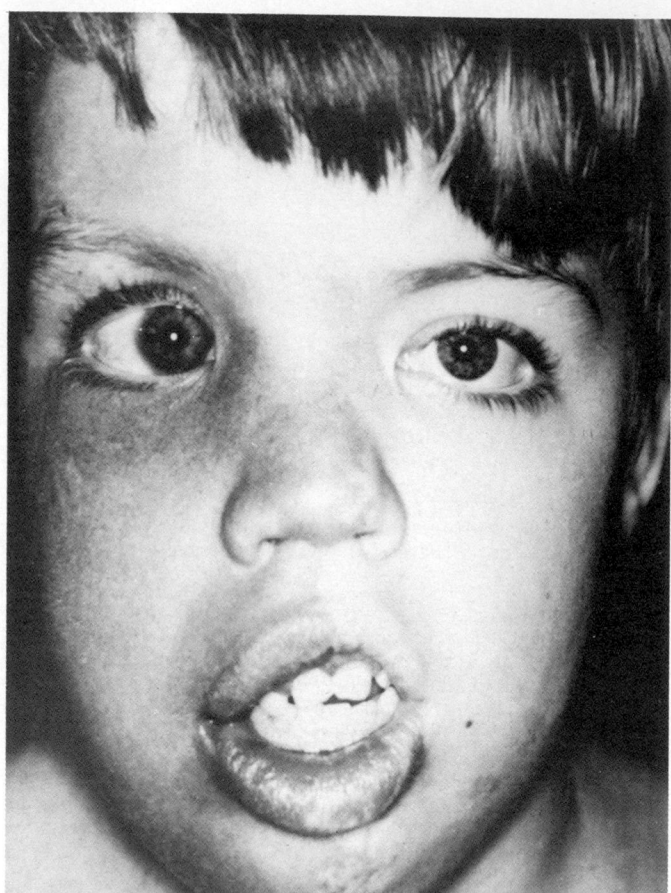

469. Sturge–Weber syndrome. Note unilateral angiomatosis and buphthalmos

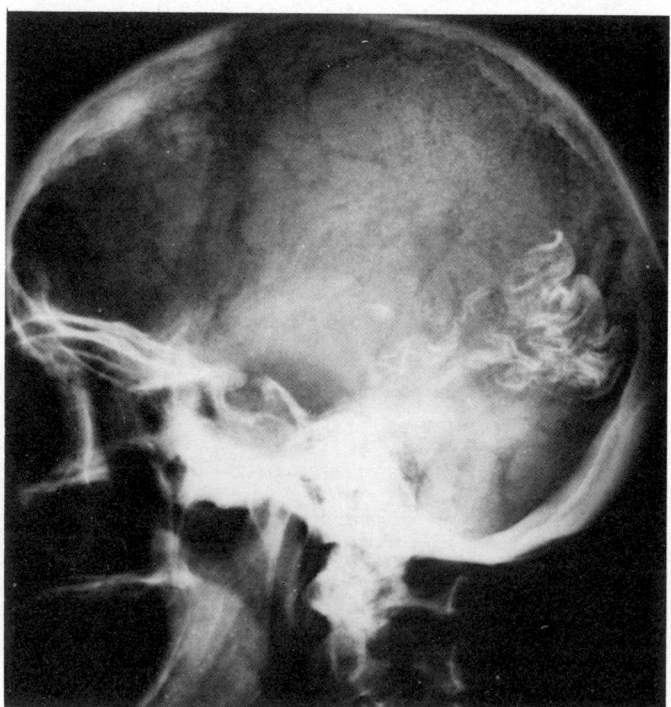

470. Intracranial calcifications of double contour "gyriform" or railroad track configuration characteristic of Sturge–Weber syndrome

SUBAORTIC STENOSIS, FIBROUS

Includes: Sténose fibreuse sous-aortique
Fibrose Subaortenstenose
Estenosis fibrosa subaórtica
Discrete subaortic stenosis
Fibromuscular subaortic stenosis
Membranous subaortic stenosis
Fibrous subaortic stenosis

Excludes: Subaortic stenosis, muscular (917)

Minimal Diagnostic Criteria: Identification, at left heart catheterization, of a pressure gradient between the left ventricular cavity and the aorta during systole that is localized to the subaortic area of the left ventricular outflow tract.

Left ventricular angiocardiography identifies the discrete area of subvalvar stenosis.

Clinical Findings: The anatomic lesion consists of a membranous diaphragm or fibrous ring encircling the left ventricular outflow tract just beneath the base of the aortic valve. The clinical differentiation between stenosis of the aortic valve and fibrous subaortic stenosis is extremely difficult and there are no clinical criteria which can be relied upon to distinguish the 2 forms of obstruction. Such differences in the clinical findings as do exist are of limited diagnostic help. Nevertheless, in the discrete form of subvalvar or fibrous subaortic stenosis, a systolic ejection sound is rarely heard and the diastolic murmur of aortic regurgitation is more common than it is in valvar aortic stenosis. Also, valvar calcification is not observed roentgenographically, even in adult patients with discrete subaortic stenosis. Dilatation of the ascending aorta is common in patients with discrete subvalvar obstruction but is usually less prominent than in patients with valvar stenosis.

Echocardiography may prove to be useful in the distinction of valvar and subvalvar stenosis. The finding by single crystal methods of a fine, high intensity echo in the left ventricular outflow tract may suggest the presence of a subaortic diaphragm. Multiple, thick echoes from a level near the annular attachment of the anterior mitral leaflet and below the sinuses of Valsalva have been observed with fibromuscular subaortic obstruction. Cross-sectional echo studies reveal persistent, prominent echoes in the subaortic left ventricle in both systole and diastole. Echocardiography also has the potential for identifying hypertrophic subaortic stenosis when it coexists with fixed subaortic stenosis and for distinguishing between the 2 forms of obstruction.

Definitive differentiation between valvar and subvalvar obstruction is best accomplished by recording pressure tracings as a catheter is withdrawn across the outflow tract and valve or by localizing the site of obstruction with selective left ventricular angiocardiography. Even then it may be difficult. Mild degrees of aortic valvar regurgitation are often observed in patients with fibrous subaortic stenosis, and are probably caused by thickening of the valve and impaired mobility of the cusps secondary to the trauma created by the high velocity jet passing through the subaortic diaphragm. Severe aortic regurgitation may result when these abnormal valve cusps are further deformed by the vegetations of bacterial endocarditis.

Complications
I **Derived:** Aortic valve insufficiency, bacterial endocarditis, congestive heart failure, syncope, arrhythmias, sudden death.
II **Associated:** Occasionally, valvar and subvalvar aortic stenosis coexist in the same patient producing a tunnel-like nar-

rowing of the left ventricular outflow tract.

Etiology: Presumably multifactorial inheritance

Pathogenesis: ?

Related Facts
I   **Sex Ratio:** M2:F1
II **Risk of Occurrence:** Unknown, but probably < 1 in 10,000 live births
III **Risk of Recurrence for**
    Patient's Sib: Unknown but probably under 2%
    Patient's Child: Unknown but probably under 2%
IV **Age of Detectability:** From birth by left heart catheterization and selective left ventricular angiocardiography
V   **Prevalence:** ?

Treatment
I   **Primary Prevention:** —
II **Secondary Prevention:** Surgical correction consists of excising the membrane or fibrous ridge. This may be expected to improve the hemodynamic state substantially and frequently may be totally corrective. In a small fraction of patients, secondary muscular hypertrophy of the outflow tract and a subaortic pressure gradient may persist following the operative relief of valvar or discrete subvalvar aortic stenosis. Ultimately, however, this form of outflow obstruction generally resolves as the secondary hypertrophy regresses.
III **Other Therapy:** —

Prognosis: The prognosis depends upon the severity of obstruction. Bacterial endocarditis or chronic trauma to the aortic valve leaflets may result in severe aortic regurgitation which may become the predominant hemodynamic lesion. In these instances, the risk of surgical correction is increased since the replacement of the aortic valve with a prosthesis may be necessary.

Detection of Carrier: —

Special Considerations: —

References:
Braunwald, E. et al: Congenital aortic stenosis. I. Clinical and hemodynamic findings in 100 patients. Circulation 27:426, 1963.
Davis, R.H. et al: Echocardiographic manifestations of discrete subaortic stenosis. Am. J. Cardiol. 33:277, 1974.
Edwards, J.E.: Congenital malformations of the heart and great vessels. In Gould, S.E. (ed.): Pathology of the Heart and Blood Vessels, 3rd Ed. Springfield: Charles C Thomas, 1968, p. 262.
Friedman, W.F. and Braunwald, E.: Congenital aortic stenosis. In Moss, A.J. and Adams, F.H. (eds.): Heart Disease in Infants, Children and Adolescents. Baltimore: Williams & Wilkins Co., 1968, p. 358.
Popp, R.L. et al: Echocardiographic findings in discrete subvalvular aortic stenosis. Circulation 49:226, 1974.
Williams, D.E. et al: Cross-sectional echocardiographic localization of the site of left ventricular outflow tract obstruction. Am. J. Cardiol. 37(2):250, 1976.

Contributors: **William F. Friedman**
Stanley E. Kirkpatrick

Editor's Computerized Descriptor: CV.

SUBAORTIC STENOSIS, MUSCULAR

Includes: Sténose sous-aortique
Muskuläre Subaortenstenose
Estenosis muscular subaórtica
Idiopathic hypertrophic subaortic stenosis
Hypertrophic obstructive cardiomyopathy
Functional obstruction of left ventricle
Pseudoaortic stenosis
Asymmetric septal hypertrophy with obstruction
Muscular subaortic stenosis

Excludes: Subaortic stenosis, fibrous (916)
Subaortic muscular hypertrophy of type II glycogen storage disease

Minimal Diagnostic Criteria: While the diagnosis may be suspected by clinical and ECG findings, nevertheless, hemodynamic and angiographic studies during left heart catheterization are required to exclude patients with cardiomyopathies other than muscular subaortic stenosis and patients with the discrete form of fibrous subaortic stenosis. A systolic intraventricular pressure gradient, either in the basal state or during provocation with isoproterenol, the Valsalva maneuver, or nitroglycerine can be demonstrated. Selective left ventricular angiography shows impingement in systole of the closed anterior leaflet of the mitral valve on the hypertrophied interventricular septum.

Clinical Findings: The disease is characterized by marked hypertrophy of the left ventricle involving especially the ventricular septum and left ventricular outflow tract. The most important landmark in the understanding of muscular subaortic stenosis was the observations, both angiographically and echocardiographically, that abnormal systolic anterior movement of the mitral valve in proximity or contact with asymmetrically hypertrophied septum created the systolic pressure gradient. The principal determinants of the severity of obstruction are the force of LV contraction, the size of the cavity during systole and the transmural pressure which distends the outflow tract during systole. Since these factors are variable, the degree of obstruction may change from moment to moment.

The discovery of a heart murmur is usually the first clinical manifestation of muscular subaortic stenosis. The most common symptoms are easy fatigability, dyspnea, palpitations, angina, dizziness and syncope. Physical findings include cardiomegaly and a left ventricular lift, often with a double or triple apical impulse. Accentuation of the atrial contraction (A) wave may be noted in the jugular venous pulse. A prominent finding is a bifid carotid pulse with a rapid upstroke. Paradoxical splitting of the second heart sound and a fourth heart sound may be present. A midsystolic ejection type murmur is always present; occasionally, the regurgitant murmur of mitral incompetence is audible.

The ECG is usually abnormal. These abnormalities include left ventricular hypertrophy with abnormally deep and broad Q waves related to gross septal hypertrophy and Wolff-Parkinson-White pattern. Radiologically, an enlarged, globular left ventricle is seen. Aortic dilatation is an uncommon finding. Evidence of right ventricular enlargement is seen in approximately half the patients.

Numerous publications exist describing the echocardiographic features of idiopathic hypertrophic subaortic stenosis. The major abnormal finding is mitral valve systolic anterior motion apposing the mitral leaflet to the thickened septum and apparently producing the subaortic obstruction during ejection. Asymmetric septal hypertrophy, ie a septum which is greater than 1.3 times thicker than the posterior left ventricular wall, is routinely demonstrated echocardiographically. Asymmetric septal hypertrophy, without abnormal motion of the mitral valve, is present in patients with the asymptomatic or nonobstructive form of this cardiomyopathy. The disease complex appears to be inherited as an autosomal dominant trait. It should be cautioned that many normal newborns, as well as patients with right ventricular outflow tract obstruction, sometimes have asymmetric septal hypertrophy.

At left heart catheterization, the obstruction can be localized to the left ventricular outflow tract by the demonstration of a pressure gradient between the left ventricular cavity and the subvalvar area. The zone of elevated pressure extends from the ventricular apex to the leaflets of the mitral valve. Variation of the magnitude of the systolic pressure gradient may occur in the course of a single hemodynamic study and distinguishes muscular subaortic stenosis from other forms of left ventricular obstruction. Analysis of the postextrasystolic pulse pressure response is a useful diagnostic test in these patients. In normal patients and in those with fixed forms of aortic stenosis the arterial pulse pressure in the cycle following a premature ventricular contraction is greater than normal. In patients with muscular subaortic stenosis, the postextrasystolic augmentation of the force of left ventricular contraction intensifies the obstruction and the arterial pulse pressure, following a premature ventricular contraction, does not exceed the pulse pressure of the control beat. A pressure gradient may be induced or intensified in these patients by isoproterenol infusion and the Valsalva maneuver. Angiographically, the site of obstruction can be seen as a radiolucent line in the frontal view representing contact of the leading edge of the anterior leaflet of the mitral valve with the hypertrophied muscular ventricular septum. In the left anterior oblique and lateral projections, the mitral leaflets do not swing posteriorly in a normal fashion but project into the outflow tract during mid and late systole.

Complications

I **Derived:** Approximately 10% of patients with muscular subaortic stenosis have a systolic pressure gradient in excess of 10 mm Hg in the outflow tract of the right ventricle. In an occasional patient, the obstruction to right ventricular outflow is more severe than on the left. Progressive clinical deterioration with the onset of angina pectoris, syncope or symptoms of congestive heart failure may occur. Arrhythmias are the most common cause of sudden, unexpected death. Bacterial endocarditis is a rare complication.

II **Associated:** Infrequently, muscular subaortic stenosis is associated with other congenital cardiovascular anomalies such as coarctation of the aorta, ventricular septal defect and a patent ductus arteriosus.

Etiology: Most recently, it has been suggested that muscular subaortic stenosis represents only 1 part of the spectrum of disease in which outflow tract obstruction may be severe, mild, or even absent. Thus, asymmetric septal hypertrophy (ASH) is now considered the characteristic anatomic abnormality that can be detected reliably and easily by either noninvasive or invasive diagnostic techniques. Conventionally, ASH is defined echocardiographically by a disproportionately thickened ventricular septum when compared to the postero-basal left ventricular free wall thickness. The current expanded clinical concept of the ASH disease spectrum includes many more patients with nonobstructive ASH than those with ASH and left ventricular outflow tract obstruction (typical muscular subaortic stenosis). The spectrum of ASH embraces 3 clinical subgroups of patients: 1) those who have no obstruction either at rest or after provocative maneuvers; 2) patients who develop obstruction after provocative maneuvers; and 3) patients who have obstruction to left ventricular outflow under resting conditions (classic muscular subaortic stenosis). It appears preferable that muscular subaortic stenosis not be considered as a clinical or physiologic entity, but rather as a form of cardiomyopathy characterized principally by asymmetric septal hypertrophy.

Family studies using echocardiography to detect disproportionate ventricular septal thickening have revealed that ASH is transmitted genetically as an autosomal dominant trait with a high degree of penetrance that occurs in an equal percentage in both sexes in preclinical and clinical forms. All clinical subtypes of the disorder may be observed in any 1 family. McK *19260

Chromosomal studies are unremarkable. In approximately one-third of patients, there is an impressive family history.

Pathogenesis: ?

Related Facts
I **Sex Ratio:** M1:F1
II **Risk of Occurrence:** Unknown but less than 0.1 in 1000 live births (less than 1% of CHD). Probably somewhat more common than discrete forms of subaortic obstruction
III **Risk of Recurrence for**
  Patient's Sib: Approaches 1 in 2
  Patient's Child: Approaches 1 in 2
IV **Age of Detectability:** From birth by echocardiography and left heart catheterization and selective left ventricular angiocardiography.
V **Prevalence:** ?

Treatment
I **Primary Prevention:** Genetic counseling, when the lesion occurs in familial aggregates
II **Secondary Prevention:** Beta adrenergic blocking agents may temporarily alleviate symptoms in some patients. Digitalis is thought by some to be contraindicated. Left ventricular myotomy, with or without resection of a portion of the hypertrophied interventricular septum, may be expected to abolish or reduce the pressure gradient and may strikingly ameliorate symptoms in the great majority of patients who are severely disabled by their disease. However, the primary myocardial disease process is not amenable to surgical correction.
III **Other Therapy:** —

Prognosis: The course in patients with muscular subaortic stenosis is extremely variable. Despite this variability, patients who are asymptomatic tend to remain so while those who are disabled at initial detection, generally deteriorate or die. Familial cases may have a higher incidence of sudden death.

Detection of Carrier: —

Special Considerations: —

References:
Abbasi, A.S. et al: Echocardiographic diagnosis of idiopathic hypertrophic cardiomyopathy without outflow obstruction. Circulation 46:897, 1972.
Clark, C.E. et al: Familial prevalence and genetic transmission of idiopathic hypertrophic subaortic stenosis. N. Engl. J. Med 289:709, 1973.
Epstein, S.E. et al: Asymmetric septal hypertrophy. Ann. Intern. Med. 81:650, 1974.
Frank, S. and Braunwald, E.: Idiopathic hypertrophic subaortic stenosis: Clincial analysis of 126 patients with emphasis on the natural history. Circulation 37:759, 1968.
Henry, W.L. et al: Asymmetric septal hypertrophy (ASH): The unifying link in the IHSS disease spectrum. Observations regarding its pathogenesis, pathophysiology and course. Circulation 47:827, 1973.

Henry, W.L. et al: Echocardiographic measurement of the left ventricular outflow gradient in idiopathic hypertrophic subaortic stenosis. N. Engl. J. Med. 88:989, 1973.

Larter, W.L. et al: The asymmetrically hypertrophied septum; further differentiation of its causes. Circulation 53:9, 1976.

Contributors: **William F. Friedman**
Stanley E. Kirkpatrick

Editor's Computerized Descriptor: CV.

SUBGLOTTIC HEMANGIOMA

Includes: Hémangiome sous-glottique
Subglottischer Hämangiom
Hemangioma subglótico
Hemangioma, subglottic

Excludes: —

Minimal Diagnostic Criteria: The clinical history and typical endoscopic appearance are considered sufficiently diagnostic for therapy without biopsy confirmation.

Clinical Findings: Because these hemangiomas are located subglottically these infants typically present with a history of dyspnea and inspiratory stridor which may become biphasic, yet the cry and voice remain clear. The fluctuating character of the respiratory distress, varying from day to day or even hour to hour, particularly with crying or exertion, is considered strongly diagnostic. The absence of marked temperature elevation, leukocytosis and pharyngeal inflammation distinguish this disease from tracheobronchitis. Dermal hemangioma, particularly of the head and neck, should prompt immediate suspicion of a similar lesion in the subglottis in any child with respiratory distress; however about half of these patients will have no external hemangioma.†

Soft tissue roentgenograms of the neck are generally nonspecific, although larger lesions may be seen on lateral views. Barium swallow may show posterior displacement of the esophagus from the air column in the subglottic area. Laryngoscopy and bronchoscopy allow visualization of the hemangioma which usually appears as a sessile mass between the true vocal cord and the lower limit of the cricoid cartilage. The color varies from pink to blue depending on the lesion's vascularity and relative depth beneath the mucosa. These hemangiomas are readily compressible, differentiating them from other tumors of the larynx. Biopsy is generally condemned as unnecessary and dangerous as hemorrhage may be very difficult to control.

Complications
I **Derived:** Acute respiratory failure or "sudden death" in about half of cases in a recent collective review of the literature.
II **Associated:** Failure to gain weight, a characteristic of chronic respiratory obstruction.

Etiology: ?

Pathogenesis: Usually a cavernous hemangioma with mature endothelium presenting on only 1 side of the subglottic area, but may circumscribe the entire lumen.

Related Facts
I **Sex Ratio:** M1:F2.
II **Risk of Occurrence:** ?†
III **Risk of Recurrence for**
   Patient's Sib: ?
   Patient's Child: ?
IV **Age of Detectability:** Usually asymptomatic at birth, however, over 90% will develop symptoms before age 3 months.
V **Prevalence:** ?

Treatment
I **Primary Prevention:** —
II **Secondary Prevention:** Systemic steroids have produced dramatic regression of tumors in 2 to 4 weeks and recurrence has been controlled by a 2nd course of steroids. Excision of the tumor by laryngofissure is reserved for those tumors requiring tracheostomy that have not regressed after 1 or 2 years.
III **Other Therapy:** Tracheostomy is necessary with moderate-

to-severe respiratory distress. Low dose irradiation is probably ineffective and may be dangerous to the developing larynx.

Prognosis: The lesions usually cease growth by 9 months, followed by gradual regression. A normal life span is expected if the patient survives infancy.

Detection of Carrier: —

†Special Considerations: The true incidence of subglottic hemangioma is difficult to determine. The autopsy gross examination of infants succumbing to an acute respiratory failure from this disease reveals no abnormality of the trachea or larynx. This is explained by the submucosal locations of these tumors, and when emptied of blood the lumen contour is restored with normal-appearing mucosa. With the recent increased awareness of this lesion, some centers advocate routine sections of the larynx and trachea in all cases of "sudden death" of unknown etiology in infants.

The association with cutaneous hemangioma and hemangioma of other organs is well documented. This includes hemangioma of the parotid gland, mediastinum, abdominal viscera, central nervous system and retina. With multiple hemangiomas there may be sufficient shunting of blood from the arterial to the venous system to cause right heart failure. Thrombocytopenia may result from the trapping of platelets within a large hemangioma.

References:
Calcaterra, T. C.: An evaluation of the treatment of subglottic hemangioma. Laryngoscope 78:1956, 1968.
Cohen, S. R.: Unusual lesions of the larynx, trachea and bronchial tree. Ann. Otol. Rhinol. Laryngol. 78:476, 1969.
Cracovaner, A. J.: Anomalies of the larynx. In Maloney, W.H. (ed.): Otolaryngology. Hagerstown: Harper and Row, 1969, p. 42.

Contributor: **Thomas C. Calcaterra**

Editor's Computerized Descriptors: Larynx, Resp., GI.

SUBGLOTTIC STENOSIS

Includes: Sténose sous-glottique
Subglottische Stenose
Estenosis subglótica
Hard stenosis
Soft stenosis
Stenosis, subglottic
Combined stenosis

Excludes: —

Minimal Diagnostic Criteria: A developmental defect of the conus elasticus or the cricoid cartilage which produces stenosis (when the infant's transverse subglottic diameter is less than 4 mm). This is suspected in the infant with stridor and cyanosis and is confirmed by endoscopic examination.

Clinical Findings: Symptoms are variable according to the degree of stenosis, associated anomalies and superimposed infection. Symptoms may begin at birth with stridor and cyanosis. Other infants will be asymptomatic until superimposed low grade infections cause recurrent bouts of respiratory difficulty commonly misdiagnosed as croup. Lateral xray of neck may show decrease in AP diameter of subglottic airway. Direct laryngoscopy and bronchoscopy are the most important studies for establishing the correct diagnosis. In the infant's larynx the subglottic region is cone-shaped and the smallest part of the larynx. The cricoid cartilage is somewhat funnel-shaped with its AP diameter being greater than that of the trachea. Later development produces the ring-shaped cricoid.

Soft stenosis: Narrowing of the normally cone-shaped conus elasticus produces a diffuse stenosis. This "hypertrophy" is composed of increased amounts of connective tissue and large dilated mucous glands with a normal epithelial covering.

Hard stenosis: Caused by the cricoid cartilage, the lumen is compressed in inward "overgrowth" of its cartilaginous walls.

Combined stenosis: A subglottic stenosis can be caused by both soft (conus elasticus) and hard (cricoid cartilage) components.

Complications
I **Derived:** Airway obstruction, exercise intolerance.
II **Associated:** —

Etiology: ?

Pathogenesis: Failure of the lateral infraglottic branchial fused masses to recanalize (soft stenosis) or recanalization after chondrification centers for the cricoid cartilage appear (Frazer); developmental arrest and formation of the stenosis from mesodermal elements (Walander).

Related Facts
I **Sex Ratio:** M1:F1
II **Risk of Occurrence:** ?
III **Risk of Recurrence for**
Patient's Sib: ?
Patient's Child: ?
IV **Age of Detectability:** Usually at or shortly after birth, but may not be detected until infant develops a respiratory infection or croup.
V **Prevalence:** ?

Treatment
I **Primary Prevention:** —
II **Secondary Prevention:** In the very mild stenosis no treatment is needed other than aggressive therapy of upper respiratory infections. Functionally significant stenosis will require a tracheotomy until laryngeal growth produces an

adequate airway. In Holinger's series of 53 infants with sub-glottic stenosis, 39 required tracheotomy because of progressive respiratory difficulty.

III Other Therapy: —

Prognosis: It is presently thought that most or all of these stenoses will "cure" themselves with growth. If the condition is severe and untreated the patient may die of acute upper airway obstruction. A marginal airway may become inadequate during a respiratory infection. If tracheotomy is required there is significant morbidity and mortality in infants and young children.

Detection of Carrier: —

Special Considerations: —

References:
Cavanagh, F.: Congenital laryngeal web. Proc. R. Soc. Med. 58:272, 1965.
Holinger, P.H. and Brown, W.T.: Congenital webs, cysts, laryngoceles, and other anomalies of the larynx. Ann. Otol. Rhinol. Laryngol. 76:744, 1967.
Holinger, P.H. et al: Congenital anomalies of the larynx. Ann. Otol. Rhinol. Laryngol. 63:581, 1954.

Contributors: **Arndt J. Duvall, III**
Roger E. Murken

***

Editor's Computerized Descriptors: Larynx, Resp.

SUCRASE-ISOMALTASE DEFICIENCY

Includes: Déficit en saccharase et en isomaltase
Sucrase-Isomaltase-Mangel
Deficiencia en sucrasa-isomaltasa
Sucrase insufficiency
Isomaltase insufficiency
Asucrosia
Anisomaltasia
Sucrose-isomaltose intolerance
Sucrase-α dextrinase insufficiency

Excludes: Secondary sucrase-isomaltase deficiency
Lactase deficiency, congenital (566)
Lactase deficiency, primary (567)

Minimal Diagnostic Criteria: Fermentative diarrhea from the earliest time of sucrose, dextrin, or starch ingestion which disappears when these foods are eliminated and which does not occur with feedings of monosaccharides or lactose. Deliberate feeding of measured doses of sucrose, isomaltose or palatinose yields flat serum glucose curve, abdominal discomfort, explosive stool of pH below 5.0. The disaccharide can usually be identified in blood, urine and stool after feeding for a tolerance test. If one is certain that the condition is congenital, these criteria may suffice if the patient's condition precludes peroral biopsy.

However, demonstration of normal intestinal histology and decreased or absent sucrase and isomaltase activity is essential in most instances.

Clinical Findings: Symptoms of fermentative diarrhea and failure to thrive begin with initial ingestion of sucrose or dextrins. This would be virtually at birth in infants on modified cow's milk formulas, or with weaning and introduction of sucrose or fruits in breast-fed infants. Severity of symptoms varies among individuals but they are usually more severe in infants and young children. In most patients sucrosuria is present on ingestion of this disaccharide. Symptoms clear as soon as the offending disaccharide is removed from the diet. Patients with intolerance to sucrose are virtually universally described as simultaneously intolerant to isomaltose, the 1-6α linked diglucose which is found at the branching points of polysaccharide molecules (dextrins, starches).

The stool is fluid and frothy from contained gas as it is passed. The pH of fresh stool is always below 5.0 if sucrose or dextrins have been ingested and it may contain reducing sugars (glucose or fructose). These monosaccharides and sucrose or isomaltose may be identified in the stool by chromatography. Ingestion of a standard dose of sucrose (1.5-2.0 gm/kg or 45-60 gm/m^2) always results in a flat 3-hour "tolerance curve" for serum glucose; the test dose almost universally produces clinical discomfort and explosive diarrhea during the 3-hour observation period.

The Zurich group initially demonstrated that all patients with sucrose intolerance were also intolerant to isomaltose. It is this defect that causes the inability to tolerate dextrins, and also starches in young infants. Since adequate supplies of isomaltose are not available to demonstrate the flat absorption curve in routine loading tests, palatinose (1-6α linked glucose and fructose), a bacterial product, is substituted. This disaccharide is split by the same α glycosidase as is isomaltose. In addition to sucrosemia and sucrosuria, patients with this deficiency of sucrase-isomaltase demonstrate isomaltose in blood and urine after dextrin and starch feedings, and also palatinose in these fluids after its ingestion for tolerance testing.

The importance of the isomaltase deficiency is variously

regarded by different authors. In our own experience, patients must remain on a sucrose-free diet for life to avoid symptoms. However, starches appear to be tolerated in reasonably normal amounts once patients are beyond the early months of life. This is probably because isomaltose makes up only approximately 10% of the average starch molecule.

Peroral biopsy specimen of the upper small intestinal mucosa is histologically normal, but contains decreased sucrase and isomaltase activities when these are compared with the activities of maltases 1 and 2 (not maltase 3, 4 and 5) and of lactase, or when assayed in relation to unit weight, or to protein content of the tissue.

Complications
I Derived: Dehydration, electrolyte and acid-base disturbance in almost 100% of cases. Failure to thrive or death in all cases, if correct diagnosis is not made and treatment instituted early enough.

II Associated: —

Etiology: Probably autosomal recessive sucrase and isomaltase deficiency.† McK *22290

Pathogenesis: Ingested sucrose or isomaltose, which results from amylolytic action on polysaccharides, are not hydrolyzed to the component monosaccharides in the upper small intestine as in normal individuals and pass undigested to the colon. In this organ these disaccharides are hydrolyzed and fermented. The resultant mixture contains 2 and 3 carbon volatile acids, glucose, fructose (if sucrose has been ingested) and often the undigested disaccharide(s). The increase in osmolarity of the colonic contents induces net flux of water to the lumen. A combination of the irritant effect of the excessive fermentation, increased colonic gas and distention of the bowel walls by the increase in fluid, results in explosive passage of the loose stool.

Related Facts
I Sex Ratio: ?
II Risk of Occurrence: ?
III Risk of Recurrence for
    Patient's Sib: Probably 1 in 4 (25%) for each offspring to be affected
    Patient's Child: Probably not increased, unless mate is carrier or homozygote
IV Age of Detectability: In early infancy, by loading with sucrose and isomaltose or palatinose and assay of enzymes in intestinal mucosal biopsy specimen.
V Prevalence: ?

Treatment
I Primary Prevention: Genetic counseling
II Secondary Prevention: Avoidance of sucrose in diet. Dextrins and starches should also be avoided in very young infants. Toddlers and older children tolerate these quite well, but sucrose is either never tolerated, or, in some instances, may begin to be taken without concomitant symptoms in the 2nd decade of life.
III Other Therapy: Fluid and electrolyte support may be necessitated during the diarrheal activity in undiagnosed infants.

Prognosis: Current indications are for normal life span if patient is diagnosed and treated. In many patients symptoms disappear with aging. In a few instances, if not recognized in infancy, patients may die of severe inanition and electrolyte disturbances.

Detection of Carrier: Although some parents have been demonstrated to have decreased sucrase-isomaltase activities in peroral biopsy specimens, the tolerance of such individuals for loading with the appropriate disaccharides is usually better than that of children. This confusing finding cannot yet clearly be interpreted to mean either that they represent heterozygote carriers or that they are affected, but have undergone the improvement in clinical symptomatology which is characteristic with growing out of childhood.

†Special Considerations: The combined deficiencies of 2 enzymes (sucrase-isomaltase) is unusual in genetic defects. No clear explanation is yet apparent. It has been suggested that a common regulator gene, or inhibitor, is shared by both enzyme molecules. More probably they indeed are not separate but represent two activity centers of the same molecule. Gray suggests that the defect be viewed for this reason as sucrase-α dextrinase deficiency, since free isomaltose is not present in the intestinal lumen.

References:
Antonowicz, I. et al: Congenital sucrase-isomaltase deficiency. Pediatrics 49:847, 1972.
Davidson, M.: Disaccharide intolerance. Pediatr. Clin. North Am. 14:93, 1967.
Gray, G.M.: Carbohydrate digestion and absorption. N. Engl. J. Med. 292:1225, 1975.
Prader, A. and Auricchio, S.: Defects of intestinal disaccharide absorption. Annu. Rev. Med. 16:345, 1965.
Townley, R.R.: Disaccharidase deficiency in infancy and childhood. Pediatrics 38:127, 1966.

Contributor: Murray Davidson

_____

Editor's Computerized Descriptor: GI.

SULFITE OXIDASE DEFICIENCY

Includes: Déficit en sulfite oxydase
Sulfitoxydase-Mangel
Deficiencia en sulfito oxidasa
Sulfocysteinuria

Excludes: —

Minimal Diagnostic Criteria: Mental retardation with progressive cerebral palsy in infancy with ectopia lentis. Abnormally large urinary excretion of S-sulpho-L-cysteine sulfite and thiosulfate. Very reduced urinary excretion of sulfate.

Clinical Findings: Progressive cerebral palsy until decerebrate. Dislocated ocular lenses.

Complications
I   **Derived:** Progressive cerebral dysfunction and early death
II **Associated:** —

Etiology: Autosomal recessive; McK *27230

Pathogenesis: Deficiency of sulfite oxidase (sulfite: oxygen oxido reductase E.C.1.8.3.1.) in liver, brain and kidney obtained at autopsy.

Related Facts
I   **Sex Ratio:** Probably M1:F1 (Only one male patient)
II   **Risk of Occurrence:** Very rare
III **Risk of Recurrence for**
     Patient's Sib: Probably 1 in 4 (25%) for each offspring to be affected
     Patient's Child: Probable death before reproductive age
IV   **Age of Detectability:** As neonate by clinical findings and urinary amino acid chromatography
V   **Prevalence:** ?

Treatment
I   **Primary Prevention:** Genetic counseling
II   **Secondary Prevention:** —
III **Other Therapy:** —

Prognosis: Patient died at 32 months. Three of 7 sibs died in infancy with pertinent data not recorded.

Detection of Carrier: ? Abnormality not present in urine of parents who were clinically normal.

Special Considerations: —

References:
Irreverre, F. et al: Sulfite oxidase deficiency; studies of a patient with mental retardation, dislocated ocular lenses, and abnormal urinary excretion of S-sulfo-L-cysteine, sulfite and thiosulfate. Biochem. Med. 1:187, 1967.
Mudd, S. H. et al: Sulfite oxidase deficiency in man; demonstration of the enzymatic defect. Science 156:1599, 1967.

Contributor: **John C. Crawhall**

Editor's Computerized Descriptors: Eye, Nerve

SUPRAVENTRICULAR TACHYCARDIAS, CONGENITAL

Includes: Tachycardie supraventriculaire congénitale
Angeborene Supraventrikuläre Tachykardie
Taquicardia supraventricular congénita
Atrial tachyarrhythmia
Supraventricular tachycardia paroxysmal
Atrial flutter, persistent and paroxysmal
Atrial fibrillation
Junctional tachycardia

Excludes: Wolff-Parkinson-White syndrome (1002)
Supraventricular tachyarrhythmias occurring later in infancy and childhood which are presumably acquired.

Minimal Diagnostic Criteria: Fast heart rate over 180/min. Irregularity of the heart rhythm with grouped beats is strongly suggestive even when the minute rate is normal. The ECG confirms the diagnosis.

Clinical Findings: Three forms of atrial tachyarrhythmias are described together because experience and theoretic considerations suggest that these 3 different arrhythmias are closely related. All 3 "entities" are rare as congenital manifestations. The congenital nature of these has been confirmed by fetal monitoring during pregnancy or labor, or recording the infant's ECG immediately after birth. In practice, tachyarrhythmias detected during the first 4 weeks of life are regarded as congenital.
Supraventricular paroxysmal tachycardia is defined as a rapid, regular atrial rate of 180-320 beats per minute originating from an ectopic atrial focus. The P waves are often not seen because they are merged in the preceding T waves. It is usually impossible to distinguish between atrial and atrioventricular junctional (nodal) tachycardia. Paroxysms usually begin suddenly and end as abruptly. T wave abnormalities may persist for several days following a paroxysm. Atrioventricular (A-V) conduction may allow each atrial beat to activate the ventricles 1:1 or block some impulses (see atrial flutter).
Atrial flutter implies atrial ectopic activity of 250-480 beats per minute. The ECG shows flutter waves, which produce a "saw-tooth pattern" in some leads. A-V conduction ratio varies: most common is a 2:1 ratio leading to a ventricular rate half of the atrial rate. In the case of 3:1 (rare), or 4:1 (second most common), and mixed ratios with up to 8:1 A-V block, the ventricular rate may be within normal limits. A-V conduction may also be of the Wenckebach type (progressive prolongation of the PR interval followed by a dropped beat which produces an irregularity of ventricular rhythm with grouped beating).
In *atrial fibrillation* the ectopic atrial impulse is excessively rapid and variable. This leads to uneven and irregular deviations of low amplitude in the ECG. The ventricular rate is also irregular. QRS complexes are usually normal, but sometimes vary in amplitude.
The distinction between these 3 forms of supraventricular tachycardias according to atrial rate is somewhat arbitrary. There are transitions from 1 form to another in 1 patient, or a mixture of 2 as seen in flutter-fibrillation. The attacks of tachycardia as well as atrial flutter may continue for longer periods (at times, months after birth). The ECG of the arrhythmia in the fetus has been described as rapid, irregular, or both, revealing atrial paroxysmal tachycardia, atrial flutter or fibrillation (which is rare without congenital heart disease).
In the fetus, paroxysms of tachycardia without other congenital heart disease, even if they last several months, usu-

ally do not affect growth-development. It has been noticed that these children appear to have a larger birthweight than the average. The condition of the child during labor is good in most cases. Rarely, intrauterine congestive heart failure can be severe enough to produce hydrops fetalis. In such cases fetal distress may be severe enough to warrant emergency cesarean section. Perinatal diagnosis and treatment of congestive heart failure is a medical emergency.

The echocardiogram in atrial fibrillation shows absence of mitral A waves, whereas those waves are present in atrial tachycardia. Left atrial dimension is increased and left ventricular dimension is decreased. After cardioversion these return toward normal, indicating improvement in cardiac function. In atrial flutter, anterior peaking of the mitral valve has been noted just after the flutter wave.

The clinical picture of supraventricular tachycardia varies considerably. The minority (about 10%) have no symptoms, whereas the majority are obviously ill with slight cyanosis and ashen grey skin, which is cold and wet. The infants are restless and dyspneic. Cardiac failure is relatively common (in contrast to adults) and mainly dependent on the duration of the tachycardia, less on its frequency. Usually, there is no heart failure in the first 24 hours of life, or in the first 24 hours of a paroxysm, but it develops in at least 50% if the tachycardia lasts 48 hours. The younger the child, the more likely is the chance to develop cardiac failure. Transient functional murmurs may appear. The xray frequently reveals signs of pulmonary venous congestion and cardiac enlargement. In the presence of congenital heart defects, the clinical picture will be influenced by the underlying malformation.

Complications

I **Derived:** Dyspnea, mild cyanosis and eventually signs of congestive heart failure with enlargement of the liver, vomiting, peripheral edema and oliguria.

II **Associated:** WPW syndrome† in approximately 12% of infants with paroxysmal supraventricular tachycardia, atrial septal defect, pulmonary atresia, Ebstein anomaly of the tricuspid valve, transposition of the great arteries, idiopathic myocardial hypertrophy, endocardial fibroelastosis and heart tumors.

Etiology: Unknown in a normal heart. Transient immaturity of the conduction tissue and inflammatory disease (myocarditis) have been suggested. In the presence of congenital heart disease: dilatation of the atria, vagal and sympathetic effects, toxic agents, hypoxemia, and electrolyte disturbances are discussed. Heart tumors, especially in the region of the sinoatrial and the A-V nodes, may lead to anatomic defects of the conduction system.

Pathogenesis: Two theories for the mechanism of supraventricular arrhythmias are: increased automaticity with origin of the beats from 1 or more ectopic atrial foci outside the sinoatrial node; and reentry as a large circus movement of the impulse within the atria, a circuit within the A-V junction or multiple small uncoordinated areas of atrial activation. Reentry can be initiated by a premature beat which encounters an area only partially recovered from the preceding beat. This has been thought to be the mechanism of atrial flutter and fibrillation, but the best demonstration is found in the tachycardia associated with the WPW syndrome. As the mechanism for atrial fibrillation, it is consistent with the rarity of the problem in infants since the available length of atrial muscle would generally be insufficient for perpetuation of multiple reentry circuits in the absence of ischemia or other cause of depressed conduction. The first theory, ie increased automaticity, is more widely accepted as the mechanism of most supraventricular tachycardias in the young.

Related Facts

I **Sex Ratio:** M3:F1
II **Risk of Occurrence:** ? Very rare
III **Risk of Recurrence for**
  Patient's Sib: ?
  Patient's Child: ?
IV **Age of Detectability:** Prenatal, from the 11th week of gestation by fetal ECG or ultrasonography
V **Prevalence:** ?

Treatment

I **Primary Prevention:** —
II **Secondary Prevention:** Digitalis is the drug of choice. Electrical cardioversion is alternate therapy and low energy levels often suffice. In atrial fibrillation, digitalis provides control of the ventricular rate. In refractory paroxysmal atrial tachyarrhythmia, long-term artificial pacemaker therapy has been used. It has been shown recently in a few cases with WPW syndrome and incapacitating tachycardia that surgical transection of a previously well-identified anomalous pathway of conduction from atria to ventricles may abolish signs of WPW syndrome and prevent further episodes of tachycardia.† Unfortunately, the abnormal conduction pathway often cannot be identified with certainty, and this form of therapy is far from established.
III **Other Therapy:** Procaineamide, quinidine, or other antiarrhythmic agents, may be successful in preventing recurrences.

Prognosis: In paroxysmal atrial tachycardia, the prognosis is usually good in young infants. The best prognosis is in males with the 1st attack occurring prior to 3 months of age. Recurrences are rare beyond 1 year after the 1st attack. The prognosis is guarded if the paroxysm is prolonged or if attacks recur repeatedly in spite of therapy. In atrial flutter, prognosis is equally favorable. Atrial fibrillation is a serious complication. It usually occurs in association with severe congenital heart disease and often has a lethal outcome. The combination of a congenital heart defect with a supraventricular tachycardia worsens the prognosis.

Detection of Carrier: Not applicable

†Special Considerations: See Wolff-Parkinson-White syndrome

References:
Bellet, S.: Clinical Disorders of the Heart Beat, 3rd Ed. Philadelphia: Lea & Febiger, 1971.
Cowan, R.H. et al: Neonatal paroxysmal supraventricular tachycardia with hydrops. Pediatrics 55:3, 1975.
DeMaria, A. et al: Effects of electroversion of atrial fibrillation on cardiac function. Echographic assessment of atrial transport, mitral movement and ventricular performance. Circulation (Suppl. IV) 46:158, 1973.
Ferrer, P.: Arrhythmias in the neonate. In Roberts, N. and Gelband, H. (eds.): Cardiac Arrythmias in the Neonate, Infant and Child. New York: Appleton-Century Crofts, 1977, pp. 265-316.
Lubbes, W.J. et al: Paroxysmal supraventricular tachycardia in infancy and childhood. Eur. J. Cardiol. 2:1, 1974.
Moller, J.H. et al: Atrial flutter in infancy. J. Pediatr. 75:643, 1959.
Nadas, A.S.: Pediatric Cardiology. Philadelphia:W.B. Saunders Co., 1963.

Contributors: **Richard L. Bucciarelli**
B. Lynn Miller
Henry J. L. Marriott

Editor's Computerized Descriptor: CV.

Includes: Syndactylie
Syndaktylie
Sindactilia
Syndactyly type I (zygodactyly)
Syndactyly type II (synpolydactyly)
Syndactyly type III (ring and little finger syndactyly)
Syndactyly type IV (Haas type and Cenani-Lenz type)
Syndactyly type V (syndactyly with metacarpal and metatarsal fusion)

Excludes: Acrocephalosyndactyly (14)
Poland syndrome (813)
Syndactyly with multifactorial inheritance
Syndactyly associated with congenital constriction rings

Minimal Diagnostic Criteria: See Clinical Findings.

Clinical Findings: In *syndactyly type I* (zygodactyly), there is usually webbing between the 3rd and 4th fingers, either complete reaching to the nails, or partial, and occasionally associated with fusion of the distal phalanges of these fingers. Other fingers are sometimes also involved but the 3rd and 4th fingers are the most commonly affected. In the feet, there is usually webbing between the 2nd and 3rd toes, either complete or partial.

In *syndactyly type II* (synpolydactyly), there is usually syndactyly of the 3rd and 4th fingers associated with polydactyly of all components or of part of the 4th finger in the web. In the feet, there is polydactyly of the 5th toe.

In *syndactyly type III* (ring and little finger syndactyly), syndactyly between the ring and the little fingers is usually complete and bilateral. The 5th finger is short with absent or rudimentary middle phalanx. Feet are usually not affected in this type. This type of syndactyly is the hand malformation in oculodentoosseous dysplasia.

In *syndactyly type IV* (Haas type) there is complete cutaneous fusion of the fingers giving the hands a cup-like appearance. In Cenani-Lenz type the complete syndactyly is associated with bizarre disorganization of metacarpals and phalanges, the radius and ulna are either fused, short, or rudimentary. Feet are similarly affected.

In *syndactyly type V*, there is an associated metacarpal and metatarsal fusion. The metacarpals and metatarsals most commonly fused are the 3rd and 4th or the 4th and 5th. Soft tissue syndactyly usually affects the 3rd and 4th fingers and the 2nd and 3rd toes. Syndactyly is usually more extensive and complete.

Complications
I **Derived:** —
II **Associated:** —

Etiology: Autosomal dominant for most types. Fusion of metacarpals 4 and 5 is inherited as an X-linked recessive trait in some families. Cenani-Lenz type of syndactyly is probably autosomal.

Pathogenesis: —

Related Facts
I **Sex Ratio:** M1:F1
II **Risk of Occurrence:** Syndactyly type I (zygodactyly) is the most common with an incidence of 1 in 3000 live births in Americans.
III **Risk of Recurrence for**
   Patient's Sib: If parent is affected, 1 in 2 (50%) for each offspring to be affected; otherwise not increased. Recurrence risk is different in the X-linked type of metacarpal-metatarsal fusion and in Cenani-Lenz type of total syndactyly with synostosis.
   Patient's Child: 1 in 2

IV **Age of Detectability:** At birth
V **Prevalence:** ?

Treatment
I   **Primary Prevention:** Genetic counseling
II **Secondary Prevention:** Surgical intervention
III **Other Therapy:** —

Prognosis: Normal life span

Detection of Carrier: —

Special Considerations: —

References:
Cenani, A. and Lenz, W.: Total Syndaktylie und totale radio-ulnare Synostose bei zwei Brüdern. Ein Beitrag zur Genetik der Syndaktylien. Z. Kinderheilkd. 101:181, 1967.
Cross, H. E. et al: Type II syndactyly. Am. J. Hum. Genet. 20:368, 1968.
Holmes, L.B. et al: Metacarpal 4-5 fusion with X-linked recessive inheritance. Am. J. Hum. Genet. 24:562, 1972.
Temtamy, S. A.: Genetic factors in hand malformations. Unpublished doctoral dissertation. Johns Hopkins University, 1966.
Temtamy, S.A. and McKusick, V.A.: The Genetics of Hand Malformations. Birth Defects: Orig. Art. Ser., D. Bergsma (ed.) New York:Alan Liss, Inc. for The National Foundation-March of Dimes, 1978, vol. XIV, no. 3.

Contributor: **Samia A. Temtamy**

Editor's Computerized Descriptor: Skel.

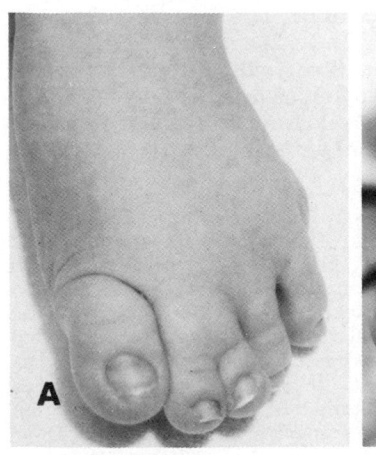 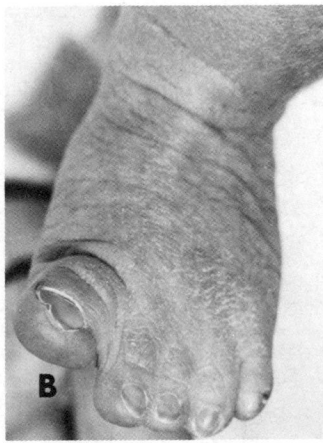

471. A) Syndactyly of 2nd and 3rd toes; B) complete soft tissue syndactyly between 2nd, 3rd, and 4th toes and partial webbing between hallux and 2nd toe

SYRINGOMYELIA

Includes: Syringomyelie
Siringomielia
Gliosis
Spinal cord cavitation

Excludes: Intramedullary spinal cord tumor
Progressive sensory neuropathy of children

Minimal Diagnostic Criteria: A disease characterized by progressive atrophy of the muscles of the upper part of body, dissociated anesthesia and trophic changes.

Clinical Findings: Syringomyelia most commonly involves the cervical enlargement, the pathologic process of cavitation most frequently originating in the posterior horn of the gray matter of the spinal cord. The symptoms and signs are the result of expanding cavitation and subsequent gliosis.

Rapidly progressive scoliosis is relatively common. Atrophy and weakness of the intrinsic hand muscles may be the first finding, but progressive wasting of arm, trunk and neck musculature follows. The upper limbs are flaccid and areflexic. The corticospinal tracts are often compressed so that spasticity, weakness, hyperreflexia and extensor plantar responses are noted in the lower limbs.

Sensory symptoms are the result of involvement of the lateral spinothalamic tracts. Analgesia is usually more prominent than tactile anesthesia. Trophic changes may be prominent. These include Charcot joints, abnormalities of perspiration, and skin ulceration. The most frequent age of presentation is in the 3rd and 4th decade.

Cervical spine xrays may show widening, particularly in the sagittal diameter. Bony erosion is rare. The CSF protein may be elevated. Myelography frequently demonstrates an abnormally enlarged spinal cord.

Complications
I **Derived:** Poser examined 245 cases of syringomyelia and found a 16% incidence of intramedullary tumors. Mild trauma to the cord has been reported to cause bleeding within the cavity and marked deterioration in function. Syringobulbia may occur due to upward extension of the process from the cervical spinal cord. This may produce bulbar signs causing aspiration, pneumonia and death.
II **Associated:** Spina bifida, Klippel-Feil syndrome, cervical ribs, Arnold-Chiari malformation, webbed fingers, abnormal hair distribution and hypospadias.

Etiology: Autosomal dominant transmission has been suggested. Most case reports present confusing clinical data and are not supported by pathologic material.

Pathogenesis: Syringomyelia may be the result of an abnormality of embryogenesis. The abnormality may be the result of arrested development of the spinal cord before complete differentiation of gray and white matter occurs. Another theory suggests that during development of the cord there is a failure of the normal migration of spongioblasts from the central canal region. These cells later develop the capability of proliferating and causing cavitation. Finally, it has been suggested that syringomyelia is the result of developmental anomalies of the intramedullary blood supply.

Related Facts
I **Sex Ratio:** M1:F1
II **Risk of Occurrence:** ?
III **Risk of Recurrence for**
    Patient's Sib: ?
    Patient's Child: ?
IV **Age of Detectability:** Between the ages of 20-40, primarily by physical examination and myelography.

V **Prevalence:** ?

Treatment
I **Primary Prevention:** —
II **Secondary Prevention:** Laminectomy and appropriate drainage of the rapidly enlarging cavity is indicated in the presence of progressive neurologic signs.
III **Other Therapy:** Proper management of trophic skin changes.

Prognosis: Generally unfavorable. Slowly progressive. Death usually occurs as the result of bulbar paralysis.

Detection of Carrier: —

Special Considerations: —

References:
Curtius, F.: Status Dysraphicus und Myelodysplasie. Fortschr. Erbpathol. 3:199, 1939.
Mulvey, B.E. and Riely, L.A.: Familial syringomyelia and status dysraphicus. Ann. Intern. Med. 16:966, 1942.
Poser, C.M.: Relationship Between Syringomyelia and Neoplasm. Springfield: Charles C Thomas, 1956.

Contributor: **Robert H. A. Haslam**

Editor's Computerized Descriptors: Skin, Sweating, Skel., Muscle, Nerve

TAPETOCHOROIDAL DYSTROPHY

Includes: Dystrophie tapéto-choroïdienne
Tapeto-choroidale Dystrophie
Distrofia tapetocoroidea
Progressive choroideremia
Progressive chorioretinal degeneration
Progressive choroidal atrophy
X-linked choroidal sclerosis†
Choroidal sclerosis, X-linked
Choroideremia

Excludes: Retinitis pigmentosa (869)
Gyrate atrophy (449)

Minimal Diagnostic Criteria: X-linked chorioretinal degeneration with at least 1 male showing the typical eyegrounds of far advanced disease.

Clinical Findings: A progressive X-linked degeneration of the choroid and retina probably beginning in the 1st few years of life. In early stages there are focal areas of choroidal atrophy with intervening exposure of choroidal vessels and a pigmentary stippling and fine atrophy in the equatorial and posterior eyegrounds similar to the changes frequently noted in carrier females. The areas of choroidal atrophy become larger and more numerous and in between the choroidal vessels become more prominent. Eventually most of the choroidal vessels disappear so that normal-appearing choroid remains only in the macula, in the far periphery and in a few small spots elsewhere. The retinal vessels may be attenuated, particularly in advanced cases. A few clumps of pigment of varying size and shape are usually seen mainly near the equatorial retina.

The visual acuity usually remains intact until at least the age of 30, but between the ages of 40 and 60 severe impairment of central acuity usually results. Severe visual field constriction and nightblindness, which is the 1st symptom of the disease, occur at a much earlier age.

Most female carriers have eyeground changes. Most commonly these are midperipheral pigmentation, localized deep in the retina, and associated spotty areas of atrophy. The pigment may show clumping, particularly near the equator and frequently is described as striated or distributed in an irradiating pattern. Pigment in the macula may be fine and mottled. The disk and retinal vessels are usually considered normal. Occasionally other types of eyegrounds are seen in the carrier which are intermediate in form between the typical carrier state and that noted in the male with far advanced disease. Functionally central visual acuity and color vision are normal until after the age of 30, visual fields show gradual loss of most peripheral field. Dark-adaptation is affected early with relentless progression and eventual severe nightblindness. ERG is subnormal in early cases with usual eventual complete disappearance of this response in advanced cases. EOG is markedly abnormal.

Complications
I Derived: —
II Associated: —

Etiology: An abiotrophy with X-linked transmission; McK *30310

Pathogenesis: Pathologic studies have been done in eyes from 2 males aged 76 and 78, 1 with glaucoma as well. In the eyes without glaucoma the bipolar cells, ganglion cells, and nerve fiber layer were normal. This would explain the usual absence of optic atrophy in this condition. The retinal vessels were also normal. However, extensive degeneration of the pigment epithelium and the receptor cells was noted.

Extensive choroidal atrophy was found with thin fibrous choroid remaining mainly in the macula and next to the ora serrata. In these areas, the walls of the choroidal vessels were thickened, and the lumina were all but obliterated. In many places the choroid and Bruch membrane had disappeared completely (eg halfway between the posterior pole and the ora serrata).

A fluorescein study done in an 18-year-old affected male showed intense fluorescence in the area of remaining visible choroid (in the macula and far periphery), faint fluorescence in areas of a few choroidal vessels and no fluorescence where choroidal vessels were absent. The findings suggested a diffuse disturbance of pigment epithelium where the choroidal vasculature remained and probably where the choroid no longer remained. An abnormality of the pigment epithelium may be the basic defect in this disease. A 21-year-old female carrier studied showed extensive diffuse spotty fluorescence characteristic of defective pigment epithelium throughout the posterior and intermediate eyegrounds. These spots had feathery borders, varied in size and brightness and formed fine, lacy, confluent fluorescent networks. Probably these fluorescent spots corresponded to areas of atrophy ordinarily seen with white light.

Related Facts
I **Sex Ratio:** M1:F rare
II **Risk of Occurrence:** ?
III **Risk of Recurrence for**
  Patient's Sib: If mother is carrier 1 in 2 (50%) for each brother to be affected and 1 in 2 for each sister to be a carrier.
  Patient's Child: Affected males' daughters are all carriers, whereas sons are uninvolved.
IV **Age of Detectability:** Detection in males usually in 1st decade. A female carrier with typical eyeground changes was seen at the age of 3 1/2 years, but because the female does not show a progressive disease it is likely that her changes are present at birth. Perhaps the initial changes seen in the male are also present at birth, but this remains to be established.
V **Prevalence:** —

Treatment
I **Primary Prevention:** Genetic counseling
II **Secondary Prevention:** —
III **Other Therapy:** —

Prognosis: Normal life span with eventual severe blindness

Detection of Carrier: Female carrier can usually be identified by typical eyeground changes described above. Occasionally more extensive eyeground changes will be seen in the female intermediate between the typical carrier state and the fully affected male. Occasionally mild functional disturbances are noted, particularly of dark-adaptation. At times an abnormality of the electrooculogram or the ERG has been reported. At least 2 females with a full form of the disease have been cited.

†Special Considerations: Frequently 1 or more males in a pedigree of known choroideremia will show typical eyegrounds of choroidal sclerosis. In fact, in the originally published pedigrees of so-called "X-linked choroidal sclerosis," there are some males with the typical eyegrounds of choroideremia. Also, female carriers of X-linked choroidal sclerosis and of choroideremia show the same eyeground findings. It is likely that these 2 conditions are the same disease.

References:
Klein, D.: Genetic approach to the nosology of retinal disorders. In Bergsma, D. (ed.): Part VIII. Eye. Birth Defects: Orig. Art. Ser., vol. VII, no. 3. Baltimore:Williams & Wilkins for The National Foundation-March of Dimes, 1971, p. 52.

Krill, A.E.: Observations; of carriers of X-chromosomal linked chorioretinal degenerations; do these support the "inactivation hypothesis"? Am. J. Ophthalmol. 64:1029, 1967.

Kurstjens, J.H.: Choroideremia and gyrate atrophy of the choroid and retina. Doc. Ophthalmol. 19:1, 1965.

McCulloch, C. and McCulloch, R.J.P.: Hereditary and clinical study of choroideremia. Trans. Am. Acad. Ophthalmol. Otolaryngol. 52:160, 1948.

Contributors: **Alex E. Krill‡**
Donald R. Bergsma

Editor's Computerized Descriptors: Vision, Eye

TAURODONTISM (MARKER)

Includes: Taurodontisme
Taurodontie
Taurodoncia (Marcador)
Hypertaurodontism
Mesotaurodontism
Hypotaurodontism

Excludes: Hypophosphatemia (517)
Shell teeth
Odontodysplasia (739)
Amelogenesis imperfecta (46)

Minimal Diagnostic Criteria: Teeth with pulp chambers enlarged in their vertical dimension.

Clinical Findings: Crowns of teeth appear normal. Condition detected radiographically. Pulp chambers are large and the bifurcation or trifurcation of molar and premolar teeth are displaced apically. The body and root of the teeth have a block rectangular shape. This is a relatively frequent trait particularly among Esquimousa Amerindians, Bantus and extinct hominids (Neanderthal). Rare in Caucasians.

Complications
I **Derived:** —
II **Associated:** X chromosome aneuploidy; other chromosome abnormalities, eg Trisomy 21 and a 22/18 translocation; scanty hair-oligodontia-taurodontia syndrome; trichodentoosseous syndrome; juvenile glaucoma with skin anomalies; microcephalic dwarfism.

Etiology: When not syndrome-associated, probably polygenic. The available completely examined kindreds are 22. Nineteen show no parents affected and none of the parents have known consanguinity. Ten of the 19 have other sibs affected. Three have what appears to be autosomal dominant transmission over 3 generations. Most likely there is genetic heterogeneity in this trait but dominant or recessive transmission is not ruled out.

Pathogenesis: Primary protein alteration unknown. The Hertwig epithelial root sheath fails to invaginate below crown to form roots in multirooted teeth resulting in teeth with large pulp chambers such that the distance from the bifurcation or trifurcation of roots to the cementoenamel junction is greater than the occlusal-cervical distance.

Related Facts
I   **Sex Ratio:**   M1:F1
II **Risk of Occurrence:**   ?
III **Risk of Recurrence for**
     Patient's Sib: Based on 22 North American Caucasian propositi and corrected for ascertainment - 20%
     Patient's Child: ?
IV **Age of Detectability:**   From 3 to 12 years of age by roentgenologic examination
V   **Prevalence:**   ? Occurs in all races. Rare in general population of the United States. Occurs in higher frequencies among Eskimos (20%) and Aleuts; in African Boskopoid and Australoid (30%), high in fossil hominid remains, particularly Neanderthal (20-60%).

Treatment
I   **Primary Prevention:** —
II **Secondary Prevention:** —
III **Other Therapy:** —

Prognosis: No effect reported on longevity†

Detection of Carrier: —

†Special Considerations: Teeth with large pulp chambers occur in hypophosphatemia, vitamin D refractory rickets (including renal types such as the Fanconi syndrome) in the shell tooth variant of dentinogenesis imperfecta, odontodysplasia and internal resorption. The anthropologic explanation for the high frequency of this trait in certain populations past and present is that it has a selective value where teeth are used as tools (skin tanning) such that the taurodont tooth is less liable to pulp exposure from attrition than the cynodont tooth.

References:
Hamner, J.E., III et al: Taurodontism: Report of a case. Oral Surg. 18:409, 1964.

Keeler, C.: Taurodont molars and shovel incisors in Klinefelter's syndrome. J. Hered. 64:234, 1973.

Shaw, J. C. M.: Taurodont teeth in the South African races. J. Anat. 62:476, 1928.

Stenvik, A. et al: Taurodontism and concomitant hypodontia in siblings. Oral Surg. 33:841, 1972.

Witkop, C. J., Jr.: Manifestations of genetic diseases in the human pulp. Oral Surg. 32:278, 1971.

Witkop, C.J., Jr.: Hereditary defects of dentin. Dent. Clin. North Am. 19:25, 1975.

Contributor: Carl J. Witkop, Jr.

Editor's Computerized Descriptor: Teeth

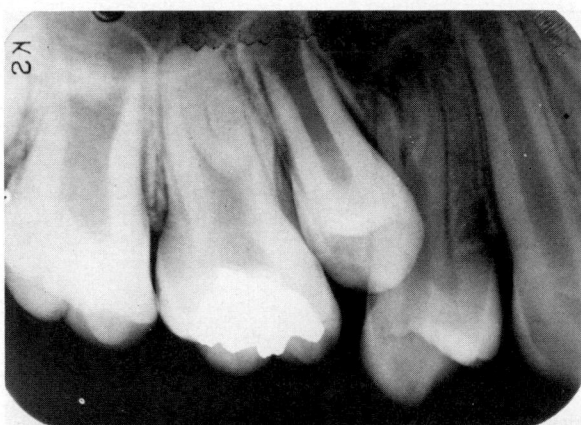

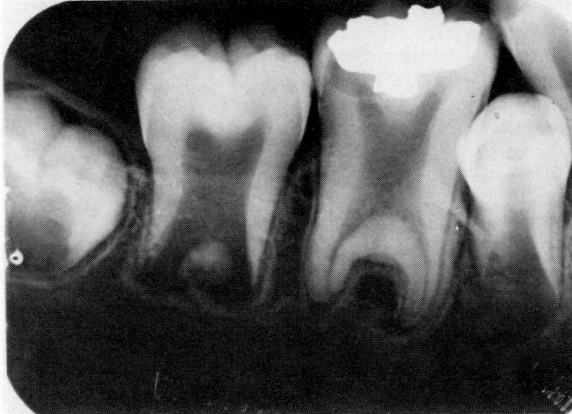

472. Taurodontism

TEETH, ANKYLOSED

Includes: Ankylose dentaire
Ankylose des zähne
Dientes anquilosados
Submerged teeth
Ankylosed teeth

Excludes: Teeth, concrescence of roots (928)
Teeth, dilacerated (929)
Dens in dente (276)
Teeth, fused (930)
Teeth, geminated (931)
Teeth, impacted (932)

Minimal Diagnostic Criteria: Occlusal surface of affected tooth is situated below the plane of occlusion and tooth lacks mobility to manual rocking.

Clinical Findings: A fusion of tooth cementum and bone, occurring anywhere along path of eruption, either before or after emergence of tooth into the mouth. Condition may affect any tooth but the mandibular 1st primary molar is most frequently involved. Ankylosis becomes clinically apparent by 1) occlusal plane of tooth beneath plane of occlusion of adjacent teeth, 2) clinical crown height less than that of adjacent teeth, and 3) immobility to manual rocking. A solid sound on percussion and radiographic evidence of partial obliteration of periodontal ligament are nonessential criteria for diagnosis. The interproximal alveolar bone height is below that of adjacent unaffected teeth.

Complications
I   **Derived:** Difficult to extract affected tooth, noneruption of succedaneous tooth, supereruption of opposing tooth/teeth, tipping of adjacent teeth, loss of arch length and possible development of malocclusion or local periodontal pathology.
II   **Associated:** Subsequent to dental caries there may be pulpal exposure, periapical infection, granuloma, cyst formation, and loss of teeth, followed by possible drifting and development of malocclusion. On occasion, ankylosis of primary teeth may be associated with congenitally missing succedaneous teeth. Lack of alveolar bone height may predispose to local periodontal pathology. Enamel opacity, hypoplasia and malformed teeth in association with ankylosed molars have been reported in the permanent dentition.

Etiology: Unknown, but genetic or congenital gap in periodontal ligament is cited as an intrinsic causative factor. Chemical or thermal irritation, disturbed local metabolism, infection, local mechanical trauma and reimplantation of evulsed tooth are cited as extrinsic causative factors.

Pathogenesis: The affected tooth has area of cemental root resorption repaired by osteoid-like tissue which is continuous with alveolar bone. Periodontal ligament may become increasingly obliterated in affected area.

Related Facts
I   **Sex Ratio:** M1:F1
II   **Risk of Occurrence:** ?
III   **Risk of Recurrence for**
     Patient's Sib: Not increased
     Patient's Child: Not increased
IV   **Age of Detectability:** Detected by clinical or radiographic examination when adjacent teeth have reached occlusal plane.
V   **Prevalence:** Reported in United States study to affect 6.9% of primary molar teeth; very rare in secondary teeth.

Treatment
I   **Primary Prevention:** Avoidance of extrinsic causative factors listed above.
II   **Secondary Prevention:** —

III Other Therapy: Extraction of affected tooth, artificial restoration of proximal and occlusal contacts, or leaving tooth undisturbed.† Affected mandibular 1st primary molars are likely to exfoliate normally and early extraction is not indicated. Affected maxillary and mandibular 2nd primary molars tend to become severely affected with marked absence of alveolar bone growth, and do not exfoliate normally. Such teeth should be extracted.

Prognosis: Treated: Excellent. If there is no succedaneous tooth, a partially restored ankylosed tooth can serve well indefinitely. Periodic replacement of the restoration may be required as changes occur in surrounding alveolar bone. Alveolar bone height will always be lower than that of adjacent unaffected teeth.

Untreated: Tooth will not erupt to the plane of occlusion and surrounding alveolar bone height will not develop. Mandibular 1st primary molars are likely to exfoliate normally. Maxillary and mandibular 2nd primary molars tend to become severely affected and tend not to exfoliate normally. In addition there may be complications as listed above. The condition does not appear to affect longevity of patient.

Detection of Carrier: —

†Special Considerations: In some instances extraction may be delayed and tooth utilized as a space maintainer until the succedaneous tooth is ready to erupt. Presence of succedaneous tooth should be established prior to extracting the affected tooth. Extraction of an ankylosed tooth usually requires vertical sectioning of the tooth and surgical removal of each section.

References:
Biederman, W.B.: The problem of the ankylosed tooth. Dent. Clin. North Am. 409:24, 1968.
Brearley, L.J. and McKibben, D.H., Jr.: Ankylosis of primary molar teeth. I. Prevalence and characteristics. II. A longitudinal study. J. Dent. Child. 40:54, 1973.
Darling, A.I. and Levers, B.G.H.: Submerged human deciduous molars and ankylosis. Arch. Oral. Biol. 18:1021, 1973.
Rule, J.T. et al: The relationship between ankylosed primary molars and multiple enamel defects. J. Dent. Child. 39:29, 1972.

Contributors: **Louise Brearley Messer**
Jay T. Cline
D. H. McKibben, Jr.

Editor's Computerized Descriptor: Teeth

TEETH, CONCRESCENCE OF ROOTS

Includes: Calescence des racines dentaires
Radikuläre Zahnverschmelzung
Concrecencia de las raíces dentarias
Concrescence of roots of teeth

Excludes: Teeth, dilacerated (929)
Teeth, geminated (931)
Teeth, impacted (932)
Teeth, ankylosed (927)
Teeth, fused (930)

Minimal Diagnostic Criteria: Two or more closely-approximated primary or secondary teeth exhibiting clinical or radiographic evidence of roots bound together with excessive cementum.

Clinical Findings: Two, or very rarely 3, closely-approximated primary or secondary teeth exhibiting roots bound together with excessive cementum. The bond may occur during or after completion of root formation. Usual location is maxillary molar area. Most commonly involves a morphologically normal 3rd molar with a distomolar or paramolar.

Complications
I **Derived:** Involved teeth may a) be delayed in eruption, b) have delay in eruption of succedaneous teeth, c) become ankylosed, d) become involved in periodontal pathology.
II **Associated:** Subsequent to dental caries there may be pulpal exposure, periapical infection, granuloma, cyst formation, loss of teeth followed by possible drifting and development of malocclusion.

Etiology: Initial event unknown; extrinsic causative factors such as local trauma, excessive occlusal trauma, local infection, and crowding of teeth followed by resorption of interdental bone, are cited.

Pathogenesis: Roots united below level of cementoenamel junction by excessive cementum with or without dentin deposition.

Related Facts
I **Sex Ratio:** Probably M1:F1
II **Risk of Occurrence:** Rare
III **Risk of Recurrence for**
Patient's Sib: ?
Patient's Child: ?
IV **Age of Detectability:** Detectable radiographically at any age as soon as cementum matrix calcifies.
V **Prevalence:** Rare

Treatment
I **Primary Prevention:** —
II **Secondary Prevention:** —
III **Other Therapy:** a) Extract involved teeth,† b) remove excessive cementum in course of periodontal treatment or c) leave tooth undisturbed.

Prognosis: Variable, depending upon extent of eruption and periodontal condition of involved teeth. If teeth fully erupted into good occlusion with healthy periodontium, prognosis excellent. Unerupted or partially erupted teeth, or involved teeth with poor periodontal health have poor prognosis. Condition only likely to affect longevity of patient if infection, dentigerous cyst or ameloblastomatous change supervenes around unerupted, involved teeth.

Detection of Carrier: —

†Special Considerations: Endodontic therapy or extraction of involved teeth may be difficult to perform.

References:
Santangelo, M. V.: Concrescence associated with a dentigerous cyst. Oral Surg. 26:769, 1968.
Shafer, W.G. et al: A Textbook of Oral Pathology, 2nd Ed. Philadelphia: W.B. Saunders, 1964, p. 37.

Stafne, E. C.: Oral Roentgenographic Diagnosis. 2nd Ed. Philadelphia:W.B. Saunders, 1963, p.21.

Contributors: **Louise Brearley Messer**
D. H. McKibben, Jr.

Editor's Computerized Descriptor: Teeth

TEETH, DILACERATED

Includes: Dents déformées par dysplasie traumatique
Dilazerierte Zähne
Dientes dilacerados

Excludes: Teeth, ankylosed (927)
Teeth, concrescence of roots (928)
Teeth, fused (930)
Teeth, geminated (931)
Teeth, impacted (932)
Teeth, supernumerary (936)
Twinning of teeth

Minimal Diagnostic Criteria: Clinical or radiographic evidence of displacement of all or part of tooth crown in relation to root.

Clinical Findings: Displacement of all or part of tooth crown in relation to root, characterized by clinically obvious malalignment of varying severity. Hard and soft tissues of the crown or root may show defective formation; the crown may show hypoplasia or hypocalcification. Radiographic appearance will depend upon severity of condition and spatial relationship of oral tissues, radiographic film and beam. The most frequently affected teeth in descending order of involvement are: 1) mandibular 3rd molars, 2) maxillary bicuspids, 3) mandibular secondary incisors and 4) maxillary secondary incisors. Primary teeth are very rarely affected.

Complications
I **Derived:** a) Psychosocial problems may arise due to unesthetic anterior affected tooth/teeth, b) dental caries may occur in hypoplastic defects, if present, c) continued root formation may be arrested, d) affected tooth or associated teeth may not erupt, e) infection, dentigerous cyst formation and ameloblastomatous change may develop in relation to an unerupted dilacerated tooth/teeth.
II **Associated:** Subsequent to dental caries there may be pulpal exposure, periapical infection, granuloma, cyst formation, and loss of teeth followed by possible drifting and development of malocclusion.

Etiology: Trauma to developing tooth prior to completion of root formation results in coronal displacement. Displacement of crown or the developing root(s) may occur 1) during traumatic intrusion or extrusion of primary teeth, 2) during removal of primary teeth, 3) in cases of tooth size-arch size discrepancy resulting in tooth crowding and 4) subsequent to pressure from adjacent pathologic processes (eg cyst).

Pathogenesis: At the point of crown-root deflection, enamel or dentin may exhibit abnormal matrix formation or calcification. Crown enamel and dentin may show hypoplasia or hypocalcification. Root apex may exhibit arrested cellular differentiation.

Related Facts
I **Sex Ratio:** M1:F1
II **Risk of Occurrence:** ?
III **Risk of Recurrence for**
   Patient's Sib: —
   Patient's Child: —
IV **Age of Detectability:** Variable, depending upon time of individual tooth formation. Condition is detectable radiographically during early crown or root formation.
V **Prevalence:** ?

Treatment
I **Primary Prevention:** a) Avoidance of trauma to unerupted or erupting teeth, b) careful surgical removal of primary teeth and c) early diagnosis and treatment of pathologic processes adjacent to dental structures.†
II **Secondary Prevention:** Orthodontic correction of tooth size-arch size deficiencies to avoid dental crowding.

III Other Therapy: a) Removal of involved tooth and fabrication of prosthetic replacement, if indicated, b) where possible, appropriate restoration of tooth structure to provide function, or c) if asymptomatic and patient-acceptable, leave undisturbed.†

Prognosis: Prognosis of condition depends upon severity of crown-root malalignment, extent of tooth eruption and condition of clinical crown. With increasing severity of any of these factors, the prognosis of involved tooth worsens. Unless pathology such as infection, dentigerous cyst formation and ameloblastomatous change develop in relation to an unerupted dilacerated tooth, the condition does not appear to interfere with longevity of patient.

Detection of Carrier: —

†Special Considerations: Endodontic therapy, if indicated, is difficult to perform satisfactorily. Root fracture may occur during extraction of involved tooth.

References:

Large, N. D.: Anomalies of the teeth and regressive alterations of the teeth. In Tiecke, R.W. (ed.): Oral Pathology, 1st Ed. New York:McGraw-Hill, 1965, p. 233.

Shafer, W. G. et al: A Textbook of Oral Pathology, 3rd Ed. Philadelphia:W.B. Saunders, 1974, p. 37.

Contributors: **Louise Brearley Messer**
Jay T. Cline
Paul O. Walker

Editor's Computerized Descriptor: Teeth

TEETH, FUSED

Includes: Fusion dentaire
Zahnverschmelzung
Dientes fusionados
Fused teeth

Excludes: Teeth, dilacerated (929)
Teeth, impacted (932)
Teeth, concrescence of roots (928)
Teeth, ankylosed (927)
Teeth, geminated (931)
Dens in dente (276)

Minimal Diagnostic Criteria: Complete or incomplete union of the crowns of 2 normally separated tooth germs resulting in confluent dentin and separate or fused root canals. Number of teeth in affected area is decreased.

Clinical Findings: Union of two normally separated tooth germs results in either complete or incomplete fusion of either crowns or roots or both. Such teeth exhibit confluent dentin and 2 separate root canals but only one root. Unless fusion is between a normal tooth and a supernumerary, the number of teeth normally in the affected area is decreased. Condition occurs in both primary and secondary dentitions and may occur between 2 normal teeth, or between a supernumerary tooth and a normal tooth. Corresponding secondary teeth may be absent.

Complications
I **Derived:** Unesthetic anterior teeth may predispose towards psychosocial concerns. Dental caries may occur in area of coronal fusion. Decrease in tooth number may produce tooth size-arch size discrepancy and possible malocclusion. Abnormal coronal morphology may predispose towards periodontal pathology.
II **Associated:** In affected children some primary and secondary teeth have been reported to be missing. Subsequent to dental caries there may be pulpal exposure, periapical infection, granuloma, cyst formation, and loss of teeth with possible drifting and resultant malocclusion.

Etiology: Unknown; but genetic expression, physical force or pressure producing contact of the coronal areas of 2 adjacent tooth buds have been cited as causative factors.

Pathogenesis: Condition thought to arise through union of coronal areas of 2 normally separated tooth germs. Depending upon stage of development of the teeth at the time of union, fusion may be either complete or incomplete.

Related Facts
I **Sex Ratio:** Probably M1:F1
II **Risk of Occurrence:** 1 in 200 in Japanese, higher in persons of Mongoloid ancestry than in Caucasians or Negroes.
III **Risk of Recurrence for**
Patient's Sib: Significantly higher than in general population
Patient's Child: ? In some cases condition reported to show a hereditary tendency.
IV **Age of Detectability:** Very variable, depending upon age of calcification of affected teeth. Detected preeruptively on radiographs or posteruptively on clinical examination.
V **Prevalence:** This condition is thought to be more common in the primary than secondary dentition. 1 in 250 in Guatemalan Indians.

Treatment
I **Primary Prevention:** —
II **Secondary Prevention:** —
III **Other Therapy:** a) Extract affected teeth,† b) esthetic restoration of crown, if possible, c) esthetic reshaping of coronally fused area of anterior teeth in order to provide appearance of 2 independent crowns, d) removal of affected part of crown, or e) leave tooth undisturbed.

Prognosis: Depends upon extent and location of coronal separation, extent of occlusal disharmony and periodontal condition of affected teeth. Completely fused teeth in good occlusion and having healthy periodontal tissues, have an excellent prognosis. Affected teeth with malocclusion or periodontal pathology have a poor prognosis. Condition does not appear to affect longevity of patient.

Detection of Carrier: —

†Special Considerations: Presence of succedaneous teeth should be ascertained prior to removing affected primary teeth. Morphology of affected teeth should be ascertained prior to attempting esthetic reshaping of crown(s) of affected anterior teeth. Endodontic therapy may be difficult if root canal is partially divided. It is not always possible to differentiate between fusion of a normal tooth with a supernumerary tooth and gemination.

References:
Gorlin, R. J. and Goldman, H. M. (eds.): Thoma's Oral Pathology, 6th Ed. St. Louis: C.V. Mosby, 1970, p. 112.
Grahner, H. and Granath, L. E.: Numerical variations in primary dentition and their correlation with the permanent dentition. Odontol. Revy. 12:348, 1961.
Levitas, T.C.: Gemination, twinning, fusion and conscrescence. J. Dent. Child. 32(2):93, 1965.
Saito, T.: A genetic study on the degenerative anomalies of deciduous teeth. Jap. J. Hum. Genet. 4:27, 1959.

Contributors: **Louise Brearley Messer**
Jay T. Cline

Editor's Computerized Descriptor: Teeth
Also see Section I, Fig. 86

TEETH, GEMINATED

Includes: Dents géminées
Zahnzwillingsbildung
Dientes geminados
Geminated teeth

Excludes: Teeth, fused (930)
Teeth, impacted (932)
Teeth, concrescence of roots (928)
Teeth, ankylosed (927)
Teeth, dilacerated (929)
Dens in dente (276)

Minimal Diagnostic Criteria: An enlarged bifid or cloven crown on a single root. Number of teeth normally in arch neither increased nor decreased.

Clinical Findings: Single tooth structure with 2 completely or incompletely separated crowns that have a single root and a single or partially divided pulp chamber. Clinical crown may exhibit hypoplasia or hypocalcification of enamel or dentin. There is a normal number of teeth in the affected area. Condition usually limited to mandibular (primary or secondary) incisors.

Complications
I **Derived:** Delayed eruption of affected or succedaneous tooth. Unesthetic anterior teeth may predispose towards psychopathology. Dental caries may occur in hypoplastic defects, if present. Abnormal coronal morphology may predispose towards malocclusion or periodontal pathology.
II **Associated:** Subsequent to dental caries there may be pulpal exposure, periapical infection, granuloma, cyst formation, and loss of teeth with possible drifting and resultant malocclusion.

Etiology: Unknown; however, in some reported cases condition appears to exhibit a hereditary tendency.

Pathogenesis: Invagination of dental lamina of tooth germ, resulting in double crown ranging in morphology from accessory cusp to bifid appearance.

Related Facts
I **Sex Ratio:** Probably M1:F1
II **Risk of Occurrence:** Rare
III **Risk of Recurrence for**
  Patient's Sib: ?
  Patient's Child: ?
IV **Age of Detectability:** Very variable, depending upon age of calcification of affected tooth. Detected preeruptively on radiographs or posteruptively on clinical examination.
V **Prevalence:** Very low

Treatment
I **Primary Prevention:** —
II **Secondary Prevention:** —
III **Other Therapy:** a) Extract affected tooth,† b) appropriate restoration of tooth crown, if possible, c) removal of minimally (?) affected part of crown, d) leave tooth undisturbed.

Prognosis: This depends upon extent and location of coronal separation, extent of occlusal disharmony and periodontal condition of affected tooth. A minimally involved tooth with good occlusion and a healthy periodontium has an excellent prognosis. Affected teeth with malocclusion or periodontal pathology have poor prognosis. Condition does not appear to affect longevity of patient.

Detection of Carrier: —

†Special Considerations: Presence of succedaneous tooth should be ascertained prior to removing affected primary tooth. Endodontic therapy may be difficult, if root canal is partially divided. It is not always possible to differentiate between gemination and a case in which there has been fusion between a normal tooth and a supernumerary tooth.

References:

Large, N. D.: Anomalies of the teeth and regressive alterations of the teeth. In Tiecke, R.W. (ed.): Oral Pathology, 1st Ed. New York: McGraw-Hill, 1965, p. 235.

Levitas, T.C.: Gemination, twinning, fusion and concrescence. J. Dent. Child. 32(2):93, 1965.

Contributors: **Louise Brearley Messer**
Jay T. Cline
Paul O. Walker

Editor's Computerized Descriptor: Teeth
Also see Section I, Fig. 87

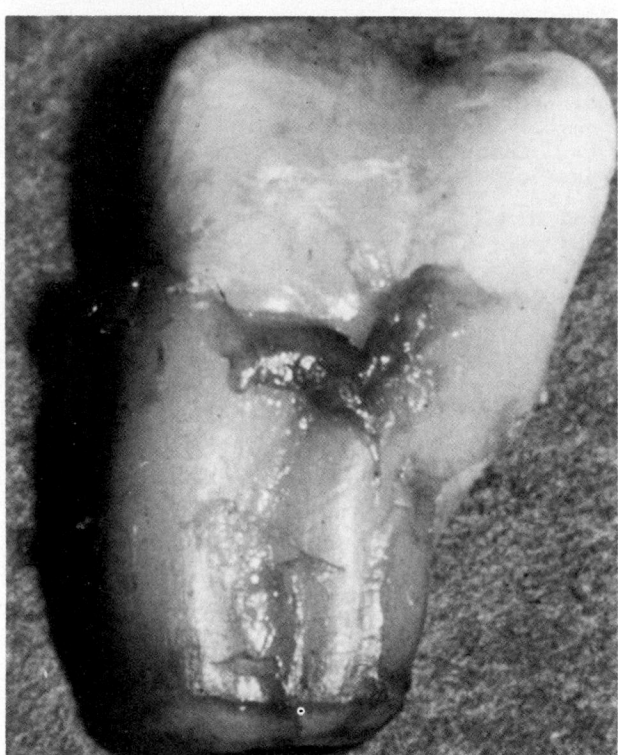

473. Geminated maxillary permanent lateral incisor

Includes: Dents incluses
Impaktierte Zähne
Dientes en inclusión
Impacted Teeth

Excludes: Teeth, geminated (931)
Teeth, fused (930)
Teeth, concrescence of roots (928)
Teeth, ankylosed (927)
Teeth, dilacerated (929)
Dens in dente (276)

Minimal Diagnostic Criteria: A clinically unerupted but radiographically apparent tooth which has failed to erupt within acceptable time limits.

Clinical Findings: An impacted tooth is clinically unerupted but visible in normal or malposed position on radiograph and may have normal or abnormal morphology. A completely impacted tooth lies entirely encased within bone; a partially impacted tooth lies partly enclosed in both hard and soft tissues. Any tooth may become impacted; teeth most commonly involved are maxillary 3rd molars (22%), mandibular 3rd molars (18%), maxillary cuspids (0.9%), followed by premolars and supernumerary teeth. The mandibular 3rd molars are more apt to exhibit severe impaction than the maxillary 3rd molars. Third molars may be sagittally positioned as follows: mesioangular, distoangular, vertical or horizontal, complicated by buccal or lingual deflection. The 3rd molars may also be inverted with the crown pointing toward the inferior border of the mandible, or with the 3rd molar situated completely within the ramus of the mandible. Maxillary cuspids may assume a variety of positions from horizontal to vertical.

Complications

I **Derived:** A completely impacted tooth may cause resorption of root structure of adjacent tooth and has been reported to be the etiologic factor in cases of periodic pain, trismus and various types of referred pain. Lack of tooth function in arch may produce loss of arch length, malocclusion or periodontal pathology of adjacent or opposing teeth. Radiolucencies of bone around crowns of impacted teeth have been reported (mandibular 3rd molars 37%, maxillary 3rd molars 15%). Dentigerous cysts may develop around these teeth, causing severe bone destruction.

II **Associated:** Partially impacted (but not completely impacted) teeth may become carious or the surrounding tissues become infected. Occasionally impacted teeth allowed to remain in situ may undergo resorption. Rarely ameloblastomas have been reported to develop from dentigerous cysts associated with impacted teeth.

Etiology: ? Abnormalities of jaw and tooth size and relationships, resulting in impeded tooth eruption, may be genetically transmitted or induced by radiation, trauma, infection or local physical barriers. Premature loss of a primary tooth may result in loss of space for the succedaneous tooth which may become impacted.

Pathogenesis: Initial event may be known. Histologic examination may reveal normal appearance of developing tooth, dysgenesis of crown or of root formation; or associated dentigerous cyst or ameloblastoma. Associated functional disorders may occur.

Related Facts
I **Sex Ratio:** Probably M1:F1
II **Risk of Occurrence:** ?
III **Risk of Recurrence for**
  Patient's Sib: Not increased
  Patient's Child: ?
IV **Age of Detectability:** Can be detected radiographically following calcification of tooth crown.

Prevalence: 1 in 6 of United States population over 20 years of age have been reported to have at least 1 impacted tooth.

Treatment

I Primary Prevention: Maintenance of a healthy primary and young permanent dentition will help prevent premature loss of primary teeth and subsequent loss of space.

II Secondary Prevention: Mechanical space maintenance to prevent loss of space after premature extraction of primary teeth.†

III Other Therapy: a) Surgical removal of impacted tooth, b) removal of physical barrier to allow tooth eruption, c) orthodontic treatment to guide impacted/associated teeth into proper occlusion or to regain lost space, or d) leave tooth undisturbed.

Prognosis: With treatment: orthodontic or surgical correction produces an excellent prognosis for the establishment and maintenance of good occlusion. Without treatment: affected tooth may stimulate bone or root resorption or be subject to infection, dentigerous cyst formation, or development of an ameloblastoma. Development of infection or dentigerous cyst formation leading to ameloblastoma may be life-threatening.

Detection of Carrier: —

†Special Considerations: Early diagnosis of impaction will assist in avoiding complications and selection of appropriate treatment.

References:

Aitasalo, K. et al: An orthopantomographic study of prevalence of impacted teeth. Int. J. Oral Surg. 1:117, 1972.

Dachi, S. F. and Howell, F. V.: A survey of 3,874 routine full-mouth radiographs. II. A study of impacted teeth. Oral Surg. 14:1165, 1961.

Winter, G. B.: Principles of Exodontia as Applied to the Impacted Mandibular Third Molar. St. Louis:American Medical Book Co., 1926.

Contributors: **Jay T. Cline**
Louise Brearley Messer
D. H. McKibben, Jr.

Editor's Computerized Descriptor: Teeth

TEETH, NATAL OR NEONATAL

Includes: Persistance des dents temporaires
Persistierendes Milchgebiss
Persistencia de dientes temporarios
Neonatal or natal teeth
Natal or neonatal teeth

Excludes: Cleidocranial dysplasia (185)
Intestinal polyposis III (536)
Odontoma

Minimal Diagnostic Criteria: Natal teeth are present in the mouth at birth. Neonatal teeth erupt from birth to 30 days after birth.

Clinical Findings: Two types are found: natal teeth (predeciduous supernumerary tooth represented by a cap of enamel and dentin); and early eruption of deciduous teeth (usually neonatal teeth). At birth natal teeth usually appear to be perched on a pad of soft tissue above gum level, whereas the neonatal teeth are covered by a cap of gum tissue. As at this stage in their development only the crown would be formed, these teeth are freely mobile and this might explain the inflamed appearance of the ragged tissue around the tooth cervical region. Natal teeth may resemble the normal deciduous teeth or the teeth may be poorly developed, differing from the normal deciduous teeth as to:

size	smaller than normal
shape	conical; deformed
color	yellowish; greyish; brownish
enamel	hypoplastic; carious

surface texture	cartilaginous
transparency	opaque
position	rotated;inclined
root formation	beginning or lack of root formation

Some neonatal teeth are supernumerary teeth while others are prematurely erupted deciduous teeth.

Complications

I Derived: Refusal on the part of the child to nurse, or ulcer of tongue or lip. Inconvenience to the mother during suckling, or ulcer of nipple.

II Associated: Natal teeth occur in cyclopia (here as a single fused tooth in the midline of the maxilla), reported in 25% of cases of chondroectodermal dysplasia but this figure is probably low. Also reported in oculomandibulodyscephaly, pachyonychia congenita and osteogenesis imperfecta.

Etiology: ? Condition reported as familial among Tlinget Indians.

Pathogenesis: ? Generally the anomaly relates to early erupting teeth of the normal deciduous set, rarely supernumerary teeth. Has been attributed to the superficial positioning of the tooth germ.

Related Facts

I Sex Ratio: M1:F1+

II Risk of Occurrence: In Britain and USA (Chicago) the incidence would appear to be in the region of 1 in 2000 live births. In Denmark the incidence appears to be at least 1 in 3000 live births. Natal teeth/neonatal teeth: 4:1. Natal and neonatal teeth in the mandible/in the maxilla: 10:1. Highest reported incidence Tlinget Indians, Alaska: 1 in 9.

III Risk of Recurrence for
    Patient's Sib: Data incomplete. Among Tlinget Indians at least 1 other sib affected in 66.7% of families studied.
    Patient's Child: ?

IV Age of Detectability: Natal teeth - at birth. Neonatal teeth - 1st-30th day of life by visual examination, supplemented in doubtful cases by xrays.

V Prevalence: ?

Treatment

I   **Primary Prevention:** —
II   **Secondary Prevention:** —
III **Other Therapy:** Extraction should not be undertaken arbitrarily on account of the risk of bleeding and because the teeth concerned may be deciduous teeth. The teeth are seldom firmly fixed and can easily be removed with forceps or by ligation. However, the following points should be observed: as far as possible no extraction until after the 10th postnatal day so as to avoid excessive hemorrhage; administration of vitamin K (according to the child's age); attention should be paid to the risk of the teeth being aspirated or swallowed.

Prognosis: Normal for life span, intelligence and function

Detection of Carrier: —

Special Considerations: —

References:

Bodenhoff, J.: Dentitio connatalis et neonatalis. Odontol. T. 67:645, 1959.
Gardiner, J. H.: Erupted teeth in the newborn. Proc. R. Soc. Med. 54:504, 1961.
Massler, M. and Savara, B. S.: Natal and neonatal teeth; review of 24 cases reported in literature. J. Pediatr. 36:349, 1950.
Mayhall, J. T.: Natal and neonatal teeth among the Tlinget Indians. J. Dent. Res. 46:748, 1967.

Contributor: **Jessie Bodenhoff**

Editor's Computerized Descriptor: Teeth

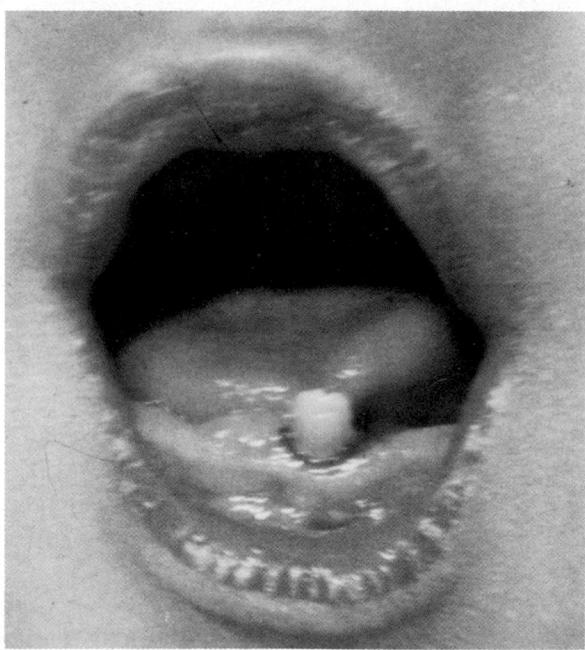

474. Natal tooth

TEETH, PEGGED OR ABSENT MAXILLARY LATERAL INCISOR

Includes: Agénésie congénitale des incisives latérales supérieures
Konisch deformierte oder Aplasie der lateralen oberen Schneidezähne
Inclusión o ausencia congénita de los incisivos laterales
Pegged or missing maxillary lateral incisor teeth and congenitally missing premolars
Hypodontia of maxillary lateral incisor teeth

Excludes: Hypodontia with Down syndrome
Hypodontia with cleft lip
Oligodontia
Pegged or congenitally missing teeth associated with syndromes
Microdontia (Marker) (660)

Minimal Diagnostic Criteria: Small maxillary lateral incisors.

Clinical Findings: The trait has variable expression such that the maxillary lateral incisor teeth may be small, peg-shaped or congenitally missing. Various degrees and combinations as to right or left side may occur within individuals and within kindreds. Teeth in both dentitions may be affected but the secondary teeth are most commonly affected.

Complications

I   **Derived:** Diastema of maxillary central incisors, or diastema between canines and central incisors. Drifting of teeth.
II   **Associated:** From 10-20% of patients with this trait also show congenital absence of premolar teeth and a higher incidence of pegged or congenitally missing 3rd molar teeth than those without the trait.

Etiology: Autosomal dominant gene in most examples.

Pathogenesis: Absence or reduction in size of tooth germ.

Related Facts

I   **Sex Ratio:** Probably M1:F1 for any expression of the gene. Observed M1:F1.4†
II   **Risk of Occurrence:** ?
III **Risk of Recurrence for**
     Patient's Sib: 1 in 2 (50%) for each offspring, if parent is affected; otherwise not increased.
     Patient's Child: 1 in 2
IV   **Age of Detectability:** Up to 8 years of age for permanent dentition
V   **Prevalence:** Caucasians: 1-3%

Treatment

I   **Primary Prevention:** — (Innocuous trait)
II   **Secondary Prevention:** —
III **Other Therapy:** Prosthetic replacement and orthodontic treatment

Prognosis: Normal life span

Detection of Carrier: —

†Special Considerations: While the trait shows an autosomal dominant inheritance pattern, the expression shows a threshold effect for missing teeth, ie below a certain size the pegged tooth gene seems to be expressed as a missing tooth and does not show smaller and smaller pegged teeth. At the other end of the continuum of tooth size, kindred studies show persons with normal sized lateral incisiors who apparently can pass the gene to offspring. The ratio between pegged and missing teeth varies by population; Swedes 1:1, U.S. Caucasians 1:1, Orientals 1:0.09. In U.S. Caucasians a 2:1 preference for the left side is reported. The author has seen several families in which both parents had pegged permanent maxillary lateral incisors and the children had severe oligodontia involving primarily agenesis of succedaneous permanent teeth. These kindreds are compatible with the hypothesis of the homozygous expression of the gene.

References:
Jöhr, A.C.: Reduktionserscheinungen an den oberen seitlichen Schneidezähnen. Arch. Klaus-Stift. Vereb.-Forsch. 9:73, 1935.

Meskin, L.H. and Gorlin, R.J.: Agenesis and peg-shaped permanent maxillary lateral incisors. J. Dent. Res. 42:1476, 1963.

Sutter, J.: L'Atteinte des incisives latérales supérieures. Étude d'une mutation à l'échelle démographique. Presse Universitaires de France, Paris, 1966.

Witkop, C.J., Jr.: Studies of intrinsic disease in isolates with observations on penetrance and expressivity of certain anatomical traits. In Pruzansky, S. (ed.): Congenital Anomalies of the Face and Associated Structures. Springfield: Charles C Thomas, 1963.

Contributor: **Carl J. Witkop, Jr.**

Editor's Computerized Descriptor: Teeth

Also see Section I, Fig. 83.

TEETH, SNOW-CAPPED

Includes: Anomalie de l'émail
Schneebedeckte Zähne
Dientes nevados

Excludes: Amelogenesis imperfecta (46)
Fluorosis

Minimal Diagnostic Criteria: White opaque enamel on incisal 1/4 of all maxillary incisor teeth†

Clinical Findings: Clinically, the occlusal in incisal 1/4 to 1/2 of crowns of teeth exhibit a white opaque hypomature enamel, the distribution of the affected teeth runs anterior-posteriorly and does not follow the developmental sequence of the crowns of the teeth. Observed in teeth of both dentitions.

Complications
I **Derived:** —
II **Associated:** —

Etiology: Possibly a gene mutation resulting in an autosomal dominantly inherited trait. Has been observed in large kindreds compatible with an autosomal dominant trait and in 10 sibships where approximately half of sibs were affected but where parents could not be examined.

Pathogenesis: Ground sections of teeth show spaces usually occupied by enamel rod sheaths in the superficial layer of enamel.

Related Facts
I **Sex Ratio:** M1:F1
II **Risk of Occurrence:** —
III **Risk of Recurrence for**
    Patient's Sib: If parent is affected 1 in 2 (50%) for each offspring to be affected; otherwise not increased
    Patient's Child: 1 in 2
IV **Age of Detectability:** Visual examination after eruption of permanent incisors from 7 to 9 years of age
V **Prevalence:** 1 in 2000 in general population of United States

Treatment
I **Primary Prevention:** Genetic counseling
II **Secondary Prevention:** —
III **Other Therapy:** —

Prognosis: Excellent, no evidence for decreased longevity

Detection of Carrier: —

†**Special Considerations:** Must be differentiated from fluorosis which has a bright sheen while snow-capped teeth are dull white and also occur in nonfluoride areas. The defect may affect any group of teeth in an anterior-posterior relationship starting from incisors, ie incisors and canine or incisors, canine, first premolars; or incisors, canine, first premolars, second premolars, etc. Sibs frequently affected.

References:
Witkop, C. J., Jr.: Genetic disease of the oral cavity. In Tiecke, R.W. (ed.): Oral Pathology. New York:McGraw-Hill, 1965, p. 786.

Witkop, C.J., Jr. and Sauk, J.J., Jr.: Defects of enamel. In Stewart, R.E. and Prescott, G.H. (eds.): Oral Facial Genetics. St. Louis:C.V. Mosby Co., 1976.

Contributor: **Carl J. Witkop, Jr.**

Editor's Computerized Descriptor: Teeth

TEETH, SUPERNUMERARY (MARKER)

Includes: Dents surnuméraires
Überzählige Zähne
Dientes supernumerarios (Marcador)
Mesiodens†
Distomolar†
Peridens†
Paramolar†
Supernumerary teeth (Marker)

Excludes: Intestinal polyposis III (536)
Cleidocranial dysplasia (185)
Odontomas

Minimal Diagnostic Criteria: The tooth or teeth must be in excess of the number of teeth in the normal dental formula as evident in the oral cavity or in appropriate radiograph.

Clinical Findings: The tooth or teeth are in excess of the number in the normal dental formula. They are present both in the primary and secondary dentitions, though they are less frequent in the primary dentition.

Though the teeth may be located anywhere in the 2 jaws, they are predominantly found in the maxilla. The most common site being between the 2 maxillary central incisors. They are also found in the 3rd molar region in the maxilla and the bicuspid region in the mandible. They may or may not be erupted in the oral cavity.

The shape is normal, conical or tuberculate. The size is usually smaller than the tooth they resemble.

Complications
I   **Derived:** When erupted, may cause malposition and malocclusion of the adjacent teeth, the reported frequency being 0.1%. When unerupted, they may cause resorption of roots of adjacent teeth or impede the normal eruption pattern. Follicle of supernumerary tooth may undergo cystic degeneration.
II **Associated:** —

Etiology: Essentially unknown. Possibly a polygenic trait in most instances. When associated with cleidocranial dysplasia and intestinal polyposis III, due to a gene mutation resulting in an autosomal dominantly inherited trait.

Pathogenesis: ?

Related Facts
I   **Sex Ratio:** M2:F1
II   **Risk of Occurrence:** ?
III **Risk of Recurrence for**
     Patient's Sib: ?
     Patient's Child: ?
IV   **Age of Detectability:** When the patient is subjected to a competent dental examination. For primary dentition: after formation of primary dentition, 3 to 4 years, by x-ray examination. For permanent dentition: after complete formation of secondary dentition, 9 to 12 years, by x-ray examination.
V   **Prevalence:** 1 in 330 to 1 in 28 in general population. In permanent dentition 1% of 48,550 complete radiographic examinations. In Scotland (Glasgow- 1935) 0.3% of 4000 school children. In U.S.A. (Kansas 1945-57) 2.4% of 3557 school children. Maxilla - 90%. Mandible - 10%.

Treatment
I   **Primary Prevention:** —
II   **Secondary Prevention:** Extraction or surgical removal
III **Other Therapy:** —

Prognosis: Excellent

Detection of Carrier: —

†Special Considerations: When the supernumerary tooth is located between the 2 maxillary central incisors, it is called a "mediodens." When it is located in the 3rd molar region, it is called a "distomolar." When the tooth erupts outside the dental arches, it is called a "peridens." When it is located buccal or lingual to one of the maxillary molars or interproximally between any of the maxillary molars, it is called a "paramolar." Supernumerary teeth occur in high frequency in cleidocranial dysplasia and intestinal polyposis III.

References:
Clayton, J. M.: Congenital dental anomalies occurring in 3,557 children. J. Dent. Child. 23:206, 1957.
Schulze, C.: Developmental abnormalities of the teeth and jaws. In Gorlin, R.J. and Goldman, H.M. (eds.): Thoma's Oral Pathology, 6th Ed. St. Louis:C.V. Mosby Co., 1970, vol. 1, p. 96.
Stevenson, W. and McKechnie, A.D.: Recurring supernumerary teeth. Oral Surg. 40:76, 1975.
Sugimura, M. et al: Mandibular distomolars. Oral Surg. 40:341, 1975.
Sykaras, S.N.: Mesiodens in primary and permanent dentitions. Oral Surg. 40:870, 1975.

Contributor: **Satish R. Rao**

Editor's Computerized Descriptor: Teeth

TEETH, THISTLE-SHAPED PULP CHAMBERS

Includes: Chambre pulpaire (en fleur de chardon)
Distelförmige Pulpa
Cámara pulpar dentaria en llama
Flame-shaped pulp chambers

Excludes: Dentin dysplasia, coronal† (277)
Taurodontism (926)
Hypophosphatemia (517)
Shell teeth

Minimal Diagnostic Criteria: Large thistle-shaped pulp chambers on radiographs.

Clinical Findings: Teeth appear normal clinically. Radiographically, they have large flame- or thistle-shaped pulp chambers that extend into the radicular part of the tooth. Pulp stones are rare.

Complications
I   **Derived:** —
II **Associated:** —

Etiology: ? Autosomal dominant

Pathogenesis: ?

Related Facts
I   **Sex Ratio:** Probably M1:F1. Actually M6:F2
II **Risk of Occurrence:** —
III **Risk of Recurrence for**
    Patient's Sib: If parent is affected 1 in 2 (50%) for each offspring to be affected; otherwise not increased.
    Patient's Child: 1 in 2
IV **Age of Detectability:** After development of roots of anterior teeth; 1-2 years of age by radiographs.
V   **Prevalence:** Rare. Two kindreds known.

Treatment
I   **Primary Prevention:** Genetic counseling
II **Secondary Prevention:** —
III **Other Therapy:** —

Prognosis: No effect reported on longevity

Detection of Carrier: —

†Special Considerations: Must be differentiated from coronal dentin dysplasia which has opalescent primary teeth, and secondary teeth with flame-shaped pulp chambers and multiple pulp stones.

References:
Witkop, C.J., Jr.: Hereditary defects in dentin. Dent. Clin. North Am. 19:25, 1975.

Contributors: **Carl J. Witkop, Jr.**
                   Albert M. Abrams

Editor's Computerized Descriptor: Teeth

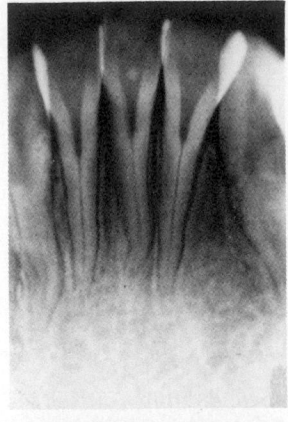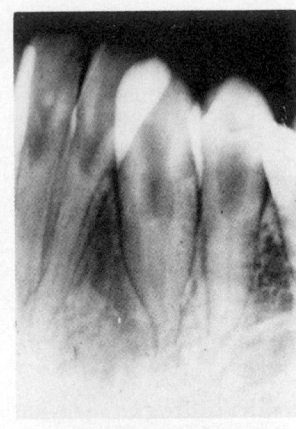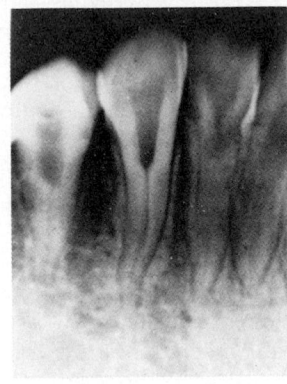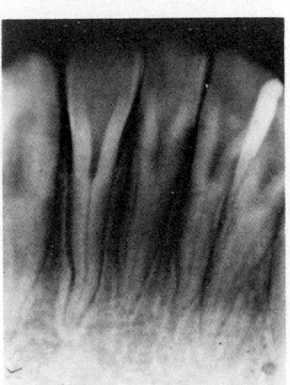

475. Thistle-shaped pulp chambers

TETRALOGY OF FALLOT

Includes: Tétralogie de Fallot
Fallotsche Tetralogie
Tetralogía de Fallot
Infracristal ventricular septal defect with overriding aorta and infundibular pulmonary atresia or stenosis
Fallot tetrad

Excludes: Pulmonary atresia with intact ventricular septum
Ventricular septal defect and pulmonary valve stenosis in the presence of a normal crista

Minimal Diagnostic Criteria: Cyanosis, systolic murmur, single second sound, normal heart size, right ventricular hypertrophy on the ECG suggest tetralogy of Fallot. A right aortic arch in addition strengthens the diagnosis. Selective right ventricular angiocardiography is confirmatory.

Clinical Findings: The pathologic anatomy of this lesion consists of the combination of a large ventricular septal defect (VSD) and narrowing of the infundibulum. The right ventricular outflow tract stenosis may occur at the ostium of the infundibulum or may consist of a diminutive infundibulum throughout with a small annulus of the pulmonary valve. Valvar stenosis occurs in association with infundibular narrowing in 25% of patients. Medial papillary muscle of the tricuspid is absent.

Since the VSD is large, variations in the physiologic state depend upon the severity of the infundibular stenosis, which is the primary regulator of pulmonary blood flow. The course may be variable. The onset of cyanosis during the 1st month of life is associated with a severe course and progressive cyanosis. Most patients demonstrate cyanosis during the first 6 months; this usually becomes accentuated over 1-3 years. Clubbing of the fingers and toes may be present in cyanotic patients after 6 months of age. A loud systolic murmur over the upper left sternal border is characteristic; with severe tetralogy and marked diminution in pulmonary blood flow, the murmur may be short and of low intensity. The second sound is single and accentuated (due to aortic valve closure). Continuous murmurs may be present after infancy and indicate collateral circulation via bronchial arteries or the presence of a patent ductus arteriosus.

Roentgenographic findings demonstrate a normal size heart with a normal to slightly enlarged heart and concavity in area of main pulmonary artery. A right aortic arch is present in 25% of patients. Left atrial enlargement is absent. With increasing degree of diminished pulmonary blood flow, pulmonary vascular markings are commensurately diminished. With marked increase in collateral blood flow through bronchial arteries, the lung fields present a reticular appearance.

ECG shows right ventricular hypertrophy and right axis deviation. Right atrial hypertrophy may be evident.

Echocardiographic findings parallel those of recognized anatomic derangement. The aorta is enlarged and aortic intercusp distance is increased. The anterior aortic wall is displaced anteriorly with respect to the ventricular septum and is not in continuity with it. This discontinuity represents an override. Additionally, the area of the discontinuity is the area of the VSD. Right ventricular anterior wall is thickened and the right ventricular outflow tract is narrow. The pulmonary valve may be found in some patients and its presence rules out a truncus arteriosus and pulmonary atresia. In other patients, the pulmonary valve is present but difficult to image. The right pulmonary artery is usually small, but may be of normal size. Left atrial

size usually reflects pulmonary blood flow.

Cardiac catheterization with selective angiocardiography confirms the presence of a VSD and clarifies the anatomy of the infundibular stenosis. Oxygen saturation data and indicator dilution curves indicate the pulmonary blood flow and degree of right-to-left shunt.

Complications
I **Derived:** Episodes of paroxysmal hyperpnea with death from severe episodes, brain abscess, bacterial endocarditis, cerebral thrombosis
II **Associated:** Down syndrome for mongolism

Etiology: Multifactorial inheritance

Pathogenesis: Due primarily to displacement of the conus septum anteriorly which produces infundibular stenosis. This results in inability to form the normal crista supraventricularis and to close the interventricular septum.

Related Facts
I **Sex Ratio:** M3:F2
II **Risk of Occurrence:** 10% of congenital heart disease
III **Risk of Recurrence for**
  Patient's Sib: Predicted risk 3.2%; Empiric risk 2.7%
  Patient's Child: Predicted risk 3.2%; Empiric risk 4.2%
IV **Age of Detectability:** From birth by selective angiocardiography
V **Prevalence:** ? 1:1000 in pediatric population

Treatment
I **Primary Prevention:** Genetic counseling
II **Secondary Prevention:** Definitive surgery with infundibulectomy and closure of ventricular defect. Surgical palliation with anastomosis of subclavian-to-pulmonary artery (Blalock-Taussig operation), anastomosis of ascending aorta to pulmonary artery (Waterston-Cooley procedure).
III **Other Therapy:** Treatment of paroxysmal hyperpnea episodes and prevention of dehydration.

Prognosis: The prognosis closely depends upon the severity of pulmonary stenosis and resultant degree of cyanosis. With palliative surgical intervention in infants, the prognosis is good. Infants who survive to undergo definitive surgical repair have good prognosis. Those who persist with marked cyanosis have marked debilitation throughout childhood and poor prognosis after adolescence.†

Detection of Carrier: —

†Special Considerations: Recent marked improvements in definitive and palliative operations have considerably improved the salvage rate of severely cyanotic infants.

References:
Chung, K.J. et al: Echocardiographic findings in tetralogy of Fallot. Am. J. Cardiol. 31:126, 1973.
Goldberg, S.J. et al: Pediatric and Adolescent Echocardiography. Chicago:Year Book Publishers, 1975.
Guntheroth, W.G.: Tetralogy of Fallot. In Moss, A.J. and Adams, F.H (eds.): Heart Disease in Infants, Children, and Adolescents. Baltimore: Williams & Wilkins, Co., 1968, p. 431.
Kirklin, J.W. et al: Early and late results after intracardiac repair of tetralogy of Fallot; 5-year review of 337 patients. Ann. Surg. 162:578, 1965.
Morgan, B.C. et al: A clinical profile of paroxysmal hyperpnea in cyanotic congenital heart disease. Circulation 31:66, 1965.

Contributor: **Madison S. Spach**

Editor's Computerized Descriptors: Resp., CV.

Includes: Thalassémie
Thalassämie
Talasemia
Cooley anemia
Microcythemia
Mediterranean anemia
Hemoglobin Lepore syndromes
Syndromes of hereditary persistence of fetal hemoglobin (some forms)

Excludes: Hematologic disease related to nutritional deficiency
Vitamin B_6 dependency (991)
Sideroblastic (siderochrestic) anemias

Minimal Diagnostic Criteria: Varies with type as indicated below and in Section III, Table XI. In general, clinically significant forms of β thalassemia are accompanied by "compensatory" changes, expressed as an increase in the percentage of hemoglobins A_2 or F. Forms of α thalassemia associated with moderate to severe clinical disease often are accompanied by the presence of abnormal hemoglobins composed entirely of non-α chains. These include hemoglobin H (β_4) and hemoglobin Bart (γ_4).†

Clinical Findings: All clinically significant forms of thalassemia are accompanied by anemia and erythrocyte microcytosis. Anemia may vary from very mild to a degree of severity sufficient to require periodic transfusions in order to sustain life. The hematologic and clinical features of some of the more common forms of thalassemia are indicated in Section III, Table XI. Also see Derived Complications. Clinical features of major forms of thalassemia by type include:

β Severe, heterozygous; possible splenomegaly and mild icterus

α_1/α_2, heterozygous; pallor, jaundice, hepatosplenomegaly

β Severe, homozygous; pallor, jaundice, bone deformities with abnormal facies, hepatosplenomegaly, usually transfusion-dependent

β Mild, homozygous; pallor, hepatosplenomegaly, jaundice; transfusions not usually required

$\beta\delta$ homozygous; mild jaundice, hepatosplenomegaly usually present

α Severe, homozygous; hydrops fetalis with severe edema, hepatosplenomegaly, congestive heart failure; stillbirth or death within first 24 hr. Hematologic changes of major forms of thalassemia by type include:

β Severe, heterozygous; erythrocyte microcytosis and hypochromia, mild-to-moderate anemia

β Mild, heterozygous; erythrocyte microcytosis and hypochromia, mild or absent anemia

$\beta\delta$ heterozygous; erythrocyte microcytosis and hypochromia, mild or absent anemia α Severe, heterozygous; erythrocyte microcytosis and hypochromia, mild anemia

α_1/α_2, heterozygous; erythrocyte hypochromia, poikilocytosis, anisocytosis; inclusion bodies demonstrable by supravital staining; moderate anemia

β Severe, homozygous; markedly abnormal red cell morphology with microcytosis and hypochromia, nucleated red cells, severe anemia β Mild, homozygous; poikilocytosis, anisocytosis, target cells; moderate anemia

$\beta\delta$, homozygous; poikilocytosis, anisocytosis, hypochromia, microcytosis; mild-to-moderate anemia

α Severe, homozygous; red cell hypochromia, anisocytosis, poikilocytosis; severe anemia

Complications
I **Derived:** *Anemia:* "Ineffective erythropoiesis" is character-

istic of severe forms of thalassemia. The bone marrow erythroid elements are greatly increased, and utilization of iron and other erythropoietic nutrients is accelerated significantly, but inadequate numbers of mature erythrocytes are released into the peripheral blood. This series of events is thought to result from intramedullary destruction of erythroid precursors. In addition to the disordered erythropoiesis in these conditions, a major hemolytic component is also present, attributed to enhanced reticuloendothelial trapping of erythrocytes as a result of inclusion body formation. The red cell inclusions represent precipitated globin material, resulting from the unbalanced synthesis of complementary (α and non-α) globin chains of hemoglobin.

Enlargement of Liver and Spleen: These changes result from several associated features of thalassemia. These include extramedullary hematopoiesis, congestive changes related to anemia and myocardial dysfunction, and proliferation of reticuloendothelial elements due to hemosiderin engorgement.

Cortical Thinning of Bone with Associated Fractures and Deformities: These changes appear to be related to the massive expansion of erythroid bone marrow.

Iron Overload: As a result of chronic anemia, patients with severe forms of thalassemia absorb considerably increased quantities of iron. For this reason, and particularly because of the large quantities of iron that are derived from blood transfusions, these patients often develop severe complications including liver dysfunction with cirrhosis, pancreatic iron loading which in some cases is associated with overt diabetes, and myocardial dysfunction which, not infrequently, leads to the development of intractable arrhythmias and death.

II **Associated:** —

Etiology: The thalassemia disorders all represent a biosynthetic defect resulting in a deficiency of synthesis of 1 or more of the globin chains of hemoglobin. DNA hybridization studies have shown that α-thalassemia disorders result from deletion of α-chain genes. The β thalassemias can apparently result from β-chain genes deletion or, in some forms, an abnormality of transcription of DNA sequences that correspond to the β-chain structural gene loci.

Pathogenesis: As a result of the genetic abnormalities that underlie these conditions, a biosynthetic deficiency of the affected globin chain occurs. A direct result of this abnormality is the underhemoglobinization of erythroid cells due to the globin deficiency. As an additional consequence a relative excess of the noninvolved globin chain is produced within the hemoglobin synthesizing cells. Because uncombined globin chains are unstable in solution, this globin material undergoes intracellular precipitation, leading to inclusion body formation. This in turn leads to greatly accelerated cellular destruction, with a major hemolytic process that greatly aggravates the primary degree of anemia.

Related Facts
I **Sex Ratio:** M1:F1
II **Risk of Occurrence:** The thalassemias occur predominantly in tropical and subtropical areas of Europe, Africa, and Asia. In regions of high gene frequency an occurrence of greater than 1 per 100 births has been documented. All forms of thalassemias are uncommon in Northern European and in Western Hemispheric native populations.
III **Risk of Recurrence for**
   Patient's Sib: 1 in 4 (25%) for each offspring to be affected.
   Patient's Child: No risk except for signs of carrier state if spouse does not carry the gene for thalassemia.
IV **Age of Detectability:** All forms of α thalassemia are fully expressed and detectable at birth. Antenatal detection in the 2nd trimester fetus has been accomplished by DNA hybridization studies using fetal cells derived from amniotic fluid.
   The β thalassemias are normally not clinically expressed until 3-6 months of age. Detection at birth and prenatal detection in 2nd trimester fetus accomplished by globin synthe-

sis studies.

V Prevalence: Highly variable depending on population group.

Treatment
I Primary Prevention: Genetic counseling
II Secondary Prevention: In the patient with severe β thalassemia periodic transfusions may be required to sustain life. By application of "hypertransfusion" regimens, whereby transfusions are administered to a sufficient degree and at frequent intervals so as to maintain a near normal hemoglobin concentration in the blood, many of the secondary complications, particularly cardiac dysfunction and skeletal changes, can be largely prevented. This form of therapy, however, serves to increase the degree of iron storage.
III Other Therapy: Treatment directed toward minimizing iron storage is coming to assume increased importance in transfusion-dependent forms of thalassemia. Desferrioxamine and other iron chelating agents are given by injection, or preferably, by long-term infusion for this purpose.

Prognosis: The application of intensive transfusion therapy in patients with severe β thalassemia has greatly improved the quality of life for these patients, but the increased iron burden that this form of therapy produces has come to represent the major cause of death of these patients, as a result of cardiac or hepatic failure. Median survival for the transfusion-dependent thalassemia patient is now approximately 20 years, but with the recent introduction of improved methods of chelation therapy, increased survival hopefully will be achieved.

Detection of Carrier: Most forms of heterozygous α and β thalassemia are accompanied by microcytosis, mild anemia, and morphologic abnormalities of the erythrocytes. "Silent-carrier" forms of these disorders have also been identified (see Table XI, Section III), and these individuals may have no apparent hematologic abnormality. Heterozygous β thalassemia can be confirmed by the findings of elevated levels of hemoglobins A_2 or F. The heterozygous forms of α thalassemia, on the other hand, typically have no abnormality of hemoglobin composition, and usually require an investigation of family members and studies of globin chain synthesis by erythroid cells in vitro for confirmation of this diagnosis. Some of the forms of hereditary persistence of fetal hemoglobin may be difficult to distinguish from heterozygous β-thalassemia syndromes.

†Special Considerations: The hemoglobin Lepore syndromes, in which an abnormal hemoglobin type is present of which the non-α chain is a hybrid molecule containing parts of the δ-and β-globin chains fused together, produce the clinical and hematologic features of a thalassemia syndrome. When present in combination with a gene for β thalassemia these syndromes may present as severe, transfusion-dependent thalassemia. The Lepore hemoglobins are identified by electrophoresis, and exhibit a mobility at alkaline pH similar to that of sickle hemoglobin.

References:
Kan, Y.W. et al: Prenatal diagnosis of homozygous β-thalassemia. Lancet 2:790, 1975.
Propper, R.D. et al: Reassessment of the use of desferrioxamine B in iron overload. N. Engl. J. Med. 294:1421, 1976.
Propper, R.D. et al: Continuous subcutaneous administration of deferoxamine in patients with iron overload. N. Engl. J. Med. 297:418, 1977.
Weatherall, D.J. and Clegg, J.B.: The Thalassemia Syndromes, 2nd Ed. Oxford: Blackwell Scientific Publications, 1972.

Contributors: **George R. Honig**
Wayne H. Borges

Editor's Computerized Descriptors: Skin, Skel., CV., Spleen, Liver
Also see Section I, Figs. 106, 107

THANATOPHORIC DYSPLASIA

Includes: Nanisme thanatophore
Thanatophorer Zwergwuchs
Enanismo tanatofórico
Thanatophoric dwarfism

Excludes: Other forms of short-limb dwarfism in newborn
Asphyxiating thoracic dysplasia (91)

Minimal Diagnostic Criteria: Severe neonatal short-limb dwarfism with characteristic radiographic features.†

Clinical Findings: Birth length, 36 to 46 cm. Limbs are very short and extend away from essentially normal size trunk with thighs abducted and externally rotated. The fingers are very short and conical shaped. Head is relatively large with prominent forehead and depressed nasal bridge. The thorax is small and respiratory distress occurs. Numerous skin folds are present. There is hypotonia and primitive reflexes are absent. Death in the first few days is usual.

Radiographic findings include vertebral bodies which have small vertical diameter with narrowest area in the middle of the body in both AP and lateral projections. The intervertebral spaces are large. The posterior vertebrae elements are well ossified. The interpediculate distance is narrowed in the mid- or lower lumbar spine. The ilia have a short vertical dimension. The transverse diameter is greater than the vertical. The inferior margin of the ilia is horizontal and the sacrosciatic notches small. The pubic and ischial bones are broad and short. The thorax is narrow in both AP and transverse diameters with short ribs whose ends are cupped. The long bones are very short, relatively broad and bowed with irregular, spur-like flaring of the metaphyses. Bones of hands and feet are very short and broad. There are no abnormal laboratory findings.

Complications
I Derived: All reported affected infants have died respiratory deaths. On autopsy, some have showed impression on spinal cord by small foramen magnum.
II Associated: —

Etiology: ? Lethal dominant mutation

Pathogenesis: Characteristic generalized disruption of growth plate

Related Facts
I Sex Ratio: Too few cases to be statistically significant
II Risk of Occurrence: ? Rare
III Risk of Recurrence for
  Patient's Sib: Negligible
  Patient's Child: Patients usually die as newborns.
IV Age of Detectability: Newborn by radiographic method
V Prevalence: Patients die as newborns or in early infancy.

Treatment
I Primary Prevention: ?
II Secondary Prevention: ?
III Other Therapy: —

Prognosis: Fatal in newborn period in all reported cases

Detection of Carrier: ?

†Special Considerations: Gross changes of thanatophoric dwarfism appear similar but more marked than those of heterozygous achondroplasia. Presumed cases of homozygous achondroplasia have gross deformity intermediate between those of thanatophoric dwarfism and heterozygous achondroplasia. No infant with changes of thanatophoric dwarfism has been born to a couple with 1 achondroplastic mate. Although several kindreds have been reported with 2 or more sibs with "thanatophoric dwarfism," analysis of their radiographs and chondroosseous histopathology has demonstrated that they are all in fact, examples of achondrogenesis, a known recessive trait. Thus all well-documented cases of thanatophoric dwarfism, to date, have been sporadic and the etiology is unknown.

References:
Langer, L.O., Jr. et al: Thanatophoric dwarfism: A condition confused with achondroplasia in the neonate, with brief comments on achondrogenesis and homozygous achondroplasia. Radiology 92:285, 1969.
Maroteaux, P. et al: Le nanisme thanatophore. Presse Méd. 75:2519, 1967.
Maroteaux, P. et al: The lethal chondrodysplasias. Clin. Orthop. 114:31, 1976.
Rimoin, D.L.: The chondrodystrophies. Adv. Hum. Genet. 5:1, 1975.

Contributors: **David L. Rimoin**
Leonard O. Langer, Jr.

Editor's Computerized Descriptors: Face, Nose, Skin, Skel., Muscle, Resp., Nerve

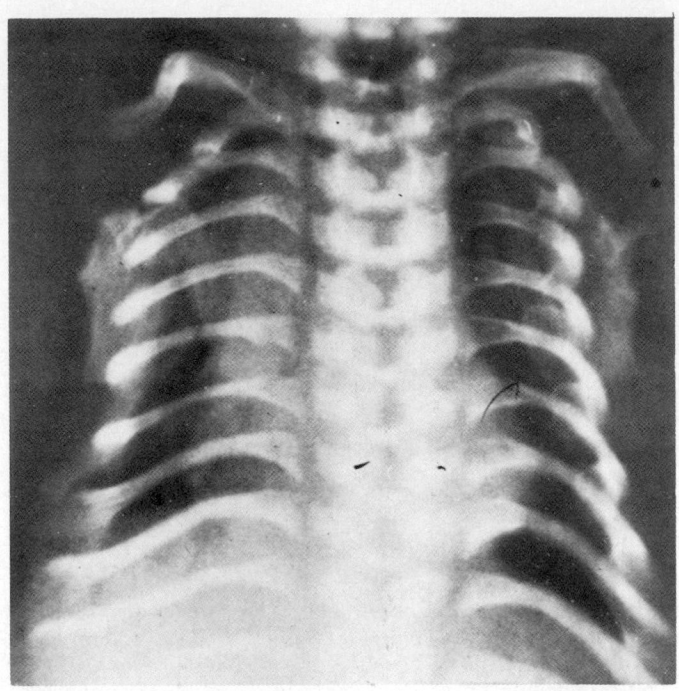

477. Note short ribs; small scapulae; relatively long, bowed clavicles

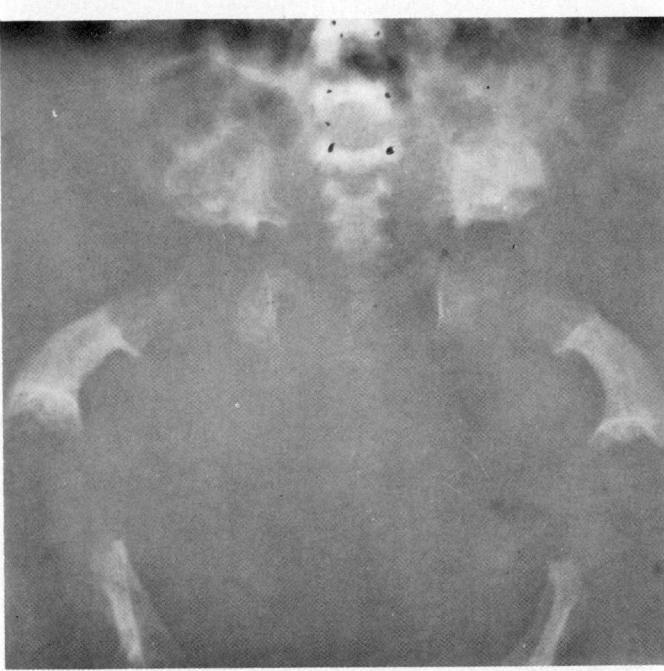

476. Squat pelvis with minute greater sciatic notches; flat acetabula; short, wide, and bowed femurs

THROMBOCYTOPENIA WITH ABSENT RADIUS

Includes: Syndrome de thrombocytopénie avec absence de radius
Thrombocytopenie-Radiusaplasie-Syndrom
Síndrome de ausencia del radio y trombocitopenia
TAR syndrome
Amegakaryocytic thrombocytopenia and bilateral absence of the radii
Congenital thrombocytopenia with aplasia of the radii
Phocomelia with congenital hypoplastic thrombocytopenia
Congenital hypoplastic thrombocytopenia with skeletal deformities
Megakaryocytopenia with radius aplasia
Radius absent and thrombocytopenia

Excludes: Fanconi anemia
Fetal thalidomide syndrome (386)
Heart-hand syndrome (455)
Chromosome eighteen trisomy syndrome (160)

Minimal Diagnostic Criteria: Thrombocytopenia < 100,000 platelets/mm³. Bilateral absence of radius.

Clinical Findings: *Hematologic:* Thrombocytopenia probably 100% at some time. More than 90% have symptoms in first 4 months of life. Megakaryocytes are small basophilic vacuolated and nongranulated when thrombocytopenia present. Thrombocytopenia is episodic, probably sometimes precipitated by stress, infections and surgery. Platelet counts, often 15-30,000 in infancy improve to almost normal range by adulthood. Platelet aggregation and survival reduced.

Leukemoid reactions - recorded in 60-70% of patients during 1st year of life. WBC greater than 35,000 with shift to left. Thrombocytopenia worse during such reactions. Often hepatosplenomegaly during leukemoid reaction.

Eosinophilia - recorded in bone marrow and peripheral smears in more than half the patients.

Anemia - probably hemolytic component, particularly during 1st year of life - frequency unknown. Anemia also related to blood loss.

Skeletal: Radius absent bilaterally in 100% of cases. Hand probably abnormal in all cases with limited extension, radial deviation, hypoplastic carpals and phalanges, but *thumbs always present.* Ulnas probably somewhat shorter and malformed in all cases, absent bilaterally in 20%, unilaterally in 8%. Humerus abnormal in at least half the cases. Absent in 5% resulting in phocomelia. Other anomalies include dislocated hips, tibial torsion, stiff knee, dislocated patella, overriding 5th toe, rib and spine anomalies, hypoplasia of mandible and maxilla, severe reduction of leg long bones (giving tetraphocomelia) reported in one family.

Cardiac anomalies: present in 30%; most common are tetralogy of Fallot and atrial septal defect.

Other anomalies: rare. Mental retardation when intracranial bleeds, glaucoma.

Complications

I   Derived: Significant symptomatic bleeding because of thrombocytopenia; death in 35-40%, almost all associated with bleeding particularly intracranial, almost all before 1 year of age; delayed motor development because of hand deformities, eventually good function, nerve compression and arthritis at older age because of hand malformation; congestive failure secondary to heart defects and anemia; abnormal dermatoglyphics present in all cases, increased frequency of simian lines, decreased flexion creases.

II   Associated: Mental retardation seen in 7% probably secondary to intracranial bleeds; milk allergy may be related and precipitate episodes of thrombocytopenia and hemolysis; diarrheal illness common during 1st year of life.

Etiology: Autosomal recessive pattern of inheritance; however no increased consanguinity or specific ethnic group involvement.† McK *27400

Pathogenesis: ? Gene action must occur early in gestation, between 4th and 8th weeks to affect radial formation, blood-forming elements and chambers of the heart. The condition may be fatal intrauterinely in some affected male embryos.

Related Facts

I   Sex Ratio: M5:F7 observed
II   Risk of Occurrence: Rare
III   Risk of Recurrence for
   Patient's Sib: 1 in 4 (25%) for each offspring to be affected. Intra-and interfamilial variability present with regard to extent of skeletal and cardiac involvement.
   Patient's Child: Not increased unless mate is a relative or also affected. Patients are fertile and no patient-to-child transmission has yet been observed.
IV   Age of Detectability: At birth
V   Prevalence: Over 70 cases are known

Treatment

I   Primary Prevention: Genetic counseling, prenatal diagnosis using xray at 18 weeks of gestation.
II   Secondary Prevention: In desired pregnancy, xrays at term for diagnosis with delivery of affected by cesarean section to avoid trauma. Avoid infections, stress and surgery during 1st year, because these may precipitate severe thrombocytopenia.
III   Other Therapy: Supportive hematologic, ie platelet transfusions, whole blood transfusions; corrective orthopedic, braces on forearms early, surgery if indicated; elimination of milk during infancy if indicated; cardiac - as may be indicated.

Prognosis: Appears to be good if the child survives the 1st year. May need strenuous supportive therapy for thrombocytopenia during the 1st year. Women have heavy menses. Probably normal life span, if patient survives childhood.

Detection of Carrier: ?

†Special Considerations: The possibility that this condition represents a genetic compound (eg one Fanconi anemia gene and one as yet undefined gene which could be lethal in homozygous states) would explain the lack of consanguinity in a rare recessive disorder. There is an interesting report from Turkey of a possibly affected man fathering a son with classic Fanconi anemia.

References:
Altay, C. et al: Fanconi's anemia in offspring of patient with congenital radial and carpal hypoplasia. N. Engl. J. Med. 293:151, 1975.
Hall, J. G. et al: Thrombocytopenia with absent radius. Medicine 48:411, 1969.
Omenn, G.S. et al: Prospects for radiographic intrauterine diagnosis - the syndrome of thrombocytopenia with absent radii. N. Engl. J. Med. 288:777, 1973.

Contributor: **Judith G. Hall**

Editor's Computerized Descriptors: Dermatoglyphic, Skel., CV.

THROMBOCYTOPENIC PURPURA AND LIPID HISTIOCYTOSIS

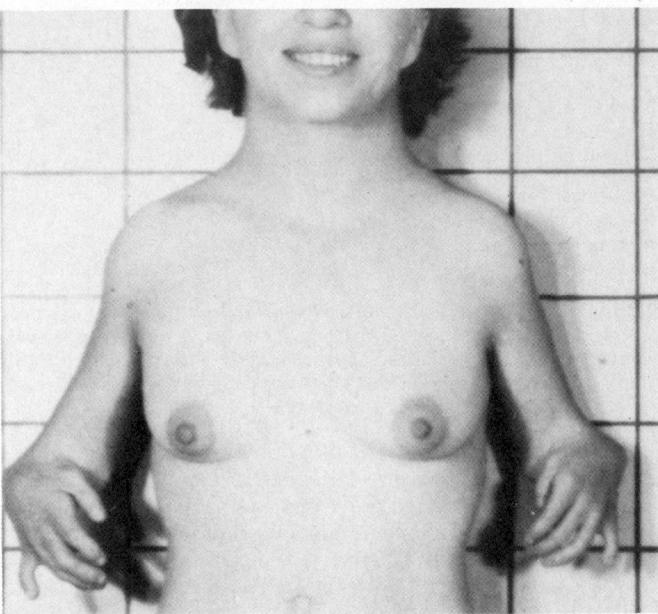

478. Symmetric short upper limbs with radial deviation of hand and hypoplastic shoulder girdle

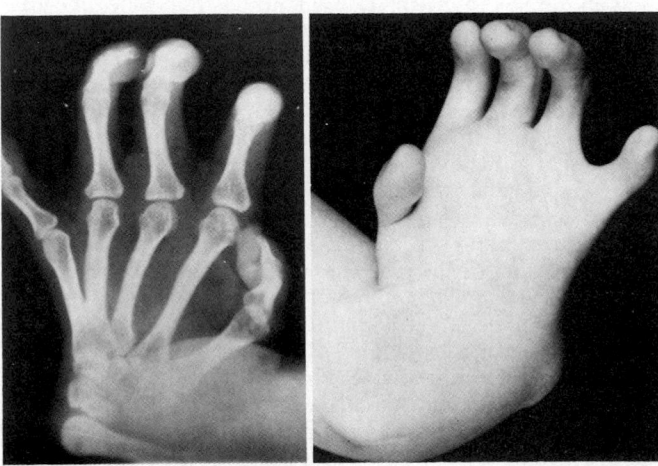

479. A) Note absent radius and middle phalanx of 5th finger; B) short forearm, radial deviation of hand, syndactyly, flexion contractures, and abduction of 5th finger

Includes: Purpura thrombocytopénique avec histiocytose
Thrombocytopenische Purpura und Histiocytose
Púrpura trombocitopénica con histiocitosis
Lipidosis with thrombocytopenia and angiomata of spleen
"Idiopathic thrombocytopenic purpura" with lipid histiocytosis of spleen

Excludes: Gaucher disease (406)
Other sphingolipidoses
Sea-blue histiocyte syndrome
Lipid histiocytosis associated with malignancy, thalassemia, or diabetes

Minimal Diagnostic Criteria: Thrombocytopenia and histologic demonstration of splenic histiocytosis.†

Clinical Findings: The general findings are those usual for chronic, so-called idiopathic thrombocytopenic purpura (ITP)- easy bruising, cutaneous petechiae and ecchymoses, epistaxis and other mucous membrane hemorrhages. The platelet count is low, tourniquet test positive and there is absent clot retraction. The serum lipids are normal. The bone marrow shows increased megakaryocytes; lipid histiocytes in the marrow are rare. The spleen is usually not enlarged clinically.

Complications
I   **Derived:**   Hemorrhage
II   **Associated:**   Risk of postsplenectomy infection

Etiology: ? Genetic substrate is likely, but unproven.† The provocative role of the administration of corticosteroids is uncertain.

Pathogenesis: Lipid-containing vacuolated histiocytes are found in the splenic pulp. By electron microscopy these are shown to contain osmiophilic lamellated inclusions in the cytoplasm.†

Related Facts
I   **Sex Ratio:**   M1:F1
II   **Risk of Occurrence:**   ? To date the incidence has been mainly in Caucasians.
III   **Risk of Recurrence for**
    Patient's Sib: ?
    Patient's Child: ?
IV   **Age of Detectability:**   Has been from 3 years to adult life, based on experience to date from examination of splenic specimens.
V   **Prevalence:**   ? †

Treatment
I   **Primary Prevention:**   —
II   **Secondary Prevention:**   —
III   **Other Therapy:**   Management of purpura or hemorrhage

Prognosis: Dependent on control of hemorrhage

Detection of Carrier: —

†Special Considerations: The process of lipid histiocytosis occurring in patients with ITP can be recognized only upon examination of the extirpated spleen, rarely on bone marrow examination. In various studies it has been reported to be present in 2-30% of splenectomized cases. Although the incidence of this phenomenon has increased sharply since the introduction of corticosteroid therapy for ITP, the true nature of this relationship is not known; it is possible that steroids enhance a metabolic block. On direct analysis, the splenic lipids are found to be generally increased, perhaps somewhat more prominently in the phospholipid fraction. Although increased destruction of formed blood elements is thought to be pertinent, a genetic predisposition for the special occurrence of lipid histiocytosis in certain patients seems likely, perhaps as a catabolic defect in lipid processing within the spleen. The principal importance in the diagnosis of this syndrome is for its separation from the other known lipidoses, with their special prognostic implications.

References:

Dollberg, L. et al: Lipid-laden histiocytes in the spleen in thrombocytopenic purpura. Am. J. Clin. Pathol. 43:16, 1965.

Hill, J.M. et al: Secondary lipidosis of spleen associated with thrombocytopenia and other blood dyscrasias treated with steroids. Am. J. Clin. Pathol. 39:607, 1963.

Landing, B.H. et al: Thrombocytopenic purpura with histiocytosis of the spleen. N. Engl. J. Med. 265:572, 1961.

Quinton, S. et al: Histiocytosis of spleen, lymph node, and bone marrow, associated with thrombocytopenia, splenomegaly and splenic angiomata. Am. J. Clin. Pathol. 47:484, 1967.

Contributor: **Lotte Strauss**

Editor's Computerized Descriptors: Nasoph., Oral, Skin

THYMIC AGENESIS

Includes: Aplasie thymique
Thymusagenesie
Agenesia del timo
DiGeorge syndrome†
Pharyngeal pouch syndrome
Thymic aplasia
Harrington syndrome
Congenital absence of the thymus and parathyroid

Excludes: Immunodeficiency, severe combined (522)
Nezelof syndrome
Agammaglobulinemia, X-linked infantile (27)
Reticular dysgenesis

Minimal Diagnostic Criteria: Congenital hypoparathyroidism, altered facies, absence of thymic shadow on radiographs, evidence of impaired cell-mediated immunity with decreased numbers of T cells. Lymph nodes showing depletion in deep cortical areas with normal germinal centers.

Clinical Findings: Neonatal hypocalcemic tetany; characteristic facial appearance: hypertelorism, antimongoloid slant of eyes, shortened philtrum, low-set ears wih notched pinnae and micrognathia; cardiac malformations mainly conotruncal and aortic arch anomalies. There is an increased susceptibility to infection manifested by chronic rhinitis, recurrent pneumonia, abscesses and septicemia. Oral candidiasis and recurrent nonspecific diarrhea are common. Patients are weak, fail to thrive and prone to sudden death. Less common features include bifid uvula, esophageal atresia, hypothyroidism, urinary tract infections and nephrocalcinosis.

Laboratory findings: 1) Evidence of hypocalcemia and hyperphosphatemia. 2) Immunologic evaluation: Cell-mediated immunity is usually depressed, as manifested by the following: Failure to develop delayed hypersensitivity, absent or delayed homograft rejection, decreased numbers of T cells (E-rosetting cells), and impaired proliferative responses to mitogens, antigens and allogenic cells. However, there have been instances when one or more of the above functions have been normal. Functions which are initially normal may later get depressed, and vice-versa, depressed immunity on rare occasions can spontaneously recover. Lymphopenia may or may not be present. B-cell numbers (Ig- bearing cells) are usually increased. Humoral immunity is intact, with normal levels of immunoglobulins and usually normal antibody response. Complement components are normal. Lymph nodes show paucity of cells in deep cortical areas and well-developed germinal centers and plasma cells. Chest radiographs show absence of thymic shadow.

Complications

I **Derived:** Convulsions, recurrent infections, nephrocalcinosis.

II **Associated:** Anomalies of the great vessels (right aortic arch; tetralogy of Fallot, coarctation of aorta). Other minor and major malformations may occur as mentioned above.

Etiology: Possibly autosomal recessive

Pathogenesis: The absence of the thymus and parathyroid glands has been attributed to a failure of embryonic differentiation of structures derived from the 3rd and 4th pharyngeal pouch endoderm and branchial cleft ectoderm.

Related Facts

I **Sex Ratio:** M1:F1

II **Risk of Occurrence:** ? Higher risk in children of women over 30 years and advanced paternal age.

III Risk of Recurrence for
Patient's Sib: Probably 1 in 4 (25%) for each offspring to be affected.
Patient's Child: Probably not increased unless mate is carrier or homozygote
IV Age of Detectability: Infancy
V Prevalence: ?

Treatment
I Primary Prevention: Genetic counseling
II Secondary Prevention: ?
III Other Therapy: A) For hypoparathyroidism, substitute function with parathormone, administer calcium, vitamin D. B) For absent thymus; transplant fetal thymus. Fetal thymus transplantation has apparently corrected the immunologic abnormality on all the occasions where this approach was used.

Prognosis: Usually failure to grow and develop normally. Neurologic impairment may result from neonatal seizures. Death by infection early in life common. Cardiac anomalies when severe, are a major cause of death.

Detection of Carrier: ?

†**Special Considerations:** The defect of the thymus is often incomplete, and the clinical findings in the DiGeorge syndrome can be very variable. Normal function of thymic-dependent lymphocytes can be present at birth but this can get progressively worse. Circulating T cells however, are almost always decreased in number. Thymic dependent lymphoid function rarely can recover. The heterogeneity of the syndrome warrants individualization of each case. In the classic DiGeorge syndrome, the success of thymus grafts is unquestionable: 6 of 7 cases thus treated are living, whereas only 11 of 35 cases not transplanted are alive. Those surviving have been patients with only partial defects, often minimal, of thymus-dependent function.

References:
Cleveland, W.W.: Immunologic reconstitution in the DiGeorge syndrome by fetal thymic transplant. In Bergsma, D. et al (eds.): Immunodeficiency in Man and Animals, Birth Defects: Orig. Art. Ser., vol. XI, no. 1. Sunderland, MA: Sinauer Asso., Inc. for The National Foundation-March of Dimes, 1975, p. 352.

DiGeorge, A.M.: Congenital absence of the thymus and its immunologic consequences: Concurrence with congenital hypoparathyroidism. In Bergsma, D. and Good, R.A. (eds.): Immunologic Deficiency Diseases in Man, Birth Defects: Orig. Art. Ser., vol. IV, no. 1. White Plains: The National Foundation-March of Dimes, 1969, p. 116.

Kretschmer, R. et al: Congenital aplasia of the thymus gland (DiGeorge syndrome). N. Engl. J. Med. 279:1295, 1968.

Lischner, H.W.: DiGeorge syndrome. J. Pediatr. 81:1042, 1972.

Pabst, M.F. et al: Partial DiGeorge syndrome with substantial cell-mediated immunity. Am. J. Dis. Child. 130:316, 1976.

Robinson, H.B.: DiGeorge's or the III-IV pharyngeal pouch syndrome: Pathology and a theory of pathogenesis. In Rosenberg, H.S. and Bolande, R.P. (eds.): Perspective in Pediatric Pathology. Chicago: Year Book Medical Publishers, 1975, vol. II, p. 173.

Contributors: **Normand Lapointe**
Savita Pahwa

Editor's Computerized Descriptors: Eye, Ear, Face, Nasoph., Skin, CV., GI., GU., Nerve, Oral, Resp.

THYMOMA AND AGAMMAGLOBULINEMIA SYNDROME

Includes: Syndrome thymome-agammaglobulinémie
Thymom-Agammaglobulinämie-Syndrom
Síndrome de timoma y agamaglobulinemia
"Acquired" agammaglobulinemia with thymoma
Agammaglobulinemia and thymoma
Hypogammaglobulinemia thymoma syndrome
Immunologic deficiency and thymoma syndrome
Thymoma with "acquired" combined immunodeficiency

Excludes: All forms of immunologic deficiency disease in absence of thymoma

Minimal Diagnostic Criteria: Anterior mediastinal mass on xray and low immunoglobulin levels.

Clinical Findings: Adults (20-77 years of age) with recurrent chronic bronchitis and bronchopneumonia, weight loss, weakness, diarrhea, stomatitis, sinusitis, GU infections, skin infections, septicemia, splenomegaly, anemia, and bleeding tendencies. Serum IgG_1 is always low or absent. Other immunoglobulins may be normal, low or absent. Antibody responses to typhoid, paratyphoid and diphtheria antigens are usually deficient. Impaired cell-mediated immunity in some patients (eg poor response of lymphocytes to phytohemagglutinin, Concanavalin A and a variety of antigens, inability to demonstrate delayed cutaneous hypersensitivity to a variety of ubiquitous antigens and sensitization with 2-4 dinitrochlorobenzene). T-lymphocyte numbers are usually normal, but may be decreased. Circulating B lymphocytes are usually absent. Antinuclear antibody and antistriated muscle antibody may be present. Xray of chest reveals an anterior mediastinal mass. Thymoma is usually benign (75% spindle cells) but may occasionally be malignant.

Complications
I Derived: Epiphenomenon: overwhelming pulmonary infections (cytomegalovirus, *Pneumocystis carinii*), and diarrhea (possibly secondary to low IgA levels on mucosal surface deficient T lymphocytes and infestation with *Giardia*).
II Associated: Myasthenia gravis, aregenerative anemia, thrombocytopenia, agranulocytosis, absence of eosinophils, eosinophilia, ulcerative colitis, pernicious anemia, astrocytoma, amyloidosis, lupus erythematosus, pulmonary tuberculosis, Cushing syndrome, Sjögren syndrome, Waldenstrom macroglobulinemia, hemolytic anemia, rheumatoid arthritis, unusual form of diabetes mellitus, pemphigus, exudative enteropathy, chronic hepatitis, adrenal gland atrophy.

Etiology: ?

Pathogenesis: No adequate explanation for the association of thymoma and immunodeficiency. Neither the appearance of the tumor nor its removal correlates well with the appearance or disappearance of any of the clinical findings except in some cases associated with aregenerative anemia which may be cured by thymectomy. Early in the clinical course when myasthenia gravis is present, thymectomy results in a cure of the myasthenia but not of the immunodeficiency. Recently, "suppressor" cell activity for immunoglobulin synthesis and secretions by B cells and plasma cells have been reported. An increased incidence of autoimmunity has been found in several family members. In one family, thymomas were found in propositus and a maternal uncle.

Related Facts
I Sex Ratio: M1:F2

II Risk of Occurrence: ?
III Risk of Recurrence for
    Patient's Sib: ?
    Patient's Child: ?
IV **Age of Detectability:** 20 years or older, usually 4th -7th decade.
V **Prevalence:** ?

Treatment
I **Primary Prevention:** —
II **Secondary Prevention:** —
III **Other Therapy:** Excision and removal of thymoma. No improvement in immunodeficiency; however, in some cases aregenerative anemia and myasthenia gravis are cured. Gamma globulin replacement therapy may be of benefit for control of the recurrent infections, particularly for chronic diarrhea.

Prognosis: An interval of 12 years has been reported between the appearance of the thymoma and immunodeficiency; however, overall prognosis is poor once the first symptoms of recurrent infection appear, there is usually a progressive deterioration of immunologic competence. Death usually results from infection but may be related to the development of associated disorders such as thrombocytopenia or diabetes. Only one patient is known to have expired with metastases.

Detection of Carrier: ?

Special Considerations: —

References:
Ammann, A.J. and Hong, R.: Immunodeficiency with thymoma (Good's syndrome). In Steihm, R. and Fulginiti, V. (eds.): Immunologic Disorders in Infants and Children. Philadelphia:W.B. Saunders Co., 1974.
Good, R. A.: Agammaglobulinemia - a provocative experiment of nature. Bull. Univ. Minn. Hosp. 26:1, 1954.

Contributor: Sudhir Gupta

Editor's Computerized Descriptors: Oral, Nasoph., Muscle, Resp., Spleen, GI., GU., Skin

---

THYROGLOSSAL DUCT REMNANT

Includes: Persistance du canal thyréoglosse
Persistierender Ductus thyreoglossus
Persistencia del conducto tirogloso
Thyroglossal duct, cyst or sinus

Excludes: Ectopic thyroid
Dermoid cyst or teratoma of head and neck (283)
Branchial cleft cysts or sinuses (117)
Suppurative lesions
Lipoma
Midline cervical cleft

Minimal Diagnostic Criteria: Lingual mass or midline neck cyst or mass moving with deglutition or tongue protrusion, with or without associated infection.

Clinical Findings: Midline or slightly lateral cystic mass or sinus in the anterior neck located anywhere from the submental to the suprasternal region. The mass also may be located in the region of the foramen cecum of the tongue. A tract from the cyst to the foramen cecum may remain patent, allowing cyst fluid to drain into the mouth. When this occurs the cyst may become smaller. However, in most cases, the duct is closed and persists as a fibrous cord which may be palpated from the neck mass to the center of the hyoid bone. A sinus opening onto the anterior neck may occasionally discharge a few drops of fluid. In approximately 50% of cases the cyst becomes infected. When the patient swallows or protrudes his tongue the cyst may appear to move upward in the neck. The thyroglossal duct cyst and tract are remnants of the embryologic descent of the developing thyroid gland from the pharynx to the neck. Rarely descent does not occur and a mass at the foramen cecum may not be a thyroglossal duct cyst, but only the thyroid tissue present. A thyroid scan should be done in the case of lingual mass. If the lingual thyroid is the only thyroid tissue in the body the only radioactive isotope uptake will be in the area of the base of the tongue. A lingual thyroglossal cyst or thyroid may obstruct an infant's or small child's airway. Histologically the cyst and duct may be lined with squamous, ciliated respiratory, pseudostratified columnar, columnar, cuboidal or transitional epithelium. More than 1 type of epithelium may be present. Subepithelial aggregations of lymphocytes may be seen. The epithelial lining may be replaced by fibrous tissue. Thyroid follicles may be seen in 2-36% of specimens. Rarely gastric or intestinal epithelium may be found lining the cyst. The contents may be mucoid, grumous or pasty.

Complications
I **Derived:** Infection, recurrence, CA, osteomyelitis of hyoid bone, airway obstruction due to large lingual cyst.
II **Associated:** —

Etiology: ?

Pathogenesis: Persistence of a cystic dilation of embryologic thyroglossal duct.

Related Facts
I **Sex Ratio:** M1:F1
II **Risk of Occurrence:** ?
III **Risk of Recurrence for**
    Patient's Sib: ?
    Patient's Child: ?
IV **Age of Detectability:** Usually in early childhood by physical examination
V **Prevalence:** 31 cases in 86,000 consecutive admissions to Mayo Clinic

Treatment

I **Primary Prevention:** —

II **Secondary Prevention:** Surgical excision of cyst and tract in continuity with middle 1/3 of hyoid bone and core of tissue to foramen cecum (Sistrunk). Treatment of infection with antibiotics. Primary excision rather than incision and drainage. No excision if lingual thyroid is present as sole thyroid tissue.

III **Other Therapy:** Tracheotomy may be needed if airway obstructed.

Prognosis: Good if adequately excised; recurrence if inadequate excision performed.

Detection of Carrier: —

Special Considerations: —

References:

Bailey, H.: Thyroglossal cysts and fistulae. Br. J. Surg. 12:579, 1925.

Butler, E.C. et al: Carcinoma of the thyroglossal duct remnant. Laryngoscope 79:264, 1969.

Gross, R.E.: The Surgery of Infancy and Childhood: Its Principles and Techniques. Philadelphia:W.B. Saunders Co., 1953, p. 936.

Sade, J. and Rosen, G.: Thyroglossal cysts and tracts: A histological and histochemical study. Ann. Otol. Rhinol. Laryngol. 77:139, 1968.

Sistrunk, W.E.: The surgical treatment of cysts of the thyroglossal tract. Ann. Surg. 71:121, 1920.

Contributor: **LaVonne Bergstrom**

Editor's Computerized Descriptors: Oral, Neck, Resp. Also see Section I, Fig. 96

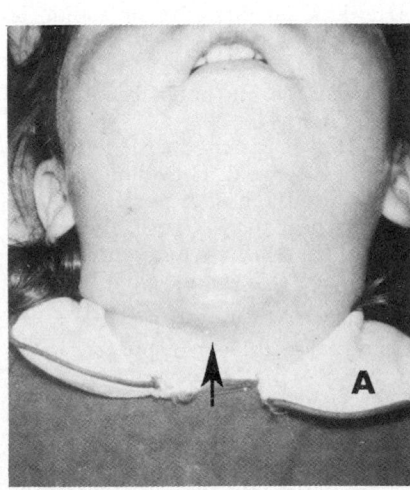
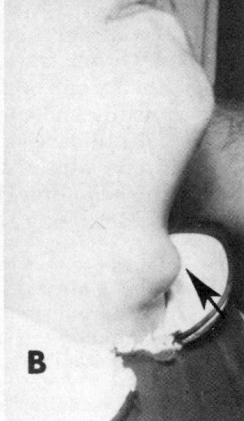

480. A) Thyroglossal duct cyst; B) lateral view

THYROID DYSGENESIS

Includes: Dysgénésie thyroïdienne
Schilddrüsen-Dysgenesie
Disgenesia tiroídea
Sporadic nongoitrous cretinism
Cretinism, athyreotic
Agoitrous cretinism
Athyrosis
Cryptothyroidism

Excludes: Goitrous cretinism
Thyrotropin deficiency
Various types of thyroid dyshormonogenesis

Minimal Diagnostic Criteria: Cord blood or filter paper spot T4 concentration < 7 g/dl and TSH concentration > 60 μU/ml. After 1 week of age, serum T4 below the range for age and TSH > 10 μU/ml. Serum T3 concentrations are variable. Thyroidal radioiodine uptake and scan may be confirmatory.

Clinical Findings: Infants with thyroid dysgenesis may have ectopic or hypoplastic thyroid tissue or total thyroid agenesis. Thus, there is a spectrum of severity of thyroid hormone deficiency. Some thyroid tissue is present in as many as 70-80% of cases. Infants with inadequate thyroid tissue are born with low (hypothyroid) circulating levels of thyroxine (T4) and high TSH concentrations. Significant but low levels of T4 usually are present in infants with residual functioning thyroid tissue, and serum TSH levels are increased. Thyroid scanning techniques are not sensitive enough to detect small volumes of residual tissue in some infants, but significant circulating concentrations of triiodothyronine (T3) during the neonatal period in the face of low serum T4 concentrations suggest the presence of residual functioning thyroid tissue.

Although signs and symptoms of hypothyroidism may occur in the newborn period, the clinical diagnosis is difficult and is made early (before 8-12 weeks) in only 30% of affected infants. Suggestive early signs and symptoms include a large posterior fontanel, prolonged "physiologic" hyperbilirubinemia, mild myxedema of the face and neck, respiratory distress in a full-term infant, hypothermia ($<$ 35.5° C rectal), bradycardia (rate < 100), constipation, lethargy, poor feeding, noisy breathing and persistent nasal stuffiness. The more classic signs and symptoms of macroglossia, abdominal distention, umbilical hernia, hypotonia, dry hair and skin, puffy facies and hoarse cry appear later in infancy and indicate prolonged hypothyroidism. In children, delayed growth, delayed skeletal maturation and delayed dental development are the most sensitive indicators of thyroid hormone deficiency. Hypofunction of a variety of organ systems may be detected by careful study but offer only nonspecific, secondary evidence for thyroid hormone deficiency. Congenital hypothyroidism leads to marked intellectual deficit and clinical brain dysfunction if thyroid replacement therapy is not begun before 3 months of age; about 80% of infants begun on treatment before this time develop normal intellect, whereas only 10% or less develop normally if treatment is delayed beyond 1 year.

Complications

I **Derived:** Mental retardation, growth retardation, delayed bone and dental maturation

II **Associated:** —

Etiology: ? The disorder is sporadic in most cases. Only a few familial cases have been described. Also a few cases have occurred after administration of therapeutic doses of radioiodine for treatment of thyrotoxicosis. In these cases the pregnancy was 10-20 weeks duration and pregnancy was not suspected.

Pathogenesis: Failure of normal embryologic development of the thyroid gland primordium. Hypoplasia may be associated with ectopy or residual gland tissue which may be located at the base of the tongue, between the base of the tongue and the hyoid bone, or between the hyoid bone and the normal position below the thyroid cartilage. Ectopic location of residual thyroid tissue occurs in 60-80% of cases. Residual tissue is hyperplastic with a high cell/colloid ratio and little visible colloid. The reduced volume of thyroid tissue results in deficiency of T4 secretion and compensatory increase in secretion of TSH from the pituitary gland. T3 secretion may be increased from the intensely stimulated residual tissue and the normal or near normal serum T3 levels offer some protection against severe thyroid hormone deficiency.

Related Facts
I   **Sex Ratio:** M1:F4
II **Risk of Occurrence:** ?
III **Risk of Recurrence for**
   Patient's Sib: Very small. There is some evidence to suggest that the risk may be increased if mother has a high titer of antithyroid antibody.
   Patient's Child: Very small.
IV **Age of Detectability:** At birth by cord blood or filter paper spot screening for T4 and TSH concentrations
V   **Prevalence:** 1 in 6000 births

Treatment
I   **Primary Prevention:** Avoidance of radioiodine treatment of thyrotoxicosis in pregnancy. Counseling for women with high thyroid antibody titer.
II **Secondary Prevention:** —
III **Other Therapy:** Treatment with thyroid hormone to prevent complications.

Prognosis: Normal life span with early diagnosis and treatment; mental deficiency and growth retardation without therapy. The prognosis for mental development is poorer the longer treatment is delayed.

Detection of Carrier: —

Special Considerations: —

References:
Dussault, J.H. et al: Thyroid function in neonatal hypothyroidism. J. Pediatr. 89:541, 1976.
Klein, A.H. et al: Improved prognosis in congenital hypothyroidism treated before age three months. J. Pediatr. 81:912, 1972.
Klein, A.H. et al: Neonatal thyroid function in congenital hypothyroidism. J. Pediatr. 89:545, 1976.

Contributor: **Delbert A. Fisher**

Editor's Computerized Descriptors: Face, Oral, Teeth, Nasoph., Speech, Neck, Skin, Hair, Skel., Muscle, Hernia not CNS, Resp., Nerve

THYROID PEROXIDASE DEFECT

Includes: Déficit en peroxidase thyroïdienne
Peroxidase-Mangel der Schilddrüse
Defecto de peroxidasa tiroídea
Some types of thyroid organification defects
Hypothyroidism, congenital
Goiter, familial

Excludes: Other thyroid nonperoxidase deficient organification defects
Deafness and goiter (249)
Hashimoto thyroiditis
Abnormal thyroglobulin synthesis
Other types of thyroid dyshormonogenesis
Thyroid dysgenesis (946)

Minimal Diagnostic Criteria: Hypothyroidism or compensated hypothyroidism, with a rapid discharge of radioiodine after administration of thiocyanate or perchlorate. In addition, in vitro demonstration of defective peroxidase activity.

Clinical Findings: Clinical heterogeneity is apparent in patients with thyroid peroxidase deficiency. One group, congenitally hypothyroid, presents in early infancy or childhood with mental, growth and skeletal retardation, and a typical cretinoid appearance. The appearance of goiter is variable but usually appears during early childhood. Clinical laboratory findings include a low serum thyroxine, and patients demonstrate a rapid discharge of radioactive iodine of variable extent from the thyroid after oral administration of thiocyanate or perchlorate. This indicates an abnormally large pool of inorganic iodide in the thyroid which is not organically bound to thyroglobulin, whereas in the normal individual virtually no iodide is dischargeable. Other conditions, such as Hashimoto thyroiditis, or a hyperactive thyroid remnant, may result in a partial perchlorate discharge and must be differentiated by other tests.

Another group of patients have presented with goiter but are clinically and chemically euthyroid. They demonstrate ·a partial radioactive iodine discharge with perchlorate or thiocyanate administration. These patients usually can be distinguished clinically from the deafness and goiter (Pendred) syndrome by the presence of normal hearing.

Complications
I   **Derived:** Mental and physical retardation due to congenital hypothyroidism.
II **Associated:** Occasionally, airway obstruction secondary to a large goiter.

Etiology: The complete defect appears to have autosomal recessive inheritance. The genetics of the partial defect, with euthyroid goiter, is unclear; though dominant inheritance has been postulated in some families. McK *27450

Pathogenesis: Thyroid peroxidase, in the presence of the necessary substrates, functions to oxidize inorganic iodide and transfer it to organically bound iodine. Two defects in peroxidase enzymatic activity have been defined. In the first, there is a quantitatively decreased activity which cannot be restored by the addition of hematin, the prosthetic group of the enzyme. This defect has been found among the group of patients with congenital hypothyroidism who also demonstrate complete in vivo perchlorate discharge.

The 2nd defect is the peroxidase apoenzyme prosthetic group defect. No in vitro peroxidase activity is present, however upon the addition of hematin, its prosthetic group, enzymatic activity is partially restored. Thus this defect appears to affect the binding site and thereby the affinity of the apoenzyme for its prosthetic group. These patients demonstrate only partial impairment of organification in vivo. These patients have shown a spectrum of severity; some compensated and euthyroid, and some hypothyroid.†

Related Facts
I **Sex Ratio:** M1:F1 in the congenital hypothyroid group. In those with euthyroid goiter there is a predominance of females.
II **Risk of Occurrence:** ?
III **Risk of Recurrence for**
 Patient's Sib: 1 in 4 (25%) for each offspring to be affected.
 Patient's Child: Not increased unless mate is carrier or homozygote.
IV **Age of Detectability:** Clinically, symptoms of hypothryoidism are usually apparent during early infancy. Goiter may be present in infancy but usually is not apparent until childhood. Serum thyroxine or TSH screening may detect hypothyroidism at birth.
V **Prevalence:** ?

Treatment
I **Primary Prevention:** Genetic counseling.
II **Secondary Prevention:** Early treatment with thyroid replacement if hypothyroid and to reduce size of the goiter.
III **Other Therapy:** Educational programs for problems of mental retardation.

Prognosis: Good in euthyroid goiter. Poor for mental development in congenital hypothyroidism, unless treated in early infancy.

Detection of Carrier: ?

†**Special Considerations:** Defects in iodide organification may result from a defect in the peroxidase enzyme as described above. In addition, a defective thyroglobulin molecule, a defective hydrogen peroxide generating system, or abnormal cytoarchitecture may also result in impaired organification. Such defects may be responsible for the organification failure in nonperoxidase deficient conditions, such as the Pendred syndrome (see Deafness and Goiter). In addition, many of the original patients described with organification defects may prove to have a peroxidase enzyme defect or a separate organification defect.

References:
Niepomniszcze, H. et al: Differentiation of two abnormalities in thyroid peroxidase causing organification defect and goitrous hypothyroidism. Metabolism 24:57, 1975.
Stanbury, J.B.: Inborn errors of the thyroid. In Steinberg, A.G. and Bearn, A.G. (eds.): Progress in Medical Genetics. New York: Grune & Stratton, 1974, vol. X, p. 55.
Stanbury, J.B.: Familial goiter. In Stanbury, J.B. et al (eds.): The Metabolic Basis of Inherited Disease, 4th Ed. New York:McGraw-Hill, 1978, p. 215.

Contributor: **Jonathan Zonana**

Editor's Computerized Descriptors: Face, Neck, Skel.

THYROTROPIN (TSH) UNRESPONSIVENESS

Includes: Insensibilité à la thyréostimuline (TSH)
Thyrotropin (TSH)-Unempfindlichkeit
Falta de respuesta a la tirotropina
Hypothyroidism, congenital

Excludes: Thyroid dysgenesis (946)
Other types of thyroid dyshormonogenesis
Thyrotropin deficiency

Minimal Diagnostic Criteria: Congenital hypothyroidism with an elevated serum TSH, a normal size thyroid, normal RAI uptake, and lack of response to exogenous thyrotropin administration.

Clinical Findings: A single patient with this defect presented at age 2 years with mental and growth retardation, cretinoid facies and other typical stigmata of congenital hypothyroidism. The thyroid was palpable but of normal size. Clinical laboratory findings included low serum thyroxine, markedly elevated serum TSH, and normal baseline radioactive iodine (RAI) uptake. Administration of exogenous TSH did not increase serum thyroxine, RAI uptake, or glandular size. Thyroid pathology showed thickening of the fibrous septa with foci of cell hypertrophy or atrophy. In vitro study of thyroid slices revealed no stimulation with the addition of TSH.

Complications
I **Derived:** Congenital hypothyroidism with accompanying mental and growth retardation.
II **Associated:** —

Etiology: ?

Pathogenesis: Thyrotropin has multiple effects on the thyroid, including stimulating cell division and thyroglobulin synthesis. An altered thyrotropin receptor site, or a defect in a subsequent step, such as a 2nd messenger system, may be responsible for this disorder.

Related Facts
I **Sex Ratio:** ?
II **Risk of Occurrence:** Very rare
III **Risk of Recurrence for**
 Patient's Sib: ?
 Patient's Child: ?
IV **Age of Detectability:** Clinically, symptoms of congenital hypothyroidism, such as growth retardation and delayed skeletal maturation, are usually apparent during the 1st half year of life. Newborn serum thyroxine or serum TSH screening may diagnose the disorder at birth.
V **Prevalence:** Very rare

Treatment
I **Primary Prevention:** ?
II **Secondary Prevention:** Early thyroxine replacement
III **Other Therapy:** Educational programs for problems of mental retardation.

Prognosis: Poor for mental and physical development if not treated early; however may be improved with early detection and therapy.

Detection of Carrier: ?

Special Considerations: —

References:
Stanbury, J.B. et al: Congenital hypothyroidism with impaired thyroid response to thyrotropin. N. Engl. J. Med. 279:1132, 1968.
Stanbury, J.B. Inborn errors of the thyroid. In Steinberg, A.G. and Bearn, A.G. (eds.): Progress in Medical Genetics. New York: Grune & Stratton, 1974, vol. X, p. 55.

Contributor: **Jonathan Zonana**

Editor's Computerized Descriptors: Face, Nerve

THYROTROPIN DEFICIENCY, ISOLATED

Includes: Déficit isolé en thyrotropine
Isolierter Thyrotropin-Mangel
Deficiencia aislada de tirotropina
Isolated TSH deficiency

Excludes: Panhypopituitary dwarfism, familial
Sporadic nonendemic cretinism
TSH deficiency associated with pseudohypoparathyroidism
Congenital thyroid aplasia
Thyroid dysgenesis (946)

Minimal Diagnostic Criteria: Documentation of low circulating TSH and thyroxine concentrations.

Clinical Findings: The severity of thyroid stimulating hormone (TSH) deficiency and secondary hypothyroidism varies; but in most cases symptoms are mild and the diagnosis is not made until adulthood. The symptoms are usually vague and not suggestive of thyroid disease, ie dizziness, weakness, constipation, angina pectoris, etc. Severely affected individuals manifesting mental retardation, hypometabolism, dry puffy skin, husky voice and delayed dental and skeletal maturation have been described, but rarely. The diagnosis is established by finding both low serum TSH and thyroxine levels.

Complications
I **Derived:** Dependent upon severity of secondary hypothyroidism. Untreated severe disease will lead to profound mental and physical retardation.
II **Associated:** —

Etiology: Almost all cases have been sporadic, but there has been at least 1 pair of female sibs reported from a consanguineous mating suggesting autosomal recessive inheritance as well.† McK *27510

Pathogenesis: Various defects in the hypothalamic-pituitary axis have been postulated and both hypothalamic and pituitary primary defects probably exist.

Related Facts
I **Sex Ratio:** M1:F1
II **Risk of Occurrence:** Very low
III **Risk of Recurrence for**
  Patient's Sib: Very low in general but autosomal recessive inheritance (risk of 25%) should be considered if consanguinity is present or more than 1 sib is affected.
  Patient's Child: Negligible
IV **Age of Detectability:** Although usually not suspected until adulthood, may be diagnosed at birth.
V **Prevalence:** Very low

Treatment
I **Primary Prevention:** Genetic counseling when appropriate†
II **Secondary Prevention:** Replacement therapy with thyroxine
III **Other Therapy:** —

Prognosis: Depends on severity of secondary hypothyroidism (see Complications)

Detection of Carrier: —

†**Special Considerations:** An isolated TSH deficiency is often a component of pseudohypoparathyroidism, an X-linked dominant disorder. For proper genetic counseling it is important to completely exclude the latter disorder.

References:
Miyai, D. et al: Familial isolated thyrotropin deficiency with cretinism. N. Engl. J. Med. 285:1043, 1971.
Odell, W.D.: Isolated deficiencies of anterior pituitary hormones, symptoms and diagnosis. JAMA 197:1006, 1966.
Rimoin, D.L. and Schimke, R.N.: Genetic Disorders of the Endocrine Glands. St. Louis: C.V. Mosby, 1971, p. 11.

Contributors: **William A. Horton**
                 David L. Rimoin

Editor's Computerized Descriptors: Teeth, Speech, Skin, Skel., Muscle, GI., Nerve

THYROXINE-BINDING GLOBULIN DEFECTS (MARKER)

Includes: Déficit en globuline lié à la thyroxine
Mangel an Thyroxin-bindendem Globulin
Defectos de la tiroxinglobulina (Marcador)
Familial increase or decrease in thyroxine-binding capacity of serum
Familial serum thyroxine-binding globulin (TBG) defects

Excludes: Chemically induced or acquired variation in thyroxine-binding capacity of serum

Minimal Diagnostic Criteria: Persistent high or low levels of TBG (or serum thyroxine) in the absence of drug administration, and demonstration of a familial pattern.

Clinical Findings: No clinical disease or associated congenital abnormality has been observed in patients with familial excess or deficiency of TBG. The abnormalities produce an increase or decrease in serum thyroid hormone concentrations and alter the pool sizes and half time of disappearance of radioiodine-labeled thyroid hormones in the extrathyroidal pools. The rates of peripheral utilization of thyroid hormones, however, are normal. Normal circulating concentrations of TBG range from about 2-5 mg/dl; values of 2-9 mg/dl are seen in the newborn. Normal serum thyroxine (T4 concentrations range from 4.5-12.5 μg/dl; values in the newborn are 7-17 μg/dl. Patients with absent TBG have T4 levels in the hypothyroid range without evidence of hypothyroidism. Patients with low levels of TBG have low or low-normal TBG levels with low or low-normal serum T4 concentrations. TBG levels in adult patients with increased TBG range from 5-10 mg/dl and T4 values from 13-25 μg/dl.

Complications
I   **Derived:** —
II **Associated:** —

Etiology: X-linked transmission of dominant or codominant biochemical defect. The defects probably represent mutations at a single X-linked locus regulating the rate of hepatic TBG synthesis. McK *31420

Pathogenesis: TBG, like glucose-6-phosphate dehydrogenase, is subject to both genetically determined increases and decreases in its concentration. The genetic defect presumably results in either an increased or decreased rate of hepatic TBG synthesis.

Related Facts
I   **Sex Ratio:**   M1:F2 (as defined by serum TBG assay)
II   **Risk of Occurrence:**   ?
III **Risk of Recurrence for**
     Patient's Sib: If affected parent is female 1 in 2 (50%) for each sib to be affected. If affected parent is male 1 in 1 (100%) for each sister to be affected; not increased for brothers.
     Patient's Child: If patient is female 1 in 2 (50%) for each offspring to be affected; if patient is male, 1 in 1 (100%) for daughters, not increased for sons.
IV   **Age of Detectability:**   For absent TBG: at birth by measuring serum thyroxine or TBG-binding capacity. For decreased or increased TBG: at 1 month by measuring serum thyroxine or TBG-binding capacity.
V   **Prevalence:**   Probably 1 in 12,000 births for TBG deficiency.

Treatment
I   **Primary Prevention:**   Not necessary
II   **Secondary Prevention:**   —
III **Other Therapy:**   —

Prognosis: Normal life span

Detection of Carrier: Reduced levels of TBG or serum thyroxine

Special Considerations: —

References:
Jones, J.E. and Seal, U.S.: X-chromosome linked inheritance of elevated thyroxine-binding globulin. J. Clin. Endocrinol. 27:1521, 1967.
Levy, R.P. et al: Radioimmunoassay of human thyroxine-binding globulin TBG. J. Clin. Endocrinol. 32:372, 1972.
Nikolai, T.F. and Seal, U.S.: X-chromosome linked familial decrease in thyroxine-binding globulin activity. J. Clin. Endocrinol. 26:845, 1966.
Nikolai, T.F.: X-chromosome linked inheritance of thyroxine-binding globulin deficiency. J. Clin. Endocrinol. 27:1515, 1967.
Refetoff, S. et al: Study of four new kindreds with inherited thyroxine-binding globulin abnormalities. J. Clin. Invest. 51:848, 1972.

Contributor: **Delbert A. Fisher**

Editor's Computerized Descriptor: —

TONGUE FOLDING OR ROLLING (MARKERS)

Includes: Capacité d'enrouler la langue
Einrollen der Zunge
Plicatura o arrollamiento lingual (Marcador)
Tongue curling

Excludes: Ankyloglossia (61)

Minimal Diagnostic Criteria: Ability to fold back the tongue or to roll the tongue so as to form a tube.

Clinical Findings: Ability to fold the tongue tip back upon itself or to roll or curl the sides of the tongue inward to form a tube. Both movements are performed by the intrinsic muscles of the tongue with no mechanical assistance. The 2 abilities are independent of one another.

Complications
I   **Derived:** —
II   **Associated:** —

Etiology: Autosomal dominant transmission for each trait independently†

Pathogenesis: Dependent upon genetic characteristics enabling unusual movement of the intrinsic muscles of the tongue†

Related Facts
I   **Sex Ratio:** M1:F1
II   **Risk of Occurrence:**   ?
III **Risk of Recurrence for**
     Patient's Sib: If parent is affected 1 in 2 (50%) for each offspring to have the trait; otherwise not increased.
     Patient's Child: 1 in 2
IV   **Age of Detectability:** Early childhood
V   **Prevalence:** In a sample of Negroid individuals it was found that 70.79% of males could roll or curl their tongues but not fold it back upon itself, that 2.10% of the males could fold but not roll their tongues, and that 10.27% could both fold and roll their tongues. In the same sample it was found that 65.25% of females could roll but not fold, that 2.44% could fold but not roll, and that 17.26% could both fold and roll their tongues.
     In a sample of various groups to determine the ability to roll the tongue, the following percentages were obtained: American Caucasians 65.62, Chinese 62.2, Dutch 65.98, Jewish, 53.33.

Treatment
I   **Primary Prevention:** Not necessary
II   **Secondary Prevention:** None needed
III **Other Therapy:** —

Prognosis: Normal for life span and intelligence with no known functional disability†

Detection of Carrier: —

†Special Considerations: No investigations have been done to establish any possible relationship between this inherited ability and speech function.

References:
Bat-Miriam, M.: A survey of some genetical characters in Ethiopian tribes. IX. Tongue folding and tongue rolling. Am. J. Phys. Anthropol. 20:198, 1962.
Hsu, T.C.: Tongue upfolding; newly reported heritable character in man. J. Hered. 39:187, 1948.
Lee, J.W.: Tongue-folding and tongue-rolling in an American Negro population sample. J. Hered. 46:289, 1955.
Liu, T. and Hsu, T.: Tongue-folding and tongue-rolling in a sample of the Chinese population. J. Hered. 40:19, 1949.
Sturtevant, A.H.: The genetics of man. In A History of Genetics. New York:Harper & Row, 1965, p.126.
Urbanowski, A. and Wilson, J.: Tongue curling. J. Hered. 38:365, 1947.

Contributor: **Darrell L. Teter**

Editor's Computerized Descriptor: Oral

952
TONGUE, CLEFT

Includes: Langue bifide
Zungenspalte
Lengua hendida
Schistoglossia
Bifid tongue
Trifid tongue
Cleft tongue

Excludes: Ankyloglossia (61)
Hypertrophied frenuli
Pseudocleft tongue
Oligophrenia, familial trembling and hand anomalies
Oro-facio-digital syndrome I (770)
Oro-facio-digital syndrome II (771)
Glossopalatine ankylosis

Minimal Diagnostic Criteria: Tongue truly cleft

Clinical Findings: True cleft of the tongue divides the tongue into 2 or more lobes, in contrast to pseudocleft tongue wherein the body is divided into 2 lobes due to a short frenum. Isolated cleft tongue may be only part of a continuum of cleft mandible. However, both occur as isolated conditions.

Complications
I   **Derived:** Does not usually interfere with speech.
II **Associated:** Cleft lip, cleft palate, cleft mandible, heart defects, polydactyly, cryptorchism, strabismus, absent hyoid, facial asymmetry, polypoid growth attached to tongue apex, cervical webbing.

Etiology: ?

Pathogenesis: Failure of fusion of lateral tongue processes during embryogenesis from a defect involving the 1st branchial arch.

Related Facts
I   **Sex Ratio:**   M5:F7, (6 with sex unreported).
II **Risk of Occurrence:**   ? Rare
III **Risk of Recurrence for**
     Patient's Sib: ?
     Patient's Child: ?
IV **Age of Detectability:**   At birth, by visual inspection
V   **Prevalence:**   ? 18 reported cases

Treatment
I   **Primary Prevention:** —
II **Secondary Prevention:** Surgical repair
III **Other Therapy:** —

Prognosis: Isolated cleft tongue does not seem to interfere with longevity. Prognosis appears to be dependent upon associated defect.

Detection of Carrier: —

Special Considerations: —

Gorlin, R. and Pindborg, J.J.: Syndromes of the Head and Neck. New York: McGraw-Hill, 1964, p. 134.
Hubinger, H.L.: Bifid tongue: Report of case. J. Oral Surg. 10:64, 1952.

Contributor: **Bernd Weinberg**

Editor's Computerized Descriptor: Oral

TONGUE, FISSURED (MARKER)

Includes: Langue fissurée
Lengua fisurada (Marcador)
Lingua fissurata types I, II, and III
Fissured tongue

Excludes: Tongue, plicated (Marker) (956)

Minimal Diagnostic Criteria: Fissures on the tongue other than the normal variation of shallow, central fissure at the insertion of the median raphe.

Clinical Findings: Many persons have 1 or 2 superficial midline fissures which are normal variations of the mucosal insertion of the median raphe of the tongue. Fissured tongue can be of several types arising from a variety of causes: *Type I*—a deep central furrow which probably represents a part of a continuum of normal midline raphe on one hand and cleft tongue at the other. *Type II*—multiple narrow fissures running parallel or obliquely at right angles to the midline raphe. *Type III*—deep, broad fissures parallel to the midline raphe in which the lingual papillae are absent and the base has a dense band of connective tissue scar. (See also Plicated Tongue.)†

Complications
I   **Derived:** —
II **Associated:** Type III fissures are associated with cleft palate.

Etiology: ? Some possibly caused by intrauterine infections.

Pathogenesis: *Type I:* Fissures represent incomplete fusion of the lateral halves of the tongue or binding of the mucosa to the central raphe of the tongue.

Type II: Unknown, but are probably acquired. When congenital they may be secondary to intrauterine infections such as syphilis and when they develop postnatally are probably associated with a wide variety of infections and malnutrition.

Type III: It is found in some patients with cleft palate including submucous clefts and is thought to be due to a misplacement of tongue-palatal shelf relationship during palatal development. Normally, initial palatal development takes place such that the palatal shelves grow downward between the lateral borders of the tongue and the cheek, then snap into a horizontal relationship with each other. These fissures appear to result from the inferior borders (which become the midline margins after snapping into horizontal relationship) of the palatal shelves developing on the surface of the tongue instead of lateral to the tongue borders.

Related Facts
I   **Sex Ratio:** M1:F1 all types
II **Risk of Occurrence:** Unknown for Types I and II. Type III occurred in 1 in 8 to patients with cleft palate in one survey.
III **Risk of Recurrence for**
    Patient's Sib: ?
    Patient's Child: ?
IV **Age of Detectability:** Type I and some Type II from infancy to adulthood by clinical examination. Type III at birth.
V   **Prevalence:** Types I and II combined 1 in 20 over all age groups. Type III, about 1 in 10 to 1 in 8 cases with cleft palate.

Treatment
I   **Primary Prevention:** —
II **Secondary Prevention:** —
III **Other Therapy:** —

Prognosis: Excellent for life and function

Detection of Carrier: —

†Special Considerations: Has different age and size distribution than plicated tongue.

References:
Gorlin, R. J.: Developmental anomalies of face and oral structures. In Gorlin, R.J. and Goldman, H.M. (eds.): Thoma's Oral Pathology, 6th Ed. St. Louis: C.V. Mosby Co., 1970, vol. I, p. 30.
Hanhart, E.: Die faltenzunge (lingua plicata) als stigma nervoser minderwertigkeit. Verh. Schweiz. Naturforsch. Ges. 115:432, 1934.
Witkop, C. J., Jr. and Barros, L.: Oral and genetic studies of Chileans, 1960. I. Oral anomalies. Am. J. Phys. Anthropol. 21:15, 1963.

Contributor: **Carl J. Witkop, Jr.**

Editor's Computerized Descriptor: Oral

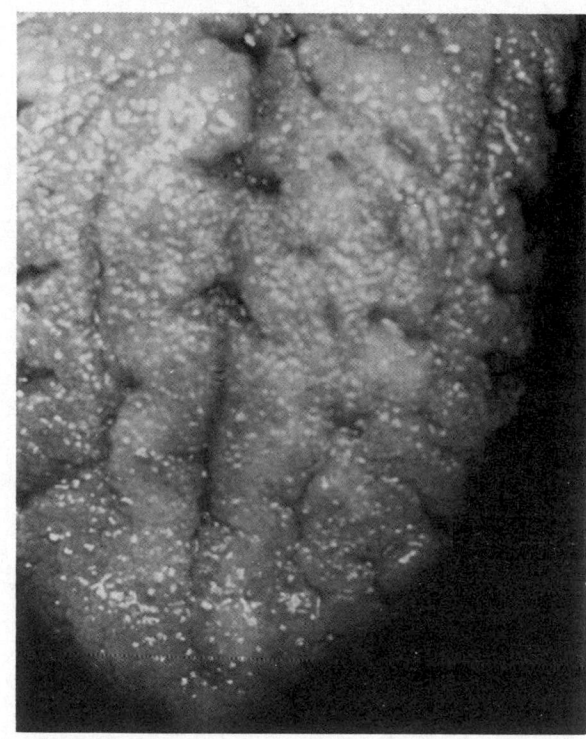

481. Fissured tongue

TONGUE, GEOGRAPHIC

Includes: Glossite exfoliatrice marginée
Landkartenzunge
Lengua geográfica
Erythema migrans lingua
Benign migratory glossitis
Wandering rash of tongue

Excludes: Glossitis, median rhomboid (417)
Glossitis of nutritional deficiencies
Lingual lesions of apthae
Erythema multiforme
Lichen planus
Pemphigus
Reiter syndrome
Syphilis
Tuberculosis

Minimal Diagnostic Criteria: Ordinarily, the diagnosis is readily made from the striking appearance of the pattern of discrete, smooth, red patches on the silver-grey, rough dorsal surface of the tongue. "Migration" or evanescence of the patches over a period of days is diagnostic in otherwise doubtful cases. Rarely, the pattern may seem static for days or weeks but even here, biopsy is seldom necessary to rule out other lesions.

Clinical Findings: Characteristic lesions are discrete, reddened, smooth, irregularly shaped patches on the dorsal and lateral surfaces of the anterior two-thirds of the tongue. The borders are often slightly raised and white or pale yellow in color. The pattern often resembles the configuration of a map; hence, the term "geographic" tongue. The lesions usually "migrate" by healing on one border while advancing on another. They tend to undergo exacerbations and regressions, and often may be completely absent for varying periods of time. About one-fourth of affected persons have symptoms (tenderness, burning); in occasional individuals, these are severe.

Complications
I **Derived:** Plicated tongue
II **Associated:** Plicated and fissured tongue, history of allergy in 40%. A few cases have been reported in which identical lesions have appeared on other areas of the oral mucosa ("stomatitis areata migrans") and even on the skin ("annulus migrans").

Etiology: Emotional stress as a contributing factor has good supporting evidence. A familial pattern seen in several surveys is best explained by a genetic factor. Nutritional deficiency and infection seem unlikely after negative results in several investigations. Local allergic reaction seems worthy of investigation.†

Pathogenesis: Lesions progress through three stages, namely: acute inflammation; chronic inflammation and desquamation; regeneration and recornification. All three may be present in different areas of a given lesion.

Microscopically, the early lesions or advancing borders of older lesions show acute inflammation of the superficial mucosa, with intercellular edema and neutrophilic infiltration of the epithelium. The central areas are noncornified, with flattened or atropic papillae and show chronic inflammation. Many lesions show a striking resemblance to pustular psoriasis. In general, other laboratory tests are of no known diagnostic value.

Related Facts
I **Sex Ratio:** M1:F1
II **Risk of Occurrence:** ? Possibly twice that of prevalence below†
III **Risk of Recurrence for**
Patient's Sib: ? †
Patient's Child: ? †
IV **Age of Detectability:** Youngest reported were infants less than one year old
V **Prevalence:** 1 in 90 to 1 in 70 for Caucasians and Negroes between 5 and 70 years of age

Treatment
I **Primary Prevention:** ?
II **Secondary Prevention:** —
III **Other Therapy:** Reassurance for cancerphobia. Soothing mouth wash for symptoms.

Prognosis: No effect on life span

Detection of Carrier: ?

†**Special Considerations:** Surveys in several countries have yielded remarkably high prevalence of geographic tongue among children. However, the populations surveyed were subject to several potentially highly important biases. Has been seen in kindreds over three generations with fathers and sons affected. A survey of families indicated that about 16% of parents and 11% of sibs of probands had geographic tongue. The study was cross-sectional and since the lesions are often evanescent, the number of primary relatives having the condition was probably considerably larger. The pattern observed is most nearly compatible with either autosomal dominant or polygenic inheritance. That infections or other environmental factors were responsible for the familial pattern of occurrence seems relatively unlikely in view of the finding that not one of the spouses of affected individuals had geographic tongue.

References:
Redman, R.S.: Prevalence of geographic tongue, fissured tongue, median rhomboid glossitis, and hairy tongue among 3,611 Minnesota schoolchildren. Oral Surg. 30:390, 1970.
Redman, R.S. et al: Psychological component in the etiology of geographic tongue. J. Dent. Res. 45:1403, 1966.
Redman, R.S. et al: Hereditary component in the etiology of benign migratory glossitis. Am. J. Hum. Genet. 24:124, 1972.
Witkop, C.J., Jr. and Barros, L.: Oral and genetic studies of Chileans, 1960. I. Oral anomalies. Am. J. Phys. Anthropol. 21:15, 1963.

Contributor: **Robert S. Redman**

Editor's Computerized Descriptor: Oral

TONGUE, PIGMENTED PAPILLAE (MARKER)

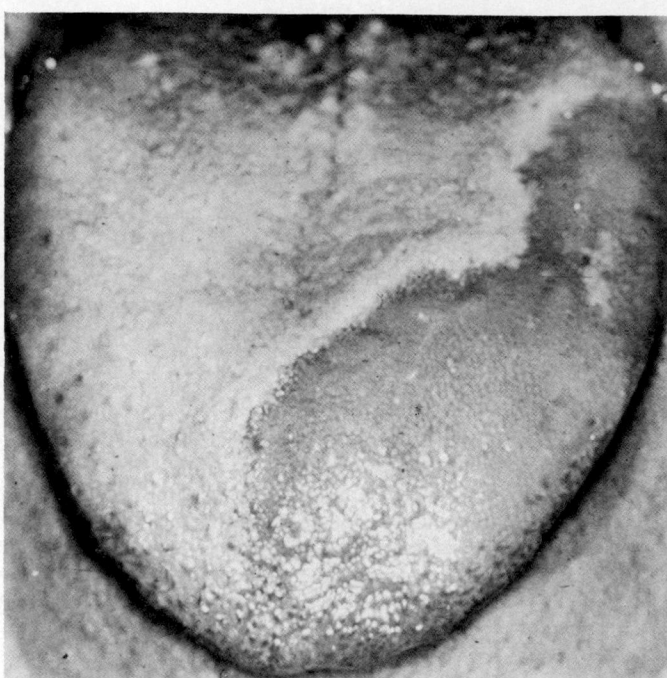

482. Geographic tongue

Includes: Papilles linguales pigmentées
Lingua nigra
Papilas linguales pigmentadas (Marcador)
Tongue, prominent pigmented papillae of

Excludes: Intestinal polyposis I & II (535)
Mucocutaneous pigmentation
Tongue pigmentation

Minimal Diagnostic Criteria: Life history of presence of pigmented fungiform papillae of tongue†

Clinical Findings: Brown to brownish-red pigmentation localized to tips of fungiform papillae. Lesions located primarily on tip and lateral margins of tongue. Occasionally, brown macules, 1-2 mm in diameter, on soft palate; distribution extending to junction of hard and soft palate. Routine blood and urine laboratory studies, serum electrolytes and x-ray films of the chest and skull are normal.

Complications
I   **Derived:** —
II **Associated:** —

Etiology: ? McK *27525

Pathogenesis: Unknown. The pigmentary defect is present at birth and persists through life. The pigmentation is limited to the fungiform papillae of the tongue with the occasional exception of pigmented macules of the soft palate. There is no correlation between this condition and the state of nutrition of the mother or the patient.

Related Facts
I   **Sex Ratio:** Undetermined (90% of cases reported have been in women.)
II **Risk of Occurrence:** ?
III **Risk of Recurrence for**
    Patient's Sib: ?
    Patient's Child: ?
IV **Age of Detectability:** Usually within first 3 months of life by clinical observation.
V. **Prevalence:** 1 in 12 African black; 1 in 50 African white, no data for U.S. population.

Treatment
I   **Primary Prevention:** —
II **Secondary Prevention:** None needed
III **Other Therapy:** —

Prognosis: Normal for life span, intelligence and function

Detection of Carrier: —

†**Special Considerations:** It is important to differentiate this marker from the Peutz-Jeghers syndrome, this being accomplished by clinical examination. To date there is no reported detrimental effect from this condition.

References:
Kaplin, E.J. and W'srand, M.B.: The clinical tongue. Lancet 1:1094, 1961.
Koplon, B.S. and Hurley, H.J.: Prominent pigmented papillae of the tongue. Arch. Dermatol. 95:394, 1967.

Contributor: **Kent F. Jacobs**

Editor's Computerized Descriptor: Oral

TONGUE, PLICATED (MARKER)

Includes: Langue plicaturée
Lingua plicata
Lengua plicada
Scrotal tongue

Excludes: Cheilitis granulomatosis
Chromosome twenty-one trisomy syndrome (171)

Minimal Diagnostic Criteria: Lingual papillae are divided into multiple groups by definite shallow fissures.

Clinical Findings: The tongue has a wrinkled or cerebriform appearance. The papillae of the tongue are divided into multiple groups or islands by definite small shallow fissures which may not be apparent without folding the tongue so the surface mucosa is stretched. The small fissures involve the dorsal mucosa including the edges of the tongue. Geographic tongue may be superimposed giving a patchy or map-like appearance with areas showing relatively short smooth appearing mucosa surrounded by longer white papillae at the borders. The 2 conditions are associated in about 20% of cases. The condition is asymptomatic.

Complications
I **Derived:** None
II **Associated:** Plicated tongue occurs in cheilitis granulomatosis (Melkersson-Rosenthal syndrome) and in about 30% of patients with chromosome twenty-one trisomy. Hanhart reported a 47% frequency in psychotic patients.

Etiology: Autosomal dominant. While many kindreds show this type of inheritance, it is not known if all examples represent an inherited type.† McK *18190

Pathogenesis: Unknown. Condition is rare before age 4 years. Cerebriform pattern becomes more pronounced around puberty.

Related Facts
I **Sex Ratio:** M1:F1
II **Risk of Occurrence:** ? Rare before age 4 years
III **Risk of Recurrence for**
   Patient's Sib: If parent is affected, 1 in 2 (50%) for each offspring to be affected; otherwise not increased.
   Patient's Child: 1 in 2
IV **Age of Detectability:** Frequency and severity of plicated tongue increases with age. Most detectable by 12 years of age by clinical examination.
V **Prevalence:** 1 in 20 to 1 in 12 in all age groups combined. Shows increasing frequency with age from about 1 in 100 in children to 1 in 8 in adults over 40.

Treatment
I **Primary Prevention:** None indicated
II **Secondary Prevention:** None indicated
III **Other Therapy:** Vitamin A has been used with questionable success.

Prognosis: Excellent. Does not reduce longevity.

Detection of Carrier: —

†**Special Considerations:** One study showed a questionable association with blood group O. More data is needed. Also an association between plicated tongue and persons with low serum vitamin A levels has not been substantiated in later studies. Autosomal dominant form associated with migraine headaches in some families.

References:
Gorlin, R. J.: Developmental anomalies of face and oral structures. In Gorlin, R.J. and Goldman, H.M. (eds.): Thoma's Oral Pathology, 6th Ed. St. Louis:C.V. Mosby Co., 1970, vol. 1, p. 30.
Hambert, E.: Die Faltenzunge (Lingua plicata) als Stigma nervöser Minderwertigkeit. Verh. Schweiz. Naturforsch. Ges. 115:432, 1934.
Witkop, C. J., Jr. and Barros, L.: Oral and genetic studies of Chi-
leans 1960. I. Oral anomalies. Am. J. Phys. Anthropol. 21:15, 1963.

Contributor: **Carl J. Witkop, Jr.**

Editor's Computerized Descriptor: Oral

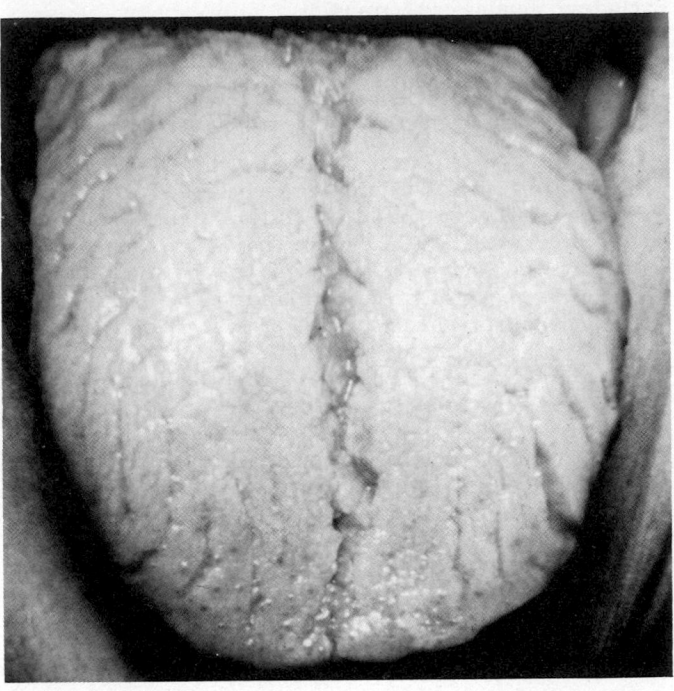

483. Plicated tongue

TORSION DYSTONIA

Includes: Maladie de Ziehen-Oppenheim
Torsionsdystonie
Distonía de torsión
Dystonia musculorum deformans

Excludes: Huntington chorea (478)
Hepatolenticular degeneration (469)
Cerebral palsy

Minimal Diagnostic Criteria: The diagnosis is a clinical one and is suspected by the appearance of dystonic posturing and the pattern of progression. The family history may be of help.†

Clinical Findings: The process is a progressive movement disorder marked by fixation of posture of the limb, part of the trunk or the head and neck. The major abnormality is a spasm of twitching and torsion of the body and limbs. The spasms are not stereotyped and all sorts of bizarre distortions of the trunk and limbs are present. The distribution may be in just 1 leg at first and then spread to involve both lower limbs, the trunk, both arms and the head and neck. Torticollis may be a 1st manifestation.

It has been suggested that there are 2 forms of the disease. An autosomal recessive form occurs primarily in Ashkenazi Jewish families. This form appears to have an earlier onset, less involvement of axial musculature and a more rapid course.

The autosomal dominant dystonia, occurring in non-Jewish families, has a later onset, a fluctuating course and more involvement of axial musculature. It is also suggested that intelligence is likely to be higher in the autosomal recessive form than in the autosomal dominant form.

Complications
I Derived: Complications are related to the progression of the disease, particularly when the patients become bedridden.
II Associated: —

Etiology: Autosomal recessive and also possible autosomal dominant; McK *12810, *22450

Pathogenesis: The basic mechanism is unknown.

Related Facts
I Sex Ratio: M1:F1
II Risk of Occurrence: 1 per 20,000 live births in Ashkenazi Jewish families; for others unknown.
III Risk of Recurrence for
  Patient's Sib: When autosomal recessive or autosomal dominant see Table I AR or AD, respectively
  Patient's Child: When autosomal recessive or autosomal dominant see Table I AR or AD, respectively. (Reproduction is unlikely.)
IV Age of Detectability: Usually apparent between ages of 10 and 15 years; sometimes earlier when autosomal recessive and later when autosomal dominant
V Prevalence: The autosomal recessive frequency in Ashkenazi Jews appears to be 1 in 40,000 with a gene frequency of 1 in 200. The autosomal dominance form is rare, < 1 in 500,000.

Treatment
I Primary Prevention: Genetic counseling
II Secondary Prevention: Surgical treatment may alleviate the movement disorder, at least for periods of time. This requires stereotactic surgery with the target area being the ventrolateral nucleus of the thalamus. There is some suggestion that L-dopa may be of some benefit but recent studies have questioned the efficacy of this drug.
III Other Therapy: —

Prognosis: The prognosis depends on the form of the disease. The life expectancy is altered now by the use of operation. In the autosomal recessive form the disease appears to be rather rapidly progressive requiring operation within a matter of months or a year or two. In the autosomal dominant form the disease runs more of an intermittent course with the progression over years rather than months.

Detection of Carrier: —

†Special Considerations: It should be pointed out that there are patients with symptomatic dystonia of other etiologies who can be confused with the hereditary forms. In addition, there are cases which do not or cannot be conveniently placed in the categories outlined for the autosomal recessive and autosomal dominant forms of the disease.

References:
Eldridge, R.: The torsion dystonias: Literature review in genetic and clinical studies. Neurology 20:1, 1970.
Zeman, W. and Dyken, P.: Dystonia musculorum deformans. Clinical, genetic and pathoanatomical studies. Psychiatr. Neurol. Neurochir. (Amst.) 70:77, 1967.

Contributor: **Guy M. McKhann**

Editor's Computerized Descriptors: Neck, Nerve, Muscle

TORUS MANDIBULARIS

Includes: Protubérance mandibulaire
Torus mandibular
Mandibular enlargement

Excludes: —

Minimal Diagnostic Criteria: A bony swelling that interrupts the smooth curvature of the lingual surface of the mandible.

Clinical Findings: An enlargement of bone on the lingual surface of the mandible above the mylohyoid line and usually opposite the cuspid and premolar teeth. They can be single- or multiple-lobed.

Complications
I **Derived:** Only if they grow so large as to interfere with mastication, speech or the wearing of a denture.
II **Associated:** —

Etiology: Autosomal dominant with variable penetrance by sex- 100% in females, 70% in males; McK *18970

Pathogenesis: ? Slowly enlarging benign growth of bone

Related Facts
I **Sex Ratio:** M0.7:F1 (70% penetrance in males)
II **Risk of Occurrence:** —
III **Risk of Recurrence for**
    Patient's Sib: If parent is affected about 1 in 3 for brothers and 1 in 2 for sisters; negligible for all sibs if patient is the result of a fresh mutation.
    Patient's Child: About 1 in 3 for sons (assuming 70% penetrance for males for autosomal dominant mutant gene) and about 1 in 2 for daughters. Above data exclude all children under 15 years of age.
IV **Age of Detectability:** Usually by 15 years of age- clinically present
V **Prevalence:** Chileans: 1 in 2000
    Peruvians: 1 in 290
    U.S. Caucasians: 1 in 13 over 15 years
    U.S. Negroes: 1 in 9
    Amerindians: 1 in 7
    Eskimos: 1 in 2.5
    Aleuts: 1 in 1.7

Treatment
I **Primary Prevention:** —
II **Secondary Prevention:** Surgical removal if interfering with oral functions
III **Other Therapy:** —

Prognosis: Excellent, do not recur after removal.

Detection of Carrier: —

Special Considerations: —

References:
Austin, J.E. et al: Palatal and mandibular tori in the negro. NY Dent. J. 31:187, 1965.
Johnson, C. C. et al: Torus mandibularis: A genetic study. Am. J. Hum. Genet. 17:433, 1965.
Suzuki, M. and Sakai, T.: A familial study of torus palatinus and torus mandibularis. Am. J. Phys. Anthropol. 18:263, 1960.

Contributor: **Clinton C. Johnson**

Editor's Computerized Descriptors: Oral, Speech

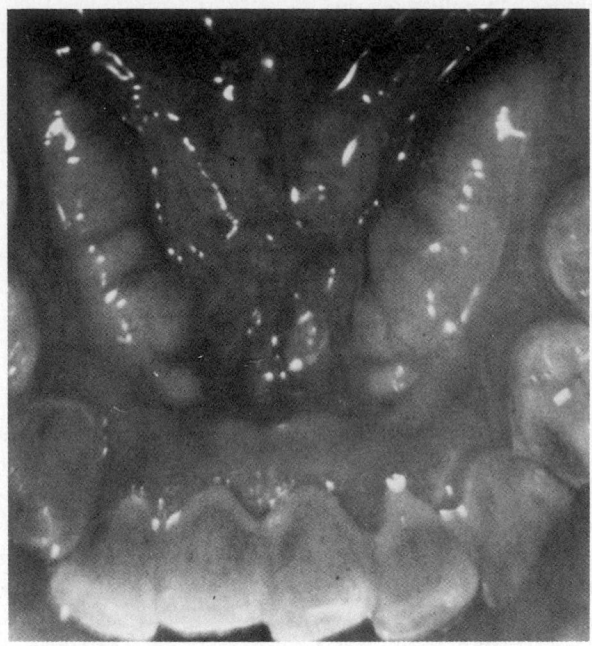

484. Torus mandibularis

TORUS PALATINUS

Includes: Protubérance palatine
Torus palatino
Palate enlargement

Excludes: —

Minimal Diagnostic Criteria: A rounded elevation in the midline of the palate with smooth edge

Clinical Findings: A slowly growing enlargement of bone on the hard palate at the junction of the midpalatal suture usually covered with normal appearing mucosa. They can be single or lobulated.

Complications
I   Derived: Only if they grow so large as to interfere with mastication, speech or the fitting of a denture
II Associated: —

Etiology: Dominant trait- questionable whether autosomal dominant or X-linked dominant, evidence also for polygenic inheritance; McK *18970

Pathogenesis: ? Gradual enlargement of bone in region of midpalatal suture

Related Facts
I   Sex Ratio: Approximately M1:F2 Caucasians, M3:F1 Amerindians
II Risk of Occurrence: ?
III Risk of Recurrence for
   Patient's Sib: When autosomal dominant or X-linked dominant, see Table I AD or X-linked D, respectively.
   Patient's Child: When autosomal dominant or X-linked dominant, see Table I AD or X-linked D, respectively.
IV Age of Detectability: Usually present by 3rd decade
V   Prevalence: 1 in 5 in midwestern Caucasian population, 1 in 50 in children

Treatment
I   Primary Prevention: Genetic counseling
II Secondary Prevention: Surgical removal if interfering with oral function or placement of denture
III Other Therapy: —

Prognosis: Excellent

Detection of Carrier: —

Special Considerations: —

References:
Gorlin, R. J.: Developmental anomalies of the face and oral structures. In Gorlin, R.J. and Goldman, H.M. (eds.): Thoma's Oral Pathology, 6th Ed. St. Louis:C.V. Mosby Co., 1970, vol. 1, p. 21.
Gould, A. W.: An investigation of the inheritance of torus palatinus and torus mandibularis. J. Dent. Res. 43:159, 1964.
King, D.R. and Moore, G.E.: The prevalence of torus palatinus. J. Oral Med. 26:113, 1971.
Kolos, S. et al: The occurrence of torus palatinus and torus mandibularis in 2,478 dental patients. Oral Surg. 6:1134, 1953.

Contributor: **Clinton C. Johnson**

Editor's Computerized Descriptors: Oral, Speech

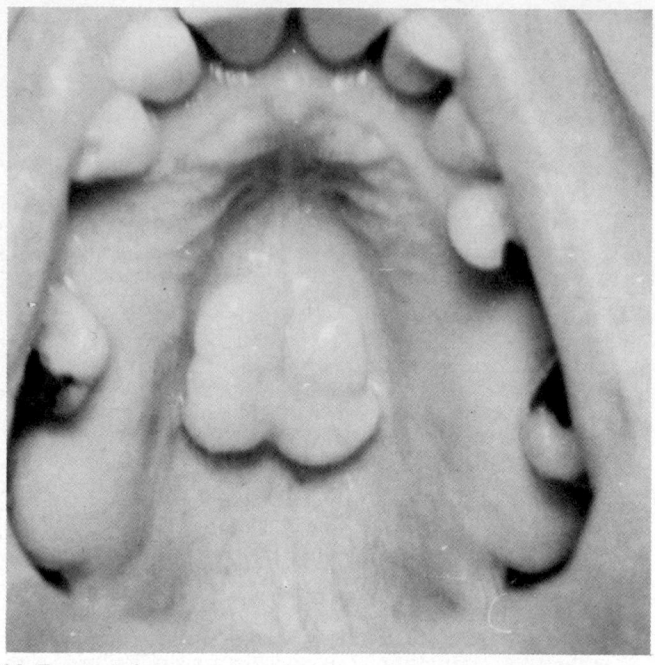

485. Torus platinus

TRACHEOESOPHAGEAL FISTULA

Includes: Fistule trachéo-oesophagienne
Tracheo-Oesophageale Fistel
Fístula tráqueoesofágica
Esophagotracheal fistula
Esophagotracheal window
"H'-type tracheoesophageal fistula

Excludes: Esophageal atresia (364)
Esophageal atresia and tracheoesophageal fistula (365)
Common tracheoesophagus
Laryngeal cleft
Laryngotracheal window

Minimal Diagnostic Criteria: Radiographic or endoscopic demonstration of isolated fistula between trachea and esophagus without esophageal atresia.

Clinical Findings: Symptoms are usually present from birth, but correct diagnosis is often delayed. Coughing or choking with swallowing, especially liquids, is the most common complaint with isolated tracheoesophageal fistula (TEF). Cyanosis is next in frequency. Recurrent respiratory infections from aspirated material are also frequent and may lead to multiple hospitalizations or courses of antibiotic therapy before the diagnosis is made. Children with this lesion almost universally have a history of abdominal distention which is most marked after crying.

Patients with the above clinical features should have a careful esophagram with the contrast material instilled into the midesophagus via a tube. This technique avoids the confusion of possible aspiration of contrast into the trachea. If a fistula is not demonstrated radiographically, bronchoscopy offers the best chance of demonstrating the isolated TEF. (The bronchoscope should be one that has a telescopic insert and allows for controlled anesthesia by a closed system during careful examination of the trachea).

The fistula most commonly is located at the level of the thoracic inlet around T-2, but double fistulas can occur. The term "H'-type, sometimes used for isolated tracheoesophageal fistula, is misleading in that the tracheal and esophageal ends of the fistula are rarely at the same level. The fistula usually extends obliquely downward from the trachea to the esophagus.

Complications
I   **Derived:** *Before corrective surgery:* Repeated contamination of the airway with ingested liquids or regurgitated gastric contents leads to varying degrees of pneumonitis. The infant forces air through the tracheoesophageal fistula into the stomach when crying, which makes regurgitation easier. The gastric distention also elevates the diaphragm and interferes with respiratory activity in the early neonatal period.
After corrective surgery: Complications are rare. Recurrence of tracheoesophageal fistula, leak from tracheal or esophageal closure leading to mediastinitis, unrecognized pneumothorax, recurrent laryngeal nerve injury causing laryngeal obstruction, esophageal stenosis, tracheal stenosis.
II **Associated:** Many anomalies are associated with tracheoesophageal fistula, as with the fistula-esophageal atresia combinations. These include in order of frequency the following: cardiac, GI, GU, imperforate anus, musculoskeletal, CNS, and face. However, the incidence of prematurity and polyhydramnios are less because the amniotic fluid is able to be ingested by the fetus.

Etiology: Failure of normal development and division of the tracheobronchial tree in the 4th embryonic week. Because of the frequency of associated anomalies which are also on the basis of an unknown embryologic insult at approximately the same time, it is felt that this is a random, generalized insult to embryogenesis. The reasons for this insult are completely unknown.

Pathogenesis: Clearly present as a lesion from the early gestational period, the difficulty begins only with postnatal oral intake. Fluids cause more difficulty than solids. Very small fistulas may allow only occasional soiling of the airway. Often the lesion is not detected until the child is several months or years of age. By this time the repetitive soiling of the airway may have led to severe bronchopulmonary disease.

Related Facts
I   **Sex Ratio:** M1:F1
II   **Risk of Occurrence:** Approximately 1 in 100,000 live births
III **Risk of Recurrence for**
     Patient's Sib: Not increased
     Patient's Child: Not increased
IV   **Age of Detectability:** Variable
V   **Prevalence:** ?

Treatment
I   **Primary Prevention:** —
II   **Secondary Prevention:** Division and suture of the tracheoesophageal fistula.†
III **Other Therapy:** —

Prognosis: Excellent once the diagnosis and treatment have been carried out.

Detection of Carrier: —

†Special Considerations: Most of these lesions may be approached surgically through the neck. These patients may have inherent peristaltic defects in the esophagus which provide some difficulty in swallowing but rarely cause clinically significant dysphagia. This amounts to tertiary contractions without effective peristalsis.

References:
Gans, S.L. and Berci, G.: Inside tracheo-esophageal fistula: New endoscopic approaches. J. Pediatr. Surg. 8:205, 1973.
Haight, C.: Congenital esophageal atresia and tracheoesophageal fistula. In Benson, C.D. et al (eds.): Pediatric Surgery. Chicago:- Year Book Medical Publishers, 1962, vol. 1, p. 266.
Holder, T. M. and Ashcraft, K. W.: Esophageal atresia and tracheoesophageal fistula. Curr. Probl. Surg., p. 1, 1966.
Kappelman, M.M. et al: H-type tracheoesophageal fistula. Diagnostic and operative management. Am. J. Dis. Child. 118:568, 1969.

Contributors: **Dale G. Johnson**
Thomas M. Holder

Editor's Computerized Descriptors: Resp., GI, GU.

TRANSGLUCURONYLASE, SEVERE DEFICIENCY

Includes: Déficience sévère en transglucuronylase
Schwere Form des Transglucuronylasemangels
Deficiencia en transglucoronilasa severa
Hepatic glucuronyl transferase deficiency type I
Jaundice without bilirubin glucuronide in bile
Crigler-Najjar syndrome

Excludes: Hyperbilirubinemia I (Marker) (487)

Minimal Diagnostic Criteria: Persistent "physiologic" jaundice of newborn in absence of hemolysis and serum bilirubin concentrations in excess of 20 mg% with no bilirubin glucuronide in bile.

Clinical Findings: Lifelong nonhemolytic unconjugated hyperbilirubinemia with serum bilirubin concentrations of approximately 15-40 mg% (mean: approximately 24 mg%).

Approximately 75% of affected individuals develop signs of kernicterus during the immediate neonatal period and may die. Survivors show varied clinical signs of kernicterus. Rarely, signs of kernicterus develop for the first time at an older age usually in association with infection.

Hepatic glucuronyl transferase activity is absent if bilirubin serves as the glucuronide receptor in vitro whereas, if other receptors, such as 4-methyl umbelliferone, o-aminophenol, etc are used, their enzyme activity is less than 10% of that found in normal controls. Urinary excretion of glucuronide after ingestion of menthol, salicylamide, n-acetyl-p-aminophenol or injection of radioactive tetrahydrocortisone is greatly reduced to about 25% of normal. Fecal urobilinogen excretion is approximately 40-50% of normal. Other conventional hematologic and liver function studies are normal. Morphologic examination of liver reveals no morphologic lesion. Bile obtained at surgery from the liver or from the duodenum intubation is pale yellow and contains only a trace of unconjugated bilirubin.

Complications
I **Derived:** Kernicterus in approximately 75% of cases with a variety of neurologic sequelae
II **Associated:** —

Etiology: Autosomal recessive transmission of enzyme defect;†
McK *21880

Pathogenesis: Severe deficiency of hepatic glucuronyl transferase

Related Facts
I **Sex Ratio:** M1:F1
II **Risk of Occurrence:** ? Rare
III **Risk of Recurrence for**
    Patient's Sib: 1 in 4 (25%) for each offspring to be affected
    Patient's Child: Not increased unless mate is carrier or homozygote
IV **Age of Detectability:** Approximately 20-30th day of life
V **Prevalence:** ? Approximately 80 cases in world literature

Treatment
I **Primary Prevention:** Genetic counseling
II **Secondary Prevention:** Exchange transfusion or plasmaphoresis during immediate newborn period may prevent kernicterus which, in general, only occurs during this time period. Exposure to ultraviolet light lowers serum bilirubin values by producing a structural change in the pigment molecule.
III **Other Therapy:** Patients should not receive drugs, such as sulfonamides, which compete with bilirubin for binding sites on plasma albumin or drugs, such as novobiocin or oleoresin aspidium, which interfere with hepatic uptake mechanisms

for organic anions. Phenobarbital administration has no effect on hyperbilirubinemia in this disorder.

Prognosis: Poor. Approximately 75% of affected individuals die during the first 5 years of life from kernicterus or infection.

Detection of Carrier: Oral menthol tolerance test (1-2 gm for young adults) is useful in distinguishing carriers from a group of controls. Menthol glucuronide excretion is quantitated in urine collected for 5 hours after menthol ingestion. Control subjects excrete $39 \pm 7.2\%$ of ingested menthol as urinary menthol glucuronide during this period. Carriers excrete only about 18% of the given dose during the test period.

†Special Considerations: Kernicterus is caused by factors other than glucuronyl transferase such as hypoxia, prematurity, sepsis, etc and therefore, is not an obligatory or specific manifestation of this disorder. Because of therapeutic implications, Type I glucuronyl transferase deficiency must be differentiated from Type II glucuronyl transferase deficiency. The Gunn strain of mutant Wistar rat has the Type I defect.

References:
Arias, I. M.: Chronic unconjugated hyperbilirubinemia without overt signs of hemolysis in adolescents and adults. J. Clin. Invest. 41:2233, 1962.
Arias, I.M. et al: Chronic nonhemolytic unconjugated hyperbilirubinemia with hepatic glucuronyl transferase deficiency: Evidence for genetic heterogeneity. Am. J. Med. 47:395, 1969.
Childs, B. et al: Glucuronic acid conjugation by patients with familial nonhemolytic jaundice and their relatives. Pediatrics 23:903, 1959.
Crigler, J. F., Jr. and Najjar, V. A.: Congenital familial nonhemolytic jaundice with kernicterus. Pediatrics 10:169, 1952.
Schmid, R. and McDonagh, A.F.: Hyperbilirubinemia. In Stanbury, J. B. et al (eds.): The Metabolic Basis of Inherited Disease, 4th Ed. New York:McGraw-Hill, 1978, p. 1221.

Contributor: **Irwin M. Arias**

Editor's Computerized Descriptors: Skin, Nerve

TRANSPOSITION OF GREAT VESSELS

Includes: Transposition complète des gros vaisseaux
Transposition der grossen Gefässe
Transposición completa de los grandes vasos
Complete transposition of great vessels
Noninverted transposition
Complete d-transposition
Single transposition of great vessels
True transposition of great vessels
Uncorrected transposition of great vessels
Great vessel transposition

Excludes: Transposition associated with a single ventricle (double inlet left ventricle)
Atretic atrioventricular (AV) valve with transposition of great vessels
Double outlet right ventricle
Inversion of ventricles (congenitally corrected transposition)

Minimal Diagnostic Criteria: In a newborn who shows: 1) cyanosis, 2) an ECG that is normal, or shows minimal signs of right ventricular hypertrophy, 3) a single second sound, 4) a normal or only questionably abnormal xray, and 5) no evidence of pulmonary disease, complete transposition is by far the most likely diagnosis. However, the confirmation of complete transposition, as well as associated anomalies, is by selective angiocardiography. Right and left ventriculography are recommended in most cases. The latter is especially important in ruling out obstructive malformations involving the subpulmonary and pulmonary valve areas. Diagnosis should never be based upon the location and course of the ascending aorta in the frontal view. At least 20% of cases will show a great vessel relationship similar to that seen in cases of ventricular inversion.

Clinical Findings: In complete transposition, there are 2 functioning ventricles. The aorta, with the coronary arteries in turn arising from it, takes origin from the right ventricle, while the pulmonary trunk takes origin exclusively from the left ventricle. The anterior leaflet of the mitral valve is in continuity with pulmonary valvar tissue. Both AV valves are patent and have the corresponding structure of the right-and left-sided valves of the normal heart. If life is maintained after birth, some communication must exist between the systemic and pulmonary circulations. These potential communications are 1) patent foramen ovale or atrial septal defect, 2) ventricular septal defect (VSD), 3) patent ductus arteriosus (PDA), 4) any combination of the foregoing, 5) bronchial arteries. The communications may be large or small. In somewhat less than half the cases, the ventricular septum is intact. The anterior-posterior relationship between the aorta and pulmonary artery varies. Commonly, the pulmonary artery is situated posterior and to the left of the aorta or lies directly behind it. Uncommonly, the 2 great vessels lie side-to-side. The right coronary artery arises above the posterior aortic valve cusp and the left coronary artery arises above the left aortic cusp; the right or anterior cusp being the noncoronary one. Theoretically, many isolated lesions may be associated with complete transposition. Certain defects tend to occur with higher degree of frequency than others. These are shunt lesions such as VSD or PDA. Less commonly, VSD and pulmonary stenosis occur. In the latter, there is a relatively high incidence of right aortic arch. Coarctation of the aorta, interruption of the aortic arch, hypoplasia of the right ventricle rarely occur with this condition.

The hemodynamic alterations vary according to the associated malformations. The pathologic arrangement of the 2 great vessels establishes the following 2 circulations: 1) the systemic venous blood enters the right atrium, proceeds to the right ventricle and passes out the aorta to the peripheral circulation where it returns to the systemic veins; 2) meanwhile, the pulmonary venous blood enters the left atrium, enters the left ventricle, then the pulmonary artery and back into the pulmonary veins. Thus, potentially there are 2 completely independent circulations. Since life depends on desaturated venous blood reaching the lungs and oxygenated blood reaching the peripheral arterial circulation, some means of communication between the 2 circulations must exist. The less the communication between the 2 circulations, the more systemic venous blood reaches the periphery without passing through the pulmonary capillary bed, and thus the more cyanotic the infant. When a large VSD or PDA is present, easy mixing between arterial and venous streams is possible. When pulmonary flow exceeds systemic flow because pulmonary vascular resistance is lower, a relatively large amount of highly oxygenated blood is available to mix with a relatively small amount of desaturated blood. Here, cyanosis may be minimal. However, in large communications, pulmonary resistance may eventually exceed systemic resistance, and the "Eisenmenger physiology" stage is reached. Pulmonary flow may also be diminished when pulmonary stenosis exists.

The typical history is that of a male infant (usually not a first-born child), who is noted to be cyanotic and tachypneic shortly after birth. Congestive heart failure follows, with hepatomegaly and increased tachypnea. The infant is often chubby, round-faced and has a higher than average birthweight. On auscultation, the first sound is followed by a short, soft systolic murmur and a loud single second sound. When a large VSD exists, the systolic murmur is of a loud regurgitant quality and both components of S_2 are noted. When pulmonary stenosis exists (usually with a VSD), the murmurs are again prominent. Congestive heart failure usually does not occur with the latter combination of defects.

The ECG usually indicates the size of the communication between the systemic and venous circulations. However, the ECG may be normal in the first 2 weeks of life. In patients with a small communication or shunt, the ECG usually reveals pure right ventricular hypertrophy. In patients with large communications, the ECG usually shows biventricular hypertrophy. Complete transposition is one form of transposition complex which shows Q waves in the left precordial leads. Left axis deviation may be present when the following lesions are associated: 1) coarctation or interruption of the aorta, 2) hypoplastic right ventricle, or 3) endocardial cushion defect.

The characteristic roentgenologic findings are prominent pulmonary vascularity of a shunt type together with a globular-shaped heart and a narrow mediastinum. The right heart in the posterior-anterior and left anterior oblique views is enlarged in nearly all cases. The left atrium is enlarged in the presence of increased flow. During the first 1 or 2 weeks of life, the heart and vasculature may appear normal or only slightly prominent. Other cyanotic or admixture lesions may mimic the roentgenologic findings in complete transposition. In cases with pulmonary stenosis and VSD, the vasculature appears normal or diminished. The cardiac silhouette often resembles tetralogy of Fallot.

The echocardiographic diagnosis of transposition of the great vessels rests on the identification of abnormal great vessel relationships, ie an anterior and rightward or midline aorta compared to a posterior pulmonary artery. Techniques for achieving this differentiation involve 1) using right and left transducer movements on single-crystal echocardiography to determine the rightward anterior great vessel, or 2) demonstrating simultaneous superimposition of 1 great vessel upon another, both in the same A-P plane, suggesting the lack of the normal spiral relationship. The latter finding has many false-positives in normal newborns. Several authors have utilized the longer preejection period and shorter ejection time parameter measured in a systematic circuit in an attempt to use valve timing to separate aortas from pulmonary arteries. Nevertheless, the diagnosis of the transposed great vessel relationship regardless of situs is most reliably made using real-time cross-sectional echocardiography.

Cardiac catheterization will determine oxygen saturations in the 4 cardiac chambers and great arteries. The peripheral oxygen saturation is uniformly higher among patients with large communications versus those with small communications, provided pulmonary vascular resistance is less than systemic vascular resistance. Determination of pulmonary artery and left ventricular pressures is important in calculating the comparable systemic vascular resistance and pulmonary vascular resistance which determines ultimate operability. Oximetry data in the calculation of shunts is not reliable since the great artery and ventricular samples are strongly influenced by streaming and bidirectional shunting at one or more levels.

Complications
I Derived: Death occurs from congestive heart failure and pneumonia in approximately 90% of cases by 1 year of age unless palliative surgery is performed; development of high pulmonary vascular resistance leading eventually to "Eisenmenger physiology" if patient survives infancy. In cases with severe pulmonary stenosis (or atresia), clubbing, hypoxic spells, etc occur.

II Associated: —

Etiology: Multifactorial inheritance

Pathogenesis: Complete transposition is thought to be due to a single embryologic error; an error which takes place in the truncus arteriosus. In the normal, there are 2 pairs of truncus swellings which actively partition the truncus. The major pair are termed dextrodorsal and sinistroventral conus swellings. The other pair (the intercalated valve swellings) form a pair of semilunar valve cusps of each great artery. It is postulated that complete (or d-) transposition is the result of the wrong truncus swellings becoming the major pair. The pulmonary and aortic intercalated valve swellings partition the truncus and align themselves, respectively, with the sinistroventral and dextrodorsal conus swellings. As a result, the aorta arises from the right ventricle anteriorly and the pulmonary artery from the left ventricle posteriorly. The conus septum develops normally, and therefore, its derivatives (the crista supraventricularis, the medial portion of the tricuspid valve, and the medial papillary muscle) are normal.

Related Facts
I Sex Ratio: Approximately M2:F1
II Risk of Occurrence: Approximately 1 in 2000 live births
III Risk of Recurrence for
    Patient's Sib: Predicted risk 2.2%; empiric risk, 1.9%
    Patient's Child: Undetermined - reproductive fitness grossly diminished
IV Age of Detectability: From birth, by selective angiocardiography.
V Prevalence: Less than 1 in 2000 in the pediatric population

Treatment
I Primary Prevention: —
II Secondary Prevention: Palliative: Creation of an atrial septal defect surgically (Blalock-Hanlon procedure) or medically by tearing the rim of the foramen ovale by passing a balloon tipped catheter (via the femoral vein) through the foramen ovale into the left atrium (Rashkind procedure). Additional procedures are surgical banding of the pulmonary artery among patients with excess blood flow to the lungs, or performance of a shunt procedure (Blalock-Taussig or Waterston-Cooley) in patients with decreased pulmonary flow.

    Corrective: The Mustard operation has been found to produce the best results and has superseded older techniques. At cardiopulmonary bypass, the atrial septum is removed and a pericardial graft is sutured into the atrium so that pulmonary venous blood is directed into the right ventricle and the systemic venous blood into the left ventricle.

III Other Therapy: Symptomatic therapy for congestive heart failure and pneumonia

Prognosis: Death occurs in approximately 90% before 6 months of age, unless adequate intracardiac shunting is surgically provided. Those who survive infancy without operation are represented by the additional anomalies, pulmonary stenosis with VSD, or develop high pulmonary vascular resistance.

Detection of Carrier: —

Special Considerations: —

References:
Elliot, L.P. et al: Complete transposition of the great vessels. I. An anatomic study of sixty cases. Circulation 27:1105, 1963.
Gramiak, R. et al: Echocardiographic diagnosis of transposition of the great vessels. Radiology 106:187, 1973.
Mustard, W.T. et al: The surgical management of transposition of the great vessels. J. Thorac. Cardiovasc. Surg. 48:953, 1964.
Paul, M.H.: Transposition of the great arteries. In Moss, A.J. and Adams, F.H. (eds.): Heart Disease in Infants, Children, and Adolescents. Baltimore: Williams & Wilkins, 1968, p. 527.
Sahn, D.J. et al: Multiple crystal cross-sectional echocardiography in the diagnosis of cyanotic congenital heart disease. Circulation 50:230, 1974.

Contributor: **Larry P. Elliott**

Editor's Computerized Descriptor: CV.

TREMOR, DUODENAL ULCERATION SYNDROME

Includes: Tremblement essentiel et ulcération duodénale
Tremor-Duodenalulcus-Syndrom
Síndrome de temblor y ulceración duodenal
Syndrome of essential tremor, congenital nystagmus, duodenal ulceration and narcolepsy-like sleep disturbance

Excludes: Essential heredofamilial tremor
Tremor of other etiology
Tremor of limbs and nystagmus
Tremor of head and nystagmus

Minimal Diagnostic Criteria: Slowly progressive "essential" tremor, "congenital" nystagmus, duodenal ulceration.

Clinical Findings: Nystagmus is present from birth or is noted in childhood (4-8 years): Rotary nystagmus at rest, intensified by lateral gaze, accompanied by refractive errors. Slowly progressive tremor starts in childhood, but more often after puberty, involving fingers, hands, shoulders and head; it is increased with fatigue or emotional upset, but temporarily alleviated by alcohol. Signs of cerebellar dysfunction may be present: Slight ataxia, unsteadiness, incoordination, clumsiness. Symptoms and signs of duodenal ulceration usually appear later in life but may precede the neurologic syndrome. Unusual need for sleep with a narcolepsy-like propensity for falling asleep is noted in some patients.

Complications
I **Derived:** Complaints and bleeding from duodenal ulceration. Physical handicap from increasing tremor and from cerebellar dysfunction. Social and mental deterioration because of alcoholism and physical disability.
II **Associated:** —

Etiology: Autosomal dominant; high penetrance and fairly uniform expressivity of the gene

Pathogenesis: ?

Related Facts
I **Sex Ratio:** M2:F1 (in the family reported)†
II **Risk of Occurrence:** ?
III **Risk of Recurrence for**
    Patient's Sib: If parent is affected 1 in 2 (50%) for each offspring to be affected; otherwise not increased
    Patient's Child: 1 in 2
IV **Age of Detectability:** Childhood or adolescence
V **Prevalence:** Rare; possibly more common in populations of Swedish-Finnish ancestry†

Treatment
I **Primary Prevention:** Genetic counseling
II **Secondary Prevention:** Dietary treatment and surgery for duodenal ulceration. Prevention of alcoholism. Physiotherapy.
III **Other Therapy:** —

Prognosis: Life expectancy usually is normal; the neurologic syndrome is slowly progressive. Some patients are incapacitated early in life by tremor, ataxia and alcoholism.

Detection of Carrier: —

†**Special Considerations:** The syndrome was seen in a family of Swedish-Finnish descent. In a few patients partial manifestations were noted, probably reflecting the heterozygous state of the mutant allele. The presence of cerebellar signs in severely affected persons may point to a possible pathogenetic relationship to the genetic cerebellar atrophies. The combination of neurologic dysfunction, duodenal ulceration and narcolepsy is explained by some disturbance of the autonomic nervous system.

References:
Neuhäuser, G. et al: Essential tremor, nystagmus and duodenal ulceration. A "new" dominantly inherited condition. Clin. Genet. 9:81, 1976.

Contributor: **Gerhard Neuhäuser**

Editor's Computerized Descriptors: Vision, Eye, GI., Nerve

TREMOR, HEREDOFAMILIAL

Includes: Tremblement hérédofamilial
Hereditärer Tremor
Temblor hereditario
Essential tremor
Tremor, autosomal dominant

Excludes: Huntington chorea (478)
Parkinson disease
Hepatolenticular degeneration (469)
Multiple sclerosis

Minimal Diagnostic Criteria: A symmetric familial tremor in an otherwise healthy individual in which medical and neurologic causes of tremor have been excluded.

Clinical Findings: A monosymptomatic tremor most commonly noted between the ages of 40 and 50 years. Although rarely documented at the age extremes, essential tremor has been noted to begin in the neonate and the elderly.

The tremor most commonly begins in the hands and arms in a symmetric fashion. It then may involve the facial muscles and tongue. If severe, dysarthria may result. The trunk and legs are least commonly involved. The tremor is more pronounced at rest. Fatigue and emotion may enhance and alcohol relieve the tremor. The tremor is of variable amplitude; the frequency 3-12 per second. The tremor may be progressive or remain unchanged throughout life. Remissions are rare. There are no associated neurologic signs in the majority of patients.

Complications
I   **Derived:** Approximately 20% eventually develop rigidity of varying degree.
II   **Associated:** —

Etiology: Autosomal dominant with complete penetrance by the age of 70; McK *19030

Pathogenesis: ? Many theories have been advanced. a) Autosomal dominant tremor is a monosymptomatic form of Parkinson disease. Larsson and Sjögren's large study did not support this view. b) Minor suggested the tremor was a triad which included fecundity and longevity. c) Marshall proposed that the tremor was physiologic but of a higher amplitude. No consistent neuropathology has been described.

Related Facts
I   **Sex Ratio:** M1:F1
II   **Risk of Occurrence:** ?
III   **Risk of Recurrence for**
    Patient's Sib: If parent is affected, 1 in 2 (50%) for each offspring to be affected; otherwise not increased.
    Patient's Child: 1 in 2
IV   **Age of Detectability:** Tremor usually evident by 5th decade
V   **Prevalence:** In Sweden it has been estimated that the gene frequency is 1 in 10,000. In the parish of Xa-sjö the gene frequency approaches 1 in 22.

Treatment
I   **Primary Prevention:** Theoretically genetic counseling†
II   **Secondary Prevention:** †
III   **Other Therapy:** If tremor is severe, appropriate job placement may be helpful.

Prognosis: Good for life span. Function affected by degree of tremor and rigidity.

Detection of Carrier: —

†**Special Considerations:** Most patients with autosomal dominant tremor do not seek medical advice. Many patients report that the tremor is mitigated by ethanol. Propanalol may be of help.

References:
Critchley, M.: Observations on essential heredofamilial tremor. Brain 72:113, 1949.
Larsson, M. and Sjögren, H.: Essential tremor; a clinical and genetic population study. Acta Psychiatr. Scand. 36(Suppl.) 144:1, 1960.

Contributor: **Robert H. A. Haslam**

Editor's Computerized Descriptor: Nerve

TRICHO-DENTO-OSSEOUS SYNDROME

Includes: Hypotrophie de l'émail, taurodontie, cheveux crépus, et sclérose de la corticale osseuse

Zahnschmelzhypoplasie, Taurodontie Kräuselhaar und Kortikalissklerose

Hipoplasia del esmalte, taurodontismo, cabello rizado y esclerosis cortical

Tooth, hair, bone and nail dysplasia

Hair, bone, nail and tooth dysplasia

Nail, hair, bone and tooth dysplasia

Bone, hair, nail and tooth dysplasia

Enamel hypoplasia and hypomaturation with taurodontism, curly hair and splitting of superficial layers of nails

Enamel hypoplasia, taurodontism, tight curly hair, and cortical sclerosteosis

Excludes: Amelogenesis imperfecta (46)

Enamel, hypoplasia (342)

Taurodontism (926)

Taurodontism associated with poly-X-chromosome genotypes

Onycholysis

Amelo-onycho-hypohidrotic syndrome (45)

Minimal Diagnostic Criteria: Hypoplasia of enamel of all teeth which have enlarged pulp chambers, the posterior teeth having a taurodont form, and with patient having tightly curly hair. Nail and bone defect not always present.

Clinical Findings: Patients with this syndrome have 5 associated features in the completely expressed syndrome.

1) Thin, brown-yellow enamel affecting both primary and secondary teeth (100%) which abrade easily and may be worn to the gums in older children. Teeth do not meet at the contact points. The enamel is thin, being about 1/4 to 1/8 normal thickness and is hypomature with a hardness less than normal enamel.

2) In addition, all teeth have very large pulp chambers (90%), the posterior teeth having an apical displacement of the bifurcation or trifurcation such that a taurodont tooth results. Tooth eruption, especially of posterior permanent teeth, may be delayed, and teeth may be congenitally missing.

3) Characteristic tightly, crinkly, curly hair of scalp and curly eyelashes (80%), especially in infancy. May become straight in later life.

4) Splitting of the superficial layers of the nails (50%). Not all nails show defect, some toenails being the only ones involved. Some nails are not brittle but have Meis lines.

5) Sclerosis of cortical bone occurs in about 30% with some affected individuals having multiple fractures. Sclerosis of base of skull, mastoids, and zones of provisional calcification in long bones.

6) Patients frequently present with single or multiple abcessed teeth from microexposures of dental pulp due to abnormal pulp horns which extend to dentinoenamel junction.

Complications

I   **Derived:** Attrition of teeth with exposure of pulp and abscess formation, premature loss of teeth

II   **Associated:** Mandibular prognathism and shallow nasal bridges are found in some families.

Etiology: Autosomal dominant; McK *13080

Pathogenesis: ? Possibly a defect in ectodermal cells involving the morpho-differentiation of tooth, hair and nail form and structure.

Related Facts

I   **Sex Ratio:** M1:F1

II   **Risk of Occurrence:** ? Very rare

III   **Risk of Recurrence for**

     Patient's Sib: 1 in 2 (50%) for each offspring to be affected; otherwise not increased

     Patient's Child: 1 in 2

IV   **Age of Detectability:** 6-12 months, at time of tooth eruption

V   **Prevalence:** Rare

Treatment

I   **Primary Prevention:** Genetic counseling

II   **Secondary Prevention:** Early restoration of teeth by jacket crowns. Later by prosthetic replacement.

III   **Other Therapy:** —

Prognosis: Does not seem to affect longevity. Premature loss of teeth in untreated case.

Detection of Carrier: —

Special Considerations: —

References:

Crawford, J.L.: Concomitant taurodontism and amelogenesis imperfecta in the American Caucasian. J. Dent. Child. 37:171, 1970.

Lichtenstein, J. et al: The tricho-dento-osseous (TDO) syndrome. Am. J. Hum. Genet. 24:569, 1972.

Robinson, G.C. et al: Hereditary enamel hypoplasia: Its association with characteristic hair structure. Pediatrics 37:498, 1966.

Contributors: **Carl J. Witkop, Jr.**
                        H. M. Worth

Editor's Computerized Descriptors: Teeth, Hair, Nails, Skel.

TRICHO-RHINO-PHALANGEAL SYNDROME, TYPE I

Includes: Syndrome tricho-rhino-phalangien de type I
Tricho-Rhino-Phalangeales Syndrom Typ I
Síndrome trico-rino-falángico tipo I

Excludes: Other forms of radiographic peripheral dysostosis
Tricho-rhino-phalangeal syndrome, Type II (967)

Minimal Diagnostic Criteria: Combination of physical and radiographic findings given below.

Clinical Findings: Small stature (variable)-adult heights have ranged from 39 (female) to 64 inches (male). Sparse slowly growing scalp hair, eyebrows heavier medially than laterally, long philtrum, pear-shaped nose (variable severity), usually deformity at proximal interphalangeal (IP) joints of hands. Cone-shaped epiphyses of fingers with premature fusion of involved epiphyses to shaft. Scattered pattern of involvement with proximal IP joints most commonly involved. There may be deviation of phalanges at involved joints. Metacarpals may be short (frontal projection). No abnormal laboratory findings.

Complications
I **Derived:** Thin hair and crooked fingers may be of cosmetic concern to affected individual, especially females. Legg-Perthes disease of dysplastic capital femoral epiphyses. One verified case, several adults with compatible residual deformity.
II **Associated:** Progressive arthritic symptoms of dorsal spine, elbows and fingers may occur in midlife.

Etiology: Majority are autosomal dominant, but a recessive form may also exist.† McK *19035

Pathogenesis: ?

Related Facts
I **Sex Ratio:** Too few cases for accurate estimate
II **Risk of Occurrence:** ?
III **Risk of Recurrence for**
   Patient's Sib: If autosomal dominant or autosomal recessive, see Table I AD or AR, respectively.
   Patient's Child: If autosomal dominant or autosomal recessive, see Table I AD or AR, respectively.
IV **Age of Detectability:** Late childhood by combination of radiographic and clinical methods
V **Prevalence:** ?

Treatment
I **Primary Prevention:** Genetic counseling
II **Secondary Prevention:** Wig if thin hair is of concern to affected individual
III **Other Therapy:** Treatment for Legg-Perthes disease if it occurs

Prognosis: Normal life expectancy

Detection of Carrier: —

†Special Considerations: There have been multiple affected sibs of both sexes with phenotypically normal parents reported. No consanguinity has been established but occurrence of 2 such affected sibs and 1 isolated case in small village suggests recessive gene. Families with affected individuals in 2 or 3 consecutive generations have been reported. There are no apparent morphologic differences between presumed recessive and dominant cases. The dominant form appears to be the most common. This syndrome must be distinguished from the TRP syndrome, type II (Langer-Giedion syndrome) which is associated with multiple cartilaginous exostoses.

References:
Giedion, A.: Cone-shaped epiphyses of the hands and their diagnostic value: The tricho-rhino-phalangeal syndrome. Ann. Radiol. (Paris) 10:322, 1967.
Giedion, A.: Die periphere Dysostose (PD) - ein Sammelbegriff. Fortschr. Rontgenstr. 110:507, 1969.
Giedion, A.: Acrodysplasias. Clin. Orthop. 114:107, 1976.

Contributors: **David L. Rimoin**
Leonard O. Langer, Jr.

Editor's Computerized Descriptors: Nose, Hair, Skel.

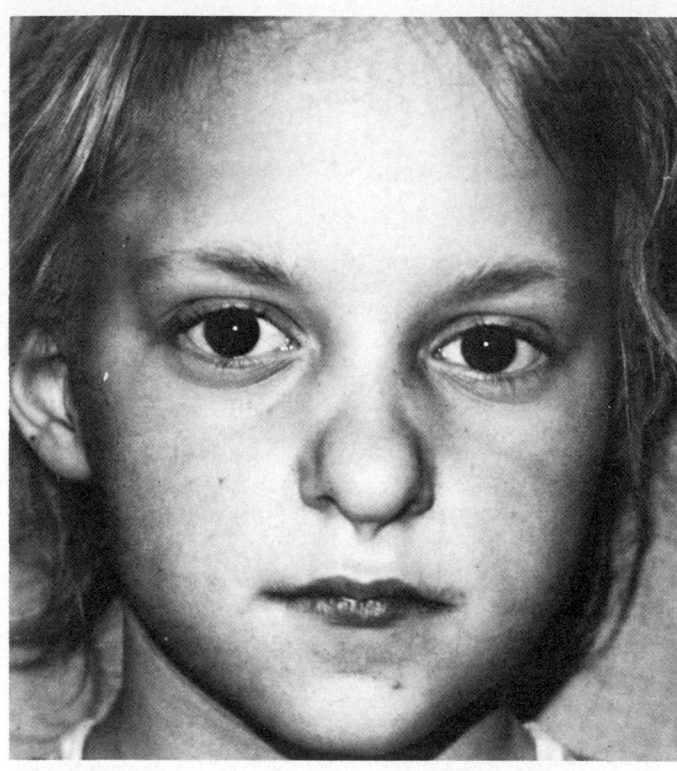

486. Note bulbous, pear-shaped nose with prominent philtrum

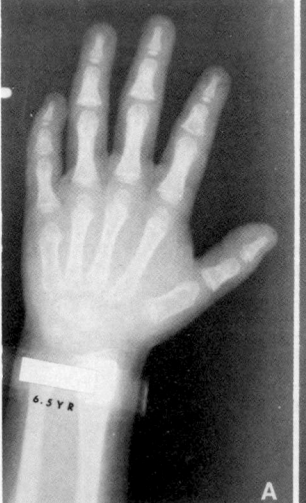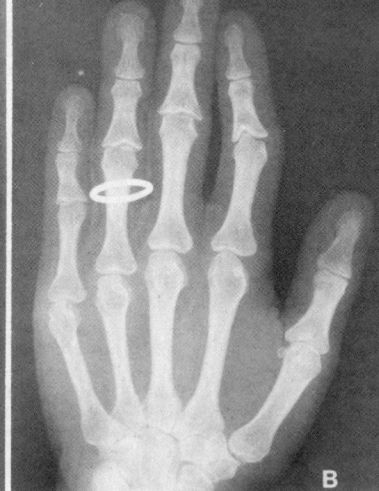

487. A) Note typical cone and ivory epiphyses in child's radiograph; B) in adult, some residual deformity from old cones is evident

TRICHO-RHINO-PHALANGEAL SYNDROME, TYPE II

Includes: Syndrome tricho-rhino-phalangien de type II
Tricho-Rhino-Phalangeales Syndrom, Typ II
Síndrome trico-rino-falángico, tipo II
Langer-Giedion syndrome
Tricho-rhino-auriculo-phalangeal multiple exostoses dysplasia
Acrodysplasia with exostoses

Excludes: Tricho-rhino-phalangeal syndrome, type I† (966)
Multiple cartilaginous exostoses† (685)

Minimal Diagnostic Criteria: Bulbous nose, cone epiphyses and multiple exostoses.

Clinical Findings: Features in all reported patients include craniofacies characterized by a bulbous, pear-shaped nose with tented alae, prominent elongated philtrum, apparent mandibular micrognathia, thin upper lip and large laterally protruding ears. Thin scalp hair, but eyebrows may be normal. Mild microcephaly not necessarily present at birth. Mild-to-moderate mental retardation and delay in onset of speech. Multiple cartilaginous exostoses with onset in childhood. The exostoses are present in the same distribution as in familial multiple exostoses. They may lead to asymmetric limb growth. Spinal curvature may be seen. Ribs may be thin. Short stature of postnatal onset. Cone-shaped epiphyses with clinobrachydactyly. Redundant or loose skin which improves with age.

Other features seen in some patients include laxity or hypermobility of joints and hypotonia, Perthes-like changes in capital femoral epiphyses, exotropia, winged scapulae, fractures, pigmented nevi increasing with age, recurrent respiratory infections, hearing deficit.

Complications
I **Derived:** Compression of nerves or vessels and limitation of movement or asymmetric growth of limbs may occur secondary to exostoses.
II **Associated:** Respiratory infections, fractures, mental retardation and developmental delay with marked delay in speech have been observed.

Etiology: ? All cases have been sporadic. No consanguinity or advanced parental age observed. Chromosomes have been normal.

Pathogenesis: Facies may be thought unusual at birth; growth delay in 1st year. The syndrome becomes diagnosable when sufficient number of epiphyses develop to note abnormalities, usually by the 3rd year. Exostoses develop and grow until puberty. Muscular hypotonia and skin laxity disappear with age.

Related Facts
I **Sex Ratio:** M6:F1
II **Risk of Occurrence:** Rare
III **Risk of Recurrence for**
    Patient's Sib: ? (1 pair of identical twins reported)
    Patient's Child: ?
IV **Age of Detectability:** Facies at birth; bone changes by 3 years of age
V **Prevalence:** Rare (7 reported cases)

Treatment
I **Primary Prevention:** ?
II **Secondary Prevention:** Orthopedic excision of impinging exostoses, special school for developmental delay with emphasis on speech development.
III **Other Therapy:** —

Prognosis: Limited by degree of mental retardation

Detection of Carrier: ?

†**Special Considerations:** It is important to distinguish this disorder from trichorhinophalangeal syndrome type I, and familial multiple exostoses because of the poorer prognosis, sporadic nature, mental retardation, and other complications seen in this condition.

References:
Hall, B.D. et al: Langer-Giedion syndrome. In Bergsma, D. (ed.): Skeletal Dysplasias. Birth Defects: Orig. Art. Ser., vol. X, no. 12. Amsterdam: Excerpta Medica for The National Foundation-March of Dimes, 1974, p. 147.
Spranger, J.W. et al: Bone Dysplasias. Philadelphia:W.B.Saunders, 1974, p. 234.

Contributor: **Judith G. Hall**

Editor's Computerized Descriptors: Ear, Face, Nose, Speech, Skin, Hair, Skel., Muscle, Resp.

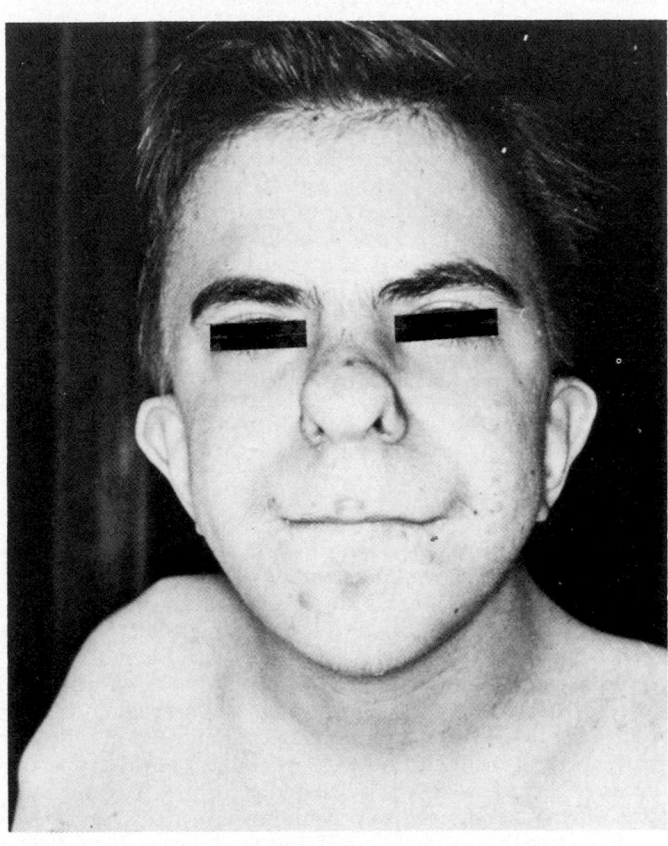

488. Note characteristic nose, bushy eyebrows, and long philtrum

TRICUSPID VALVE ATRESIA

Includes: Atrésie de la valvule tricuspide
Tricuspidalatresie
Atresia de la válvula tricuspídea
All cases in which the atrioventricular (AV) valve of the right
atrium is atretic†
Atresia of tricuspid valve

Excludes: Tricuspid valve stenosis (970)
Hypoplasia of tricuspid valve and right ventricle in conjunction
with pulmonary valve atresia
Cases of ventricular inversion in which the valve of the left atrium,
while tricuspid, is atretic

Minimal Diagnostic Criteria: Although tricuspid atresia is a great mimicker of other forms of cyanotic heart disease, the following findings are virtually pathognomonic in a patient who exhibits cyanosis: reversed Q loop in the horizontal plane (deeper Q waves in lead V_5 than V_6), diminished vascularity by xray and left axis deviation and the 2 aforementioned signs, plus the added roentgenologic finding of juxtaposition of the atrial appendages.

A selective right atriogram is the procedure of choice to confirm the diagnosis. All cases reveal the typical sequence of opacification: right atrium, left atrium, left ventricle. In cases with normally related great vessels and transposition with noninversion, there is a clear zone just below and medial to the lower margin of the right atrium, termed "right ventricular window." In patients with inversion, the right ventricular window is absent because the right ventricle is located superiorly and anteriorly. A selective left ventriculogram is recommended for precise location of the origin of the great arteries, type of obstruction to pulmonary flow if present, contractile state of the left ventricle, position of the right ventricle, and size of ventricular septal defect.

Clinical Findings: Despite considerable variation in the anatomic and physiologic manifestations from case to case, certain features are common to all. These are: atresia of the AV valve of the right atrium, patent atrial septum, an enlarged mitral orifice, a hypertrophied left ventricle which functions as a single ventricle, a rudimentary and essentially nonfunctioning right ventricle. Tricuspid atresia is divided into 2 main categories according to the relationship of the aorta and the pulmonary trunk, those with normally related great vessels and those with transposition of the great vessels. Tricuspid atresia with transposition may be subdivided into 2 additional categories, those with and without inversion of the ventricles. Regardless from which morphologic ventricle the pulmonary trunk arises, obstruction to pulmonary flow occurs under the following circumstances: atresia of the pulmonary valve with the pulmonary arteries perfused through a patent ductus arteriosus or via bronchial arteries, stenosis of the pulmonary valve, a narrowed subpulmonary tract, or a combination of the latter two. Among cases with normally related great vessels, obstruction to pulmonary flow may occur because of a small ventricular septal defect. Lastly, patients with transposition may exhibit the additional abnormality, double outlet right ventricle. The aorta is anterior and arises from a rudimentary right ventricle, while the pulmonary trunk arises partially or entirely from the right ventricle. Regardless, the left AV valve tissue is not in continuity with either semilunar valve. Juxtaposition of the atrial appendages-levoposition of the right atrial appendage-occurs in a relatively high percentage of cases with transposition and noninversion. A right aortic arch is present in 7-8% of cases. Dextrocardia or dextroversion, with atria in situs solitus position, also occurs with increased frequency especially where there is shunt vascularity.

The hemodynamic alterations, and consequently the clinical manifestations, will vary according to the magnitude of pulmonary flow, position of the great vessels and type of ventricular arrangement, inversion or noninversion. Whatever the anatomic type, in all cases of tricuspid atresia there is a right-to-left shunt at the atrial level. The right atrium becomes enlarged and hypertrophied since it functions as the sole pumping chamber for blood from the venae cavae. It pushes all the systemic venous blood through either a forced-open foramen ovale or through an atrial septal defect. The right ventricle is usually so diminutive as to be functionally ineffective. Consequently, the left ventricle becomes the single propelling chamber for delivery of blood into both great arteries. As the left atrium is the common mixing chamber into which all the saturated (pulmonary venous) and desaturated (systemic venous) blood is poured, the peripheral arterial saturation depends on the relative amounts of each. Other factors that diminish peripheral arterial saturation are ventricular failure and obstruction to aortic flow.

The presence of cyanosis, the ECG and the thoracic roentgenogram are the vital clinical data. The auscultatory findings are of little help. Cyanosis is common to most patients. Those with decreased pulmonary flow may exhibit hypoxic spells as well. In patients with increased pulmonary flow, cyanosis may be clinically absent. Congestive heart failure often occurs during infancy, especially when pulmonary flow is increased. Older children exhibit the usual stigmata of the cyanotic child, such as clubbing, growth retardation and frequent bouts of bronchitis. ECG evidence of left axis deviation is present in at least 90% of the cases. The exceptions are usually patients with excess pulmonary flow in whom a normal axis may be present. Usual signs are left ventricular hypertrophy and diminished or absent signs of right ventricular activity. Pure right ventricular hypertrophy is never seen. Patients with normally related great vessels show Q waves in the left precordial leads, whereas those with transposition rarely show Q waves in the left precordial leads. The presence of deeper Q waves in the lead V_5 than V_6 in a cyanotic patient is virtually pathognomonic of tricuspid atresia with normally related great vessels. The thoracic roentgenogram is extremely variable, and may mimic virtually any form of cyanotic heart disease. The pulmonary flow may be excessive (uncommon), normal (rare), or diminished (common). The classic and most common variety resembles tetralogy of Fallot. There are certain roentgen findings, when occurring in a cyanotic patient, that are suggestive of tricuspid atresia: juxtaposition of the atrial appendages, dextroversion or dextrocardia (in whom the atria are situs solitus), and right aortic arch which occurs in approximately 7-8% of cases.

The echocardiogram shows an absent tricuspid valve (although motion of the right atrial floor can be confused as valve), dilation of the left ventricular cavity, a small right ventricular cavity and a thickened right ventricular anterior wall. Caution must be exercised as this is a diagnosis of exclusion.

Cardiac catheterization will confirm the presence of a right-to-left shunt at the atrial level, degree of peripheral arterial desaturation, and often the presence or absence of obstruction to pulmonary flow, if the catheter is placed within the pulmonary trunk.

Complications

I Derived: Death from congestive heart failure and pneumonia, clubbing, severe hypoxic spells, growth retardation and frequent bouts of bronchitis.

II Associated: —

Etiology: Presumably multifactorial inheritance.

Pathogenesis: The formation of the right AV valve probably occurs during the 4th intrauterine week. Although embryogenesis is not fully understood, normal rotation of the ventricular septum probably fails and the right AV orifice is sacrificed, so that the embryologic AV valve results in an enlarged mitral valve at the expense of an atretic tricuspid valve.

Related Facts
I Sex Ratio: Approximately M1:F1
II Risk of Occurrence: Approximately 1 in 5000 live births
III Risk of Recurrence for
  Patient's Sib: Predicted risk 1.4%; empiric risk 1.0%
  Patient's Child: ? Reproductive fitness is grossly diminished.
IV Age of Detectability: From birth, by selective angiocardiography
V Prevalence: < 1 in 5000 in the pediatric population

Treatment
I Primary Prevention: Genetic counseling
II Secondary Prevention: In patients with obstruction to pulmonary flow, procedures are aimed at increasing pulmonary blood flow, which can be accomplished by a side-to-side anastomosis of the ascending aorta to the right pulmonary artery (Waterson-Cooley shunt) or by the creation of a subclavian artery-pulmonary artery shunt (Blalock-Taussig operation). In older children, an anastomosis between the superior vena cava and the distal right pulmonary artery (Glenn procedure) is preferred by some. Those patients with excess flow to the pulmonary arteries may require a banding to decrease pulmonary flow and prevent hyperresistant changes occurring in the vasculature. Some of these, plus patients with only a moderate degree of obstruction to pulmonary flow, may be managed medically. A few such patients reach adult age.
III Other Therapy: Symptomatic therapy for congestive heart failure and pneumonia.

Prognosis: The prognosis closely depends upon the anatomic type and in particular, the magnitude of pulmonary blood flow. Most patients, regardless of type, expire during infancy unless palliative surgery is performed. Those with some form of severe pulmonary stenosis expire owing to severe hypoxia and those with excess pulmonary flow expire secondary to congestive heart failure, pneumonia, etc. Those patients who survive infancy without palliation do so because they developed high pulmonary vascular resistance, or there is only a moderate degree of obstruction to pulmonary flow, regardless of origin of the pulmonary trunk.

Detection of Carrier: —

†Special Considerations: This includes cases with ventricular inversion in which the atretic right AV valve is bicuspid or mitral-like and the functioning left AV valve is tricuspid. Thus, the term "tricuspid atresia" is retained for all cases in which the AV valve of the right atrium is atretic, regardless of its anatomy.

References:
Diehl, A.M.: Tricuspid atresia. In Moss, A.J. and Adams, F.H. (eds.): Heart Disease in Infants, Children, and Adolescents. Baltimore: Williams & Wilkins Co., 1968.
Elliott, L.P. et al: The roentgenology of tricuspid atresia. Semin. Roentgenol. 3:399, 1968.
Glenn, W.W. et al: Circulatory bypass of the right side of the heart. VI. Shunt between superior vena cava and distal right pulmonary artery: Report of clinical application in 38 cases. Circulation 31:172, 1965.
Meyer, R.A., and Kaplan, S.: Echocardiography in the diagnosis of hypoplasia of the left or right ventricles in the neonate. Circulation. 46:55, 1972.

Contributors: **Larry P. Elliott**
Irvin F. Hawkins, Jr.

Editor's Computerized Descriptors: Resp., CV.

TRICUSPID VALVE INSUFFICIENCY

Includes: Insuffisance tricuspidienne
Tricuspidal insuffizienz
Insuficiencia tricuspídea
Tricuspid regurgitation
Tricuspid incompetence

Excludes: Tricuspid insufficiency secondary to Ebstein anomaly
Endocardial cushion defects (347)
Tricuspid insuffiency associated with acquired tricuspid insufficiency secondary to rheumatic heart disease, trauma, bacterial or fungal endocarditis
Transient neonatal tricuspid valve insufficiency

Minimal Diagnostic Criteria: Angiocardiography is the procedure of choice with cine- or biplane angiograms from the right ventricle demonstrating reflux into the right atrium. The normally inserted tricuspid valve distinguishes this lesion from Ebstein anomaly. Other diagnoses within the differential include pulmonary stenosis or atresia with tricuspid insufficiency with a normally sized right ventricle.

Clinical Findings: The pathologic anatomy in congenital tricuspid insufficiency varies. It may be due to a primary malformation (dysplasia) of the valve, shortened chordae tendineae, or defective papillary muscles with fibrosis. In some cases, the septal cusp remains adherent to the ventricular septum.

Isolated congenital tricuspid insufficiency is an extremely rare cardiac lesion. The most common presenting signs and symptoms include dyspnea, cyanosis, cardiomegaly and right-sided congestive heart failure. A pulsatile, enlarged liver and neck vein distention with prominent v waves have been observed.

A loud pansystolic murmur is invariably heard along the lower right or left sternal border with transmission to the back. The increase in intensity on inspiration suggests that the murmur is of tricuspid origin. An associated mid and late diastolic rumble represents relative tricuspid stenosis.

The roentgenographic findings are dependent on the severity of the lesion. In the symptomatic patient, the usual findings include massive cardiac enlargement with either normal or diminished vascularity of the lung fields. The right atrium is huge and, in postmortem studies, is 2-3 times the normal size. The right ventricular cavity is also increased in size.

The ECG commonly shows tall, peaked P waves, particularly in lead II, right axis deviation, and a q^R or $rs^{R'}$ pattern over the right precordium, indicating right atrial enlargement and right ventricular hypertrophy. Also seen in some cases is a right bundle branch block pattern.

The echocardiogram in the Ebstein abnormality is described elsewhere (see Ebstein Anomaly). In tricuspid insufficiency it shows a dilated right ventricle and septal motion may be paradoxic.

Selective right ventricular angiocardiography demonstrates reflux of contrast material into the right atrium during ventricular systole. A right-to-left atrial shunt through a patent foramen ovale is often an associated finding.

The right atrial mean pressure is invariably elevated; and the right atrial pressure pulse has a systolic plateau with a prominent V wave and a rapid y descent. In the symptomatic neonate, right ventricular pressure is often at systemic levels, and is associated with pulmonary hypertension.

Complications
I   **Derived:** Most infants improve with digitalis, diuretics, and

oxygen as the pulmonary vascular resistance falls. Follow-up of many of these children has shown relatively normal hemodynamics with mild tricuspid insufficiency.
II   **Associated:** Not determined

Etiology: ?

Pathogenesis: Uncertain, but probably due to the abnormal or incomplete elaboration of the septal cusp of the tricuspid valve. This may be adherent to the septum or possess only very short chordae tendineae.

Related Facts
I   **Sex Ratio:** M1:F1 probable
II   **Risk of Occurrence:** Extremely rare. Less than 20 cases reported in the world literature.
III   **Risk of Recurrence for**
    Patient's Sib: ?
    Patient's Child: ?
IV   **Age of Detectability:** From birth by selective angiocardiography
V   **Prevalence:** ?

Treatment
I   **Primary Prevention:** —
II   **Secondary Prevention:** Those instances of functional tricuspid insufficiency revert to normal when the underlying abnormality is corrected. Oxygen, which dilates the pulmonary vascular bed and thus results in a lowering of pulmonary vascular resistance, has a role in management. Surgical intervention has rarely been attempted, and usually has a fatal outcome.
III   **Other Therapy:** Symptomatic therapy for right-sided congestive heart failure including digitalization and diuretics, and oxygen.

Prognosis: —

Detection of Carrier: ?

Special Considerations: —

References:
Ahn, A.J. and Segal, B.L.: Isolated tricuspid insufficiency: Clinical features, diagnosis and management. Prog. Cardiovasc. Dis. 9:166, 1966.
Gŏldberg, S.J. et al: Pediatric and Adolescent Echocardiography. Chicago:Year Book Medical Publishers, 1975.
Reisman, M. et al: Congenital tricuspid insufficiency: A cause of massive cardiomegaly and heart failure in the neonate. J. Pediatr. 66:869, 1965.

Contributors: **William E. Hellenbrand**
Michael A. Berman
Norman S. Talner

Editor's Computerized Descriptors: Resp., CV., Liver

TRICUSPID VALVE STENOSIS

Includes: Sténose tricuspidienne
Tricuspidalstenose
Estenosis tricuspídea
Congenital narrowing of tricuspid orifice as a consequence of either a small annulus or thickened valve leaflets

Excludes: Acquired tricuspid stenosis secondary to rheumatic heart disease or right atrial myxomas
Functional or relative tricuspid stenosis due to increased flow in cases with large atrial level shunts
Tricuspid valve atresia (968)
Ebstein anomaly (332)

Minimal Diagnostic Criteria: The clinical, radiologic, ECG, and echocardiographic manifestations of tricuspid stenosis with right ventricular hypoplasia are often identical, with tricuspid atresia. Cardiac catheterization with selective angiocardiography are confirmatory for the diagnosis.

Clinical Findings: Isolated tricuspid stenosis is extremely rare, with only 6 proven cases reported in the literature. With moderate-to-severe tricuspid stenosis right atrial hypertension occurs, resulting in hypertrophy and dilatation of the chamber. Atrial dilatation promotes continued patency of the foramen ovale which allows for right atrial decompression. A large atrial communication may transfer the burden of right atrial overload to the left heart as systemic venous blood gains access to the systemic circulation. The majority of children with congenital tricuspid stenosis have diminished pulmonary flow and may present in early infancy with cyanosis, initially only when the infant is straining or crying. Cyanotic spells associated with paroxysmal dyspnea may occur in these patients within the first 6 months of life. The large right-to-left atrial communication may bypass the right ventricle in toto and, therefore, there is insufficient flow across the tricuspid valve to produce a detectable murmur. Where right atrial to right ventricular blood flow is of sufficient magnitude, atrial contraction may be reflected as a presystolic precordial impulse at the left sternal border, a jugular venous a wave, or a hepatic presystolic pulsation. A short mid-to-late diastolic rumble can rarely be appreciated. Other murmurs will reflect the associated lesions, particularly pulmonary stenosis, ventricular septal defect, and patent ductus arteriosus.

Roentgenograms of the chest reveal decreased pulmonary vascularity and signs of an enlarged right atrium. The plain films cannot be distinguished from the trilogy of Fallot, Ebstein malformation of the tricuspid valve, and certain forms of tricuspid atresia.

The ECG demonstrates a normal or right axis with right atrial and left ventricular hypertrophy. Dominance by left ventricular forces could result from the presence of right ventricular hypoplasia.

The echocardiogram shows decreased amplitude of the tricuspid valve in diastole, a decreased E-F slope of valve motion, a small right ventricular cavity and thickened right ventricular anterior wall. In severe forms, the tricuspid valve motion may be absent and thus be indistinguishable from tricuspid atresia.

Cardiac catheterization helps to confirm the diagnosis of tricuspid stenosis as well as to rule out any associated defects. Passage of the catheter from the right atrium to the right ventricle on occasion may be difficult since the preferred pathway is into the left atrium. Simultaneous right atrial and right ventricular tracings should demonstrate a diastolic pressure difference, but such simultaneous records are rarely obtained. Generally, pullback tracings from the right ventricle to the right atrium are used for detection of the abnormality.

Selective right atrial and right ventricular angiocardiography are the procedure(s) of choice, in conjunction with echocardiography, for demonstrating the abnormality and associated defect(s). Frequently, the right atrial injection will show thickening of the valve and demonstrate the right-to-left atrial shunt.

Complications
I **Derived:** Systemic venous congestion manifested by peripheral edema and ascites. Infrequently, a superior vena caval type of syndrome may develop.
II **Associated:** —

Etiology: ?

Pathogenesis: Tricuspid stenosis is probably due to partial fusion of the tricuspid valve primordia at an early age.

Related Facts
I **Sex Ratio:** M?:F?
II **Risk of Occurrence:** 1 in 1000 cases of autopsied congenital heart disease.
III **Risk of Recurrence for**
    Patient's Sib: ?
    Patient's Child: ?
IV **Age of Detectability:** From birth, with selective angiocardiography
V **Prevalence:** ? Very rare

Treatment
I **Primary Prevention:** —
II **Secondary Prevention:** Tricuspid stenosis may be corrected by valvotomy or prosthetic valvar replacement. Associated lesions must be considered individually. Patients with right ventricular hypoplasia or other lesions, which are not amenable to surgical corrections, may benefit from either a superior vena cava to right pulmonary artery anastomosis or a systemic to pulmonary artery anastomosis.
III **Other Therapy:** The use of an atrial-to-pulmonary artery conduit or right artial-right ventricular outflow conduit has also been suggested.

Prognosis: Influenced primarily by the severity of the stenosis, and usually by the severity of the associated intracardiac abnormalities.

Detection of Carrier: ?

Special Considerations: —

References:
Bopp, R.K. et al: Surgical considerations for treatment of congenital tricuspid atresia and stenosis with particular reference to vena cava-pulmonary artery anastomosis. J. Thorac. Cardiovasc. Surg. 43:97, 1962.
Gasul, G.M. et al: Tricuspid stenosis and isolated hypoplasia of the right ventricle. In Heart Disease in Children: Diagnosis and Treatment. Philadelphia:J.P. Lippincott, 1966, p. 686.
Goldberg, S.J. et al: Pediatric and Adolescent Echocardiography. Chicago:Year Book Medical Publishers, 1975.
Medd, W.E. et al: Isolated hypoplasia of the right ventricle and tricuspid valve in siblings. Br. Heart J. 23:25, 1961.

Contributors: **William E. Hellenbrand**
                    Michael A. Berman
                    Norman S. Talner

Editor's Computerized Descriptor: CV.

TRUE HERMAPHRODITISM

Includes: Hermaphrodisme vrai
Echter Hermaphroditismus
Hermafroditismo
Hermaphroditism
Hermaphroditismus vera

Excludes: Chromosome 45,X/46,XY mosaicism (173)
All disorders of sexual differentiation without demonstrable ovarian follicles and testicular tubules or spermatozoa
All other forms of male pseudohermaphroditism
All forms of female pseudohermaphroditism

Minimal Diagnostic Criteria: Histologically verified ovarian follicles and seminiferous tubules or spermatozoa. A 46,XX/46,XY or 46,XX/47,XXY complement does not alone warrant the diagnosis.

Clinical Findings: True hermaphrodites have both ovarian and testicular tissue, specifically 1) histologically verified ovarian follicles or proof of their prior existence (eg corpora albicantia); fibrous stroma will not suffice; and 2) testicular tubules or spermatozoa; Leydig or hilar cells will not suffice. The diagnosis is applied irrespective of chromosome complement. Somatic anomalies are usually absent.

Most true hermaphrodites are 46,XX but a few are 46,XY, 46,XX/46,XY, or 46,XX/47,XXY. Their external genitalia are usually ambiguous or predominantly male with evidence of androgen insufficiency (eg hypospadias or bifid scrotum). About 70% are reared as males. A vagina and well-differentiated uterus are usually present. Fallopian tubes are less likely to be normal.

Gonadal tissue may be organized into separate ovary and testis, or, more often, combined into 1 or more ovotestes. Relative locations of ovarian and testicular tissue may be 1) bilateral, both ovarian and testicular tissue present on each side, usually in the form of ovotestes; 2) unilateral, both ovarian and testicular tissue present only on 1 side, with gonadal tissue of a single type present on the contralateal side; or 3) alternate, ovarian tissue present on 1 side and testicular tissue present on the opposite side. The greater the proportion of testicular tissue in an ovotestis, the greater the likelihood of gonadal descent. In 80% of the ovotestes the testicular and ovarian components exist in end-to-end fashion; thus, most testes can be detected externally because testicular tissue is softer and darker than ovarian tissue. In 20% of ovotestes the testicular tissue is limited to the hilar region. A vas deferens may be present near a testis or ovotestis; if so, no fallopian tube is usually present on that side. Fallopian tubes adjacent to ovotestes often show occlusion of the fimbriated end. Spermatozoa are rarely present but oocytes are often present. Leydig cell hyperplasia occurs in about one-third of cases, and seminiferous tubules may contain many Sertoli cells.

Endocrine features at puberty depend upon the extent of testicular or ovarian tissue present, but true hermaphrodites are more likely to feminize than to virilize. Most patients with a uterus menstruate. If the uterus is not connected to the urogenital sinus, hematometrocolpos may develop. In some true hermaphrodites with predominantly male external genitalia menstruation has occurred in the form of cylic hematuria. Squamous metaplasia of the endocervix is relatively common. The above description applies in general to true hermaphrodites; however, some data suggest that the phenotypes associated with different karyotypes may be dissimilar.†

Complications
I   Derived: Puberal virilization in individuals reared as females; puberal feminization in individuals reared as males. Neoplastic transformation of intraabdominal or inguinal testes has been reported.
II   Associated: None consistently present.

Etiology: True hermaphrodites are etiologically heterogeneous. 46,XX/46,XY or 46,XX/47,XXY true hermaphroditism presumably results from chimerism or mosaicism. The etiology of 46,XY true hermaphroditism is unknown, but phenotypic similarities with 46,XX/46,XY true hermaphrodites suggest that many apparent 46,XY true hermaphrodites may have undetected 46,XX cells. There is 1 report of X-chromatin negative sibs with true hermaphroditism, but more extensive cytogenetic studies were not available.

The presence of testicular tissues in individuals lacking a Y (ie 46,XX true hermaphrodites) could be explained in at least 4 ways. 1) Undetected mosaicism or chimerism, 46,XY cells thus being present but not detected. 2) Translocation of Y-linked testicular determinants to an X chromosome. 3) Translocation of Y-linked testicular determinants to an autosome. 4) A mutant gene(s). Each may be applicable in certain cases. H-Y antigen, which is either closely linked to or the actual gene product of the Y-testicular determinant, has been detected in 46,XX true hermaphrodites. This and other evidence suggests that in some 46,XX true hermaphrodites a portion of the Y chromosome containing the H-Y locus (and the testicular determinants) has become translocated to an X or to an autosome. However, translocation involving H-Y antigen cannot alone explain 46,XY true hermaphroditism because it fails to explain the coexisting ovarian development. 46,XX true hermaphroditism is usually not heritable, but in 3 families multiple sibs had 46,XX true hermaphroditism. The presence of both XX males and XX true hermaphrodites in more than 1 generation of another family cannot be explained by recessive factors.

Pathogenesis: The cellular pathogenesis depends upon the etiology of true hermaphroditism. 46,XX/46,XY true hermaphroditism presumably results from admixtures of 46,XX and 46,XY germ cells. Translocation of testicular determinants from the Y to an X or an autosome could explain the presence of testicular tissue in indiviudals who apparently lack a Y chromosome. However, such an explanation fails to account for the presence of both ovarian and testicular tissue. Likewise, even if sex-reversal gene(s) exist, their mechanism of action is unknown.

Related Facts
I   Sex Ratio: Not applicable
II   Risk of Occurrence: Rare
III   Risk of Recurrence for
Patient's Sib: Usually negligible. However, in families in which 46,XX true hermaphroditism appears to be inherited in autosomal recessive fashion, the recurrence risk is presumably 1 in 8 for all sibs, and 1 in 4 for 46,XX sibs.
Patient's Child: Patients are infertile, except for 1 purported case. If true hermaphrodites are fertile, their offspring are not likely to be affected.
IV   Age of Detectability: Usually at birth because of genital ambiguity, but some patients with relatively normal external genitalia may not be detected until puberty, at which time they fail to show normal secondary sexual development. Occasionally 46,XX/46,XY true hermaphroditism is suspected by recognizing iridal heterochromia or by detecting 2 populations of erythrocytes during blood grouping analyses.
V   Prevalence: Rare

Treatment
I   Primary Prevention: Genetic counseling is appropriate in selected instances.
II   Secondary Prevention: Genital reconstruction. Extirpation

of cryptorchid testes may be appropriate to prevent neoplastic transformation. Administration of hormones may be necessary.

III Other Therapy: —

Prognosis: Normal life span, provided neoplasia does not occur; infertility.

Detection of Carrier: No information; usually not applicable

†Special Considerations: True hermaphroditism is usually not diagnosed before surgical exploration. Thus, an infant with genital ambiguity is best considered to have a form of female or male pseudohermaphroditism. True hermaphroditism should be considered only after other diagnoses seem inappropriate. However the diagnosis may be suspected if one observes 1) chimerism, 2) a gonad the tissue of which shows 2 consistencies (a softer testicular portion and a firmer ovarian portion), 3) squamous metaplasia of the endocervix, or 4) a fallopian tube with fimbrial occlusion.

References:
Armendares, S. et al; Familial true hermaphroditism in three siblings. Humangenetik 20;99, 1976.
Jones, H.W., Jr. and Scott, W.M.; Hermaphroditism, Genital Anomalies, and Related Endocrine Disorders, 2nd Ed. Baltimore; Williams and Wilkins, 1971.
Simpson, J.L.; Disorders of Sexual Differentiation; Etiology and Clinical Delineation. New York: Academic Press, 1976.
Simpson, J.L.: True hermaphroditism, etiology and phenotypic considerations. In Bergsma, D. and Summitt, R.L. (eds.): Sex Differentiation and Chromosomal Abnormalities. Birth Defects: Orig. Art. Ser., vol. XIV, no. 6C. New York: Alan R. Liss, Inc. for the National Foundation-March of Dimes, 1978.
Van Niekerk, W.A.: True Hermaphroditism. New York: Harper and Row, 1974.
Wachtel, S.S. et al: Possible role for H-Y antigen in the primary determination of sex. Nature (London) 257:235, 1975.
Wachtel, S.S. et al: Serologic detection of a Y-linked gene in XX males and XX true hermaphrodites. N. Engl. J. Med. 295:750, 1976.

Contributor: **Joe Leigh Simpson**

Editor's Computerized Descriptor: GU.

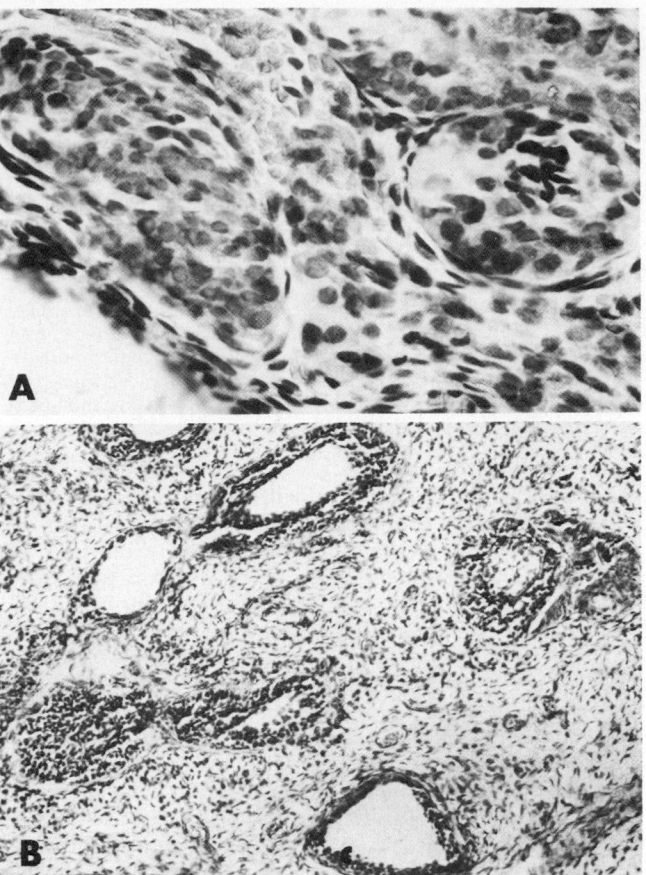

489. A) Neonatal biopsy of right gonad: immature well-formed testicular tubules and regressing Leydig cells in interstitium; B) left gonad: loose, poorly differentiated ovarian stroma; solid and vesicular follicles. Note single tubulofollicular structure

TRUNCUS ARTERIOSUS

Includes: Persistencia del tronco arterioso
Persistent truncus arteriosus types I,II,III & IV
Truncus arteriosus communis persistens

Excludes: Pseudotruncus arteriosus (tetralogy of Fallot with pulmonary atresia)
Hemitruncus
Aortico-pulmonary septal defect (83)

Minimal Diagnostic Criteria: Angiocardiography is the procedure of choice to confirm the diagnosis. Either selective ascending thoracic "aortography" or right ventriculography will delineate the anatomic abnormalities. Since in this malformation there is a certain degree of maldevelopment of the conus septum, the latter procedure will characteristically show absence of a well-developed right ventricular infundibulum.

Clinical Findings: The pathologic anatomy of this lesion is characterized by the presence of a large single arterial vessel at the base of the heart (without any remnant of either an atretic aorta or pulmonary trunk) from which the aortic arch, pulmonary and coronary arteries originate. The truncal valve is usually tricuspid but may be bicuspid or have 4 or more cusps. A large subvalvar ventricular septal defect is always present.

Four basic anatomic types have been described according to the site of origin of the arteries supplying the lungs. In the most common, type I, the pulmonary arteries arise from the left inferior aspect of the common arterial trunk by means of a short main stem. Less frequently, the pulmonary arteries arise close together from the dorsal wall (type II) or independently from either side of the truncus (type III). In the rare and controversial type IV, the pulmonary arteries are absent and the lungs are supplied by bronchial arteries arising from the descending aorta. It may be impossible to differentiate this type with certainty from tetralogy of Fallot with atresia of the pulmonary trunk. A right aortic arch is present in approximately 25% of the cases. Associated extracardiac anomalies are common.

The hemodynamic alterations and consequently the clinical manifestations will vary according to the magnitude of pulmonary blood flow. In the common types, with large unobstructed pulmonary arteries arising from the arterial trunk, pulmonary blood flow is greatly increased. This is the case in infants and small children with low resistance in the pulmonary vascular bed. They present with the physical findings of a large extracardiac left-to-right shunt. Cyanosis is only minimal or absent and the infants usually have congestive heart failure, frequent respiratory infections and growth retardation. A loud systolic murmur along the lower left sternal border is always present. It is characteristically preceded by a constant ejection click and ends before the second sound. The second sound is described as loud and single but "splitting" is not uncommon. A diastolic apical flow murmur is frequently present. Early diastolic murmurs of truncal valve insufficiency may also be present. Continuous, machinery-type murmurs are rare. With the development of a high pulmonary vascular resistance, the left-to-right shunt gradually diminishes, the patient becomes progressively more cyanotic and the apical diastolic flow murmur disappears. In the few instances of small or stenotic arteries to the lungs (pulmonary or bronchial) pulmonary blood flow is markedly reduced and the clinical features, from early infancy, are similar to those seen in cyanotic tetralogy of Fallot.

The roentgenographic findings depend on which hemo-dynamic situation is present. In the usual case, with a large left-to-right shunt, cardiomegaly and prominent pulmonary vascularity are the rule. In the presence of a right aortic arch these findings are highly suggestive of persistent truncus arteriosus. If the pulmonary vascular resistance increases, the magnitude of the left-to-right shunt progressively diminishes. Consequently the cardiomegaly and pulmonary plethora decrease. In the few cases with decreased pulmonary blood flow due to small arterial supply to the lungs, as in the so-called type IV, the plain roentgenographic findings will be similar to those seen in severe cases of tetralogy of Fallot.

The ECG commonly shows normal mean QRS axis for age, atrial enlargement and biventricular hypertrophy. With high resistance in the pulmonary vascular bed, right axis deviation and right ventricular hypertrophy are usually present.

Abnormalities of the tetralogy/truncus group are characterized echocardiographically by the demonstration of preservation of mitral-aortic continuity with a lack of septal aortic continuity; that is, aortic override. Echocardiographic differentiation between tetralogy and truncus requires the demonstration of a pulmonary valve. As this is often difficult to do in severe tetralogy, it is a hazardous differential diagnosis. Both lesions often have concomitant thickening of the right ventricular wall and enlargement of the right ventricular cavity. In many patients with truncus arteriosus, the degree of override is greater, and at times multiple abnormal truncal valve cusp echoes may be imaged to aid in the differential diagnosis.

Cardiac catheterization will usually confirm the presence of high flow, high pressure, intra-and extracardiac, bidirectional shunt. Oximetry data are not reliable, since right ventricular, pulmonary artery, and aortic samples are strongly influenced by streaming. A left-to-right shunt at the ventricular level may go undetected, and aortic oxygen saturation may exceed pulmonary artery saturation.

Complications
I **Derived:** Truncal valve insufficiency, death from congestive heart failure and pneumonia, frequent development of high pulmonary vascular resistance leading eventually to the "Eisenmenger physiology."
II **Associated:** A high incidence of extracardiac congenital anomalies has been reported (up to 50%) particularly when a left aortic arch is present. Most common are absence or hypoplasia of 1 kidney, absent gallbladder, hypoplastic lung, and cleft palate or bony abnormalities.

Etiology: Present evidence supports multifactorial inheritance.

Pathogenesis: Most likely due to failure of division of the embryonic truncus arteriosus with consequent abnormal development of the truncoconal area, resulting in a single semilunar valve and a subvalvar ventricular septal defect. The difference between the described anatomic types may well result from the lack of development of the truncus septum alone (type I) or in association with nondevelopment of the aorticopulmonary septum (types II and III). Type IV could theoretically be the result of an associated complete failure of development of the 6 aortic arches bilaterally.

Related Facts
I **Sex Ratio:** M2:F1
II **Risk of Occurrence:** ? Approximately 1 in 200 cases of congenital heart defects
III **Risk of Recurrence for**
Patient's Sib: Predicted risk and empiric risk for truncus or developmentally related lesion 1 in 100
Patient's Child: ?
IV **Age of Detectability:** From birth by selective angiocardiography
V **Prevalence:** Near 1 in 33,000

Treatment
I Primary Prevention: —

II Secondary Prevention: Palliative banding of the pulmonary arteries to prevent the development of pulmonary vascular changes. Repair of the ventricular septal defect and construction of a pulmonary trunk with a valved external conduit.

III Other Therapy: Symptomatic therapy for congestive heart failure and pneumonia.

Prognosis: The prognosis closely depends upon the anatomic type and in particular, the magnitude of the pulmonary blood flow. It is generally poor in infants with excessive blood flow to the lungs. Most of these die within the 1st year. The few patients who survive infancy develop high pulmonary vascular resistance and have only a small increase in pulmonary blood flow. They have a better short-term prognosis with a relatively normal life during childhood.

Detection of Carrier: —

Special Considerations: —

References:

Chung, K.J. et al: Echocardiography in truncus arteriosus. Circulation 48:381, 1973.

McNamara, D.G. and Sommerville, R.J.: Truncus arteriosus. In Moss, A.J. and Adams, F.H. (eds.): Heart Disease in Infants, Children, and Adolescents. Baltimore: Williams & Wilkins Co., 1968. p. 637.

Morris, D.C. et al: Echocardiographic diagnosis of tetralogy of Fallot. Am. J. Cardiol. 36:911, 1975.

Victorica, B.E. et al: Persistent truncus arteriosus in infancy: A study of 14 cases. Am. Heart J. 77:13, 1969.

Wallace, R.B. et al: Complete repair of truncus arteriosus defects. J. Thorac. Cardiovasc. Surg. 47:95, 1969.

Contributor: **Benjamin E. Victorica**

Editor's Computerized Descriptors: Resp., CV.

TRYPSINOGEN DEFICIENCY

Includes: Déficit en trypsinogène
Trypsinogenmangelkrankheit
Deficiencia de tripsinógeno
Isolated trypsinogen deficiency

Excludes: Enterokinase deficiency
Generalized pancreatic exocrine insufficiency

Minimal Diagnostic Criteria: Demonstration of trypsinogen deficiency is required. Basal-and secretin-stimulated duodenal aspirates will contain subnormal activities of peptidases but normal amylase and lipase. After incubation with enterokinase there is no increase in trypsin activity. After incubation with bovine trypsin, there is normal activity of carboxypeptidase, chymotrypsin and elastase, but no augmentation of tryptic activity. The maneuvers indicate an absence of pancreatic trypsinogen.†

Clinical Findings: The 3 reported patients presented in infancy with failure to thrive, hypoproteinemia, edema, and anemia—the pattern of protein-calorie malnutrition. Generalized malabsorption was evident in each. There was no evidence for serum protein loss in urine or stool. Fecal nitrogen and fat excretion were increased. Pancreatic exocrine function was characteristically disturbed.

Complications

I Derived: Protein malabsorption; hypoproteinemia; edema; secondary pancreatic exocrine dysfunction; generalized malabsorption; failure to grow and gain weight; and anemia.

II Associated: —

Etiology: ? McK *27600

Pathogenesis: Normal trypsinogen is secreted by the pancreas and is converted within the intestinal lumen to trypsin. Trypsin, in turn, activates other propeptidases to their active enzymatic forms. Deficiency of trypsinogen results in subnormal activities of all peptidases. Lipase and amylase are secreted as active enzymes and are not deficient in trypsinogen deficiency disease.

Related Facts

I Sex Ratio: M2:F1

II Risk of Occurrence: ?

III Risk of Recurrence for
    Patient's Sib: ?
    Patient's Child: ?

IV Age of Detectability: Infancy

V Prevalence: ? 3 reported cases

Treatment

I Primary Prevention: —

II Secondary Prevention: Provision of pancreatic enzymes by per oral replacement; elemental diets are useful in providing nutrition in infancy.

III Other Therapy: —

Prognosis: Excellent

Detection of Carrier: —

†Special Considerations: Confusion may occur in 2 circumstances: 1) The severely malnourished infant with generalized pancreatic exocrine dysfunction and subnormal activities of all exocrine enzymes. 2) Trypsinogen activation may be accomplished by incubation with bovine trypsin (4° C for 16 hours) in some patients. This test is not reliable and should not be used to diagnose absence of trypsinogen. Enterokinase alone should be used in the incubation as a pro-enzyme activator.

References:

Morris, M.D. and Fisher, D.A.: Trypsinogen deficiency disease. Am. J. Dis. Child. 114:203, 1967.

Townes, P.L.: Trypsinogen deficiency disease. J. Pediatr. 66:275, 1965.

Townes, P.L. et al: Further observations on trypsinogen deficiency disease: Report of a second case. J. Pediatr. 71:220, 1967.

Contributor: **Peter F. Whitington**

Editor's Computerized Descriptor: Skin

TRYPTOPHAN MALABSORPTION

Includes: Malabsorption de tryptophane
Malabsorción de triptófano
Blue diaper syndrome

Excludes: Intestinal malabsorption syndromes
Hartnup disorder† (453)
Phenylketonuria† (808)

Minimal Diagnostic Criteria: Severe prolonged hypercalcemia which can be provoked by L-tryptophan. Excess tryptophan in feces.

Tryptophan derivatives increased in urine (eg indole acetic acid, indolelactic acid, indolylacetyl glutamine, indole acetamide and indican); these derivatives are of intestinal origin, secondary to retention of tryptophan in the intestinal lumen.

Blue staining of diapers caused by indigotin presumably formed by enzymatic conversion of indolic compounds in urine. The source of the urinary enzyme(s) may be from damaged renal tissue.

Normal plasma tryptophan concentration and less-than-normal rise following oral L-tryptophan load (100 mg/kg).

Renal clearance of tryptophan normal under endogenous conditions.

Clinical Findings: A syndrome characterized by hypercalcemia and nephrocalcinosis, associated with defect in intestinal absorption of L-tryptophan. Two brothers had a similar clinical course involving failure to thrive, recurrent unexplained fever, infections, irritability and constipation. Bluish discoloration of the diapers was observed continuously from early infancy. The first-born died after a mastoidectomy; the second was alive at 44 months. The vitamin D intake was 1400 units daily in both patients (maximum RDA: 400 units), but no clinical signs of the infantile hypercalcemia syndrome were apparent.

Complications
I   **Derived:** Hypercalcemia, producing nephrocalcinosis. The defect in tryptophan absorption is, in some way as yet undetermined, correlated with the occurrence of hypercalcemia.
II **Associated:** —

Etiology: Limited evidence suggests autosomal recessive or X-linked recessive biochemical defect.

Pathogenesis: Proposed deficiency of substrate-specific intestinal membrane transport system for L-tryptophan.

Related Facts
I   **Sex Ratio:** In the only reported pedigree there were 2 affected male sibs, 1 female sib with no symptoms, but "occasionally blue diapers," and 1 normal male sib.
II   **Risk of Occurrence:**   ?
III **Risk of Recurrence for**
     Patient's Sib: If autosomal recessive or X-linked recessive, see Table I AR or X-linked R, respectively.
     Patient's Child: If autosomal recessive or X-linked recessive, see Table I AR or X-linked R, respectively.
IV   **Age of Detectability:**   ?
V   **Prevalence:**   ?

Treatment
I   **Primary Prevention:** —
II   **Secondary Prevention:** Reduced protein intake; advisable to limit vitamin D intake to 400 units/day. Treatment for hypercalcemia, avoidance of dietary alkali and high milk intake is prudent.
III **Other Therapy:** —

Prognosis: Limited if hypercalcemia is complicated by nephrocalcinosis.

Detection of Carrier: Both parents in the only reported pedigree were free of abnormal biochemical manifestations or clinical symptoms.

†**Special Considerations:** The indoluria may resemble that present in Hartnup disease, but a specific hyperaminoaciduria distinguishes the latter trait. Indoluria also occurs in phenylketonuria, apparently because phenylalanine competes with tryptophan for intestinal absorption. In neither primary disease is there hypercalcemia. Tryptophan malabsorption and indoluria accompany many forms of intestinal malabsorption.

References:

Drummond, K. N. et al: The blue diaper syndrome: Familial hypercalcemia with nephrocalcinosis and indicanuria; a new familial disease with definition of the metabolic abnormality. Am. J. Med. 37:928, 1964.

Michael, A. F. et al: Tryptophan metabolism in man. J. Clin. Invest. 43:1730, 1964.

Contributor: **Charles R. Scriver**

————————————

Editor's Computerized Descriptors: GI., GU., Nerve

TUBEROUS SCLEROSIS

Includes: Sclérose tubéreuse
Tuberöse Sklerose
Esclerosis tuberosa
Epiloia
Bourneville syndrome
Adenoma sebaceum, seizures and mental retardation
Seizures, adenoma sebaceum and mental retardation
Mental retardation, seizures and adenoma sebaceum

Excludes: Neurofibromatosis (712)

Minimal Diagnostic Criteria: There are many variations of the disease even within the same family. The presence of adenoma sebaceum, seizures and mental retardation is the classic symptom complex.

Clinical Findings: Tuberous sclerosis is a multisystem disease characterized by the triad of adenoma sebaceum, epilepsy and mental retardation. Many variations have been documented. The infant may present with infantile spasms and white nevi. The nevi are differentiated from vitiligo by the presence of melanocytes in the white nevi. Tuberous sclerosis is frequently recognized in the preschool child. The most common symptom is epilepsy. Although the seizures are primarily major motor, focal, psychomotor and petit-mal, variants have been observed. Mental retardation of a moderate to severe degree occurs in 75% of the cases. Skin lesions are present in the majority.

Adenoma sebaceum, shagreen plaques, subungual fibroma, depigmented patches, subcutaneous nodules and café-au-lait spots occur in decreasing frequency. Phakomas have been noted in as many as 70%. Patients who have survived to the 3rd decade tend to be of normal intelligence. Attention is brought to their disease secondary to the complications of tuberous sclerosis.

Skull xrays demonstrate intracranial calcification in approximately 50%. They are most frequently found in the region of the basal ganglia. A pneumoencephalogram may show the typical "candle guttering" of the lateral ventricles produced by the subependymal protrusion of glial nodules.

Radiographs of the hands reveal cystic areas of rarefaction, particularly in the phalanges. A chest xray rarely demonstrates symmetric coarse markings which appear as multiple cysts. Occasionally an IVP will suggest a renal mass lesion. The EEG is not characteristic.

Biopsy of an adenoma sebaceum demonstrates a benign hamartomatous tumor which is composed of many cellular elements, including sebaceous glands, smooth muscle and hair follicles.

Complications

I **Derived:** Infrequently, the cerebral glial nodules undergo malignant transformation. More commonly the nodules may by their position or growth cause obstruction and an increase in intracranial pressure. Optic atrophy may be the end result. The rupture of a cyst within the lung parenchyma may produce a pneumothorax. More commonly, progressive dyspnea, hemoptysis and pulmonary hypertension occur if the lung is involved. Tumors located within the kidney can cause obstruction leading to pyelonephritis and uremia. Rhabdomyoma of the heart can result in congestive heart failure.

II **Associated:** —

Etiology: Autosomal dominant. (It has been estimated that as many as 85% of the cases are the result of new mutations.) McK *19110

Pathogenesis: ?

Related Facts
I **Sex Ratio:** M1:F1
II **Risk of Occurrence:** ?
III **Risk of Recurrence for**
   Patient's Sib: If parent is affected, 1 in 2 (50%); otherwise not increased.
   Patient's Child: 1 in 2. (It should be noted that the most severe cases do not reproduce because of death at an early age.)
IV **Age of Detectability:** 2-5 years by physical examination and appropriate radiographs.
V **Prevalence:** 1 in 100,000 in all populations and ethnic groups studied.

Treatment
I **Primary Prevention:** Genetic counseling
II **Secondary Prevention:** Anticonvulsants for the treatment of seizures. Occasional surgical removal of a strategically placed glial nodule. Treatment of the complications.
III **Other Therapy:** —

Prognosis: Tends to be slowly progressive. The majority die by 25 years of age. However, the disease is compatible with normal intelligence and long life.

Detection of Carrier: —

Special Considerations: —

References:
Borberg, A.: Clinical and genetic investigations into tuberous sclerosis and Recklinghausen's neurofibromatosis; contribution to elucidation of interrelationship and eugenics of syndromes. Acta Psychiatr. Neurol. (Suppl.) 71:3, 1951.
Bundey, S. and Evans, K.: Tuberous sclerosis; a genetic study. J. Neurol. Neurosurg. Psychiatry 32:591, 1969.

Contributor: **Robert H. A. Haslam**

———————————

Editor's Computerized Descriptors: Skin, Nails, Skel., Resp., GU., Nerve

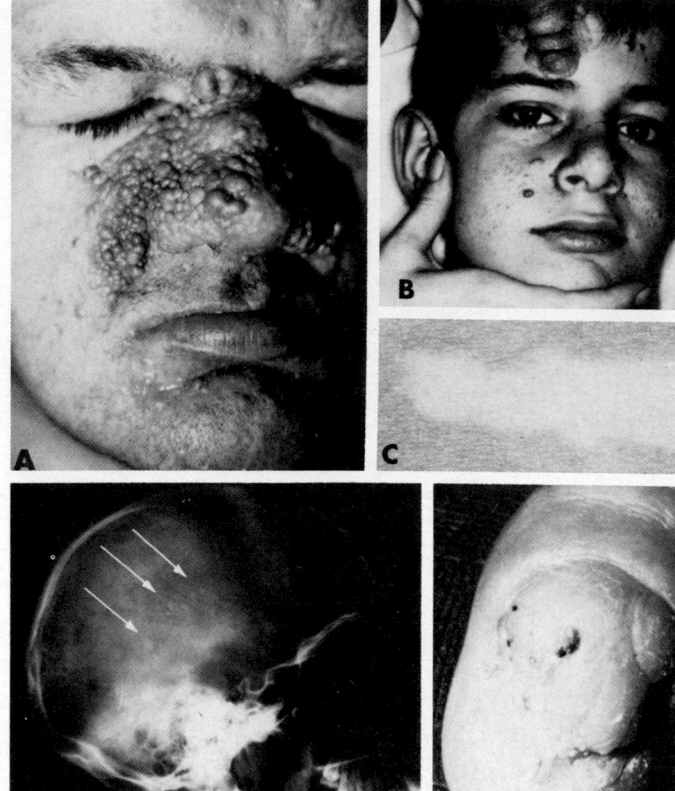

490. A) Angiofibromas; B) polypoid fibrous masses of forehead; C) patch of vitiligo; D) skull radiograph showing intracranial calcifications; E) subungual fibroma

TUBULAR STENOSIS

Includes: Rétrécissement du canal médullaire
Tubuläre Stenose
Estenosis tubular
Kenny-Caffey disease
Dwarfism and cortical thickening of tubular bones

Excludes: Pseudohypoparathyroidism (830)
Osteopetrosis (779, 780)
Silver syndrome (887)
Diaphyseal dysplasia (290)

Minimal Diagnostic Criteria: Low birthweight, proportionate dwarfism, narrow long bones with internal thickening of cortical walls and diminished medullary cavity, retarded bone maturation, episodes of hypocalcemia, normal mentation

Clinical Findings: A mother and son have been described. Short stature of prenatal onset occurred in the son who attained a height of only 31 inches by the age of 3 years 3 months. The mother was 48 inches tall at 38 years of age. Both were normally proportioned. Xrays showed narrow long bones with thick cortical walls, and diminished medullary cavities; the ribs and clavicles were also affected. Transient hypocalcemia with hyperphosphatemia occurred in both patients. The mother had a documented episode of hypocalcemia with tetany postoperatively as an adult. The son had symptomatic hypocalcemia in infancy. Delayed closure of the fontanel occurred in the mother and all bones showed retarded maturation in the son. There was no mental retardation in either patient.

Complications
I **Derived:** Episodic hypocalcemia especially during infancy or postoperatively
II **Associated:** Both patients were also myopic.

Etiology: Assumed autosomal dominant, however, X-linked dominant is not excluded. McK *12700

Pathogenesis: ? Excessive hypocalcitonin was considered as a possible factor but has not yet been investigated.†

Related Facts
I **Sex Ratio:** M1:F1
II **Risk of Occurrence:** ? Very rare; reported cases were Caucasians
III **Risk of Recurrence for**
   Patient's Sib: If autosomal dominant and if parent is affected, 1 in 2 (50%) for each offspring to be affected; otherwise not increased.
   Patient's Child: 1 in 2 if autosomal dominant
IV **Age of Detectability:** Infancy
V **Prevalence:** ?

Treatment
I **Primary Prevention:** Genetic counseling
II **Secondary Prevention:** —
III **Other Therapy:** Appropriate calcium or vitamin D therapy for hypocalcemia.†

Prognosis: Apparently good for normal life span and intelligence. There is risk of infantile and postoperative hypocalcemia.

Detection of Carrier: —

†Special Considerations: The 2 known patients refused more complete study. The investigation of hypocalcitonin in any future cases was considered to be of great interest. No adverse effect on either fertility (in the mother) or mental ability was apparent.

References:
Caffey, J.: Congenital stenosis of medullary spaces in tubular bones and calvaria in two proportionate dwarfs - mother and son; coupled with transitory hypocalcemic tetany. Am. J. Roentgenol. Radium Ther. Nucl. Med. 100:1, 1967.
Kenny, F.M. and Linarelli, L.: Dwarfism and cortical thickening of tubular bones. Am. J. Dis. Child. 111:201, 1966.
Wilson, M.G. et al: Dwarfism and congenital medullary stenosis (Kenny syndrome). In Bergsma, D. (ed.): Skeletal Dysplasias. Birth Defects: Orig. Art. Ser., vol. X, no. 12. Amsterdam: Excerpta Medica for the National Foundation-March of Dimes, 1974, p. 128.

Contributor: **David C. Siggers**

Editor's Computerized Descriptors: Vision, Skel.

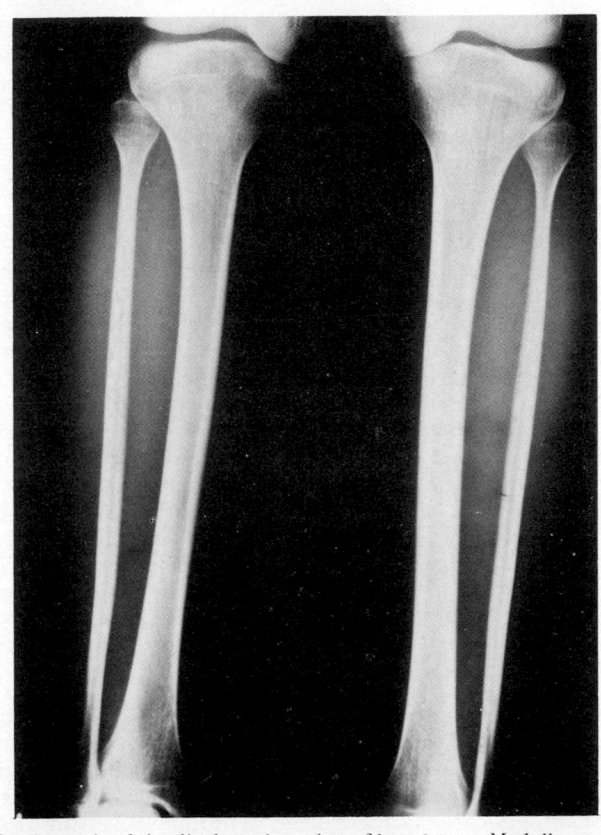

491. Stenosis of the diaphyseal portion of long bones. Medullary canals severely constricted; in the fibula, almost obliterated

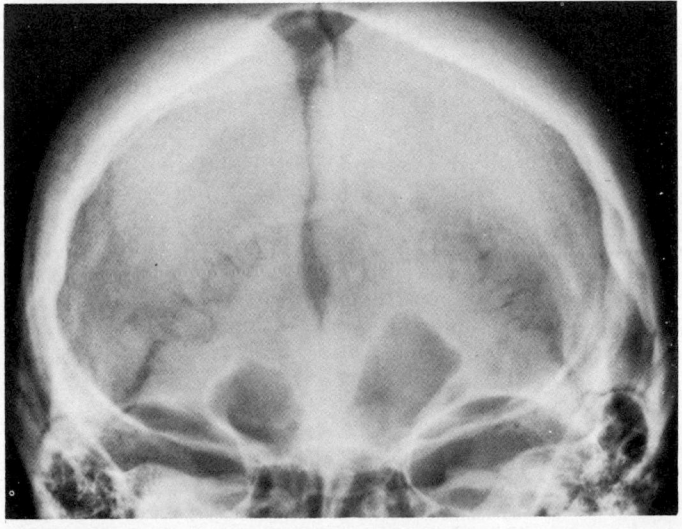

492. Markedly thickened bony calvaria with wide open anterior fontanel and unfused metopic suture

TURNER SYNDROME

Includes: Syndrome de Ullrich-Turner
Síndrome de Ullrich-Turner
Ullrich-Turner-syndrome
XO syndrome
Monosomy X
Short stature and sexual infantilism

Excludes: Noonan syndrome (720)
Gonadal dysgenesis, XY type (437)
Gonadal dysgenesis, XX type (436)
Chromosome 45,X/46,XY mosaicism (173)

Minimal Diagnostic Criteria: Edema or webbing of the neck in a newborn female should suggest the Turner syndrome. Short stature, a left-sided cardiac lesion or coarctation of the aorta in a prepuberal female should alert the observer to the diagnosis of the Turner syndrome, with or without webbing of the neck, and whether or not peripheral lymphedema has persisted. Any female with delayed adolescence or primary amenorrhea, especially associated with short stature, should be suspect.

The Turner syndrome, in light of currently available knowledge, is defined not on the basis of clinical phenotype, but strictly on cytogenetic grounds. While other patients may have some of the somatic features seen in the Turner syndrome, and while gonadal dysgenesis can occur in other individuals, including some without a chromosome abnormality, a diagnosis of the Turner syndrome requires the demonstration of partial or complete monosomy X. Thus, the diagnosis depends on chromosome analysis, and investigation of cells from multiple tissue sources may be necessary. The diagnosis of the Turner syndrome is inappropriate in the absence of complete or partial monosomy for the X chromosome. Sex chromatin studies (X- and Y-chromatin) can provide an indirect indication of the sex chromosome complement of any patient and are an important adjunct to chromosome analysis.†

Clinical Findings: The features usually considered characteristic of the Turner syndrome are shortness of stature, atypical facies, webbed neck, shield chest, cubitus valgus, sexual infantilism, primary amenorrhea and sterility. Among 388 cases of the Turner syndrome resulting from complete monosomy X, short stature was documented in 98% of cases. The mean adult height among 173 cases tabulated is 140.8 cm. Of 271 patients, 96% had primary amenorrhea, and several of the remaining experienced early secondary amenorrhea. Greater than 99% of affected females are sterile. Failure of sex development in adolescence, attributable to gonadal dysgenesis, occurs in 94% of adult patients with complete monosomy X. Peripheral lymphedema occurs at some time in life in approximately 40%, webbed neck in 54%, cubitus valgus in 56%, epicanthal folds in 30%, a low posterior nuchal hairline in 73%, shield chest in 60%, and documented cardiac or vascular lesion in 15%. Coarctation of the aorta and ventricular septal defect are said to be the most frequent cardiovascular lesions encountered. Unexplained hypertension occurs in approximately 27% of patients with complete monosomy X, an anomaly of the urinary tract in 38%, hypoplasia or hyperconvexity of nails in 73%, short metacarpals (usually the 4th metacarpal) or metatarsals in 44%, and an increased number of pigmented cutaneous nevi in 60%. While mental retardation has not been ordinarily considered a feature of the Turner syndrome, 36 of 223 patients (16%) with complete monosomy X, on whom information was available, in 4 series were found to be mentally subnormal. Thus, it appears that the risk of mental retardation in the Turner syndrome is significantly increased over that in the general population. A highly arched palate has been described in 39% of cases with complete monosomy X, a short neck in 71%, defective visual acuity in 22%, decreased hearing in 53%, micrognathia in 40%, and pectus excavatum in 38%. Obviously, no single one of these features is seen in every affected patient, and by the same token, no single patient exhibits all of the clinical features. Less commonly encountered but nevertheless significant features include hypoplastic, inverted nipples; loose posterior nuchal skin in infancy; ptosis of the eyelids; hypertelorism; vertebral anomalies; minor abnormalities in some long bones; osteoporosis in adult patients; and altered spatial orientation even in the absence of mental retardation. Dermatoglyphic features include distal displacement of the axial triradius, large patterns with an increased total digital ridge count, and hypothenar patterns. A transverse palmar crease is seen more often than in the general population.

Complications

I   Derived: Psychologic problems may stem from such features as sexual infantilism, short stature, primary amenorrhea and sterility. Cardiac defects and hypertension may produce additional problems.

An increased risk of gonadal neoplasia is not ordinarily considered a complication of the Turner syndrome. However, in those cases with a karyotype 45,X/46,XY, the addition of a Y-bearing cell line does predispose the patient to gonadal neoplasia.

II Associated: An increased incidence of (possibly autoimmune) thyroiditis, diabetes mellitus and collagen-vascular disease has been reported.

Etiology: As mentioned in Minimal Diagnostic Criteria, the cytogenetic abnormality necessary to make a diagnosis of the Turner syndrome is monosomy for the short arm of the X chromosome. The most frequent karyotype (57%) in the Turner syndrome is 45,X; ie complete monosomy X. A 45,X karyotype may coexist with other karyotypes in the same individual. Such mosaic individuals may have a 45,X/46,XX karyotype, in which case the effects of complete monosomy X may be mitigated by the presence of the normal 46,XX cell line. Other types of mosaicism may occur, but the common denominator still is the presence in some cells of monosomy for the short arm of X. Structural abnormalities producing partial or complete monosomy for the short arm of X may produce the Turner syndrome. Monosomy for all or a portion of the *long* arm of X, while it may produce gonadal dysgenesis, does not ordinarily produce the somatic features of the Turner syndrome.

Karyotypes found in patients with the Turner syndrome include the following:

Karyotype	Explanation	Percentage of Cases
45,X	Complete monosomy X	57
46,X,i(Xq) and mosaics which include i(Xq) cell line	Isochromosome of the long arm of the X chromosome (monosomy Xp)	17
Mosaics 45,X/46,XX; 45,X/47,XXX; etc.	Mosaic monosomy X	12

| Mosaic 45,X/46,XY | Mosaic monosomy X with Y-bearing cell line | 4 |
| Other (del(Xp), r(X), mosaics) | Xp monosomy, ring X | 10 |

Pathogenesis: Monosomy X may arise by nondisjunction in gametogenesis in the mother or father, or may be the result of postfertilization errors in mitosis. A lack of maternal age effect on the incidence of monosomy X militates against an error in meiosis I in oogenesis, in contrast to the situation in autosomal trisomy. The fact that in testable cases, the paternal-derived X chromosome is more often missing than the maternal X favors a meiotic error in spermatogenesis or a loss of the paternal X through an error in mitosis of the zygote. The frequency of mosaicism also suggests a postfertilization mitotic error as the mechanism involved, as does the frequency of assoication between X monosomy and twinning in the same family.

The mechanism whereby the absence of the short arm of or all of an X chromosome produces the Turner syndrome is unknown. It is apparent that monosomy X is a highly lethal abnormality, since cytogenetic investigation of the products of spontaneous abortion has shown that at least 95% of 45,X fetuses conceived do not survive pregnancy.

The investigation of 45,X abortuses has revealed that ovarian differentiation of the bipotential primitive gonad does begin, and that germ cells do migrate into the gonadal ridges. However, these primary oocytes apparently degenerate shortly after formation of primordial follicles, probably because of faulty follicle formation. This might be visualized as abnormally rapid progress of the process of attrition of germ cells which normally spans the reproductive life of the normal 46,XX female. Obviously, the occurrence of secondary sex development, menses and fertility in occasional 45,X females indicates that normal follicle formation can occur, and that perhaps there is a spectrum of rates at which attrition of germ cells occurs in the Turner syndrome. In most of those patients who experience menarche, secondary amenorrhea occurs at an early age.

Patients with 45,X/46,XY mosaicism may virilize to some extent at puberty, and may show clitoridal enlargement from birth. This is apparently attributable to the influence of the Y-bearing cell line. The pathogenesis of gonadal tumors in such individuals is poorly understood.

Related Facts
I Sex Ratio: M0:F1
II Risk of Occurrence: A minimum estimate of 1 in 10,000 live female births has a 45,X karyotype.
III Risk of Recurrence for
  Patient's Sib: Virtually zero unless identical twin.
  Patient's Child: More than 99% of affected patients are sterile. Among 35 liveborn children of 25 women with proved Turner syndrome, 5 of those also had the Turner syndrome. Each had a mosaic karyotype which included a 45,X cell line. Three other offspring had 21 trisomy and, in all, 12 of the 35 had some type of congenital malformation.
IV Age of Detectability: In the newborn period, if infant has webbed neck or lymphedema. In childhood, on basis of short stature and cardiovascular malformation. In adolescence, on basis of short stature, primary amenorrhea and sexual infantilism. Some patients are diagnosed later on the basis of secondary amenorrhea at a young age. The diagnosis should be suspected on the basis of any of these features; sex chromatin studies on a buccal smear and chromosome analysis should be undertaken.
V Prevalence: As mentioned, while the incidence of the 45,X

karyotype is 1 in 10,000 live births, at least 95% of all 45,X conceptions are spontaneously aborted. Thus, at least 1 in 500 females conceived has a 45,X karyotype. If the 45,X Turner syndrome accounts for 57% of all cases of the Turner syndrome, then at least 1 in 5,700 liveborn females has the Turner syndrome on the basis of some form of monosomy for the short arm of the X chromosome. It is interesting to note that while the 45,X karyotype is the most common single abnormal karyotype found in the products of spontaneous abortion, sex chromosome mosaics and structural abnormalities of the X chromosome are rare in such samples.

Treatment
I Primary Prevention: —
II Secondary Prevention: Cyclic estrogen substitution therapy should be initiated in the 2nd decade of life in patients with sexual infantilism and primary amenorrhea. This therapy should be continued at least until the expected age of menopause. Such therapy should, however, be delayed, if possible, until ultimate height is attained and no further growth potential remains. Delay in onset of estrogen substitution therapy, while desirable because of the effect of estrogens on epiphyseal fusion, may not be possible for psychologic reasons. Some authorities recommend the use of anabolic steroids for several years prior to the onset of estrogen therapy in an effort to enhance height. Surgical intervention may be necessary for ptosis of the eyelids, cardiovascular anomalies, renal anomalies (including hypertension), and webbing of the neck. Corrective lenses for visual defect, hearing aid for hearing defect, orthodontic treatment for dental malocclusion. Supportive counseling/psychotherapy may be necessary because of short stature, sexual infantilism, amenorrhea and sterility.

Laparotomy and removal of any remaining gonadal structure is indicated in patients with a 45,X/46,XY karyotype. This should be done as soon as the diagnosis is made because gonadal tumors have been reported in the 1st decade of life in such children.
III Other Therapy: Psychotherapy for feelings of inadequacy and inferiority, withdrawal and neurotic depression

Prognosis: Presumably normal life span if hypertension does not supervene, if cardiovascular defect is absent or is successfully repaired, and if gonadal neoplasia (in 45,X/46,XY mosaicism) does not shorten life.

Detection of Carrier: —

†Special Considerations: The clinical features enumerated for the Turner syndrome are based on tabulation of cases with 45,X karyotype. As mentioned previously, the occurrence of a 46,XX cell line in a patient with 45,X/46,XX mosaicism mitigates the effects of monosomy X, since the frequency of sexual maturation, menses and fertility is greater in mosaic patients than in nonmosaic monosomy X. In addition, the mean ultimate height of mosaic patients is significantly greater than in patients with nonmosaic monosomy X. A recent report reveals a total of 58 pregnancies in 25 women with cytologically documented Turner syndrome. Four of the 25 women were 45,X; 9 were 45,X/46,XX; 4 were 45,X/47,XXX; and 8 were 45,X/46,XX/47,XXX. Thus, fertility, although extremely rare, is possible in patients with the Turner syndrome.

In nonmosaic patients with a 46,X,i(Xq) karyotype the phenotype is not significantly different from that seen in nonmosaic monosomy X. The severity of the phenotypic alterations in 46,X,r(X) and 46,X,del(Xp) patients may roughly correlate with the extent of deletion of the short arm of X.

The result of a deletion of the long arm of the X chromosome (46,X,del(Xq) or 46,X,i(Xp)) is unclear. While an isochromosome of the short arm of the X chromosome has been reported, some question remains regarding the true identity of such chromosomes. The banding pattern of the X chromosome is such that the differentiation of an i(Xp) from a del(Xq) may be difficult. A long arm X deletion does produce gonadal dysgenesis with its resultant sexual infantilism, amenorrhea and sterility. While the majority of patients with Xq deletions do not exhibit somatic features of the Turner syndrome, some reports have dealt with patients with Xq deletions who were short of stature and had somatic features of the Turner syndrome. One might question the presence of an undetected 45,X cell line in those patients and whether they have been studied using banding techniques. According to the review by Simpson, about half of patients with nonmosaic del(Xq) are short of stature, and 20% or less have other Turner phenotypic features. The mean ultimate height in that series was 152.5 cm. compared with 141 cm. in patients with 45,X.

References:

Buczkowski, K. and Mikkelsen, M.: Fluorescence and autoradiographic studies in patients with Turner's syndrome and 46,XXp- and 46,XXq- karyotypes. J. Med. Genet. 10:350, 1973.

Carr, D.H.: Chromosomes and abortion. In Harris, H. and Hirschhorn, K. (eds.): Advances in Human Genetics. New York: Plenum Press, 1971, vol. 2, p. 201.

Hamerton, J.L.: Human Cytogenetics. vol. II. Clinical Cytogenetics. New York: Academic Press, 1971.

Jirásek, J.E.: Principles of reproductive embryology. In Simpson, J.L. (ed.): Disorders of Sexual Differentiation. Chicago:Year Book Publishers, 1977, p. 52.

Palmer, C.G. and Reichmann, A.: Chromosomal and clinical findings in 100 females with Turner syndrome. Hum. Genet. 35:35, 1976.

Simpson, J.L. Disorders of Sexual Differentiation. Chicago: Year Book Publishers, 1977.

Wilroy, R.S. et al: Phenotype-karyotype correlations in 81 patients with the Turner syndrome. Clin. Res. 25:74A, 1977.

Contributor: **Robert L. Summitt**

Editor's Computerized Descriptors: Eye, Face, Oral, Skin, Hair, Skel., CV., Lymphatic, GU., Nails, Neck, Dermatoglyphic

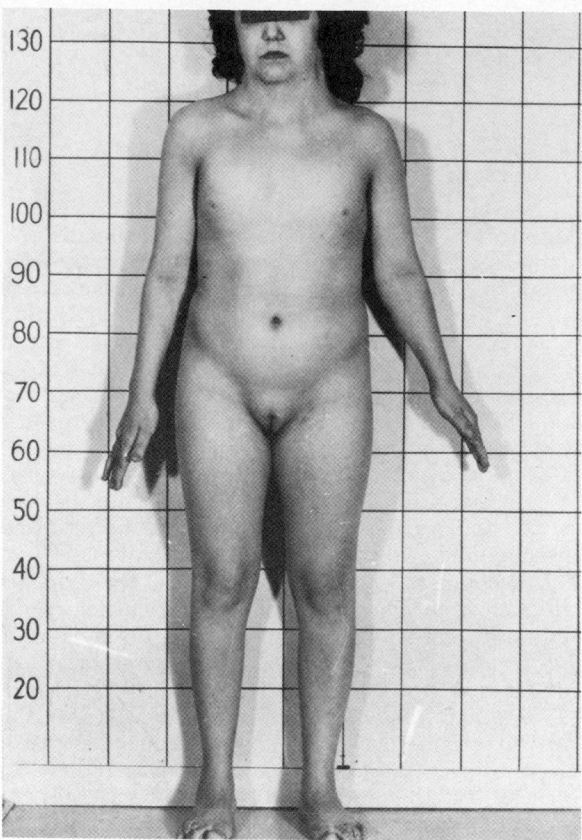

493. Turner syndrome with 45,X karyotype. Note webbed neck, shield-like chest, cubitus valgus, and sexual infantilism

TYROSINEMIA

Includes: Tyrosinémie
Tyrosinämie
Tirosinemia
Tyrosinosis
Hereditary tyrosinemia and tyrosyluria†

Excludes: Transient tyrosinemia and tyrosyluria of newborn
Tyrosinemia and tyrosyluria associated with disease states such as hepatic disease, scurvy, and thyrotoxicosis

Minimal Diagnostic Criteria: The persistent elevation of plasma tyrosine levels above 3 mg/100 ml, normal or slightly elevated plasma phenylalanine levels, ie phenylalanine/tyrosine ratio less than 1.0 and urinary hyperexcretion of tyrosyl compounds (p-hydroxyphenyllactic acid, > p-hydroxyphenylpyruvic acid, p-hydroxyphenylacetic acid) in the fasting state.†

Clinical Findings: There are 2 variant patterns.

The *acute form* of hereditary tyrosinemia is represented by most of the reported cases. Onset of symptoms occurs in early infancy (2-7 months), demise is rapid and usually occurs under 1 year of age. The presenting symptoms frequently are general manifestations such as temperature elevation, lethargy, and irritability; but failure to thrive has been the presenting complaint in nearly all cases. Hepatomegaly with or without abdominal distention, or hepatic cirrhosis, has been found in more than 80% of patients. Vomiting, edema, ascites, and peculiar odor occur in at least half of the cases. Anemia, jaundice, melena, splenomegaly, hematuria, diarrhea, and ecchymosis are noted in nearly one-third of patients, often in the terminal stage.

The *chronic form* of hereditary tyrosinemia has been reported in a relatively small number of patients. Symptoms develop secondary to renal tubular dysfunction and patients present with rickets and a less severe degree of hepatic cirrhosis. These patients have died under 10 years of age; exceptions are cited of a 20-year-old patient and several cases recently reported to have benefited from dietary treatment.

Mental retardation and neurologic abnormalities are not constant findings.

Biochemical determinations in patients with acute or chronic hereditary tyrosinemia show elevated plasma levels of tyrosine above 3 mg/100 ml, with range of 3-12 mg/100 ml, (normal: < 1 mg/100 ml) and constant hyperexcretion of tyrosyl compounds (p-hydroxyphenyllactic acid, p-hydroxyphenylpyruvic acid and p-hydroxyphenylacetic acid) in the fasting state.

The plasma phenylalanine levels are usually not elevated.

Other significant urinary findings are a generalized aminoaciduria, hyperphosphaturia and the presence of reducing substances such as glucose, fructose, galactose or lactose.

Hypophosphatemia, reduced prothrombin-proconvertin index, hypoglycemia and elevated methionine in serum are frequent laboratory findings, particularly in terminal stages of hepatic failure.

Roentgenograms demonstrate the characteristic bony changes of rickets.

Complications

I Derived: Hepatic cirrhosis resulting in hepatic failure and death in over 80% of cases; complex renal tubular defect producing a generalized aminoaciduria; hypophosphatemic rickets, more common in chronic form of hereditary tyrosinemia; coagulation defect evidenced by ecchymosis, melena, hematuria and prothrombin abnormality in about one-third of the cases.

II Associated: Hepatoma diagnosed at autopsy in several reported cases.

Etiology: Probably autosomal recessive†; McK *27670

Pathogenesis: Probable deficiency of liver enzyme p-hydroxyphenylpyruvic acid oxidase resulting in tyrosyluria and tyrosinemia.†

Related Facts

I Sex Ratio: M1:F1 based on limited number of reported cases

II Risk of Occurrence: 1 in 1500 live births in an isolate French Canadian population; reliable data is not available for other populations.

III Risk of Recurrence for
  Patient's Sib: Probably 1 in 4 (25%) for each offspring to be affected
  Patient's Child: Only 1 patient was reported to have reached adult reproductive age. Probably not increased unless mate is carrier or homozygote.

IV Age of Detectability: Acute form: hyperexcretion of tyrosyl compounds in urine and elevated plasma tyrosine has been reported as early as 2-3 weeks in 1 patient with a known affected sib.
  Chronic form: onset of symptoms reported as early as 6 months but most cases detected between 1 and 3 years.

V Prevalence: 1 in 3700 in the French Canadian isolate population; insufficient data available on other populations.

Treatment

I Primary Prevention: Genetic counseling

II Secondary Prevention: Low phenylalanine - low tyrosine diets have been tried in several patients and preliminary findings indicate measurable improvements in biochemical and clinical aspects of the disorder.

III Other Therapy: Supportive and symptomatic treatment for GI disturbances, electrolyte imbalance, hypoglycemia, anemia, bleeding, and possibly rickets.

Prognosis: Untreated patients:
  Acute form: Most patients die before 1 year of age and frequently within 1 month after onset of symptoms.
  Chronic form: Only 1 patient is reported to have survived beyond 10 years of age.
  Treated patients on restricted phenylalanine-tyrosine diets may have an increased life expectancy, but data on long-term follow-up is not yet available.

Detection of Carrier: ?

†Special Considerations: Tyrosinemia, tyrosinosis and tyrosyluria have been interchangeably used in the literature to describe conditions with increased tyrosine in blood and urine, but it has become increasingly clear that a number of different conditions are described under these names. Some are probably true inborn errors of metabolism and some represent maturational delay. Only about 60 cases of "hereditary tyrosinemia" appear in the literature to date and most of these have been published within the last 3 years. This represents a limiting factor in totally evaluating the disorder, since very basic questions regarding etiology and pathogenesis remain unanswered.

However, there is evidence that these cases represent an inherited metabolic defect resulting in an altered tyrosine metabolism. Specific data are not available to answer whether or not the observed impairment of enzyme activity (p-hydroxyphenylpyruvic acid oxidase) is the primary expression of the abnormal gene. Finding acute and chronic cases in a single family further strengthens the hypothesis that we are dealing with one disease process, which has variable clinical manifestations.

The one case of "tyrosinosis" reported by Medes appears

to represent a different inborn error of metabolism with the enzymatic block resulting in hyperexcretion of p-hydroxyphenylpyruvic acid, which increased in amounts greater than the excretion of other tyrosyl compounds as dietary tyrosine was added. The site of the block has not been clearly identified, but appears to be different than that found in patients with "hereditary tyrosinemia." Medes' patient had myasthenia gravis, but was essentially unaffected by the biochemical abnormality (tyrosinosis) and no other case has been reported.

Tyrosinemia of the newborn also presents with elevated plasma tyrosine, normal or slightly elevated phenyalanine and tyrosyluria. This is a transient disorder which appears to have no significant clinical sequelae. The elevation of tyrosine and tyrosyluria in this condition occurs within the first 2 weeks of life and usually persists for 1-2 months, but may persist for longer periods. The alteration of tyrosine metabolism seen in this condition is indicative of delayed maturation of liver enzyme systems and not a true inborn error of metabolism. It is more apt to occur in immature infants ingesting high-protein formula without supplemental vitamin C. Administration of high doses of vitamin C results in rapid return to normal of elevated plasma tyrosine levels.

References:

Hsia, D. Y.: Symposium: Treatment of amino acid disorders. Am. J. Dis. Child. 113:1, 1967.
Scriver, C.R. et al: Conference on hereditary tyrosinemia. Can. Med. Assoc. J. 97:1045, 1967.
Shear, C.S. et al: Tyrosinosis and tyrosinemia. In Nyhan, W.L. (ed.): Amino Acid Metabolism and Genetic Variation. New York: McGraw-Hill Inc., 1967, p. 97.

Contributor: **Carol S. Shear**

Editor's Computerized Descriptors: Skin, Skel., Spleen, GI., Liver, Nerve

UHL ANOMALY

Includes: Anomalie de Uhl
Aplasie der rechten Ventrikel (Uhl)
Anomalía de Uhl
Aplasia of right ventricular myocardium
Parchment right ventricle

Excludes: Ebstein anomaly (332)
Hypoplastic right ventricle
Endomyocardial fibrosis of right ventricle (354)

Minimal Diagnostic Criteria: The diagnosis may be suspected clinically from the marked cardiomegaly, reduced pulmonary vascular markings, feeble heart tones without any significant murmurs and the above ECG findings. It is established by angiocardiography which demonstrates the enormous but thin-walled and poorly contracting right ventricle devoid of trabeculae, and the normal location of the tricuspid orifice.

Clinical Findings: The pathologic anatomy is characterized by enormous dilatation of the heart, chiefly of the right atrium and right ventricle, and virtual absence of muscle fibers in the wall of the right ventricle. The right atrium is dilated and thick-walled due to hypertrophy and endocardial fibroelastosis. The foramen ovale is often patent; the tricuspid valve is normal. The wall of the grossly dilated right ventricle is thin, translucent and parchment-like, ranging in thickness from 1-2 mm. Its endocardial surface is opaque white due to fibroelastosis. The trabeculae are deficient and flat, the papillary muscles and chordae tendineae are thin and delicate. The crista supraventricularis is likewise flat and hypoplastic. On microscopic examination, the right ventricular wall consists solely of a thickened endocardial layer, showing fibroelastosis, and a subjacent epicardial layer with increased fatty and connective tissue. No intervening muscle fibers are observed between these 2 layers except, occasionally, a few islands of myocardial cells in areas adjoining the pulmonary ring, tricuspid annulus or diaphragmatic surface. The pulmonary valve is normal but the pulmonary trunk and main branches appear hypoplastic. The left atrium and left ventricle are normal or may reveal hypertrophy with fibroelastosis. The coronary vessels appear normal, as do the systemic and pulmonary veins. The positional relationship of the pulmonary trunk and aorta is also normal. The basic physiologic abnormality consists of failure of the right ventricle to function as a pump for the pulmonary circulation. It behaves as a passive reservoir for blood coming from the right atrium, and as such, is a constantly overloaded chamber, which accounts for its enormously dilated state. Pumping is accomplished by right atrial contraction, and cardiac output is accordingly low.

The clinical picture is characterized by heart failure in infancy or early childhood, marked cardiomegaly, feeble heart tones with gallop rhythm and the absence of murmurs. The increased cardiac dullness is unaccompanied by any significant precordial heave or apical impulse. Heart failure is chiefly right-sided, manifested by hepatomegaly, peripheral edema and clear lung fields.

The chest roentgenograms reveal an enormous cardiac shadow with reduced pulmonary vascular markings. In the frontal projection, there is increased convexity of the right heart border due to right atrial enlargement, and extension of the left heart border up to the lateral chest wall due to the pronounced dilatation of the right ventricle. The pulmonary artery segment is inconspicuous. In the lateral as well as in the right and left anterior oblique projections, there is marked extension of the cardiac borders anteriorly and posteriorly, giving an impression of combined ventricular enlargement. The prominent posterior heart border is, however, due mainly to the posterior displacement of the heart from the right heart dilatation.

The ECG commonly shows broad, peaked and tall P waves due to right atrial enlargement, and small amplitude QRS complexes in the chest lead tracings without a definite ventricular hypertrophy pattern. In addition, the vectorcardiogram may reveal counterclockwise posteriorly oriented horizontal QRS vector loops with the initial forces directed leftwards and anteriorly.

The echocardiographic findings in the Uhl anomaly include increased right ventricular dimension, delayed tricuspid closure and a prolapse-like appearance of the mitral valve (pansystolic flat to posterior systolic motion). The major differentiation between this and the Ebstein anomaly is an atrial systole-coincident diastolic opening of the pulmonary valve. In Ebstein disease, the septal motion may be paradoxic, whereas the septal motion in the Uhl anomaly has been reported to be normal. The right ventricular anterior wall is thin in each.

The right atrial presystolic "a" wave is high and of approximately the same magnitude as the right ventricular and pulmonary arterial systolic pressures. Slight systemic arterial oxygen unsaturation may be present if right-to-left shunting across a patent foramen ovale is present. Angiocardiography is diagnostic. It characteristically reveals gross enlargement of the right ventricle with generalized thinness of its wall, absence of trabeculae, normal location of the tricuspid orifice and prolonged emptying time. Small shunting across a patent foramen ovale may or may not be demonstrated following opacification of the right atrium. The pulmonary trunk and main branches appear hypoplastic.

Complications
I **Derived:** The cardiac abnormality results in congestive heart failure and death in infancy or early childhood. The presence of an additional abnormality of the left ventricle such as endocardial fibroelastosis or myofibrosis may promote earlier onset of these terminal events.
II **Associated:** —

Etiology: ?

Pathogenesis: ? It has been proposed that the lesion is due to a primary congenital defect of the primordium of the right ventricular myocardium.

Related Facts
I **Sex Ratio:** M?:F?
II **Risk of Occurrence:** Less than 1 in 100,000 births (under 0.1% of CHD)
III **Risk of Recurrence for**
  Patient's Sib: ?
  Patient's Child: ?
IV **Age of Detectability:** From birth, by cardiac catheterization and angiocardiography
V **Prevalence:** ?

Treatment
I **Primary Prevention:** —
II **Secondary Prevention:** Superior vena cava - right pulmonary artery anastomosis, in those with heart failure but without associated left ventricular myocardial disease, to decompress the right heart and improve the pulmonary circulation.
III **Other Therapy:** Symptomatic therapy for congestive heart failure.

Prognosis: Poor. In the usual cases where there is almost total absence of the right ventricular myocardium, death from heart failure occurs during infancy. Survival for several years is possible when the myocardial defect is not that extensive.

Detection of Carrier: —

Special Considerations: —

References:
Arcilla, R.A. and Gasul, B.M.: Congenital aplasia or marked hypoplasia of the myocardium of the right ventricle (Uhl's anomaly): Clinical angiocardiographic and hemodynamic findings. J. Pediatr. 58:381, 1961.
Cumming, G.R. et al: Congenital aplasia of the myocardium of the right ventricle (Uhl's anomaly). Am. Heart J. 70:671, 1965.
French, J.W. et al: Echocardiographic findings in Uhl's anomaly: Demonstration of diastolic pulmonary valve opening. Am. J. Cardiol. 36:349, 1975.

Contributor: **René A. Arcilla**

Editor's Computerized Descriptors: Resp., CV.

ULNAR DRIFT WITH DIGITAL WEBS AND CONTRACTURES

Includes: Deviation cubitale des doigts et palmures
Ulnare Abweichung mit Schwimmhauten und Kontrakturen
Desviación cubital con membranas inter-digitales y contracturas
Digitotalar dysmorphism
Ulnar drift syndrome

Excludes: Windmill vane syndrome
Cranio-carpo-tarsal dysplasia (223)

Minimal Diagnostic Criteria: Ulnar deviation of hands with flexion contractures of digits.

Clinical Findings: Features include soft tissue webbing between thumbs and palms, flexion contractures of interphalangeal joints of 1 or more fingers, ulna deviation of hands and fingers. Fully expressed at birth with little if any progression thereafter. A South African kindred has associated short stature and rockerbottom feet caused by vertical talus. Individual patients have had lateral drift of toes, scoliosis, simian lines.

Roentgenographic examination shows only positional deformities without bony abnormalities.

Complications
I   **Derived:** Limitation of use of digits
II **Associated:** —

Etiology: Autosomal dominant

Pathogenesis: ?

Related Facts
I   **Sex Ratio:** M1:F1
II   **Risk of Occurrence:** ?
III **Risk of Recurrence for**
     Patient's Sib: 1 in 2 (50%) for each offspring to be affected; otherwise not increased.
     Patient's Child: 1 in 2
IV   **Age of Detectability:** At birth
V   **Prevalence:** ?

Treatment
I   **Primary Prevention:** Genetic counseling
II   **Secondary Prevention:** Surgical release of soft tissue webbing and flexion contractures.
III **Other Therapy:** Physical therapy

Prognosis: Normal life expectancy; degree of incapacitation dependent on severity of hand deformity.

Detection of Carrier: No carrier state

Special Considerations: —

References:
Sallis, J.G. and Beighton, P.: Dominantly inherited digito-talar dysmorphism. J. Bone Joint Surg. (Br.) 54B:509, 1972.
Stevenson, R.E. et al: Dominantly inherited ulnar drift. In Bergsma, D. (ed.): New Chromosomal and Malformation Syndromes. Birth Defects: Orig. Art. Ser., vol. XI, no. 5. Miami: Symposia Specialists for The National Foundation-March of Dimes, 1975, p. 75.

Contributor: Roger E. Stevenson

Editor's Computerized Descriptors: Dermatoglyphic, Skel., Skin

ULNAR-MAMMARY SYNDROME, TYPE PALLISTER

Includes: Syndrome cubito-mammaire
Pallister Syndrom
Síndrome cúbito-mamario tipo Pallister

Excludes: Mesomelic dysplasia, Reinhardt-Pfeiffer type (648)
Mesomelic dysplasia, Nievergelt type (647)

Minimal Diagnostic Criteria: Combination of absent or duplicated ulnar ray structures with hypoplastic/absent apocrine and mammary glands.

Clinical Findings: This is a complex malformation syndrome with variable expression, characteristically involving a combination of upper limb and mammary gland defects. The abnormalities of the upper limbs may be quite asymmetric. They include clinodactyly, camptodactyly, hexadactyly and shortness/absence of phalanges/metacarpals of the ulnar digits, of carpal bones and of the ulna, but the thumb, radius, humerus and shoulder girdle may also be involved. The apocrine-mammary defects include absence of body odor and axillary sweating, and hypoplasia/absence of mammary glands and nipples. Associated anomalies include renal malformations, absence of teeth, bifid uvula, scoliosis and imperforate hymen.

Complications
I   **Derived:** Physical limitations due to upper limb defects; inability to nurse; renal disease and urinary tract infection; imperforate hymen.
II **Associated:** Scoliosis, absence of teeth

Etiology: Probably autosomal dominant

Pathogenesis: ?

Related Facts
I   **Sex Ratio:** M1:F1
II   **Risk of Occurrence:** Small
III **Risk of Recurrence for**
  . **Patient's Sib:** If parent is affected 1 in 2 (50%) for each offspring to be affected; otherwise not increased
     Patient's Child: 1 in 2
IV   **Age of Detectability:** At birth
V   **Prevalence:** Rare

Treatment
I   **Primary Prevention:** Genetic counseling
II   **Secondary Prevention:** —
III **Other Therapy:** Orthopedic surgery for upper limb malformations; plastic surgery for breast and nipple absence/hypoplasia; hymenotomy; orthodontic procedures.

Prognosis: Good

Detection of Carrier: Variability of gene expression may be such that very minimally affected persons may have severely affected offspring.

Special Considerations: —

References:
Gonzalez, C.A. et al: Studies of malformation syndromes of man 42B: Mother and son affected with the ulnar-mammary syndrome type Pallister. Europ. J. Pediatr. 123:225, 1976.
Pallister, P.D. et al: Studies of malformation syndromes in man 42: A pleiotropic dominant mutation affecting skeletal, sexual and apocrine-mammary development. In Bergsma, D. (ed.): Cytogenetics, Environment and Malformation Syndromes. Birth Defects: Orig. Art. Ser. vol. XII, no. 5. New York: Alan R. Liss, Inc. for The National Foundation-March of Dimes, 1976, pp. 247-254.

Contributor: Jürgen Herrmann

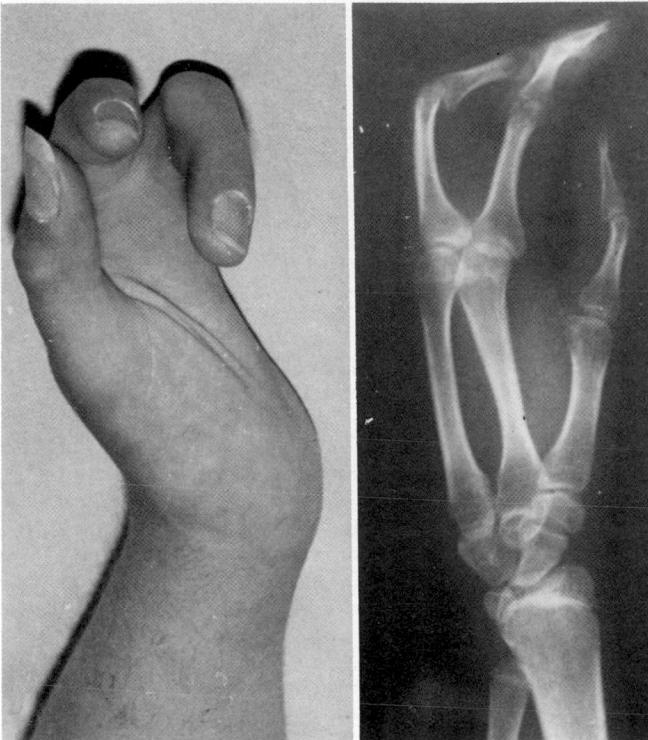

494. Hypoplasia of distal ulna and absence of ulnar ray derivatives including lateral carpals, 4th and 5th metacarpals, and phalanges

URTICARIA, DEAFNESS AND AMYLOIDOSIS

Includes: Amylose avec urticare et surdité
Urticaria, Taubheit und Amyloidose
Urticaria, sordera y amiloidosis
Deafness, urticaria and amyloidosis
Amyloidosis, deafness and urticaria

Excludes: Familial Mediterranean fever†

Minimal Diagnostic Criteria: "Aguey bouts" with characteristic skin rash, progressive perceptive deafness, nephropathy, typical perireticulin amyloidosis and autosomal dominant inheritance.

Clinical Findings: During adolescence "aguey bouts" (chills, fever, malaise) make their appearances and recur continually thereafter. Over the next 2-4 decades perceptive deafness appears and progresses; finally nephropathy appears and leads to death. The "aguey bouts" recur every 3 weeks or so, lasting 24 to 48 hours. They are accompanied by malaise, a geographic urticarial rash, no particular alteration of leukocytes, but hyperglobulinemia and raised ESR. With deafness, comes loss of libido and some skin thickening. Nephropathy is of the sclerotic amyloid variety, combining predominantly azotemic manifestations with substantial proteinuria. Amyloidosis is also present in other parts of the body in the pattern of distribution characteristic of typical (ie perireticulin) amyloidosis plus pulmonary parenchymal involvement. The changes in the ear include degeneration of the organ of Corti and vestibular sensory epithelium, atrophy of the cochlear nerve, and ossification of the basilar membrane, but do not include amyloidosis.

Complications
I   **Derived:** Loss of libido and eventually uremic renal failure in all but 1 case
II **Associated:** Pes cavus, short metacarpals and short stature in all subjects, glaucoma in two.

Etiology: Autosomal dominant; McK *19190

Pathogenesis: ?

Related Facts
I   **Sex Ratio:** M1:F1
II **Risk of Occurrence:** ? Very low
III **Risk of Recurrence for**
    Patient's Sib: If parent is affected 1 in 2 (50%) for each offspring to be affected; othewise not increased.
    Patient's Child: 1 in 2
IV **Age of Detectability:** Early adolescence, clinical appraisal of "aguey bouts" which are initial manifestations. Full syndrome not established before the 3rd decade.
V   **Prevalence:** ? Very low

Treatment
I   **Primary Prevention:** Genetic counseling
II **Secondary Prevention:** Hearing aids, auditory and speech training, and lip-reading may be helpful.
III **Other Therapy:** Eventually usual supportive therapy for renal failure

Prognosis: Usually death from uremia during the 6th decade

Detection of Carrier: —

†**Special Considerations:** Three other families with this condition, and 4 sporadic examples have been described. In addition, 1 family has been described with what appears to be an incomplete variant, comprising all the features of the clinical syndrome but lacking amyloidosis. Finally, a family with dominantly inherited familial Mediterranean fever, which included no deafness or urticaria, has been

reported by Bergman and Warmenius.

In the urticaria, deafness and amyloidosis syndrome deafness always develops and the condition is transmitted as an autosomal dominant. It thus differs from familial Mediterrenenan fever which does not include deafness and is autosomal recessive. It also differs from the other forms of hereditary but dominantly nephropathic amyloidosis, and all the other types of hereditary amyloidosis, in a number of details which are thoroughly reviewed in the recent paper by Alexander and Atkins.

References:

Alexander, F. and Atkins, E.L.: Familial renal amyloidosis - case reports, literature review and classification. Am. J. Med. 59:121, 1975.

Andersen, V. et al: Deafness, urticaria and amyloidosis: A sporadic case with a chromosomal aberration. Am. J. Med. 42:449, 1967.

Bergman, F. and Warmenius, S.: Familial perireticulin amyloidosis in a Swedish family. Am. J. Med. 45:601, 1968.

Black, J.T.: Amyloidosis, deafness, urticaria and limb pains: A hereditary syndrome. Ann. Intern. Med. 70:989, 1969.

De Castro Torres, A. and Garcia, J.M.P.: Urticaria, sordera y amiloidosis. Estudio de un caso con immunofluorescencia directa. Actas Dermo-Sifilograficas 66:505, 1975.

Guenel, J. et al: Un cas d'amylose genetique associant: Urticaire, surdite, arthralgies et atteinte renale (syndrome de Muckle). 1971 Rapport de la Reunion commune des Societes de Nephrologie italienne et francaise, Lyon. Seance Fevrier 1971.

Heller, H. et al: Familial Mediterranean fever. Arch. Intern. Med. 102:50, 1958.

Kennedy, D.D. et al: Amyloidosis presenting as Urticaria. Br. Med. J. 1:31, 1966.

Lagrue, G. et al: Syndrome de Muckle et Wells. Cinquieme observation familiale. Nouv. Presse Med. 1:2223, 1972.

Muckle, T.J. and Wells, M.V.: Urticaria, deafness and amyloidosis: A new heredo-familial syndrome. Q. J. Med. 31:235, 1962.

Perrottet, C. et al: Surdite, urticaire, arthrites, hypogonadisme et insuffisance renale. Le syndrome de Muckle et Wells. Schweiz. Rundschau Med. (Praxis) 63:651, 1974.

Prost, A. et al: Rhumatisme intermittent revelateur d'un syndrome familial arthrites - eruption urticarienne - surdite: Syndrome de Muckle et Wells sans amylose renale. Rev. Rhum. Mal. Osteoartic 43:201, 1976.

Contributor: **Thos. J. Muckle**

Editor's Computerized Descriptors: Hearing, Ear, Skin, Skel., GU.

USHER SYNDROME

Includes: Syndrome d'Usher
Síndrome de Usher
Retinitis pigmentosa and congenital deaf-mutism
Retinitis pigmentosa-dysacusis syndrome

Excludes: Retinitis pigmentosa with noncongenital or progressive hearing loss
Hallgren syndrome†
Phytanic acid storage disease (810)

Minimal Diagnostic Criteria: Association of congenital deaf-mutism with retinitis pigmentosa

Clinical Findings: The association of deaf-mutism and retinitis pigmentosa (RP) was first pointed out in the 19th century but is named after Usher who established the hereditary nature of the disorder in 1913. Although the classic form of the disease is not associated with vestibular problems or mental retardation, there have been large family studies with these findings in some patients, and it is not yet clear whether those cases represent a different genetic entity.† There are many patients with retinitis pigmentosa who have mild-to-moderate hearing loss but that is not referred to as Usher syndrome. The congenital deafness of the Usher syndrome varies among patients from moderate to profound but does not appear to be progressive.

The features of retinitis pigmentosa are no different from the autosomal recessive form, with onset in the 1st or 2nd decade and a moderate rate of progression. The mutism is secondary to the congenital deafness and the features are identical to other forms of congenital nerve deafness.

Complications
I **Derived:** Cataracts, macular degeneration
II **Associated:** Vestibular disturbances, mental retardation, psychoses†

Etiology: Autosomal recessive gene which may be pleiotropic. All affected members of 1 family are similar but some families have additional vestibular problems or mental retardation. McK *27690

Pathogenesis: Because there is a close association between the embryologic development of the inner ear and retina, a common mechanism may be responsible.

Related Facts
I **Sex Ratio:** M1:F1
II **Risk of Occurrence:** ?
III **Risk of Recurrence for**
   Patient's Sib: 1 in 4 (25%) for each offspring to be affected
   Patient's Child: Not markedly increased unless mate is carrier or homozygote
IV **Age of Detectability:** The deafness is noted shortly after birth but the visual problems are usually not noted until the 2nd decade.
V **Prevalence:** Reported as 1.8-3.5 per 100,000 in Europe. About 10% of all retinitis pigmentosa patients have severe hearing loss while the frequency of retinitis pigmentosa in congenital deaf-mutism has been reported as 1-20%; generally 5-10% affected with RP is found in large, nonisolated populations of congenitally deaf individuals.

Treatment
I **Primary Prevention:** Genetic counseling
II **Secondary Prevention:** —
III **Other Therapy:** Appropriate therapy for deafness such as hearing aid, lip reading, sign language, speech therapy. Visual aids include night vision pocketscope, visual field widener, and protective sunglasses.

Prognosis: Apparently normal life span

Detection of Carrier: —

†**Special Considerations:** The association of vestibular problems is probably common in the Usher syndrome. In 1959 Hallgren made an analysis of the association of RP, deafness, ataxia, and mental abnormality. He defined a syndrome including all these elements. Until further evidence is brought forth, it appears reasonable to distinguish between the syndromes (both of which are inherited autosomal recessively) as follows: Usher syndrome: congenital deafness, RP, $\pm$ vestibular ataxia; Hallgren syndrome: congenital deafness, RP, vestibulocerebellar ataxia, and mental abnormality.

References:
Franceschetti, A. et al: Chorioretinal Heredodegenerations. Springfield: Charles C Thomas, 1974.

Kloepfer, H.W. et al: The hereditary syndrome of congenital deafness and retinitis pigmentosa (Usher's syndrome). Laryngoscope 76:850, 1966.

McCay, V.: Usher's syndrome-deafness and progressive blindness. J. Chronic. Dis. 22:133, 1969.

Merin, S. and Auerbach, E.: Retinitis pigmentosa. Surv. Ophthalmol. 20:303, 1976.

Usher, C.H.: Bowman's lecture on a few hereditary eye affections. Trans. Ophthalmol. Soc. U.K. 55:164, 1935.

Contributors: **Alex E. Krill‡**
Mitchel L. Wolf
Donald R. Bergsma

Editor's Computerized Descriptors: Vision, Eye, Hearing

VAGINAL ATRESIA

Includes: Atrésie vaginale
Scheidenatresie
Atresia de la vagina
One form of "congenital absence of vagina"

Excludes: Hymen, imperforate (483)
Müllerian aplasia† (682)
All forms of female pseudohermaphroditism
All forms of male pseudohermaphroditism
Renal, genital and middle ear anomalies (860)

Minimal Diagnostic Criteria: Atresia of the lower vagina in a female (46,XX) with a normal upper vagina, uterus, external genitalia, and ovaries.

Clinical Findings: The lower one-fifth to one-third of the vagina is replaced by 2-3 cm of fibrous tissue. The remaining (superior) portion of the vagina is well differentiated. External genitalia are normal for females, and the uterine cervix and corpus, fallopian tubes, and ovaries are likewise normal. Usually somatic anomalies are not present, although renal anomalies have been reported. At puberty female secondary sexual development is normal except for absence of menses.

Complications
I   **Derived:**   Menstrual products cannot pass because of the atretic lower vagina. Hydrometrocolpos may lead to amenorrhea as well as abdominal pain or palpable masses as a result of accumulation of fluid.
II **Associated:**   Renal anomalies have been reported.

Etiology: ? Familial aggregates are relatively rare, but perhaps common enough to be consistent with multifactorial etiology.

Pathogenesis: The caudal portion of the vagina is formed from invagination of the urogenital sinus, whereas the cephalad portion is of müllerian origin. In vaginal atresia the urogenital sinus presumably fails to contribute the caudal portion of the vagina.

Related Facts
I   **Sex Ratio:**   M0:F1
II   **Risk of Occurrence:**   Rare
III **Risk of Recurrence for**
     Patient's Sib: ? Probably not greater than 2-5% for female sib to be affected, assuming multifactorial etiology.
     Patient's Child: No more than 2-5% for a female child to be affected, assuming multifactorial etiology.
IV   **Age of Detectability:**   Usually at puberty because hydrometrocolpos causes primary amenorrhea. Occasionally mucocolpos occurs in neonates.
V   **Prevalence:**   Rare. Occurs in perhaps 5-10% of females said to have "absence of the vagina."

Treatment
I   **Primary Prevention:**   Genetic counseling
II   **Secondary Prevention:**   Surgical extirpation of the fibrous tissue. The thickness of atretic portion precludes simple incisional drainage.
III **Other Therapy:**   —

Prognosis: Normal life span; normal fertility

Detection of Carrier: —

†**Special Considerations:**   Vaginal atresia should be differentiated from müllerian aplasia, a condition in which the cephalad portion of the vagina and the uterus are absent. Some authors group both these conditions under "congenital absence of vagina." In addition, an autosomal recessive trait characterized by vaginal atresia, renal hypoplasia or agenesis, and middle ear anomalies has been described.

References:
Dennison, W.M. and Bacsich, P.: Imperforate vagina in the newborn: Neonatal hydrocolpos. Arch. Dis. Child. 36:156, 1961.

Jones, H.W., Jr. and Scott, W.M.: Hermaphroditism, Genital Anomalies, and Related Endocrine Disorders, 2nd Ed. Baltimore: Williams & Wilkins, 1971.

Simpson, J.L.: Disorders of Sexual Differentiation: Etiology and Clinical Delineation. New York: Academic Press, 1976.

Winter, J.S.D. et al: A familial syndrome of renal, genital and middle ear anomalies. J. Pediatr. 71:88, 1968.

Contributor: **Joe Leigh Simpson**

Editor's Computerized Descriptor: GU.

VAGINAL SEPTUM, TRANSVERSE

Includes: Cloison vaginale transversale
Transversales septum vaginae
Septum vaginal transverso
Transverse vaginal septum

Excludes: Müllerian fusion, incomplete (684)
Müllerian aplasia (682)
Hymen, imperforate (483)
Longitudinal vaginal septum†
Vaginal atresia (984)

Minimal Diagnostic Criteria: Transverse vaginal septum, with or without a perforation, in a 46,XX individual with normal ovaries, normal external genitalia, and otherwise normal müllerian derivatives.

Clinical Findings: Transverse septa are usually located near the junction of the upper third and lower two-thirds of the vagina; however, septa may be present in the middle or lower third. These septa are about 1 cm thick and may or may not have a perforation. A perforation, if present, is usually central in location; however, it may occasionally be eccentric. The external genitalia, uterine cervix, uterine corpus, fallopian tubes, and ovaries are normal. No somatic abnormalities are present. At puberty normal secondary sexual development occurs.

Complications
I   **Derived:** If no perforation is present, mucus and menstrual fluid cannot be expelled and, hence, hydrometrocolpos may develop. Coital difficulties or abnormalities of the 2nd stage of labor have been reported.
II   **Associated:** Polydactyly and cardiac anomalies have been associated with transverse vaginal septum, but usually no associated anomalies are present.

Etiology: An autosomal recessive allele is probably responsible for transverse vaginal septa in the Amish. In other ethnic groups heritable tendencies have not been verified.

Pathogenesis: Vaginal septa probably result from failure of the urogenital sinus derivatives and the müllerian duct derivatives to fuse or canalize properly in order to form a normal vagina. Although this explanation is accepted by most investigators, the situation may be more complex because some data suggest that abnormal mesodermal proliferation may occur.

Related Facts
I   **Sex Ratio:** M0:F1
II   **Risk of Occurrence:** Rare
III   **Risk of Recurrence for**
   Patient's Sib: In the Amish 1 in 4 for 46,XX sibs: 1 in 8 for all sibs. In other ethnic groups similar risk figures may or may not be appropriate.
   Patient's Child: Some forms could be inherited in polygenic/multifactorial fashion, in which case a patient's child has a small (?2-5%) chance of being affected.
IV   **Age of Detectability:** Usually at puberty because hydrometrocolpos causes primary amenorrhea; occasionally mucolcolpos is noted at birth. Occasionally affected patients are detected because of coital difficulties or abnormalities during labor.
V   **Prevalence:** ?

Treatment
I   **Primary Prevention:** Genetic counseling
II   **Secondary Prevention:** Surgical extirpation or creation of an opening in the septum if no perforation is present; enlargement of the perforation may be necessary if the opening is very small.
III   **Other Therapy:** —

Prognosis: Normal life span

Detection of Carrier: —

†**Special Considerations:** Longitudinal vaginal septa-sagittal or coronal-have been reported, but these septa represent an entity different from transverse vaginal septa. Longitudinal septa rarely produce clinical problems.

References:

Jones, H.W., Jr. and Scott, W.M.: Hermaphroditism, Genital Anomalies and Related Endocrine Disorders, 2nd Ed. Baltimore: Williams & Wilkins, 1971.

McKusick, V.A. et al: Recessive inheritance of a congenital malformation syndrome. JAMA 204:113, 1968.

Sarto, G.E. and Simpson, J.L.:Abnormalities of the müllerian and wolffian duct systems. In Summitt, R.E. and Bergsma, D. (eds.): Sex Differentiation and Chromosomal Abnormalities. Birth Defects: Orig. Art. Ser. vol XIV, no. 6C. New York: Alan R. Liss Inc. for the National Foundation-March of Dimes, 1978, p. 37.

Simpson, J.L.: Disorders of Sexual Differentiation: Etiology and Clinical Delineation. New York: Academic Press, 1976.

Contributor: **Joe Leigh Simpson**

Editor's Computerized Descriptors: Skel., CV., GU.

986
VAN DEN BOSCH SYNDROME
980-500

Includes: Syndrome de Van den Bosch
Síndrome de Van den Bosch

Excludes: X—linked mental retardation
Ectodermal dysplasia, anhidrotic (333)
Tapetochoroidal dystrophy (925)

Minimal Diagnostic Criteria: Anhidrosis, mental retardation, choroideremia, acrokeratosis verruciformis and winged scapulae.

Clinical Findings: Anhidrosis associated with, a) mental deficiency, b) delayed somatic growth, c) ophthalmologic abnormalities, (horizontal nystagmus, myopia, choroideremia, abnormal retinogram), d) winged scapulae e) acrokeratosis verruciformis, f) bronchial and skin infections.

Complications
I **Derived:** Hyperthermia, intolerance to heat, bronchial and skin infections.
II **Associated:** —

Etiology: This apparently X-linked recessive condition has been observed in 2 brothers of a single Dutch kindred. McK *31450

Pathogenesis: ?

Related Facts
I **Sex Ratio:** M1:F0
II **Risk of Occurrence:** Rare
III **Risk of Recurrence for**
    Patient's Sib: If mother is a carrier 1 in 2 (50%) for each brother to be affected and 1 in 2 (50%) for each sister to be a carrier.
    Patient's Child: 1 in 1 (100%) for carrier daughters; not increased for sons unless wife is carrer.
IV **Age of Detectability:** Neonate
V **Prevalence:** ?

Treatment
I **Primary Prevention:** Genetic counseling
II **Secondary Prevention:** Avoid high environmental temperature, encourage hydration; special education as needed.
III **Other Therapy:** —

Prognosis: ?

Detection of Carrier: Altered sweat pores in carrier mother?

Special Considerations: —

References:

Van Den Bosch, J.: A new syndrome in three generations of a Dutch family. Ophthalmologica 137:422, 1959.

Contributor: **R.S. Wilroy, Jr.**

Editor's Computerized Descriptors: Vision, Eye, Skin, Sweating, Skel., Resp., Nerve

VATER ASSOCIATION

Includes: Anomalies vertébro-ano-trachéo-radiales
Asociación Vater
Duhamel anomalad
Imperforate anus/polydactyly
Vertebral anomalies syndrome
Cravet association
Vactel association
Vacterl syndrome

Excludes: Heart-hand syndrome (455)
Anus-hand-ear syndrome (72)

Minimal Diagnostic Criteria: Recognition of any 1 of the 5 major anomalies comprising the VATER association should alert one to the possibility of the presence of other associated anomalies. This has not, however, been recognized as a concise syndrome.

Clinical Findings: The term VATER Association refers to the principal features of this disorder, ie *V*ertebral defects, *A*nal atresia, *T-E* fistula with esophageal atresia, *R*enal defects and *R*adial limb dysplasia. Other features are cardiac defects, single umbilical artery, prenatal growth deficiency, genital anomalies, large fontanels, minor defects of the external ear and lower limb dysplasia. The vast majority of affected individuals have normal intelligence. The vertebral anomalies include bifid vertebrae, hemivertebrae and sacral anomalies. Rectourethral and rectovaginal fistulas are commonly found in association with high anorectal agenesis. Radial limb dysplasia includes any defect involving the radial side of the arm, ie hypoplasia of the thumb, triphalangeal thumb, radial polydactyly, and radial aplasia. Ventricular septal defect is the most common cardiac anomaly.

Complications
I   **Derived:** Scoliosis, chronic urinary tract infection, aspiration pneumonia, congestive heart failure, growth deficiency.
II **Associated:** See Clinical Findings.

Etiology: ?

Pathogenesis: Although unknown, the most likely possibility is a single primary defect in germinal center or disk morphogenesis leading to disorganization of the primitive streak and thereby migration of early caudal mesoderm giving rise to many of the various anomalies comprising this pattern of malformation.

Related Facts
I   **Sex Ratio:** M1:F1
II   **Risk of Occurrence:** ?
III **Risk of Recurrence for**
     Patient's Sib: ? Presumably of low magnitude, although careful evaluation of sibs has not been undertaken.
     Patient's Child: ?
IV   **Age of Detectability:** At birth
V   **Prevalence:** ?

Treatment
I   **Primary Prevention:** ?
II   **Secondary Prevention:** Surgery for associated malformations.
III **Other Therapy:** ?

Prognosis: Though patients may fail to thrive and may have developmental delay early in life because of associated anomalies, prognosis for normal intelligence is usually excellent. Therefore, vigorous attempts toward surgical rehabilitation should be instituted.

Detection of Carrier: —

Special Considerations: —

References:

Barry, J.E. and Auldist, A.W.: The VATER association- One end of a spectrum of anomalies. Am. J. Dis. Child. 128:769, 1974.
Quan, L. and Smith, D.W.: The VATER association. J. Pediatr. 82:104, 1973.
Temtamy, S.A. and Miller, J.D.: Extending the scope of the VATER association: Definition of the VATER syndrome. J. Pediatr. 85:345, 1974.

Contributor: **Kenneth Lyons Jones**

_____

Editor's Computerized Descriptors: Ear, Skel., CV., GI., GU.

VENTRICULAR DIVERTICULUM

Includes: Diverticule ventriculaire
Kammerdivertikel
Divertículo ventricular
Diverticulum of left ventricle
Diverticulum of right ventricle

Excludes: Ventricular aneurysm

Minimal Diagnostic Criteria: The cardinal diagnostic feature of diverticulum of the left ventricle is that of a herniated, pulsating mass palpable just below the xiphoid. Selective right or left atriograms or pulmonary arteriograms are preferred to confirm the presence of a communicating diverticulum.

Clinical Findings: Anatomically, the diverticulum of the left ventricle is most frequently located at the apex. The wall of the diverticulum is either muscular or fibrous. The 1 reported case involving the right ventricle also had its origin at the apex.

A congenital diverticulum of the left ventricle is frequently associated with midline defects of the diaphragm and anterior abdominal wall. These permit its projection into the epigastric region. Associated cardiac defects have been reported in both types.

Hemodynamic data are rare. In 1 case, systolic pressure within the diverticulum of the left ventricle was reported as twice that of the systolic pressure within the left ventricle. Thus, the diverticulum was a muscular chamber acting to overcome the outflow obstruction of the communicating orifice.

The cardinal manifestation of diverticulum of the left ventricle, when present at birth or early infancy, is that of a herniated pulsating mass palpable just below the xiphoid. In the absence of associated cardiac defects, usually no murmurs are audible; however, systolic murmurs and thrills may be noted in the area of the mass.

Chest roentgenographic findings and ECGs reflect principally the associated cardiac defects.

Complications
I   **Derived:** Sudden death from rupture of the diverticulum, thromboembolism, bacterial endocarditis.
II **Associated:** Defects of the pericardium, midline defects of the diaphragm and anterior abdominal wall are almost always present with diverticulum of the left ventricle. Omphalocele has also been noted with this entity. A broad spectrum of associated cardiac anomalies includes atrial and ventricular septal defects, single ventricle, tricuspid atresia, patent ductus arteriosus and coarctation of the aorta.

Etiology: ?

Pathogenesis: ?

Related Facts
I   **Sex Ratio:** ? M1:F1 on the basis of 25 cases
II   **Risk of Occurrence:** Less than 1 in 200,000 births (less than 0.05% CHD)
III **Risk of Recurrence for**
     Patient's Sib. ?
     Patient's Child: ?
IV   **Age of Detectability:** From birth by physical examination or selective angiocardiography
V   **Prevalence:** ?

Treatment
I   **Primary Prevention:** —
II   **Secondary Prevention:** Resection of the diverticulum as early as possible after confirming the diagnosis.
III **Other Therapy:** Repair of the midline defects as necessary. Medical or surgical management of associated cardiac de-

fects as indicated.

Prognosis: The majority of patients with undiagnosed diverticulum of the left ventricle die within the first 6 months of life. In the absence of associated cardiac defects, these patients, once successfully surgically repaired, should have normal lives. In those patients with associated cardiac anomalies, the prognosis is further limited by the type and physiology of these lesions.

Detection of Carrier: —

Special Considerations: —

References:
Cumming, G.R.: Congenital diverticulum of the right ventricle. Am. J. Cardiol. 23:294, 1969.
Dumas, P.A. and Schiebler, G.L.: Miscellaneous congenital cardiovascular abnormalities. In Gellis, S.S. and Kagen, B.M. (eds.): Current Pediatric Therapy-4. Philadelphia: W.B. Saunders, 1970, p. 226.
Keith, J.D. et al (eds.): Heart Disease in Infancy and Childhood, 2nd Ed. New York: Macmillan Co., 1967.
Neill, C.A.: Extopia cordis and cardiac diverticulum. In Watson, H. (ed.): Paediatric Cardiology. St. Louis: C.V. Mosby Co., 1968, p. 674.
Taussig, H.B.: Congenital Malformations of the Heart, 2nd Ed. Cambridge: Harvard University Press, 1960, vol. II.

Contributor: **Gerold L. Schiebler**

Editor's Computerized Descriptor: GI.

VENTRICULAR SEPTAL DEFECT

Includes: Anomalie du septum ventriculaire
Ventrikelseptumdefekt
Defecto del tabique inter-ventricular
Membranous septal defect
Aneurysm of membranous septum with one or more perforations
Defects in various portions of muscular septum
Infracristal ventricular septal defect with overriding aorta without infundibular stenosis (Eisenmenger complex)
Supracristal ventricular septal defect

Excludes: Tetralogy of Fallot (938)
Endocardial cushion defects (347)

Minimal Diagnostic Criteria: For patients with small defects who are asymptomatic and have normal xray and ECG, the hallmark of diagnosis is the characteristic VSD murmur. For symptomatic patients and those who have evidence of abnormal hemodynamic overloads, cardiac catheterization is the procedure of choice to confirm the diagnosis and establish the hemodynamic state.†

Clinical Findings: The position of single or multiple defects of the ventricular septum is variable; however, the associated hemodynamic changes are due primarily to the size of the defect. Clinical assessment should be made on the basis of size of the defect, the magnitude of the left-to-right shunt, and the resistance to blood flow through the lungs. The spectrum of clinical findings can be divided into 3 categories: small ventricular septal defects, moderate-to-large defects with large pulmonary blood flow and moderate elevation of pulmonary vascular resistance, and large ventricular septal defects with marked elevation of pulmonary vascular resistance and normal-to-diminished pulmonary blood flow.

Small Ventricular Defects have minimal hemodynamic changes and clinical manifestations are inapparent. A harsh holosystolic murmur and thrill along the lower left sternal border is the characteristic finding. Components of the second sound are usually normal. The roentgenographic findings demonstrate a normal sized heart with normal-to-slight increase in pulmonary vascularity. The ECG usually is normal or has early biventricular hypertrophy pattern. Some patients, however, demonstrate left axis deviation which possibly is due to an associated anomaly of the left ventricular conduction system. An unruptured aneurysm of the membranous septum causes no symptoms unless large enough to obstruct right ventricular outflow.

Moderate-to-Large Ventricular Defect with increased pulmonary blood flow and moderate elevation of pulmonary vascular resistance: The clinical manifestations are primarily determined by the magnitude of pulmonary blood flow. Congestive heart failure occurs in approximately one-third of these patients between 3-6 months of age. After 12-16 months of age, large left-to-right shunts are usually tolerated without severe heart failure. The usual systolic murmur is located along the left sternal border and is usually decrescendo in nature. An early faint diastolic blow in the pulmonic area is rarely present as a result of pulmonary insufficiency. There is an apical diastolic murmur of increased mitral flow across the mitral valve. The second sound is loud and single in those patients with high pulmonary artery pressure; splitting of the second sound indicates that pulmonary artery pressure is below systemic level. The roentgenogram demonstrates cardiomegaly and increased pulmonary vascularity commensurate with the magnitude of the left-to-right shunt. In infants, associated pulmonary venous congestion may be evi-

dent. Left atrial enlargement usually is present. The ECG demonstrates combined ventricular hypertrophy and left atrial enlargement as a rule. In infants under 6 months of age with cardiomegaly, left axis deviation may serve as a major index of left ventricular hypertrophy.

Large Ventricular Septal Defect with high pulmonary vascular resistance and approximately normal pulmonary blood flow: The major hemodynamic overload is right ventricular hypertension, which is tolerated well throughout early childhood. There are no symptoms throughout infancy and cyanosis is rare until later childhood. Growth proceeds normally. There is no VSD murmur; however, there is frequently a pulmonic ejection murmur in the second left interspace which may be associated with an early diastolic blow of pulmonary insufficiency. The second sound is loud and single. Apical diastolic murmurs are absent. The roentgenographic findings demonstrate a normal to minimally enlarged heart, right ventricular hypertrophy, prominent main pulmonary artery segment and increased hilar markings. There is pronounced contrast between the prominent central pulmonary arterial vessels and the diminished markings in the outer third of the lung field in some cases. The ECG demonstrates right ventricular hypertrophy and right axis deviation. Left atrial and left ventricular hypertrophy are absent. Cardiac catheterization will confirm the presence of a defect, the magnitude of shunting present, the pulmonary vascular resistance and the work load on the left ventricle. Oxygen saturation data and indicator dilution curves are important in assessing systemic and pulmonary blood flow, detection of the site of shunt and evaluating bidirectional shunts. Angiocardiography, although not mandatory, is helpful to visualize the site of the defect, especially to confirm multiple muscular communications, and to determine left heart volumes.

While some cross-sectional studies have reported visualization of ventricular septal defects, it is quite uncommon to echocardiographically detect the presence of a VSD using single-crystal systems. Lack of defect visualization is a function of septal alignment, the position of the defect within the septum and the width of the echo beam. However, the defect can occasionally be seen in tetralogy of Fallot, truncus arteriosus or double outlet right ventricle. The echocardiographic findings in ventricular septal defect are a manifestation of flow dynamics. Left atrial enlargement is usually present in large defects with high flow, but it may be absent with high resistance-low flow ventricular septal defects. If the latter situation exists (Eisenmenger syndrome), abnormal thickening of the right ventricular anterior wall and an unusual pulmonary valve motion pattern which resembles the shape of the letter "W" is noted and the normal "A" dip of the pulmonary valve motion trace is missing. The latter are the typical pulmonary valve findings in pulmonary hypertension.

Complications
I **Derived:** Death from congestive heart failure and pneumonia, especially in infancy, bacterial endocarditis with small defects, development of high pulmonary vascular resistance. Aortic insufficiency occasionally occurs.
II **Associated:** —

Etiology: Multifactorial inheritance

Pathogenesis: Failure of closure of subaortic portion of ventricular septum with anomalous development of any one or several components, ie embryonic muscular septum, the endocardial cushions and conal swellings. Muscular defects may be due to failure of increasing muscle mass to obliterate intratrabecular spaces.†

Related Facts

I **Sex Ratio:** M1:F1
II **Risk of Occurrence:** 1 in 400 full-term live births; slightly higher in prematures
III **Risk of Recurrence for**
   Patient's Sib: Predicted risk 5.0%; empiric risk 4.4%.
   Patient's Child: Predicted risk 5.0%; empiric risk 4.0%
IV **Age of Detectability:** From birth by cardiac catheterization. Murmur usually present by 3 weeks
V **Prevalence:** Approximately 1 in 400 in pediatric population

Treatment

I **Primary Prevention:** Genetic counseling
II **Secondary Prevention:** Definitive surgery: recommended for moderate and large defects with increased pulmonary blood flow.
III **Other Therapy:** Medical therapy for congestive heart failure and pneumonia.

Prognosis: Patients with small defects have excellent prognosis. Without proper medical or surgical therapy, infants with heart failure have poor prognosis. Those who survive infancy with large defects and high pulmonary pressure have good prognosis during childhood. However, some with high pulmonary artery pressure develop further increases in pulmonary vascular resistance.

Detection of Carrier: —

†**Special Considerations:** The natural history of ventricular defects may involve dynamic changes in the physiologic state of the patient with time. Also, it is the most common congenital heart defect. Small defects present little physiologic overload and these patients do well. Also, up to 30% of small ventricular defects may spontaneously close during infancy. Infants with large defects and marked increase in pulmonary blood flow may follow 1 of several courses between the age of 6 months to 4 years: the defect may become smaller and thereby diminish the left-to-right shunt; the size of the defect may remain constant with little change in pulmonary vascular resistance and thereby, the patient may maintain marked increased pulmonary blood flow with associated overload on the left ventricle. After 12-18 months of age, congestive heart failure may spontaneously improve in the face of an unchanging pulmonary blood flow; in patients with large defects and marked pulmonary blood flow, hypertrophy of the infundibulum may occur with development of pulmonary hypertension; large defects may not change in size and pulmonary vascular resistance may gradually increase with ultimate reduction in pulmonary blood flow. It is this latter group which may progress from the infant picture of large pulmonary blood flow and heart failure to the childhood state of markedly elevated pulmonary resistance (Eisenmenger syndrome). Note: Eisenmenger *syndrome* clinically refers to a physiologic state in which the pulmonary vascular resistance is equal to or exceeds that of the systemic vascular resistance: Eisenmenger *complex* refers specifically to a particular type of large ventricular septal defect which embryologically results from a hypoplasia of the conus septum.

References:
Goldberg, S.J. et al: Pediatric and Adolescent Echocardiography. Chicago: Year Book Medical Publishers, 1975.
Hoffman, J.I. and Rudolph, A.M.: The natural history of ventricular septal defects in infancy. Am. J. Cardiol. 16:634, 1965.
Rudolph, A.M.: The effects of postnatal circulatory adjustments in congenital heart disease. Pediatrics 36:763, 1965.
Sahn, D.J. et al: Echocardiographic detection of large left-to-right shunts and cardiomyopathies in infants and children. Am. J. Cardiol. 38:73, 1976.
Spach, M.S. et al: Defects of the ventricular septum. In Moss, A.J. and Adams, F.H. (eds.): Heart Disease in Infants, Children, and Adolescents. Baltimore: Williams & Wilkins, 1968, p. 311.

Contributor: **Madison S. Spach**

Editor's Computerized Descriptors: Resp., CV.

VISCERA, FATTY METAMORPHOSIS

Includes: Métamorphose graisseuse des viscéres
Familiäre fettige Metamorphose der Viscera
Metamorfosis grasosa visceral familiar
Familial jaundice, hepatosteatosis, and kernicterus
Familial steatosis of liver and kidney
Peremans disease
Fatal neonatal hepatic steatosis
Fatty metamorphosis of viscera

Excludes: Secondary fatty metamorphosis of viscera
Reye syndrome
Buhl disease
Niemann-Pick disease (717)
Other sphingolipidoses

Minimal Diagnostic Criteria: For the first involved infant in a family, the presence of the clinical syndrome and characteristic autopsy findings establish the diagnosis. In other sibs the clinical pattern alone may justify defense of this diagnosis.

Clinical Findings: Sixteen patients have been described from 4 families, in 4 separate publications. The infants appear normal at birth, but become lethargic, hypotonic, and icteric between the 1st and 14th day of life, and die rapidly thereafter. One child presented with this picture at 19 months of age. There are abnormal hepatic function and hemostatic tests; hypoglycemia and hypocalcemia may be present (and respond variably to therapy). Some infants have had respiratory distress and vomiting. Heart block has been described.

At autopsy there is severe fatty metamorphosis of the liver, kidney, heart, and skeletal muscle. The brain, in some instances, has shown severe bilirubin staining of nuclei.†

Complications
I **Derived:** —
II **Associated:** —

Etiology: ? Possibly autosomal recessive. In 1 family with 6 involved sibs, the parents were 2nd cousins. In another family an X-linked disorder was suggested (5 males were affected, 2 males were not affected, and 2 females were well).

Pathogenesis: The rapid onset of multiple organ dysfunction and the extreme degree of triglyceride accumulation in the viscera suggest a massive metabolic aberration, but the specific pathogenesis is unknown. Features such as the hyperbilirubinemia and the hypoglycemia are diffiuclt to assess. Infection is presumably not causative.

Related Facts
I **Sex Ratio:** Unclear; 5 affected males were reported in each of 2 publications
II **Risk of Occurrence:** ? Probably very low
III **Risk of Recurrence for**
Patient's Sib: ? Very high in 3 reports
Patient's Child: All affected patients have died in infancy
IV **Age of Detectability:** Usually in newborn period
V **Prevalence:** ?

Treatment
I **Primary Prevention:** Genetic counseling
II **Secondary Prevention:** Vigorous supportive measures, including exchange transfusion and parenteral alimentation, are indicated in the hope of maintaining the child while intrinsic adjustments are accomplished.
III **Other Therapy:** —

Prognosis: The syndrome is uniformly fatal, based on presently available patient reports.

Detection of Carrier: ?

†Special Considerations: This disorder is not be be confused with the picture of lesser accumulations of cytoplasmic neutral fat in the organs of newborn infants dying from a variety of unrelated disorders which have hypoxia as the common feature. It also differs from Buhl disease in which the fatty changes are related to the effects of sepsis, and Reye syndrome in which encephalopathy is associated with triglyceride steatosis of the liver, kidney, and myocardium.

More extensive study of affected infants during life, and more sophisticated autopsy studies, will hopefully delineate a basic pathogenetic mechanism.

References:
Peremans, J. et al: Familial metabolic disorder with fatty metamorphosis of the viscera. J. Pediatr. 69:1108, 1966.
Räsänen, O. et al: Fatal familial steatosis of the liver and kidney in two siblings. Z. Kinderheilkd. 110:267, 1971.
Reye, R.D. et al: Encephalopathy and fatty degeneration of the viscera; a disease entity in childhood. Lancet 2:749, 1963.
Satran, L. et al: Fatal neonatal hepatic steatosis, a new familial disorder. J. Pediatr. 75:39, 1969.
Wadlington, W.B. and Riley, H.D.: Familial disease characterized by neonatal jaundice and probable hepatosteatosis and kernicterus: A new syndrome? Pediatrics 51:192, 1973.

Contributors: **Blaise E. Favara
Sandra Stenmark**

Editor's Computerized Descriptors: Muscle, Resp., CV., GI., Liver, Skin, Nerve

VITAMIN B₆ DEPENDENCY

Includes: Pyridoxin-dépendance
Vitamin B$_6$ Abhängigkeit
Dependencia a la vitamina B$_6$
Pyridoxine dependency
Vitamin B$_6$ dependency with convulsions†

Excludes: Vitamin B$_6$ deficiency states

Minimal Diagnostic Criteria: There is, as yet, no specific biochemical or enzymatic phenotype to characterize this convulsive trait. Diagnosis must rest at present on immediate control of seizures with pyridoxine HC1, 10-50 mg IM, IV or po, positive family history, and no objective evidence for vitamin B$_6$ deficiency.

Clinical Findings: The familial convulsive disorder, which was first called "pyridoxine dependency," has been reported in at least 14 pedigrees. Symptoms appear in the perinatal period. Convulsions in utero have been described, but most patients developed grand mal seizures in first week of life; occasionally onset is delayed for several weeks after birth. Hyperirritability, hyperacusis and feeding difficulties accompany the seizures. The usual anticonvulsant drugs are ineffective; pyridoxine (or other forms of vitamin B$_6$), given by any route, is the only agent which will control seizures. Electroencephalography can be used to monitor the effect of pyridoxine therapy; the response appears within minutes after administration of the vitamin. The majority of known patients are now severely retarded, or have died for want of proper treatment; early treatment with pyridoxine is compatible with normal growth and development. The most important negative features of the syndrome are the absence of any cause or evidence for vitamin B$_6$ deficiency, or other causes for a convulsive disorder.

Complications
I   **Derived:**   Retarded development or death
II **Associated:**   —

Etiology: A mutation affecting the enzymatic synthesis of a neuroregulatory (inhibitor) compound. First-cousin consanguinity in parents of proband in one pedigree supports likelihood of autosomal recessive transmission. McK *26610

Pathogenesis: Endogenous metabolism of vitamin B$_6$ and synthesis of its active coenzyme, pyridoxal-5-phosphate, from dietary precursors (eg pyridoxine) is normal. Deficiency of vitamin B$_6$ is not the cause of the trait. The immediate clinical response indicates adequate cellular uptake of the vitamin, as well as an intact B$_6$-dependent function awaiting activation. The exaggerated nutritional requirement for the vitamin to sustain normal activity of a particular cellular protein enzyme constitutes the pharmacologic dependency for vitamin B$_6$. It is believed that the mutation alters the normal relation of glutamic acid decarboxylase (the apoenzyme) with pyridoxal-5-phosphate (the coenzyme); the product of this enzyme's activity is gamma-aminobutyric acid, a presynaptic neuro-inhibitor.

Related Facts
I   **Sex Ratio:**   M1:F1
II   **Risk of Occurrence:**   ?
III **Risk of Recurrence for**
     Patient's Sib: Probably 1 in 4 (25%) for each sib
     Patient's Child: Not increased unless mate is heterozygote or homozygote
IV   **Age of Detectability:**   In perinatal period
V   **Prevalence:**   ? But probably more frequent than suspected

Treatment

I   **Primary Prevention:**   Genetic counseling
II **Secondary Prevention:**   Coenzyme supplementation: Vitamin B$_6$ as pyridoxine HC1, 2-50 mg/day; dose must be titrated for individual patient. Dependency is permanent.
III **Other Therapy:**   Febrile conditions and infections may temporarily increase vitamin B$_6$ requirement.

Prognosis: Can be excellent if treated early enough; this may even mean treating the mother with pyridoxine during pregnancy to prevent manifestation of the trait in utero. Late diagnosis and treatment has an 80% risk of retarded development or death.

Detection of Carrier: ?

†**Special Considerations:** The hereditary nutritional state, broadly termed "vitamin B$_6$ dependency," is a heterogeneous trait involving several distinctive and inherited abnormalities of different apoenzymes. In each case, it is possible that the normal relationship of the apoenzyme with its coenzyme is altered. Precedence for this concept is found in the mutations which affect the pyridoxal-5-phosphate binding site on the B$_6$-requiring enzyme, tryptophan synthetase, in Neurospora crassa. Since the original proposal by Scriver that "vitamin B$_6$ dependency with convulsions" is a phenotype reflecting the effect of mutation on one catabolic reaction (probably glutamate decarboxylation), rather than a primary abnormality of vitamin B$_6$ metabolism affecting many apoenzymes, other traits have been proposed as additional forms of "vitamin B$_6$ dependency." Thus, hereditary cystathioninuria, xanthurenicaciduria, and some forms of familial pyridoxine-responsive anemia can each be interpreted as inherited abnormalities of a specific enzyme. Discovery of many other forms of vitamin B$_6$ dependency can be anticipated in view of the many B$_6$-requiring enzyme reactions in amino acid, carbohydrate and fatty acid metabolism, hyper-β-alaninemia, and some forms of homocystinuria may be further examples. The basis for pyridoxine responsiveness in each trait requires further investigation. The recent discovery of glutamic acid decarboxylase in mammalian kidney (it was previously thought to be in brain only) may assist the investigation of the convulsive trait.

References:
Scriver, C. R.: Vitamin B$_6$ deficiency and dependency in man. Am. J. Dis. Child. 113:109, 1967.
Scriver, C. R.: Vitamin B$_6$ dependency syndromes; their larger significance. Pediatrics 37:553, 1966.
Scriver, C. R. and Whelan, D. T.: Glutamic acid decarboxylase (GAD) in mammaliam tissue outside the central nervous system, and its possible relevance to hereditary vitamin B$_6$ dependency with seizures. Ann. N.Y. Acad. Sci. 166:83, 1969.
Yoshida, T. et al: Vitamin B$_6$-dependency of glutamic acid decarboxylase in the kidney from a patient with vitamin B$_6$ dependent convulsions. Tohoku J. Exp. Med. 104:195, 1971.

Contributor: **Charles R. Scriver**

Editor's Computerized Descriptors: GI., Nerve

VITAMIN B$_{12}$ MALABSORPTION

Includes: Malabsorption de la vitamine B$_{12}$
Malabsorción de la vitamina B$_{12}$
Malabsorption of vitamin B$_{12}$ (two types)
Juvenile pernicious anemia
Gastric intrinsic factor deficiency
Ileal B$_{12}$ transport deficiency
Cobalamin malabsorption

Excludes: Acquired pernicious anemia due to deficiency of extrinsic factor
Blind loop syndrome or Diphyllobothrium latum infestation
Folic acid malabsorption
Transcobalamin II deficiency

Minimal Diagnostic Criteria: Demonstration of vitamin B$_{12}$ deficiency by abnormal Schilling test, reduced serum vitamin B$_{12}$ concentration or excretion of methylmalonic acid in the urine. Patients with isolated inherited deficiency of intrinsic factor will respond to ingestion of normal gastric juice. Patients with B$_{12}$ malabsorption due to specific ilial "receptor site" defect will respond only to parenteral administration of vitamin B$_{12}$.

Clinical Findings: Megaloblastic anemia noted during the first 1-3 years of life (100%): 1 group of children lacks gastric intrinsic factor; a 2nd group has an immunologically identifiable, functionally defective intrinsic factor; the 3rd group lacks the ileal transport mechanism for vitamin B$_{12}$.†

Complications
I   **Derived:** Combined system disease of the CNS
II **Associated:** Proteinuria noted in nearly 50% of patients with ileal transport defect.

Etiology: Autosomal recessive transmission for defect affecting either the synthesis of gastric intrinsic factor or the specific vitamin B$_{12}$ transport system in the terminal ileum. McK *26110

Pathogenesis: Deficiency of vitamin B$_{12}$ leads to megaloblastic anemia, methylmalonic aciduria and CNS disease.

Related Facts
I   **Sex Ratio:** M1:F1
II   **Risk of Occurrence:** ?
III **Risk of Recurrence for**
     Patient's Sib: 1 in 4 (25%) for each offspring to be affected
     Patient's Child: Not increased unless mate is carrier or homozygote
IV   **Age of Detectability:** 1-2 years
V   **Prevalence:** ?

Treatment
I   **Primary Prevention:** Genetic counseling
II   **Secondary Prevention:** Parenteral administration of vitamin B$_{12}$ (1 µg/day)
III **Other Therapy:** Blood transfusions; physical therapy, nutritional support

Prognosis: Good, if treatment initiated before permanent CNS damage ensues.

Detection of Carrier: Not well-defined; both parents of single patient with ileal transport defect reported to have moderate impairment of vitamin B$_{12}$ absorption without anemia.

†Special Considerations: Existence of such patients provides strong evidence for single gene control of synthesis of gastric intrinsic factor and of ileal "receptor" in vitamin B$_{12}$ transport process; must be distinguished from inherited deficiency of folic acid absorption.

References:
Donaldson, R.H.: Mechanisms of malabsorption of cobalamin. In Babior, B.M. (ed.): Cobalamin Biochemistry and Pathophysiology. New York:John Wiley & Sons, 1975, p. 335.
Grasbeck, R. et al: Selective vitamin B$_{12}$ malabsorption and proteinuria in young people. Acta. Med. Scand. 167:289, 1960.
McIntyre, O.R. et al: Pernicious anemia in childhood. N. Engl. J. Med. 272:981, 1965.
Mohamed, S.D. et al: Juvenile familial megaloblastic anaemia due to selective malabsorption of vitamin B$_{12}$: A family study and a review of the literature. Q. J. Med. 35:433, 1966.

Contributor: **Leon E. Rosenberg**

Editor's Computerized Descriptor: Nerve

VITILIGO

987-500

Includes: Achromia, primary
Leukoderma, primary

Excludes: Albinism
Albinism-cutaneous without deafness (31)
Nevus anemicus
Ash leaf macule of tuberous sclerosis
Depigmentation from secondary causes
Oculocutaneous albinism and deafness

Minimal Diagnostic Criteria: Acquired progressive primary melanin depigmentation of the skin.

Clinical Findings: Peripherally enlarging, progressive, sharply demarcated melanin depigmentation in otherwise normal skin over any portion of the body. Usually symmetric over the hands, face, neck, trunk, and body folds. The involvement can be localized or generalized with a convex configuration and a hyperpigmented border. Vitiliginous skin is sunlight-sensitive and burns rather than tans.

Complications
I **Derived:** Sunburn of depigmented skin. Cosmetic deficit; more apparent in darker races
II **Associated:** Alopecia areata, leukoderma acquisitum centrifugum (halo nevus), Addison disease, diabetes mellitus, hyperthyroidism, hypothyroidism, pernicious anemia.

Etiology: Probably autosomal dominant with variable penetrance†

Pathogenesis: Melanin depigmentation develops insidiously. May remain static or progress. May rarely involute spontaneously. There is a lack of melanin in the epidermis resulting in a milk-white coloration. Electron microscopy reveals that the melanocyte population is reduced or absent in the depigmented epidermis.†

Related Facts
I **Sex Ratio:** M1:F1
II **Risk of Occurrence:** About 1 in 100
III **Risk of Recurrence for**
  Patient's Sib: If autosomal dominant and if parent is affected, < 1 in 2 (50%) for each offspring to be affected; otherwise not increased.
  Patient's Child: If autosomal dominant, < 1 in 2
IV **Age of Detectability:** Onset before age 20 in more than 50% of cases
V **Prevalence:** About 1 in 100. Higher prevalence observed in darker races because of marked contrast by depigmented skin.

Treatment
I **Primary Prevention:** ? Genetic counseling
II **Secondary Prevention:** —
III **Other Therapy:** Sunlight protection with topical sun screens, cosmetics to camouflage the lesions and topical or systemic methoxypsoralen to promote repigmentation.

Prognosis: Normal for life span and intelligence. Depigmentation can be disfiguring. May have increased risk of skin cancer, due to lack of protection to sunlight.

Detection of Carrier: —

†**Special Considerations:** Both alopecia areata and leukoderma acquisitum centrifugum are found with greater frequency than would be expected in patients with vitiligo. Although the cause of vitiligo is not known, the increased incidence of autoantibodies and the occurrence of vitiligo in cases of solitary or multiple glandular insufficiencies, such as Addison disease, diabetes mellitus, hypothyroidism, and pernicious anemia, are suggestive of a possible end-organ autoimmune etiology.

References:
Lerner, A.B.: Vitiligo. J. Invest. Dermatol. 32:285, 1959.
McGregor, B. et al: The association of vitiligo and multiple glandular insufficiencies. JAMA 219:724, 1972.
Rook, A. et al: Textbook of Dermatology. Philadelphia:F.A. Davis, 1969, p. 1145.

Contributor: **Harry Irving Katz**

Editor's Computerized Descriptor: Skin

VITREOUS, PERSISTENT HYPERPLASTIC PRIMARY

Includes: Hyperplasie persistante du corps vitré
Persistieren des primitiven Glaskörpers
Humor vítreo primario hiperplástico persistente
Persistent tunica vasculosa lentis
Persistent fetal fibrovascular sheath of lens
Persistence of hyaloid artery

Excludes: Retinal dysplasia (866)
Retrolental fibroplasia (872)
Retinoblastoma (870)

Minimal Diagnostic Criteria: The presence of a retrolental fibrovascular mass.

Clinical Findings: This entity is usually detected immediately after birth on the basis of the white pupil (leukocoria) and these eyes are usually removed because of suspected retinoblastoma. This condition occurs in full-term infants, is unilateral and there is always some degree of microphthalmos. The anterior chamber is shallow and the blood vessels on the iris are prominent. A dehiscence in the posterior lens capsule may be present or a complete cataract may exist. Characteristically, there is a retrolental fibrovascular mass into which the ciliary processes are pulled. The hyaloid artery is sometimes observable clinically.

Complications
I **Derived:** Vitreous hemorrhage, retinal detachment, secondary glaucoma, cataract, phthisis bulbi.
II **Associated:** —

Etiology: ?

Pathogenesis: Persistence of the entire hyaloid system with hyperplasia of its associated tissue. Dysplastic retina is often seen within the retina on histopathologic examination.

Related Facts
I **Sex Ratio:** M?:F?
II **Risk of Occurrence:** ? Rare
III **Risk of Recurrence for**
  Patient's Sib: ?
  Patient's Child: ?
IV **Age of Detectability:** At birth
V **Prevalence:** ? Rare

Treatment
I **Primary Prevention:** —
II **Secondary Prevention:** Attempts have been made to intervene surgically and some success has been reported.
III **Other Therapy:** —

Prognosis: Normal for life span and intelligence; poor for vision in the affected eye.

Detection of Carrier: —

Special Considerations: —

References:
Duke-Elder, S.: System of Ophthalmology. In Congenital Deformities, vol. III, pt. 2. St. Louis: C.V. Mosby, 1964.
Gass, J.D.: Surgical excision of persistent hyperplastic primary vitreous. Arch. Ophthalmol. 83:163, 1970.
Reese, A.B.: Tumors of the Eye, 2nd Ed. New York: Harper and Row, Hoeber Medical Division, 1963.

Contributor: **Morton E. Smith**

Editor's Computerized Descriptor: Eye

VON HIPPEL-LINDAU SYNDROME

Includes: Syndrome de von Hippel-Lindau
Síndrome de von Hippel-Lindau
Hemangiomatosis, multiple

Excludes: Cerebellar tumor

Minimal Diagnostic Criteria: The diagnosis is made by a positive family history for retinal or cerebellar hemangioblastoma or the presence of a retinal and CNS hemangioblastoma occurring in the same patient.

Clinical Findings: Patients with von Hippel-Lindau disease present because of symptoms due to retinal or CNS hemangioblastomas. The age of onset varies, but is most common in the 4th decade.

The retinal lesions are most frequent in the peripheral retina and are, therefore, asymptomatic but may be seen at the disk border or macula, producing complaints of visual disturbance.

The lesion typically is raised, red and globular. It is fed by a dilated arteriole and drained by a tortuous vein. The retinal hemangioblastomas may undergo calcification and ossification. The retinal lesions are multiple in about 1/3 of the patients.

Hemangioblastomas involving the CNS are most common in the posterior fossa. The tumor may be situated in the cerebellar hemispheres, vermis or medulla. They may be multiple; most are cystic. An intermittent occipital headache is a frequent early symptom. Vomiting, vertigo, ataxia, nystagmus, dysarthria and dysmetria are common findings. Bizarre mental changes may accompany the increase in intracranial pressure.

The spinal cord is frequently involved, primarily in the cervical and thoracic segments. The hemangioblastoma is usually intramedullary and posterior producing initial complaints of loss of sensation and proprioception. A spastic paraparesis develops with progressive cord compression.

Approximately 15% of cerebellar hemangioblastomas are associated with polycythemia. A skull xray may show signs of increased intracranial pressure. A vertebral angiogram is the study of choice to demonstrate a posterior fossa hemangioblastoma. A myelogram and selective angiogram will identify a spinal cord tumor. IVP and renal angiography are used to demonstrate renal or adrenal lesions.

Complications
I **Derived:** The retinal lesions are usually progressive. Exudation occurs at the site of the tumor causing retinal detachment and eventual blindness. Cataracts and glaucoma may occur as well. The posterior fossa hemangioblastomas produce hydrocephaly by distortion of the aqueduct of Sylvius. Herniation of the cerebellar tonsils can result. Syringomyelia has occasionally been noted in association with a spinal cord hemangioblastoma. Hypertensive crises may complicate a pheochromocytoma and renal carcinomas may metastasize.
II **Associated:** Renal, pancreatic, hepatic, and epididymal cysts, renal carcinoma, pheochromocytoma

Etiology: Autosomal dominant; McK *19330

Pathogenesis: ? †

Related Facts
I **Sex Ratio:** M1:F1
II **Risk of Occurrence:** ?
III **Risk of Recurrence for**
  Patient's Sib: If parent is affected, 1 in 2 (50%) for each offspring to be affected; otherwise not increased.

Patient's Child: 1 in 2
IV **Age of Detectability:**   Usually by the 4th decade by a positive family history and the presence of retinal and CNS hemangioblastomas
V **Prevalence:**   ?

Treatment
I **Primary Prevention:**   Genetic counseling
II **Secondary Prevention:**   If a retinal tumor is found, photocoagulation is the treatment of choice. Diathermy is used if the lesion is extensive. Enucleation may be necessary. Treatment of the CNS lesions is surgical. Consideration should be given to surgical removal of a tumor before irreversible damage has occurred.
III **Other Therapy:**   Once a diagnosis has been made, the patient's entire family should be carefully examined. This should include regular examination of the retina by indirect ophthalmoscopy, neurologic examination and perhaps yearly IVPs.

Prognosis: Usually slowly progressive. Patients tend to die from increased intracranial pressure secondary to the CNS hemangioblastomas.

Detection of Carrier: —

†Special Considerations: The finding of polycythemia in some patients with von Hippel-Lindau disease is of considerable interest. It has been shown that the cyst fluid from some cerebellar hemangioblastomas has a definite erythropoietic stimulator effect, measured by the red cell incorporation of Fe^{59} in these patients.

The kidney is known to be the principal site of erythropoietin production. Some cystic renal carcinomas produce erythropoietin. Histologically cerebellar hemangioblastomas and renal carcinomas have many similarities. The reappearance of polycythemia following successful removal of a CNS hemangioblastoma might, therefore, suggest a recurrence of the CNS tumor or the development of a renal cell carcinoma.

References:
Hennessy, T.G. et al: Cerebellar hemangioblastoma: Erythropoietic activity by radioiron assay. J. Nucl. Med. 8:606, 1967.
Melmon, K.L. and Rosen, S.W.: Lindau's disease: A review of the literature and study of a large kindred. Am. J. Med. 36:595, 1964.
Walsh, F.B. and Hoyt, W.F.: Clinical Neuro-Ophthalmology, 3rd Ed. Baltimore:Williams & Wilkins, 1969, vol. 3.

Contributor: **Robert H.A. Haslam**

Editor's Computerized Descriptors: Eye, Vision, GI., Nerve

VON WILLEBRAND DISEASE

Includes: Maladie de von Willebrand
Mb. von Willebrand
Enfermedad de von Willebrand
Pseudohemophilia

Excludes: Hemophilia A (461)

Minimal Diagnostic Criteria: Prolonged bleeding time (template method) and decreased Factor VIII activity are the most commonly accepted criteria. Factor VIII antigenic activity is reduced to an equal degree. Platelet aggregation is inhibited by ristocetin when Factor VIII antigen is below 30%. The results of all of these studies are variable in a single individual and among affected members of a family. The bleeding time may sporadically become normal in a patient who usually has a prolonged bleeding time. Depressed baseline Factor VIII activity may be elevated into the normal range by stress or pregnancy.

Clinical Findings: Epistaxis and excessive bleeding after minor mouth injuries, lacerations, and loss of deciduous teeth, as well as bruising after mild trauma. Patients with lowest activities of Factor VIII have the greatest tendency to easy bruising, periarticular hemorrhages, and other manifestations characteristic of classic hemophilia (Hemophilia A).

Complications
I **Derived:**   Increased risk of bleeding following surgery, dental procedures and acute trauma
II **Associated:**   Hepatitis from transfusions. Development of antibodies to Factor VIII reduces effectiveness of Factor VIII transfusion in less than 10% of patients.

Etiology: Autosomal dominant; McK *19340

Pathogenesis: Decreased synthesis of Factor VIII and Factor VIII-associated von Willebrand factor which is necessary for normal bleeding time and platelet aggregation.

Related Facts
I **Sex Ratio:**   M1:F1
II **Risk of Occurrence:**   ? Dependent upon criteria
III **Risk of Recurrence for**
   Patient's Sib: If parent is affected 1 in 2 (50%) for each offspring to be affected, but manifestations within a single family can vary markedly.
   Patient's Child: 1 in 2, but manifestations within a single family can vary markedly.
IV **Age of Detectability:**   Probably at birth, though more often only when accidental injury precipitates bleeding episodes, as in early childhood.
V **Prevalence:**   Dominant inheritance of a prolonged bleeding time per se is not rare.

Treatment
I **Primary Prevention:**   Genetic counseling, but manifestations in most cases are mild and variable.
II **Secondary Prevention:**   Cryoprecipitated Factor VIII, fresh frozen plasma, and stored plasma all will elevate circulating Factor VIII levels (usually more than can be accounted for by the activity of the amount of Factor VIII administered) and reduce the risk of bleeding following surgical and dental procedures. Aspirin prolongs the bleeding time and should be avoided. Factor VIII concentrate raises the level of Factor VIII but does not correct the bleeding time.
III **Other Therapy:**   Treatment with any of the agents above may be required to stop persistent bleeding, most frequently epistaxis. If one dose does not suffice, treatment intervals of 24 hours can be employed since severity of bleeding is generally correlated with Factor VIII activity, and the response of the Factor VIII level to therapy is frequently more prolonged than the average T 1/2 of 12 hours observed in classic hemophilia. The correction in bleeding time and platelet function is shorter, with a T 1/2 closer to 12 hours.

Prognosis: Few patients are substantially handicapped by the defect and little excessive bleeding in female patients is likely with childbirth.

Detection of Carrier: Screening procedures include template bleeding time, level of Factor VIII procoagulant activity, Factor VIII antigen, and von Willebrand factor, and platelet aggregation with ristocetin, not all of which are abnormal in all patients.

Special Considerations: —

References:
Biggs, R. and Macfarlane, R. G. (eds.): Treatment of Haemophilia and Other Coagulation Disorders. 2nd Ed. Philadelphia: F.A. Davis, 1976.

Brinkhous, K.M. and Hemker, H.C. (eds.): Handbook of Hemophilia. Amsterdam: Excepta Medica, 1975.

Contributors: **Marion A. Koerper**
Louis K. Diamond

Editor's Computerized Descriptors: Skin, Nasoph.

Includes: Syndrome de Waardenburg
Síndrome de Waardenburg
Klein-Waardenburg syndrome

Excludes: Albinism-cutaneous without deafness (31)
Albinism-cutaneous and deafness (30)
Vogt-Koyanagi syndrome

Minimal Diagnostic Criteria: The most consistent finding in this syndrome is lateral displacement of the medial canthi and lacrimal ducts. If this is present, plus any of the below listed findings, the diagnosis of Waardenburg syndrome should seriously be considered. There is, however, an overlap between this syndrome and other syndromes with nerve deafness, heterochromia and albinism and they may all represent a single entity.

Clinical Findings: Common features include lateral displacement of the inner canthi or the inferior lacrimal puncta, 95-99%; prominence of the root of the nose, 75%; hyperplasia of the medial portion of the eyebrows, 50%; heterochromium iridium or iris bicolor, 45%; and congenital sensorineural deafness, varying from one report of 92% penetrance to the Waardenburg 20% penetrance. In a pedigree totaling 22 affected family members, the risk of recurrence of congenital deafness was 2% with marked intrafamilial variability. White forelock or early greying occurs in 17-45% of cases. Patients with a hypochromic iris may have a homolateral brunet fundus. If unilateral iris bicolor is present, the homolateral fundus is associated with a unilateral bicolor or marked pigmentary mottling. Other clinical findings include a thin nose with flaring alae nasae, "cupid bow" configuration of the lips, ocular hypertelorism, dacrocystitis, ptosis, lack of frontonasal angle, prominent mandible, cleft or high-arched palate, vitiligo, and minor skeletal abnormalities. Marked degeneration of the organ of Corti, atrophy of spiral ganglion cells and of stria vascularis have been observed.

Complications
I   **Derived:** Sensorineural deafness, infection of tear ducts, learning difficulties due to deafness
II   **Associated:** —

Etiology: Autosomal dominant with variable penetrance. Within a family, all degrees of severity may be encountered. McK *19350

Pathogenesis: ?

Related Facts
I   **Sex Ratio:** M1:F1
II   **Risk of Occurrence:** 1 in 4000 live births
III **Risk of Recurrence for**
     Patient's Sib: If parent is affected, 1 in 2 (50%) for each sib; otherwise not increased.
     Patient's Child: 1 in 2
IV   **Age of Detectability:** The diagnosis may be made in infancy by observing the clinical manifestations. The white forelock which has been reported at birth, may disappear by 3 months and return in early childhood.
V   **Prevalence:** ?

Treatment
I   **Primary Prevention:** Genetic counseling
II   **Secondary Prevention:** Hearing aid, lip-reading, special schooling, sign language or hearing conservation when hearing loss is unilateral. Repair of cleft palate may be necessary.
III **Other Therapy:** —

Prognosis: For life: No effect upon life expectancy. For intelligence: Mental retardation has been rarely reported but may be suspected because of unrecognized severe deafness which can lead to mutism. For function: As noted, deafness may lead to mutism and its complications. Also, cleft palate can lead to functional problems.

Detection of Carrier: The affected patient is heterozygous for the dominant mutant gene. Close examination of the apparently unaffected individual may reveal minimal expression of the mutant gene.

Special Considerations: —

References:

DiGeorge, A.M. et al: Waardenburg's syndrome: A syndrome of heterochromia of the irides, lateral displacement of the medial canthi and lacrimal puncta, congenital deafness, and other characteristic associated defects. Trans. Am. Acad. Ophthalmol. Otolaryngol. 64:816, 1960.

Pantke, O.A. and Cohen, M.M., Jr.: The Waardenburg syndrome. In Bergsma, D. (ed.): Part XI. Orofacial Structures. Birth Defects: Orig. Art. Ser. vol. VII, no. 7. Baltimore:Williams and Wilkins Co. for The National Foundation-March of Dimes, 1971, p. 147.

Reed, W. B. et al: Pigmentary disorders in association with congenital deafness. Arch. Dermatol. 95:176, 1967.

Rugel, S. J. and Keats, E. U.: Waardenburg's syndrome in six generations of one family. Am. J. Dis. Child. 109:579, 1965.

Waardenburg, P. J.: New syndrome combining developmental anomalies of the eyelids, eyebrows and nose root with pigmentary defects of the iris and head hair and with congenital deafness. Am. J. Hum. Genet. 3:195, 1951.

Contributor: **Murray Feingold**

Editor's Computerized Descriptors: Eye, Hearing, Nose, Hair

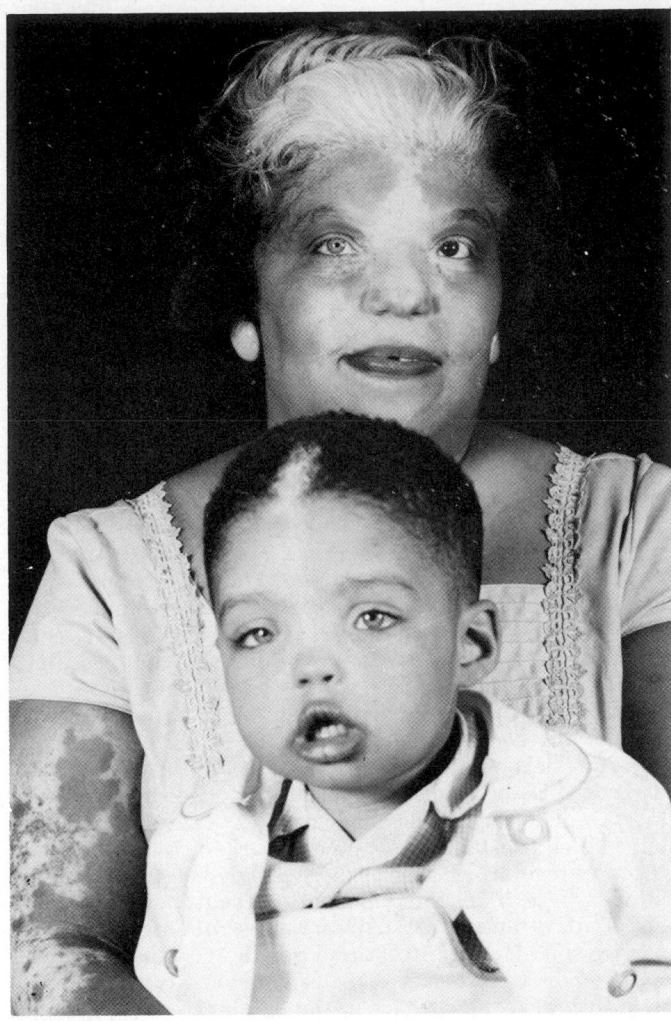

495. Son has bilaterally blue irides; mother's right eye is blue; both have distopia cathorum and patchy depigmentation of skin of limbs

Includes: Progéria à début tardif
Síndrome de Werner
Progeria adultorum

Excludes: Progeria (825)
Poikiloderma congenita
Scleroderma

Minimal Diagnostic Criteria: These include arrest of growth at puberty, development of cataracts in the 2nd or 3rd decade, premature greying and balding, scleroderma-like involvement of limbs, marked diminution of muscle mass and subcutaneous tissue of limbs, chronic slowly healing ulcerations over pressure points of feet and ankles, beak-shaped nose; premature development of arteriosclerosis, diabetes mellitus, hypogonadism, and localized soft tissue calcifications.

Clinical Findings: Features first become apparent between 15 and 30 years of age with habitus of premature aging, shortness of stature, beaked nose, premature greying of hair with alopecia, diabetes mellitus, and cataract formation starting at an early age. There is atrophy with loss of subcutaneous tissue and tightness of the limbs. Circumscribed keratosis and ulcers develop on the skin, persisting over pressure points on the limbs. Poor muscular development and localized soft tissue calcifications are noted in the limbs. Ocular findings, usually noted in the 2nd or 3rd decade, include bilateral juvenile cataracts, macular degeneration, retinitis pigmentosa and chorioretinitis. Diabetes mellitus and hypogonadism are the 2 most frequent endocrine abnormalities. Endocrine studies have failed to establish any other disorder. Sterility, impotence, irregular or absent menses, loss of libido, high-pitched voice, mild gynecomastia, and neuter or scanty pubic, axillary and trunk hair are present. Intelligence is described in 22 cases; 10 of these were noted to be retarded. Xrays reveal osteoporosis, osteomyelitis-type lesions, neurotrophic bone changes in the feet, gross foot deformities, osteoarthritis of peripheral joints, and spondylotic deformities of the spine. Signs of generalized arteriosclerosis are prominent with diminished or absent peripheral pulses in the lower limbs, and angina with myocardial infarction is seen.

Complications
I   **Derived:** Myocardial infarction, congestive heart failure, ulcerations of limbs, blindness secondary to cataracts
II **Associated:** —

Etiology: Autosomal recessive; McK *27770

Pathogenesis: Pathologically 14 patients have shown generalized arteriosclerosis and coronary artery disease. Hearts have revealed calcification of coronary arteries and valves, and either typical myocardial infarction or multifocal myocardial fibrosis. Endocrine organs have shown no specific histologic changes except testicular atrophy. Microscopic changes in skin have included atrophy of the epidermis, thickening of the corium with fibrous tissue, and atrophy or rete pegs. A striking increase in the incidence of neoplasia has been noted pathologically (melanotic sarcoma, sarcoma of the uterus, fibroliposarcoma, hepatoma, carcinoma of the female breast, and osteogenic sarcoma). Many resemblances to progeria in children suggest that the Werner syndrome may represent a later expression of progeria. Many resemblances to experimental progeria in rats (from chronic administration of dihydrotachysterol) suggest that the progeria-like syndrome in the rat may represent an animal model for this disease. However, attempts to implicate abnormal calcium metabolism in the Werner syndrome have failed. Suggesting an aberration in connective tissue metabolism are the scleroderma-type skin lesions and sclerotic lesions in other organs; a high incidence of mesenchymal tumors. Tissue culture studies indicate a striking diminution of the growth potential of fibroblasts in vitro, suggesting that this is a manifestation of senescence at the cellular level.

Related Facts
I   **Sex Ratio:** M1:F1
II   **Risk of Occurrence:** ? The condition has been observed in Caucasians, Orientals, and Negroes; and has been reported in North and South America, Europe, Middle East, Japan; particularly in Caucasians of Jewish ancestry.
III **Risk of Recurrence for**
     Patient's Sib: 1 in 4 (25%) for each sib
     Patient's Child: Not increased unless mate is heterozygote or homozygote. (Fertility is diminished, 0.4 known children per patient on the average.)
IV   **Age of Detectability:** Detectable clinically at age 15 to 30 years
V   **Prevalence:** 130 cases have been reported in world's literature since 1904.

Treatment
I   **Primary Prevention:** Genetic counseling
II   **Secondary Prevention:** Cataracts are surgically resected when mature. Diabetes mellitus is usually mild and responds to diet or oral hypoglycemic therapy. Accepted methods of treatment are indicated for arteriosclerotic heart disease, cutaneous ulcers, and malignancy.
III **Other Therapy:** —

Prognosis: For life: Patients survive to the 4th and 5th decades, and a few to the 6th and 7th decades. Death is usually caused by malignancy or arteriosclerotic heart disease. For intelligence: No effect upon intelligence. For function: Onset occurs between age 15 and 30 years with a slow insidious course, with necessity for hospitalization beginning 15 to 20 years after the onset. Generalized arteriosclerosis and scleroderma-type skin changes are irreversible and progressive.

Detection of Carrier: Increased frequency of premature greying in relatives suggests that heterozygotes may have partial expression.

Special Considerations: —

References:
Epstein, C.J. et al: Werner's syndrome; a review of its symptomatology, natural history, pathologic features, genetics and relationship to the natural aging process. Medicine (Baltimore) 45:177, 1966.
Fleischmajer, R. and Nedwich, A.: Werner's syndrome. Am. J. Med. 54:111, 1973.
Goldstein, S. and Niewiarowski, S.: Increased procoagulant activity in cultured fibroblasts from progeria and Werner's syndromes of premature aging. Nature 260:711, 1976.
Martin, G.M. et al: Replicative life span of cultivated human cells. Lab. Invest. 23:86, 1970.
Thannhauser, S.J.: Werner's syndrome (progeria of adult) and Rothmund's syndrome; 2 types of closely related heredofamilial atrophic dermatoses with juvenile cataracts and endocrine features; critical study of 5 new cases. Ann. Intern. Med. 23:559, 1945.
Tokunaga, M. et al: Postmortem study of a case of Werner's syndrome. J. Am. Geriatr. Soc. 24:407, 1976.
Zucker-Franklin, D. et al: Werner's syndrome: An analysis of ten cases. Geriatrics 23:123, 1968.

Contributor: **William Reichel**

Editor's Computerized Descriptors: Eye, Nose, Skin, Hair, Skel., Muscle, CV., Nerve, GU.

WILLIAMS SYNDROME

Includes: Syndrome d'hypercalcémie précoce
Syndrom der frühkindlichen Hyperkalzämie
Síndrome de hipercalcemia precoz
Idiopathic infantile hypercalcemia syndrome
Hypercalcemia, peculiar facies, supravalvular aortic stenosis syndrome
Early hypercalcemia syndrome

Excludes: Idiopathic infantile hypercalcemia without any associated facial or cardiac anomalies
Aortic stenosis, supravalvar (78)

Minimal Diagnostic Criteria: Peculiar facies with full lips, with or without growth and mental deficiency, aortic or pulmonary arterial stenosis.

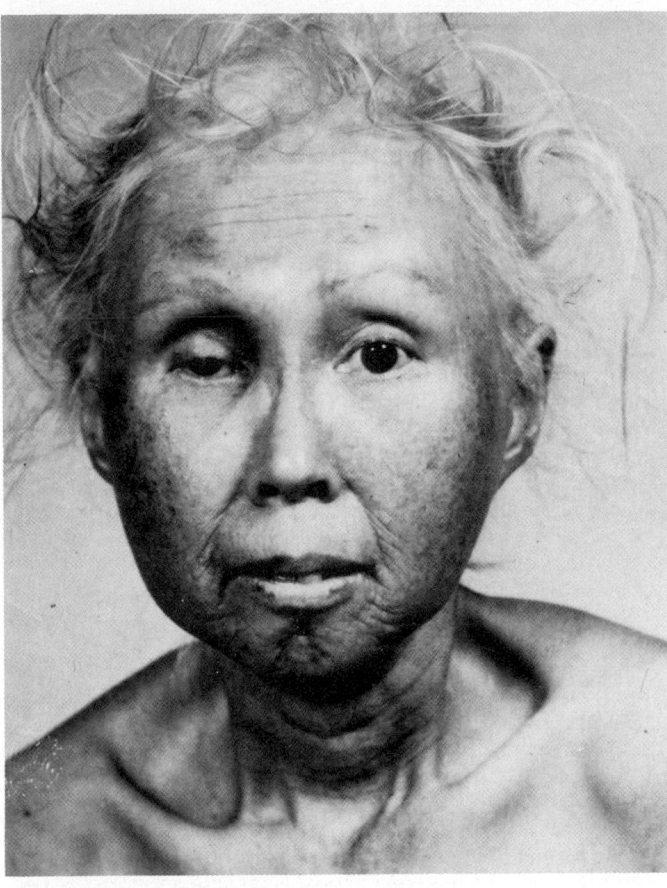

496. Werner syndrome at age 48

Clinical Findings: More frequent features include: 1) short stature, sometimes low birthweight (median of 2.7 kg with range of 1.5-4.0 kg); 2) mental retardation moderate to severe, IQ most commonly 40-70; 3) broad maxilla and mouth with full prominent "cupid's bow" upper lip, anteverted small nose, full pouting cheeks and open mouth with tendency toward inner epicanthic folds, small mandible, prominent ears and unusual stellate patterning in the iris; and 4) supravalvular aortic stenosis or hypoplasia, peripheral pulmonary artery stenosis, or septal defect in about half the patients.

Occasional features include raucous voice, strabismus, craniosynostosis, partial anodontia, inguinal hernia, kyphosis, kyphoscoliosis (21%), mitral insufficiency, elevated serum cholesterol and hypercalcemia in infancy most commonly within the first 8-18 months of life with symptoms and signs such as hypotonia, constipation, anorexia, vomiting, polyuria, polydipsia, renal insufficiency, vicarious calcification and transient facial palsy.

Complications
I   **Derived:** —
II **Associated:** —

Etiology: ? Usually a sporadic occurrence. McK *18550

Pathogenesis: ?

Related Facts
I   **Sex Ratio:**   No striking predilection for male vs female
II   **Risk of Occurrence:**   ? Rare
III **Risk of Recurrence for**
     Patient's Sib: Usually sporadic in families
     Patient's Child: Usually sporadic in families
IV   **Age of Detectability:**   Birth to early childhood
V   **Prevalence:**   ?

Treatment
I   **Primary Prevention:** —
II   **Secondary Prevention:**   When hypercalcemia still exists, elimination of vitamin D from the diet, plus drastic limitation of calcium intake to 25-100 mg per day. For severe hypercalcemia, hydrocortisone analog therapy should be considered on a temporary basis.
III **Other Therapy:** —

Prognosis: The prognosis is variable. No average life span can be stated from existing data.

Detection of Carrier: —

Special Considerations: —

References:
Forbes, G.B. et al: Vitamin D and infantile hypercalcemia. Pediatrics 42:203, 1968.
Fraser, D. et al: A new look at infantile hypercalcemia. Pediatr. Clin. North Am. 13:503, 1966.
Jones, K.L. and Smith, D.W.: The Williams elfin facies syndrome, a new perspective. J. Pediatr. 86:718, 1975.

Contributor: **David W. Smith**

Editor's Computerized Descriptors: Eye, Ear, Face, Nose, Skel., Muscle, Hernia not CNS, CV., GI., GU., Nerve

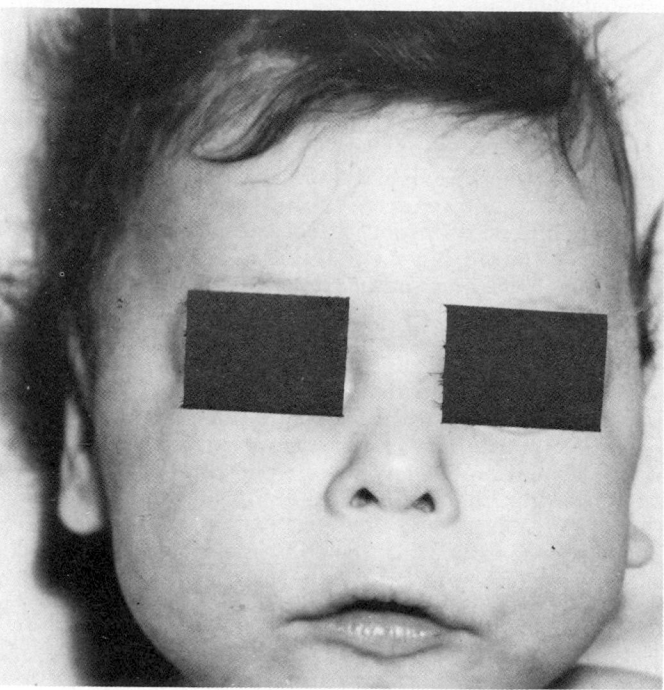

497. Note long philtrum, full cheeks, and anteverted nares

WINCHESTER SYNDROME

Includes: Syndrome de Winchester
Síndrome de Winchester
Winchester-Grossman syndrome
Winchester disease

Excludes: Other forms of carpotarsal and multicentric osteolysis

Minimal Diagnostic Criteria: Short stature, joint stiffening with severe flexion contractures, peripheral corneal opacities, skin thickening, radiographic features of progressive carpotarsal osteolysis, and progressive destruction of small joints. Light and electron microscopic evaluation of a biopsy of thickened skin confirm the diagnosis.

Clinical Findings: The Winchester syndrome begins before age 2, heralded by the onset of fairly symmetric polyarthralgias of major and minor joints and swelling and painful limitation of motion, but erythema or constitutional symptoms are absent. Intermittent polyarthralgias continue throughout childhood, and lead to joint stiffening and flexion contractures of the fingers, elbows, hips, knees, and ankles. Areas of skin become thickened and gradually hyperpigmented and hypertrichotic, and 3 of 5 patients have had coarsened facial features.† Peripheral corneal opacities become evident by midchildhood. Linear growth is retarded from early childhood, leading to dwarfism. Although motor development may be retarded due to arthralgias, intelligence is normal.

Skeletal radiographs reveal generalized osteoporosis and progressive osteolysis of carpal and tarsal bones which may lead to complete resorption by the 2nd decade. Progressive intra- and periarticular erosions of small joints can simulate severe rheumatoid arthritis and lead to bony ankylosis.

Skin biopsies of affected areas have revealed fibroblastic hyperplasia; and, at a later age, abnormal collagen bundle architecture in the deep dermis. Characteristic ultrastructural dilation of mitochondria is observed in fibroblasts. The carpal bones appear to be replaced by dense fibrous tissue, and sections of bone disclose a paucity of trabeculae; growth plates appear to be normal.

Complications
I   **Derived:** Severe and progressive flexion contractures at major and minor joints leading to immobile claw hands and inability to ambulate which produces almost complete disability.
II   **Associated:** Easy fractures due to osteoporosis.

Etiology: Autosomal recessive; McK *27795

Pathogenesis: ? The observed contractures, skin thickening, abnormal dermal collagen, and corneal opacities may be due to abnormal fibroblast function, and the dwarfism, osteolysis and osteoporosis to excessive resorption of bone.

Related Facts
I   **Sex Ratio:**   M1:F1; actual M1:F4 in 5 cases
II   **Risk of Occurrence:**   ? Recorded cases have occurred in Puerto Rican and Mexican families
III   **Risk of Recurrence for**
   Patient's Sib: 1 in 4 (25%) for each offspring to be affected
   Patient's Child: Not increased unless mate is carrier or homozygote
IV   **Age of Detectability:**   Usually by age 1, before age 2.
V   **Prevalence:**   Rare

Treatment
I   **Primary Prevention:**   Genetic counseling
II   **Secondary Prevention:**   Serial casting or other orthopedic procedures to reduce and alleviate flexion contractures may

be of some benefit.
III Other Therapy: —

Prognosis: Complete functional disability; normal intelligence.

Detection of Carrier: —

†Special Considerations: The coarsened facies, thickened skin, corneal clouding, dwarfism and contractures may suggest a mucopolysaccharide storage disease or one of the mucolipidoses. However, the absence of mucopolysaccahariduria and the presence of rheumatoid-like small joint destruction and carpotarsal osteolysis serve to distinguish the Winchester syndrome from these conditions, as does the absence of lysosomal vacuolization in fibroblasts and chondrocytes. The Winchester syndrome may be distinguished from juvenile rheumatoid arthritis by the lack of prominent constitutional symptoms, negative serologies and by the extra-skeletal manifestations.

References:

Brown, S.I. and Kawabara, T: Peripheral corneal opacification and skeletal deformities. A newly recognized acid mucopolysaccaridosis simulating rheumatoid arthritis. Arch. Ophthalmol. 83:667, 1970.
Hollister, D.W. et al: The Winchester syndrome: A nonlysosomal connective tissue disease. J. Pediatr. 84:701, 1974.
Winchester, P. et al: A new acid mucopolysaccaridosis with skeletal deformities simulating rheumatoid arthritis. Am. J. Roentgenol. Radium Ther. Nucl. Med. 106:121, 1969.

Contributor: **David W. Hollister**

Editor's Computerized Descriptors: Eye, Face, Skin, Skel.

WL SYMPHALANGISM-BRACHYDACTYLY SYNDROME

Includes: Syndrome de symphalangisme et brachydactylie
WL Symphalangie-Brachydaktylie Syndrom
Síndrome de braquidactilia-sinfalangismo tipo WL
Multiple synostoses and conduction deafness

Excludes: Proximal symphalangism (most cases)
Dominant symphalangism and conduction deafness
Several syndromes with primarily distal symphalangism

Minimal Diagnostic Criteria: The hand and foot malformations with characteristic facies and hearing loss.

Clinical Findings: This pleiotropic syndrome is characterized by proximal symphalangism, brachydactyly, absence of distal portions of digits, dermatoglyphic abnormalities, shortness of 1st metacarpals/metatarsals, synostosis of carpal/tarsal bones, dislocation of the head of the radius, conductive hearing deficit, and a particular facial appearance. The face is long and narrow with a prominent, long, hemicylindrical nose and a thin upper lip. The hearing deficit is apparently due to ankylosis of the stapes. Patients are of normal height but may have abnormal body proportions due to short arms. The syndrome shows considerable intrafamilial variability. In early infancy symphalangism may be apparent clinically (stiffness, absence of flexion and extension creases at the joint) but not roentgenographically.

Complications
I   Derived: Syndactyly; limited joint mobility in fingers, wrists, elbows and feet; gait abnormalities.
II Associated: Strabismus

Etiology: Autosomal dominant

Pathogenesis: ?

Related Facts
I   Sex Ratio: M1:F1
II   Risk of Occurrence: Small
III Risk of Recurrence for
     Patient's Sib: 1 in 2 (50%) for each offspring to be affected, if parent is affected; otherwise not increased.
     Patient's Child: 1 in 2
IV   Age of Detectability: At birth
V   Prevalence: Rare

Treatment
I   Primary Prevention: Genetic counseling
II   Secondary Prevention: The abnormalities of the arms, hands, and feet do not usually require surgical procedures. Patients with symphalangism should have a hearing evaluation (may need to be repeated) to rule out a hearing deficit and a roentgenographic skeletal survey to rule out further skeletal abnormalities. Hearing aids, stapedectomy and insertion of a prosthesis may improve hearing.
III Other Therapy: —

Prognosis: Symphalangism, carpal synostoses and hearing loss are slowly progressive.

Detection of Carrier: —

Special Considerations: —

References:

Herrmann, J.: Symphalangism and brachydactyly syndrome: Report of the *WL* symphalangism-brachydactyly syndrome: Review of literature and classification. In Bergsma, D. (ed.): Limb Malformations. Birth Defects: Orig. Art. Ser., vol X, no. 5. Miami: Symposia Specialists for The National Foundation-March of Dimes, 1974, p. 23.

Konigsmark, B.W. and Gorlin, R.J.: Dominant symphalangism and conduction deafness. In Genetic and Metabolic Deafness. Philadelphia: W.B. Saunders Co., 1976, p. 159.

Maroteaux, P. et al: La maladie des synostoses multiples. Nouv. Presse Med. 1:3041, 1972.

Contributor: **Jürgen Herrmann**

Editor's Computerized Descriptors: Hearing, Ear, Face, Nose, Dermatoglyphic, Skel.

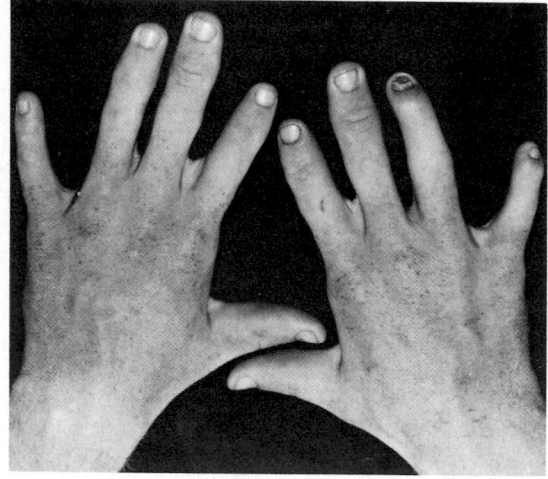

498. Note proximal symphalangism and brachydactyly

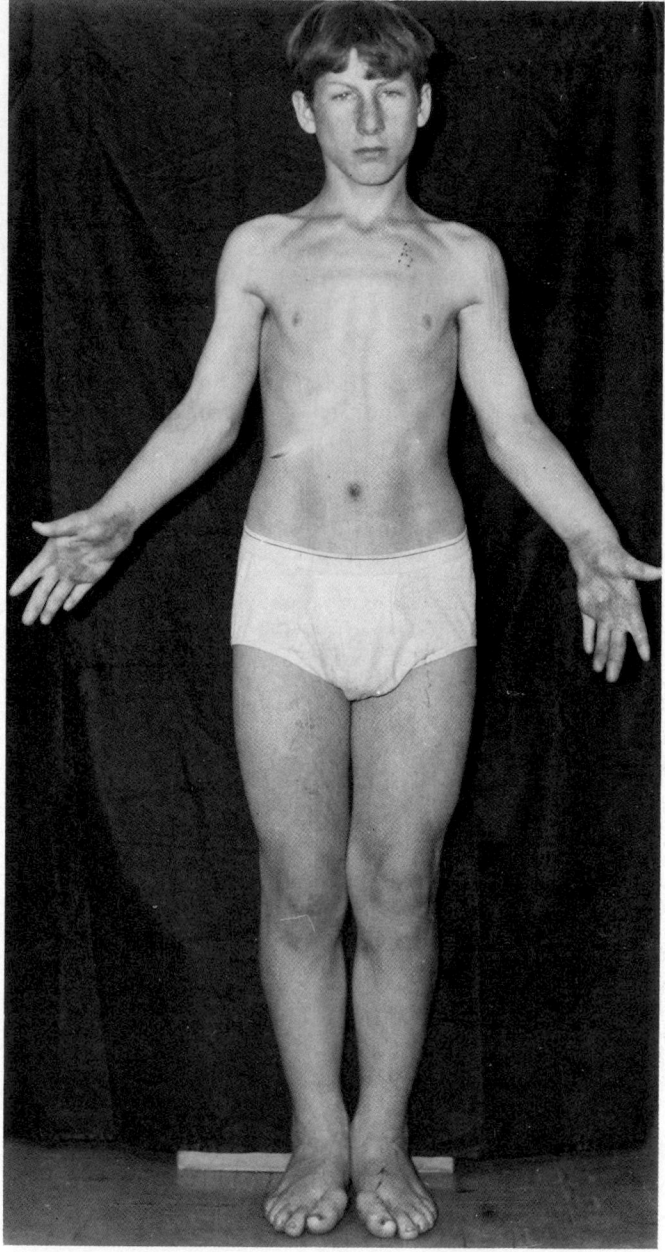

499. Characteristic facial features with long nose and thin upper lip. Note skeletal defects

WOLFF-PARKINSON-WHITE SYNDROME

Includes: Syndrome de Wolff-Parkinson White
Síndrome de Wolff-Parkinson-White
Anomalous atrioventricular (AV) conduction
Accelerated AV conduction
Ventricular preexcitation

Excludes: Supraventricular tachycardias, congenital (922)
Short PR interval-normal QRS syndrome
Lown-Ganong-Levine syndrome

Minimal Diagnostic Criteria: The ECG findings during sinus rhythm of a short PR interval and a prolonged QRS complex (both compared to normal limits for age) with the QRS widened in its initial portion by a slurred onset termed a delta wave. The delta wave is almost always directed abnormally leftward, whether anterior or posterior, and is therefore positive in lead V_6. The WPW pattern shows a phasic variation in degree "concertina effect" or intermittency in approximately 40% of cases. Comparison of the ECG during normal AV conduction with that during preexcitation reveals a constant P-J interval (the J point is the junction of the end of the QRS complex with the beginning of the ST segment), but a shorter PR interval and a longer QRS complex during preexcitation. Rarely preexcitation presents with a normal PR interval when there is associated first degree heart block. The WPW syndrome has been classified by ECG as WPW type A, when an R wave is the sole or dominant QRS deflection in lead V_1, and WPW type B when the dominant QRS deflection in lead V_1 is negative. The delta wave is positive in lead V_1 in type A, but may be either negative or biphasic in type B. Cases which fulfill the criteria of neither type A nor type B are generally best termed atypical. With the use of vectorcardiographic tracings the WPW syndrome has been classified according to the direction of the initial slow portion of the QRS, the delta vector-type A when the mean delta is anterior and type B when it is directly to the left or posterior. The WPW syndrome may either simulate or obscure bundle branch block, ventricular hypertrophy or myocardial infarction patterns. In the presence of WPW conduction any additional ECG diagnosis must be made with reservation. Digitalis, antiarrhythmic agents, and drugs that mimic or block the effects of the autonomic nervous system have been shown to influence the degree of preexcitation. An atropine test is sometimes employed to abolish the WPW pattern transiently, permitting the ECG to be of more assistance in diagnosis of associated cardiopathy.

The echocardiogram in the WPW syndrome (type A) shows later septal and earlier left ventricular posterior wall systolic motion as compared to normal. The amplitude and duration of the premature left ventricular posterior wall contraction can be related to the prominence of the delta wave. Right ventricular anterior wall contraction has a prolonged onset as compared to normal. In type B WPW syndrome, the septal systolic contraction pattern can have a double notch, in contrast to the normal single notch, and can be followed by double anterior thrusts of the left ventricular posterior wall (near the apex).

Clinical Findings: Originally described as a specific ECG pattern in individuals with otherwise normal hearts but subject to paroxysms of tachycardia, Wolff-Parkinson-White (WPW) syndrome has since been employed to denote the ECG abnormality with or without paroxysmal tachycardia. There may be no clinical findings in the absence of paroxysmal tachycardia or in between bouts. However, there is an increased incidence of soft ejection systolic murmurs and an increased intensity of S_1. Abnormal splitting of the first and second heart sounds has been noted. The frequent association of congenital heart disease and the occasional association of acquired heart disease also have been confirmed since the original description. In hospital practice, the WPW syndrome is found with approximately equal frequency in patients with paroxysmal tachycardia and in those with evident or suspected heart disease.

Complications

I **Derived:** Congenital supraventricular tachycardias, paroxysmal atrial tachycardia, atrial flutter or atrial fibrillation occurs in approximately 13% of asymptomatic individuals in whom the WPW syndrome is an incidental finding. Conversely, approximately 12% of infants with a congenital supraventricular tachycardia will have the WPW syndrome. Type A WPW is more commonly associated with arrhythmias than type B. In some cases, the paroxysmal tachycardia is of major clinical significance, and the decrease in cardiac output may cause heart failure (especially in infants), faintness, cerebral insufficiency and even death. Ventricular fibrillation has been documented in several patients, and may evolve from atrial fibrillation.

II **Associated:** Although WPW occurs more commonly as an isolated defect, it has been found in association with many types of cardiac defects. Ebstein anomaly of the tricuspid valve accounts for approximately 30% of the reported cases of WPW with associated congenital heart defects (only WPW type B has been found with the Ebstein anomaly). Other associated defects include inversion of the ventricles (corrected transposition), primary myocardial disease (sometimes familial), hypoplastic left heart syndrome, subaortic stenosis, endocardial fibroelastosis, ventricular septal defect, patent ductus arteriosus, coarctation of the aorta, tetralogy of Fallot, or idiopathic hypertrophic subaortic stenosis. The only known associated extra-cardiac abnormalities are those of the CNS. These are of various types including seizures and mental retardation.

Etiology: ? The congenital nature is supported by the fact that the WPW pattern is often detected in infancy, plus its association with congenital heart disease and its occasional familial distribution. Although WPW is found occasionally in association with acquired heart disease, a congenital predisposition or an intermittent form of WPW cannot be excluded in these cases. Autosomal dominant families have been reported.

Pathogenesis: A functional and, in some instances, a structural, anomalous pathway between the atria and the ventricles permits rapid conduction relative to normal AV conduction of an atrial impulse with premature excitation of a portion of the ventricular myocardium near the atria. Activation of this area proceeds slowly through common ventricular myocardium accounting for the slurring of the initial portion of the QRS complex-the delta wave. In most cases of WPW the remainder of the ventricles undergo a dual activation, and the resulting QRS is a fusion beat and is relatively normal. In other instances there is a more advanced degree of preexcitation, and the terminal portions of the QRS are also distorted. In a few recent cases ECG and surgical evidence has been obtained to support a structural aberrant pathway across the AV valvar ring, a muscular "bundle of Kent." Such muscular bridges have been demonstrated pathologically in a few, but not all, cases of WPW syndrome examined by histologic techniques. In the other cases, different aberrant routes are operative; and the abnormally rapid conduction passes near or through a portion of the AV node via fibers of James and Mahaim. There appear to be several mechanisms which may produce the WPW syndrome.

The congenital supraventricular tachycardias that are

associated with the WPW syndrome appear to be on the basis of a reentry mechanism. An impulse may descend from the atria via the normal AV pathway to activate the ventricles prematurely, and then ascend retrogradely through the anomalous pathway to reactivate the atria and continue at a rapid rate with a narrow QRS due to normal AV conduction. Less commonly, the reentry circuit operates with the impulse descending through the anomalous pathway and ascending through the normal AV pathway, and shows the broad QRS of ventricular preexcitation during the tachycardia.

Related Facts
I **Sex Ratio:** M1.8:F1
II **Risk of Occurrence:** 1 in 330 to 1 in 2500 live births with no known predilection for any specific group. Found in approximately 1 in 200 cases of congenital heart disease.
III **Risk of Recurrence for**
  Patient's Sib: ?
  Patient's Child: ?
IV **Age of Detectability:** From birth, by ECG
V **Prevalence:** About 1 in 5000 general population

Treatment
I **Primary Prevention:** —
II **Secondary Prevention:** Preexcitation per se does not produce symptoms and does not require treatment as long as the heart rate is normal. However, when supraventricular tachycardias complicate the WPW syndrome, they require treatment and, in the case of infants or a severely symptomatic patient of any age, may constitute a medical emergency.† In most cases the acute episode of tachycardia can be controlled by the usual antiarrhythmic drugs, including digitalis. Cardioversion has been employed successfully. Digitalis, propranolol, or quinidine have proven effective in preventing recurrent tachycardia in most cases. In refractory paroxysmal atrial tachyarrhythmia, artificial pacemaker therapy has been used sucessfully to interrupt the tachycardia in appropriately selected cases. In a few cases with incapacitating tachycardia, it has been shown recently that surgical transection of a previously well-identified anomalous pathway of conduction from atria to ventricles may abolish the signs of WPW syndrome and prevent further episodes of tachycardia. Unfortunately, the abnormal conduction pathway often cannot be identified with certainty, and this form of therapy is reserved for severely symptomatic cases.
III **Other Therapy:** —

Prognosis: In the absence of associated cardiac defects and paroxysmal tachycardia, it has been suggested that the WPW syndrome should be considered a variation of the normal pattern, and that it may be compatible with a normal life span. When associated supraventricular tachycardia occurs in infancy, recurrences after 18 months of age are rare. While most individuals follow this benign course, there are rare instances of symptomatic paroxysmal tachycardia with the initial episode in childhood or adulthood. Associated supraventricular tachycardia is more apt to be fatal when associated with other cardiac defects.

Detection of Carrier: —

†**Special Considerations:** See Supraventricular Tachycardias, Congenital.

References:
Berkman, N.L. and Lamb, L.E.: The Wolff-Parkinson-White electrocardiogram: A follow-up study of 5 to 28 years. N. Engl. J. Med. 278:492, 1968.
DeMaria, A.N. et al: Alterations in ventricular contraction pattern in the Wolff-Parkinson-White syndrome—Detection by echocardiography. Circulation 53:249, 1976.
Gallagher, J.J. et al: Wolff-Parkinson-White syndrome: The problem, evaluation and surgical correction. Circulation 51:767, 1975.
Giardiana, A.C.V. et al: Wolff-Parkinson-White syndrome in infants and children: A long-term follow-up study. Br. Heart J. 24:451, 1972.
Lev, M. et al: Mahaim and James fibers as a basis for a unique variety of preexcitation. Am. J. Cardiol. 36:880, 1975.
Schiebler, G.L. et al: The Wolff-Parkinson-White syndrome in infants and children: A review and a report of 28 cases. Pediatrics 24:585, 1959.
Swiderski, J. et al: The Wolff-Parkinson-White syndrome in infancy and childhood. Br. Heart J. 24:561, 1972.

Contributor: **B. Lynn Miller**

Editor's Computerized Descriptor: CV.

WOLMAN DISEASE

Includes: Maladie de Wolman
Wolmansche Krankheit
Enfermedad de Wolman
Primary familial xanthomatosis with involvement and calcification of adrenals

Excludes: Niemann-Pick disease (717)
Lipogranulomatosis (598)
Analphalipoproteinemia (48)
Cholesteryl ester storage disease (151)
Partial diffuse intrahepatic biliary atresia

Minimal Diagnostic Criteria: The diagnosis can be considered certain in a small infant with hepatosplenomegaly, enlarged and calcified adrenals, foam cells in the marrow, and vacuolization of lymphocytes.

Substantiation of the diagnosis depends on demonstration of tissue triglyceride and cholesterol ester accumulation in characteristic foam cells, with distribution beyond the liver (involving spleen, lymph nodes, adrenal, thymus, etc). Further support is provided by demonstrating a specific lipase deficiency in the liver, leukocytes, and cultured skin fibroblasts.

Clinical Findings: Characteristically, infants present with poor weight gain, vomiting and loose frequent stools in the early weeks of life. Symmetrically enlarged, calcified adrenals can be seen on x-ray examination of the abdomen. Chronic nutritional failure becomes increasingly severe in spite of all special management efforts (handicapped by foam cell infiltration in the intestinal villi), and the patients die by 2-9 months with wasting and infection. Neuromuscular development is retarded, but mostly in a secondary fashion, with neuronal changes of limited distribution when present at all (retina, sympathetic ganglia, myenteric plexi). There is moderate enlargement of the liver and spleen, organs where the fundamental lipid-laden foam cell diathesis is well visualized: neutral fat accumulation is major, as is also cholesterol (80-90% esterified). Liver cholesterol levels have varied from 3-9% of the net weight, and spleen figures from 1-3%; phospholipid levels are normal. Foam cells are found in the bone marrow, and there is prominent vacuolization of the circulating agranulocytes. The possibility has now been raised that some children with this same basic syndrome may have a considerably later expression of the GI symptoms, longer survival and less evident calcification of the adrenals.

Complications
I **Derived:** The major secondary difficulties deriving from the basic handicap are the chronic nutritional failure and possibly some degree of adrenocortical insufficiency. In this situation a positive balance for nutriments and electrolytes, with a margin for support of general development, is extremely difficult to achieve.
II **Associated:** On several occasions, serum α-lipoprotein levels have been found to be very low, although not comparable to those in analphalipoproteinemia.

Etiology: Autosomal recessive inheritance. The fatty acids which are bound to the cholesterol and triglycerides are not remarkable. Cholesterol has been shown to be the only sterol accumulated in the tissues; a recent study reports the presence of oxygenated steryl esters. In extensive experiments, Patrick and Lake have shown deficiency of lysosomal acid esterase activity, which would be relevant to tissue accumulation of both triglycerides and cholesterol esters. These findings have been confirmed, but the assay is not widely performed. McK *27800

Pathogenesis: The inborn defect leading to lipid aggregation in foam cells understandably produces the observed organomegaly (liver and spleen). That the cellular abnormality is so evident in the intestinal mucosa is puzzling, but the presence of this infiltration certainly handicaps the nutritional situation. The involvement of the liver and adrenals so prominently in this disease seems to correlate with the liver's special concern in cholesterol metabolism and the role of the adrenal cortex in sterol conversion. Perhaps the nervous system is more spared in this lipidosis because of the slow and well-monitored metabolism of cholesterol in cortical gray matter.

Related Facts
I **Sex Ratio:** M1:F1
II **Risk of Occurrence:** Rare
III **Risk of Recurrence for**
   Patient's Sib: 1 in 4 (25%) for each offspring to be affected
   Patient's Child: Not increased unless mate is carrier or homozygote. To date all patients die in childhood.
IV **Age of Detectability:** For the usual infant patient it is probably very early, on clinical grounds. Calcification of the adrenals has been detected within the first few days of life on several occasions, and should be visible on abdominal xrays of the mother in late pregnancy. Prenatal diagnosis (lipase studies on cultured fetal cells) is theoretically possible.
V **Prevalence:** Low, with several dozen children identified to date. No predilection in any particular group.

Treatment
I **Primary Prevention:** Genetic counseling
II **Secondary Prevention:** Very unsatisfactory to date. Simplified, high-calorie, high-protein feedings, or low-residue feedings, have not been adequate to allow reasonable weight gain, and have been limited by the diarrhea and vomiting. Adrenal corticosteroid supplements have been regularly used. No useful effects have been identified from the use of cholestyramine, d-thyroxine, clofibrate, or medium-chain triglycerides. More recently, an attempt has been made to maintain an infant with Wolman disease on complete parenteral alimentation, using a central venous catheter (thus bypassing the intestinal mucosal handicap). A positive nitrogen balance, and small weight gain, were achieved, but blood stream infection limited the continuation of this technique. Further efforts in this direction can be considered.
III **Other Therapy:** —

Prognosis: The usual (infant) patients have expired, in spite of all therapeutic efforts, at from 1 1/2-9 months of age, rarely a few months longer. Reports now exist of children with milder symptoms, of later onset, who are surviving into middle or late childhood.

Detection of Carrier: Detection of partial reduction in acid lipase activity in cultured skin fibroblasts in parents of a Wolman disease infant, has been reported; such work remains at present on an experimental basis.

Special Considerations: —

References:
Crocker, A.C. et al: Nutritional support, including intravenous alimentation for the infant with Wolman's disease. In Volk, B.W. and Aronson, S.M. (eds.): Sphingolipids, Sphingolipidoses and Allied Disorders. New York: Plenum Press, 1972, p. 661.
Crocker, A.C. et al: Wolman's disease; three new patients with a recently described lipidosis. Pediatrics 35:627, 1965.
Patrick, A.D. and Lake, B.D.: Deficiency of an acid lipase in Wolman's disease. Nature 222:1067, 1969.
Wolman, M. et al: Primary familial xanthomatosis with involvement and calcification of the adrenals: Report of two more cases in siblings of a previously described infant. Pediatrics 28:742, 1961.

Contributor: **Allen C. Crocker**

Editor's Computerized Descriptors: Spleen, GI., Liver

XERODERMA AND MENTAL RETARDATION

Includes: Xeroderma avec retard mental
Xerodermische Idiotie
Xeroderma con retardo mental
DeSanctis-Cacchione syndrome
Mental retardation and xeroderma

Excludes: Xeroderma pigmentosum (1005)
Other photodermatoses with neurologic disease

Minimal Diagnostic Criteria: Xeroderma pigmentosum, microcephaly, dwarfism

Clinical Findings: Characterized by photophobia and other evidence of xeroderma pigmentosum plus mental retardation, microcephaly, dwarfism, retarded bone age, choreoathetosis, cerebellar ataxia, poor sexual maturation, sensorineural deafness and shortening of Achilles tendon.

Complications
I   **Derived:** —
II **Associated:** —

Etiology: Autosomal recessive; McK *27880

Pathogenesis: Uncertain whether this is a more severe form of xeroderma pigmentosum or a different genotype. No DNA repair after ultraviolet light. Necropsy reveals cerebral and olivopontocerebellar atrophy. Atypical nuclei of pancreatic islet cells and liver cells. Reduced 17-ketosteroid and 17-hydroxycorticosteroid levels.

Related Facts
I   **Sex Ratio:** M1:F1
II   **Risk of Occurrence:** Extremely rare
III **Risk of Recurrence for**
     Patient's Sib: 1 in 4 (25%) for each offspring to be affected
     Patient's Child: Not increased unless mate is carrier or homozygote.
IV   **Age of Detectability:** Photophobia as neonate. Skin changes at 3-5 years.
V   **Prevalence:** Extremely rare

Treatment
I   **Primary Prevention:** Genetic counseling
II   **Secondary Prevention:** Avoidance of sun, use of topical fluorouracil to remove premalignant lesions. Early excision of tumors.
III **Other Therapy:** As may be indicated

Prognosis: Poor for life span, intelligence and function

Detection of Carrier: ?

Special Considerations: —

References:
Cleaver, J.E.: Defective repair replication of DNA in xeroderma pigmentosum. Nature 218:652, 1968.
Reed, W.B. et al: Xeroderma pigmentosum: Clinical and laboratory investigation of its basic defect. JAMA 207:2073, 1969.
Reed, W.B. et al: Xeroderma pigmentosum with neurological complications. Arch. Dermatol. 91:224, 1965.

Contributor: **William B. Reed‡**

Editor's Computerized Descriptors: Eye, Hearing, Skin, Skel., Nerve , GU.

XERODERMA PIGMENTOSUM

Includes: Xeroderma pigmentoso
Autosomal recessive xeroderma pigmentosum
Angioma pigmentosum et atrophicum
Pigmented epitheliomatosis
Lentigo maligna
Kaposi dermatoses

Excludes: Xeroderma and mental retardation (1004)
Autosomal dominant (milder type) xeroderma pigmentosum
Other photodermatoses with malignancy

Minimal Diagnostic Criteria: Photosensitivity and photophobia, early development of skin cancers.†

Clinical Findings: Early photosensitivity and photophobia to ultraviolet range of light, development of premalignant and malignant skin lesions in light damaged areas (senile keratoses, keratoacanthoma, angiomas, basal and squamous cell carcinomas, malignant melanoma and rarely fibrosarcoma). Lip is dangerous area. Development of keratitis and scarring of cornea, and malignant tumors of conjunctiva and eyelids. Hyperpigmentation, depigmentation.

Complications
I   **Derived:** —
II **Associated:** —

Etiology: Autosomal recessive; McK *27870

Pathogenesis: Failure to repair DNA damage after ultraviolet exposure. This demonstrated in cultured fibroblasts and lymphocytes and in vivo epidermis. Endonuclease probably missing to remove damaged DNA. Endonuclease deficiency may lead to carcinogenesis. Only 10-20% repair of DNA in xeroderma pigmentosum.†

Related Facts
I   **Sex Ratio:** M1:F1
II   **Risk of Occurrence:** Rare in U.S.A., high in Arabic countries where consanguinity is high.
III **Risk of Recurrence for**
     Patient's Sib: 1 in 4 (25%) for each offspring to be affected
     Patient's Child: Not increased unless mate is carrier or homozygote
IV   **Age of Detectability:** Photophobia as neonate; skin changes at 3-5 years.
V   **Prevalence:** ? Highest in inbred groups - Arabs, Jews, Japanese, rare in Negroes and Europeans.

Treatment
I   **Primary Prevention:** Genetic counseling
II   **Secondary Prevention:** Avoidance of sun, use of topical fluorouracil to remove premalignant lesions. Early excision of tumors.
III **Other Therapy:** —

Prognosis: Poor, death before 20 from cancer or infection.

Detection of Carrier: ?

†Special Considerations: Parents with single mutant gene can repair DNA after exposure to sun. There are families with easily damaged skin from sun exposure which is inherited as autosomal dominant, but this is not the severe autosomal recessive xeroderma pigmentosum.

References:
Cleaver, J.E.: Defective repair replication of DNA in xeroderma pigmentosum. Nature 218:652, 1968.
Cockayne, E.A.: Inherited Abnormalities of Skin and Its Appendages. London:Oxford University Press, 1963.
Haddida, E. et al: Xeroderma pigmentosum (a propos de 48 observations personnels). Ann. Dermatol. Syphiligr. (Paris) 90:467, 1963.
Siegelman, M.H. and Sutow, W.W.: Xeroderma pigmentosum; report of 3 cases. J. Pediatr. 67:625, 1965.

Contributor: **William B. Reed‡**

Editor's Computerized Descriptors: Eye, Skin

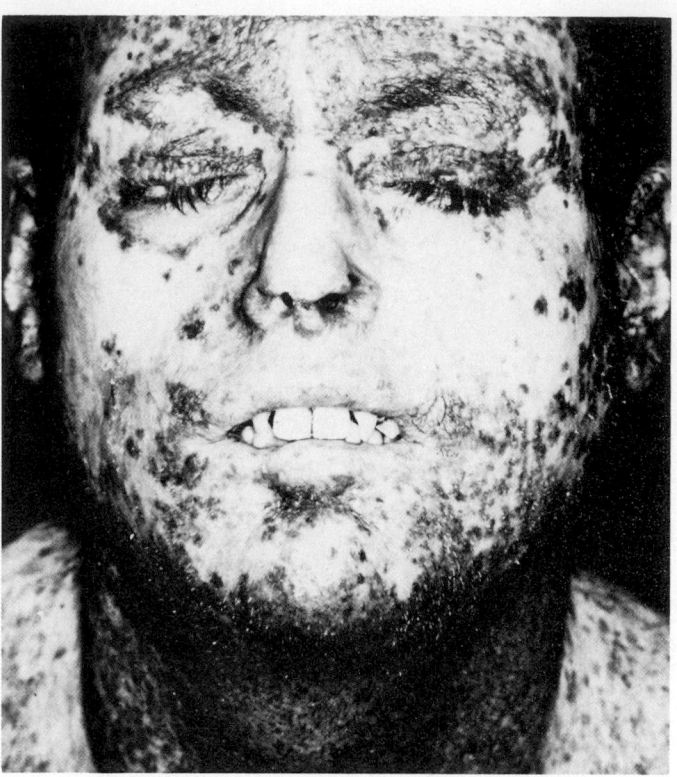

501. Marked skin changes of xeroderma pigmentosum

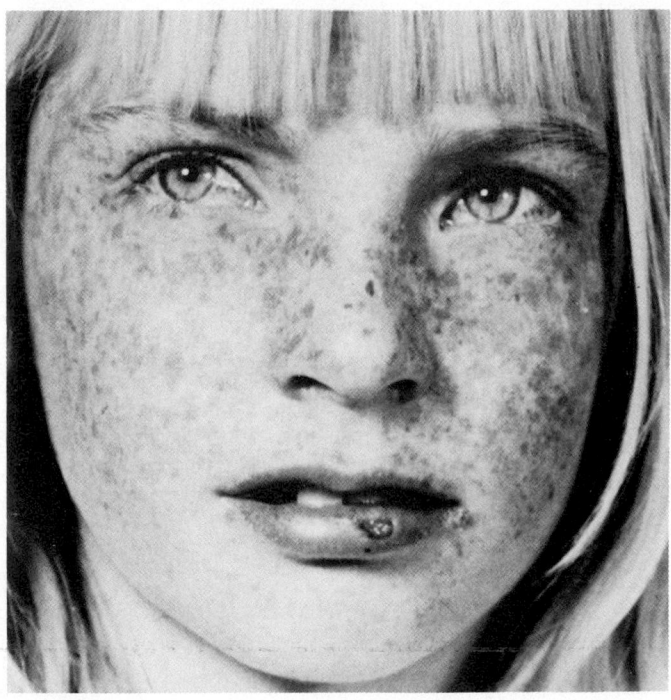

500. Mild skin changes of xeroderma pigmentosum

Section III
TABLES AND DIAGRAMS

TABLE I
MODES OF MENDELIAN INHERITANCE, RELATED SEX RATIOS AND RISKS OF RECURRENCE*

Code	Mode of transmission	Sex ratio		Risk of recurrence for
AR	Autosomal recessive	M1:F1	Patient's sib:	1 in 4(25%) for each offspring to be affected
			Patient's child:	Not increased unless mate is carrier or homozygote
AD	Autosomal dominant	M1:F1	Patient's sib:	If parent is affected 1 in 2 (50%) for each offspring to be affected; otherwise not increased
			Patient's child:	1 in 2
AD-85% ± penetrance	Autosomal dominant with about 85% penetrance	M1:F1	Patient's sib:	If parent is affected < 1 in 2 (< 50%) for each offspring to be affected; otherwise not increased
			Patient's child:	< 1 in 2
AD-60% ± penetrance	Autosomal dominant with about 60% penetrance	M1:F1	Patient's sib:	If parent is affected 1 in 3 (30%) for each offspring to be affected, 1 in 2 for inheriting mutant gene; otherwise not increased
			Patient's child:	1 in 3 (30%) for each offspring to be affected, 1 in 2 for inheriting mutant gene
AD-possibly	Autosomal dominant possibly	M1:F1 probable	Patient's sib:	? If parent is affected 1 in 2 (50%) for each offspring to be affected; otherwise not increased
			Patient's child:	? 1 in 2
X-linked R	X-linked recessive (rare)	M1:F0	Patient's sib:	If mother is a carrier 1 in 2 (50%) for each brother to be affected and 1 in 2 (50%) for each sister to be a carrier
			Patient's child:	1 in 1 (100%) for carrier daughters; not increased for sons unless wife is a carrier
X-linked D	X-linked dominant (rare)	M1:F2	Patient's sib:	If affected parent is female 1 in 2 (50%) for each sib to be affected. If affected parent is male 1 in 1 (100%) for each sister to be affected; not increased for brothers
			Patient's child:	If patient is female 1 in 2 (50%) for each offspring to be affected; if patient is male 1 in 1 (100%) for daughters, not increased for sons

*This Table was designed as a reference to shorten those entries which involve phenotypic expressions having more than one mode of mendelian inheritance. This Table is a concise summary only; and hence is incomplete, eg more complete data are given concerning transmission of phenotype than to transmission of mutant genes. For more complete and specific information about human genetics the reader is referred to the references cited below. Not only heterogeneity and fresh mutations must always be carefully considered but also variable penetrance and expressivity. Lack of search for, or recognition of, minimal phenotypic expressions has caused confusion in autosomal dominant inheritance. Biochemical tests, with or without cell culturing, are increasingly helpful especially in identifying persons with minimal expressivity or carriers.

References:

McKusick, V.A.: *Human Genetics.* 2nd Ed., Prentice-Hall, Englewood Cliffs, N.J., 1969.

Stern, C.: *Principles of Human Genetics.* 3rd Ed., W. H. Freeman and Co., San Francisco, 1973.

TABLE II

METABOLIC DISORDERS WHERE SPECIFIC ENZYME DEFECTS HAVE BEEN DESCRIBED

Disease	Compendium Birth Defect no.	Disease	Compendium Birth Defect no.
Acatalasemia	6	Lactose malabsorption	
Acid maltase deficiency	11	Lesch-Nyhan syndrome	588
Acid phosphatase deficiency		L-glyceric aciduria	616
Adenine phosphoribosyl transferase deficiency		Lysinemia	616
Adenosine deaminase deficiency		Maple syrup urine disease	628
Adenosine triphosphatase deficiency		Metachromatic leukodystrophies	651
Albinism-oculocutaneous, tyrosinase negative	34	Methemoglobinemia	
Alkaptonuria	37	Methylcrotonylglycinuria	
Argininemia	86	Methylmalonic acidemia	658
Argininosuccinic aciduria	87	Mucopolysaccharidosis I-H	674
Brancher deficiency	116	Mucopolysaccharidosis I-S	675
Carnosinemia	126	Mucopolysaccharidosis II	676
Citrullinemia	174	Mucopolysaccharidosis III	677
Cystathioninuria	236	Myophosphorylase deficiency	698
Disaccharide intolerance		Niemann-Pick disease	717
Fabry disease	373	Nucleoside phosphorylase deficiency	729
Fructose-1-phosphate aldolase deficiency	395	Oroticaciduria	772
Fructose-1,6-diphosphatase deficiency	396	Pentosuria (marker)	804
Fructosuria (marker)	397	Phenylketonuria	808
Galactokinase deficiency	402	Phosphofructokinase deficiency	
Galactosemia	403	Phosphoglycerate kinase deficiency	
Gaucher disease	406	Phosphohexose isomerase deficiency	
Globoid cell leukodystrophy	415	Phytanic acid storage disease	810
Glucose-6-phosphate dehydrogenase deficiency	420	Porphyria, erythropoietic	821
Glutathione peroxidase deficiency		Propionic acidemia	826
Glutathione reductase deficiency		Pyroglutamic acidemia	849
Glycogenosis, type I	425	Pyroglutamic aciduria	
Glycogenosis, type III	426	Pyruvate decarboxylase deficiency	
Glycogenosis, type VI	427	Pyruvate kinase deficiency	852
G_{M1}-gangliosidosis, type 1	431	Saccharopinuria	
G_{M2}-gangliosidosis with hexosaminidase A and B deficiency	433	Steroid 11 β-hydroxylase deficiency	902
		Steroid 17 α-hydroxylase deficiency	903
G_{M2}-gangliosidosis with hexosaminidase A deficiency	434	Steroid 17, 20-desmolase deficiency	904
		Steroid 18-hydroxylase deficiency	905
Goitrous cretinism		Steroid 18-hydroxysteroid dehydrogenase deficiency	906
G-phosphogluconate dehydrogenase deficiency		Steroid 20-22 desmolase deficiency	907
Hexokinase deficiency		Steroid 21-hydroxylase deficiency	908
Histidinemia	472	Steroid 3 β-hydroxysteroid dehydrogenase deficiency	909
Homocystinuria	474	Sulfite oxidase deficiency	921
Hydroxyprolinemia (marker)	482	Thiolase deficiency	
Hyperammonemia	485	Transglucuronylase, severe deficiency	961
Hyperoxaluria		Triosephosphate isomerase deficiency	
Hyperprolinemia (marker)	502	2,3-diphosphoglycerate mutase deficiency	
Hypervalinemia	509	Tyrosinemia	978
Hypophosphatasia	516	Wolman disease	1003
Isovalericacidemia	547	Xanthinuria	
Juvenile G_{M1}-gangliosidosis, type II		Xanthurenic aciduria	
Juvenile G_{M2}-gangliosidosis, type III			

TABLE III
METABOLIC DISORDERS WHERE VARIANTS HAVE BEEN DESCRIBED

Disease	Compendium Birth Defect no.	Disease	Compendium Birth Defect no.
Acatalasemia	6	Homocystinuria	474
Albinism		Hydroxykynureninuria	
Citrullinemia	174	Hyperammonemia	485
Cystathionuria	236	Iminoglycinuria (marker)	520
Cystinosis	238	Lesch-Nyhan syndrome	588
Cystinuria	239	Maple syrup urine disease	628
Galactosemia	403	Metachromatic leukodystrophies	651
Gaucher disease	406	Methylcrotonylglycinuria	
Glucose-6-phosphate dehydrogenase deficiency	420	Methylmalonic acidemia	658
Glycogenosis, type VI	427	Niemann-Pick disease	717
G_{M1}-gangliosidosis	431, 432	Oroticaciduria	772
G_{M2}-gangliosidosis	433, 434	Phenylketonuria	808
Hereditary methemoglobinemia		Propionic acidemia	826
Histidinemia	472	Pyruvate kinase deficiency	852

TABLE IV
METABOLIC DISORDERS TRANSMITTED AS AUTOSOMAL
RECESSIVES WHERE HETEROZYGOTES CAN BE DETECTED BY
DIRECT MEASUREMENT

Disease	Compendium Birth Defect no.	Disease	Compendium Birth Defect no.
Acatalasemia	6	Hereditary disaccharide intolerance	
Acid maltase deficiency	11	Hereditary methemoglobinemia	
Acid phosphatase deficiency		Hexokinase deficiency	
Adenine phosphoribosyl transferase deficiency		Histidinemia	472
Alpha$_1$-antitrypsin deficiency	39	Homocystinuria	474
Argininemia	86	Hypervalinemia	509
Argininosuccinic aciduria	87	Hypophosphatasia	516
Brancher deficiency	116	Iminoglycinuria (marker)	520
Citrullinemia	174	L-glyceric aciduria	
Cystinosis	238	Lysinemia	616
Cystinuria	239	Maple syrup urine disease	628
Galactokinase deficiency	402	Metachromatic leukodystrophies	651
Galactosemia	403	Mucolipidosis II	672
Gaucher disease	406	Mucopolysaccharidosis I-H	674
Glucose-galactose malabsorption	419	Mucopolysaccharidosis I-S	675
Glycogenosis, type I	425	Oroticaciduria	772
Glycogenosis, type III	426	Pentosuria (marker)	804
Glycogenosis, type VI	427	Phosphofructokinase deficiency	
G_{M1}-gangliosidosis	431, 432	Phosphohexose isomerase deficiency	
G_{M2}-gangliosidosis	433, 434	Pyruvate decarboxylase deficiency	
Goitrous cretinism		Pyruvate kinase deficiency	852
Hemochromatosis, idiopathic	460	Triosephosphate isomerase deficiency	
		2, 3-diphosphoglycerate mutase deficiency	

TABLE V
METABOLIC DISORDERS TRANSMITTED AS AUTOSOMAL RECESSIVES WHERE HETEROZYGOTES CAN BE DETECTED BY LOADING TESTS

Disease	Compendium Birth Defect no.	Loading material
Cystathioninuria	236	Methionine
Hartnup disorder	453	Tryptophan
Hepatolenticular degeneration	469	Cu^{64} by mouth
Hydroxykynureninuria		Tryptophan
Ornithine transcarboxylase deficiency		Protein
Phenylketonuria	808	Phenylalanine
Transglucuronylase, severe deficiency	961	Menthol
Tyrosinemia	978	Phenylalanine

TABLE VI
METABOLIC DISORDERS TRANSMITTED AS X-LINKED RECESSIVES WHERE HETEROZYGOTES CAN BE DETECTED BY DIRECT MEASUREMENT

Disease	Compendium Birth Defect no.
Diabetes insipidus, vasopressin-resistant	287
Fabry disease	373
Glucose-6-phosphate dehydrogenase deficiency	420
Granulomatous disease of males, chronic	443
Lesch-Nyhan syndrome	588
Mucopolysaccharidosis II	676
Muscular dystrophy, childhood pseudohypertrophic	689
Phosphoglycerate kinase deficiency	

TABLE VII
METABOLIC DISORDERS WHICH CAN BE SCREENED FOR DURING NEWBORN PERIOD

Disease	Compendium Birth Defect no.
A. Bacterial inhibition assay	
Galactokinase deficiency	402
Galactosemia	403
Histidinemia	472
Maple syrup urine disease	628
Phenylketonuria	808
B. By paper chromatography for amino acids	
I. Conditions detected by excess in the blood and urine	
Argininemia	86
Carnosinemia	126
Citrullinemia	174
Cystinosis	238
Histidinemia	472
Homocystinuria	474
Hydroxyprolinemia (marker)	482
Hyperbeta-alaninemia	486
Hyperglycinemia, nonketotic	492
Hyperprolinemia (marker)	502
Hypersarcosinemia	503
Hypervalinemia	509
Lysine intolerance	
Lysinemia	616
Maple syrup urine disease	628
Methylmalonic acidemia	658
Phenylketonuria	808
Propionic acidemia	826
Saccharopinuria	
Tyrosinemia	978
II. Conditions detected by excess in the urine only	
Argininosuccinic aciduria	87
Cystathioninuria	236
Cystinuria	239
Hartnup disorder	453
Hyperdibasic-aminoaciduria	491
Iminoglycinuria (marker)	520
Oculo-cerebro-renal syndrome	736
C. NADP reduction	
Galactosemia	403
Glucose-6-phosphate dehydrogenase deficiency	420
Glutathione reductase deficiency	
Pyruvate kinase deficiency	852
D. Other methods	
Adenosine deaminase deficiency	
G_{M2}-gangliosidosis with hexosaminidase A deficiency	434
Lesch-Nyhan syndrome	588
Metachromatic leukodystrophies	651
Methylcrotonylglycinuria	
Mucopolysaccharidosis I-H	674
Mucopolysaccharidosis I-S	675
Mucopolysaccharidosis II	676
Mucopolysaccharidosis III	677
Mucopolysaccharidosis IV	678
Mucopolysaccharidosis VI	679
Nucleoside-phosphorylase deficiency	729

TABLE VIII
METABOLIC DISORDERS WHICH CAN BE DETECTED IN LEUKOCYTES OR FIBROBLASTS

Disease	Compendium Birth Defect no.	Leukocytes		Fibroblasts	
		Homozygote	Heterozygote	a	b
Acatalasemia	6	+		+	+
Acid maltase deficiency	11	+	+*	+	+
Acid phosphatase deficiency		+	+*	+	
Adenosine deaminase deficiency				+	
Argininosuccinic aciduria	87	+			
Brancher deficiency	116		+		
Citrullinemia	174			+	
Cystathioninuria	236	+		+	
Cystic fibrosis	237			+	
Cystinosis	238	+	+	+	+
Fabry disease	373	+	+	+	+‡
Galactosemia	403	+	+	+	+
Gaucher disease	406	+		+	+
Glucose-6-phosphate dehydrogenase deficiency	420	+	+	+	+‡
Glutathione reductase deficiency		+			
Glycogenosis, type III	426	+	+	+	
Glycogenosis, type VI	427	+	+	+	
G_{M1}-gangliosidosis, type 1	431	+	+	+	
G_{M1}-gangliosidosis, type 2	432	+	+	+	
G_{M2}-gangliosidosis, types 1, 2	433, 434	+	+	+	+
Granulomatous disease of males, chronic	443	+	+‡		
Hexokinase deficiency		−			
Histidinemia	472			+	
Homocystinuria	474	+		+	
Hypervalinemia	509	+		+	
Hypophosphatasia	516	−			
Isovalericacidemia	547	+			
L-glyceric aciduria		+	+		
Lesch-Nyhan syndrome	588	+		+	+‡
Lysinemia	616			+	
Maple syrup urine disease	628	+	+	+	+
Metachromatic leukodystrophies	651	+		+	+
Methylcrotonylglycinuria				+	+
Methylmalonic acidemia	658	+		+	
Mucolipidosis II	672			+	+
Mucopolysaccharidosis I-H	674	+		+	+
Mucopolysaccharidosis I-S	675	+		+	
Mucopolysaccharidosis II	676	+		+	+‡
Mucopolysaccharidosis III	677	+		+	
Mucopolysaccharidosis IV	678	+		+	
Mucopolysaccharidosis VI	679	+		+	
Niemann-Pick disease	717	+		+	
Nucleoside-phosphorylase deficiency	729			+	
Oroticaciduria	772	+	+	+	+
Phosphoglycerate kinase deficiency		+			
Phosphohexose isomerase deficiency		+			
Phytanic acid storage disease	810			+	
Porphyria, erythropoietic	821			+	
Propionic acidemia	826	+		+	
Pyruvate decarboxylase deficiency				+	
Pyruvate kinase deficiency	852	−			
Triosephosphate isomerase deficiency		+	+	+	

a   Homozygote
b   Heterozygote
*   Following stimulation with PHA
‡   Two cell populations confirming Lyon hypothesis
+   Abnormality present
−   Abnormality absent

TABLE IX
METABOLIC DISORDERS WHICH THEORETICALLY CAN AND WHICH HAVE BEEN DETECTED PRENATALLY

Condition	Compendium Birth Defect no.	Amniotic fluid alone		Cultivated amniotic fluid cells	
		Possible	Detected	Possible	Detected
Acid maltase deficiency	11	+		+	+
Acid phosphatase deficiency				+	+
Adenosine deaminase deficiency				+	
Argininemia	86			+	
Argininosuccinic aciduria	87			+	
Brancher deficiency	116			+	
Cystathioninuria	236			+	
Cystinosis	238			+	
Fabry disease	373			+	
Galactokinase deficiency	402			+	+
Galactosemia	403			+	+
Gaucher disease	406			+	
Glucose-6-phosphate dehydrogenase deficiency	420			+	
Glycogenosis, type III	426			+	
G_{M1}-gangliosidosis, type 1	431			+	
G_{M2}-gangliosidosis with hexosaminidase A deficiency	434	+	+	+	+
Homocystinuria	474			+	
Hyperammonemia	485	+			
Hypervalinemia	509			+	
Lesch-Nyhan syndrome	588			+	+
Maple syrup urine disease	628			+	+
Metachromatic leukodystrophies	651			+	+
Methylcrotonylglycinuria		+		+	
Methylmalonic acidemia	658	+	+	+	+
Mucolipidosis II	672			+	
Mucopolysaccharidosis I-H	674			+	+
Mucopolysaccharidosis II	676			+	+
Mucopolysaccharidosis III, A and B				+	+
Niemann-Pick disease	717			+	
Oroticaciduria	772			+	
Phytanic acid storage disease	810			+	
Propionic acidemia	826	+	+	+	+

TABLE X
METABOLIC DISEASES WHERE SPECIFIC FORMS OF THERAPY ARE AVAILABLE

Disease	Compendium Birth Defect no.	Elimination diet or drug	Substitution therapy	Drug treatment
Adenosine deaminase deficiency			Bone marrow transplantation	
Argininosuccinic aciduria	87	+		
Cystathioninuria	236	+	B_6	
Cystinuria	239			Penicillinamine
Diabetes insipidus, vasopressin-resistant	287			
Disaccharide intolerance		+		
Fructose-1-phosphate aldolase deficiency	395	+		
Fructose-1,6-diphosphatase deficiency	396			
Galactokinase deficiency	402	+		
Galactosemia	403	+		
Glucose-galactose malabsorption	419	+		
Glucose-6-phosphate dehydrogenase deficiency	420	+		
Goitrous cretinism			Thyroid	
Gout	441			Probenecid, allopurinol
Hartnup disorder	453		Nicotinamide	
Hemochromatosis, idiopathic	460	+		
Hepatolenticular degeneration	469			Penicillinamine
Homocystinuria	474	+	B_6	
Hydroxykynureninuria		+	Niacin	
Hypervalinemia	509	+		
Hypophosphatemia	517		Vitamin D	
Juvenile diabetes mellitus	549		Insulin	
Lactose malabsorption		+		
Lesch-Nyhan syndrome	588			Allopurinol
Lysine intolerance		+		
Lysinemia	616	+		
Maple syrup urine disease	628	+		
Methemoglobinemia				Methylene blue
Methylcrotonylglycinuria		+	Biotin	
Methylmalonic aciduria	658	+	B_{12}	
Normokalemic periodic paralysis			NaCl	
Oroticaciduria	772			Uridine
Paralysis, hypokalemic periodic	795		K	
Phenylketonuria	808	+		
Pituitary diabetes insipidus			Pitressin	Chlorpropamide
Propionic acidemia	826	+	Biotin	
Transglucuronylase, severe deficiency	961			Phototherapy
Tyrosinemia	978	+		
Vitamin B_6 dependency	991	+	B_6	
Xanthurenic aciduria		+	B_6	

TABLE XI
CLINICAL AND HEMATOLOGIC FEATURES OF THE MAJOR FORMS OF THALASSEMIA

Type	Hemoglobin findings	Hematologic changes	Clinical features
Heterozygous			
β Severe (high A_2)	A_2, 3.5%–7.5% F, 1%–6%	Erythrocyte microcytosis and hypochromia, mild-to-moderate anemia	Possible splenomegaly and mild icterus
β Mild (high A_2)	A_2, 3.5%–7.5%	Erythrocyte microcytosis and hypochromia, mild or absent anemia	Usually none
β Silent carrier	A_2 and F, normal (F-containing cells sometimes detectable by slide elution test)	Hematologically normal	None
$\beta\delta$ (high F)	A_2, normal or low F, 5%–20%	Erythrocyte microcytosis and hypochromia, mild or absent anemia	Usually none
α Severe (α_1)	Adult: normal Newborn: Barts, 5%–10%	Erythrocyte microcytosis and hypochromia, mild anemia	Usually none
α Mild (α_2) (α Silent carrier)	Adult: normal Newborn: Barts, 1%–2%	Usually normal	Usually none
α_1/α_2 Heterozygous	H (β_4), 5%–25% Barts (γ_4), 1%–3%	Erythrocyte hypochromia, poikilocytosis, anisocytosis; inclusion bodies demonstrable by supravital staining; moderate anemia	Pallor, jaundice, hepatosplenomegaly
Homozygous			
β Severe (high A_2)	F, 30%–95%	Markedly abnormal red cell morphology with microcytosis and hypochromia, nucleated red cells, severe anemia	Pallor, jaundice, bone deformities with abnormal facies, hepatosplenomegaly, usually transfusion-dependent
β Mild (high A_2)	F, 40%–80%	Poikilocytosis, anisocytosis, target cells; moderate anemia	Pallor, hepatosplenomegaly, jaundice; transfusions not usually required
$\beta\delta$ (high F)	F, 100%	Poikilocytosis, anisocytosis, hypochromia, microcytosis; mild-to-moderate anemia	Mild jaundice, hepatosplenomegaly usually present
α Severe (α_1)	Barts, 80%–90% A and F, absent	Red cell hypochromia, anisocytosis, poikilocytosis; severe anemia	Hydrops fetalis with severe edema, hepatosplenomegaly, congestive heart failure; stillbirth or death within first 24 hr.

TABLE XII
CLEFT LIP WITH OR WITHOUT CLEFT PALATE, DERIVED COMPLICATIONS AND FREQUENCIES

Defect	Percent
Absence of philtrum	?
Flattening of nose and flaring of ala nasae	?
Defect in nasal septum	?
Absence, duplication, malposition of microforms of anterior teeth especially the maxillary lateral incisor	?
Anterior-posterior deficiency of mid-third of face	30
Broad nasopharyngeal widths	25
Short mandible	(statistical)
Short mandibular ramus	(statistical)
Increased gonial angle	(statistical)
Increased mandibular width	(statistical)
When alveolus is cleft	
Median primary fissural tooth	50
Median permanent fissural tooth	25
Distal primary fissural tooth	75
Distal permanent fissural tooth	45
Agenesis of primary teeth	15
Agenesis of permanent teeth	45
Without alveolar cleft	
Primary and permanent supernumerary teeth	50
Agenesis of permanent teeth	10
Hypodontia of teeth other than cleft area	40 (more common in maxilla)
Difficulty in nursing, breathing and swallowing	?
Speech defects	?
Death usually from respiratory causes in untreated cases or from associated defects	?

TABLE XIII
CLEFT LIP WITH OR WITHOUT CLEFT PALATE, ASSOCIATED COMPLICATIONS AND FREQUENCIES

Defect	Percent with CL/P*
Autosomal Dominant	
CL/P or CP and lip pits or mounds	67
CL/P or CP and filiform fusion of eyelids, may have lip pits	80
CL/P, ectrodactyly-ectodermal dysplasia-clefting syndrome	80
CL/P or CP with enlarged parietal foramina	Rare
CL/P or CP with congenital neuroblastoma	Rare
CL/P or CP, popliteal pterygium syndrome	90
CL/P or CP and basal cell nevus syndrome	5
CL/P or CP and Waardenburg syndrome	3
CL/P hypohidrosis, thin wiry hair and dystrophic nails (Rapp-Hodgkin s.)	70–80
CL/P and oculo-dento-osseous dysplasia	Rare
CL/P and Robinow syndrome (possible autosomal recessive forms)	Rare
CL/P and hypertelorism-hypospadias syndrome	Uncommon
Incomplete CL/submucous CP and Pallister-W syndrome	70–80
Autosomal Recessive	
CL/P or CP, Meckel syndrome	90–100
CL/P or CP and ablepharon	10
CL/P, Roberts syndrome	100
CL/P, pseudothalidomide syndrome	Uncommon
CL/P, ocular hypertelorism, microtia, ectopic kidney, congenital heart and growth deficiency	90–100
CL/P, oro-cranio-digital syndrome	100
CL/P tetraperomelia, large deformed pinna, ectodermal dysplasia and oligophrenia (Freire-Maia s.)	Uncommon
Environmentally Induced Cleft Lip/Palate Syndromes	
CL/P and ring constrictions	Uncommon
CL/P and fetal hydantoin syndrome	Uncommon
CL/P or CP and fetal trimethadione syndrome	Uncommon
Unknown Genesis Syndromes	
CL/P or CP and oculo-auriculo-vertebral dysplasia	7*
CL/P or CP and median cleft face syndrome	30*
CL/P or CP and thoracopagus twins	10
CL/P or CP, forearm bone aplasia	2
CL/P or CP, congenital heart disease	2
CL/P or CP anencephaly	10
CL/P or CP and encephalomeningocele	?
CL/P or CP and congenital oral teratoma	50
CL/P clefting ectropion syndrome	100
CL/P with microbrachycephaly, craniostenosis oligophrenia and malformed limbs (Herrmann s. II, possibly Freire-Maia s.)	?
CL/P with Pilotto syndrome	?
CL/P with mandibulofacial dysostosis, and limb deficiencies (Wildervanck-Smith s.)	?
CL/P and hypogonadotropic hypogonadism	Rare
CL/P and hypophyseal dwarfism	Rare

(Continued)

TABLE XIII
CLEFT LIP WITH OR WITHOUT CLEFT PALATE, ASSOCIATED COMPLICATIONS AND FREQUENCIES (Continued)

Defect	Percent with CL/P*
CL/P and sacral agenesis	Rare
CL/P with cleft larynx and laryngeal web	Rare
CL/P and proboscis lateralis	10
Premaxillary agenesis	100
Median CL/P and short rib-polydactyly syndrome, Majewski type	100
Chromosomal Defects	
CL/P or CP and 1q+	50?
CL/P or CP and 3p–, q+	30
CL/P or CP and 4p–	66
CL/P or CP and 5p–	?
CL/P and 9p+	?
CL/P or CP and 10p+	?
CL/P or CP and 11p+	?
CL/P or CP and 13+	60
CL/P or CP and 18+	15
CL/P or CP and 18p– (agenesis premaxilla)	Rare
CL/P or CP and 18q–	30
CL/P or CP and 21+	0.5
CL/P or CP and 21q–	?
CL/P or CP and 49,XXXXY	15
Triploidy	30
Translocations, various types	20–40

*Possible genetic forms
s = Syndrome
CL/P = Cleft lip with or without cleft palate

TABLE XIV
CLEFT PALATE, ASSOCIATED COMPLICATIONS AND FREQUENCIES

Syndrome or Defect	Percent with cleft palate
Autosomal Dominant	
CL/P or CP and lip pits or mounds	67
CL/P or CP and filiform fusion of eyelids	100
CL/P or CP with enlarged parietal foramina	?
CL/P or CP with popliteal pterygium syndrome	90–100
CL/P or CP and congenital neuroblastoma	?
CL/P or CP and basal cell nevus syndrome	3–7
CL/P or CP and Waardenburg syndrome	1–2
CL and acrocephalosyndactyly 42% also have bifid uvula, and 26% also have Byzantine arch	32
CP and Marfan syndrome	?
CP, arthro-ophthalmopathy	20–30
CP and mandibulofacial dysostosis	30
CP and spondyloepiphyseal dysplasia congenita	35
CP, camptodactyly and clubfoot	Rare
CP and hydrocephaly, Dandy-Walker malformation, hip dislocation, malformed ears (Aase-Smith S.)	?
CP brachial plexus neuritis syndrome	30
CP lateral synechiae syndrome	90–100
CP and Kniest dysplasia	40
CP and cleidocranial dysplasia (submucous cleft and high-arched palate common)	2–5
CP, ectrodactyly	90–100
CP and micrognathia, dysplastic ears, ectro-and syndactyly, C/S oligophrenia (submucous cleft common) (Fontaine s.)	50
CP and Larsen syndrome (recessive forms also)	50
CP and acrocephalosyndactyly	?
CP and small head size, large ears, short stature, hypoplastic distal phalanges, proximally placed thumbs (Say s.)	100
Autosomal Recessive	
CL/P or CP and ablepharon	10
CL/P or CP and Meckel syndrome	90–100
CP and chondrodysplasia punctata, rhizomelic type	3
CP and diastrophic dysplasia	25–50
CP and Smith-Lemli-Opitz syndrome	5
CP and multiple pterygium syndrome	90–100
CP and stapes fixation and oligodontia	100
CP and cerebro-costo-mandibular syndrome	100
CP or branchio-skeleto-genital syndrome	100
CP and campomelic dysplasia (Maroteaux s.) genetic heterogeneity	?
CP de la Chapelle syndrome	100
CP, craniostenosis, microcephaly, arthrogryposis, and adduced thumbs (Christian s.I.)	100

(Continued)

Syndrome or Defect	Percent with cleft palate	Syndrome or Defect	Percent with cleft palate
CP, Dubowitz syndrome (submucous cleft, bifid uvula and high-arched palate most common defect)	?	CL/P or CP and oculo-auriculo-vertebral dysplasia	7
CP, short stature, oligophrenia (Katcher-Hall s.)	90–100	CP and Beckwith-Wiedemann syndrome	Rare
		CP and cervico-oculo-acoustic syndrome	Common
		CP and Charlie M. syndrome	?
		CP and acanthosis nigricans and cutis gyratum	?
CP and Larsen syndrome (possible dominant forms)	50	CP and Coffin-Siris syndrome	10
CP, persistent truncus arteriosus, abnormal right pulmonary artery, intrauterine death (Lowry-Miller s.)	100	CL and femoral hypoplasia – unusual facies syndrome	?
		CL and Hanhart syndrome	11
CP and Marden-Walker syndrome	Uncommon	CL and micrognathia, wormian bones, congenital heart defect, dislocated hips, absent tibiae, bowed fibulae, preaxial polydactyly (feet) simian creases, ulnar deviation of fingers (Ho s.)	?
CP and micromelic dwarfism, small mandible, cleft vertebra	70		
CP and rhizomelic dwarfism, dysplastic ears, thick leathery skin, soft tissue calcifications (Nance-Sweeney chondrodysplasia)	Rare		
CP and oro-facio-digital syndrome II	Rare	CP and Klippel-Feil syndrome	5
CP and Nager acrofacial dysostosis. ? if recessive	10	CP and de Lange syndrome	?
		CP and Walden syndrome	?
CP, microcephaly, short stature, oligophrenia, almond-shaped deep-set eyes, bulbous nasal tip, clinodactyly of toes, wrist defect (Palant s.)	100	CP and oral teratoma	?
		CP and buccopharyngeal membrane	50
		CP, micrognathia and glossoptosis	?
CP, growth retardation, flexion contractures of hands, simian creases, small fingers and nails, ureteral stenosis, coarse facies, lethal in infancy (Rudiger s.)	100	CP and oral duplication	60
		Chromosomal Defects	
		CL/P or CP chromosome 1q+	50
X-linked syndromes		CP chromosome 3p+	50
CP and oro-facio-digital syndrome I	80	CL/P or CP chromosome 3p–,q+	30
CP and oto-palato-digital syndrome (XD-lethal in male)	90–100	CL/P or CP chromosome 4p–	66
		CL/P or CP chromosome 5p–	?
CP (uvula) and familial nephrosis, deafness, urinary tract and digital anomalies	20	CP (bifid uvula) chromosome 7p–	?
		CP chromosome 7q+	?
CP and micrognathia, talipes equinovarus, atrial septal defect and persistence of left superior vena cava	100	CL/P or CP chromosome 10p+	?
		CP chromosome 10q+	?
		CL/P or CP chromosome 11p+	?
CP, short stature (Gareis-Smith s.)	100	CP chromosome 11q+	?
CP submucous connective tissue dysplasia syndrome	80–90	CL/P or CP chromosome 13+	60
		CP chromosome 13q+p	Uncommon
		CP chromosome 13q–	Uncommon
		CP chromosome 14q+	50
Environmentally Induced Syndromes		CL/P or CP chromosome 18+	15
CL/P or CP and fetal thalidomide syndrome	Rare	CL/P or CP chromosome 18p–	Rare
CP and fetal aminopterin syndrome	Uncommon	CL/P or CP chromosome 18q–	30
CP and fetal alcohol syndrome	Uncommon	CL/P or CP chromosome 21+	0.5
		CL/P or CP chromosome 21q–	?
Unknown Genesis Syndromes		CP chromosome 22+	30
CL/P or CP and median cleft face syndrome	30	CP chromosome 22q+	?
CL/P or CP and encephalomeningocele	?	CP XO	?
CL/P or CP and thoracopagus twins	10	CL/P or CP 49,XXXXY	5
CL/P or CP and forearm bone aplasia	?	Triploidy	30
CL/P or CP and congenital heart disease	2	Many translocation syndromes	20–40
CL/P or CP and anencephaly	10		

CL/P = cleft lip with or without cleft palate

TABLE XV
FREQUENCY OF CLEFT LIP AND/OR PALATE UNDER VARIOUS CONDITIONS

	Percent affected
In sibs of propositi with and without associated anomalies	
Females without associated anomalies	5.17
Females with associated anomalies	1.33
Males without associated anomalies	4.00
Males with associated anomalies	1.36
Total without associated anomalies	4.44
Total with associated anomalies	1.35
With bilateral and unilateral cleft lip and/or palate	
Female–bilateral	8.59
Female–unilateral	4.10
Male–bilateral	5.50
Male–unilateral	3.70
Total–bilateral	6.71
Total–unilateral	3.83
In sibs of male and female propositi	
Females	4.67
Males	3.61
Influence of family history of cleft lip and/or palate on frequency of cleft lip and/or palate in sibs of propositi	
No family history	2.24
Occurrence of CL(P) in fourth-degree relative	3.69
Occurrence of CL(P) in third-degree relative	6.90
Occurrence of CL(P) in second-degree relative	9.91
Occurrence of CL(P) in parent	15.55
Frequency of isolated cleft palate in families of patients with this anomaly	
Sibs when neither parent has CP	1.96
Sibs when one parent has CP	13.64
Parents	1.48
Children	8.70
Grandparents	0.18
Aunts and uncles	0.32
First cousins	0.09

TABLE XVI
ADULT SKELETAL ELEMENTS OF THE FACE DERIVED FROM THE FRONTONASAL PROMINENCE AND THE BRANCHIAL ARCHES*

Median Plane Facial Skeletal Elements Derived from the Frontonasal Prominence	Skeletal Elements of the Face Derived from the Branchial Arches
Frontal bones	Temporal bone, in part, and ossicles
Cristal galli	
Ethmoid bone	Zygomatic arch
Nasal bones	Maxillary bone
Vomer and cartilaginous nasal septum	Mandible
Premaxillary bone	Hard palate
Anterior primary palatine triangle	

*The table includes only the frontonasal derivatives which are unpaired and in the median plane, or paired and which meet in the median plane. The bones of branchial arch origin which meet in the median plane are the mandible and hard palate.

TABLE XVII
NATURAL APPOSITIONS OR JUNCTIONS OF THE FACE ALONG WHICH CLEFTS OCCUR

Natural Junction	Clinical Type of Cleft
Nasomedial processes with each other	Median notch or cleft of upper lip / Median cleft of nose (bifid nose)
Nasomedial processes with maxillary processes	Ordinary lateral cleft lip
Nasolateral processes with maxillary process (along line of nasooptic furrow)	Oblique facial cleft (and possibly dystopia canthorum and lateral displacement of the lacrimal punctum)
Maxillary-mandibular processes of first branchial arch	Horizontal facial cleft (macrostomia)
Mandibular-hyoid arch junction	Pits, sinus tracts, clefts and other ear malformations
Maxillary-frontonasal prominence junction at lateral aspect of lower eyelid	Colobomas of lower lid
Mandibular processes with each other at midline	Clefts or pits of the lower lip and median cleft mandible

TABLE XVIII
SYNDROMES WITH A PROMINENT OR FORWARD BULGING FOREHEAD, AS DISTINGUISHED FROM HIGH, FLAT OR BROAD FOREHEADS WHICH DO NOT BULGE FORWARD AS IN ACROCEPHALOPOLYSYNDACTYLY

Cerebrohepatorenal syndrome – **139**
Chondrodysplasia punctata, Conradi-Hünermann type – **153**
Chromosome 4p– syndrome – **164**
Craniotelencephalic dysplasia
Diaphyseal dysplasia – **290**
Ectodermal dysplasia, anhidrotic – **333**
Elastic tissue deficiency and hypertelorism
Hydrocephaly – **481**
Hypercalcemia
Lissencephaly syndrome – **603**
Meningoencephalocele
Oculocerebral syndrome
Oculomandibulofacial syndrome – **738**
Osteopetrosis, dominant – **779**
Osteopetrosis, recessive – **780**
Otopalatodigital syndrome – **786**

Some types of anatomic or metabolic megalencephaly, ie mucopolysaccharidoses and gangliosidoses

TABLE XIX
SYNDROMES WITH LARGE SUTURES AND FONTANELS OR DELAYED CLOSURE

Frequent in:

Cerebrohepatorenal syndrome — **139**
Chromosome 18 trisomy syndrome — **160**
Chromosome 13 trisomy syndrome — **168**
Chromosome 21 trisomy syndrome — **171**
Cleidocranial dysplasia (but some have sagittal synostosis) — **185**
Craniofacial dysostosis with diaphyseal hyperplasia — **226**
Fetal aminopterin syndrome — **380**
Hypophosphatasia — **516**
Oculomandibulofacial syndrome — **738**
Progeria — **825**
Pyknodysostosis, (Lamy and Maroteaux type) — **846**
Thyroid dysgenesis — **946**
Tubular stenosis — **976**

Occasional in:

Broad thumb-hallux syndrome — **119**
Chondrodysplasia punctata, Conradi-Hünermann type — **153**
Otopalatodigital syndrome — **786**

TABLE XX
CONDITIONS WHICH MAY CAUSE THE ILLUSION OF HYPERTELORISM EVEN THOUGH THE ACTUAL INTERORBITAL DISTANCE AS MEASURED ON PA RADIOGRAPHS MAY BE SMALL OR NORMAL

Blepharophimosis
Cryptophthalmos
Dystopia canthorum
Epicanthal folds
External strabismus
Flat nasal bridge
Microphthalmos
Small face with normally spaced eyes
Small nose
Symblepharon
Widely spaced eyebrows

TABLE XXI
GENETIC FORMS OF PITUITARY DWARFISM

	Congenital Absence of Pituitary	Familial Panhypo-pituitarism	Isolated hGH Deficiency I	Isolated hGH Deficiency II	Laron-type Dwarfism	Pygmies
Inheritance:	AR	AR	AR	AD	AR	?
Clinical Features:						
Birthweight	N	N	N	N	N	N
Craniofacial disprop.	+	+	+	+	+	−
Truncal obesity	+	+	+	+	+	−
Wrinkled skin	?	+	+	−	?	−
Hypoglycemic attacks	+	+	+	−	+	−
Sexual development	−	−	N	N	N	N
Thyroid function	↓	N/↓	N	N	N	N
Adrenal function	↓	N/↓	N	N	N	N
Plasma hGH:						
Fasting concentration	↓	↓	↓	↓	↑	N
Response to stimuli	↓	↓	↓	↓	N	N
Sulfation Factor:						
Before hGH therapy	↓	↓	↓	?	↓	N
After hGH therapy	N	N	N	?	↓	N
Carbohydrate Metabolism:						
Insulin hypersensitivity	+	+	+	−	+	+
Glucose intolerance	?	+	+	+	+	−
Insulin release	↓	↓	↓	↑	↓	↓
Response to hGH Therapy:						
Plasma FFA	?	+	+	↓	↓	↓
Nitrogen retention	?	+	+	?	↓	↓
Insulin release	?	+	+	+	?	↓
Growth	?	+	+	+	↓	?

TABLE XXII
BIOLOGIC MOTHER

Drugs ingested during patient's prenatal life

Aminopterin, **380**
Diphenylhydantoin, (phenytoin, dilantin, mephenytoin, phenantoin, mesantoin, ethotoin, peganone), **382**
Excess alcohol, (ethanol), **379**
Iodides, **435**
Propylthiouracil (PTU), **435**
Tetracycline, **341**
Thalidomide, **386**
Trimethadione, (tridione, paradione, paramethadione), **388**
Warfarin, (prothromadin, coumadin, panwarfarin), **389**

Exposed to infection or radiation during patient's prenatal life

Cytomegalovirus, **381**
Early, active syphilis, **385**
Maternal radiation dose of 100 rad or more, **383**
Rubella, **384**
Toxoplasmosis, **387**
Unspecified infection, **274**

TABLE XXIII
RETARDATION

Growth

1, 16, 24, 27, 94, 100, 148, 158, 159, 161, 162, 163, 164, 166, 170, 172, 188, 189, 223, 238, 242, 249, 299, 302, 304, 305, 347, 379, 381, 384, 385, 388, 389, 423, 425, 427, 431, 440, 485, 491, 509, 524, 534, 542, 543, 544, 586, 593, 616, 658, 678, 679, 697, 717, 736, 769, 772, 785, 825, 826, 851, 864, 873, 906, 946, 947, 948, 986, 1000

Motor

10, 22, 166, 227, 424, 425, 432, 557, 588, 629, 638, 689, 803, 873, 895, 1000, 1003

Delayed developmental milestones

25, 107, 115, 119, 121, 162, 169, 379, 398, 406, 413, 415, 431, 433, 434, 482, 491, 512, 513, 598, 643, 674, 680, 686, 689, 717, 741, 850, 891

Mental

1, 14, 16, 22, 29, 40, 44, 78, 86, 87, 97, 100, 104, 105, 106, 112, 118, 119, 126, 137, 138, 142, 143, 148, 154, 159, 160, 162, 163, 165, 166, 168, 170, 171, 172, 174, 179, 182, 189, 190, 220, 224, 225, 227, 229, 236, 239, 242, 243, 249, 250, 251, 254, 262, 266, 299, 302, 304, 306, 327, 333, 337, 342, 376, 379, 380, 381, 382, 383, 384, 385, 387, 388, 389, 401, 403, 408, 410, 412, 413, 421, 422, 424, 431, 432, 440, 453, 458, 472, 474, 478, 481, 482, 485, 492, 503, 505, 506, 509, 512, 513, 525, 526, 542, 543, 544, 547, 554, 555, 556, 562, 578, 588, 593, 616, 628, 629, 632, 635, 638, 657, 658, 659, 670, 671, 673, 676, 677, 689, 702, 713, 717, 720, 721, 724, 727, 730, 732, 736, 741, 754, 755, 759, 769, 772, 773, 783, 791, 808, 823, 826, 830, 843, 849, 850, 851, 860, 875, 881, 885, 891, 921, 947, 948, 949, 967, 975, 978, 986, 991, 998, 999, 1004

Psychomotor

44, 139, 157, 161, 164, 167, 398, 473, 514, 672, 823

TABLE XXIV
BIRTH DEFECTS WHICH MAY INVOLVE THE EYE

Eye as a unit

1, 2, 3, 12, 13, 14, 15, 16, 18, 27, 30, 31, 32, 34, 35, 36, 37, 41, 43, 47, 48, 52, 57, 58, 59, 60, 67, 70, 84, 90, 93, 94, 97, 101, 102, 105, 106, 111, 115, 118, 119, 121, 122, 126, 130, 131, 132, 133, 136, 139, 140, 142, 143, 147, 153, 154, 155, 158, 159, 160, 162, 163, 164, 165, 166, 167, 168, 169, 170, 171, 172, 176, 177, 179, 182, 183, 188, 189, 190, 191, 195, 198, 201, 205, 206, 207, 208, 209, 210, 211, 212, 213, 214, 215, 216, 221, 223, 225, 226, 227, 228, 229, 230, 231, 234, 238, 242, 243, 247, 250 252, 253, 261, 262, 265, 270, 281, 282, 283, 284, 296, 299, 302, 307, 309, 310, 318, 337, 338, 343, 344, 355, 356, 371, 372, 373, 375, 376, 377, 378, 379, 381, 382, 384, 385, 387, 388, 389, 394, 395, 398, 399, 400, 401, 402, 403, 406, 408, 413, 414, 431, 433, 434, 439, 440, 443, 449, 451, 457, 469, 473, 474, 475, 479, 480, 481, 488, 494, 495, 497, 504, 505, 506, 512, 513, 515, 526, 530, 534, 538, 539, 544, 548, 549, 550, 552, 553, 554, 555, 557, 560, 563, 564, 565, 570, 574, 578, 579, 580, 583, 584, 585, 586, 587, 591, 593, 595, 598, 603, 616, 620, 621, 622, 627, 629, 630, 632, 634, 635, 636, 637, 638, 639, 640, 651, 657, 661, 662, 663, 667, 671, 672, 673, 674, 675, 676, 678, 679, 680, 692, 695, 697, 699, 702, 703, 705, 706, 708, 712, 713, 716, 717, 720, 721, 722, 724, 726, 727, 732, 733, 734, 735, 736, 737, 738, 740, 744, 745, 746, 749, 750, 751, 752, 753, 754, 755, 756, 757, 758, 759, 761, 762, 763, 764, 765, 771, 775, 776, 777, 779, 780, 783, 785, 786, 788, 789, 791, 803, 808, 810, 811, 818, 820, 821, 822, 823, 824, 825, 830, 832, 834, 844, 845, 847, 850, 856, 865, 866, 867, 868, 869, 870, 871, 872, 875, 876, 880, 881, 885, 889, 891, 893, 897, 915, 921, 925, 943, 952, 963, 975, 977, 983, 986, 994, 995, 997, 998, 999, 1000, 1004, 1005

Vision

1, 2, 12, 32, 34, 35, 36, 41, 43, 57, 59, 70, 90, 101, 103, 143, 155, 179, 182, 188, 189, 195, 196, 197, 198, 199, 201, 206, 207, 209, 210, 211, 212, 215, 224, 229, 242, 250, 251, 253, 261, 270, 350, 355, 381, 384, 386, 387, 388, 389, 394, 399, 408, 414, 415, 433, 449, 474, 479, 515, 538, 539, 550, 552, 557, 578, 579, 583, 584, 585, 591, 593, 621, 630, 637, 663, 675, 699, 713, 718, 719, 720, 721, 732, 733, 734, 736, 740, 745, 749, 750, 753, 755, 757, 758, 759, 763, 764, 777, 780, 783, 810, 834, 865, 867, 869, 870, 871, 893, 897, 925, 963, 976, 983, 986, 1004, 1005

Nystagmus

32, 34, 35, 36, 41, 43, 57, 94, 118, 136, 143, 147, 159, 188, 191, 195, 198, 225, 227, 281, 344, 377, 413, 433, 530, 593, 621, 651, 671, 733, 745, 746, 751, 752, 755, 759, 765, 803, 810, 850, 963, 986, 995

Eyeball small

84, 140, 155, 160, 163, 166, 167, 168, 172, 182, 242, 281, 283, 284, 384, 387, 389, 413, 440, 457, 544, 550, 585, 634, 635, 661, 662, 721, 733, 737, 738, 783, 866, 872, 994

Drooping of upper eyelid

1, 48, 111, 118, 155, 158, 160, 162, 166, 167, 172, 229, 281, 299, 371, 377, 382, 388, 475, 548, 574, 692, 695, 697, 702, 720, 735, 750, 751, 752, 753, 754, 788, 834, 889, 891, 977

Palpebral fissures

1 13, 119, 121, 139, 154, 159, 162, 163, 164, 165, 166, 168, 170, 171, 190, 223, 227, 262, 395, 401, 544, 603, 627, 632, 720, 735, 786, 791

Epicanthic fold

13, 16, 97, 101, 119, 121, 139, 155, 158, 162, 163, 165, 170, 172, 183, 231, 299, 337, 338, 356, 382, 388, 395, 401, 505, 544, 554, 629, 638, 672, 720, 732, 791, 856, 891, 977, 997, 999

Cataract

41, 43, 57, 101, 131, 132, 133, 139, 140, 153, 154, 170, 182, 189, 250, 261, 388, 389, 402, 403, 449, 479, 515, 544, 550, 585, 634, 635, 637, 638, 661, 663, 697, 702, 703, 708, 721, 732, 735, 736, 783, 785, 810, 830, 845, 865, 866, 869, 994, 998

Hypertelorism

1, 14, 16, 97, 101, 118, 119, 122, 139, 158, 163, 164, 166, 190, 223, 225, 228, 229, 261, 281, 338, 382, 389, 401, 504, 506, 544, 570, 586, 587, 595, 629, 634, 635, 720, 722, 724, 726, 727, 732, 737, 754, 786, 856, 875, 876, 880, 943

Hypotelorism

163, 166, 168, 231, 355, 473, 634

Retina and macula

2, 32, 34, 35, 36, 41, 43, 47, 70, 90, 93, 121, 136, 140, 159, 163, 182, 189, 195, 201, 238, 242, 261, 338, 373, 384, 399, 400, 431, 433, 434, 449, 474, 479, 534, 549, 550, 557, 578, 583, 598, 620, 621, 622, 630, 640, 661, 671, 675, 676, 699, 713, 716, 717, 721, 732, 733, 734, 740, 745, 756, 763, 764, 776, 783, 810, 820, 822, 832, 865, 866, 867, 868, 869, 870, 871, 872, 897, 925, 983, 998

Strabismus

1, 35, 43, 59, 101, 118, 119, 142, 143, 158, 159, 163, 164, 166, 170, 171, 182, 188, 223, 225, 227, 229, 242, 243, 250, 252, 261, 281, 344, 371, 376, 377, 382, 388, 394, 395, 401, 406, 457, 504, 505, 512, 513, 544, 548, 616, 632, 667, 699, 702, 712, 733, 735, 744, 745, 750, 751, 752, 753, 754, 755, 779, 780, 791, 823, 834, 867, 870, 881, 889, 891, 952, 999

TABLE XXV
BIRTH DEFECTS WHICH MAY INVOLVE THE EAR

Ear as a unit

1, 12, 13, 28, 55, 72, 85, 88, 97, 98, 104, 121, 122, 139, 140, 141, 142, 145, 150, 157, 158, 159, 160, 161, 162, 163, 164, 165, 166, 167, 168, 170, 171, 172, 182, 183, 190, 225, 227, 229, 231, 232, 241, 242, 244, 247, 248, 249, 250, 254, 262, 263, 266, 272, 274, 285, 293, 312, 313, 314, 315, 316, 317, 318, 320, 321, 322, 323, 324, 325, 326, 327, 328, 329, 330, 331, 370, 374, 376, 377, 378, 385, 388, 389, 409, 457, 505, 506, 510, 523, 526, 530, 544, 555, 562, 587, 591, 592, 596, 603, 619, 627, 629, 632, 634, 636, 662, 664, 667, 706, 712, 720, 727, 728, 735, 754, 771, 773, 775, 777, 786, 787, 821, 823, 856, 860, 883, 943, 967, 982, 987, 999, 1001

Hearing

10, 12, 14, 27, 30, 41, 55, 70, 72, 89, 97, 114, 123, 141, 142, 145, 150, 159, 162, 168, 173, 182, 183, 189, 206, 207, 224, 228, 229, 243, 244, 245, 246, 247, 248, 249, 250, 251, 252, 253, 254, 255, 256, 257, 258, 259, 260, 261, 262, 263, 264, 265, 266, 267, 268, 269, 270, 271, 272, 273, 274, 275, 315, 318, 324, 326, 327, 330, 331, 333, 337, 370, 376, 377, 381, 384, 385, 386, 387, 388, 389, 394, 415, 436, 450, 451, 457, 497, 506, 508, 530, 550, 554, 557, 558, 562, 578, 586, 592, 627, 664, 667, 671, 674, 675, 676, 678, 679, 706, 708, 721, 732, 735, 759, 771, 773, 776, 777, 780, 784, 785, 786, 787, 810, 860, 863, 880, 982, 983, 997, 1001, 1004

Sensorineural hearing loss

10, 30, 41, 72, 89, 123, 150, 206, 207, 243, 245, 246, 247, 248, 249, 251, 252, 253, 255, 256, 257, 258, 259, 260, 261, 262, 263, 265, 266, 267, 268, 270, 271, 272, 274, 275, 330, 381, 384, 385, 386, 387, 394, 436, 450, 497, 508, 530, 550, 557, 558, 578, 586, 664, 708, 721, 732, 773, 784, 787, 810, 863, 982, 997, 1004

Conductive hearing loss

10, 27, 97, 141, 150, 159, 183, 229, 244, 247, 250, 254, 264, 318, 324, 326, 327, 330, 331, 337, 370, 377, 394, 506, 530, 557, 558, 592, 627, 664, 667, 706, 771, 773, 786, 787, 860, 1001

Mixed hearing loss

247, 263, 264, 530

TABLE XXVI
BIRTH DEFECTS WHICH MAY INVOLVE THE FACE, FACIAL BONES, NOSE, OR NASOPHARYNX

Face

1, 9, 10, 13, 14, 16, 17, 18, 28, 29, 78, 90, 97, 101, 102, 104, 105, 111, 112, 114, 118, 121, 122, 137, 138, 139, 140, 144, 146, 147, 153, 154, 155, 156, 157, 158, 159, 160, 161, 162, 163, 164, 165, 166, 167, 168, 170, 171, 176, 177, 178, 179, 180, 182, 185, 189, 190, 220, 223, 224, 225, 226, 227, 228, 229, 231, 242, 247, 257, 280, 281, 284, 291, 299, 302, 303, 312, 313, 318, 326, 333, 337, 352, 355, 360, 374, 375, 376, 380, 381, 382, 388, 390, 391, 394, 395, 398, 401, 412, 413, 425, 426, 427, 431, 439, 440, 447, 451, 457, 469, 470, 473, 497, 505, 506, 510, 511, 536, 539, 542, 543, 548, 554, 555, 557, 570, 576, 578, 587, 594, 595, 596, 599, 603, 616, 626, 627, 629, 630, 631, 632, 634, 635, 636, 638, 644, 646, 652, 662, 664, 671, 672, 673, 674, 675, 676, 677, 678, 679, 680, 702, 711, 720, 724, 727, 735, 737, 738, 746, 749, 754, 769, 770, 771, 775, 777, 779, 784, 788, 791, 818, 823, 825, 830, 846, 847, 856, 873, 874, 875, 876, 880, 881, 882, 883, 887, 891, 897, 900, 939, 940, 941, 943, 946, 947, 948, 952, 958, 967, 977, 999, 1000, 1001

Maxilla

14, 16, 97, 104, 112, 118, 159, 161, 162, 163, 167, 178, 189, 223, 225, 226, 227, 229, 291, 302, 352, 382, 388, 439, 440, 555, 626, 632, 791, 876, 941, 977,

Mandible

10, 13, 14, 18, 90, 97, 104, 121, 122, 137, 138, 139, 140, 155, 158, 159, 160, 161, 162, 163, 164, 165, 166, 168, 170, 180, 182, 189, 190, 226, 227, 231, 242, 247, 281, 291, 299, 302, 312, 381, 388, 394, 395, 401, 412, 451, 457, 497, 576, 603, 616, 626, 627, 629, 634, 638, 646, 678, 720, 727, 735, 738, 754, 775, 825, 847, 856, 881, 891, 941, 943, 967, 977, 999

Nose

1, 9, 10, 13, 14, 16, 22, 102, 105, 112, 119, 121, 122, 140, 153, 157, 158, 159, 161, 162, 163, 164, 166, 167, 168, 170, 171, 172, 189, 190, 223, 226, 227, 228, 229, 231, 234, 242, 261, 263, 281, 283, 299, 302, 305, 333, 375, 382, 385, 386, 388, 389, 395, 401, 409, 431, 444, 504, 506, 555, 557, 570, 587, 593, 595, 603, 627, 629, 634, 635, 674, 676, 679, 722, 723, 724, 725, 726, 728, 732, 737, 738, 754, 770, 771, 786, 791, 821, 825, 856, 860, 875, 876, 880, 881, 883, 891, 893, 940, 943, 966, 967, 997, 998, 999, 1001

Nasopharynx

27, 70, 117, 119, 180, 190, 224, 225, 228, 229, 237, 271, 283, 285, 307, 343, 369, 370, 385, 389, 401, 406, 412, 425, 426, 443, 506, 521, 522, 524, 575, 606, 627, 635, 644, 655, 664, 672, 674, 676, 681, 692, 706, 707, 723, 724, 725, 726, 727, 735, 790, 794, 795, 797, 810, 824, 942, 943, 944, 946, 996

TABLE XXVII
BIRTH DEFECTS WHICH MAY INVOLVE THE ORAL CAVITY TEETH, SPEECH, OR NECK

Oral Cavity

6, 15, 22, 25, 28, 37, 61, 88, 90, 97, 104, 111, 113, 118, 119, 121, 122, 138, 139, 143, 156, 157, 158, 159, 160, 163, 164, 165, 166, 168, 171, 172, 176, 177, 178, 179, 180, 181, 182, 183, 184, 185, 220, 223, 225, 226, 227, 229, 230, 242, 247, 261, 264, 279, 281, 283, 291, 293, 307, 329, 337, 338, 352, 360, 364, 365, 375, 376, 378, 380, 381, 382, 389, 390, 394, 401, 407, 408, 409, 410, 411, 412, 413, 417, 431, 443, 451, 469, 470, 494, 505, 506, 522, 535, 536, 538, 542, 543, 544, 557, 570, 574, 576, 578, 593, 596, 599, 609, 618, 627, 629, 630, 634, 635, 636, 644, 662, 664, 667, 674, 676, 681, 696, 714, 720, 727, 732, 735, 737, 749, 754, 760, 769, 770, 771, 786, 789, 790, 791, 799, 818, 823, 846, 874, 875, 876, 878, 883, 897, 944, 945, 946, 951, 952, 953, 954, 955, 956, 959, 977, 981

Teeth

6, 16, 17, 22, 44, 45, 46, 78, 102, 105, 118, 156, 158, 163, 177, 178, 179, 183, 185, 189, 225, 226, 229, 242, 261, 262, 276, 277, 278, 279, 280, 281, 291, 302, 310, 333, 337, 340, 341, 342, 346, 385, 388, 394, 407, 408, 410, 412, 439, 440, 451, 457, 474, 493, 494, 511, 515, 516, 526, 539, 554, 557, 593, 607, 613, 617, 618, 626, 627, 631, 632, 634, 660, 667, 674, 676, 678, 703, 720, 728, 732, 735, 737, 738, 739, 749, 750, 754, 770, 771, 775, 777, 780, 784, 791, 806, 821, 823, 825, 830, 843, 846, 847, 873, 891, 926, 927, 928, 929, 930, 931, 932, 933, 934, 935, 936, 937, 946, 949, 965, 981, 999

Speech

12, 64, 93, 94, 97, 103, 117, 118, 123, 127, 138, 155, 157, 162, 163, 171, 180, 184, 223, 233, 242, 247, 263, 264, 266, 269, 270, 273, 299, 302, 303, 315, 376, 388, 401, 413, 422, 438, 447, 450, 469, 472, 478, 506, 508, 562, 572, 573, 574, 575, 577, 598, 599, 618, 628, 651, 689, 722, 732, 736, 742, 744, 745, 746, 747, 803, 818, 823, 825, 855, 891, 908, 946, 949, 958, 959, 967, 995, 999

Neck

9, 70, 103, 111, 117, 127, 140, 155, 157, 158, 163, 166, 171, 181, 188, 242, 247, 249, 257, 283, 329, 350, 389, 391, 412, 435, 515, 525, 542, 543, 575, 636, 676, 678, 702, 720, 727, 809, 830, 896, 898, 945, 946, 947, 948, 952, 957

TABLE XXVIII
BIRTH DEFECTS WHICH MAY INVOLVE SKIN, HAIR, OR NAILS

Skin

5, 9, 12, 13, 15, 18, 24, 25, 26, 27, 30, 31, 33, 34, 35, 36, 37, 45, 47, 51, 54, 55, 56, 88, 89, 94, 101, 102, 104, 105, 107, 112, 113, 119, 121, 122, 129, 131, 140, 141, 143, 153, 154, 157, 158, 159, 160, 161, 164, 165, 166, 168, 171, 189, 190, 203, 221, 233, 235, 242, 245, 258, 259, 265, 275, 281, 282, 292, 299, 301, 303, 307, 313, 333, 334, 337, 338, 339, 340, 346, 351, 352, 359, 361, 362, 373, 381, 382, 384, 385, 387, 388, 391, 393, 395, 398, 403, 406, 411, 412, 413, 416, 425, 431, 440, 442, 443, 444, 447, 448, 453, 456, 459, 460, 466, 470, 474, 481, 488, 489, 494, 495, 499, 500, 501, 505, 506, 508, 514, 522, 523, 524, 526, 533, 534, 535, 536, 539, 543, 551, 558, 560, 561, 565, 578, 586, 587, 593, 598, 599, 600, 601, 603, 608, 609, 614, 615, 630, 633, 634, 641, 642, 644, 647, 648, 667, 672, 676, 693, 700, 703, 709, 710, 712, 715, 716, 717, 720, 738, 741, 754, 763, 770, 777, 781, 788, 789, 792, 808, 810, 811, 812, 813, 818, 819, 820, 821, 822, 825, 827, 832, 833, 846, 874, 875, 883, 884, 886, 887, 890, 908, 915, 924, 939, 940, 943, 946, 949, 967, 973, 975, 977, 978, 982, 986, 993, 998, 1000, 1004, 1005

Skin hyperpigmentation

12, 24, 25, 26, 30, 129, 143, 189, 281, 346, 352, 362, 384, 391, 406, 460, 474, 526, 539, 560, 586, 644, 703, 712, 763, 821, 822, 825, 887, 975, 1000, 1004, 1005

Skin depigmentation

26, 30, 33, 34, 35, 36, 105, 143, 160, 171, 242, 281, 337, 346, 413, 442, 526, 821, 975, 993, 1004, 1005

Sweating

5, 37, 44, 102, 179, 189, 237, 259, 261, 281, 333, 351, 398, 448, 493, 545, 703, 788, 793, 820, 822, 885, 894, 924, 981, 986

Hair

1, 3, 13, 15, 26, 30, 31, 34, 35, 36, 38, 49, 67, 99, 102, 105, 119, 121, 143, 153, 154, 155, 163, 166, 171, 179, 189, 227, 229, 242, 259, 281, 292, 296, 299, 302, 319, 333, 334, 337, 355, 362, 371, 372, 388, 410, 412, 413, 437, 438, 440, 493, 507, 511, 526, 554, 556, 578, 587, 595, 603, 608, 614, 616, 623, 627, 629, 632, 635, 643, 644, 653, 657, 670, 674, 676, 677, 702, 703, 720, 735, 737, 738, 754, 770, 791, 808, 821, 822, 825, 855, 875, 900, 903, 908, 909, 946, 965, 966, 967, 977, 997, 998, 1000

Nails

15, 16, 21, 27, 37, 38, 45, 65, 66, 102, 131, 156, 160, 168, 179, 252, 259, 262, 281, 334, 337, 362, 382, 409, 411, 511, 558, 559, 570, 589, 609, 615, 621, 703, 704, 788, 789, 811, 821, 825, 833, 846, 874, 880, 965, 975

TABLE XXIX
BIRTH DEFECTS WHICH MAY INVOLVE THE SKELETAL SYSTEM

Skeletal system

1, 8, 9, 10, 13, 14, 16, 17, 18, 19, 20, 21, 22, 25, 27, 28, 29, 37, 39, 47, 51, 52, 55, 65, 66, 69, 72, 73, 85, 88, 89, 90, 91, 94, 97, 98, 100, 101, 103, 104, 105, 106, 112, 114, 115, 118, 119, 121, 122, 128, 129, 137, 138, 139, 140, 142, 145, 150, 153, 154, 155, 156, 157, 158, 159, 160, 161, 162, 163, 164, 165, 166, 167, 168, 169, 170, 171, 172, 173, 174, 175, 177, 178, 179, 180, 181, 182, 183, 185, 187, 188, 189, 190, 193, 202, 216, 221, 222, 223, 224, 225, 226, 227, 228, 229, 230, 231, 238, 239, 242, 244, 247, 250, 257, 259, 261, 262, 263, 264, 265, 270, 274, 280, 281, 282, 283, 290, 292, 293, 295, 299, 301, 302, 303, 304, 305, 306, 308, 310, 311, 325, 329, 335, 336, 337, 338, 343, 345, 346, 352, 358, 364, 370, 373, 374, 375, 376, 377, 379, 380, 381, 382, 383, 384, 385, 386, 387, 388, 389, 390, 391, 392, 393, 394, 398, 401, 403, 406, 408, 409, 411, 412, 413, 423, 424, 425, 426, 431, 440, 441, 443, 445, 447, 450, 451, 455, 458, 459, 460, 470, 474, 477, 478, 480, 481, 491, 492, 494, 496, 497, 498, 499, 501, 505, 506, 508, 510, 515, 516, 517, 526, 531, 532, 536, 539, 542, 543, 544, 555, 556, 557, 560, 562, 570, 572, 574, 576, 578, 586, 587, 588, 592, 593, 598, 599, 601, 602, 603, 616, 621, 627, 629, 630, 632, 634, 635, 638, 641, 642, 644, 646, 647, 648, 649, 650, 651, 652, 653, 654, 655, 656, 658, 659, 662, 664, 667, 670, 671, 672, 673, 674, 675, 676, 677, 678, 679, 680, 682, 685, 687, 689, 691, 696, 700, 703, 704, 711, 712, 720, 722, 724, 727, 728, 730, 735, 737, 738, 749, 750, 754, 759, 763, 765, 769, 770, 771, 774, 775, 776, 777, 778, 779, 780, 781, 782, 783, 785, 786, 788, 791, 798, 801, 802, 803, 808, 810, 812, 813, 814, 817, 818, 821, 823, 824, 825, 826, 828, 830, 843, 846, 847, 853, 854, 856, 859, 864, 873, 874, 875, 876, 880, 881, 882, 883, 884, 885, 886, 887, 891, 893, 894, 895, 896, 897, 898, 899, 900, 901, 902, 908, 915, 923, 924, 939, 940, 941, 946, 947, 948, 949, 952, 960, 965, 966, 967, 975, 976, 977, 978, 980, 981, 982, 985, 986, 987, 998, 999, 1000, 1001, 1004

Brachycephaly

10, 16, 118, 139, 168, 171, 185, 225, 226, 227, 229, 242, 305, 370, 398, 440, 510, 554, 556, 578, 635, 738, 893

Macrocephaly > 2 SD for age

9, 10, 115, 122, 137, 188, 227, 302, 480, 481, 644, 674, 676, 711, 776, 780, 825, 876, 940

Microcephaly < 2 SD for age

97, 104, 119, 138, 140, 154, 158, 159, 160, 161, 163, 164, 165, 166, 167, 168, 170, 171, 174, 180, 182, 189, 226, 227, 229, 242, 281, 299, 306, 337, 379, 381, 382, 383, 384, 387, 388, 424, 492, 506, 578, 587, 603, 634, 638, 659, 662, 727, 737, 759, 769, 783, 808, 875, 881, 885, 891, 967, 1004

Scaphocephaly

20, 112, 162, 227, 230, 231, 370, 401, 517, 629, 630, 672, 674, 676, 891

Stature short > 2 SD below appropriate mean

8, 9, 10, 16, 19, 20, 98, 100, 105, 112, 114, 119, 121, 122, 153, 155, 156, 161, 163, 171, 185, 188, 189, 190, 223, 224, 226, 227, 239, 242, 250, 281, 293, 299, 302, 303, 306, 308, 310, 358, 379, 381, 382, 384, 385, 388, 389, 394, 425, 426, 445, 447, 470, 506, 510, 516, 517, 542, 543, 554, 557, 578, 632, 638, 646, 647, 648, 649, 650, 652, 653, 654, 655, 656, 667, 671, 673, 674, 679, 680, 685, 703, 720, 738, 754, 775, 776, 777, 782, 798, 823, 828, 830, 843, 846, 876, 881, 882, 885, 887, 891, 893, 896, 897, 898, 899, 902, 908, 940, 947, 966, 967, 976, 977, 980, 982, 998, 999, 1000, 1004

Tall > 2 SD above appropriate mean

85, 90, 137, 556, 578, 670

Kyphosis

103, 140, 166, 189, 281, 293, 352, 398, 474, 629, 632, 672, 674, 679, 720, 782, 899, 999

Kyphoscoliosis

85, 122, 155, 157, 190, 557, 593, 630, 652, 656, 672, 712, 759, 777, 798, 999

Lordosis

20, 103, 250, 290, 292, 352, 394, 412, 557, 644, 646, 678, 687, 689, 754, 828

Scoliosis

19, 88, 101, 122, 140, 153, 163, 185, 250, 270, 281, 290, 293, 388, 394, 412, 474, 644, 685, 704, 720, 735, 750, 823, 828, 847, 881, 895, 924, 967

Ectrodactyly

65, 242, 281, 336, 337, 375, 451, 459, 592, 700, 813, 818, 875

Polydactyly

8, 17, 22, 55, 85, 89, 91, 121, 139, 156, 157, 158, 160, 166, 168, 171, 172, 178, 181, 223, 229, 242, 281, 379, 392, 450, 556, 578, 634, 644, 649, 662, 737, 814, 817, 880, 883, 884, 887, 923, 952, 966, 980, 981, 987

Brachydactyly

1, 8, 13, 16, 19, 20, 21, 22, 114, 121, 156, 158, 160, 171, 189, 190, 224, 229, 242, 262, 281, 293, 306, 358, 382, 389, 392, 398, 409, 413, 445, 459, 506, 578, 621, 667, 700, 737, 786, 813, 818, 823, 828, 846, 874, 875, 887, 923, 940, 941, 967, 981, 1001

Syndactyly

1, 13, 14, 22, 55, 97, 121, 158, 160, 163, 168, 169, 172, 177, 179, 229, 242, 259, 293, 337, 374, 376, 393, 506, 554, 574, 578, 605, 616, 634, 662, 737, 754, 769, 813, 817, 818, 874, 880, 885, 887, 891, 923

TABLE XXX
BIRTH DEFECTS WHICH MAY INVOLVE THE MUSCULAR SYSTEM

Muscular defects

2, 11, 12, 26, 47, 48, 80, 88, 89, 93, 100, 107, 113,
115, 116, 118, 121, 122, 124, 125, 134, 139, 140, 143,
152, 155, 158, 159, 160, 161, 163, 165, 166, 170, 171,
172, 175, 188, 221, 242, 270, 275, 288, 289, 290, 292,
295, 352, 376, 382, 398, 403, 406, 421, 425, 429, 430,
432, 434, 450, 455, 457, 460, 486, 491, 492, 499, 505,
508, 543, 560, 568, 578, 587, 590, 603, 628, 629, 630,
632, 638, 641, 644, 651, 664, 671, 678, 686, 687, 688,
689, 690, 691, 692, 694, 695, 696, 697, 698, 700, 701,
702, 736, 754, 755, 759, 776, 783, 785, 794, 795, 796,
810, 813, 820, 822, 823, 847, 849, 850, 851, 864, 873,
891, 895, 897, 901, 924, 940, 944, 946, 949, 967, 990,
998, 999

TABLE XXXI
BIRTH DEFECTS WHICH MAY INVOLVE THE RESPIRATORY SYSTEM

Respiratory defects

24, 27, 39, 51, 74, 75, 76, 77, 79, 80, 91, 92, 96,
107, 117, 120, 121, 122, 138, 139, 140, 152, 156, 165,
180, 181, 183, 187, 189, 200, 203, 218, 237, 242, 257,
261, 263, 283, 285, 286, 288, 289, 297, 298, 332, 333,
338, 347, 363, 365, 366, 367, 368, 369, 381, 384, 385,
387, 396, 401, 403, 406, 443, 451, 457, 470, 471, 499,
513, 515, 521, 522, 525, 528, 531, 539, 541, 543, 549,
557, 570, 571, 572, 573, 574, 575, 576, 577, 581, 598,
601, 605, 606, 610, 611, 612, 628, 630, 634, 665, 674,
676, 678, 680, 702, 706, 714, 717, 722, 727, 731, 754,
760, 766, 767, 768, 777, 800, 805, 810, 816, 820, 825,
835, 836, 837, 838, 839, 842, 856, 859, 860, 879, 883,
884, 895, 914, 918, 919, 938, 940, 944, 945, 946, 947,
960, 967, 968, 969, 972, 975, 979, 982, 986, 989, 990

Dyspnea or stridor

39, 75, 80, 91, 107, 122, 140, 180, 200, 257, 261,
283, 289, 347, 363, 365, 368, 383, 384, 401, 406, 451,
499, 515, 519, 557, 570, 571, 572, 574, 576, 577, 598,
674, 676, 722, 727, 766, 805, 810, 837, 856, 883, 884,
914, 918, 919, 940, 946, 990

Cyanosis

24, 39, 76, 79, 91, 165, 189, 242, 283, 286, 289,
297, 332, 338, 365, 401, 403, 513, 541, 610, 665, 727,
766, 768, 825, 837, 842, 919, 938, 960, 969, 972, 989

TABLE XXXII
BIRTH DEFECTS WHICH MAY INVOLVE HEART OR VESSELS

CV system

11, 14, 24, 26, 28, 37, 39, 47, 51, 53, 55, 64, 69,
73, 74, 76, 77, 78, 79, 80, 82, 83, 88, 91, 92, 95,
96, 97, 104, 108, 109, 116, 121, 123, 127, 138, 139,
154, 156, 157, 159, 160, 161, 162, 163, 164, 165, 166,
167, 168, 170, 171, 172, 173, 176, 181, 182, 186, 204,
217, 218, 236, 242, 263, 265, 285, 286, 297, 298, 300,
332, 335, 338, 346, 347, 348, 351, 353, 354, 364, 379,
381, 382, 384, 385, 386, 387, 388, 389, 398, 401, 404,
420, 424, 440, 441, 450, 454, 455, 460, 464, 466, 468,
474, 484, 505, 506, 508, 528, 530, 531, 532, 540, 541,
544, 546, 570, 578, 581, 586, 587, 590, 592, 593, 603,
606, 610, 629, 630, 632, 634, 662, 665, 666, 667, 668,
669, 672, 673, 674, 675, 678, 680, 689, 695, 697, 698,
702, 712, 720, 727, 731, 735, 748, 754, 767, 768, 776,
777, 785, 795, 800, 805, 810, 816, 820, 822, 825, 829,
832, 835, 836, 837, 838, 839, 842, 856, 860, 874, 879,
883, 885, 888, 895, 902, 903, 916, 917, 922, 938, 939,
941, 943, 946, 952, 960, 968, 969, 972, 977, 979, 985,
987, 989, 990, 998, 999, 1002

Blood vessel defects

24, 28, 53, 55, 74, 80, 81, 82, 88, 95, 121,
138, 139, 154, 156, 157, 159, 160, 161, 162, 163, 164,
165, 166, 167, 168, 170, 171, 172, 176, 182, 217, 219,
242, 263, 300, 338, 347, 379, 381, 384, 388, 389, 401,
404, 440, 455, 464, 468, 474, 505, 506, 527, 530, 532,
544, 570, 578, 586, 593, 603, 606, 630, 632, 634, 662,
667, 673, 675, 678, 680, 720, 735, 754, 777, 807, 816,
829, 832, 835, 841, 842, 856, 860, 874, 879, 885, 888,
916, 941, 952, 962, 972, 977, 985, 987, 999, 1002

TABLE XXXIII
BIRTH DEFECTS WHICH MAY INVOLVE THE LIVER OR SPLEEN

Liver

7, 27, 39, 48, 87, 104, 110, 116, 121, 124, 139, 143,
149, 151, 160, 189, 222, 237, 340, 381, 384, 385, 387,
395, 398, 403, 406, 409, 424, 425, 426, 427, 430, 431,
432, 433, 443, 446, 452, 458, 460, 463, 465, 466, 467,
468, 469, 487, 489, 491, 499, 500, 501, 503, 525, 544,
568, 587, 598, 603, 605, 606, 634, 662, 671, 674, 676,
677, 679, 680, 717, 748, 780, 820, 842, 859, 888, 939,
961, 969, 978, 990, 1003

Hepatomegaly

48, 87, 104, 110, 121, 139, 151, 189, 340, 381, 384,
385, 387, 395, 403, 406, 409, 424, 425, 426, 427, 430,
431, 433, 443, 458, 489, 491, 499, 500, 501, 603, 671,
674, 676, 680, 717, 780, 842, 939, 978, 1003

Hepatosplenomegaly
143, 503, 677, 679

Splenomegaly

48, 110, 151, 189, 340, 381, 384, 385, 387, 403, 406,
409, 420, 431, 433, 442, 458, 468, 489, 491, 499, 500,
501, 521, 603, 671, 672, 674, 676, 680, 717, 780, 821,
852, 886, 892, 939, 944, 978, 1003

TABLE XXXIV
BIRTH DEFECTS WHICH MAY INVOLVE THE GI SYSTEM

Gastrointestinal

2, 9, 10, 12, 14, 15, 23, 24, 25, 26, 27, 28, 40, 48, 54, 55, 62, 63, 69, 72, 74, 75, 86, 92, 100, 104, 107, 110, 112, 113, 121, 138, 139, 140, 148, 149, 160, 161, 162, 163, 167, 168, 174, 188, 192, 193, 194, 237, 240, 265, 275, 289, 299, 300, 329, 335, 338, 346, 347, 350, 351, 362, 363, 364, 365, 366, 367, 368, 369, 376, 386, 388, 395, 401, 403, 404, 405, 406, 412, 419, 420, 421, 422, 424, 425, 426, 451, 460. 466, 467, 468, 469, 471, 485, 489, 491, 499, 506, 509, 513, 514, 515, 521, 522, 523, 524, 525, 528, 529, 531, 532, 533, 534, 535, 536, 537, 542, 544, 545, 547, 549, 566, 567, 569, 571, 574, 577, 578, 597, 603, 604, 605, 606, 628, 633, 634, 645, 653, 657, 662, 671, 672, 677, 681, 693, 697, 702, 727, 729, 748, 754, 766, 793, 808, 812, 816, 820, 822, 823, 826, 829, 832, 848, 850, 851, 852, 856, 859, 863, 873, 877, 884, 885, 886, 888, 891, 892, 894, 900, 905, 906, 909, 910, 911, 912, 913, 914, 918. 920, 943, 944, 946, 949, 960, 963, 974, 978, 981, 987, 988, 990, 991, 995, 999, 1003

Diarrhea

2, 15, 24, 27, 48, 112, 148, 265, 299, 350, 351, 403, 419, 491, 514, 515, 522, 523, 524, 525, 531, 533, 534, 535, 566, 567, 569, 657, 729, 812, 820, 885, 920, 943, 944, 978, 1003

Vomiting

12, 23, 24, 26, 40, 54, 62, 86, 100, 107, 174, 188, 193, 194, 265, 275, 299, 300, 346, 366, 395, 403, 421, 422, 471, 485, 489, 491, 509, 531, 532, 534, 537, 547, 566, 569, 628, 697, 793, 808, 826, 829, 848, 850, 863, 891, 905, 906, 909, 910, 911, 912, 913, 978, 990, 995, 999, 1003

TABLE XXXV
BIRTH DEFECTS WHICH MAY INVOLVE THE GU SYSTEM

The GU system

29, 30, 37, 42, 47, 49, 50, 68, 69, 70, 72, 88, 91, 93, 97, 101, 104, 105, 116, 118, 119, 121, 125, 128, 138, 139, 140, 148, 155, 156, 157, 159, 160, 161, 162, 163, 164, 166, 167, 168, 169, 170, 171, 173, 181, 189, 192, 193, 194, 222, 229, 236, 238, 239, 240, 242, 254, 255, 258, 264, 287, 292, 294, 300, 301, 302, 303, 305, 329, 337, 350, 364, 373, 375, 383, 385, 386, 388, 389, 391, 395, 401, 408, 412, 418, 436, 437, 438, 440, 441, 442, 443, 447, 458, 460, 469, 474, 483, 490, 498, 499, 502, 505, 506, 508, 517, 518, 520, 529, 531, 532, 535, 536, 544, 556, 571, 574, 578, 580, 586, 587, 588, 590, 603, 605, 616, 629, 632, 634, 635, 662, 681, 682, 683, 684, 693, 698, 702, 704, 708, 710, 711, 720, 727, 730, 732, 736, 741, 748, 754, 755, 785, 810, 815, 818, 823, 825, 829, 831, 855, 856, 857, 858, 859, 860, 861, 862, 863, 864, 873, 876, 877, 881, 883, 884, 885, 886, 887, 891, 894, 895, 902, 903, 904, 908, 909, 943, 944, 952, 960, 971, 974, 975, 977, 981, 984, 985, 987, 999

TABLE XXXVI
BIRTH DEFECTS WHICH MAY INVOLVE THE NERVOUS SYSTEM

Nervous system

2, 7, 10, 12, 13, 15, 24, 25, 27, 40, 44, 48, 59, 63, 69, 74, 75, 80, 86, 87, 89, 93, 94, 97, 101, 103, 104, 112, 113, 117, 118, 121, 123, 126, 127, 135, 136, 137, 139, 143, 145, 147, 150, 152, 154, 157, 158, 160, 161, 164, 166, 168, 174, 180, 181, 182, 186, 187, 188, 191, 203, 220, 221, 224, 227, 228, 229, 234, 239, 248, 251, 255, 262, 265, 266, 270, 274, 275, 283, 292, 295, 303, 307, 310, 314, 340, 344, 345, 346, 351, 363, 368, 373, 375, 376, 377, 378, 379, 380, 381, 384, 385, 387, 389, 395, 396, 398, 401, 402, 403, 406, 410, 413, 415, 421, 422, 423, 424, 425, 431, 432, 433, 434, 450, 451, 453, 460, 469, 472, 473, 474, 478, 480, 481, 485, 486, 492, 497, 498, 499, 502, 503, 508, 509, 512, 513, 514, 515, 517, 519, 521, 524, 526, 530, 531, 547, 550, 554, 556, 571, 572, 575, 578, 579, 588, 593, 598, 602, 603, 628, 629, 634, 635, 638, 642, 643, 651, 657, 658, 659, 664, 670, 671, 672, 675, 676, 677, 678, 686, 689, 690, 692, 693, 695, 696, 697, 702, 703, 712, 713, 717, 726, 727, 730, 736, 741, 742, 743, 744, 745, 746, 747, 748, 750, 752, 753, 754, 755, 759, 763, 777, 779, 780, 782, 791, 794, 795, 803, 805, 808, 810, 820, 822, 823, 824, 825, 826, 830, 832, 849, 850, 851, 859, 873, 880, 881, 886, 894, 895, 915, 921, 924, 940, 943, 949, 957, 961, 963, 964, 974, 975, 978, 991, 992, 995, 999, 1004

Structural defects of CNS

10, 69, 103, 104, 121, 139, 157, 158, 160, 161, 168, 182, 186, 188, 220, 227, 234, 283, 292, 375, 380, 381, 387, 389, 401, 473, 478, 480, 481, 485, 517, 526, 531, 571, 578, 593, 602, 603, 629, 634, 635, 642, 678, 693, 727, 742, 743, 744, 745, 746, 747, 748, 754, 780, 824, 859, 881, 894, 924

Neurologic dysfunction

2, 7, 94, 103, 126, 135, 187, 188, 203, 255, 344, 398, 402, 406, 421, 478, 515, 519, 547, 578, 579, 588, 598, 638, 671, 675, 697, 712, 717, 742, 777, 782, 810, 820, 822, 850, 894, 921, 957, 961, 963, 978, 992, 1004

Behavioral or psychologic defect

12, 15, 86, 93, 112, 135, 152, 203, 221, 229, 239, 255, 307, 314, 381, 384, 406, 415, 422, 423, 453, 469, 472, 478, 485, 492, 498, 509, 556, 588, 598, 603, 635, 675, 676, 677, 713, 730, 808, 820, 822, 823, 850, 886, 974, 978, 991

Altered consciousness or mentation

12, 40, 80, 86, 87, 93, 103, 123, 127, 145, 174, 248, 255, 310, 396, 406, 424, 432, 460, 478, 485, 512, 530, 547, 598, 628, 651, 658, 676, 677, 702, 713, 730, 744, 805, 820, 822, 826, 949, 995,

Altered reflexes

2, 48, 139, 143, 265, 275, 295, 303, 307, 413, 486, 492, 499, 515, 578, 628, 629, 671, 686, 689, 693, 695, 696, 736, 742, 743, 746, 750, 755, 759, 808, 810, 823, 850, 895, 924, 940

(Continued)

TABLE XXXVI (Continued)

Seizures

24, 25, 44, 87, 118, 126, 135, 139, 143, 158, 164,
166, 174, 186, 188, 203, 224, 227, 229, 255, 262, 340,
381, 387, 389, 395, 396, 398, 403, 406, 410, 415, 424,
425, 431, 432, 433, 434, 469, 473, 478, 486, 492, 498,
499, 502, 512, 513, 514, 515, 517, 530, 578, 593, 603,
628, 638, 643, 657, 658, 659, 670, 671, 672, 695, 712,
713, 717, 741, 754, 759, 791, 808, 820, 822, 826, 830,
849, 850, 851, 873, 915, 943, 961, 975, 991

Ataxia

2, 12, 13, 87, 93, 94, 136, 188, 255, 344, 432,
485, 508, 547, 638, 651, 671, 713, 717, 742, 743, 744,
745, 746, 747, 755, 759, 803, 849, 850, 851, 963, 995
1004

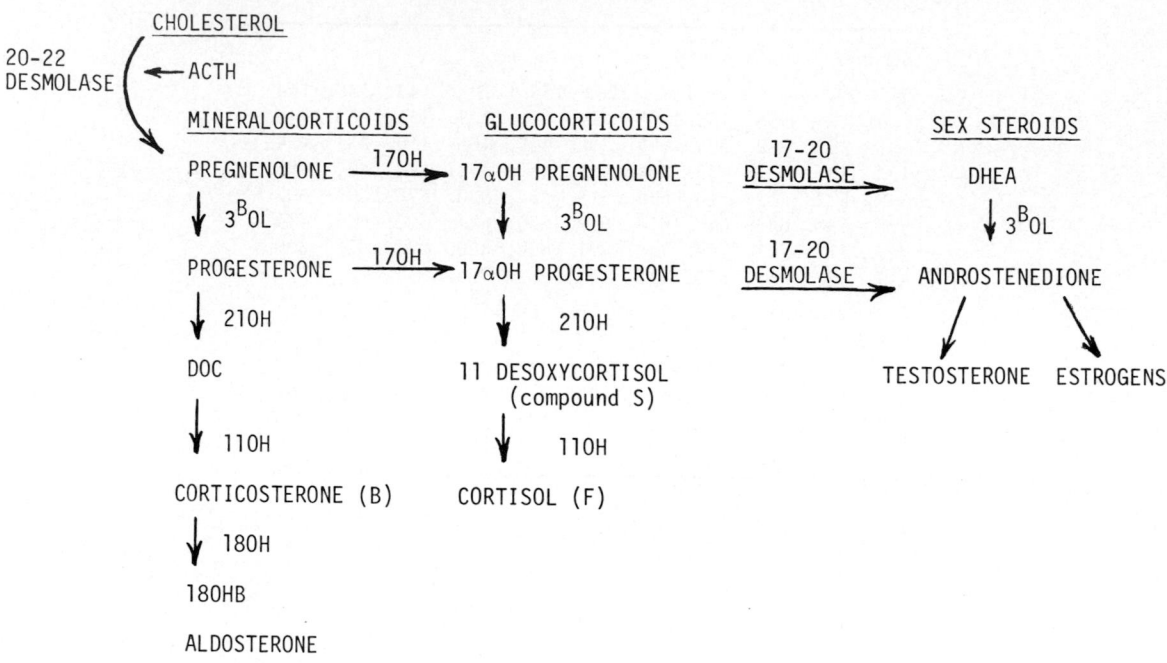

DIAGRAM I
SIMPLIFIED SCHEME OF STEROIDOGENESIS IN THE ADRENAL GLAND

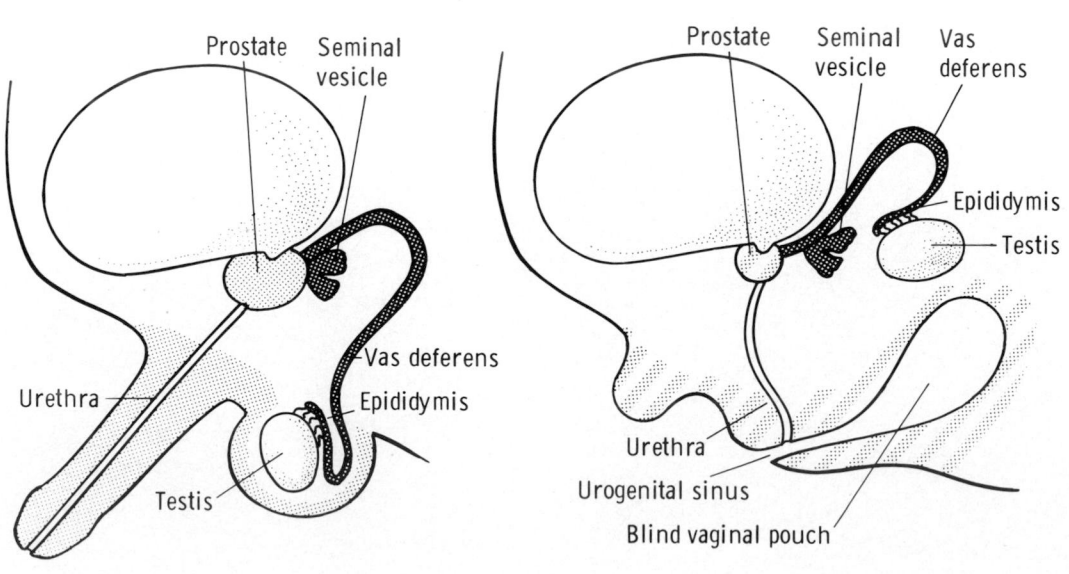

DIAGRAM II
ROLE OF TESTOSTERONE AND DIHYDROTESTOSTERONE
IN SEXUAL DIFFERENTIATION IN UTERO

DIAGRAM III

HYPOSPADIAS ASSOCIATED WITH MATERNAL TREATMENT WITH PROGESTINS

POSITION OF MEATUS	AGENT	DOSE mg/day	WEEK OF GESTATION (2 6 10 14 18 22)
	MEDROXYPROGESTERONE	10	
	NOR-ETHISTERONE	5	
	UNKNOWN	?	
	HYDROXYPROGESTERONE CAPROATE	250 (i m)	
	NOR-ETHISTERONE	10	
	MEDROXYPROGESTERONE	5	
	NOR-ETHISTERONE	5	
	METHYLESTRADIOL	0.3	
	NOR-ETHISTERONE	10	
	ETHINYLESTRADIOL	0.02	
	NOR-ETHISTERONE	20	

DIAGRAM IV

GONADAL DYSGENESIS AND ITS VARIANTS

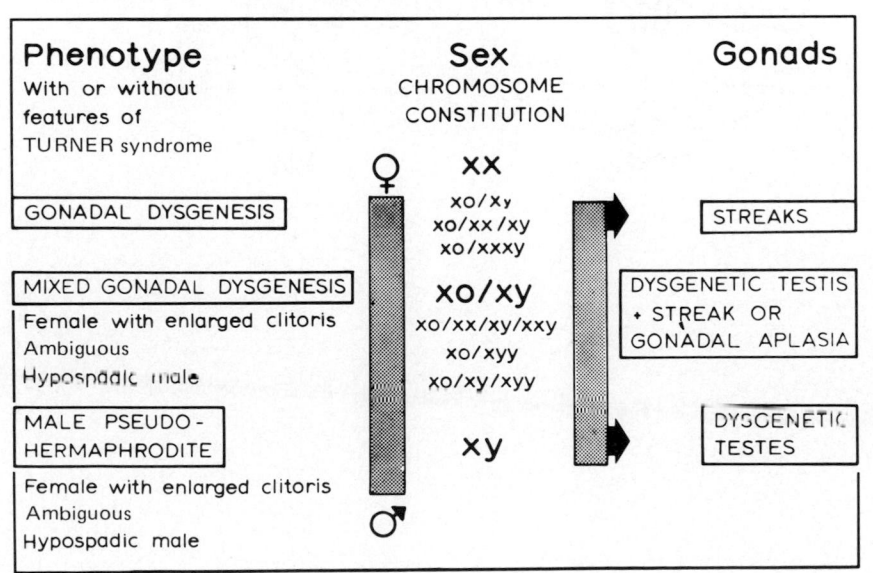

Phenotype With or without features of TURNER syndrome	Sex CHROMOSOME CONSTITUTION	Gonads
GONADAL DYSGENESIS	XX / xo/xy / xo/xx/xy / xo/xxxy	STREAKS
MIXED GONADAL DYSGENESIS — Female with enlarged clitoris, Ambiguous, Hypospadic male	xo/xy / xo/xx/xy/xxy / xo/xyy / xo/xy/xyy	DYSGENETIC TESTIS + STREAK OR GONADAL APLASIA
MALE PSEUDO-HERMAPHRODITE — Female with enlarged clitoris, Ambiguous, Hypospadic male	xy	DYSGENETIC TESTES

DIAGRAM V

EXTERNAL GENITAL DIFFERENTIATION IN THE HUMAN FETUS

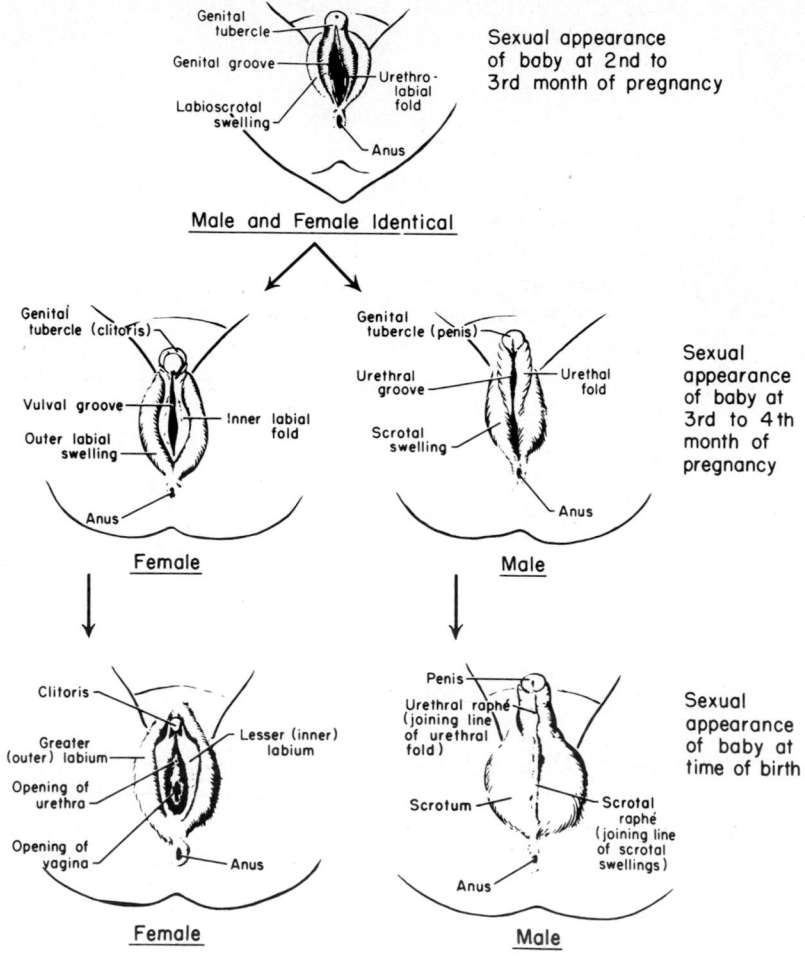

Genital tubercle

Genital groove

Labioscrotal swelling

Urethro-labial fold

Anus

Sexual appearance of baby at 2nd to 3rd month of pregnancy

Male and Female Identical

Genital tubercle (clitoris)

Vulval groove

Outer labial swelling

Inner labial fold

Anus

Female

Genital tubercle (penis)

Urethral groove

Scrotal swelling

Urethal fold

Anus

Male

Sexual appearance of baby at 3rd to 4th month of pregnancy

Clitoris

Greater (outer) labium

Opening of urethra

Opening of vagina

Lesser (inner) labium

Anus

Female

Penis

Urethral raphé (joining line of urethral fold)

Scrotum

Anus

Scrotal raphé (joining line of scrotal swellings)

Male

Sexual appearance of baby at time of birth

DIAGRAM VI

SEXUAL DIFFERENTIATION IN THE HUMAN FETUS

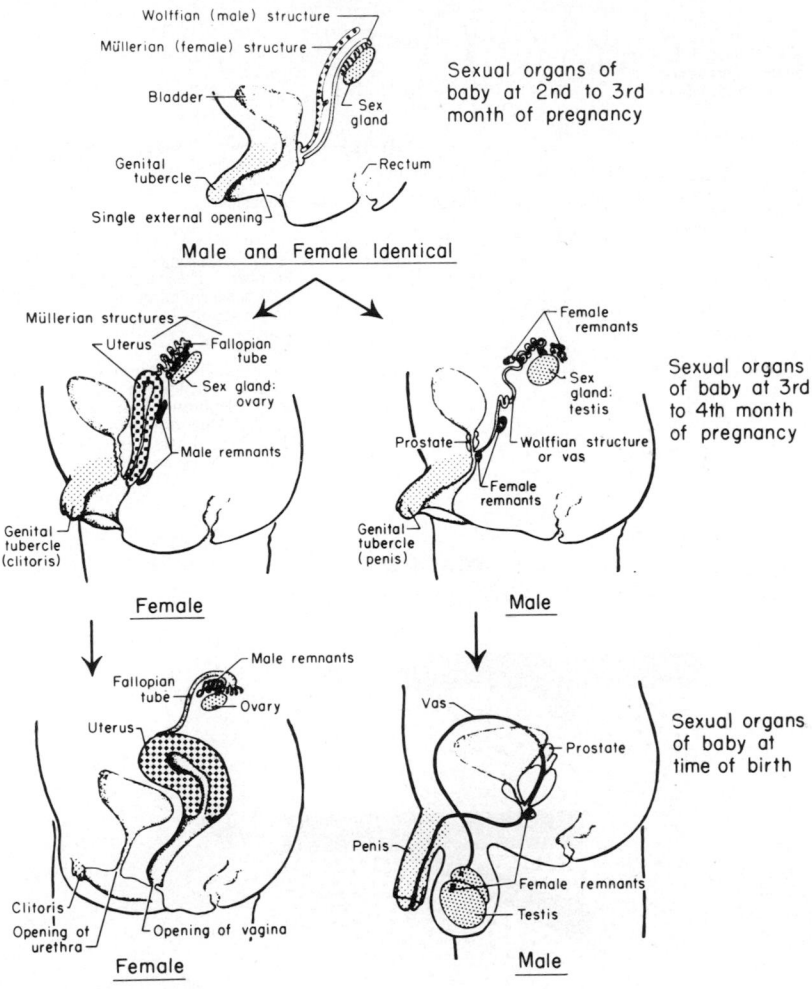

Wolffian (male) structure

Müllerian (female) structure

Bladder

Sex gland

Genital tubercle

Rectum

Single external opening

Sexual organs of baby at 2nd to 3rd month of pregnancy

Male and Female Identical

Müllerian structures

Uterus

Fallopian tube

Sex gland: ovary

Male remnants

Genital tubercle (clitoris)

Female

Female remnants

Sex gland: testis

Prostate

Wolffian structure or vas

Female remnants

Genital tubercle (penis)

Male

Sexual organs of baby at 3rd to 4th month of pregnancy

Male remnants

Fallopian tube

Ovary

Uterus

Clitoris

Opening of urethra

Opening of vagina

Female

Vas

Prostate

Penis

Female remnants

Testis

Male

Sexual organs of baby at time of birth

DIAGRAM VII

ALLOTRANSPLANTATION IN GENETIC DISEASES

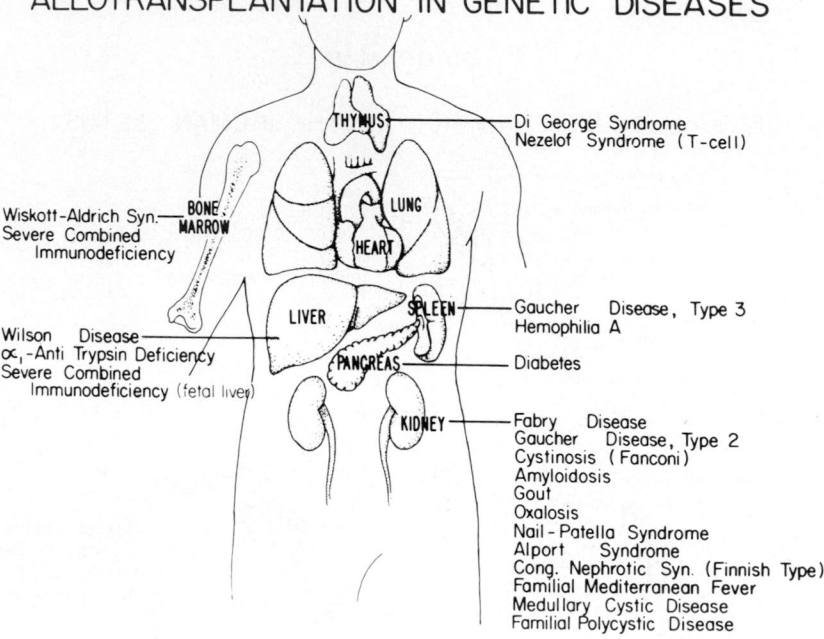

THYMUS — Di George Syndrome / Nezelof Syndrome (T-cell)

Wiskott-Aldrich Syn. / Severe Combined Immunodeficiency — BONE MARROW

LUNG

HEART

Wilson Disease / α_1-Anti Trypsin Deficiency / Severe Combined Immunodeficiency (fetal liver) — LIVER

SPLEEN — Gaucher Disease, Type 3 / Hemophilia A

PANCREAS — Diabetes

KIDNEY — Fabry Disease / Gaucher Disease, Type 2 / Cystinosis (Fanconi) / Amyloidosis / Gout / Oxalosis / Nail-Patella Syndrome / Alport Syndrome / Cong. Nephrotic Syn. (Finnish Type) / Familial Mediterranean Fever / Medullary Cystic Disease / Familial Polycystic Disease

DIAGRAM VIII
HAIR PATTERNING

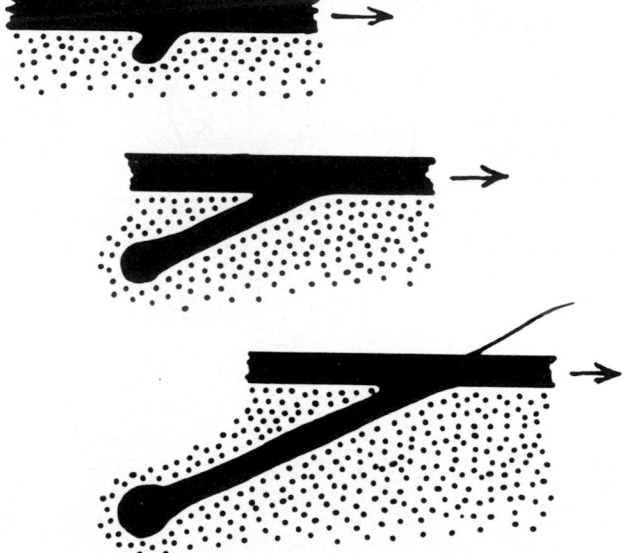

Hair follicles over scalp begin their downgrowth into the loose underlying mesenchyme at 10 fetal weeks. The slope of each hair follicle and thereby the hair directional pattern is determined by the direction of growth stretch (arrows) exerted on the surface skin by the development of underlying tissues. The scalp hair patterning relates to the growth in size and form of the underlying brain during the period 10–16 weeks. By 18 weeks when hairs are extruded onto the surface, their patterning is set.

DIAGRAM IX
HAIR PATTERNING

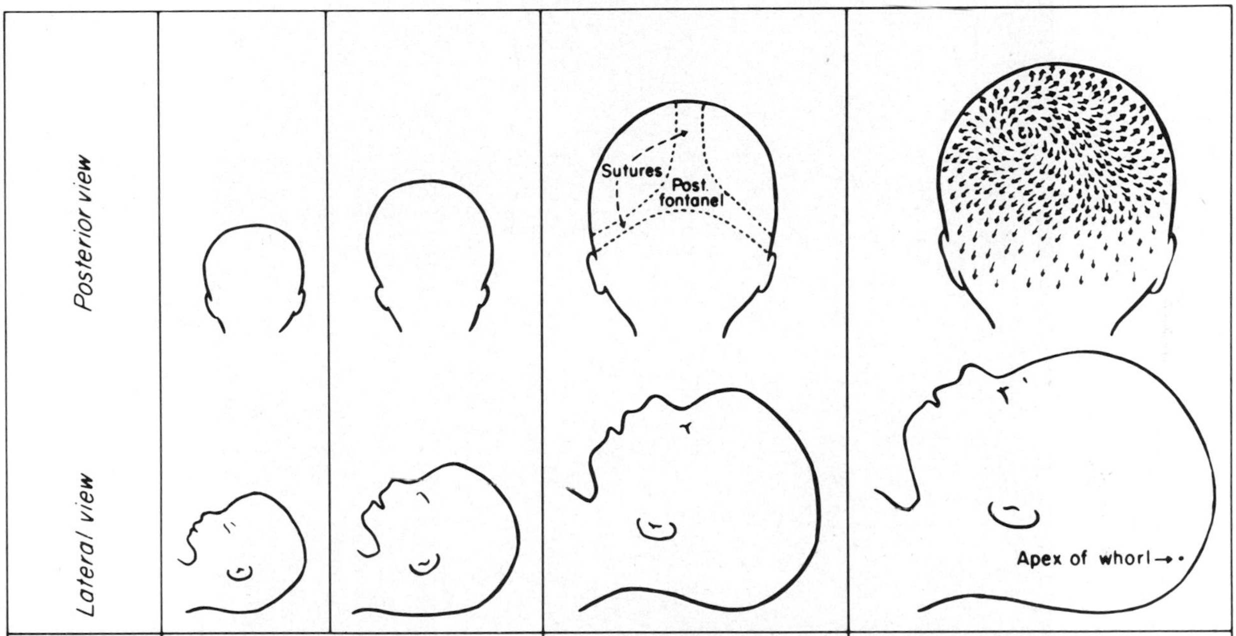

Hair	Early hair follicles with sloping downgrowth		Hair being produced	Surface hair patterning evident
Gestational age	11 weeks	12 ½ weeks	16 ½ weeks	18 weeks
C-R length	71 mm	83 mm	122 mm	145 mm

The rapid dome-like outgrowth of the upper head during the period of hair follicle downgrowth is evident in these proportionate tracings from fetuses.

DIAGRAM X
HAIR PATTERNING

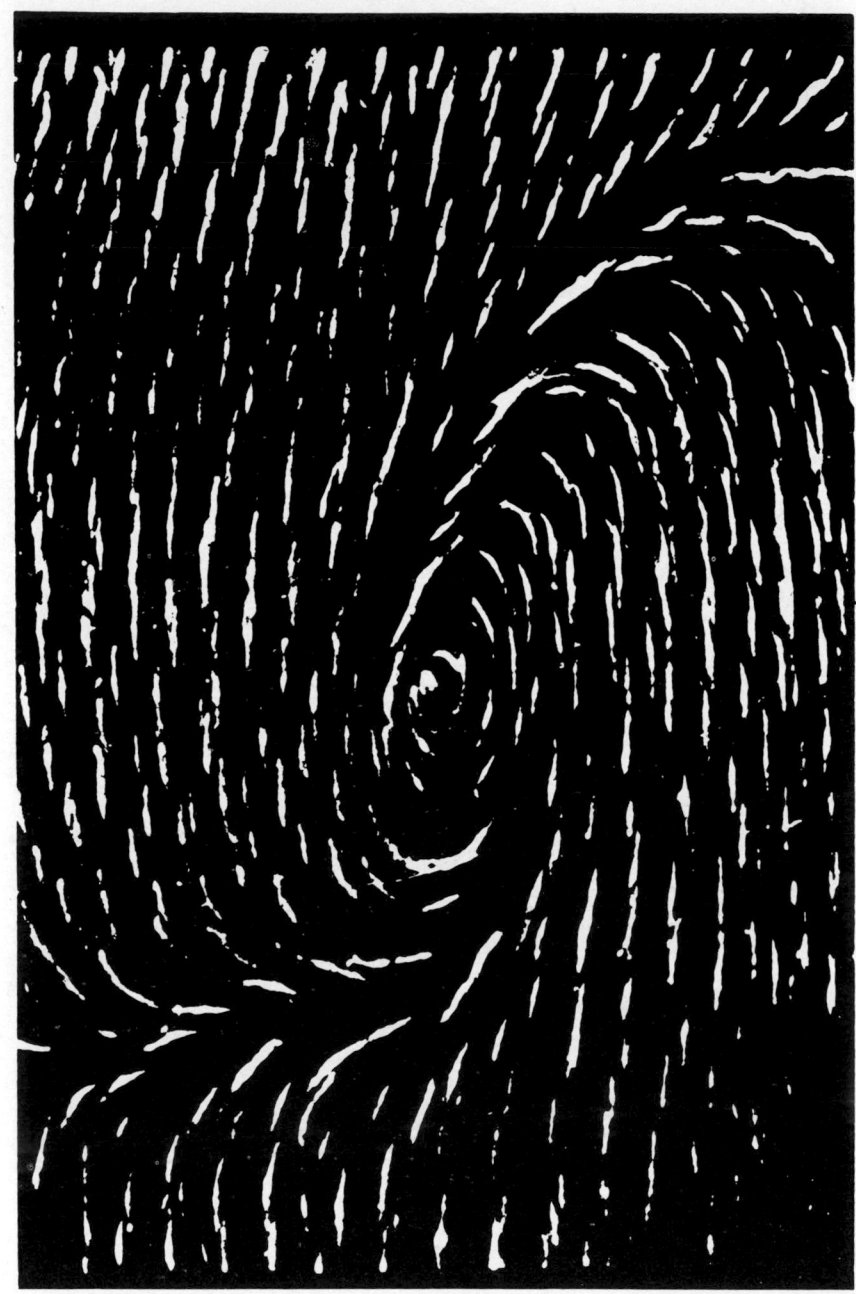

Parietal hair whorl at 18 weeks. This appears to be the focal fixed point from which the skin is under stretch by the dome-like outgrowth of the brain between 10−16 weeks.

Figure Credits

Aarskog, D., Diagrams III, IV
Abrams, A., 475
Agatston, H.J., 33
Allderdice, P.W., 177
American Journal of Diseases of Children (© AMA)
  151 **105**:588, 1963
  267 **123**:254, 1972
  455 **107**:49, 1964
American Journal of Human Genetics (U. of Chicago Press)
  175 **19**:586, 1967
  177 **20**:500, 1969
Annales de Génétique
  169 **10**:221, 1967
  170 **7**:17, 1964
Annales de Radiologie
  453 **16**:19, 1973
Annales Paediatrici (Basel)
  204 **199**:393, 1962
Annals of Internal Medicine
  449–452 **84(4)**:393, 1976
Archives of Dermatology (© AMA)
  295 **101**:669, 1970
Archives of Neurology (© AMA)
  143 **8**:318, 1963
Armstrong, H.B., 188
Aurbach, G.D., 433, 434
Ayerst Laboratory, 1, 7, 16, 25, 26, 29, 30, 33, 35, 36, 40–42, 52
Baller, F., 208
Bannerman, R.M., 463
Bart, B.J., 246, 425 (left), 501
Bartsocas, C.S., 391
Beaudet, A., Jr., 196
Becker, P.E., 411
Beighton, P., 166, 412, 449–452
Bergsma, D.R., 2, 3, 5, 8, 19–21
Bergstrom, L.V., 79, 93, 94, 96
Berman, P., 111
Bianchine, J.W., 181, 248, 414, 470
Bixler, D., 293, 421, 422
Borges, W., 106–108, Table XI
Bowen, P., 116, 159, 188, 256B
Brown, A.C., 344–346
Brown, K.S., 38
Brown, R., 24
Buckingham, R.A., 77, 78
Bulletin of The Johns Hopkins Hospital (© Johns Hopkins Press)
  159, 256B **114**:402, 1964
Buyse, M., 157, 252, 441
Carter, C.H., 214
Char, F., 174
Chase, L.R., 144, 145
Clinical Genetics
  160 **5**:294, 1974
  446 **5**:1, 1974
Coccaro, P.J., 286
Cogan, D.G., 399
Cohen, M.M., Jr., 134, 137, 139, 147, 189, 190, 192, 206, 210
  249–251, 270, 271, 287, 332, 386, 394, 400, 401, 405, 427B,
  428, 443, 469, 481, 490
Confina Neurologica (Basel)
  290 **23**:1, 1963
Curth, H.O., 112
Dallaire, L., 306
Danks, D.M., 267
Debauchez, C., 170
DeBlanc, G.D., 318

DeFraites, F., 427A
DeMyer, W., 290, 340, Tables XVI–XX
Dental Clinics of North America
  475 **19**:27, 1975
Desnick, R.J., Diagram VII
Dieker, H., 328, 329
Dorst, J.P., 296, 298
Doyle, P.J., 319
Drescher, E., 272, 273
Drews, R., 53, 54
Duhamel, B., 126
Durand, P., 268
Eastman Kodak ©, 109
Elsahy, N.I., 150
English, G.M., 318
Epstein, C.J., 496
Evans, P.Y., 6, 11–13, 15, 17, 18, 22, 27, 28, 31, 32, 43, 45–47,
  55, 59, 61, 65, 71, 75, 76, 92, 95
Excerpta Medica International Congress Series No. 55, Proc. XII
  Int. Cong. Derm.
  112 p. 331, 1962
Feingold, M., 67, 73, 74, 97, 207
Ferguson-Smith, M.A., 98, 493
Forsius, H., 444
Franceschetti, A.T., 259–261
Francke, U., 173
François, J., 127
Fraser, F.C., 247
Fraser, G.R., 215
Fraumeni, J.F., Jr., 288
Frenkel, J.K., 265
Fulginiti, V.A., 302
Gans, J.A., 1
Georgetown University Medical Center, 6, 11–13, 15, 17, 18, 22,
  27, 28, 31, 32, 43, 45–47, 55, 59, 61, 65, 71, 75, 76, 92, 95
Georg Thiem Verlag
  77, 78 "Atlas of Otorhinolaringology and Broncheoesophagology"
Gerber, P.H., 244
German, J., 70
Gier, R.E., 336, 337
Göbel, P., 465
Goldberg, M.F., 309, 397, 454
Goldstein, J.L., 292
Goodman, R.M., 120–122
Goodwin, B. (artist), 343
Gordon, H., 327
Gorlin, R.J., 128, 255, 278, 283, 291, 325, 326, 392, 393 (left),
  402
Gray, B.H., 280
Gutmann, L., 143
Hall, B.D., 284, 285, 388, 488
Hall, J.G., 297, 478, 479
Harrison, R., 10
Herrmann, J., 138, 158, 193–195, 289, 310, 311, 357, 358, 494,
  498, 499
Hoefnagel, R., 124, 136, 417, 418, 427C
Holder, T., 258
Holmes, L.B., 223
Honig, G.R., Table XI
Horven, I., 320
Houghton Mifflin Co., Boston
  212, 243 Winchester, A.M.: "Genetics: A Survey of the Principles
  of Heredity," 1966
Houston, F.M., 387
Howard, N., 262

Imbrie, J.D., 319
Imperato-McGinley, J., 435, 436, Diagram II
Jirásek, J.E., 301
Joab, N., 169
Jorgenson, R.J., 119A, 146, 168, 183, 187, 227, 229, 230, 238, 245, 307, 343, 356, 364, 375, 416, 474, 484
Journal of Bone and Joint Surgery
    412 58B:343, 1976
Journal of Pediatrics
    278 56:778, 1960
Kaufman, R.L., 144, 145, 236, 237
Keene, H.J., 330
Kelly, T.E., 185, 186, 362
Kenyon, K.R., 367
Keutel, J., 231
Knox, D., 255F
Kolker, A., 39, 68, 275
Kontras, S.B., 279
Kopits, S.E., 431
Kowlesser, M., 129
Krill, A.E., 4, 60, 63
Lamy, M.E., 355
Langer, L.O., Jr., 113
Lemli, L., 143
Lousiana State University, Department of Ophthalmology, 41, 42
Lowry, R.B., 316, 317, 489
Manhattan Eye, Ear and Throat Hospital, 50, 56
Masson et Cie, Paris
    126 Duhamel, B.: "Morphogenese Pathologique," 1966
Maumenee, A.E., 200, 201
McGuire, W.P., 14
McKusick, V.A., 115–118, 119B, 125, 133, 148, 149, 167, 181, 191, 197, 199, 202, 209, 211, 221, 222A, 224–226, 232, 235, 257, 277, 303–305, 308, 313, 321, 333–335, 341, 342, 347, 351–354, 360, 361, 365, 366, 369–371, 379, 381–385, 390, 404, 408, 413, 415, 425 (right), 429, 430, 437, 438, 442, 456, 495, Table I
Meskin, L., 90, 161
Messer, L.B., 473
Miller, O.J., 175, 176
Minas, T.F., 23
Minerva Pediatrica
    268 19:2187, 1967
Morillo-Cucci, G., 184
Nager, G.T., 110; 407
National Eye Institute, 2, 3, 5
National Institute of Dental Research, 38
National Institutes of Health, 24, 34, 44, 49, 51, 62
Neuhauser, E.D.B., 314
Neurology (© The New York Times Media Co., Inc.)
    340 17:961, 1967
Nichols, B.L., 198, 368
Nyhan, W., Tables II–X
Okun, E., 37
Opitz, J.M., 256A&C, 269, 294, 338, 339, 458B, 471B
Oral Surgery, Oral Medicine and Oral Pathology
    330 17:683, 1964
    472 18:409, 1964
Pallister, P.D., 409, 410
Passarge, E., 156, 453
Passmore, J.W., 16
Patterson, J.H., 322, 323
Pearlman, J.T., 52
Pearson, C.M., 376–378
Pediatrics
    288 40:886, 1967
    468 48:756, 1971
Pergamon Press Ltd., Oxford
    390 McKusick, V.A.: "Medical Genetics," 1961–1963
Perlman, A., 414
Pfeiffer, R., 205
Phelps, C., 34
Pillary, V.K., 445
Plastic and Reconstructive Surgery
    150 48:542, 1971
Podos, S.M., 9

Poznanski, A.K., 486, 487
Preus, M., 152, 153, 160
Pruzansky, S., 180
Radiology
    114 92:285, 1969
Rahn, E.K., 64
Reed, W.B., 254, 500
Reisner, S., 393 (right)
Rimoin, D.L., 114, 154, 203, 216–218, 233, 234, 239–242, 282, 300, 432, Table XXI
Robinow, M., 299, 363, 447
Rossier, A., 169
Rubinstein, J.H., 151
Rudd, N., 262
Ryan, T., 426
Scheinberg, H.I., 57, 58
Schimke, R.N., 155, 324, 420
Scott, C.I., Jr., 281, 372, 373, 423, 424, 459, 460
Seigel, J.M., 274
Sharkey, R., 100, 171, 179, 312, 440, 448, 480
Shearer, R.V., 7
Sheehan, V., 172
Siggers, D.S., 476, 477
Silver, H., 455
Sly, S., 374
Smith, D.W., 178, 263, Diagrams VIII–X
Smith, G.F., 213
Smith, M.E., 66
Sperling, M.A., 466, 467, 468, Diagram I
Spranger, J., 162, 163, 315, 359, 461, 462, 464
Sreebny, L., 482
Stevenson, R., 36
Stransky, E., 204
Sugar, H.S., 40
Sugarman, G.I., 164
Summitt, R.L., 140, 331, 348, 349, 389, 395, 396, 457, 458A, 471A, 497
Suskind, R., 295
Temtamy, S.A., 131, 132, 148, 149, 403, 439
The National Foundation, 69, 182
Thomas, Charles C, Springfield, Ill.
    214 Carter, C.H.: "Handbook of Mental Retardation Syndromes," 2nd Ed., 1970
Touloukian, R., 135
Townes, P.L., 228
Tucker, A., 141
Tulane University School of Medicine, 25, 26
Vachier, E., 446
Van Mierop, L.H., 142, 419
Via, W.F., Jr., 253
Visekul, C., 165
Walton, J.N., 380
Warburg, M., 222B, 264, 266
Weilbacher, S. (artist), 255F
Weyers, H., 123
Wilkins, L., Diagrams V, VI
Williams & Wilkins Co., Baltimore
    265 Frenkel, J.K.: Toxoplasmosis. In Marcial-Rojas, M.A. (ed.): "Pathology of Protozoal and Helminthic Diseases," 1971, pp 254–290
Wills Eye Hospital, 29, 30, 35
Wilson, M.G. 491, 492
Winchester, A.M., 212, 243
Witkop, C.J., Jr., 48, 72, 80–91, 99, 101–105, 130, 219, 220, 276, 398, 406, 472, 483, 485, Tables XII–XIV
Wood, B.P., 350
Woolf, C.M., Table XV
Year Book Medical Publishers, Inc., Chicago
    258 Holder, T.M. et al: Esophageal atresia and tracheo-esophageal fistula. In Ravitch, M.M. (ed.): "Current Problems in Surgery" © 1966
Young, L.W., 350
Zeitschrift für menschliche Vererbungs- und Konstitutionslehre
    208 29:782, 1950
Zeligman, I., 387

Author Index

Aarskog, D., **1**
Abele, D.C., **416**
Aberfeld, D.C., **155**
Abrams, A.M., **937**
Acquarelli, M.J., **797**
Aebi, H., **6**
Aleck, K., **672, 680, 782**
Alford, C.A., Jr., **385**
Allderdice, P.W., **167**
Alström, C.H., **41**
Ammann, A.J., **729**
Anast, C.S., **499, 514, 515, 873**
Arcilla, R.A., **53, 979**
Arias, I.M., **487, 961**
Armstrong, H.B., **179**
Ashcraft, K.W., **363, 364, 366, 367, 368, 369, 471**
Austin, J.H., **651**
Aziz, K.U., **581**

Baird, H.W., **393**
Barness, L.A., **485**
Barnhart, R.A., **70**
Barrett, J.L., **551**
Bart, B.J., **608, 609**
Bart, R.S., **558**
Bartoshesky, L.E., **895**
Beighton, P., **233, 507**
Bennhold, H., **47**
Bergren, W.R., **152, 403**
Bergsma, D.R., **43, 59, 130, 201, 234, 356, 371, 400, 479, 504, 548, 563, 565, 623, 705, 740, 750, 751, 752, 753, 834, 844, 869, 925, 983**
Bergstrom, L., **70, 97, 232, 247, 272, 273, 312, 313, 314, 315, 316, 317, 318, 320, 321, 324, 325, 326, 327, 328, 329, 330, 331, 377, 378, 448, 450, 508, 530, 562, 601, 619, 664, 724, 787, 799, 945**
Berman, M.A., **665, 666, 669, 969, 970**
Bernstein, J.M., **248**
Bieber, F.R., **266**
Bingol, N., **518, 859**
Bishop, H.C., **288**
Black, J.A., **305**
Blackfield, H.M., **374**
Blaine, R.W., **890**
Bland, J.H., **792**

Blass, J.P., **697, 850, 851**
Blizzard, R.M., **435**
Bloomer, W.E., **611**
Bodenhoff, J., **933**
Böök, J.A., **493**
Borges, W.H., **886, 939**
Bourland, B.J., **766**
Bowen, P., **179**
Breg, W.R., **163**
Bucciarelli, R.L., **83, 922**
Buyse, M., **578**

Calcaterra, T.C., **918**
Caplan, R.M., **599**
Carter, C.O., **423**
Carter, V.H., **561**
Cassidy, S.B., **157**
Cederbaum, S.D., **86, 697, 850, 851**
Červenka, J., **177, 319, 596,**
Christian, J.C., **505**
Clatworthy, H.W., Jr., **110, 149, 404, 463, 464, 465, 466, 467, 468, 604, 605, 606**
Clawson, C.C., **143**
Clendenning, W.E., **101**
Cleve, H., **446**
Cline, J.T., **340, 739, 927, 929, 930, 931, 932**
Cogan, D., **191**
Cohen, M.M., Jr., **28, 55, 104, 111, 182, 337, 375, 595, 618, 626, 627, 636**
Cohen, M.M., Sr., **594, 806**
Comings, D.E., **31, 827**
Cooper, L.Z., **384**
Cortner, J.A., **624, 625**
Crawhall, J.C., **106, 921**
Cremers, C.W.R.J., **12, 72, 89, 183, 206, 250, 253, 255, 258, 261, 262, 263, 265, 268, 275, 506, 592, 732, 759, 785, 863**
Crocker, A.C., **598, 717, 1003**
Cross, H.E., **32, 57, 58, 131, 132, 133, 413, 583, 584, 585, 733, 845**
Cunningham-Rundles, C., **525**
Curth, H.O., **5, 105, 526, 703**
Dahlberg, A.A., **607**
Dancis, J., **509, 547, 628**
Davidson, M., **566, 567, 920**
Davidson, R.G., **624, 625**
DeBusk, F., **825**

All index numbers refer to the Birth Defect Number — NOT page number.

DeGroot, L.J., 257
Dennis, N.R., 423
Derlacki, E.L., 150
Desnick, R.J., 373
DeWind, L.T., 257
Diamond, L.K., 4, 51, 420, 461, 462, 852, 996
Diamond, L.S., 874
Dolowitz, D.A., 267, 269, 708
Donnell, G.N., 152, 403
Downs, M.P., 271
Doyle, P.J., 577
‡Drescher, E., 411
Durand, P., 569
Duvall, A.J., III, 919

Edwards, J.E., 82
Eldjarn, L., 849
Elliott, L.P., 286, 541, 962, 968
Ellis, E.F., 92, 240
Ellsworth, R.M., 620, 721, 756, 757, 867, 870, 871, 872
Elsahy, N.I., 118
Engel, E., 157
English, G.M., 117, 283, 573, 575, 726
Erich, J.B., 725
Escher, F., 244
Eskritt, N.R., 65, 66
Esterly, J.R., 614
Evans, D.A.P., 7
Ewing, J.A., 741

Falls, H.F., 136, 195, 196, 197, 198, 199, 865
Favara, B.E., 990
Feingold, M., 457, 735, 997
Feinmesser, M., 252
Fenton, R.S., 722
Ferguson-Smith, M.A., 359
Fineman, R.M., 665
Fisher, D.A., 946, 950
Fitch, N., 629
Folger, G.M., Jr., 348, 349, 353, 354
Fonkalsrud, E.W., 300, 888
Fox, S.A., 296
Francke, U., 161, 162
Fraser, D., 516
Fraser, F.C., 334
Fraser, G.R., 123, 249, 550
Fraumeni, J.F., Jr., 458
Fredrickson, D.S., 48
Freeman, J.M., 137, 344, 643
Frichot, B.C., III, 56
Friedman, W.F., 78, 80, 81, 108, 916, 917
Frimpter, G.W., 236
Froesch, E.R., 395

Gaethe, G., 811
Gans, S.L., 545
Gardner, D.W., 499, 514, 515, 873
Gatti, R.A., 524
Gebhart, R.N., 797
Gentry, W.C., Jr., 259, 412
German, J.L., III, 112
Gerritsen, T., 503
Gessner, I.H., 286, 297, 298
Ghadimi, H., 472, 616

Giammona, S.T., 237
Giblett, E.R., 452
Gier, R.E., 631
Gilbert, E.F., 187
Gittinger, J.W., 752
Gitzelmann, R., 357, 396, 402
Goldberg, M.F., 18, 205, 207, 208, 209, 210, 211, 212, 213, 214, 215, 216, 282, 309, 552, 553, 637, 868
Goltz, R., 281
Good, R.A., 27, 94, 143, 521, 525
Goodman, R.M., 615
Goodman, S.I., 421, 422
Goodman, T.F., Jr., 416
Goodman, W.S., 722
Gorlin, R.J., 176, 440, 586, 730, 737, 770, 786
Graham, T.P., Jr., 64, 217, 218, 219
Grosfeld, J.L., 110, 149, 404, 463, 464, 465, 466, 467, 468, 604, 605, 606
Guerrero, J.R., 200, 527
Guggenheim, P., 706
Gupta, S., 54, 944

Hagan, P.J., 708
Halasz, N.A., 612
Hall, J.G., 85, 88, 226, 231, 389, 555, 828, 900, 941, 967
Hanson, J.W., 382, 388
Hardcastle, B., 727
Haslam, R.H.A., 103, 135, 295, 376, 712, 924, 964, 975, 995
Hastings, N., 532
Hatch, F.T., 489, 488, 495, 496, 500, 501
Hawkins, I.F., Jr., 968
Hays, D.M., 531
Hayward, J.R., 61
Hecht, F., 160, 165, 166, 168
Hellenbrand, W.E., 665, 666, 669, 969, 970
Herrmann, J., 138, 451, 470, 554, 791, 875, 981, 1001
Hildyard, V.H., 530
Hillman, R.E., 40
Hintz, R.L., 473
Hognestad, S., 246
Holder, T.M., 363, 364, 365, 366, 367, 368, 369, 471, 960
Holinger, P.H., 572, 576
Hollister, D.W., 16, 21, 128, 129, 346, 390, 391, 641, 779, 780, 847, 898, 1000
Holmes, L.B., 285
Hong, R., 523
Honig, G.R., 886, 939
Horton, W.A., 8, 9, 26, 303, 304, 336, 338, 345, 438, 447, 777, 853, 901, 949
Hudson, C.D., 225, 511
Hussels-Maumenee, I., 90, 621, 893
Ickenroth, A.M., 12, 206, 255, 268, 506, 592, 732, 759
Imbrie, D., 577

Jacobs, K.F., 444, 448, 955
Jellum, E., 849
Jirásek, J.E., 181, 790
Johnson, C.C., 958, 959
Johnson, D.G., 289, 365, 960

Johnson, W.C., **144**
Johnson, W.J., **708**
Johnston, P.W., **633**
Jones, K.L., **190, 379, 987**
Jorgenson, R.J., **102, 613, 738**
Joseph, H.L., **789**
Juberg, R.C., **769**
Kaitila, I.I., **19, 20, 646, 647, 648, 649**
Kalmus, H., **809**
Katz, H.I., **993**
Kay, D., **117**
Kean, B.H., **387**
Keene, H.J., **607**
Keyes, G.G., **17, 146**
Kimball, A.C., **387**
Kirkpatrick, S.E., **78, 80, 81, 108,
  916, 917**
Kitano, Y., **411**
Koerper, M.A., **4, 461, 462, 996**
Kogut, M.D., **397**
Kohlschütter, A., **44**
Kohut, R.I., **274**
‡Konigsmark, B.W., **245, 256, 270, 742,
  743, 744, 745, 746, 747**
Kozlowski, K.S., **652, 653, 654, 655, 899**
‡Krill, A.E., **43, 400, 479, 622, 719,
  734, 740, 869, 925, 983**
Krugman, S., **384**
Lachman, R.S., **122, 308, 310, 345,
  557, 650**
Langer, L.O., Jr., **10, 510, 940, 966**

Lapointe, N., **943**
Laurell, C.-B., **39**
Leadholm, B.C., **313**
Lees, R.S., **488**
Levin, L.S., **613, 784**
Levy, R.I., **495**
Lichtenstein, J.R., **311, 685, 777,
  778, 781**
Linde, L.M., **73, 96**
Lucas, R.V., Jr., **204, 528, 807,
  841, 842**

McCarter, T.J., **276**
McCrory, W.M., **708, 710**
McGee, B.J., **157**
McKhann, G.M., **115, 307, 415, 433, 434,
  478, 713, 803, 957**
McKibben, D.H., Jr., **340, 927, 928, 932**
McKusick, V.A., **156, 832, 881**
McNamara, D.G., **63, 74, 76, 200, 527,
  546, 766**
Magenis, E., **168**
Marden, P.M., **593, 629**
Maroteaux, P., **91, 358, 497**
Marriott, H.J.L., **454, 922**
Masuda, Y., **141**
Medansky, R.S., **589**
Mehregan, A.H., **339**
Mengel, M.C., **254**
Mentzer, W.C., Jr., **420, 852**
Meskin, L., **184, 617**
Messer, L.B., **340, 739, 927, 928,
  929, 930, 931, 932**
Meyer, I., **760**

Mikhail, G.R., **819**
Miller, B.L., **286, 454, 610, 922, 1002**
Miller, D.R., **370, 723, 724, 787, 878**
Miller, M.E., **812**
Miller, O.J., **158, 159, 169, 170, 171,
  172, 242**
Miller, R.H., **335, 582**
Miller, R.W., **383**
Miller, S.H., **374**
Mininberg, D.T., **518**
Mohandas, N., **2**
Moller, J.H., **109, 731, 836, 837, 838,
  839, 840**
Morris, M.E., **280**
Morrow, G., III, **87, 174**
Moynahan, E.J., **670**
Muckle, T.J., **982**
Muller, S.A., **38, 99**
Mullins, C.E., **63, 74, 200, 527, 546**
Murken, R.E., **919**

Nance, W.E., **266**
Neblett, L.M., **251, 571**
Neuhäuser, G., **93, 227, 632, 638, 783, 963**
Newell, R.C., **127**
Nichols, B.L., **202**
Nora, A.H., **805, 835**
Nora, J.J., **75, 77, 805, 835**
Norum, R.A., **301, 477, 630, 774, 854**
Nyhan, W.L., **37, 441, 492, 588, 658,
  772, 808, 826**

Obenshain, S.S., **513**
O'Brien, J.S., **431, 432**
Opitz, J.M., **22, 121, 401, 556, 603
  634, 754**
O'Reilly, R.J., **522, 523, 524**
Orti, E., **42, 815**
Owsley, J.Q., Jr., **374**

Pahwa, S., **943**
Patrick, A.D., **422**
Paul, M.H., **581**
Pearson, C.M., **11, 116, 124, 125, 134,
  686, 687, 688, 689, 690, 691, 692,
  694, 695, 696, 698, 700, 701, 702,
  794, 795, 796**
Perry, T.L., **126, 474**
Pfandler, U., **243**
Pfeiffer, R.A., **544**
Philippart, M., **398, 406**
Pickett, L.K., **62, 405, 529, 545, 645, 748**
Pillay, V.K., **749**
Podos, S.M., **736**
Polgar, G., **802**
Posner, P., **610**
Preus, M., **140**
‡Puretić, B., **644**
Puretić, S., **644**

Qazi, Q.H., **42, 815**

Rahn, E.K., **3, 60, 67, 84, 355, 372, 475,
  661, 662, 663, 699, 718, 758, 889**
Rao, S.R., **291, 660, 843, 936**
Reaven, G.M., **495, 500, 501**
Redman, R.S., **417, 954**
‡Reed, W.B., **30, 333, 1004, 1005**

Refetoff, S., 257
Reichel, W., 998
Rice, J.S., 113
Riemenschneider, T.A., 73
Rimoin, D.L., 10, 16, 21, 26, 122, 128, 129, 302
    303, 304, 308, 310, 390, 391, 438,
    447, 498, 510, 557, 641, 650, 771,
    779, 780, 788, 847, 896, 898, 940,
    949, 966
Riopel, D.A., 767, 768
Robinow, M., 876
Rosenberg, L.E., 148, 239, 287, 419, 490,
    858, 861, 862, 892, 992
Rowe, N.H., 711
Rubinstein, J.H., 119
Saddi, R., 460
Sagel, I., 859,
Sando, I., 141
Sauk, J.A., Jr., 711
Schapira, G., 460
Scheinberg, I.H., 469
Schiebler, G.L., 83, 332, 540, 541, 988
Schimke, R.N., 350, 351, 352
Schneider, J.A., 238
Schulman, J.D., 422
Schwartz, R., 513
Schwartz, S.A., 94
Scott, C.I., Jr., 98, 185, 290, 293, 445,
    560, 570, 673, 775, 846
Scriver, C.R., 294, 418, 453, 482, 486,
    491, 502, 516, 517, 520, 657, 736,
    830, 864, 974, 991
Sedano, H.O., 17, 223, 494, 818
Selmanowitz, V.J., 715
Shapiro, L.J., 672, 680, 782
Shear, C.S., 978
Shibuya, M., 709, 856, 857
Shinefield, H.R., 381
Shohet, S.B., 2
Shulman, K., 52, 186, 188, 220, 230, 292,
    343, 480, 481, 602, 642, 659,
    693, 712, 894, 915
Sidbury, J.B., Jr., 425, 426, 427, 428,
    429, 430
Sieber, W.K., 848, 910, 911, 912, 913, 914
Siggers, D.C., 392, 455, 459, 704, 882, 976
Silver, H.K., 887
Silverman, F.N., 221
Simell, O.G., 148, 491
Simpson, J.,385
Simpson, J.L., 29, 50, 68, 173, 436, 437,
    483, 682, 683, 684, 831, 855, 971,
    984, 985
Singer, W., 895
Singleton, G.T., 727
Sloan, H.R., 151, 580
Smith, D.W., 891, 999
Smith, M.E., 284, 414, 439, 564, 579, 591,
    639, 640, 716, 755, 761, 762, 763,
    764, 765, 866, 994
Smith, R.O., Jr., 574, 707, 824
Smithwick, E.M., 442, 443, 714
Snyderman, S., 628
Spach, M.S., 938, 989

Sperling, M.A., 23, 24, 25, 100, 222, 484,
    590, 829, 902, 903, 904, 905, 906,
    907, 908, 909
Spranger, J.W., 153, 154, 224, 228, 306,
    394, 656, 671, 776, 798, 880,
    883, 884, 897
Steinberg, A.G., 71, 476
Steinberg, D., 810
Stenmark, S., 990
Stevenson, R.E., 674, 675, 676, 677, 678,
    679, 980
Stewart, J.M., 264, 450, 667, 860
Stokke, O., 849
Stone, O.J., 559
Strauss, L., 942
Sugar, J., 205, 207, 208, 209, 210, 211, 212,
    213, 214, 215, 216, 552, 553, 637, 868
Suhr, M.P., 152
Summitt, R.L., 49, 50, 189, 587, 720, 831,
    855, 977
Sutton, H.E., 95
Sveger, T., 39
Sweetman, L., 107
Swinyard, C.A., 386
Talner, N.S., 665, 666, 669, 969, 970
Temtamy, S.A., 13, 14, 114, 813, 814,
    817, 923
Teree, T.M., 424
Teter, D.L., 951
Thorne, E.G., 600
Tocci, P.M., 519
Toomey, K., 346
Touloukian, R.J., 69, 192, 193, 194, 535,
    877
Touster, O., 804
Trodahl, J.N., 821
Tschudy, D.P., 203, 362, 820, 821, 822
Uitto, J., 777
Ulstrom, R.A., 104, 512
Vandersteen, P.R., 361
Van Doren Hough, J., 773
Van Mierop, L.H.S., 92, 332, 347, 541, 816
Vargo, T.A., 546
Via, W.F., Jr., 342
Vickers, R.A., 360
Victorica, B.E., 668, 800, 972
Wadlington, W.B., 147
Waldmann, T.A., 534
Waldron, C.A., 539
Walker, P.O., 929, 931
Wallman, I.S., 341
Wara, D.W., 729
Warburton, D., 164
Ward, P.H., 260
Warkany, J., 380
Wasserman, E., 518, 859
Watson, D.G., 79
Watson, W., 833
Way, G.L., 75, 77
Weil, W.B., Jr., 549
Weinberg, B., 952
Wells, B.T., 15
Weyler, W., Jr., 107

White, J.G., **33**
Whitington, P.F., **533, 597, 793, 885, 973**
Wildervanck, L.S., **142**
Williams, R.L., **76**
Wilroy, R.S., Jr., **299, 635, 986**
Wilson, C.J., **456**
Winchester, A.M., **241, 322, 323**
Witkop, C.J., Jr., **33, 34, 35, 36, 44, 45,
46, 118, 178, 180, 229, 277, 278,
279, 280, 407, 408, 409, 410, 411,
412, 413, 511, 538, 660, 681, 784,
843, 926, 934, 935, 937, 953,
956, 965**

Wolf, M.L., **43, 399, 400, 449, 479, 622,
719, 734, 740, 869, 983**
Wood, R.P., II, **145, 235, 536, 728**
Woolley, M.M., **537**
Worth, H.M., **965**
Wyandt, H.E., **165, 166**
Wyss, S.R., **6**

Zelkowitz, P.S., **120, 801, 879**
Zellweger, H., **139, 823**
Zinkham, W.H., **568**
Zonana, J., **175, 302, 542, 543, 947, 948**

Index

A

AARSKOG SYNDROME, 1
Abdomen
  distention of, 9, 10, 27, 54, 148, 192,
    194, 240, 365, 403, 406, 425, 426,
    532, 566, 567, 569, 597, 884, 900,
    946, 960, 978
  distention of in neonatal period, 193,
    531, 566, 567, 569
  mass in, 149, 194, 240, 532, 604, 605,
    645, 848, 912, 914, 988
  scaphoid, 289
  scaphoid lower, 910
Abdominal pain or tenderness, 54, 203, 240,
  265, 420, 469, 495, 534, 549, 566,
  567, 569, 645, 684, 820, 822, 886,
  892, 903
Abdominal wall
  defect of, 104, 193, 335, 405, 467, 671,
    748
  spasm of, 489
Abducens
  decreased function, 188
  paralysis, 376
Abduzensparese, 889
Aberfeld syndrome, 155
Aberrant bronchus, 611
Aberrant hepatic arterial supply, 464
Aberrant lacrimal gland, 564
Aberrant left pulmonary artery, 766
Aberrant lobe of lung, 611
Aberrant right ventricular muscle bands,
  731
ABETALIPOPROTEINEMIA, 2
Abgang des Pulmonalarterie von Ductus
  Botalli, 768
Abiotrophic ophthalmoplegia externa, 752
Abiotrophies of inner ear, 315
Ablatio falciformis congenita, 867
Ablépharie, 3
ABLEPHARON, 3
Abnormal facies, myopia and short stature,
  261
ABNORMAL FIBRINOGENS, 4
Abrikossoff tumor, 360
Absence congénitale de bêta-lipoprotéines,
  2
Absence congénitale de valvules pulmonaires,
  836
Absence de dermatoglyphes, 393
Absence de phagocytose, 812
Absence de transférrine, 95
Absence defect of limbs, scalp and skull,
  459
Absence des conduits lacrymaux, 705
Absence du lobe de l'oreille, 320
Absence du segment hépatique de la veine
  cave inférieure, 528
Absence du tragus, 312
Absence of
  anal sphincter, voluntary control of, 693
  anterior axillary skin fold, 813
  annulus tympanicus, 97

anus, 69, 72, 160, 167, 329, 364, 401,
  544, 574, 578, 634, 727, 754, 884,
  885, 960, 987
auditory meatus, 225, 506
auditory meatus, unilateral, 457, 735
beard, 438, 855
brain, 283, 380
breasts, 42, 93
calvaria, 634
caruncle, 130
carpal bones, 455, 981
cerebral cortex, 480
cerebrum, 727
choroid, at birth, 986
clavicle, 185
color vision, total, 198, 253, 755
corneal endothelium, 140
corpus callosum, 157, 158, 161, 220, 227,
  473, 578, 635, 754
dental pulp chamber, 277, 278, 280
deep tendon reflexes, 2, 139, 307, 628,
  629, 743, 750, 759, 810, 850, 895
deep tendon reflexes in ankle or knee,
  265
deep tendon reflexes in lower limb,
  693, 746
deep tendon reflexes in upper limb,
  924
ear, 457, 664
earlobe, 162, 320, 323, 326
eparterial bronchus, 816
epididymus, 49, 855
ethmoid sinus, 723, 797
extensor pollicis brevis, 175
extensor pollicis longis, 175
eyeball, 67, 168, 281, 634, 662, 735, 824
eyebrow, 3, 623, 670
eyebrow, focally without scarring, 38
eyebrow, lateral 3rd of, 105
eyelash, complete, 3, 623
eyelash, focally without scarring, 38
eyelash, medial to cleft, 627
eye lens, 84
eyelid, 3
fallopian tube, 49, 50, 682
fallopian tube, unilateral, 173
femur, 451, 875
fenestra cochleae, 664
fenestra, vestibuli, 592
fibula, 875
fingernail, at birth, 409
finger, 5th, 875
fingers, all except one, 336
fingers, one or more, 65, 242, 281, 336,
  337, 451, 459, 592, 700, 813, 818
foot, 451
forearm, 451
frontal sinus, 797
fungiform papilla on tongue, 307
gallbladder, 401, 404
great toe, 875
gyri of brain, 139, 578, 603
hair, axillary, 437, 903
hair, lanugo or downy, 105

hair on torso and limb at birth, 670
hair, pubic, 437, 903
half-nose, 722
hallux, 875
hand, 451
humerus, 875, 941
hyoid bone, 28, 952
incus, 592, 664, 860
internal auditory meatus, 562
interphalangeal flexion creases of
  finger, 89, 160
iridal pattern, 205
iris, 57, 281, 284
kidney, bilateral, 856, 860
kidney, unilateral, 337, 603, 634, 682,
  857, 860
labia majora, 88, 818
labia minora, 823
labyrinth of inner ear, 562
lacrimal canaliculus, complete or incomplete, 563
lacrimal punctum, 337, 371, 563
lateral nasal wall, 824
left or both aortic fourth arches, 76
lenticular process of incus, 247
light reflex in retinal blood vessels, 34, 35
liver, 463
lower limb, 451
lower lip sulcus, 17
lunula, 362
lymphatic vessels, 615
lymph nodes, 522, 524
mammary gland, 981
mandible, 28, 312
mandibular central incisor, 17, 771, 791
mandibular lateral incisor, 17, 291, 770,
  791
maxillary central incisor, 771, 791
maxillary lateral incisor, 177, 229, 291,
  770, 791, 934
maxillary sinus, 723, 735, 797
meibomian glands, 296
metacarpal, 459, 592, 875
metacarpals of ulnar digits, 981
metatarsal, 875
molar, 3rd, 934
motion of toe, 114
moustache, 105
mouth, 28
müllerian derivatives, 49, 68
nail, 65, 66, 262, 281, 409, 511, 609,
  704, 821, 880
nail, at birth, 409, 511
nail, part of, 65, 66
nails, totally, 65
nasal bones, 261
nasal septum, 727
nipple, unilateral, 42
nipples, 981
nose, 234, 722
nose, tip of, 635
olfactory lobe, 634
oocytes in gonad, 173
oropharyngeal lymphoid patches, 522

All index numbers refer to the Birth Defect Number — NOT page number.

ovary, 29
paranasal sinus, 723, 735, 797
parathyroid, 515
patella, 157, 704
pectoralis major, 455
penis, 876
petrous portion of temporal bone, 562
phalanges, middle of toes, 413, 737
phalanges of ulnar digits, 981
phalanx, distal, of finger, 21, 114, 1001
phalanx, distal, of toes, 21, 846, 1001
phalanx of finger, one or more, 65, 242,
    281, 336, 337, 451, 459, 692, 700,
    813, 818
phalanx of 2nd toe, 22
phalanx of 5th finger, 262, 875, 923
phalanx of 5th toe, 262
philtrum, 162, 395, 401, 473
pigment in retina, 32, 34
premolar teeth, 493, 784, 934
primitive reflexes, 139, 628, 940
prostate, 908
pupillary reflexes, 721, 865
radius, 160, 168, 231, 592, 853, 875, 941,
    987
retinal pigment, 32, 34
salivary gland, 627, 664
scalp hair, 13, 153, 154, 526, 623, 703,
    738, 770, 825, 998
scalp hair, focal at birth, 608
scalp hair, total, acquired, 15
scalp hair with scarring, 179
scalp hair without scarring, 259
scrotum, 818
semicircular canals, 142
seminal vesicles, 49, 855
sensation in finger or toe, 265
sexual characteristics, secondary, 29,
    68, 105, 438, 902, 903
skin, multiple areas, 281
skin creases of joints, 88, 470
skin on lower limb at birth, 609
speech, 103, 562, 732
sphenoid sinus, 797
spleen, 606, 727
stapedius reflex, 377
stapedius reflex ipsilateral to palsy,
    378
stapes, 592
sulci of brain, 603
sweating, 33, 986
sweating, axillary, 981
sweating on lower limb, 984
teeth, one or more, 6, 105, 178, 179,
    183, 333, 337, 439, 440, 451, 511,
    738, 930, 965, 999
testicular enlargement at puberty, 908
testis, 29, 68
thumb, 160, 167, 231, 455, 649, 875
thumbnail, 609
thymus gland, 522, 655
thyroid, 181, 946
tibia, 875
toenail, at birth, 409
toenail, great, 609
toes, all, 375
toes, all except one, 336
toes, one or more, 336, 337, 375, 451,
    459, 700, 818
tongue, 28
tooth enamel, 46
tragus, 312
ulna, 853, 875, 941, 981

ulnar ray structure, 981
upper limb, 451, 875
usual lymph nodes, 522, 524
uterine cervix, 49, 682
uterine corpus, 682
uterine horn, 684
uterus, 49, 50, 908
uveal pigment, 143
vagina, upper part, 682
vas deferens, 49, 855
voice, 572, 574, 575, 577
vulva, 908, 909, 971
yellow pigment in retinal macula, 32
zonules of eye lens, 584
Absent atrial septum, 96
Absent fingerprints, 393
Absent hepatic segment of inferior vena
    cava, 528
Absent inferior vena cava, 528
Absent pulmonary valve, 836
Acalasia esofágica, 363
Acanthocytosis, 2
ACANTHOSIS NIGRICANS, 5
ACATALASEMIA, 6
Acatalasemia Type I (Japanese variant of
    low specific activity), 6
Acatalasemia Type II (Swiss variant of low
    stability), 6
Acatalasia, 6
Accelerated AV conduction, 1002
Accessory hepatic lobes, 467
Accessory lung arising from bronchial tree,
    esophagus, or stomach, 611
ACETYLATOR POLYMORPHISM (MARKER),
    7
Achalasie, 363
Achalasie oesophagienne, 363
Achondrogénèse type I, 9
Achondrogénèse type II, 8
ACHONDROGENESIS, LANGER–SALDINO
    TYPE, 8
ACHONDROGENESIS, PARENTI-
    FRACCARO TYPE, 9
ACHONDROPLASIA, 10
Achromatism, 198
Achromatopsia with amblyopia, 198
Achromia, primary, 993
ACID MALTASE DEFICIENCY, 11
Acidémia metilmalónica, 658
Acidémie isovalérique, 547
Acidémie méthylmalonurique, 658
Acidémie pyroglutamique, 849
Acidose rénale, 862
Acidose rénale tubulaire et surdité neuro-
    sensorielle, 863
Acidosis renal tubular (distal), 862
Acidosis renal tubular (proximal), 858
Acidosis renal tubular y sordera neuro-
    sensorial, 863
Acidura α-metil acetoacética, 40
Acidurie glutarique, 421
Acondrogénesis tipo I, 9
Acondrogénesis tipo II, 8
Acondroplasia, 10
ACOUSTIC NEUROMATA, 12
ACPS type I, 13
ACPS type II, 13
ACPS type III, 13
Acquired agammaglobulinemia, 521
Acquired agammaglobulinemia with thymoma,
    944
Acrania, 52
Acrocéfalopolisindactilia, 13

Acrocéfalosindactilia, 14
ACROCEPHALOPOLYSYNDACTYLY, 13
ACROCEPHALOSYNDACTYLY, 14
Acrocephalosyndactyly, Herrmann-Opitz
    type, 14
Acrocephalosyndactyly, Summitt type, 14
Acrocephalosyndactyly, Waardenburg type,
    14
ACRODERMATITIS ENTEROPATHICA,
    15
ACRODYSOSTOSIS, 16
Acrodysplasia with exostoses, 967
ACROFACIAL DYSOSTOSIS, 17
Acromégalie avec cutis verticis gyrata et
    leucome de la cornée, 18
ACROMEGALOID PHENOTYPE, CUTIS
    VERTICIS AND GYRATA-
    CORNEAL LEUKOMA, 18
Acromegaloider Habitus-Cutis verticis gyrata
    und Hornhaut-Leukom, 18
ACROMESOMELIC DYSPLASIA,
    CAMPAILLA–MARTINELLI TYPE,
    19
ACROMESOMELIC DYSPLASIA,
    MAROTEAUX TYPE, 20
ACRO-OSTEOLYSE, DOMINANT TYPE,
    21
Acroosteolysis without neuropathy, 21
ACROPECTOROVERTEBRAL DYSPLASIA,
    22
Acylcholine acyl-hydrolase EC 3.1.1.8.,
    152
Adducted thumbs, 175
Adenolipomatosis, 601
Adenoma, hereditary pleiomorphic
    salivary, 878
Adenoma sebaceum, seizures and mental
    retardation, 975
Adiposidad-hipertermia-oligomenorrea y
    tumefacción de la parótida, 730
Adolescent or young adult renal tubular
    acidosis and slowly progressive
    sensorineural deafness, 863
Adrenal gland, defect of, 181, 502
Adrenal hyperplasia, congenital: 17α-
    hydroxylase deficiency, 903
Adrenal hyperplasia, congenital: 3β-
    hydroxysteroid dehydrogenase de-
    ficiency, 909
Adrenal hyperplasia, congenital: 11β-
    hydroxylase deficiency, 902
Adrenal hyperplasia, congenital: 20–22
    desmolase deficiency, 907
Adrenal hyperplasia, congenital: 21-
    hydroxylase deficiency, 908
ADRENAL HYPOALDOSTERONISM OF
    INFANCY, TRANSIENT ISOLATED,
    23
ADRENAL HYPOPLASIA CONGENITAL
    autosomal recessive form, 24
    X-linked form, 24
Adrenal 18-hydroxylase deficiency, 905
Adrenal 18-hydroxysteroid dehydrogenase
    deficiency, 906
ADRENOCORTICAL UNRESPONSIVE-
    NESS TO ACTH, HEREDITARY,
    25
ADRENOCORTICOTROPIC HORMONE
    DEFICIENCY, ISOLATED, 26
Adrenogenital syndrome, 908
    salt-losing form, 908
    non-salt losing form, 908
    simple virilizing form, 908

Adrenogenital syndrome with hypertension, 902
Adult hemochromatosis, 460
Adult lactase deficiency, 567
Adult lactose intolerance, 567
Adult liver fibrosis and cirrhosis, 39
Adult pseudohypertrophic muscular dystrophy, 687
Adynamia episodica hereditaria, 794
Afaquia, 84
African cardiopathy, 353, 354
Agalactokinase, 402

Agamaglobulinemia ligada al sexo, 27
Agamaglobulinemia linfopénica autosómica recesiva, 522
Agammaglobulinemia and thymoma, 944
AGAMMAGLOBULINEMIA, X–LINKED INFANTILE, 27
Agammaglobulinémie liée au sexe, 27

Agammaglobulinémie lymphopénique, 522
Aganglionic megacolon, 192
Aganglionose colique, 192
Aganglionosis del colon, 192
Agenesia del cuerpo calloso, 220
Agenesia del pericardio, 805
Agenesia del timo, 943
Agenesia hepática, 463
Agenesia renal bilateral, 856
Agenesia renal unilateral, 857
Agénésie congénitale des incisives latérales supérieures, 934
Agénésie de la rate, 92
Agénésie de l'oreille, 232
Agénésie des corpus callosum, 220
Agénésie des sinus de la face, 797
Agénésie du corps calleux, 220
Agénésie hépatique, 463
Agénésie partielle de l'oreille avec plicature de l'hélix, 331
Agénésie péricardique, 805
Agénésie rénale bilatérale, 856
Agénésie rénale unilatérale, 857
Agenesis of corpus callosum, 220
Agenesis of inner ear, 562
Agenesis of paranasal sinuses, unilateral, 797
Agenesis of pericardium, 805
Aging premature, 998
Aglossia-adactylia syndrome, 451
Aglossia congenita, 451
Aglycogenosis, 424

AGNATHIA, MICROSTOMIA AND SYNOTIA, 28
Agoitrous cretinism, 946
AGONADIA, 29
AHF deficiency, 461
AHG deficiency, 461
AHOP syndrome, 730
Ahornsirupkrankheit, 628
Ahotutuo, 886
Aislamiento de la arteria subclavia de la aorta, 546
Akatalasaemie, 6
Akromesomele Dysplasie, Typ Campailla Martinelli, 19
Akromesomele Dysplasie, Typ Maroteaux, 20
Akroosteolyse, 21
Akrozephalopolysyndaktylie, 13
Akrozephalosyndaktylie, 14
Akute intermittierende Porphyrie, 820
Akzessorisch Leberlappen, 467
Akzessorischer Lungenlappen, 611

Alaninuria, 851
Albers-Schönberg disease, 779, 780
Albinism, cutaneous and deaf-mutism, 30
ALBINISM-CUTANEOUS AND DEAFNESS, 30
ALBINISM-CUTANEOUS WITHOUT DEAFNESS, 31
Albinism, hemorrhagic diathesis and pigmented reticuloendothelial cells, 33
ALBINISM-OCULAR, 32
ALBINISM-OCULOCUTANEOUS, HERMANSKY-PUDLAK TYPE, 33
ALBINISM-OCULOCUTANEOUS, TYROSINASE NEGATIVE, 34
ALBINISM-OCULOCUTANEOUS, TYROSINASE POSITIVE, 35
ALBINISM-OCULOCUTANEOUS, YELLOW MUTANT, 36
Albinism, tyrosinase negative oculocutaneous, 34
Albinism, tyrosinase positive oculocutaneous, 35
Albinism, yellow mutant oculocutaneous, 36
Albinisme avec surdi-mutité, 30
Albinisme cutané sans surdité, 31
Albinisme oculaire, 32
Albinisme oculaire cutané, mutant jaune, 36
Albinisme oculocutané avec absence de tyrosinase, 34
Albinisme oculocutané avec tyrosinase, 35
Albinisme oculocutané, Hermansky-Pudlak type, 33
Albinismo cutáneo sin sordera, 31
Albinismo cutáneo y sordomudez, 30
Albinismo ocular, 32
Albinismo óculocutáneo, Hermansky-Pudlak tipo, 33
Albinismo óculocutáneo mutante amarillo, 36
Albinismo óculocutáneo tirosinasa negativa, 34
Albinismo óculocutáneo tirosinasa positiva, 35
Albinismus mit Schwerhörigkeit, 30
Albinismus ohne Schwerhörigkeit, 31
Albinismus Okulokutaner, Hermansky-Pudlak typ, 33
Albrecht syndrome, 269
Albright-Butler syndrome, 862
Albright hereditary osteodystrophy, 830
Alcaptonuria, 37
Aldosterone unresponsiveness, 829
Alkalosis with diarrhea, 148
ALKAPTONURIA, 37
Alkinetic or atonic "drop" seizures, 135
Allotypes, antibodies to human, 71
Allotypes chez l'homme, 476
Alopecia adnata, 623
ALOPECIA AREATA, 38
Alopecia areata, 38, 259, 281
Alopecia, male or female pattern, 99
Alopecia totalis, 38
Alopecia universalis, 38
Alopécie en aires, 38
Alotipos humanos (Marcadores), 476
ALPHA–METHYL-ACETOACETIC ACIDURIA, 40
α-Methyl-β-hydroxybutyric aciduria, 40
ALPHA$_1$–ANTITRYPSIN DEFICIENCY, 39
Alpha 1,4-glucosidase deficiency, 11
Alphalipoprotein deficiency, 48
Alport syndrome, 708
Alström-Hallgren syndrome, 41

ALSTRÖM SYNDROME, 41
Alveolar ridge,
  broad, 22, 388, 891
  cyst in alveolus, 118, 407, 408, 412, 617, 929, 931, 932, 965
  granuloma of alveolus, 276, 929, 931
  lymphangioma of, 613
  periapical abscess in alveolus, 276, 279, 929, 965
  short, 554
  v-shaped maxillary, 225
Altered consciousness or mentation (see Section III, Table XXXVI)
Altered reflexes (see Section III, Table XXXVI)
Alymphocytosis, 524
AMASTIA, 42
AMAUROSIS CONGENITA OF LEBER, 43
  types I and II, 43
Amaurotic familial idiocy, all three types, 713
Amegakaryocytic thrombocytopenia and bilateral absence of the radii, 941
AMELO–CEREBRO–HYPOHIDROTIC SYNDROME, 44
AMELOGENESIS IMPERFECTA, 46
Amelogenesis imperfecta nonhereditaria segmentalis, 739
Amelogenesis imperfecta with onycholysis, hypohidrosis, rough skin and seborrhea of scalp, 45
Amelogenesis imperfecta, 9 types, 46
Ameloonychodyshidrotic syndrome, 45
AMELO–ONYCHO–HYPOHIDROTIC SYNDROME, 45
Ameloonycholyticdyshidrotic syndrome, 45
Amenorrhea, primary, 49, 303, 350, 436, 437, 438, 483, 823, 903, 984
Aminoaciduria dicarboxilica, 294
Amino-acidurie-hyperdibasique, 491
Aminopterin damage in utero, 380
Amish albinism, 36
Amnion nodosum, 856
Amniotic bands, 874
Amniotic fluid
  decreased, 856
  increased, 9, 62, 148, 153, 160, 187, 300, 364, 603, 910
Amputation (deletion) du bras court du chromosome 18, 158
Amputation (deletion) du bras long du chromosome 18, 159
Amusie, 273
Amyloidosis, deafness and urticaria, 982
Amylopectinosis, 116
Amylose avec urticare et surdité, 982
Amyoplasia congenita, 88
Anabolic idiopathic hypoalbuminemias, 47
Anal aganglionosis, 192
Anal atresia and iris coloboma, 544
Anal atresia or stenosis, 69
Anal membrane, 69
Analatresie, dreigliedrige Daumen, abstehende Ohren, Innenohr-Schwerhörigkeit, 72
ANALBUMINEMIA, 47
ANALPHALIPOPROTEINEMIA, 48
Ancestry
  Amish, 156
  Arab, 420
  Ashkenazic Jewish, 112, 406, 717, 804
  Azore-Portugese, 598
  Black race, 420, 613
  Brazilian, 8

Filipino, **420**
Finnish, **148, 491, 963**
French Canadian, **491, 717**
Japanese, **6**
Jewish, **397**
Kurd, **420**
Lebanese, **804**
Mediterranean basin, **420**
Oriental, **420**
Scandinavian, **810, 963**
Swiss, **418**
Ugandan, **353, 354**
Andersen disease, **116**
Androgen-genetic regional alopecia, **99**
ANDROGEN INSENSITIVITY SYNDROME, COMPLETE, **49**
ANDROGEN INSENSITIVITY SYNDROME, INCOMPLETE, **50**
Androgenetic alopecia, **99**
Anectine apnea, **152**
Anemia falciforme, **886**
ANEMIA, HYPOPLASTIC CONGENITAL, **51**
Anémie drépanocytaire, **886**
ANENCEPHALY, **52**
Aneurisma de la carótida interna del oído medio, **530**
Aneurisma del seno aórtico de Valsalva, **53**
ANEURYSM OF AORTIC SINUS OF VALSALVA, **53**
Aneurysm of membranous septum with one or more perforations, **989**
Aneurysm of middle ear, **530**
Aneurysm of vein of Galen, **186**
Aneurysm serpentina of external ear, **313**
Aneurysma der a. carotis im Bereich des Mittelohrs, **530**
Aneurysma des Sinus Valsalva, **53**
Anévrisme de l'oreille moyenne, **530**
Angeborene anosmie, **70**
Angeborene Fazialisparese, **377**
Angeborene generalisierte Muskelhypoplasie, **686**
Angeborene Glaukom, **414**
Angeborene hereditäre Hornhautdystrophie, **207**
Angeborene hypoplastische Anämie, **51**
Angeborene Lid-Ektropie, **371**
Angeborene Linsenektopia, **584**
Angeborene Lues, **385**
Angeborene Nebennieren-Hyperplasie: 3 β-Hydroxysteroid-Dehydrogenase-Mangel, **909**
Angeborene Nebennieren-Hyperplasie 11 β-Hydroxylase-Mangel, **902**
Angeborene Nebennieren-Hyperplasie 17 α-Hydroxylase-Mangel, **903**
Angeborene Nebennieren-Hyperplasie 20-22 Desmolase-Mangel, **907**
Angeborene Nebennieren-Hyperplasie 21-Hydroxylase-Mangel, **908**
Angeborene Nebennieren-Hypoplasie, **24**
Angeborene Nephrose, **709**
Angeborene oculäre motorische Apraxie, **191**
Angeborene Pigmentation der Papille, **639**
Angeborene Ptose, **834**
Angeborene Supraventrikuläre Tachykardie, **922**
Angeborene Toxoplasmose, **387**
Angeborene Zwerchfellhernie, **289**
Angeborener, familiärer Hyperparathyreoidismus, **499**
Angeborener isolierter Lipasemangel, **597**

Angeborener kompletter atrioventrikulärer Block, **454**
Angeborener Laktasemangel, **566**
Angewachsen Ohrläppchen, **323**
ANGIOEDEMA, HEREDITARY, **54**
Angioid streaks with skin changes, **832**
Angiokeratoma corporis diffusum universale, **373**
Angioma cavernosum of external ear, **313**
Angioma pigmentosum et atrophicum, **1005**
Angiomatose cutanée et digestive, **113**
ANGIO–OSTEOHYPERTROPHY SYNDROME, **55**
ANHIDROSIS, **56**
Anhidrosis hypotrichotica, **333**
Anhidrotische ektodermale Dysplasie, **333**
Anhydrose, **56**
ANIRIDIA, **57**
ANISOCORIA, **58**
Anisomaltasia, **920**
ANISOMETROPIA, **59**
Ankle
    calcaneovalgus deformity of, **882**
    decreased range of motion of, **128, 311, 560**
    dorsiflexed, **85**
    fixed, **1001**
    flexion contracture of, **470**
    increased range of motion of, **90**
    large, **90, 873**
    valgus deformity of, **85, 653, 685**
    varus deformity of, **510, 882**
    unspecified defect of, **649**
Ankyloblépharie, **60**
ANKYLOBLEPHARON, **60**
Ankyloblepharon filiforme adnatum, **60**
ANKYLOGLOSSIA, **61**
Ankyloglossum superior syndrome, **451**
Ankylose dentaire, **927**
Ankylose des zähne, **927**
Ankylosed teeth, **927**
Annular corneal dystrophy, **215**
Annular grooves, **874**
ANNULAR PANCREAS, **62**
Ano imperforado, pulgares trifalángicos, orejas en asa y pérdida de la audición neurosensorial, **72**
Anoftalmia, **67**
Anomaler Ursprung der A. subclavia, **546**
Anomalía de Uhl, **979**
Anomalía total del drenaje venoso pulmonar, **842**
Anomalía venosa hepática, **468**
Anomalías carpo-tarsales, paladar hendido, oligodoncia y sordera for fijación del estribo, **183**
Anomalías de la carúncula, **130**
Anomalías de la unión corticosteroide globulina, **222**
Anomalías de la vesícula biliar, **404**
Anomalías de las arterias hepáticas, **464**
Anomalías de las manos y sordera neurosensorial, **450**
Anomalías del tabique interauricular, **96**
Anomalías renales, genitales y del oído medio, **860**
Anomalie cutanée et unguéale-épidermolyse, **609**
Anomalie de la deshalogénation des iodotyrosines, **543**
Anomalie de la veine hépatique, **468**
Anomalie de l'émail, **935**
Anomalie de Uhl, **979**

Anomalie des gros vaisseaux (aorte et artère pulmonaire) qui prennent leur origine dans le ventricule droit communication interventrículaire antérieure, **297**
Anomalie des gros vaisseaux (aorte et artère pulmonaire) qui prennent leur origine dans le ventricule droit communication interventrículaire postérieure, **298**
Anomalie du nez et de la cloison nasale, **722**
Anomalie du septum aortico-pulmonaire, **83**
Anomalie du septum ventriculaire, **989**
Anomalie du transport de l'iode, **542**
Anomalie partielle des veines pulmonaires, **841**
Anomalien der a. hepatica, **464**
Anomalien des Kortikoid-bindenden Globulins, **222**
Anomalies artérielles hépatiques, **464**
Anomalies de la caroncule, **130**
Anomalies de la globuline transporteuse du cortisol (CBG-transcortine), **222**
Anomalies de la trompe d'eustache, **370**
Anomalies de la vésicule biliaire, **404**
Anomalies des mains-surdité de perception, **450**
Anomalies du carpe et du tarse, fissure palatine, oligodontie et surdité par ankylose de l'etrier, **183**
Anomalies du fibrinogéne, **4**
Anomalies of caruncle, **130**
Anomalies rénale génitale et de l'orielle moyenne, **860**
Anomalies vertébro-ano-trachéo-radiales, **987**
Anomalous atrioventricular (AV) conduction, **1002**
Anomalous closure of embryonic cleft, **733**
Anomalous muscle bundle of right ventricle, **731**
Anomalous origin of both coronary arteries from pulmonary artery, **64**
ANOMALOUS ORIGIN OF CONTRALATERAL SUBCLAVIAN ARTERY, **63**
ANOMALOUS ORIGIN OF CORONARY ARTERIES FROM PULMONARY ARTERY, **64**
Anomalous origin of left coronary artery from pulmonary artery, **64**
Anomalous origin of left subclavian artery from right aortic arch, **63**
Anomalous origin of right coronary artery from pulmonary artery, **64**
Anomalous origin of right subclavian artery from left aortic arch, **63**
Anomalous panleukocytic granulation, **143**
Anomalous shortened chordae tendineae, **666**
Anoniquia hereditaria, **66**
Anoniquia y ectrodactilia, **65**
Anonychia, **66**
ANONYCHIA AND ECTRODACTYLY, **65**
ANONYCHIA, HEREDITARY, **66**
Anonychia totalis congenital, **66**
Anonychie avec ectrodactylie, **65**
Anonychie héréditaire, **66**
Anonychie mit Ektrodaktylie, **65**
Anoperineal fistula, **69**
ANOPHTHALMIA, **67**
Anophthalmia and digital anomalies, **662**
ANORCHIA, **68**

ANORECTAL MALFORMATIONS, 69
Anorquia, 68
ANOSMIA, CONGENITAL, 70
Anosmia, isolated, 70
Anotia, 664
Anquiloblefarón, 60
Anquiloglosia, 61
Anterior chamber cleavage syndrome, 439
Anterior duodenal portal vein, 468
Anterior megalophthalmos, 637
Anterior nasal atresia, 723
Anterior tunica vasculosa lentis persistence, 845
Anterolateral diaphragmatic hernia, 289
Anthelix
   crumpled, 85
   partially obliterates concha, 85
   prominent, 97, 157, 159, 161, 162, 328, 330
Anthélix saillant, 330
ANTIBODIES TO HUMAN ALLOTYPES (MARKERS), 71
Anticorps contre les allotypes, 71
Anticuerpos contra los alotipos humanos (Marcadores), 71
Anthélix auriculaire prominente, 330
Antikörper gegen menschliche Allotypen, 71
Antimongolism, 170
Antral atresia, 910
Anus
   absence of voluntary control of anal sphincter, 693
   anterior distortion of anal orifice, 877
   duplication of, 194, 677
   ectopic site, 69
   imperforate, 69, 72, 160, 167, 329, 364, 401, 544, 574, 578, 634, 727, 754, 884, 885, 960, 987
   mucoid discharge from, 535
   palpable fecal mass at end of exam finger, 192
   small in size but normal in location, 69
   unspecified defect of, 193
   white folded soft hyperplastic lesions of anal mucosa, 681
ANUS–HAND–EAR SYNDROME, 72
AOP syndrome, 730
AORTA, COARCTATION, 73
Aorta (also see each part of CV system and Section III, Table XXXII)
   coarctation of, 182, 455, 593, 720, 977
   cystic medial necrosis of, 977
   dissection of, 338
   poststenotic dilatation of ascending, 80, 916
   prominent ascending, 82
   separate origin of left internal and external carotids from, 121
Aortenisthmusstenose, 73
Aortenklappen-Atresie, 79
Aortic aneurysm, 630, 977
Aortic arch
   anomalies, 74, 384
   inconspicuous, 74
AORTIC ARCH, CERVICAL, 74
AORTIC ARCH, DOUBLE, 75
AORTIC ARCH INTERRUPTION, 76
AORTIC ARCH, RIGHT, 77
Aortic atresia, 79
Aortic coarctation, 73
Aortic pulmonary lobe, 612
Aortic septal defect, 83
AORTIC STENOSIS, SUPRAVALVAR, 78
Aortic valve
   insufficiency, 630, 673, 675, 678, 680, 777

stenosis, 632, 720
AORTIC VALVE ATRESIA, 79
Aortic valve, bicuspid, 108
AORTIC VALVE STENOSIS, 80
AORTIC VALVE, TETRACUSPID, 81
AORTICO-LEFT VENTRICULAR TUNNEL, 82
Aorticopulmonary fenestration, 83
Aorticopulmonary fistula, 83
Aorticopulmonary window, 83
AORTICO–PULMONARY SEPTAL DEFECT, 83
Aorto-linksventrikuläre Tunnelung, 82
Aortopulmonaler Septumdefekt, 83
Aortopulmonary defect, 83
Apert-Crouzon disease or Vogt cephalo-dactyly, 14
Apert syndrome, 14
APHAKIA, 84
Apical cardiac impulse, double or triple, 917
Aplasia cutánea, 608
Aplasia cutis circumscripta, Blasenbildung und Nagelanomalien, 609
Aplasia cutis congenita, 608
Aplasia cutis congenita circumscripta, 608
Aplasia de los conductos de Müller, 682
Aplasia del laberinto, 562
Aplasia of right ventricular myocardium, 979
Aplasia of tibia with polydactyly and absent thumbs, 649
Aplasia retineana, 865
Aplasie cutanée, 608
Aplasie der labyrinths, 562
Aplasie der Nasennebenhöhlen, 797
Aplasie der rechten Ventrikel (Uhl), 979
Aplasie des Ohrläppchens, 320
Aplasie labyrinthique, 562
Aplasie radiale, 853
Aplasie rétinienne, 865
Aplasie thymique, 943
Aplasie von Uterus und Vagina, 682
Apnea, 24, 152, 283, 513, 571
Appelt-Gerken-Lenz syndrome, 875
Apraxie oculomotrice congénitale, 191
Arachnodactylie avec contractions, 85
Arachnodactyly, 85, 166, 183, 557, 629, 630
ARACHNODACTYLY, CONTRACTURAL, 85
Aracnodactilia con contracturas, 85
Arche aortique cervicale, 74
Arche aortique double, 75
Arco aórtico cervical, 74
Arco aórtico derecho, 77
Arco aórtico doble, 75
Arcuate uterus, 684
Arginase deficiency, 86
ARGININEMIA, 86
ARGININOSUCCINIC ACIDURIA, 87
Argininosuccinuria, 87
Arhinencephaly, 473
Arnold-Chiari deformity, 103, 693
Arrhinencephalia unilateralis, 824
Artère coronaire unique, 219
Artère pulmonaire anormale partie de l'aorte ascendante, 767
Artère pulmonaire anormale partie du canal artériel, 768
Arteria coronaria única, 219
Arteriosus
   patent ductus, 121, 139, 161, 176, 182, 384, 401, 440, 455, 720
   truncus, 389
Arteriovenöse Fehlbildungen des Zentral-nervensystem, 186

Arteriovenöse Fistel des äusseren Ohr, 313
Arteriovenöse Koronarfistel, 218
Arteriovenous aneurysm of external ear, 313
Arteriovenous fistula, 55
Arteriovenous malformations, spinal, cortical, cerebellar, 186
Artery
   carotid, occlusion of, 474
   coronary, calcification of, 217
   rupture of, 338, 832
   single umbilical, 160, 634, 856, 987
   stenosis of peripheral pulmonary, 263, 720, 999
ARTHRO–OPHTHALMOPATHY, 90
Arthrochalasis multiplex congenita, 338
Arthrogrypose de la main et surdité de per-ception, 89
Arthrogrypose der Hand mit Innenohr-Schwerhörigkeit, 89
Arthrogrypose multiple congénitale, 88
ARTHROGRYPOSIS, 88
Arthrogryposis multiplex congenita, 88
ARTHROGRYPOTIC HAND ANOMALY AND SENSORINEURAL DEAFNESS, 89
Arthroosteoonychodysplasia, 704
Artrogriposis múltiple congénita, 88
Artro-oftalmopatía, 90
Ascher syndrome, 111
Ascites, 395, 403, 460, 469, 710, 717, 978
   chylous, 534, 645
Asexual ateleotic dwarfism, 303
Asociación Vater, 987
Asphyxia, 181, 575
ASPHYXIATING THORACIC DYSPLASIA, 91
Asphyxierende Thoraxidystrophie, 91
ASPLENIA SYNDROME, 92
Astigmatism, 591, 637
   asymmetric myopic astigmatism, 552
   hyperopic astigmatism, 1
   myopic astigmatism, 90, 479, 757
Astrocytoma including optic nerve glioma, 188
Asucrosia, 920
Asymmetric gonadal dysgenesis, 173
Asymmetric septal hypertrophy with obstruc-tion, 917
Ataxia (see Section III, Table XXXVI)
   cerebellar, progressive, 12, 93, 94, 743, 745, 746, 849, 850, 1004
   gait, 188, 759
   intermittent, 547
   limb, 746
   progressive, 136, 742, 744, 745
   spinocerebellar, progressive, 508
   telangiectasia, Louis-Bar, 13
   truncal, 188, 746
   with onset in adulthood, 742, 743, 744, 746, 747
   with onset in childhood, 651, 747
   with onset in early infancy, 94
Ataxia and tapetoretinal degeneration, 136
Ataxia cerebelosa y degeneración corio-retineana, 136
ATAXIA–HYPOGONADISM SYNDROME, 93
ATAXIA–TELANGIECTASIA, 94
Ataxie cérébelleuse avec dégénérescence chorio-rétinienne, 136
Athetosis, gingival fibromatosis, depig-mentation, microphthalmia, and oligophrenia, 413
Athyrosis, 946
Atopic dermatitis and neural hearing loss, 245

ATRANSFERRINEMIA, 95
Atresia biliar, 110
Atresia, bronchial, 120
Atresia coanal posterior, 727
Atresia de la vagina, 984
Atresia de la válvula aórtica, 79
Atresia de la válvula pulmonar, 837
Atresia de la válvula tricuspídea, 968
Atresia del canalículo lacrimal, 563
Atresia del conducto auditivo externo, 97
Atresia del esófago con fístula traqueo-
    esofágica, 365
Atresia esofágica, 364
Atresia gástrica, 910
Atresia laríngea, 571
Atresia mitral, 665
Atresia nasal anterior, 723
Atresia o estenosis del colon, 193
Atresia o estenosis duodenal, 300
Atresia of anterior nares, 723
Atresia of aortic valve, 79
Atresia of canaliculus and punctum, 563
Atresia of foramina of Luschka and
    Magendie, 481
Atresia of larynx types I, II, and III, 571
Atresia of nasolacrimal ducts, 705
Atresia of posterior nares, 727
Atresia of pulmonary valve, 837
Atresia of tricuspid valve, 968
Atrésie bronchique, 120
Atrésie choanal postérieure, 727
Atrésie de la valvule tricuspide, 968
Atrésie de l'estomac, 910
Atrésie de l'oesophage avec fistule trachéo-
    oesophagienne, 365
Atrésie des canaux lacrymaux, 563
Atrésie des valvules aortiques, 79
Atrésie des valvules pulmonaires, 837
Atrésie de voies biliaires, 110
Atrésie du conduit auditif externe, 97
Atrésie et hypoplasie auriculaire, 664
Atrésie laryngée, 571
Atrésie mitrale, 665
Atrésie nasale antérieure, 723
Atrésie oesophagienne, 364
Atrésie ou sténose colique, 193
Atrésie ou sténose duodénale, 300
Atrésie ou sténose intestinale, 531
Atrésie vaginale, 984
Atrial fibrillation, 922
Atrial flutter, persistent and paroxysmal,
    922
Atrial septal defect at fossa ovalis, 96
ATRIAL SEPTAL DEFECTS, 96
Atrial tachyarrhythmia, 922
Atriodigital dysplasia, 455
Atrioventricularis communis, 347
Atrofia girata, 449
Atrofia muscular espinal, 895
Atrofia olivopontocerebelosa con degener-
    ación retineana, 745
Atrofia olivopontocerebelosa dominante con
    oftalmoplegia y demencia, 744
Atrofia olivopontocerebelosa dominante (tipo
    Menzel), 742
Atrofia olivopontocerebelosa dominante (tipo
    Schut-Haymaker), 743
Atrofia olivopontocerebelosa esporádica, 746
Atrofia olivopontocerebelosa recesiva (tipo
    Fickler-Winkler), 747
Atrofia óptica de Leber, 579
Atrofia óptica infantil heredo familiar, 755
Atrophia gyrate choroideae et retinae, 449
Atrophie gyrée de la chorio-rétine, 449
Atrophie musculaire spinale, 895
Atrophie olivopontocérébelleuse, 746

Atrophie olivopontocérébelleuse avec
    dégénérescence rétinienne, 745
Atrophie olivopontocérébelleuse avec ophtal-
    moplégie et démence, 744
Atrophie olivopontocérébelleuse dominante
    (type Menzel), 742
Atrophie olivopontocérébelleuse dominante
    (type Schut-Haymaker), 743
Atrophie olivopontocérébelleuse récessive, de
    type Fickler-Winkler, 747
Atrophie optique associée à la surdi-mutité,
    253
Atrophie optique de Leber, 579
Atrophie optique hérédo-familiale infantile,
    755
Atypical retinitis pigmentosa (some forms),
    201
Atypische Plasma-Cholinesterase, 152
Atypischer Abgang der aa. subclaviae, 63
Atypischer Ursprung der Koronararterien
    aus der Pulmonararterie, 64
Atypischer Ursprung der linken Pulmonal-
    arterie von der rechten a. pulmonalis,
    766
Auditory canal
    atresia of, 97, 159, 315, 664, 823, 860
    bony nodules on wall of, 318
    defect of, 97, 370, 627
    fistula or pit near usual position of
        external auditory meatus, 664
    narrow, 247, 664, 667
    oblique, 667
Auditory meatus, external
    atresia of, 255, 457, 506, 735
    bleeding, profuse after mild trauma,
        530
    bleeding spontaneously, 457, 530
    skin covers, 97, 457
Auditory meatus, internal defect of, 142,
    562
Auditory ossicles
    displacement of, 97, 250
    disruption of, 318
    small, 506
Aural exostoses, 318
AURICULO-OSTEODYSPLASIA, 98
Auriculotemporal syndrome, 448
Ausencia de huellas dactilares, 393
Ausencia de la válvula pulmonar, 836
Ausencia de los senos paranasales, 797
Ausencia del lóbulo de la oreja, 320
Ausencia del segmento hepático de la vena
    cava inferior, 528
Ausencia del trago, 312
Ausencia localizada de piel, vesiculización
    y anomalías ungüeales, 609
Äussere Fehlbildungen von Nase und Nasen-
    septum, 722
Äussere Ophthalmoplegie und Myopie, 750
Automatisms and psychopathic behavior, 135
Autosomal dominant multiple hemivertebrae,
    896
Autosomal dominant nightblindness, 719
Autosomal dominant optic atrophy, 755
Autosomal recessive hereditary lymphocyto-
    plasmic dysgenesis, 522
Autosomal recessive multiple hemivertebrae,
    900
Autosomal recessive nightblindness, 719
Autosomal recessive optic atrophy, 755
Autosomal recessive primary or essential
    lymphocytothesis, 522
Autosomal recessive vitamin D-dependency
    (ARVDD), 873
Autosomal recessive xeroderma pigmentosum,
    1005

Axenfeld anomaly, 439
Azygous continuation of inferior vena cava,
    528
Azygous vein, large, 816

B

Baelz syndrome, 144
BALDNESS, COMMON, 99
Baller-Gerold syndrome, 231
Balloon or billowing mitral valve, 668
Band keratitis, 553
Band-shaped keratopathy, 553
Bandförmige Keratopathie, 553
Bardet-Biedl syndrome, 578
Barlow syndrome, 668
Bart-Pumphrey syndrome, 558
BARTTER SYNDROME, 100
BASAL CELL NEVUS SYNDROME, 101
Basal ganglion dysfunction, 820, 822
BASAN SYNDROME, 102
BASILAR IMPRESSION, PRIMARY, 103
Bassen-Kornzweig syndrome, 2
"Bat ear," 326
Batten-Vogt syndrome, 713
BBB syndrome, 505
Beals-Hecht syndrome, 85
Bec-de-lièvre-avec ou sans fente palatine,
    178
BECKWITH-WIEDEMANN SYNDROME,
    104
Béguez César-Steinbrinck-Chédiak-Higashi
    syndrome, 143
Behaarte Ohren, 319
Behavior
    destructive, bizarre or psychopathic
        135, 422, 588, 676
    self-mutilating, 422, 588
Behavioral or psychomotor defect (see
    Section III, Table XXXVI)
Behr syndrome (complicated optic atrophy),
    755
Beiderseitige Nierenagenesie, 856
Beidseitiges Acusticus-Neurinom, 12
Bell palsy, 224, 228, 376, 377, 378, 664, 727,
    779, 780, 880, 999
Benign acanthosis nigricans, 5
Benign adult form of osteopetrosis, 779
Benign cystinosis, 238
Benign epiphyseal osteochondroma, 311
Benign mellituria, 861
Benign migratory glossitis, 954
Benign symmetric lipomatosis, 601
Benign X-linked recessive muscular dys-
    trophy, 687
BERLIN SYNDROME, 105
Best disease, 622
β-glucuronidase deficiency, 680
β-hydroxyisovaleric aciduria, 107
β-ketothiolase deficiency, 40
Betalipoprotein deficiency, 2
BETA-MERCAPTOLACTATE-CYSTEINE
    DISULFIDURIA (MARKER), 106
BETA-METHYL-CROTONYL-GLYCIN-
    URIA, 107
Biber-Haab-Dimmer degeneration, 211
Bicornuate uterus, 684
BICUSPID AORTIC VALVE, 108
BICUSPID PULMONARY VALVE, 109
Bicuspid pulmonary valve with or without
    a raphe, 109
Bidermoma of head or neck, 283
Bifid nose, 724
Bifid tongue, 952

Bifid uvula, 184
Bikuspidale Aortenklappe, 108
Bikuspidale Pulmonalklappe, 109
Bilateral acoustic neurofibromata, 12
Bilateral aortic arch with left or right
    descending aorta, 75
Bilateral conductive deafness and absent
    incus-stapes junction, 244
Bilateral hyperopia with marked difference
    between eyes, 59
Bilateral myopia with marked difference
    between eyes, 59
Bile duct
    obstruction of, 110
    obstruction of common, 532
Bile duct cyst, 149
BILIARY ATRESIA, 110
Bilobed gallbladder, 404
Bing-Siebenmann dysplasia, 315
Biologic mother (see Section III, Table
    XXII)
Biotin-responsive β-methylcrotonylglycin-
    uria, 107
Bird-headed dwarfism, 881
Birthmark, 715
Birthweight
    high for gestational age and for ethnic
        group, 856
    low for gestational age and for ethnic
        group (see also Intrauterine growth
        retardation), 9, 160, 161, 163, 164,
        166, 167, 168, 169, 170, 242, 299,
        300, 305, 379, 381, 384, 385, 388,
        389, 603, 823, 999
    low for shortened gestational age
        and for ethnic group, 382
Bixler syndrome, 506
Bladder (see Gallbladder or Urinary bladder)
Bléfarocalasia, labio doble y tiroidea notóxica
    tumefacción, 111
Blepharochalasis, dédoublement de la lèvre et
    goitre non toxique, 111
Blepharochalasis, Doppellippe und Struma,
    111
BLEPHAROCHALASIS, DOUBLE LIP AND
    NONTOXIC THYROID
    ENLARGEMENT, 111
Blindness (see also Vision Section III, Table
    XXIV), 2, 224, 415, 433, 578, 593,
    621, 675, 736, 759, 780
    at birth, 101, 865
    at birth in male, 721
    secondary to corneal vascularization, 408
    temporary during summer in early life,
        538
    terminal after 5th–6th decade, 538
    with onset before 1 year, 43, 783
    with onset before 7 years, 759
    with onset in 5th decade, 408
Blindness for color
    confusion with yellow and blue shades,
        199, 755
    pastel color confusion, 197
    subnormal appreciation of green, 195, 196
    subnormal appreciation of red, 195, 197
    total, 198, 253, 755
Blistering, localized absence of skin and nail
    abnormalities, 609
Bloc cardiaque complet d'origine congénitale,
    454
Bloch-Sulzberger syndrome, 526
Blood group incompatibility during patient's
    prenatal life, 340
Blood pressure
    decreased, 47

decreased in left or right arm, 546
increased, 26, 91, 351, 441, 484, 578, 590,
    712, 776, 902, 903
labile hypertension, 351, 820, 822
postural hypotension, 820, 822
pulmonary venous hypertension, 92, 666
systolic pressure gradient between radial
    and femoral pulse, 73
widely different systemic arterial pulse
    pressure, 82, 466, 800
Blood vessel defects (see Section III, Table
    XXXII)
BLOOM SYNDROME, 112
Bloqueo aurículo-ventricular completo
    congéntio, 454
Blue diaper syndrome, 974
Blue monocone-monochromatic color blind-
    ness, 195
Blue rubber bleb nevus of skin and gastro-
    intestinal tract, 113
BLUE RUBBER BLEB NEVUS SYNDROME,
    113
Bochdalek hernia, 289
Bocio causado por bociógenos, 435
Boder-Sedgwick syndrome, 94
Body habitus
    eunuchoid, 438
    small for gestational age, 977
    stocky, 305
    thin, 39, 265, 352, 759
Bone (also see by name, group or part and
    Section III, Table XXIX)
    increased fractures with prenatal onset,
        777
    increased fragility of, 310, 325, 391, 776,
        847, 967
Bone, hair, nail, and tooth dysplasia, 965
Bony changes characteristic of rickets, 516,
    593, 873
Bony choanal atresia, anterior, 723
Bony choanal atresia, posterior, 727
Böök syndrome, 493
Bound-β-alanine metabolism, disorders of,
    126
Bourneville syndrome, 975
Bowed lower leg, 250, 704, 798, 828, 897
Bowel and bladder, dysfunction, 877
Bowel paralysis, 894
Bowen syndrome, 139
Brachycephaly (see Section III, Table
    XXIX)
BRACHYDACTYLY, 114
Brachydactyly (see also Section III, Table
    XXIX)
Brachydactyly and fibula dysplasia, 392
Brachydactyly and macular coloboma, 621
Brachydactyly, peculiar facies and mental
    retardation syndrome, 119
Brachydactyly type A₁ (Farabee type), 114
Brachydactyly type A₂ (brachymesophalangy
    II, Mohr-Wreidt type), 114
Brachydactyly type A₃ (brachymesophalangy
    V, clinodactyly), 114
Brachydactyly type B, 114
Brachydactyly type C, 114
Brachydactyly type D ("stub thumb"), 114
Brachydactyly type E (brachymesophalangy
    and brachymetapody), 114
Brailsford syndrome, 678
Brain
    absence of, 283, 380
    asymmetric, 578
    cerebral cortex, absent, 480
    cerebral cortex convolutions thickened,
        139, 578

cerebrocortical atrophy, 485, 744
cerebrum absent, 727
forebrain, failure to divide, 158, 168,
    473
gyri absent, 139, 578, 603
large ventricles, 481
midline defect of, 139, 158, 401
olfactory lobe absent, 634
olivopontocerebellar atrophy, 742, 743,
    744, 745, 746, 747
small, 220
spongoid, 881
sulci absent, 603
BRAIN, SPONGY DEGENERATION, 115
Branched-chain ketoaciduria, 628
Branched-chain ketonuria, 628
BRANCHER DEFICIENCY, 116
Branchial cleft cysts, Bailey type IV, 706
BRANCHIAL CLEFT CYSTS OR SINUSES,
    117
Branchial cleft fistula, 117
BRANCHIO–SKELETO–GENITAL
    SYNDROME, 118
Branchiogene Zyste, branchiogene Sinus, 117
Braquidactilia, 114
Breast fibroadenomas, hypertrichosis and
    gingival fibromatosis, 412
Breath sounds
    absence of, at base of lung, 39
    decreased at base of lung, 39
    decreased in left lower lobe, 120
    decreased on side of diaphragmatic
        hernia, 289
    pulmonary parenchymal amyloidosis,
        982
Breech delivery, 754, 823, 856
Brides, sillons (amniotiques), 874
Brièveté des tendons fléchisseurs des doigts
    avec incapacité d'ouverture complète-
    ment de la bouche, 882
"Broad beta" syndrome, 495
BROAD THUMB–HALLUX SYNDROME,
    119
Broad thumbs syndrome, 119
BRONCHIAL ATRESIA, 120
Bronchial atresia of posterior apical seg-
    ment left upper lobe, 120
Bronchiectasis, sinusitis and dextrocardia,
    285
Bronchitis, 522, 606, 986
    chronic, 706, 944
    recurrent, 263
    subacute, 706
Bronchus
    aberrant, 611
    absence of eparterial, 816
    atresia of, 120, 860
    bronchoesophageal fistula, 571
    bronchogenic cyst, 805
    pattern defect, 612
Bronze diabetes, 460
Brushfield spots, 121, 139, 171
Bruton agammaglobulinemia, 27
Bulbar symptoms, 344, 820, 822
Bürger-Grütz syndrome, 489
Buttocks, protuberant, 10

C

C SYNDROME, 121
Caffey disease, 221
Calasia esofágica, 366
Calcinose des artères coronaires, 217

Calcinosis de las coronarias, 217
Calescence des racines dentaires, 928
Calvaria (also see Section III, Table XXIX)
    anterior bifid cranium, 635
    asymmetric, 158, 227, 230, 408, 505,
        593, 887
    bifid cranium, 724
    bony defect in midline of, 343
    bulging areas of, 555
    craniofacial deformity secondary to bony
        mass, 390
    defect of, with midline herniation of
        meninges, 642
    defect of, with neural tissue exposed, 52
    deforming overgrowth of, 887
    hemicrania, 283
    midline mass of, 353
    oval shape of, 85
    pointed, vertical index above, 77
    progression of defect of, during infancy,
        227
    round, 281
    small on side of facial angioma, 915
    small (see Section III, Table XXIX)
    soft membranous, 77
    triangular shape of, 121, 162, 167, 470
    trilobed, 555
    wormian bones in, 825
Calvicie común, 99
Calvitie commune, 99
Cámara pulpar dentaria en llama, 937
Campomelic dwarfism, 122
CAMPOMELIC DYSPLASIA, 122
Camptodactyly, 22, 85, 89, 114, 139, 140,
    157, 160, 165, 166, 168, 379, 393,
    450, 556, 603, 634, 635, 644, 650,
    737, 791, 981
Camptodactyly and limited jaw excursion,
    882
Camptodactyly, facultative, 882
Camptomelic syndrome, 122
Camurati-Engelmann syndrome, 290
Canalicules lacrymaux surnuméraires, 844
Canaliculi and puncta, supernumerary, 844
Canalículos y orificios lacrimales super-
    numerarios, 844
Canavan disease, 115
Cancer endocrinien multiple I, 350
Cancer endocrinien multiple II, 351
Cancer endocrinien multiple III, 352
Canine teeth
    globe-shaped crown of, 784
    malposition of, 493
    pit in center of, 276
Capacité d'enrouler la langue, 951
Capillary hemangioma, 715
Capillary lymphangiomas of orbit, 765
Capillary nevus, 715
Capsular and polar cataracts, 133
Capsulolenticular cataract, 133
Carbamyl phosphate synthetase deficiency,
    485
Carbohydrate-induced hyperlipemia, 500
Cardiac limb syndrome, 455
CARDIOAUDITORY SYNDROME, 123
Cardiocutaneous syndrome, 586
Cardioduodenal duct, 912
Cardiomelic syndrome, 455
Cardiopatía congénita, sordera y mal-
    formaciones esqueléticas, 667
Cardiopathie congénitale, surdité et mal-
    formations squelettiques, 667
Cardiospasm, 363
Cardiovascular inflammation, 37, 97, 236,
    387, 398, 441, 460, 531, 748, 883

Cardiovascular system (see parts and Section
    III, Table XXXII)
CARNITINE DEFICIENCY OF MUSCLE,
    PRIMARY, 124
CARNITINE PALMITYL TRANSFERASE
    DEFICIENCY, 125
Carnitinpalmityl-Transferase-Mangel, 125
CARNOSINEMIA, 126
Carotid artery aneurysm, 530
Carotid artery, common origin of brachio-
    cephalic and contralateral, 200
Carotid artery, occlusion of, 474
CAROTID BODY TUMOR, 127
Carpal osteochondroma, 311
CARPAL–TARSAL OSTEOLYSIS AND
    CHRONIC PROGRESSIVE
    GLOMERULOPATHY, 128
CARPAL–TARSAL OSTEOLYSIS, RE-
    CESSIVE, 129
Carpenter syndrome, 13
Carpopedal spasm, 515
Carpotarsal and cranial dystrophy, 223
Carpotarsale Anomalien, Gaumenspalte,
    Oligodontie und Schwerhörigkeit mit
    Stapes-Fixation, 183
Cartilage-hair hypoplasia, 653
CARUNCLE ABERRATIONS, 130
Cat cry syndrome, 163
Cat eye syndrome, 544
Catación de la feniltiocarbamida
    (Marcador), 809
Cataract (also see Section III, Table XXIV)
    present at birth, 106, 261, 635, 708
    with juvenile onset, 155, 261, 403,
        550
CATARACT AND ICHTHYOSIS, 131
Cataractes corticales et nucléaires, 132
Cataractes polaires et capsulaires, 133
CATARACTS, CORTICAL AND NUCLEAR,
    132
CATARACTS, POLAR AND CAPSULAR,
    133
Cataratas corticales y nucleares, 132
Cataratas polar y capsular, 133
Cauda equina lipoma, 602
Cavernous lymphangiomas of orbit, 765
Cavernous transformation of portal vein, 468
CBG-transcortin, 222
Cebocephaly, 234
Cécité aux couleurs, 198
Cécité pour le bleu et le jaune, 199
Cecum, free floating, 121
Cefalocele orbitario, 762
Ceguera al color amarillo-azul, 199
Ceguera al color total, 198
Ceguera-monocónica-monocromática al color
    azul, 195
Ceguera nocturna, 718
Ceguera nocturna estacionaria, 719
Celiac disease, 423
Celiac sprue, 423
CENTRAL CORE DISEASE, 134
Central crystalline corneal dystrophy, 216
Central cystoid dystrophy, 622
Central exudative detachment of retina, 622
Central nervous system arteriovenous mal-
    formation, 186
Central nervous system neoplasms, 188
Central neurofibromatosis, 12
CENTRALOPATHIC EPILEPSY, 135
Centronuclear myopathy, 695
CEREBELLAR ATAXIA AND CHORIO-
    RETINAL DEGENERATION, 136
Cerebellar-macular abiotrophy, 745

Cerebellar signs, 2, 255, 344, 406, 579, 717,
    810, 820, 822, 963
Cerebral artery, occlusion of, 832
CEREBRAL GIGANTISM, 137
Cerebral G_{M1}-gangliosidosis, 431
Cerebral palsy, spastic, 588
Cerebral sclerosis, degenerative diffuse-
    Scholz type, 651
Cerebral sclerosis – diffuse Krabbe type, 415
Cerebral sclerosis I, 803
Cerebral white matter, spongy degeneration,
    115
CEREBRO–COSTO–MANDIBULAR
    SYNDROME, 138
CEREBRO–HEPATO–RENAL SYNDROME,
    139
Cerebromacular degeneration, 713
Cerebro-oculo-facio-ossäres Syndrom, 140
CEREBRO–OCULO–FACIO–SKELETAL
    SYNDROME, 140
Cerebroside lipidosis, 406
Cerebroside sulfatidosis, 651
Cerebrosidosis, 406
Cerebrovascular defect, 121, 186, 187, 777,
    825, 832, 859
Ceruloplasmin deficiency, 469
CERUMEN VARIATION (MARKER), 141
Ceruminalformen, 141
Cervical aortic arch, 74
Cervical cyst or sinus, 117
Cervical lipomatosis, familial benign, 601
Cervical spina bifida with meningocele,
    642, 727
Cervical spine
    short, 900
    with block vertebrae, 130, 142, 481, 667
Cervical teratomas, 283
Cervical, thoracic (complete or incomplete)
    and thoracoabdominal ectopia cordis,
    335
CERVICO–OCULO–ACOUSTIC SYN-
    DROME, 142
Cervicooculofacial dystrophy, 142
CESD, 151
Chalasie, 366
Chalasoderma, 233
Chambre pulpaire (en fleur de chardon), 937
Charcot-Marie-Tooth disease with optico-
    acoustic degeneration, 268
Chédiak anomaly, syndrome or disease, 143
CHÉDIAK–HIGASHI SYNDROME, 143
Chédiak-Steinbrinck anomaly, disease or
    syndrome, 143
Cheeks
    full, broad, 13, 223, 470, 775, 999
    sagging, 629
Cheilite glandulaire, 144
CHEILITIS GLANDULARIS, 144
Cheilitis glandularis apostematosa, 144
Cheilopalatoschisis, 178
Cheiloschisis, 178
Chéloïde, 551
Chemisch induzierte Struma, 435
CHEMODECTOMA OF MIDDLE EAR, 145
Chemodectoma of neck, 127
Chémodectomie de l'oreille moyenne, 145
Cherry red spot – myoclonus syndrome, 671
Cherub dwarfs, 293
Cherubism, 539
Chest
    asymmetry of, 338, 887
    barrel, 306, 897
    broad, 629, 898
    defect of, 156, 270, 532, 685

Chest – *Continued*
  funnel (pectus excavatum), 1, 85, 118,
      190, 394, 412, 474, 554, 572, 576,
      629, 630, 676, 754, 777, 802
  keeled (pectus carinatum), 22, 85, 155,
      190, 257, 306, 394, 474, 629, 630,
      678, 777, 801
  large, 898
  long and narrow in infancy, 656
  midline defect of anterior thoracic wall,
      335
  narrow, costal angle below 90°, 10, 91,
      883, 884, 940
  pear-shaped, 825
  proximally keeled with distal funnel
      chest, 720
  reduced mobility of, 91, 470, 700
  small in all dimensions, 156
  short, 940
Chicken breast, 801
Childhood pseudohypertrophic muscular
      dystrophy, 689
Chin
  depression on, 223
  fissure on, 146
  protruding, 10, 394, 626
  rests on chest, 900
  round dimple on, 146
  small, 155, 394, 881
  trembling of, 147
Chin cleft, 146
Chin dimple, 146
CHIN FISSURE, 146
Chin groove or furrow, 146
Chin, quivering, 147
CHIN, TREMBLING, 147
CHLORIDE DIARRHEA, CONGENITAL,
      148
Choanal atresia, anterior, 723
Choanal atresia, posterior, 727
CHOLEDOCHAL CYST, 149
Choledochocele, 149
Choledochus-zyste, 149
Cholesteatom, 150
CHOLESTEATOMA OF TEMPORAL
      BONE, 150
Cholesteatome de l'os temporal, 150
Cholesterinester-Speicherkrankheit, 151
CHOLESTERYL ESTER STORAGE
      DISEASE, 151
CHOLINESTERASE, ATYPICAL, 152
CHONDRODYSPLASIA PUNCTATA,
      CONRADI-HÜNERMANN TYPE, 153
Chondrodysplasia punctata, rhizomele
      form, 154
CHONDRODYSPLASIA PUNCTATA,
      RHIZOMELIC TYPE, 154
Chondrodysplasie léthale avec polydactylie,
      type Majewski, 883
Chondrodysplasie léthale avec polydactylie,
      type Saldino-Noonan, 884
Chondrodysplasie métaphysaire avec in-
      suffisance pancréatique exocrine et
      neutropénie cyclique, 885
Chondrodysplasie métaphysaire avec thymo-
      lymphopénie, 655
Chondrodysplasie métaphysaire dominante,
      type Schmid, 654
Chondrodysplasie métaphysaire récessive
      autosomique, type McKusick, 653
Chondrodysplasie métaphysaire type Jansen,
      652
Chondrodysplasie ponctuée, type Conradi-
      Hünermann, 153

Chondrodysplasie ponctuée, type rhizomélique,
      154
Chondrodysplasie spondylométaphysaire,
      type Kozlowski, 899
Chondrodystrophia calcificans, 153
Chondrodystrophia foetalis, 10
CHONDRODYSTROPHIC MYOTONIA, 155
Chondrodystrophie epiphysaire, 311
Chondrodystrophy, 10
Chondrodystrophy with clubfeet, 293
CHONDROECTODERMAL DYSPLASIA,
      156
Chondromes du pavillon de l'oreille, 317
Chondroosteodystrophy, 678
Chonechondrosternon, 802
Chorea, progressive, 478
Chorea Huntington, 478
Choreiform movements, 94, 421, 478, 588,
      638, 742, 1004
Chorioretinal degeneration and ataxia, 136
Chorioretinitis, toxoplasmic, 387
Choroid
  atrophy of, 479, 732, 925
  blood vessel changes, 925
  calcification of, 494
  cleft of, 457, 544, 585, 593, 733
  cleft of uvea, 585
  degeneration of, 449
  inflammation of, 381, 387, 998
  sclerosis of, 136
Choroidal sclerosis, X-linked, 925
Choroideremia, 925
Christ-Siemens-Touraine syndrome, 333
Christmas disease factor deficiency, 462
Chromatophore nevus of Naegeli, 703
Chromosome E1-trisomy syndrome, 160
CHROMOSOME EIGHT TRISOMY
      SYNDROME, 157
CHROMOSOME EIGHTEEN p− SYN-
      DROME, 158
CHROMOSOME EIGHTEEN q− SYN-
      DROME, 159
CHROMOSOME EIGHTEEN TRISOMY
      SYNDROME, 160
CHROMOSOME ELEVEN q PARTIAL
      TRISOMY SYNDROME, 161
CHROMOSOME ELEVEN q− SYN-
      DROME, 162
CHROMOSOME FIVE p− SYNDROME,
      163
CHROMOSOME FOUR p− SYNDROME,
      164
CHROMOSOME FOURTEEN q DISTAL
      PARTIAL TRISOMY SYNDROME
      165
CHROMOSOME FOURTEEN q PROXIMAL
      PARTIAL TRISOMY SYNDROME,
      166
Chromosome partial 17 trisomy, 160
CHROMOSOME THIRTEEN q− SYN-
      DROME, 167
CHROMOSOME THIRTEEN TRISOMY
      SYNDROME, 168
CHROMOSOME TRIPLOIDY SYNDROME,
      169
Chromosome trisomy 17 syndrome, 160
Chromosome trisomy 17-18 syndrome, 160
CHROMOSOME TWENTY–ONE MONO-
      SOMY, 170
CHROMOSOME TWENTY–ONE TRISOMY
      SYNDROME, 171
CHROMOSOME TWENTY–TWO MONO-
      SOMY, 172

Chromosome 13r syndrome, 167
Chromosome 18r syndrome (most cases),
      159
CHROMOSOME 45,X/46,XY MOSAICISM,
      173
Chronic diffuse alopecia, 99
Chronic familial granulomatosis, 443
Chronic granulomatous disease of child-
      hood, 443
Chronic osteopathy with hyperphosphatasia,
      776
Chronic progressive external ophthalmo-
      plegia, 752
Chronic progressive keratoatrophoderma,
      819
Chronische Granulomatose beim männlichen
      Geschlecht, 443
Chronische Granulomatose beim weiblichen
      Geschlecht, 442
Chvostek sign, positive, 515, 873
Chwechweechwe, 886
Chylous ascites, 534
Cicatricial keloids, 551
Ciclopía, 234
Cilindromas del cuero cabelludo, 235
Circumvallate placenta syndrome, 187
Cirsoid aneurysm of external ear, 313
Cistationinuria, 236
Cistinosis, 238
Cistinuria, 239
CITRULLINEMIA, 174
Citrullinuria, 174
CLASPED THUMBS, 175
Class III skeletal malocclusion, 626
Classic hemophilia, 461
Classic X-linked recessive muscular dystrophy,
      689
Clavicle
  absence of, 185
  defect of, 98, 160, 161, 455, 901
  short, 455, 825
  short lateral portion of, 846
Cleft ear lobe, 321
Cleft, facial lateral, 374
Cleft, facial oblique, 375
Cleft larynx, posterior, 577
CLEFT LIP OR PALATE AND FILIFORM
      FUSION OF EYELIDS, 176
CLEFT LIP OR PALATE AND LIP PITS
      OR MOUNDS, 177
CLEFT LIP–PALATE, ECTODERMAL
      DYSPLASIA AND SYNDACTYLY,
      179
Cleft lip-palate, ectodermal dysplasia, hand-
      foot anomalies and oligophrenia, 179
Cleft lip-palate, popliteal pterygium, digital
      and genital anomalies, 818
Cleft lip-palate with split hand or foot, 337
CLEFT LIP WITH OR WITHOUT
      CLEFT PALATE, 178
Cleft, maxillary median alveolar, 631
Cleft of soft and hard palate, 180
Cleft of soft palate, 180
CLEFT PALATE, 180
Cleft palate and cleft lip, 178
CLEFT PALATE AND PERSISTENCE
      OF BUCCOPHARYNGEAL MEM-
      BRANE, 181
CLEFT PALATE, MICROGNATHIA AND
      GLOSSOPTOSIS, 182
CLEFT PALATE, STAPES FIXATION AND
      OLIGODONTIA, 183
Cleft tongue, 952
CLEFT UVULA (MARKER), 184

Cleidocranial dysostosis, 185
CLEIDOCRANIAL DYSPLASIA, 185
Clinical anophthalmia, 67
Clinodactyly, 22, 72, 85, 121, 157, 158,
    162, 163, 166, 171, 172, 223, 229,
    242, 281, 634, 635, 769, 770, 771, 769
    791, 887, 966, 980, 981
Clitoris
    hypertrophy of, 104, 139, 173, 388, 389,
        437, 587, 818, 909, 971
    hypoplasia of, 876
    marked hypertrophy of, 908
    progressive hypertrophy of, 908
Cloaca exstrophy of, persisting, 193
Cloison vaginale transversale, 985
Clorurorrea, 148
Cloverleaf skull syndrome, 555
Clumsiness (also see Coordination)
    of fine motor movements of upper
        limb, 803
    progressive, 86
CNS ARTERIOVENOUS MALFORMA-
    TION, 186
CNS DEPRESSION, HEMORRHAGE,
    SKELETAL SYNDROME, 187
CNS NEOPLASMS, 188
CNS tumors, 12, 101, 113, 345, 346, 351,
    712, 763, 995
Coarctación de la arteria pulmonar, 835
Coarctation de l'aorte, 73
Coarctation of abdominal aorta, 73
Coarctation of lower thoracic aorta, 73
Coartación de la aorta, 73
Cobalamin malabsorption, 992
Cochlea, defect of, 142, 315, 777, 982
Cochlear deafness, myopia and oligo-
    phrenia, 251
COCKAYNE SYNDROME, 189
Coelonychie, 559
COFFIN–LOWRY SYNDROME, 190
Coffin syndrome, 190
COFS syndrome, 140
COGAN CONGENITAL OCULAR MOTOR
    APRAXIA, 191
Coiloniquia, 559
Colesteatoma del hueso temporal, 150
Colinesterasa plasmática atipíca, 152
Coloboma de la mácula y braquidactilia, 621
Colobomas oculares, 733
Colobome maculaire et brachydactylie, 621
Colobomes de l'iris, de la rétine, 733
Colon absence, 193
COLON AGANGLIONOSIS, 192
Colon agenesis, 193
COLON ATRESIA OR STENOSIS, 193
COLON DUPLICATION, 194
Colon polyposis, 535
Colonic "cyst," 194
Color blindness (see Blindness)
COLOR BLINDNESS, BLUE MONOCONE-
    MONOCHROMATIC, 195
COLOR BLINDNESS, RED–GREEN
    DEUTAN SERIES, 196
COLOR BLINDNESS, RED–GREEN
    PROTAN SERIES, 197
COLOR BLINDNESS, TOTAL, 198
COLOR BLINDESS, YELLOW–BLUE, 199
Coma, 40, 87, 174, 424, 460, 485, 512, 530,
    547, 628, 658, 820, 822, 826
    as newborn, 396
    in fasting state or with fever, 396
    intermittent, 547
Combined hyperlipidemia, 496
Combined hyperlipoproteinemia, 496

Combined stenosis, 919
Commissural lip pits (isolated trait), 596
Common atrium, 96
COMMON ORIGIN OF BRACHIO-
    CEPHALIC AND CONTRALATERAL
    CAROTID ARTERY, 200
Common variable immunodeficiency, 521
Communicating hydrocele, 529
Communication interauriculaire, 96
Complement C′1 esterase inhibitor deficiency,
    54
Complement C′1 esterase inhibitor dysfunc-
    tion, 54
Complement C5 deficiency, 812
Complete atrioventricular (A-V) block, 454
Complete d-transposition, 962
Complete transposition of great veins, 842
Complete transposition of great vessels, 962
Componente del grupo específico Gc
    (Marcador), 446
Concrescencia de las raíces dentarias, 928
Concrescence of roots of teeth, 928
Condrodisplasia espóndilometafisaria, tipo
    Kozlowski, 899
Condrodisplasia metafisaria con timolinfo-
    penia, 655
Condrodisplasia metafisaria, tipo Jansen, 652
Condrodisplasia metafisaria, tipo McKusick,
    653
Condrodisplasia metafisaria, tipo Schmid,
    654
Condrodisplasia punctata, tipo Conradi-
    Hünermann, 153
Condrodisplasia punctata, tipo rizomiélica,
    154
Conductive deafness with malformed low-
    set ears, 254
Conductive hearing loss (see Section III,
    Table XXV)
Conducto nasolacrimal impermeable, 705
Cone monochromatism, 195
CONE–ROD DEGENERATION, 201
Conexión anómala de las venas pulmonares
    parcial, 841
Congenital absence of hemidiaphragm, 289
Congenital absence of nails, 66
Congenital absence of one pulmonary artery
    with blood supplied to the affected
    lung by means of a ductus arteriosus,
    768
Congenital absence of testes, 68
Congenital absence of the thymus and
    parathyroid, 943
Congenital absence of uterus and vagina, 682
Congenital absence or deficiency of muscle
    between the pleura and peritoneum,
    288
Congenital adrenal hypoplasia associated
    with congenital hypoplasia of the
    pituitary gland, 24
Congenital agammaglobulinemia, 27
Congenital alactasia, 566
Congenital amaurosis of retinal origin, 43
Congenital amputations, 874
Congenital anhidrosis, 56
Congenital anterior staphyloma, 439
Congenital aortic sinus aneurysm with or
    without rupture, 53
Congenital aplasia of pylorus, 910
Congenital asymmetry, 458
Congenital atresia of nasopharynx, 181
Congenital atresia of the subclavian artery,
    546
Congenital bicuspid aortic valve, 108

Congenital bilateral absence of kidneys, 856
Congenital bilateral facial palsy, 377
Congenital bilateral pseudoglioma of
    retina with recessive X-linked in-
    heritance, 721
Congenital blepharoptosis, 834
Congenital bowing of the limbs, 122
Congenital buphthalmos, 414
Congenital cataracts, 132
Congenital cholesteatoma, 150
Congenital chondrosternal prominence,
    801
Congenital complete heart block, 454
Congenital complete sinoatrial block, 454
Congenital contractural arachnodactyly, 85
Congenital croup, 576
Congenital cystic dilation of common duct,
    149
Congenital cysts of larynx, 572
Congenital cysts of the nasopharynx, 706
Congenital cytomegalic inclusion disease,
    381
Congenital defects of eustachian tube, 370
Congenital diaphragm of esophagus, 369
Congenital dislocation of lacrimal gland, 564
Congenital dysfibrinogenemia, 4
Congenital dysphagocytosis, 443
Congenital ectopia lentis, 584
Congenital ectopic lens and pupil, 583
Congenital ectropion of conjuctiva, 371
Congenital ectropion of lids, 371
Congenital endothelial dystrophy of cornea,
    208
Congenital entropion of lid, 372
Congenital erythroid hypoplastic anemia, 51
Congenital esophageal stricture, 369
Congenital gastric diverticulum, 911
Congenital generalized cutaneous elasto-
    lysis, 233
Congenital gigantism of peroxidase granules,
    143
Congenital goiter, 435
Congenital granular cell myoblastoma, 360
Congenital granular cell tumor, 360
Congenital hereditary absence of breast
    tissue and nipple either unilateral or
    bilateral, with no associated endo-
    crine or chromosomal disorder, 42
Congenital hereditary corneal dystrophy,
    207
Congenital hereditary endothelial dys-
    trophy, 207
Congenital hereditary lymphedema, 614
Congenital hereditary stationary dystrophy,
    207
Congenital Horner syndrome, 475
Congenital hyperparathyroidism, 499
Congenital hypertrichosis lanuginosa, 507
Congenital hypertrophic pyloric stenosis,
    848
Congenital hypoplastic thrombocytopenia
    with skeletal deformities, 941
Congenital isolated lipase deficiency, 597
Congenital laryngeal atresia, 571
Congenital laryngeal chondromalacia, 576
Congenital lysinuria, 491
Congenital macular degeneration, 622
Congenital medial sclerosis of coronary
    arteries, 217
Congenital median fissure of nose, 724
Congenital mesodermal dysmorphodys-
    trophy, brachymorphic type, 893
Congenital microphakia and spherophakia,
    663

Congenital mitral valve insufficiency, 668
Congenital myopia, 699
Congenital myotonia, 701
Congenital narrowing of tricuspid orifice as a consequence of either a small annulus or thickened valve leaflets, 970
Congenital nephrotic syndrome, 709
Congenital nonspherocytic hemolytic anemia associated with G6PD deficiency, 420
Congenital nonspherocytic hemolytic anemias associated with diminished activity or kinetic abnormalities of erythrocyte pyruvate kinase, 852
Congenital oculodermal melanocytosis, 716
Congenital optic atrophy, 755
Congenital pancreatic aplasia, 885
Congenital pancreatic lipase deficiency, 597
Congenital partial atresia of larynx, 571
Congenital partial facial palsy, 377
Congenital partial or complete absence of the pericardium, 805
Congenital pericardial defects, 805
Congenital pharyngopalatinal diaphragm, 181
Congenital pigmentary cirrhosis, 460
Congenital pigmentation of optic disk, 639
Congenital posterior cleft of larynx and trachea with persistent esophagotrachea, 577
Congenital pronation, 854
Congenital red cell aregenerative anemia, 51
Congenital relaxation of diaphragm, 288
Congenital retinal cyst, 871
Congenital retinal degeneration, 43
Congenital retinal septum, 867
Congenital rhabdomyoma, 360
Congenital rubella, 384
Congenital sinuses of external ear, 329
Congenital stridor, 576
Congenital "subclavian steal" syndrome, 546
Congenital syngnathism, 181
Congenital telangiectatic erythema and stunted growth, 112
Congenital thrombocytopenia with aplasia of the radii, 941
Congenital thymic dysplasia, 524
Congenital underdevelopment of the lashes, 623
Congenital unilateral facial palsy, 377
Congenital vascular veils in the vitreous, 871
Congenital virilizing adrenal hyperplasia, 908
Congenital vitelliform cysts of macula, 622
Conical cornea, 552
CONJOINED TWINS, 202
Conjunctiva
    bluish-grey spots on palpebral, 716
    conjunctivitis, 15, 355, 413, 515, 821
    cystine crystal deposits on slit-lamp exam, 238
    gelatinous peripheral plaques on, 538
    malignant tumor of, 1004, 1005
    marked dryness of, 885
    persistent, 102
    pterygia in, 47
    purulent, 27
    yellow connective tissue thickening in, 47, 406, 591
Conjunctival dermoid, 591
Conjunctival vessels
    aneurysmal dilatation of, 373
    subconjunctival lipoma, 735
    telangiectasia of, 94
    tortuous, 373

Conradi-Hünermann syndrome, 153
Constipation, 542, 672, 754, 820, 822, 848, 949, 974, 999
    as neonate, 69, 531
    chronic, 192
    fecal soiling absent in infancy or childhood (also see Obstipation), 192
    in infancy, 193
Constitutional granular gigantism, 143
Constitutional hepatic dysfunction, 487
Constricciones anulares congénitas, 874
Constrictive cardiopathy, 353, 354
Contracture de Dupuytren, 301
Contractures, multiple with arachnodactyly, 85
Cooley anemia, 939
Coordination
    decreased, 12, 93, 137, 188, 191, 671, 713, 743, 963
    defect of motor and power, 384, 638
Copper retention, 469
Coproporfiria hereditaria, 203
COPROPORPHYRIA, 203
Coproporphyrie héréditaire, 203
COR TRIATRIATUM, 204
Cor triatriatum sinistrum, 204
Cor triatum, 204
Cor triloculare, 182
Cor triloculare biatriatum, 286
Cord cyst associated with posterior mediastinal cyst, 894
Corea de Huntington, 478
Cornea
    cataract at birth, 738
    central anterior adhesions, 845
    conical protrusion of, 43, 552, 777, 865
    cystine crystal deposits on slit-lamp exam, 238
    desquamation of, 215
    diameter over 13 mm, 637, 638
    dryness of, 378
    erosions of, 209, 212, 214
    erosions of 1–2 mm, 214
    granulation of, 736
    infiltration of, 48
    inflammation of, 372, 385, 515, 553, 821, 1004, 1005
    large, 1, 414, 637, 672
    limbus sclerization of, 205
    macules on, 212
    recurrent painful erosions of, 211
    recurrent painful erosions with onset before puberty, 214, 215
    reflexes diminished, 12, 211, 212, 215, 265, 560
    rupture of, 338
    scarring of, 210, 593, 736, 1004, 1005
    small, 155, 242, 732, 735, 737
    spheric protrusion of, 43, 865
    stroma of diffusely edematous, 206
    stroma of diffusely thickened at birth, 207
    vascularization of, 413, 593
    Vogt limbal girdles, 216
Cornea, conical, 552
Cornea, enlarged, 637
Cornea guttata, 208
CORNEA PLANA, 205
Corneal clouding
    circumlimbal, 603
    diffuse, 678
    edema with, 139, 140, 213, 281, 384, 398, 414, 672, 675, 679, 680
    irregular, 212
    progressive, 207, 674, 679

CORNEAL DYSTROPHY AND SENSORINEURAL DEAFNESS, 206
Corneal endothelium
    partial detachment of, 140
    vesicles on, 213
CORNEAL DYSTROPHY, CONGENITAL HEREDITARY, 207
Corneal dystrophy, crystalline, 216
Corneal dystrophy, disturbed eruption of teeth and gingival fibromatosis, 408
CORNEAL DYSTROPHY, ENDOTHELIAL, 208
CORNEAL DYSTROPHY, GRANULAR, 209
CORNEAL DYSTROPHY, JUVENILE EPITHELIAL, 210
CORNEAL DYSTROPHY, LATTICE, 211
CORNEAL DYSTROPHY, MACULAR, 212
CORNEAL DYSTROPHY, POLYMORPHOUS POSTERIOR, 213
CORNEAL DYSTROPHY, RECURRENT EROSIVE, 214
CORNEAL DYSTROPHY, REIS-BÜCKLERS, 215
CORNEAL DYSTROPHY, SCHNYDER CRYSTALLINE, 216
Corneal opacity
    arcus juvenilis, 216, 488, 495
    arcus senilis, 216
    blue-white, 206
    by slit lamp, 673
    central, 282, 439
    curtain-like, affecting upper half of cornea, 408
    diffuse, 205, 206, 373
    multiple in axial corneal stroma, 209
    peripheral, 205, 1000
    progressive, 18, 57
    punctate, 210
    ring-like or annular in region of Bowman membrane, 215
    staphylomatous, 439
    total, 205
    traumatic, 372
    unspecified, 552, 661, 671, 680, 749, 757, 783
    white, 18, 843
Corneal opacities and gingival fibromatosis, 408
Cornée plane, 205
Cornelia de Lange syndrome, 242
Coronal dentin dysplasia, 277
CORONARY ARTERIAL CALCINOSIS, 217
Coronary arteries, anomalous origin from pulmonary artery, 64
CORONARY ARTERIOVENOUS FISTULA, 218
Coronary artery, calcification of, 217
Coronary artery-cameral shunt, 218
Coronary artery sclerosis, 217
CORONARY ARTERY, SINGLE, 219
Coronary calcification of infancy, 217
CORPUS CALLOSUM AGENESIS, 220
Corrected transposition of great vessels or arteries, 540
Cortical and nuclear cataracts, 132
CORTICAL HYPEROSTOSIS, INFANTILE, 221
CORTICOSTEROID–BINDING GLOBULIN ABNORMALITIES, 222
Cough, 39, 75, 117, 200, 283, 573, 805, 960
Coumadin embryopathy, 389
Cowden disease, 412

Crâne en feuille de trèfle, 555
Cráneosinostosis, 230
Cranial base
  flattened, **121, 777**
  foramen magnum small, **10, 103**
  short, **10, 14, 180, 227**
Cranial meningoceles, **642**
Cranial meningoencephaloceles, **343**
Cranial nerve involvement, **97, 127, 145, 150, 188, 224, 228, 310, 376, 377, 378, 451, 497, 530, 578, 664, 727, 743, 779, 780, 820, 823, 880, 999**
Cranial sutures
  delayed closure of, **139**
  depression of coronal or lambdoidal, **226**
  palpable at birth, **230**
  premature closure of, **13, 225, 230, 380, 516, 555, 634, 754, 999**
  ridging of all, **230**
  ridging of lambdoidal, **227**
  ridging of metopic, **121**
  ridging of posterior portion of sagittal suture, **227**
  separated after age 1 yr, **188**
  wide separation of, **139, 846**
CRANIO–CARPO–TARSAL DYSPLASIA, **223**
CRANIODIAPHYSEAL DYSPLASIA, **224**
CRANIOFACIAL DYSOSTOSIS, **225**
CRANIOFACIAL DYSOSTOSIS WITH DIAPHYSEAL HYPERPLASIA, **226**
CRANIOFACIAL DYSSYNOSTOSIS, **227**
Craniofaciale Dysostosie mit diaphysärer Hyperplasie, **226**
CRANIOMETAPHYSEAL DYSPLASIA, **228**
CRANIO–OCULO–DENTAL SYNDROME, **229**
Craniorachischisis, **52**
Craniostenosis, **13, 225, 230, 380, 516, 555, 634, 754, 999**
Craniosynostose avec aplasie radiale, **231**
CRANIOSYNOSTOSIS, **230**
Craniosynostosis-craniofacial dysostosis syndrome with mental retardation and other malformations, **227**
CRANIOSYNOSTOSIS–RADIAL APLASIA SYNDROME, **231**
Cranium bifidum, **343**
Crater-like cavities in optic disk, **756**
Cravet association, **987**
Cretinism, athyreotic, **946**
Crétinisme acquis, **435**
Cri du chat syndrome, **163**
Crigler-Najjar syndrome, **961**
Criptotia, **232**
Crouzon syndrome, **225**
Crown-pubis length decreased, **306, 394, 671, 798, 897, 898, 899**
Cry
  abnormal, **163**
  excessive, **64, 163, 689**
  high-pitched, **163, 628, 736, 891**
  hoarse, **401, 946**
  weak, **163**
Cryptophthalmus, **3**
Cryptothyroidism, **946**
CRYPTOTIA, **232**
Crystalline corneal dystrophy, **216**
Cubitus valgus, **98, 139, 308, 685, 704, 720, 791, 977**
Cumarin-Embryopathie, **389**
Cup ear, **314**
Cutaneous, cartilaginous and corneal lesions, **282**

CUTIS LAXA, **233**
Cyanosis (see Section III, Table XXXI)
Cyclic neutropenia, **714**
CYCLOPIA, **234**
CYLINDROMAS OF SCALP, **235**
Cylindromatosis, **235**
Cylindrome du cuir chevelu, **235**
Cystathionine synthase deficiency, **474**
Cystathioninemia, **236**
CYSTATHIONINURIA, **236**
Cystic arteriovenous malformations, **186**
Cystic artery anomalies, **404**
CYSTIC FIBROSIS, **237**
Cystic fibrosis of pancreas, **237**
Cystic hamartoma of liver, **604**
Cystic hygroma of mesentery, **645**
Cystic lymphangiomas of orbit, **765**
Cystic teratoma, **760**
Cystine-lysine-arginine-ornithinuria, **239**
Cystine storage disease, **238**
CYSTINOSIS, **238**
CYSTINURIA, **239**
Cystinuria and dibasic aminoaciduria, **239**
Cystinuria I, II, III, **239**
Cystinuria without dibasic aminoaciduria, **490**
Cystinurie, **239**
CYSTS OF SPLEEN, **240**
Cytomegalovirus infection, **381**
Cytomegalovirus in utero, **381**

D

D Trisomy syndrome, **168**
Daltonisme-protanomalie-protanopie, **197**
Dandy-Walker syndrome, **481**
DARWIN TUBERCLE (MARKER), **241**
Darwinscher Höcker, **241**
Davies disease, **353, 354**
DE LANGE SYNDROME, **242**
Deaf-mutism and cutaneous albinism, **30**
DEAF-MUTISM, SEMILETHAL, **243**
Deafness (also see Section III, Table XXV)
DEAFNESS AND ABSENT INCUDO–STAPEDIAL JUNCTION, **244**
DEAFNESS AND ATOPIC DERMATITIS, **245**
Deafness and cataract with muscular atrophy and skeletal defects, **785**
DEAFNESS AND DIABETES, **246**
DEAFNESS AND EAR PITS, **247**
DEAFNESS AND EPISODIC VERTIGO, **248**
Deafness and functional heart disease, **123**
DEAFNESS AND GOITER, **249**
DEAFNESS AND METAPHYSEAL DYSOSTOSIS, **250**
DEAFNESS AND MYOPIA, **251**
DEAFNESS AND ONYCHODYSTROPHY, **252**
DEAFNESS AND PROGRESSIVE OPTIC NERVE ATROPHY, **253**
DEAFNESS-CONDUCTIVE, AND MALFORMED LOW-SET EARS, **254**
Deafness, congenital unilateral, **274**
DEAFNESS, DIABETES, PHOTOMYOCLONUS AND NEPHROPATHY, **255**
DEAFNESS, DOMINANT LOW-FREQUENCY, **256**
DEAFNESS, GOITER AND PERIPHERAL RESISTANCE TO THYROID HORMONE, **257**
DEAFNESS, HYPERPROLINURIA AND ICHTHYOSIS, **258**

DEAFNESS, KERATOPACHYDERMIA AND DIGITAL CONSTRICTIONS, **259**
Deafness, knuckle pads and leukonychia, **558**
DEAFNESS, LOW-TONE, **260**
Deafness, mitral insufficiency and skeletal malformations, **667**
DEAFNESS, MYOPIA, CATARACT AND SADDLE NOSE, **261**
DEAFNESS, ONYCHODYSTROPHY AND DIGITAL ANOMALIES, **262**
Deafness-optic atrophy syndrome, **253**
DEAFNESS, PERIPHERAL PULMONARY STENOSES AND BRACHYTELEPHALANGY, **263**
DEAFNESS, RENAL AND DIGITAL ANOMALIES, **264**
Deafness, sensorineural and hand muscle wasting, **450**
Deafness, sensorineural, ataxia and hyperuricemia, **508**
DEAFNESS-SENSORINEURAL, DIVERTICULITIS, AND NEUROPATHY, **265**
DEAFNESS-SENSORINEURAL, DYSTONIA AND RETARDATION, **266**
DEAFNESS-SENSORINEURAL, MID-FREQUENCY, **267**
DEAFNESS-SENSORINEURAL, POLYNEUROPATHY AND OPTIC ATROPHY, **268**
DEAFNESS-SENSORINEURAL, PROGRESSIVE HIGH-TONE, **269**
DEAFNESS-SENSORINEURAL, RECESSIVE EARLY-ONSET, **270**
DEAFNESS-SENSORINEURAL, RECESSIVE PROFOUND, **271**
Deafness, severe isolated congenital, **271**
DEAFNESS, STREPTOMYCIN–SENSITIVITY, **272**
DEAFNESS, TUNE (MARKER), **273**
DEAFNESS, UNILATERAL INNER EAR, **274**
Deafness, urticaria and amyloidosis, **982**
DEAFNESS, VITILIGO AND MUSCLE WASTING, **275**
Deafness with onycho-osteo dystrophy and mental retardation (DOOR syndrome), **262**
Deafness with preauricular pits or sinuses, **247**
Death
  during 1st mo of life, **122, 153, 169, 187, 555, 587, 883, 884, 939, 940, 990, 991**
  during 1st wk of life, **9, 24, 875, 883**
  during 1st yr of life, **138, 139, 154, 406, 555, 587, 655, 780, 1003**
  early, **40, 121, 174, 202, 406, 431, 432, 486, 547, 598, 628, 658, 671, 697, 780, 824, 850, 907, 978, 1003**
  sudden, **805, 810**
  sudden, of infant, **123, 918**
Decreased corticosteroid-binding globulin, **222**
Défaut de réabsorption rénale du bicarbonate, **858**
Défaut des coussins endocardiques, **347**
Défaut héréditaire de l'émail, **46**
Defective T-cell and normal B-cell immunity in nucleoside-phosphorylase deficiency, **729**
Defecto de la fagocitosis relacionado con el plasma, **812**

Defecto de peroxidase tiroídea, 947
Defecto de reabsorción renal de bicarbonato, 858
Defecto del tabique aórtico pulmonar, 83
Defecto del tabique inter-ventricular, 989
Defecto del transporte del yodo, 542
Defectos de la nariz y del tabique nasal, 722
Defectos de la tiroxinglobulina (Marcador), 950
Defectos de la trompa de eustaquio, 370
Defectos de las almohadillas endocárdicas, 347
Defectos del radio, 853
Defects in various portions of muscular septum, 989
Defekte der Endokardpolster, 347
Déficience en pyruvate déshydrogénase, 851
Déficience sévère en transglucuronylase, 961
Deficiencia aislada de gonadotropina, 438
Deficiencia aislada de hormona adrenocorticotrópica, 26
Deficiencia aislada de hormona de crecimiento, 447
Deficiencia aislada de tirotropina, 949
Deficiencia congénita aislada de lipasa, 597
Deficiencia congénita en lactasa, 566
Deficiencia de brancher, 116
Deficiencia de carnitina palmitil transferase, 125
Deficiencia de enteroquinasa intestinal, 533
Deficiencia de epimerase, 357
Deficiencia de fructosa-1-fosfato aldolasa, 395
Deficiencia de fructose-1,6-difosfatasa, 396
Deficiencia de glucógeno-sintetasa, 424
Deficiencia de iodotirosina deiodonasa, 543
Deficiencia de nucleósido fosforilasa, 729
Deficiencia de piruvato carboxilasa con acidemia láctica, 850
Deficiencia de piruvato deshidrogenasa, 851
Deficiencia de tripsinógeno, 973
Deficiencia de 17 esteroide 20 desmolasa, 904
Deficiencia en galactoquinasa, 402
Deficiencia en glucosa-6-fosfato dehidrogenasa, 420
Deficiencia en inmunoglobulina A, 525
Deficiencia en maltasa ácida, 11
Deficiencia en miofosforilasa, 698
Deficiencia en piruvato quinasa, 852
Deficiencia en sucrasa-isomaltasa, 920
Deficiencia en sulfito oxidasa, 921
Deficiencia en transglucoronilasa severa, 961
Deficiencia inmunológica linfopénica ligada al sexo, 524
Deficiencia inmunológica tardía, 521
Deficiencia primaria de lactasa, 567
Deficiencia primaria muscular de carnitina, 124
Deficiencia suprarrenal de 18-hidroxilasa, 905
Deficiencia suprarrenal de 18-hidroxisteroide dehidrogenasa, 906
Deficient radial rays and phocomelia, 853
Déficit congénital isolé en lipase, 597
Déficit congénital en lactase, 566
Déficit de la 18-hydroxylase surrénalienne, 905
Déficit de la 18-hydroxystéroïde-deshydrogénase surrénalienne, 906
Déficit en carnitine palmityl transférase, 125
Déficit en enterokinase, 533
Déficit en enzyme branchante (glycogénose type IV), 116

Déficit en épimérase, 357
Déficit en fructose-1-phosphate aldolase, 395
Déficit en fructose-1,6-diphosphatase hépatique, 396
Déficit en galactokinase, 402
Déficit en globuline lié à la thyroxine, 950
Déficit en glucose-6-phosphate déhydrogénase, 420
Déficit en glycogène synthétase, 424
Déficit en immunoglobuline A, 525
Déficit en lecithine – cholestérol acyl transférase, 580
Déficit en maltase acide, 11
Déficit en myophosphorylase, 698
Déficit en nucléoside-phosphorylase, 729
Déficit en peroxidase thyroïdienne, 947
Déficit en pyruvate carboxylase avec acidémie, 850
Déficit en pyruvate-kinase, 852
Déficit en saccharase et en isomaltase, 920
Déficit en stéroïde 17-20-desmolase, 904
Déficit en sulfite oxydase, 921
Déficit en trypsinogène, 973
Déficit immunologique lymphopénique lié au sexe, 524
Déficit immunologique tardif (acquis), 521
Déficit isolé en gonadotropine, 438
Déficit isolé en hormone adrénocorticotrope, 26
Déficit isolé en hormone de croissance, 447
Déficit isolé en thyrotropine, 949
Déficit musculaire en carnitine, 124
Déficit primaire en lactase, 567
Deformación de Sprengel, 901
Deformidad craneana tri-lobulada, 555
Deformity with mesomelic dwarfism, 308
Degeneración de conos y bastones, 201
Degeneración esponjosa de la substancia blanca cerebral, 115
Degeneración hepatolenticular, 469
Degeneración hialoidea retineana de Wagner, 479
Degeneración macular congénita, 622
Degeneración óptico-cócleo-dentata, 759
Degeneration der Opticus-, cochlearis-, Dentatun- und Schleifensysteme, 759
Dégénération hyaloide de la rétine, 479
Degeneration von Zäpfchen und Stäbchen, 201
Dégénérescence des cones et bâtonnets, 201
Dégénérescence hépato-lenticulaire, 469
Dégénérescence spongieuse de la substance blanche, 115
Dégénéresence systématisée optico-cochléodentelée, 759
Dehydration, 23, 25, 148, 152, 238, 398, 419, 421, 566, 569, 829, 848, 863, 864, 886, 905, 907, 908, 909, 910, 920
Dehydrogenase deficiency, glucose-6-phosphate, 420
Delayed biochemical maturation of 18-oxidation, 23
Delayed developmental milestones (see Section III, Table XXIII)
Delayed healing of skin, 4, 338
Délétion du bras court du chromosome 4, 164
Délétion du bras long du chromosome 13, 167
DENS IN DENTE, 276
DENTIN DYSPLASIA, CORONAL, 277
DENTIN DYSPLASIA, RADICULAR, 278
Dentin dysplasia, type I, 278

Dentin dysplasia, type II, 277
Dentin dysplasia with sclerotic bone and skeletal anomalies, 280
Dentinogénèse imparfaite, 279
DENTINOGENESIS IMPERFECTA, 279
DENTINO–OSSEOUS DSYPLASIA, 280
Dento-auriculaire, 784
Dentocranioocular syndrome, 229
Dents déformées par dysplasie traumatique, 929
Dents géminées, 931
Dents incluses, 932
Dents surnuméraires, 936
Dependencia a la vitamina B_6, 991
Depigmentation, gingival fibromatosis, microphthalmia, oligophrenia and athetosis, 413
Dépôts cristallins dans la cornée, 216
Depression, 203, 255, 730, 820, 822
DERMAL HYPOPLASIA, FOCAL, 281
Dermatochalasia, 233
Dermatoglyphics, 1, 18, 29, 89, 102, 119, 137, 139, 140, 142, 157, 159, 161, 163, 164, 168, 170, 171, 190, 229, 242, 262, 275, 379, 382, 393, 399, 450, 554, 556, 603, 632, 634, 667, 720, 754, 814, 823, 874, 891, 980
Dermatolipom, 284
Dermatomegaly, 233
Dermatorrhexis cutis hyperelastica, 338
DERMO–CHONDRO–CORNEAL DYSTROPHY OF FRANÇOIS, 282
Dermoid cyst of stomach, 914
DERMOID CYST OR TERATOMA OF HEAD AND NECK, 283
Dermoid cysts of nose of both skin and dural origin, 722
Dermoid cysts, orbital and periorbital, 761
Dermoid of the cornea, 591
Dermoid Zysten oder Teratome von Kopf und Hals, 283
Dermoide der Mundhöhle, 760
Dermoide du limbe, 591
Dermoide limbal, 591
Dermoids of the head and neck, 283
Dermoids, oral, 760
DERMOLIPOMA, 284
DeSanctis-Cacchione syndrome, 1004
Descemet membrane
    many tiny excrescences on, 208
    unspecified defect of, 439
    vesicles on, 213
Desmolase deficiency, 907
Desviación cubital con membranas interdigitales y contracturas, 980
Deutanformen der Rot-Grün Blindheit, 196
Deutéranomalie, 196
Deuteranopia, 196
Developmental cyst, 760
Deviation cubital des doigts et palmures, 980
DEXTROCARDIA, BRONCHIECTASIS AND SINUSITIS SYNDROME, 285
Dextroposición del tabique inter-ventricular y ventrículo izquierdo a doble entrada, 286
Dextroposition des Kammerseptumsdoppelte Einstrombahn des linken Ventrikels, 286
Dextroposition du septum ventriculaire, 286
DEXTROPOSITION OF VENTICULAR SEPTUM AND DOUBLE INLET LEFT VENTRICLE, 286
Di- and trihexosyl ceramide lipidosis, 373
Diabète insipide pitresso-résistant, 287

Diabète sucré juvénile, 549
Diabète sucré juvénile avec atrophie optique
  et surdité, 550
Diabetes insípida nefrogénica, 287
Diabetes insipidus and optic atrophy, 550
DIABETES INSIPIDUS, VASOPRESSIN–
  RESISTENT, 287
Diabetes mellitus and optic atrophy, 550
Diabetes mellitus juvenil, 549
Diabetes mellitus juvenil, atrofia óptica
  y sordera, 550
Diamond-Blackfan syndrome, 51
Diapers
  blue-stained, 974
  oil-stained, 597
Diaphragm abnormally high, 288
DIAPHRAGM, EVENTRATION, 288
Diaphragm, herniation of stomach above,
  471
Diaphragmatic esophageal hiatus hernia, 471
DIAPHRAGMATIC HERNIA, 289
Diaphysäre Dysplasie, 290
Diaphyseal aclasis, 685
Diaphyseal and cranial dysplasia, 224
DIAPHYSEAL DYSPLASIA, 290
Diarrhea, congenital chloride, 148
Diarrhea (see Section III, Table XXXIV)
Diarrhée chlorée, 148
Diastema de los incisivos medianos (Marcador),
  291
Diastema der Mittleren Schneidezähne, 291
DIASTEMA, MEDIAN INCISAL (MARKER),
  291
DIASTEMATOMYELIA, 292
Diastème de la möelle (épinière), 292
Diastème des incisives médianes, 291
Diastrophic dwarfism, 293
DIASTROPHIC DYSPLASIA, 293
Diastrophischer Zwergwuchs, 293
DICARBOXYLIC AMINOACIDURIA, 294
Diencephalic parotitis, 730
Dientes anquilosados, 927
Dientes dilacerados, 929
Dientes en inclusión, 932
Dientes fusionados, 930
Dientes geminados, 931
Dientes nevados, 935
Dientes supernumerarios (Marcador), 936
Diffuse capillary or cavernous hemangioma
  of liver, 466
DiGeorge syndrome, 943
Digit (also see Finger, Toe, Thumb, Joints,
  and Section III, Table XXIX)
  absence of one or more (see Ectro-
    dactyly)
  amputation of, due to gangrene or sepsis,
    259
  asymmetric length of, 185
  ball-like toe with grooves at attachment,
    8
  broad, 308, 578
  clubbed, 409, 938
  completely webbed hand, 14
  cylindrical, 570
  extra digit, poorly formed, 22, 187,
    262, 662, 814
  extra digit, well formed, 814
  irregular, asymmetric shortening, 162
  knobby, 557
  long, 85, 166, 183, 557, 629
  mild shortening of, 358
  mitten syndactyly, 14
  narrow, 85
  overlapping, 159, 160, 168
  partial absence, 874, 1001

polydactyly (see Section III, Table
  XXIX)
polysyndactyly, 13, 22, 771, 923
prenatal amputation of, 874
progressive shortening of, 21
prominent tip of, 409
short distal phalanx, 66, 156, 263
spatulated distal phalanx, 66
stocking syndactyly, 14
syndactyly (also see Section III, Table
  XXIX)
  fenestrated soft tissue, 874
  of 2nd and 3rd fingers, 229
  osseous, 14, 22, 874, 923
  tapered, 66, 159, 166, 190, 940
  thick, 1, 158, 190
  unilateral shortening of, 813
Digital and renal anomalies and deafness,
  264
Digital anomalies and microphthalmia, 662
Digital constrictions, keratopachydermia and
  deafness, 259
Digital, ear, nose anomalies, gingival fibro-
  matosis, and hepatosplenomegaly, 409
Digitofacial-mental retardation syndrome,
  119
Digitotalar dysmorphism, 980
Dilantin syndrome, 382
Dilazerierte Zähne, 929
Diplegia espástica, 295
Diplegia facial congénita, 376
Diplegia, infantile spastic, 295
DIPLEGIA, SPASTIC, 295
Diplégie faciale congénitale, 376
Diplégie spastique, 295
Diplomyelia with bony spur, 292
Direkter Abgang der a. vertebralis aus der
  Aorta, 527
Disautonomía, 307
Discondrostosis, 308
Discoria, 309
Discrete subaortic stenosis, 916
Disgenesia ovárica familiar, 436
Disgenesia tiroídea, 946
Disinostosis cráneo facial, 227
Dislocation of ocular lens, 584
Disorder of uric acid metabolism and central
  nervous system function, 588
Disorientation, 820
Disosteoesclerosis, 310
Disostosis acrofacial, 17
Disostosis cráneo-facial, 225
Disostosis craneo-facial con hiperplasia
  diafisaria, 226
Disostosis mandíbulofacial, 627
Disostosis metafisaria, retardo mental y
  sordera de conducción, 250
Displasia acromesomiélica tipo, Campailla-
  Martinelli, 19
Displasia acromesomielica, tipo Maroteaux, 20
Displasia acro-péctoro-vertebral, 22
Displasia cleidocraniana, 185
Displasia condroectodérmica, 156
Displasia cráneo-carpo-tarsal, 223
Displasia cráneo-diafisial, 224
Displasia cráneo metafisial, 228
Displasia de la dentina coronaria, 277
Displasia de la dentina radicular, 278
Displasia de la retina, 866
Displasia del peroné y braquidactilia, 392
Displasia dentino ósea, 280
Displasia diafisiaria, 290
Displasia ectodérmica anhidrótica, 333
Displasia epifisaria hemimélica, 311
Displasia epifisaria múltiple, 358

Displasia espóndilocostal, 896
Displasia espóndiloepifisaria congénita, 897
Displasia espóndiloepifisaria tardía, 898
Displasia espóndilotoraxica, 900
Displasia fibrosa monostótica, 390
Displasia fibrosa polióstica, 391
Displasia frontometafisaria, 394
Displasia hidrótica ectodérmica, 334
Displasia mesénquimatica de Puretić, 644
Displasia mesomiélica, tipo Langer, 646
Displasia mesomiélica, tipo Nievergelt, 647
Displasia mesomiélica, tipo Reinhardt-
  Pfeiffer, 648
Displasia mesomiélica, tipo Werner, 649
Displasia óculo-aurículo-vertebral, 735
Displasia oftalmo-mandíbulomélica, 749
Displasia pseudoacondroplástica, 828
Displasia pulpar, 843
Displasia toráxica asfixiante, 91
Displasias del oído interno, 315
Displasie pulpaire, 843
Disqueratosis intraepitelial, 538
Disseminated lipogranulomatosis, 598
Distal muscular dystrophy, 690
Distelförmige Pulpa, 937
DISTICHIASIS, 296
Distichiasis congenita, 296
Distichiasis congenita vera, 296
Distomolar, 936
Distonía de torsión, 957
Distonía, sordera neurosensorial y posible
  deterioro intelectual, 266
Distorted limb dwarfism, 798
Distrofia corneana congénita hereditaria, 207
Distrofia corneana de Reis-Bücklers, 215
Distrofia corneana en enrejado, 211
Distrofia corneana endotelial, 208
Distrofia corneana erosiva recurrente, 214
Distrofia corneana posterior polimórfica, 213
Distrofia corneana y pérdida de la audición
  neurosensorial progresiva, 206
Distrofia cristalina-corneana de Schnyder,
  216
Distrofia dermo-condro-corneana de
  François, 282
Distrofia epitelial de la córnea, 210
Distrofia granular de la córnea, 209
Distrofia macular de la córnea, 212
Distrofia muscular distal, 690
Distrofia muscular escápulo-pélvica, 691
Distrofia muscular óculofaringea, 692
Distrofia muscular pseudohipertrófica del
  adulto, 687
Distrofia muscular pseudohipertrófica infantil,
  689
Distrofia muscular pseudohipertrófica re-
  cesiva autosómica, 688
Distrofia tapetocoroidea, 925
Disturbance of histidine metabolism, 472
Disturbed eruption of teeth, corneal dys-
  trophy and gingival fibromatosis, 408
Diverticula of canaliculus, 844
Diverticule de l'estomac, 911
Diverticule de l'oesophage, 367
Diverticule de Meckel, 633
Diverticule ventriculaire, 988
Divertículo de Meckel, 633
Divertículo del esófago, 367
Divertículo gástrico congénito, 911
Divertículo ventricular, 988
Diverticulum of common bile duct, 149
Diverticulum of gallbladder, 404
Diverticulum of larynx, 575
Diverticulum of left ventricle, 988
Diverticulum of right ventricle, 988

Division palatine, micrognathie et glosso-
    ptosis, 182
Division palatine ou bec-de-lièvre et fossettes
    des lèvres, 177
Doggennase, 724
Dominant erblicher Hörverlust nieder-
    frequenter Bereiche, 256
Dominant osteopetrosis, 779
Dominante olivopontozerebellare Atrophie
    mit ophthalmoplegie und Demenz,
    744
Dominante olivopontozerebellare Atrophie,
    Typ Menzel, 742
Dominante olivopontozerebellare Atrophie,
    Typ Schut-Haymaker, 743
Dominante olivopontozerebellare Atrophie
    und Retina degeneration, 745
Dominanter Zwergwuchs Typ Levi, 305
Dominantly inherited dwarfism of Levi, 305
Donohue syndrome, 587
Doppellippe, 594
Doppelnase, 725
Doppelte Ausstrombahn des rechten
    Ventrikels mit anterior gelegenem
    Ventrikelseptumdefekt, 297
Doppelte Ausstrombahn des rechten
    Ventrikels mit posterior gelegenem
    Ventrikelseptumdefekt, 298
Doppelter Aortenbogen, 75
Double, aortic arch, 75
Double inlet left ventricle with ventricular
    inversion, 286
Double inlet left ventricle without ventric-
    ular inversion, 286
Double lip, blepharochalasis and nontoxic
    thyroid enlargement, 111
Double outlet left ventricle with intact
    ventricular septum and atresia of right
    ventricular infundibulum, 581
Double outlet left ventricle with ventricu-
    lar septal defect, 581
Double outlet left ventricle with ventricular
    septal defect and pulmonary stenosis,
    581
DOUBLE OUTLET RIGHT VENTRICLE
    WITH ANTERIOR VENTRICULAR
    SEPTAL DEFECT, 297
DOUBLE OUTLET RIGHT VENTRICLE
    WITH POSTERIOR VENTRICU-
    LAR SEPTAL DEFECT, 298
"Double uterus," 684
Down syndrome, 171
Doyne honeycombed retinal degeneration,
    734
Drepanocytic anemia, 886
Drooping of upper eyelid (see Section III,
    Table XXIV)
    at birth, 834
    at puberty, 111
    at rest, 548
    bilateral, 750
    intermittent, 48, 155
    ipsilateral to facial nerve palsy, 377
    pseudoptosis, 155, 889
    unilateral, 155
    with 2° hypertrophy, 788
Drug, adverse reaction, 7, 420, 820, 864
Drugs ingested by biologic mother during
    patient's prenatal life (see Section
    III, Table XXII)
Drusen ocular, 734
Duane retraction syndrome, 889
DUBOWITZ SYNDROME, 299
Duchenne muscular dystrophy, 689
Duhamel anomalad, 987

Dünndarmatresie (–stenose), 531
DUODENAL ATRESIA OR STENOSIS,
    300
Duodenal duplication, 532
Duplicación del colon, 194
Duplicación del esófago, 368
Duplicación gástrica, 912
Duplicación intestinal, 532
Duplicación nasal, 725
Duplication colique, 194
Duplication de l'estomac, 912
Duplication de l'oesophage, 368
Duplication intestinale, 532
Duplication of distal 11q, 161
Duplication of distal 14q, 165
Duplication of gallbladder, 404
Duplication of nose, 725
Duplication of proximal 14q, 166
Duplicité labiale, 594
Duplikation der Magen, 912
Duplikation des Oesophagus, 368
DUPUYTREN CONTRACTURE, 301
Durch Ankylose von Hammer und Amboss
    bedingte Schalleitungsschwerhörigkeit,
    244
Dwarfism and cortical thickening of tubular
    bones, 976
Dwarfism, diastrophic, 293
DWARFISM, LARON, 302
DWARFISM, PANHYPOPITUITARY, 303
DWARFISM, PITUITARY WITH ABNOR-
    MAL SELLA TURCICA, 304
Dwarfism, polydactyly and dysplastic nails,
    156
Dwarfism, Seckel, 881
DWARFISM, SNUB–NOSE, 305
DYGGVE–MELCHIOR–CLAUSEN
    SYNDROME, 306
DYSAUTONOMIA, 307
Dyscephalia oculomandibulofacialis, 738
Dyscephaly with congenital cataract and
    hypotrichosis, 738
Dyschondroplasia, 345
Dyschondroplasia and hemangiomatosis
    (some cases), 346
DYSCHONDROSTEOSIS, 308
DYSCORIA, 309
Dyscrania pygophalangea, 662
Dysencephalia splanchnocystica, 634
Dysfibrinogenämie, 4
Dysgammaglobulinemia, 521
Dysgammaglobulinemia type IV, 525
Dysgénésie ovarienne, 436
Dysgénésie thyroïdienne, 946
Dysgenesis mesostromal, 439
Dysgenesis neuroepithelialis retinae, 43
Dysgenesis of inner ear, 315
Dyskeratosis, intraepithelial, 538
Dyskorie, 309
Dysontogenetic cyst, 760
DYSOSTEOSCLEROSIS, 310
Dysostose acro-faciale, 17
Dysostose cranio-faciale, 225
Dysostose cranio-oculo-digitale, 769
Dysostose mandibulofaciale, 627
Dysostose métaphysaire, deficience mentale
    et surdité de conduction, 250
Dysostosis, acrofacial, 17
Dysostosis acrofacialis, 17
Dysostosis craniofacialis, 225
Dysostosis enchondralis meta epiphysaria
    (Catel-Hempel type), 155
Dysostosis mandibulofacialis, 627
Dysphagia, 12, 63, 74, 75, 103, 117, 127,
    180, 181, 275, 283, 363, 368, 401,
    503, 572, 575, 692, 702, 794, 795,

Dysplasia cleidocranialis, 185
Dysplasia, craniodiaphyseal, 224
Dysplasia, craniometaphyseal, 228
Dysplasia, diaphyseal, 290
DYSPLASIA EPIPHYSEALIS HEMIMELICA,
    311
Dysplasia epiphysealis punctata (congenita),
    153
Dysplasia epiphysialis multiplex, 358
Dysplasia, osteodental, 185
Dysplasia pulpae, 843
Dysplasia spondyloepiphysaria congenita,
    897
Dysplasia spondyloepiphysaria tarda, 898
Dysplasie acromésomélique, type Campailla-
    Martinelli, 19
Dysplasie acromésomélique, type Maroteaux,
    20
Dysplasie acropectoro-vertébrale, 22
Dysplasie chondro-ectodermique, 156
Dysplasie cléidocranienne, 185
Dysplasie cranio-carpo-tarsienne, 223
Dysplasie cranio-diaphysaire, 224
Dysplasie cranio-métaphysaire, 228
Dysplasie de la dentine coronaire, 277
Dysplasie de la radiculaire, 278
Dysplasie de la dentition et de l'os, 280
Dysplasie der Innenohr, 315
Dysplasie diaphysaire, 290
Dysplasie du péroné et brachydactylie, 392
Dysplasie ectodermique anhydrotique, 333
Dysplasie ectodermique hydrotique, 334
Dysplasie épiphysaire hémimélique, 311
Dysplasie fibreuse monostotique, 390
Dysplasie fibreuse polyostotique, 391
Dysplasie frontométaphysaire, 394
Dysplasie mésenchymale-syndrome de
    Puretić, 644
Dysplasie mésomélique, type Langer, 646
Dysplasie mésomélique, type Nievergelt, 647
Dysplasie mésomélique, type Reinhardt-
    Pfeiffer, 648
Dysplasie métaphysaire de Pyle, 847
Dysplasie oculo-auriclo vertébrale, 735
Dysplasie oculo-dento-osseuse, 737
Dysplasie oculo-mandibulaire, 749
Dysplasie polyépiphysaire dominante, 358
Dysplasie pseudo-achondroplastique, 828
Dysplasie rétinienne, 866
Dysplasie spondylo-costale, 896
Dysplasie spondylo–épiphysaire congénitale,
    897
Dysplasie spondylo-épiphysaire tardive, 898
Dysplasie spondylo-thoracique, 900
Dysplasie thoracique asphyxiante, 91
Dysplasie tibiale avec anomalies digitales,
    649
Dysplasies de l'oreille interne, 315
Dysplastic retina, 866
Dyspnea (see Section III, Table XXXI)
Dyssynostose cranio-faciale, 227
Dystonia musculorum deformans, 957
Dystonie, Schalleitungs-Schwerhörigkeit,
    möglicherweise geistige Retardierung,
    266
Dystonie, surdité sensorielle, déficit intellect-
    uel inconstant, 266
Dystrophia dermato-chondro-cornealis
    (François), 282
Dystrophia myotonica, 702
Dystrophie cervico-oculo-faciale, 142
Dystrophie cornéenne et surdité de per-
    ception progressive, 206
Dystrophie cornéenne congénitale héréditaire,
    207

Dystrophie cornéenne (en réseau), 211
Dystrophie cornéenne érosive, à rechutes, 214
Dystrophie cornéenne type Reis-Bücklers, 215
Dystrophie dermo-chondro-cornéenne de François, 282
Dystrophie endothéliale de la cornée, 208
Dystrohpie épithéliale de la cornée, 210
Dystrophie granulaire de la cornée, 209
Dystrophie maculaire de la cornée, 212
Dystrophie maculaire ponctuée, 400
Dystrophie musculaire distal, 690
Dystrophie musculaire oculopharyngée, 692
Dystrophie musculaire pseudohypertrophique de l'enfant, 689
Dystrophie musculaire pseudohypertrophique (de transmission autosomique), 688
Dystrophie myotonique, 702
Dystrophie polymorphe postérieure de la cornée, 213
Dystrophie tapéto-choroidienne, 925
Dysversion of optic disk, 757

E

Ear (also see parts of external ear, Hearing loss and Section III, Table XXV)
    cauliflower-like deformity of, 293
    crumpled, 85, 664
    cup-ear, 254, 314, 388
    defect of overall structure of, 1, 88, 157, 158, 162, 163, 166, 167, 168, 505, 526, 634, 662, 727, 735, 754, 987
    deficient cartilage, 374
    displaced, 316
    dysplastic, 13, 121, 142, 160, 164, 182 227, 231, 313, 327, 374, 389, 592, 603, 627, 636, 823, 883, 943
    folded, 229, 254
    large, 97, 140, 157, 158, 167, 170, 263, 313, 326, 587, 619, 775, 856, 967,
    lop-ear, 72, 158, 247
    pink-blue discoloration of, 313
    posteriorly rotated, 121, 227, 325, 327, 388, 603, 754
    preauricular fistula, 247, 627, 735
    preauricular pit, 164, 247, 329, 596
    preauricular tag, 163, 247, 374, 457, 544, 591, 627, 629, 664, 735
    protruding, 190, 263, 388, 967, 999
    pulsatile, 313
    small, 97, 98, 121, 168, 171, 229, 231, 247, 326, 327, 331, 457, 506, 664, 860
    unilateral posterior displacement of, 735
    unilaterally undifferentiated, 157
EAR, ABSENT TRAGUS, 312
EAR, ARTERIOVENOUS FISTULA, 313
Ear, arteriovenous fistula of external, 313
EAR, CUPPED, 314
Ear, defect of middle (also see parts of middle ear), 316, 377, 664
Ear, dysgenesis of, 664
EAR, DYSPLASIAS, INNER, 315
EAR, ECTOPIC PINNA, 316
Ear, endolymphatic duct and sac, defect of inner, 315
Ear, enlarged scapha and lobule, 619
EAR, EXCHONDROSIS (MARKER), 317
Ear, exchondrosis of pinna, 317
EAR EXOSTOSES, 318
Ear, floppy helix of, 326
EAR, HAIRY, 319

EAR LOBE, ABSENT, 320
EAR LOBE, CLEFT, 321
EAR LOBE PIT (MARKER), 322
EAR LOBES, ATTACHED (MARKER), 323
EAR LOBES, HYPERTROPHIC THICKENED, 324
EAR, LONG, NARROW, POSTERIORLY ROTATED, 325
EAR, LOP, 326
EAR, LOW–SET, 327
Ear malformations and lateral (or branchial) cervical fistulas and deafness, 247
Ear, middle, tumor of, 12, 145, 150, 318, 664, 712
EAR, MOZART (MARKER), 328
Ear, nose, digital anomalies, gingival fibromatosis, and hepatosplenomegaly, 409
Ear pits and external ear malformations with deafness, 247
EAR PITS (MARKER), 329
EAR, PROMINENT ANTHELIX, 330
EAR, SMALL WITH FOLDED–DOWN HELIX, 331
Ear wax grey or brown, 141
Ear, with folded-down helix (incompletely developed), 331
Eardrum
    pink flush, 787
    pulsating red bulge behind, 530
Earlobe (also see Ear)
    at right angle to head, 157, 314
    attachment of, 323
    disproportionately large, 157, 324, 619
    elongated, 98
    fibrotic in center of, 324
    hypoplastic, 162, 320
    longitudinal cleft of, 321
    pit 1 mm deep in, 322
    thickened, 244, 324
    unspecified defect in, 98, 376, 664
    vertical groove in, 104
Early hypercalcemia syndrome, 999
Early-onset alactasia, 566
Early-onset lymphedema, 614
Ears, malformed and low-set, with conductive deafness, 254
EBSTEIN ANOMALY, 332
Ebstein anomaly of tricuspid valve, 332
Echter Hermaphroditismus, 971
Ectodermal dysplasia and cleft lip, 179
ECTODERMAL DYSPLASIA, ANHIDROTIC, 333
Ectodermal dysplasia, Berlin type, 105
ECTODERMAL DYSPLASIA, HIDROTIC, 334
Ectodermal dysplasia with hypotrichosis, hypohidrosis, defective teeth and unusual dermatoglyphics, 102
Ectodermal polydysplasia, 333
ECTOPIA CORDIS, 335
Ectopia del cristalino y de la pupila, 583
Ectopia lentis et pupillae, 583
Ectopia of macula, 620
Ectopic anus, 69
Ectopic gallbladder, 404
Ectopic pinealomas, 188
Ectopic placement of pinna, 316
Ectopie cardiaque, 335
Ectopie des glandes lacrymales, 564
Ectopie du cristallin et de la pupille, 583
Ectopie du pavillon de l'oreille, 316
Ectrodactilia, 336
Ectrodactilia, displasia ectodérmica y síndrome de acrofisuras, 337

Ectrodactyly, 65, 242, 281, 336, 337, 375, 451, 459, 592, 700, 813, 818, 875
Ectrodactyly and anonychia, 65
ECTRODACTYLY–ECTODERMAL DYSPLASIA–CLEFTING SYNDROME, 337
Ectropion congénital, 371
Ectropión congénito de los párpados, 371
Eczema, thrombocytopenia, diarrhea, and infection syndrome, 523
Edentate hypertrichosis, 507
Edwards syndrome, 160
EEC syndrome, 337
EHLERS–DANLOS SYNDROME, 338
18-Hydroxylase-Mangel, 905
18-Hydroxysteroid-Dehydrogenease-Mangel, 906
Einengung des rechten Ventrikels oder seiner Ausflussbahn, 731
Einrollen der Zunge, 951
Einseitige Nierenangenesie, 857
Einseitige Schallempfindungsschwerhörigkeit, 274
Ekchondrose des Ohrläppchens, 317
Ektodermale Dysplasie mit fehlendes Papillarmuster, Nagelveranderungen und Vierfingerfurche, 102
Ektopie der Ohrmuschel, 316
Ektopie der Tränendrüse, 564
Ektrodactylie, 336
Ektrodaktylie-Ektodermale Dysplasie-Spaltsyndrom, 337
Ekzem-Thrombozytopenie-Diarrhoe-Syndrom, 523
Elastoma intrapapillare perforans verruciforme Miescher, 339
Elastose perforante serpigneuse, 339
Elastosis dystrophica, 832
ELASTOSIS PERFORANS SERPIGINOSA, 339
Elbow
    crepitation of, 121
    decreased extension of, 89, 477, 704, 854
    decreased flexion of, 477, 560, 854
    decreased pronation-supination of, 20, 89, 450, 455, 648, 704, 854
    decreased range of motion of, 10, 16, 20, 85, 98, 128, 129, 510, 646, 647, 674, 675, 828, 847
    decreased supination of, 647
    extension contracture of, 20, 88, 749
    fixation of forearm in pronation, 854
    flexion contracture of, 88, 121, 242, 450, 470, 1000
    increased carrying angle of, 98, 139, 308, 685, 704, 720, 791, 977
    prenatal onset of contracture of, 629
    prenatal onset of dislocation of, 570
    webbing of, 704

Eldridge syndrome, 251
Ellis-van Creveld syndrome, 156
Elsahy-Waters syndrome, 118
Embriopatía por radiación, 383
Embriopatía por talidomida, 386
Embriopatía por warfarina, 389
Embryofetales Alkohol Syndrom, 379
Embryoma of head or neck, 283
Embryopathie causée par le thalidomide, 386
Embryopathie due à la radioactivité, 383
Embryopathie due à l'hydantoïne, 382
Embryopathie due à la warfarine, 389
Embryopathie due à le triméthadione, 388

Embryopathies et foetopathies dues à l'aminophtérine, 380
EMG syndrome, 104
Emotional instability, 307, 384, 472, 478, 823
Emphysème familial, 39
ENAMEL AND DENTIN DEFECTS FROM ERYTHROBLASTOSIS FETALIS, 340
ENAMEL AND DENTIN DEFECTS FROM TETRACYCLINE, 341
Enamel and dentin staining from erythropoietic porphyria, 821
Enamel hypocalcification, onycholysis and hypohidrosis, 45
ENAMEL, HYPOPLASIA, 342
Enamel hypoplasia and hypomaturation with taurodontism, curly hair and splitting of superficial layers of nails, 965
Enamel hypoplasia, taurodontism, tight curly hair, and cortical sclerosteosis, 965
Enamel shelf, 340
Enanismo de Laron, 302
Enanismo diastrófico, 293
Enanismo familiar hipofisario con silla turca anormal, 304
Enanismo metatrófico, 656
Enanismo panhipopituitario, 303
Enanismo parastremático, 798
Enanismo tanatofórico, 940
Enanismo tipo "Cabeza de Pájaro," 881
Enanismo tipo "nariz aplastada, 305
Encefalocele, 343
Encefalopatía necrotizante, 344
Encephalocele, 375, 481, 635
   meningoencephalocele, 380, 635
   occipital, 634
Encephalocele, orbital, 762
Encephalochoristoma nasofrontalis, 726
Encephalofacial angiomatosis, 915
Encephalomyelopathy, 344
ENCEPHALOPATHY NECROTIZING, 344
Encephalotrigeminal angiomatosis, 915
Enchondromatose avec hémangiomes, 346
Enchondromatose mit Hemangiomen (Maffucci), 346
ENCHONDROMATOSIS, 345
ENCHONDROMATOSIS AND HEMANGIOMAS, 346
ENDOCARDIAL CUSHION DEFECTS, 347
Endocardial cushion defects, complete type, 347
Endocardial cushion defects, partial type, with interatrial and interventricular communication, 347
Endocardial cushion defects, partial type, with interatrial communication, 347
Endocardial cushion defects, partial type, with interventricular communication, 347
Endocardial cushion defects, partial type, with isolated cleft of the anterior cusp of the mitral valve, 347
Endocardial cushion defects, partial type, with left ventricular to right atrial communication, 347
ENDOCARDIAL FIBROELASTOSIS OF LEFT VENTRICLE, 348
ENDOCARDIAL FIBROELASTOSIS OF RIGHT VENTRICLE, 349
Endocardial fibrosis, 885
ENDOCRINE NEOPLASIA I, MULTIPLE, 350

ENDOCRINE NEOPLASIA II, MULTIPLE, 351
ENDOCRINE NEOPLASIA III, MULTIPLE, 352
Endogenous hypertriglyceridemia, 500
Endokard-Fibroelastose des linken Ventrikels, 348
Endokard-Fibroelastose des rechten Ventrikels, 349
Endolymphatic hydrops, 248
Endomykardfibrose des linken Ventrikels, 353
Endomykardfibrose des rechten Ventrikels, 354
ENDOMYOCARDIAL FIBROSIS OF LEFT VENTRICLE, 353
ENDOMYOCARDIAL FIBROSIS OF RIGHT VENTRICLE, 354
Endophytum type retinoblastoma, 870
Endostosis cranii, 498
Endothelial corneal dystrophy, 208
Endotheliale Hornhautdystrophie, 208
Endothelioma capitis of Kaposi, 235
Enfermedad de Ebstein, 332
Enfermedad de Fabry, 373
Enfermedad de Gaucher, 406
Enfermedad de Hartnup, 453
Enfermedad de Kyrle, 561
Enfermedad de Niemann-Pick, 717
Enfermedad de Norrie, 721
Enfermedad de Oguchi, 740
Enfermedad de Pyle, 847
Enfermedad de Sturge-Weber, 915
Enfermedad de von Willebrand, 996
Enfermedad de Wolman, 1003
Enfermedad del grupo central de miofibrillas de la fibra muscular esquelética, 134
Enfermedad granulomatosa crónica del varón, 443
Enfermedad poliquística del hígado, 605
Enfermedad renal poliquística tipo adulto, 859
Enfermedad urinaria a jarabe de arce, 628
Enfisema familial, 39
Enteric cyst, 532
Enterocystoma, 532
Enterogenous cyst, 532
Enteropatía causada por el gluten, 423
Entropion, 372
Entropión del párpado, 372
Entropion des Augenlids, 372
Enzephalozele, 343
Ependymoma, 188
EPIBLEPHARON, 355
Epibulbar dermoid, 591
Epicanthic fold (see Section III, Table XXIV)
EPICANTHUS, 356
Epicanthus inversus, 356
Epicanthus palpebris, 356
Epicanthus supraciliaris, 356
Epicanthus tarsalis, 356
Epicanto, 356
Epidermoid cyst, 760
Epignathus, 283
Epikanthus, 356
Epilepsia centropática, 135
Épilepsie d'origine centrale, 135
Epilepsy, centralopathic, 135
Epilepsy, centrencephalic, 135
Epiloia, 975
EPIMERASE DEFICIENCY (MARKER), 357
Epimerase-Mangel, 357
Epiphyseal changes and high myopia, 90
EPIPHYSEAL DYSPLASIA, MULTIPLE, 358
Episodic vertigo and hearing loss, 248

Epitelioma escamoso múltiple autocicatrizante, 359
Epitheliale Hornhautdystrophie, 210
Epithelioma adenoids cysticum, 235
Epithélioma multiple à cellules squameuses, 359
EPITHELIOMA, MULTIPLE SELF-HEALING SQUAMOUS, 359
Epulis, 360
EPULIS, CONGENITAL, 360
Erblicher, progressiver Hörnervlust für hohe Frequenzen, 269
Eritema palmo-plantar, 792
Eritroqueratoderma variable, 361
Erythema migrans lingua, 954
Erythema nuchae, 715
Erytheme palmare hereditarium, 792
Erythéme palmo-plantaire, 792
Erythroblastosis fetalis and staining of enamel and dentin, 340
Erythrocyte malate dehydrogenase supernatant, 625
Erythrodontia, 821
Erythrogenesis imperfecta, 51
Erythrokeratoderma figurata variabilis, 361
Erythrokeratoderma progressiva, 361
ERYTHROKERATODERMIA, VARIABLE, 361
Erythrokeratodermia variabilis Mendes da Costa, 361
ERYTHROPOIETIC PROTOPORPHYRIA, 362
Erythropoietic uroporphyria, 821
Esclerosis a células globoides, 415
Esclerosis cerebral I, 803
Esclerosis tuberosa, 975
Esclerosteosis, 880
Esferocitosis, 892
ESOPHAGEAL ACHALASIA, 363
ESOPHAGEAL ATRESIA, 364
ESOPHAGEAL ATRESIA AND TRACHEOESOPHAGEAL FISTULA, 365
ESOPHAGEAL CHALASIA, 366
Esophageal cyst, 368
ESOPHAGEAL DIVERTICULUM, 367
ESOPHAGEAL DUPLICATION, 368
Esophageal hiatus hernia, 471
Esophageal lobe, 611
ESOPHAGEAL STENOSIS, 369
Esophageal web or veil, 396
Esophagotracheal fistula, 960
Esophagotracheal window, 960
Esophagus
   achalasia of, 275
   atresia of, 160, 531, 571, 943, 987
   blind upper, 365
   cleft in anterior wall of, 577
   dilated, 913
   dilated proximal third of, 369
   gastroesophageal reflux, 366, 401, 471
   indentation in right lateral wall of, 75
   large posterior indentation of, 74
   narrowing of middle third of, 369
   obstructed, 364
   stricture of, 471
   varices in, 149, 468
   web in middle third of, 369
Essential fructosuria, 397
Essential hereditary osteolysis, 128
Essential nightblindness, 719
Essential osteolysis and nephropathy, 128
Essential tremor, 964
Estenosis aórtica supravalvular, 78
Estenosis de la válvula aórtica, 80
Estenosis de la válvula pulmonar, 839

Estenosis de la vena pulmonar, 204
Estenosis del esófago, 369
Estensosis fibrosa subaórtica, 916
Estenosis infundibular del ventrículo derecho, 731
Estenosis mitral, 669
Estenosis muscular subaórtica, 917
Estenosis nasofaríngea, 707
Estenosis o atresia intestinal, 531
Estenosis pilórica, 848
Estenosis pulmonar periférica múltiple, sordera mixta, braquitelefalangia y calcificación de los cartílagos, 263
Estenosis subglótica, 919
Estenosis tricuspídea, 970
Estenosis tubular, 976
Ethmocephaly, 203
Eulenburg disease, 796
Eunuchoid habitus, 93, 438
Euryopia, 504
Eustachian tube atresia, 370
Eustachian tube cysts, 370
EUSTACHIAN TUBE DEFECTS, 370
Eustachian tube, defect of, 316
Eustachian tube tumors, 370
Eventración del diafragma, 288
Eventration diaphragmatique, 288
Eversion of sacculus, 573
Eversion of ventricle, 573
Exchondrosis of pinna, 317
Excrétion urinaire du disulfide β mercaptolactate-cystéine, 106
Exencephaly, 52
Exocondrosis del pabellón auricular (Marcador), 317
Exogenous hypertriglyceridemia, 489
Exomphalos, 748
Exomphalos-Makroglossie-Gigantismus-Syndrom, 104
Exophytum type retinoblastoma, 870
Exostoses de l'oreille, 318
Exostoses of external auditory canal, 318
Exostosis auriculares, 318
Expanded rubella syndrome, 384
Exstrophy of the cloaca, 193
Extensor pollicis brevis or longus, aplasia or hypoplasia, 175
External ankyloblepharon, 60
External ear aneurysm by anastomosis, 313
External ear arteriovenous fistula, 313
External genitalia, unspecified defect of, 166, 173, 883, 987
External ophthalmoplegia and myopia, 750
External ophthalmoplegia congenita, 751
Extra lobe sequestration, 612
Extraadenoidal cysts, 706
Extrahepatic biliary atresia with discontinuity of bile duct (correctable), 110
Extralobäre Lungensequestration, 612
Extrapulmonic lobe, 611
Exudative central detachment, 622
Eye (see parts and Section III, Table XXIV)
Eye absent, 67
Eye lens
  abnormal zonules, 733, 584
  anterior conical projection, 585, 708
  cleft of, 585, 732, 733
  dislocation, 281, 474, 583, 584, 630, 663, 893, 921
  lenses and pupils displaced in opposite directions, 583
  posterior conical projection, 585, 708
  retrolental fibroplasia, 620
  ring reflex on slit-lamp examination, 585

small, 630, 663, 893
  spheric, 630, 663, 708, 893
  thickened anterior cortex, 585
Eye lens cataract (also see Section III, Table XXIV)
  anterior polar, 133, 250, 585
  capsular, 133
  embryonic nuclear, 132
  nuclear, 402
  posterior polar, 133, 201, 585, 736
  present at birth, 106, 261, 635, 708
  secondary, 449
  variably shaped, 132
  white plaque in, 845
Eye, muscle weakness, 142, 188, 229, 344, 376, 735, 744, 751, 752, 753, 834, 889
Eye, orbital roof (also see Supraorbital ridge)
  bony defect, 712
  trunk-like process attached, 824
Eye, socket (also see Eye, orbital roof)
  fused, 234
  hyperostosis, 318
  large, 765
  low position of, 735
  shallow, 67, 226, 389
  small, 52
  structural anomaly, 375, 565
  surrounded by deep furrow, 105
Eye, undersized, 661
Eyeball (also see Section III, Table XXIV)
  atrophy, 550, 737
  coloboma, 101, 159, 281, 284, 574, 634
  deep-set, 159, 629
  defect of, 169, 526, 697, 821
  defect of ocular tissue, 733
  fused, 158, 168, 234
  pain in, 126, 212, 870
  protrusion of, 52, 221, 225, 226, 283, 355, 539, 555, 557, 712, 761, 762, 763, 764, 765, 775, 779, 825, 875
  retracted, 142, 189, 223, 736
  seemingly shrunken, 783, 872
  small (see Section III, Table XXIV)
  unilaterally small, 457
Eyeball, tumor (also see Orbital tumor and Periorbital tumor)
  epibulbar dermoid, 735
  lipodermoid, 593
  pink-white, 591
  upper temporal quadrant, 284
  yellow-white, 284
Eyelashes, accessory, 296
Eyelashes, underdeveloped, 623
Eyelid (also see Drooping of upper lid and Section III, Table XXIV)
  absent, 3
  blepharochalasis, 170
  cleft of, 162, 247, 375, 627, 635, 735, 824
  epiblepharon, 355, 395, 401
  eversion of, 371
  eversion of tarsus, 811, 821
  fusion and cleft lip or palate, 176
  fusions, 60, 176, 177, 179, 818
  inability to close completely, 371
  inability to close completely with postnatal onset, 378
  inability to open to normal extent, 223, 299, 371, 629, 834
  inflammation of, 443, 706
  inversion of tarsus, 372
  protrusion of lower, 552
  puffy, 139

reduced ability to close, 371
  skin continuous over eyeball, 3
  small, 389
  spasmodic winking, 414, 515
  thickened, 190, 788
  tumor of, 142, 247, 457, 635, 712, 1004, 1005
  underdeveloped lower, 375
  upper easily everted, 338
  upper elevates on inspiration, 548
  upper protruding over lower, 634
  white plaques on, 538
  yellow plaques on, 488, 495
EYELID ECTROPION, CONGENITAL, 371
EYELID ENTROPION, 372

F

F syndrome, 22
Fabry-Anderson disease, 373
FABRY DISEASE, 373
Face (also see parts and Section III, Table XXVI)
  aged appearance before puberty, 189
  asymmetric face, 157, 163, 167, 227, 229, 281, 284, 326, 391, 735, 952
  bird-like, 257
  chubbiness over cheeks, 154, 223, 303, 355, 425, 426, 427, 447, 539
  coarse, 18, 644, 671, 672, 673, 675, 676, 677, 679, 680, 788, 1000
  coarse face at birth, 672
  coarse face with onset in infancy, 676
  craniofacial disproportion, 302, 825, 846, 887
  craniofacial dysostosis, 470
  cretinoid, 542, 543, 947, 948
  fixed, mask-like, 155, 223, 376, 629, 746
  flat, 122, 153, 154, 155, 168, 171, 557, 823, 897
  long, 630, 1001
  midline depression of, 635, 874
  narrow, 112, 163, 630, 881, 1001
  pinched, lethargic, 189, 412
  prominent facial bones, 168, 313
  round, moon, 114, 139, 163, 170, 447, 554, 557, 830, 900
  small, 122, 155
  swollen, edematous, 9, 946
  triangular, 78, 587, 777, 876, 887
  unusual appearance of, 158, 190, 224, 391, 394, 470, 555, 603, 652, 775, 779, 880, 883, 939, 999
Face, diffuse symmetric lipomatosis of, 601
Facial and cranial dysostosis, 225
Facial angioma with epsilateral small calvaria, 915
FACIAL CLEFT, LATERAL, 374
FACIAL CLEFT, OBLIQUE, 375
Facial diplegia, 823
FACIAL DIPLEGIA, CONGENITAL, 376
Facial diplegia (6th and 7th cranial nerves), 376
Facial hypoplasia unilateral, 457
Facial nerve paralysis present at birth, 376, 377
FACIAL PALSY, CONGENITAL, 377
FACIAL PALSY, LATE-ONSET, 378
Faciodigitogenital syndrome, 1
Factor VIII deficiency, 461
Factor IX deficiency, 462
Failure to thrive (also see Inanition, Malnutrition and Weight loss), 27, 62,

Failure to thrive – *Continued*
121, 138, 139, 154, 167, 237, 363,
366, 368, 376, 379, 381, 385, 388,
389, 395, 419, 423, 431, 471, 491,
499, 533, 534, 566, 569, 576, 587,
593, 598, 603, 643, 655, 717, 780,
812, 825, 829, 850, 858, 863, 885,
891, 905, 918, 920, 943, 973, 974,
978
Fainting, 80, 123, 127, 805
Fairbank disease, 358
Fallopian tube
fallopian tube with male gender, 683, 904
rudimentary, 29, 682
small, 437
Fallot tetrad, 938
Fallotsche Tetralogie, 938
Falta de respuesta a la tirotropina, 948
Falta de respuesta suprarrenal al ACTH
hereditaria, 25
Familial Addison disease, 25
Familial aldosterone deficiency with en-
zyme defect, 905, 906
Familial anhidrosis, 56
Familial cerebelloolivary degeneration with
late development of rigidity and
dementia, 744
Familial chronic obstructive lung disease, 39
Familial colloid bodies, 734
Familial combined hyperlipoproteinemia,
496
Familial congenital peripheral facial paralysis,
377
Familial cylindroma of scalp, 235
Familial deficiency of postheparin lipo-
lytic activity, 489
Familial drusen, 734
Familial dwarfism with high plasma im-
munoreactive human growth hormone
(hGH), 302
Familial emphysema, 39
Familial high density lipoprotein deficiency,
48
Familial hypomagnesemia, 514
Familial hypophosphatemia (X-linked), 517
Familial increase or decrease in thyroxine-
binding capacity of serum, 950
Familial isolated glucocorticoid deficiency,
25
Familial jaundice, hepatosteatosis, and
kernicterus, 990
Familial lymphedema with onset after child-
hood, 615
Familial multiple primary self-healing squa-
mous cell epithelioma, 359
Familial nephrotic syndrome occurring post-
natally, 710
Familial neurovisceral lipidosis, 431
Familial ovarian dysgenesis, 436
Familial pancreatitis, 793
Familial perineal hypospadias (Van Wyck
and Grumbach), 831
Familial periodic paralysis, 795
Familial plasma cholesteryl ester deficiency,
580
Familial polyposis coli, 535
Familial serum thyroxine-binding globulin
(TBG) defects, 950
Familial spastic diplegia, 295
Familial steatosis of liver and kidney, 990
Familial telecanthus with associated
anomalies, 505
Familiäre fettige Metamorphose der Viscera,
990
Familiäre Nephrose, 710

Familiäre Ovarialdysgenesie, 436
Familiäre statische Ophthalmoplegie, 751
Familiäre symmetrischelipome, 600
Familiärer Emphysem, 39
Familiärer Glukokortikoid-supprimierbarer
Hyperaldosteronismus, 484
Familiärer hypophysärer Zwergwuchs mit
abnormer sella turcica, 304
Familiärer, periodisch auftretender Schwindel
und Hörverlust, 248
Fanconi-Syndrom, 864
Farber disease, 598
Farsightedness (also see Astigmatism and
Refractive error), 1, 229, 250, 777
Fat-induced hyperlipemia, 489
Fatal granulomatous disease of females, 442
Fatal granulomatous disease of males, 443
Fatal neonatal hepatic steatosis, 990
Fatty metamorphosis of viscera, 990
Favism, 420
Favre microfibrillary vitreoretinal dystrophy,
479
Fecal soiling absent (also see Obstipation),
192
Feeding difficulties, 24, 25, 40, 121, 138,
139, 140, 161, 163, 167, 299, 347,
376, 401, 406, 424, 451, 499, 506
509, 513, 603, 628, 823, 991
Fehlbildungen der Carunculi lacrimales, 130
Fehlbildungen der Eustachischen Röhre, 370
Fehlbildungen der v. hepatica, 468
Fehlbildungen von Anus und Rektum, 69
Fehlbildungen von Gehörknöchelchen und
Mittelohr, 773
Fehlen der Pulmonalklappe, 836
Fehlen von Fingerbeerenmustern, 393
Fehlendes hepatisches Segment der Vena
cava inferior, 528
Fehr corneal dystrophy, 212
Female pseudohermaphroditism, 908
Female pseudo-Turner syndrome, 720
Female Turner syndrome with normal XX
sex karyotype, 720
Feminizing male pseudohermaphroditism
(Jones), 50
Feminizing testes syndrome, 49
Femur
absence of, 451, 875
bowing of, 122
dislocation of, 98
dislocation of femoral head, 881
long, 122
short, 154, 875
Fenilcetonuria, 808
Fenotipo acromegaloide, cutis verticis
gyrata y leucoma corneano, 18
Fente alvéolaire médiane du maxillaire
supérieur, 631
Fente du lobe de l'oreille, 321
Fente palatine, 180
Fente palatine avec persistance de la mem-
brane bucco-pharyngée, 181
Fertile eunuch syndrome, 438
Fertility decreased, 29, 68, 93, 112, 243,
303, 436, 437, 438, 556, 682, 702,
720, 823, 855, 902, 903, 904, 907,
909, 971
Fetal activity
decreased, 160, 470, 486, 754, 895
decreased in 3rd trimester of pregnancy,
823
FETAL ALCOHOL SYNDROME, 379
Fetal aminopterin damage, 380
FETAL AMINOPTERIN SYNDROME, 380

FETAL CYTOMEGALOVIRUS SYN-
DROME, 381
Fetal damage from hydantoin anticonvul-
sants, 382
Fetal damage from oxazolidine anticonvul-
sants, 388
Fetal damage from 4-amino-pteroyl-glutamic
acid, 380
Fetal face syndrome, 876
FETAL HYDANTOIN SYNDROME, 382
FETAL RADIATION SYNDROME, 383
FETAL RUBELLA SYNDROME, 384
FETAL SYPHILIS SYNDROME, 385
FETAL THALIDOMIDE SYNDROME, 386
FETAL TOXOPLASMOSIS SYNDROME,
387
FETAL TRIMETHADIONE SYNDROME,
388
FETAL WARFARIN SYNDROME, 389
Fetales Hydantoin-Syndrom, 382
Fetales Trimethadion-Syndrom, 388
Fetalgesicht-Minderwuchs Syndrom, 876
Fett-induzierte Hyperlipämie, 489
Fettsucht-Hyperthermie-Oligomenorrhoe-
Parotis-Schwellung, 730
FG syndrome, 754
Fibrinogens, abnormal, 4
Fibrocytic disease of pancreas, 237
Fibrodysplasia ossificans progressiva, 700
Fibro-élastose du ventricule droit, 349
Fibro-élastose du ventricule gauche, 348
Fibroelastosis endocárdica del ventrículo
derecho, 349
Fibroelastosis endocárdica del ventrículo
izquierdo, 348
Fibromatose gingivale, 407
Fibromatose gingivale, anomalie de
l'éruption dentaire et dystrophie
cornéenne, 408
Fibromatose gingivale-anomalies des doigts,
des oreilles et du nez avec hépato-
splénomégalie, 409
Fibromatose gingivale avec hypertrichose,
410
Fibromatose gingivale dépigmentation
microphthalmie, oligophrénie et
athétose, 413
Fibromatose gingivale et fibromes hyalines
mutliples, 411
Fibromatose gingivale hypertrychose et
fibroádenomes mammaires, 412
Fibromatosis gingivae, 407
Firbomatosis gingivae, gestörter Zahndurch-
bruch und Hornhautdystrophie, 408
Fibromatosis gingivae, Hypertrichose und
Fibroadenome der Mammae, 412
Fibromatosis gingivae mit Fehlbildungen
von Fingern, Ohr, Nase und Hepato-
splenomegalie, 409
Fibromatosis gingivae mit hypertrichose,
410
Fibromatosis gingivae mit multiplem hy-
alinen Fibromen, 411
Fibromatosis gingivae, Pigmentmangel,
Mikrophthalmie, Oligophrenie und
Athetose, 413
Fibromatosis gingival, 407
Fibromatosis gingival, alteración de la
erupción dentaria y distrofia cornea,
408
Fibromatosis gingival con depigmentación,
microftalmia, oligofrenia y atetosis,
413
Fibromatosis gingival con fibromas hialinos
múltiples, 411

Fibromatosis gingival con hipertricosis, 410
Fibromatosis gingival, hipertricosis y fibro-adenomas mamarios, 412
Fibromatosis gingival y anomalías auriculares y nasales con hepatoesplenomelia, 409
Fibromatosis hyalinica multiplex juvenilis, 411
Fibromatosis, palmar, 301
Fibromuscular atresia of antrum, 910
Fibromuscular subaortic stenosis, 916
Fibroplasia retrolental, 872
Fibroplasie rétro-cristallinienne, 872
Fibrose Dysplasie, 390
Fibrose endomyocardiaque du ventricule droit, 354
Fibrose endomyocardiaque du ventricule gauche, 353
Fibrose Subaortenstenose, 916
Fibrosis endomiocárdica del ventrículo derecho, 354
Fibrosis endomiocárdica del ventrículo izquierdo, 353
Fibrosis quística, 237
FIBROUS DYSPLASIA, MONOSTOTIC, 390
FIBROUS DYSPLASIA, POLYOSTOTIC, 391
Fibrous subaortic stenosis, 916
Fibula
    absence of, 875
    angulation of shaft, 648
    bowing of, 648
    dislocation of proximal head, 649
    disproportionately long shaft of, 10, 510
    short, 19, 20, 122, 392, 646, 648, 875
FIBULA DYSPLASIA AND BRACHY-DACTYLY, 392
Fifth phacomatosis, 101
Finger (also see Digit, Phalanx and Section III, Table XXIX)
    absence of, all except one, 336
    absence of distal phalanx, 21, 114, 1001
    absence of 5th, 875
    absence of, one or more (see Ectro-dactyly)
    absence of phalanges of ulnar digits, 981
    absence of phalanx of 5th, 262, 923
    brachydactyly (see Section III, Table XXIX)
    broad, 578
    broad distal phalanx of, 119
    clubbed, 409
    curved 2nd, 121
    defect of distal phalanx, 263
    defect of shape or size, 821
    duplication of index, 814
    extra bone in soft tissue, 22
    extra index, 814
    extra on radial side of hand, 649, 814, 883, 987
    extra on ulnar side of hand, 17, 156, 578, 634, 814, 817, 883, 884
    knobby, 557
    lateral deviation at proximal interpha-langeal joint, 89
    lateral deviation of all, 450
    long, 85, 166, 557, 629
    marked shortening of, 114
    medial curvature of, 158, 172
    medial deviation of all, 392
    medial deviation of 2nd, 22
    medial deviation of 2nd and 3rd, 880
    mitten syndactyly, 14
    overlapping, 160, 168
    permanently flexed 5th, 556, 644
    permanently flexed 4th and 5th, 737

    permanent flexion of, 139, 157, 160, 166, 168, 379, 981
    prenatal amputation, 874
    progressive shortening of, 21
    short distal phalanx of index, 22
    short distal phalanx of 5th, 242
    short 5th, 1, 171, 242, 506, 875, 887, 923
    short middle phalanx of, 13, 19, 114, 823
    short middle phalanx of index, 22, 392
    short middle phalanx of 5th, 171, 242, 621, 700, 923
    syndactyly including 4th, 229
    syndactyly, partial of 3rd and 4th, 13, 169, 754, 817, 923
    syndactyly, partial of 4th and 5th, 737
    syndactyly to proximal interphalangeal joints, 293
    synostosis, 14, 874, 923
    thick, 158, 190
    toe-like, 8, 445
    unilateral shortening of, 813
Finger flexor tendons, short, 882
FINGERPRINTS ABSENT, 393
First arch syndrome, 457
Fissure labiale et palatine-dysplasie ecto-dermique-anomalies des extrémities-oligophrénie, 179
Fissure labio-palatine avec blépharophi-mosis, 176
Fissure latérale, 374
Fissure médiane de la lèvre supérieure, 595
Fissure médiane labio-mandibule-linguale, 636
Fissure mentonnière, 146
Fissure oblique de la face, 375
Fissured tongue, 953
Fístula arterio-venosa coronaria, 218
Fístula arteriovenosa del oído externo, 313
Fistula auris congenita, 329
Fistula of lacrimal sac, 565
Fistula of palate, 790
Fístula palatina (Marcador), 790
Fistula tráqueoesofágica, 960
Fistule artério-veineuse de l'oreille externe, 313
Fistule coronaire artério-veineuse, 218
Fistule des voies lacrymales, 565
Fistule laryngo-trachéo-oesophagienne, 577
Fistule palatine, 790
Fistule trachéo-oesophagienne, 960
Fisura alveolar mediana del maxilar, 631
Fisura del mentón, 146
Fisura facial lateral, 374
Fisura facial oblicua, 375
Fisura labial o palatina con fóveas labiales, 177
Fisura labial o palatina con fusión filiforme de los párpados, 176
Fisura labio-palatina-displasia ectodérmica-anomalías de manos y pies y oligo-frenia, 179
Fisura laringo-tráqueo-esofágica, 577
Fisura mediana del labio inferior, de la mandíbula y de la lengua, 636
Fisura mediana del labio superior, 595
Fisura palatina y persistencia de la mem-brana bucofaríngea, 181
5α-reductase deficiency, 831
5-oxoprolinuria, 849
Flame-shaped pulp chambers, 937
Flank, mass in, 859
Fleck form pigmentation, 639
Floating gallbladder, 404

Flowing hyperostosis, 641
Fontanel
    abnormal position of anterior, 722
    bulging anterior, 403
    delayed closure of, 118, 139, 185, 846, 976
    delayed closure of anterior, 775, 825, 846
    large anterior, 401
    large posterior, 946
    premature closure of anterior, 121
    prenatal onset of large, 480
    rapidly growing tumor of anterior, 711
    tense, 481
Food, adverse reaction, 423, 453, 513, 657
Foot, as a unit
    abducted, 647
    adducted, 648
    broad, 1, 8, 250, 445, 510, 893, 940
    central ray deficiency of, 336, 337
    central ray deficiency with syndactyly of, 336
    defect of, 282, 998, 1001
    disproportionate shortness of, 823
    foot drop, 143
    long, 137, 189, 587
    metatarsus adductus, 1, 139
    metatarsus varus, 791
    plantarflexed, inverted and abducted, 161, 170, 570, 629, 662
    rockerbottom, 140, 159, 160, 980
    short, 8, 16, 20, 250, 358, 445, 510, 893, 940
    square, 20
    talipes, 88, 97, 158, 159, 160, 164, 170, 178, 180, 182, 223, 293, 338, 376, 380, 634, 649, 754, 874, 881, 882, 897
    talipes cavus, 265, 352, 474, 676, 791, 810, 982
    talipes calcaneovalgus, 139
    talipes calcaneovarus, 164, 647
    talipes equinus, 560
    talipes planus, 19, 72, 106, 163, 290, 338, 560, 630, 648, 678, 786, 791, 823, 882
    talipes valgus, 8, 290, 445, 560, 570, 823
Foramen magnum small, 10, 103
Foramen of Morgagni hernia, 289
Foramen ovale patent, 139, 182, 401
Forbes-Albright syndrome, 350
Forbes disease, 426
Forearm, as a unit
    bowing of, 308, 685, 749
    lateral bony protuberance of, 647
    lateral bowing of, 648
    progressive shortening of, 128
    short, 16, 380, 853
Forebrain, failure to divide, 158, 168, 473
Forehead
    broad domed, 158, 754, 777
    flat, 14
    frontal bossing, 10, 97, 137, 139, 158, 185, 190, 227, 333, 398, 431, 510, 570, 638, 738, 779, 846, 847, 873, 876, 940
    high, 14, 139, 165, 231, 299, 603, 754, 791
    low, 168
    sloping, 140, 299, 634
    small frontal region of, 629
    swelling of, 228
Forma semiletal de sordomúdez, 243
45/X,46,XY mosaicism, 173
Fossettes auriculaires, 329

Fossettes de la macule, 756
Fossettes labiales, 596
Fotomioclonus, diabetes mellitus, sordera
    neurosensorial, nefropatía, y dis-
    función cerebral, 255
Four-cusped aortic valve, 81
Fovea mentalis, 146
Fóveas auriculares (Marcador), 329
Fóveas del disco óptico, 756
Fóveas o montículos labiales (Marcador),
    596
Fractures, 310, 345, 346, 391, 406, 474,
    499, 516, 712, 777, 779, 780, 782,
    783, 859, 873, 939, 965, 1000
    increase of, 310, 391, 474, 712, 777,
        782, 783, 859, 939, 965, 1000
    pathologic, 345, 346, 406, 499, 516,
        779, 780, 873
Fragilitas ossium, 777
Franceschetti-Jadassohn syndrome, 703
François dyscephaly, 738
Fredrickson type I hyperlipoproteinemia,
    489
Fredrickson type II hyperlipoproteinemia,
    488
Fredrickson type III hyperlipoproteinemia,
    495
Fredrickson type IV hyperlipoproteinemia,
    500
Fredrickson type V hyperlipoproteinemia,
    501
Freeman-Sheldon syndrome, 223
Frenulum, lingual
    abnormally attached, 291
    hypertrophied, 634, 770, 771
    multiple labial, 121, 735, 770
    prominent, 156
Frères Siamois, 202
Frey syndrome, 448
Frontal bone (see Forehead)
FRONTOMETAPHYSEAL DYSPLASIA,
    394
Frontonasal dysplasia, 635
Fructose intolerance, 395
FRUCTOSE–1–PHOSPHATE ALDOLASE
    DEFICIENCY, 395
FRUCTOSE–1,6–DIPHOSPHATASE
    DEFICIENCY, 396
Fructosemia, 395
FRUCTOSURIA (MARKER), 397
Frühmanifeste Osteopetrose, 779
Frühmanifeste recessive Taubheit, 270
Frühmanifestes Lymphödem, 614
Fruktose-1-Phosphat-Aldolase Mangel, 395
Fruktose-1,6-Diphosphatasemangel, 396
Fruktosurie, 397
Fuchs endothelial dystrophy, 208
FUCOSIDOSIS, 398
Functional obstruction of left ventricle, 917
Fundo albino puntato, 399
FUNDUS ALBIPUNCTATUS, 399
Fundus albipunctatus cum hemeralopia, 399
FUNDUS FLAVIMACULATUS, 400
Fundus flavimaculatus with macular de-
    generation, 400
Funnel chest, 802
Fused teeth, 930
Fusion dentaire, 930
Fusión incompleta de los conductose de
    Müller, 684
Fussionsstörung der Müllerschen Gänge, 684

G

G SYNDROME, 401

Gait
    clumsy, 190, 478
    defect of, 223, 292, 775
    difficult, 818
    on knees, 560
    progressive defect, 295
    spastic, 270, 295
    unsteady, 103
    waddling, 290, 306, 358, 391, 560, 654,
        687, 689, 828, 899
    wide-based, 190, 270, 290
GALACTOKINASE DEFICIENCY, 402
Galactose-glucose malabsorption, 419
Galactose-1-phosphate uridyl transferase
    deficiency, 403
GALACTOSEMIA, 403
Galactosemia-Duarte and Negro variants,
    403
Galaktokinasemangel, 402
Galaktosämie, 403
Gallbladder
    absence of, 401, 404
    biliary atresia, 160, 544, 606, 888
    biliary cirrhosis, 149
    gallstones in, 362, 403, 420, 852, 886
    gallstones, bilirubin, 892
    gallstones, double row of, 404
    obstruction of bile duct, 110
    obstruction of common bile duct, 532
    variable defects of, 404
GALLBLADDER ANOMALIES, 404
Gallenblasen-Fehlbildungen, 404
Gallengangsatresie, 110
Gamma globulin (Gm) antigen, 476
Gamma-glutamyl transpeptidase deficiency,
    422
Ganglion nodosum tumor, 127
Gangliosidose G_{M2} avec déficit en hexos-
    aminidase A, 434
Gangliosidose G_{M2} avec déficit en hexos-
    aminidase A et B, 433
Gangliosidose-type I, 431
Gangliosidose-type II, 432
Gangliosidosis G_{M1} tipo 1, 431
Gangliosidosis G_{M1} tipo 2, 432
Gangliosidosis G_{M2} con deficiencia de hexos-
    aminidasa A, 434
Gangliosidosis G_{M2} con deficiencia de hexos-
    aminidasa A y B, 433
Gardner syndrome, 536
Gargoylism, 674
Gastric atresia, 910
Gastric enterocystoma, 912
Gastric intrinsic factor deficiency, 992
Gastric peristaltic waves, visible, 848
Gastric teratoma, 914
Gastroesophageal reflux without radio-
    graphically or surgically demonstrable
    hiatus hernia, 366
Gastrointestinal malignancy, 521, 535, 536
Gastrointestinal system (see parts and
    Section III, Table XXXIV)
GASTROSCHISIS, 405
Gastrosquisis, 405
GAUCHER DISEASE, 406
Gaumenfistel, 790
Gaumenspalte, 180
Gaumenspalte und persistierende bucco-
    pharingeale Membran, 181
Gc, 446
Gehörgangsatresie, 97
Gehörgangs-Exostosen, 318
Gelb-blau Blindheit, 199
Gemeinsamer Ursprung der A. brachio-
    cephalica und der gegenseitigen A.
    carotis, 200

Gemelos siameses, 202
Geminated teeth, 931
Generalized gangliosidosis, type 1, 431
Genital, renal and middle ear anomalies, 860
Genital system (see parts and Section III,
    Table XXXV)
Genitalia (also see parts and Section III,
    Table XXXV)
    ambiguous at birth, 907, 908
    ambiguous, external, 29, 50, 173, 388,
        634, 902, 903, 904, 971
    duplication of external, 194, 684
    female internally, with male gender and
        ambiguous external genitalia, 634
    hyperpigmented external, 30, 37, 908
    internally consisting of wolffian and
        müllerian duct derivatives, 971
    small external, 93, 303
    small internal, 93
Genetic epilepsy, 135
Genetic variant of soluble malate dehydro-
    genase, 625
Genito-oculo-oligophrenic-dento-skeleto
    syndrome (GOODS), 118
Genitourinary system, unspecified defect of,
    69, 375, 458, 505, 532, 662, 748,
    856, 857, 881
Genu recurvatum, 651
Genu valgum, 106, 156, 185, 216, 290, 352,
    474, 630, 647, 654, 672, 675, 679,
    749, 798, 828, 847, 897
Genu varum, 250, 704, 798, 828, 897
Germinomas, 188
Geschlechtsgebundene Agammaglobulin-
    ämie, 27
Geschlechtsgebundener lymphopenischer
    Immunkörpermangel, 524
Gespaltene Uvula, 184
Gespaltenes Ohrläppchen, 321
Gestation
    terminated as spontaneous abortion
        (< 20 wks and <20 gm), 412, 684
    terminated as stillbirth, 9, 153, 340, 412,
        516, 555, 780, 875, 884, 939
    time shortened (> 20 wks and < 35 wks-
        premature birth), 9, 148, 169, 856,
        864, 872
Giant cyst of the retina, 871
Gicht, 441
Gigantism, 85, 556, 578, 670
Gigantism, cerebral, 137
Gilbert disease, 487
Gilbert-Dreyfus syndrome, 50
Gingiva
    firm, hard, 407, 408, 410, 411
    gangrenous lesions in, 6
    gingivitis, 494, 714
    hyperpigmentation or stippling of, 25,
        407
    hyperplasia of, 407, 409, 410, 411, 412
    localized and bilaterally symmetrically
        enlarged, 407
    noninflammatory enlargement of, 279,
        408, 413, 431, 644, 876
    papilloma on, 281
    smooth round mass in, 360
GINGIVAL FIBROMATOSIS, 407
GINGIVAL FIBROMATOSIS AND
    CORNEAL DYSTROPHY, 408
GINGIVAL FIBROMATOSIS AND
    DIGITAL ANOMALIES, 409
GINGIVAL FIBROMATOSIS AND
    HYPERTRICHOSIS, 410
GINGIVAL FIBROMATOSIS AND
    MULTIPLE HYALINE FIBROMAS,
    411

GINGIVAL FIBROMATOSIS, COWDEN TYPE, 412
GINGIVAL FIBROMATOSIS, DEPIGMENTATION AND MICROPHTHALMIA, 413
Gingival fibromatosis, depigmentation, microphthalmia, oligophrenia and athetosis, 413
Gingival fibromatosis, digital, ear, nose anomalies and hepatosplenomegaly, 409
Gingival fibromatosis, disturbed eruption of teeth and corneal dystrophy, 408
Gingival fibromatosis, hypertrichosis and fibroadenomas of breasts, 412
Gitlin form of alymphopenic immunologic deficiency, 524
Gitterförmige Hornhautdystrophie, 211
Glándula lacrimal ectópica, 564
GLAUCOMA, CONGENITAL, 414
Glaucoma, infantile, 414
Glioma nasal, 726
Glioma opticum, 763
Glioma orbitario, 763
Gliome de l'orbite, 763
Gliome nasal, 726
Gliosis, 924
Globodontia with high frequency hearing loss, 784
GLOBOID CELL LEUKODYSTROPHY, 415
Glomangiomas, 416
Glomus caroticum tumor, 127
Glomus jugulare of middle ear, 145
Glomus jugulare tumor, 145
GLOMUS TUMORS, MULTIPLE, 416
Glomus tympanicum tumor, 145
Glositis mediana romboidea, 417
Glossite exfoliatrice marginée, 954
GLOSSITIS, MEDIAN RHOMBOID, 417
Glossopalatine ankylosis, microglossia, hypodontia and limb anomalies, 451
Glossopalatine ankylosis syndrome, 451
Glottic atresia, 571
Glottic cysts, 572
Glottic web, 574
Glucocerebrosidosis, 406
Glucogenosis, tipo I, 425
Glucogenosis, tipo II, 11
Glucogenosis, tipo III, 426
Glucogenosis, tipo IV, 116
Glucogenosis, tipo V, 698
Glucogenosis, tipo VI, 427
Glucogenosis, tipo VII, 428
Glucogenosis, tipo VIII, 429
Glucogenosis, tipo IX, 430
GLUCOGLYCINURIA (MARKER), 418
GLUCOSE-GALACTOSE MALABSORPTION, 419
GLUCOSE-6-PHOSPHATE DEHYDROGENASE DEFICIENCY, 420
Glucosuria renal (Marcador), 861
Glukoglyzinurie, 418
Glukose-Galaktose-Malabsorption, 419
Glukose-6-phosphat Dehydrogenase-Mangel, 420
GLUTARIC ACIDURIA, 421
Glutathionase deficiency, 422
Glutathione synthetase deficiency, 849
Glutathionmangel, 422
GLUTATHIONURIA, 422
GLUTEN-INDUCED ENTEROPATHY, 423
Glycinosis, 826
Glycogen deficiency syndrome with visceral fatty metamorphosis, 424
Glycogen storage disease, type I, 425
Glycogen storage disease, type II, 11

Glycogen storage disease, type III, 426
Glycogen storage disease, type IV, 116
Glycogen storage disease, type V, 698
Glycogen storage disease, type VI, 427
Glycogen storage disease, type VII, 428
Glycogen storage disease, type VIII, 429
Glycogen storage disease, type IX, 430
GLYCOGEN SYNTHETASE DEFICIENCY, 424
GLYCOGENOSIS, TYPE I, 425
Glycogenosis, type II, 11
GLYCOGENOSIS, TYPE III, 426
Glycogenosis, type IV, 116
Glycogenosis, type V, 698
GLYCOGENOSIS, TYPE VI, 427
GLYCOGENOSIS, TYPE VII, 428
GLYCOGENOSIS, TYPE VIII, 429
GLYCOGENOSIS, TYPE IX, 430
Glycolipid lipidosis, 373
Glycosurie rénale, 861
Glykogen-Synthetase-Mangel, 424
Glykogenose, Typ I, 425
Glykogenose, Typ II, 11
Glykogenose, Typ III, 426
Glykogenose, Typ IV, 116
Glykogenose, Typ V, 698
Glykogenose, Typ VI, 427
Glykogenose, Typ VII, 428
Glykogenose, Typ VIII, 429
Glykogenose, Typ IX, 430
Gm antigen type, 476
G_{M1}-gangliosidosis of late onset without bony deformities, 432
G_{M1}-GANGLIOSIDOSIS, TYPE 1, 431
G_{M1}-GANGLIOSIDOSIS, TYPE 2, 432
G_{M2}-GANGLIOSIDOSIS WITH HEXOSAMINIDASE A AND B DEFICIENCY, 433
G_{M2}-GANGLIOSIDOSIS WITH HEXOSAMINIDASE A DEFICIENCY, 434
Goiter, 249, 257, 350, 412, 435, 542, 543, 809, 947
Goiter and sensorineural deafness, 249
Goiter, familial, 542, 543, 947
GOITER, GOITROGEN-INDUCED, 435
Goiter, nontoxic, 111
Goiter with high levels of serum thyroid hormones, deafness and stippled epiphyses, 257
Goitrogen-induced goiter, 435
Goldenhar syndrome, 735
Goltz-Gorlin syndrome, 281
Gonadal agenesis, 29
GONADAL DYSGENESIS, XX TYPE, 436
GONADAL DYSGENESIS, XY TYPE, 437
Gonadal interstitial cell hyperplasia, 104
Gonadal tissue, presence of both ovarian and testicular, 971
Gonadenaplasie, 29
GONADOTROPIN DEFICIENCY, ISOLATED, 438
Gonflement fibreux des maxillaires, 539
GONIODYSGENESIS, 439
Gonosomal intersexuality, 173
Gonosomale Intersexualität, 173
GORLIN-CHAUDHRY-MOSS SYNDROME, 440
Gorlin-Psaume syndrome, 770
Gorlin syndrome, 101
Gota, 441
GOUT, 441
Goutte, 441
Gowers form of dystrophy, 690
Grand mal epilepsy, 135
Granular cell neurofibroma, 360
Granular cell perineural fibroblastoma, 360

Granular cell pseudotumor, 360
Granular cell schwannoma, 360
Granular corneal dystrophy, 209
Granular neuroma, 360
Granuläre Hornhautdystrophie, 209
Granulation anomaly of leukocytes, 143
Granulocellular rhabdomyoma, 360
Granulomatosis crónica de las mujeres, 442
GRANULOMATOUS DISEASE OF FEMALES, CHRONIC, 442
GRANULOMATOUS DISEASE OF MALES, CHRONIC, 443
GRANULOSIS RUBRA NASI, 444
Grasp reflex retained into childhood, 413
Great arteries, inversion of ventricles with transposition of, 540
Great vessel transportation, 388, 455, 962
Grebe chondrodysplasia, 445
Grebe disease, 445
GREBE SYNDROME, 445
Gregg syndrome, 384
Greig syndrome, 504
Groenblad-Strandberg syndrome, 832
Groenouw type I corneal dystrophy, 209
Groenouw type II corneal dystrophy, 212
GROUP-SPECIFIC COMPONENT (MARKER), 446
Group-specific protein, 446
Growth, accelerated in childhood, 104, 391
GROWTH HORMONE DEFICIENCY, ISOLATED, 447
Growth retardation (see Section III, Table XXIII)
Grubenpapillen, 756
Gruber syndrome, 634
Gruppenspezifische Eiweisskomponente, 446
Guérin-Stern syndrome, 88
Günther disease, 821
GUSTATORY SWEATING, 448
Gyratacorneal leukoma, acromegaloid phenotype and cutis verticis, 18
GYRATE ATROPHY, 449
G6PD deficiency, 420

H

"H"-type tracheoesophageal fistula, 960
Haemangiomatosis cutis et visceralis cavernosa, 113
Hair, axillary (also see Hair color, differentiating characteristics, special body parts and Section III, Table XXVIII)
    decreased, 26, 49, 438
    early development of, 908
Hair, bone, nail and tooth dysplasia, 965
Hair, color
    change of, 36
    blond or light-colored, 143, 337, 720, 808, 875
    darkening of, 35
    frosted-grey sheen of, 143
    hyperpigmented, black, 410, 412
    pigment reduced, 413
    prematurely grey, 163, 493, 997, 998
    white, 30, 34, 35, 36, 657
    white developing yellow cast with sun exposure, 34
    white forelock, 31, 997
    white scalp hair with pigmented patches, 30
Hair, differentiating characteristics
    coarse, 412
    dry, 737, 946
    fragile, 334, 643
    kinky, 720, 965

Hair, differentiating characteristics —
  Continued
    lanugo or downy, 105, 670, 720
    short, 670
    slow growth of, 102, 302
    thin, 334, 413, 511
Hair, ear
    long coarse hairs on helix, 319
    tongue-shaped preauricular tuft of
      hair, 627
Hair, excessive and gingival enlargement,
    410
Hair, eyebrow
    cleft of, 735
    confluent, 242, 388, 616, 632
    depigmented medial portion of, 31
    hypoplastic, 67, 102, 105, 653
    hypoplastic lateral third of, 299
    long, thick and bushy throughout, 119,
      242, 644
    long, thick and bushy medial portion of,
      966, 997
    loss of, in early childhood, 825
    markedly elevated arch of, 119
Hair greying, premolar aplasia and hyper-
    hidrosis, 493
Hairy cyst on head or neck, 283
Hairy pinnae, 319
Half nose plus proboscis, 722
Hallermann-Streiff syndrome, 738
Hallux (also see Digit, Toe and Joints)
    absence of (see Ectrodactyly), 875
    angulation deformity of, 119
    bifurcation of distal phalanx of, 119,
      264, 621
    broad, 325, 578, 621, 754
    broad distal phalanx of, 114, 119
    bulbous distal phalanx of, 264
    duplication of, 13, 621, 817
    duplication of proximal phalanx of, 119
    polysyndactyly of, 771
    short, 160, 190, 700, 875
    short distal phalanx of, 114, 264, 817
    syndactyly with 2nd toe, 22
    turned outward, 19, 229
    turned upward, 160
Hämangiom der orbita, 764
Hämangiomatose der Leber, 466
Hamartoma del hígado, 604
Hamartoma of CNS, 188
Hamartoma of liver, 604
Hamartoma, venous, 113
Hamartome hépatique, 604
Hammer toe, 89, 140, 393
Hämochromatose, 460
Hämophilie A, 461
Hämophilie B, 462
Hand Fehlbildung und Innenohrschwerhörig-
    keit, 450
Hand, as a unit
    broad, 1, 20, 171, 250, 389, 510, 893,
      940
    central ray deficiency of, 281, 336, 337
    claw-like, 281, 672, 1000
    clubbed, 380, 574, 749
    clubhand with deviation to ulnar side,
      223
    contracture of web space of, 301
    decreased range of motion of, 557
    defect of, 282, 727, 1001
    defect of metacarpophalangeal joint, 129
    duplication of ulnar ray structure of, 981
    hyperextensible metacarpophalangeal
      joints, 409
    inability to make a fist, 557
    inability to make a tight fist, 156

    long, 137, 189, 190, 587
    marked shortness of, 8, 823
    radial deviation of, 231, 647, 941
    radial ray deficiency of, 336
    short, 1, 16, 20, 171, 242, 250, 302,
      358, 389, 445
    tremor of, 472, 963
    trident-like, 10
    ulnar deviation of, 160, 270, 749, 980
HAND MUSCLE WASTING AND SENSORI-
    NEURAL DEAFNESS, 450
Hand writing, deterioration of, 266
HANHART SYNDROME, 451
Hapsburg jaw, 626
HAPTOGLOBIN (MARKER), 452
Harelip, 178
Harrington syndrome, 943
HARTNUP DISORDER, 453
Hartnupsche Krankheit, 453
Head, backward tilting of, 75, 413, 752, 753
Head held in extensor position, 406
Head, increased transillumination, 480, 481
Head tilt, 188
Hearing loss (see also Ear and Section III,
    Table XXV)
    bilateral, 183, 206, 244, 249, 252, 260,
      265, 550
    conductive, due to middle ear malforma-
      tion (also see Section III, Table
      XXV), 330, 331, 377, 664
    fluctuating, 248
    inability to recognize pitch, 273
    marked (71 + db), 89, 97, 123, 142,
      150, 243, 247, 249, 252, 253, 257,
      261, 265, 268, 269, 272, 275, 315,
      562, 592, 784
    mild (27 — 40 db), 254, 258, 550
    mixed, 247, 263, 264, 530
    moderate (41 — 70 db), 89, 245, 246,
      247, 254, 258, 261, 272, 550, 784
    nonprogressive, 245, 249, 251, 260,
      267, 269, 785
    paralleled onset of loss of libido, 982
    present at birth, 70, 142, 243, 244, 245,
      249, 251, 252, 256, 257, 259, 269,
      315, 377, 450, 983
    sensorineural (see Section III, Table
      XXV)
    slow progression of, 246, 267, 708
    unilateral, 89, 248, 274, 457, 592
Hearing loss and nephritis, 708
Hearing loss, familial low-frequency, 256
Hearing loss, hereditary progressive high-
    tone type, 269
Hearing loss, low-frequency, 260
Heart (also see Section III, Table XXXII)
HEART BLOCK, CONGENITAL
    COMPLETE, 454
Heart disease, glycogen, 11
Heart failure
    acute onset, 217, 922
    acyanotic, 82, 298, 348, 767, 922
    by xray or percussion, 51, 76, 80, 104,
      218, 286, 297, 298, 347, 348, 353,
      398, 581, 672, 800, 805, 922, 968,
      969, 972, 989
    congestive, 11, 39, 53, 64, 76, 79, 80,
      82, 116, 204, 217, 286, 297, 298,
      347, 348, 353, 384, 420, 460, 581,
      665, 666, 689, 695, 698, 767, 825,
      836, 838, 842, 922, 939, 969, 972,
      979, 989
    cyanotic, 92, 297, 541, 968
    left heart, 353
    moderate, 79, 968
    onset after 1 yr of age, 353

    onset before 1 yr of age, 64, 79, 186,
      217, 298, 347, 348, 466, 581, 666,
      767, 838, 842, 969, 972, 979, 989
    right heart, 204, 332, 354, 838
    severe, 979
    unspecified heart failure, 51, 332, 541

HEART–HAND SYNDROME, 455
Heart, hemosiderosis of, 95
Heart murmur
    abrupt onset of, 53
    at apex, 298, 347, 348, 353, 669, 917,
      989
    at 4th left intercostal space at sternal
      border, 218, 347, 581, 969
    at 3rd left intercostal space at sternal
      border, 80, 298, 731, 836, 972, 989
    at 2nd left intercostal space at sternal
      border, 78, 96, 297, 347, 731, 800,
      835, 836, 838, 839, 842, 916, 989
    at left sternal border, 53, 79, 82, 83, 96,
      286, 347, 836, 838, 842, 938, 989
    at 3rd right intercostal space at sternal
      border, 80
    at 2nd right intercostal space at sternal
      border, 78, 82, 916
    blowing quality of, 82, 204, 347
    bruit, 186
    bruit over spine, 186
    continuous, 53, 218, 800
    crescendo-decrescendo configuration
      to, 800
    decrescendo configuration to, 83, 989
    diastolic, 82, 83, 96, 298, 347, 669, 836,
      838, 842, 916, 972, 989
    early timing of diastolic, 838
    early timing of systolic, 353
    ejection configuration to (diamond-
      shaped), 78, 80, 83, 96, 108, 109,
      347, 454, 581, 665, 731, 835, 838,
      839, 916, 917, 989
    flow quality of (rumble), 96, 298, 347,
      669
    harsh quality of, 78, 80, 82, 286, 297,
      298, 347, 839, 916, 989
    high-pitched quality of, 347, 835
    late timing of diastolic, 669
    late timing of systolic, 668
    low-pitched quality of, 669
    mid timing of diastolic, 96, 669
    mid timing of systolic, 73, 917
    murmur intensity grade II (soft),
      109, 204, 837
    murmur intensity grade III (moderately
      loud), 109
    murmur intensity grade IV (loud), 78, 80,
      82, 347, 581, 916, 938, 969, 972
    murmur intensity grade V (loud), 347
    pansystolic configuration to (holosystolic),
      347, 581, 666, 917, 969, 989
    posteriorly, 73
    regurgitant, 666, 668, 916, 917
    soft quality of, 842, 1002
    systolic, 64, 73, 78, 79, 80, 82, 83, 96,
      108, 109, 204, 286, 297, 298, 332,
      347, 348, 353, 454, 541, 581, 665,
      666, 668, 731, 768, 835, 836, 837,
      838, 839, 842, 916, 917, 938, 969,
      972, 989
    transmission to carotid (carotid bruit),
      78, 80, 916
    transmission to lung fields, 838
    transmission to jugular notch (supra-
      sternal notch), 78, 80, 916
    unspecified heart murmur, 53, 587,
      674, 805

Heart position
    complete displacement of, from thorax, 335
    dextrocardia, 92, 182, 285, 468, 606, 629, 888
    midline position of, 401
    partial displacement of, from thorax, 335
    unspecified malposition of, 805
Heart, septal defect
    atrial, 139, 156, 157, 161, 182, 381, 384, 388, 455, 632, 720, 941, 999
    ventricular, 53, 138, 157, 161, 162, 182, 379, 384, 388, 455, 632, 754, 999
Heart thrill
    diastolic at left sternal border, 82
    diastolic on palpation, 82
    over precordium, 78, 80, 916
    systolic at lower left sternal border, 218, 298, 989
    systolic at upper left sternal border, 839
    systolic on palpation, 82, 286, 298, 347, 666, 800, 839
    systolic over aortic area, 82
    transmitted to carotid, 78, 80, 916
    transmitted to jugular notch, 78, 80, 190, 916
Heart upper limb syndrome, 455
Heart valve closure sounds on auscultation
    accentuated 3rd heart sound, 332, 348, 666, 842, 979
    aortic heart paradoxical splitting of (2nd sound), 80, 916, 917
    aortic valve accentuated closure sound, 78, 540, 938
    ejection click to heart sound, aortic or pulmonic, 80, 108, 839, 842, 916, 972
    feeble heart sounds, 979
    fourth heart sound prominent, 332, 348, 842, 979
    loud single 2nd heart sound, aortic or pulmonic, 581, 989
    mid-systolic click to heart sound, 668
    mitral valve accentuated closure sound (1st sound), 669
    opening snap to heart sound, 669
    pulmonic heart fixed splitting of sound (2nd sound closely or widely split), 96, 286, 297, 298, 332, 347, 581, 731, 835, 838, 839, 842, 989
    pulmonic valve, absence of closure sound, 838
    pulmonic valve, accentuated closure sound (loud component of 2nd heart sound), 204, 286, 297, 298, 581, 666, 669, 800, 835, 838, 842, 989
    pulmonic valve, diminished closure sound (feeble 2nd sound), 839
    single 2nd heart sound, aortic or pulmonic, 80, 286, 297, 541, 768, 837, 916, 938, 972
    tricuspid valve accentuated closure sound (1st sound), 842
    tricuspid valve variable closure sound (1st sound), 454
    widely split components of 1st sound, 332
Heat intolerance, 5, 56, 102, 189, 237, 333, 703, 986
Helix (also see Ear)
    auditory meatus covered by, 314
    concha covered by, 326
    crus of helix fused to crura of anthelix, 328
    folded, 97, 388, 720
    helical pit, 329

hypoplastic, 85, 98, 159, 161, 314, 330, 331, 664
large scapha of, 619
poorly developed scapha of, 326
Hemangiectatic hypertrophy, 55
HEMANGIOMA AND THROMBOCYTO-PENIA SYNDROME, 456
Hemangioma de la órbita, 764
Hemangioma of lids and orbit, 764
Hemangioma, subglottic, 918
Hemangiomata and enchondromatosis, 346
Hémangiomatose hépatique, 466
Hemangiomatosis generalized cavernous, 113
Hemangiomatosis hepática, 466
Hemangiomatosis, multiple, 995
Hemangiomatous macroglossia, 618
Hémangiome de l'orbite, 764
Hémangiome sous-glottique, 918
Hematoporphyria congenita, 821
Héméralopie, 718
Héméralopie stationnaire, 719
Hémi-hypertrophie, 458
Hemicrania, 52
Hemifacial hypertrophy, 458
HEMIFACIAL MICROSOMIA, 457
Hemifaziale Mikrosomie, 457
Hemigigantism, 458
HEMIHYPERTROPHY, 458
HEMIMELIA AND SCALP–SKULL DEFECTS, 459
Hemimelic skeletal dysplasias, 311
Hemimelie, 459
Hemiparesis, 186, 188, 255, 474, 886
Hemitruncus arteriosus, 767
HEMOCHROMATOSIS, IDIOPATHIC, 460
Hemofilia A, 461
Hemofilia B, 462
Hemoglobin-binding α_2 globulins, 452
Hemoglobin-binding β_2 globulins, 452
Hemoglobin Lepore syndromes, 939
Hemolytic disease of newborn, 340
HEMOPHILIA A, 461
HEMOPHILIA B, 462

Hemorrhage
    increased after circumcision, 4, 462
    increased after injury or surgery, 4, 462, 996
    increased after loss of deciduous tooth, 996
    into mucous membrane, 942
    into skin or joints spontaneously or after injury or surgery, 461, 462
    spontaneous within joints, 461, 996
    spontaneous within organs, 461
    transient purpura, 826
    uncontrolled bleeding after eruption of deciduous tooth, 461
    uncontrolled bleeding after injury or surgery, 461
    unspecified bleeding defect, 406, 990
    within skin after slight injury, 403, 406, 461, 462, 978

HEPATIC AGENESIS, 463
HEPATIC ARTERIAL ANOMALIES, 464
Hepatic cholesteryl ester storage disease, 151
HEPATIC CYST, SOLITARY, 465
Hepatic cyst, unilocular, 465
Hepatic cysts, multiple, 605
Hepatic fructose-1,6-diphosphatase deficiency, 396
Hepatic glucuronyl transferase deficiency type I, 961

Hepatic hamartoma, 604
HEPATIC HEMANGIOMATOSIS, 466
Hepatic infantile hemangioendothelioma, 466
HEPATIC LOBES, ACCESSORY, 467
Hepatic lobes anomalous, 467
Hepatic situs inversus, 606
HEPATIC VENOUS ANOMALIES, 468
HEPATOLENTICULAR DEGENERATION, 469
Hepatomegaly (see Section III, Table XXXIII)
Hepatosplenomegaly (also see Section III, Table XXXIII), 143, 503, 677, 679
Hepatosplenomegaly, gingival fibromatosis, digital, ear, and nose anomalies, 409
Hereditäre ACTH-Unempfindlichkeit der Nebennierenrinde, 25
Hereditäre Anonychie, 66
Hereditäre Koproporphyrie, 203
Hereditäre Mischtumoren der Speichel-drüsen, 878
Hereditäre Nephritis und Schalleitungs-schwerhörigkeit, 708
Hereditäre Pankreatitis, 793
Hereditärer lokalisierter Pruritus, 827
Hereditärer Tremor, 964
Hereditäres angioneurotisches Ödem, 54
Hereditäres palmo-plantares erythem, 792
Hereditary angioneurotic edema, 54
Hereditary chronic nephritis, 708
Hereditary congenital ophthalmoplegia, 751
Hereditary constitutional giant granulations of leukocytes, 143
Hereditary coproporphyria, 203
Hereditary crystalline corneal dystrophy, 216
Hereditary cutaneomandibular polyoncosis, 101
Hereditary deep corneal dystrophy, 213
Hereditary differences of taste threshold to bitter compounds containing the N–C=S group, 809
Hereditary dysplasia of bone with kypho-scoliosis, contractures and abnormally shaped ears, 85
Hereditary dystopic lipidosis, 373
Hereditary ectodermal dystrophy, 334
Hereditary epithelial corneal dystrophy, 210
Hereditary gigantism of cytoplasmic organelles, 143
Hereditary hyperglycinemia, 492
Hereditary hyperparathyroidism, 350
Hereditary hypoaldosteronism due to 18-oxidation defect, 905, 906
Hereditary interstitial pyelonephritis, 708
Hereditary koilonychia, 559
Hereditary lactase deficiency (insufficiency), 566
Hereditary midfrequency nerve loss, 267
Hereditary multicentric osteolysis with recessive transmission, 129
Hereditary multiple leiomyoma of skin, 890
Hereditary multiple lipomata, 600
Hereditary onychial dysplasia, 66
Hereditary palmo-plantar erythema, 792
Hereditary palpebromaxillary synergy, 548
Hereditary parathyroid hyperplasia, 499
Hereditary pseudovitamin D-deficiency rickets (PDR), 873
Hereditary quivering of chin, 147
Hereditary recurrent erosive corneal dys-trophy, 214
Hereditary retinal aplasia, 43
Hereditary spherocytosis, 892
Hereditary tyrosinemia and tyrosyluria, 978

Hereditary vitamin D-dependent rickets, 873

Hereditary vitelliruptive macular degeneration, 622

Heredodegeneration of inner ear, 315

Heredofamiliäre Opticusa trophie infantile Form, 755

Heredopathia atactica polyneuritiformia, 810

Heredoretinopathy congenitalis monohybrida, recessiva autosomalis, 43

Hermafroditismo, 971

Hermansky-Pudlak syndrome, 33

Hermaphrodisme vrai, 971

Hermaphroditism, 971

Hermaphroditismus vera, 971

Hernia (excepting CNS)
  abdominal, 13, 104, 338, 405, 531
  diaphragmatic, 104, 289, 382, 727
  hiatus, 727
  inguinal, 1, 13, 49, 155, 158, 161, 162, 163, 170, 305, 337, 388, 470, 505, 557, 587, 603, 630, 674, 676, 680, 683, 999
  inguinal, containing testis, 49
  inguinal, containing uterus and fallopian tubes, 683
  umbilical, 13, 155, 158, 160, 161, 168, 180, 388, 440, 467, 505, 531, 542, 543, 557, 587, 674, 676, 680, 748, 946
  unspecified hernia, excepting CNS, 675, 678, 679, 777

Hernia, congenital diaphragmatic, 289

Hernia hiatal, 471

Hernia inguinal, 529

Hernia, inguinal direct or indirect, 529

Hernia uteri inguinale syndrome, 683

Hernie diphragmatique congénitale, 289

Hernie hiatale, 471

Hernie inguinale, 529

HERRMANN–OPITZ ARTHROGRYPO-SIS SYNDROME, 470

Heterotopia de la mácula, 620

Heterotopia of macula, 620

HHHO, 823

HIATUS HERNIA, 471

Hiatushernie, 471

Hidranencefalía, 480

Hidrocefalía, 481

Hidrotische ektodermale Dysplasie, 334

Hidroxiprolinemia, 482

"High" and "low" imperforate anus, 69

High scapula, 901

High sinus venosus type defect with or without partial pulmonary venous connection, 96

Himen imperforado, 483

Hip
  coxa vara (femoral neck angle decreased to approach 90°), 185, 250, 380, 654, 672, 885
  coxa valga (femoral neck angle increased to approach 180°), 140, 185, 308, 775, 786, 825
  decreased range of motion of, 98, 358, 674, 898
  decreased rotary motion of, 88
  dislocation of, 88, 90, 98, 140, 161, 182, 379, 388, 544, 823
  dislocation of hip on weight bearing, 293
  flexed, 88
  flexion contracture of, 1000
  flexion contracture of hip in late infancy, 413

prenatal onset of contracture of, 629

prenatal onset of dislocation of, 97, 158, 570

Hiper-beta-alaninemia, 486

Hiper-diabásico-aminoaciduria, 491

Hiperaldosteronismo, 484

Hiperamonemia, 485

Hiperbilirubinemia (Marcador), 487

Hipercistinuria (Marcador), 490

Hipercolesteremia, 488

Hiperglicinemia cetónica, 826

Hiperglicinemia no cetónica, 492

Hiperhidrosis, encanecimiento prematuro y aplasia de los premolares, 493

Hiperlipoproteinemia combinada, 496

Hiperlipoproteinemia tipo III, 495

Hiperostosis cortical generalizada, 497

Hiperostosis cortical infantil, 221

Hiperostosis frontal interna, 498

Hiperparatiroidismo neonatal familiar, 499

Hiperplasia suprarrenal congénita deficiencia de 3β-hidroxisteroide dehidrogenasa, 909

Hiperplasia suprarrenal congénita deficiencia de 11β-hidroxilasa, 902

Hiperplasia suprarrenal congénita deficiencia de 17α-hidroxilasa, 903

Hiperplasia suprarrenal congénita deficiencia de 20-22 desmolasa, 907

Hiperplasia suprarrenal congénita deficiencia de 21-hidroxilasa, 908

Hiperprebeta-lipoproteinemia, 500

Hiperprebeta-lipoproteinemia e hiperquilo-micronemia, 501

Hiperprolinemia (Marcador), 502

Hiperquilomicronemia, 489

Hipersarcosinemia, 503

Hipertelorismo, 504

Hipertelorismo, microtia, hendidura facial y sordera de conducción, 506

Hipertricosis de las orejas, 319

Hipertricosis lanuginosa, 507

Hiperuricemia-sordera y ataxia, 508

Hipervalinemia, 509

Hipoaldosternosimo aislado transitorio de la infancia, 23

Hipocalcificación del esmalte, onicolisis e hipodrosis, 45

Hipocondroplasia, 510

Hipodoncia con disgenesia de las uñas, 511

Hipofosfatasia, 516

Hipofosfatemia, 517

Hipoglicemia inducida por la leucina, 513

Hipoglicemia neonatal, 512

Hipomagnesemia primaria, 514

Hipoparatiroidismo infantil ligado al X, 515

Hipoplasia de las extremidades superiores, arritmia cardíaca, oído externo malformado y sordera de conducción, 592

Hipoplasia del esmalte, 342

Hipoplasia del esmalte, taurodontismo, cabello rizado y esclerosis cortical, 965

Hipoplasia del esmalte y la dentina y decoloración por tetraciclinas, 341

Hipoplasia del nervio óptico, 758

Hipoplasia dérmica focal, 281

Hipoplasia gástrica, 913

Hipoplasia muscular universal congénita, 686

Hipoplasia pancreática, disfunción de la médula ósea y displasia metafisaria, 885

Hipoplasia suprarrenal congénita, 24

Hipoplasia y pigmentación del esmalte y la dentina por eritroblastosis fetal, 340

Hipospadia pseudovaginal perineoescrotal, 831

Hipospadias, 518

Hirntumoren, 188

Hirschsprung disease, 192

Hirsutism and gingival enlargement, 410

Histidine metabolism disturbance, 472

HISTIDINEMIA, 472

HMC syndrome, 506

Holes in optic disk, 756

Holmes heart, 286

HOLOPROSENCEPHALY, 473

Holt-Oram syndrome, 455

HOMOCYSTINURIA, 474

Homogentisic aciduria, 37

Homozygous sickle hemoglobinopathy, 886

Homozystinurie, 474

HORNER SYNDROME, 475

Hornhautdystrophie mit progressiver Innenohr-Schwerhörigkeit, 206

HUMAN ALLOTYPES (MARKERS), 476

HUMERORADIAL SYNOSTOSIS, 477

Humerus
  absence of, 875, 941
  defect of, 455, 941, 981
  marked shortening of, 10
  short, 154, 226, 592, 853, 875

Humor vítreo primario hiperplástico presistente, 994

Hunger, constant, 823

Hunter syndrome, 676

HUNTINGTON CHOREA, 478

Hurler-Pfaundler syndrome, 674

Hurler syndrome, 674

Hutchinson-Gilford syndrome, 825

Hutchinson incisors, 342

Hutchinson-Tay choroiditis, 734

Hyaline fibromas and gingival fibromatosis, 411

Hyalinosis cutis et mucosae, 599

HYALOIDEORETINAL DEGENERATION OF WAGNER, 479

Hydradenoma, 235

HYDRANENCEPHALY, 480

Hydrocele, 529

Hydrocephalus, 186, 481
  noncommunicating, 188
  due to atrophy of brain, 603

HYDROCEPHALY, 481

Hydroxylysine deficient collagen disease, 338

HYDROXYPROLINEMIA, 482

Hydrozephalie, 481

Hymen
  bulging, 483
  imperforate, 483, 981

HYMEN, IMPERFORATE, 483

Hymen imperforatus, 483

Hyper-bêta-alaninémie, 486

Hyperacetylation, 7

Hyperactivity, 381, 509
  intermittent, 603

HYPERALDOSTERONISM, FAMILIAL GLUCORTICOID SUPPRESSIBLE, 484

Hyperaldostéronisme familial suppressible par les glucocorticoïdes, 484

HYPERAMMONEMIA, 485

HYPERBETA–ALANINEMIA, 486

Hyperbêta-lipoprotéinémie, 500

Hyperbetaalaninämie, 486

Hyperbetalipoproteinemia, 488

Hyperbêtalipoprotéinémie avec hyperchylo-micronémie, **501**
HYPERBILIRUBINEMIA I (MARKER), **487**
Hyperbilirubinemia unconjugated, **487**
Hypercalcemia, peculiar facies, supravalvular aortic stenosis syndrome, **999**
HYPERCHOLESTEREMIA, **488**
Hypercholesteremic xanthomatosis, **488**
HYPERCHYLOMICRONEMIA, **489**
HYPERCYSTINURIA (MARKER), **490**
HYPERDIBASIC–AMINOACIDURIA, **491**
Hyperextension of entire body, **340, 603**
Hyperglycinemia, ketotic, **826**
HYPERGLYCINEMIA, NONKETOTIC, **492**
Hyperglycinemia with hypooxaluria, **492**
Hyperglycinémie, **826**
Hyperglycinémie san cétose, **492**
Hyperglycinuria of DeVries et al, **520**
HYPERHIDROSIS, PREMATURE HAIR GREYING AND PREMOLAR APLASIA, **493**
Hyperkalemic periodic paralysis, **794**
Hyperkaliämische Paresen, **794**
Hyperkeratose palmoplantaire et périodonto-clasie, **494**
Hyperkeratosis eccentrica, **819**
Hyperkeratosis follicularis et parafollicularis in cutem penetrans, **561**
HYPERKERATOSIS PALMOPLANTARIS AND PERIODONTOCLASIA, **494**
Hyperkeratosis penetrans, **561**
Hyperlipämie Typ V n. Fredrickson, **501**
Hyperlipidemia I, **489**
Hyperlipidemia II, **488**
Hyperlipidemia III, **495**
Hyperlipidemia IV, **500**
Hyperlipidemia V, **501**
Hyperlipidémie combinée, **496**
Hyperlipoproteinämie III, **495**
HYPERLIPOPROTEINEMIA, COMBINED, **496**
Hyperlipoproteinemia I, **489**
Hyperlipoproteinemia II, **488**
HYPERLIPOPROTEINEMIA III, **495**
Hyperlipoproteinemia IV, **500**
Hyperlipoproteinemia V, **501**
Hyperlipoprotéinémie type III, **495**
Hyperlysinemia, **616**
Hyperlysinuria with hyperammonemia, **491**
Hyperopia (also see Astigmatism and Refractive error), **1, 229, 250, 777**
Hyperostose corticale généralisée, **497**
Hyperostose cortical infantile, **221**
Hyperostose endostale, **497**
Hyperostose frontale interne, **498**
Hyperostoses of auditory canal, **318**
Hyperostosis calvariae interna, **498**
Hyperostosis corticalis deformans, **776**
HYPEROSTOSIS CORTICALIS GENERALISATA, **497**
HYPEROSTOSIS FRONTALIS INTERNA, **498**
Hyperostosis generalisata with striation, **778**
HYPERPARATHYROIDISM, NEONATAL FAMILIAL, **499**
Hyperphenylalanemia, **808**
Hyperphosphatasia (hereditary, chronic, familial), **776**
Hyperplasia of caruncle, **130**
Hyperplasie congénitale des surrénales par déficit en 3β-hydroxystéroïde-deshydrogénase, **909**
Hyperplasie congénitale des surrénales par déficit en 11β-hydroxylase, **902**

Hyperplasie congénitale des surrénales par déficit en 17α-hydroxylase, **903**
Hyperplasie congéntale des surrénales par déficit en 20-22 desmolase, **907**
Hyperplasie congénitale des surrénales par déficit en 21-hydroxylase, **908**
Hyperplasie diaphysaire avec dysostose cranio-faciale, **226**
Hyperplasie persistante du corps vitré, **994**
Hyperplastic form of chondrodystrophy, **656**
Hyperpnea, compensatory, **678**
HYPERPREBETA–LIPOPROTEINEMIA, **500**
HYPERPREBETA–LIPOPROTEINEMIA AND HYPERCHYLOMICRONEMIA, **501**
HYPERPROLINEMIA (MARKER), **502**
Hyperprolinemia type I, **502**
Hyperprolinemia type II, **502**
HYPERSARCOSINEMIA, **503**
Hypertaurodontism, **926**
HYPERTELORISM, **504**
Hypertelorism (see Section III, Table XXIV)
HYPERTELORISM–HYPOSPADIAS SYNDROME, **505**
HYPERTELORISM, MICROTIA, FACIAL CLEFTING AND CONDUCTIVE DEAFNESS, **506**
Hypertélorisme, **504**
Hypertélorisme, microtie et la fissure de la lèvre et du palais, **506**
Hypertelorismus, **504**
Hypertelorismus-Hypospadie-Syndrom, **505**
Hypertelorismus, Microtie und Lippe und Gaumenspalten, **506**
Hypertensive congenital adrenal hyperplasia, **903**
Hypertrichose congénitale-hirsutisme, **507**
Hypertrichose des oreilles, **319**
Hypertrichosis, gingival fibromatosis and fibroadenomas of breasts, **412**
HYPERTRICHOSIS LANUGINOSA, **507**
Hypertrichosis of the dog-man, **507**
Hypertrichosis pinnae auris, **319**
Hypertrichosis universalis congenita, **507**
Hypertrophic ear lobes, **324**
Hypertrophic obstructive cardiomyopathy, **917**
Hypertrophic pyloric stenosis, **848**
Hypertrophie des lobes de l'oreille, **324**
Hypertrophische (fleischige) Ohrläppchen, **324**
Hyperuricämie-Schwerhörigkeit-Ataxie, **508**
HYPERURICEMIA, DEAFNESS AND ATAXIA, **508**
Hyperuricemia, primary, **441**
HYPERVALINEMIA, **509**
Hyperzystinurie, **490**
Hypoacetylation, **7**
Hypoaldostéronisme isolé et transitoire du nourrison, **23**
Hypocalcemic, hypophosphatemic rickets with aminoaciduria, **873**
Hypocalcification de l'émail avec onycholyse et hypohydrose, **45**
Hypoceruloplasminemia, **469**
HYPOCHONDROPLASIA, **510**
HYPODONTIA AND NAIL DYSGENESIS, **511**
Hypodontia-mesoectodermal dysgenesis of iris and cornea, **439**

Hypodontia of maxillary lateral incisor teeth, **934**
Hypodontie avec dysgénésie des ongles, **511**
Hypodontie und Nageldysgenesie, **511**
Hypogammaglobulinemia, **521**
Hypogammaglobulinemia and retinal telangiectasia, **868**
Hypogammaglobulinemia thymoma syndrome, **944**
Hypogenital dystrophy with diabetic tendency, **823**
Hypoglossia-hypodactylia syndrome, **451**
HYPOGLYCEMIA, FAMILIAL NEONATAL, **512**
HYPOGLYCEMIA, LEUCINE–INDUCED, **513**
Hypoglycémie induit par la leucine, **513**
Hypoglycémie néo-natale, **512**
Hypohidrosis, hypodontia, hypotrichosis syndrome, **333**
Hypohidrosis, onycholysis and enamel hypocalcification, **45**
Hypohidrotic ectodermal dysplasia, **333**
Hypokalemic periodic paralysis, **795**
Hypokaliämische Paresen, **795**
HYPOMAGNESEMIA, PRIMARY, **514**
Hypomagnesémie essentielle, **514**
Hypomelia-hypotrichosis-facial hemangioma syndrome, **875**
Hypoparathyroïde infantile liée au sexe, **515**
HYPOPARATHYROIDISM, X–LINKED INFANTILE, **515**
Hypophosphatämie, **517**
HYPOPHOSPHATASIA, **516**
HYPOPHOSPHATEMIA, **517**
Hypoplasia cutis circumscripta, **281**
Hypoplasia of caruncle, **130**
Hypoplasia of inner ear, **315**
Hypoplasia of iris with rudimentary root, **57**
Hypoplasia of optic nerve, **758**
Hypoplasia of ulna and fibula, **648**
Hypoplasie congénitale des surrénales, **24**
Hypoplasie de l'émail, **342**
Hypoplasie de l'émail et de la dentine associés à une érythroblastose fétale, **340**
Hypoplasie de l'émail et de la dentine coloration des dents par les tétracyclines, **341**
Hypoplasie der Magen, **913**
Hypoplasie der oberen Extremitäten, Ohrfehlbildungen mit Taubheit, und kardialer arrythmie, **592**
Hypoplasie dermique en foyers, **281**
Hypoplasie des n. opticus, **758**
Hypoplasie du nerf optique, **758**
Hypoplasie faciale uniltérale avec microsomie, **457**
Hypoplasie gastrique, **913**
Hypoplasie musculaire généralisée congénitale, **686**
Hypoplastic anemia, congenital, **51**
Hypoplastic lung with systemic arterial supply and venous drainage, **879**
Hyposmia, **70**
HYPOSPADIAS, **518**
Hypospadias–dysphagia syndrome, **401**
Hypospadias–hypertelorism syndrome, **505**
Hypospadias périnéo-scrotal, **831**
Hypospadias with or without chordee, **518**
Hypospadie, **518**
Hypotaurodontism, **926**
Hypotelorism, **163, 166, 168, 231, 355, 473, 634**

Hypothalamic dysfunction, 820, 822
Hypothyroidism, congenital, 542, 543, 947, 948
Hypotonia and craniofacial dysmorphia, 139
Hypotonia and weakness, 134
Hypotonia, hypomentia, hypogonadism and obesity, 823
Hypotrophie de l'émail, taurodontie, cheveux crépus, et sclérose de la corticale osseuse, 965
Hypoxanthine guanine phosphoribosyl transferase deficiency, 588

I

I-cell disease, 672
Ichthyosis and cataract, 131
Ichthyosis, epilepsy and oligophrenia, 741
Idiopathic familial hyperlipemia, 489
Idiopathic hyperglycinemia, 492
Idiopathic hypertrophic osteoarthropathy, 788
Idiopathic hypertrophic subaortic stenosis, 917
Idiopathic infantile hypercalcemia syndrome, 999
Idiopathic juvenile osteoporosis, 782
Idiopathic lymphedema, 615
Idiopathic recurrent myoglobinuria, 125
"Idiopathic thrombocytopenic purpura" with lipid histiocytosis of spleen, 942
IgA-Mangel, 525
Ileal atresia or stenosis, 531
Ileal B₁₂ transport deficiency, 992
Ileal duplication, 532
Íleo meconial aislado, 545
Ileum
    atresia of, 727
    duplication of terminal, 194
Ileus meconial, 545
Iliac horns, 704
IMIDAZOLE AMINOACIDURIA (MARKER), 519
Imidazolurie, 519
IMINOGLYCINURIA (MARKER), 520
Iminoglyzinurie, 520
IMMUNODEFICIENCY, COMMON VARIABLE, 521
IMMUNODEFICIENCY, SEVERE COMBINED, 522
IMMUNODEFICIENCY WITH WISKOTT-ALDRICH SYNDROME, 523
IMMUNODEFICIENCY, X-LINKED SEVERE COMBINED, 524
Immunodeficiency, X-linked severe dual system, 524
IMMUNOGLOBULIN A DEFICIENCY, 525
Immunologic deficiency and thymoma syndrome, 944
Impacted teeth, 932
Impaktierte Zähne, 932
Imperforate anus, 69
Imperforate anus/polydactyly, 987
Imperforate hymen, 483
Imperforation de l'anus, triphalangie du pouce, décollement du pavillon de l'oreille et surdité de perception, 72
Imperforation de l'hymen, 483
Impresión basilar primaria, 103
Impression basilaire primitive, 103
Inability to utilize long-chain fatty acids as a source of energy in muscle, 125
Inactivación de la isoniácida (Marcador), 7

Inactivation de l'isoniazide, 7
Inanition, (also see Weight loss, Failure to thrive and Malnutrition), 403, 535, 566, 588, 1003
Incapacidad auditiva para la afinación, 273
Incarcerated hernia, 529
Incisor teeth
    duplicated maxillary lateral incisor, 229
    peg-shaped mandibular incisor, 17
    peg-shaped maxillary lateral incisor, 177, 229, 934
Incisura mentalis Types I, II, III, & IV, 146
Inclusión o ausencia congénita de los incisivos laterales, 934
Incompetence of pulmonary valve, 838
Incomplete feminizing testes syndrome, 50
Incomplete male pseudohermaphroditism type 1 (Wilson and Goldstein), 50
Incomplete male pseudohermaphroditism, type 2 (Wilson and Goldstein), 831
Incomplete oculocutaneous albinism, 143
Incomplete pyloric diaphragm, 910
Incomplete testicular feminization syndrome, 50
Incomplete tricuspid aortic valve, 80
INCONTINENTIA PIGMENTI, 526
Incontinentia pigmenti achromians, 526
Increased corticosteroid-binding globulin, 222

Incus
    connective tissue fibers at distal end of, 324
    defect of, 28, 247, 324, 331, 627, 664, 771, 773, 786, 860
    fails to articulate with stapes, 244, 324, 331, 664
    fused to bony atretic plate, 664
    long crus shaped like a hook, 244
Indentations of upper lip, 178
INDEPENDENT ORIGIN OF IPSILATERAL VERTEBRAL ARTERY, 527
Index finger (see Digit, Finger, Phalanx, and Joint)
Infantile
    pyloric stenosis, 162, 388, 754
    spasms, 126, 135, 713
Infantile cerebellar atrophy with retinal degeneration, 745
Infantile hypoglycemosis, familial, 512
Infantile kortikale Hyperostose, 221
Infantile recessive optic atrophy, 755
Infantile renal tubular acidosis and congenital sensorineural deafness, 863
Infección por citomegalovirus, 381
Infection of biologic mother during patient's prenatal life (see Section III, Table XXII)
Infections, 22, 27, 75, 94, 112, 139, 140, 143, 154, 200, 206, 285, 347, 398, 403, 406, 425, 426, 431, 442, 443 521, 522, 523, 524, 598, 644, 655, 658, 672, 714, 717, 729, 730, 772, 812, 826, 851, 885, 886, 912, 943, 944, 974
Inferior epiblepharon, 355
INFERIOR VENA CAVA, ABSENT HEPATIC SEGMENT, 528
Infracristal ventricular septal defect with overriding aorta and infundibular pulmonary atresia or stenosis, 938
Infracristal ventricular septal defect with overriding aorta without infundibular stenosis (Eisenmenger complex), 989

Infrahepatic interruption of inferior vena cava, 528
Inguinal area, mass in, 529
INGUINAL HERNIA, 529
Inherited copper toxicosis, 469
Inkomplete testikuläre Feminisierung, 50
Innenohr-Schwerhörigkeit, Polyneuropathie und Opticusatrophie, 268
Innenohrschwerhörigkeit, Dünndarm-Divertikulose und Neuropathie, 265
Innenohrschwerhörigkeit, Myopie und Oligophrenie, 251
Inner ear, aplasia, 562
Inner ear dysplasia, 315
Insensibilité à la thyréostimuline (TSH), 948
Insensibilité surrénalienne congénitale à l'ACTH, 25
Insertion basse des oreilles, 327
Insuffisance de la valvule pulmonaire, 838
Insuffisance mitrale, 666
Insuffisance tricuspidienne, 969
Insuficiencia de la válvula pulmonar, 838
Insuficiencia mitral, 666
Insuficiencia tricuspídea, 969
Intermediate (late-onset) cystinosis, 238
Intermittent branched-chain ketonuria, 628
Internal ankyloblepharon, 60
INTERNAL CAROTID ARTERY ANEURYSM OF MIDDLE EAR, 530
Internal chondromatosis, 345
Interrupción del arco aórtico, 76
Interruption de la crosse aortique, 76
Intersexualidad gonosómica, 173
Intersexualité par aberration des gonosomes, 173
INTESTINAL ATRESIA OR STENOSIS, 531
Intestinal bleeding, 113, 139, 194, 368, 460, 469, 532, 535, 536, 633, 832, 912, 914
INTESTINAL DUPLICATION, 532
INTESTINAL ENTEROKINASE DEFICIENCY, 533
INTESTINAL LYMPHANGIECTASIA, 534
Intestinal malrotation, 537
Intestinal monosaccharide intolerance, 419
Intestinal obstruction (also see Obstipation), 62, 69, 149, 162, 192, 194, 237, 289, 300, 386, 388, 401, 529, 531, 536, 545, 603, 633, 645, 727, 748, 754, 888, 912, 914
    in neonatal period, 62, 192, 531

INTESTINAL POLYPOSIS I & II, 535
INTESTINAL POLYPOSIS III, 536
INTESTINAL ROTATION, INCOMPLETE, 537
Intestinal tract, air in, 365
Intestinal volvulus, 121, 193, 531, 532, 537, 645, 888
Intestinale Duplikation, 532
Intestinale Lymphangiektasie, 534
Intestinaler Enterokinasemangel, 533
Intestine
    abnormal fixation of, 104, 748
    ascending colon within mesentery of ileum, 121
    carcinoma in duplicated segment of intestine, 532
    cecum, free floating, 121
    colon, duplication of, 194
    diverticulum of small, 160, 265, 401, 412, 513

duodenal stenosis or atresia, 300, 386, 401, 603
duodenal ulcer, 62, 963
duplication of small, 531
duplication of colon, 194
ileum, atresia of, 727
ileum, duplication of terminal, 194
lymphangiectasia, small intestinal, 55
malabsorption, small intestinal, 653
malrotation of, 28, 104, 160, 168, 300, 405, 531, 537, 606, 748, 888
meconium ileus, 237
meconium, inspissated, 545
perforation of, 7, 338, 529, 531, 633
polyps, multiple, in colon or rectum, 412, 535
polyps, multiple, in small intestine, 535, 536
unspecified defect of, 14, 69
Intolérance au lactose, 569
Intolerancia a la lactosa, 569
Intraadenoidal cysts, 706
Intraarticular osteochondroma of the astragalus, 311
Intracranial hemorrhage, 121, 186, 187, 777, 825, 832, 859
INTRAEPITHELIAL DYSKERATOSIS, 538
Intrahepatic biliary atresia, 110
Intrahepatic cystic dilatation of bile ducts, 149
Intraoral bands with cleft uvula, 181
INTRAOSSEOUS FIBROUS SWELLING OF JAWS, 539
Intraspinal hemorrhage, 186
Intraspinal lipomas, 602
Intrauterine and neonatal enamel hypoplasia, 342
Intrauterine growth retardation (also see Birthweight, low for gestational age and ethnic group), 112, 139, 152 158, 382, 769, 881, 887, 891, 977
Intrauterine healed clefts, 178
Intrauteriner Aminopterin Schaden, 380
Inv antigen type, 476
Invagination dentaire, 276
Inversion der Ventrikel mit Transposition der grossen Gefässe, 540
Inversion der Ventrikel ohne Transposition der grossen Gefässe, 541
Inversion des ventricules avec transposition des gros vaisseaux, 540
Inversion des ventricules sans transposition des gros vaisseaux, 541
Inversion du disque optique, 757
INVERSION OF VENTRICLES WITH TRANSPOSITION OF GREAT ARTERIES, 540
Inversion of ventricles without reversal of arterial trunks, 541
INVERSION OF VENTRICLES WITHOUT TRANSPOSITION OF GREAT ARTERIES, 541
Inversión ventricular con transposición de los grandes vasos, 540
Inversión ventricular sin transposición de los grandes vasos, 541
Inverted transposition, 540
Iodide goiter, 435
IODIDE TRANSPORT DEFECT, 542
Iodide trapping defect, 542
Iodotyrosine dehalogenase deficiency, 543
IODOTYROSINE DEIODINASE DEFICIENCY, 543

Ipsilateral vertebral artery directly from aortic arch rather than from subclavian artery, 527
Iridocorneal mesodermal dysgenesis, 439
Iridogoniodysgenesis, 439
IRIS COLOBOMA AND ANAL ATRESIA SYNDROME, 544
Iron-binding β-globulin deficiency, 95
Iron retention, 460
Irritability, 15, 86, 406, 423, 485, 492, 598, 808, 820, 850, 886, 974, 978, 991
with onset at 4–6 mos, 221, 415
Islet cells, hypofunction of, 702
Iris stroma
hyperplastic, 845
hypoplastic, 732
Iris (also see Section III, Table XXIV)
adhesions to posterior embryotoxon of, 439
aniridia, 57, 281, 284
anterior adhesions of, 451, 845
atrophy of, 479, 637, 735
blood vessels prominent, 732, 872, 994
Brushfield spots, 121, 139, 171
cleft of, 162, 164, 168, 169, 242, 544, 585, 636, 732, 733, 735, 824
dark blue, in adulthood, 36
deep blue, bilaterally, 657, 808
deep blue, in infancy, 35
deep blue, in opaque light, 34
forward curling eversion of pigment layer, 721
heterochromia of, 30, 31, 475, 716, 732, 997
hypoplasia of, 439, 638, 721
patterning abnormal, 205, 999
posterior adhesions of, 451, 721, 845, 872
stroma, hyperplastic, 845
stroma, hypoplastic, 732
translucent, 32, 34, 35, 36
tremulousness of, 630, 638
unilateral cleft of, 457
Isolated congenital hypotrichosis, 623
Isolated congenitally enlarged tongue, 618
Isolated FSH deficiency, 438
Isolated hemihypertrophy, 458
Isolated IgA deficiency, 525
Isolated infundibular pulmonary stenosis, 731
Isolated LH deficiency, 438
ISOLATED MECONIUM ILEUS, 545
Isolated trypsinogen deficiency, 973
Isolated TSH deficiency, 949
Isolated ventricular inversion, 541
ISOLATION OF SUBCLAVIAN ARTERY FROM AORTA, 546
Isolation of subclavian artery types I, II, and III, 546
Isolierter ACTH-Mangel, 26
Isolierter Gonadotropin-Mangel, 438
Isolierter Thyrotropin-Mangel, 949
Isolierter Wachtumshormon-Mangel, 447
Isomaltase insufficiency, 920
Isoniazid inactivation, 7
Isoniazid-Inaktivierung, 7
Isovaleriazidämie, 547
ISOVALERICACIDEMIA, 547
Ivory exostoses of ear canal, 318

J

Jaffe-Lichtenstein disease, 390

Jansky-Bielschowsky syndrome, 713
Jarcho-Levin syndrome, 900
Jaundice, 48, 110, 121, 139, 143, 148, 149, 300, 340, 395, 403, 460, 469, 487, 603, 717, 821, 849, 878, 886, 939, 946, 961, 978, 990
hyperbilirubinemia, physiologic, 946
persistent, physiologic, 961
persisting beyond 6 wks of age, 403
recurrent, 149
Jaundice chronic benign, 487
Jaundice without bilirubin glucuronide in bile, 961
Jaw excursion, limitation of, 882
JAW–WINKING SYNDROME, 548
Jejunal atresia or stenosis, 531
Jejunal duplication, 532
Jervell and Lange-Nielsen syndrome, 123
Jodthyrosin-Dejodinase-Mangel, 543
Joint (also see specific named joints)
arthritic changes, 308
arthritis, gouty, 441, 508, 859
arthrogryposis, 375, 895
atrophic, 924
contractures of, 85, 88, 157, 375, 470, 560, 598, 644, 895
decreased range of motion, 37, 153, 154, 155, 157, 189, 306, 358, 394, 398, 470, 474, 517, 557, 641, 652, 672, 673, 677, 680, 700, 754, 774, 798, 825, 893, 1000
dislocation of, 678
dislocation, prenatal onset of, 570
dislocation, recurrent, 338
fixed, 37
fixed in extension of, 88, 1001
fixed in flexion, 88, 160, 1001
fusiform swelling of, 644
increased range of motion (hyperextension of), 1, 121, 338, 352, 678, 728, 754, 774, 777, 783, 828, 967
large, 557, 825
loose body within, 774
marked decrease in range of motion of, 598
progressive contracture of, 598, 644
progressive decrease in range of motion of, 673
stiff, 644, 679, 825, 1000
stiff, with onset in childhood, 675
stiffness, progressive, 641
Joint, interphalangeal
decreased range of motion at interphalangeal joints of fingers, 557, 650, 980
decreased range of motion at proximal interphalangeal joint of finger, 85
decreased range of motion of finger, 647, 749
defect of distal interphalangeal joint of finger, 373
defect of interphalangeal joint of finger, 129, 966
extension contracture of finger, 89, 450
fixed fused finger, 114
flexion contracture at metacarpophalangeal joint, 301
flexion contracture at proximal interphalangeal joint of finger, 301
flexion contracture of finger, 88, 89, 121, 140, 160, 223, 393, 450, 470, 641, 882, 1000
flexion contracture of finger, present at birth, 450

Joint (see also specific named joints) –
  Continued
  flexion of distal interphalangeal joint, 1
  hyperextensible fingers, 105, 250
  increased range of motion at interpha-
    langeal joint of finger, 190
  lateral deviation of finger at proximal
    interphalangeal joint, 89
  marked increase of range of motion at
    proximal interphalangeal joint of
    finger, 1
  stiff proximal, 1001
  trigger position of index, 160
Joint, phalangeal
  decreased range of motion of, 157, 674,
    675
  increased range of motion of, 653
Junctional tachycardia, 922
Juvenile acanthosis nigricans, 5
Juvenile cirrhosis, 39
JUVENILE DIABETES MELLITUS, 549
JUVENILE DIABETES MELLITUS, OPTIC
  ATROPHY AND DEAFNESS, 550
Juvenile epithelial corneal dystrophy, 210
Juvenile epithelial degeneration of cornea,
  210
Juvenile hemochromatosis, 460
Juvenile hyaline fibromatosis, 411
Juvenile or infantile coronary sclerosis, 217
Juvenile osteoporosis, 782
Juvenile Paget disease, 776
Juvenile paradentose, 806
Juvenile periodontosis, 806
Juvenile pernicious anemia, 992
Juvenile retinoschisis, X-linked, 871
Juveniler Diabetes mellitus, 549
Juveniler Diabetes mellitus, Optikus-
  atrophie und Taubheit, 550
Juxtavagal tumor, 127

K

Kahlköpfigkeit, 99
Kalzinose der Koronararterien, 217
Kammerdivertikel, 988
Kampomeles Syndrom, 122
Kaposi dermatoses, 1005
Kardioauriculäres Syndrom, 123
Kardiomeler Syndrom, 455
Karnosinämie, 126
Karpo-tarsale Osteolyse, 128
Kartagener syndrome, 285
Kasabach-Merritt Syndrom, 456
Katarakt-Ichthyosis-Syndrom, 131
Katzenaugen-Syndrom, 544
Katzenschreisyndrom, 163
Kearns-Sayre-Shy-Daroff syndrome, 752
Kehlkopfatresie, 571
Kehlkopfmembran, 574
Kehlkopfzysten, 572
KELOID, 551
Kenny-Caffey disease, 976
Keratoakanthom Typ Ferguson-Smith, 359
Kératocone, 552
KERATOCONUS, 552
Keratoma hereditarium mutilans, 259
Keratomegalia, 637
Keratopachydermia, digital constrictions
  and deafness, 259
Kératopathie en bande, 553
KERATOPATHY, BAND–SHAPED, 553
Kératose palmaire-leuconychie-surdité, 558
Keratosis follicularis serpiginosa, 339

Keratosis palmoplantaris und Periodonto-
  klasie, 494
Keratosis rubra figurata, 361
Keratosulfaturia, 678
Ketosis-prone diabetes mellitus, 549
Ketotische Form der Hyperglyzinämie, 826
KGB SYNDROME, 554

Kidney
  abnormal rotation or position of, 506, 682,
    977
  aplasia of, 337, 603, 634, 682, 857,
    860
  cyst in, 578, 883, 884
  dilation of urinary collecting system,
    629
  duplicated renal pelvis, 264, 401
  duplication of, 162
  duplication of urinary collecting sys-
    tem, 720
  glomerulonephritis, 255, 578, 708
  horseshoe, 159, 160, 544, 977
  hydronephrosis, 97, 157, 162, 337, 578,
    720, 727
  hypoplasia of, 571, 720, 977
  immature, 121
  in pelvis, 682
  large, 104, 458, 859
  mixed kidney lesions, 160, 168, 544
  multiple cysts throughout, 138, 168, 605,
    634, 662
  nephritis, 385
  nephropathy, 383, 704
  nephrosis, 128, 264, 385
  partial agenesis of, 977
  pelvic, 682
  pyelonephritis, 255, 578
  renal calculi, 37, 258, 441
  renal colic, 239, 859
  renal dysfunction, progressive, 239,
    441, 736
  renal defect, unspecified, 140, 157, 163,
    173, 229, 386, 388, 886, 908, 960,
    981, 984, 987
  renal excretion, decreased, 710
  renal failure, chronic, 258
  renal function decrease with adult on-
    set, 373, 508, 859
  renal function decrease with onset in
    2nd or 3rd decade, 708
  renal function, progressive loss of, 708
  renal hypertension, 474, 977
  renal insufficiency, 91, 116, 128, 239,
    578, 580, 862, 864, 999
  renal mass, 975
  renal tubular acidosis, 395, 736, 863,
    864
  renal tubular necrosis, acute, 125, 698
  unilateral hypoplasia of, 860
  urinary cystine stones, 239
  unspecified structural defect of, 170,
    300, 329, 364, 977
  uremia, 238, 441, 578

Kidney, adult polycystic disease of, 859
Kidney, congenital solitary, 857
Kidneys, absence of, 856
Kinky hair disease, 643
Kinngrübchen, 146
KLEEBLATTSCHÄDEL ANOMALY,
  555
Klein-Waardenburg syndrome, 997
KLINEFELTER SYNDROME, 556
Klippel-Trénaunay-Syndrom, 55

Knee
  decreased range of motion of, 85,
    129, 311, 560, 774
  dislocation of, 704
  dislocation of knee on weight bearing,
    293
  flexion contracture of, 1000
  genu recurvatum, 651
  genu valgum, 106, 156, 185, 216, 290,
    352, 474, 630, 647, 654, 672, 675,
    679, 749, 798, 828, 847, 897
  genu varum, 250, 704, 798, 828, 897
  increased range of motion of, 90, 774
  knee fixed in position, 88
  large, 90
  loose body within knee joint, 774
  prenatal onset of contracture of, 629
  prenatal onset of dislocation of, 570
Kniepterygium-Syndrom, 818
KNIEST DYSPLASIA, 557
Kniest-Syndrom, 557
Knöchelpolster, leukonychie und Taubheit,
  558
Knock-knee, 106, 156, 185, 216, 290, 352,
    474, 630, 647, 654, 672, 675, 679,
    749, 798, 828, 847, 897
KNUCKLE PADS, LEUKONYCHIA AND
  DEAFNESS, 558
Kohlenhydrat-induzierte Hyperlipämie, 500
Kohlschütter syndrome, 44
KOILONYCHIA, 599
Kolon-Duplikation, 194
Kolonatresie oder-stenose, 193
Kombinierte Hyperlipoproteinämie, 496
Komplette Farbenblindheit, 198
Komplette Lungenvenen-Transposition, 842
Kongenitale Pachyonychie, 789
Konisch deformierte oder Aplasie der lateralen
  oberen Schneidezähne, 934
Kontrakturelle Arachnodaktylie, 85
Koronare Dentin-Dysplasie, 277
Krabbe disease, 415
Kranio-okulo-dentales Syndrom, 229
Kraniodiaphysäre Dysplasie, 224
Kraniofaziale Dyssynostose, 227
Kraniokarpotarsale Dysplasie, 223
Kraniometaphysäre Dysplasie, 228
Kraniosynostose, 230
Kristalline Form der Hornhautdystrophie
  (Schnyder), 216
Kryptotie, 232
Kufs disease, 713
Kugelberg-Welander disease, 895
KUSKOKWIM SYNDROME, 560
Kyphoscoliosis (also see Scoliosis, and
  Section III, Table XXIX)
  progressive, 656
Kyphosis (also see Section III, Table XXIX)
  lumbar, 398, 679
  marked, 189, 672
  thoracic, 103, 189
  thoracolumbar, 674
KYRLE DISEASE, 561
Kyste bronchogénique, 117
Kyste du cholédoque, 149
Kyste hépatique solitaire, 465
Kyste neuro-entérique, 894
Kystes dermoïdes de la tête et du cou, 283
Kystes dermoïdes orbitaires et périorbitaires,
  761
Kystes laryngés, 572
Kystes mésentériques, 645
Kystes nasopharyngiens, 706
Kystes spléniques, 240

L

L'association phocomélie-ectrodactylie, malformations des oreilles avec surdité, arythmie sinusale, 592
Labia (majora or minora)
  completely fused, 908, 909, 971
  containing testis, 49, 50
  hypoplasia of, 29, 160, 440
  labia minora hypoplasia of, 823, 876
  labia minora prominent, 587
  partially fused, 903, 908, 909, 971
  resembling cleft scrotum, 50, 908
Labile diabetes mellitus, 549
Labio doble, 594
Labio leporino con o sin paladar hendido, 178
LABYRINTH APLASIA, 562
Labyrinth of inner ear, defect of, 315, 562
Labyrinthine otosclerosis, 787
Labyrinthine otosclerosis with fixed stapes footplate, 787
Lacrimal canaliculi
  impatent, 229, 337, 563, 565, 705
  impatent at junction with nasal mucosa, 705
  supernumerary, 844
LACRIMAL CANALICULUS ATRESIA, 563
Lacrimal caruncle, defect of, 130
Lacrimal duct impatency, 705
Lacrimal gland
  displaced, 564
  hyperplastic, 111
LACRIMAL GLAND, ECTOPIC, 564
Lacrimal passage ectasia, 565
Lacrimal punctum
  lateral displacement of, 732, 997
  supernumerary, 844
Lacrimal sac
  drainage opens onto skin, 565
  inflammation of, 337, 565, 705
  mucocele of, 705
LACRIMAL SAC FISTULA, 565
Lacrimal system, inflammation of, 337, 844
Lacrimation
  decreased, 102, 163, 307, 378, 475
  increased, 337, 355, 371, 414, 563, 705
LACTASE DEFICIENCY, CONGENITAL, 566
LACTASE DEFICIENCY, PRIMARY, 567
LACTATE DEHYDROGENASE ISO-ZYMES, 568
Lactate déshydrogénase, 568
Lactato deshidrogenasa, 568
Lactic acidemia without hypoxemia, 850
Lactic and pyruvic acidemia with carbo-hydrate sensitivity, 851
Lactic and pyruvic acidemia with episodic ataxia and weakness, 851
LACTOSE INTOLERANCE, 569
Laktat Dehydrogenase, 568
Laktoseintoleranz, 569
Lakuregebee, 886
Lamellar cataract, 132
Landkartenzunge, 954
Lane disease, 792
Langer-Giedion syndrome, 967
Langes, schmales, dorsal rotiertes Ohr, 325
Langue bifide, 952
Langue fissurée, 953
Langue plicaturée, 956
Laringocele, 575
Laringomalacia, 576

Laron dwarfism, 302
Laron Zwergwuchs, 302
LARSEN SYNDROME, 570
Laryngeal aerocele, 575
LARYNGEAL ATRESIA, 571
LARYNGEAL CYSTS, 572
Laryngeal hernia, 575
Laryngeal mucocele, 575
Laryngeal pouch, 575
Laryngeal pyocele, 575
Laryngeal stridor, congenital, 576
Laryngeal tumors, 352, 572, 573, 575, 918
LARYNGEAL VENTRICLE PROLAPSE, 573
LARYNGEAL WEB, 574
LARYNGO-TRACHEO-ESOPHAGEAL CLEFT, 577
Laryngo-tracheo-ösophageale Spalte, 577
LARYNGOCELE, 575
Laryngoceles: internal, external or com-bined, 575
LARYNGOMALACIA, 576
Laryngozele, 575
Larynx, 163, 257, 352, 401, 406, 571, 572, 573, 574, 575, 576, 577, 599, 634, 883, 918, 919
  aryepiglottic fold, abnormal and flutters on inspiration, 576
  arytenoid, abnormal and flutters on inspi-ration, 576
  cricoid cartilage abnormal for size or shape, 919
  epiglottis, abnormal and flutters on in-spiration, 576
  epiglottis, cleft, 634
  epiglottis, short, 401, 634, 883
  eversion of saccular mucosa of, 573
  glottic atresia in, 571
  hypoplasia of, 401
  membranous web in, 574
  obstruction of, 599
  saccular dilatation of appendix of, 575
Larynx, congenital flaccid, 576

Late infantile systemic lipidosis, 432
Late-occurring immunologic deficiency, 521
Late-onset alactasia, 567
Late-onset lymphedema, 615
Lateral nasal proboscis, 824
Laterale Gesichtsspalte, 374
Lattice corneal dystrophy, 211
Laurence-Moon-Biedl-Bardet syndrome, 578
LAURENCE-MOON-BIEDL SYNDROME, 578
Laurence-Moon syndrome, 578
LCAT deficiency, 580
Leber Hamartom, 604
LEBER OPTIC ATROPHY, 579
Leberaplasie, 463
Lebersche congenitale Atrophie, 43
Lebersche Opticusatrophie, 579
Lecithin-Cholesterin-Acyl-Transferase Mangel, 580
LECITHIN:CHOLESTEROL ACYL TRANSFERASE DEFICIENCY, 580
Lecitina: deficiencia de colesterol acil trans-ferasa, 580
Left atrial herniation, 805
Left common carotid artery arising from innominate artery, 200
LEFT VENTRICLE, DOUBLE OUTLET, 581

LEFT VENTRICLE, SINGLE PAPILLARY MUSCLE, 582
Left ventricular endocardial fibrosis fibro-elastosis, 348
Left ventricular endocardial sclerosis, 348
Left ventricular primary myocardial hyper-trophy with endocardial fibroelastosis, 348
Left ventricular subendocardial fibroelastosis, 348
Leigh disease, 344
Leiner disease, 812
Leinersche Krankheit, 812
Leiomioma cutáneo múltiple, 890
Leiomyoma, multiple of skin, 890
Leiomyomatosis cutis, 890
Léiomyome multiple de la peau, 890
Leistenbruch, 529
Lengua fisurada (Marcador), 953
Lengua geográfica, 954
Lengua hendida, 952
Lengua plicada, 956
Lens, (see Eye, lens)
LENS AND PUPIL, ECTOPIC, 583
LENS, ECTOPIC, 584
LENTICONUS, 585
Lenticular cataract, 132
LENTIGINES SYNDROME, MULTIPLE, 586
Lentiginose profuse ou diffuse, 586
Lentiglobus, 585
Lentigo maligna, 1005
Lenz microphthalmia, 662
Leopard syndrome, 586
LEPRECHAUNISM, 587
Léri dyschondrosteosis, 308
Leri-Weill disease, 308
LESCH-NYHAN SYNDROME, 588
Lesión fetal por aminopterina, 380
Lethal syndrome of microcephaly with multiple congenital anomalies, 140
Lethargy, 492, 978
Leucine-induced hypoglycemia, 513
Leucine-sensitive hypoglycemia, 513
Leucine-sensitive hypoglycemia of in-fancy, familial, 512
Leucodistrofias metacromáticas, 651
Leucodystrophie métachromatique, 651
Leucokératose esfobrante des muqueuses, 681
Leuconiquia, 589
Leuconychie, 589
Leukemogenesis, 383
Leukoderma, primary, 993
LEUKONYCHIA, 589
Leukonychia, knuckle pads, and deafness, 558
Leukonychia partialis, striata, and totalis, 589
Leukoplakische epitheliale Naevi, 681
Leuzin-induzierte Hypoglykämie, 513
Libido
  decreased, 102, 556
  loss of, 460, 982
Lichen acuminatus, 811
Lichen ruber acuminatus, 811
LIDDLE SYNDROME, 590
Lightwood syndrome, 862
Limb (also see parts and Joints)
  absence of, 451, 875
  absence, partial (also see Phocomelia), 242, 459, 941
  anterior dislocation of lower, 121

Limb (also see parts and Joints) –
  Continued
  asymmetry of, 129, 153, 190, 391, 641,
    712, 887, 967, 981
  bowing of, 10, 122, 290, 391, 510, 557,
    648, 654, 783, 798
  bowing of lower, marked, 777
  bowing or angulation, unilateral, 641
  bowing, progressive, 776
  contractures of lower, 759, 803
  decreased arm span, 685
  decreased motion of lower, 818
  defect of, 231, 455, 856, 987
  deformity of, progressive, 345
  deformity, severity of increased distally,
    88
  deformity of upper, secondary to
    fracture, 391
  "diamond" configuration of lower, 88
  difficulty using upper, 469
  flexion contracture of, 140, 431
  fracture of lower, 391
  gigantism of, 641, 648
  hypertrophy of, 55, 458, 712, 998
  lateral bony protuberance of lower, 647
  long, disproportionately, 189
  long unilaterally, 641
  long and narrow, 474, 630, 696
  lower more shortened than upper, 445
  medial bony protuberance of lower, 647
  micromelia, 293
  obesity of, 8, 445
  obesity of, proximal, 823
  paralysis of lower, variable, 693
  phocomelia, 242, 455, 884, 941
  severity of deformity increased distally,
    88
  short, 9, 91, 231, 242, 250, 303, 346,
    592, 876, 883, 1001
  short, disproportionate lower, 510, 641
  short, disproportionate with short distal
    segment, 19, 20, 156, 646
  short, disproportionate with short middle
    segment, 19, 308, 646, 647, 648, 649
  short, disproportionate prenatally with
    absent proximal segment, 967
  short, disproportionate prenatally with
    lower limbs more affected than upper
    limbs, 8
  short, markedly, 121, 884
  short, progressively from proximal to
    distal segments, 445
  short, proportionate, 171, 345
  short proximal portion of, 10, 470,
    941
  short upper limb to one half its normal
    length, 875
  spasticity of lower, 803, 924
  straight lower, 20
  symmetric defect, 875, 981
  thin, 105, 825, 895
  upper more severely affected than lower,
    875
Limb-girdle muscular dystrophy, 691
LIMB–OTO–CARDIAC SYNDROME, 592
LIMBAL DERMOID, 591
LINEAR NEVUS SEBACEOUS SYNDROME,
  593
Linfangiectasia intestinal, 534
Linfangioma de los bordes alveolares
  dentarios, 613
Linfangioma orbitario, 765
Linfedema de instalación precoz, 614
Linfedema tardío, 615
Lingua fissurata types I, II, and III, 953

Lingua nigra, 955
Lingua plicata, 956
Lip, (also see Section III, Tables XII and
  XIII)
  cleft of, 158, 159, 160, 164, 168, 176,
    177, 178, 179, 220, 242, 281, 337,
    375, 380, 382, 401, 473, 505, 506,
    578, 634, 662, 724, 737, 769, 818,
    874, 875, 883, 952
  cleft, median of lower, 636, 771
  cleft, median of upper, 595, 636, 770,
    771, 791
  drooping of lower, 626, 702
  double lower, 594
  double upper, 111, 554, 594
  everted, 190, 333, 511, 629
  large lower, 144
  mound on lower, 177
  mucocele of lower, 144
  papillomas on, 412
  pit or fistula on commissure, 596
  pit or fistula on lower, 176, 177, 596,
    818
  pit or fistula on upper, 596
  puckered, 121
  retracted lower, 161
  squamous cell carcinoma of lower,
    144
  thick, 190, 352, 587, 599, 674, 676,
    679, 754
  thin, 887
  thin upper, 102, 162, 242, 967, 1001
LIP, DOUBLE, 594
Lip, enlargement of lower, 144
LIP, MEDIAN CLEFT OF UPPER, 595
Lip pits and cleft lip or palate, 177
LIP PITS OR MOUNDS (MARKER), 596
LIPASE DEFICIENCY, CONGENITAL ISO-
  LATED, 597
Lipid fibroma, 360
Lipidose à ester du cholestérol, 151
Lipidosis, sulfatide, 651
Lipidosis with thrombocytopenia and angi-
  omata of spleen, 942
Lipochrome histiocytosis of females, 442
Lipodermoid, 284
Lipofuschinose du système nerveux, 713
Lipofuscinosis neuronal ceroidea, 713
Lipoglycoproteinosis, 599
LIPOGRANULOMATOSIS, 598
Lipoid adrenal hyperplasia, 907
LIPOID PROTEINOSIS, 599
Lipoid thesaurismosis, 360
LIPOMAS, FAMILIAL SYMMETRIC, 600
Lipomatose de la face et du cou, 601
Lipomatose von Gesicht und Hals, 601
Lipomatosis de la cara y del cuello, 601
LIPOMATOSIS OF FACE AND NECK, 601
Lipomatosis simétrica familiar, 600
Lipome dermoïde, 284
LIPOMENINGOCELE, 602
Lipomes symétriques familiaux, 600
Lipomucopolysaccharidosis, 671
Lippen-Kiefer-Gaumenspalte, ektodermale
    Dysplasie, Hand-und Fussfehlbildungen,
    Oligophrenie, 179
Lippen-oder Gaumenspalte und filiforme
    Fusion der Augenlider, 176
Lippen-oder Gaumenspalte und Lippen-
    grübchen, 177
Lippengrübchen, 596
Lippenspalte mit oder ohne Gaumenspalte,
  178
Lisinemia, 616
LISSENCEPHALY SYNDROME, 603

Liver (also see Section III, Table XXXIII)
  abnormal fixation, 748
  absence of, 463
  cirrhosis of, 237, 395, 460, 525, 939,
    978
  cirrhosis of, with onset in infancy, 116
  cyst, 465
  cyst, multiple, 605, 662
  cyst, unspecified, 634, 859
  ectopic, 467
  failure of, 460
  hepatitis, 7, 39, 381, 384, 385, 387,
    469, 568
  hepatoblastoma, 458
  hepatomegaly (also see Section III,
    Table XXXIII)
    decrease in, after puberty, 426, 430
    pulsatile, 969
  hepatosplenomegaly, 143, 503, 677, 679
  infectious hepatitis, 27
  portal hypertension, 149, 460, 465, 468,
    469, 605
  progressive enlargement of, in 1st 6 mos,
    466
  progressive failure of, with onset in in-
    fancy, 116
  systolic bruit or thrill over, 466
  transposed, 606, 888
  unspecified defect of, 446, 452, 748
Liver, cholesteryl ester storage, 151
Liver cyst, solitary but multilocular, 465
Liver cysts, multiple, 605
LIVER HAMARTOMA, 604
LIVER, POLYCYSTIC DISEASE, 605
LIVER TRANSPOSITION, 606

Lobe aberrant du poumon, 611
Lobes des oreilles attachés, 323
Lobes hépatiques accesoires, 467
LOBODONTIA, 607
Lobstein syndrome, 777
Lobster claw deformity, 336
Lóbulo de la oreja fisurado, 321
Lóbulo pulmonar aberrante, 611
Lóbulos auriculares engrosados e hiper-
    tróficos, 324
Lóbulos de las orejas pegadas (Marcador),
    323
Lóbulos hepáticos accesorios, 467
LOCALIZED ABSENCE OF SKIN, 608
LOCALIZED ABSENCE OF SKIN, BLISTER-
    ING AND NAIL ABNORMALITIES,
    609
Localized arrested tooth development, 739
Localized myositis ossificans, 700
Löffelohr, 314
LONG QT SYNDROME WITHOUT DEAF-
    NESS, 610
Lordosis (also see Section III, Table XXIX)
  cervical, 103
  lumbar, 20, 250, 290, 352, 412, 557,
    646, 678, 687, 689, 754, 828
  lumbosacral spine, curvature of, 292
  marked, 290, 646
  thoracic, 394
Lösliche Malatdehydrogenase, 624, 625
Louis-Bar syndrome, 94
Low-set ear, 327
Low sinus venosus type defect, 96
Low-tone deafness, 260
Lowe syndrome, 736
L-transposition with situs solitus, 540

Lubs syndrome, 50
Luette bifide, 184
Lumbosacral lipoma, 602

Lung
  atelectasis on side of eventration of
    diaphragm, 288
  emphysema, 39, 120, 836
  hypoplasia of left lung, 401
  hypoplasia of lung, 289, 634, 856
  hypoplasia of right lung, 401, 879
  immature, 121
  lack of segmentation, 401
  pulmonary agenesis on side of hemi-
    facial microsomia, 457
  pulmonary anomaly, 531
  pulmonary bleeding, 611, 612, 767
  rales, 39
LUNG, ABERRANT LOBE, 611
LUNG LOBE SEQUESTRATION, 612
Luxación congénita del cristalino, 584
Luxation congénitale du cristallin, 584
L-xylulosuria, 804
Lymph nodes
  absence of usual nodes, 522, 524
  inflammation of cervical nodes, 443
  large, 48, 143, 521, 717
  large cervical, 443, 539
  large submandibular, 539
  small, 655
Lymphangiectasie intestinale, 534
Lymphangiom der Zahnleisten, 613
LYMPHANGIOMA OF ALVEOLAR
    RIDGES, 613
Lymphangioma of mesentery, 645
Lymphangiomatous macroglossia, 618
Lymphangiome de l'orbite, 765
Lymphangiome gingival, 613
Lymphatic cyst of mesentery, 645
Lymphatic vessels
  absent or small, 615
  large, 615
  lymphangiectasia, small intestinal, 55
  lymphedema of skin on foot, 977
  lymphedema, peripheral, 720
  obstruction of thoracic duct and
    chylous ascites, 534
Lyphedema forme tarde, 615
Lymphedema praecox, 615
LYMPHEDEMA I, 614
LYMPHEDEMA II, 615
Lymphocytophisis, 524
Lymphoédème à début tardif, 615
Lymphoédème congénitale, 614
Lymphopenic agammaglobulinemia, auto-
  somal recessive, 522
LYSINEMIA, 616
Lysinuric protein intolerance, 491
Lysyl hydroxylase deficiency, 338

M

Mâchoires à clignotement, 548
Macrocephaly (see Section III, Table
    XXIX)
MACRODONTIA, 617
Macrogenitosomia praecox, 908
MACROGLOSSIA, 618
Macroglossia, omphalocele and viscero-
  megaly syndrome, 104
Macrostomia, 374
MACROTIA, 619
Macula (also see Section III, Table XXIV)
MACULA, HETEROTOPIC, 620
MACULAR COLOBOMA AND BRACHY-
    DACTYLY, 621
Macular corneal dystrophy, 212

Macular cysts, 622
Macular degeneration and fundus flavi-
  maculatus, 400
MACULAR DEGENERATION, VITELLI-
    RUPTIVE, 622
Macular pseudocysts, 622
Maculocerebral degeneration, 713
MADAROSIS, 623
Maffucci syndrome, 346
Magenatresie, 910
Magendivertikulum, 911
Magnocellular nevus, 639
Major motor seizures, 25, 135, 188, 791,
  975
Makrodontie, 617
Makroglossie, 618
Makula-Kolobom und Brachydaktylie, 621
Makuläre Hornhautdystrophie, 212
Malabsorbtion de la méthionine, 657
Malabsorción de la glucosa-galactosa, 419
Malabsorción de la vitamine B$_{12}$, 992
Malabsorción del glucosa-galactosa, 419
Malabsorción del triptófano, 974
Malabsorption de la vitamine B$_{12}$, 992
Malabsorption de tryptophane, 974
Malabsorption du glucose et du galactose, 419
Malabsorption of vitamin B$_{12}$ (two types),
  992
Malabsorption, small intestinal, 653
Maladie coéliaque, 423
Maladie d'Ebstein, 332
Maladie d'Oguchi, 740
Maladie de Best, 622
Maladie de Fabry, 373
Maladie de Fanconi, 864
Maladie de Gaucher, 406
Maladie de Hartnup, 453
Maladie de Kyrle, 561
Maladie de Leber, 43
Maladie de Minkowski-Chauffard, 892
Maladie de Niemann-Pick, 717
Maladie de Norrie, 721
Maladie de Pendred, 249
Maladie de Sturge-Weber, 915
Maladie de Tangier, 48
Maladie de von Willebrand, 996
Maladie de Wolman, 1003
Maladie de Ziehen-Oppenheim, 957
Maladie des inclusions cytomégaliques, 381
Maladie des urines à odeur de sirop
    d'érable, 628
Maladie granulomatéine chronique observée
    chez les femmes, 442
Maladie granulomateuse chronique atteignant
  les garçons, 443
Maladie polykystique du foie, 605
MALATE DEHYDROGENASE, MITO-
    CHONDRIAL (MARKER), 624
MALATE DEHYDROGENASE, SOLUBLE
    (MARKER), 625
Malato deshidrogenasa mitocondrial
    (Marcador), 624
Malato deshidrogenasa soluble (Marcador),
  625
Malattia levantinese, 734
Male gender with female escutcheon, 438
Male gender with feminization, 971
Male habitus, premature development of
    mature, 908
Male pseudohermaphroditism due to steroid
    17,20-desmolase deficiency, 904
Male pseudo-precocious puberty, 720
Male, secondary gonadal atrophy in young,
  460
Male Turner syndrome, 720

Malformación artrogripótica de la mano
  y sordera neurosensorial, 89
Malformaciones anorectales, 69
Malformaciones de los huesesillos auriculares
  y del oído medio, 773
Malformation artério-veineuse, 186
Malformations ano-rectales, 69
Malformations des osselets et de l'oreille
  moyenne, 773
Malico-déhydrogénase mitochondriale, 624
Malico-déhydrogénase soluble, 625
Malignant congenital osteopetrosis, 780
Malleus
  defect of, 28, 247, 627, 664, 773, 786
  fused to atretic plate, 664
  fused to incus, 97
  fused to tympanic plate, 97
Malnutrition (also see Failure to thrive, Inanition and Weight loss), 39, 192, 39ɔ,
  566, 569, 717, 973
  at birth, 913
Malrotation, 537
Malrotation of midgut, 537
Malrotation of pancreas, 62
Mammary gland
  breast, aberrant tissue, 815
  breast, enlargement, rapid or slow, 412
  breast, failure of development, 437, 438,
    903
  breasts, huge with premalignant giant
    fibroadenomas, 412
  female gender with large breasts for age,
    587
  galactorrhea, 350
  gynecomastia, 47, 93, 556, 855, 902
  nipples, illusion of widely spaced, 720
  nipples small, 171, 242, 981
  nipples supernumerary, 815
  nipples widely spaced, 121, 140
  polymastia, 574
  rapid growth of breast with onset at puber-
    ty or first pregnancy, 412
Mandible (also see Section III, Table XXVI)
  ankylosis of condyles of, 229, 451, 749
  asymmetric ramus of, 735
  broad, 470
  cleft, 17, 636, 952
  concave lower border of, 627
  condyle adjacent to mastoid process, 664
  cyst of, midline, 291
  exostoses on lingual surface of, 958
  flat angle of, 506
  large, 228, 847
  obtuse gonial angle of, 180, 626, 846, 847
  prominent, 18, 159
  pseudoprognathism, 14, 112, 161, 162,
    178, 352, 941
  small, 159
  smooth, round mass on, 360
  swelling of angles of, 539
  thickening of, 190, 318, 413, 497, 737,
    880
  tumors of, 101, 118, 280, 536, 539, 711
  unilateral hypoplasia of condyle of, 457,
    735
Mandibular cleft, median, 636
Mandibular enlargement, 958
MANDIBULAR PROGNATHISM, 626
MANDIBULOFACIAL DYSOSTOSIS, 627
Mangel an Thyroxin-bindendem Globulin,
  950
MAPLE SYRUP URINE DISEASE, 628
Marble bone disease, 779, 780
Marcus Gunn phenomenon, 548
MARDEN–WALKER SYNDROME, 629

MARFAN SYNDROME, 630
Marie-Sainton disease, 185
Marked backward motion of knee, 651
Maroteaux-Lamy syndrome, 679
Marshall syndrome, 261
Masculinizing male hermaphroditism (Jones), 831
Masculinizing male pseudohermaphroditism (Jones), 831
Maumenee syndrome, 207
Maxilla (also see Section III, Table XXVI)
    broad, 470, 791
    cleft of, 178
    cleft of premaxilla, 631
    cyst of, midline, 291
    defect of, 28
    hypoplastic zygomatic arch of, 112, 627, 735
    large, 390
    pseudoprognathism, 14, 112, 161, 162, 178, 352, 941
    smooth, round mass on, 360
    tumors of, 101, 118, 280, 536, 711
    unilateral hypoplasia of, 457
MAXILLA, MEDIAN ALVEOLAR CLEFT, 631
Maxillopalpebral synkinesis, 548
Mb. Fabry, 373
Mb. Gaucher, 406
Mb. Hirschsprung, 192
Mb. Krabbe, 415
Mb. Norrie, 721
Mb. Oguchi, 740
Mb. Pelizaeus-Merzbacher, 803
Mb. Pyle, 847
Mb. Sturge-Weber, 915
Mb. Tangier, 48
Mb. von Willebrand, 996
McArdle disease, 698
McCune-Albright syndrome, 391
MCDONOUGH SYNDROME, 632
MECKEL DIVERTICULUM, 633
MECKEL SYNDROME, 634
Meckelsches Divertikel, 633
Meconium
    ileus, 237
    inadequate passage of, in neonatal period, 192
    inspissated, 545
    in urine, 69
Meconium ileus, isolated, 545
MEDIAN CLEFT FACE SYNDROME, 635
Median cleft of nose "doggennose," 724
Median cleft of upper lip, 595
MEDIAN CLEFTS OF LOWER LIP, MANDIBLE AND TONGUE, 636
Median incisal diastema, 291
Median rhomboid, glossitis, 417
Mediane Overkieferspalte, 631
Mediastinal defects
    abdominal viscera displaced into lower lateral mediastinum, 289
    mediastinal shift contralateral to eventration of diaphragm, 288
    round mass in posterior mediastinum continuous with esophagus, 368
Mediterranean anemia, 939
Medullary thyroid carcinoma and pheochromocytoma syndrome, 351
Medullary thyroid carcinoma syndrome, 351
Medulloblastoma, 188
Meesmann corneal dystrophy, 210
Megaesophagus, 363
Megakaryocytopenia with radius aplasia, 941

MEGALOCORNEA, 637
MEGALOCORNEA–MENTAL RETARDATION SYNDROME, 638
Meige type lymphedema, 615
Mekoniumileus, isoliert, 545
MELANOCYTOMA, 639
Mélanose oculaire, 716
Mélanose oculaire congénitale, 640
Melanosis bulbi congenitalis, 640
Melanosis ocular, 716
MELANOSIS OCULI, CONGENITAL, 640
Melnick-Needles syndrome, 775
MELORHEOSTOSIS, 641
Melorheostosis Leri, 641
Meloschisis, 375
Membrana laríngea, 574
Membranous choanal atresia, anterior, 723
Membranous choanal atresia, posterior, 727
Membranous septal defect, 989
Membranous subaortic stenosis, 916
MEN I syndrome, 350
MEN II syndrome, 351
MEN III syndrome, 352
Mendes da Costa syndrome, 361
Ménière disease, familial, 248
Meningeal capillary angiomatosis, 915
MENINGOCELE, 642
Meningocele, 635
    cervical spina bifida with, 642, 727
Meningocele, orbital, 762
Meningomyelocele, 160, 481, 693
Meningozele, 642
MENKES SYNDROME, 643
Menschliche Allotypen, 476
Menstruation
    amenorrhea, 469
    amenorrhea, primary, 93, 682, 720, 977
    amenorrhea, secondary, 720
    delayed, 720, 823
    oligomenorrhea, 730
    pelvic discomfort during, 971
    vaginal bleeding before puberty, 391
    vaginal bleeding in infancy, 391
    very irregular, 412, 702, 823
Mental deterioration, 86, 93, 103, 406, 432, 478, 598, 651, 676, 702, 713, 730, 744
    progressive, 86, 255, 310, 406, 478, 677
Mental retardation (see Section III, Table XXIII)
Mental retardation and xeroderma, 1004
Mental retardation, seizures and adenoma sebaceum, 975
Mental retardation with osteocartilaginous anomalies, 190
Mentation (see Section III, Tables XXIII and XXXVI)
Mentón trémulo, 147
MESENCHYMAL DYSPLASIA OF PURETIĆ, 644
Mesenchymal hamartoma of liver, 604
Mesenterial Zysten, 645
MESENTERIC CYSTS, 645
Mesiodens, 936
Mesoectodermal dysgenesis of anterior segment, 439
Mesoectodermal dysgenesis of iris and cornea, 439
Mesoectodermal dysplasia, 156
Mesomele Dysplasie, Typ Langer, 646
Mesomele Dysplasie, Typ Nievergelt, 647
Mesomele Dysplasie, Typ Reinhardt-Pfeiffer, 648
Mesomele Dysplasie, Typ Werner, 649
Mesomelic dwarfism and Madelung deformity, 308

Mesomelic dwarfism, Nievergelt type, 647
Mesomelic dwarfism of the hypoplastic ulna, fibula, mandible type, 646
Mesomelic dwarfism, type Robinow, 876
Mesomelic dwarfism with hemivertebrae and small genitalia, 876
MESOMELIC DYSPLASIA, LANGER TYPE, 646
MESOMELIC DYSPLASIA, NIEVERGELT TYPE, 647
MESOMELIC DYSPLASIA, REINHARDT-PFEIFFER TYPE, 648
MESOMELIC DYSPLASIA, WERNER TYPE, 649
Mesotaurodontism, 926
Metabolic craniopathy, 498
Metacarpal bones
    broad, 308
    fusion of, 231
    fusion of 3rd and 4th, 923
    fusion of 4th and 5th, 923
    fusion of 5th and 6th, 17
    long, 629
    long 2nd, 185
    mild shortening of, 1000
    short, 16, 20, 21, 66, 101, 114, 121, 163, 189, 231, 306, 308, 358, 392, 570, 875, 966, 982
    short metacarpals of ulnar digits, 981
    short 1st, 160, 242, 700, 853, 1001
    short 4th, 830
    short 5th, 830
METACHONDROMATOSIS, 650
Metachromatic form of diffuse cerebral sclerosis, 651
METACHROMATIC LEUKODYSTROPHIES, 651
Metacondromatosis, 650
Metamorfosis grasosa visceral familiar, 990
Métamorphose graisseuse des viscéres, 990
Metaphysäre Chondrodysplasie, geistige Retardierung und Schalleitungs-Schwerhörigkeit, 250
Metaphysäre Chondrodysplasie mit Thymolymphopenie, 655
Metaphysäre Chondrodysplasie, Typ Jansen, 652
Metaphysäre Chondrodysplasie, Typ McKusick, 653
Metaphysäre Chondrodysplasie, Typ Schmid, 654
METAPHYSEAL CHONDRODYSPLASIA, TYPE JANSEN, 652
METAPHYSEAL CHONDRODYSPLASIA, TYPE MCKUSICK, 653
METAPHYSEAL CHONDRODYSPLASIA, TYPE SCHMID, 654
METAPHYSEAL CHONDRODYSPLASIA WITH THYMOLYMPHOPENIA, 655
Metaphyseal dysostosis, type Jansen, 652
Metaphyseal dysostosis, type Schmid, 654
Metaphyseal dysostosis with Swiss type agammaglobulinemia, 655
Metaphyseal dysplasia, familial, 847
Metatarsal bones
    extra, 649, 885
    fusion of 3rd to 1st and 2nd, 22
    fusion of 3rd and 4th, 923
    fusion of 4th and 5th, 22, 923
    fusion of 5th and 6th, 17
    long, 629
    partial duplication of 1st, 22
    partial duplication of 2nd, 22
    short, 20, 21, 163, 810, 875
    single broad metatarsal associated with great toe and 2nd toe, 22

short 1st, **183, 1001**
short 4th and 5th, **830**
Metatropic dwarfism, **656**
METATROPIC DYSPLASIA, **656**
Metatropic dysplasia, type II, **557**
Metatropischer Zwergwuchs, **656**
METHIONINE MALABSORPTION
    SYNDROME, **657**
METHYLMALONIC ACIDEMIA, **658**
Methylmalonic aciduria, **658**
Michel malformation of inner ear, **562**
Micrencephaly, **220**
    spongoid, **881**
Microcefalia, **659**
MICROCEPHALY, **659**
Microcephaly (see Section III, Table XXIX)
Microcystic renal disease, **709**
Microcythemia, **939**
MICRODONTIA (MARKER), **660**
Microencephaly, **659**
Microesferofaquia, **663**
Microftalmia, **661**
Microftalmia con anomalías digitales, **662**
Microgastria, **913**
Micrognathia and glossoptosis syndrome, **182**
Microphtalmie, **661**
Microphtalmie avec anomalies digitales, **662**
MICROPHTHALMIA, **661**
MICROPHTHALMIA AND DIGITAL
    ANOMALIES, **662**
Microphthalmia, gingival fibromatosis,
    depigmentation, oligophrenia and
    athetosis, **413**
Microphthalmos, **661**
Microsomía hemifacial, **457**
MICROSPHEROPHAKIA, **663**
Microstomia, agnathia and synotia, **28**
MICROTIA–ATRESIA, **664**
Microtia, facial clefting, hypertelorism, **506**
Middle ear and ossicle malformations, **773**
Middle ear aneurysm of internal carotid
    artery, **530**
Middle ear chemodectoma, **145**
Middle ear, genitourinary anomalies, **860**
Middle ear malformations with hearing loss,
    773
Midfrequency sensorineural deafness, **267**
Midsystolic click-late systolic murmur syn-
    drome, **668**
Migeon syndrome, **25**
Mikrodontie, **660**
Mikrophthalmie, **661**
Mikrophthalmie und Fingerderformitäten,
    662
Mikrosphärophakie, **663**
Mikrotie und Atresie, **664**
Mikrozephalie, **659**
Mikulicz disease, **799**
Milestones, delayed (see Section III,
    Table XXIII)
Milroy disease, **614**
Milzzysten, **240**
Miopatía con acidemia láctica, **697**
Miopatía miotubular, **695**
Miopatía mitocondrial, **694**
Miopatía por alteración enzimológica
    parcial vermiforme de la fibra muscular
    esquelética, **696**
Miopía, **699**
Miopía, catarata, nariz en silla de montar,
    hipertelorismo, estatura baja y pérdida
    de la audición neurosensorial de
    moderada a severa, **261**
Miopía, telecanto secundario (hipertelorismo)
    y pérdida severa de la audición
    neurosensorial, **732**

Miosis and partial ptosis, **475**
Miositis osificante, **700**
Miotonía congénita, **701**
Miotonía distrófica, **702**
Mitochondrale Myopathie, **694**
Mitochondrial malate dehydrogenase,
    genetic variant of, **624**
Mitochondrial myopathy, **694**
Mitral Insuffizienz, **666**
Mitral regurgitation due to isolated cleft
    posterior leaflet of mitral valve, **666**
Mitral valve
    insufficiency, **347, 630, 667, 999**
    stenosis, **381**
MITRAL VALVE ATRESIA, **665**
MITRAL VALVE INSUFFICIENCY, **666**
MITRAL VALVE INSUFFICIENCY, DEAF-
    NESS AND SKELETAL MALFORMA-
    TIONS, **667**
MITRAL VALVE PROLAPSE, **668**
MITRAL VALVE STENOSIS, **669**
Mitralklappen-Atresie, **665**
Mitralstenose, **669**
Mittlere Unterlippen-Unterkiefer-Zungen
    spalte, **636**
Mittlere Unterlippenspalte, **595**
Mixed cyst on head or neck, **283**
Mixed gonadal dysgenesis, **173**
Mixed hearing loss (see Section III, Table
    XXV)
Mixed porphyria, **822**
Mixed tumor, salivary gland, **878**
Möbius syndrome, **376**
Mohr syndrome, **771**
Molar tooth
    central pit on occlusal surface, **276**
    duplicated pulp chamber of, **784**
    globe-shaped crown on, **784**
    impacted 3rd, **932**
    peg-shaped 3rd, **934**
    single large root, **607**
    single pulp chamber with small root, **926**
    variable crown or cusp, **607**
Mollities ossium, **777**
Mondini-Alexander malformation of inner
    ear, **315**
Mongolism, **171**
Monochromasie, **195**
Monochromatische Blau-Blindheit, **195**
Monodermoma of head or neck, **283**
Monosomie G de type I, **170**
Monosomie G de type II, **172**
Monosomie partielle 11q, **162**
Monosomy-G syndrome type I, **170**
Monosomy-G syndrome type II, **172**
Monosomy X, **977**
Morgagni-Stewart-Morel syndrome, **498**
Morquio syndrome, **678**
Morquio-Ullrich syndrome, **678**
Mosaic gonadal dysgenesis, **173**
Mosaic 21 syndrome, **171**
Motor retardation (see Section III, Table
    XXIII)
Mouth
    cleft of, **374, 375**
    corners turned downward, **158, 159,
        164, 242, 603, 876, 887, 943**
    deep furrows around, **105**
    large, **121, 190, 375, 457, 469, 543, 557,
        627, 735, 754, 876**
    limited opening of, **160, 882**
    opens on upward gaze, **548**
    small, **28, 155, 160, 223, 451, 506, 578,
        627, 629**
    triangular, **754, 823, 876**

Movements
    extreme slowness of, **746**
    involuntary, **421**
    purposeless, **808**
MOYNAHAN SYNDROME, **670**
Mozart ear (Marker), **328**
Mozart-Ohr, **328**
MPS I, **674**
MPS II, **676**
MPS III, **677**
MPS IV, **678**
MPS V, **675**
MPS VI, **679**
Mucolipidose de type I, **671**
Mucolipidose de type II, **672**
Mucolipidose de type III, **673**
MUCOLIPIDOSIS I, **671**
MUCOLIPIDOSIS II, **672**
MUCOLIPIDOSIS III, **673**
Mucopolisacaridosis Tipo I, **674, 675**
Mucopolisacaridosis Tipo II, **676**
Mucopolisacaridosis Tipo III, **677**
Mucopolisacaridosis Tipo IV, **678**
Mucopolisacaridosis Tipo V, **675**
Mucopolisacaridosis Tipo VI, **679**
Mucopolisacaridosis Tipo VII, **680**
Mucopolysaccharidose de type I, **674, 675**
Mucopolysaccharidose de type II, **676**
Mucopolysaccharidose de type III, **677**
Mucopolysaccharidose de type IV, **678**
Mucopolysaccharidose de type V, **675**
Mucopolysaccharidose de type VI, **679**
Mucopolysaccharidose de type VII, **680**
"Mucopolysaccharidosis F," **398**
MUCOPOLYSACCHARIDOSIS I-H, **674**
MUCOPOLYSACCHARIDOSIS I-S, **675**
MUCOPOLYSACCHARIDOSIS II, **676**
MUCOPOLYSACCHARIDOSIS III, **677**
MUCOPOLYSACCHARIDOSIS IV, **678**
MUCOPOLYSACCHARIDOSIS VI, **679**
MUCOPOLYSACCHARIDOSIS VII, **680**
Mucosa plegada, blanca displásica, **681**
MUCOSA, WHITE FOLDED DYSPLASIA,
    681
Mucosal neuroma syndrome, **352**
Muco-viscidose-fibrose kystique du pancréas,
    237
Mucoviscidosis, **237**
Mulberry molars, **342**
MÜLLERIAN APLASIA, **682**
MÜLLERIAN DERIVATIVES IN MALES,
    PERSISTENT, **683**
MÜLLERIAN FUSION, INCOMPLETE, **684**
MULTIPLE CARTILAGINOUS EXOSTOSES,
    685
Multiple choristomas, convulsions and
    mental retardation, **593**
Multiple circumscribed lipomas, **600**
Multiple compact osteomata, **318**
Multiple congenital articular rigidities, **88**
Multiple congenital dislocations with unusual
    facies and skeletal abnormalities, **570**
Multiple enchondromatosis, **345**
Multiple endocrine adenomatosis, type I,
    350
Multiple endocrine adenomatosis type II,
    351
Multiple endocrine adenomatosis, type IIb,
    352
Multiple epiphysäre Dysplasie, **358**
Multiple exostoses, **685**
Multiple familial benign nodular intraepi-
    dermal basal cell epithelioma, **235**
Multiple glomus tumors, **416**
Multiple hamartoma syndrome, **412**

Multiple hemangiomas of skin and internal organs, 113
Multiple Kartilaginäre Exostosen, 685
Multiple leiomyomas of skin, 890
Multiple lentigines syndrome, 586
Multiple peripheral pulmonary stenosis, mixed deafness, brachytelephalangy, calcification of cartilages, 263
Multiple symmetric lipomatosis, 600
Multiple synostoses and conduction deafness, 1001
Murray syndrome, 411
Muscle atrophy (also see Muscle by body parts, characteristics and Section III, Table XXX), 48, 88, 107, 155, 275, 508, 629, 630, 644, 695, 696, 759, 785, 810
    musculature poorly developed, 88, 163, 290
    overlying bone defect, 641
    replaced by fat, 88
    with onset after puberty, 687, 688, 691, 702
    with onset in childhood, 134, 686, 689, 690, 691, 702
    with onset in infancy, 134, 686
Muscle defect, general (also see Section III, Table XXX)
    nonprogressive, 125, 134, 686, 691, 694, 695, 696, 698, 701, 794, 795, 796
    rapid progression of, 11, 116, 689, 700
    slow progression of, 124, 125, 688, 694, 695, 696, 698, 794, 795
Muscle fatigability or weakness
    increased, 47, 80, 290, 429, 430, 794
    overlying bone defect, 641
    unspecified weakness, 2, 26, 48, 100, 143, 290, 398, 432, 590, 697, 810, 822, 847, 851, 873, 895, 944, 949
MUSCLE HYPOPLASIA, CONGENITAL UNIVERSAL, 686
Muscle papillaire unique du ventricule gauche, 582
Muscle paralysis
    hypokalemic, periodic, 100
    ketosis, 125
    transient, flaccid, induced by cold, 794, 795, 796
    transient, flaccid, induced by emotion, infection or anesthesia, 794, 795
    transient, flaccid, induced by exercise, 125
    transient, flaccid, induced by food, 795
    transient, flaccid, induced by hunger, 794
    transient, flaccid, induced by high fat diet, 125
    transient, flaccid, induced by rest after exercise, 698, 794, 795
    transient, flaccid, induced by starvation with ketosis, 125
Muscle phosphorylase deficiency, 698
Muscle strength, general
    decrease in, 430, 460, 508, 671, 776, 820, 864
    generalized decrease in strength with onset in infancy, 686, 694
    mainly distal decrease in early childhood, 690, 702
    mainly proximal decrease, 124, 125, 687, 688, 691, 692, 698, 794, 795, 796, 895
    mainly proximal decrease with onset in early childhood, 688, 689
    mainly proximal decrease with onset in infancy, 11, 116, 134, 694, 695, 696

symmetric decrease in, 895
Muscle tone (also see Section III, Table XXX)
    decreased, 93, 107, 115, 122, 134, 158, 159, 163, 171, 172, 188, 352, 398, 403, 421, 425, 486, 491, 492, 499, 543, 578, 587, 603, 638, 651, 686, 689, 695, 696, 736, 754, 783, 850, 873, 891, 895, 940, 946, 967, 990, 999
    decreased in infancy, 434, 897
    episodic decrease in, 628, 794, 795, 796
    hypotonia produced by cold or exercise, 125, 698, 794, 795, 796
    hypotonia produced by food, hunger or emotion, 125, 794, 795
    increased, 158, 160, 165, 166, 170, 242, 406, 492, 755
    increased in lower limb, 161, 295
    increased in upper limb, 161
    intermittent hypertonia, 115
    lack of, 139, 823
    marked decrease, 139, 823
    myotonia, constant, 701, 702
    rigidity, 432, 469, 478, 515, 603, 743, 744, 746, 964
    unspecified decreased muscle tone, 165, 671, 823
    unspecified delayed relaxation of muscle, 155
Muscle volume
    allusory increase, 687, 688, 689, 691
    increased, 155, 701
Muscle weakness, 2, 26, 48, 100, 143, 290, 398, 432, 590, 697, 810, 822, 847, 851, 873, 895, 944, 949
Muscle weakness overlying bone defect, 641
Muscles, diaphragmatic
    abdominal viscera displaced into thoracic cavity, 289
    diaphragmatic hernia, 104, 382, 727
    diaphragmatic paralysis with 2° scapular involvement, 221
    elevated position of diaphragm, 288
    paradoxical motion of leaf of diaphragm, 288
Muscles of face or neck
    atrophy of neck muscle, 924
    hypoplasia of, ipsilateral to microtia, 664
    persistent weakness of cervical muscles, 152
    unilateral hypoplasia of, 457
    weakness of, 12, 697
Muscles of foot
    atrophy of, around ankle, 560
    compensatory hypertrophy of, around ankle, 560
    marked atrophy of, 275
Muscles of hand
    atrophy of, 270, 924
    decreased strength in distribution of ulnar nerve, 89, 450
    decreased tone of, 152
    marked atrophy of, 275
    nonprogressive atrophy of hypothenar, 89, 450
    nonprogressive atrophy of interosseous, 89, 450
    nonprogressive atrophy of thenar, 89, 450
    small extensor pollicis brevis or longis, 175
    weakness of, 270, 924
Muscles of shoulder and upper limb
    atrophy of upper limb, 270, 629
    aplasia of sternal head of pectoralis major, 813

difficulty in lifting arms over head, 691
    small pectoralis major, 376
    weakness in shoulder girdle, 691
    unspecified defect of shoulder girdle or upper arm, 901
Muscles of trunk
    atrophy of, 924
    defect of diastasis recti, 118, 121, 163, 505, 587, 632
    hypotonia in, 161
Muscles, intercostal, weakness of, 152
Muscles of pelvic girdle and lower limb
    atrophy around knee, 560
    atrophy of lower limb, 270, 292, 629, 998
    compensatory hypertrophy around knee, 560
    marked atrophy of lower limb, 275
    weakness in pelvic girdles, 691
    weakness of lower limb, 292, 678, 924
Muscular central core disease, 134
MUSCULAR DYSTROPHY, ADULT PSEUDOHYPERTROPHIC, 687
MUSCULAR DYSTROPHY, AUTOSOMAL RECESSIVE PSEUDOHYPER-TROPHIC, 688
Muscular dystrophy, Becker, 687
MUSCULAR DYSTROPHY, CHILDHOOD PSEUDOHYPERTROPHIC, 689
MUSCULAR DYSTROPHY, DISTAL, 690
MUSCULAR DYSTROPHY, LIMB-GIRDLE, 691
MUSCULAR DYSTROPHY, OCULO-PHARYNGEAL, 692
Muscular macroglossia, 618
Muscular subaortic stenosis, 917
Muscular system (see Muscle by body parts, characteristics, and Section III, Table XXX)
Músculo papilar único del ventrículo izquierdo, 582

Muskeldystrophie, Typ Duchenne, 689
Muskeldystrophie, Typ Welander, 690
Muskuläre Subaortenstenose, 917
Mutilating keratoderma, 259
MYELOMENINGOCELE, 693
Myeloschisis, 292, 693

Myoblastic myoma, 360
Myoblastoma, 360
Myoclonic petit mal, 135
Myoclonic variant of cerebral lipoidosis, 713

Myoepithelial tumor, 360
Myogenic stiff ptosis, 834
Myogenic xanthoma, 360
Myopathic ophthalmoplegia externa, 752
Myopathie avec acidémie lactique, 697
Myopathie (forme des ceintures), 691
Myopathie mit Laktatacidämie, 697
Myopathie mitochondriale, 694
Myopathie myotubulaire, 695
Myopathie némaline, 696
Myopathie pseudo-hypertrophique de l'adulte, 687
Myopathy, megaconial, 694
MYOPATHY, MITOCHONDRIAL, 694
MYOPATHY, MYOTUBULAR, 695
MYOPATHY, NEMALINE, 696
MYOPATHY WITH LACTIC ACIDEMIA, 697
MYOPHOSPHORYLASE DEFICIENCY, 698
Myophosphorylase Mangel, 698
MYOPIA, 699

Myopia (also see Astigmatism, Nearsightedness and Refractive error)
high-grade nearsightedness, **35, 261, 750**
major refractive error, **757**
nearsightedness, **90, 155, 182, 229, 242, 384, 449, 474, 557, 585, 630, 663, 720, 732, 893, 897, 976, 986**
nearsightedness from birth, **699**
nearsightedness with onset before puberty, **251, 699**
Myopia and external ophthalmoplegia, **750**
Myopia, cataract, saddle nose, hypertelorism, short stature, and moderate-to-severe sensorineural hearing loss, **261**
Myopia, cochlear deafness and intellectual impairment, **251**
Myopia unilateral, **59**
Myopie, **699**
Myopie, cataracte, ensellure nasale profonde, hypertélorisme, nanisme, et surdité de perception d'intensité variable, **261**
Myopie, hypertélorisme et surdité de perception sévère, **732**
Myopie, Katarakt, Sattelnase, Hypertelorismus, Kleinwuchs, Innenohrschwerhörigkeit, **261**
Myopie, Telecanthus (Hypertelorismus) und Innenohrschwerhörigkeit, **732**
MYOSITIS OSSIFICANS, **700**
Myositis ossificans, progressive, **700**
Myotone Dystrophie, **702**
Myotonia atrophica, **702**
MYOTONIA CONGENITA, **701**
Myotonia congenita intermittens, **796**
MYOTONIC DYSTROPHY, **702**
Myotonic myopathy, dwarfism, chondrodystrophy, ocular and facial abnormalities, **155**
Myotonie congénitale, **701**
Myotubular myopathy, **695**
Myotubuläre Dystrophie, **695**

N

Nachtblindheit, **718**
NAEGELI SYNDROME, **703**
Naevi à cellules basales, **101**
Naevus flammeus, **715**
Nagel-Patella-Syndrom, **704**
Nail abnormalities, localized absence and blistering of skin, **609**
Nail absent, **66**
Nail dysgenesis and hypodontia, **511**
Nail dystrophy and sensorineural deafness, **252**
Nail, hair, bone and tooth dysplasia, **965**
Nails (also see Section III, Table XXVIII)
brittle or splitting, **704, 811, 965**
broad, **16**
clubbing of, **27, 788**
color change of, **37, 281, 558, 589, 615, 811, 965**
concave or spoon-shaped, **281, 511, 559**
defect of, **15, 38, 65, 102, 160, 168, 281, 334, 337, 382, 615, 703, 825, 833, 880**
deformed, **156, 179, 252, 259, 409, 609, 621**
depigmented, **37, 281, 558, 589, 615, 811, 965**
dystrophic, **15, 38, 65, 102, 156, 160, 168, 179, 252, 259, 281, 334, 337, 382, 409, 609, 615, 621, 703, 825, 833, 880**

elliptical, **21**
everted edges of, **559**
fibromas in nailbed, **975**
fissured center of, **559**
flat, **846**
grooved, **281**
hyperkeratosis of, **45**
infection of nailbed, **334**
narrow, **704**
new growth in nailbed, **411**
pitted, **38, 833**
ridged, **38, 102, 259, 811**
separation from nailbed at distal portion of, **45, 833**
slow growing, **511**
small, **16, 21, 66, 102, 156, 262, 511, 570, 621, 825**
smooth, **45**
smooth surface, **264**
thickened, **131, 334, 789**
thin, **511, 559**
NAIL–PATELLA SYNDROME, **704**
Nanisme à nez camus, **305**
Nanisme à tête d'oiseau, **881**
Nanisme de type Laron, **302**
Nanisme diastrophique, **293**
Nanisme métatropique, **656**
Nanisme panhypopituitaire, **303**
Nanisme parastrématique, **798**
Nanisme pituitaire avec anomalie de la selle turcique, **304**
Nanisme thanatophore, **940**
Nanophthalmia, **661**
Nape nevus, **715**
Nariz de dogo, **724**
Nasal and nasopharyngeal tumors, **237, 283, 285, 343, 370, 726**
Nasal bridge
flat (depressed), **10, 13, 14, 105, 121, 122, 153, 157, 158, 159, 168, 171, 172, 242, 261, 302, 305, 333, 382, 385, 388, 395, 401, 504, 557, 570, 587, 593, 674, 732, 786, 880, 893, 940**
midline pit or fistula of, **283**
obtuse frontonasal angle, **627**
prominent, **22, 112, 119, 140, 164, 167, 168, 170, 229, 231, 555, 738, 754, 825, 856, 860, 997, 998, 1001**
Nasal cavity
choanal atresia, **389, 627, 724, 727**
obstruction of, **224, 228, 726, 727**
reduced nasal airway, **707**
Nasal crease, **728**
Nasal dermoids, **283**
Nasal duplication, **725**
Nasal glioma, **726**
Nasal groove, familial transverse, **728**
Nasal septum
deviated, **225, 229, 271**
duplicated, **724**
extends below wings of nostril, **119**
has slit-like openings, **725**
nasal columella, broad or short, **724**
thick, **190**
Nasengliom, **726**
NASOLACRIMAL DUCT IMPATENCY, **705**
Nasopharyngeal atresia, **707**
NASOPHARYNGEAL CYSTS, **706**
NASOPHARYNGEAL STENOSIS, **707**
Nasopharyngeal teratomas, **283**
Nasopharyngeal Zysten, **706**
Nasopharynx (also see Section III, Table XXVI)
agenesis of adenoid, **27, 655**

attachment of soft palate to posterior, **707**
cyst in wall of, **706**
shallow, **707**
soft tissue membrane in, **727**
wide, **180**
Natal or neonatal teeth, **933**
Nathalie Syndrom, **785**
Natural earring holes, **322**
Nausea, **12, 26, 102, 188, 395, 428, 793**
after fructose ingestion, **395**
induced by exercise, **428**
Nearsightedness (also see Myopia), **35, 90, 155, 182, 229, 242, 251, 261, 384, 449, 474, 557, 585, 630, 663, 699, 720, 732, 750, 757, 893, 897, 976, 986**
Neck (also see glands by name and Section III, Table XXVII)
branchial arch cyst, **117**
branchial arch fistula, **117, 247, 329**
branchial arch sinus, **117**
broad, **720, 896**
cleft of anterior midline structures of, **636**
cyst between hyoid bone and thyroid gland, **575**
cyst that moves upward when swallowing, **945**
limited movement of, **103**
short, **9, 103, 140, 155, 157, 158, 163, 166, 171, 242, 389, 676, 678, 720, 830, 896, 898**
sinus at or near midline of, **945**
stiffness of, **103, 188**
torticollis, **957**
tumor of, **117, 127, 283**
webbed, **51, 158, 382, 578, 586, 720, 977**
Neck veins (also see Heart)
accentuated jugular A waves, **917**
cannon A waves of, **454**
neck vein distended, **454, 969**
prominent V waves of, **969**
Necrotizing, infantile subacute encephalopathy, **344**
Nefritis hereditaria y sordera neural, **708**
Nefropatía, pérdida de la agudeza auditiva neuro-sensorial hiperprolinuria e ictiosis, **258**
Nefrosis congénita, **709**
Nefrosis familiar, **710**
Neill-Dingwall syndrome, **189**
Nekrotisierende Enzephalopathie, **344**
Nemaline myopathy, **696**
Neonatal familial primary hyperparathyroidism, **499**
Neonatal hemochromatosis, **460**
Neonatal hepatitis, **39**
Neonatal hypomagnesemia with selective malabsorption of magnesium, **514**
Neonatal nephrosis, **709**
Neonatal or natal teeth, **933**
Neonatal seborrheic diathesis, **812**
Neoplasia endócrina múltiple tipo I, **350**
Neoplasia endócrina múltiple tipo II, **351**
Neoplasia endócrina múltiple tipo III, **352**
Neoplasmas del SNC, **188**
Neoplasms of CNS, **188**
NEPHRITIS AND NERVE DEAFNESS, HEREDITARY, **708**
Nephritis with hearing loss, **708**
Nephrogenic diabetes insipidus, **287**
Nephropathic cystinosis, **238**
Néphropathie héréditaire avec surdité, **708**

Nephropathie, Innenohrschwerhörigkeit, Hyperprolinurie und Ichthyose, 258

Néphropathie, surdité neurosensorielle, hyperprolinurie et ichtyose, 258

Nephropathy with deafness, hereditary, 708

NEPHROSIS, CONGENITAL, 709

NEPHROSIS, FAMILIAL, 710

Nerve malformations of middle ear, 773

Nervous system (see parts, functions, and Section III, Tables XXIII and XXXVI)

Neugeborenen Hypoglykämie, 512

Neural hearing loss and hereditary atopic dermatitis, 245

Neurenteric cyst of spinal cord, 894

Neurenterische Rückenmarkszysten, 894

Neurodegenerative disease, 643

NEUROECTODERMAL PIGMENTED TUMOR, 711

Neuroepithelioma adenoids, 235

NEUROFIBROMATOSIS, 712

Neurogenic flaccid ptosis, 834

Neurologic defect unspecified, general, 135, 187, 578, 777, 782, 961, 978, 992

Neurologic dysfunction (see parts of body and Section III, Tables XXIII and XXXVI)
  acute attacks of, 203, 820, 822
  progressive, 2, 103, 126, 398, 406, 519, 547, 598, 671, 697, 850, 894, 921

Neuroma acústico bilateral, 12

Neuromes auditifs bilatéraux, 12

NEURONAL CEROID–LIPOFUSCINOSES, 713

Neuronal storage disease with curvilinear bodies, 713

Neuropathy
  peripheral, 7, 671
  sensory, peripheral, 93, 143, 265, 270, 398, 810, 820

NEUTROPENIA, CYCLIC, 714

Nevi flammei, 715

Nevi, linear sebaceous, 593

Nevoid basal cell carcinoma syndrome, 101

NEVUS FLAMMEUS, 715

Nevus fuscocaeruleus maxillofacialis, 716

NEVUS OF OTA, 716

Nevus sebaceous of Jadassohn, 593

Nevus telangiectatica, 715

Nevus varicosus osteohypertrophicus, 55

New neurocutaneous syndrome, 593

Nez bifide, 725

Nez de dogue, 724

Nez latérale, 824

Nicht-ketotische Form der Hyperglyzinämie, 492

Nicotinamide adenine dinucleotide and oxi-doreductase, 568

NIEMANN–PICK DISEASE, 717

Niemann-Picksche Krankheit, 717

Nightblindness
  nyctalopia, 270, 578, 718, 719, 740, 810, 869, 925, 983
  progressive, 449
  stationary from birth, 399

NIGHTBLINDNESS, STATIONARY, 719

Nipples (see Mammary gland)

Noack syndrome, 13

Nodular macroglossia, 618

Nodular myolysis, 360

Nonchromaffin paragangliomata of middle ear, 145

Noncongenital isolated lactase deficiency (insufficiency), 567

"Noncorrectable" extrahepatic biliary atresia, 110

Noninverted transposition, 962

Nonketotic hyperglycinemia, 492

Nonne-Milroy type hereditary lymphedema, 614

Nonopalescent opalescent dentine, 278

Nonpapillary hyalinizing hydradenoma, 235

Nonparasitic hepatic cyst, 465

Nonplasmatic autosomal recessive thymic alymphoplasia or alymphocytosis, 522

Nonrotation of midgut, 537

Nontumorous primary aldosteronism, 484

NOONAN SYNDROME, 720

NORRIE DISEASE, 721

Nose (also see Nasal parts, tip of nose, and Section III, Table XXVI)
  bifid at birth, 506
  broad, 162, 164, 166, 724
  calcified cartilage of, 263
  cylindrical structure, 234, 1001
  defect of, 726, 821, 825
  duplication of bony structure of, 725
  flat, 9, 16, 105, 431, 724, 883
  hemangioma of, 386
  large, 881
  long, 1001
  midline cleft, 635, 943
  midline nasal groove, 635
  short, 1, 16, 161, 162, 876, 883
  small, 16, 223, 242, 281, 389, 722, 738, 825, 999
  small cartilage of, 738
  small nasal bones, 261
  soft cartilage of, 409
  thin (narrow), 189, 737, 738, 997
  two separate, 725

NOSE AND NASAL SEPTUM DEFECTS, 722

NOSE, ANTERIOR ATRESIA, 723

NOSE, BIFID, 724

NOSE, DUPLICATION, 725

Nose, ear, digital anomalies, gingival fibro-matosis, and hepatosplenomegaly, 409

NOSE, GLIOMA, 726

NOSE, POSTERIOR ATRESIA, 727

Nose, red skin and papules on, 444

NOSE, TRANSVERSE GROOVE (MARKER), 728

Nostril
  anteverted, 16, 162, 190, 227, 261, 395, 401, 603, 891, 999
  narrow, 223, 737
  single, 158, 168, 634
  small, 121
  unilateral stenosis or narrowness of, 723

Notch or cleavage of caruncle, 130

Nougaret nightblindness, 719

Nuclear cataract, 132

Nuclear facial palsy, 377

Nuclear hypoplasia congenital (6th and 7th cranial nerves), 376

NUCLEOSIDE–PHOSPHORYLASE DE-FICIENCY, 729

Nuidudui, 886

Nukleosidphosphorylase-Mangel, 729

Nyctalopia, 718

Nyssen and van Bogaert syndrome, 759

Nystagmus (also see Section III, Table XXIV)
  at birth or onset in childhood, 963
  coarse, 413
  horizontal, 147, 413, 755, 986
  jerky, 413
  lateral, 147, 413, 755, 986
  rotatory, 803, 963

O

Oast-house urine disease, 657

Obésité, hyperthermie oligomenorrhée et tuméfaction de la parotide, 730

Obesity, 106, 441, 447, 496, 498, 578, 730
  limb, 8, 455
  potbelly, 27
  protuberant buttocks, 10
  proximal limb, 823
  truncal, 302, 823

OBESITY, HYPERTHERMIA, OLIGO-MENORRHEA AND PAROTID SWELLING, 730

Obesity with onset in infancy, 41, 533

Obstipation, 192
  as neonate, 193, 531

OBSTRUCTION WITHIN RIGHT VEN-TRICLE OR ITS OUTFLOW TRACT, 731

Occipital bone
  bossing of, 160, 185, 227, 401, 603, 900
  flattened, 171, 227
  midline mass of, 343
  presence of only basal portion of, 52
  prominent shelf of, 777
  small, 227

Occipito-facial-cervico-thoracic-abdomino-digital dysplasia, 900

Ochronosis, 37

Ochronotic arthritis, 37

OCULAR AND FACIAL ANOMALIES WITH PROTEINURIA AND DEAFNESS, 732

Ocular anterior chamber
  deep, 637, 638
  dysplasia of, 84, 439
  exudate of, 140
  glaucoma of, 57, 101, 139, 182, 206, 261, 384, 387, 414, 474, 479, 553, 583, 591, 638, 663, 712, 736, 737, 872
  incomplete cleavage of angle, 140
  shallow, 205, 721, 994
  underdeveloped filtration angle, 732
  unspecified defect of, 637

OCULAR COLOBOMAS, 733

OCULAR DRUSEN, 734

Ocular hypertelorism (see Section III, Table XXIV)

Ocular hypotelorism, 163, 166, 168, 231, 355, 473, 634

Ocular lymphangioma, 765

Ocular melanocytosis, 640

Ocular motor apraxia, congenital, 191

Ocular muscular dystrophy, 692

Ocular myopathy, 752

Ocular nerve dysfunction, external, 1, 702, 712, 744, 745, 750, 779

Ocular retraction syndrome, 889

OCULO–AURICULO–VERTEBRAL DYSPLASIA, 735

OCULO–CEREBRO–RENAL SYNDROME, 736

Oculocraniodental syndrome, 229

Oculo-cranio-somatic neuromuscular disease with ragged-red fibers, 752

Oculocutaneous pigmentation syndrome, 716

Oculodentodigital dysplasia, 737

OCULO–DENTO–OSSEOUS DYSPLASIA, 737

Oculomandibulodyscephaly, 738

OCULO–MANDIBULO–FACIAL SYN-DROME, 738

Oculomotor nerve paralysis, 779
Oculopharyngeal muscular dystrophy, 692
Oculopharyngeal myopathy, 692
Oculopupillary syndrome, 475
Oculosympathetic syndrome, 475
ODONTODYSPLASIA, 739
Odontogenesis imperfecta, 739
Odontogenic dysplasia, 739
Oédème angioneurotique héréditaire, 54
Oesophagusatresie, 364
Oesophagusatresie mit tracheo-oesophagealer
    fistel, 365
Oesophagusdivertikel, 367
Oesophagusstenose, 369
OFD I syndrome, 770
OFD II syndrome, 771
Offener Ductus arteriosus, 800
Oftalmoplejía estática familiar, 751
Oftalmoplejía externa y miopía, 750
Oftalmoplejía progresiva, 752
Oftalmoplejía total con ptosis y miosis, 753
OGUCHI DISEASE, 740
Oguchi disease types 1, 2A, and 2B, 740
Ohr, kleines mit umgeschlagener Helix, 331
Ohr, prominente Anthelix, 330
Ohrgrübchen, 329
Ohrläppenchen-Fistel, 322
Okuläre Drusen, 734
Okuläre Kolobome, 733
Okulärer Albinismus, 32
Okuloaurikulovertebrale Dysplasie, 735
Okuol-dento-ossäres Dysplasie, 737
Okulokutaner Albinismus – gelbe mutante,
    36
Okulomandibulofazialen Syndrom, 738
Okulopharyngeale Form der Muskeldystrophie,
    692
Okulozerebrorenales Syndrom, 736
Olfaction loss, congenital, 70
Oligophrenia, cochlear deafness and myopia,
    251
OLIGOPHRENIA, EPILEPSY AND
    ICHTHYOSIS SYNDROME, 741
Oligophrenia, gingival fibromatosis, depig-
    mentation, microphthalmia, and
    athetosis, 413
OLIVOPONTOCEREBELLAR ATROPHY,
    DOMINANT MENZEL TYPE, 742
OLIVOPONTOCEREBELLAR ATROPHY,
    DOMINANT SCHUT–HAYMAKER
    TYPE, 743
OLIVOPONTOCEREBELLAR ATROPHY,
    DOMINANT WITH OPHTHALMO-
    PLEGIA, 744
Olivopontocerebellar atrophy, 742, 743, 744,
    745, 746, 747
OLIVOPONTOCEREBELLAR ATROPHY,
    DOMINANT WITH RETINAL DE-
    GENERATION, 745
OLIVOPONTOCEREBELLAR ATROPHY,
    LATE–ONSET, 746
OLIVOPONTOCEREBELLAR ATROPHY,
    RECESSIVE FICKLER–WINKLER
    TYPE, 747
Olivopontocerebellar atrophy I, 742
Olivopontocerebellar atrophy II, 747
Olivopontocerebellar atrophy III, 745
Olivopontocerebellar atrophy IV, 743
Olivopontocerebellar atrophy V, 744
Ollier syndrome, 345
Omphalocele (see Hernia, umbilical)
Omphalocele, visceromegaly and macroglossia
    syndrome, 104
Omphalomesenteric duct, 633
One form of "congenital absence of vagina,"
    984

Onicodistrofia, pulgares trifalángicos,
    orejas recortadas y périda de la
    audición neurosensorial, 262
Onychodysplasie, triphalangie des pouces et
    des gros orteils, retard mental, épilep-
    sie et surdité de perception, 262
Onychodystrophie, dreigliedrige Daumen
    und Zehen, geistige Retardierung,
    Krampfänfalle, angebornene Innen-
    ohrschwerhörigkeit, 262
Onychodystrophy, triphalangeal thumbs, and
    halluces, mental retardation, seizures,
    and congenital sensorineural deafness,
    262
Onycholysis, hypohidrosis and enamel hypo-
    calcification, 45
Onychoosteodysplasia, 704
Opalescent dentin, 279
Ophiasis, 38
Ophtalmoplégie avec ptosis et miosis, 753
Ophtalmoplégie externe avec myopie, 750
Ophtalmoplégie familiale, 751
Ophtalmoplégie progressive, 752
Ophthalmoarthropathy, 90
OPHTHALMO–MANDIBULO–MELIC
    DYSPLASIA, 749
OPHTHALMOPLEGIA EXTERNA AND
    MYOPIA, 750
Ophthalmoplegia externa, complete or in-
    complete, 751
OPHTHALMOPLEGIA, FAMILIAL STATIC,
    751
Ophthalmoplegia plus, 752
OPHTHALMOPLEGIA, PROGRESSIVE
    EXTERNAL, 752
Ophthalmoplegia totalis, 751
OPHTHALMOPLEGIA TOTALIS WITH
    PTOSIS AND MIOSIS, 753
Opisthotonus, 340, 603
Opitz-Frias syndrome, 401
OPITZ–KAVEGGIA FG SYNDROME, 754
Opitz trigonocephaly syndrome, 121
Optic atrophy and pigmentary stippling, 43
OPTIC ATROPHY, INFANTILE HEREDO-
    FAMILIAL, 755
Optic atrophy, juvenile diabetes and deaf-
    ness, 550
Optic atrophy, nerve deafness and distal
    neurogenic amyotrophy, 268
Optic disk (also see Optic nerve)
    atrophy of, 389, 414, 579, 755
    cleft in, 121, 620
    deep physiologic cup, 414, 733, 758
    edema of, 188, 230, 676, 763, 764
    elevated or flat, 579
    misshapen or mottled, 738
    pallor of, 41, 253, 480, 579, 758, 865
    pallor of, bilateral, 755
    pallor of, temporal, 755
    pallor of, waxy, 869, 983
    pigmented nevus of, 639
    pit in, 733, 756
    tilted, 757
Optic disk fossae, 756
Optic disk, melanocytoma, 639
OPTIC DISK PITS, 756
OPTIC DISK, SITUS INVERSUS, 757
Optic nerve (also see Optic disk)
    abnormally shaped, 661
    atrophy of, 43, 115, 140, 154, 189, 227,
        228, 229, 230, 253, 270, 281, 310,
        344, 389, 474, 479, 661, 759, 763,
        779, 780, 975
    edema of, 579
    small, 661, 758
    tumor of, 712

Optic nerve glioma, 763
OPTIC NERVE HYPOPLASIA, 758
Optic nerve paralysis, 779
OPTICO–COCHLEO–DENTATE DE-
    GENERATION, 759
Opticus-atrophie in Kombination mit Taub-
    heit, 253
Oral anticoagulant embryopathy, 389
Oral cavity (also see parts and Section III,
    Table XXVII)
    chewing difficulty, 390, 749
    closed by band or septum, 28, 181
    elevated floor, 618, 760
    feeling of fullness, 760
    inability to move jaw, 749
    progressive gangrenous lesions, 6
ORAL DERMOIDS, 760
Oral mucosa
    blistering, 609
    dry, 823
    hyperkeratotic papillomas, 412
    hyperplastic mucous glands in, 111
    leukoplakia of, 789
    neuroma, 352
    patches of hyperpigmentation in, 37,
        535
    soft, white, hyperplastic and folded onto
        itself, 681
    stomatitis, 15, 443, 494, 944
    thickened palatal mucosa, 593
    ulcerated, 143
    white shaggy plaque on, 538
ORBITAL AND PERIORBITAL DERMOID
    CYSTS, 761
ORBITAL CEPHALOCELES, 762
ORBITAL GLIOMA, 763
ORBITAL HEMANGIOMA, 764
Orbital hydrencephalocele, 762
ORBITAL LYMPHANGIOMA, 765
Orbital tumor, (also see Periorbital tumor),
    565, 591, 762
Orbitale und periorbitale Dermoidzysten,
    761
Orbitale Zephalozele, 762
Orbitales Lymphangiom, 765
Oreille de Mozart, 328
Oreille en cupule, 314
Oreilles allongées en rotation postérieure,
    325
Oreilles flasques, 326
Oreja colgante, 326
Oreja de Mozart (Marcador), 328
Oreja en copa, 314
Oreja implantada baja, 327
Oreja pequeña con hélix doblada, 331
Orejas largas, estrechas y con rotación
    posterior, 325
Orengua, 886
Organ of Corti, defect of, 315, 982
Organic brain syndrome, 203, 820, 822
Origen anormal de la arteria vertebral, 527
Origen anormal de las coronarias en la
    arteria pulmonar, 64
Origen común del tronco braquiocefálico
    y de la carótida interna, 200
Origen contralateral de las arterias sub-
    clavias, 63
Origen de la arteria pulmonar en el conducto
    arterioso, 768
Origen de la arteria pulmonar en la aorta
    ascendente, 767
Origen de la arteria pulmonar izquierda en la
    arteria pulmonar derecha, 766
Origin of a pulmonary artery from the con-
    tralateral (to aortic arch) ductus
    arteriosus, 768

Origin of a pulmonary artery from the ipsilateral (to aortic arch) ductus arteriosus, 768

Origin of both great vessels from right ventricle with posterior ventricular septal defect, 298

Origin of both great vessels from right ventricle with subpulmonic ventricular septal defect, 297

ORIGIN OF LEFT PULMONARY ARTERY FROM RIGHT PULMONARY ARTERY, 766

Origin of one pulmonary artery from ascending aorta, anterior or posterior, right or left, 767

ORIGIN OF PULMONARY ARTERY FROM ASCENDING AORTA, 767

ORIGIN OF PULMONARY ARTERY FROM DUCTUS ARTERIOSUS, 768

Origine anormale de l'artère vertébrale, 527

Origine anormale des coronaires naissant de l'artère pulmonaire, 64

Origine commune du tronc brachio-céphalique et de l'artère carotide gauche, 200

Origine contra-latérale de l'artère sous-clavière, 63

Origine de l'artère pulmonaire gauche dans l'artère pulmonaire droite, 766

Ornithine transcarbamylase deficiency, 485

Ornithinemia, 485

Ornithuria with retinal degeneration, 449

ORO–CRANIO–DIGITAL SYNDROME, 769

Orodigitofacial dysostosis, 770

ORO–FACIO–DIGITAL SYNDROME I, 770

ORO–FACIO–DIGITAL SYNDROME II, 771

Orokraniodigitales Syndrom, 769

OROTICACIDURIA, 772

Osseo-dentine Dysplasie, 280

Osseous syndactyly, 14, 22, 874, 923

OSSICLE AND MIDDLE EAR MALFORMATIONS, 773

Osteitis condensans, generalisata, 781

Osteoarthropathy, idiopathic hypertrophic, 788

Osteochalasia desmalis familiaris, 776

Ostéochondrite disséquante, 774

OSTEOCHONDRITIS DISSECANS, 774

Osteochondroma of the distal femoral epiphysis, 311

Osteodermatopoikilosis, 781

Osteodisplasia auricular, 98

Osteodisplastia, 775

Osteodysplasia enostotica, 781

OSTEODYSPLASTY, 775

Ostéodystrophie, 830

OSTEOECTASIA, 776

Osteoectasia with macrocranium (with hyperphosphatasia), 776

OSTEOGENESIS IMPERFECTA, 777

Osteogenesis imperfecta congenita, 777

Osteogenesis imperfecta tarda, 777

Osteoktasie, 776

Osteolisis carpo-tarsal, 128

Osteolisis carpo-tarsal recesiva, 129

Ostéolyse carpo-tarsienne, 128

Ostéolyse carpo-tarsienne (récessive), 129

Ostéolysis and proteinuria, 128

Osteopathia condensans disseminata, 781

Osteopathia hyperostotica sclerotisans multiplex infantilis, 290

OSTEOPATHIA STRIATA, 778

Ostéopathie striée, 778

Osteopatía estrida, 778

Osteopetrosa generalisata, 780

Ostéopétrose à manifestation précoce, 779

Ostéopétrose à manifestation tardive, 780

OSTEOPETROSIS, DOMINANT, 779

Osteopetrosis precoz, 779

OSTEOPETROSIS, RECESSIVE, 780

Osteopetrosis tardìa, 780

Osteopetrosis with late manifestation, 779

Osteopoecilia, 781

OSTEOPOIKILOSIS, 781

OSTEOPOROSIS, JUVENILE IDIOPATHIC, 782

OSTEOPOROSIS–PSEUDOGLIOMA SYNDROME, 783

Osteoporosis with ocular pseudoglioma, 783

Osteopsathyrosis idiopathica, 777

Osteosclerosis fragilis generalisata, 780

Osteosis eburnisans monomelica, 641

Ostium primum type atrial septal defect, persistent ostium primum, 347

Ostium secundum, 96

Otas Nävus, 716

Otitis media, 22, 27, 145, 206, 263, 285, 318, 370, 510, 524, 530, 644, 672, 706, 729, 786

Oto-dentales Syndrom, 784

OTO–OCULO–MUSCULO–SKELETAL SYNDROME, 785

OTO–PALATO–DIGITAL SYNDROME, 786

Otocephaly, 28

OTODENTAL DYSPLASIA, 784

Otodental syndrome, 784

Otoesclerosis, 787

Otomandibular dysostosis, 457

OTOSCLEROSIS, 787

Oval shape of calvaria, 85

Ovarian dysgenesis, familial, 436

Ovary
    adenocarcinoma of, 101
    bilateral streak, 436, 437
    cysts, large follicular, 391
    cyst of, 412, 587
    large, 903
    ovotestis, 971
    small atrophic, 529
    streak gonad with hilar cells, 173
    streak gonad with mesonephric remnants, 173
    tumor of, 535
    unilateral streak, 173
    unspecified defect of ovary, 860

P

Pabellón de la oreja ectópico, 316

PACHYDERMOPERIOSTOSIS, 788

PACHYONYCHIA CONGENITA, 789

Pachyonychia congenita types I, II, and III, 789

Pain, indifference to, 307, 450

Paladar hendido, 180

Paladar hendido, micrognatia y glosoptosis, 182

Palate, hard (also see Section III, Tables XII, XIII, and XIV)
    bilateral cleft of, 875
    cleft of, 90, 118, 122, 138, 157, 158, 159, 160, 164, 165, 166, 168, 172, 176, 177, 178, 179, 180, 181, 182, 185, 220, 225, 229, 230, 242, 261, 293, 329, 337, 375, 380, 381, 382, 401, 451, 470, 505, 506, 544, 557, 570, 578, 627, 629, 634, 635, 662, 664, 727, 737, 769, 770, 771, 786, 818, 874, 883, 897, 952, 953
    cysts at junction with maxilla and premaxilla, 59
    deep broad furrow, 121, 953
    defect of, 28, 88, 727
    fissured, 283
    flat, 121, 163, 226
    highly arched, 22, 118, 119, 121, 139, 157, 163, 166, 171, 182, 185, 223, 227, 229, 261, 381, 394, 412, 413, 627, 629, 630, 667, 696, 720, 732, 735, 754, 771, 823, 977
    lobed bony swelling of, 536, 959
    narrow, 160, 163, 171, 172, 227, 242, 720, 846, 977
    partial median cleft of, 791
    submucous cleft of, 97, 180, 184
    wide, 163

Palate, soft
    brown to brownish-red macules on, 955
    cleft of, 176, 178, 180, 181, 182, 183, 230, 293, 634
    fistula at junction with pharynx in anterior pillars, 790
    fistula in, 247
    weakness of, 376

Palate enlargement, 959

PALATE FISTULA (MARKER), 790

Palatoschisis, 180

Pallister Syndrom, 981

PALLISTER–W SYNDROME, 791

Pallor, 51, 403, 513, 886, 939

Palmar fibromatosis, 301

PALMO–PLANTAR ERYTHEMA, 792

Palmure laryngée, 574

Palpebral fissure (also see Section III, Table XXIV)
    long, 371
    narrow, 140, 155, 160, 168, 379, 395, 401
    narrows in adduction, 889
    short, 155, 166, 299, 371, 632
    unilaterally low-placed, 457
    widens in abduction, 889

Pancreas
    annular, 62, 300
    cysts, multiple, 605, 662, 859, 884
    cyst, single, 884
    hypofunction of islet cells, 702
    large, 104
    inflammation of, 62, 489, 532
    insufficiency, 237

Pancreatic fibrosis, 237

Pancreatic hypoplasia, bone marrow dysfunction and metaphyseal dysplasia, 885

PANCREATITIS, HEREDITARY, 793

Panhypopituitarismus, 303

Pankreas annulare, 62

Pankreasdysplasie, Knochenmarksdysfunktion und metaphysäre Dysplasie, 885

Papilas linguales pigmentadas (Marcador), 955

Papilles linguales pigmentées, 955

Papilloma of choroid plexus, 188

Papilloma-Leáge and Psaume syndrome, 770

Papillon-Lefèvre syndrome, 494

Paquidermoperiostosis, 788

Paquioniquia congénita, 789

Parachute mitral valve, 582
Paradione syndrome, 388
Parálisis congénita del sexto par, 889
Parálisis facial congénita, 377
Parálisis facial de comienzo tardío, 378
Parálisis periódica hipercaliémica, 794
Parálisis periódica hipocaliémica, 795
Paralysie de la sixième paire, 889
Paralysie faciale à début tardif, 378
Paralysie facial congénitale, 377
Paralysie périodique hyperkaliémique, 794
Paralysie périodique hypokaliémique, 795
PARALYSIS, HYPERKALEMIC PERIODIC, 794
PARALYSIS, HYPOKALEMIC PERIODIC, 795
Paralysis of sixth nerve, congenital, 889
Paramedian pits of lower lip (isolated trait), 596
Paramolar, 936
PARAMYOTONIA CONGENITA, 796
Paranasal sinus
    hypoplasia of, 225, 635, 735
    infection of, 27, 285, 521, 606, 706, 726, 944
PARANASAL SINUSES, ABSENT, 797
Paranasal sinuses, panagenesis, 797
Paranoia, 478
Paraparesis, spastic, 995
Paraplegia, 678
Paraplegia with sudden onset, 186
Parasternal hernia, 289
PARASTREMMATIC DYSPLASIA, 798
Parastremmatischer Zwergwuchs, 798
Parathyroid
    hypofunction of, 70, 515
    large, 391
    tumor of, 350
Parchment right ventricle, 979
Paresthesia, 48, 810, 820, 822, 995
Parietal bone
    bossing bilateral, 554
    lateral ridging of, 401
    midline mass of, 343
Parodontopathia acroectodermalis, 494
Parotidite ponctuée, 799
Parotiditis punctata, 799
Parotitis associated with Sjögren syndrome, 799
Parotitis of childhood, chronic recurrent, 799
Parotitis punctata, 799
PAROTITIS, PUNCTATE, 799
Partial absence of optic nerve, 758
Partial agenesis of corpus callosum, 220
Partial anomalous pulmonary venous connection, 841
Partial anomalous pulmonary venous return, 879
Partial anomalous venous return, 841
Partial chromosome 4 deletion syndrome, 164
Partial deficiencies of hypoxanthine guanine phosphoribosyl transferase, 441
Partial iodide transport defect, 542
Partial idotyrosine deiodinase deficiency, 543
Partial monosomy G, 170
Partial monosomy of distal 11q, 162
Partial transposition of great veins, 841
Partial 13 trisomy, 168
Partielle Lungenvenenfehlmündung, 841
Partielle Trisomie 11q, 161
Passagerer, isolierter Hypoaldosteronismus des Säuglingsalters, 23
Patau syndrome, 168

Patella
    dislocation of, 941
    lateral dislocation of, 308, 704
    small, 157, 560, 649, 704
PATENT DUCTUS ARTERIOSUS, 800
Pecho excavado, 802
Pectum recurvatum, 802
PECTUS CARINATUM, 801
Pectus carinatum, 22, 85, 155, 190, 257, 306, 394, 474, 629, 630, 678, 777, 801
PECTUS EXCAVATUM, 802
Pectus excavatum, 1, 85, 118, 190, 394, 412, 474, 554, 572, 576, 629, 630, 676, 754, 777, 802
Pegged or missing maxillary lateral incisor teeth and congenitally missing premolars, 934
PELIZAEUS–MERZBACHER SYNDROME, 803
Pelvis
    defect of, 171, 189, 685
    narrow, 122, 140, 157
    small, 160, 557
    tilted, 882
Pendred syndrome, 249
Penis
    chordee, 401, 518
    clitoris-like, 50
    fibrous contracture of, 301
    glans penis deformed downward, 401, 518
    partially deficient foreskin on ventral aspect of, 518
PENTOSURIA (MARKER), 804
Pérdida de la audición a las frequencias bajas dominante, 256
Peremans disease, 990
Perforaciones naturales de los pabellones auriculares (Marcador), 322
Perforation du pavillon de l'oreille, 322
PERICARDIUM AGENESIS, 805
Peridens, 936
Perikard-Agenesie, 805
Perineal anus, 69
Periodic neutropenia, 714
Periodic paralysis, hyperpotassemic, 794
Periodic paralysis, hypopotassemic, 795
Periodontoclasia and hyperkeratosis palmoplantaris, 494
PERIODONTOSIS, JUVENILE, 806
Peripheral dysostosis, nasal hypoplasia and mental retardation syndrome (PNM), 16
Peripheral iodotyrosine deiodinase deficiency, 543
Periphere Pulmonalstenose, Kombinierte Schwerhörigkeit, Brachytelephalangie, Knorpelverkalkungen, 263
Peromelia and micrognathia, 451
Peroxidase-Mangel der Schilddrüse, 947
Persistance de la membrane pupillaire, 845
Persistance de la veine cave supérieure gauche unie à l'atrium droit par l'intermédiaire du sinus coronarien, 807
Persistance des dents temporaires, 933
Persistance du canal artériel, 800
Persistance du canal thyréoglosse, 945
Persistence of hyaloid artery, 994
Persistence of oviducts in males, 683
Persistence of third aortic arch, 74
Persistencia de dientes temporarios, 933
Persistencia de la membrana pupilar, 845

Persistencia de la vena cava superior izquierda comunicada con la aurícula derecha por medio del seno coronario, 807
Persistencia del canal arterial, 800
Persistencia del conducto tirogloso, 945
Persistencia del tronco arterioso, 972
Persistent common atrioventricular canal, 347
Persistent ductus arteriosus, 800
Persistent fetal fibrovascular sheath of lens, 994
Persistent frontonasal process, 722
PERSISTENT LEFT SUPERIOR VENA CAVA CONNECTED TO CORONARY SINUS, 807
Persistent left superior vena cava connecting to right atrium via coronary sinus, 807
Persistent truncus arteriosus types I, II, III, and IV, 972
Persistent tunica vasculosa lentis, 994
Persistenz der linken Vena cava superior mit Verbindung zum rechten Vorhof über den Sinus coronarius, 807
Persistieren des primitiven Glaskörpers, 994
Persistierende Pupillarmembran, 845
Persistierender Ductus thyreoglossus, 945
Persistierendes Milchgebiss, 933
Peter anomaly, 439
Petit mal automatism, 135
Petit mal-grand mal epilepsy, 135
Petit mal lapse ("absence"), 135
Petrous pyramid cholesteatoma, 150
Peutz-Jeghers syndrome, 535
Pfeiffer syndrome, 14
Phalangeal hypoplasia and gingival fibromatosis, 409
Pharyngeal cyst or fistula, 117
Pharyngeal muscular dystrophy, 692
Pharyngeal pouch syndrome, 943
Pharyngoesophageal diverticulum, 367
Phenylalanine hydroxylase deficiency, 808
PHENYLKETONURIA, 808
PHENYLTHIOCARBAMIDE TASTING (MARKER), 809
Phenylthiurea sensitivity, 809
Pheochromocytoma, medullary thyroid carcinoma and multiple neuroma syndrome, 352
Phocomelia with congenital hypoplastic thrombocytopenia, 941
Photomyoclonie, diabète sucré, surdité de perception, néphropathie, et encéphalopathie, 255
Photomyoklonus, Diabetes mellitus, Innenohr-Schwerhörigkeit, Nephropathie, zerebrale Dysfunktion, 255
PHYTANIC ACID STORAGE DISEASE, 810
Phytansäure-Speicherkrankheit, 810
Pi phenotype ZZ, SZ, −Z and − , 39
Picnodisostosis, 846
Piebaldism with white forelock, 31
Piebaldness, 31
Piebalds, 31
Pierre Robin-Syndrom, 182
Pigeon breast, 801
Pigmentación congénita del disco óptico, 639
Pigmentary retinal degeneration, 869
Pigmentary retinal lipoid neuronal heredodegeneration, 713
Pigmentary retinitis with congenital amaurosis, 43

Pigmentation congénitale du disque (optique), 639
Pigmented epitheliomatosis, 1005
Pigmented lipid histiocytosis, 443
Pigmentierter neuroektodermaler Tumor, 711
Pitiriasis rubra pilaris, 811
Pits of upper lip, 596
Pityriasis pilaris, 811
PITYRIASIS RUBRA PILARIS, 811
Placenta circumvallata, 187
Plagiocephaly, 230
PLASMA-ASSOCIATED DEFECT OF PHAGOCYTOSIS, 812
Plasma cholinesterase, atypical, 152
Plasma thromboplastin component (PTC) deficiency, 462
Platybasie, 103
Pleoconial myopathy, 694
Plicatura o arrollamiento lingual (Marcador), 951
Plicature rétinienne, 867
Pliegue retineano, 867
PNM, 16
Pol-und Kapsel-Katarakte, 133
Poland syndactyly, 813
POLAND SYNDROME, 813
Polar and capsular cataracts, 132
Polidactilia, 814
Polimastia, 815
Poliposis del colon, 535
Polisindactilia, 817
Polisplenia, 816
Polycorie cholesterolique, 151
Polycystic disease of kidneys with liver involvement, 605
Polycystic renal disease, adult type, 859
Polydactylie avec syndactylie, 817
POLYDACTYLY, 814
Polydactyly and chondrodystrophy, 156
Polydactyly of index finger and polysyndactyly, 814
Polydystrophia oligophrenia, 677
Polykystose rénale du type adulte, 859
POLYMASTIA, 815
Polymorphe hintere Hornhautdystrophie, 213
Polymorphous posterior corneal dystrophy, 213
Polyosteochondrite (Turpin et Coste), 358
Polyostotic fibrous dysplasia, skin pigmentation and sexual precocity, 391
Polyostotisch Fibröse Dysplasie, 391
Polypose colique, 535
Polyposis coli, 535
Polyposis I and II, intestinal, 535
Polyposis III, intestinal, 536
POLYSPLENIA SYNDROME, 816
POLYSYNDACTYLY, 817
Polythelia, 815
Pompe disease, 11
Pompesche Krankheit, 11
POPLITEAL PTERYGIUM SYNDROME, 818
Porfiria aguda intermitente, 820
Porfiria eritropoyética congénita, 821
Porfiria variegada, 822
POROKERATOSIS, 819
Porokeratosis of Mibelli, 819
Poroqueratosis, 819
Porphyria, 203
PORPHYRIA, ACUTE INTERMITTENT, 820
Porphyria, congenital erythropoietic, 821
Porphyria erythropoetica (Günther), 821
PORPHYRIA, ERYTHROPOIETIC, 821

PORPHYRIA, VARIEGATE, 822
Porphyrie aigüe intermittente, 820
Porphyrie érthropoïètique congénitale, 821
Portal vein
    atresia, 468
    cavernous transformation, 468
    preduodenal, 468, 606
Portal-vein atresia, 468
Port-wine stain, 715
Postaxial polydactyly, types A and B, 814
Postductal coarctation, 73
Posterior embryotoxon, 439
Posterior marginal dysplasia of cornea, 439
Posterior marginalis dysplasia, 439
Posterior nasal atresia, 727
Posterolateral diaphragmatic hernia, 289
Postoperative psychologic disturbance, 152
Posture, stooped, 118
Posturing
    dystonic, 421
    progressive dystonic, 266
    unusual, 266
Potassium-losing nephropathy with low aldosterone, 590
Potbelly, 27
Potter syndrome, 856
Pouce en griffe, 175
PPSH, 831
Prader-Labhart-Willi syndrome, 823
PRADER–WILLI SYNDROME, 823
Preauricular appendages and deafness, 247
Preauricular pits, 329
Preaxial polydactyly, 814
Preaxial polydactyly of toes associated with syndactyly, 817
Precordial bulge on left, 82, 96
Preductal coarctation, 73
Preduodenal portal vein, 468
Prehelicine fistula, 329
Premature alopecia, 99
Premature lambdoid suture closure, 230
Premolar aplasia, hyperhidrosis and canities, 493
Premolar teeth
    accentuated buccal cusp of, 607
    globe-shaped crown of, 784
    pit in occlusal surface of, 276
Prenatal amputation of limb, 376, 874
Prenatal onset of increase of fractures, 777
Prepyloric atresia, 910
Prepyloric membrane, 910
Presence of aberrant gland tissue without nipple or areola, 815
Presence of complete supernumerary mammary glands, 815
Primaquine sensitive anemia, 420
Primäre Hypomagnesiämie, 514
Primärer Carnitinmangel der Muskulatur, 124
Primärer Laktasemangel, 567
Primary aphakia, 84
Primary basilar impression, 103
Primary cholesteatoma, 150
Primary enterokinase deficiency, 533
Primary essential lymphopenia (X-linked), 524
Primary familial hyperuricemia, 441
Primary familial xanthomatosis with involvement and calcification of adrenals, 1003
Primary hypomagnesemia with secondary hypocalcemia, 514
Primary infantile hypomagnesemia, 514
Primary lactase deficiency, 567
Primary macroglossia, 618
Primary micro-orchidism, 556

Primary noninflammatory lymphedema, 615
Proboscis lateral, 824
PROBOSCIS LATERALIS, 824
Procollagen peptidase deficiency, 338
Progenia, 626
PROGERIA, 825
Progéria à début tardif, 998
Progeria aultorum, 998
Progerie, 825
Progeronanism, 825
Prognathisme, 626
Prognatismo mandibular, 626
Progonoma, 711
Progressive arthroophthalmopathy, 90
Progressive chorea, 478
Progressive chorioretinal degeneration, 925
Progressive choroidal atrophy, 925
Progressive choroideremia, 925
Progressive cone-rod degeneration, 201
Progressive diaphyseal dysplasia, 290
Progressive extraocular muscular dystrophy, 752
Progressive high-tone nerve loss, 269
Progressive lenticular degeneration, 469
Progressive muscular dystrophy of childhood, 689
Progressive ophthalmoplegia, 752
Progressive septic granulomatous disease, 443
Prolaps des Kehlkopfdeckels, 573
Prolapse of laryngeal ventricle, 573
Prolapso de la válvula mitral, 668
Prolapso del ventrículo laríngeo, 573
Prolapsus du ventricule laryngée, 573
Prolapsus mitral, 668
Prolonged obstructive jaundice, 39
PROPIONIC ACIDEMIA, 826
Proprioception, loss of, 2, 995
Propylthiouracil (PTU) goiter, 435
Protanformen der Rot-Grün Blindheit, 197
Protanopia, 197
Protein intolerance, 491
Protein-losing enteropathy with dilated intestinal lymphatics, 534
Protéines de groupe, 446
Protéinose lipoidique, 599
Proteinosis lipodea, 599
Proteinuria and osteolysis, 128
Protocoproporphyria, 822
Protoporfiria eritropoyética, 362
Protoporphyria, erythropoietic, 362
Protubérance mandibulaire, 958
Protubérance palatine, 959
Proximal renal tubular acidosis, 858
Prurito localizado hereditario, 827
PRURITUS, HEREDITARY LOCALIZED, 827
PSEUDOACHONDROPLASTIC DYSPLASIA, 828
Pseudoachondroplastic spondyloepiphyseal dysplasia, 828
Pseudoaortic stenosis, 917
Pseudocholinesterase defect, 152
Pseudohemophilia, 996
Pseudohipoaldosteronismo, 829
Pseudohipoparatiroidismo, 830
Pseudo-Hurler polydystrophy, 673
Pseudohypertrophic muscular dystrophy, 688
Pseudohypertrophic muscular dystrophy, adult type, 687
Pseudohypertrophische Muskel-dystrophie, autosomal-rezessive Form, 688
Pseudohypertrophische Muskeldystrophie Typ Becker, 687
Pseudohypoadrenocorticism, 100

PSEUDOHYPOALDOSTERONISM, 829
PSEUDOHYPOPARATHYROIDISM, 830
Pseudohypoparathyroidism, Type 1
    (PHP-1), 830
Pseudohypoparathyroidism, Type 2
    (PHP-2), 830
Pseudohypophosphatasia, 516
Pseudometatropic dwarfism, 557
Pseudopolydystrophy, 673
Pseudoprognathism, 14, 112, 161, 162, 178,
    352, 941
Pseudo-pseudohypoparathyroidism, 830
PSEUDOVAGINAL PERINEOSCROTAL
    HYPOSPADIAS, 831
PSEUDOXANTHOMA ELASTICUM, 832
PSORIASIS VULGARIS, 833
Psychologic disturbance, postoperative, 152
Psychomotor retardation (see Section III,
    Table XXIII)
Psychosis, 498
    acute or chronic, 820, 822
    intermittent, 453

Ptérygium poplité, 818
Pterygoid-levator synkinesis, 548
Ptosis and miosis with ophthalmoplegia
    totalis, 753
PTOSIS, CONGENITAL, 834
Ptosis with superior rectus weakness, 834

Pulgar en gancho, 175
Pulmonalinsuffizienz, 838
Pulmonalklappen-Atresie, 837
Pulmonalstenose, 839
PULMONARY ARTERY COARCTATION,
    835
Pulmonary artery stenosis, 835
Pulmonary artery stenosis or atresia, 182,
    384, 632
Pulmonary atresia with hypoplastic right
    ventricle, 837
Pulmonary atresia with normal aortic root,
    837
Pulmonary branch stenosis, 835
Pulmonary infundibular stenosis, 586, 720
Pulmonary regurgitation due to intrinsic ab-
    normality of pulmonary valve, 838
Pulmonary valvar stenosis with intact ven-
    tricular septum, 839
Pulmonary valvar stenosis with normal
    aortic root, 839
PULMONARY VALVE ABSENT, 836
PULMONARY VALVE ATRESIA, 837
Pulmonary valve atresia with intact ven-
    tricular septum, 837
Pulmonary valve, bicuspid, 109
PULMONARY VALVE INCOMPETENCE,
    838
PULMONARY VALVE STENOSIS, 839
Pulmonary valve, stenosis, 381, 384, 586,
    720
PULMONARY VALVE, TETRACUSPID,
    840
Pulmonary vascular sling, 766
PULMONARY VENOUS CONNECTION,
    PARTIAL ANOMALOUS, 841
PULMONARY VENOUS CONNECTION,
    TOTAL ANOMALOUS, 842
PULPAL DYSPLASIA, 843
Pulsating venous aneurysm of external ear,
    313
Pulse rate
    absence of femoral, 73, 998
    bifid, carotid, 917
    bounding radial, 466, 800
    bradycardia, 454, 805, 946
    diminished femoral, 73, 998

diminished femoral pulse when supra-
    clavicular mass is compressed, 74
    intermittent tachycardia, 332
    paroxysmal fast radial pulse, 1002
    tachycardia, 51, 332, 424, 697, 820, 822,
        922
    weak diminished quality to radial, 546
PUNCTA AND CANALICULI, SUPER-
    NUMERARY, 844
Punctate epiphyseal dysplasia, 153
Punto de Darwin auricular (Marcador), 241
Pupil
    abnormalities, 309
    asymmetric, 583
    constricted, 475, 637, 753
    dilation of, 57, 721
    eccentric, 242
    imperforate pupillary membrane, 737,
        845
    increased sensitivity of pupil to
        methacholine as adult, 163
    inequality greater than 20%, 58
    irregularly shaped, 309, 583
    malposition of, 583, 593, 750
    sluggish, 344, 751
    sunsetting, 302, 481
    tissue remnants in pupillary space,
        121, 140, 732, 845
Pupillary light reflex
    red, 32, 34, 35, 36
    white, 866, 870, 994
PUPILLARY MEMBRANE PERSISTENCE,
    845
Pupillary reflexes, 43, 721, 865
Pure testicular dysgenesis, 437
Puretić syndrome, 644
Purpura thrombocytopénique avec histio-
    cytose, 942
Púrpura trombocitopénica con histocitosis,
    942
Pustular psoriasis, 833
PXE, 832
PYKNODYSOSTOSIS, 846
PYLE DISEASE, 847
Pyloric atresia, 910
PYLORIC STENOSIS, 848
Pylorusstenose, 848
Pyramidal signs, 344, 579
Pyridoxine dependency, 991
PYROGLUTAMIC ACIDEMIA, 849
Pyrroloporphyria, 820
Pyruvat-Dehydrogenase-Mangel, 851
PYRUVATE CARBOXYLASE DE-
    FICIENCY WITH LACTIC ACIDEMIA,
    850
PYRUVATE DEHYDROGENASE DE-
    FICIENCY, 851
PYRUVATE KINASE DEFICIENCY, 852
Pyruvatkarboxylase-Mangel mit Laktat-
    acidämie, 850
Pyruvatkinasemangel, 852

Q

Quadricuspid aortic valve, 81
Quadricuspid pulmonary valve, 840
Queilitis glandular, 144
Queloide, 551
Quemodectoma del oído medio, 145
Queratocono, 552
Queratopatía en bandas, 553
Queratosis palmar, leuconiquia y sordera,
    558
Queratosis palmoplantar y periodontoclasia,
    494

Quere Nasenfurche, 728
Quiste del colédoco, 149
Quiste dermoide o teratoma de la cabeza y
    cuello, 283
Quiste hepático solitario, 465
Quiste neurentérico de la médula espinal,
    894
Quistes dermoides orales, 760
Quistes dermoides orbitarios y periorbitarios,
    761
Quistes esplénicos, 240
Quistes laríngeos, 572
Quistes mesentéricos, 645
Quistes nasofaríngeos, 706
Quistes o senos de las hendiduras
    branquiales, 117

R

Rachitisme vitamino dépendant, 873
Racial lactase deficiency, 567
Radial aplasia, 853
RADIAL DEFECTS, 853
Radial dysplasia, 853
Radial hemimelia, 853
Radiation embryopathy, 383
Radiation of biologic mother during
    patient's prenatal life, 383
Radiation teratogenesis, 383
Radicular dentin dysplasia, 278
Radius
    anterior dislocation of radial head, 225
    bowing of, 19, 20, 646, 648, 685, 775,
        791
    defect of, 16, 455, 853, 981, 987
    dislocation of, 98, 769, 786
    dislocation of proximal radial head, 20,
        647
    dislocation of radial head, 121,
        221, 242, 648, 1001
    partial absence of, 231
    short, 19, 20, 166, 646, 769, 853, 875,
        923
Radikuläre Zahnverschmelzung, 928
RADIOULNAR SYNOSTOSIS, 854
Radius absent and thrombocytopenia, 941
Radius defekte, 853
Rand-und Kern-Katarakte, 132
Rapid izoniazid (INH) inactivation, 7
Raquitismo vitamino D-dependiente, 873
Recessive carpal-tarsal osteolysis, 129
Recessive early-onset neural deafness, 270
Recessive myopia and hearing loss, 251
Recessive optic atrophy, hearing loss and
    juvenile diabetes, 550
Recessive osteopetrosis, 780
Recessive profound sensorineural deafness,
    271
Rechtsaortenbogen, 77
Rectal aganglionosis, 192
Rectal atresia or stenosis, 193
Rectal duplication, 194
Rectoperineal fistula, 69, 72
Rectum
    empty on rectal exam, 192
    mass in, 194
    prolapse of, 535
    prolapse, recurrent, 237
Recurrent erosive corneal dystrophy, 214
Recurrent facial nerve paralysis, 378, 999
Red-green deutan series color blindness, 196
Red-green protan series color blindness, 197
Red palms, 792
Reduplication of stomach, 912

Reflexes
  absence of deep tendon, 2, 139, 265, 307, 628, 629, 693, 743, 746, 750, 759, 810, 850, 895, 924
  absence of primitive (Moro, root, stepping), 139, 628, 940
  decreased deep tendon, 49, 139, 143, 303, 307, 486, 578, 671, 686, 689, 695, 696, 736, 823, 895
  grasp or sucking reflex retained into childhood, 413
  increased deep tendon, 275, 295, 413, 492, 499, 515, 578, 671, 743, 755, 759, 808, 924
  sucking absent or poor, 121, 139, 823
  swallowing, absent or poor, 139, 823
Reflux oesophagien, 366
Refractive error (also see Astigmatism, Hyperopia, Myopia)
  major, 757
  uncorrectable, 188
  unspecified type, 963
Refsum disease, 810
Regional odontodysplasia, 739
Regurgitation, 364, 365
  of old food, 367, 369
  unspecified, 363, 366, 368
REIFENSTEIN SYNDROME, 855
Reis-Bücklers corneal dystrophy, 215
Reis-Bücklersche Hornhautdystrophie, 215
Reissner membrane, defect of, 315
Renal (see Kidney)
RENAL AGENESIS, BILATERAL, 856
RENAL AGENESIS, UNILATERAL, 857
Renal and digital anomalies and deafness, 264
Renal aplasia, unilateral, 857
Renal artery, occlusion of, 474
RENAL BICARBONATE REABSORPTIVE DEFECT, 858
RENAL DISEASE, POLYCYSTIC ADULT TYPE, 859
RENAL, GENITAL AND MIDDLE EAR ANOMALIES, 860
Renal glycosuria A and B, 861
RENAL GLYCOSURIA (MARKER), 861
Renal iminoglycinuria, 520
RENAL TUBULAR ACIDOSIS, 862
RENAL TUBULAR ACIDOSIS AND SENSORINEURAL DEAFNESS, 863
Renal tubular bicarbonate-losing syndrome, 858
RENAL TUBULAR SYNDROME, FANCONI, 864
Renale Glucosurie, 861
Renale tubuläre Azidose, 862
Renaler Bikarbonat-Resorptions-Defekt, 858
Respiration (also see Breath Sounds, Respiratory, each part and Section III, Table XXXI)
  airway obstruction, 74, 283, 367, 543, 945, 947
  choking on feedings, 139, 401, 577
  chronic lung disease, 237
  defect of, unspecified, general, 628, 777
  paradoxical respiration, 895
  reduced pulmonary ventilation, 702, 760
  use of accessory muscles of, 39
Respiratory failure, 39, 187
Respiratory obstruction
  caused by lipomas in neck, 601
  total, 572
Respiratory paralysis, 203, 820

Respiratory infection
  bronchitis, 522, 606, 986
  bronchitis chronic, 706, 944
  bronchitis recurrent, 263
  bronchitis subacute, 706
  pneumonia, 27, 51, 381, 384, 387, 522, 577, 714
  pneumonia alba, 385
  pneumonia aspiration, 187, 365, 366, 367, 368, 369, 471, 960
  pneumonia recurrent, 27, 363, 754, 879
  pulmonary infection, 138, 470, 611, 612
  recurrent, 120, 237, 333, 525, 680, 895, 967
Respiratory system (see Section III, Table XXXI)
Respiratory tumor
  cyst of lung, 630
  cystic areas in lung with air-fluid levels, 120
  cysts throughout lung, 605, 859
Respiratory vasculature
  increased, 79, 96, 218, 286, 297, 298, 347, 581, 665, 800, 842, 968, 989
  decreased, 92, 581, 612, 731, 835, 837, 839, 938, 968, 969, 979
  prominent, 838, 972
Retardation (see Section III, Table XXIII for items listed below)
  delayed developmental milestones
  growth
  mental
  motor
  psychomotor
Reticular pigmented dermatosis, 703
Retina (also see Section III, Table XXIV)
  bilateral pigmented macular cleft, 621
  blond retina in pigmented races, 32, 35
  bone spicule pigmentation of, 43, 201
  cleft, 242, 733
  coalescent cysts of Blessig, 871
  dark grey, 716
  degeneration of, 2, 41, 43, 70, 136, 189, 201, 449, 578, 675, 713, 810, 865, 983, 998
  depigmentation, 34, 35, 36, 201, 479, 550, 578
  detached, 90, 182, 266, 338, 474, 479, 557, 583, 630, 661, 675, 721, 732, 783, 866, 870, 872, 879
  fold in, 620, 721, 867, 872
  hemorrhage of, 140, 622, 763, 764, 832, 872
  hyperpigmentation of, 479, 865, 869, 925, 983
  mixed defects of, 159
  red-orange, 32
  retinoschisis, 479, 871
  scalloped plaques, 449
  scarring, 622, 872
  tapetoretinal degeneration, typical, 2, 70, 136, 578, 713, 810, 865, 869, 983, 998
  unilateral slate grey, 640
  velvety pigment, 449
  white dots in, 399
  yellow flecks in, 400
  yellow-white lesions in, 734
Retina-Aplasie, 865
Retina-Falte, 867
RETINAL APLASIA, 865
Retinal blood vessels
  angioid retinal streaks, 832
  artery spasm, 820, 822

  decreased number of, 140
  dilatation of, 41, 189, 373, 868, 869, 872, 925, 983
  narrowing of, 449, 872
  pulled into fold, 867
  sludge phenomenon in, 47
  tortuosity of, 163, 373, 872
  vascular changes of diabetes, 549
Retinal degeneration associated with spinocerebellar ataxia, 745
RETINAL DYSPLASIA, 866
RETINAL FOLD, 867
Retinal macula (also see Section III, Table XXIV)
  abnormal position of, 620
  atrophic degeneration of, 400, 776
  cherry red spot, 431, 433, 434, 671, 717
  cystic degeneration of, 871
  degeneration of, 93, 136, 622, 734, 745, 756, 869, 998
  edema of, 534
  enlargement of, 745
  exudative lesion, 622
  focal hyperpigmentation, 195, 745
  pallor of, 745
  white plaques on, 734
RETINAL TELANGIECTASIA AND HYPOGAMMAGLOBULINEMIA, 868
Retinal tumors
  cysts, 479
  hamartoma, 975
  grey mass in periphery, 872
  pink tumor with many surface blood vessels, 870
  protuberant retina, 733
  pseudotumors, 721
  retinoblastoma, 167, 995
  yellow-orange cystic lesion, 622
Retinale Dysplasie, 866
Rétinite pigmentaire, 869
RETINITIS PIGMENTOSA, 869
Retinitis pigmentosa and congenital deaf-mutism, 983
Retinitis pigmentosa-dysacusis syndrome, 983
Retinitis pigmentosa sine pigmenta, 869
RETINOBLASTOMA, 870
Retinopathy of prematurity, 872
RETINOSCHISIS, 871
Retinosquisis, 871
Retour veineux pulmonaire anormal total, 842
Rétrécissement du canal médullaire, 976
Rétrécissement mitral, 669
RETROLENTAL FIBROPLASIA, 872
Retrolental fibroplasia, 620
Retrosternal diaphragmatic hernia, 289
Rezessiv erbliche Carpo-tarsale Osteolyse, 129
Rezessive Schalleitungsschwerhörigkeit, 271
Rezidivierende erosive Hornhautdystrophie, 214
Rh hump, 340
Rheumatoid agglutinators (Raggs), 71
Rib, defect of, 121, 157, 735, 941
Rib gap defects with micrognathia, 138
RICKETS, VITAMIN D-DEPENDENT, 873
Rieger syndrome, 439
Riggs type nyctalopia, 719
Right aortic arch types I, II and III, 77

Right aortic arch with or without retro-
esophageal anomalous subclavian
artery, 77
Right common carotid artery originating
from left innominate artery in cases
with a right-sided aortic arch, 200
Right ventricular endocardial fibrosis fibro-
elastosis, 349
Right ventricular primary myocardial hyper-
trophy with endocardial fibro-
elastosis, 349
Right ventricular subendocardial fibro-
elastosis, 349
Riley-Day syndrome, 307
RING CONSTRICTIONS, 874
Ringförmige Strikturen, 874
Ring-like corneal dystrophy, 215
ROBERTS SYNDROME, 875
Robin anomaly, 182
Robinow-Silverman-Smith syndrome, 876
ROBINOW SYNDROME, 876
Rod body myopathy, 696
Rod-cone dystrophy, 869
Rod monochromatism, 198
Rokitansky-Küster-Hauser syndrome, 682
Roman-Ward syndrome, 610
Romano-Ward syndrome, 610
Rootless teeth, 278
Rosenberg-Chutorian syndrome, 268
Rotación intestinal incompleta, 537
Rotation intestinale incompléte, 537
Rötelnembryopathie, 384
Round
calvaria, 281
face (moon), 114, 139, 163, 170, 447,
554, 557, 830, 900
Rubella embryopathy, 384
Rubella malformation syndrome, 384
Rubéole congénitale, 384
Rubinstein-Taybi syndrome, 119
Rud syndrome, 741
Rudimentary uterine horn, 684
Ruiter-Pompen-Wyers syndrome, 373
Ruptured omphalocele, 748
Russell-Silver syndrome, 887
Rutherford syndrome, 408

S

SACROCOCCYGEAL TERATOMA, 877
Saethre-Chotzen syndrome, 14
Sakati syndrome, 13
Sakrococcygeal teratome, 877
Salivary gland
chronic drooling, 469, 754
decreased salivation, 378, 799
excessive salivation, 364, 365
hypoplasia of, 664
parotid mass, 878
swelling of parotid, 799
SALIVARY GLAND, MIXED TUMOR, 878
Salivary gland virus infection, 381
Salmon patch, 715
Sandhoff disease, 433
Sanfilippo syndrome, 677
(SC) Pseudothalidomide syndrome, 875
Scalp cylindroma types I and II, 235
Scalp-skull and limbs, absence defect of,
459
Scaphocephaly, 230 (see also Section III,
Table XXIX)
Scapula
abnormal rotation of, 901

close to midline, 901
defect of, 98, 455, 884
elevation of, 257, 394, 586, 712, 901,
967, 986
round, 884
small, 122, 185, 455, 884, 901
Scapula elevata, 901
Schalleitungsschwerhörigkeit mit vor-
wiegendem Ausfall mittlerer
Frequenzen, 267
Schalleitungsschwerhörigkeit und de-
formierte, tiefsitzende Ohren, 254
Scheibe cochleosaccular degeneration of
inner ear, 315
Scheidenatresie, 984
Scheie syndrome, 675
Schilddrüsen-Dysgenesie, 946
Schistoglossia, 952
Schizencephaly with head enlarge-
ment, 480
Schizophrenia, 229
Schlaffe Ohrmuschel, 326
Schlichting syndrome, 213
Schmelz-dentinhypoplasie mit Tetra-
zyklinverfarbung, 341
Schmelz-dentinverfarbung durch Erythro-
blastosis Fetalis, 340
Schneebedeckte Zähne, 935
Schnyder crystalline corneal dystrophy, 216
Schräge Gesichtsspalte, 375
Schubert-Bornschein type nyctalopia, 719
Schulter-Beckengürtelform der Muskel-
dystrophie, 691
Schusterbrust, 802
Schwalbe line, prominent, 439
Schwartz-Jampel syndrome, 155
Schwere Form des Transglucuronylase-
mangels, 961
SCIMITAR SYNDROME, 879
Sclera
blue, 777
dark pigmentation, 37, 716
exposed, 733
posterior staphyloma, 732
rupture of, 338
scleral rims exposed, 539
unilateral focal pigmentation, 640
Sclerocornea, 205
Sclérose cérébrale à cellules globoïdes, 415
Sclérose cérébrale-type I, 803
Sclérose tubéreuse, 975
SCLEROSTEOSIS, 880
Sclerotic bone disease, 290
Scoliosis (also see Section III, Table
XXIX)
progressive, 293
thoracolumbar, 644
with onset in infancy, 153
Scrotal tongue, 956
Scrotum
bifid, 50, 167, 578, 818, 831, 855, 909
hooded, 1, 401
hydrocele persistent, 529
inguinal mass in, 529
labioscrotal fold, incomplete fusion of,
29, 401
labioscrotal fusion posterior, 173
prominent raphe, 168
small, 105, 159, 823
unrugated, 438
Seborrheic alopecia, 99
SECKEL SYNDROME, 881
Secondary or apparent aphakia, 84
Secuestración del lóbulo pulmonar, 612

SED, 898
SED congenita, 897
Seizures (see Section III, Table XXXVI)
focal, 188, 851, 961, 975
refractory to usual anticonvulsant medication, 486, 713, 991
with onset during infancy, 434, 492,
975
with onset in childhood, 44, 118, 478,
713, 915
with onset in neonatal period, 396, 492,
514, 991
Seizures, adenoma sebaceum and mental
retardation, 975
Selective anosmia, 70
Self-healing multiple squamous epithelioma,
359
Self-mutilation, 422, 588
Semicircular canals, defect of, 142, 249,
272, 315, 385, 728, 982
Semilethale Form der Taubstummheit,
243
Seminiferous tubule dysgenesis, 556
Senile nanism, 825
Senile retinoschisis, autosomal recessive,
871
Sensation
absence of, 48, 265, 270, 693, 894,
924
loss of temperature, 810
moderate loss of position and pain,
743, 810
Sensibilité gustative à la thio-urée, 809
Sensorineural deafness and corneal dystrophy,
206
Sensorineural deafness associated with dia-
betes, 246
Sensorineural deafness, profound, 271
Sensorineural deafness, short stature,
vitiligo, muscle wasting and
achalasia, 275
Sensorineural hearing loss (also see Section
III, Table XXV)
Sensorineural unilateral hearing loss, 274
Sensory peripheral neuropathy, 93, 143,
265, 270, 398, 810, 820
Séparation de l'artère sous-clavière et de
l'aorte, 546
Septum vaginal transverso, 985
Séquestration d'un lobe pulmonaire, 612
Serum carnosinase deficiency, 126
Serum normal agglutinants (SNaggs), 71
17-Ketosteroid reductase deficiency
(some cases), 831
17-20-Desmolase-Mangel, 904
Severe infantile myopia, 699
Severe, recurrent, or persistent neonatal
and infantile hypoglycemia, familial,
512
Sex, external characteristics of opposite,
903
Sexual ateleotic dwarfism, 447
Sexual development, precocious, 391, 887
Sexual infantilism, 437, 438, 616, 741,
977
regressive with onset at puberty, 460
Sexual maturation
altered, 908, 971
deficient pubertal, 70, 460, 556, 578,
785, 823, 825, 855, 903, 909, 977
delayed, 302, 305, 447, 578, 823
eunuchoid habitus, 93, 438
female gender with virilization, 498, 902,
908, 971

Sexual maturation – *Continued*
  male gender with feminization, 971
  male gender with mild virilization, 909
  male habitus, premature development
    of mature, 908
  male, secondary gonadal atrophy in young,
    460
  poor, 437, 438, 616, 741, 977
  sex, external characteristics of opposite,
    903
  sexual development precocious, 391, 887
  sexual infantilism, 437, 438, 616, 741,
    977
  sexual infantilism, regressive with onset
    at puberty, 460
  sexual maturation altered, 908, 971
  virilization at puberty, 173
SHORT FINGER–FLEXOR–TENDONS
    AND INABILITY TO OPEN
    MOUTH FULLY, 882
SHORT RIB–POLYDACTYLY SYN-
    DROME, MAJEWSKI TYPE, 883
SHORT RIB–POLYDACTYLY SYN-
    DROME, SALDINO–NOONAN
    TYPE, 884
Short stature (see Section III, Table XXIX)
Short stature and sexual infantilism, 977
Short stature, characteristic facies, mental
    retardation, macrodontia and skeletal
    anomalies, 554
Short stature, elongated ear lobe, elbow-hip
    dislocation, 98
Shortened or defective valve tissue, 666
Shoulder
  decreased abduction at, 901
  decrease of rotary motion of shoulder
    joint, 88
  decreased range of motion of, 674, 675
  dislocation of, 570
  drooping, 185
  flexion contractures of, 413
  hyperextensible, 185
  hunched, 691, 898
  narrow, 157, 185, 825
  that can tough anteriorly, 185
  tumor of shoulder which destroys bone,
    711
Schwachman-Diamond-Oski-Kaw syn-
    drome, 885
SCHWACHMAN SYNDROME, 885
Shy-Magee disease, 134
Sialangiectasis, 799
Sialectasis, 799
Sialidosis, 671
Sialorrhoea hereditaria, 448
Siamese twins, 202
Siamesische Zwillinge, 202
Sichelzellanämie, 886
SICKLE CELL ANEMIA, 886
Siderophilin, 95
Sífilis congénita, 385
Sillon nasal transversal, 728
SILVER SYNDROME, 887
Simple anhidrosis, 56
Simple iris coloboma, 57
Simple recessive optic atrophy, 755
Sincinesia máxilo-palpebral, 548
Sindactilia, 923
Sindactilia de Poland, 813
Síndrome amielo-cerebro hipohidrótico, 44
Síndrome asplénico, 92
Síndrome C, 121
Síndrome campomiélico, 122
Síndrome cardioauditivo, 123
Síndrome cardiomélico, 455

Síndrome cerebro-costo-mandibular, 138
Síndrome cerebro-hepato-renal, 139
Síndrome cerebro-óculo-facio esquelético,
    140
Síndrome cérvico-óculo-acústico, 142
Síndrome cráneo-óculo-dental, 229
Síndrome cúbito-mamario tipo Pallister, 981
Síndrome de Aarskog, 1
Síndrome de Aberfeld, 155
Síndrome de Alström, 41
Síndrome de angio-osteohipertrófico, 55
Síndrome de artrogriposis de Herrmann-
    Opitz, 470
Síndrome de ausencia del radio y trombo-
    citopenia, 941
Síndrome de Bartter, 100
Síndrome de Basan, 102
Síndrome de Berlín, 105
Síndrome de Bloom, 112
Síndrome de braquidactilia-sinfalangismo
    tipo WL, 1001
Síndrome de cataratas e ictiosis, 131
Síndrome de Chédiak-Higashi, 143
Síndrome de Cockayne, 189
Síndrome de Coffin-Lowry, 190
Síndrome de coloboma y atresia anal, 544
Síndrome de costillas cortas y polidactilia
    tipo Majewski, 883
Síndrome de costillas cortas y polidactilia
    tipo Saldino-Noonan, 884
Síndrome de cráneosinostosis y aplasia
    radial, 231
Síndrome de-Lange, 242
Síndrome de dextrocardia, bronquiectasias y
    sinusitis, 285
Síndrome de Dubowitz, 299
Síndrome de Dyggve-Melchior-Clausen, 306
Síndrome de eczema, trombocitopenia y
    diarrea infecciosa, 523
Síndrome de Ehlers-Danlos, 338
Síndrome de esferofaquia y braquimorfia,
    893
Síndrome de Fanconi, 864
Síndrome de feminización testicular in-
    completo, 50
Síndrome de fisura media del rostro, 635
Síndrome de Gardner, 536
Síndrome de Gorlin-Chaudhry-Moss, 440
Síndrome de Grebe, 445
Síndrome de Hanhart, 451
Síndrome de hemangioma y trombocito-
    penia, 456
Síndrome de hernia uterina, 683
Síndrome de Herrmann-Pallister-Tiddy-
    Opitz tipo KGB, 554
Síndrome de hipercalcemia precoz, 999
Síndrome de hipertelorismo e hipospadias,
    505
Síndrome de hipogonadismo y ataxia, 93
Síndrome de Horner, 475
Síndrome de Klinefelter, 556
Síndrome de Kniest, 557
Síndrome de Kuskokwim, 560
Síndrome de la delección 5p, 163
Síndrome de la delección 18p, 158
Síndrome de la delección 18q, 159
Síndrome de la monosomía G tipo I, 170
Síndrome de la monosomía G tipo II, 172
Síndrome de la trimetadiona fetal, 388
Síndrome de la trisomía 8, 157
Síndrome de la trisomía 13, 168
Síndrome de la trisomía 18, 160
Síndrome de la trisomía 21, 171
Síndrome de Larsen, 570
Síndrome de Laurence-Moon-Biedl, 578

Síndrome de lentigos múltiples, 586
Síndrome de Lesch-Nyhan, 588
Síndrome de Liddle, 590
Síndrome de lisencefalía, 603
Síndrome de malabsorción de la metionina,
    657
Síndrome de Marden-Walker, 629
Síndrome de Marfan, 630
Síndrome de McDonough, 632
Síndrome de Meckel, 634
Síndrome de Menkes, 643
Síndrome de Mohr, 771
Síndrome de Moynahan, 670
Síndrome de Naegeli, 703
Síndrome de Nathalie, 785
Síndrome de nevus a células basales, 101
Síndrome de nevus sebáceos lineares, 593
Síndrome de nevus vesiculosos azulados, 113
Síndrome de Noonan, 720
Síndrome de oligofrenia, epilepsia,
    ictiosis, 741
Síndrome de Pallister tipo W, 791
Síndrome de placenta circumvalada, 187
Síndrome de Prader-Willi, 823
Síndrome de pseudogliomas y osteoporosis,
    783
Síndrome de pterigión poplíteo, 818
Síndrome de pulgar y dedo gordo del pie
    ancho, 119
Síndrome de QT largo sin sordera, 610
Síndrome de Reifenstein, 855
Síndrome de retardo mental y megalocórnea,
    638
Síndrome de Roberts, 875
Síndrome de rostro fetal, 876
Síndrome de scimitar, 879
Síndrome de Silver, 887
Síndrome de Smith-Lemli-Opitz, 891
Síndrome de Swyer, 437
Síndrome de temblor y ulceración duodenal,
    963
Síndrome de timoma y agamaglobulinemia,
    944
Síndrome de triploidía, 169
Síndrome de trisomía parcial del cromo-
    soma 11q, 161
Síndrome de trisomía parcial del cromo-
    soma 14q tipo I, 166
Síndrome de trisomía parcial del cromo-
    soma 14q tipo II, 165
Síndrome de Ullrich-Turner, 977
Síndrome de Usher, 983
Síndrome de Van den Bosch, 986
Síndrome de visceromegalía, onfalocele y
    macroglosia, 104
Síndrome de von Hippel-Lindau, 995
Síndrome de Waardenburg, 997
Síndrome de Werner, 998
Síndrome de Winchester, 1000
Síndrome de Wolff-Parkinson-White, 1002
Síndrome del cromosoma 4p–, 164
Síndrome del cromosoma 11q, 162
Síndrome del cromosoma 13q–, 167
Síndrome del testículo feminizante, 49
Síndrome fetal por alcohol, 379
Síndrome FG, 754
Síndrome G, 401
Síndrome génito-branquio-esquelético, 118
Síndrome hidantoínico fetal, 382
Síndrome óculocerebrorenal, 736
Síndrome óculomandíbulofacial, 738
Síndrome óculo-óseo-dentario, 737
Síndrome ónico-patelar, 704
Síndrome oro-cráneo-digital, 769
Síndrome oro-facio-digital I, 770

Síndrome oto-pálato-digital, 786
Síndrome otodentario, 784
Síndrome trico-rino-falángico tipo I, 966
Síndrome trico-rino-falángico, tipo II, 967
Single left or right coronary artery, 219
Single or recurrent episodes of Bell palsy, 378
Single transposition of great vessels, 962
Single ventricle with rudimentary outflow chamber, 286
Singuläre Koronararterie, 219
Singulärer Papillarmuskel des linken Ventrikels, 582
Sinostosis húmeroradial, 477
Sinostosis radial cubital, 854
Sinuses, absence of frontal, 797
Sipple syndrome, 351
Siringomielia, 924
Situs inversus (complet, partiel), 888
Situs inversus del disco óptico, 757
Situs inversus der Leber, 606
Situs inversus der Papille, 757
Situs inversus intestinalis, 888
Situs inversus visceral, 888
SITUS INVERSUS VISCERUM, 888
Six-fingered dwarfism, 156
SIXTH NERVE PARALYSIS, 889
Skeletal changes, progressive, 516, 675, 678
Skeletal frame (also see Section III, Table XXIX)
    asymmetric, 281, 458
    long trunk, 157, 303
    lower body segment greater than upper, 556
    narrow trunk, 157
    proportionate, 88
    small, 105, 157
    short trunk, 121, 783
    tall, prenatally, 137
    tall with long limbs, 90
Skeletal malformations, heart disease and conductive hearing loss, 667
Skeletal system (see parts and Section III, Table XXIX)
Skin color (also see Differentiating characteristics, Skin lesions, Hair, Nails, and Section III, Table XXVIII)
    banal bronze tan, 460
    brown round flat areas with rete ridges, 586
    café-au-lait spots, 12, 352, 391, 539, 712, 763, 887, 975
    depigmentation (see Section III, Table XXVIII)
    erythema nodosum, 27
    erythematous, 27, 34, 35, 36, 107, 129, 131, 361, 362, 641
    fair, 808
    flush of, 102, 351, 474
    freckling, heavy, 712
    hyperpigmentation (see Section III, Table XXVIII)
    malar flush, 474
    salmon pink serpiginous, 54
    slate grey, 143
    violaceous hue, 712
    yellow-brown, diffuse, 406
    yellow pallor, 406
Skin depigmentation (see Section III, Table XXVIII)
Skin differentiating characteristics (also see Section III, Table XXVIII)
    aged appearance of, 825
    atrophy of, 644, 738
    coarse, rough, 45

delayed healing of, 4, 338
dimple, 292
dry, 45, 56, 102, 131, 171, 333, 543, 808, 825, 946, 949
dull, 825
easy bruisability of, 338, 406, 462, 942, 996
excessive oiliness, 788
fragile, 338, 822
glossy, 88, 825
gyrate convolutions, 18
hemorrhagic spots or excess bleeding, 4, 187, 456, 777, 942
hyperextensible, lax, 190, 233, 338
hypersensitivity to sunlight, 203, 362, 453, 821, 1004, 1005
hypoplasia, 825
inelastic, 811
large open pores, 788
photosensitivity of, 822
pock-like scarring, 599
redundant or excessive folds, 121, 161, 190, 233, 587, 940, 967
shiny, 641
soft, 447
streaks on, 281
sweating defect of, 5, 44, 179, 189, 259, 261, 281, 333, 351, 398, 448, 493, 703, 788, 820, 822, 924
tense, 641
thickened, 131, 362, 398, 644, 672, 676, 822, 825, 982, 1000
thin, 777
tight, 88, 672, 825
waxy appearance, 88
webbing between pelvis and heel, 818
webbing intracrural, 88
webbing of neck, 51, 158, 382, 578, 720
webbing of skin on sides of neck, 586, 977
wrinkled excessively, 447, 825
Skin hyperpigmentation (see Section III, Table XXVIII)
SKIN LEIOMYOMAS, MULTIPLE, 890
Skin lesions (also see Section III, Table XXVIII)
    acne, 908
    angiokeratoma (also see hemangioma), 373, 398
    blister, gelatinous, 644
    bullae (also see rash), 526, 822
    carcinoma, 101, 1004, 1005
    cyst, dermoid, 536
    cyst, epidermoid, 101, 536
    eczema, 27, 159, 299, 333, 522, 523, 524
    edema, 47, 54, 153, 265, 340, 362, 395, 403, 431, 460, 514, 533, 534, 709, 710, 883, 884, 886, 939, 949, 973, 977
    fibroma, 101, 536, 977
    fibrosarcoma, 536, 1004, 1005
    granulomatous lesion, 443
    gyrate convolutions of scalp, 18
    hemangioma (also see angiokeratoma), 55, 113, 121, 346, 456, 466, 634
    ichthyosis, 131, 153, 154, 258, 741, 810
    keratosis, 703, 1004, 1005
    lichenoid infiltration, 644
    linear scleroderma, 641
    lipoma, 101, 505, 536, 600, 601, 874
    lymphedema, 154, 614, 615, 874, 977
    macules, 384
    milia, 101, 393, 770

myxedema, 946
nevus, 104, 119, 337, 505, 539, 560, 593, 715, 975, 977
nodule, 282, 411, 416, 425, 489, 644, 676, 717, 832, 890
papilloma, 281, 412
papular thickening, 362
papule, 131, 143, 281, 339, 359, 551, 561, 598, 599, 819, 822
plaque, 275, 551, 599, 811, 819, 975
psoriasis, 15, 833
rash, 362, 381, 384, 385, 387, 522, 808
scar, 189, 338, 359, 362, 777, 821, 822
soft tissue swelling, 221
streak, 281
telangiectasia, 94, 281, 373, 601, 644
tumor (also see Skin lesions – carcinoma, fibroma, fibrosarcoma, and cysts), 12, 235, 712
ulceration, 609, 700, 821, 822, 924
verrucose lesion, 412, 526, 599, 819, 986
vesicle, 821, 822
vesiculobullous, 15
vitiligo, 275
xanthoma, 425, 488, 489, 495, 500, 501, 598, 717

Skin lesions, papular, 339
Skin, localized absence, 608
Skin, localized absence, blistering and nail abnormalities, 609
Sklerosteose, 880
Skull (see Section III, Table XXIX)
Sliding hernia, 529
Smelling loss, congenital, 70
SMITH–LEMLI–OPITZ SYNDROME, 891
SNC-malformación arteriovenosa, 186

Solitäre Leberzyste, 465
Some cases of incomplete androgen insensitivity syndrome, 855
Some causes of hydrometrocolpos, 483
Some forms of atypical cystinuria, 86
Some types of thyroid organification defects, 947

Sordera a los tonos bajos, 260
Sordera, anomalías renales y digitales, 264
Sordera coclear, miopía y oligofrenia, 251
Sordera con foveas auriculares, 247
Sordera de conducción bilateral y ausencia de la articulación yunque-estribo, 244
Sordera de conducción y orejas malformadas de implantación baja, 254
Sordera del oído interno unilateral, 274
Sordera-epífisis punteaday bocio y PBI elevado, 257
Sordera, estatura baja, vitíligo, emaciación muscular y acalasia, 275
Sordera neural recesiva precoz, 270
Sordera neurosensorial a las frecuencias medias, 267
Sordera neurosensorial, diverticulitis del intestino delgado y neuropatía, 265
Sordera neurosensorial, polineuropatía y atrofia óptica, 268
Sordera neurosensorial profunda recesiva, 271
Sordera por sensibilidad a la estreptomicina, 272
Sordera progresiva hereditaria para las frecuencias elevadas, 269
Sordera, queratopaquidermia y constricciones digitales, 259
Sordera y atrofia del nervio óptico progresiva, 253

Sordera y bocio, 249
Sordera y dermatitis atópica, 245
Sordera y diabetes, 246
Sordera y ónicodistrofia, 252
Sorsby syndrome, 621
Sotos syndrome, 137
South African genetic porphyria, 822
Spasm
    carpopedal, 515
    infantile, 126, 135, 713
Spastic díplegia, hereditary, 295
Spastic quadriplegia, 86, 154, 398, 743,
    759

Spasticity
    progressive, 432
    with onset before age 1 yr, 415
    with onset during infancy, 492

Spastische Diplegie, 295
Spätmanifeste Fazialisparese, 378
Spätmanifeste Osteopetrose, 780
Spätmanifester Immunokörpermangel, 521
Spätmanifestes Lymphödem, 615
Sphärophakie-Brachymorphie-Syndrom, 893
Sphärozytose, 892
Speech (also see Voice, and Section III,
        Table XXVII)
    delayed, 138, 157, 162, 247, 263, 264,
        266, 422, 450, 803, 823, 967
    indistinct, 12, 93, 97, 123, 155, 157, 180,
        266, 269, 270, 376, 388, 450, 469,
        472, 478, 618, 651, 722, 742, 744,
        745, 746, 747, 818, 958, 959, 995
    scanning, 742, 744, 746, 747
    slow, 94
    slurred, 223, 508
Sphenoid bone, defect of, 28, 712
Spherocytic anemia congenital, 892

SPHEROCYTOSIS, 892
SPHEROPHAKIA–BRACHYMORPHIA
        SYNDROME, 893
Sphingomyelin lipidosis, 717
Spielmeyer-Vogt disease, 713
Spina bifida, 182, 230, 329, 735
    aperta, 481
    cervical, 247
    lumbosacral, 292, 602
    occulta, 101, 157, 159, 162, 281, 901
    spina bifida occulta of L5, 22
    spina bifida occulta of S1, 22
    thoracic, 292
Spina bifida cystica with paralysis, 693
Spina bifida cystica without neurologic
        deficit, 642
Spinal cord
    cleft, 292, 693
    compression of, 10, 517, 678
    large, 924
    rootlet irritation of, 10, 678
Spinal cord cavitation, 924
SPINAL CORD, NEURENTERIC CYST,
        894
Spinal dysraphism syndrome, 602
SPINAL MUSCULAR ATROPHY, 895
Spleen
    absence of, 606, 727
    cyst, 240, 859
    polysplenia, 816
    ruptured, 406, 892
    splenomegaly (see Section III, Table
        XXXIII)
Splenic agenesis, 92
Splenic cysts, 240
Split-hand deformity, 336
Split hand or foot with cleft lip, 337

Split notocord syndrome, 292
SPONDYLOCOSTAL DYSPLASIA, 896
SPONDYLOEPIPHYSEAL DYSPLASIA
        CONGENITA, 897
SPONDYLOEPIPHYSEAL DYSPLASIA
        TARDA, 898
Spondylokostale Dysplasie, 896
SPONDYLOMETAPHYSEAL CHONDRO-
        DYSPLASIA, TYPE KOZLOWSKI,
        899
SPONDYLOTHORACIC DYSPLASIA, 900
Spondylothorakale Dysplasie, 900
Spongiöse Dystrophie der weissen Hirn-
        substanz, 115
Spongy degeneration of brain, 115
Spontaneous keloids, 551
Spoon nails, 559
Sporadic nongoitrous cretinism, 946
Sporadische olivopontocerebellare
        Atrophie, 746
"Spotted bones," 781
Spotted corneal dystrophy, 212
SPRENGEL DEFORMITY, 901
Sprengelsche Difformität, 901
Stance, wide-based, 825
Stanesco dysostosis, 226
Stapes
    defect of, 28, 247, 331, 627, 664, 773,
        786
    fixed footplate, 97, 183, 315, 664, 667,
        1001
    fused, 787
Stargardt disease, 400
Starvation, 910
Stationäre Nachtblindheit, 719
Stature (also see Section III, Table XXIX)
    disproportionate, short prenatally, with
        short limbs, 8, 9, 10, 16, 153, 154,
        156, 293, 940
    disproportionate, short, with short limbs,
        19, 20, 122, 226, 308, 358, 557, 646,
        647, 648, 649, 652, 653, 685, 828
    disproportionate, short prenatally, with
        short trunk (decreased crown-pubis
        length), 896, 900
    disproportionate short trunk (decreased
        crown-pubis length), 306, 394, 671,
        798, 897, 898, 899
    markedly short, 828
    proportionate, short, 185, 302, 303, 382,
        447, 738, 976
    short (see Section III, Table XXIX)
    short, markedly, 828
    tall, 85, 90, 137, 556, 578, 670

Steinert disease, 702
Sténose aortique supra-valvulaire, 78
Sténose de la'artère pulmonaire, 835
Sténose de l'oesophage, 369
Sténose des valves aortiques, 80
Sténose des valvules pulmonaires, 839
Sténose du pylore, 848
Sténose fibreuse sous-aortique, 916
Sténose nasopharyngée, 707
Sténose sous-aortique, 917
Sténose sous-glottique, 919
Sténose tricuspidienne, 970
Sténose ventriculaire droite, 731
Sténoses pulmonaire multiples, surdité
        mixte, brachytéléphalangie calci-
        fication des cartilages, 263
Stenosis at the conus elasticus, 571
Stenosis of anterior nares, 723
Stenosis of aortic valve, 80
Stenosis of aqueduct of Sylvius, 481
Stenosis of ostium infundibulum, 731

Stenosis of the common pulmonary vein,
        204
Stenosis, subglottic, 919
Stenotic bicuspid aortic valve, 80
Sternum (also see pectus carinatum and
        excavatum)
    defect of, 182, 632
    long xiphoid process of, 121
    short, 121, 160, 242
STEROID 3β–HYDROXYSTEROID DE-
        HYDROGENASE DEFICIENCY,
        909
STEROID 11β–HYDROXYLASE DE-
        FICIENCY, 902
STEROID 17α–HYDROXYLASE DE-
        FICIENCY, 903
STEROID 17, 20–DESMOLASE DE-
        FICIENCY, 904
STEROID 18–HYDROXYLASE DE-
        FICIENCY, 905
STEROID 18–HYDROXYSTEROID DE-
        HYDROGENASE DEFICIENCY,
        906
STEROID 20–22 DESMOLASE DEFICIENCY,
        907
STEROID 21–HYDROXYLASE DE-
        FICIENCY, 908
Stickler syndrome, 90
Stilling-Türk-Duane syndrome, 889
Stippled epiphyses, deafness and goiter
        with high levels of serum thyroid
        hormone, 257
Stomach
    distended, 300, 910
    displaced, 528
    failure of rotation, 913
    failure to differentiate into fundus,
        body and pyloric areas, 913
    gastric perforation, 823, 911
    gastrocolic fistula, 912
    herniation above diaphragm, 471
    intussusception of gastric wall, 535, 911
    polyps, multiple in, 412
    pyloric stenosis, infantile, 162, 388, 754
STOMACH ATRESIA, 910
STOMACH DIVERTICULUM, 911
STOMACH DUPLICATION, 912
STOMACH HYPOPLASIA, 913
STOMACH TERATOMA, 914
Störung des Jod-Transports, 542
Strabismus (also see Section III, Table
        XXIV)
    alternating, 250, 791
    convergent, 159, 182, 223, 261, 394
    divergent, 163, 225, 504, 667
    pseudostrabismus, 620
    vertical, 261

Strahlenembryopathie, 383
Strangulated hernia, 529
Streeter dysplasia, 874
Streptomycin-sensitivity deafness, 272
Stridor (see Section III, Table XXXI)
Structural defect of CNS (see Section III,
        Table XXXVI)
STURGE–WEBER SYNDROME, 915
SUBAORTIC STENOSIS, FIBROUS, 916
SUBAORTIC STENOSIS, MUSCULAR,
        917
Subarachnoid hemorrhage, 859
Subclavian artery, anomalous origin of
        contralateral, 63
Subclavian artery, isolation from aorta, 546
Subcostosternal hernia, 289
SUBGLOTTIC HEMANGIOMA, 918

SUBGLOTTIC STENOSIS, 919
Subglottic stenosis, hard, 919
Subglottic stenosis, soft, 919
Subglottic web, 574
Subglottischer Hämangiom, 918
Subluxation of lens, 584
Submerged teeth, 927
Submucous cleft palate, 180
Succinylcholine apnea, 152
Sucking reflex
   absent, 139
   poor, 121, 139, 823
   retained into childhood, 413
Sucrase-α- dextrinase insufficiency, 920
Sucrase insufficiency, 920
SUCRASE–ISOMALTASE DEFICIENCY,
   920
Sucrose-isomaltose intolerance, 920
Sudación asociada a la gustación, 448
Sudation gustative, 448
Sulcus mentalis, 146
SULFITE OXIDASE DEFICIENCY, 921
Sulfitoxydase-Mangel, 921
Sulfocysteinuria, 921
Superior epiblepharon, 355
Supernumerary caruncle, 130
Supernumerary nipples without obvious
   glandular tissue, 815
Supernumerary puncta and canaliculi, 844
Supernumerary teeth (Marker), 936
Supraaortic stenosis, 78
Supraclavicular pulsating mass, 74
Supracristal ventricular septal defect, 989
Supraglottic web, 574
Supraorbital ridge (also see Eye, Orbital
   roof)
   prominent, 190, 847
   shallow, 139, 168, 227
Supravalvar aortic stenosis, 78
Supravalvular pulmonary stenosis, 835
Supravalvuläre Aortenstenose, 78
Supravalvuläre Pulmonalstenose, 835
Supraventricular tachycardia paroxysmal,
   922
SUPRAVENTRICULAR TACHYCARDIAS,
   CONGENITAL, 922
Surco nasal transverso, 728
Surdi-mutité semiléthale, 243
Surdité, anomalies rénales et digitales, 264
Surdité avec onycho-dystrophie, 252
Surdité causée par la streptomycine, 272
Surdité cochléaire, myopie et oligophrénie,
   251
Surdité de conduction-insertion basse des
   oreilles, 254
Surdité de conduction par malformation
   des osselets, 244
Surdité de perception, polynéurite et
   atrophie optique, 268
Surdité de perception pour less ondes de
   fréquence moyenne, 267
Surdité de perception précoce, 270
Surdité de perception (unilatérale), 274
Surdité, dermatite atopique, 245
Surdité, diabète, 246
Surdité, épiphyses ponctuées, goitre avec
   élévation du taux sanguin en hor-
   mones thyroïdien, 257
Surdité, fossettes auriculaires, 247
Surdité héréditaire progressive pour les tons
   aigus, 269
Surdité kératopachydermie, constrictions
   digitales, 259
Surdité, nanisme, vitiligo, hypotrophie
   musculaire et achalasie, 275

Surdité neurosensorielle, diverticulite in-
   testinale et neuropathie, 265
Surdité pour les basses fréquences, 260
Surdité pour les sons graves, 256
Surdité sévere récessive neurosensorielle, 271
Surdocardiac syndrome, 123
Surélévation de l'omoplate, 901
Sutural cataract, 132
Suxamethonium sensitivity, 152
Swallowing reflex
   absent, 139
   poor, 139, 823
Sweating (also see Section III, Table XXVIII)
Sweating, gustatory, 448
Sweating, increased, 424
Sweaty feet syndrome, 547
Swedish genetic porphyria, 820
Swiss-cheese cartilage syndrome, 557
Swiss-type agammaglobulinemia, auto-
   somal recessive, 522
Swiss type agammaglobulinemia, X-linked,
   524
Swyer syndrome, 437
Symbrachydactyly with ipsilateral aplasia
   of sternal head of pectoralis major
   muscle, 813
Syncope and QT prolongation without
   deafness, 610
Syndactylie de type Poland, 813
SYNDACTYLY, 923
Syndactyly (see Section III, Table XXIX)
Syndactyly type I (zygodactyly), 923
Syndactyly type II (synpolydactyly), 923
Syndactyly type III (ring and little finger
   syndactyly), 923
Syndactyly type IV (Haas type and Cenani-
   Lenz type), 923
Syndactyly type V (syndactyly with meta-
   carpal and metatarsal fusion), 923
Syndacktylie, 923
Syndrom der ballonierenden Mitralklappe,
   668
Syndrom der breiten Daumen und Gross-
   zehen, 119
Syndrom der frühkindlichen Hyperkalzämie,
   999
Syndrom der multiplen endocrinen Tumoren
   I, 350
Syndrom der multiplen endocrinen Tumoren
   II, 351
Syndrom der multiplen endocrinen Tumoren
   III, 352
Syndrom der multiplen Lentigines, 586
Syndrom der Placenta circumvallata, 187
Syndrom des eingeschlagenen Daumens, 175
Syndrom des langen QT ohne Taubheit, 610
Syndrom des Lineären Naevus sebaceus, 593
Syndrom von Ataxie und Hypogonadismus,
   93
Syndrom von Hyperhydrose, vorzeitig ergrautem
   Haar und Aplasie der Prämolaren,
   493
Syndrom von Megalocornea und geistiger
   Retardierung, 638
Syndrom von Osteoporose und Pseudo-
   gliom, 783
Syndrome amélocérébrohypohydrotique,
   44
Syndrome branchio-squeletto-génital, 118
Syndrome C, 121
Syndrome campomélique, 122
Syndrome cardiomélique, 455
Syndrome cataracte-ichtyose, 131
Syndrome cérébro-costo-mandibulaire, 138
Syndrome cérébro-hépato-rénal, 139

Syndrome cérébro-oculo-facio-squelettique,
   140
Syndrome colobome-atrésie anale, 544
Syndrome cranio-oculo-dentaire, 229
Syndrome cubito-mammaire, 981
Syndrome d'Aberfeld, 155
Syndrome d'Alström, 41
Syndrome d'ataxie et hypogonadisme, 93
Syndrome d'Edwards, 160
Syndrome d'Ehlers-Danlos, 338
Syndrome d'hypercalcémie précoce, 999
Syndrome d'imprégnation alcoolique de
   foetus, 379
Syndrome d'ostéoporose et pseudogliome,
   783
Syndrome d'Usher, 983
Syndrome de Aarskog, 1
Syndrome de Bartter, 100
Syndrome de Basan, 102
Syndrome de Berlin, 105
Syndrome de Bloom, 112
Syndrome de Chédiak-Higashi, 143
Syndrome de Cockayne, 189
Syndrome de Coffin-Lowry, 190
Syndrome de Cornelia de Lange, 242
Syndrome de délétion 5p, 163
Syndrome de Dubowitz, 299
Syndrome de Dyggve-Melchior-Clausen, 306
Syndrome de féminisation testiculaire, 49
Syndrome de féminisation testiculaire in-
   complète, 50
Syndrome de figure foetale, 876
Syndrome de Gardner, 536
Syndrome de Gorlin-Chaudhry-Moss, 440
Syndrome de Grebe, 445
Syndrome de Hanhart, 451
Syndrome de hernie utérine, 683
Syndrome de Horner, 475
Syndrome de Jervell-Nielsen, 123
Syndrome de Klinefelter, 556
Syndrome de Kniest, 557
Syndrome de l'acide phytanique, 810
Syndrome de l'arche aortique droite, 77
Syndrome de la rivière Kuskokwim, 560
Syndrome de Larsen, 570
Syndrome de Laurence-Moon-Biedl, 578
Syndrome de Lesch-Nyhan, 588
Syndrome de Liddle, 590
Syndrome de Marden-Walker, 629
Syndrome de Marfan, 630
Syndrome de McDonough, 632
Syndrome de Meckel, 634
Syndrome de mégalocornée et retard mental,
   638
Syndrome de Menkes, 643
Syndrome de Mohr, 771
Syndrome de Moynahan, 670
Syndrome de Naegeli, 703
Syndrome de naevus sébacé, 593
Syndrome de Nathalie, 785
Syndrome de Noonan, 720
Syndrome de Prader-Willi, 823
Syndrome de Reifenstein, 855
Syndrome de Roberts, 875
Syndrome de Rokitansky-Küster-Hauser,
   682
Syndrome de Rubinstein-Taybi, 119
Syndrome de scimitar, 879
Syndrome de Silver, 887
Syndrome de Smith-Lemli-Opitz, 891
Syndrome de sphérophakie-brachymorphie,
   893
Syndrome de Swyer, 437
Syndrome de symphalangisme et brachy-
   dactylie, 1001

Syndrome de thrombocytopénie avec absence de radius, 941
Syndrome de thrombocytopénie avec hémangiome, 456
Syndrome de Ullrich-Turner, 977
Syndrome de Van den Bosch, 986
Syndrome de von Hippel-Lindau, 995
Syndrome de Waardenburg, 997
Syndrome de Winchester, 1000
Syndrome de Wiskott-Aldrich, 523
Syndrome de Wolff-Parkinson-White, 1002
Syndrome dextrocardie-bronchiectasies, 285
Syndrome G, 401
Syndrome hyperhidrose-blanchîment précoce des cheveux-aplasie des prémolaires, 493
Syndrome hypertélorisme-hypospadias, 505
Syndrome hyperuricémie-surdité-ataxie, 508
Syndrome oculo-cérébro renal, 736
Syndrome oculo-mandibulo faciale, 738
Syndrome of bilateral left-sidedness, 816
Syndrome of bilateral right-sidedness, 92
Syndrome of cerebellar ataxia and hypo-gonadotropic hypogonadism, 93
Syndrome of congenital asymmetry, short stature and variations in sexual development, 887
Syndrome of essential tremor, congenital nystagmus, duodenal ulceration and narcolepsy-like sleep disturbance, 963
Syndrome of mental retardation, seizures, hypotonic cerebral palsy and megalocornea, 638
Syndrome of pseudogliomatous blindness, osteoporosis and mild mental retardation, 783
Syndrome oligophrénie-épilepsie ichtyose, 741
Syndrome oro-facio-digital I, 770
Syndrome ostéo-angio-hypertrophique, 55
Syndrome oto-palato-digital, 786
Syndrome QT long sans surdité, 610
Syndrome thymome-agammaglobulinémia, 944
Syndrome tricho-rhino-phalangien de type I, 966
Syndrome tricho-rhino-phalangien de type II, 967
Syndrome W, 791
Syndromes of hereditary persistence of fetal hemoglobin (some forms), 939
Synkinetic ptosis, 548
Synopthalmia, 234
Synostose huméro-radiale, 477
Synostose radiale cubitale, 854
Synostosis of digits, 14, 22, 874, 923
Synotia, agnathia and microstomia, 28
Syphilis, congenital, 385
Syphonoma, 235
SYRINGOMYELIA, 924
Systematized mesodermal dysplasia, 644
Systemic elastorrhexis, 832
Systemic familial mesenchymosis of Puretić et al, 644
Systemic G$_{M2}$-gangliosidosis, 433
"Systemic hyalinosis" Ishikawa-Hori, 644

T

Tachycardie supraventriculaire congénitale, 922

Tachypnea, 91, 107, 288, 347, 365, 396, 549
Takahara syndrome, 6
Talasemia, 939
Tall, prenatally, 137
Tall stature greater than 2 SD above appropriate mean, 85, 90, 137, 556, 578, 670
Tall with long limbs, 90
Tangier disease, 48
TAPETOCHOROIDAL DYSTROPHY, 925
Tapetoretinal degeneration, 869
Tapetoretinal degeneration and ataxia, 136
Tapetoretinal degeneration (some forms), 201
Tapetoretinal degeneration, typical, 2, 70, 136, 578, 713, 810, 865, 983, 993
Tapetoretinal dystrophy, 869
Taquicardia supraventricular congénita, 922
TAR syndrome, 941
Tarsomegaly, 311
Taste blindness, 809

Taubheit durch Streptomycin-Empfindlichkeit, 272
Taubheit, Kleinwuchs, Vitiligo, Muskelhypotrophie und Achalasie, 275
Taubheit-multicentrische Ossifikation der Epiphysen, hohes eiweissgebundenes Jod, 257
Taubheit, renale und digitale Fehlbildungen, 264
Taubheit und atopische Dermatitis, 245
Taubheit und Diabetes mellitus, 246
Taubheit und Nageldystrophie, 252
Taubheit und Ohrgrübchen, 247
Taubheit und Struma, 249
Taurodoncia (Marcador), 926
Taurodontie, 926
TAURODONTISM (MARKER), 926
Taussig-Bing syndrome, 297
Tay-Sachs disease, 434

Teeth (also see parts, kinds of teeth and Section III, Table XXVII)
  abnormally shaped, 276, 739, 927
  brittle, 302
  conical, 276, 333, 408, 439, 936
  crossbite, 178, 626
  crowded, 225, 226, 474, 554, 617, 667, 825
  delayed eruption, 105, 185, 242, 302, 310, 410, 739, 780, 784, 825, 830, 928, 931, 946, 949, 965
  delayed loss of, 407, 493, 846
  displaced, 278, 394, 474, 539, 674, 825, 846, 929, 936
  excessive attrition, 277, 341, 965
  extra, 178, 185, 738, 933, 936
  impacted teeth, multiple, 45, 46, 118, 394, 407, 408, 617, 739, 784, 929, 932, 936
  impacted tooth, single, 45, 46, 394, 407, 408, 739, 784, 928, 929, 932, 936
  imperfect, 281, 388, 739, 770, 846
  inclined or tipped, 178, 927, 933
  large, 554, 617
  malocclusion, 16, 163, 225, 346, 457, 617, 618, 627, 632, 720, 739, 750, 754, 775, 784, 825, 847, 927, 930, 932, 936
  migrating, 102, 278, 279, 280, 410, 494, 806, 933, 934
  open bite, 46, 720, 735, 749
  premature loss of deciduous, 102, 278, 279, 280, 410, 494, 516, 806

premature loss of permanent, 102, 278, 279, 280, 410, 494, 806
rotated, 825, 933
sensitive to temperature change, 46
shovel-shaped, 607
small, 226, 291, 394, 593, 607, 660, 674, 739, 823, 933, 934, 936
spacing variants of, 46, 242, 281, 291, 607, 631, 676, 934
tuberculate, 385, 936
TEETH, ANKYLOSED, 927
Teeth, carnivore-like, 607
TEETH, CONCRESCENCE OF ROOTS, 928
TEETH, DILACERATED, 929
Teeth, enlarged, 617
TEETH, FUSED, 930
TEETH, GEMINATED, 931
Teeth, ghost, 739
TEETH, IMPACTED, 932
TEETH, NATAL OR NEONATAL, 933
TEETH, PEGGED OR ABSENT MAXILLARY LATERAL INCISOR, 934
TEETH, SNOW-CAPPED, 935
TEETH, SUPERNUMERARY (MARKER), 936
TEETH, THISTLE-SHAPED PULP CHAMBERS, 937
Telangiectasia and ataxia, 94
Telangiectasia retineana e hipogamaglobulinemia, 868
Télangiectasie rétinienne et hypogammaglobulinémie, 868
Telangiektasie der Retina und Hypogammaglobulinämie, 868
Telecanthus, 356
Telecanthus-hypospadias syndrome, 505
Telecanthus with associated abnormalities, 505
Tembloe hereditario, 964
Temporal bone
  absence or hypoplasia of petrous portion, 562
  bulging, 777
  cholesteatoma of petrous pyramid of, 150
  narrow, 190, 603
  small mastoid process of, 664
Tendones flexores cortos de los dedos e incapacidad para abrir la boca en forma completa, 882
Teratoid cyst, 760
Teratoid tumor of head or neck, 283
Teratologic syndrome of visceral heterotaxy, 92
Teratom der Magen, 914
Teratoma, 760
Teratoma gástrico, 914
Teratoma sacrococcygeal (benign or malignant), 877
Teratoma sacrocoxígeo, 877
Teratomas of the orbit, 283
Tératome gastrique, 914
Tératome sacrococcygienne, 877
Tesaurismosis de ácido fitánico, 810
Tesaurismosis hepática de ésteres del colesterol, 151
Testicular feminization syndrome, complete, 49
Testikuläre Feminisierung, 49
Testis
  deficient spermatogonia, 49
  delayed descent of, 119
  gonad unilateral streak and a contralateral testis, 173

histologically normal before puberty, 49
in inguinal canal, 831, 855
interstitial fibrosis of, 855
Leydig cell hyperplasia in, 49, 855
Leydig cell hypoplasia in, 438
male gender with hypogenitalism, 13, 302
small, 47, 105, 155, 438, 529, 556, 634, 702, 855
sperm decreased, 438
testicular enlargement, nodular, 908
testicular germinal cell hypoplasia, 169
undescended, 1, 13, 88, 104, 119, 121, 139, 159, 160, 163, 167, 168, 170, 173, 189, 242, 254, 305, 337, 408, 438, 544, 578, 586, 587, 603, 632, 634, 635, 683, 720, 736, 754, 818, 823, 857, 891, 903, 908, 909, 952
with female gender, 49
Tetracuspid pulmonary valve, 840
Tetracycline discoloration of enamel and dentin, 341
TETRALOGY OF FALLOT, 938
Tetralogy of Fallot with absent pulmonary valve, 836
Tetraphocomelia with cleft lip and palate (and penis or clitoris hypertrophy), 875
THALASSEMIA, 939
Tetrology of Fallot, 182, 388, 720, 941
Thalidomide embryopathy, 386
Thalidomide external ear malformation, 664
Thanatophorer Zwergwuchs, 940
Thanatophoric dwarfism, 940
THANATOPHORIC DYSPLASIA, 940
Thickening and deformities of chordae tendineae, 666
Third degree atrioventricular block, 454
Thomsen disease, 701
Thoracic dysplasia, asphyxiating, 91
Thorax en carène, 801
Thorax en entonnoir, 802
Thoraxdysplasie-Polydaktylie-Syndrom Typ Majewski, 883
Thoraxdysplasie-Polydaktylie-Syndrom Typ Saldino-Noonan, 884
3β-H5D deficiency, 909
3β-hydroxysteroid dehydrogenase and isomerase deficiency, 909
Thrombocytopenia and hemangioma syndrome, 456
THROMBOCYTOPENIA WITH ABSENT RADIUS, 941
THROMBOCYTOPENIC PURPURA AND LIPID HISTIOCYTOSIS, 942
Thrombocytopenie-Radiusaplasie-Syndrom, 941
Thrombocytopenische Purpura und Histiocytose, 942
Thumb (also see Digit, Finger, Joints, and Section III, Table XXIX)
absence of, 160, 167, 231, 455, 649, 875
angulation deformity of, 119
bifurcation of distal phalanx, 22, 264, 621, 817
broad, 22, 119, 325, 570, 621, 754
decreased extension of, 175
defect of, 22, 114, 981
distally placed, 769
duplication of, 13, 51, 72, 621, 814
duplication of finger-like, 72, 814
finger-like (triphalangism), 51, 72, 262, 382, 455, 544
flexed across palm, 85, 175
fixed, 769

in same plane as fingers, 455
large, 13
medially placed, 280
narrow, 85, 172
proximally placed, 293
radial deviation of distal phalanx, 817
short, 231, 455, 700, 769, 853, 875, 881, 987
short distal phalanx of, 114, 264, 817
soft tissue syndactyly of thumb and palm, 980
syndactyly with index finger, 22
Thumb extensors, aplasia or hypoplasia, 175
Thumb polydactyly, 814
Thumbs clasped, 175
THYMIC AGENESIS, 943
Thymic alymphoplasia, 524
Thymic aplasia, 943
THYMOMA AND AGAMMAGLO-BULINEMIA SYNDROME, 944
Thymoma with "acquired" combined immunodeficiency, 944
Thymusagenesie, 943
Thymus gland
absence of, 522, 655
large, for age, 104
small, 139
Thyroglossal duct, cyst or sinus, 945
THYROGLOSSAL DUCT REMNANT, 945
Thyroid
atrophy of, 946, 948
ectopic, 946
goiter, 249, 257, 350, 412, 435, 542, 543, 809, 947
goiter, nontoxic, 111
hypofunction of, 412, 702, 946
infection of, 412, 525
large, 391, 435, 542, 543, 948
tumor of, 350, 412
THYROID DYSGENESIS, 946
THYROID PEROXIDASE DEFECT, 947
Thyroidal deiodination deficiency, 543
THYROTROPIN DEFICIENCY, ISOLATED, 949
Thyrotropin (TSH)-Unempfindlichkeit, 948
THYROTROPIN (TSH) UNRESPONSIVE-NESS, 948
THYROXINE–BINDING GLOBULIN DEFECTS (MARKER), 950
Tibia
absence of, 875
anterior dislocation onto femur, 570
bowed anteriorly (saber shin), 385, 777
bowed midportion of, 648
bowing of, 122, 712, 775
disproportionately short, 883
long, 122
short, 19, 646, 648, 649, 875
Tiefsitzende Ohren, 327
Tiefton-Schwerhörigkeit, 260
Tinnitus, 12, 145, 248, 530, 787
Tip of nose (also see Nose)
bifid, 595, 724, 771
broad, 16, 166, 168, 506, 771, 791, 891
bulbous, 168, 226, 966, 967
dimple at, 16
pug nose, 157, 893
upturned, 242, 629, 876
Tirosinemia, 978
Toe (also see Digit, Hallux, Joints, and Section III, Table XXIX)

absence of 1 or more (see Ectrodactyly)
crowding of, 754
curved 5th, 72
decreased range of motion, 450
decreased range of motion at interphalangeal joints, 650
duplication of 2nd, 817
extra on fibular side of foot, 17, 22, 121, 578, 634, 814
extra on tibial side of foot, 649
flexion deformity of proximal interphalangeal joints of, 85
fusion of middle and distal phalanges of 3rd–5th, 262
hammer, 89, 140, 393
lateral deviation of, 392
mediodorsal curvature of 4th, 769
overlapping, 159
partial soft tissue syndactyly of toes 2 and 3, 172, 923
short, 16, 20, 114, 121, 392, 459, 578, 667, 700, 818, 1001
short distal phalanx of, 19, 21, 262, 409, 786, 846
shortening marked of, 8, 114, 445
stocking syndactyly, 14
syndactyly of, 13, 22, 55, 97, 121, 179, 259, 337, 376, 393, 578, 634, 662, 817, 818, 885
syndactyly of 4th and 5th, 229
syndactyly of 2nd and 3rd, 229, 506, 554, 603, 634, 769, 887, 891, 923
synostosis, 14, 874, 923
widely spaced, between 1st and 2nd, 171

Tomato tumor, 235

Tongue
bifid, 281, 634, 636, 735, 770, 952
cleft of anterior tip of, 401
cystic mass connected to lingual foramen, 945
decreased mobility of, 61, 177, 636
deep central furrow of, 953
downward displacement of, 182
fissured, 953, 954, 956
geographic, 954, 956
glossitis, 15, 618
hamartoma of, 662, 770
large, 171, 618, 754
leukoplakia of, 789
papilloma of, 281, 634
paralysis of, 376
plicated, 954, 956
polypoid growth at apex of, 952
posteriorly positioned, 28
protruding, 171, 754
scalloped edge on, 789
small, 28, 376, 451, 576
sublingual mass, 760
taste impaired, 378
tender or burning, 954
tongue-tie, 61, 574, 599, 770
trifid, 770
ulceration of, 618
unusual mobility of, 338, 951

TONGUE, CLEFT, 952
Tongue curling, 951
TONGUE, FISSURED (MARKER), 953
TONGUE FOLDING OR ROLLING (MARKERS), 951
TONGUE, GEOGRAPHIC, 954
Tongue gigantism, 618
Tongue, median cleft, 636
TONGUE, PIGMENTED PAPILLAE (MARKER), 955

TONGUE, PLICATED (MARKER), 956
Tongue, prominent pigmented papillae of, 955
Tongue-tie, 61
Tonsil
   agenesis, bilateral, 27, 522, 524, 655, 790
   agenesis ipsilateral to microtia, 664
   agenesis, unilateral, 790
   small, 524
   teratoid tumor of, 664
Tooth and nail syndrome, 511
Tooth cementum
   excessive, 928
   fused to bone, 927
Tooth crown
   bulbous shape of, 279
   exaggerated cingulum of, 276, 607
   fractured, 739
   fused with crown of adjacent tooth, 930
   moth-eaten appearance, 46
   ovoid shape of, 843
   small, 607
Tooth dentin
   confluent with that of adjacent tooth, 930
   contains porphyrins, 821
   hypocalcification of, 739, 931
   hypoplasia of, 739, 931
   radicular type of dysplasia of, 118
Tooth enamel
   abrades easily, 279
   contains porphyrins, 821
   fractures easily, 46, 279, 777
   hypocalcification of, 45, 739, 931
   hypomaturation of, 342, 784, 935
   hypoplasia of, 46, 678, 873
   soft, 46
   variable color of, 45, 46, 262, 277, 279, 302, 340, 341, 703, 732, 777, 784, 821, 927, 933, 935, 965
Tooth, hair, bone and nail dysplasia, 965
Tooth pulp chamber
   dental pulp stones in, 276, 277, 739, 843
   enlarged in all dimensions, 279, 739
   enlarged in apical dimensions, 926, 965
   necrotic, 276, 607
   obliterated, 118, 279
   small, 279
   variably shaped, 118, 277, 278, 280, 843, 937
Tooth root
   block-shaped, 926
   diverged roots of central incisors, 631
   fused with root of adjacent tooth, 928, 930
   large root canal, 843
   resorption of, 407, 932
   short, 118, 277, 278, 279, 280, 739, 843, 929
   thin or dilacerated, 279
Tórax en quilla, 801
TORSION DYSTONIA, 957
Torsion of trunk or limbs, 957
TORUS MANDIBULARIS, 958
Torus palatino, 959
TORUS PALATINUS, 959
Total anomalous hepatic venous return, 468
Total anomalous pulmonary venous return, 842

Total cataract, 132
Touraine-Solente-Golé syndrome, 788
Townes syndrome, 72
Toxoplasmose congénitale, 387
Toxoplasmosis congénita, 387
Toxoplasmosis, infantile, 387
Trachea
   airway obstruction, 117
   cleft in posterior wall of, 577
   tracheobronchial tree, defect of, 156
   tracheoesophageal atresia, 571
      fistula, 160, 300, 364, 365, 571, 727, 960, 987
   tracheomalacia, 557
Tracheal lobe, 611
TRACHEOESOPHAGEAL FISTULA, 960
Tracheoesophageal fistula and esophageal atresia, 365
Tragus, unspecified defect of, 664
Tragus-Aplasie, 312
Tränengangsatresie, 563
Tränengangsstenose, 705
Tränensackfistel, 565
Transferrin variant markers, 95
TRANSGLUCURONYLASE, SEVERE DEFICIENCY, 961
Transient adrenocortical insufficiency of infancy, 23
"Transitional" cases presenting some clinical manifestations of both classic incontinentia pigmenti and Naegeli syndrome, 703
Translocation 21 syndrome, 171
Transposición completa de los grandes vasos, 962
Transposición del hígado, 606
Transposition complète des gross vaisseaux, 962
Transposition der grossen Gefässe, 962
Transposition du foie, 606
TRANSPOSITION OF GREAT VESSELS, 962
Transposition of liver, 606
Transversales septum vaginae, 985
Transverse nasal groove (Marker), 728
Transverse nasal stripe, 728
Transverse vaginal septum, 985
Traumatic keloids, 551
Treacher Collins syndrome, 627
Tremblement essentiel et ulcération duodénale, 963
Tremblement hérédofamilial, 964
Tremor, 2, 93, 188, 344, 469, 472, 547, 671, 742, 744, 745, 746, 747, 759, 791, 895, 957, 963, 964
   autosomal dominant, 964
   coarse, 744, 895
   increased with fatigue, 963, 964
   intention, 188, 469, 744, 759
   of facial muscles or tongue, 964
   of hands, 472, 963
   of head, 746, 747, 963
   of trunk, 746, 964
   while at rest, 469, 744
   with onset in childhood, 963
TREMOR, DUODENAL ULCERATION SYNDROME, 963
Tremor-Duodenalulcus-Syndrom, 963
TREMOR, HEREDOFAMILIAL, 964
Trémulation du menton, 147
Treponema pallidum in utero, 385
Triangular shape of calvaria, 121, 162, 167, 470
Trias fragilitis ossium hereditaria, 777

TRICHO–DENTO–OSSEOUS SYNDROME, 965
Tricho-rhino-auriculo-phalangeal multiple exostoses dysplasia, 967
TRICHO–RHINO–PHALANGEAL SYNDROME, TYPE I, 966
TRICHO–RHINO–PHALANGEAL SYNDROME, TYPE II, 967
Trichterbrust, 802
Tricuspid incompetence, 969
Tricuspid regurgitation, 969
TRICUSPID VALVE ATRESIA, 968
Tricuspid valve, downward displacement, 332
TRICUSPID VALVE INSUFFICIENCY, 969
TRICUSPID VALVE STENOSIS, 970
Tricuspidal insuffizienz, 969
Tricuspidalatresie, 968
Tricuspidalstenose, 970
Tridermal gastric teratoma, 914
Tridermic teratoma of stomach, 914
Tridermoma of head or neck, 283
Tridione syndrome, 388
Trifid tongue, 952
Trigeminal nerve, decreased function of, 188
Trilobed calvaria, 55
Trilogy of Fallot, 839
Triple nares, 722
Triploid/diploid mosaicism, 169
Triploidie, 169
Trisomie 8, 157
Trisomie 13, 168
Trisomie 13–15, 168
Trisomie 18, 160
Trisomie 21, 171
Trisomie distal 14q, 165
Trisomie proximale 14q, 166
Trisomy D1 syndrome, 168
Trisomy G syndrome, 171
Trisomy-8/normal diploid mosaicism, 157
Trisomy 13–15 syndrome, 168
Tritanomaly, 199
Tritanopia, 199
Trousseau sign, positive, 515, 873
True agonadism, 29
True cholesteatoma, 150
True esophageal diverticulum, 367
TRUE HERMAPHRODITISM, 971
True Klinefelter syndrome, 556
True median cleft, 595
True or primary anophthalmos, 67
True transposition of great vessels, 962
Truncal obesity, 302, 823
TRUNCUS ARTERIOSUS, 972
Truncus arteriosus communis persistens, 972
Trunk
   long, 157, 303
   narrow, 157
   short, 121, 783
TRYPSINOGEN DEFICIENCY, 973
Trypsinogenmangelkrankheit, 973
TRYPTOPHAN MALABSORPTION, 974
Tubercule de Darwin, 241
TUBEROUS SCLEROSIS, 975
Tubular male pseudohermaphroditism, 683
TUBULAR STENOSIS, 976
Tubuläre Azidose und Innenohrschwerhörigkeit, 863
Tubuläre Stenose, 976
Tumefacción fibrosa intraósea mandibular, 539

Tumeur du cortuseule carotidien, 127
Tumeur mixte des glandes salivaires, 878
Tumeur neuro-ectodermique pigmentée, 711
Tumeurs du système nerveux central, 188
Tumeurs glomiques multiples, 416
Tumor, bulging into perineum, 877
Tumor del cuerdo carotìdeo, 127
Tumores múltiples de los glomos, 416
Tumor mixto hereditario de las glándulas salivares, 878
Tumor neuroectodérmico pigmentado, 711
Tumors of nervous system
   astrocytoma, 12
   cavernous hemangioma of CNS, 113
   glioma of CNS, 345, 346, 351, 712
   hemangioblastoma of CNS, 995
   medulloblastoma, 101
   menigioma, 12, 351
   neuroma of CNS, 712
Tune deafness (Marker), 273
Túnel aórtico-ventricular izquierdo, 82
Tunnel aortico-ventriculaire gauche, 82
Turban tumors of scalp, 235
Turbantumoren, 235
Turner phenotype with normal karyotype, 720
TURNER SYNDROME, 977
Turricephaly, 230
Two-chambered right ventricle, 731
Type III, A, ii vitamin D refractory rickets with aminoaciduria (classification of Fraser and Slater), 873
Typical iris colobomas, ciliary body, choroid, retina, optic nerve, 733
Typical retinoschisis, autosomal dominant, 871
Typus degenerativus Amstelodamensis, 242
Tyrosinämie, 978
Tyrosinase negative oculocutaneous albinism, 34
Tyrosinase-negativer okulo-kutaner Albinismus, 34
Tyrosinase positive oculocutaneous albinism, 35
Tyrosinase-positiver okulo-kutaner Albinismus, 35
TYROSINEMIA, 978
Tyrosinosis, 978

U

"U"-shaped hearing loss, 267
Überzählige Tränenpunktchen und-gänge, 844
Überzählige Zähne, 936
UHL ANOMALY, 979
Ullrich-Noonan syndrome, 720
Ullrich syndrome, 720
Ullrich-Turner syndrome, 977
Ulna
   bowing of, 231
   bowing of midportion of, 20
   defect of, 16, 455, 941
   dislocation of proximal ulnar head, 647
   dorsal dislocation of, 308
   prominent styloid process of, 510
   short, 19, 231, 510, 685, 791, 875, 923, 941, 981
Ulnar drift syndrome, 980
ULNAR DRIFT WITH DIGITAL WEBS AND CONTRACTURES, 980

ULNAR-MAMMARY SYNDROME, TYPE PALLISTER, 981
Ulnare Abweichung mit Schwimmhauten und Kontrakturen, 980
Ulnofibular dysplasia, Reinhardt-Pfeiffer type, 648
Umbilical hernia, 748
Umbilical ring widely open, 104, 671, 748
Uncorrected transposition of great vessels, 962
Unicommissural aortic valve stenosis, 80
Unilateral dental malformation, 739
Unilateral hyperopia, 59
Unilateral hypertrophy, 458
Unilateral inner ear deafness, 274
Univentricular heart, 286
Unsteadiness, 963
Unterbrechung des Aortenbogens, 76
Upper limb cardiovascular syndrome, 455
Urbach-Wiethe syndrome, 599
Ureter
   dilation of, 732
   duplication of, 264
   hydroureter, 337, 571, 578
   hypoplasia of, 634
   obstruction of, 264
   stenosis of, 574
   ureteral reflux, 157
   ureteral reflux bilateral, 732
Urethra
   atresia of, 571
   duplication of, 194
   epispadias, 156
   hypospadias, 97, 118, 159, 160, 162, 164, 167, 168, 170, 242, 388, 401, 505, 578, 586, 855, 891, 903, 971
   opens into vagina, 173
   rectourethral fistula, 401, 885, 987
   severe displacement of urethral meatus, 401, 831, 855
   urethral meatus displaced to coronal sulcus (1st degree), 401, 518
   urethral meatus displaced to perineum (4th degree), 50, 518, 909
   urethral meatus displaced to scrotum (3rd degree), 518, 831
   urethral meatus displaced to shaft of penis (2nd degree), 173, 518, 909
Uridine diphosphate galactose 4'-epimerase deficiency, 357
Urinary bladder
   calculi, 441
   dysfunction of, 292
   exstrophy of, 193
   large thick, 104
   loss of voluntary control of, 693
   obstruction of neck, 264
   paralysis of, 693, 894
   unspecified defect of, 755
Urinary system (see parts and Section III, Table XXXV)
Urinary tract
   generalized dilatation of, 754
   infection of, 239, 264, 603, 943
   obstructive uropathy, 192, 239, 720
   unspecified defect of, 161, 531, 720
   urinary tract calculi, 236, 588
   urogenital sinus in perineum, 578, 831, 971
Urogenital-und Mittelohrfehlbildungen, 860
Ursprung beider grosser Arterien aus dem linken Ventrikel, 581
Ursprung des Pulmonalarterie von der Aorta ascendens, 767

URTICARIA, DEAFNESS AND AMYLOIDOSIS, 982
Urticaria, sordera y amiloidosis, 982
Urticaria, Taubheit und Amyloidose, 982
USHER SYNDROME, 983
Uterine hernia syndrome, 683
Uterine inguinal hernia syndrome, 683
Uterus
   bicornuate, 104, 168, 571, 578
   fibroid tumor of, 412
   hydrometrocolpos at menarche, 860
   hyperplastic, 104
   infantile, 173, 438, 904
   infantile müllerian derivatives, 436
   rudimentary müllerian, 682
   rupture of, 684
   small, 437
   unspecified defect of, 173, 860
   variable defects of, 884
   with male gender, 683
Uterus arcuatus, 684
Uterus bicornus, 684
Uterus bicornus unicollis, 684
Utérus bifide, 684
Uterus bilocularis, 684
Uterus bipartitus, 684
Uterus didelphys, 684
Uterus-Hernie, 683
Uterus pseudodidelphys, 684
Uterus subseptus, 684
Uterus unicornus, 684
Uveal pigment, decreased, 143
Uvula
   broad, 22, 791
   brown to brownish-red macules on, 955
   cleft of, 118, 164, 172, 177, 178, 181, 184, 225, 264, 401, 505, 574, 720, 735, 981
   long, 22
   short, 401
Uvula, cleft, 184
Úvula hendida (Marcador), 184

V

Vactel association, 987
Vacterl syndrome, 987
Vagina
   atresia of, 544, 578, 857, 860
   atresia of lower, 984
   fistula, rectovaginal, 72, 987
   fistula, vesicovaginal, 571
   mucosa, white folded soft hyperplastic lesions of, 681
   septate, 578, 634, 684
   short, 49, 682, 903
   that ends blindly, 682
   transverse vaginal septum, 985
   urogenital orifice leading inferiorly to, 173
   vaginal orifices paired in perineum, 684
   vaginal pouch in perineum, 831
VAGINAL ATRESIA, 984
VAGINAL SEPTUM, TRANSVERSE, 985
Valvar aortic stenosis, 80
Valve aortique tétracuspide, 81
Valve pulmonaire tétracuspide, 840
Válvula aórtica bicúspide, 108
Válvula aórtica tetracuspídea, 81
Válvula pulmonar bicúspide, 109
Válvula pulmonar tetracuspídea, 840

Valvuläre Aortenstenose, 80
Valvule aortique bicuspidé, 108
Valvule pulmonaire bicuspidé, 109
Van Buchen syndrome, 497
VAN DEN BOSCH SYNDROME, 986
Van der Woude syndrome, 177
Variación del cerumen (Marcador), 141
Variant form of Swiss type agammaglob-
    ulinemia, 655
Variations dans le cerumen, 141
Vascular collapse, 24, 829
Vascular malformations of middle ear, 773
Vas deferens and epididymis
    blind-ended, 68
    epididymis rudimentary, 29
    epididymis, tumor of, 711
    thickened, 529
Vasopressin-resistant diabetes mellitus, 287
Vasopressin-resistenter Diabetes insipidus,
    287
VATER ASSOCIATION, 987
Vein of Galen aneurysm, 186
Vena cava
    anomalous right pulmonary vein drain-
        ing into inferior, 879
    persistence of left superior, 182
Venous return to heart, anomalous, 401
Ventricular cyst of larynx, 575
VENTRICULAR DIVERTICULUM, 988
Ventricular inversion without transposition of
    great arteries, 541
Ventricular preexcitation, 1002
VENTRICULAR SEPTAL DEFECT, 989
Ventricular septal defect of the endocardial
    cushion defect type, 347
Ventricular septal defect with absent pulmon-
    ary valve, 836
Ventricular septal defect with double outlet
    right ventricle, 297
Ventricule gauche à double issue, 581
Ventrículo derecho a doble salida con
    comunicación interventricular
    anterior, 297
Ventrículo derecho a doble salida con
    comunicación interventricular
    posterior, 298
Ventrículo izquierdo a doble salida, 581
Ventrikelseptumdefekt, 989
Verkürzte Beugesehnen der Finger und
    Unterkieferkontraktur, 882
Vermehrte Ausscheidung dibasischer
    Aminosäuren, 491
Vertebra, unspecified defect of, 29, 69,
    101, 157, 281, 506, 554, 682, 720,
    735, 960, 987
Vertebral anomalies syndrome, 987
Vertebral column (also see Section III,
    Table XXIX)
    anterior curvature (see kyphosis)
    asymmetry of, 887
    cervical spine with block vertebrae, 103,
        142, 481, 667
    decreased range of motion of, 898
    decreased rotary motion of, 896
    defect of, 680, 941
    defect of cervical spine, 178
    fused, 103, 142, 481, 667
    lateral curvature (see scoliosis)
    localized widening of, 924
    progressive decreased range of motion
        of, 896
    rigid, 516, 998
    short cervical spine, 900
Vertige épisodique avec surdite, 248
Vertigo, 12, 145, 248, 530, 949, 995

Vértigo episódico y sordera familiar, 248
Vestibular hydrops, 248
Vierklappiges Aortenostium, 81
Vierklappiges Pulmonalostium, 840
Virilization
    at puberty, 173
    female gender with, 498, 902, 908, 971
    male gender with mild, 909
VISCERA, FATTY METAMORPHOSIS,
    990
Visceral malrotation, partial, 92, 816
Viscéromégalie, omphalocèle et macro-
    glossie, 104
Visceromegaly, 104
Visceromegaly, umbilical hernia and macro-
    glossia, 104
Vision (see Section III, Table XXIV)
Visual acuity, decreased (also see Blindness)
    at birth, 206, 755, 867
    hemianopsia, 188
    in legally blind range, 621
        in male, 195, 925
    markedly after 4th decade, 449
    no improvement with age, 34
    progressive, 70, 713, 745, 780
    rapid deterioration, 550, 579
    reduced vision, 32, 350, 763, 764
    sudden loss centrally in 2nd–3rd
        decades, 579
    with onset before 1 year, 43, 755
    with onset before puberty, 43, 211, 755
    with onset after 20 years, 209, 211, 253,
        925
Visual field
    concentric narrowing, 810
    constricted, 869, 925, 983
    defect of, 757, 763
    hemianopsia, 188
Viszeraler Situs inversus, 888
Vitamin B$_6$ Abhängigkeit, 991
VITAMIN B$_6$ DEPENDENCY, 991
Vitamin B$_6$ dependency with convulsions,
    991
VITAMIN B$_{12}$ MALABSORPTION, 992
Vitamin-D-abhängige Rachitis (Prader), 873
Vitamin D-resistant rickets, 517
Vitamin K-antagonist embryopathy, 389
Vitelliform, macular degeneration, 622
Vitelline duct, remnant, 633
Vitelline macular degeneration, 622
Vitelliruptive Makuladegeneration, 622
VITILIGO, 993
Vitium cordis congenitum, Taubheit und
    Skelett Fehlbildungen, 667
Vitreoretinal dysplasia with recessive X-
    linked inheritance, 721
Vitreoretinal dystrophy, 871
Vitreous
    altered posterior hyaloid membrane, 479
    exudate of, 140
    detachment of, 479
    floaters in, 870
    hemorrhage in, 872
    liquefaction of, 479
    posterior detachment of, 871
VITREOUS, PERSISENT HYPERPLASTIC
    PRIMARY, 994
Vogelkopf-Zwerguchs, 881
Vogt cephalodactyly, 14
Vohwinkel syndrome, 259
Voice (also see Speech)
    high-pitched, 299, 302, 303, 413, 438,
        447, 744, 825
    hoarse, 117, 127, 242, 299, 401, 572,
        573, 574, 575, 577, 598, 599, 949

    loss of, 572, 574, 575, 577
    low-pitched, 171, 184, 233, 855, 908
    nasal, 118, 270
    raucous, 401, 999
Vomiting (also see Section III, Table
    XXXIV)
    after 1 mo of age immediately after
        feeding, 193, 471
    as newborn, 531, 909. 913
    bile-stained, 62, 194, 537
    bile stained in early infancy, 300
    hematemesis, 346, 913
von Gierke disease, 425
VON HIPPEL–LINDAU SYNDROME, 995
von Recklinghausen disease, 712
VON WILLEBRAND DISEASE, 996
Voorhoeve disease, 778
Vordere Nasengangsatresie, 723
Vorhofseptum-Defekte, 96
Vrolik disease, 777
VSR syndrome, 470

                    W

W syndrome, 791
WAARDENBURG SYNDROME, 997
Wackelkinn, 147
Wandering rash of tongue, 954
Warfarin embryopathy, 389
Webbing, popliteal, 818
Weight gain, absent or decreased, 424, 1003
Weight loss, (also see Inanition, Failure to
    thrive, and Malnutrition)
Weight low by 2SD, 174
Weill-Marchesani syndrome, 893
Welander type of muscular atrophy, 690
Werdnig-Hoffman disease, 895
Wermer syndrome, 350
WERNER SYNDROME, 998
Whistling face syndrome, 223
White folded dysplasia of mucosa, 681
White forelock without deafness, 31
White sponge nevus, 681
Wiedemann-Beckwith syndrome, 104
Wildermuth ear, 330
Wildervanck syndrome, 142
WILLIAMS SYNDROME, 999
Wilson disease, 469
Winchester disease, 1000
Winchester-Grossman syndrome, 1000
WINCHESTER SYNDROME, 1000
Wing of nostril
    flared, 587, 997
    grooved, 728
    narrow, 102, 737, 875
    notched, 281, 375, 635, 967
    thickened, 676, 679
Wiskott-Aldrich syndrome, 523
WL SYMPHALANGISM–BRACHDACTYLY
    SYNDROME, 1001
Wolf syndrome, 164
WOLFF–PARKINSON–WHITE SYNDROME,
    1002
WOLMAN DISEASE, 1003
Wolmansche Krankheit, 1003
Wrist
    contracture of, 89
    decreased extension of, 89, 121, 470, 941
    decreased range of motion of, 128, 308
        450, 649
    defect of, 129
    dislocation of, 678
    fixed, 1001
    flexed, 88

increased range of motion of, 90
large, 90, 672, 873
Madelung deformity of, 19, 308
ulnar deviation of, 89, 646, 648

X

X-Chromosomaler infantiler Hypopara-
   thyreoidismus, 515
X-linked and kinky hair, 643
X-linked choroidal sclerosis, 925
X-linked congenital nightblindness with
   myopia, 719
X-linked form of spondyloepiphyseal
   dysplasia, 898
X-linked lymphopenic immunologic deficiency,
   524
X-linked neonatal hypoparathyroidism, 515
X-linked primary hyperuricemia, 588
X-linked recessive form of lymphopenic hy-
   pogammaglobulinemia, 524
X-linked recessive lymphopenic agammaglo-
   bulinemia, 524
X-linked severe dual system immunodeficiency,
   524
X-linked thymic epithelial hypoplasia, 524

XERODERMA AND MENTAL RETARDA-
   TION, 1004
Xeroderma avec retard mental, 1004
Xeroderma con retardo mental, 1004
XERODERMA PIGMENTOSUM, 1005
Xerodermische Idiotie, 1004
XO syndrome, 977
XX form of pure gonadal dysgenesis, 436
XX gonadal dysgenesis, 436
XY form of pure gonadal dysgenesis, 437
XY gonadal dysgenesis, 437

Y

Y-shaped fissure of chin, 146
Yellow-blue color blindness, 199
Yellow mutant oculocutaneous albinism, 36
Yellow nail syndrome with familial late-onset
   lymphedema, 615

Z

Zahndysplasie, 739
Zahnschmelzhypoplasie, 342

Zahnschmelzhypoplasie, Onycholyse und
   Hypohidrose, 45
Zahnschmelzhypoplasie, Taurodontie
   Kräuselhaar und Kortikalissklerose,
   965
Zahnverschmelzung, 930
Zahnzwillingsbildung, 931
Zellweger syndrome, 139
Zentralfibrillen-Myopathie, 134
Zentrenzephale Epilepsie, 135
Zerebellëre Ataxie und Chorioretinale De-
   generation, 136
Zerebraler Gigantismus, 137
Zervico-Oculo-Acusticus Syndrom, 142
Zervikaler Aortenbogen, 74
Zollinger-Ellison syndrome, 350
Zonular cataract, 132
Zungenspalte, 952
Zwerchfell-Eventration, 288
Zyklische Neutropenie, 714
Zyklopie, 234
Zystathioninurie, 236
Zystenleber, 605
Zystennieren-Erwachsenenform, 859
Zystinurie, 239
Zystische Pankreasfibrose, 237
Zytomegalie, 381